72805
20
AE027076

CLINICAL PHARMACY

Volume 7, Number 1
January 1988

NON-CIRCULATING UNTIL
FEB 4
MEDICAL LIBRARY
THE MARY IMOGENE BASSETT HOSPITAL

Lovastatin

Sulbactam: A β-lactamase inhibitor

AMERICAN SOCIETY OF HOSPITAL PHARMACISTS

When it comes to taking their medicine, some patients need—

SPECIAL DELIVERY

INTENSOL™

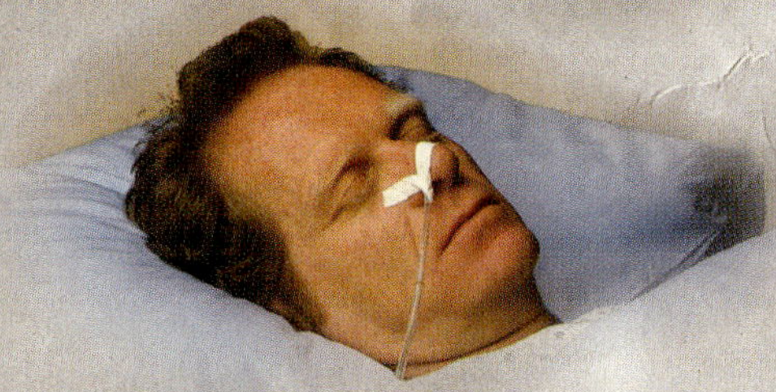

For patients who have difficulty with tablets

The nasogastric patient

The elderly or debilitated patient

The cancer patient on high or variable doses

The pediatric patient

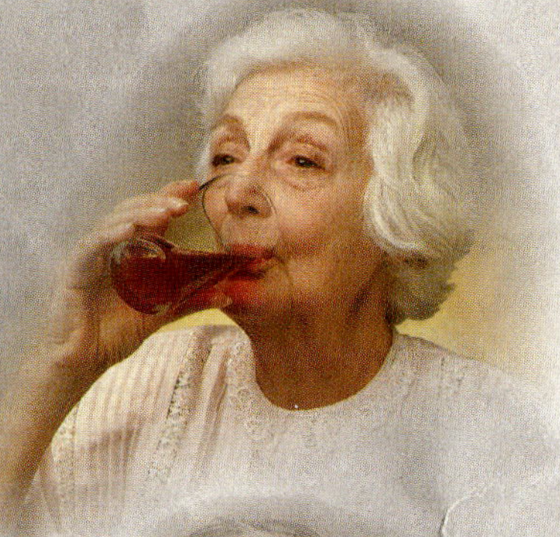

Concentrated oral solutions

Intensols are highly concentrated medications—Chlorpromazine, Dexamethasone, DHT, Hydrochlorothiazide, Prednisone, Thioridazine, to name a few—in low volume solutions.

Easier than swallowing tablets

Intensols can be mixed with juice or semisolid foods, or even administered through nasogastric tubing.

Most Intensols have no flavor, so medications taste like the food or liquid they are mixed with. Each bottle comes with a calibrated dropper for easy dosage titration.

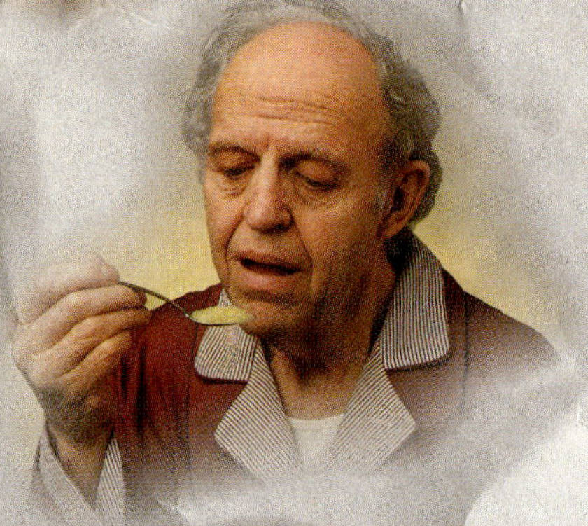

Easy to dispense

- Every dose is accurate.
- Ends the need to crush or break tablets—yielding inexact doses.
- Enhances patient compliance.
- Eliminates pharmacy compounding.

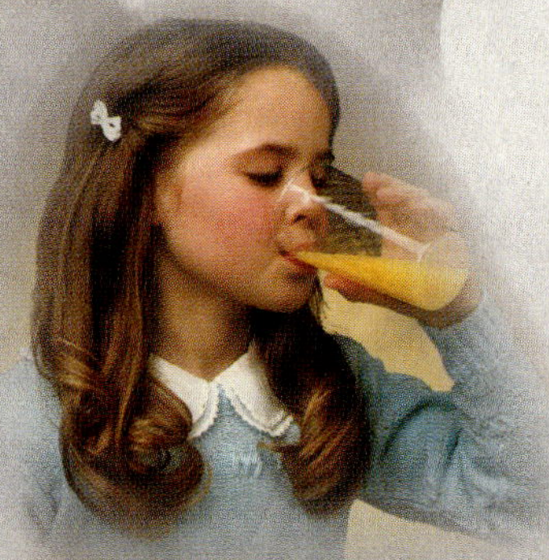

INTENSOLS...

A SPECIAL DELIVERY SYSTEM for special patients.

Roxane Laboratories, Inc.
Columbus, Ohio 43216

Intensols for your special patients

To find out more about INTENSOLS for your patients, fill out the following and mail to: Roxane Laboratories, Inc., PO Box 16532, Columbus, Ohio 43216.

Name ____________

Address ____________

Specialty ____________

January 1988 Volume 7, Number 1 Coden: CPHADV ISSN: 0278-2677

CLINICAL PHARMACY

7 **News**

FDA approves marketing of second fluoroquinolone, ciprofloxacin . . . Study suggests role for trimetrexate in AIDS-associated *Pneumocystis carinii* pneumonia . . . Studies refute efficacy of corticosteroids in severe sepsis . . . FDA divides drugs and biologics evaluation unit . . . Distribution of ivermectin for onchocerciasis announced by Merck . . . Efficacy of *Haemophilus influenzae* vaccine reassessed . . . Research fellowships and grants offered for 1988–1989

14 **Therapy Consultation**

Treatment of stomatitis associated with antineoplastic-drug therapy

18 **Letters**

Routine monitoring of serum vancomycin concentrations: The answer lies in the middle, Jeffrey F. B. Sayers, Robert Shimasaki . . . Notice to readers, Frederick P. Zeller, Karen J. Klamerus

Drug Reviews

21 **Lovastatin: A new cholesterol-lowering agent**
James M. McKenney

37 **Sulbactam: A β-lactamase inhibitor**
Jean K. Noguchi and Mark A. Gill

Research

52 **Pharmacokinetics of leucovorin calcium after intravenous, intramuscular, and oral administration**
Brian W. McGuire, Luisa L. Sia, Philip T. Leese, Manuel L. Gutierrez, and E. L. Robert Stokstad

58 **Effect of sucralfate on theophylline absorption in healthy volunteers**
Kimberly A. Cantral, Larry J. Schaaf, Paul W. Jungnickel, and Howard P. Monsour

Research Note

62 **Estimation of creatinine clearance in malnourished patients**
Alan H. Lau, Steven I. Berk, Theresa Prosser, and Terry Stonich

Drug Experience

66 **Bromate poisoning from ingestion of professional hair-care neutralizer**
Jane N. Lue, Cary E. Johnson, and Deborah L. Edwards

70 **Treatment of oral candidiasis with amphotericin B solution**
Renée Brandell, Sandra L. Chase, and John R. Cohn

ASHP Report

73 **Procedure for submission of manuscripts to journals published by the American Society of Hospital Pharmacists**

75 **CP Continuing Education**

77 **Current Literature**

Drug Reaction Alerts . . . Book Review: *Cancer Chemotherapy by Infusion* (*Lokich*), Rebecca S. Finley . . . Books Received

80 **Advertising Index**

CLINICAL PHARMACY

Editor
William A. Zellmer

Managing Editor
C. Richard Talley

Associate Editor, Manuscript Development
Jane L. Miller

Associate Editor, Redaction
Nancy Tarleton Landis

Assistant Editors, Manuscript Development
Cynthia A. Knapp
Catherine A. Nichols

Assistant Editor, Redaction
Susan S. McLaughlin

Production Manager
Martha S. McDonald

Assistant Production Manager
Wende B. Mack

Editorial Assistant
Nancy K. Hughitt

Editorial Office
4630 Montgomery Avenue
Bethesda, MD 20814
301-657-3000

Editorial Board
David M. Angaran, M.S.
Steven L. Barriere, Pharm.D.
Stephen G. Bryant, Pharm.D.
Barry L. Carter, Pharm.D.
Burke A. Cunha, M.D.
Joseph T. DiPiro, Pharm.D.
Larry Ereshefsky, Pharm.D.
William R. Garnett, Pharm.D.
Robert J. Ignoffo, Pharm.D.
John W. Jenne, M.D.
Edward P. Krenzelok, Pharm.D.
Calvin Kunin, M.D.
Gary R. Matzke, Pharm.D.
Frans W. H. M. Merkus, Ph.D.
Jay M. Mirtallo, M.S.
John E. Murphy, Pharm.D.
Milap C. Nahata, Pharm.D.
Stephanie J. Phelps, Pharm.D.
John J. Piecoro, Jr., Pharm.D., M.S.
Richard Quintiliani, M.D.
John H. Rodman, Pharm.D.
Keith A. Rodvold, Pharm.D.
Fred Salter, Pharm.D.
Gerald E. Schumacher, Pharm.D., Ph.D.
Catherine Angell Sohn, Pharm.D.
Robert L. Talbert, Pharm.D.

Consulting Editors
Randal L. Batenhorst, Pharm.D.; Larry A. Bauer, Pharm.D.; Rosemary R. Berardi, Pharm.D.; John Bosso, Pharm.D.; Daniel T. Casto, Pharm.D.; Robert J. Cipolle, Pharm.D.; Joseph F. Dasta, M.Sc.; Michael N. Dudley, Pharm.D.; Lawrence J. Hak, Pharm.D.; David W. Hawkins, Pharm.D.; J. Heyward Hull, Pharm.D.; Martin J. Jinks, Pharm.D.; Cary E. Johnson, Pharm.D.; H. William Kelly, Pharm.D.; Jeffrey R. Koup, Pharm.D.; Thomas C. Majerus, Pharm.D.; Anthony S. Manoguerra, Pharm.D.; James M. McKenney, Pharm.D.; Donald S. North, Pharm.D.; Vaughn W. Payne, Pharm.D.; Donald G. Perrier, Ph.D.; Ronald E. Polk, Pharm.D.; Robert P. Rapp, Pharm.D.; Nathan Rawls, Pharm.D.; David R. Rush, Pharm.D.; Steven L. Sheaffer, Pharm. D.; John K. Siepler, Pharm.D.; Ralph E. Small, Pharm.D.; Glen L. Stimmel, Pharm.D.; Timothy R. Sykes, Pharm.D.; Scott L. Traub, Pharm.D.; William Troutman, Pharm.D.; Peter H. Vlasses, Pharm.D.; Barbara G. Wells, Pharm.D.; Dennis West, M.S.; Michael E. Winter, Pharm.D.

Copyright © 1988, American Society of Hospital Pharmacists, Inc. All rights reserved.

Instructions to Authors

CLINICAL PHARMACY, a forum for the drug therapeutics information that pharmacists need to perform their clinical roles, gives priority to (1) studies that objectively evaluate drug effects in human trials, (2) evaluative review articles on the clinical uses of new drugs, and (3) evaluations of the current status of drug therapy in selected diseases. Contributions to the following sections are invited:

Drug Reviews: Detailed, analytical reviews on the clinical use of specific drugs, with preference given to new drugs and to evaluative rather than descriptive literature reviews.

Therapy Reviews: Articles that focus primarily on a disease state (rather than on a drug or drug class) and its treatment. These reviews foster an understanding of the pathophysiology of a disease and the related treatment.

Research: Reports of well-conducted original research on drug effects in humans.

Research Notes: Short research reports, such as updates on previously published work, confirmations of previous findings, or original research of modest scope.

Grand Rounds: Patient case reports and literature reviews combined in a way that gives them high educational value.

Drug Experience: Straightforward reports, with selected literature references, of unusual drug experiences.

Therapy Consultation: Brief advice, in a question-and-answer format, on how to handle specific drug-therapy problems. Readers are invited to submit questions, which the editor will forward to appropriate consultants for answering.

Letters: Short comments on previously published work or about potential problems, apparent trends, or controversies in drug therapy or clinical research.

Commentaries: Well-reasoned expressions of opinion on drug-therapy or clinical-research issues.

The editors have the sole authority to decide in which section to publish an accepted manuscript.

Manuscripts are subject to review by qualified outside reviewers, as well as by the editors, and will be accepted for publication only if they are believed to represent an important contribution to the literature. All papers submitted for publication must be accompanied by a completed copy of a manuscript checklist. The checklist, which generally conforms to the Uniform Requirements for Manuscripts Submitted to Biomedical Journals, appears on pages 73–74 of the January 1988 issue. Authors of especially important original work may request "fast-track" review of their papers. Authors may suggest appropriate reviewers for their papers.

Accepted materials become the permanent and sole property of ASHP and may not be published or reprinted elsewhere without written permission from both the author and the editor.

The editors reserve the right to revise all materials submitted, if necessary. The publisher assumes no responsibility for the statements and opinions advanced by contributors to CLINICAL PHARMACY.

Under the terms of the Copyright Revision Act of 1976 (Public Law 94-553) it is necessary to have the rights of the authors transferred to the publisher in order to provide for the widest possible dissemination of professional and scientific literature. Accordingly, all transmittal letters accompanying manuscripts submitted for publication, including contributions for the Letters column, must contain the following language: "In consideration of the American Society of Hospital Pharmacists (ASHP) taking action in reviewing and editing my (our) submission, the author(s) undersigned hereby transfer(s), assign(s), or otherwise convey(s) all ownership rights in the submission and all copyright ownership to ASHP. In the event that such work is not published by ASHP, all said rights shall be released." We regret that we cannot consider manuscripts for publication that are not accompanied with transmittal letters containing the above language signed by all authors.

Authors must certify in their letter of transmittal that none of the material in their manuscript has been published previously nor is under consideration or been accepted for publication elsewhere. If this certification cannot be made, suitable explanation must be offered.

Six copies of all manuscripts should be submitted. Manuscripts should be typewritten with double spacing (including tables) on one side of good quality, 21.6 × 27.9-cm white paper, and with margins of at least 2.5 cm. For guidance on style, authors should consult the manuscript checklist, recent issues of CLINICAL PHARMACY, and the *Council of Biology Editors Style Manual*, fifth edition. *The American Heritage Dictionary of the English Language* and the AMA's *Manual for Authors and Editors* contain helpful advice on correct usage.

Galley proofs are sent to authors for inspection against the original manuscript and for correction. Unnecessary alterations in galley proof must be avoided. An order form for reprints is sent to the corresponding author after galley proofs have been cleared.

CLINICAL PHARMACY (ISSN 0278-2677) is published monthly by the American Society of Hospital Pharmacists, 4630 Montgomery Avenue, Bethesda, MD 20814. Joseph A. Oddis, Executive Vice President. Second class postage is paid at Bethesda, MD, and at additional mailing offices. **Postmaster: Send address changes to: *Clinical Pharmacy,* 4630 Montgomery Avenue, Bethesda, MD 20814.**

Annual Subscription Rate:	*USA*	*Non-USA*
ASHP Member	$40	$45
ASHP Student Members and Residents	$30	$35
Institutions and Nonmembers	$63	$68

The cost of single copies is $10. Airmail delivery outside of the continental United States is available for an additional charge of $72 per year. Requests to replace missing issues free of charge are honored only up to six months after date of issue.

Advertising for CLINICAL PHARMACY is accepted in accordance with the Statement of Advertising Policy of the American Society of Hospital Pharmacists (see *Am J Hosp Pharm.* 1987; 44:1146). For additional information, contact the Advertising Representative (William McCausland Associates, Inc., P.O. Box 189, Pitman, NJ 08071. Phone 609-589-5454, FAX 609-582-7611.)

All articles published, including editorials, letters, and book reviews, represent the opinions of the authors and do not reflect the official policy of the American Society of Hospital Pharmacists or the institution with which the author is affiliated, unless this is specified.

Microfilm and microfiche editions are available for purchase. Contact University Microfilms, 300 N. Zeeb Road, Ann Arbor, MI 48106.

Articles in CLINICAL PHARMACY are abstracted and indexed in *Current Contents, Clinical Sciences, Excerpta Medica, Index Medicus, Inpharma, International Pharmaceutical Abstracts,* and *Reactions.*

February 1988 Volume 7, Number 2 Coden: CPHADV ISSN: 0278-2677

CLINICAL PHARMACY

85 **News**

Recombinant tissue-plasminogen activator approved by FDA . . . Efficacy of intravenous streptokinase after myocardial infarction confirmed; labeled indications expanded . . . Study shows gemfibrozil reduces risk of coronary heart disease . . . Ganciclovir shows promise against cytomegalovirus, but data are insufficient for approval recommendation . . . Periodic dressing changes of peripheral venous catheter sites not indicated, study shows . . . CDC advises on detection and control of antibiotic-resistant *Neisseria gonorrhoeae*

93 **Therapy Consultation**

Metronidazole for pseudomembranous colitis

95 **Letters**

Anabolic steroid use as an AIDS risk factor, Walter J. McClain, Kathryn K. Bucci . . . Wanted: Insightful authors of review articles, John H. Rodman

Drug Review

97 **Nicardipine, nitrendipine, and bepridil: New calcium antagonists for cardiovascular disorders**
Guy R. Hasegawa

Therapy Reviews

109 **Rocky Mountain spotted fever**
Claudia A. Kamper, Katherine Hammond Chessman, and Stephanie J. Phelps

117 **Pathophysiology and treatment of the anemia of renal failure**
Curtis A. Johnson and Michael I. S. Chester

123 **Management of hypophosphatemia**
Charles W. Lloyd and Cary E. Johnson

Research

129 **Comparison of equal-weight oral dosages of verapamil hydrochloride and diltiazem hydrochloride in patients with mild to moderate hypertension**
John W. Hollifield, James J. Heusner, Mary DesChamps, James Gray, Daniel A. Spyker, Karl E. Peace, and Brian Dickson

135 **Comparative bioavailability of two oral sustained-release procainamide products**
Brian A. Baker, John R. Reynolds, Louis Gleckel, Edward A'Zary, and Monty M. Bodenheimer

Research Notes

139 **Effect of diphenoxylate with atropine sulfate on the bioavailability of quinidine sulfate in healthy subjects**
John J. Ponzillo, Joseph M. Scavone, Robert P. Paone, George P. Lewis, Carolyn M. Rayment, and William E. Fitzsimmons

142 **Effect of temperature on in vitro measurement of quinidine free fraction**
Catherine N. Verme, Thomas M. Ludden, and Steven C. Harris

146 **Association between depression and propranolol use in ambulatory patients**
David Bartels, Michael Glasser, Arthur Wang, and Patrick Swanson

150 **Comparison of 16-meq and 20-meq daily potassium supplement regimens**
Bonita L. Roohk, Fred L. Meister, Mary K. Hewett, and John A. Rumsfeld

Drug Experience

153 **Phenytoin-induced pseudolymphoma with mycosis fungoides manifestations**
L. Evans Cooke, Thomas C. Hardin, and Dan J. Hendrickson

158 **CP Continuing Education**

160 **Current Literature**

Drug Reaction Alerts . . . Book Reviews: *Avery's Drug Treatment: Principles and Practice of Clinical Pharmacology and Therapeutics, Third Edition* (*Speight*), Michael J. Melby . . . *Guide to Planning and Managing Multiple Clinical Studies* (*Spilker*), Mark C. Norris and Ghassem E. Larijani . . . Books Received

162 **Advertising Index**

CLINICAL PHARMACY

Editor
William A. Zellmer

Managing Editor
C. Richard Talley

Associate Editor, Manuscript Development
Jane L. Miller

Associate Editor, Redaction
Nancy Tarleton Landis

Assistant Editors, Manuscript Development
Cynthia A. Knapp
Catherine A. Nichols

Assistant Editor, Redaction
Susan S. McLaughlin

Production Manager
Martha S. McDonald

Assistant Production Manager
Wende B. Mack

Editorial Assistant
Nancy K. Hughitt

Editorial Office
4630 Montgomery Avenue
Bethesda, MD 20814
301-657-3000

Editorial Board
David M. Angaran, M.S.
Steven L. Barriere, Pharm.D.
Stephen G. Bryant, Pharm.D.
Barry L. Carter, Pharm.D.
Burke A. Cunha, M.D.
Joseph T. DiPiro, Pharm.D.
Larry Ereshefsky, Pharm.D.
William R. Garnett, Pharm.D.
Robert J. Ignoffo, Pharm.D.
John W. Jenne, M.D.
Edward P. Krenzelok, Pharm.D.
Calvin Kunin, M.D.
Gary R. Matzke, Pharm.D.
Frans W. H. M. Merkus, Ph.D.
Jay M. Mirtallo, M.S.
John E. Murphy, Pharm.D.
Milap C. Nahata, Pharm.D.
Stephanie J. Phelps, Pharm.D.
John J. Piecoro, Jr., Pharm.D., M.S.
Richard Quintiliani, M.D.
John H. Rodman, Pharm.D.
Keith A. Rodvold, Pharm.D.
Fred Salter, Pharm.D.
Gerald E. Schumacher, Pharm.D., Ph.D.
Catherine Angell Sohn, Pharm.D.
Robert L. Talbert, Pharm.D.

Consulting Editors
Randal L. Batenhorst, Pharm.D.; Larry A. Bauer, Pharm.D.; Rosemary R. Berardi, Pharm.D.; John Bosso, Pharm.D.; Daniel T. Casto, Pharm.D.; Robert J. Cipolle, Pharm.D.; Joseph F. Dasta, M.Sc.; Michael N. Dudley, Pharm.D.; Lawrence J. Hak, Pharm.D.; David W. Hawkins, Pharm.D.; J. Heyward Hull, Pharm.D.; Martin J. Jinks, Pharm.D.; Cary E. Johnson, Pharm.D.; H. William Kelly, Pharm.D.; Jeffrey R. Koup, Pharm.D.; Thomas C. Majerus, Pharm.D.; Anthony S. Manoguerra, Pharm.D.; James M. McKenney, Pharm.D.; Donald S. North, Pharm.D.; Vaughn W. Payne, Pharm.D.; Donald G. Perrier, Ph.D.; Ronald E. Polk, Pharm.D.; Robert P. Rapp, Pharm.D.; Nathan Rawls, Pharm.D.; David R. Rush, Pharm.D.; Steven L. Sheaffer, Pharm. D.; John K. Siepler, Pharm.D.; Ralph E. Small, Pharm.D.; Glen L. Stimmel, Pharm.D.; Timothy R. Sykes, Pharm.D.; Scott L. Traub, Pharm.D.; William Troutman, Pharm.D.; Peter H. Vlasses, Pharm.D.; Barbara G. Wells, Pharm.D.; Dennis West, M.S.; Michael E. Winter, Pharm.D.

Copyright © 1988, American Society of Hospital Pharmacists, Inc. All rights reserved.

Instructions to Authors

Clinical Pharmacy, a forum for the drug therapeutics information that pharmacists need to perform their clinical roles, gives priority to (1) studies that objectively evaluate drug effects in human trials, (2) evaluative review articles on the clinical uses of new drugs, and (3) evaluations of the current status of drug therapy in selected diseases. Contributions to the following sections are invited:

Drug Reviews: Detailed, analytical reviews on the clinical use of specific drugs, with preference given to new drugs and to evaluative rather than descriptive literature reviews.

Therapy Reviews: Articles that focus primarily on a disease state (rather than on a drug or drug class) and its treatment. These reviews foster an understanding of the pathophysiology of a disease and the related treatment.

Research: Reports of well-conducted original research on drug effects in humans.

Research Notes: Short research reports, such as updates on previously published work, confirmations of previous findings, or original research of modest scope.

Grand Rounds: Patient case reports and literature reviews combined in a way that gives them high educational value.

Drug Experience: Straightforward reports, with selected literature references, of unusual drug experiences.

Therapy Consultation: Brief advice, in a question-and-answer format, on how to handle specific drug-therapy problems. Readers are invited to submit questions, which the editor will forward to appropriate consultants for answering.

Letters: Short comments on previously published work or about potential problems, apparent trends, or controversies in drug therapy or clinical research.

Commentaries: Well-reasoned expressions of opinion on drug-therapy or clinical-research issues.

The editors have the sole authority to decide in which section to publish an accepted manuscript.

Manuscripts are subject to review by qualified outside reviewers, as well as by the editors, and will be accepted for publication only if they are believed to represent an important contribution to the literature. All papers submitted for publication must be accompanied by a completed copy of a manuscript checklist. The checklist, which generally conforms to the Uniform Requirements for Manuscripts Submitted to Biomedical Journals, appears on pages 73–74 of the January 1988 issue. Authors of especially important original work may request "fast-track" review of their papers. Authors may suggest appropriate reviewers for their papers.

Accepted materials become the permanent and sole property of ASHP and may not be published or reprinted elsewhere without written permission from both the author and the editor.

The editors reserve the right to revise all materials submitted, if necessary. The publisher assumes no responsibility for the statements and opinions advanced by contributors to Clinical Pharmacy.

Under the terms of the Copyright Revision Act of 1976 (Public Law 94-553) it is necessary to have the rights of the authors transferred to the publisher in order to provide for the widest possible dissemination of professional and scientific literature. Accordingly, all transmittal letters accompanying manuscripts submitted for publication, including contributions for the Letters column, must contain the following language: "In consideration of the American Society of Hospital Pharmacists (ASHP) taking action in reviewing and editing my (our) submission, the author(s) undersigned hereby transfer(s), assign(s), or otherwise convey(s) all ownership rights in the submission and all copyright ownership to ASHP. In the event that such work is not published by ASHP, all said rights shall be released." We regret that we cannot consider manuscripts for publication that are not accompanied with transmittal letters containing the above language signed by all authors.

Authors must certify in their letter of transmittal that none of the material in their manuscript has been published previously nor is under consideration or been accepted for publication elsewhere. If this certification cannot be made, suitable explanation must be offered.

Six copies of all manuscripts should be submitted. Manuscripts should be typewritten with double spacing (including tables) on one side of good quality, 21.6 × 27.9-cm white paper, and with margins of at least 2.5 cm. For guidance on style, authors should consult the manuscript checklist, recent issues of Clinical Pharmacy, and the *Council of Biology Editors Style Manual*, fifth edition. *The American Heritage Dictionary of the English Language* and the AMA's *Manual for Authors and Editors* contain helpful advice on correct usage.

Galley proofs are sent to authors for inspection against the original manuscript and for correction. Unnecessary alterations in galley proof must be avoided. An order form for reprints is sent to the corresponding author after galley proofs have been cleared.

Clinical Pharmacy (ISSN 0278-2677) is published monthly by the American Society of Hospital Pharmacists, 4630 Montgomery Avenue, Bethesda, MD 20814. Joseph A. Oddis, Executive Vice President. Second class postage is paid at Bethesda, MD, and at additional mailing offices. **Postmaster: Send address changes to: *Clinical Pharmacy*, 4630 Montgomery Avenue, Bethesda, MD 20814.**

Annual Subscription Rate:	*USA*	*Non-USA*
ASHP Member	$40	$45
ASHP Student Members and Residents	$30	$35
Institutions and Nonmembers	$63	$68

The cost of single copies is $10. Airmail delivery outside of the continental United States is available for an additional charge of $72 per year. Requests to replace missing issues free of charge are honored only up to six months after date of issue.

Advertising for Clinical Pharmacy is accepted in accordance with the Statement of Advertising Policy of the American Society of Hospital Pharmacists (see *Am J Hosp Pharm.* 1987; 44:1146). For additional information, contact the Advertising Representative (William McCausland Associates, Inc., P.O. Box 189, Pitman, NJ 08071. Phone 609-589-5454, FAX 609-582-7611.)

All articles published, including editorials, letters, and book reviews, represent the opinions of the authors and do not reflect the official policy of the American Society of Hospital Pharmacists or the institution with which the author is affiliated, unless this is specified.

Microfilm and microfiche editions are available for purchase. Contact University Microfilms, 300 N. Zeeb Road, Ann Arbor, MI 48106.

Articles in Clinical Pharmacy are abstracted and indexed in *Current Contents, Clinical Sciences, Excerpta Medica, Index Medicus, Inpharma, International Pharmaceutical Abstracts*, and *Reactions*.

March 1988 Volume 7, Number 3

Coden: CPHADV ISSN: 0278-2677

CLINICAL PHARMACY

166 **News**

FDA's drug review process is focus of attention in 1987; agency approves 27 new products . . . Immunization of younger children possible with new *Haemophilus influenzae* vaccine . . . More potent inactivated poliovirus vaccine approved by FDA; CDC to review vaccination policies in 1988 . . . Serotonin-uptake inhibition accounts for activity of new antidepressant . . . Studies suggest possible role for sucralfate in critically ill patients . . . Rule on nonprescription first-aid antibiotics finalized by FDA

184 **Therapy Consultation**

Management of vancomycin-induced "red-man syndrome"

Drug Review

187 **Guanfacine hydrochloride: A centrally acting antihypertensive agent**
Laura A. Cornish

Therapy Review

198 **Drug dosing during continuous arteriovenous hemofiltration**
Susan K. Bickley

Research

207 **Intrapatient variation of aminoglycoside pharmacokinetics in critically ill surgery patients**
David W. Fuhs, Henry J. Mann, Carol Ann M. Kubajak, and Frank B. Cerra

214 **Effect of infusion pump fill-stroke flow interruption on response to sodium nitroprusside in surgical patients**
Henry J. Mann, David W. Fuhs, and Frank B. Cerra

219 **Efficacy of individualized phenytoin sodium loading doses administered by intravenous infusion**
Francine G. Dela Cruz, Michele Z. Kanter, James H. Fischer, and Jerrold B. Leikin

224 **Glipizide pharmacokinetics in young and elderly volunteers**
Kelly A. Kobayashi, Larry A. Bauer, John R. Horn, Kent Opheim, Francis Wood, Jr., and Wayne A. Kradjan

228 **Effect of food and gastric acidity on absorption of orally administered ketoconazole**
Parichat Lelawongs, Joseph A. Barone, John L. Colaizzi, Alice T. M. Hsuan, Witold Mechlinski, Robert Legendre, and Joseph Guarnieri

Research Note

235 **Effects of diltiazem hydrochloride on glucose tolerance in persons at risk for diabetes mellitus**
Barbara J. Jones, James M. McKenney, Jackson T. Wright, Jr., and Robert P. Goodman

Commentary

239 **Selection of a human growth hormone product**
Kelly J. Burch and Mariela Alvarado-Hughes

241 **CP Continuing Education**

243 **Current Literature**

Drug Reaction Alerts . . . Book Reviews: *Cardiovascular Drug Therapy* (*Hunyor*), Daniel E. Hilleman . . . *Drug Treatment of the Rheumatic Diseases, Third Edition* (*Hart*), Stephen L. Dahl . . . *Pharmacokinetics and Pharmacodynamics: Research and Analysis* (*Smith, Kroboth, Juhl*), David A. Graves . . . *Pharmacology in Medicine: Principles and Practice* (*Pradhan, Maickel, Dutta*), Jon W. Banning . . . *Problems in Pediatric Drug Therapy, Second Edition* (*Pagliaro, Pagliaro*), Karin E. Zenk . . . Books Received

246 **Advertising Index**

CLINICAL PHARMACY

Editor
William A. Zellmer

Managing Editor
C. Richard Talley

Associate Editor, Manuscript Development
Jane L. Miller

Associate Editor, Redaction
Nancy Tarleton Landis

Assistant Editors, Manuscript Development
Cynthia A. Knapp
Catherine A. Nichols

Assistant Editor, Redaction
Susan S. McLaughlin

Production Manager
Martha S. McDonald

Assistant Production Manager
Wende B. Mack

Editorial Assistant
Nancy K. Hughitt

Editorial Office
4630 Montgomery Avenue
Bethesda, MD 20814
301-657-3000

Editorial Board
David M. Angaran, M.S.
Steven L. Barriere, Pharm.D.
Stephen G. Bryant, Pharm.D.
Barry L. Carter, Pharm.D.
Burke A. Cunha, M.D.
Joseph T. DiPiro, Pharm.D.
Larry Ereshefsky, Pharm.D.
William R. Garnett, Pharm.D.
Robert J. Ignoffo, Pharm.D.
John W. Jenne, M.D.
Edward P. Krenzelok, Pharm.D.
Calvin Kunin, M.D.
Gary R. Matzke, Pharm.D.
Frans W. H. M. Merkus, Ph.D.
Jay M. Mirtallo, M.S.
John E. Murphy, Pharm.D.
Milap C. Nahata, Pharm.D.
Stephanie J. Phelps, Pharm.D.
John J. Piecoro, Jr., Pharm.D., M.S.
Richard Quintiliani, M.D.
John H. Rodman, Pharm.D.
Keith A. Rodvold, Pharm.D.
Fred Salter, Pharm.D.
Gerald E. Schumacher, Pharm.D., Ph.D.
Catherine Angell Sohn, Pharm.D.
Robert L. Talbert, Pharm.D.

Consulting Editors
Randal L. Batenhorst, Pharm.D.; Larry A. Bauer, Pharm.D.; Rosemary R. Berardi, Pharm.D.; John Bosso, Pharm.D.; Daniel T. Casto, Pharm.D.; Robert J. Cipolle, Pharm.D.; Joseph F. Dasta, M.Sc.; Michael N. Dudley, Pharm.D.; Lawrence J. Hak, Pharm.D.; David W. Hawkins, Pharm.D.; J. Heyward Hull, Pharm.D.; Martin J. Jinks, Pharm.D.; Cary E. Johnson, Pharm.D.; H. William Kelly, Pharm.D.; Jeffrey R. Koup, Pharm.D.; Thomas C. Majerus, Pharm.D.; Anthony S. Manoguerra, Pharm.D.; James M. McKenney, Pharm.D.; Donald S. North, Pharm.D.; Vaughn W. Payne, Pharm.D.; Donald G. Perrier, Ph.D.; Ronald E. Polk, Pharm.D.; Robert P. Rapp, Pharm.D.; Nathan Rawls, Pharm.D.; David R. Rush, Pharm.D.; Steven L. Sheaffer, Pharm. D.; John K. Siepler, Pharm.D.; Ralph E. Small, Pharm.D.; Glen L. Stimmel, Pharm.D.; Timothy R. Sykes, Pharm.D.; Scott L. Traub, Pharm.D.; William Troutman, Pharm.D.; Peter H. Vlasses, Pharm.D.; Barbara G. Wells, Pharm.D.; Dennis West, M.S.; Michael E. Winter, Pharm.D.

Copyright © 1988, American Society of Hospital Pharmacists, Inc. All rights reserved.

Instructions to Authors

CLINICAL PHARMACY, a forum for the drug therapeutics information that pharmacists need to perform their clinical roles, gives priority to (1) studies that objectively evaluate drug effects in human trials, (2) evaluative review articles on the clinical uses of new drugs, and (3) evaluations of the current status of drug therapy in selected diseases. Contributions to the following sections are invited:

Drug Reviews: Detailed, analytical reviews on the clinical use of specific drugs, with preference given to new drugs and to evaluative rather than descriptive literature reviews.

Therapy Reviews: Articles that focus primarily on a disease state (rather than on a drug or drug class) and its treatment. These reviews foster an understanding of the pathophysiology of a disease and the related treatment.

Research: Reports of well-conducted original research on drug effects in humans.

Research Notes: Short research reports, such as updates on previously published work, confirmations of previous findings, or original research of modest scope.

Grand Rounds: Patient case reports and literature reviews combined in a way that gives them high educational value.

Drug Experience: Straightforward reports, with selected literature references, of unusual drug experiences.

Therapy Consultation: Brief advice, in a question-and-answer format, on how to handle specific drug-therapy problems. Readers are invited to submit questions, which the editor will forward to appropriate consultants for answering.

Letters: Short comments on previously published work or about potential problems, apparent trends, or controversies in drug therapy or clinical research.

Commentaries: Well-reasoned expressions of opinion on drug-therapy or clinical-research issues.

The editors have the sole authority to decide in which section to publish an accepted manuscript.

Manuscripts are subject to review by qualified outside reviewers, as well as by the editors, and will be accepted for publication only if they are believed to represent an important contribution to the literature. All papers submitted for publication must be accompanied by a completed copy of a manuscript checklist. The checklist, which generally conforms to the Uniform Requirements for Manuscripts Submitted to Biomedical Journals, appears on pages 73–74 of the January 1988 issue. Authors of especially important original work may request "fast-track" review of their papers. Authors may suggest appropriate reviewers for their papers.

Accepted materials become the permanent and sole property of ASHP and may not be published or reprinted elsewhere without written permission from both the author and the editor.

The editors reserve the right to revise all materials submitted, if necessary. The publisher assumes no responsibility for the statements and opinions advanced by contributors to CLINICAL PHARMACY.

Under the terms of the Copyright Revision Act of 1976 (Public Law 94-553) it is necessary to have the rights of the authors transferred to the publisher in order to provide for the widest possible dissemination of professional and scientific literature. Accordingly, all transmittal letters accompanying manuscripts submitted for publication, including contributions for the Letters column, must contain the following language: "In consideration of the American Society of Hospital Pharmacists (ASHP) taking action in reviewing and editing my (our) submission, the author(s) undersigned hereby transfer(s), assign(s), or otherwise convey(s) all ownership rights in the submission and all copyright ownership to ASHP. In the event that such work is not published by ASHP, all said rights shall be released." We regret that we cannot consider manuscripts for publication that are not accompanied with transmittal letters containing the above language signed by all authors.

Authors must certify in their letter of transmittal that none of the material in their manuscript has been published previously nor is under consideration or been accepted for publication elsewhere. If this certification cannot be made, suitable explanation must be offered.

Six copies of all manuscripts should be submitted. Manuscripts should be typewritten with double spacing (including tables) on one side of good quality, 21.6 × 27.9-cm white paper, and with margins of at least 2.5 cm. For guidance on style, authors should consult the manuscript checklist, recent issues of CLINICAL PHARMACY, and the *Council of Biology Editors Style Manual*, fifth edition. *The American Heritage Dictionary of the English Language* and the AMA's *Manual for Authors and Editors* contain helpful advice on correct usage.

Galley proofs are sent to authors for inspection against the original manuscript and for correction. Unnecessary alterations in galley proof must be avoided. An order form for reprints is sent to the corresponding author after galley proofs have been cleared.

CLINICAL PHARMACY (ISSN 0278-2677) is published monthly by the American Society of Hospital Pharmacists, 4630 Montgomery Avenue, Bethesda, MD 20814. Joseph A. Oddis, Executive Vice President. Second class postage is paid at Bethesda, MD, and at additional mailing offices. **Postmaster: Send address changes to: *Clinical Pharmacy,* 4630 Montgomery Avenue, Bethesda, MD 20814.**

Annual Subscription Rate:	*USA*	*Non-USA*
ASHP Member	$40	$45
ASHP Student Members and Residents	$30	$35
Institutions and Nonmembers	$63	$68

The cost of single copies is $10. Airmail delivery outside of the continental United States is available for an additional charge of $72 per year. Requests to replace missing issues free of charge are honored only up to six months after date of issue.

Advertising for CLINICAL PHARMACY is accepted in accordance with the Statement of Advertising Policy of the American Society of Hospital Pharmacists (see *Am J Hosp Pharm.* 1987; 44:1146). For additional information, contact the Advertising Representative (William McCausland Associates, Inc., P.O. Box 189, Pitman, NJ 08071. Phone 609-589-5454, FAX 609-582-7611.)

All articles published, including editorials, letters, and book reviews, represent the opinions of the authors and do not reflect the official policy of the American Society of Hospital Pharmacists or the institution with which the author is affiliated, unless this is specified.

Microfilm and microfiche editions are available for purchase. Contact University Microfilms, 300 N. Zeeb Road, Ann Arbor, MI 48106.

Articles in CLINICAL PHARMACY are abstracted and indexed in *Current Contents, Clinical Sciences, Excerpta Medica, Index Medicus, Inpharma, International Pharmaceutical Abstracts,* and *Reactions.*

April 1988 Volume 7, Number 4 Coden: CPHADV ISSN: 0278-2677

CLINICAL PHARMACY

253 **News**

Record number of orphan drug designations granted in 1987 . . . Primary prevention study finds cardiovascular benefit with aspirin therapy . . . Panel cites deficiencies in cholesterol testing, urges national laboratory standardization . . . Study shows photoaged skin improves with topical tretinoin . . . Experimental antineoplastic regimen granted treatment IND status . . . Second AIDS vaccine enters clinical trials

265 **Therapy Consultation**

Choice of diluents for intrathecal drug administration

269 **Letters**

Suspected gentamicin allergy could be sulfite sensitivity, Dennis J. Mikolich, William W. McCloskey . . . Magnesium gluconate can be used as oral supplement, Harry Wong

269 **Corrections**

Drug Reviews

271 **Comparison of famotidine with cimetidine and ranitidine**
Rosemary R. Berardi, Roberta M. Tankanow, and Timothy T. Nostrant

285 **Use of cephalosporins with enhanced antianaerobic activity for treatment and prevention of anaerobic and mixed infections**
Joseph T. DiPiro and J. Russell May

Research

303 **Delivery of gentamicin by a controlled-release infusion system versus a minibag system**
Dee Marie Munoz, Elaine R. Green, Margaret M. Chrymko, Joseph M. Mylotte, and Jack G. Kitrenos

307 **Simulated effect of gentamicin assay errors on calculated pharmacokinetic values**
Eric G. Boyce and Carol B. Pugh

Research Notes

314 **Evaluation of lithium-tetracycline interaction**
Martha P. Fankhauser, James L. Lindon, Brigid Connolly, and Walter J. Healey

317 **Effect of ranitidine and cimetidine on ibuprofen pharmacokinetics**
David W. Stephenson, Ralph E. Small, John H. Wood, Hayes E. Willis, Steven M. Johnson, H. Thomas Karnes, and Kusuma Rajasekharaiah

Drug Experience

322 **Continuous infusion of midazolam hydrochloride to control status epilepticus**
Catherine B. Crisp, Richard Gannon, and Frederic Knauft

326 **CP Continuing Education**

329 **Current Literature**

Drug Reaction Alerts . . . Books Received

330 **Advertising Index**

CLINICAL PHARMACY

Editor
William A. Zellmer

Managing Editor
C. Richard Talley

Associate Editor, Manuscript Development
Jane L. Miller

Associate Editor, Redaction
Nancy Tarleton Landis

Assistant Editors, Manuscript Development
Cynthia A. Knapp
Catherine A. Nichols

Assistant Editor, Redaction
Susan S. McLaughlin

Production Manager
Martha S. McDonald

Assistant Production Manager
Wende B. Mack

Editorial Office
4630 Montgomery Avenue
Bethesda, MD 20814
301-657-3000

Editorial Board
David M. Angaran, M.S.
Steven L. Barriere, Pharm.D.
Stephen G. Bryant, Pharm.D.
Barry L. Carter, Pharm.D.
Burke A. Cunha, M.D.
Joseph T. DiPiro, Pharm.D.
Larry Ereshefsky, Pharm.D.
William R. Garnett, Pharm.D.
Robert J. Ignoffo, Pharm.D.
John W. Jenne, M.D.
Edward P. Krenzelok, Pharm.D.
Calvin Kunin, M.D.
Gary R. Matzke, Pharm.D.
Frans W. H. M. Merkus, Ph.D.
Jay M. Mirtallo, M.S.
John E. Murphy, Pharm.D.
Milap C. Nahata, Pharm.D.
Stephanie J. Phelps, Pharm.D.
John J. Piecoro, Jr., Pharm.D., M.S.
Richard Quintiliani, M.D.
John H. Rodman, Pharm.D.
Keith A. Rodvold, Pharm.D.
Fred Salter, Pharm.D.
Gerald E. Schumacher, Pharm.D., Ph.D.
Catherine Angell Sohn, Pharm.D.
Robert L. Talbert, Pharm.D.

Consulting Editors
Randal L. Batenhorst, Pharm.D.; Larry A. Bauer, Pharm.D.; Rosemary R. Berardi, Pharm.D.; John Bosso, Pharm.D.; Daniel T. Casto, Pharm.D.; Robert J. Cipolle, Pharm.D.; Joseph F. Dasta, M.Sc.; Michael N. Dudley, Pharm.D.; Lawrence J. Hak, Pharm.D.; David W. Hawkins, Pharm.D.; J. Heyward Hull, Pharm.D.; Martin J. Jinks, Pharm.D.; Cary E. Johnson, Pharm.D.; H. William Kelly, Pharm.D.; Jeffrey R. Koup, Pharm.D.; Thomas C. Majerus, Pharm.D.; Anthony S. Manoguerra, Pharm.D.; James M. McKenney, Pharm.D.; Donald S. North, Pharm.D.; Vaughn W. Payne, Pharm.D.; Donald G. Perrier, Ph.D.; Ronald E. Polk, Pharm.D.; Robert P. Rapp, Pharm.D.; Nathan Rawls, Pharm.D.; David R. Rush, Pharm.D.; Steven L. Sheaffer, Pharm. D.; John K. Siepler, Pharm.D.; Ralph E. Small, Pharm.D.; Glen L. Stimmel, Pharm.D.; Timothy R. Sykes, Pharm.D.; Scott L. Traub, Pharm.D.; William Troutman, Pharm.D.; Peter H. Vlasses, Pharm.D.; Barbara G. Wells, Pharm.D.; Dennis West, M.S.; Michael E. Winter, Pharm.D.

Copyright © 1988, American Society of Hospital Pharmacists, Inc. All rights reserved.

Instructions to Authors

Clinical Pharmacy, a forum for the drug therapeutics information that pharmacists need to perform their clinical roles, gives priority to (1) studies that objectively evaluate drug effects in human trials, (2) evaluative review articles on the clinical uses of new drugs, and (3) evaluations of the current status of drug therapy in selected diseases. Contributions to the following sections are invited:

Drug Reviews: Detailed, analytical reviews on the clinical use of specific drugs, with preference given to new drugs and to evaluative rather than descriptive literature reviews.

Therapy Reviews: Articles that focus primarily on a disease state (rather than on a drug or drug class) and its treatment. These reviews foster an understanding of the pathophysiology of a disease and the related treatment.

Research: Reports of well-conducted original research on drug effects in humans.

Research Notes: Short research reports, such as updates on previously published work, confirmations of previous findings, or original research of modest scope.

Grand Rounds: Patient case reports and literature reviews combined in a way that gives them high educational value.

Drug Experience: Straightforward reports, with selected literature references, of unusual drug experiences.

Therapy Consultation: Brief advice, in a question-and-answer format, on how to handle specific drug-therapy problems. Readers are invited to submit questions, which the editor will forward to appropriate consultants for answering.

Letters: Short comments on previously published work or about potential problems, apparent trends, or controversies in drug therapy or clinical research.

Commentaries: Well-reasoned expressions of opinion on drug-therapy or clinical-research issues.

The editors have the sole authority to decide in which section to publish an accepted manuscript.

Manuscripts are subject to review by qualified outside reviewers, as well as by the editors, and will be accepted for publication only if they are believed to represent an important contribution to the literature. All papers submitted for publication must be accompanied by a completed copy of a manuscript checklist. The checklist, which generally conforms to the Uniform Requirements for Manuscripts Submitted to Biomedical Journals, appears on pages 73–74 of the January 1988 issue. Authors of especially important original work may request "fast-track" review of their papers. Authors may suggest appropriate reviewers for their papers.

Accepted materials become the permanent and sole property of ASHP and may not be published or reprinted elsewhere without written permission from both the author and the editor.

The editors reserve the right to revise all materials submitted, if necessary. The publisher assumes no responsibility for the statements and opinions advanced by contributors to Clinical Pharmacy.

Under the terms of the Copyright Revision Act of 1976 (Public Law 94-553) it is necessary to have the rights of the authors transferred to the publisher in order to provide for the widest possible dissemination of professional and scientific literature. Accordingly, all transmittal letters accompanying manuscripts submitted for publication, including contributions for the Letters column, must contain the following language: "In consideration of the American Society of Hospital Pharmacists (ASHP) taking action in reviewing and editing my (our) submission, the author(s) undersigned hereby transfer(s), assign(s), or otherwise convey(s) all ownership rights in the submission and all copyright ownership to ASHP. In the event that such work is not published by ASHP, all said rights shall be released." We regret that we cannot consider manuscripts for publication that are not accompanied with transmittal letters containing the above language signed by all authors.

Authors must certify in their letter of transmittal that none of the material in their manuscript has been published previously nor is under consideration or been accepted for publication elsewhere. If this certification cannot be made, suitable explanation must be offered.

Six copies of all manuscripts should be submitted. Manuscripts should be typewritten with double spacing (including tables) on one side of good quality, 21.6 × 27.9-cm white paper, and with margins of at least 2.5 cm. For guidance on style, authors should consult the manuscript checklist, recent issues of Clinical Pharmacy, and the *Council of Biology Editors Style Manual*, fifth edition. *The American Heritage Dictionary of the English Language* and the AMA's *Manual for Authors and Editors* contain helpful advice on correct usage.

Galley proofs are sent to authors for inspection against the original manuscript and for correction. Unnecessary alterations in galley proof must be avoided. An order form for reprints is sent to the corresponding author after galley proofs have been cleared.

Clinical Pharmacy (ISSN 0278-2677) is published monthly by the American Society of Hospital Pharmacists, 4630 Montgomery Avenue, Bethesda, MD 20814. Joseph A. Oddis, Executive Vice President. Second class postage is paid at Bethesda, MD, and at additional mailing offices. **Postmaster: Send address changes to: *Clinical Pharmacy,* 4630 Montgomery Avenue, Bethesda, MD 20814.**

Annual Subscription Rate:	*USA*	*Non-USA*
ASHP Member	$40	$45
ASHP Student Members and Residents	$30	$35
Institutions and Nonmembers	$63	$68

The cost of single copies is $10. Airmail delivery outside of the continental United States is available for an additional charge of $72 per year. Requests to replace missing issues free of charge are honored only up to six months after date of issue.

Payments to ASHP are not deductible as charitable contributions for federal income tax purposes. However, they may be deductible under other provisions of the Internal Revenue Code.

Advertising for Clinical Pharmacy is accepted in accordance with the Statement of Advertising Policy of the American Society of Hospital Pharmacists (see *Am J Hosp Pharm.* 1987; 44:1146). For additional information, contact the Advertising Representative (William McCausland Associates, Inc., P.O. Box 189, Pitman, NJ 08071. Phone 609-589-5454, FAX 609-582-7611.)

All articles published, including editorials, letters, and book reviews, represent the opinions of the authors and do not reflect the official policy of the American Society of Hospital Pharmacists or the institution with which the author is affiliated, unless this is specified.

Microfilm and microfiche editions are available for purchase. Contact University Microfilms, 300 N. Zeeb Road, Ann Arbor, MI 48106.

Articles in Clinical Pharmacy are abstracted and indexed in *Current Contents, Clinical Sciences, Excerpta Medica, Index Medicus, Inpharma, International Pharmaceutical Abstracts,* and *Reactions.*

May 1988 Volume 7, Number 5 Coden: CPHADV ISSN: 0278-2677

CLINICAL PHARMACY

334 **News**

Report supports FDA's bioequivalence evaluation criteria, advocates more stringent statistical testing . . . FDA approves treatment IND protocol for trimetrexate . . . Focus of new FDA division is AIDS, opportunistic infections . . . FDA challenges Alzheimer's disease study findings . . . Study suggests limited role for comprehensive toxicology testing in drug overdoses

344 **Therapy Consultation**

Topical cromolyn sodium for recurrent aphthous ulcers

Therapy Review

351 **Parenteral nutrition in pediatric patients**
Emily B. Cochran, Stephanie J. Phelps, and Richard A. Helms

Research

367 **Accuracy of tobramycin delivery by four i.v. infusion methods**
Roy A. Pleasants, William T. Sawyer, Dennis M. Williams, William R. McKenna, John M. Brown, and J. Robert Powell

374 **Effect of four intravenous infusion methods on tobramycin pharmacokinetics**
Roy A. Pleasants, William T. Sawyer, Dennis M. Williams, William R. McKenna, and J. Robert Powell

Research Note

380 **Pharmacokinetic and pharmacodynamic comparison of mezlocillin and ticarcillin**
Robert G. Deeter, Steven L. Barriere, and Robert Fekety

Commentary

385 **Aminoglycosides: A reassessment of their therapeutic role**
Steven L. Barriere

Grand Rounds

391 **Death of a child associated with multiple overdoses of acetaminophen**
Kathryn V. Blake, David Bailey, Gary M. Zientek, and Leslie Hendeles

Drug Experience

398 **Neutropenia associated with oral acyclovir and multiple antibacterial agents in a patient with acquired immunodeficiency syndrome**
Mary Lynn McPherson and Karen I. Plaisance

402 **CP Continuing Education**

405 **Current Literature**

Drug Reaction Alerts . . . Book Review: *Drug Use in Respiratory Disease* (*Wilson*), Cary E. Johnson

406 **Advertising Index**

CLINICAL PHARMACY

Editor
William A. Zellmer

Managing Editor
C. Richard Talley

Associate Editor, Manuscript Development
Jane L. Miller

Associate Editor, Redaction
Nancy Tarleton Landis

Assistant Editors, Manuscript Development
Cynthia A. Knapp
Catherine A. Nichols

Assistant Editor, Redaction
Susan S. McLaughlin

Production Manager
Martha S. McDonald

Assistant Production Manager
Wende B. Mack

Editorial Office
4630 Montgomery Avenue
Bethesda, MD 20814
301-657-3000

Editorial Board
David M. Angaran, M.S.
Steven L. Barriere, Pharm.D.
Stephen G. Bryant, Pharm.D.
Barry L. Carter, Pharm.D.
Burke A. Cunha, M.D.
Joseph T. DiPiro, Pharm.D.
Larry Ereshefsky, Pharm.D.
William R. Garnett, Pharm.D.
Robert J. Ignoffo, Pharm.D.
John W. Jenne, M.D.
Edward P. Krenzelok, Pharm.D.
Calvin Kunin, M.D.
Gary R. Matzke, Pharm.D.
Frans W. H. M. Merkus, Ph.D.
Jay M. Mirtallo, M.S.
John E. Murphy, Pharm.D.
Milap C. Nahata, Pharm.D.
Stephanie J. Phelps, Pharm.D.
John J. Piecoro, Jr., Pharm.D., M.S.
Richard Quintiliani, M.D.
John H. Rodman, Pharm.D.
Keith A. Rodvold, Pharm.D.
Fred Salter, Pharm.D.
Gerald E. Schumacher, Pharm.D., Ph.D.
Catherine Angell Sohn, Pharm.D.
Robert L. Talbert, Pharm.D.

Consulting Editors
Randal L. Batenhorst, Pharm.D.; Larry A. Bauer, Pharm.D.; Rosemary R. Berardi, Pharm.D.; John Bosso, Pharm.D.; Daniel T. Casto, Pharm.D.; Robert J. Cipolle, Pharm.D.; Joseph F. Dasta, M.Sc.; Michael N. Dudley, Pharm.D.; Lawrence J. Hak, Pharm.D.; David W. Hawkins, Pharm.D.; J. Heyward Hull, Pharm.D.; Martin J. Jinks, Pharm.D.; Cary E. Johnson, Pharm.D.; H. William Kelly, Pharm.D.; Jeffrey R. Koup, Pharm.D.; Thomas C. Majerus, Pharm.D.; Anthony S. Manoguerra, Pharm.D.; James M. McKenney, Pharm.D.; Donald S. North, Pharm.D.; Vaughn W. Payne, Pharm.D.; Donald G. Perrier, Ph.D.; Ronald E. Polk, Pharm.D.; Robert P. Rapp, Pharm.D.; Nathan Rawls, Pharm.D.; David R. Rush, Pharm.D.; Steven L. Sheaffer, Pharm. D.; John K. Siepler, Pharm.D.; Ralph E. Small, Pharm.D.; Glen L. Stimmel, Pharm.D.; Timothy R. Sykes, Pharm.D.; Scott L. Traub, Pharm.D.; William Troutman, Pharm.D.; Peter H. Vlasses, Pharm.D.; Barbara G. Wells, Pharm.D.; Dennis West, M.S.; Michael E. Winter, Pharm.D.

Copyright © 1988, American Society of Hospital Pharmacists, Inc. All rights reserved.

Instructions to Authors

CLINICAL PHARMACY, a forum for the drug therapeutics information that pharmacists need to perform their clinical roles, gives priority to (1) studies that objectively evaluate drug effects in human trials, (2) evaluative review articles on the clinical uses of new drugs, and (3) evaluations of the current status of drug therapy in selected diseases. Contributions to the following sections are invited:

Drug Reviews: Detailed, analytical reviews on the clinical use of specific drugs, with preference given to new drugs and to evaluative rather than descriptive literature reviews.

Therapy Reviews: Articles that focus primarily on a disease state (rather than on a drug or drug class) and its treatment. These reviews foster an understanding of the pathophysiology of a disease and the related treatment.

Research: Reports of well-conducted original research on drug effects in humans.

Research Notes: Short research reports, such as updates on previously published work, confirmations of previous findings, or original research of modest scope.

Grand Rounds: Patient case reports and literature reviews combined in a way that gives them high educational value.

Drug Experience: Straightforward reports, with selected literature references, of unusual drug experiences.

Therapy Consultation: Brief advice, in a question-and-answer format, on how to handle specific drug-therapy problems. Readers are invited to submit questions, which the editor will forward to appropriate consultants for answering.

Letters: Short comments on previously published work or about potential problems, apparent trends, or controversies in drug therapy or clinical research.

Commentaries: Well-reasoned expressions of opinion on drug-therapy or clinical-research issues.

The editors have the sole authority to decide in which section to publish an accepted manuscript.

Manuscripts are subject to review by qualified outside reviewers, as well as by the editors, and will be accepted for publication only if they are believed to represent an important contribution to the literature. All papers submitted for publication must be accompanied by a completed copy of a manuscript checklist. The checklist, which generally conforms to the Uniform Requirements for Manuscripts Submitted to Biomedical Journals, appears on pages 73–74 of the January 1988 issue. Authors of especially important original work may request "fast-track" review of their papers. Authors may suggest appropriate reviewers for their papers.

Accepted materials become the permanent and sole property of ASHP and may not be published or reprinted elsewhere without written permission from both the author and the editor.

The editors reserve the right to revise all materials submitted, if necessary. The publisher assumes no responsibility for the statements and opinions advanced by contributors to CLINICAL PHARMACY.

Under the terms of the Copyright Revision Act of 1976 (Public Law 94-553) it is necessary to have the rights of the authors transferred to the publisher in order to provide for the widest possible dissemination of professional and scientific literature. Accordingly, all transmittal letters accompanying manuscripts submitted for publication, including contributions for the Letters column, must contain the following language: "In consideration of the American Society of Hospital Pharmacists (ASHP) taking action in reviewing and editing my (our) submission, the author(s) undersigned hereby transfer(s), assign(s), or otherwise convey(s) all ownership rights in the submission and all copyright ownership to ASHP. In the event that such work is not published by ASHP, all said rights shall be released." We regret that we cannot consider manuscripts for publication that are not accompanied with transmittal letters containing the above language signed by all authors.

Authors must certify in their letter of transmittal that none of the material in their manuscript has been published previously nor is under consideration or been accepted for publication elsewhere. If this certification cannot be made, suitable explanation must be offered.

Six copies of all manuscripts should be submitted. Manuscripts should be typewritten with double spacing (including tables) on one side of good quality, 21.6 × 27.9-cm white paper, and with margins of at least 2.5 cm. For guidance on style, authors should consult the manuscript checklist, recent issues of CLINICAL PHARMACY, and the *Council of Biology Editors Style Manual*, fifth edition. *The American Heritage Dictionary of the English Language* and the AMA's *Manual for Authors and Editors* contain helpful advice on correct usage.

Galley proofs are sent to authors for inspection against the original manuscript and for correction. Unnecessary alterations in galley proof must be avoided. An order form for reprints is sent to the corresponding author after galley proofs have been cleared.

CLINICAL PHARMACY (ISSN 0278-2677) is published monthly by the American Society of Hospital Pharmacists, 4630 Montgomery Avenue, Bethesda, MD 20814. Joseph A. Oddis, Executive Vice President. Second class postage is paid at Bethesda, MD, and at additional mailing offices. **Postmaster: Send address changes to: *Clinical Pharmacy*, 4630 Montgomery Avenue, Bethesda, MD 20814.**

Annual Subscription Rate:	*USA*	*Non-USA*
ASHP Member	$40	$45
ASHP Student Members and Residents	$30	$35
Institutions and Nonmembers	$63	$68

The cost of single copies is $10. Airmail delivery outside of the continental United States is available for an additional charge of $72 per year. Requests to replace missing issues free of charge are honored only up to six months after date of issue.

Payments to ASHP are not deductible as charitable contributions for federal income tax purposes. However, they may be deductible under other provisions of the Internal Revenue Code.

Advertising for CLINICAL PHARMACY is accepted in accordance with the Statement of Advertising Policy of the American Society of Hospital Pharmacists (see *Am J Hosp Pharm.* 1987; 44:1146). For additional information, contact the Advertising Representative (William McCausland Associates, Inc., P.O. Box 189, Pitman, NJ 08071. Phone 609-589-5454, FAX 609-582-7611.)

All articles published, including editorials, letters, and book reviews, represent the opinions of the authors and do not reflect the official policy of the American Society of Hospital Pharmacists or the institution with which the author is affiliated, unless this is specified.

Microfilm and microfiche editions are available for purchase. Contact University Microfilms, 300 N. Zeeb Road, Ann Arbor, MI 48106.

Articles in CLINICAL PHARMACY are abstracted and indexed in *Current Contents, Clinical Sciences, Excerpta Medica, Index Medicus, Inpharma, International Pharmaceutical Abstracts*, and *Reactions*.

June 1988 Volume 7, Number 6 Coden: CPHADV ISSN: 0278-2677

CLINICAL PHARMACY

413 **News**

Guidelines for authors of biomedical journal articles revised . . . Marketing of intravenous enalaprilat approved by FDA . . . Preliminary findings suggest APSAC reduces mortality after myocardial infarction . . . Information sheets for institutional review boards available from FDA . . . Conference for health-statistics data users set

422 **Therapy Consultation**

Use of H_2 histamine antagonists in allergic disorders

423 **Letters**

Midazolam sedation and amnesia in elective cardioversion, Daniel W. Krichbaum, Imtiaz Hamid

Drug Review

424 **Clinical use of systemic antifungal agents**
John M. Benson and Milap C. Nahata

Research

439 **Heparin sodium versus 0.9% sodium chloride injection for maintaining patency of indwelling intermittent infusion devices**
Robert A. Hamilton, Jeannine M. Plis, Carol Clay, and Lawrence Sylvan

444 **False-positive serum digoxin concentrations determined by three digoxin assays in patients with liver disease**
Julie Frisolone, Lynne M. Sylvia, Jeffrey Gelwan, Somnath Pal, and Crescens Pellechia

449 **Endogenous digoxin-like immunoreactivity in elderly patients with normal serum creatinine concentrations**
Thomas E. Lackner, Brad W. C. Lau, Curtis Parvin, and Roland Valdes, Jr.

454 **Continuous i.v. infusion versus multiple bolus doses of metoclopramide for prevention of cisplatin-induced emesis**
William A. Agostinucci, Richard H. Gannon, Grant R. Golub, Robert S. Martin, Peter K. Schauer, and Emelie B. Dinonno

Research Notes

457 **Effect of pentoxifylline and its metabolites on three theophylline assays**
Ira A. Cohen, Cary E. Johnson, Laurie Wesolowicz, and Kathleen Converse–Swastek

462 **Accuracy and time requirements for use of three rapid theophylline assay methods**
G. Dennis Clifton, Mark E. West, Bernard A. Hunt, and N. K. Burki

467 **Intraoperative serum, bile, and gallbladder-wall concentrations of cefmetazole in patients undergoing cholecystectomy**
Matthew K. Ito, Mark A. Gill, Frank C. Chenella, Thomas V. Berne, Albert E. Yellin, Peter N. R. Heseltine, and Maria D. Appleman

Commentaries

469 **Thrombolysis for acute myocardial infarction: Does a greater incidence of reperfusion justify preferential use of an agent?**
Paul E. Nolan, Jr.

473 **Thrombolysis for acute myocardial infarction: Is proof of a reduction in mortality critical to drug selection?**
Jeffrey A. Green

478 **CP Continuing Education**

480 **ASHP CE Instructions and Enrollment Form**

481 **Current Literature**

Drug Reaction Alerts . . . Books Received

482 **Advertising Index**

CLINICAL PHARMACY

Editor
William A. Zellmer

Managing Editor
C. Richard Talley

Associate Editor, Manuscript Development
Jane L. Miller

Associate Editor, Redaction
Nancy Tarleton Landis

Assistant Editors, Manuscript Development
Cynthia A. Knapp
Catherine A. Nichols

Assistant Editor, Redaction
Susan S. McLaughlin

Production Manager
Martha S. McDonald

Assistant Production Manager
Wende B. Mack

Editorial Office
4630 Montgomery Avenue
Bethesda, MD 20814
301-657-3000

Editorial Board
David M. Angaran, M.S.
Steven L. Barriere, Pharm.D.
Stephen G. Bryant, Pharm.D.
Barry L. Carter, Pharm.D.
Burke A. Cunha, M.D.
Joseph T. DiPiro, Pharm.D.
Larry Ereshefsky, Pharm.D.
William R. Garnett, Pharm.D.
Robert J. Ignoffo, Pharm.D.
John W. Jenne, M.D.
Edward P. Krenzelok, Pharm.D.
Calvin Kunin, M.D.
Gary R. Matzke, Pharm.D.
Frans W. H. M. Merkus, Ph.D.
Jay M. Mirtallo, M.S.
John E. Murphy, Pharm.D.
Milap C. Nahata, Pharm.D.
Stephanie J. Phelps, Pharm.D.
John J. Piecoro, Jr., Pharm.D., M.S.
Richard Quintiliani, M.D.
John H. Rodman, Pharm.D.
Keith A. Rodvold, Pharm.D.
Fred Salter, Pharm.D.
Gerald E. Schumacher, Pharm.D., Ph.D.
Catherine Angell Sohn, Pharm.D.
Robert L. Talbert, Pharm.D.

Consulting Editors
Randal L. Batenhorst, Pharm.D.; Larry A. Bauer, Pharm.D.; Rosemary R. Berardi, Pharm.D.; John Bosso, Pharm.D.; Daniel T. Casto, Pharm.D.; Robert J. Cipolle, Pharm.D.; Joseph F. Dasta, M.Sc.; Michael N. Dudley, Pharm.D.; Lawrence J. Hak, Pharm.D.; David W. Hawkins, Pharm.D.; J. Heyward Hull, Pharm.D.; Martin J. Jinks, Pharm.D.; Cary E. Johnson, Pharm.D.; H. William Kelly, Pharm.D.; Jeffrey R. Koup, Pharm.D.; Thomas C. Majerus, Pharm.D.; Anthony S. Manoguerra, Pharm.D.; James M. McKenney, Pharm.D.; Donald S. North, Pharm.D.; Vaughn W. Payne, Pharm.D.; Donald G. Perrier, Ph.D.; Ronald E. Polk, Pharm.D.; Robert P. Rapp, Pharm.D.; Nathan Rawls, Pharm.D.; David R. Rush, Pharm.D.; Steven L. Sheaffer, Pharm. D.; John K. Siepler, Pharm.D.; Ralph E. Small, Pharm.D.; Glen L. Stimmel, Pharm.D.; Timothy R. Sykes, Pharm.D.; Scott L. Traub, Pharm.D.; William Troutman, Pharm.D.; Peter H. Vlasses, Pharm.D.; Barbara G. Wells, Pharm.D.; Dennis West, M.S.; Michael E. Winter, Pharm.D.

Copyright © 1988, American Society of Hospital Pharmacists, Inc. All rights reserved.

Instructions to Authors

CLINICAL PHARMACY, a forum for the drug therapeutics information that pharmacists need to perform their clinical roles, gives priority to (1) studies that objectively evaluate drug effects in human trials, (2) evaluative review articles on the clinical uses of new drugs, and (3) evaluations of the current status of drug therapy in selected diseases. Contributions to the following sections are invited:

Drug Reviews: Detailed, analytical reviews on the clinical use of specific drugs, with preference given to new drugs and to evaluative rather than descriptive literature reviews.

Therapy Reviews: Articles that focus primarily on a disease state (rather than on a drug or drug class) and its treatment. These reviews foster an understanding of the pathophysiology of a disease and the related treatment.

Research: Reports of well-conducted original research on drug effects in humans.

Research Notes: Short research reports, such as updates on previously published work, confirmations of previous findings, or original research of modest scope.

Grand Rounds: Patient case reports and literature reviews combined in a way that gives them high educational value.

Drug Experience: Straightforward reports, with selected literature references, of unusual drug experiences.

Therapy Consultation: Brief advice, in a question-and-answer format, on how to handle specific drug-therapy problems. Readers are invited to submit questions, which the editor will forward to appropriate consultants for answering.

Letters: Short comments on previously published work or about potential problems, apparent trends, or controversies in drug therapy or clinical research.

Commentaries: Well-reasoned expressions of opinion on drug-therapy or clinical-research issues.

The editors have the sole authority to decide in which section to publish an accepted manuscript.

Manuscripts are subject to review by qualified outside reviewers, as well as by the editors, and will be accepted for publication only if they are believed to represent an important contribution to the literature. All papers submitted for publication must be accompanied by a completed copy of a manuscript checklist. The checklist, which generally conforms to the Uniform Requirements for Manuscripts Submitted to Biomedical Journals, appears on pages 73–74 of the January 1988 issue. Authors of especially important original work may request "fast-track" review of their papers. Authors may suggest appropriate reviewers for their papers.

Accepted materials become the permanent and sole property of ASHP and may not be published or reprinted elsewhere without written permission from both the author and the editor.

The editors reserve the right to revise all materials submitted, if necessary. The publisher assumes no responsibility for the statements and opinions advanced by contributors to CLINICAL PHARMACY.

Under the terms of the Copyright Revision Act of 1976 (Public Law 94-553) it is necessary to have the rights of the authors transferred to the publisher in order to provide for the widest possible dissemination of professional and scientific literature. Accordingly, all transmittal letters accompanying manuscripts submitted for publication, including contributions for the Letters column, must contain the following language: "In consideration of the American Society of Hospital Pharmacists (ASHP) taking action in reviewing and editing my (our) submission, the author(s) undersigned hereby transfer(s), assign(s), or otherwise convey(s) all ownership rights in the submission and all copyright ownership to ASHP. In the event that such work is not published by ASHP, all said rights shall be released." We regret that we cannot consider manuscripts for publication that are not accompanied with transmittal letters containing the above language signed by all authors.

Authors must certify in their letter of transmittal that none of the material in their manuscript has been published previously nor is under consideration or been accepted for publication elsewhere. If this certification cannot be made, suitable explanation must be offered.

Six copies of all manuscripts should be submitted. Manuscripts should be typewritten with double spacing (including tables) on one side of good quality, 21.6 × 27.9-cm white paper, and with margins of at least 2.5 cm. For guidance on style, authors should consult the manuscript checklist, recent issues of CLINICAL PHARMACY, and the *Council of Biology Editors Style Manual*, fifth edition. *The American Heritage Dictionary of the English Language* and the AMA's *Manual for Authors and Editors* contain helpful advice on correct usage.

Galley proofs are sent to authors for inspection against the original manuscript and for correction. Unnecessary alterations in galley proof must be avoided. An order form for reprints is sent to the corresponding author after galley proofs have been cleared.

CLINICAL PHARMACY (ISSN 0278-2677) is published monthly by the American Society of Hospital Pharmacists, 4630 Montgomery Avenue, Bethesda, MD 20814. Joseph A. Oddis, Executive Vice President. Second class postage is paid at Bethesda, MD, and at additional mailing offices. **Postmaster: Send address changes to: *Clinical Pharmacy*, 4630 Montgomery Avenue, Bethesda, MD 20814.**

Annual Subscription Rate:	*USA*	*Non-USA*
ASHP Member	$40	$45
ASHP Student Members and Residents	$30	$35
Institutions and Nonmembers	$63	$68

The cost of single copies is $10. Airmail delivery outside of the continental United States is available for an additional charge of $72 per year. Requests to replace missing issues free of charge are honored only up to six months after date of issue.

Payments to ASHP are not deductible as charitable contributions for federal income tax purposes. However, they may be deductible under other provisions of the Internal Revenue Code.

Advertising for CLINICAL PHARMACY is accepted in accordance with the Statement of Advertising Policy of the American Society of Hospital Pharmacists (see *Am J Hosp Pharm*. 1987; 44:1146). For additional information, contact the Advertising Representative (William McCausland Associates, Inc., P.O. Box 189, Pitman, NJ 08071. Phone 609-589-5454, FAX 609-582-7611.)

All articles published, including editorials, letters, and book reviews, represent the opinions of the authors and do not reflect the official policy of the American Society of Hospital Pharmacists or the institution with which the author is affiliated, unless this is specified.

Microfilm and microfiche editions are available for purchase. Contact University Microfilms, 300 N. Zeeb Road, Ann Arbor, MI 48106.

Articles in CLINICAL PHARMACY are abstracted and indexed in *Current Contents, Clinical Sciences, Excerpta Medica, Index Medicus, Inpharma, International Pharmaceutical Abstracts*, and *Reactions*.

July 1988 Volume 7, Number 7 Coden: CPHADV ISSN: 0278-2677

CLINICAL PHARMACY

488 **News**

National committee recommends greater flexibility in stepped-care treatment of hypertension . . . Procedures for reporting childhood-vaccine injuries announced . . . FDA amends standards for nonsterile neomycin sulfate to specify oral use only . . . FDA requires stronger warnings, imposes no limits on isotretinoin use

493 **Therapy Consultation**

Catecholamine selection for vasopressor-dependent patients

497 **Letters**

Status of injectable calcium antagonists, David M. Angaran . . . Applicability of phenytoin predictive formulas to long-term-care facility residents, Paul J. Drinka, Jan Miller, Susan K. Voeks

Drug Review

501 **Update on pentamidine for the treatment of *Pneumocystis carinii* pneumonia**
Francine R. Salamone and Burke A. Cunha

Editorials

511 **Infectious complications of AIDS**
Steven L. Barriere

512 **What is the role of parenteral nutrition in AIDS?**
Alan W. Hopefl

Grand Rounds

514 **Treatment of *Pneumocystis carinii* pneumonia in patients with AIDS**
Cindy J. Wordell and Stephen P. Hauptman

528 **Management of cryptococcal meningitis in patients with AIDS**
Jan Sahai

536 **Parenteral nutrition in the management of gastrointestinal Kaposi's sarcoma in a patient with AIDS**
Douglas D. Janson and Kathleen M. Teasley

545 **Treatment of nontuberculous mycobacterial infections in pediatric patients**
Robert H. Levin and Ann M. Bolinger

552 **CP Continuing Education**

555 **Current Literature**

Drug Reaction Alerts . . . Books Received

556 **Advertising Index**

CLINICAL PHARMACY

Editor
William A. Zellmer

Managing Editor
C. Richard Talley

Associate Editor, Manuscript Development
Jane L. Miller

Associate Editor, Redaction
Nancy Tarleton Landis

Assistant Editors, Manuscript Development
Cynthia A. Knapp
Catherine A. Nichols

Assistant Editor, Redaction
Susan S. McLaughlin

Editorial Production Coordinator
Wende B. Mack

Editorial Office
4630 Montgomery Avenue
Bethesda, MD 20814
301-657-3000

Editorial Board
Steven L. Barriere, Pharm.D.
Stephen G. Bryant, Pharm.D.
Barry L. Carter, Pharm.D.
Burke A. Cunha, M.D.
Joseph T. DiPiro, Pharm.D.
Larry Ereshefsky, Pharm.D.
William R. Garnett, Pharm.D.
Robert J. Ignoffo, Pharm.D.
John W. Jenne, M.D.
Edward P. Krenzelok, Pharm.D.
Calvin Kunin, M.D.
Gary R. Matzke, Pharm.D.
Frans W. H. M. Merkus, Ph.D.
Jay M. Mirtallo, M.S.
John E. Murphy, Pharm.D.
Milap C. Nahata, Pharm.D.
Stephanie J. Phelps, Pharm.D.
John J. Piecoro, Jr., Pharm.D., M.S.
Richard Quintiliani, M.D.
John H. Rodman, Pharm.D.
Keith A. Rodvold, Pharm.D.
Fred Salter, Pharm.D.
Gerald E. Schumacher, Pharm.D., Ph.D.
Catherine Angell Sohn, Pharm.D.
Robert L. Talbert, Pharm.D.

Consulting Editors
Randal L. Batenhorst, Pharm.D.; Larry A. Bauer, Pharm.D.; Rosemary R. Berardi, Pharm.D.; John Bosso, Pharm.D.; Daniel T. Casto, Pharm.D.; Robert J. Cipolle, Pharm.D.; Joseph F. Dasta, M.Sc.; Michael N. Dudley, Pharm.D.; Lawrence J. Hak, Pharm.D.; David W. Hawkins, Pharm.D.; J. Heyward Hull, Pharm.D.; Martin J. Jinks, Pharm.D.; Cary E. Johnson, Pharm.D.; H. William Kelly, Pharm.D.; Jeffrey R. Koup, Pharm.D.; Thomas C. Majerus, Pharm.D.; Anthony S. Manoguerra, Pharm.D.; James M. McKenney, Pharm.D.; Donald S. North, Pharm.D.; Vaughn W. Payne, Pharm.D.; Donald G. Perrier, Ph.D.; Ronald E. Polk, Pharm.D.; Robert P. Rapp, Pharm.D.; Nathan Rawls, Pharm.D.; David R. Rush, Pharm.D.; Steven L. Sheaffer, Pharm. D.; John K. Siepler, Pharm.D.; Ralph E. Small, Pharm.D.; Glen L. Stimmel, Pharm.D.; Timothy R. Sykes, Pharm.D.; Scott L. Traub, Pharm.D.; William Troutman, Pharm.D.; Peter H. Vlasses, Pharm.D.; Barbara G. Wells, Pharm.D.; Dennis West, M.S.; Michael E. Winter, Pharm.D.

Copyright © 1988, American Society of Hospital Pharmacists, Inc. All rights reserved.

Instructions to Authors

CLINICAL PHARMACY, a forum for the drug therapeutics information that pharmacists need to perform their clinical roles, gives priority to (1) studies that objectively evaluate drug effects in human trials, (2) evaluative review articles on the clinical uses of new drugs, and (3) evaluations of the current status of drug therapy in selected diseases. Contributions to the following sections are invited:

Drug Reviews: Detailed, analytical reviews on the clinical use of specific drugs, with preference given to new drugs and to evaluative rather than descriptive literature reviews.

Therapy Reviews: Articles that focus primarily on a disease state (rather than on a drug or drug class) and its treatment. These reviews foster an understanding of the pathophysiology of a disease and the related treatment.

Research: Reports of well-conducted original research on drug effects in humans.

Research Notes: Short research reports, such as updates on previously published work, confirmations of previous findings, or original research of modest scope.

Grand Rounds: Patient case reports and literature reviews combined in a way that gives them high educational value.

Drug Experience: Straightforward reports, with selected literature references, of unusual drug experiences.

Therapy Consultation: Brief advice, in a question-and-answer format, on how to handle specific drug-therapy problems. Readers are invited to submit questions, which the editor will forward to appropriate consultants for answering.

Letters: Short comments on previously published work or about potential problems, apparent trends, or controversies in drug therapy or clinical research.

Commentaries: Well-reasoned expressions of opinion on drug-therapy or clinical-research issues.

The editors have the sole authority to decide in which section to publish an accepted manuscript.

Manuscripts are subject to review by qualified outside reviewers, as well as by the editors, and will be accepted for publication only if they are believed to represent an important contribution to the literature. All papers submitted for publication must be accompanied by a completed copy of a manuscript checklist. The checklist, which generally conforms to the Uniform Requirements for Manuscripts Submitted to Biomedical Journals, appears on pages 73–74 of the January 1988 issue. Authors of especially important original work may request "fast-track" review of their papers. Authors may suggest appropriate reviewers for their papers.

Accepted materials become the permanent and sole property of ASHP and may not be published or reprinted elsewhere without written permission from both the author and the editor.

The editors reserve the right to revise all materials submitted, if necessary. The publisher assumes no responsibility for the statements and opinions advanced by contributors to CLINICAL PHARMACY.

Under the terms of the Copyright Revision Act of 1976 (Public Law 94-553) it is necessary to have the rights of the authors transferred to the publisher in order to provide for the widest possible dissemination of professional and scientific literature. Accordingly, all transmittal letters accompanying manuscripts submitted for publication, including contributions for the Letters column, must contain the following language: "In consideration of the American Society of Hospital Pharmacists (ASHP) taking action in reviewing and editing my (our) submission, the author(s) undersigned hereby transfer(s), assign(s), or otherwise convey(s) all ownership rights in the submission and all copyright ownership to ASHP. In the event that such work is not published by ASHP, all said rights shall be released." We regret that we cannot consider manuscripts for publication that are not accompanied with transmittal letters containing the above language signed by all authors.

Authors must certify in their letter of transmittal that none of the material in their manuscript has been published previously nor is under consideration or been accepted for publication elsewhere. If this certification cannot be made, suitable explanation must be offered.

Six copies of all manuscripts should be submitted. Manuscripts should be typewritten with double spacing (including tables) on one side of good quality, 21.6 × 27.9-cm white paper, and with margins of at least 2.5 cm. For guidance on style, authors should consult the manuscript checklist, recent issues of CLINICAL PHARMACY, and the *Council of Biology Editors Style Manual*, fifth edition. *The American Heritage Dictionary of the English Language* and the AMA's *Manual for Authors and Editors* contain helpful advice on correct usage.

Galley proofs are sent to authors for inspection against the original manuscript and for correction. Unnecessary alterations in galley proof must be avoided. An order form for reprints is sent to the corresponding author after galley proofs have been cleared.

CLINICAL PHARMACY (ISSN 0278-2677) is published monthly by the American Society of Hospital Pharmacists, 4630 Montgomery Avenue, Bethesda, MD 20814. Joseph A. Oddis, Executive Vice President. Second class postage is paid at Bethesda, MD, and at additional mailing offices. **Postmaster: Send address changes to: *Clinical Pharmacy*, 4630 Montgomery Avenue, Bethesda, MD 20814.**

Annual Subscription Rate:	*USA*	*Non-USA*
ASHP Member	$40	$45
ASHP Student Members and Residents	$30	$35
Institutions and Nonmembers	$63	$68

The cost of single copies is $10. Airmail delivery outside of the continental United States is available for an additional charge of $72 per year. Requests to replace missing issues free of charge are honored only up to six months after date of issue.

Payments to ASHP are not deductible as charitable contributions for federal income tax purposes. However, they may be deductible under other provisions of the Internal Revenue Code.

Advertising for CLINICAL PHARMACY is accepted in accordance with the Statement of Advertising Policy of the American Society of Hospital Pharmacists (see *Am J Hosp Pharm.* 1987; 44:1146). For additional information, contact the Advertising Representative (William McCausland Associates, Inc., P.O. Box 189, Pitman, NJ 08071. Phone 609-589-5454, FAX 609-582-7611.)

All articles published, including editorials, letters, and book reviews, represent the opinions of the authors and do not reflect the official policy of the American Society of Hospital Pharmacists or the institution with which the author is affiliated, unless this is specified.

Microfilm and microfiche editions are available for purchase. Contact University Microfilms, 300 N. Zeeb Road, Ann Arbor, MI 48106.

Articles in CLINICAL PHARMACY are abstracted and indexed in *Current Contents, Clinical Sciences, Excerpta Medica, Index Medicus, Inpharma, International Pharmaceutical Abstracts,* and *Reactions.*

August 1988 Volume 7, Number 8 Coden: CPHADV ISSN: 0278-2677

CLINICAL PHARMACY

560 **News**

National Cancer Institute announces new study findings on breast-cancer treatment. . .Fourth histamine antagonist, nizatidine, reaches U.S. market. . .Preliminary study suggests role for clonidine in smoking cessation. . .Overview of studies shows benefit of perioperative heparin use

563 **Therapy Consultation**

Treatment of acetaminophen overdose when oral acetylcysteine therapy is not tolerated

570 **Letters**

Sodium thiosulfate unproven as bromate antidote, Newell E. McElwee, Thomas E. Kearney; Cary E. Johnson

Drug Review

574 **Mitoxantrone: A novel anthracycline derivative**
Jim Koeller and Melody Eble

Therapy Review

582 **Drug therapy of hypertensive crises**
Janice L. Stumpf

Commentaries

592 **Reassessment of the value of lowering serum cholesterol**

592 **Questioning the wisdom of widespread intervention**
Dustan G. Labreche

604 **Defending cholesterol-reduction efforts**
Robert L. Talbert

605 **The questions are when and how to treat, not whether to treat, hypercholesterolemia**
James M. McKenney

608 **Aminoglycoside pharmacokinetic monitoring: An integral part of patient care?**
Keith A. Rodvold, Humphrey Zokufa, and John C. Rotschafer

Drug Experience

614 **Reversal of iatrogenic diazepam overdose with flumazenil**
Emeka O. C. Ume and Adrian W. Gelb

616 **Histamine-like reaction after a single intravenous dose of rifampin**
Patty Fan-Havard, Milap C. Nahata, William J. Barson, Henry Bartkowski, and Edward Kosnik

620 **Theophylline toxicity after iodine 131 treatment for hyperthyroidism**
Cary E. Johnson and Ira A. Cohen

622 **Use of fluconazole in a patient with documented malabsorption of ketoconazole**
Richard H. Drew, John R. Perfect, and Harry A. Gallis

624 **CP Continuing Education**

627 **Current Literature**

Drug Reaction Alerts. . .Book Reviews: *Psychotropic Drug Handbook, 5th Edition* (*Perry, Alexander, Liskow*), Peter G. Dorson. . .*Manual of Antibiotics and Infectious Diseases, Sixth Edition* (*Conte, Barriere*), George G. Zhanel. . .Books Received

630 **Advertising Index**

CLINICAL PHARMACY

Editor
William A. Zellmer

Managing Editor
C. Richard Talley

Associate Editor, Manuscript Development
Jane L. Miller

Associate Editor, Redaction
Nancy Tarleton Landis

Assistant Editors, Manuscript Development
Guy R. Hasegawa
Cynthia A. Knapp
Catherine A. Nichols

Assistant Editor, Redaction
Susan S. McLaughlin

Editorial Production Coordinator
Wende B. Mack

Advertising Production Coordinator
Nasrine L. Sabi

Editorial Assistant
Margery M. Wiltamuth

Editorial Office
4630 Montgomery Avenue
Bethesda, MD 20814
301-657-3000

Editorial Board
Steven L. Barriere, Pharm.D.
Stephen G. Bryant, Pharm.D.
Barry L. Carter, Pharm.D.
Burke A. Cunha, M.D.
Joseph T. DiPiro, Pharm.D.
Larry Ereshefsky, Pharm.D.
William R. Garnett, Pharm.D.
Robert J. Ignoffo, Pharm.D.
John W. Jenne, M.D.
Edward P. Krenzelok, Pharm.D.
Calvin Kunin, M.D.
Gary R. Matzke, Pharm.D.
Frans W. H. M. Merkus, Ph.D.
Jay M. Mirtallo, M.S.
John E. Murphy, Pharm.D.
Milap C. Nahata, Pharm.D.
Stephanie J. Phelps, Pharm.D.
John J. Piecoro, Jr., Pharm.D., M.S.
Richard Quintiliani, M.D.
John H. Rodman, Pharm.D.
Keith A. Rodvold, Pharm.D.
Fred Salter, Pharm.D.
Gerald E. Schumacher, Pharm.D., Ph.D.
Catherine Angell Sohn, Pharm.D.
Robert L. Talbert, Pharm.D.

Consulting Editors
Randal L. Batenhorst, Pharm.D.; Larry A. Bauer, Pharm.D.; Rosemary R. Berardi, Pharm.D.; John Bosso, Pharm.D.; Daniel T. Casto, Pharm.D.; Robert J. Cipolle, Pharm.D.; Joseph F. Dasta, M.Sc.; Michael N. Dudley, Pharm.D.; Lawrence J. Hak, Pharm.D.; David W. Hawkins, Pharm.D.; J. Heyward Hull, Pharm.D.; Martin J. Jinks, Pharm.D.; Cary E. Johnson, Pharm.D.; H. William Kelly, Pharm.D.; Jeffrey R. Koup, Pharm.D.; Thomas C. Majerus, Pharm.D.; Anthony S. Manoguerra, Pharm.D.; James M. McKenney, Pharm.D.; Donald S. North, Pharm.D.; Vaughn W. Payne, Pharm.D.; Donald G. Perrier, Ph.D.; Ronald E. Polk, Pharm.D.; Robert P. Rapp, Pharm.D.; Nathan Rawls, Pharm.D.; David R. Rush, Pharm.D.; Steven L. Sheaffer, Pharm. D.; John K. Siepler, Pharm.D.; Ralph E. Small, Pharm.D.; Glen L. Stimmel, Pharm.D.; Timothy R. Sykes, Pharm.D.; Scott L. Traub, Pharm.D.; William Troutman, Pharm.D.; Peter H. Vlasses, Pharm.D.; Barbara G. Wells, Pharm.D.; Dennis West, M.S.; Michael E. Winter, Pharm.D.

Copyright © 1988, American Society of Hospital Pharmacists, Inc. All rights reserved.

Instructions to Authors

CLINICAL PHARMACY, a forum for the drug therapeutics information that pharmacists need to perform their clinical roles, gives priority to (1) studies that objectively evaluate drug effects in human trials, (2) evaluative review articles on the clinical uses of new drugs, and (3) evaluations of the current status of drug therapy in selected diseases. Contributions to the following sections are invited:

Drug Reviews: Detailed, analytical reviews on the clinical use of specific drugs, with preference given to new drugs and to evaluative rather than descriptive literature reviews.

Therapy Reviews: Articles that focus primarily on a disease state (rather than on a drug or drug class) and its treatment. These reviews foster an understanding of the pathophysiology of a disease and the related treatment.

Research: Reports of well-conducted original research on drug effects in humans.

Research Notes: Short research reports, such as updates on previously published work, confirmations of previous findings, or original research of modest scope.

Grand Rounds: Patient case reports and literature reviews combined in a way that gives them high educational value.

Drug Experience: Straightforward reports, with selected literature references, of unusual drug experiences.

Therapy Consultation: Brief advice, in a question-and-answer format, on how to handle specific drug-therapy problems. Readers are invited to submit questions, which the editor will forward to appropriate consultants for answering.

Letters: Short comments on previously published work or about potential problems, apparent trends, or controversies in drug therapy or clinical research.

Commentaries: Well-reasoned expressions of opinion on drug-therapy or clinical-research issues.

The editors have the sole authority to decide in which section to publish an accepted manuscript.

Manuscripts are subject to review by qualified outside reviewers, as well as by the editors, and will be accepted for publication only if they are believed to represent an important contribution to the literature. All papers submitted for publication must be accompanied by a completed copy of a manuscript checklist. The checklist, which generally conforms to the Uniform Requirements for Manuscripts Submitted to Biomedical Journals, appears on pages 73–74 of the January 1988 issue. Authors of especially important original work may request "fast-track" review of their papers. Authors may suggest appropriate reviewers for their papers.

Accepted materials become the permanent and sole property of ASHP and may not be published or reprinted elsewhere without written permission from both the author and the editor.

The editors reserve the right to revise all materials submitted, if necessary. The publisher assumes no responsibility for the statements and opinions advanced by contributors to CLINICAL PHARMACY.

Under the terms of the Copyright Revision Act of 1976 (Public Law 94-553) it is necessary to have the rights of the authors transferred to the publisher in order to provide for the widest possible dissemination of professional and scientific literature. Accordingly, all transmittal letters accompanying manuscripts submitted for publication, including contributions for the Letters column, must contain the following language: "In consideration of the American Society of Hospital Pharmacists (ASHP) taking action in reviewing and editing my (our) submission, the author(s) undersigned hereby transfer(s), assign(s), or otherwise convey(s) all ownership rights in the submission and all copyright ownership to ASHP. In the event that such work is not published by ASHP, all said rights shall be released." We regret that we cannot consider manuscripts for publication that are not accompanied with transmittal letters containing the above language signed by all authors.

Authors must certify in their letter of transmittal that none of the material in their manuscript has been published previously nor is under consideration or been accepted for publication elsewhere. If this certification cannot be made, suitable explanation must be offered.

Six copies of all manuscripts should be submitted. Manuscripts should be typewritten with double spacing (including tables) on one side of good quality, 21.6 × 27.9-cm white paper, and with margins of at least 2.5 cm. For guidance on style, authors should consult the manuscript checklist, recent issues of CLINICAL PHARMACY, and the *Council of Biology Editors Style Manual*, fifth edition. *The American Heritage Dictionary of the English Language* and the AMA's *Manual for Authors and Editors* contain helpful advice on correct usage.

Galley proofs are sent to authors for inspection against the original manuscript and for correction. Unnecessary alterations in galley proof must be avoided. An order form for reprints is sent to the corresponding author after galley proofs have been cleared.

CLINICAL PHARMACY (ISSN 0278-2677) is published monthly by the American Society of Hospital Pharmacists, 4630 Montgomery Avenue, Bethesda, MD 20814. Joseph A. Oddis, Executive Vice President. Second class postage is paid at Bethesda, MD, and at additional mailing offices. **Postmaster: Send address changes to: *Clinical Pharmacy,* 4630 Montgomery Avenue, Bethesda, MD 20814.**

Annual Subscription Rate:	*USA*	*Non-USA*
ASHP Member	$40	$45
ASHP Student Members and Residents	$30	$35
Institutions and Nonmembers	$63	$68

The cost of single copies is $10. Airmail delivery outside of the continental United States is available for an additional charge of $72 per year. Requests to replace missing issues free of charge are honored only up to six months after date of issue.

Payments to ASHP are not deductible as charitable contributions for federal income tax purposes. However, they may be deductible under other provisions of the Internal Revenue Code.

Advertising for CLINICAL PHARMACY is accepted in accordance with the Statement of Advertising Policy of the American Society of Hospital Pharmacists (see *Am J Hosp Pharm.* 1987; 44:1146). For additional information, contact the Advertising Representative (William McCausland Associates, Inc., P.O. Box 189, Pitman, NJ 08071. Phone 609-589-5454, FAX 609-582-7611.)

All articles published, including editorials, letters, and book reviews, represent the opinions of the authors and do not reflect the official policy of the American Society of Hospital Pharmacists or the institution with which the author is affiliated, unless this is specified.

Microfilm and microfiche editions are available for purchase. Contact University Microfilms, 300 N. Zeeb Road, Ann Arbor, MI 48106.

Articles in CLINICAL PHARMACY are abstracted and indexed in *Current Contents, Clinical Sciences, Excerpta Medica, Index Medicus, Inpharma, International Pharmaceutical Abstracts,* and *Reactions.*

September 1988 Volume 7, Number 9
Coden: CPHADV ISSN: 0278-2677

CLINICAL PHARMACY

634 **News**

Pediatrics academy issues recommendations on use of *Haemophilus influenzae* type b conjugate vaccine . . . Study finds similar reperfusion rates with intravenous APSAC and intracoronary streptokinase in acute myocardial infarction . . . Guidelines issued on treatment of pediatric bacterial meningitis . . . Wider use of clomipramine approved by FDA . . . FDA requires new, permanent Reye's syndrome warning on aspirin products

640 **Therapy Consultation**

Use of tamoxifen in stage I breast cancer

Drug Reviews

647 **Teicoplanin: An investigational glycopeptide antibiotic**
Randy D. Pryka, Keith A. Rodvold, and John C. Rotschafer

659 **Lisinopril: A nonsulfhydryl angiotensin-converting enzyme inhibitor**
Teresa A. Noble and Kim M. Murray

670 **Use of ipratropium bromide in obstructive lung disease**
Katherine V. Mann, Ann L. Leon, and Karen J. Tietze

Research

681 **Predicting need for pharmacokinetic consultation follow-up using discriminant analysis**
Diane E. Beck, Edwin L. Bradley, and John A. Farringer

Research Note

688 **Predictability of unbound antiepileptic drug concentrations in children treated with valproic acid and phenytoin**
Michael V. Miles, O. Carter Snead III, and Michael D. Thorn

Commentary

694 **How many subjects are required for a study?**
Jerry W. McLarty

Grand Rounds

697 **Diagnosis and treatment of neuroleptic malignant syndrome**
Rawley M. Guerrero and Kenneth A. Shifrar

702 **CP Continuing Education**

704 **Current Literature**

Drug Reaction Alerts . . . Book Reviews: *Immunology, Immunopathology, and Immunity* (Sell), Michael D. Parr . . . *Therapeutic Pharmacology* (*Appelt, Appelt*), Norman L. Katz . . . Books Received

706 **Advertising Index**

CLINICAL PHARMACY

Editor
William A. Zellmer

Managing Editor
C. Richard Talley

Associate Editor, Manuscript Development
Jane L. Miller

Associate Editor, Redaction
Nancy Tarleton Landis

Assistant Editors, Manuscript Development
Guy R. Hasegawa
Cynthia A. Knapp
Catherine A. Nichols

Assistant Editor, Redaction
Susan S. McLaughlin

Editorial Production Coordinator
Wende B. Mack

Advertising Production Coordinator
Nasrine L. Sabi

Editorial Assistant
Margery M. Wiltamuth

Editorial Office
4630 Montgomery Avenue
Bethesda, MD 20814
301-657-3000

Editorial Board
Steven L. Barriere, Pharm.D.
Stephen G. Bryant, Pharm.D.
Barry L. Carter, Pharm.D.
Burke A. Cunha, M.D.
Joseph T. DiPiro, Pharm.D.
Larry Ereshefsky, Pharm.D.
William R. Garnett, Pharm.D.
Robert J. Ignoffo, Pharm.D.
John W. Jenne, M.D.
Edward P. Krenzelok, Pharm.D.
Calvin Kunin, M.D.
Gary R. Matzke, Pharm.D.
Frans W. H. M. Merkus, Ph.D.
Jay M. Mirtallo, M.S.
John E. Murphy, Pharm.D.
Milap C. Nahata, Pharm.D.
Stephanie J. Phelps, Pharm.D.
John J. Piecoro, Jr., Pharm.D., M.S.
Richard Quintiliani, M.D.
John H. Rodman, Pharm.D.
Keith A. Rodvold, Pharm.D.
Fred Salter, Pharm.D.
Gerald E. Schumacher, Pharm.D., Ph.D.
Catherine Angell Sohn, Pharm.D.
Robert L. Talbert, Pharm.D.

Consulting Editors
Randal L. Batenhorst, Pharm.D.; Larry A. Bauer, Pharm.D.; Rosemary R. Berardi, Pharm.D.; John Bosso, Pharm.D.; Daniel T. Casto, Pharm.D.; Robert J. Cipolle, Pharm.D.; Joseph F. Dasta, M.Sc.; Michael N. Dudley, Pharm.D.; Lawrence J. Hak, Pharm.D.; David W. Hawkins, Pharm.D.; J. Heyward Hull, Pharm.D.; Martin J. Jinks, Pharm.D.; Cary E. Johnson, Pharm.D.; H. William Kelly, Pharm.D.; Jeffrey R. Koup, Pharm.D.; Thomas C. Majerus, Pharm.D.; Anthony S. Manoguerra, Pharm.D.; James M. McKenney, Pharm.D.; Donald S. North, Pharm.D.; Vaughn W. Payne, Pharm.D.; Donald G. Perrier, Ph.D.; Ronald E. Polk, Pharm.D.; Robert P. Rapp, Pharm.D.; Nathan Rawls, Pharm.D.; David R. Rush, Pharm.D.; Steven L. Sheaffer, Pharm. D.; John K. Siepler, Pharm.D.; Ralph E. Small, Pharm.D.; Glen L. Stimmel, Pharm.D.; Timothy R. Sykes, Pharm.D.; Scott L. Traub, Pharm.D.; William Troutman, Pharm.D.; Peter H. Vlasses, Pharm.D.; Barbara G. Wells, Pharm.D.; Dennis West, M.S.; Michael E. Winter, Pharm.D.

Copyright © 1988, American Society of Hospital Pharmacists, Inc. All rights reserved.

Instructions to Authors

CLINICAL PHARMACY, a forum for the drug therapeutics information that pharmacists need to perform their clinical roles, gives priority to (1) studies that objectively evaluate drug effects in human trials, (2) evaluative review articles on the clinical uses of new drugs, and (3) evaluations of the current status of drug therapy in selected diseases. Contributions to the following sections are invited:

Drug Reviews: Detailed, analytical reviews on the clinical use of specific drugs, with preference given to new drugs and to evaluative rather than descriptive literature reviews.

Therapy Reviews: Articles that focus primarily on a disease state (rather than on a drug or drug class) and its treatment. These reviews foster an understanding of the pathophysiology of a disease and the related treatment.

Research: Reports of well-conducted original research on drug effects in humans.

Research Notes: Short research reports, such as updates on previously published work, confirmations of previous findings, or original research of modest scope.

Grand Rounds: Patient case reports and literature reviews combined in a way that gives them high educational value.

Drug Experience: Straightforward reports, with selected literature references, of unusual drug experiences.

Therapy Consultation: Brief advice, in a question-and-answer format, on how to handle specific drug-therapy problems. Readers are invited to submit questions, which the editor will forward to appropriate consultants for answering.

Letters: Short comments on previously published work or about potential problems, apparent trends, or controversies in drug therapy or clinical research.

Commentaries: Well-reasoned expressions of opinion on drug-therapy or clinical-research issues.

The editors have the sole authority to decide in which section to publish an accepted manuscript.

Manuscripts are subject to review by qualified outside reviewers, as well as by the editors, and will be accepted for publication only if they are believed to represent an important contribution to the literature. All papers submitted for publication must be accompanied by a completed copy of a manuscript checklist. The checklist, which generally conforms to the Uniform Requirements for Manuscripts Submitted to Biomedical Journals, appears on pages 73–74 of the January 1988 issue. Authors of especially important original work may request "fast-track" review of their papers. Authors may suggest appropriate reviewers for their papers.

Accepted materials become the permanent and sole property of ASHP and may not be published or reprinted elsewhere without written permission from both the author and the editor.

The editors reserve the right to revise all materials submitted, if necessary. The publisher assumes no responsibility for the statements and opinions advanced by contributors to CLINICAL PHARMACY.

Under the terms of the Copyright Revision Act of 1976 (Public Law 94-553) it is necessary to have the rights of the authors transferred to the publisher in order to provide for the widest possible dissemination of professional and scientific literature. Accordingly, all transmittal letters accompanying manuscripts submitted for publication, including contributions for the Letters column, must contain the following language: "In consideration of the American Society of Hospital Pharmacists (ASHP) taking action in reviewing and editing my (our) submission, the author(s) undersigned hereby transfer(s), assign(s), or otherwise convey(s) all ownership rights in the submission and all copyright ownership to ASHP. In the event that such work is not published by ASHP, all said rights shall be released." We regret that we cannot consider manuscripts for publication that are not accompanied with transmittal letters containing the above language signed by all authors.

Authors must certify in their letter of transmittal that none of the material in their manuscript has been published previously nor is under consideration or been accepted for publication elsewhere. If this certification cannot be made, suitable explanation must be offered.

Six copies of all manuscripts should be submitted. Manuscripts should be typewritten with double spacing (including tables) on one side of good quality, 21.6 × 27.9-cm white paper, and with margins of at least 2.5 cm. For guidance on style, authors should consult the manuscript checklist, recent issues of CLINICAL PHARMACY, and the *Council of Biology Editors Style Manual*, fifth edition. *The American Heritage Dictionary of the English Language* and the AMA's *Manual for Authors and Editors* contain helpful advice on correct usage.

Galley proofs are sent to authors for inspection against the original manuscript and for correction. Unnecessary alterations in galley proof must be avoided. An order form for reprints is sent to the corresponding author after galley proofs have been cleared.

CLINICAL PHARMACY (ISSN 0278-2677) is published monthly by the American Society of Hospital Pharmacists, 4630 Montgomery Avenue, Bethesda, MD 20814. Joseph A. Oddis, Executive Vice President. Second class postage is paid at Bethesda, MD, and at additional mailing offices. **Postmaster: Send address changes to: *Clinical Pharmacy*, 4630 Montgomery Avenue, Bethesda, MD 20814.**

Annual Subscription Rate:	*USA*	*Non-USA*
ASHP Members	$43	$48
ASHP Student Members and Residents	$32	$40
Institutions and Nonmembers	$67	$72

The cost of single copies is $10. Airmail delivery outside of the continental United States is available for an additional charge of $75 per year. Requests to replace missing issues free of charge are honored only up to six months after date of issue.

Payments to ASHP are not deductible as charitable contributions for federal income tax purposes. However, they may be deductible under other provisions of the Internal Revenue Code.

Advertising for CLINICAL PHARMACY is accepted in accordance with the Statement of Advertising Policy of the American Society of Hospital Pharmacists (see *Am J Hosp Pharm.* 1987; 44:1146). For additional information, contact the Advertising Representative (William McCausland Associates, Inc., P.O. Box 189, Pitman, NJ 08071. Phone 609-589-5454, FAX 609-582-7611.)

All articles published, including editorials, letters, and book reviews, represent the opinions of the authors and do not reflect the official policy of the American Society of Hospital Pharmacists or the institution with which the author is affiliated, unless this is specified.

Microfilm and microfiche editions are available for purchase. Contact University Microfilms, 300 N. Zeeb Road, Ann Arbor, MI 48106.

Articles in CLINICAL PHARMACY are abstracted and indexed in *Current Contents, Clinical Sciences, Excerpta Medica, Index Medicus, Inpharma, International Pharmaceutical Abstracts*, and *Reactions*.

October 1988 Volume 7, Number 10 Coden: CPHADV ISSN: 0278-2677

CLINICAL PHARMACY

710 **News**

Future applications of biotechnology explored by ACCP speakers, Jane L. Miller. . .Biotechnology-based drug products grow in importance. . .CDC updates influenza recommendations for 1988–1989 season. . .Study supports previous findings of colchicine activity in primary biliary cirrhosis. . . New AIDS reference service available through National Library of Medicine. . .FDA issues consumer warning, announces crackdown on bogus Retin A products. . .Papers sought for National Conference on High Blood Pressure Control

718 **Therapy Consultation**

Treatment of metronidazole-resistant cases of vaginal trichomoniasis

720 **Letters**

Phlebitis associated with vancomycin therapy, James C. Garrelts, Dale F. Smith, Jr., Dan Ast, Joanne LaRocca, Jerry D. Peterie. . .Aseptic meningitis associated with muromonab-CD3 therapy, Martha E. Joy, Marcia L. Michals, Daniel M. Canafax. . .Diminishing bioavailability of oral leucovorin calcium, Joseph G. Rossi; Richard Steffan, Joseph De Vito, Brian W. McGuire

Drug Review

725 **Therapeutic evaluation of omeprazole**
Marijke H. Adams, John D. Ostrosky, and Craig F. Kirkwood

Therapy Review

746 **Management and prevention of bacterial diarrhea**
Jeanette Suarez and Francine R. Salamone

Research

760 **Postinfusion phlebitis after intravenous push versus intravenous piggyback administration of antimicrobial agents**
James C. Garrelts, Dan Ast, Joanne LaRocca, Dale F. Smith, Jr., and Jerry D. Peterie

Grand Rounds

766 **Sulindac-induced toxic epidermal necrolysis**
Ralph E. Small and William R. Garnett

Drug Experience

772 **Rebound hypertension after discontinuation of transdermal clonidine**
Gary E. Schmidt and Arthur A. Shuna

775 **CP Continuing Education**

778 **Current Literature**

Drug Reaction Alerts. . .Book Reviews: *Basic Clinical Pharmacokinetics, Second Edition* (*Winter, Koda-Kimble, Young*), John E. Murphy, David R. Collette. . . *Clinical Pharmacokinetics: The MCQ Approach* (*Curry*), Donald P. Hill, Jr., Michael E. Burton. . .Books Received

780 **Advertising Index**

CLINICAL PHARMACY

Editor
William A. Zellmer

Managing Editor
C. Richard Talley

Associate Editor, Manuscript Development
Jane L. Miller

Associate Editor, Redaction
Nancy Tarleton Landis

Assistant Editors, Manuscript Development
Guy R. Hasegawa
Cynthia A. Knapp
Catherine A. Nichols

Assistant Editor, Redaction
Susan S. McLaughlin

Editorial Production Coordinator
Wende B. Mack

Advertising Production Coordinator
Nasrine L. Sabi

Editorial Assistant
Margery M. Wiltamuth

Editorial Office
4630 Montgomery Avenue
Bethesda, MD 20814
301-657-3000

Editorial Board
Steven L. Barriere, Pharm.D.
Stephen G. Bryant, Pharm.D.
Barry L. Carter, Pharm.D.
Burke A. Cunha, M.D.
Joseph T. DiPiro, Pharm.D.
Larry Ereshefsky, Pharm.D.
William R. Garnett, Pharm.D.
Robert J. Ignoffo, Pharm.D.
John W. Jenne, M.D.
Edward P. Krenzelok, Pharm.D.
Calvin Kunin, M.D.
Gary R. Matzke, Pharm.D.
Frans W. H. M. Merkus, Ph.D.
Jay M. Mirtallo, M.S.
John E. Murphy, Pharm.D.
Milap C. Nahata, Pharm.D.
Stephanie J. Phelps, Pharm.D.
John J. Piecoro, Jr., Pharm.D., M.S.
Richard Quintiliani, M.D.
John H. Rodman, Pharm.D.
Keith A. Rodvold, Pharm.D.
Fred Salter, Pharm.D.
Gerald E. Schumacher, Pharm.D., Ph.D.
Catherine Angell Sohn, Pharm.D.
Robert L. Talbert, Pharm.D.

Consulting Editors
Randal L. Batenhorst, Pharm.D.; Larry A. Bauer, Pharm.D.; Rosemary R. Berardi, Pharm.D.; John Bosso, Pharm.D.; Daniel T. Casto, Pharm.D.; Robert J. Cipolle, Pharm.D.; Joseph F. Dasta, M.Sc.; Michael N. Dudley, Pharm.D.; Lawrence J. Hak, Pharm.D.; David W. Hawkins, Pharm.D.; J. Heyward Hull, Pharm.D.; Martin J. Jinks, Pharm.D.; Cary E. Johnson, Pharm.D.; H. William Kelly, Pharm.D.; Jeffrey R. Koup, Pharm.D.; Thomas C. Majerus, Pharm.D.; Anthony S. Manoguerra, Pharm.D.; James M. McKenney, Pharm.D.; Donald S. North, Pharm.D.; Vaughn W. Payne, Pharm.D.; Donald G. Perrier, Ph.D.; Ronald E. Polk, Pharm.D.; Robert P. Rapp, Pharm.D.; Nathan Rawls, Pharm.D.; David R. Rush, Pharm.D.; Steven L. Sheaffer, Pharm. D.; John K. Siepler, Pharm.D.; Ralph E. Small, Pharm.D.; Glen L. Stimmel, Pharm.D.; Timothy R. Sykes, Pharm.D.; Scott L. Traub, Pharm.D.; William Troutman, Pharm.D.; Peter H. Vlasses, Pharm.D.; Barbara G. Wells, Pharm.D.; Dennis West, M.S.; Michael E. Winter, Pharm.D.

Copyright © 1988, American Society of Hospital Pharmacists, Inc. All rights reserved.

Instructions to Authors

CLINICAL PHARMACY, a forum for the drug therapeutics information that pharmacists need to perform their clinical roles, gives priority to (1) studies that objectively evaluate drug effects in human trials, (2) evaluative review articles on the clinical uses of new drugs, and (3) evaluations of the current status of drug therapy in selected diseases. Contributions to the following sections are invited:

Drug Reviews: Detailed, analytical reviews on the clinical use of specific drugs, with preference given to new drugs and to evaluative rather than descriptive literature reviews.

Therapy Reviews: Articles that focus primarily on a disease state (rather than on a drug or drug class) and its treatment. These reviews foster an understanding of the pathophysiology of a disease and the related treatment.

Research: Reports of well-conducted original research on drug effects in humans.

Research Notes: Short research reports, such as updates on previously published work, confirmations of previous findings, or original research of modest scope.

Grand Rounds: Patient case reports and literature reviews combined in a way that gives them high educational value.

Drug Experience: Straightforward reports, with selected literature references, of unusual drug experiences.

Therapy Consultation: Brief advice, in a question-and-answer format, on how to handle specific drug-therapy problems. Readers are invited to submit questions, which the editor will forward to appropriate consultants for answering.

Letters: Short comments on previously published work or about potential problems, apparent trends, or controversies in drug therapy or clinical research.

Commentaries: Well-reasoned expressions of opinion on drug-therapy or clinical-research issues.

The editors have the sole authority to decide in which section to publish an accepted manuscript.

Manuscripts are subject to review by qualified outside reviewers, as well as by the editors, and will be accepted for publication only if they are believed to represent an important contribution to the literature. All papers submitted for publication must be accompanied by a completed copy of a manuscript checklist. The checklist, which generally conforms to the Uniform Requirements for Manuscripts Submitted to Biomedical Journals, appears on pages 73–74 of the January 1988 issue. Authors of especially important original work may request "fast-track" review of their papers. Authors may suggest appropriate reviewers for their papers.

Accepted materials become the permanent and sole property of ASHP and may not be published or reprinted elsewhere without written permission from both the author and the editor.

The editors reserve the right to revise all materials submitted, if necessary. The publisher assumes no responsibility for the statements and opinions advanced by contributors to CLINICAL PHARMACY.

Under the terms of the Copyright Revision Act of 1976 (Public Law 94-553) it is necessary to have the rights of the authors transferred to the publisher in order to provide for the widest possible dissemination of professional and scientific literature. Accordingly, all transmittal letters accompanying manuscripts submitted for publication, including contributions for the Letters column, must contain the following language: "In consideration of the American Society of Hospital Pharmacists (ASHP) taking action in reviewing and editing my (our) submission, the author(s) undersigned hereby transfer(s), assign(s), or otherwise convey(s) all ownership rights in the submission and all copyright ownership to ASHP. In the event that such work is not published by ASHP, all said rights shall be released." We regret that we cannot consider manuscripts for publication that are not accompanied with transmittal letters containing the above language signed by all authors.

Authors must certify in their letter of transmittal that none of the material in their manuscript has been published previously nor is under consideration or been accepted for publication elsewhere. If this certification cannot be made, suitable explanation must be offered.

Six copies of all manuscripts should be submitted. Manuscripts should be typewritten with double spacing (including tables) on one side of good quality, 21.6 × 27.9-cm white paper, and with margins of at least 2.5 cm. For guidance on style, authors should consult the manuscript checklist, recent issues of CLINICAL PHARMACY, and the *Council of Biology Editors Style Manual,* fifth edition. *The American Heritage Dictionary of the English Language* and the AMA's *Manual for Authors and Editors* contain helpful advice on correct usage.

Galley proofs are sent to authors for inspection against the original manuscript and for correction. Unnecessary alterations in galley proof must be avoided. An order form for reprints is sent to the corresponding author after galley proofs have been cleared.

CLINICAL PHARMACY (ISSN 0278-2677) is published monthly by the American Society of Hospital Pharmacists, 4630 Montgomery Avenue, Bethesda, MD 20814. Joseph A. Oddis, Executive Vice President. Second class postage is paid at Bethesda, MD, and at additional mailing offices. **Postmaster: Send address changes to: *Clinical Pharmacy,* 4630 Montgomery Avenue, Bethesda, MD 20814.**

Annual Subscription Rate:	*USA*	*Non-USA*
ASHP Members	$43	$48
ASHP Student Members and Residents	$32	$40
Institutions and Nonmembers	$67	$72

The cost of single copies is $10. Airmail delivery outside of the continental United States is available for an additional charge of $75 per year. Requests to replace missing issues free of charge are honored only up to six months after date of issue.

Payments to ASHP are not deductible as charitable contributions for federal income tax purposes. However, they may be deductible under other provisions of the Internal Revenue Code.

Advertising for CLINICAL PHARMACY is accepted in accordance with the Statement of Advertising Policy of the American Society of Hospital Pharmacists (see *Am J Hosp Pharm.* 1987; 44:1146). For additional information, contact the Advertising Representative (William McCausland Associates, Inc., P.O. Box 189, Pitman, NJ 08071. Phone 609-589-5454, FAX 609-582-7611.)

All articles published, including editorials, letters, and book reviews, represent the opinions of the authors and do not reflect the official policy of the American Society of Hospital Pharmacists or the institution with which the author is affiliated, unless this is specified.

Microfilm and microfiche editions are available for purchase. Contact University Microfilms, 300 N. Zeeb Road, Ann Arbor, MI 48106.

Articles in CLINICAL PHARMACY are abstracted and indexed in *Current Contents, Clinical Sciences, Excerpta Medica, Index Medicus, Inpharma, International Pharmaceutical Abstracts,* and *Reactions.*

November 1988 Volume 7, Number 11 Coden: CPHADV ISSN: 0278-2677

CLINICAL PHARMACY

785 **News**

FDA approves marketing of diclofenac. . .Study suggests added benefit from combined aspirin–streptokinase therapy after myocardial infarction. . . FDA approves treatment IND protocols for selegiline and pentostatin. . .Design of future thrombolytic studies explored by speaker. . . Reimbursement for contraception counseling, initial pregnancy test included in isotretinoin program

791 **Therapy Consultation**

Conversion from oral to intravenous verapamil therapy

792 **Letters**

Storing extra calibration curves in the TDx assay system, David E. Nix, Charles A. Peloquin

Drug Review

795 **Biological mechanisms and cardiovascular effects of omega-3 fatty acids**
Bruce A. Mueller and Robert L. Talbert

Therapy Review

808 **Combination drug therapy for ventricular arrhythmias**
Daniel W. Krichbaum

Research

820 **Clindamycin pharmacokinetics and tissue penetration after head and neck surgery**
Gary P. Stoehr, Victor L. Yu, Jonas T. Johnson, Edward J. Antal, Raymond J. Townsend, and Robin Wagner

825 **Lack of endogenous crossreactivity with three digitoxin radioimmunoassays in adults with renal insufficiency**
Bruce A. Mueller, Henry I. Bussey, Daniel T. Casto, N. Kathryn Lowder, Nancy J. Sugarek, and Karl F. Cremer

Research Notes

828 **Effect of influenza vaccine on serum concentrations of total and free phenytoin**
Christopher D. Smith, Michael A. Bledsoe, Roger Curran, Lawrence Green, and Jack Lewis

832 **Efficacy of 0.9% sodium chloride injection with or without heparin sodium for maintaining patency of intravenous catheters in children**
Thomas P. Lombardi, Berit Gundersen, Lorna O. Zammett, J. Ken Walters, and Barbara A. Morris

Commentary

837 **1988 Report of the Joint National Committee on Detection, Evaluation, and Treatment of High Blood Pressure: A commentary**
Arthur A. Schuna

Drug Experience

842 **Morphine concentrations in plasma, ascitic fluid, and nasogastric aspirate fluid during high-dose intravenous morphine infusion**
Paul R. Hutson, Terry J. Baumann, Robert R. Lavoie, and Michael R. Mullane

846 **Probable anaphylactoid reaction to a pyrethrin pediculocide shampoo**
Charles A. Culver, Joanne J. Malina, and Robert L. Talbert

851 **CP Continuing Education**

853 **Current Literature**

Drug Reaction Alerts. . .Book Review: *The Merck Manual, Fifteenth Edition* (*Berkow*), David W. Hawkins

854 **Advertising Index**

CLINICAL PHARMACY

Editor
William A. Zellmer

Managing Editor
C. Richard Talley

Associate Editor, Manuscript Development
Jane L. Miller

Associate Editor, Redaction
Nancy Tarleton Landis

Assistant Editors, Manuscript Development
Guy R. Hasegawa
Cynthia A. Knapp
Catherine Nichols Klein

Assistant Editor, Redaction
Susan S. McLaughlin

Editorial Production Coordinator
Wende B. Mack

Advertising Production Coordinator
Nasrine L. Sabi

Editorial Assistant
Margery M. Wiltamuth

Editorial Office
4630 Montgomery Avenue
Bethesda, MD 20814
301-657-3000

Editorial Board
Steven L. Barriere, Pharm.D.
Stephen G. Bryant, Pharm.D.
Barry L. Carter, Pharm.D.
Burke A. Cunha, M.D.
Joseph T. DiPiro, Pharm.D.
Larry Ereshefsky, Pharm.D.
William R. Garnett, Pharm.D.
Robert J. Ignoffo, Pharm.D.
John W. Jenne, M.D.
Edward P. Krenzelok, Pharm.D.
Calvin Kunin, M.D.
Gary R. Matzke, Pharm.D.
Frans W. H. M. Merkus, Ph.D.
Jay M. Mirtallo, M.S.
John E. Murphy, Pharm.D.
Milap C. Nahata, Pharm.D.
Stephanie J. Phelps, Pharm.D.
John J. Piecoro, Jr., Pharm.D., M.S.
Richard Quintiliani, M.D.
John H. Rodman, Pharm.D.
Keith A. Rodvold, Pharm.D.
Fred Salter, Pharm.D.
Gerald E. Schumacher, Pharm.D., Ph.D.
Catherine Angell Sohn, Pharm.D.
Robert L. Talbert, Pharm.D.

Consulting Editors
Randal L. Batenhorst, Pharm.D.; Larry A. Bauer, Pharm.D.; Rosemary R. Berardi, Pharm.D.; John Bosso, Pharm.D.; Daniel T. Casto, Pharm.D.; Robert J. Cipolle, Pharm.D.; Joseph F. Dasta, M.Sc.; Michael N. Dudley, Pharm.D.; Lawrence J. Hak, Pharm.D.; David W. Hawkins, Pharm.D.; J. Heyward Hull, Pharm.D.; Martin J. Jinks, Pharm.D.; Cary E. Johnson, Pharm.D.; H. William Kelly, Pharm.D.; Jeffrey R. Koup, Pharm.D.; Thomas C. Majerus, Pharm.D.; Anthony S. Manoguerra, Pharm.D.; James M. McKenney, Pharm.D.; Donald S. North, Pharm.D.; Vaughn W. Payne, Pharm.D.; Donald G. Perrier, Ph.D.; Ronald E. Polk, Pharm.D.; Robert P. Rapp, Pharm.D.; Nathan Rawls, Pharm.D.; David R. Rush, Pharm.D.; Steven L. Sheaffer, Pharm. D.; John K. Siepler, Pharm.D.; Ralph E. Small, Pharm.D.; Glen L. Stimmel, Pharm.D.; Timothy R. Sykes, Pharm.D.; Scott L. Traub, Pharm.D.; William Troutman, Pharm.D.; Peter H. Vlasses, Pharm.D.; Barbara G. Wells, Pharm.D.; Dennis West, M.S.; Michael E. Winter, Pharm.D.

Copyright © 1988, American Society of Hospital Pharmacists, Inc. All rights reserved.

Instructions to Authors

CLINICAL PHARMACY, a forum for the drug therapeutics information that pharmacists need to perform their clinical roles, gives priority to (1) studies that objectively evaluate drug effects in human trials, (2) evaluative review articles on the clinical uses of new drugs, and (3) evaluations of the current status of drug therapy in selected diseases. Contributions to the following sections are invited:

Drug Reviews: Detailed, analytical reviews on the clinical use of specific drugs, with preference given to new drugs and to evaluative rather than descriptive literature reviews.

Therapy Reviews: Articles that focus primarily on a disease state (rather than on a drug or drug class) and its treatment. These reviews foster an understanding of the pathophysiology of a disease and the related treatment.

Research: Reports of well-conducted original research on drug effects in humans.

Research Notes: Short research reports, such as updates on previously published work, confirmations of previous findings, or original research of modest scope.

Grand Rounds: Patient case reports and literature reviews combined in a way that gives them high educational value.

Drug Experience: Straightforward reports, with selected literature references, of unusual drug experiences.

Therapy Consultation: Brief advice, in a question-and-answer format, on how to handle specific drug-therapy problems. Readers are invited to submit questions, which the editor will forward to appropriate consultants for answering.

Letters: Short comments on previously published work or about potential problems, apparent trends, or controversies in drug therapy or clinical research.

Commentaries: Well-reasoned expressions of opinion on drug-therapy or clinical-research issues.

The editors have the sole authority to decide in which section to publish an accepted manuscript.

Manuscripts are subject to review by qualified outside reviewers, as well as by the editors, and will be accepted for publication only if they are believed to represent an important contribution to the literature. All papers submitted for publication must be accompanied by a completed copy of a manuscript checklist. The checklist, which generally conforms to the Uniform Requirements for Manuscripts Submitted to Biomedical Journals, appears on pages 73–74 of the January 1988 issue. Authors of especially important original work may request "fast-track" review of their papers. Authors may suggest appropriate reviewers for their papers.

Accepted materials become the permanent and sole property of ASHP and may not be published or reprinted elsewhere without written permission from both the author and the editor.

The editors reserve the right to revise all materials submitted, if necessary. The publisher assumes no responsibility for the statements and opinions advanced by contributors to CLINICAL PHARMACY.

Under the terms of the Copyright Revision Act of 1976 (Public Law 94-553) it is necessary to have the rights of the authors transferred to the publisher in order to provide for the widest possible dissemination of professional and scientific literature. Accordingly, all transmittal letters accompanying manuscripts submitted for publication, including contributions for the Letters column, must contain the following language: "In consideration of the American Society of Hospital Pharmacists (ASHP) taking action in reviewing and editing my (our) submission, the author(s) undersigned hereby transfer(s), assign(s), or otherwise convey(s) all ownership rights in the submission and all copyright ownership to ASHP. In the event that such work is not published by ASHP, all said rights shall be released." We regret that we cannot consider manuscripts for publication that are not accompanied with transmittal letters containing the above language signed by all authors.

Authors must certify in their letter of transmittal that none of the material in their manuscript has been published previously nor is under consideration or been accepted for publication elsewhere. If this certification cannot be made, suitable explanation must be offered.

Six copies of all manuscripts should be submitted. Manuscripts should be typewritten with double spacing (including tables) on one side of good quality, 21.6 × 27.9-cm white paper, and with margins of at least 2.5 cm. For guidance on style, authors should consult the manuscript checklist, recent issues of CLINICAL PHARMACY, and the *Council of Biology Editors Style Manual*, fifth edition. *The American Heritage Dictionary of the English Language* and the AMA's *Manual for Authors and Editors* contain helpful advice on correct usage.

Galley proofs are sent to authors for inspection against the original manuscript and for correction. Unnecessary alterations in galley proof must be avoided. An order form for reprints is sent to the corresponding author after galley proofs have been cleared.

CLINICAL PHARMACY (ISSN 0278-2677) is published monthly by the American Society of Hospital Pharmacists, 4630 Montgomery Avenue, Bethesda, MD 20814. Joseph A. Oddis, Executive Vice President. Second class postage is paid at Bethesda, MD, and at additional mailing offices. **Postmaster: Send address changes to: *Clinical Pharmacy,* 4630 Montgomery Avenue, Bethesda, MD 20814.**

Annual Subscription Rate:	*USA*	*Non-USA*
ASHP Members	$43	$48
ASHP Student Members and Residents	$32	$40
Institutions and Nonmembers	$67	$72

The cost of single copies is $10. Airmail delivery outside of the continental United States is available for an additional charge of $75 per year. Requests to replace missing issues free of charge are honored only up to six months after date of issue.

Payments to ASHP are not deductible as charitable contributions for federal income tax purposes. However, they may be deductible under other provisions of the Internal Revenue Code.

Advertising for CLINICAL PHARMACY is accepted in accordance with the Statement of Advertising Policy of the American Society of Hospital Pharmacists (see *Am J Hosp Pharm.* 1987; 44:1146). For additional information, contact the Advertising Representative (William McCausland Associates, Inc., P.O. Box 189, Pitman, NJ 08071. Phone 609-589-5454, FAX 609-582-7611.)

All articles published, including editorials, letters, and book reviews, represent the opinions of the authors and do not reflect the official policy of the American Society of Hospital Pharmacists or the institution with which the author is affiliated, unless this is specified.

Microfilm and microfiche editions are available for purchase. Contact University Microfilms, 300 N. Zeeb Road, Ann Arbor, MI 48106.

Articles in CLINICAL PHARMACY are abstracted and indexed in *Current Contents, Clinical Sciences, Excerpta Medica, Index Medicus, Inpharma, International Pharmaceutical Abstracts,* and *Reactions.*

December 1988 Volume 7, Number 12 Coden: CPHADV ISSN: 0278-2677

CLINICAL PHARMACY

858 **News**

Study demonstrates efficacy of clozapine in treatment-resistant schizophrenia . . . Topical minoxidil approved by FDA

865 **Therapy Consultation**

Treatment of acute agitation in the elderly

867 **Letters**

Hearing loss associated with muromonab-CD3 therapy, Marcia Michals, John P. Roberts, Daniel Canafax

Drug Review

869 **Propafenone: A new antiarrhythmic agent**
Moses S. S. Chow, Cynthia Lebsack, and Daniel Hilleman

Therapy Review

878 **Effect of antimicrobial therapy on bowel flora**
K. Dale Hooker and Joseph T. DiPiro

Research Notes

889 **Serum fibronectin and somatomedin-C as nutritional markers in adults receiving total parenteral nutrition**
Douglas A. Powers, Valerie L. Franse, Rex O. Brown, Ann Hinson, and George S. M. Cowan, Jr.

894 **Predicting human-albumin replacement dosages in hypoalbuminemic patients receiving total parenteral nutrition**
Dana J. Reid, Rex O. Brown, Kathryn L. Vehe, Douglas A. Powers, and R. Wayne Luther

897 **Lack of correlation between objective indicators and clinical-response scores during antimicrobial therapy for acute pulmonary exacerbations of cystic fibrosis**
John A. Bosso and Kay B. Walker

901 **Additive and synergistic bactericidal activity contributed by desacetylcefotaxime during cefotaxime therapy**
Emory S. Moore, Mayra Jimenez, Steven L. Barriere, Marisa L. Cimino, and F. Robert Fekety

Drug Experience

906 **Use of conjugated estrogens to control gastrointestinal tract bleeding in two patients with chronic renal failure**
Shiv Seth and Teresa M. Geier

ASHP Report

910 **Acknowledgment to reviewers**

911 **CP Continuing Education**

913 **CP Continuing Education Enrollment Form**

914 **Current Literature**

Drug Reaction Alerts . . . Books Received

915 **Advertising Index**

916 **Annual Index**

CLINICAL PHARMACY

Editor
William A. Zellmer

Managing Editor
C. Richard Talley

Associate Editor, Manuscript Development
Jane L. Miller

Associate Editor, Redaction
Nancy Tarleton Landis

Assistant Editors, Manuscript Development
Guy R. Hasegawa
Catherine Nichols Klein
Cynthia A. Knapp

Assistant Editor, Redaction
Susan S. McLaughlin

Editorial Production Coordinator
Wende B. Mack

Advertising Production Coordinator
Nasrine L. Sabi

Editorial Assistant
Margery M. Wiltamuth

Editorial Office
4630 Montgomery Avenue
Bethesda, MD 20814
301-657-3000

Editorial Board
Steven L. Barriere, Pharm.D.
Stephen G. Bryant, Pharm.D.
Barry L. Carter, Pharm.D.
Burke A. Cunha, M.D.
Joseph T. DiPiro, Pharm.D.
Larry Ereshefsky, Pharm.D.
William R. Garnett, Pharm.D.
Robert J. Ignoffo, Pharm.D.
John W. Jenne, M.D.
Edward P. Krenzelok, Pharm.D.
Calvin Kunin, M.D.
Gary R. Matzke, Pharm.D.
Frans W. H. M. Merkus, Ph.D.
Jay M. Mirtallo, M.S.
John E. Murphy, Pharm.D.
Milap C. Nahata, Pharm.D.
Stephanie J. Phelps, Pharm.D.
John J. Piecoro, Jr., Pharm.D., M.S.
Richard Quintiliani, M.D.
John H. Rodman, Pharm.D.
Keith A. Rodvold, Pharm.D.
Fred Salter, Pharm.D.
Gerald E. Schumacher, Pharm.D., Ph.D.
Catherine Angell Sohn, Pharm.D.
Robert L. Talbert, Pharm.D.

Consulting Editors
Randal L. Batenhorst, Pharm.D.; Larry A. Bauer, Pharm.D.; Rosemary R. Berardi, Pharm.D.; John Bosso, Pharm.D.; Daniel T. Casto, Pharm.D.; Robert J. Cipolle, Pharm.D.; Joseph F. Dasta, M.Sc.; Michael N. Dudley, Pharm.D.; Lawrence J. Hak, Pharm.D.; David W. Hawkins, Pharm.D.; J. Heyward Hull, Pharm.D.; Martin J. Jinks, Pharm.D.; Cary E. Johnson, Pharm.D.; H. William Kelly, Pharm.D.; Jeffrey R. Koup, Pharm.D.; Thomas C. Majerus, Pharm.D.; Anthony S. Manoguerra, Pharm.D.; James M. McKenney, Pharm.D.; Donald S. North, Pharm.D.; Vaughn W. Payne, Pharm.D.; Donald G. Perrier, Ph.D.; Ronald E. Polk, Pharm.D.; Robert P. Rapp, Pharm.D.; Nathan Rawls, Pharm.D.; David R. Rush, Pharm.D.; Steven L. Sheaffer, Pharm. D.; John K. Siepler, Pharm.D.; Ralph E. Small, Pharm.D.; Glen L. Stimmel, Pharm.D.; Timothy R. Sykes, Pharm.D.; Scott L. Traub, Pharm.D.; William Troutman, Pharm.D.; Peter H. Vlasses, Pharm.D.; Barbara G. Wells, Pharm.D.; Dennis West, M.S.; Michael E. Winter, Pharm.D.

Copyright © 1988, American Society of Hospital Pharmacists, Inc. All rights reserved.

Instructions to Authors

CLINICAL PHARMACY, a forum for the drug therapeutics information that pharmacists need to perform their clinical roles, gives priority to (1) studies that objectively evaluate drug effects in human trials, (2) evaluative review articles on the clinical uses of new drugs, and (3) evaluations of the current status of drug therapy in selected diseases. Contributions to the following sections are invited:

Drug Reviews: Detailed, analytical reviews on the clinical use of specific drugs, with preference given to new drugs and to evaluative rather than descriptive literature reviews.

Therapy Reviews: Articles that focus primarily on a disease state (rather than on a drug or drug class) and its treatment. These reviews foster an understanding of the pathophysiology of a disease and the related treatment.

Research: Reports of well-conducted original research on drug effects in humans.

Research Notes: Short research reports, such as updates on previously published work, confirmations of previous findings, or original research of modest scope.

Grand Rounds: Patient case reports and literature reviews combined in a way that gives them high educational value.

Drug Experience: Straightforward reports, with selected literature references, of unusual drug experiences.

Therapy Consultation: Brief advice, in a question-and-answer format, on how to handle specific drug-therapy problems. Readers are invited to submit questions, which the editor will forward to appropriate consultants for answering.

Letters: Short comments on previously published work or about potential problems, apparent trends, or controversies in drug therapy or clinical research.

Commentaries: Well-reasoned expressions of opinion on drug-therapy or clinical-research issues.

The editors have the sole authority to decide in which section to publish an accepted manuscript.

Manuscripts are subject to review by qualified outside reviewers, as well as by the editors, and will be accepted for publication only if they are believed to represent an important contribution to the literature. All papers submitted for publication must be accompanied by a completed copy of a manuscript checklist. The checklist, which generally conforms to the Uniform Requirements for Manuscripts Submitted to Biomedical Journals, appears on pages 73–74 of the January 1988 issue. Authors of especially important original work may request "fast-track" review of their papers. Authors may suggest appropriate reviewers for their papers.

Accepted materials become the permanent and sole property of ASHP and may not be published or reprinted elsewhere without written permission from both the author and the editor.

The editors reserve the right to revise all materials submitted, if necessary. The publisher assumes no responsibility for the statements and opinions advanced by contributors to CLINICAL PHARMACY.

Under the terms of the Copyright Revision Act of 1976 (Public Law 94-553) it is necessary to have the rights of the authors transferred to the publisher in order to provide for the widest possible dissemination of professional and scientific literature. Accordingly, all transmittal letters accompanying manuscripts submitted for publication, including contributions for the Letters column, must contain the following language: "In consideration of the American Society of Hospital Pharmacists (ASHP) taking action in reviewing and editing my (our) submission, the author(s) undersigned hereby transfer(s), assign(s), or otherwise convey(s) all ownership rights in the submission and all copyright ownership to ASHP. In the event that such work is not published by ASHP, all said rights shall be released." We regret that we cannot consider manuscripts for publication that are not accompanied with transmittal letters containing the above language signed by all authors.

Authors must certify in their letter of transmittal that none of the material in their manuscript has been published previously nor is under consideration or been accepted for publication elsewhere. If this certification cannot be made, suitable explanation must be offered.

Six copies of all manuscripts should be submitted. Manuscripts should be typewritten with double spacing (including tables) on one side of good quality, 21.6 × 27.9-cm white paper, and with margins of at least 2.5 cm. For guidance on style, authors should consult the manuscript checklist, recent issues of CLINICAL PHARMACY, and the *Council of Biology Editors Style Manual*, fifth edition. *The American Heritage Dictionary of the English Language* and the AMA's *Manual for Authors and Editors* contain helpful advice on correct usage.

Galley proofs are sent to authors for inspection against the original manuscript and for correction. Unnecessary alterations in galley proof must be avoided. An order form for reprints is sent to the corresponding author after galley proofs have been cleared.

CLINICAL PHARMACY (ISSN 0278-2677) is published monthly by the American Society of Hospital Pharmacists, 4630 Montgomery Avenue, Bethesda, MD 20814. Joseph A. Oddis, Executive Vice President. Second class postage is paid at Bethesda, MD, and at additional mailing offices. **Postmaster: Send address changes to: *Clinical Pharmacy*, 4630 Montgomery Avenue, Bethesda, MD 20814.**

Annual Subscription Rate:	*USA*	*Non-USA*
ASHP Members	$43	$48
ASHP Student Members and Residents	$32	$40
Institutions and Nonmembers	$67	$72

The cost of single copies is $10. Airmail delivery outside of the continental United States is available for an additional charge of $75 per year. Requests to replace missing issues free of charge are honored only up to six months after date of issue.

Payments to ASHP are not deductible as charitable contributions for federal income tax purposes. However, they may be deductible under other provisions of the Internal Revenue Code.

Advertising for CLINICAL PHARMACY is accepted in accordance with the Statement of Advertising Policy of the American Society of Hospital Pharmacists (see *Am J Hosp Pharm.* 1987; 44:1146). For additional information, contact the Advertising Representative (William McCausland Associates, Inc., P.O. Box 189, Pitman, NJ 08071. Phone 609-589-5454, FAX 609-582-7611.)

All articles published, including editorials, letters, and book reviews, represent the opinions of the authors and do not reflect the official policy of the American Society of Hospital Pharmacists or the institution with which the author is affiliated, unless this is specified.

Microfilm and microfiche editions are available for purchase. Contact University Microfilms, 300 N. Zeeb Road, Ann Arbor, MI 48106.

Articles in CLINICAL PHARMACY are abstracted and indexed in *Current Contents, Clinical Sciences, Excerpta Medica, Index Medicus, Inpharma, International Pharmaceutical Abstracts*, and *Reactions*.

News

FDA approves marketing of second fluoroquinolone, ciprofloxacin

An oral formulation of ciprofloxacin hydrochloride (Cipro, Miles Pharmaceuticals) was approved recently by FDA. It is the second fluoroquinolone antimicrobial agent to be marketed in the United States. Ciprofloxacin was reviewed in the February 1987 issue of *Clinical Pharmacy*.

Of the new fluoroquinolones, ciprofloxacin has one of the broadest spectrums of antimicrobial activity: it is active in vitro against many gram-positive and gram-negative bacteria, including *Staphylococcus aureus, Pseudomonas aeruginosa*, Enterobacteriaceae, *Haemophilus influenzae, Neisseria* spp., *Branhamella catarrhalis*, and various gastrointestinal pathogens.

Oral ciprofloxacin hydrochloride is about 70% bioavailable. Administration with food may delay drug absorption. Ciprofloxacin distributes widely into body fluids and tissues, with a steady-state volume of distribution of 2–3 L/kg. The drug is concentrated in prostate and bile and achieves therapeutic concentrations in sputum, bone, peritoneal fluid, and female pelvic tissue. Ciprofloxacin is eliminated primarily by the kidneys; tubular secretion appears to be important. The terminal half-life is about four hours in healthy volunteers.

Studies have demonstrated the efficacy of oral ciprofloxacin in the treatment of complicated and uncomplicated urinary-tract infections and gonococcal infections. Although *Chlamydia trachomatis* is susceptible in vitro, single-dose therapy with ciprofloxacin has been ineffective in eradicating chlamydial infections. Clinical trials indicate that ciprofloxacin may be useful for bowel decontamination and for the treatment of gastrointestinal infections. Ciprofloxacin has been used successfully in open clinical trials involving patients with soft-tissue infections, osteomyelitis, bacteremia, and respiratory-tract infections caused by susceptible organisms.

FDA-approved labeling indications include infectious diarrhea, lower-respiratory-tract infections, skin and skin structure infections, bone and joint infections, and urinary-tract infections caused by susceptible organisms. The usual adult dosages are 250–500 mg (of ciprofloxacin) orally every 12 hours for urinary-tract infections and 500–750 mg orally every 12 hours for infections of the respiratory tract, bones, joints, skin, and skin structures. The recommended dosage for infectious diarrhea is 500 mg orally every 12 hours. The usual duration of therapy is 7 to 14 days; however, 5 to 7 days of treatment may be adequate for infectious diarrhea, and bone and joint infections may require 4 to 6 weeks of therapy. The dosage should be adjusted for patients with renal impairment.

Adverse reactions to ciprofloxacin are generally infrequent and mild. Gastrointestinal disturbances are the most common complaints. Transiently elevated liver-function-test values and serum creatinine concentrations have been reported infrequently. Ciprofloxacin appears to have less effect on serum theophylline concentrations than enoxacin, which has been reported to elevate theophylline concentrations, resulting in toxicity. Coadministration of aluminum- and magnesium-containing antacids may markedly reduce the absorption of oral ciprofloxacin.

Cipro is available as 250-, 500-, and 750-mg tablets in bottles of 50 and unit dose packages of 100. The costs are $1.40, $1.50, and $2.90 per 250-, 500-, and 750-mg tablet, respectively.

Study suggests role for trimetrexate in AIDS-associated *Pneumocystis carinii* pneumonia

Treatment of AIDS-associated *Pneumocystis carinii* pneumonia with trimetrexate plus leucovorin is well tolerated and is effective for many patients, according to a recent preliminary study of 49 patients.[1] A Phase III trial is scheduled to begin shortly; the study will be conducted by the National Institute of Allergy and Infectious Diseases through the AIDS Treatment Evaluation Units. Trimetrexate is a potent inhibitor of the protozoan dihydrofolate reductase. Because *P. carinii* organisms lack the ability to use preformed folates, leucovorin can be administered concomitantly to protect against trimetrexate-induced myelosuppression. Trimetrexate is also under investigation as an antineoplastic agent.

Participants in the uncontrolled study included 16 patients who had not tolerated or had not responded to a seven-day course of pentamidine or trimethoprim–sulfamethoxazole (group 1), 16 patients with untreated *P. carinii* pneumonia who had not tolerated or had not responded to sulfonamides during a previous episode of *P. carinii* pneumonia (group 2), and 17 patients who received the study regimen as initial therapy and had no history of intolerance or lack of response to sulfonamides (group 3). Of the 49 episodes of *P. carinii* pneumonia, 23 were recurrent infections. All patients received trimetrexate 30 mg/sq m intravenously daily for 21 days and leucovorin 20 mg/sq m intravenously or orally every six hours for 23 days. Group 3 patients also received sulfadiazine 1 g orally every six hours for 21 days.

Response rates for groups 1 through 3 were 69%, 63%, and 71%, respectively; corresponding survival rates were 69%, 88%, and 77%. The contribution of sulfadiazine to

Continued on page 11

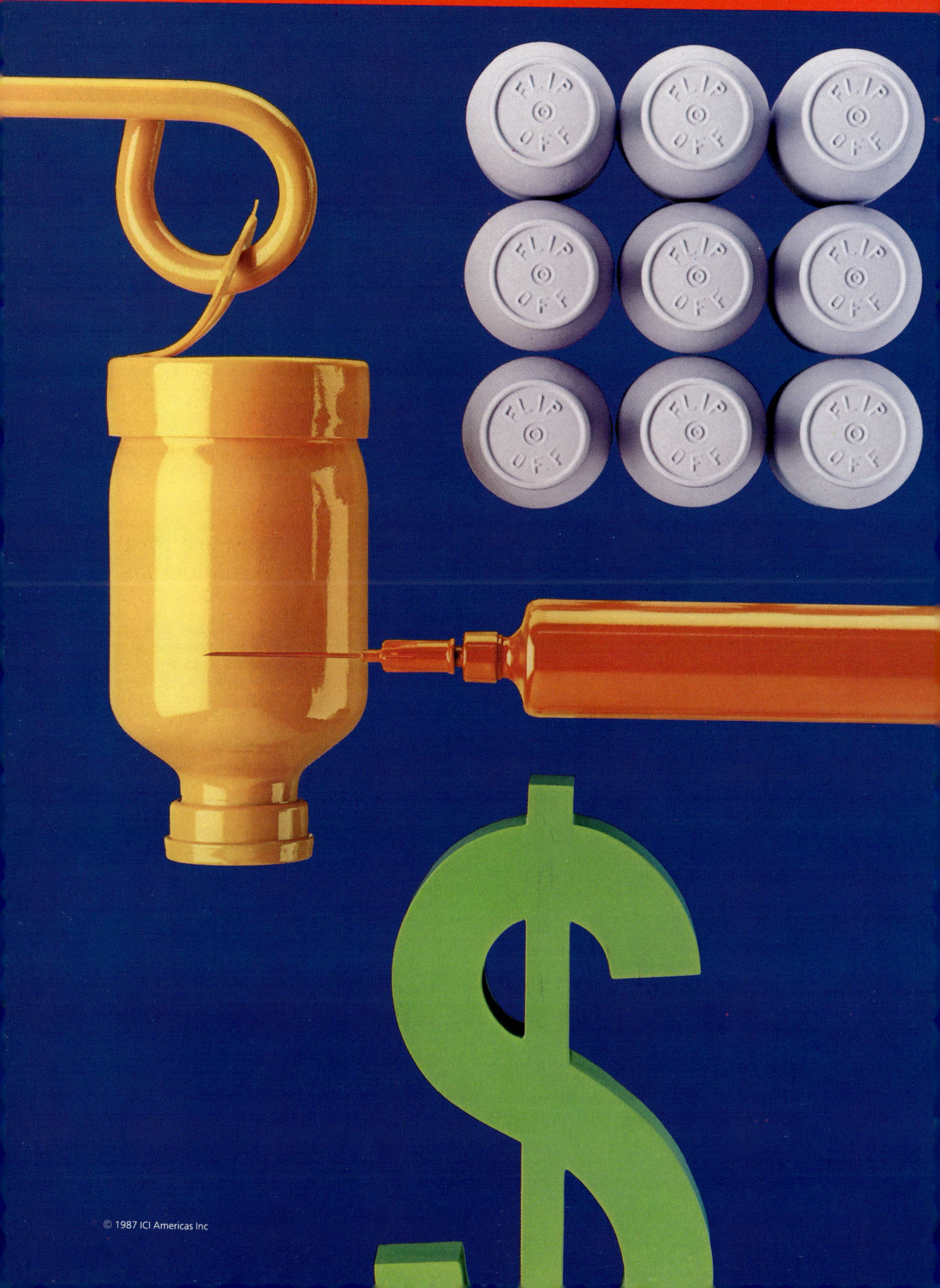

© 1987 ICI Americas Inc

Continued from page 7

efficacy or toxicity could not be determined. Neutropenia was reported in eight patients, thrombocytopenia in five patients, and transient increases in aminotransferase concentrations in four patients. Reduction of the trimetrexate dosage to 15 mg/sq m/day for an average of four days typically led to an increase in the neutrophil or platelet count within three days. Correlation of laboratory abnormalities with treatment was difficult because values were frequently abnormal at the outset of therapy.

Response to trimetrexate–leucovorin therapy appears to be similar to that reported for other regimens; however, patient populations and assessment methods vary greatly. Direct comparisons are needed to determine trimetrexate's therapeutic role.

1. Allegra CJ, Chabner BA, Tuazon CU et al. Trimetrexate for the treatment of *Pneumocystis carinii* pneumonia in patients with the acquired immunodeficiency syndrome. *N Engl J Med.* 1987; 317:978–85.

Studies refute efficacy of corticosteroids in severe sepsis

High-dose corticosteroid therapy is not beneficial in the treatment of severe sepsis, according to results of two multicenter, prospective, randomized, double-blind, placebo-controlled studies published recently in *The New England Journal of Medicine.*[1,2]

In the first study, 382 patients who met predetermined diagnostic criteria for severe sepsis and septic shock received either placebo or methylprednisolone 30 mg/kg (as the sodium succinate salt) every six hours for four doses.[1] Treatment was begun within two hours after diagnosis. Methylprednisolone-treated patients tended to have more genitourinary infections; significantly more patients receiving placebo had multiple sites of infection. Overall, there were no significant differences between the two groups in prevention of shock, resolution of shock, or mortality at 14 days. The mortality rates at 14 days were 34% and 25%, respectively, for the methylprednisolone and placebo groups. Among patients who initially had elevated serum creatinine concentrations, the mortality rate was higher with methylprednisolone therapy (52%) than with placebo administration (17%). Significantly more deaths were attributed to secondary infections in the methylprednisolone group (34%) than in the placebo group (7%).

The second study involved 223 patients with suspected sepsis and a normal sensorium who received either placebo or methylprednisolone 30 mg/kg (as the sodium succinate salt) intravenously followed by a nine-hour constant infusion of 5 mg/kg/hr (maximum dose, 10 g).[2] Treatment was begun an average of 2.8 hours after diagnosis. Mortality rates at 14 days were not significantly different between the placebo (22%) and methylprednisolone (21%) groups overall or in the subgroups of patients with positive culture results, negative culture results, gram-negative bacteremia, gram-negative infections, or gram-positive bacteremia. The percentages of placebo- and methylprednisolone-treated patients who developed complications were similar. Resolution of secondary infections within the 14-day study period occurred more frequently in the placebo group.

Both research groups concluded that high-dose corticosteroid therapy does not have a role in the treatment of patients with sepsis.

1. Bone RC, Fisher CJ, Clemmer TP et al. A controlled clinical trial of high-dose methylprednisolone in the treatment of severe sepsis and septic shock. *N Engl J Med.* 1987; 317:653–8.
2. The Veterans Administration Systemic Sepsis Cooperative Study Group. Effect of high-dose glucocorticoid therapy on mortality in patients with clinical signs of systemic sepsis. *N Engl J Med.* 1987; 317:659–65.

FDA divides drugs and biologics evaluation unit

FDA's Center for Drugs and Biologics, the unit responsible for reviewing all new drug and biological products, was divided in October into two units: the Center for Drug Evaluation and Research, now under the direction of Carl C. Peck, M.D., and the Center for Biologics Evaluation and Research, now headed by Paul D. Parkman, M.D. The combined biologics and drug evaluation unit had been in existence since 1982.

According to Otis R. Bowen, Secretary of Health and Human Services, the pressures generated by AIDS and the drug review process made these two programs unmanageable in a single unit. FDA's drug approval process had come under increasing criticism in recent months, particularly over the agency's handling of tissue-plasminogen activator.

Activities of the Center for Drug Evaluation and Research will focus on the drug review process. Evaluation of new and investigational drug applications, development and implementation of standards for nonprescription drugs, postmarketing drug surveillance, monitoring of prescription drug advertising, and analysis of accidental poisoning and toxicity data are responsibilities of this division. The dominant focus of the Center for Biologics Evaluation and Research is coordination of AIDS-related activities, including research, vaccine studies, and blood testing technologies. Biologics licensing and control programs are under the purview of this division. Both units will handle biotechnology products.

Distribution of ivermectin for onchocerciasis announced by Merck

Merck & Co., Inc., has announced plans to donate supplies of ivermectin (Mectizan) to qualified health programs worldwide for the treatment of onchocerciasis, a parasitic disease that is also known as river blindness. Distribution of ivermectin will involve a cooperative effort of Merck and the World Health Organization. Onchocerciasis is most prevalent in West and Central Africa, areas of the Middle East, and in Central and South America. It is one of the leading causes of blindness in developing countries.

The larvae are transmitted to humans by blackfly bites and develop into adult worms in the subcutaneous tissue. The microfilariae (embryos) produced by the adult worms migrate throughout the body, causing inflammatory lesions and subsequent scarring. The most serious tissue damage occurs in the eye. Studies suggest that administration of single doses of ivermectin once or twice yearly may adequately control onchocerciasis. Dermal microfilarial counts are reduced to near zero within a month after single oral 200-μg/kg doses of ivermectin; six months after treatment, counts gradually increase to 2–10% of the pretreatment density. Previously, the only treatments for onchocerciasis were suramin and diethylcarbamazine. Both of these drugs must be given as multiple-dose regimens and require close medical supervision; thus, they are poorly suited to mass use.

Efficacy of *Haemophilus influenzae* vaccine reassessed

In response to postmarketing reports of invasive *Haemophilus influenzae* disease in children vaccinated with *H. influenzae* type b vaccine, the Centers for Disease Control (CDC) has re-evaluated its recommendations for vaccination and has concluded that a change in vaccination strategies is not warranted.[1] Vaccine efficacy was reviewed and reports of invasive disease occurring within seven days after vaccination were discussed at a workshop convened by FDA in April of this year.[2] Preliminary data from five studies—a nonrandomized, prospective cohort study of 122,000 children and four small case-control studies—were presented. Analysis of the data available at that time indicated that four of these studies were "not inconsistent" with the 90% efficacy rate found in an earlier randomized, prospective study conducted in Finland; the fifth study, a case-control study, failed to demonstrate a beneficial effect of vaccination. Analysis of the cases of invasive disease occurring soon after vaccination was hindered by insufficient data. The workshop's recommendation was that current CDC guidelines for vaccination should be followed.

1. Immunization Practices Advisory Committee. Update: prevention of *Haemophilus influenzae* type b disease. *MMWR*. 1987; 36:529.
2. Anon. FDA workshop on *Haemophilus* b polysaccharide vaccine—a preliminary report. *MMWR*. 1987; 36:529–31.

Research fellowships and grants offered for 1988–1989

Three research fellowships and five research awards will be offered for the 1988–1989 academic year by the Research Institute of the American College of Clinical Pharmacy (ACCP). The fellowships include the Merck Research Fellowship in Cardiovascular, Infectious Disease, Rheumatology, or Pain Control Therapeutics; the Miles Pharmaceuticals Research Fellowship in Infectious Disease or Cardiovascular Therapeutics; and a newly funded Sandoz Pharmaceuticals Research Fellowship in Immunology Therapeutics. Combined applications from prospective preceptors (ACCP full members only) and fellows (ACCP members or associate members) are required. Awards of $5000 each are being offered to support research in the areas of pharmacotherapy (Glaxo), central nervous system pharmacotherapy (Mead Johnson Laboratories), pulmonary pharmacotherapy (Schering Laboratories), cost-effectiveness (The Upjohn Company), and innovative clinical practice (Upjohn). Grant recipients must be ACCP members or associate members.

The deadline for submission of fellowship and research award applications is February 1. Further information can be obtained from ACCP, 3101 Broadway, Suite 350, Kansas City, MO 64111; 816-531-2177.

News Briefs

• Clinical testing of **tetrahydroaminoacridine (THA) in Alzheimer's disease** has been halted, at least temporarily, because of hepatic enzyme abnormalities in several patients; a two-year study involving approximately 300 patients at 17 medical centers in the United States was begun recently.

• A two-year contract from the Centers for Disease Control to establish and operate a **national clearinghouse for information on AIDS** has been awarded to Aspen Systems Corporation, a health-information management company in Rockville, Maryland; the clearinghouse will answer questions about AIDS, make referrals for additional information, and distribute government-approved publications.

• **"What You Should Know About AIDS,"** an eight-page brochure that answers commonly asked questions about AIDS, is available from the United States Public Health Service, "America Responds to AIDS," P.O. Box 23961, Washington, DC 20026-3961.

• FDA has amended the **standards for allergenic products** to state that nonstandardized methods of labeling potency based on protein nitrogen units (PNUs) or ratios of allergen weight to extracting fluid volume should be replaced "as soon as practical" by a unit that measures allergenic activity.

• New guidelines available from FDA for professional and patient **labeling of estrogen products** include new information on the benefits and risks of estrogen therapy, use of estrogen therapy for postmenopausal osteoporosis, and use of progestogens in combination with estrogens.

• An article entitled **"Managing Glucose Testing in the Hospital,"** published in the September 25, 1987, issue of the *Journal of the American Medical Association*, relates three hospitals' experiences with bedside testing of blood glucose concentrations and describes a program for quality assurance.

• A report entitled **"Guidelines for the Use of Enteral Nutrition in the Adult Patient"** has been developed by the American Society for Parenteral and Enteral Nutrition; the report was published in the September–October 1987 issue of the *Journal of Parenteral and Enteral Nutrition*.

Upcoming Specialty Meetings

Congress of the International Anesthesia Research Society (62nd) . . . San Diego, CA . . . March 5–9 . . . contact: E. A. Moffitt, M.D., 3645 Warrensville Center Road, Cleveland, OH 44122; 216-295-1124.

American Society for Clinical Pharmacology and Therapeutics . . . San Diego, CA . . . March 9–11 . . . contact: E. Galasso, 1719 Gallagher Road, Norristown, PA 19401; 215-825-3838.

People count on you for the latest drug therapy information. You can count on Clinical Pharmacy to provide it.

Clinical Pharmacy . . . the monthly journal that brings you the most current drug therapy information available.

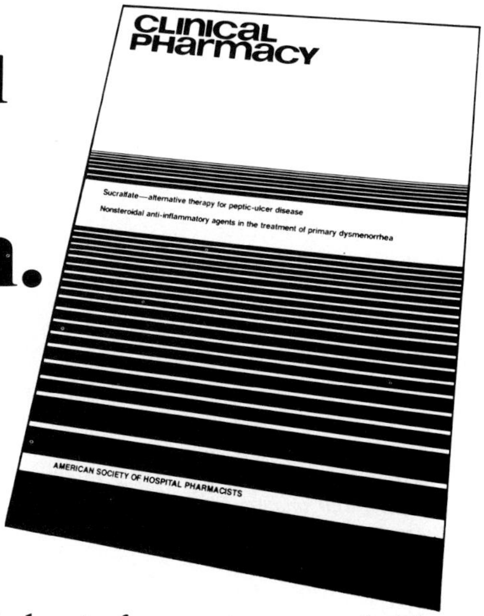

There aren't enough hours in your day to uncover all the information available on new drugs, current therapies, the latest research results. That's why there's *Clinical Pharmacy*.

Each month, *Clinical Pharmacy* provides you—

- an analysis of new drugs and new drug therapy
- current perspectives on existing drug therapies
- reviews of the latest drug literature
- reports on clinical research
- news from FDA and clinical centers around the country

For as little as $40 a year!*

Clinical Pharmacy keeps you current on the drugs and research you want to know about.

New drugs recently featured include:

- mupirocin
- flecainide and encainide
- midazolam hydrochloride
- quinolone antimicrobials

**This low annual fee applies to ASHP members only! Foreign, ASHP Student and Nonmember rates vary.*

Original research recently featured . . .

- accuracy of four dosing methods for vancomycin
- minimum urine collection periods for accurate determination of creatinine clearance

Subscribing to *Clinical Pharmacy* is money and time well spent! Here are *just* three reasons why:

1. CP's Drug Tracking System. The *CP* staff identifies important new drugs and follows them through FDA approval. The result—articles on new drugs even before they reach the market.

2. CP's Editorial Expertise. Twenty-five clinical practitioners, researchers and educators advise the *CP* editorial staff on trends, developments and findings making an impact on drug therapy. The result—well-written, accurate reviews that analyze the appropriate therapy for major diseases.

3. CP's Continuing Education Opportunities. *CP* offers selected articles for continuing education (CE) credit. The American Society of Hospital Pharmacists is accredited by the American Council on Pharmaceutical Education as a CE provider. You can test your grasp of the material whether or not you're seeking CE credits.

Many turn to you for answers on the best drug therapies . . . latest research results . . . potential side effects.

Clinical Pharmacy can help you meet that challenge.

Order Form ☐ Please enter by subscription to *Clinical Pharmacy* at the rate I've noted below.

☐ Enclosed is my check for $ ________ . (Checks must be drawn on a U.S. bank and payable to ASHP.)

Charge $ ________ to my: ☐ MasterCard ☐ VISA Acct. # ____________________ Exp. ____________ (month/year)

Signature ______________________________

☐ My purchase order # ______________________ is attached; please issue an invoice and add postage and handling.

Name ______________________________

Institution ______________________________

ASHP I.D. # ______________________

Address ______________________________

City ________ State ______________ Zip ________

CP Rates

ASHP Member	$40/year
ASHP Student/Resident	$30/year
Nonmember	$63/year

(Outside the USA, please add $5)

Send to:
ASHP Publication
Record Dept.
4630 Montgomery Ave
Bethesda, MD 20814

Therapy Consultation

The Therapy Consultation *section provides brief advice, in question-and-answer format, on how to handle specific drug-therapy problems. Readers are invited to submit questions, which will be referred to a consultant for an answer. The problems should not be highly specialized or unusual, nor should they be mundane. Questions are answered briefly, based largely on the judgment and personal experience of the consultant, although selected references may be cited to substantiate the consultant's advice.*

Assistance in identifying Therapy Consultation *topics is provided by the drug information centers at the following institutions: Albert B. Chandler Medical Center and College of Pharmacy, University of Kentucky, Lexington; Arizona Health Sciences Center, Tucson; Medical College of Virginia Hospitals, Richmond; University of California Medical Center, San Diego; and University of Michigan Medical Center, Ann Arbor.*

Treatment of stomatitis associated with antineoplastic-drug therapy

Question: A woman who is being treated with doxorubicin, fluorouracil, and cyclophosphamide for breast cancer developed severe stomatitis after a course of therapy. What can be done to relieve her discomfort and prevent infection?

Response: Stomatitis is a frequent complication of antineoplastic-drug therapy and is a result of the cytotoxic effects of antineoplastic agents on rapidly proliferating, nonmalignant cells including bone marrow and gastrointestinal epithelial cells. Stomatitis may be caused directly by destruction of the oral mucosal cells, resulting in inflammation and dryness that can lead to severe oral ulcers. Stomatitis may also result from microbial invasion of the oral mucosa, facilitated by drug-induced neutropenia. This patient may develop oral ulcers so painful that she cannot eat, swallow, or even speak. Additionally, life-threatening systemic infection can result from the entry of microorganisms into the bloodstream through inflamed oral mucosa. Thus, the goals of treatment are to provide pain relief and to promote healing while preventing the development of systemic infection.[1]

The treatment of stomatitis caused by antineoplastic agents is based almost entirely on anecdotal information; the only controlled research is in the area of fungal stomatitis. There is no evidence that commonly used symptomatic treatments are effective, but many have been reported to provide subjective relief.

Intitial treatment of this patient's stomatitis should include promotion of oral hygiene with the use of saline–alkaline mouthwash. This is made by dissolving sodium chloride crystals and sodium bicarbonate powder in water. At least four times daily, the patient should swish the mouthwash in the mouth for two or three minutes and then spit it out. This preparation is also soothing to the oral mucosa.[1]

One of the most important aspects of the treatment of severe stomatitis is to provide pain relief. Cold substances such as popsicles and ice chips seem to provide adequate relief for many patients with mild or moderate stomatitis. Use of these agents alone is unlikely to provide adequate pain relief for the patient described.

Because this patient's stomatitis is severe, a topical anesthetic is indicated. The available agents include diphenhydramine hydrochloride (Benadryl or Benylin, Warner–Lambert), dyclonine hydrochloride (Dyclone, Astra), and lidocaine hydrochloride (Xylocaine, Astra).

Lidocaine and dyclonine are commercially available in viscous solutions that coat the oral mucosa. Lidocaine hydrochloride 2% and dyclonine hydrochloride 0.5% or 1% are effective in doses of 5 mL swished and spat out at least four times daily; unfortunately, they are unpalatable, and their anesthetic action interferes with the pharyngeal phase of swallowing, making eating difficult or impossible.[1]

Diphenhydramine is an effective topical anesthetic that does not interefere with swallowing. However, it may cause sedation if ingested, and commercially available oral solutions have low viscosity and contain up to 14% alcohol, which can be painful and drying to the already inflamed mucosa. In compounding mouthwashes, therefore, injectable diphenhydramine should be used to avoid alcohol, and kaolin–pectin or antacid suspension can be added to increase the viscosity of the final product.[1] If diphenhydramine mouthwash is used, the patient should be instructed to swish the equivalent of 12.5 mg of diphenhydramine hydrochloride in her mouth for three minutes four times daily, then spit it out. If a sedative effect is desired, the patient may be instructed to swallow the product.

Sucralfate is currently being studied as an aid in healing of stomatitis and is thought to work by binding to the inflamed areas of stomatitis, protecting them from further insult. Sucralfate 1 g, given as 10–15 mL of slurry, is swished in the mouth for two minutes and then spat out or swallowed four to six times daily.[2,3] Small, uncontrolled studies have shown that this preparation is effective in providing symptomatic relief in patients with existing stomatitis. The data also suggest that it may speed the healing of mouth ulcers or, alternatively, may decrease the number of mouth ulcers that develop.[2,3] This theory remains to be tested in a controlled clinical trial.

Continued on page 17

Continued from page 14

If the patient is neutropenic, use of an antifungal agent to prevent or treat local fungal infection should be considered. Available antifungal agents include nystatin oral suspension (5 mL swished and spat out or swallowed four times daily), nystatin vaginal tablets used as lozenges four times daily, and clotrimazole troches (10 mg dissolved in the mouth five times daily).[4,5] In addition, nystatin troches (200,000–400,000 units dissolved in the mouth four to five times daily) were marketed recently. These agents are equally effective; drug selection depends on patient tolerance. Nystatin suspension is unpalatable to some patients, and it contains 50% sucrose, which can have a detrimental effect on dentition. Nystatin vaginal tablets and troches and clotrimazole troches have prolonged contact time with oral mucosa; clotrimazole and nystatin troches are more palatable than nystatin tablets, which have a bitter taste. In addition to their efficacy in the treatment of local infection, there is some suggestion in the literature that these agents may aid in prevention of systemic fungal infection in neutropenic patients.[4,5]

Antibacterial agents such as tetracycline and neomycin have been used as mouthwashes in an attempt to prevent local and systemic bacterial infections. Since there are no data to suggest that they are effective, there is no indication for their use.

Combination mouthwashes containing two or more of the agents described above are commonly used for the treatment of stomatitis. Although this practice seems reasonable, there are no data available on either the stability or the efficacy of these combination products. For this reason, the use of combination preparations cannot be recommended at this time.

1. Lucarelli CD. Chemotherapy-induced oral mucositis: causes and treatment. *Cancer Chemother Update.* 1984; 2:1–4.
2. Ferraro JM. Sucralfate suspension for mouth ulcers. *Drug Intell Clin Pharm.* 1985; 19:480. Letter.
3. Solomon MA. Oral sucralfate suspension for mucositis. *N Engl J Med.* 1986; 315:459–60. Letter.
4. Quintiliani R, Owens NJ, Quercia RA et al. Treatment and prevention of oropharyngeal candidiasis. *Am J Med.* 1984; 77 (Suppl 4D):44–8.
5. Meunier-Carpentier F. Chemoprophylaxis of fungal infections. *Am J Med.* 1984; 76:652–6.

Betty J. Kinzie, Pharm.D.
Clinical Pharmacist–Oncology and Clinical Assistant Professor
University of Michigan Medical Center and College of Pharmacy, University of Michigan
Ann Arbor, MI 48109

A handy sized pocket reference is now available from ASHP®

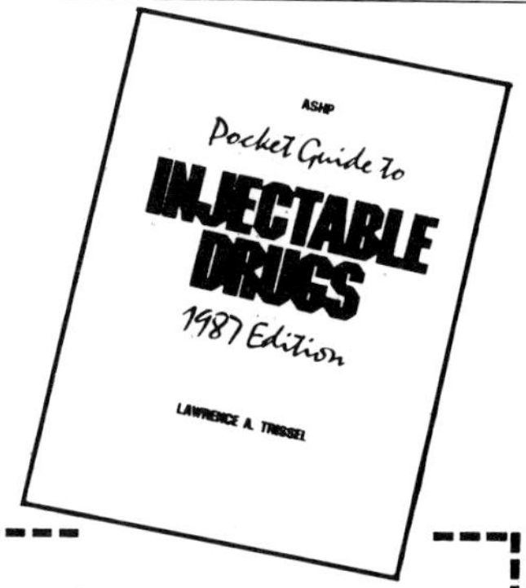

Order Form Order your copy of the *Pocket Guide* today.

Please send me ______ copies of P249, ***Pocket Guide to Injectable Drugs*, 1987 Edition**, at $15 each.

☐ Enclosed is my check for $ __________ .
(Checks must be drawn on a U.S. bank and payable to ASHP.)

☐ Enclosed is our purchase order # __________ ; please issue an invoice and add postage and handling.

OR Charge $ ________ to my: ☐ MasterCard ☐ VISA

Acct. # ____________ Exp. ________ month/year

Signature ____________

Name ____________

Institution ____________

ASHP I.D.# ____________

Address ____________

City ________ State ______ Zip ______

Send to: ASHP Publication Records Dept., 4630 Montgomery Avenue
Bethesda, MD 20814

© 1987 American Society of Hospital Pharmacists

This popular reference provides comprehensive coverage of injectable drugs used in admixtures.

Based on the acclaimed ***Handbook on Injectable Drugs***, the ***Pocket Guide*** gives you the necessary information to make on-the-spot decisions about injectable drug therapy. Its unique format provides quick answers to the most commonly asked questions.

The 1987 edition features 100 monographs on injectable drug products.

Monographs cover information on:
- *dosage*
- *administration*
- *preparation*
- *stability*
- *compatibility*

The ***Pocket Guide*** will give you quick answers to the most commonly asked questions on injectable drug products. Indexing to the ***Handbook*** will help to resolve complex problems.

New drugs in this edition are:
- *bleomycin sulfate*
- *cefotaxime sodium*
- *cisplatin*
- *codeine phosphate*
- *corticotropin*
- *doxorubicin HCl*
- *fluorouracil*
- *hydrocortisone sodium phosphate*
- *hydromorphone HCl*
- *hydroxyzine HCl*
- *methotrexate sodium*
- *metronidazole*
- *moxalactam disodium*
- *nalbuphine HCl*
- *nitroglycerin*
- *oxytocin*
- *perphenazine*
- *secobarbital sodium*
- *vancomycin HCl*

"ASHP is a service mark of the American Society of Hospital Pharmacists, Inc.; Registered in the U.S. Patent and Trademark Office."

Letters

Routine monitoring of serum vancomycin concentrations: The answer lies in the middle

We read with interest the Commentaries on the routine monitoring of serum vancomycin concentrations in the August issue of *Clinical Pharmacy*.[1,2] Edwards and Pancorbo[1] defended the position that since routine monitoring of serum vancomycin concentrations is not indicated in most clinical situations, it should be reserved for cases in which the patient has severe renal impairment, the culture and sensitivity testing demonstrates elevated minimum inhibitory concentrations, or there is poor therapeutic response. Rodvold et al.[2] defended routine monitoring of serum vancomycin concentrations for all patients. In consideration of these polar viewpoints, we would like to describe our experience with the vancomycin monitoring program at our institution.

All patients for whom vancomycin is prescribed are monitored. Estimated peak and trough serum vancomycin concentrations are calculated using the multiple-infusion equations of Sawchuk and Zaske,[3] in which the elimination rate constant is represented by the equation

$$k = 0.000954\,(CL_{cr}) + 0.0036$$

and volume of distribution (V) is 0.66 L/kg. Once actual serum concentrations have been determined, all pharmacokinetic variables are calculated using the multiple-infusion equations. A dosage adjustment is recommended for any patient who has an estimated or actual serum vancomycin concentration higher or lower than accepted therapeutic values.

A 13-month audit of our program from July 1986 to July 1987 identified 207 courses of vancomycin therapy. Of these, 77 were prescribed for patients undergoing dialysis, 16 were prescribed for surgical prophylaxis in penicillin-allergic patients, and 114 were prescribed for the treatment of acute infections. A total of 33 patients who were being treated for acute infections required dosage adjustments (3 increases in dosage and 30 decreases). The total duration of therapy was 467 days. Of the 30 decreases in dosage, 16 were based on 42 serum concentration determinations and 14 were adjusted on the basis of estimated concentrations. Of the three increases in dosage, one was based on two serum concentration determinations and two were adjusted on the basis of estimated concentrations. Since the hospital cost for each assay is $20, the total cost of the 44 actual serum vancomycin concentration determinations was $880. The net impact of the adjusted dosages, based on reduced drug acquisition costs for decreased dosages ($4435.90) minus increased costs for increased dosages ($238.38) minus laboratory costs ($880.00), was a savings in drug costs of $6363.16.

In our opinion, the solution to the controversy over routine monitoring of serum vancomycin concentrations falls somewhere between the viewpoints of Edwards and Pancorbo and Rodvold et al. We agree that not all patients require routine monitoring of serum vancomycin concentrations. However, when monitoring is performed, it can be both useful and cost-justifiable.

1. Edwards DJ, Pancorbo S. Routine monitoring of serum concentrations: waiting for proof of its value. *Clin Pharm*. 1987; 6:652–4. Commentary.
2. Rodvold KA, Zokufa H, Rotschafer JC. Routine monitoring of serum vancomycin concentrations: can waiting be justified? *Clin Pharm*. 1987; 6:655–8. Commentary.
3. Sawchuk RJ, Zaske DE. Pharmacokinetics of dosing regimens which utilize multiple intravenous infusions: gentamicin in burn patients. *J Pharmacokinet Biopharm*. 1976; 4:183–95.

JEFFREY F. B. SAYERS, PHARM.D., Antimicrobial/Pharmacokinetic Specialist
ROBERT SHIMASAKI, PHARM.D., Drug Information Specialist

Veterans Administration Medical Center, Sepulveda
Sepulveda, CA 91343

Notice to readers

Following publication of our paper entitled "Controversies in the use of transdermal nitroglycerin systems" in the August 1987 issue of *Clinical Pharmacy*, the editor brought to our attention a reader inquiry. Based upon this and our own review of the publication, we learned that some statements in this review article were quoted verbatim from other published papers or were used with slight modification of the sentence structure, without use of quotation marks or technically proper referencing. The corresponding references (numbers 7, 24, 28, 45, 49, and 54) were, however, listed at the end of the article. In many cases, the appropriate paper was cited, either as the sole citation or as one of several; however, in no instance was there any indication that sentences or phrases in our article were being quoted verbatim. We regret this problem inasmuch as there was never any intention to pass off any data or findings as our own but simply to correctly state such data and findings.

We have doubled our efforts in conforming to the high publishing standards of ASHP.

FREDERICK P. ZELLER, PHARM.D., Assistant Professor
KAREN J. KLAMERUS, PHARM. D., Assistant Professor

Department of Pharmacy Practice
College of Pharmacy
University of Illinois at Chicago
833 South Wood Street, Room 244
Chicago, IL 60612

Drug Reviews

Lovastatin: A new cholesterol-lowering agent

James M. McKenney

Abstract: The chemistry, pharmacology, pharmacokinetics, clinical efficacy, dosage and administration, and adverse effects of lovastatin are reviewed.

Lovastatin is the first agent marketed in a new class of pharmacologic compounds called the 3-hydroxy-3-methylglutaryl coenzyme A (HMG CoA) reductase inhibitors. By competitively inhibiting HMG CoA reductase, the drug disrupts the biosynthesis of cholesterol in hepatic and peripheral cells. This increases the synthesis of low-density-lipoprotein (LDL) receptors and thereby increases the uptake of LDL cholesterol from the plasma. In doses of 20 to 80 mg daily, lovastatin decreases total and LDL cholesterol concentrations 25 to 45%. It also substantially reduces concentrations of triglycerides, very-low-density-lipoprotein (VLDL) cholesterol, and apolipoprotein B and slightly increases high-density-lipoprotein (HDL) cholesterol concentrations. Lovastatin is effective in patients with heterozygous familial and nonfamilial (polygenic) hypercholesterolemia but is ineffective in patients with homozygous familial hypercholesterolemia. It is also effective in combination with bile acid sequestrants, nicotinic acid, and gemfibrozil. Administration of lovastatin once daily in the evening (to enhance compliance) or twice daily is recommended to maximize the drug's cholesterol-lowering effects.

Headache and gastrointestinal complaints are the most common adverse effects. Treatment has been withdrawn from 1.9% of patients receiving the drug because of elevated aminotransferase concentrations. The relationship of lovastatin to the development of lens opacities requires further evaluation.

Lovastatin is highly effective in the treatment of primary hypercholesterolemia and represents an important therapeutic advance. Safety with long-term use and effect on coronary heart disease remain to be established.

Index terms: Antilipemic agents; Combined therapy; Dosage; Gemfibrozil; Hypercholesterolemia; Lovastatin; Mechanism of action; Niacin; Pharmacokinetics; Toxicity
Clin Pharm. 1988; 7:21–36

Lovastatin (formerly called mevinolin) was recently approved by the Food and Drug Administration for the treatment of primary hypercholesterolemia. Lovastatin will be a major advance in the treatment of hypercholesterolemia if it is shown to lack serious toxicity with long-term use. Although other cholesterol-lowering agents are available, they are poorly accepted by patients or produce relatively modest effects. Lovastatin has become available at a time when there is growing national emphasis on the treatment of high blood cholesterol levels. Lovastatin is the first agent marketed in a new class of pharmacologic compounds called the 3-hydroxy-3-methylglutaryl-coenzyme A (HMG CoA) reductase inhibitors. Other agents in this class, including pravastatin from Squibb and simvastatin from Merck, are currently undergoing clinical evaluation in the United States. Lovastatin is marketed under the trade name Mevacor by Merck Sharp & Dohme.

The purpose of this paper is to review the available information on the pharmacology and therapeutics of lovastatin. In addition, the rationale for treating hypercholesterolemia, the transport and synthesis of cholesterol, the place of lovastatin in the treatment of hypercholesterolemia, approaches to patient monitoring, and formulary considerations will be discussed.

Rationale for Treatment

The impetus to treat high blood cholesterol levels is mounting, and the need is great for effective agents that are easy for patients to take. Thus, the release of lovastatin comes at an opportune time.

An elevated serum cholesterol concentration has long been recognized as a major risk factor for coronary heart disease (CHD), the number-one

James M. McKenney, Pharm.D., is Professor of Pharmacy, School of Pharmacy, Medical College of Virginia–Virginia Commonwealth University, Richmond, VA 23298.

Copyright © 1988, American Society of Hospital Pharmacists, Inc. All rights reserved. 0278-2677/88/0101-0021$04.00.

killer of Americans. Thirty-five years ago, Enos et al.[1] reported that 77% of 300 young, apparently healthy, asymptomatic men who were casualties during the Korean War had grossly visible lesions in their coronary arteries at autopsy. The authors speculated that these lesions may have been associated with a high blood cholesterol concentration. Population studies demonstrated a direct relationship between cholesterol levels and the incidence of CHD.[2] Any notion that a high cholesterol concentration was due to unique ethnic traits was dispelled when it was observed that the Japanese, who have low cholesterol levels and low rates of CHD, developed progressive increases in cholesterol levels and coronary heart disease as they moved to Honolulu and then to the San Francisco Bay area.[3] Prospective epidemiologic studies in the United States, such as the Framingham Heart Study,[4] the Pooling Project,[5] and the Multiple Risk Factor Intervention Trial (MRFIT),[6] have demonstrated that the relationship between cholesterol levels and risk of developing CHD is continuous throughout the range of cholesterol levels and curvilinear (as serum cholesterol concentrations increase above 200 mg/dL, the risk is compounded).

What was unknown until recently was whether treatment to lower cholesterol levels could prevent or reverse this relationship. The report of the Coronary Primary Prevention Trial (CPPT) provided the first evidence that effective drug treatment could decrease deaths caused by CHD.[7,8]

The CPPT was a large, multicenter trial involving 3806 men aged 35 to 59 who had initial blood cholesterol concentrations above 265 mg/dL and no evidence of CHD. These men were randomized to receive a diet low in saturated fats and resin placebo or a low-saturated-fat diet and cholestyramine. After a minimum of seven years, the diet-cholestyramine group had a 24% reduction in deaths caused by CHD, a 19% decrease in nonfatal myocardial infarctions, 25% fewer positive exercise-tolerance tests, 20% fewer episodes of angina, and 21% fewer coronary-artery bypass surgeries. The reduction in CHD deaths and nonfatal myocardial infarctions combined was significant (one-sided test of significance at an alpha level of 0.05).

Recent evidence also suggests that lowering blood cholesterol levels with drugs can not only prevent CHD but may even reverse the atherosclerotic process.[9-11] Blankenhorn et al.[9] reported that combination therapy with diet, colestipol, and niacin, which reduced cholesterol levels an average of 24%, slowed the progression and produced regression of angiographically determined coronary atherosclerosis in men with bypass grafts.

This evidence means that the question is no longer whether to treat hypercholesterolemia but when and how to treat it. The National Cholesterol Education Program, which has been formed to relay this important message about cholesterol first to professionals and then to the public, has announced guidelines for the diagnosis and treatment of high blood cholesterol concentrations. Lovastatin is an important part of these recommendations. Lovastatin was judged to be a highly effective cholesterol-lowering agent, but the lack of data on long-term safety and effects on CHD endpoints prompted the program's panel to classify lovastatin as a second-line agent.

Figure 1. Structural formula of lovastatin and its active metabolite, showing the inactive prodrug in the lactone form (left) and the active inhibitor in the hydroxyacid form.

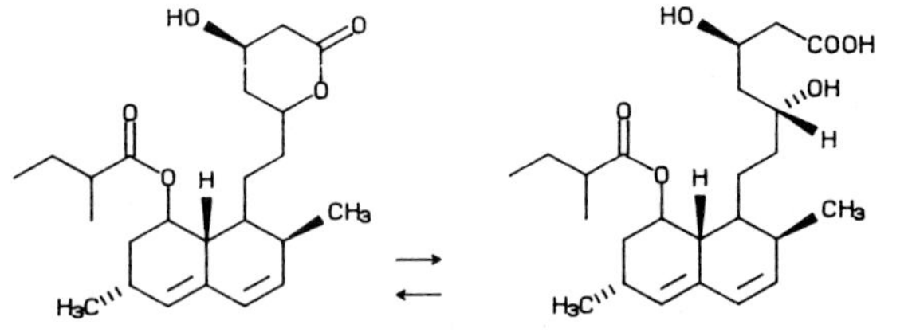

Chemistry

Lovastatin is a chemical modification of a fermentation product of the microorganism *Aspergillus terreus*. Its chemical name is [1S-[1α(R*), 3α, 7β, 8β (2S*,-4S*), 8aβ]]-1,2,3,7,8,8a-hexahydro-3,7-dimethyl-8-[2-(tetrahydro-4-hydroxy-6-oxo-2H-pyran-2-yl)-ethyl]-1-naphthalenyl 2-methyl-butanoate. It has a molecular formula of $C_{24}H_{36}O_5$ and a molecular weight of 404.55. Its structural formula is displayed in Figure 1. It is insoluble in water, sparingly soluble in ethanol, soluble in acetone, dimethylformamide, and methanol, and is freely soluble in chloroform.

The first compound with sterol-synthesis-inhibiting properties from the *A. terreus* strain, compactin, was isolated by Endo and associates in Tokyo in 1976.[12] Lovastatin was isolated by Alberts and colleagues at Merck Sharp & Dohme from a different mold in 1979.[13] Lovastatin differs from compactin by a methyl group in the 3 position and is often referred to as 3-methyl compactin.

Lovastatin is a prodrug existing in an inactive lactone form. On administration, it is hydrolyzed to the active hydroxyacid form L-154,819 (Figure 1).

Pharmacology

Lovastatin exerts its cholesterol-lowering effect indirectly by inhibiting HMG CoA reductase, the enzyme responsible for the rate-limiting conversion of acetyl CoA to mevalonate. To understand this mechanism and the implications it has in the treatment of hypercholesterolemia, it is important to first understand cholesterol transport and biosynthesis. These processes are summarized below.

Several excellent reviews that offer a more complete description of lipid physiology and the pathogenesis of atherosclerosis have been published recently.[14–17]

Cholesterol Transport. Cholesterol is an essential component of cell membranes and supports hormone synthesis in the adrenal gland and gonads. All cells have the capacity to synthesize cholesterol; cellular synthesis accounts for 60 to 80% of the cholesterol found in the plasma. The remaining 20 to 40% is mostly derived from the diet.[18,19]

The general process of cholesterol transport in the body is shown in Figure 2. Cholesterol and triglycerides from the diet are incorporated into chylomicron particles in the intestine and enter the body via the exogenous pathway. Some of the triglycerides are removed from the chylomicron particle by lipoprotein lipase in the capillaries of adipose tissue. The remaining particle, the chylomicron remnant, is taken up by special receptors on the hepatic cell.

The cholesterol deposited in the hepatic cell may be degraded into bile acids and secreted into the intestine through enterohepatic circulation. Some of the cholesterol combines with triglycerides from endogenous sources to form very-low-density lipoprotein (VLDL) particles in the liver, which are secreted into the circulation. Triglycerides are removed from the core of the VLDL particle through the action of lipoprotein lipase to form first intermediate-density lipoproteins (IDLs) and then smaller, cholesterol-rich low-density lipoproteins (LDLs). LDL is the major lipoprotein transporting cholesterol in plasma. It is also the lipoprotein that is most strongly associated with the development of atherosclerosis.[21]

LDL particles are removed from the plasma via LDL receptors on hepatic and extrahepatic cells.[22,23] The liver, adrenal gland, and ovaries have the highest concentration of LDL receptors and thus take up and degrade the largest amount of cholesterol (up to 75%).[23] These receptors were recently described by Brown and Goldstein,[18] who received the Nobel prize for their work. The number of these receptors and their affinity for the LDL particle determine how much LDL cholesterol will remain in the circulation. The longer LDL particles remain in the circulation, the more likely they will become involved in the atherosclerotic process.

Two patient groups with genetically determined hypercholesterolemia help illustrate the importance of LDL receptors. Patients with heterozygous familial hypercholesterolemia have half the normal number of these receptors and as a consequence have serum cholesterol concentrations in the range of 300 to 500 mg/dL and develop premature coronary heart disease.[15] Patients with homozygous familial hypercholesterolemia have none (or very few) of these receptors and consequently develop cholesterol concentrations well above 600 mg/dL and rarely survive their 20th birthday.[15]

High-density-lipoprotein (HDL) particles provide a major mechanism for removing cholesterol from peripheral cells.[22] This so-called "good cholesterol" delivers cholesterol esters to hepatic cells, where they are removed, degraded into bile acids, and secreted into the intestine. The HDL level is inversely related to the incidence of CHD.[21]

Cholesterol Biosynthesis and LDL Receptors. Once the LDL particle is trapped in the cell through endocytosis, it is transported to the lysosome, where the cholesterol ester is hydrolyzed to cholesterol. This pool of cholesterol combines with any endogenous cholesterol and controls a number of enzyme systems that, in turn, determine the level of cholesterol in the plasma. As depicted in

Figure 2. The exogenous and endogenous cholesterol transport pathways. HDL = high-density lipoprotein; LDL = low-density lipoprotein; IDL = intermediate-density lipoprotein; LCAT = lecithin–cholesterol acyltransferase; E, C, B-48, and B-100 = apolipoproteins. Reprinted with permission from reference 20.

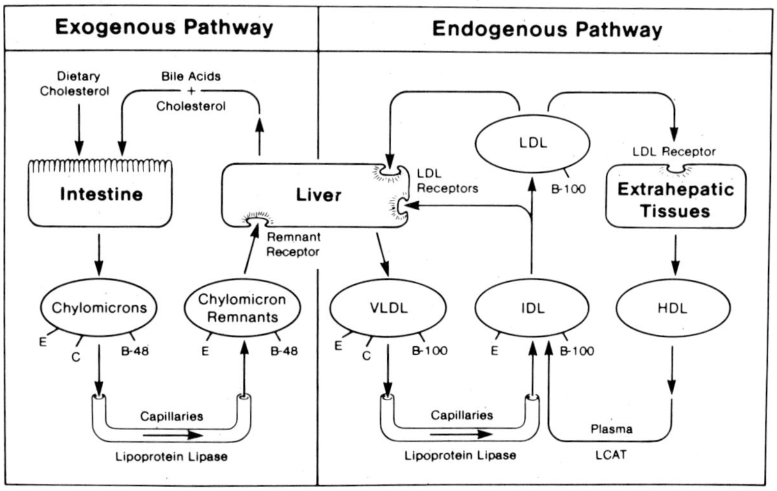

Figure 3. Low-density-lipoprotein (LDL) cholesterol catabolism by nonhepatic tissues. HMG CoA = 3-hydroxy-3-methylglutaryl-coenzyme A; CE = cholesteryl esters. Reprinted with permission from reference 24.

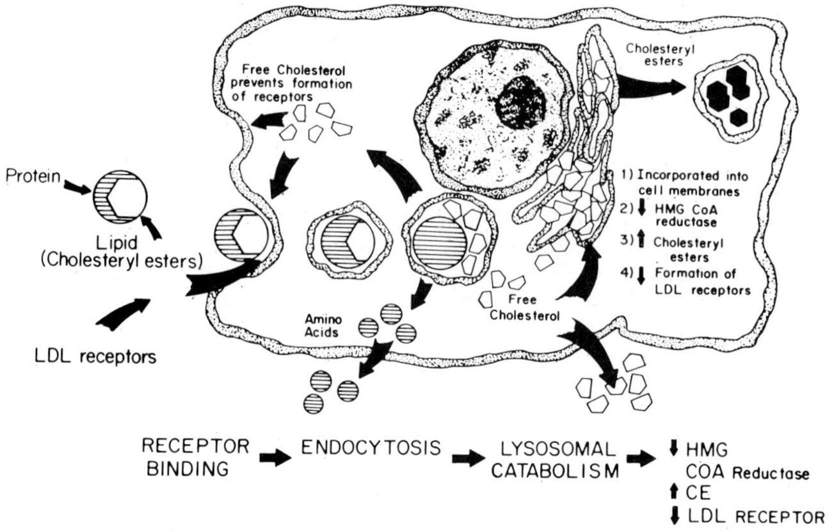

Figure 3, rising levels of cholesterol in the pool inhibit the synthesis of new LDL receptors, thus reducing the uptake of LDL into the cell and increasing the level of circulating cholesterol. An increase in this pool also inhibits the in vivo synthesis of cholesterol by decreasing the activity of HMG CoA reductase. The pool also activates acylcholesterol acyltransferase, which increases the esterification of free cholesterol for storage in the cell.

Proposed Mechanism of Action of Lovastatin. Lovastatin inhibits HMG CoA reductase, which is responsible for the conversion of 3-hydroxy-3-methylglutaryl coenzyme A (HMG CoA) to mevalonate, a precursor of several sterols, including cholesterol (Figure 4).[12,18] HMG CoA can readily be metabolized back to acetyl CoA, which is the precursor of other compounds in the body. Thus, accumulation of toxic intermediates would not be anticipated. The inhibition of HMG CoA reductase by lovastatin is competitive and incomplete, thus allowing for biologically necessary amounts of mevalonate to be available for cholesterol synthesis.[13,25] Thus, adverse reactions caused by loss of cholesterol for steroidogenesis and cell-membrane formation would not be anticipated. However, because in vivo synthesis is responsible for 60 to 80% of the cholesterol pool, lovastatin has the potential to profoundly reduce cholesterol levels, much more so than alterations in the fat content of the diet.

The inhibition of cholesterol biosynthesis reduces the cholesterol pool in hepatic and peripheral cells, which stimulates the synthesis of LDL receptors and thereby increases the uptake of LDL particles. The ultimate result of these mechanisms is a reduction of the plasma cholesterol concentration. Some of the studies that help confirm these mechanisms are reviewed below.

Figure 4. The biosynthetic pathway of cholesterol. Acetyl CoA = acetyl coenzyme A; HMG CoA = 3-hydroxy-3-methylglutaryl coenzyme A.

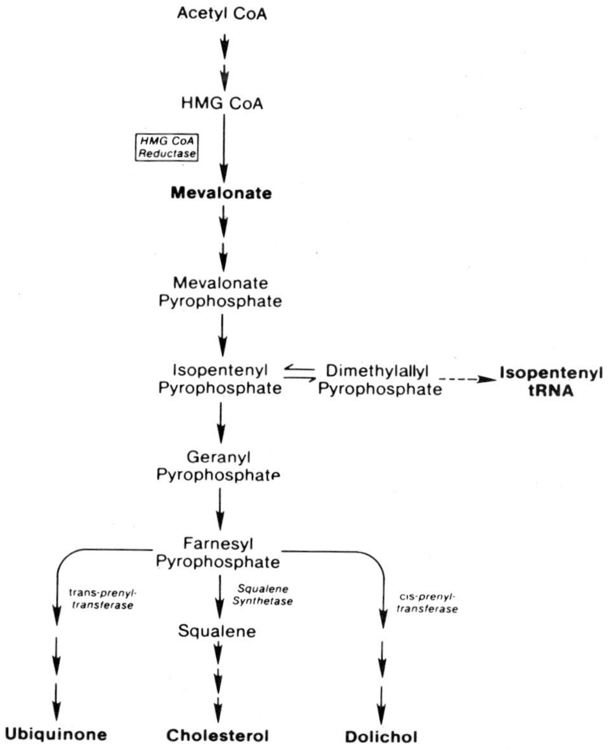

Effect on Cholesterol Biosynthesis. Inhibition of the synthesis of cholesterol by lovastatin has been demonstrated in vitro in a variety of cell types.[26,27] Experiments with liver cells from rats[13] and mononuclear leukocytes from patients with familial hypercholesterolemia[28] that had been incubated with acetate labeled with radioactive carbon (^{14}C) and lovastatin have shown significantly less output of ^{14}C-labeled cholesterol. The percentage of inhibition of cholesterol synthesis increases as the lovastatin concentration increases but never reaches 100%, in part because additional reductase enzyme is synthesized to compete with it. When tissue cells were incubated in vitro with mevalonate labeled with radioactive hydrogen (^{3}H)—mevalonate is a product of the HMG CoA reductase reaction—and lovastatin, cholesterol synthesis was not altered. These studies demonstrate that lovastatin inhibits the conversion of HMG CoA to mevalonate without interfering with the subsequent steps in the biosynthesis of cholesterol (Figure 4).

The reduction in mevalonate and cholesterol produced by lovastatin apparently stimulates the synthesis of HMG CoA reductase.[25] Studies of leukocytes from patients with familial hypercholesterolemia demonstrate that HMG CoA reductase activity is increased 40 to 50% in the presence of lovastatin.[28] This enzyme induction is blunted by an increase in dietary cholesterol, and in rats enzyme induction can be suppressed with the administration of mevalonate.[25] The induction of HMG CoA reductase activity disappears within two days of discontinuing lovastatin as levels of mevalonate and cholesterol, which are potent regulators of the enzyme's activity, increase.[29] Since lovastatin is a competitive inhibitor of HMG CoA reductase, increased synthesis of the enzyme may modulate the inhibition of cholesterol synthesis with lovastatin. Further investigation is needed to determine whether these relationships can be extrapolated to humans.

Plasma concentrations of mevalonic acid between 0700 and 0900 and mean 24-hour urinary concentrations of mevalonic acid have been shown to correlate with the rate of whole body cholesterol synthesis.[30] This has made it possible to evaluate the effect of lovastatin on cholesterol synthesis in humans without the introduction of isotopes. In these studies, the plasma mevalonic acid concentration decreased by 78% for up to six hours after administration of a single 100- or 200-mg dose of lovastatin.[31] The maximum inhibition was seen four to six hours after the dose; less than half of the inhibition was evident 24 hours after dosing. When lovastatin doses of 6.25, 12.5, 25, and 50 mg were administered orally twice daily for four weeks to eight healthy adult male volunteers, a dose-related reduction in the urinary mevalonic acid concentration at 24 hours was demonstrated. The lowest dose produced 80% of the reduction of the plasma LDL concentration seen with the highest dose, suggesting a flat dose–response relationship in healthy subjects.

Effect on LDL Receptors. Lovastatin probably exerts its effect on plasma cholesterol ultimately by increasing the number of LDL receptors. When the pool of cholesterol in the cell is reduced because the synthesis of cholesterol is inhibited by lovastatin, the number of LDL receptors available for binding with circulating LDL cholesterol particles increases.[32] This results in a fall in plasma cholesterol levels.

Several investigators have shown that LDL receptor activity is increased in human tissue cells cultured with acetate labeled with radioactive carbon (^{14}C) in the presence of lovastatin.[28,33] The intensity of this effect apparently abates after several days under these in vitro conditions, suggesting that the initial effect on LDL receptors may not be sustained.

These observations have been extended to humans with heterozygous familial hypercholesterolemia.[34] Six patients with heterozygous familial hypercholesterolemia were given LDL labeled with radioactive iodine (^{131}I) intravenously before and during treatment with lovastatin. After lovastatin administration, LDL levels declined 27%, and the fractional catabolic rate for LDL (taken as a measure of the number of LDL receptors) increased 37%.

When this study was repeated in patients with nonfamilial (polygenic) hypercholesterolemia, LDL levels were reduced 20 to 31%, but the fractional catabolic rate was only minimally increased.[35] This suggests that lovastatin does not appreciably increase the number of LDL receptors in these patients. The reason for this finding is not obvious. Perhaps the fractional catabolic rate is an insensitive measure of the number of receptors. Patients with nonfamilial hypercholesterolemia may not have a deficiency of LDL receptors, as seen in patients with familial hypercholesterolemia[32]; instead, they may have LDL receptors that are saturated with LDL cholesterol and are unable to increase the rate of LDL clearance beyond a certain point.[22] In these patients, lovastatin may not appreciably increase the number of receptors but may act in other, as yet undefined, ways. It has also been proposed that lovastatin may enhance the binding of the apolipoprotein B protein on VLDL remnants with the LDL receptor and so may preferentially promote the removal of VLDL particles from the plasma.[36] This would leave fewer VLDL particles for conversion to LDL and thereby result in a drop in plasma LDL cholesterol concentrations. Further study of these and other proposed mechanisms is required.

Effect on Tissue Lipids. One of the concerns with drugs that inhibit cholesterol synthesis is that levels of cholesterol and other essential sterols might be reduced so much that synthesis of the cell membrane and production of hormones by the adrenal gland would be seriously impaired. In a series of experiments carried out by the manufacturer, the cholesterol content of various tissues from rats and dogs treated with lovastatin was determined.[a] The result was that "no tissue examined showed any decrease in this essential membrane component. This included liver, brain, testis, ovary, mesenteric lymph node, and lens."[37] The cholesterol content in liver cells of dogs was unchanged; ubiquinone levels were decreased. No abnormal sterols were seen. In rats, there was a 14% decrease in cholesterol content in stomach tissue; the cholesterol content of other tissues was unchanged by lovastatin therapy.

Grundy and Bilheimer[37] extended these evaluations to humans. They compared the fecal excretion of neutral and acidic steroids in five heterozygous familial hypercholesterolemia patients taking lovastatin 40 mg orally daily for 20 to 40 days with steroid excretion during placebo therapy. They found modest reductions in these steroids, but levels were never below values seen in healthy subjects. They concluded that lovastatin did not appear to cause total body depletion of vital stores of cholesterol.

Effect on Atherosclerosis. A beneficial effect of lovastatin-induced cholesterol lowering on atherosclerotic plaque formation is assumed but has not been demonstrated. If reducing the plasma cholesterol concentration is the determining factor in plaque regression, lovastatin should be effective. The 24% reduction in LDL cholesterol achieved by Blankenhorn et al.[9] with diet, cholestyramine, and niacin produced plaque regression; this effect should be achievable with lovastatin monotherapy. Studies evaluating the efficacy of lovastatin on the development of atherosclerosis have already begun, and results should be available about 1990.

Animal studies have demonstrated a reduction of atherosclerosis with lovastatin. Kritchevsky et al.[38] evaluated two groups of eight rabbits each that were fed an atherogenic diet; one group was treated with oral lovastatin. Results showed significantly lower cholesterol levels and less severe atherosclerosis in the lovastatin-treated group. Whether this suggests a similar benefit in humans is not known. Further studies, especially in humans, are needed.

Pharmacokinetics

Most of the pharmacokinetic data available for lovastatin are derived from studies conducted by the manufacturer. These studies used a reverse isotope dilution method that measured the ^{14}C-labeled parent drug lovastatin and the active metabolite L-154,819[a] and an HMG CoA enzyme inhibition assay that measured lovastatin equivalents (as hydroxyacids) in the general circulation.[39] A high-performance liquid chromatographic assay for lovastatin has been described recently.[40]

When ^{14}C-labeled lovastatin is administered orally to humans, less than 5% of the labeled dose is available to the general circulation as active inhibitors.[a] Approximately 30% of a dose is absorbed, but most of it is extracted on first pass through the liver.

Lovastatin is a prodrug and exists in an inactive lactone form when administered to humans (Figure 1). The drug undergoes rapid conversion to its principal active metabolite, a β-hydroxyacid form, L-154,819.[a] Lovastatin may be further metabolized to active and inactive metabolites. The principal phase 1 biotransformations involve hydroxylation and dehydrogenation. In humans, three other lactone–hydroxyacid metabolite pairs have been identified; all of the hydroxyacid metabolites have HMG CoA reductase inhibitory activity. Currently identified metabolites account for 80% of the total HMG CoA reductase inhibitory activity detected in the plasma after a dose.

Peak levels of the drug based on the enzyme-inhibition assay occur approximately three to four hours after a single oral dose; the drug is still detectable 24 hours after a single dose.[a] Area under the concentration–time curve (AUC) and maximum concentration (C_{max}) increase proportionally with the dose, suggesting linear pharmacokinetics (Table 1). After two to three once-daily doses, enzyme inhibition increases to a steady-state level of activity that is approximately 50% greater than that seen with a single dose.

The major active metabolite is cleared rapidly. Total body clearance was reported to be between 300 and 1250 mL/min in four patients. Elimination half-lives were between 1.1 and 1.7 hours.

Food appears to increase the bioavailability of lovastatin approximately 50% based on area under the concentration–time curve measurements of active metabolites. Since the drug was administered with food during its premarketing clinical trials without sequelae, it is recommended that doses be taken with the evening meal.

Lovastatin and the principal active metabolite are highly bound to plasma proteins in humans.[a]

Table 1.
Lovastatin Pharmacokinetics in Healthy Volunteers[a]

Dose	C_{max} (ng equivalents/mL)	t_{max} (hr)	AUC_{0-24} (ng equivalents · hr/mL)
Single Oral Dose in mg (n = 12)			
60	24.6 ± 24.5	4.1 ± 2.2	135 ± 118
90	26.4 ± 24.8	3.0 ± 1.1	227 ± 231
120	39.4 ± 37.1	3.5 ± 1.9	291 ± 279
60, with food	46.7 ± 31.0	2.6 ± 1.0	233 ± 180
Multiple Oral Doses of 80 mg Once Daily (n = 10)			
Initial dose	17.6 ± 15.0	2.4 ± 1.0	126 ± 81
Seventh dose	26.2 ± 17.7	2.2 ± 0.8	216 ± 161

[a] Values given as mean ± S.D. C_{max} = maximum concentration, t_{max} = time to maximum concentration, AUC = area under the concentration–time curve from time zero to 24 hours.

The average unbound fraction is 1.6% for lovastatin and 4.3% for L-154,819. Saturation of these binding sites has not been detected with concentrations attained with the usual therapeutic doses of the drug.

The drug is primarily eliminated via biliary excretion.[a] Up to 83% of an oral ^{14}C-labeled dose of lovastatin may be recovered in feces; less than 10% is found in the urine.

Lovastatin has not been evaluated in patients with liver or kidney disease.

Studies in Healthy Volunteers

The results of studies evaluating the efficacy of lovastatin are shown in Table 2. Initial Phase II evaluations in healthy subjects demonstrated that lovastatin produces substantial reductions in plasma lipoproteins.[41,42] Total and LDL cholesterol levels were reduced by approximately 35%, even with the smallest dose (6.25 mg orally twice daily). The difference between the response to the smallest dose and the largest dose (50 mg orally twice daily) was not significant. This response to small doses and the flat dose–response relationship later proved to be specific for healthy subjects; patients with primary hypercholesterolemia required slightly higher doses for a similar cholesterol reduction and demonstrated a clearer dose–response relationship.

The reduction in cholesterol levels was evident in these studies in healthy volunteers after the

Table 2.
Results of Lovastatin Efficacy Trials

Study	No. Subjects	Study Design	Drug[a] and Dose	Percentage Change in Lipid Concentration[b] TC	LDL-C	HDL-C	TG
Healthy Volunteers							
Tobert et al.[41]	24	Placebo run-in, randomized, placebo controlled, double-blind, seven-day treatment period	P	−4			
			L 5 mg b.i.d.	−14			
			L 15 mg b.i.d.	−25			
			L 50 mg b.i.d.	−24			
Tobert et al.[42]	59	Placebo run-in, randomized, placebo controlled, double-blind, 28-day treatment period	P		−3		
			L 6.25 mg b.i.d.		−35		
			L 12.5 mg b.i.d.		−35		
			L 25 mg b.i.d.		−38		
			L 50 mg b.i.d.		−45		
			L 25 mg each morning		−25		
Patients with Familial Hypercholesterolemia (FH)							
Illingworth and Sextron[43]	13	Drug-free run-in, open-label, sequential dose assignment, 42-day treatment period	L 5 mg b.i.d.	−17	−20	−8	−6
			L 10 mg b.i.d.	−24	−28	+2	−11
			L 20 mg b.i.d.	−30	−35	0	−31
			L 40 mg b.i.d.	−33	−38	+2	−34
Havel et al.[45]	100	Placebo run-in, randomized, placebo controlled, double-blind, multicenter, 42-day treatment period	P	−2	−2	0	+7
			L 5 mg b.i.d.	−15	−20	+18	+5
			L 10 mg b.i.d.	−23	−29	+8	−8
			L 20 mg b.i.d.	−27	−33	+12	−17
			L 40 mg b.i.d.	−34	−42	+8	−15
Patients with Nonfamilial (Polygenic) Hypercholesterolemia (NonFH)							
Hoeg et al.[46]	18 NonFH, 6 FH	Diet run-in, randomized, crossover, placebo controlled, double-blind, 30-day treatment period	P	−7	−5	−8	−22
			L 20 mg b.i.d.	−29	−34	+6	−36
Tikkanen et al.[47]	40 NonFH and FH patients	Unknown	NonFH: L 40 mg/day		−39	+18	
			L80 mg/day		−42	+16	
			FH: L 40 mg/day		−30	+18	
			L 80 mg/day		−40	+11	
Lovastatin Study Group[49]	100	Placebo run-in, randomized, placebo controlled, double-blind, multicenter, three consecutive six-week treatment periods	P	+5	+9	+1	−3
			L 5 mg b.i.d.	−21	−25	+6	−19
			L 10 mg b.i.d.	−18	−24	+4	−15
			L 20 mg b.i.d.	−29	−34	+11	−23
			L 40 mg b.i.d.	−32	−39	+13	−27
Patients with Homozygous Familial Hypercholesterolemia							
Uauy et al.[44]	3	Open label	L 2 mg/kg/day	−5	−2	−19	−4
Patients with Combined Hypercholesterolemia and Hypertriglyceridemia							
East et al.[48]	8	Diet run-in, open-label, assignment to two treatment groups for eight weeks each, crossover	G 600 mg b.i.d.+ Col 10 g b.i.d.	−16	−12	+21	−40
			G 600 mg b.i.d.+ L 20 mg b.i.d.	−27	−21	+35	−57

[a] P = placebo, L = lovastatin, G = gemfibrozil, Col = colestipol hydrochloride. All drugs were administered orally.

[b] TC = total cholesterol, LDL-C = low-density-lipoprotein cholesterol, HDL-C = high-density-lipoprotein cholesterol, TG = triglyceride.

third day of therapy and reached a plateau after 14 days of therapy. The single daily dose was inferior to all of the twice-daily regimens (Table 2).

The effects of lovastatin on HDL and VLDL cholesterol in these studies of healthy volunteers were not clinically important. Plasma cortisol and testosterone concentrations and urinary 17-hydroxy and 17-keto steroid levels were not significantly altered with lovastatin therapy.

Effectiveness in Familial Hypercholesterolemia

Heterozygous Familial Hypercholesterolemia. Patients with heterozygous familial hypercholesterolemia (FH) characteristically have very high cholesterol concentrations (usually in the upper 10th percentile for age and sex), may have tendon xanthomas, and have a family history of CHD consistent with an autosomal dominant inheritance pattern. Heterozygous FH is estimated to affect 1 out of 500 people in the general population and frequently causes those afflicted to have serious CHD by their 50th birthday. The basis of their disease is the presence of only one gene for LDL receptors and thus only half the number of receptors to clear LDL cholesterol particles from the plasma. Since inhibition of cholesterol synthesis within the cell would be expected to increase the number of LDL receptors,[18] therapy with lovastatin is ideally suited for these patients.

Studies indicate that lovastatin is effective in heterozygous FH patients.[43,45] As illustrated in Table 2, total and LDL cholesterol levels can be reduced profoundly with lovastatin in a dose-dependent fashion. These changes were sustained for 12 or more weeks. Each of the patients in the study by Illingworth and Sextron[43] had a reduction in LDL levels with sequential increases in lovastatin doses, but there was considerable variation in the magnitude of the individual patient response. For example, the reduction in LDL levels ranged from approximately 20% to more than 50% from baseline with the maximum 80-mg daily lovastatin dose.

Changes in HDL and triglyceride levels were equally variable but tended to move in the direction of increases in HDL and decreases in triglyceride levels, especially with higher doses of lovastatin. Apolipoprotein levels were not reported.

Homozygous Familial Hypercholesterolemia. Patients with homozygous FH lack both genes for LDL receptors and thus are unable to clear LDL cholesterol from their plasma.[14] Therapy with drugs that depend on stimulation of LDL receptor synthesis should not be very effective in these patients.

Uauy et al.[44] studied three children with homozygous FH who were given 2 mg/kg/day of lovastatin and who experienced virtually no change in lipoprotein levels (see Table 2). The change in the fractional clearance of LDL from baseline to after initiation of lovastatin therapy was not significant, indicating no change in the number of LDL receptors.

East et al.[50] recently described a child with homozygous FH who underwent a liver transplant and had a subsequent 81% reduction in LDL levels. Because the child's lipoprotein levels were still significantly elevated, therapy with 10 mg of lovastatin twice daily was initiated, which resulted in an additional 49% reduction in the LDL level, to values in the normal range.

Effectiveness in Nonfamilial (Polygenic) Hypercholesterolemia

Patients with nonfamilial (polygenic) hypercholesterolemia (nonFH) are the largest group requiring management of high blood cholesterol concentrations. Based on a National Institutes of Health Consensus Statement, 25% of Americans have an elevated serum cholesterol concentration requiring management.[51] A small number of these patients will have heterozygous FH[28]; a rare patient may have homozygous FH. The majority will have polygenic hypercholesterolemia. These patients are thought to have elevated cholesterol levels because of two major factors—diet and heredity.[22] Because of the very high saturated-fat diet of our Western society, the LDL receptor mechanisms for removing cholesterol from the plasma are thought to be saturated, and their synthesis is thought to be suppressed. However, since cholesterol levels do not rise equally in all patients with the same dietary indiscretions, genetic factors are thought to play a part, thus the term polygenic hypercholesterolemia. Most nonFH patients will be adequately managed with a low-saturated-fat diet. However, approximately one third of these patients or 10 million Americans will require drug therapy in addition to their diet for control. Lovastatin is an alternative to conventional lipid-lowering drug therapy in these patients.

The results of studies evaluating the efficacy of lovastatin in nonFH and FH patients are summarized in Table 2. These results indicate that lovastatin is effective in these patients.[46,47,49]

Lovastatin has been shown to produce a dose-dependent reduction in total and LDL cholesterol levels with daily oral doses of 10 to 80 mg.[46,47,49] The reductions found over this dosage range for total and LDL cholesterol levels ranged from 21 and 25%, respectively, with the lowest dose to 32 and 39%, respectively, with the highest dose. The multicenter trial found that the magnitude of the reduction in the plasma cholesterol concentration with the smallest dose (25%) was proportionately greater than that achieved with the largest dose (39%).[49] With respect to treating patients, this suggests that it would be best to initiate therapy with the lowest dose and slowly titrate doses upward as needed.

Lovastatin was reported to have increased HDL cholesterol levels approximately 5 to 10% in these studies.[46,47,49] However, the increase in HDL failed to achieve significance in the large multicenter trial, probably because of the large variance in the data.[49] Hoeg et al.[46] reported that 16 of the 18 nonFH patients in their study had an increase in the plasma HDL concentration. Some of these patients had substantial increases (up to 23%); others had little change. Tikkanen et al.[47] found that the increase in HDL in a subgroup of their study patients was due to a selective increase in the HDL_2 fraction without any change in the HDL_3 fraction. Since HDL_2 is thought to be more antiatherogenic than HDL_3,[52] this finding may have important implications if confirmed in other studies.

The reductions in triglycerides and VLDL with lovastatin in these trials were similar to the reduction found in LDL.[46,47,49] Reductions ranged from a low of 15% and 2% to a high of 36% and 41% in triglycerides and VLDL, respectively. The dose–response relationship with these changes was less obvious than that found for LDL reductions. These results suggest that lovastatin may be useful in treating not only primary hypercholesterolemia but also combined hypercholesterolemia and hypertriglyceridemia.

Lovastatin has also been found to substantially reduce apolipoprotein B levels.[35,46,49] Since each LDL particle contains one molecule of apolipoprotein B,[53] lovastatin apparently reduces apolipoprotein B levels by reducing the overall concentration of LDL particles. Some investigators believe that apolipoprotein B levels are strongly correlated with CHD risk.[54] Levels of the major apolipoproteins carried by HDL, apolipoprotein AI and apolipoprotein AII, are slightly increased with lovastatin therapy.[46,49]

These data also show that lovastatin produces maximal to near-maximal response to a given dose after two to four weeks of therapy. Response to a dose administered for at least 18 weeks is very consistent. For example, twice-daily oral doses of 20 mg produced reductions in LDL levels of 34, 38, and 34% at the end of three successive six-week treatment periods.

When therapy with lovastatin is rapidly withdrawn, cholesterol levels quickly return to pretreatment levels. There appears to be no rebound phenomenon. This quick reversal of effect may be due to the induction by lovastatin of the HMG CoA reductase enzyme, which rapidly activates synthesis of cholesterol upon withdrawal of the inhibiting drug.

These data also demonstrate that dose increases and decreases lead to the establishment of a new response plateau. Thus, reduction of a dose after initial therapy should not be accompanied by a carryover effect. A dose reduction as may be seen with noncompliance would lead to a new, lower level of control.

Effectiveness in Familial Combined Hyperlipidemia

One of the most prevalent genetic forms of dyslipidemia is familial combined hyperlipidemia, which may be manifested by increased levels of both triglycerides and cholesterol.[55,56] These patients can often be treated with diet alone, but some will require drug therapy, most commonly with nicotinic acid or fibric acid derivatives.[57,58] Because lovastatin substantially reduces plasma cholesterol and triglyceride levels, it may also be effective in the treatment of these patients when used alone or in combination with other lipid-lowering agents.

Only one study has evaluated lovastatin in patients with familial combined hyperlipidemia.[48] As presented in Table 2, East et al.[50] evaluated the combinations of gemfibrozil, a fibric acid derivative with predominate triglyceride-lowering effect, plus colestipol, an anion-exchange resin, and gemfibrozil plus lovastatin each for eight weeks in eight patients with this lipid disorder. Both regimens substantially reduced lipid levels. The reduction in cholesterol and triglyceride levels with the lovastatin–gemfibrozil combination (27% and 57%, respectively) was superior to the reduction achieved with the gemfibrozil–colestipol combination (16% and 40%, respectively). However, the small sample size limits the conclusions that can be drawn from these data.

Unfortunately, the incidence of myositis may be higher in patients receiving lovastatin in combination with gemfibrozil (see section on adverse reactions).

Effectiveness in Other Patient Groups

One of the methods of treating severe FH has been distal ileal bypass surgery, in which the section of the bowel primarily responsible for bile acid reabsorption is removed. This enhances the fecal excretion of bile acids, increases the conversion of bile acids in the liver, increases the number of LDL receptors on hepatic cells, and reduces the plasma LDL concentration. Illingworth and Connor[59] describe a patient who continued to have seriously high cholesterol levels after this procedure. When this patient was treated with 40 to 80 mg of lovastatin orally daily, the LDL cholesterol concentration was reduced 43 to 49% and the HDL cholesterol concentration was increased 32 to 61%. These changes were maintained for six months without adverse biochemical changes.

Nephrotic syndrome is frequently associated with difficult-to-treat hypercholesterolemia and coronary heart disease. Vega and Grundy[60] tried lovastatin 20 mg orally twice daily for one month in three patients with nephrotic syndrome. Total cholesterol concentrations were reduced an average of 32%. In two of the patients, LDL cholesterol concentrations were reduced an average of 50%. In the third patient, the LDL concentration was reduced only 18%, but the triglyceride concentration was reduced 53% and the HDL concentration was increased 92%.

Use Alone and in Combination with Other Lipid-Lowering Drugs

Decisions to treat patients with lovastatin should be based on, among other things, its comparative efficacy alone and in combination with other lipid-lowering drugs. The information currently available on these comparisons is summarized in Table 3.

Combining lovastatin with a resin increases the reduction in total and LDL cholesterol concentrations 15 to 25% compared with the reduction achieved with lovastatin alone.[61–63] This additive cholesterol-lowering effect also occurs when lovastatin is combined with niacin and, to a lesser extent, with probucol.[63]

The effects on lipoproteins with these combinations are strongly influenced by the lipoprotein effects of the individual agents being added to lovastatin. For example, when used alone, resins substantially reduce LDL levels, modestly increase HDL levels, and often raise triglyceride levels.[56] Illingworth[61] reported that when resins are administered with lovastatin, the LDL concentration is reduced an additional 13%, HDL levels are minimally increased, and the reduction in triglyceride levels achieved with lovastatin alone is substantially blunted. When probucol is administered with lovastatin, Lees et al.[63] reported that the LDL concentration is reduced an additional 8%, the HDL concentration is reduced a substantial 33%, and triglyceride levels are minimally increased. These authors also reported that niacin in combination with lovastatin produced the most desirable lipoprotein changes—lowering of total and LDL cholesterol levels, lowering of triglyceride levels, and elevation of HDL cholesterol levels.[63] Hoeg et al.[64] reported that neomycin in combination with lovastatin provides modest, clinically unimportant additional effects on lipoproteins.

When used alone, lovastatin appears to lower plasma cholesterol levels more than cholestyramine,[65] probucol,[65] and neomycin[64] (Table 3). Based on dose–reponse data, at least 90% of patients treated with either bile acid sequestrants, nicotinic acid, or lovastatin can achieve a sustained reduction in total and LDL cholesterol concentrations of

Table 3.
Results of Trials Using Lovastatin Alone and in Combination with Other Lipid-Lowering Agents

Study	No. Subjects[a]	Study Design	Drug[b] and Dose	Percentage Change in Lipid Concentration[c]			
				TC	LDL-C	HDL-C	TG
Studies with Resins							
Illingworth[61]	12 FH	Three-week diet lead-in, open-label, sequential drug assignment: L for five to nine weeks then L + Col for six to nine weeks	L 40 mg b.i.d.	−33	−38		−25
			L + Col 20 g/day	−45	−64		+6
Grundy et al.[62]	10 FH	Drug-free lead-in, open-label, combination therapy for five to six weeks	L 20 mg b.i.d. + Col 10 g/day	−43	−52	+29	−1
Lees et al.[63]	30 FH	Open-label	L	−30	−38	0	−26
			L + R	−47	−56	0	−5
			L	−32	−37	−5	−26
			L + P	−40	−42	−36	−17
			L	−35	−41	−3	−17
			L + N	−47	−55	+8	−30
Merck Sharp & Dohme[65]	88 Mix	Diet lead-in, randomized, placebo controlled, L blinded, 12-week study	L 20 mg b.i.d.	−27	−32	+9	−21
			L 40 mg b.i.d.	−34	−42	+8	−21
			C 12 g b.i.d.	−17	−23	+8	+11
Studies with Probucol							
Merck Sharp & Dohme[65]	97 Mix	Diet lead-in, randomized, placebo controlled, L blinded, 14-week study	L 40 mg once daily	−25	−32	+9	−18
			L 80 mg once daily	−30	−37	+11	−17
			L 40 mg b.i.d.	−33	−40	+12	−25
			P 500 mg b.i.d.	−10	−8	−23	+1
Studies with Neomycin							
Hoeg et al.[64]	21 Mix	Three-month diet lead-in, open-label, sequential assignments: L for one month, Neo for two months, L + Neo for one month	L 20 mg b.i.d.	−24	−31	+15	−17
			Neo 1 g b.i.d.	−11	−10	−9	0
			L + Neo	−28	−34	−9	−10

[a] FH = familial hypercholesterolemia, Mix = some patients with familial hypercholesterolemia and some with nonfamilial hypercholesterolemia.

[b] L = lovastatin, Col = colestipol hydrochloride, Neo = neomycin sulfate, R = resin, P = probucol, N = niacin, C = cholestyramine. All drugs were administered orally.

[c] TC = total cholesterol, LDL-C = low-density-lipoprotein cholesterol, HDL-C = high-density-lipoprotein cholesterol, TG = triglycerides.

more than 10%.[66] Comparisons made among lovastatin and other therapies by the manufacturer during premarketing clinical trials suggest that resin therapy comes the closest to replicating the lipoprotein changes seen with lovastatin (i.e., reduced total and LDL cholesterol levels and raised HDL cholesterol levels), although the magnitude of these changes is less.[65] Presumably, the same is true for niacin, but a parallel comparison has not been made. Independent verification of these results is needed.

Dosage and Administration

Scheduling Doses. Studies have shown that plasma concentrations of mevalonic acid reflect the degree of cholesterol synthesis in humans.[30] Plasma mevalonic acid concentrations during a 24-hour period have a diurnal rhythm, with peak concentrations three to five times above the nadir occurring between 2400 and 0300. This suggests that cholesterol synthesis is greatest during these early morning hours and that administering a drug that inhibits cholesterol synthesis just before this period may show optimal effects. Studies evaluating the timing of lovastatin doses confirm this hypothesis.

Tobert et al.[42] reported that 25 mg of lovastatin administered orally every morning to 59 healthy volunteers produced a 25% reduction in LDL cholesterol concentrations, which was significant, but that this reduction was inferior to the 35% reduction achieved with lovastatin 12.5 mg orally twice daily. When studying different schedules for administering the same total daily dose of lovastatin in 12 patients with heterozygous FH, Illingworth[67] reported that total and LDL cholesterol concentrations were reduced 30% and 36%, respectively, on a twice-daily dosing schedule, 21% and 27%, respectively, with a once-every-morning dosing schedule, and 27% and 32%, respectively, with a once-every-evening dosing schedule. The large multicenter efficacy trial of lovastatin in nonFH patients showed a similar trend.[49] In the crossover evaluation, patients had a 21% reduction in LDL cholesterol concentrations with a dosage of 40 mg orally every evening and a 29% reduction with a dosage of 20 mg twice daily.[49] In the parallel group comparisons, LDL cholesterol concentrations were reduced 21 and 31% in the two groups receiving every-evening doses and 32 and 38% in the two other groups receiving lovastatin twice daily.[49]

These data demonstrate that evening dosing produces a clinically important reduction in LDL cholesterol levels that is superior to the reduction seen with morning dosing. However, these data also demonstrate that the evening dosing regimen is consistently, although minimally, inferior to the twice-daily regimen. To enhance compliance, it would be advisable to initiate therapy with every-evening dosing and to use the twice-daily dosing regimen to enhance the therapeutic effect in those patients who require it.

Dosing. Patient studies have demonstrated a clear relationship between 10- to 80-mg daily doses of lovastatin and the degree of reduction of total and LDL cholesterol levels.[41–43,45–47,49] The lowest dose (5 mg orally twice daily), for example, produces a substantial 20 to 25% reduction in LDL cholesterol concentrations; the highest dose (40 mg orally twice daily) reduces LDL cholesterol concentrations 38 to 42%.[43]

It is unfortunate that the product will be available only in 20-mg unscored tablets, since this negates the use of a 5- or 10-mg twice-daily regimen. Given this constraint, it would be advisable to initiate therapy with 20 mg orally every evening and to increase doses in 20-mg increments by adding tablets in the morning or evening. Since doses greater than 80 mg daily have not been evaluated, patients whose conditions are not controlled on this maximum dose should be considered for combination therapy with either a bile acid sequestrant or nicotinic acid. Dose changes may be made at monthly intervals.

Adverse Drug Reactions

One of the first drugs designed to alter cholesterol synthesis in humans, triparanol (MER 29), caused serious adverse reactions, including cataracts, accelerated atherosclerosis, and cutaneous adverse effects, and had to be withdrawn from clinical investigation.[68,69] These reactions were apparently related to triparanol's inhibition of late steps in cholesterol synthesis and the subsequent accumulation of desmosterol and other toxic sterol intermediates. Since lovastatin inhibits an early step in cholesterol synthesis and since inhibited substances may participate in other synthetic pathways in the body, accumulation of toxic products would not be expected with lovastatin.[12]

Most of the information on the adverse reactions associated with lovastatin comes from the clinical trials conducted by the manufacturer.[a,65] This information was collected on a total of 919 patients and healthy volunteers who received the drug in company-sponsored studies and 259 patients who received it from investigators who had their own investigational new drug license. The drug has been administered for up to four years to some of these patients.[70]

The adverse reactions reported in 613 patients receiving lovastatin, 88 patients receiving resin therapy, and 97 patients receiving probucol during controlled trials are listed in Table 4. Headache and gastrointestinal complaints were the most prevalent findings with lovastatin; gastrointestinal symptoms were more prevalent with resin therapy. Six of these 613 patients who received lovasta-

Table 4.
Percentage of Patients Having Adverse Drug Reactions to Lovastatin and Other Lipid-Lowering Agents during Clinical Trials

Reaction	Lovastatin (*n* = 613)	Placebo (*n* = 82)	Cholesty-ramine (*n* = 88)	Probucol (*n* = 97)
Gastrointestinal				
Constipation	4.9	...	34.1	2.1
Diarrhea	5.5	4.9	8.0	10.3
Dyspepsia	3.9	...	13.6	3.1
Flatus	6.4	2.4	21.6	2.1
Abdominal pain and cramps	5.7	2.4	5.7	5.2
Heartburn	1.6	...	8.0	...
Nausea	4.7	3.7	9.1	6.2
Musculoskeletal				
Muscle cramps	1.1	...	1.1	...
Myalgia	2.4	1.2	...	...
Nervous System				
Dizziness	2.0	1.2	...	1.0
Headache	9.3	4.9	4.5	8.2
Skin				
Rash and pruritus	5.2	...	4.5	...
Special Senses				
Blurred vision	1.5	...	1.0	6.2
Dysgeusia	0.8	...	1.1	...
Laboratory Tests[a]				
ALT increases	3.1	1.2	3.4	2.1
AST increases	2.1	1.2	2.3	2.1
CPK increases	11	...	9	2

[a] ALT = alanine aminotransferase (formerly called SGPT), AST = aspartate aminotransferase (formerly called SGOT), CPK = creatine phosphokinase.

tin during controlled clinical trials (1%) and 46 of the total 919 patients (5%) who received lovastatin alone or in combination experienced a serious nonfatal adverse event, including myocardial infarction and coronary-artery bypass surgery.[a] In addition, the investigator or study monitor considered single cases of peripheral neuropathy, hepatitis B, breast cancer, and seizure to be possibly related to the drug.

Three of the 613 patients receiving lovastatin alone during controlled trials discontinued therapy because of an adverse experience (0.5%).[65] An additional five patients receiving lovastatin in combination with other lipid-lowering drugs were withdrawn from therapy because of an adverse experience. The reactions precipitating these discontinuations were fatigue, diarrhea, nausea, hepatitis, insomnia, and rash.

Liver Dysfunction. The most common clinical laboratory abnormalities in the 613 patients who received lovastatin during controlled trials were increases in aspartate aminotransferase (AST, formerly called SGOT), alanine aminotransferase (ALT, formerly called SGPT), and creatine phosphokinase (CPK) (Table 4).[65] When all patients who received only lovastatin are considered, increases in ALT, AST, and CPK levels were seen in 7.3%, 5.9%, and 5.1% of patients, respectively. Approximately 1.9% of all who received the drug were withdrawn from it because aminotransferase concentrations increased above three times the upper limit of normal and persisted or spiked.[70] After cessation of therapy, elevations returned to pretreatment levels in all patients after several weeks. Rechallenge with lovastatin in some of these patients resulted in elevations in about half. Spikes occurred 3 to 15 months after therapy began. None of the patients developed jaundice or symptoms. Alkaline phosphatase levels remained normal in most patients, suggesting a hepatocellular, rather than a cholestatic, mechanism.[70] A biopsy in one patient showed mild focal hepatitis.[a]

Merck Sharp & Dohme recommends that liver-function studies be performed every four to six weeks during the first 15 months of therapy with lovastatin and periodically thereafter and that therapy be discontinued if aminotransferase levels rise above three times the upper limit of normal and are persistent. Moderate elevations may be transient but should prompt close monitoring and evaluation of patient symptoms. Patients who have liver disease or abuse alcohol should probably not be treated with lovastatin.

Lens Opacities. The relationship of lovastatin to lens opacities has received much attention during the drug's clinical evaluations. Part of the concern comes from the previous experience with triparanol.[69] In addition, the lens is rich in cholesterol, and inhibitors of its local synthesis in rats have resulted in cataract formation.[71]

Slit-lamp ophthalmologic examinations at baseline and at least once during treatment of 431 patients who received lovastatin for up to 18 months revealed that 34% had an opacity at baseline and 32% had one after therapy.[65,72] Thirty-four patients had lens opacities at the end of the study but not at the beginning, while 45 patients had lens opacities at the beginning but not at the end.[65] Whether these changes are related to lovastatin administration, other causes, or imprecise detection methodology is unknown. The opacities that were detected were predominately cortical. No patient who developed a new lens opacity experienced loss of visual acuity, and no patient was withdrawn from lovastatin therapy because of the opacity. Information on whether these opacities will progress with continued therapy and eventually result in symptoms is not available and will have to await the results of further ongoing studies.

Until more is known about the long-term nature of this finding, the manufacturer recommends baseline and annual slit-lamp examinations.[65]

Testicular Function. Testicular function is unaffected by lovastatin.[65] Semen volume and sperm concentration are not altered; sperm motility may be slightly decreased. Luteinizing hormone, follicle-stimulating hormone, serum testosterone, and prolactin concentrations all appear unaffected by lovastatin.

Adrenal Cortical Response. Since the biosynthesis of adrenal corticosteroids in humans depends on a supply of cholesterol, the possibility that inhibition of cholesterol biosynthesis could cause a deleterious effect has been evaluated. No adverse effects of lovastatin on corticotropin-stimulated plasma cortisol concentrations have been found.[73]

Myositis. Approximately 0.5% of patients receiving lovastatin therapy have been reported to develop myositis, characterized by symptoms of myalgias and very high CPK levels.[65] The incidence appears to be higher in patients given lovastatin with gemfibrozil (up to 5%) and in transplant patients receiving immunosuppressant therapy with cyclosporine and steroids (up to 30%).[a] The mechanism of this effect is not understood. Patients should be withdrawn from lovastatin therapy if symptoms of muscle tenderness and pain and elevated CPK levels occur. Until more is known regarding the effect of concomitant therapy, lovastatin should be used with caution in patients receiving gemfibrozil or immunosuppressant therapy.

Drug Interactions

The manufacturer has investigated several potential drug interactions with lovastatin.[a] Long-term administration of lovastatin compared with placebo did not alter the pharmacokinetics of antipyrine, suggesting that the metabolism of drugs by microsomal hepatic enzymes is not affected by lovastatin.[65] A single-dose study in 12 healthy volunteers showed no alteration in the pharmacokinetics of propranolol with concurrent administration of lovastatin.[a] A multidose placebo-controlled study in 12 hypercholesterolemic patients did not demonstrate a clinically important effect of lovastatin on plasma digoxin concentrations.[65] Four hypercholesterolemic patients experienced no change in response to long-term warfarin therapy when given sequentially increasing doses of lovastatin.[a]

Use in Pregnancy

There is no experience with the use of lovastatin in pregnancy. Because cholesterol is an important component in steroid synthesis and cell-wall formation, drugs that inhibit its synthesis could produce deleterious effects on fetal development. Toxicologic studies in rats with lovastatin doses greater than 500 times the maximum dose used in humans have revealed skeletal malformations in the offspring.[65] No fetal abnormalities were seen in rats and rabbits fed lower doses of lovastatin.

Because of the theoretical considerations and teratogenic effects seen in animal studies, lovastatin should not be given to pregnant or breast-feeding women. The drug may be given to a woman of childbearing potential so long as she is using a highly effective method of birth control and consents to the potential risk of therapy. Women who wish to become pregnant should be withdrawn from lovastatin therapy. They may be kept off of therapy for the duration of the pregnancy, since the risks of doing so are minimal and the teratogenic risks of other lipid-lowering drugs have not been carefully studied.

Use in Pediatrics

The safety and efficacy of lovastatin in pediatric patients has not been established. The drug has been given to children with homozygous FH without adverse reactions but also without important therapeutic effect.[44] Lovastatin was also given to a child with homozygous FH after liver transplantation to successfully control cholesterol levels.[49]

Because of the importance of cholesterol in steroid synthesis and cell-wall formation, lovastatin should not be used in children. In selected cases, when the hypercholesterolemia is threatening the child's life and the potential benefit of lovastatin outweighs the potential harm from adverse effects, lovastatin therapy may be justified.

Patient Education

Patients receiving lovastatin should understand the goals of therapy and follow the effects of lovastatin therapy on their cholesterol levels. Giving patients this opportunity will help reinforce the importance of compliance with prescribed doses to maintain long-term control.

Lovastatin-treated patients need instruction on scheduling doses. The rationale of dosing in the evening needs to be thoroughly explained so that the patient will be more attentive to this schedule. The patient also needs to know what to do if a dose is missed. In reality, occasional missed doses will probably make little difference. Frequent lapses in therapy could be important. To promote good compliance, it would be advisable to instruct patients to administer missed doses when they remember them.

Patients need to be warned about some of the potential adverse reactions associated with the drug. Since liver-function studies and ophthalmologic studies are to be obtained periodically during the initial phase of therapy, the patient needs to understand the nature of these adverse reactions. Patients should be encouraged to disclose any symptoms that are out of the ordinary, including muscle pain and tenderness, fever, malaise, and anorexia. Patients may also be advised to take lovastatin with food to increase bioavailability and possibly minimize gastrointestinal symptoms.

Monitoring Lovastatin Therapy

The therapeutic effects of lovastatin may be measured using either total or LDL cholesterol levels. Since LDL cholesterol is most strongly correlated with CHD risk,[4] a lipoprotein profile should be used to establish therapeutic response. However, because of the convenience and lower cost of determining total serum cholesterol concentrations, these values may be used for long-term monitoring.

According to the National Cholesterol Education Program's adult treatment panel, the minimum goal of therapy in hypercholesterolemic patients without coronary heart disease or risk factors for coronary heart disease is to reduce total cholesterol concentrations to less than 240 mg/dL and LDL concentrations to less than 160 mg/dL.[74] For patients with coronary heart disease or risk factors, the total cholesterol concentration should be reduced at least to less than 200 mg/dL, and the LDL concentration should be reduced to less than 130 mg/dL. These are minimum goals that may be exceeded. Lipid measurements may be made at the end of four weeks of continuous lovastatin therapy with a given dose and repeated at least once before the dose is adjusted. When two consecutive measurements indicate that the goal of therapy has been reached, repeat measurements every 6 to 12 months to establish long-term control are advisable.

Adverse reactions should be diligently monitored, especially during initial therapy. Careful review of symptoms to detect myositis, hepatitis, and other adverse reactions should be done at each follow-up visit. Liver-function tests should be evaluated during every follow-up visit for the first 15 months of therapy. CPK levels should also be determined at baseline and whenever symptoms of muscle pain or tenderness are present or periodically in patients at higher risk (for example, those on immunosuppressant therapy). Baseline and yearly slit-lamp evaluations by an ophthalmologist are also recommended.

Place of Lovastatin in the Treatment of Hypercholesterolemia

Diet is the primary treatment modality for hypercholesterolemia. The National Cholesterol Education Program recommends that drug therapy be initiated only if the phase 1 diet and the more restrictive phase 2 diet have failed to achieve the goal of therapy.[74] If the patient has been reasonably compliant with intensive dietary therapy for six months and cholesterol levels are still elevated, drug therapy may then be initiated.

Bile acid sequestrants and nicotinic acid are considered the drugs of first choice for the treatment of hypercholesterolemia by the National Cholesterol Education Program.[74] This is primarily because both drugs have been used in trials that demonstrated reduction in coronary heart disease and have a long-term safety profile.

Lovastatin should be used in patients who are unable to tolerate resin or nicotinic acid therapy or when these agents alone are unable to control the patient's cholesterol levels. As greater experience is gained with lovastatin, especially with its long-term effects on the liver and eyes and its effect on coronary heart disease, it could well become first-line therapy in the treatment of hypercholesterolemia.

Cost

Lovastatin is available as a 20-mg tablet in a unit-of-use bottle of 60 or unit dose packages of 100. The retail direct cost per 20-mg tablet is approximately $1.25. The total cost of therapy, however, with ophthalmologic evaluations, laboratory monitoring, and periodic physician evaluations will be considerably more than simply the cost of the drug.

Formulary Considerations

Lovastatin is recommended for addition to the formulary for the treatment of hypercholesterolemia. Existing drugs for hypercholesterolemia should be retained on the formulary since these provide complimentary mechanisms for treating hypercholesterolemia. Professional educational programs to thoroughly review the efficacy and safety of lovastatin and its place in the treatment of dyslipidemias are strongly recommended. Periodic drug-use evaluations are also advisable since this drug may be a major item in the pharmacy budget.

Conclusion

Lovastatin has the potential for revolutionizing the treatment of hypercholesterolemia. It appears capable of reducing total and LDL cholesterol levels more profoundly than any other lipid-lowering drug currently available; the drug also substantially reduces apolipoprotein B, triglyceride, and VLDL levels and modestly increases HDL levels. Lovastatin is effective in combination with other lipid-lowering drugs. Since lovastatin is easier for patients to take than other drugs, compliance may be improved. The big questions that remain are whether it can alter the course of atherosclerosis and whether it will cause serious adverse reactions with long-term use. The answers to these questions will require more experience and study. Until then, restrained use and careful monitoring of treated patients are recommended.

---

[a] Tobert JA, Merck Sharp & Dohme Research Laboratories. Personal communication. 1987 Feb 12.

References

1. Enos WF, Holmes RH, Beyer J. Coronary disease among United States soldiers killed in action in Korea. *JAMA*. 1953; 152:1090–3.
2. Keys A. Coronary heart disease in seven countries. *Circulation*. 1970; 41(Suppl 1):1–211.
3. Reed D, Katsuhiko Y, Kagan A. Lipids and lipoproteins as predictors of coronary heart disease, stroke, and cancer in the Honolulu Heart Program. *Am J Med*. 1986; 80:871–8.
4. Kannel WB, Castelli W, Gordon T et al. Serum cholesterol, lipoproteins, and risk of coronary heart disease: The Framingham Study. *Ann Intern Med*. 1971; 74:1–12.
5. Anon. Relationship of blood pressure, serum cholesterol, smoking habits, relative weight and ECG abnormalities to incidence of major coronary events: final report of the pooling project research group. *J Chronic Dis*. 1978; 31:201–306.
6. Stamler J, Wentworth D, Neaton J. Is the relationship between serum cholesterol and risk of death from coronary heart disease continuous and graded? *JAMA*. 1986; 256:2823–8.
7. Lipid Research Clinics Program. The lipid research clinics coronary primary prevention trial results. I. Reduction in incidence of coronary heart disease. *JAMA*. 1984; 251:351–64.
8. Lipid Research Clinics Program. The lipid research clinics coronary primary prevention trial results. II. The relationship of reduction in incidence of coronary heart disease to cholesterol lowering. *JAMA*. 1984; 251:365–74.
9. Blackenhorn D, Nessim S, Johnson R et al. Beneficial effects of combined colestipol–niacin therapy on coronary atherosclerosis and coronary venous bypass grafts. *JAMA*. 1987; 257:3233–40.
10. Brensike JF, Levy RI, Kelsey SF et al. Effects of therapy with cholestyramine on progression of coronary arteriosclerosis: results of the NHLBI type II coronary intervention study. *Circulation*. 1984; 69:313–24.
11. Levy RI, Brensike JF, Epstein SE et al. The influence of changes in lipid values induced by cholestyramine and diet on progression of coronary artery disease: results of the NHLBI type II coronary intervention study. *Circulation*. 1984; 69:325–37.
12. Endo A. HMG-CoA reductase inhibitors. In: Kritchevsky D, Holmes WL, Paoletti R, eds. Drugs affecting lipid metabolism. VIII. New York: Plenum Press; 1983:295–310.
13. Alberts AW, Chen J, Kuron G et al. Mevinolin: a highly potent competitive inhibitor of hydroxymethylglutaryl-coenzyme A reductase and a cholesterol-lowering agent. *Proc Natl Acad Sci*. 1980; 77:3957–61.
14. Grundy SM. Cholesterol and coronary heart disease. A new era. *JAMA*. 1986; 256:2849–58.
15. Schaefer EJ, Levy RI. Pathogenesis and management of lipoprotein disorders. *N Engl J Med*. 1985; 312:1300–10.
16. Ross R. The pathogenesis of atherosclerosis—an update. *N Engl J Med*. 1986; 314:488–500.
17. Goldstein JL, Brown MS. Familial hypercholesterolemia: a genetic receptor disease. *Hosp Pract*. 1985; 20 (Nov 15):35–46.
18. Brown MS, Kovanen PT, Goldstein JL. Regulation of plasma cholesterol by lipoprotein receptors. *Science*. 1981; 212:628–35.
19. Dietschy JM, Wilson JD. Regulation of cholesterol metabolism. *N Engl J Med*. 1970; 282:1179–83.
20. Goldstein JL, Kita T, Brown MS. Defective lipoprotein receptors and atherosclerosis. Lessons from the animal counterpart of familial hypercholesterolemia. *N Engl J Med*. 1983; 309:288–96.
21. Gordon T, Castelli WP, Hjortland MC et al. The prediction of coronary heart disease by high density and other lipoproteins: an historical perspective. In: Rifkind B, Levy R, eds. Hyperlipidemia—diagnosis and therapy. New York: Grave & Stratton Inc.; 1977:71–8.
22. Brown MS, Goldstein JL. A receptor-mediated pathway for cholesterol homeostasis. *Science*. 1986; 232:34–47.
23. Brown MS, Goldstein JL. How LDL receptors influence cholesterol and atherosclerosis. *Sci Am*. 1984; 251:2–10.
24. Gotto AM, Jackson RL. Plasma lipoproteins and atherosclerosis. *Atherosclerosis Rev*. 1978; 3:231–41.
25. Kita T, Brown MS, Goldstein JL. Feedback regulation of 3-hydroxy-3-methylglutaryl coenzyme A reductase in livers of mice treated with mevinolin, a competitive inhibitor of the reductase. *J Clin Invest*. 1980; 66:1094–100.
26. Tsujita Y, Kurada M, Shimada Y et al. CS-514, a competitive inhibitor of 3-hydroxy-3-methylglutaryl coenzyme A reductase: tissue-selective inhibition of sterol synthesis and hypolipidemic effect on various animal species. *Biochem Biophys Acta*. 1986; 877:50–60.
27. Brown MS, Faust JR, Goldstein JL. Induction of 3-hydroxy-3-methylglutaryl coenzyme A reductase activity in human fibroblasts incubated with compactin (ML-236B), a competitive inhibitor of the reductase. *J Biol Chem*. 1978; 253:1121–8.
28. Hagemenas FC, Lindsay S, Illingworth DR. Influence of mevinolin on cholesterol homeostasis in mononuclear leukocytes from patients with familial hypercholesterolemia. *Arteriosclerosis*. 1986; 6:543a. Abstract.
29. Brown MS, Goldstein JL. Multivalent feedback regulation of HMG CoA reductase, a control mechanism coordinating isoprenoid synthesis and cell growth. *J Lipid Res*. 1980; 21:505–17.
30. Parker TSD, McNamara DJ, Brown C et al. Mevalonic acid in human plasma: relationship of concentration and circadian rhythm to cholesterol synthesis rates in man. *Proc Natl Acad Sci*. 1982; 79:3037–41.
31. Parker TS, McNamara DJ, Brown CD et al. Plasma mevalonate as a measure of cholesterol synthesis in man. *J Clin Invest*. 1984; 74:795–804.
32. Brown MS, Goldstein JL. Lipoprotein receptors in the liver control signals for plasma cholesterol traffic. *J Clin Invest*. 1983; 72:743–7.
33. Traber MG, Kayden HJ. Inhibition of cholesterol synthesis by mevinolin stimulates low density lipoprotein receptor activity in human monocyte-derived macrophages. *Atherosclerosis*. 1984; 52:1–11.
34. Bilheimer DW, Grundy SM, Brown MS et al. Mevinolin and colestipol stimulate receptor-mediated clearance of low density lipoprotein from plasma in familial hypercholesterolemia heterozygotes. *Proc Natl Acad Sci*. 1983; 80:4124–8.
35. Grundy SM, Vega GL. Influence of mevinolin on metabolism of low density lipoproteins in primary moderate hypercholesterolemia. *J Lipid Res*. 1985; 26:1464–75.
36. Vega GL, Grundy SM. In vivo evidence for reduced binding of low density lipoproteins to receptors as a cause of primary moderate hypercholesterolemia. *J Clin Invest*. 1986; 78:1410–4.
37. Grundy SM, Bilheimer DW. Inhibition of 3-hydroxy-3-methylglutaryl-CoA reductase by mevinolin in familial hypercholesterolemia heterozygotes: effects on cholesterol balance. *Proc Natl Acad Sci*. 1984; 81:2538–42.
38. Kritchevsky D, Tepper SA, Klurfeld DM. Influence of mevinolin on experimental atherosclerosis in rabbits. *Pharmacol Res Commun*. 1981; 13:921–6.
39. Shapiro DJ, Nordstrom JL, Mitschelin JJ et al. Microassay for 3-hydroxy-3-methylglutaryl CoA reductase in rat liver and in L-cell fibroblasts. *Biochem Biophys Acta*. 1974; 370:369–77.
40. Stubbs RJ, Schwartz M, Bayne WF. Determination of mevinolin and mevinolinic acid in plasma and bile by reversed-phase high-performance liquid chromatography. *J Chromatogr*. 1986; 383:438–43.
41. Tobert JA, Hitzenberger G, Kukovetz WR et al. Rapid and substantial lowering of human serum cholesterol by mevinolin (MK-803), an inhibitor of hydroxymethylglutaryl-coenzyme A reductase. *Atherosclerosis*. 1982; 41:61–5.
42. Tobert JA, Bell GD, Birtwell J et al. Cholesterol-lowering effect of mevinolin, an inhibitor of 3-hydroxy-3-methylglutaryl-coenzyme A reductase, in healthy volunteers. *J Clin*

Invest. 1982; 69:913–9.
43. Illingworth DR, Sextron GJ. Hypocholesterolemic effects of mevinolin in patients with heterozygous familial hypercholesterolemia. *J Clin Invest*. 1984; 74:1972–8.
44. Uauy R, Vega GL, Bilheimer DW et al. Effect of lovastatin and LDL kinetics in homozygous familial hypercholesterolemia (FH). *Pediatr Res*. 1987; 24:349A. Abstract.
45. Havel RJ, Hunninghake DB, Illingworth DR et al. A multicenter study of lovastatin (mevinolin) in the therapy of heterozygous familial hypercholesterolemia. *Ann Intern Med*. 1987; 107:609–15.
46. Hoeg JM, Maher MB, Zech LA et al. Effectiveness of mevinolin on plasma lipoprotein concentrations in type II hyperlipoproteinemia. *Am J Cardiol*. 1986; 57:933–9.
47. Tikkanen MJ, Helve E, Nikkila EA. Treatment of familial and nonfamilial hypercholesterolemia with mevinolin. *Arteriosclerosis*. 1986; 6:550a. Abstract.
48. East CS, Bilheimer DW, Grundy SM. Combination drug therapy for treatment of patients with familial combined hyperlipidemia resulting in combined hypertriglyceridemia and hypercholesterolemia. *Arteriosclerosis*. 1986; 6:544a. Abstract.
49. The Lovastatin Study Group. II. Therapeutic response to lovastatin (mevinolin) in nonfamilial hypercholesterolemia. A multicenter study. *JAMA*. 1986; 256:2829–34.
50. East C, Grundy SM, Bilheimer DW. Normal cholesterol levels with lovastatin (mevinolin) therapy in a child with homozygous familial hypercholesterolemia following liver transplantation. *JAMA*. 1986; 256:2843–8.
51. Anon. Consensus conference statement. Lowering blood cholesterol to prevent heart disease. *JAMA*. 1985; 253:2080–6.
52. Ballantyne FC, Clark RS, Simpson HS et al. High-density and low-density lipoprotein subfractions in survivors of myocardial infarction and in control subjects. *Metabolism*. 1982; 31:433–7.
53. Elovson J, Jacobs JC, Schumaker VN et al. Molecular weights of apoprotein B obtained from low-density lipoprotein (apoprotein B-PI) and from rat very low-density lipoprotein (apoprotein B-PIII). *Biochemistry*. 1985; 24:1569–78.
54. Kukita H, Hiwada K, Kokubu T. Serum apolipoprotein AI, AII and B levels and their discriminative values in relatives of patients with coronary artery disease. *Atherosclerosis*. 1984; 51:261–7.
55. Goldstein JL, Hazzard WR, Schrott HG et al. Hyperlipidemia in coronary heart disease. I. Lipid levels in 500 survivors of myocardial infarction. *J Clin Invest*. 1973; 52:1533–43.
56. Goldstein JL, Schrott HG, Hazzard WR et al. Hyperlipidemia in coronary heart disease. II. Genetic analysis of lipid levels in 176 families and delineation of a new inherited disorder, combined hyperlipidemia. *J Clin Invest*. 1973; 52:1544–68.
57. Perry RS. Contemporary recommendations for evaluating and treating hyperlipidemia. *Clin Pharm*. 1986; 5:113–27.
58. LaRosa JC. Drug therapy for lipid disorders. *Postgrad Med*. 1987; 82:103–11.
59. Illingworth DR, Connor WE. Hypercholesterolemia persisting after distal ileal bypass: response to mevinolin. *Ann Intern Med*. 1984; 100:850–1.
60. Vega AL, Grundy SM. Mevinolin effectively treats hyperlipidemia of the nephrotic syndrome. *Arteriosclerosis*. 1986; 6:551a. Abstract.
61. Illingworth DR. Mevinolin plus colestipol in therapy for severe heterozygous familial hypercholesterolemia. *Ann Intern Med*. 1984; 101:598–604.
62. Grundy SM, Vaga GL, Bilheimer DW. Influence of combined therapy with mevinolin and interruption of bile-acid reabsorption on low density lipoproteins in heterozygous familial hypercholesterolemia. *Ann Intern Med*. 1985; 103:339–43.
63. Lees AM, Stein SW, Lees RS. Therapy of hypercholesterolemia with mevinolin and other lipid-lowering drugs. *Arteriosclerosis*. 1986; 6:544a. Abstract.
64. Hoeg JM, Maher MB, Bailey KR et al. The effects of mevinolin and neomycin alone and in combination on plasma lipid and lipoprotein concentrations in type II hyperlipoproteinemia. *Atherosclerosis*. 1986; 60:209–14.
65. Merck Sharp & Dohme. Mevacor package insert. West Point, PA; 1987 Aug.
66. Tikkanen MJ, Nikkila EA. Current pharmacologic treatment of elevated serum cholesterol. *Circulation*. 1987; 76:529–33.
67. Illingworth DR. Comparative efficacy of once versus twice daily mevinolin in the therapy of familial hypercholesterolemia. *Clin Pharmacol Ther*. 1986; 40:338–43.
68. Achor RW, Winklemann RK, Perry HO. Cutaneous side effects from the use of triparanol (MER-29). *Mayo Clin Proc*. 1961; 36:217–8.
69. Laughlin RC, Carey TF. Cataracts in patients treated with triparanol. *JAMA*. 1962; 181:339–40.
70. Tobert JA. New developments in lipid-lowering therapy: the role of inhibitors of hydroxymethylglutaryl coenzyme A reductase. *Circulation*. 1987; 76:534–8.
71. Cenedella RJ, Bierkamper GG. Mechanism of cataract production by 3-beta(2-diethylaminoethoby) androst-5-en-17-one hydrochloride, U18666A: an inhibitor of cholesterol biosynthesis. *Exp Eye Res*. 1979; 28:673–88.
72. Hunninghake DB, Miller VT, Palmer RH et al. Inhibitors of cholesterol synthesis and cataracts. *JAMA*. 1987; 257:1602. Letter.
73. Illingworth DR, Corbin D. The influence of mevinolin on the adrenal cortical response to corticotropin in heterozygous familial hypercholesterolemia. *Proc Natl Acad Sci*. 1985; 82:6291–4.
74. National Cholesterol Education Program. Report of the expert panel on detection, evaluation, and treatment of high cholesterol in adults. *Arch Intern Med*. 1988; 148:(in press).

Sulbactam: A β-lactamase inhibitor

JEAN K. NOGUCHI AND MARK A. GILL

Abstract: The chemistry, pharmacology, microbiology, pharmacokinetics, clinical efficacy, and adverse effects of sulbactam are reviewed.

Sulbactam is a competitive, irreversible β-lactamase inhibitor. Its binding to penicillin-binding proteins imparts weak intrinsic antibacterial activity. Synergy of sulbactam with β-lactam antibiotics is most marked in bacterial species in which β lactamase is a major mechanism of resistance. Sulbactam sodium is available in combination with ampicillin sodium for injection in a 1:2 ratio of sulbactam to ampicillin. Sultamicillin, an oral prodrug that is hydrolyzed to equimolar amounts of ampicillin and sulbactam, is in clinical trials. Ampicillin and sulbactam have similar pharmacokinetic properties.

Sulbactam–ampicillin appears to be most useful for the treatment of polymicrobial aerobic or anaerobic infections and uncomplicated gonorrhea. Persistence, relapse, and superinfections have been reported after sulbactam–ampicillin treatment of urinary-tract and respiratory-tract infections. The combination is not effective against pseudomonal infections. Sulbactam–ampicillin is generally well tolerated.

By restoring or expanding the activity of older, well-established β-lactam antibiotics, sulbactam offers a new approach to the management of bacterial infections; the minimal toxicity of sulbactam–ampicillin makes the combination appealing for the treatment of gram-negative nonpseudomonal and anaerobic infections.

Index terms: Ampicillin; Ampicillin sodium; Antibiotics; Cephalosporins; Drugs; Drug administration routes; Gonorrhea; Mechanism of action; Penicillins; Pharmacokinetics; *Pseudomonas* infections; Respiratory-tract infections; Spectinomicin; Sulbactam; Sulbactam sodium; Sultamicillin; Toxicity; Urinary-tract infections
Clin Pharm. 1988; 7:37–51

Bacterial resistance to benzylpenicillin was described even before the drug was accepted as a useful antibiotic. Recognition of β-lactamase enzymes as primary mediators of resistance has led to the evolution of two basic methods to overcome their effect: (1) modifying the β-lactam nucleus to produce antibiotics that are stereochemically stable to enzyme effect and (2) designing drugs to inhibit β-lactamase action. Each of these techniques restores β-lactam-antibiotic activity at bacterial target proteins, thus augmenting antibacterial effect. In some cases (e.g., cefoxitin, methicillin), both principles have been applied in a single molecule.

The concept of β-lactamase inhibitors as potential enhancers of penicillin activity was described as early as 1950. A trial of methicillin plus penicillin G in the treatment of a penicillin-resistant gram-negative urinary-tract infection was reported in 1967.[1] Interest in β-lactamase inhibitors was rekindled in the late 1970s, with the discoveries of clavulanic acid and sulbactam. These two drugs represent a unique therapeutic approach, because they can potentially restore the activities of older penicillins, such as ampicillin, which have been cast aside because of the development of resistance.

According to Wise,[2] a good β-lactamase inhibitor is (1) active at concentrations attainable in body fluids, (2) active against a wide range of β-lactamase enzymes from gram-positive and gram-negative, aerobic and anaerobic organisms, (3) similar in pharmacology to its β-lactam-antibiotic partner in healthy and diseased patients, (4) free from toxicity, and (5) not too costly. The inhibitor itself should also resist hydrolysis by β lactamases, and it should not induce β-lactamase-enzyme production. This article will characterize and evaluate sulbactam's properties in these areas. Sulbactam sodium was marketed recently in the United States in combination with ampicillin sodium for injection (Unasyn, Pfizer Inc.). An oral prodrug, sultamicillin, is under investigation.

Chemistry

Chemically, sulbactam is 3,3-dimethyl-7-oxo-4-thia-1-azabicyclo (3,2,0)-heptane-2-carboxylic acid 4,4-dioxide, [2*S*-(2α,5α)] (Figure 1). Its molecular weight is 232 ($C_8H_{10}NO_5S$). Sulbactam is a water-soluble, white to off-white crystalline solid.

In vitro, sulbactam is extremely stable in solution at 37 °C, with a half-life of >100 hours at concentrations of 100 and 1000 μg/mL in various buffers and in human serum and urine.[3] Sulbactam is not a naturally occurring compound; it was syn-

JEAN K. NOGUCHI, PHARM.D., is Assistant Professor of Clinical Pharmacy, and MARK A. GILL, PHARM.D., is Associate Professor of Clinical Pharmacy, School of Pharmacy, University of Southern California, Los Angeles.

Address reprint requests to Dr. Gill at the School of Pharmacy, University of Southern California, 1985 Zonal Avenue, Los Angeles, CA 90033.

The assistance of Alfred Chin, Pharm.D., in preparing this manuscript is acknowledged.

This is **article 680-204-8801** in the **ASHP Continuing Education System;** it qualifies for 1.0 hour of continuing-education credit. See page 75 for learning objectives and test questions.

Copyright © 1988, American Society of Hospital Pharmacists, Inc. All rights reserved. 0278-2677/88/0101-0037$03.75.

Figure 1. Chemical structures of sulbactam (top) and sultamicillin.

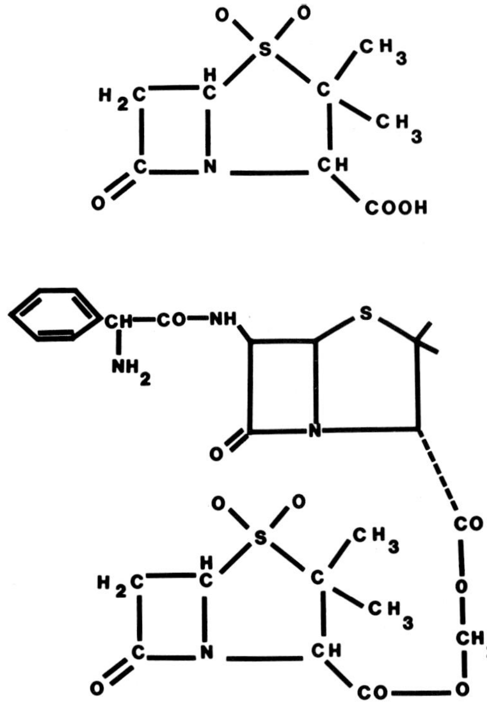

thesized by researchers at Pfizer Central Research.[3]

When reconstituted with water for injection, sulbactam sodium–ampicillin sodium for injection demonstrates stability similar to that of ampicillin sodium.[4] Further dilution of sulbactam sodium and ampicillin sodium in concentrations ranging from sulbactam 1 mg/mL and ampicillin 2 mg/mL up to sulbactam 15 mg/mL and ampicillin 30 mg/mL resulted in physical compatibility, with <10% degradation of the sulbactam component after eight hours at room temperature in the following solutions: sterile water for injection, 0.9% sodium chloride injection, 5% dextrose injection, 5% dextrose and 0.45% sodium chloride injection, lactated Ringer's injection, 0.167 M sodium lactate injection, and 10% invert sugar injection. The stability of ampicillin was not altered in the presence of sulbactam. Sulbactam was more stable than ampicillin under all studied conditions; reconstitution and storage limitations of sulbactam sodium–ampicillin sodium are thus determined by the stability of the ampicillin component.

A similar evaluation of sulbactam sodium–ampicillin sodium after reconstitution with sterile water for injection, 0.5% lidocaine hydrochloride injection, and 2% lidocaine hydrochloride injection, showed no difference in stability among the three diluents.[4]

Sultamicillin is a novel formulation designed for oral use.[5] The combination of sulbactam and ampicillin as a double ester linked by a methylene group (Figure 1) results in a mutual prodrug. During enteral absorption, hydrolysis to equimolar amounts of the two active drugs allows simultaneous delivery to the systemic circulation, with enhanced and more reliable absorption than after administration of the simple salts.

Other names for sulbactam include penicillanic acid sulfone (or sulphone) and CP-45,899 (CAS registry number 68373-14-8). The sodium salt is also known as CP-45,899-2, and the pivoxyl ester is known as CP-47,904. Sultamicillin is CP-49,952 (CAS registry number 76497-13-7).

Pharmacology

Beta-lactam antibiotics may be hydrolyzed by four classes of enzymes.[6] Beta lactamases hydrolyze the cyclic lactam ring. Esterases remove the acetyl group of certain cephalosporins (e.g., cephalothin, cefotaxime). Of minor clinical importance, amino acid acylases (or amidases) remove acyl side chains. Finally, a specific group of dehydropeptidases inactivate the carbapenem compounds (e.g., imipenem).

By far the most important enzymes, both clinically and microbiologically, are the β lactamases. Production is widespread among aerobic and anaerobic, gram-positive and gram-negative bacteria, as well as some algae, yeasts, and mammalian tissues.[7] Beta-lactamase production may be constitutive or induced, with genetic information transferred in a chromosomal-mediated manner or via plasmids (R factors).

Beta lactamases should not be considered homogeneous, but rather a diverse group of enzymes with variable structures and activities. Gram-positive bacteria produce only a few types, which are categorized into four groups (A–D) according to serologic data.[8,9] In contrast, the β lactamases of gram-negative species are numerous, diverse, and ever changing. The Richmond–Sykes classification of gram-negative β lactamases identifies five classes (I–V), based on substrate activities. Sulbactam inhibits the β lactamases of group A (gram-positive) bacteria and classes II–V (gram-negative) bacteria. The drug has relatively little activity against class I enzymes,[10,11] which may be explained by sulbactam's inability to reach the enzyme's catalytic site or by a different affinity pattern of the enzyme receptor sites.

It is important to recognize that stability of an antibiotic to β lactamase does not imply clinical efficacy nor does clinical efficacy imply β-lactamase resistance. To be active against a microorganism, a β-lactam antibiotic must (1) penetrate the cell to reach the target protein; (2) bind to the target protein and exert its action; and (3) withstand enzymatic breakdown.[7] Addition of a β-lactamase inhibitor will prevent hydrolysis of the β-lactam ring but will not alter cell penetration or target protein binding, nor will it prevent antibiotic degradation by other types of enzymes. Some bacteria (e.g., *Bacteroides fragilis* and *Haemophilus influenzae*) derive most of their antibiotic resistance from the production of β lactamases. On the other hand, many gram-negative bacteria possess a permeability barrier that inhibits antibiotic penetration into the periplasmic space, complementing the activity of β lactamase. If penetration to target proteins is impaired, inhibition of β-lactamase activity may not markedly alter antibiotic susceptibility. Thus, β-lactamase inhibition may have an unpredictable effect on antibiotic activity. Tests performed in cell-free β-lactamase preparations may be misleading, and results should not be extrapolated to intact bacteria.

Some drugs have both inhibitor and antibiotic properties. Cefoxitin, cefamandole, aztreonam, moxalactam, methicillin, and the isoxazoyl penicillins (e.g., cloxacillin, oxacillin) are all β-lactamase inhibitors to varying degrees.

Beta-lactamase inhibitors may be reversible or irreversible, and competitive or noncompetitive. Sulbactam best fits the competitive, irreversible model.[12] The interaction of β-lactamase enzyme and inhibitor may be diagrammed as follows[12]:

$$E + I \rightleftarrows E{\cdot}I \rightarrow E{-}I'$$

where E = enzyme (β lactamase), I = inhibitor, $E{\cdot}I$ = reversible enzyme–inhibitor complex, and $E{-}I'$ = modified enzyme–inhibitor complex incapable of subsequent reaction. The inhibitor (sulbactam) in native form is poorly reactive. Binding at the active site on the β-lactamase enzyme results in conversion into highly reactive sulbactam fragments ($E{\cdot}I$). The fragments then form covalent bonds at another site on the enzyme in a virtually irreversible reaction ($E{-}I'$). Sulbactam is sometimes called a "suicide inhibitor" because the inactivation process renders both the inhibitor and enzyme incapable of all further action.

The degree and nature of β-lactamase inhibition is concentration dependent. Sulbactam has a much higher affinity for reactive sites on the enzyme than most β-lactam antibiotics.[10] Further studies of the sulbactam–β-lactamase interaction have demonstrated a first-order reaction at low inhibitor concentrations and a zero-order reaction at high concentrations. Inhibition is also time-dependent; binding of sulbactam is more intense after prolonged exposure. This property allows classification of sulbactam as a "progressive inhibitor." [10]

Hydrolysis of sulbactam by β lactamases of various species has been shown to be minimal.[13] Furthermore, incubation with sublethal concentrations of β-lactam antibiotics has shown sulbactam to be a poor inducer of β-lactamase production.[13] These two properties contribute to the overall effectiveness of β-lactamase inhibition.

A second property of sulbactam separate from its β-lactamase-inhibitor activity is its affinity for penicillin-binding proteins. Penicillin-binding proteins are membrane-bound proteins involved in cell-wall synthesis, and the target proteins for β-lactam-antibiotic activity. At least six types of penicillin-binding proteins have been identified. Sulbactam has demonstrated affinity for penicillin-binding protein types 1a and 2.[13] After incubation for one hour at a sulbactam concentration of 8–256 μg/mL there was inhibition of *Escherichia coli* division, with formation of long filaments.[14] Raising the sulbactam concentration to ≥256 μg/mL resulted in spheroplast formation and bacteriolysis. Antibacterial activity against *Neisseria gonorrhoeae* and *Acinetobacter calcoaceticus* is thought to be due in part to this weak penicillin-like activity. In addition, some investigators postulate that the synergistic effect of sulbactam with β-lactam antibiotics may result from a combination of its abilities to inhibit β lactamase and bind to penicillin-binding proteins.[13]

The spectrum of β lactamases inhibited by sulbactam is similar to that for clavulanic acid, and both compounds are classified as "suicide-type" β-lactamase inhibitors. However, clavulanic acid may itself be hydrolyzed by β lactamases and may induce β-lactamase production under certain conditions.[15] Additionally, sulbactam binds to penicillin-binding proteins, allowing a penicillin-like action on certain bacteria. Thus, although studies have shown sulbactam to be two to five times less potent on a weight basis than clavulanic acid, it has several theoretical advantages that merit further consideration.

Microbiology

In the first major description of sulbactam, English et al.[3] compared its activities with those of clavulanic acid. Testing in cell-free β-lactamase preparations showed similar activity profiles. Subsequent testing with intact bacteria confirmed sulbactam's β-lactamase-inhibiting properties in a variety of gram-positive and gram-negative species. Combination with β-lactam antibiotics potentiated the activities of both agents, as evidenced by a reduction in the minimum inhibitory concentrations (MICs) (Table 1). Synergy is most marked in species in which β-lactamase production is a major mechanism of resistance (e.g., *Staphylococcus aureus, Haemophilus influenzae,* and *Bacteroides fragilis*) and more pronounced in β-lactamase-producing strains as compared with non-β-lactamase-producing strains.

Antibiotic-to-inhibitor ratios of 2:1, 1:1, or 1:2 have resulted in optimal in vitro bactericidal activity.[11,16,17] Early animal studies further supported the potential activity of these ratios. Correlation of this

Table 1.
Minimum Inhibitory Concentration of Sulbactam and Ampicillin, Alone or in Combination

Organism	Minimum Inhibitory Concentration (μg/mL) Sulbactam	Ampicillin	Sulbactam + Ampicillin	Reference[a]
Streptococcus pyogenes	50	0.025	0.025 + 0.025	3
Streptococcus faecalis	>50	1.56	1.56 + 1.56	3
Staphylococcus aureus				
Ampicillin-susceptible	200	0.05	0.05 + 0.05	3
Methicillin-susceptible	100–≥200	100–≥200	1.6–6.25 + 1.6–6.25	3, 11, 16, 17
Methicillin-resistant	ND[b]	>128	16 + 16	17
Staphylococcus epidermidis	>50–≥200	25–64	1.6–3.12 + 1.6–6.25	3, 16, 17
Neisseria gonorrhoeae				
Ampicillin-susceptible	0.15–0.8	0.07–0.10	0.05–0.07 + 0.05–0.07	3, 16
Ampicillin-resistant	1.2–12.5	≥10	0.31–2.5 + 0.31–2.5	3, 17
Branhamella catarrhalis	100	12.5	0.4 + 0.4	17
Haemophilus influenzae				
Ampicillin-susceptible	100	0.2–0.39	0.025–0.39 + 0.025–0.39	3, 16
Ampicillin-resistant	>64–200	64–>400	1.0–3.12 + 1.0–3.12	3, 11, 17
Escherichia coli				
Ampicillin-susceptible	25	3.12	3.12 + 3.12	3
Ampicillin-resistant	25–64	100–>400	6.2–25 + 6.2–25	3, 16, 17
	200	4000	100 + 2000	3
Klebsiella pneumoniae	50–64	50–>128	3.1–8.0 + 3.1–8.0	3, 16, 17
Enterobacter cloacae	100–>128	200–>400	12.5–>64 + 12.5–>64	3, 16, 17
Enterobacter aerogenes	64	128	16 + 16	17
Proteus mirabilis	50	0.39	0.39 + 0.39	3
Morganella morganii	50–200	50–200	3.12 + 3.12	3, 16
Proteus species	100–>128	>128–>400	3.12–8.0 + 3.12–8.0	3, 16, 17
Serratia marcescens	100	200	12.5 + 12.5	3
Serratia species	>128	>128	32 + 32	17
Pseudomonas aeruginosa	>400	1000	100 + 25	3
Providencia alcalifaciens	100	50	12.5 + 12.5	3
Citrobacter species	>128–200	100–>128	12.5–32 + 6.25–32	3, 17
Salmonella species	100	400	12.5 + 6.25	3
Shigella species	>400	200	6.2 + 6.2	16
Bacteroides fragilis	12.5–50	25–800	0.78–12.5 + 1.6–12.5	3, 11, 16, 17

[a] In reference 3, minimum inhibitory concentrations of sulbactam and ampicillin were determined individually. In references 11, 16, and 17, the minimum inhibitory concentration of a 1:1 sulbactam–ampicillin mixture was determined.
[b] ND = not determined.

information with the pharmacokinetic profiles of the two drugs has resulted in the use of an ampicillin-to-sulbactam ratio of 2:1 in most clinical trials.

Broth- or agar-dilution methods for MIC determination generally use inocula of 10^4 colony-forming units (CFU) (agar) to 10^6 CFU (broth), sulbactam-to-ampicillin ratios of 1:2, and the following breakpoints: susceptible ≤8 μg/mL, intermediate 16 μg/mL, and resistant ≥32 μg/mL (as ampicillin).[18] Disks containing 10 μg each of sulbactam and ampicillin have been suggested for use in in vitro susceptibility studies.[19] For *Staph. aureus* and gram-negative bacteria, zone diameter breakpoints of susceptible ≥14 mm, intermediate 12–13 mm, and resistant ≤11 mm, corresponding to an MIC breakpoint of about 16 μg/mL, are advised for ampicillin–sulbactam disk testing.

Gram-positive Bacteria. Among β lactamases produced by gram-positive bacteria, those of *Staph. aureus* are clinically the most important. Approximately 80–90% of *Staph. aureus* strains produce β lactamases that confer resistance to penicillin G. These enzymes preferentially hydrolyze penicillins over cephalosporins and are highly inducible; induction may increase production by as much as 1000-fold.

Ampicillin- and methicillin-susceptible strains of *Staph. aureus* (corresponding to non-penicillinase-producing and penicillinase-producing strains, respectively) demonstrate marked susceptibility to combinations of ampicillin and sulbactam. As expected, synergy is more pronounced with the penicillinase-producing strains (methicillin-susceptible in Table 1).

Although most strains of methicillin-resistant *Staph. aureus* (MRSA) produce β lactamase, the mechanism for methicillin resistance is not thought to be related to elaboration of this enzyme. Thus, the apparent susceptibility of MRSA strains to the ampicillin–sulbactam combination (Table 1) was an unexpected finding. Favorable results using a simulated in vivo model led to recommendations for trials in animals.[20] However, this suggestion must be tempered by previous experience with other β-lactam antibiotics, such as the cephalosporins. Although active against MRSA in vitro, these drugs have failed in clinical trials.

Other gram-positive bacteria known to produce

β lactamases include species of *Nocardia* and *Bacillus*. The susceptibility of 12 strains of *Nocardia asteroides* to various antibiotics was studied.[21] Although 11 of 12 strains were found to elaborate β lactamase, sulbactam 10 μg/mL had virtually no synergistic effect in combination with ampicillin or various other antibiotics.

Gram-negative Bacteria. In contrast to those of gram-positive bacteria, the β lactamases of gram-negative bacteria are numerous, diverse, and constantly adapting to their environment. Recent evaluations have indicated not only that carrier rates are increasing but also that the epidemiology of enzyme production is changing. In the past, enzymes of Richmond–Sykes class III (also called TEM-type β lactamases) were the most important in clinical resistance. Current studies suggest this class may be decreasing in importance with the development of antibiotics stable to their hydrolytic activity.[9] Furthermore, until recently, the majority of clinically important enzymes were plasmid mediated. Chromosomal-mediated enzymes are now emerging in clinical isolates, possibly in response to exposure to antibiotics designed to resist plasmid-mediated enzymes. Thus, as bacteria are "stressed" by exposure to antibiotics, they may adapt by inducing the formation of larger quantities of β lactamase, or by producing different types. This adaptability allows the β lactamases of gram-negative bacteria to remain a constant threat in the treatment of infections.

As a single agent, sulbactam has very weak intrinsic antibacterial activity. The only major exception to this is *N. gonorrhoeae*. In vitro MIC values for ampicillin-susceptible (i.e., non-penicillinase-producing) strains have ranged from 0.15–0.8 μg/mL (Table 1).[3,11,16,17,22] When tested in penicillinase-producing strains of *N. gonorrhoeae*, sulbactam MICs were higher (1.2–12.5 μg/mL), although still within the range of clinically achievable concentrations. Combination with ampicillin results in marked synergy in penicillinase-producing strains of *N. gonorrhoeae*, with essentially no change in the MICs of non-penicillinase-producing strains. Limited data also suggest intrinsic activity of sulbactam against *Neisseria meningitidis*, *A. calcoaceticus*, and *Pseudomonas acidovorans*.[16]

An unfortunate aspect of the activity profile of the sulbactam–ampicillin combination is its relative lack of efficacy against species of *Pseudomonas* and *Enterobacter*. To a lesser extent, this has also been noted with species of *Serratia*, *Citrobacter*, and *Providencia*.

Studies of multiple-drug-resistant gram-negative bacteria have had variable results. The activities of ampicillin, mezlocillin, and several cephalosporins were evaluated, alone and in combination with sulbactam.[23] Marked and consistent synergy of the ampicillin–sulbactam combination was seen only with *H. influenzae* and *B. fragilis*. On the other hand, synergy (defined as a ≥ fourfold reduction in the MICs or MBCs of both agents) was seen in none of the tested strains of *E. coli*, *Enterobacter aerogenes*, *Enterobacter cloacae*, *Serratia marcescens*, *Citrobacter diversus*, *Pseudomonas aeruginosa*, or *Ps. maltophilia*. Synergy was inconsistent with strains of *Klebsiella pneumoniae*, *Morganella morganii*, and *Providencia stuartii*. Possible explanations for the lack of synergy include a permeability barrier to bacterial entry of the antibiotic or sulbactam (thought to be the major mechanism), an inefficacy of sulbactam against the β lactamases of these species, or hydrolysis of sulbactam by the β lactamases. Another investigator noted an increase in ceftazidime MICs for several strains of *Ps. aeruginosa* after the addition of sulbactam.[24]

Observations regarding the effect of inoculum size on sulbactam efficacy are relevant and potentially clinically important in certain infections (e.g., meningitis). At an inoculum of 10^5 CFU, MIC reductions of most penicillin derivatives by sulbactam were variable, but significant, when tested for all organisms except *Ps. aeruginosa*.[25] In contrast, when the inoculum size was increased to 10^7 CFU, the synergistic effect was retained only for strains of *B. fragilis*. MIC reduction after the addition of sulbactam was less marked for strains of *H. influenzae* and totally eliminated for *Staph. aureus*, *Staph. epidermidis*, and *E. coli*.

Branhamella catarrhalis is a relatively common pathogen in upper-respiratory-tract infections. Isolation of β-lactamase-producing strains has increased dramatically in the past 10 years. In the United States, as many as 80–87% of strains may produce β lactamase.[26] In β-lactamase-producing strains, the addition of sulbactam at 1 μg/mL resulted in a 44-fold reduction in the MIC of penicillin G and a 19-fold reduction in the MIC of amoxicillin.[26,27]

Haemophilus ducreyi (etiologic organism of chancroid) was found to be generally susceptible to ampicillin.[28] Most but not all ampicillin-resistant strains produced β lactamase. Addition of sulbactam resulted in a reduction in the ampicillin MIC for 90% of the ampicillin-resistant strains tested (MIC_{90}), from ≥16 to 0.25 μg/mL.

The activity of sulbactam against various species of *Campylobacter* has been evaluated by two investigators.[29,30] Combining sulbactam with ampicillin (or several other β-lactam antibiotics) did not result in a potentiation of antibiotic effect, which suggests that antibiotic resistance of *Campylobacter* species is probably not related to β-lactamase production.

Synergy of the ampicillin–sulbactam combination was seen in 23 of 33 *Legionella* strains, with partial synergy in 7 of 33; this effect was most marked and consistent with strains of *Legionella pneumophila*.[31] However, the role of β lactamases in the antibiotic resistance of *Legionella* species is not as pronounced as that for other gram-negative aerobes.[31] The intracellular location of the bacteria is another potential etiologic factor for poor efficacy. This conclusion limits the theoretical role of sulbactam in treating *Legionella* infections.

Anaerobic Bacteria. Beta-lactamase production has been demonstrated in species of *Bacteroides, Fusobacterium,* and *Clostridium.* Ninety percent of *Bacteroides* species causing infections in the gastrointestinal tract produce β lactamase[8] and are thus resistant to penicillin G. In a survey of anaerobic β lactamases, only one enzyme (from a *B. fragilis* isolate) was resistant to sulbactam among enzymes from strains of *Bacteroides, Fusobacterium,* and *Clostridium.*[32] Wexler et al.[33] observed a $\geq$ fourfold reduction in ampicillin MIC after combination with sulbactam in 86% of 70 strains of *B. fragilis,* 37% of other *Bacteroides* species, 6% of *Fusobacterium* species, and essentially no species of *Clostridium* (including *Clostridium difficile*) and other gram-positive cocci and rods. Sulbactam alone had a dose-dependent antibacterial effect, with inhibition of 10.3% of *B. fragilis* strains at 16 μg/mL, 93% at 32 μg/mL, and 100% at a concentration of 64 μg/mL. Variation in the susceptibility patterns of *Bacteroides* species when tested against various antibiotics suggested that the weighting of various subspecies may affect outcome in antibiotic susceptibility studies.

In vitro evaluations of sulbactam in combination with various penicillins,[3,11,22,23,25,34-36] cephalosporins,[16,23-25,37-43] and aztreonam,[24] have also been conducted. However, these studies will not be discussed in this report because of a lack of corresponding clinical trials.

Pharmacokinetics

Interpretation of pharmacokinetic data is hindered by uncertainty as to whether the ratio of β-lactam antibiotic to inhibitor or a certain minimum concentration of one or both drugs is more important in overall clinical efficacy.

Comparison of the pharmacokinetics of sulbactam and ampicillin (Table 2) shows similar values for the two drugs (with the exception of the rate constants k_{12} and k_{21}). Rogers measured a correlation coefficient (Pearson estimate) for the half-lives of the two drugs in the same subject of 0.898.[45] This suggests that doses may be adjusted proportionately in different disease states and with varying degrees of renal dysfunction.

Crossover studies[46,48-51] and comparisons with previously reported data[45-48] have been performed in both healthy subjects and patients with renal dysfunction to study potential pharmacokinetic interactions of sulbactam with ampicillin, penicillin G, and cefoperazone. No alteration in the pharmacokinetics of either sulbactam or the β-lactam antibiotics was observed. Similar pharmacokinetic characteristics and lack of interactions make sulbactam and ampicillin excellent candidates for coadministration.

Absorption. Preliminary animal studies showed poor oral absorption of sulbactam (19%) when administered as the sodium salt.[52] This led to the development of sulbactam esters for oral administration, with most studies evaluating the sultamicillin formulation. Sultamicillin is rapidly hydrolyzed during enteral absorption by esterases in the intestinal epithelium, releasing equimolar quantities of sulbactam and ampicillin. No intact sultamicillin was measured in the blood 15 minutes after an oral dose[53]; this suggests that only the two active parent drugs are delivered to the systemic circulation. The bioavailability of sulbactam and ampicillin after oral administration of sultamicillin has been estimated at 80% for both components.[45] Administration of sultamicillin 750 mg to fasting healthy volunteers and patients has resulted in peak serum concentrations at about one hour of 9.1–9.7 μg/mL for ampicillin and 6.4–8.9 μg/mL for sulbactam.[45,54,55] Data suggest little to no alteration in absorption by administration with food.[49,53]

Peak serum concentrations of 13 and 28 μg/mL were measured at 0.5 hour after the i.m. administration of sulbactam 500 and 1000 mg, respectively.[46] Compared to i.v. administration of the same doses, i.m. absorption of sulbactam was assessed to be rapid and complete. Injection with 0.5% lidocaine hydrochloride did not affect the pharmacokinetics of i.m. sulbactam or ampicillin.[56]

Table 2.
Pharmacokinetics of Sulbactam and Ampicillin in Healthy Volunteers

Pharmacokinetic Variable[a]	Sulbactam	Ampicillin	Reference
Volume of central compartment (L)	7.34–11.73	10.9–13.4	44–47
Beta-phase volume of distribution (L)	22.8–28.6	25.0	45, 46
Steady-state volume of distribution (L/kg)	0.240–0.320	0.279–0.297	44–46
k_{12} (hr^{-1})	0.9	0.401	44, 46
k_{21} (hr^{-1})	1.8	0.73	44, 46
k_{10} (hr^{-1})	1.4	1.71	44, 46
Beta-phase half-life (hr)	0.97–1.41	0.85–1.3	44–48
Total clearance (mL/min)	201–266	296–348	44–47
Renal clearance (mL/min)	169–204	251–319	44–47
Fractional urinary recovery (per 24 hr)	0.83–0.85	0.76–0.92	45–47

[a] k_{12} = rate constant associated with movement of drug from compartment 1 to compartment 2; k_{21} = rate constant associated with movement of drug from compartment 2 to compartment 1, k_{10} = rate constant associated with elimination of drug from compartment 1.

Distribution and Tissue Penetration. Most studies of i.v. sulbactam administration suggest a two-compartment open model.[45–47,57,58]

After equal doses, serum concentrations of sulbactam are about 1.3–1.5 times higher than those of ampicillin.[47] Infusion of sulbactam 1 g plus ampicillin 2 g i.v. over 15 minutes in healthy volunteers has resulted in extrapolated peak serum concentrations of approximately 60 μg/mL (sulbactam) and 120 μg/mL (ampicillin).[56] Halving the dose resulted in a proportionate decrease in serum concentrations. Similar values have been obtained in surgical[58] and postpartum[57] patients.

Sulbactam undergoes an initial rapid distribution phase, with a distribution-phase rate constant of 3.52–3.66 hr^{-1} (distribution-phase half-life of 11–12 minutes).[45,58] Protein binding of sulbactam to human serum using ultrafiltration has been measured at 38%,[56] with ampicillin protein binding estimated at 15–25%.[59]

The pharmacokinetics of sulbactam has been evaluated in several subsets of patients. In a comparison of appendectomy patients and healthy volunteers, no significant differences in distribution were noted except for a higher steady-state volume of distribution (V_{ss}) in the appendectomy patients.[58] This difference was considered to be of limited clinical importance. Pharmacokinetic variables in postpartum women were not significantly different from those in healthy volunteers and surgical patients.[57] A higher V_{ss} and lower peak serum concentration were seen in subjects with cystic fibrosis, while the V_{ss} (reported in liters per kilogram) in children without cystic fibrosis was comparable to that in healthy adults.[60]

Wright and Wise[50] measured sulbactam distribution volumes in patients with varying degrees of renal dysfunction, reporting an overall mean of 9.0 liters. No significant differences were measured among patients having estimated glomerular filtration rates ranging from <5 to 100 mL/min, although a trend towards a larger distribution volume with diminishing renal function was observed.

Distributive pharmacokinetic values of ampicillin (Table 2) are similar to those of sulbactam, which makes ampicillin a good candidate for coadministration with sulbactam. However, this does not imply that specific tissue distribution will be comparable, since these are derived variables without anatomic specificity.

Tissue Penetration. Penetration into tissues, including gallbladder,[61] intestinal mucosa,[62,63] appendix,[64] myometrium,[65] salpinx,[65] ovary,[65] and prostate,[66] has been shown to be good, with tissue concentrations about 60–100% of simultaneous serum concentrations (Table 3). An interesting exception is prostate tissue, where tissue sulbactam concentrations were an average of 2.6 times higher than serum concentrations. This high degree of tissue entry was not observed with ampicillin, and the authors postulated a possible active transport mechanism for sulbactam into prostate tissue.[66]

Sulbactam entry into body fluids, including maxillary sinus aspirate,[67] middle-ear effusion,[68] common bile,[61] gallbladder bile,[61] peritoneal fluid,[51,64,69] and blister fluid,[47] has also been demonstrated (Table 3).

In general, the penetration of sulbactam and ampicillin into cerebrospinal fluid (CSF) is similar and proportional to the degree of meningeal inflammation. In adult patients with normal menin-

Table 3.
Penetration of Sulbactam and Ampicillin into Tissues and Fluids

Reference	Fluid/Tissue	Drug[a]	Concentration[b] Sulbactam	Concentration[b] Ampicillin	% Penetration[c] Sulbactam	% Penetration[c] Ampicillin
47	Blister fluid	0.5 S + 0.5 A	10.3 (3.2–19.2)	5.7 (2.0–8.1)	163	177
69	Peritoneal fluid	0.5 S + 0.5 A	12.3 (6.6–20)	6.2 (3.4–11)	101	70
64	Peritoneal fluid	7.5 S + 15 A[d]	9.2 (3.1–24)	29.7 (10.5–72)		
	Appendix	Same	4.4 (0.7–10)	6.1 (2.9–11.1)		
67	Maxillary sinus aspirate	0.75 SA	0.3 (0.2–0.53)	0.3 (0.1–0.65)	17	11
68	Middle-ear effusion	50 SA[d]	1.12 (0.35–2.7)	1.54 (0.2–5.2)	32	32
61	Common bile	0.5 S + 1.0 A	(~0–20)	(~40–175)		
	Gallbladder bile	Same	4.3	15.9	22	79
	Gallbladder tissue	Same	6.3	7.7	32	38
62	Intestinal mucosa	0.5 S + 0.5 A	13.9 (0–28.5)	8.3 (0–28.4)	107	50
63	Intestinal mucosa	1.0 S + 2.0 A	11.0 (3.2–17.1)	19.0 (2.2–39.0)	60	63
	Feces	Same	7.5 (0–29.0)	10.5 (0–27.6)		
66	Prostate	0.5 S + 1.0 A	17.0 (5.2–46.2)	1.30 (0.4–9.3)	258	19
65	Myometrium	1.0 S + 2.0 A	13.8 (4.7–26.9)	26.9 (8.9–53.6)	57	52
	Salpinx	Same	22.5 (19.6–25.3)	28.5 (16.0–41.0)		
	Ovary	Same	16.2 (14.5–17.8)	22.6 (17.7–27.5)		

[a] Amount expressed in grams, except where noted; S = sulbactam, A = ampicillin, SA = sultamicillin.
[b] Concentration, expressed in micrograms per milliliter or micrograms per gram. Range is given in parentheses.
[c] Calculated as fluid or tissue concentration/serum concentration × 100.
[d] Expressed in milligrams per kilogram.

ges, sulbactam was not detected in CSF until four hours after administration of a single dose of 1 g i.m.[70] In contrast, adult patients with bacterial meningitis had detectable concentrations as early as one to two hours, which declined over four hours.[71] In a comparison of single versus multiple doses of sulbactam, accumulation was not seen.[71] Penetration of sulbactam into CSF in children has also been evaluated.[72]

Penetration of sulbactam into sputum was poor after oral administration of sulbactam pivoxyl[73] and sultamicillin.[55] However, the large numbers of patients with nondetectable sputum concentrations may have been due to the poor sensitivity of the assay used. Saliva concentrations were also nondetectable.[45]

Studies of sulbactam and ampicillin in peripartum and nursing women have shown that both drugs readily cross the placenta, with concentrations in umbilical-cord blood approaching those in serum one hour after dosing.[56] The urine of neonates born to mothers who had received the two drugs had measurable amounts of both, although at concentrations that were less than what would be expected in maternal urine. Sulbactam was also detected in breast milk after i.v. doses of 0.5–1 g every six hours.[57] Estimated exposure to the nursing infant of a mother receiving sulbactam was <1% of the typical oral dose; coupled with the poor absorption of the sodium salt, exposure to the nursing infant would be minimal.

Elimination. There are no reported qualitative or quantitative descriptions of sulbactam metabolites. The primary route of elimination of sulbactam is renal (Table 2). The high renal clearance suggests active renal tubular secretion, as with penicillins and cephalosporins.[45,46] Urine concentrations of sulbactam >200 μg/mL and ampicillin >400 μg/mL were measured after a single 500-mg dose of sultamicillin.[53]

Administration of sulbactam to surgical patients has produced varying results. The half-life in appendectomy patients was similar to that in healthy volunteers, with a slightly larger total clearance.[58] Another investigator reported a half-life of 0.97 hour in patients undergoing abdominal surgery.[51] Kager et al.[62,63] found longer half-lives of 1.8–2.2 hours in surgical patients but did not report the renal function of the older patient population (mean age, 72 years).

Elimination in postpartum women was similar to that in healthy volunteers.[57] In patients with gonorrhea, sulbactam had a half-life of 1.12 hours after the second of two 0.5-g i.m. doses.[74]

In preterm newborns tested at less than one to six days of age, the half-lives of sulbactam and ampicillin were 7.9 and 9.4 hours, respectively.[75] The oldest child, tested at six days of age, had a sulbactam half-life of two hours. Half-life prolongation at birth, with rapid reduction in the first week of life, is probably due to reduced renal function in premature newborns and is consistent with the pharmacokinetic profile of ampicillin. Evaluation in infants from 11 to 18 months has shown sulbactam and ampicillin half-lives of 0.92 and 0.83 hours, respectively. Total clearance in healthy children was comparable to that in adults. In subjects with cystic fibrosis total clearance was 2.2 times higher than that in healthy children.[60]

No accumulation of sulbactam with repetitive dosing has been noted in studies of healthy volunteers,[46,48] surgical patients,[58] and premature newborns.[75]

Wright and Wise[50] demonstrated a lengthening of sulbactam half-life from 1.1 hours in patients with glomerular filtration rates (GFRs) of 30–100 mL/min to 21.3 hours in patients with GFRs of <5 mL/min. This was associated with a rise in ampicillin half-life from 1.8 to 19 hours in the same two GFR ranges. The ratio of serum concentrations of the two drugs remained essentially constant over the entire range of GFRs, suggesting this combination may be a good choice for patients with renal insufficiency and supporting the similarities in their renal elimination.

Prolongation of the half-life of sulbactam by concomitant administration of probenecid has been demonstrated,[74,76] which further supports the concept of sulbactam's elimination by tubular secretion.

Clinical Trials

The first clinical trial of sulbactam (combined with ampicillin) was reported in 1982,[77] in 18 patients with non-life-threatening infections. All 11 patients found to have ampicillin-resistant pathogens responded favorably, and the drug was well tolerated. Based on these results, further evaluation of the combination was believed to be appropriate.

Gonococcal Infections. Although initial in vitro studies suggested that sulbactam had intrinsic activity against *Neisseria gonorrhoeae*, early trials using the drug alone were disappointing. Microbiologic cure rates of 30% and 55% were observed in two clinical trials in patients with uncomplicated gonococcal infections.[74,78]

Subsequent studies using injectable sulbactam plus ampicillin or penicillin G (with oral probenecid)[18,78–80] have shown much higher microbiologic cure rates ranging from 96 to 100%. In trials using the oral sultamicillin formulation, doses of sultamicillin ≥2 g with probenecid 1 g have resulted in cure rates of 94–97% in men and women with uncomplicated gonococcal urethritis.[81,82]

In general, microbiologic failures have been associated with MIC values for ampicillin or penicillin G in the higher range (≥0.25 μg/mL to 0.8 or 1.0 μg/mL). Penicillinase production has not altered outcome. The potential utility of sulbactam in uncomplicated gonococcal urethritis involves three considerations: (1) it is efficacious against penicillinase-producing strains in an oral regimen, whereas other current therapies require injections; (2) the injectable form may be a cost-effective alternative to spectinomycin and the third-generation cephalosporins in the management of infections caused by penicillinase-producing strains; (3) the emergence of penicillin- and spectinomycin-resistant strains of *N. gonorrhoeae* is particularly worrisome, and the possible utility of sulbactam in this situation may merit further investigation.[78]

Skin, Soft-Tissue, and Bone Infections. Trials have been conducted in patients with gram-positive and gram-negative, aerobic and anaerobic bacterial isolates. Two randomized, double-blind trials of sulbactam plus ampicillin versus clindamycin with or without an aminoglycoside in patients with serious soft-tissue infections have been reported.[83,84] Clinical outcome in the two treatment groups was similar, with success (defined as clinical cure or improvement) in 87–93% of sulbactam–ampicillin-treated patients and 80–81% of clindamycin–aminoglycoside-treated patients. Bacterial persistence, colonization, and superinfection were more common in the clindamycin–aminoglycoside groups. The sulbactam–ampicillin combination was judged safe and efficacious, but it was noted that this regimen did not always eliminate the need for aminoglycoside therapy.

In noncomparative open trials of sulbactam plus either ampicillin or penicillin G,[85,86] complete resolution or clinical and bacteriologic improvement was observed in 84–93% of patients. Isolation of penicillin- or ampicillin-resistant bacterial isolates did not alter clinical or microbiologic outcome.

In elderly diabetics with skin and soft-tissue infections, 47% of 15 courses of sulbactam plus ampicillin and 64% of 14 courses of flucloxacillin plus ampicillin resulted in cure or marked improvement.[87] The overall lower response rate in this study was attributed to the high prevalence of serious underlying disease, with the two regimens judged comparable.

Respiratory Infections. Randomized controlled trials of sulbactam in adults with upper- or lower-respiratory-tract infections are lacking. Some of the open trials in respiratory infections have had disappointing results, especially with regard to bacteriologic outcome. Patients have completed treatment courses but demonstrated persistence, reinfection, or colonization of organisms in sputum. Despite these disappointing bacteriologic results, many patients have demonstrated favorable responses on clinical criteria.

Pilot studies of sulbactam plus ampicillin (as sultamicillin or sulbactam pivoxyl plus bacampicillin) were conducted in patients with acute purulent exacerbations of chronic bronchitis.[55,73] Clinical resolution was observed in 63–86% of patients at the end of treatment, declining to 50–79% one week later.

Mehtar et al.[88] evaluated patients with intrathoracic infections (pneumonia, bronchopneumonia, empyema) in an open trial of intravenous sulbactam plus ampicillin, followed by oral sultamicillin. Ampicillin-resistant organisms were isolated from 13 of 14 patients. Clinical and bacteriologic response was seen in 93% of patients. One patient with *Klebsiella aerogenes* pneumonia developed *Ps. aeruginosa* colonization at the completion of therapy. Analysis of data showed the MIC for this organism had increased during sulbactam–ampicillin therapy.

In an open trial of sultamicillin in adults with acute maxillary sinusitis,[67] 11 of 13 patients had remission of all signs and symptoms.

Urinary-Tract Infections. Clinical trials involving patients with urinary-tract infections have yielded disappointing results. None of the studies reported to date has included patients with complicated or upper-urinary-tract infections. In an early trial, a single dose of sulbactam 1 g plus ampicillin 2 g i.v. was evaluated in adult women with uncomplicated urinary-tract infections.[89] At a seven-day follow-up examination, only 3 of 13 patients had sterile urine. In 8 of 10 patients whose treatment failed, cultures revealed organisms susceptible to both sulbactam and ampicillin, before and after therapy. The cause of clinical and bacteriologic failure in this trial was not determined.

Two regimens of sultamicillin were evaluated in elderly hospitalized patients with documented ampicillin-resistant lower-urinary-tract infections.[54] Clinical response was seen in 93–100% of patients. Bacteriologic evaluation showed short- and long-term cure rates of 59–79.5% and 19–54%, respectively. Reasons for failure included persistence of the original organism, relapse, and superinfection. The selection of an elderly, hospitalized patient population with known antimicrobial-resistant infection may partly explain the poor long-term response observed in this study.

The investigators of one study reported high prostate concentrations of sulbactam and suggested that sulbactam may be useful in treating prostatic infections, but this finding has not been confirmed by other investigators.[65]

Intra-abdominal Infections. A double-blind randomized trial compared sulbactam plus ampicillin versus clindamycin plus gentamicin in gangrenous or perforated appendicitis.[90] A significant difference in clinical response was observed, with a complication rate of 13% in the sulbactam–ampicillin group and no complications in the clindamycin–gentamicin group. Analysis of data in patients receiving sulbactam–ampicillin revealed isolation of *Pseudomonas* species in five of eight failures but in only 12 of 57 cures ($p = 0.01$). Susceptibility testing showed a strong association with recovery of sulbactam–ampicillin-resistant *Pseudomonas* species in patients whose treatment failed. The authors concluded that the combination of clindamycin plus gentamicin remained the treatment of choice in patients with perforated or gangrenous appendicitis.

Preliminary results of a trial comparing the same drug combinations in serious intra-abdominal infections showed clinical cure, improvement, and failure rates of 78, 9, and 13%, respectively, for sulbactam–ampicillin and 89, 8, and 3%, respectively, for clindamycin–gentamicin.[91] Another open, noncomparative trial of sulbactam–ampicillin in intra-abdominal infections demonstrated a clinical cure in 28 of 29 patients.[88] Microbiologic results in these two studies include a total absence of *Pseudomonas* isolation in one trial and a lack of synergy of sulbactam and ampicillin against *Pseudomonas* species in the other. Thus, although both authors concluded that the sulbactam–ampicillin regimen was efficacious, the findings in the Yellin et al.[90] study should be recognized.

Pelvic Infections. Clinical trials showing a high cure rate, equivalence to the comparative regimens, and a low incidence of adverse drug reactions support the potential usefulness of the sulbactam–ampicillin combination in gynecologic infections. Several small randomized trials[92–95] conducted in patients with a variety of acute, polymicrobial gynecologic infections were summarized by Hemsell.[96] Although prospective and randomized, the majority were unblinded, open trials. Sulbactam plus ampicillin was compared with several regimens, including clindamycin plus gentamicin, metronidazole plus gentamicin, or cefoxitin alone. Clinical and short-term microbiologic response rates were similar in all treatment groups, ranging from 92 to 96%. Persistence, reinfection, or relapse was caused predominantly by *Chlamydia trachomatis* (a pathogen resistant to sulbactam–ampicillin). Similar results were reported in an open trial of sulbactam–ampicillin in patients with pelvic infections.[97]

Surgical Prophylaxis. Prophylactic regimens of sulbactam and ampicillin have been evaluated in a spectrum of surgical patients. Studies in small numbers of elderly patients undergoing colorectal surgery have documented safety and efficacy in preventing postoperative infection. In two open trials,[62,63] a dose of sulbactam 1 g plus ampicillin 2 g was found to be more efficacious than 0.5 g of each drug in reducing the numbers of anaerobic and aerobic isolates. A comparative trial of sulbactam–ampicillin versus cefoxitin showed equivalent efficacy.[98] Overgrowth of yeast or *Pseudomonas* species or both occurred in all trials but was not thought to be clinically important.

Men undergoing transurethral surgery were given sulbactam plus ampicillin, or cefoxitin.[66] Evaluation at 1–3, 5–7, and 30 days showed a similar rate of infection (overall approximately 2.5–3%) in the two treatment groups.

The efficacy of prophylactic sulbactam–ampicillin has been studied in a variety of gynecologic procedures. In a placebo-controlled, double-blind trial in patients undergoing first-trimester abortion by vacuum aspiration, patients given a single dose of sulbactam–ampicillin had a significantly lower rate of early but not late infection.[99] Lack of efficacy in late infections was thought to be due to the high prevalence of *C. trachomatis* in these patients.

Houang et al.[100] evaluated prophylactic sulbactam plus ampicillin against metronidazole plus ampicillin in a placebo-controlled trial. Patients undergoing abdominal or vaginal hysterectomy who received either drug regimen had a significantly lower incidence of postoperative wound, pelvic, and vaginal infections and fever (2–4%) compared with those receiving placebo (24–30%). Between the two active drug regimens, there was no significant difference in postoperative infection. In other gynecologic procedures, a trend favoring drug prophylaxis was observed, but the difference was not significant.

Pediatric Infections. Studies of sulbactam have been performed in a variety of pediatric infectious diseases. A trial comparing sulbactam plus ampicillin versus metronidazole plus cefotaxime in children with acute appendicitis revealed no significant difference in efficacy between the two regimens.[64] In an open, randomized trial comparing sulbactam plus ampicillin versus chloramphenicol plus ampicillin in infants and children with bacterial meningitis, clinical failure and complication rates in the two groups were comparable.[72] Further, good in vitro activity was demonstrated, as assessed by cerebrospinal fluid bactericidal titers and indices.

In an open trial, a 95% clinical response rate was seen in patients treated for epiglottitis, primarily caused by *H. influenzae* type b.[101] This rate was judged comparable to that in previous studies using ampicillin plus chloramphenicol and better than ampicillin alone. In nine children with septic arthritis or osteomyelitis, or both, treatment with injectable sulbactam–ampicillin followed by oral sultamicillin was effective and well tolerated.[102] After an average of 33 days of therapy, all patients fulfilled criteria for clinical and microbiologic cure on both short-term (at the conclusion of therapy) and long-term (four to six months) evaluation. Peak serum bactericidal titers ranged from 1:8 to 1:512 on injectable therapy and 1:<4 to 1:256 on oral therapy.

Various ratios of sulbactam and ampicillin or penicillin G were evaluated in 23 children with urinary-tract infection, suppurating cervical adenitis, or lobar pneumonia.[103] There was no difference in clinical response among patients receiving sulbactam–ampicillin in ratios of 1:2 or 1:3 and those receiving sulbactam–penicillin G in ratios of 1:1.2 or 1:1.8.

Sultamicillin has been evaluated in patients with streptococcal pharyngitis,[104] acute otitis media with effusion,[105] and cystic fibrosis or other chronic pulmonary disease.[106] All studies demonstrated favorable clinical and microbiologic response, although patient populations were small. Poor drug tolerance because of diarrhea (42% of patients) and an unpalatable taste (22% of patients) limited the potential utility of sultamicillin in one trial.[105]

Adverse Effects and Drug Interactions

Sulbactam is generally well tolerated. A notable aspect of its adverse-effect profile is the lack of bleeding disorders and nephrotoxicity. Lees et al.[18] pooled data of 1287 patients from 39 therapeutic and 6 prophylactic trials, estimating an incidence of 10% for clinical adverse effects (e.g., pain on injection, diarrhea). The incidence of laboratory-test abnormalities was not specified, although liver-function abnormalities were seen in as many as 6.9%.

Adverse Reactions. The most common adverse effect was pain at the injection site, occurring in 4.5% of patients. This occurred primarily after i.m. injection, but phlebitis and pain may also occur with i.v. use. Pain on i.m. injection may be minimized by administration with 0.5% lidocaine hydrochloride.[18,74,79]

Among patients receiving oral sultamicillin, diarrhea is the most common and troublesome adverse effect, occurring in approximately 10–15% of patients. It may also be seen with i.v. or i.m. administration, with the pooled data of Lees et al.,[18] suggesting an incidence of 1.6% after i.v. or i.m. injection. The severity ranges from mild to severe. Most patients are able to continue treatment; their conditions improve during or shortly after completion of therapy. There was at least one reported case of diarrhea associated with *C. difficile* toxin,[67] requiring oral then i.v. vancomycin therapy. Other reported gastrointestinal adverse effects include nausea, vomiting, abdominal pain, dry mouth, and bitter taste.

As a β-lactam compound, sulbactam would be expected to demonstrate cross-reactivity in patients who are allergic to β-lactam antibiotics. Thus, it is contraindicated in patients with histories of hypersensitivity reactions to β lactams. Hypersensitivity reactions, including skin rash, urticaria, pruritus, fever, and anaphylaxis, have been observed. It should be recognized that it is impossible to distinguish allergic reactions to sulbactam from those to the β-lactam antibiotic. Lees et al.[18] noted skin disorders (type unspecified) in 1.2% of patients.

Reported central nervous system effects include dizziness, confusion, fatigue, malaise, headache, and lightheadedness. Other clinical adverse effects include fever, chills, tinnitus, tachycardia, hypertension, breathlessness, and chest pain or tightness. In studies using active drugs in comparative regimens, the incidence of these reactions was generally similar in the treatment groups.

Overgrowth of resistant organisms, including species of fungus (*Candida, Torulopsis*) and gram-negative aerobic bacilli (*Pseudomonas, Enterobacter, Klebsiella*), has been observed. Patients should be monitored for superinfections (usually *Candida* or *Pseudomonas*) during therapy.

Laboratory Abnormalities. In the pooled survey of Lees et al.,[18] the most frequent laboratory abnormalities were elevations of aspartate aminotransferase (formerly called SGOT) in 6.2% and alanine aminotransferase (formerly called SGPT) in 6.9% of patients. An association with intra-abdominal infections was noted, without relationship to duration of therapy or patient age. Elevated concentrations of bilirubin and alkaline phosphatase have also been reported. Most have been described as mild, although increases of 50% above baseline have been reported. Decreases in alanine aminotransferase, total bilirubin, and alkaline phosphatase have also been reported.

Most investigators have characterized liver function abnormalities as clinically unimportant and probably related to underlying disease in the patient. However, hepatotoxic effects of sulbactam were noted in early animal studies after prolonged high-dose therapy.

Early studies showed diffuse hepatocellular glycogen deposits in rats and dogs given high doses for prolonged periods.[107] This was associated with an elevation in liver enzymes and hepatomegaly. Exogenous glucagon challenge in dogs elicited no change in glucose mobilization after a single dose, but a blunted blood glucose response was seen after 35 days of treatment. Other aspects of carbohydrate metabolism were not altered. Histologic and chemical liver abnormalities were found to be related to dose and duration, with marked changes after doses of 800 mg/kg i.v. for 28–30 days. Recovery to baseline was seen 3–10 weeks after discontinuation of the drug. Clinical trials in humans were considered safe because much lower doses for shorter durations were anticipated. To date, similar deposits have not been reported in humans treated with sulbactam, although patients with pre-existing liver dysfunction have been excluded from the majority of trials.

Early clinical studies excluded patients with diabetes mellitus, hypoglycemia, or glycogen-storage disease because of the possible effect of sulbactam on glucose physiology. Chiodini et al.[87] studied the effect of sulbactam on glucose mobilization and regulation in patients with types I and II diabetes mellitus, concluding that sulbactam was unlikely to adversely affect diabetic control when given in standard doses for short to intermediate durations.

The most common hematologic abnormality has been eosinophilia. White blood cell counts have both increased and decreased during therapy, probably in relation to the underlying infection.

Use in Pregnancy. There are no studies evaluating the safety of sulbactam in pregnant or perinatal women. Genetic studies in animals showed no mutagenic activity at either the chromosomal or subchromosomal level. In an early study in rats given sulbactam 200–800 mg/kg i.m. daily, growth was partially inhibited in the mothers at the end of gestation, but no effect was observed on the remainder of the pregnancy, fertility, or lactation.[107] Offspring viability, survival, growth, and development were normal. Further, there were no drug-related abnormalities found during postmortem examination of the offspring.[107]

Drug Interactions. The combination of probenecid and sulbactam may result in higher serum concentrations and more prolonged elimination of sulbactam.[74,76]

Availability and Cost

Sulbactam is marketed under the trade name Unasyn as a combination of ampicillin and sulbactam. Vials or bottles contain either 1.5 g or 3 g, as ampicillin 1 g (as the sodium salt) plus sulbactam 0.5 g (as the sodium salt) or ampicillin 2 g plus sulbactam 1 g. The costs of the 1.5- and 3-g doses are $4.90 and $9.25, respectively.[a]

Sultamicillin remains in the research phase; submission of a new drug application is scheduled for 1988.[a]

Dosage and Administration

Sulbactam sodium–ampicillin sodium may be administered by i.v. or i.m. injection. For i.v. use, the dose can be infused slowly undiluted over at least 10–15 minutes or diluted to 50–100 mL and infused over 15–30 minutes. Adult doses of ampicillin 1–2 g plus sulbactam 0.5–1 g every six hours are advised, with a total daily dose of sulbactam no greater than 4 g. In patients with impaired renal function, the same dosage (in grams) may be given, using the guidelines shown in Table 4.

Table 4.
Dosing Guidelines for Sulbactam Sodium–Ampicillin Sodium in Patients with Impaired Renal Function[a]

Creatinine Clearance (mL/min/1.73 sq m)	Ampicillin or Sulbactam Half-life (hr)	Dosage Interval (hr)
≥30	1	6 or 8
15–29	5	12
5–14	9	24

[a] From reference 108.

FDA-Approved Labeling

Injectable sulbactam–ampicillin is indicated for skin and skin-structure infections caused by β-lactamase-producing strains of *Staph. aureus, E. coli,*[b] *Klebsiella* spp.,[b] *Proteus mirabilis,*[b] *B. fragilis,*[b] *Enterobacter* spp.,[b] and *A. calcoaceticus*[b]; intra-abdominal infections caused by β-lactamase-producing strains of *E. coli, Klebsiella* spp. (including *K. pneumoniae*[b]), *Enterobacter* spp.,[b] and *Bacteroides* spp. (including *B. fragilis*); and gynecologic infections caused by β-lactamase-producing strains of *E. coli*[b] and *Bacteroides* spp.[b] (including *B. fragilis*[b]).

Formulary Considerations

Sulbactam has demonstrated an ability to restore or enhance the activity of ampicillin, a safe, well-established β-lactam antibiotic. The combination appears to have its greatest potential use in the treatment of polymicrobial aerobic or anaerobic infections and in uncomplicated gonorrhea. Injectable sulbactam–ampicillin merits addition to hospital formularies for the management of these infections. However, because of the paucity of blinded, randomized, comparative trials, its ultimate place in the current spectrum of antibiotics is not clear. Potential limitations in the treatment of respiratory-tract and urinary-tract infections are suggested by clinical trials to date. The following aspects should be considered in formulary decisions:

1. Sulbactam has a low toxicity level.
2. In theory, sulbactam could become an alternative to aminoglycosides in treating gram-negative infections. However, its lack of efficacy against *Pseudomonas* species, both in vitro and in clinical trials, is a potentially important limitation.
3. The cost of an average daily dose (Unasyn 12 g, equivalent to sulbactam 4 g plus ampicillin 8 g) is $37. This is comparable to or less than that of other drugs used in polymicrobial infections, such as clindamycin or cefoxitin.[109] Sulbactam–ampicillin is thus a potentially cost-effective addition to hospital formularies.
4. If marketed, the sultamicillin formulation would represent a therapeutic advantage as an oral agent in penicillinase-producing uncomplicated gonococcal infections and as sequential therapy after intravenous treatment of infections requiring long-term therapy. The availability of an oral form would be an unusual feature; recently marketed extended-spectrum penicillins and cephalosporins are not available in oral form.

Conclusion

Sulbactam is a "suicide-type" β-lactamase inhibitor with minimal intrinsic antibacterial activity.

When combined with β-lactam antibiotics, the activity of the antibiotic is enhanced. Sulbactam joins clavulanic acid as the second "suicide-type" inhibitor to be commercially available. Both have activity against a broad spectrum of β-lactamase enzymes. Although less active on a weight basis than clavulanic acid, sulbactam has the advantageous properties of stability to hydrolysis, lack of enzyme induction, and ability to bind to penicillin-binding proteins. The novel oral form, sultamicillin, incorporates equimolar quantities of sulbactam and ampicillin in a readily absorbed mutual prodrug.

Clinical trials of sulbactam combined with ampicillin have demonstrated activity in a number of infectious diseases in both adults and children. The minimal toxicity of this drug makes it appealing for the treatment of gram-negative nonpseudomonal and anaerobic infections. By restoring or expanding the activity of older, well-established antibiotics, sulbactam offers a new approach to the management of bacterial infections. Its potential use in combination with other β-lactam antibiotics offers interesting prospects for the future.

[a] Kelly JP Jr, Pfizer Laboratories Division. Personal communication. 1987 May 29.

[b] Efficacy for such organisms in the labeled organ systems was studied in fewer than 10 infections.

References

1. Sabath LD, Elder HA, McCall CE et al. Synergistic combinations of penicillin in the treatment of bacteriuria. *N Engl J Med.* 1967; 277:232–8.
2. Wise R. Beta-lactamase inhibitors. *J Antimicrob Chemother.* 1982; 9(Suppl B):31–40.
3. English AR, Retsema JA, Girard AE et al. CP-45,899, a beta-lactamase inhibitor that extends the antibacterial spectrum of beta-lactams: initial bacteriological characterization. *Antimicrob Agents Chemother.* 1978; 14:414–9.
4. Mushinsky RF, Reynolds ML, Nicholson CA et al. Stability of sulbactam/ampicillin in diluents for parenteral administration. *Rev Infect Dis.* 1986; 8(Suppl 5):S523–S527.
5. Baltzer B, Binderup E, von Daehne W et al. Mutual prodrugs of beta-lactam antibiotics and beta-lactamase inhibitors. *J Antibiot.* 1980; 33:1183–92.
6. Sykes RB. The classification and terminology of enzymes that hydrolyze beta-lactam antibiotics. *J Infect Dis.* 1982; 145:762–5.
7. Hamilton-Miller JMT. Beta-lactamases and their clinical significance. *J Antimicrob Chemother.* 1982; 9(Suppl B):11–9.
8. Bauernfeind A. Classification of beta-lactamases. *Rev Infect Dis.* 1986; 8(Suppl 5):S470–S481.
9. Bush K, Sykes RB. Characterization and epidemiology of beta-lactamases. In: Peterson PK, Verhoef J, eds. The antimicrobial agents annual—2. New York, NY: Elsevier Science Publishing Co., Inc.; 1987:371–82.
10. Fu KP, Neu HC. Comparative inhibition of beta-lactamases by novel beta-lactam compounds. *Antimicrob Agents Chemother.* 1979; 15:171–6.
11. Retsema JA, English AR, Girard AE. CP-45,899 in combination with penicillin or ampicillin against penicillin-resistant *Staphylococcus, Haemophilus influenzae,* and *Bacteroides. Antimicrob Agents Chemother.* 1980; 17:615–22.
12. Bush K, Sykes RB. Beta-lactamase inhibitors in perspective. *J Antimicrob Chemother.* 1983; 11:97–107.
13. Labia R, Morand A, Lelievre V et al. Sulbactam: biochemical factors involved in its synergy with ampicillin. *Rev Infect Dis.* 1986; 8(Suppl 5):S496–S502.
14. Greenwood D, Eley A. In vitro evaluation of sulbactam, a penicillanic acid sulphone with beta-lactamase inhibitory properties. *J Antimicrob Chemother.* 1982; 10:117–23.
15. Acar JF, Minozzi C. Role of beta-lactamases in the resistance of gram-negative bacilli to beta-lactam antibiotics. *Rev Infect Dis.* 1986; 8(Suppl 5):S482–S486.
16. Aswapokee N, Neu HC. A sulfone beta-lactam compound which acts as a beta-lactamase inhibitor. *J Antibiot.* 1978; 31:1238–44.
17. Retsema JA, English AR, Girard A et al. Sulbactam/ampicillin: in vitro spectrum, potency, and activity in models of acute infection. *Rev Infect Dis.* 1986; 8(Suppl 5):S528–S534.
18. Lees L, Milson JA, Knirsch AK et al. Sulbactam plus ampicillin: interim review of efficacy and safety for therapeutic and prophylactic use. *Rev Infect Dis.* 1986; 8(Suppl 5):S644–S650.
19. Barry AL, Jones RN, Thornsberry C. Interpretive standards and quality control limits for susceptibility tests with ampicillin–sulbactam combination disks. *J Clin Microbiol.* 1984; 19:134–9.
20. Kazmierczak A, Duez JM, Pechinot A et al. In vitro bactericidal activity of sulbactam plus ampicillin against methicillin-resistant *Staphylococcus aureus. Rev Infect Dis.* 1986; 8(Suppl 5):S549–S554.
21. Kitzis MD, Gutmann L, Acar JF. In vitro susceptibility of *Nocardia asteroides* to 21 beta-lactam antibiotics, in combination with three beta-lactamase inhibitors, and its relationship to the beta-lactamase content. *J Antimicrob Chemother.* 1985; 15:23–30.
22. Wise R, Andrews JM, Bedford KA. Clavulanic acid and CP-45,899: a comparison of their in vitro activity in combination with penicillins. *J Antimicrob Chemother.* 1980; 6:197–206.
23. Fass RJ. Inconsistency of synergy between the beta-lactamase inhibitor CP-45,899 and beta-lactam antibiotics against multiply drug-resistant Enterobacteriaceae and *Pseudomonas* species. *Antimicrob Agents Chemother.* 1981; 19:361–3.
24. Bolivar R, Weaver SS, Bodey GP. Activity of beta-lactamase inhibitors in combination with new beta-lactam antibiotics against resistant gram-negative organisms. *Diagn Microbiol Infect Dis.* 1984; 2:255–60.
25. Aldridge KE, Sanders CV, Marier RL. Variation in the potentiation of beta-lactam antibiotic activity by clavulanic acid and sulbactam against multiply antibiotic-resistant bacteria. *J Antimicrob Chemother.* 1986; 17:463–9.
26. Philippon A, Riou JY, Guibourdenche M et al. Detection, distribution and inhibition of *Branhamella catarrhalis* beta-lactamases. *Drugs.* 1986; 31(Suppl 3):64–9.
27. Farmer T, Reading C. Inhibition of the beta-lactamases of *Branhamella catarrhalis* by clavulanic acid and other inhibitors. *Drugs.* 1986; 31(Suppl 3):70–8.
28. Jones BM, Hafiz S, Duerden BI. Susceptibility of *Haemophilus ducreyi* to ampicillin and sulbactam in vitro. *Antimicrob Agents Chemother.* 1986; 29:1110–2.
29. Fliegelman RM, Petrak RM, Goodman LJ et al. Comparative in vitro activities of twelve antimicrobial agents against *Campylobacter* species. *Antimicrob Agents Chemother.* 1985; 27:429–30.
30. Van der Auwera P, Scorneaux B. In vitro susceptibility of *Campylobacter jejuni* to 27 antimicrobial agents and various combinations of beta-lactams with clavulanic acid or sulbactam. *Antimicrob Agents Chemother.* 1985; 28:37–40.
31. Jones RN, Thornsberry C, Wilson HW et al. The in vitro activity of sulphones alone and in combination with ampicillin or amoxicillin against *Legionella pneumophila* and other *Legionella* spp. including beta-lactamase studies. *Diagn Microbiol Infect Dis.* 1985; 3:179–83.
32. Nord CE. Mechanisms of beta-lactam resistance in anaerobic bacteria. *Rev Infect Dis.* 1986; 8(Suppl 5):S543–S548.
33. Wexler HM, Harris B, Carter WT et al. In vitro efficacy of

sulbactam combined with ampicillin against anaerobic bacteria. *Antimicrob Agents Chemother.* 1985; 27:876–8.
34. Neu HC, Fu KP. Synergistic activity of piperacillin in combination with beta-lactamase inhibitors. *Antimicrob Agents Chemother.* 1980; 18:582–5.
35. Calderwood SB, Gardella A, Philippon AM et al. Effects of azlocillin in combination with clavulanic acid, sulbactam, and *N*-formimidoyl thienamycin against beta-lactamase-producing, carbenicillin-resistant *Pseudomonas aeruginosa. Antimicrob Agents Chemother.* 1982; 22:266–71.
36. Neu HC. Synergistic activity of mecillinam in combination with the beta-lactamase inhibitors clavulanic acid and sulbactam. *Antimicrob Agents Chemother.* 1982; 22:518–9.
37. Jones RN, Wilson HW, Thornsberry C et al. In vitro antimicrobial activity of cefoperazone–sulbactam combinations against 554 clinical isolates including a review and beta-lactamase studies. *Diagn Microbiol Infect Dis.* 1985; 3:489–99.
38. Fu KP, Neu HC. Synergistic activity of cefoperazone in combination with beta-lactamase inhibitors. *J Antimicrob Chemother.* 1981; 7:287–92.
39. Jones RN, Barry AL, Thornsberry C et al. The cefoperazone–sulbactam combination: in vitro qualities including beta-lactamase stability, antimicrobial activity, and interpretive criteria for disk diffusion tests. *Am J Clin Pathol.* 1985; 84:496–504.
40. Souza Dias MB, Jacobus NV, Tally FP. In vitro activity of cefoperazone–sulbactam against *Bacteroides* species. *J Antimicrob Chemother.* 1986; 18:467–71.
41. Crosby MA, Gump DW. Activity of cefoperazone and two beta-lactamase inhibitors, sulbactam and clavulanic acid, against *Bacteroides* spp. correlated with beta-lactamase production. *Antimicrob Agents Chemother.* 1982; 22:398–405.
42. Yu PKW, Washington JA. Bactericidal activity of cefoperazone with CP-45,899 against large inocula of beta-lactamase-producing *Haemophilus influenzae. Antimicrob Agents Chemother.* 1981; 20:63–5.
43. Fu KP, Kimble EF, Zoganas H et al. Synergistic activity of cefsulodin combined with cefoxitin and sulbactam against *Bacteroides* species. *J Antimicrob Chemother.* 1984; 13:257–65.
44. Lewis GP, Jusko WJ. Pharmacokinetics of ampicillin in cirrhosis. *Clin Pharmacol Ther.* 1975; 18:475–84.
45. Rogers HJ, Bradbrook ID, Morrison PJ et al. Pharmacokinetics and bioavailability of sultamicillin estimated by high performance liquid chromatography. *J Antimicrob Chemother.* 1983; 11:435–45.
46. Foulds G, Stankewich JP, Marshall DC. Pharmacokinetics of sulbactam in humans. *Antimicrob Agents Chemother.* 1983; 23:692–9.
47. Brown RM, Wise R, Andrews JM et al. Comparative pharmacokinetics and tissue penetration of sulbactam and ampicillin after concurrent intravenous administration. *Antimicrob Agents Chemother.* 1982; 21:565–7.
48. Hartley S, Wise R. A three-way crossover study to compare the pharmacokinetics and acceptability of sultamicillin at two dose levels with that of ampicillin. *J Antimicrob Chemother.* 1982; 10:49–55.
49. Ginsburg CM, McCracken GH, Olsen K et al. Pharmacokinetics and bactericidal activity of sultamicillin in infants and children. *J Antimicrob Chemother.* 1985; 15:345–51.
50. Wright N, Wise R. The elimination of sulbactam alone and combined with ampicillin in patients with renal dysfunction. *J Antimicrob Chemother.* 1983; 11:583–7.
51. Wise R, Donovan IA, Andrews JM et al. Penetration of sulbactam and ampicillin into peritoneal fluid. *Antimicrob Agents Chemother.* 1983; 24:290–2.
52. English AR, Girard D, Haskell SL. Pharmacokinetics of sultamicillin in mice, rats, and dogs. *Antimicrob Agents Chemother.* 1984; 25:599–602.
53. Foulds G, Stankewich JP, Knirsch AK et al. The pharmacokinetics of sultamicillin in man. Paper presented to 22nd Interscience Conference on Antimicrobial Agents and Chemotherapy. Miami Beach, FL: 1982 Oct 5. Abstract 519.
54. Ball AP, Fox C, Ghosh D. Sultamicillin (CP-49,952): evaluation of two dosage schedules in urinary infection. *J Antimicrob Chemother.* 1984; 14:395–401.
55. Davies BI, Maesen FPV, van Noord JA. Clinical, bacteriological and pharmacokinetic results from an open trial of sultamicillin in patients with acute exacerbations of chronic bronchitis. *J Antimicrob Chemother.* 1984; 13:161–70.
56. Foulds G. Pharmacokinetics of sulbactam/ampicillin in humans: a review. *Rev Infect Dis.* 1986; 8(Suppl 5):S503–S511.
57. Foulds G, Miller RD, Knirsch AK et al. Sulbactam kinetics and excretion into breast milk in postpartum women. *Clin Pharmacol Ther.* 1985; 38:692–6.
58. Gill MA, Kern JW, Chenella FC et al. Pharmacokinetics of parenteral sulbactam in patients with appendicitis. *Ther Drug Monit.* 1984; 6:428–31.
59. Aminopenicillins. In: McEvoy GK, ed. American Hospital Formulary Service Drug Information 87. Bethesda, MD: American Society of Hospital Pharmacists, Inc; 1987:235–48.
60. Schaad UB, Guenin K, Straehl P. Single-dose pharmacokinetics of intravenous sulbactam in pediatric patients. *Rev Infect Dis.* 1986; 8(Suppl 5):S512–S517.
61. Morris DL, Ubhi CS, Robertson CS et al. Biliary pharmacokinetics of sulbactam plus ampicillin in humans. *Rev Infect Dis.* 1986; 8(Suppl 5):S589–S592.
62. Kager L, Liljeqvist L, Malmborg AS et al. Effects of ampicillin plus sulbactam on bowel flora in patients undergoing colorectal surgery. *Antimicrob Agents Chemother.* 1982; 22:208–12.
63. Kager L, Malmborg AS, Sjostedt S et al. Concentrations of ampicillin plus sulbactam in serum and intestinal mucosa and effects on the colonic microflora in patients undergoing colorectal surgery. *Eur J Clin Microbiol.* 1983; 2:559–63.
64. Foster MC, Kapila L, Morris DL et al. A randomized comparative study of sulbactam plus ampicillin vs. metronidazole plus cefotaxime in the management of acute appendicitis in children. *Rev Infect Dis.* 1986; 8(Suppl 5):S634–S638.
65. Schwiersch U, Lang N, Wildfeuer DA. Concentration of sulbactam and ampicillin in serum and the myometrium. *Drugs.* 1986; 31(Suppl 2):26–8.
66. Dorflinger T, Madsen PO. Antibiotic prophylaxis in transurethral surgery: a comparison of sulbactam–ampicillin and cefoxitin. *Infection.* 1985; 13:66–9.
67. Jones S, Yu VL, Johnson JT et al. Pharmacokinetic and therapeutic trial of sultamicillin in acute sinusitis. *Antimicrob Agents Chemother.* 1985; 28:832–3.
68. Reilly JS, Kim HK, Rohn DD. Concentrations of sultamicillin in serum and middle ear fluid of children with chronic otitis media with effusion. *Ann Otol Rhinol Laryngol.* 1983; 92(Suppl 107):44–5.
69. Houang ET, Colley N, Chapman M. Penetration of sulbactam–ampicillin and clavulanic acid–amoxicillin into the pelvic peritoneum. *Antimicrob Agents Chemother.* 1985; 28:165–6.
70. Hanninen P, Rossi T. Penetration of sulbactam into cerebrospinal fluid of patients with viral meningitis or without meningitis. *Rev Infect Dis.* 1986; 8(Suppl 5):S609–S611.
71. Stahl JP, Bru JP, Fredj G et al. Penetration of sulbactam into the cerebrospinal fluid of patients with bacterial meningitis receiving ampicillin therapy. *Rev Infect Dis.* 1986; 8(Suppl 5):S612–S616.
72. Rodriguez WJ, Khan WN, Puig J et al. Sulbactam/ampicillin vs chloramphenicol/ampicillin for the treatment of meningitis in infants and children. *Rev Infect Dis.* 1986; 8(Suppl 5):S620–S629.
73. Davies BI, Maesen FPV, Jevons S et al. Combination of sulbactam pivoxyl and bacampicillin in acute exacerbations of chronic bronchitis. *J Antimicrob Chemother.* 1982; 10:445–52.
74. Caine VA, Foulds G, Handsfield HH. Therapeutic trial and pharmacokinetics of sulbactam for uncomplicated gonorrhea in men. *Antimicrob Agents Chemother.* 1984; 26:683–5.
75. Sutton AM, Turner TL, Cockburn F et al. Pharmacokinetic

study of sulbactam and ampicillin administered concomitantly by intraarterial or intravenous infusion in the newborn. *Rev Infect Dis*. 1986; 8(Suppl 5):S518–S522.
76. Emmerson AM, Cox DA, Lees LJ. Pharmacokinetics of sulbactam and ampicillin following oral administration of sultamicillin with probenecid. *Eur J Clin Microbiol*. 1983; 2:340–4.
77. Plouffe JF. Treatment of infections caused by ampicillin-resistant pathogens with a combination of ampicillin and CP-45,899. *Antimicrob Agents Chemother*. 1982; 21:519–20.
78. Crider SR, Kilpatrick ME, Harrison WO et al. A comparison of penicillin G plus a beta-lactamase inhibitor (sulbactam) with spectinomycin for treatment of urethritis caused by penicillinase-producing *Neisseria gonorrhoeae*. *Sex Transm Dis*. 1984; 11:314–7.
79. Houang ET. Single dose intramuscular sulbactam and ampicillin in treating acute uncomplicated gonorrhoea. *Genitourin Med*. 1985; 61:209. Letter.
80. Kim JH, Choi KH, Kim YT et al. Treatment of infections due to multiresistant *Neisseria gonorrhoeae* with sulbactam/ampicillin. *Rev Infect Dis*. 1986; 8(Suppl 5):S599–S603.
81. Atia WA, Emmerson AM, Holmes D. Sultamicillin in the treatment of gonorrhoea caused by penicillin sensitive and penicillinase producing strains of *Neisseria gonorrhoeae*. *Br J Vener Dis*. 1983; 59:293–7.
82. Farthing C, Thin RN, Smith S et al. Two regimens of sultamicillin in treating uncomplicated gonorrhoea. *Genitourin Med*. 1985; 61:44–7.
83. Stromberg BV, Reines HD, Hunt P. Comparative clinical study of sulbactam and ampicillin and clindamycin and tobramycin in infections of soft tissues. *Surg Gynecol Obstet*. 1986; 162:575–8.
84. Reinhardt JF, Johnston L, Ruane P et al. A randomized, double-blind comparison of sulbactam/ampicillin and clindamycin for the treatment of aerobic and aerobic–anaerobic infections. *Rev Infect Dis*. 1986; 8(Suppl 5):S569–S575.
85. Nichols RL, Smith JW, Adinolfi MF et al. Inhibition of beta-lactamase-induced resistance in soft-tissue infections. *Arch Surg*. 1985; 120:36–42.
86. Loffler L, Bauernfeind A, Keyl W et al. An open, comparative study of sulbactam plus ampicillin vs. cefotaxime as initial therapy for serious soft tissue and bone and joint infections. *Rev Infect Dis*. 1986; 8(Suppl 5):S593–S598.
87. Chiodini PL, Toop MJ, Odugbesan O et al. Sulbactam/ampicillin: effects on glucose metabolism in diabetics with soft tissue infection. *J Antimicrob Chemother*. 1985; 16:643–7.
88. Mehtar S, Croft RJ, Hilas A. A non-comparative study of parenteral ampicillin and sulbactam in intra-thoracic and intra-abdominal infections. *J Antimicrob Chemother*. 1986; 17:389–96.
89. Bailey RR, Peddie BA. Single dose sulbactam/ampicillin for uncomplicated urinary tract infections. *NZ Med J*. 1985; 98:21. Letter.
90. Yellin AE, Heseltine PNR, Berne TV et al. The role of *Pseudomonas* species in patients treated with ampicillin and sulbactam for gangrenous and perforated appendicitis. *Surg Gynecol Obstet*. 1985; 161:303–7.
91. Study Group on Intraabdominal Infections. A randomized controlled trial of ampicillin plus sulbactam vs. gentamicin plus clindamycin in the treatment of intraabdominal infections: a preliminary report. *Rev Infect Dis*. 1986; 8(Suppl 5):S583–S588.
92. Gunning J. A comparison of parenteral sulbactam/ampicillin versus clindamycin/gentamicin in the treatment of pelvic inflammatory disease. *Drugs*. 1986; 31(Suppl 2):14–7.
93. Senft HH, Stiglmayer R, Eibach HW et al. Sulbactam/ampicillin versus cefoxitin in the treatment of obstetric and gynaecological infections. *Drugs*. 1986; 31(Suppl 2):18–21.
94. Bruhat MA, Pouly JL, LeBoedec G et al. Treatment of acute salpingitis with sulbactam/ampicillin: comparison with cefoxitin. *Drugs*. 1986; 31(Suppl 2):7–10.
95. Crombleholme W, Landers D, Ohm-Smith M et al. Sulbactam/ampicillin versus metronidazole/gentamicin in the treatment of severe pelvic infections. *Drugs*. 1986; 31(Suppl 2):11–3.
96. Hemsell DL. Sulbactam/ampicillin for treatment of polymicrobial pelvic infections. *Drugs*. 1986; 31(Suppl 2):22–5.
97. Giamarellou H, Trouvas G, Aviami A et al. Efficacy of sulbactam plus ampicillin in gynecologic infections. *Rev Infect Dis*. 1986; 8(Suppl 5):S579–S582.
98. De la Hunt MN, Karran SJ, Chir M. Sulbactam/ampicillin compared with cefoxitin for chemoprophylaxis in elective colorectal surgery. *Dis Colon Rectum*. 1986; 29:157–9.
99. Krohn KT. Effect of prophylactic administration of sulbactam/ampicillin on the rate of postoperative endometritis after first-trimester abortion. *Rev Infect Dis*. 1986; 8(Suppl 5):S576–8.
100. Houang ET, Watson C, Howell R et al. Ampicillin combined with sulbactam or metronidazole for single-dose chemoprophylaxis in major gynaecological surgery. *J Antimicrob Chemother*. 1984; 14:529–35.
101. Wald E, Reilly JS, Bluestone CD et al. Sulbactam/ampicillin in the treatment of acute epiglottitis in children. *Rev Infect Dis*. 1986; 8(Suppl 5):S617–S619.
102. Aronoff SC, Scoles PV, Makley JT et al. Efficacy and safety of sequential treatment with parenteral sulbactam/ampicillin and oral sultamicillin for skeletal infections in children. *Rev Infect Dis*. 1986; 8(Suppl 5):S639–S643.
103. Syriopoulou V, Bitsi M, Theodoridis C et al. Clinical efficacy of sulbactam/ampicillin in pediatric infections caused by ampicillin-resistant or penicillin-resistant organisms. *Rev Infect Dis*. 1986; 8(Suppl 5):S630–S633.
104. Aronoff SC, Klinger JD, O'Brien CA et al. A double-blinded comparative study of sultamicillin and potassium penicillin V in the treatment of childhood streptococcal pharyngitis. *J Antimicrob Chemother*. 1984; 14:261–5.
105. Kaleida PH, Bluestone CD, Blatter MM et al. Sultamicillin (ampicillin–sulbactam) in the treatment of acute otitis media in children. *Ped Infect Dis*. 1986; 5:33–8.
106. Pressler T, Pedersen SS, Christiansen L et al. Sultamicillin—a new antibiotic in the treatment of persistent lower respiratory tract infections caused by *Haemophilus influenzae*. *J Antimicrob Chemother*. 1986; 17:529–33.
107. Pfizer Inc. Investigators reference manual, sulbactam parenteral. Groton, CT: Pfizer Inc; 1981.
108. Pfizer Inc. Unasyn package insert. New York, NY; 1987 Aug.
109. Ampicillin/sulbactam (Unasyn). *Med Lett Drugs Ther*. 1987; 29:79–81.

Research

Pharmacokinetics of leucovorin calcium after intravenous, intramuscular, and oral administration

BRIAN W. MCGUIRE, LUISA L. SIA, PHILIP T. LEESE, MANUEL L. GUTIERREZ, AND E. L. ROBERT STOKSTAD

Abstract: The pharmacokinetics of leucovorin was evaluated after intravenous, intramuscular, and oral administration in a randomized crossover study of 37 healthy men.

A single 25-mg dose of leucovorin calcium was administered intravenously, intramuscularly, or orally to the subjects. Blood samples were obtained immediately before and at 13 time points up to 24 hours after the leucovorin dose. The three treatment phases were separated by one-week intervals. Bioavailability was assessed by measuring over 24 hours the blood concentrations of total folates, the parent compound 5-formyltetrahydrofolate, and the metabolite 5-methyltetrahydrofolate, using differential microbiologic assays with *Lactobacillus casei* and *Streptococcus faecalis*.

Both intravenous and intramuscular administration produced rapid increases in serum concentrations of biologically active folates; these rises were sustained over time and were still detectable at 24 hours after drug administration. The bioavailability of intravenous and intramuscular doses was comparable based on area under the serum concentration–time curve, although for intramuscular administration, the peak concentration was lower and the time to peak concentration was longer. The initial rise in serum folate with intravenous and intramuscular dosing represented 5-formyltetrahydrofolate; this fell concomitantly with the appearance of 5-methyltetrahydrofolate. Oral leucovorin was 92% bioavailable compared with intravenous administration and produced a predictably different pattern of circulating folates, 5-methyltetrahydrofolate being the predominant form. Terminal elimination half-life, apparent volume of distribution, and clearance of total folate were not significantly different among the three treatments.

Based on measured serum concentrations of total reduced folates, the bioavailability of leucovorin calcium is similar after intramuscular and intravenous administration; oral administration of leucovorin calcium produces a distinct pattern of serum folate concentrations, but the percentage of drug available is comparable to that with intravenous and intramuscular administration.

Index terms: Aromatic elixir; Blood levels; Drug administration routes; Drugs, availability; Drugs, body distribution; Equivalency; Excretion; Half-life; Leucovorin; Leucovorin calcium; Metabolism; Methyltetrahydrofolate; Pharmacokinetics; Vitamins; Water for injection
Clin Pharm. 1988; 7:52–8

Leucovorin, also known as folinic acid, citrovorum factor, or 5-formyltetrahydrofolate (5-formyl-THF), is one of several biologically active forms of the reduced vitamin folic acid. Various dosage forms of leucovorin calcium are commercially available and are indicated for the treatment of certain folic acid deficiencies but are used primarily to counteract the hematologic toxicities of folic acid antagonists such as methotrexate.

The various active forms of tetrahydrofolate play an integral role in single-carbon transfers between a variety of metabolites. The net effect of leucovorin administration, whether oral or by injection, is expansion of the body's total reduced folate pool and subsequent use in many biochemical processes including de novo nucleotide synthesis, amino acid metabolism, and other reactions involving one-carbon donors and acceptors.

BRIAN W. MCGUIRE, PH.D., is Project Manager, Clinical Research Department, Alpha Therapeutic Corporation, Los Angeles, CA. LUISA L. SIA, PH.D., is Senior Research Statistician, Department of Statistical Design and Analysis, Medical Research Division, American Cyanamid Company, Pearl River, NY. PHILIP T. LEESE, M.D., is Medical Director, Quincy Research Center, Kansas City, MO. MANUEL L. GUTIERREZ, M.D., is Associate Director, Department of Clinical Development, Lederle Laboratories Division, American Cyanamid Company. E. L. ROBERT STOKSTAD, PH.D., is Professor Emeritus, Department of Nutritional Sciences, University of California, Berkeley.

Address reprint requests to Professional Medical Services, Lederle Laboratories, North Middletown Rd., Pearl River, NY 10965.

The technical work of D. Caesar, J. Eatherton, and S. Meachum is acknowledged.

Sponsored by the Department of Clinical Development, Lederle Laboratories Division of American Cyanamid.

Copyright © 1988, American Society of Hospital Pharmacists, Inc. All rights reserved. 0278-2677/88/0101-0052$01.75.

In the context of leucovorin "rescue" of methotrexate, by providing reduced folates, leucovorin bypasses the enzymatic block at dihydrofolate reductase that methotrexate elicits. As a whole, however, competitive and noncompetitive mechanisms have been implicated in the rescue phenomenon by leucovorin at the enzymatic and transport levels.[1]

Preclinical studies on the potentiation of fluorouracil by reduced folates have been conducted, and early clinical trials using high doses (up to 500 mg/sq m) of leucovorin calcium are in progress.[2,3] The active metabolite of fluorouracil, 5-fluorodeoxyuridilic acid, competitively inhibits the folate-requiring enzyme thymidylate synthesis, which functions in nucleic acid synthesis. When high concentrations of the reduced folate cofactor are present, the enzyme is sequestered in an inactive covalent ternary complex with the cofactor and 5-fluorodeoxyuridilic acid.[2]

This study was designed to examine the pharmacokinetics of leucovorin after intravenous, intramuscular, and oral administration in healthy men.

Methods

Drug Administration and Sample Collection. A total of 42 healthy adult male volunteers participated in the randomized, three-way crossover study; of these, 36 were original subjects, and 6 were dropout replacements. The study was approved by the institutional review committee of Quincy Research Center. All subjects gave written informed consent before participation.

Subjects were screened for inclusion by means of a medical history, a physical examination, and a battery of laboratory tests including blood chemistries, hematology, and urinalysis. The mean age of the 42 subjects was 29 years (range, 20–42 years); body weight averaged 71 kg (range, 56–89 kg).

The subjects fasted from the evening before until four hours after administration of 25 mg of leucovorin (as the free acid) the next morning. Leucovorin calcium cryodesiccated powder, a racemic mixture of the D,L-diastereoisomers of the compound, was used. The injectable drug (Leucovorin Calcium for Injection, Lederle, lot 745-305) was reconstituted with bacteriostatic water for injection to a final concentration of leucovorin free acid 10 mg/mL. The cryodesiccated powder for oral administration (Leucovorin Calcium for Oral Solution, Lederle, lot 4700-81-D01) was reconstituted with Aromatic Elixir, USP, to a final concentration of 1 mg/mL. The intramuscular injection (2.5 mL) was administered into the gluteus maximus muscle. The intravenous bolus injection (also 2.5 mL) was administered via a peripheral arm vein. The oral dose (25 mL) was followed by 215 mL of water to rinse the medication cup and facilitate total ingestion. As a match for this liquid consumption, the subjects receiving leucovorin by injection were given 240 mL of water orally.

Blood samples (10 mL each) were obtained immediately before and at 10, 20, 30, and 45 minutes and at 1, 1.5, 2, 2.5, 3, 5, 8, 12, and 24 hours after drug administration. The three treatment phases were separated by one-week intervals.

The whole-blood samples were collected into red-top Vacutainer tubes (Terumo Medical Corporation, Elkton, MD), allowed to clot fully, and then centrifuged at 4 °C (2500 rpm) for 15 minutes. The sera were decanted into Sarstedt polypropylene screw-top tubes (Sarstedt Inc., Princeton, NJ), to which sodium ascorbate (as an antioxidant) was added, to achieve a final concentration of 5 mg of ascorbate per milliliter of serum. The samples were stored at −10 °C to −20 °C.

Assay Procedures. Reduced folates in the serum samples were measured through growth response of two folate-dependent microorganisms, *Lactobacillus casei* and *Streptococcus faecalis.* The bacterium *L. casei* displays a growth response to the natural L-stereoisomer of all known pteroylmonoglutamates (unreduced folic acid and all oxidation levels of tetrahydrofolate); *Strep. faecalis* responds to all of these but 5-methyl-THF, one major metabolite of the parent compound leucovorin (5-formyl-THF). Since plasma folate is almost exclusively reduced tetrahydrofolate (predominantly 5-methyl-THF), unreduced folic acid being a very minor constituent, the *L. casei* activity alone measures total reduced folate. The difference between *L. casei* and *Strep. faecalis* activities corresponds to 5-methyl-THF, and the *Strep. faecalis* growth-promoting form itself represents predominantly 5-formyl-THF. The various other derivatives of tetrahydrofolate (for example, 5,10-methylene-THF and 5,10-methenyl-THF) represent different oxidation states of the single-carbon moiety and are intracellular coenzyme forms not normally found in plasma.

Lactobacillus casei ATCC 7469 and *Streptococcus faecalis* ATCC 8043 were obtained from the American Type Culture Collection, maintained in stab cultures, and transferred to the liquid inoculum media as required. The glycerol-cryoprotected inoculum was prepared according to the procedure of Wilson and Horne.[4] The assay medium was based on that in the general procedure of Waters and Mollin[5] and modified as described by Tamura et al.,[6] by the use of an enzymic casein hydrolysate as the amino acid source (Roberts and Snell[7]).

The sera were extracted by autoclaving for 10 minutes at 105 °C a 1:20 dilution in 0.05 M phosphate, pH 5.7, containing ascorbic acid 1.5 mg/mL. The folate standard used was 5-formyltetrahydrofolate, which promotes equal growth of both *L. casei* and *Strep. faecalis.* This was prepared from folinic acid calcium salt (Sigma Chemicals, St. Louis, MO) and was standardized by ultraviolet spectrophotometry using the molecular extinction coefficient of 28,200 at 282 nm for 5-formyl-THF at pH 13. Results were expressed as quantities of 5-formyl-THF (molecular weight, 473). The general procedures for the microbiological assay have been described previously.[6]

The 5-formyl-THF standard response curve included six concentrations of 5-formyl-THF, ranging from 0.062 ng/mL to 2 ng/mL per 5-mL tube of growth medium. This concentration range corresponded to five 1:2 serial dilutions. Unknown samples and the standard serum extract (after appropriate preliminary dilutions) were diluted in a similar manner to give six dilutions. By using this wide range of dilutions, it was possible to get at least three tubes on the workable part of the response curve.

The limits of sensitivity of these microbiologic assays extend down to approximately 0.3 ng of folate per milliliter of serum (6×10^{-10} M). The reproducibility was measured by determining the standard deviation and coefficient of variation (CV) for 250-ng/mL standard serum extracts, which were included with each day's assay. This standard extract was prepared by adding 0.025 mg of D,L-5-formyl-THF to 100 mL of a pooled sample of serum. This provided 250 ng/mL of 5-formyl-THF in addition to the endogenous folate present (approximately 10 ng/mL). This pooled serum was extracted in a 1:20 dilution with buffer using the same procedure used for subjects' serum samples. Aliquots of the extract were frozen and stored until used. For the *L. casei* assay the CV was 4.9%; for the *Strep. faecalis* assay the CV was 5.6%. The average (±S.D.) measured concentration of 5-formyl-THF in the standard serum extracts ($n = 102$) was 263 ± 13.6 ng/mL.

Data Analysis. The three serum folate fractions studied included total folates (*L. casei* activity), 5-formyl-THF or leucovorin (*Strep. faecalis* activity), and the major metabolite 5-methyl-THF (the arithmetic difference of the two). For all samples obtained after leucovorin administration, the concentrations were adjusted for nonzero baseline values by subtracting the predose concentration value from each measured value. Pharmacokinetic variables calculated from the serum folate data included area under the serum concentration–time curve from time zero to 24 hours (AUC_{0-24}) and from time zero to infinity ($AUC_{0-\infty}$), peak concentration (C_{max}), time to peak concentration (t_{max}), terminal elimination half-life ($t_{1/2}$), apparent volume of distribution (V), and total clearance (CL).

The terminal elimination rate constant (k) was computed using the last three nonzero concentrations of the baseline-adjusted data. Least-squares regression technique was applied to the log transformation of these data. When one or more of the 8-, 12-, or 24-hour time points were below quantifiable limits of the assay, k was not calculated. Terminal elimination half-life was calculated as $t_{1/2} = ln(2)/k$. The trapezoidal rule was used in computing AUC_{0-24}. The AUC extrapolation to infinity was calculated as follows:

$$AUC_{0-\infty} = AUC_{0-t} + C_t/k$$

where C_t = the last detectable serum concentration at time t, usually 24 hours. When the baseline-adjusted concentration at 8, 12, or 24 hours was below detection, the AUC_{0-24} value was used for $AUC_{0-\infty}$.

Apparent volume of distribution was calculated for each subject as $V = CL/k$, where CL = dose/$AUC_{0-\infty}$. Since leucovorin consists of equal amounts of the D,L-diastereoisomers (of which only the latter is biologically active and detectable by the microbiologic assay), dose in these calculations was one half that actually administered. Apparent absolute bioavailability (F) of the oral dose was computed as the following ratio:

$$F = AUC_{0-\infty_{oral}}/AUC_{0-\infty_{i.v.}}$$

Crossover analysis of variance (ANOVA) was used to compare the three treatments; the linear model included treatment route, period, and subject as factors. Pairwise comparisons were carried out using Tukey's least-significant-difference t test with the ANOVA error term, which took into account period and subject variability. The a priori level of significance for all comparisons was $p < 0.05$.

The statistical power of this study for detecting a 20% difference in $AUC_{0-\infty}$ between treatments at the 5% alpha level was greater than 99% for all three folate fractions (total, 5-formyl-THF, and 5-methyl-THF).

Results

Of the 42 study participants, 34 completed all three treatment phases and 3 completed two treatment phases; data from these 37 subjects were analyzed. Of 108 sets of folate concentration data, 106 had detectable total folate concentrations through 24 hours after the dose. Inspection of the log serum concentration–time curves showed a biphasic decline in serum folate concentrations, with evidence of an earlier phase at three to eight hours. Only the terminal elimination half-life was calculated. Mean pharmacokinetic values for the three folate fractions after intravenous, intramuscular, and oral administration of leucovorin calcium are shown in Table 1.

As illustrated in Figure 1, the instantaneous rise in total folates after intravenous administration of leucovorin calcium represented predominantly the parent 5-formyl-THF, peaking at 1259 ng/mL. The sharp drop of plasma 5-formyl-THF in the first hour coincided with the appearance of the metabolite 5-methyl-THF, which after one hour became

Table 1.
Leucovorin Pharmacokinetics after Intravenous, Intramuscular, and Oral Administration[a,b]

Folate Fraction	C_{max} (ng/mL)[c]	t_{max} (min)[d]	$t_{1/2}$ (hr)[e]	AUC_{0-24} (ng·hr/mL)[f]	$AUC_{0-\infty}$ (ng·hr/mL)[g,h]	CL (mL/min)	V (L)[e]
Intravenous Leucovorin Calcium[i]							
Total folates	1259 ± 205	10 ± 0	6.6 ± 2.1[j]	2252 ± 409	2345 ± 444	91.2 ± 17.6	50.3 ± 17.5[j]
5-Formyl-THF	1206 ± 211	10 ± 0	9.3 ± 2.8[k]	780 ± 160	792 ± 162	270 ± 56.1	221 ± 82.5[k]
5-Methyl-THF	258 ± 55	78 ± 42	6.5 ± 2.3[j]	1477 ± 327	1563 ± 366	...	...
Intramuscular Leucovorin Calcium[l]							
Total folates	436 ± 123	52 ± 36	6.5 ± 2.0[k]	2274 ± 427	2392 ± 489	91.0 ± 19.4	49.4 ± 14.9[j]
5-Formyl-THF	360 ± 114	28 ± 9	8.8 ± 3.5[j]	733 ± 180	759 ± 212	292 ± 75.8	218 ± 83.2[k]
5-Methyl-THF	226 ± 52	169 ± 54	6.4 ± 2.0[k]	1547 ± 348	1649 ± 406	...	...
Oral Leucovorin Calcium[i]							
Total folates	393 ± 96	140 ± 32	6.0 ± 1.9[k]	2063 ± 587	2149 ± 612	...	...
5-Formyl-THF	51 ± 50	73 ± 35	9.5 ± 4.6[m]	135 ± 80	140 ± 81	...	...
5-Methyl-THF	367 ± 87	142 ± 29	6.0 ± 1.9[k]	1929 ± 542	2012 ± 567	...	...

[a] All data are reported as mean ± S.D.

[b] C_{max} = peak concentration; t_{max} = time to peak concentration; $t_{1/2}$ = terminal elimination half-life; AUC_{0-24} and $AUC_{0-\infty}$ = area under the serum concentration–time curve from time zero to 24 hours and from time zero to infinity, respectively; CL = total clearance; V = apparent volume of distribution.

[c] Significant difference in C_{max} values for all three folate fractions (overall ANOVA). Significant difference between intravenous and intramuscular values for total folates and 5-formyl-THF and between intravenous and oral values for all three folate fractions (paired comparison using least-squares-difference t test with the ANOVA error term).

[d] Significant difference in t_{max} values for all three folate fractions (overall ANOVA). Significant difference between intravenous and intramuscular values and between intravenous and oral values for all three folate fractions (paired comparison using least-squares-difference t test with the ANOVA error term).

[e] Sample size for $t_{1/2}$ and V is smaller than that of the other variables because some subjects had one or more concentrations between 8 and 24 hours that were below the assay's limit of detection.

[f] Significant difference in AUC_{0-24} values for 5-formyl-THF and 5-methyl-THF (overall ANOVA). Significant difference between intravenous and oral values for 5-formyl-THF and 5-methyl-THF (paired comparison using least-squares-difference t test with the ANOVA error term).

[g] Significant difference in $AUC_{0-\infty}$ values for 5-formyl-THF and 5-methyl-THF (overall ANOVA). Significant difference between intravenous and oral values for 5-formyl-THF and 5-methyl-THF (paired comparison using least-squares-difference t test with the ANOVA error term).

[h] When one or more baseline-adjusted concentrations at 8, 12, or 24 hours were zero, AUC_{0-24} was used for $AUC_{0-\infty}$.

[i] n = 35 unless stated otherwise.

[j] n = 32.

[k] n = 34.

[l] n = 36 unless stated otherwise.

[m] n = 25.

the predominant circulating form. The appearance of 5-methyl-THF was delayed (mean t_{max} = 1.3 hours), and its presence was prolonged: At 24 hours, concentrations of the metabolite above baseline were still detectable (8.0 ng/mL).

The concentration–time curves for intramuscular drug administration followed the intravenous patterns closely (Figure 2). The mean total folate peak concentration (436 ng/mL) was predictably blunted compared with intravenous administration and occurred later (mean t_{max} = 52 minutes; Table 1). As was the case with intravenous administration, the initial rise was due to the parent compound 5-formyl-THF. The concentration of 5-methyl-THF increased over time as a proportion of the total, until at 1.5 hours it represented half of the total circulating folates. The presence of this metabolite was prolonged and was still detectable at 24 hours (9.8 ng/mL).

Oral leucovorin administration elicited a mean peak total folate concentration of 393 ng/mL at 140 minutes postadministration (Figure 3, Table 1). In contrast to the rise in folates after i.v. and i.m. administration, the rise seen here was due predominantly to the metabolite 5-methyl-THF. There was a slight early rise of parent 5-formyl-THF, preceding the rise of total folates. This contrasted sharply with the proportion of the two forms observed after i.v. and i.m. administration, in which initially the parent compound was the predominant form.

Concentration–time curves of total folates for the different treatments are superimposed in Figure 4. Although the point-by-point changes in serum concentrations over time differed between intravenous and intramuscular administration, there were no significant differences between the two modes of treatment in the AUCs of total folate, 5-formyl-THF, or 5-methyl-THF (Table 1). In both the intravenous and intramuscular routes of administration, although 5-formyl-THF displayed a higher peak concentration than did 5-methyl-THF, the AUC for the latter was about twofold greater because of the prolonged concentrations of this metabolite in the circulation and the rapid uptake and metabolism of the former (Figures 1 and 2). Because of the extensive degrees of folate interconversion and tissue exchange of administered leucovorin with endogenous folates, the estimations necessary to perform the CL and V_{ss} calculations for the metabolite 5-methyl-THF are not reliable, and therefore these are not presented. Clearance of 5-formyl-THF after i.v. and i.m. administration was approximately threefold that of total folate because of its rapid tissue uptake and conversion to 5-meth-

Figure 1. Serum folate concentrations after intravenous injection of leucovorin 25 mg (n = 35), shown from 0 to 8 hours. Δ = total folates, O = 5-formyltetrahydrofolate, □ = 5-methyltetrahydrofolate.

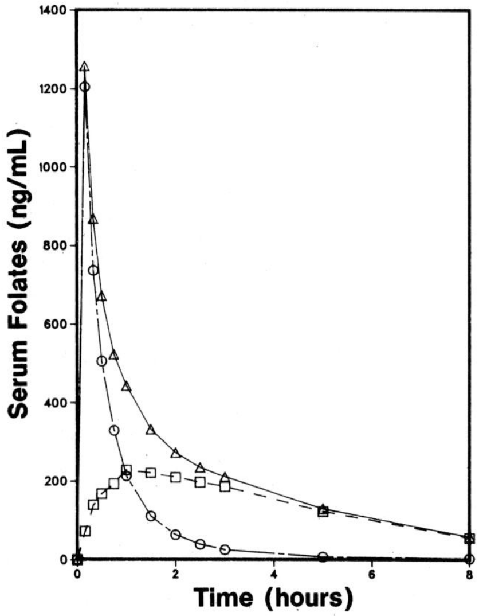

Figure 2. Serum folate concentrations after intramuscular injection of leucovorin 25 mg (n = 36), shown from 0 to 8 hours. Δ = total folates, O = 5-formyltetrahydrofolate, □ = 5-methyltetrahydrofolate.

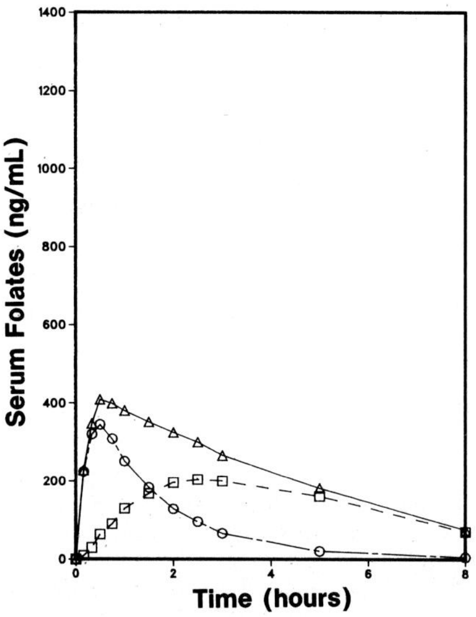

Figure 3. Serum folate concentrations after oral administration of leucovorin 25 mg (n = 36), shown from 0 to 24 hours. Δ = total folates, O = 5-formyltetrahydrofolate, □ = 5-methyltetrahydrofolate.

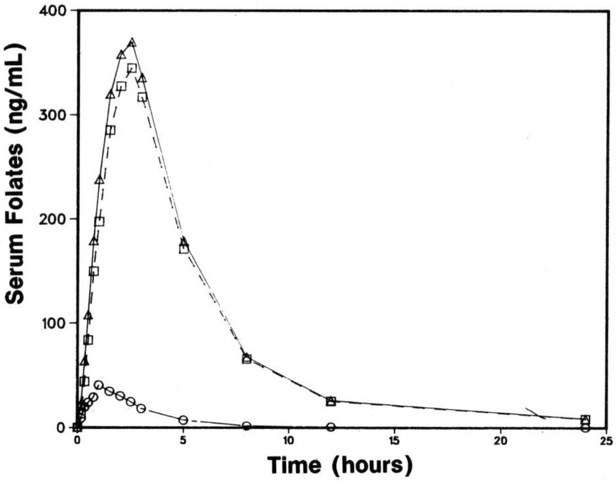

Figure 4. Comparison of the concentrations of total circulating folates achieved between 0 and 8 hours after administration of leucovorin 25 mg intravenously (Δ), intramuscularly (O), and orally (□).

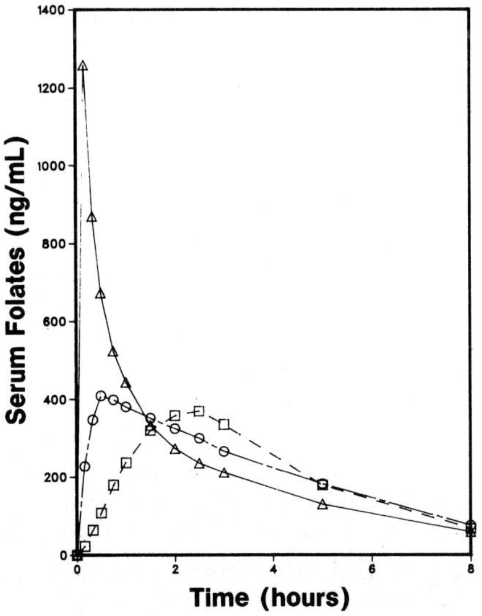

yl-THF, which constitutes a major portion of the total folate fraction. The V of the parent compound was more than fourfold that of the total folate fraction.

For the intravenous and intramuscular routes of administration, values of $t_{1/2}$ for the three folate fractions and V and CL for the total folate and N-formyl-THF fractions were not significantly different.

Bioavailability of the oral leucovorin elixir was estimated to be 92% by comparing mean total folate $AUC_{0-\infty}$ with that of intravenously administered drug. When the subjects' oral-to-i.v. $AUC_{0-\infty}$ ratios were calculated individually, a mean availability of 93% for oral administration was derived. Pharmacokinetic differences between the oral and intravenous administration routes are summarized in Table 1.

Period Effects. Analysis of variance of AUC showed a "period" or residual effect, which consisted of a trend toward successively higher values through periods one, two, and three, increasing an average of 6% per period. This effect was most marked in the AUCs of total folate and 5-methyl-THF after intravenous or intramuscular administration. The importance of this phenomenon is unknown, but it was not an artifact of the assay. The trend toward incrementally higher folate AUCs through time may be due to saturation of intracellular folate stores; i.e., once the initial leucovorin administration(s) repleted tissue folate pools or saturated membrane or cytoplasmic binding sites, or both, cellular uptake of subsequent leucovorin doses was inhibited and thus blood concentrations were prolonged, giving rise to the effects observed.

Discussion

This study demonstrated the comparable bioavailability of 25-mg doses of leucovorin calcium injection given intravenously and intramuscularly to healthy subjects. There were no significant differences between the two treatments in the AUC measurements, terminal elimination half-lives, clearances, or apparent volumes of distribution of the folate fractions.

Others have reported $t_{1/2}$ values somewhat shorter than those reported here (6 to 65 hours) for total folate.[8,9,10] In this study, folates from the leucovorin administration were still well above the quantifiable limits of the microbiologic assays through 24 hours, and after baseline adjustment, concentrations were still elevated in most subjects. These $t_{1/2}$ values, derived from the k during the 8- to 24-hour interval after drug administration, reflect the elimination rather than the distribution phase and are therefore greater than those in previous reports.

The peak concentration and time to peak concentration displayed predictable differences between intravenous and intramuscular treatment that were attributable to the nature of each mode of administration. In terms of producing rapid and sustained plasma concentrations of reduced folates, both injection routes were equally effective; in terms of providing the highest plasma concentrations in the shortest time, the intravenous route was superior. As anticipated based on prior studies, the initial predominant circulating form is the parent compound 5-formyl-THF; this is replaced in time by the major metabolite 5-methyl-THF. Because of the persistence through time of the latter form, it represents approximately two thirds of the AUC of total reduced folates over the 24-hour postadministration period.

Evidence in previous investigations points to the appearance of the metabolite 5-methyl-THF after injection of radioactively labeled tetrahydrofolates as representing not a direct conversion of administered drug but instead a displacement or "flushing" of preformed metabolite from the tissues.[11,12] Our study cannot distinguish between these two mechanisms, but the results are not inconsistent with such an exchange with the tissue pools of folate.

Oral administration of leucovorin produced a distinct pattern of circulating folates. The total folate fraction peaked later in time than when leucovorin was given intravenously or intramuscularly, produced a peak concentration of lesser magnitude, and consisted predominantly of 5-methyl-THF. This metabolic conversion is known to take place in the intestinal mucosa at the time of absorption from the lumen.[11,13] Therefore, the initially appearing folate form is the metabolite of leucovorin. Concentrations of the parent leucovorin are detectable but constitute less than 7% of the AUC of total reduced folate. The earlier rise and peak of 5-formyl-THF compared with the total folate fraction (73 versus 140 minutes) and lack of conversion to 5-methyl-THF may be explained by uptake of a small amount of administered drug proximal to the small intestine, thereby bypassing presystemic intestinal metabolism. The total folate AUC resulting from oral leucovorin administration was approximately 92% of the corresponding intramuscular or intravenous value. This effect might be due merely to efficiency of intestinal absorption or to a first-pass effect of traversing the portal circulation through the liver. This percentage of absolute bioavailability is consistent with the results of other studies at the same dose[8] and at much smaller doses.[13]

Conclusion

Based on measured serum concentrations of total reduced folates, the bioavailability of leucovorin calcium is similar after intramuscular or intravenous administration; oral administration of leucovorin calcium produces a distinct pattern of serum folate concentrations, but at the dosage studied, the percentage of drug available is comparable to that with intravenous and intramuscular administration.

References

1. Matherly LH, Fry DW, Goldman D. Role of methotrexate polyglutamylation and cellular energy metabolism in inhibition of methotrexate binding to dihydrofolate reductase by 5-formyltetrahydrofolate in Ehrlich ascites tumor cells in vitro. *Cancer Res.* 1983; 43:2694–9.
2. Danenberg PV, Langerbach RJ, Heidelberger C. Structures of reversible and irreversible complexes of thymidylate synthetase and fluorinated pyrimidine nucleotides. *Biochemistry.* 1974; 13:926–33.
3. Madajewicz S, Petrelli N, Rustum YM et al. Phase I–II trial of high-dose calcium leucovorin and 5-fluorouracil in advanced colorectal cancer. *Cancer Res.* 1984; 44:4667–9.
4. Wilson SD, Horne DW. Use of glycerol-cryoprotected *Lactobacillus casei* for microbiological assay of folic acid. *Clin Chem.* 1982; 28:1198.
5. Waters AH, Mollin DL. Studies of the folic acid activity of human serum. *J Clin Pathol.* 1961; 14:335–44.
6. Tamura T, Shin YS, Williams MA et al. *Lactobacillus casei* response to pteroylglutamates. *Anal Biochem.* 1972; 49:517–21.
7. Roberts EC, Snell EE. An improved medium for microbiological assays with *Lactobacillus casei. J Biol Chem.* 1946; 163:499–509.
8. Straw JA, Szapary D, Wynn WT. Pharmacokinetics of the

diastereoisomers of leucovorin after intravenous and oral administration to normal subjects. *Cancer Res.* 1984; 44:3114–9.
9. Mehta BM, Gisolfi AL, Hutchison DJ et al. Serum distribution of citrovorum factor and 5-methyltetrahydrofolate following oral and IM administration of calcium leucovorin in normal adults. *Cancer Treat Rep.* 1978; 62:345–50.
10. Campbell J, Rustum YM, Canobbio L et al. Metabolic modulation of 5-fluorouracil (FU) by thymidine (TdR) and citrovorum factor (CF). *Proc 13th Int Congr Chemother.* 1983; 221:17–22.
11. Perry J, Chanarin I. Intestinal absorption of reduced folate compounds in man. *Br J Haematol.* 1970; 18:329–39.
12. Pratt RF, Cooper BA. Folates in plasma and bile of man after feeding folic acid-^{3}H and 5-formyltetrahydrofolate (folinic acid). *J Clin Invest.* 1971; 50:455–62.
13. Nixon PF, Bertino JR. Effective absorption of oral formyltetrahydrofolate in man. *N Engl J Med.* 1972; 286:175–9.

Effect of sucralfate on theophylline absorption in healthy volunteers

KIMBERLY A. CANTRAL, LARRY J. SCHAAF, PAUL W. JUNGNICKEL, AND HOWARD P. MONSOUR

Abstract: The effect of oral administration of sucralfate concurrently with a single oral dose of non-sustained-release theophylline was studied in eight healthy male volunteers.

A two-way, randomized, crossover study design was used. During the control phase, each subject received a single 5-mg/kg dose of a non-sustained-release theophylline product. During the treatment phase, a 1-g sucralfate tablet was ingested four times a day for two days before the theophylline dose, with the theophylline dose, and six hours after the dose. Plasma samples were collected at frequent intervals for 24 hours after theophylline dosing.

Plasma theophylline concentrations, determined by high-performance liquid chromatography, were similar in the absence and presence of sucralfate. No significant differences in theophylline half-life or mean residence time between the control and treatment phases were observed. A significant decrease in the area under the plasma drug concentration–time curve was observed in the presence of sucralfate. However, the magnitude of this change was minimal and unlikely to be clinically important.

In these healthy subjects, the concomitant administration of sucralfate with a single dose of non-sustained-release theophylline did not alter the rate or extent of theophylline absorption to a clinically important degree.

Index terms: Absorption; Blood levels; Drug interactions; Gastrointestinal drugs; Half-life; Pharmacokinetics; Respiratory smooth-muscle relaxants; Sucralfate; Theophylline
Clin Pharm. 1988; 7:58–61

Sucralfate is an aluminum salt of a sulfated disaccharide, which was developed for the treatment of peptic-ulcer disease.[1] When exposed to the acidic environment of the stomach, it becomes a highly condensed, anionic substance that is able to electrostatically bind with positively charged protein molecules on the ulcer crater, forming a stable complex.[2] This barrier inhibits the diffusion of acid across the mucosal surface,[3] and has been shown to adsorb pepsin[3] as well as bile salts.[2]

The barrier to diffusion, as well as the binding capabilities of sucralfate, have led to the speculation that altered absorption may occur when other medications are administered concurrently. Several studies have been performed to assess this theoretical interaction. No significant effect on bioavailability seems to occur when digoxin,[4,5] quinidine,[4] propranolol,[4] aspirin,[6–8] acetaminophen,[9] ibuprofen,[10] warfarin,[11] or chlorpropamide[12] is coadministered with sucralfate. Lacz et al.,[4] in a series of bioavailability studies in dogs, reported a decrease in relative bioavailability of phenytoin when sucralfate was administered concurrently. In double-blind, placebo-controlled, crossover studies in humans, Smart and associates,[13] as well as Hall and associates,[14] reported reductions in the absorption of phenytoin when it was administered with sucralfate.

A preliminary study in dogs suggests that the administration of sucralfate does not affect the absorption of single doses of aminophylline.[4] In contrast, Fleischmann et al.[15] recently demonstrated in

KIMBERLY A. CANTRAL, PHARM.D., is Clinical Pharmacy Resident; LARRY J. SCHAAF, PH.D., is Assistant Professor of Pharmaceutical Sciences, College of Pharmacy; PAUL W. JUNGNICKEL, M.S., is Assistant Professor of Pharmacy Practice, College of Pharmacy; and HOWARD P. MONSOUR, M.D., is Gastroenterology Fellow, University of Nebraska Medical Center.

Address reprint requests to Dr. Schaaf at the College of Pharmacy, University of Nebraska Medical Center, 42nd and Dewey Ave., Omaha, NE 68105.

The assistance of David E. Cantral, M.D., Lane Hawley, Pharm.D. candidate, Vijay Bhargava, Ph.D., and Thomas G. Tape, M.D., is acknowledged.

Presented in the Clinical Research Forum, 22nd Annual ASHP Midyear Clinical Meeting, Atlanta, GA, December 9, 1987.

Copyright © 1988, American Society of Hospital Pharmacists, Inc. All rights reserved. 0278-2677/88/0101-0058$01.00.

humans that the administration of sucralfate reduced the extent of theophylline absorption as measured by the area under the plasma drug concentration–time curve.

Gastrointestinal absorption of many drugs has been reported to be reduced by the prompt administration of activated charcoal. Berlinger et al.[16] reported enhanced theophylline clearance with the oral administration of activated charcoal. It has been suggested that activated charcoal may enhance the diffusion of theophylline from the systemic circulation to the gastrointestinal tract by maintaining an active concentration gradient.[17] Since sucralfate produces a viscous barrier on the gastric lining and has binding and adsorption characteristics, an effect similar to that observed with activated charcoal may occur when sucralfate is administered concomitantly with theophylline.

The purpose of this study was to determine whether sucralfate has an effect on the bioavailability and resulting serum concentrations of theophylline when a rapid-release theophylline product and sucralfate are administered concomitantly to healthy volunteers.

Methods

Study Population. The study group included eight nonsmoking, healthy male volunteers, ranging in age from 21 to 37 years (mean, 26.4 years) and weighing 52 to 85 kg (mean, 73 kg). After giving written informed consent, each volunteer underwent a comprehensive medical evaluation, including a medical history, complete physical exam, electrocardiogram, and routine laboratory tests. No prescription or nonprescription medications were allowed during the study period. All xanthine-containing foods and beverages were eliminated from the diets of the participants 48 hours before and during the two separate testing periods. The protocol was reviewed and approved by the university's institutional review board.

Treatment Groups. The study was conducted using a two-way, randomized, crossover design. Subjects were randomly assigned to either the control or treatment group. After a one-week washout period, the participants were "crossed over," thus allowing each subject to act as his own control. Each subject fasted overnight and for three hours after the dose of theophylline on the morning of each study day. Standard meals were provided at three and nine hours after the theophylline dose.

On the morning of the control phase of the study, the subjects received a 5-mg/kg oral dose of non-sustained-release anhydrous theophylline (Slo-Phyllin, W. H. Rorer Inc., lot 64042) with 240 mL of water. During the treatment phase of the study, the subjects ingested a 1-g sucralfate tablet (Carafate, Marion Laboratories, lot P6087) four times a day (one hour before meals and at bedtime) for two days before the theophylline dose, with the theophylline dose, and six hours after the dose.

Sampling. An indwelling venous catheter fitted with a three-way stopcock was placed into a forearm vein before the dose of theophylline, and venous blood samples (5 mL) were collected just before drug administration and at the following intervals after theophylline dosing: 0.25, 0.5, 0.75, 1, 1.5, 2, 4, 6, 8, 10, 12, and 24 hours. Blood samples were placed in heparinized tubes, and plasma was separated as soon as possible by centrifugation. All plasma samples were frozen at −20 °C until the time of analysis (within one month). The catheters were flushed with 1 to 2 mL of a dilute solution of heparin sodium (10 units/mL) after each blood sample was drawn to maintain patency. To prevent possible sample dilution, 1 to 2 mL of blood was withdrawn and discarded before the actual blood samples were obtained.

Plasma samples were analyzed for theophylline using a modification of the high-performance liquid chromatographic method of Peng et al.[18] Plasma (100 μL) containing the internal standard β-hydroxyethyltheophylline (150 μL of a 6.25-μg/mL aqueous solution) was extracted with 2 mL of ethyl acetate. The organic phase was separated, placed in a fresh conical glass tube, and evaporated to dryness under a gentle stream of nitrogen at 42 °C. Samples were then reconstituted with 100 μL of mobile phase, and a 20-μL aliquot was injected onto the column. The mobile phase consisted of 5% acetonitrile in double-distilled water. Theophylline and the internal standard were separated using a reverse-phase phenyl column (phenyl analytical; 5 μm, 15 cm × 4.5 mm internal diameter; IBM Instruments, Inc., Danbury, CT 06810) with a mobile-phase flow rate of 1.5 mL/min. Both were detected at 275 nm using a variable-wavelength ultraviolet detector. The retention times for theophylline and the internal standard were 4.9 and 5.9 minutes, respectively. Calibration curves of peak-height ratio versus theophylline concentration were prepared daily by analyzing drug-free plasma to which known quantities of theophylline were added. The standard curves were linear over the range of 0.5 to 12 μg/mL. The between-day coefficients of variation (eight replications) at 1, 4, and 10 μg/mL were 6.3%, 1.2%, and 1.2%, respectively.

Pharmacokinetic and Statistical Analysis. The theophylline plasma-concentration-versus-time data were analyzed separately for each subject using model-independent area methods.[18,19] The terminal elimination rate constant (k) was calculated from the slope of the terminal log-linear phase using least-squares regression analysis. The half-life ($t_{1/2}$) was determined by $t_{1/2} = 0.693/k$. The area under the plasma drug concentration–time curve (AUC) was calculated using the linear trapezoidal rule. The area from the last measured time to infinity was calculated by dividing the concentration on the regression line at that time (C_t) by the elimination rate constant. The area under the first moment curve (AUMC) was also calculated using the linear trapezoidal rule. The area from the last measured time to infinity for the first moment curve was calculated by using the formula $(t)(C_t/k) + C_t/k^2$.[20] The mean residence time (MRT) was calculated by dividing AUMC by AUC.[20] MRT represents the average time a theophylline molecule is present in the body (including time of absorption, distribution, and elimination) when administered orally. Assuming that theophylline disposition does not change (distribution and elimination) in the presence or absence of sucralfate, any change in MRT will reflect a change in absorption rate (i.e., an increase in MRT would suggest a decrease in the rate of absorption).

The calculated pharmacokinetic variables for theophylline with and without sucralfate were analyzed using a modified Wilcoxon rank sum test for paired data.[21] A p value of 0.05 or less was considered to be statistically significant.

Results

The mean plasma theophylline concentrations versus time, with and without sucralfate, are shown in Figure 1. Serum concentrations increased rapidly after oral administration and reached maximum values after 1 to 1.5 hours. It is apparent from Figure 1 that serum theophylline concentrations observed after concomitant administration of sucralfate were similar to those observed when theophylline was administered alone. The pharmacokinetic data and their statistical significance are summarized in Table 1. A significant decrease in AUC was found when theophylline was administered with sucralfate. No significant differences were found for $t_{1/2}$ (statistical test performed on k) or for MRT.

Discussion

The occurrence of peptic ulcers or gastritis in patients with asthma or chronic obstructive pulmonary disease is not uncommon. Although it has been argued that these complications may result from the medications used in this population (e.g., theophylline and corticosteroids) rather than from the basic underlying disease, antiulcer therapies are commonly prescribed for these patients. Available data on the possible interaction between theophylline and sucralfate are limited. Since theophylline has a relatively narrow therapeutic range, alterations in the absorption or elimination process, or both, by concurrently administered sucralfate could result in treatment failure.

Figure 1. Plot of mean plasma theophylline concentrations versus time in the absence (solid line) and presence (broken line) of sucralfate.

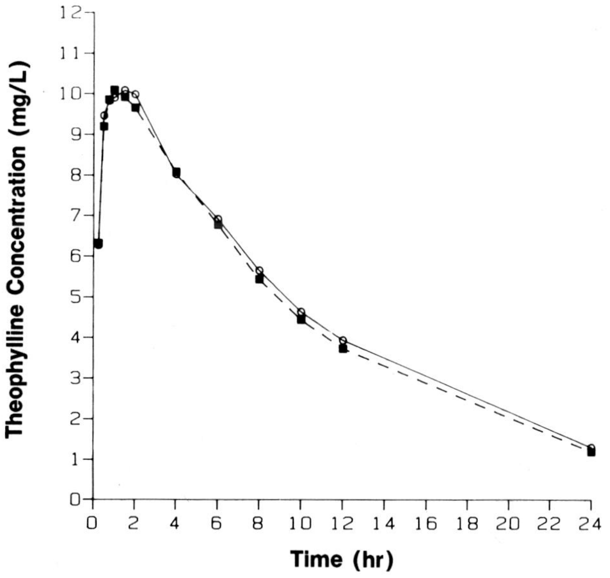

Table 1.
Theophylline Absorption and Elimination Data in the Absence (T) and Presence (T + S) of Sucralfate

Subject No.	$t_{1/2}$ (hr)[a]		AUC (μg/mL/hr)[b]		MRT (hr)[c]	
	T	T + S	T	T + S	T	T + S
1	6.5	6.5	113.3	112.2	9.4	9.3
2	7.6	6.5	139.6	113.3	10.9	9.4
3	5.5	5.4	124.4	118.7	8.2	8.2
4	6.4	6.0	98.8	97.4	8.9	8.8
5	12.0	10.8	177.0	171.6	17.6	15.6
6	7.3	7.1	103.7	95.7	10.6	10.6
7	7.9	8.2	135.0	133.7	11.2	11.4
8	7.4	6.9	140.2	133.2	10.8	10.0
Mean ± S.D.	7.3[d] ± 1.5[e]	6.9[d] ± 1.3[e]	129.0 ± 25.1	122.0 ± 24.5[f]	11.0 ± 2.9	10.0 ± 2.3

[a] Elimination half-life. Statistical test performed on the elimination rate constant values.
[b] Area under the theophylline plasma concentration–time curve from time 0 to infinity.
[c] Mean residence time.
[d] Harmonic mean.
[e] "Pseudo" standard deviation.[22]
[f] Significantly different in the absence versus the presence of sucralfate.

Sulcralfate, as expected, did not significantly affect the elimination characteristics of theophylline, as evidenced by the lack of change in half-life values during the two study phases. Thus, the assumption that differences in MRT between trial phases reflect differences in the rate of absorption appears valid. The absence of significant differences in MRT suggests that sucralfate has essentially no effect on the rate of theophylline absorption. Although a significant decrease in the extent of absorption, as determined by AUC, was observed when the subjects were given sucralfate, the magnitude of the reduction was minimal and unlikely to be clinically important.

Although a preliminary study in dogs suggested that administration of sucralfate does not affect the absorption of single doses of aminophylline,[4] Fleischmann et al.[15] recently demonstrated that the administration of sucralfate 1 g 30 minutes before the administration of a 350-mg dose of sustained-release theophylline reduced the extent of theophylline absorption by an average of 40%. In contrast, our study used a rapid-release theophylline product. This may explain the different results obtained by the two studies.

Although the current study suggests that concomitant administration of sucralfate does not alter the rate or extent of theophylline absorption, extrapolation of these results to the clinical setting must be done with caution for several reasons. First, subjects in our study were healthy volunteers, not patients with peptic-ulcer disease. Since sucralfate binds preferentially to ulcer sites, one might expect less binding of the sucralfate to the gastric mucosa in our study population than might be seen in actual patients. As a result, this difference in binding potential may result in a greater decrease in theophylline absorption when the combination is used in patients with peptic-ulcer disease. Second, theophylline was administered as a single dose in the current study; thus, definitive conclusions regarding the effect of coadministered sucralfate on steady-state theophylline concentrations cannot be made. Last, theophylline was administered as a rapid-release product in the current investigation. However, most patients who are treated with theophylline receive a sustained-release product. Because such products release drug in the gastrointestinal tract for a prolonged period of time, a greater opportunity for an interaction between theophylline and sucralfate may exist.

Conclusion

The concomitant administration of sucralfate with a rapid-release theophylline product in eight healthy male volunteers did not alter the rate or extent of theophylline absorption to a clinically important degree. Whether these results will be confirmed using a sustained-release theophylline product, and how coadministration of sucralfate might affect steady-state theophylline concentrations, will require further investigation. This potential interaction should also be studied in patients with peptic-ulcer disease.

References

1. Nagashima R. Development and characteristics of sucralfate. *J Clin Gastroenterol.* 1981; 3(Suppl 2):103–10.
2. Garnett WR. Sucralfate—alternative therapy for peptic ulcer disease. *Clin Pharm.* 1982; 1:307–14.
3. Bighley LD, Giesling D. Sucralfate: a new concept in ulcer therapy. In: Peptic ulcer disease: an update. Third International Symposium on Gastroenterology. New York: Biomedical Information Corporation; 1979:307–9.
4. Lacz JP, Groschang AG, Geising DH et al. The effect of sucralfate on drug absorption in dogs. *Gastroenterology.* 1982; 82:1108. Abstract.
5. Giesing DH, Lanman RC, Dimmitt DC et al. Lack of effect of sucralfate on digoxin pharmacokinetics. *Gastroenterology.* 1983; 84:1165. Abstract.
6. Lau AH, Chang CW, Schlesinger PK et al. Evaluation of a potential drug interaction between sucralfate and aspirin. *Clin Pharmacol Ther.* 1986; 39:151–5.
7. Graham DY, Sackman JW, Giesing DH et al. In vitro adsorption of bile salts and aspirin to sucralfate. *Dig Dis Sci.* 1984; 29:402–6.
8. Tesler MA, Lim ES. Protection of gastric mucosa by sucralfate from aspirin-induced erosions. *J Clin Gastroenterol.* 1981; 3(Suppl 2):175–9.
9. Kamali F, Fry JR, Smart HL et al. A double-blind placebo controlled study to examine effects of sucralfate on paracetamol absorption. *Br J Clin Pharmacol.* 1985; 19:113–4. Letter.
10. Pugh MC, Small RE, Garnett WR et al. Effect of sucralfate on ibuprofen absorption in normal volunteers. *Clin Pharm.* 1984; 3:630–3.
11. Neuvonen PJ, Jaaddola A, Totterman J et al. Clinically significant sucralfate-warfarin interaction is not likely. *Br J Clin Pharmacol.* 1985; 20:178–80. Letter.
12. Letendre PW, Carlson JD, Seifert RD et al. Effect of sucralfate on the absorption and pharmacokinetics of chlorpropamide. *J Clin Pharmacol.* 1986; 26:622–25.
13. Smart HL, Somerville KW, Williams J et al. The effects of sucralfate upon phenytoin absorption in man. *Br J Clin Pharmacol.* 1985; 20:238–40.
14. Hall TG, Cuddy PG, Glass CJ et al. Effect of sucralfate on phenytoin bioavailability. *Drug Intell Clin Pharm.* 1986; 20:607–10.
15. Fleischmann R, Bozler G, Boekstegers P. Bioverfugbarkeit von Theophylline unter Ulkustherapeutika. *Verh Dtsch Ges Inn Med.* 1984; 90(II):1876–9.
16. Berlinger WG, Spector R, Goldberg MJ et al. Enhancement of theophylline clearance by activated charcoal. *Clin Pharmacol Ther.* 1983; 33:351–4.
17. Berg MJ, Berlinger WJ, Goldberg MJ. Acceleration of the body clearance of phenobarbital by oral activated charcoal. *N Engl J Med.* 1982; 307:642–4.
18. Peng GW, Smith V, Peng A et al. A rapid and sensitive method for determination of theophylline in plasma and saliva by high pressure liquid chromatography. *Res Commun Chem Pathol Pharmacol.* 1976; 15:341–50.
19. Gibaldi M, Perrier D, eds. Pharmacokinetics. 2nd ed. New York: Marcel Dekker, 1982:409–17.
20. D'Angio R, Mayersohn M, Conrad KA et al. Cimetidine absorption in humans during sucralfate coadministration. *Br J Clin Pharmacol.* 1986; 21:515–20.
21. Lam F, Longnecker M. A modified Wilcoxon rank sum test for paired data. *Biometrika.* 1983; 70:510–3.
22. Lam F, Hung C, Perrier D. Estimation of variance for harmonic mean half-lives. *J Pharm Sci.* 1985; 74:229–31.

Research Note

Estimation of creatinine clearance in malnourished patients

ALAN H. LAU, STEVEN I. BERK,
THERESA PROSSER, AND TERRY STONICH

Clin Pharm. 1988; 7:62-5

Rapid determination of renal function is often needed for patient assessment and drug dosing. Urinary creatinine clearance is an indicator of kidney function; creatinine clearance is determined by measuring creatinine in urine collected over a 24-hour period. Disadvantages of using this measure of kidney function are that the test results are not available readily and the accuracy of the measurement depends on the completeness of urine collection in the 24-hour period. Various methods have been developed in the last two decades for estimating urinary creatinine clearance from serum creatinine concentration.[1,2] These methods provide instant estimation of kidney function without the need for laborious urine collection, and they are now used extensively in determining drug dosages.

The accuracy of methods for rapid creatinine clearance estimation depends on normal production and elimination of creatinine. In morbidly obese patients, none of the commonly used methods for creatinine clearance estimation is accurate because of the patients' larger than normal muscle mass and their higher urinary excretion of creatinine.[3] In contrast, malnourished patients are expected to have smaller muscle mass, which would result in a diminished rate of creatinine production.[4] Because the various methods for rapid creatinine clearance estimation are used frequently, and because up to 50% of hospitalized patients suffer from protein–calorie malnutrition,[5,6] it is important to examine the validity of these methods for creatinine clearance estimation in malnourished patients. Errors in predicted renal function may result in excessive drug administration; this may cause serious toxicities, especially when agents such as aminoglycosides or antineoplastic drugs are used. We evaluated the accuracy and precision of seven methods for rapid creatinine clearance estimation in hospitalized patients with protein–calorie malnutrition.

Methods. *Subjects.* Fifty-two hospitalized patients with protein–calorie malnutrition were enrolled in the study. Each patient fulfilled at least one of the following criteria for nutritional assessment:

1. Somatic protein mass less than 85% of lean body weight (LBW); LBW is determined as follows[7]:

   LBW (male) = 50.0 kg + 2.3 kg/each inch over 5 feet

   LBW (female) = 45.5 kg + 2.3 kg/each inch over 5 feet
2. Assessment of visceral protein mass: serum albumin concentration below 3.5 mg/dL
3. Assessment of immune competence: total lymphocyte count (TLC) below 1000/cu mm (This criterion was not used in patients who had received recent antineoplastic drug treatment.)

Excluded from the study were patients who had changing renal function, defined as fluctuation of serum creatinine concentration of more than 0.5 mg/dL 24 hours before and after the study period. Also excluded were patients with muscular diseases. None of the patients received cefoxitin, cephalothin, cephacetrile, cephaloglycin, or cephaloridine during the study. High concentrations of these medications have been reported to cause falsely elevated values of creatinine when the alkaline picrate assay is used for creatinine determination.[8-10] Cimetidine was also reported to increase serum creatinine concentration through competition for secretion by the kidney tubules[11]; however, blood urea concentrations were not observed to be elevated. Patients receiving cimetidine were therefore excluded from our study if their serum creatinine concentrations were elevated without a corresponding increase in serum urea nitrogen.

Sample Collection. The nursing staff collected urine for a 24-hour period from each patient; no samples were collected from patients who were uncooperative or incontinent. One of the investigators inspected the 24-hour urine specimens to verify the reported urine output during the collection period. Creatinine concentrations in the urine and in serum specimens obtained in the morning

ALAN H. LAU, PHARM.D., is Associate Professor and STEVEN I. BERK, PHARM.D., is Clinical Assistant Professor, Department of Pharmacy Practice, College of Pharmacy, University of Illinois at Chicago (UIC). THERESA PROSSER, PHARM.D., is Assistant Professor, Division of Clinical Pharmacy, St. Louis College of Pharmacy, St. Louis, MO; at the time of this study, she was a Pharm.D. student, College of Pharmacy, UIC. TERRY STONICH, PHARM.D., is Clinical Assistant Professor, Department of Pharmacy Practice, College of Pharmacy, UIC.

Address reprint requests to Dr. Lau at the Department of Pharmacy Practice, College of Pharmacy, University of Illinois at Chicago, 833 South Wood Street, Room 244, Chicago, IL 60612.

The assistance of Anita Lorenzo, Pharm.D., in establishing the criteria for patient selection, is acknowledged.

Presented in part at the 20th Annual ASHP Midyear Clinical Meeting, New Orleans, LA, December 10, 1985.

Copyright © 1988, American Society of Hospital Pharmacists, Inc. All rights reserved. 0278-2677/88/0101-0062$01.00.

during the urine collection period were determined by Astra 8 Automatic Analyzer Systems (Beckman Instruments Inc., Fullerton, CA), using the Jaffé rate colorimetry method to determine the rate of alkaline picrate–creatinine complex formation. The assay had a within-run precision of 3%.

Calculations. Urinary creatinine clearance (CL_{cr}) was determined by the following equation:

$$CL_{cr} = UV/P$$

where U = urinary creatinine concentration, V = volume of urine during the collection period, and P = serum creatinine concentration.

Creatinine clearance was also estimated by the seven methods listed in the appendix, using the patients' serum creatinine concentrations and lean body weights. If actual body weight was less than lean body weight, actual body weight was used. All of the calculated creatinine clearance values were normalized to the patients' lean body weight or surface area.

Data Analysis. The estimated creatinine clearance values obtained by each method were compared with those determined from the 24-hour urine collection. The effect of renal function on the accuracy of the individual methods was evaluated by separating the observed creatinine clearance values into three renal function categories: less than 30 mL/min, between 30 and 70 mL/min, and greater than 70 mL/min. The effect of nutritional status on the validity of the methods was assessed by categorizing the results according to the patients' serum albumin concentrations.

The percent prediction errors (%PE) and percent absolute prediction errors (%APE) were calculated to evaluate the bias and precision, respectively, of the individual methods,[18] as follows:

%PE = [(Predicted value − Measured value)/Measured value] × 100

%APE = [(| Predicted value − Measured value |)/Measured value] × 100

The mean and standard deviation of the two types of prediction errors were then determined to allow comparison among the methods. Thus, the standard deviation represented the variability of the prediction error for each method.

Analysis of variance (ANOVA) was conducted, and least significant difference (LSD) was used to determine if there was a significant difference in %PE and %APE among the seven methods. The LSD was determined according to the following formula:

$$LSD = t_{\alpha[v]} \sqrt{2(MS)/n}$$

where $t_{\alpha[v]}$ is the t value for the degree of freedom v and level of significance α, MS is the within-cells mean square.[19] The mean prediction errors for two methods were considered significantly different if the difference between the two means exceeded the calculated LSD value. The a priori level of significance for all statistical tests was $p < 0.05$.

Results. Urinary creatinine clearance values were determined in 52 patients (25 men and 27 women). The mean ± S.D. total body weight of the patients was 59.2 ± 12.6 kg and the mean ± S.D. surface area was 1.63 ± 0.19 sq m. Of the 52 patients, 9 patients fulfilled one of the three criteria used to determine protein–calorie malnutrition, 28 patients fulfilled two criteria, and 15 patients fulfilled all of the three criteria. The mean ± S.D. urinary creatinine clearance of the patients was 25.4 ± 38.3 mL/min. Thirteen patients had creatinine clearance values greater than 70 mL/min, 23 patients had creatinine clearance values between 30 and 70 mL/min, and 16 patients had creatinine clearance values less than 30 mL/min.

The mean ± S.D. measured and predicted creatinine clearance values, percent prediction errors, and percent absolute prediction errors, by renal function group, are shown in Table 1. The mean predicted creatinine clearance values obtained by most of the seven methods were higher than the measured creatinine clearance values in all three renal function groups. The overestimation became more marked in the patients with poor renal function, as reflected by the increasing mean %PE and mean %APE in these patients.

Table 1.
Prediction Error and Absolute Prediction Error for Creatinine Clearance Determinations[a]

Method[b]	Predicted CL_{cr} (mL/min)	% Prediction Error	% Absolute Prediction Error
CL_{cr} > 70 mL/min (n = 13)			
Measured	108.0 ± 30.7		
BJ	125.4 ± 38.6	25.6 ± 40.6	36.8 ± 29.7
CG	109.3 ± 29.3	4.1 ± 27.5	19.7 ± 18.9
HA	157.7 ± 40.6	50.4 ± 37.4	50.4 ± 37.4
J1	135.2 ± 43.5	28.4 ± 36.3	35.0 ± 29.4
J2	113.1 ± 26.1	7.9 ± 24.0	19.6 ± 15.0
MA	114.9 ± 31.1	9.4 ± 28.7	20.2 ± 21.9
SN	108.6 ± 25.7	8.3 ± 24.1	18.3 ± 17.1
CL_{cr} 30–70 mL/min (n = 23)			
Measured	52.0 ± 13.5		
BJ	87.1 ± 22.3	76.4 ± 52.9	77.7 ± 50.8
CG	62.7 ± 22.7	22.2 ± 34.5	33.3 ± 23.5
HA	89.3 ± 32.0	76.7 ± 56.1	76.7 ± 56.1
J1	83.6 ± 23.1	67.0 ± 47.4	70.1 ± 42.5
J2	67.2 ± 23.0	31.9 ± 38.3	40.6 ± 28.3
MA	65.7 ± 23.7	28.2 ± 36.4	37.2 ± 26.6
SN	64.2 ± 23.6	25.2 ± 36.7	36.0 ± 25.5
CL_{cr} <30 mL/min (n = 16)			
Measured	17.6 ± 6.5		
BJ	42.0 ± 17.9	146.5 ± 68.5	146.4 ± 68.5
CG	30.4 ± 16.3	75.3 ± 63.1	78.9 ± 58.3
HA	45.2 ± 25.1	160.5 ± 92.9	160.5 ± 92.9
J1	34.6 ± 18.7	95.9 ± 59.4	96.0 ± 59.4
J2	31.9 ± 18.0	82.6 ± 63.4	84.5 ± 60.6
MA	30.9 ± 17.2	77.0 ± 64.1	80.1 ± 59.9
SN	32.8 ± 18.2	89.2 ± 66.0	90.1 ± 64.6

[a] CL_{cr}, % PE, and % APE are expressed as mean ± S.D.
[b] Appendix describes prediction methods.

ANOVA revealed a significant difference among the mean %PE values for the seven methods; similar differences among the mean %APE values were also found. Least significant differences (LSDs) for %PE and %APE were calculated for each renal function group and for patients grouped by serum albumin concentration (>2.6 mg/dL and ≤2.6 mg/dL), as shown in Table 2. According to these LSD values, method HA had higher mean %PE and mean %APE than the other six methods for patients with creatinine clearance values greater than 70 mL/min. Although the mean %PE and mean %APE for methods BJ and J1 were also higher than the remaining four methods, the LSD values did not reveal a significant difference between these methods.

For patients with creatinine clearance values between 30 and 70 mL/min, the LSD values for mean %PE revealed a significant difference between the methods of BJ, HA, and J1, and those of CG, J2, MA, and SN. Similarly, significantly higher mean %APE values were also observed for methods BJ, HA, and J1. For patients with creatinine clearance values less than 30 mL/min, both the mean %PE and mean %APE for the methods of BJ and HA were significantly greater than the values for the other five methods.

Overall, methods CG, J2, MA, and SN have smaller mean %PE and mean %APE than methods BJ, HA, and J1 in all three renal function groups. The first four methods (CG, J2, MA, and SN) therefore had less bias and better precision in predicting urinary creatinine clearance values than did the latter three methods.

When the performances of the seven methods were evaluated according to the patients' serum albumin concentration categories (Table 3), both the mean %PE and %APE for all seven methods were greater in the patients with serum albumin concentrations of less than 2.6 mg/dL. Increased bias and diminished precision were therefore observed in the patients with low serum albumin concentrations, which is indicative of their poor nutritional status. The LSD values again demonstrated a significantly larger %PE and %APE for the methods of BJ and HA in both serum albumin concentration groups.

Discussion. Our patients' renal function and their extent of malnutrition were observed to affect the accuracy of creatinine clearance prediction. All of the prediction methods demonstrate the greatest accuracy for urinary creatinine clearance prediction when the patient's renal function is good (creatinine clearance greater than 70 mL/min). Methods CG, J2, MA, and SN were the most accurate for patients in all renal function categories; the other methods had prediction errors of 25–50% in patients with good renal function and 67–77% and 95–160% in patients with moderate and severe renal dysfunction, respectively.

Table 2.
Least Significant Difference (LSD) Values for % Prediction Error and % Absolute Prediction Error by Patient Characteristics

Patient Characteristic	LSD for %PE	LSD for %APE
Creatinine clearance >70 mL/min	25.0	19.9
Creatinine clearance 30–70 mL/min	25.6	22.3
Creatinine clearance <30 mL/min	48.3	47.1
Serum albumin concentration >2.6 mg/dL	32.8	30.5
Serum albumin concentration ≤2.6 mg/dL	31.4	28.7

Table 3.
Statistical Evaluation of Creatinine Clearance Estimations in Patients with High and Low Serum Albumin Concentrations

Method[a]	% Prediction Error[b]	% Absolute Prediction Error[b]
Albumin Concentration >2.6 mg/dL (n = *20)*		
BJ	78.9 ± 74.3	82.0 ± 70.7
CG	16.9 ± 39.4	27.3 ± 32.7
HA	74.7 ± 67.0	74.7 ± 67.0
J1	49.8 ± 47.0	52.0 ± 44.3
J2	28.5 ± 42.8	35.7 ± 36.6
MA	20.9 ± 39.7	28.9 ± 34.0
SN	24.6 ± 44.8	31.1 ± 40.3
Albumin Concentration ≤2.6 mg/dL (n = *32)*		
BJ	93.1 ± 70.1	96.1 ± 65.7
CG	44.8 ± 56.2	54.2 ± 46.9
HA	109.1 ± 83.8	109.1 ± 83.8
J1	76.6 ± 56.8	80.1 ± 51.6
J2	49.6 ± 57.6	57.1 ± 49.9
MA	49.5 ± 56.2	57.0 ± 48.4
SN	52.1 ± 60.4	60.3 ± 52.0

[a] Appendix describes prediction methods.
[b] Expressed as mean ± S.D.

The reduced production of creatinine in protein–calorie malnutrition may be responsible for the error of creatinine clearance estimation. In our patients, the mean urinary creatinine excretion was 12.8 mg/kg/24 hr, which is lower than the 15–25 mg/kg/24 hr expected in subjects with adequate nutritional status. Forbes and Bruining reported that urinary creatinine excretion was proportional to lean body mass.[20] Schiller et al.[21] made similar observations in patients with malnutrition; urinary creatinine excretion was found to increase progressively as the nutritional status of their patients began to improve. Because creatinine production in malnourished patients is reduced, the serum creatinine concentration is expected to be lower than normal. Since serum creatinine concentration is used in the denominator of all the equations evaluated in this study, the estimated creatinine clearance values were higher than expected. The magnitude of the error was highest in the patients with poor renal function.

Reduced urinary creatinine excretion has been observed in renal failure.[22] Muscle wasting and biochemical disturbances found in uremia are thought to be responsible for the decreased creatinine production. Increased nonrenal elimination of creatinine may also contribute to the increased discrepancy between the predicted and the observed urinary creatinine clearances in renal failure.[23]

Serum albumin concentration is a measure of nutritional status; all the seven creatinine clearance estimation methods that we evaluated were more accurate in patients with serum albumin concentrations >2.6 mg/dL. As the patient becomes more malnourished, the reliability of these estimation methods diminishes further.

Other factors that affect the accuracy of renal function estimation methods include morbid obesity,[3] hepatic diseases,[24] and acute illnesses.[25] None of the malnourished patients that we evaluated was morbidly obese. However, some of the patients had mild liver dysfunction and others suffered from acute diseases. Nonetheless, our patient population should represent a cross-section of patients with protein-calorie malnutrition commonly seen in an acute-care hospital.

In patients who have only a mild degree of protein-calorie malnutrition and in whom relatively normal renal function is expected, predictions by methods CG, J2, MA, and SN should be comparable in accuracy to predictions in patients with adequate nutritional status.[26] For malnourished patients in whom poor renal function is expected, a 24-hour urine collection for creatinine clearance determination is indicated. Similarly, the urine collection method is necessary for all patients who have substantial protein-calorie malnutrition.

Conclusion. In malnourished patients, commonly used methods for predicting creatinine clearance may overestimate renal function. Thus, use of CL_{cr} estimates as a basis for determining drug dosages in these patients may result in drug toxicities.

References

1. Lott RS, Hayton WL. Estimation of creatinine clearance from serum creatinine concentration—a review. *Drug Intell Clin Pharm.* 1977; 12:140–50.
2. Bjornsson TD. Use of serum creatinine concentrations to determine renal function. *Clin Pharmacokinet.* 1979; 4:200–22.
3. Dionne RE, Bauer LA, Gibson GA et al. Estimating creatinine clearance in morbidly obese patients. *Am J Hosp Pharm.* 1981; 38:841–4.
4. Bistrian BR, Blackburn GL, Sherman M et al. Therapeutic index of nutritional depletion in the hospitalized patients. *Surg Gynecol Obstet.* 1975; 141:512–6.
5. Bistrian BR, Blackburn GL, Hallowell E et al. Protein status of general surgical patients. *JAMA.* 1974; 230:858–60.
6. Bistrian BR, Blackburn GL, Vitale J et al. Prevalence of malnutrition in general medical patients. *JAMA.* 1976; 235:1567–70.
7. Devine BJ. Clinical pharmacy case studies—gentamicin therapy. *Drug Intell Clin Pharm.* 1974; 8:650–5.
8. Swain RR, Briggs SL. Positive interference with the Jaffé reaction by cephalosporin antibiotics. *Clin Chem.* 1977; 23:1340–2.
9. Durham SR, Bignell AHC, Wise R. Interference of cefoxitin in the creatinine estimation and its clinical relevance. *J Clin Pathol.* 1979; 32:1148–51.
10. Allen LC, Michalko KM, Coons C. More on cephalosporin interference with creatinine determinations. *Clin Chem.* 1982; 28:555–6.
11. Dubb JW, Stote RM, Familiar RG et al. Effects of cimetidine on renal function in normal man. *Clin Pharmacol Ther.* 1978; 24:76–83.
12. Cockcroft DW, Gault MH. Prediction of creatinine clearance from serum creatinine. *Nephron.* 1976; 16:31–41.
13. Hallynck T, Soep HH, Thomis J et al. Prediction of creatinine clearance from serum creatinine concentration based on lean body mass. *Clin Pharmacol Ther.* 1981; 30:414–21.
14. Jelliffe RW. Estimation of creatinine clearance when urine cannot be collected. *Lancet.* 1971; 1:975–6.
15. Jelliffe RW. Creatinine clearance: bedside estimate. *Ann Intern Med.* 1973; 79:604–5.
16. Mawer GE, Knowles BR, Lucas BB et al. Computer-assisted prescribing of kanamycin for patients with renal insufficiency. *Lancet.* 1972; 1:12–5.
17. Kampmann J, Siersbaek-Nielsen JM. Rapid evaluation of creatinine clearance. *Acta Med Scand.* 1974; 196:517–20.
18. Sheiner LB, Beal SL. Some suggestions for measuring predictive performance. *J Pharmacokinet Biopharm.* 1981; 9:503–12.
19. Sokal RR, Rohlf FJ. Biometry. San Francisco: W. H. Freeman; 1981.
20. Forbes GB, Bruining GJ. Urinary creatinine excretion and lean body mass. *Am J Clin Nutr.* 1976; 29:1359–66.
21. Schiller WR, Long CL, Blakemore WS. Creatinine and nitrogen excretion in seriously ill and injured patients. *Surg Gynecol Obstet.* 1979; 149:561–6.
22. Enger E, Blegen EM. The relationship between endogenous creatinine clearance and serum creatinine in renal failure. *Scand J Clin Lab Invest* 1964; 16:273–80.
23. Jones JD, Burnett PC. Creatinine metabolism in humans with decreased renal function: creatinine deficit. *Clin Chem.* 1974; 20:1204–12.
24. Cocchetto DM, Tschanz C, Bjornsson TD. Decreased rate of creatinine production in patients with hepatic diseases: implications for estimation of creatinine clearance. *Ther Drug Monit.* 1983; 5:161–8.
25. Chrymko MM, Schentag JJ. Creatinine clearance predictions in acutely ill patients. *Am J Hosp Pharm.* 1981; 38:837–40.
26. Hull JH, Hak LJ, Koch GG et al. Influence of range of renal function and liver disease on predictability of creatinine clearance. *Clin Pharmacol Ther.* 1981; 29:516–21.

Appendix—Methods for Urinary Creatinine Clearance Estimation

1. Bjornsson (BJ) Use nomogram in reference 2
2. Cockcroft and Gault (CG) (reference 12)
   Male: $CL_{cr} = [(140 - \text{age in yr}) \times LBW]/72\ Scr$
   Female: $CL_{cr} = 0.85 \times CL_{cr}$ (male)
3. Hallynck (HA) (reference 13)
   $CL_{cr} = E/Scr$, where E (urinary creatinine excretion rate) is obtained from graph
4. Jelliffe (J1) (reference 14)
   Male: $CL_{cr} = 100/(Scr - 12)$
   Female: $CL_{cr} = 80/(Scr - 7)$
5. Jelliffe (J2) (reference 15)
   Male: $CL_{cr} = [98 - 0.8\ (\text{age in yr} - 20)]/\ Scr$
   Female: $CL_{cr} = 0.90 \times CL_{cr}$ (male)
6. Mawer (MA) (reference 16)
   Male: Creatinine output $(OP)m = Wt\ (29.3 - 0.203\ \text{age in yr})$
   Female: Creatinine output $(OP)f = Wt\ (25.3 - 0.175\ \text{age in yr})$
   Adjusted output $(AOP) = OP\ (1 - 0.03\ Scr)$
   $CL_{cr} = [100\ (AOP)]/[Scr\ (1440)]$
7. Siersbaek-Nielsen (SN)
   Use nomogram in reference 17

Drug Experience

Straightforward reports of unusual drug experiences are included in this section. These may be confirmations of previously reported drug experiences or brief apparent first reports. While selected references may be cited, the purpose of a Drug Experience report is not to present an extensive review of the literature.

A related section, Grand Rounds, includes papers that are well-documented patient case reports with a thorough review of the important literature to help put the case in perspective.

Bromate poisoning from ingestion of professional hair-care neutralizer

JANE N. LUE, CARY E. JOHNSON, AND DEBORAH L. EDWARDS

Clin Pharm. 1988; 7:66–70

Eleven cases of bromate poisoning were reported in the United States in the 1940s and 1950s when potassium bromate was marketed as a neutralizer in home permanent cold wave hair kits.[1–7] As a result, manufacturers subsequently substituted less toxic neutralizing agents such as perborate and hydrogen peroxide in the home permanent kits, and the reports of bromate poisoning were reduced to one in 1975.[8] However, case reports of bromate poisoning have increased, with five case reports in black children being described in recent literature.[9,10] The following case report, as well as the previous five case reports, involved ingestion of bromate found in "for-professional-use-only" neutralizer products. These products can be obtained from wholesale–retail vendors of beauty supplies that often sell special hair-care products to the public. The objective of this report is to inform practitioners of the clinical features and management of bromate poisoning by professional hair-care neutralizer.

JANE N. LUE, M.S., PHARM.D., is Resident in Hospital Pharmacy, Hermann Hospital, University of Texas, Houston; at the time of this report she was a Doctor of Pharmacy candidate, College of Pharmacy, The University of Michigan, Ann Arbor. CARY E. JOHNSON, PHARM.D., is Associate Professor of Pharmacy, College of Pharmacy, The University of Michigan, and Clinical Pharmacist–Pediatrics, University of Michigan Medical Center. DEBORAH L. EDWARDS, M.S., is Associate Director, Pharmacy Education, Charlotte Area Health Education Center, and Pediatric Clinical Pharmacist, Department of Pediatrics, Charlotte Memorial Hospital, Charlotte, NC; at the time of this report she was Clinical Pharmacist–Pediatrics, and Clinical Assistant Professor of Pharmacy, College of Pharmacy, The University of Michigan.

Address reprint requests to Dr. Johnson at the College of Pharmacy, The University of Michigan, 428 Church Street, Ann Arbor, MI 48109-1065.

Presented at the 44th ASHP Annual Meeting, Washington, DC, June 4, 1987.

Copyright © 1988, American Society of Hospital Pharmacists, Inc. All rights reserved. 0278-2677/88/0101-0066$01.25.

Case Report. A 21-month-old black boy was given approximately 6 oz of a professional cold wave neutralizer, California Curl (Morrow, San Diego, CA), to drink by his four-year-old cousin. When the mother found the child and the empty bottle, she immediately administered milk to induce vomiting. The patient was then taken, along with the empty bottle of neutralizer, to the emergency room of a local hospital. A poison control center was consulted regarding the ingredients of the neutralizer; however, the product's contents could not be conclusively identified until the manufacturer could be contacted the next morning. The only information available was that neutralizers generally contain either hydrogen peroxide, perborate, or bromate. Empiric therapy with activated charcoal 10 g orally every four hours was begun while further information from the poison control center was sought.

On admission, results of the physical examination were normal. The patient weighed 10.7 kg, and his blood pressure was 100/50 mm Hg. Results of laboratory tests revealed the following values: white blood cell count, 28,700/cu mm with no left shift; hemoglobin, 10.5 g/dL; hematocrit, 31.8%; and platelet count, 559,000/cu mm. Serum electrolyte concentrations were within normal limits, except for a bicarbonate concentration of 18.1 meq/L; values for blood urea nitrogen (BUN) and serum creatinine were 32 mg/dL and 1.7 mg/dL, respectively. The patient had been anuric since the time of ingestion. A Foley catheter was inserted, and a 20-mL sample of urine was obtained. Urinalysis results showed a specific gravity of 1.04, pH 6.5, proteinuria (3+), and trace amounts of glucose and ketones. Urine electrolyte concentrations were as follows: sodium, 48 meq/L; potassium, 72 meq/L; and chloride, 136 meq/L. The urine urea nitrogen concentration was 61 mg/dL. The calculated fractional excretion of sodium was 26.5%, indicating acute renal failure. In an attempt to maintain urinary output, three doses of intravenous furosemide 5 mg were administered at 30-minute intervals, resulting in a total urine production of 40 mL.

The next morning, information was received from the poison control center via the manufacturer that California Curl contained 7% sodium bromate. The recommendations for management of bromate poisoning were provided, as follows: (1) administration of an emetic agent, (2) gastric lavage with 2% sodium bicarbonate, (3) administration of 1% sodium thiosulfate solution by intravenous drip in a total dose of 100 to 500 mL or 10 to 50 mL of a 10% solution given intravenously over ½ to 1 hour, and (4) supportive management of acute renal failure and anemia. Subsequently, 20 mL of 10% sodium thiosulfate solution was infused intravenously over one hour. Laboratory studies revealed metabolic acidosis (blood pH 7.29; bicarbonate, 15 meq/L; and urine pH 5.0). Lactated Ringer's injection and sodium bicarbonate were administered intravenously to increase the blood pH to 7.34. Another finding was severe anemia (hemoglobin, 7.9 g/dL; hematocrit, 24.4%). Evaluation of red blood cell morphology showed the presence of anisocytes, poikilocytes, and Burr cells. A transfusion of packed red blood cells 10 mL/kg was administered. Because of continued anuria, the child was transferred on the evening of the second hospital day to The University of Michigan Medical Center for initiation of peritoneal dialysis.

On admission, physical examination revealed a lethargic boy with decreased bilateral muscle tone. The initial laboratory data were as follows: sodium, 129 meq/L; potassium, 4.6 meq/L; chloride, 94 meq/L; bicarbonate, 12 meq/L; BUN, 72 mg/dL; creatinine, 4.5 mg/dL; white blood cell count, 25,000/cu mm with segmented neutrophils 69%, band neutrophils 5%, lymphocytes 19%, and monocytes 7%; platelet count, 551,000/cu mm; hemoglobin, 5.68 g/dL; and hematocrit, 19.2%. Calcium and phosphorus concentrations were within normal limits and aminotransferase concentrations were slightly elevated. Anuria continued with a total urine output of 9 mL after intravenous administration of one dose of furosemide 10 mg. Urinalysis results disclosed moderate bacteriuria, proteinuria (3+), glucosuria (2+), hematuria (2+), and ketonuria (1+). Urine osmolarity was 280 mOsm/L. Peritoneal dialysis was initiated and continued for seven days.

During the first three days of hospitalization, the hematocrit, hemoglobin, and blood pressure continued to fall, and three transfusions of packed red blood cells 10 mL/kg were administered. The lactate dehydrogenase concentration was 1069 IU/L, and hemolysis was suspected. Fluid intake was restricted to 600 mL per day. Spontaneous voiding resumed on the sixth day after ingestion, after 144 hours of anuria and four days of dialysis. The peritoneal catheter was removed two days later when the child's urine output exceeded 100 mL per day. At this time his BUN was 87 mg/dL, and the creatinine concentration was 6.1 mg/dL. His urine output steadily increased, and intravenous fluid was administered accordingly. He entered a transient phase of high-output renal failure; however, this condition resolved, and he was discharged to home 14 days after the ingestion. Laboratory values on discharge were hemoglobin, 9.2 g/dL; hematocrit, 27.6%; white blood cell count, 13,000/cu mm; BUN, 49 mg/dL; and creatinine, 1.3 mg/dL.

Results of laboratory tests conducted during a return visit one month after ingestion showed continued mild renal failure, with a creatinine clearance 20% below the predicted normal range. The laboratory value for BUN was 20 mg/dL, and the creatinine concentration was 0.6 mg/dL. At this time, the patient's anemia had resolved, and there was no apparent hearing loss.

Discussion. Permanent cold wave setting solutions containing bromates consist of (1) a thioglycollate hair-care lotion that changes sulfur–sulfur bonds of keratins to sulfur–hydrogen bonds, thus making hair flexible, and (2) either a 2–4% potassium bromate solution or a 10–20% sodium bromate solution, which is a strong oxidizing agent that oxidizes the sulfur–hydrogen bond to the original sulfur–sulfur bond, thus stabilizing the curling of the hair[11] (Table 1).

Bromate is absorbed unchanged[5] from the gastrointestinal tract and is primarily excreted unchanged in the urine[13] at a slow rate. Although not well established, the estimated toxic dose of potassium bromate in children is 240–500 mg/kg of body weight.[11] All of the previous case reports involved ingestion of potassium bromate (Table 2). In this case, approximately 12.6 g of sodium bromate (molecular weight, 151) was ingested. This is equivalent, on a weight-to-weight basis, to 13.9 g or 1300 mg of potassium bromate (molecular weight, 167) per kilogram of body weight. This quantity is three to six times the estimated toxic dose in children, although sodium bromate has been found to be less toxic than potassium bromate in an animal model.[14] Serum bromide concentrations have not correlated with the degree of toxicity, and serum bromate concentrations have not been reported.[9,10]

Toxic Effects of Bromate. Ingestion of bromate is followed by nausea, vomiting, severe abdominal pain, and diarrhea in varying degrees of severity beginning 30 minutes to 2 hours after ingestion.[11] These effects have been attributed to the caustic actions of hydrobromic acid produced by the chemical reaction between gastric acid and the bromate ion.[14] Hematologic effects of bromate toxicity have included anemia and hemolysis. Anemia was reported in four pediatric cases,[1–3,10] and hemolytic anemia occurred in one case (Table 2).[9] Severe ane-

Table 1.
Selected Bromate-Containing Neutralizers in Permanent Wave Preparations

Product	Manufacturer	Form	Contents[a]
Bio Wave permanent wave neutralizer	Redken	Lotion	Sodium (or potassium), bromate 10–25%, surfactant 0–1%, phosphates 0–1%, protein 0–2%, clouding agents 0–5%, water greater than 50%
Curl & Condition permanent wave neutralizer	Redken	Lotion	Sodium (or potassium) bromate 10–25%, surfactants 0–1%, phosphates 0–1%, protein 0–2%, clouding agents 0–5%, water greater than 50%
RK Trichoperm Style support neutralizer	Redken	Lotion	Sodium bromate 15–18%, surfactant 0–1%, phosphates 0–1%, protein 0–2%, water greater than 50%
Revlon hair preparation neutralizer	Revlon	Lotion	Sodium bromate 10%, conditioning agents, surfactants, emulsifiers, fragrance, water
Trichoperm permanent wave neutralizing lotion	Redken	Lotion	Sodium bromate 15–18%, surfactants 0–1%, phosphates 0–1%, protein 0–2%, clouding agents 0–5%, water
California Curl	Morrow	Lotion	Sodium bromate 7%, urea 1.5%, lanolin 2%, surfactants 0–1%, water

[a] Information on California Curl was obtained from the manufacturer; all other information was obtained from reference 12.

mia also developed in our patient, although the evidence for hemolysis was inconclusive.

Central nervous system effects have included seizures, which have been reported in three cases,[1,2,9] and a transient loss of consciousness, which has been reported in one case.[5] Long-term sequelae have not been reported.

Although the toxic manifestations described above are considered reversible, hearing loss and renal failure are potentially irreversible sequelae of bromate poisoning.[10] Case reports in which the patient died were primarily associated with acute renal failure.[1,11,15] Of the 17 pediatric cases reported, 12 patients developed acute renal failure, resulting in one death (Table 2). A total of 22 adult intoxications have been reported in the foreign literature, which were associated with suicide attempts by professional hairdressers who ingested professional cold wave neutralizers.[11,15] Of these 22 adult patients, 20 developed acute renal failure, and 9 died of this complication.[11,15] In many of the adult cases, recovery of renal function was not complete, and in some patients chronic renal failure developed, requiring hemodialysis.[16] Sections of the kidney obtained from a pediatric patient who died three days after ingesting bromate showed acute tubular necrosis evidenced by flattening and desquamation of the renal tubular epithelium.[9] Serial renal biopsies from the adult patients who had chronic renal failure demonstrated interstitial fibrosis and infiltration by lymphocytes,[8,15] destruction of basement membrane,[17] and hyalinization of glomeruli.[18]

Metabolic acidosis, which has been reported in many cases of bromate toxicity,[3,9,10] occurred in this case. It can be associated with the destruction of the carbonic anhydrase system in the renal tubules, as evidenced by low serum bicarbonate concentrations and elevated urine pH.

Permanent sensorineural hearing loss occurred within 4 to 16 hours in 20 adult patients[11,15] and within 7 days to 3 months in two children.[8,9] Although no obvious sequelae were described in most of the other pediatric cases, hearing function was not specifically described. Several substances are known to have a profound effect on both the kidney and the inner ear. These include the aminoglycoside antibiotics, furosemide, and ethacrynic acid. Quick et al.[8] demonstrated antigenic similarities between the stria vascularis of the cochlea and the renal tubules. Physiologically, the kidney and the inner ear both manifest highly efficient systems for the transport of water and electrolytes across cellular barriers. The patient in this case had

Table 2.
Summary of Pediatric Cases of Bromate Toxicity

Reference	Age (yr)	Race and Sex[a]	Amount of Bromate Ingested	Product (Manufacturer)	Vomiting/ Diarrhea[b]	ARF[c]	Abnormal Urinary Sediments[b]	Anemia[b]	Neurological Symptoms and Other Complications	Outcome
1	1½	M			+/−	+ (24)	+	+	Generalized seizures	Patient died
2	2½	M	120 mL	Toni (Revlon)	+/+	+ (16)	+	+	Seizures	Normal
3	3	WM			+/+	+	+	+	Metabolic acidosis	Mild renal failure
	2½	WF	60–90 mL		+/−	+ (48)	+		Metabolic acidosis	Normal renal function
	3	WF	1–1.5 g		+/−	−	−			Normal renal function
	8	M	60 mL		+/−	−	−			
4	14	WF	14 g	Toni (Revlon)	+/−	+ (12)	+	−		Normal renal function
5	3	M	4 g	Toni (Revlon)	+/+	+	+		Loss of consciousness, depressed respiration	Normal physical examination on follow-up
6	4	M			+/−	−	−			No follow-up
7	2	M	3.5 g	Toni (Revlon)	+/+	−	+	−		Normal renal function
	1¾	WF		Richard Hudnut	+/−	+ (72)	+	−		Full recovery
8	6	M	0.5 g		+/+	+ (12)				Permanent renal failure and deafness
9	1½	BF		Professional Preference (Fe. Davis Co.)	+/+	+ (3)	+	+	Seizures, metabolic acidosis, hemolytic uremic syndrome	Permanent renal failure and deafness, renal tubular acidosis
10	2	BM	Mouthful	Soft & Free (M & M Products Co.)	+/−	+ (6)		−		Normal hearing
	1½	BM	30 mL	Cosmopolitan Curl (Bronner Bros.)	+/−	+ (0.5)	+	−		Normal hearing
	1½	BM		Cosmopolitan Curl (Bronner Bros.)	+/−	−	−	−	Metabolic acidosis	No follow-up
	1½	BM	60–90 mL	Soft & Free (M & M Products Co.)	−/−	+	+	+	Metabolic acidosis	Normal hearing

[a] Race indicated if this information was supplied.
[b] + = Finding present; − = finding absent.
[c] ARF = acute renal failure; time of onset in hours after ingestion is given in parentheses.

no apparent hearing loss one month after bromate ingestion.

Treatment. Immediate gastric acid neutralization by lavage with sodium bicarbonate dissolved in water may remove unabsorbed bromate and prevent or reduce formation of hydrobromic acid.[2] Although intravenous sodium thiosulfate is an antidote for bromate poisoning by reducing bromate to the bromide ion, which is much less toxic,[10] it should not be included in gastric lavage because it reacts with bromate, in the presence of gastric acid, to form highly toxic and irritating hydrogen sulfide.[5] The therapeutic value of hemodialysis in reducing or preventing nephrotoxicity or ototoxicity has not been established, but it should be considered in treating patients with bromate poisoning if it is begun within 24 hours of ingestion of a large quantity of bromate.[10]

The current guidelines for management of bromate ingestion can be summarized as follows: (1) induce vomiting, (2) perform gastric lavage with 2% sodium bicarbonate, (3) administer 1% sodium thiosulfate solution by intravenous drip in a total dose of 100 to 500 mL or administer 10 to 50 mL of a 10% solution intravenously over 30 minutes to 1 hour, (4) correct dehydration and electrolyte or acid–base disturbances with appropriate intravenous solutions, (5) correct anemia with transfusions of packed red blood cells as necessary, and (6) in case of acute renal failure with oliguria or anuria that is unresponsive to intravenous furosemide, initiate peritoneal dialysis or hemodialysis.

Need for Product Labeling. The "for-professional-use-only" neutralizers are exempt from the packaging and labeling regulations of the Fair Packaging and Labelling Act, which requires accurate labeling of the contents of consumer products. Because the chemical contents of these products are not listed on the package and are not included in toxicology references, confusion and delay in specific medical management occurred in this case and two other reported pediatric cases.[9,10] In this case, the ingested substance could only be identified via the manufacturer, and the identification was delayed for 34 hours after ingestion. Earlier administration of the antidote, sodium thiosulfate, and initiation of peritoneal dialysis may have reduced the severity and duration of anemia, metabolic acidosis, and acute renal failure in this 21-month-old boy. To facilitate appropriate treatment in cases of intoxication with these professional neutralizing solutions, legislation requiring explicit labeling with product ingredients and precautions is needed, and 24-hour telephone numbers should be provided on every product label so that product information can be readily obtained. Tighter control of distribution of these products to the public should be developed and enforced. Additionally, these products should be listed in current toxicology references.

Conclusion. This case illustrates the need for early recognition and appropriate treatment of bromate intoxication as a result of ingestion of a "for-professional-use-only" hair-curling neutralizer.

References

1. Dunsky I. Potassium bromate poisoning. *Am J Dis Child.* 1947; 74:730–4.
2. Thompson HC, Westfall SW. Potassium bromate poisoning: report of a case due to ingestion of a "cold wave" neutralizer. *J Pediatr.* 1949; 34:362–4.
3. Kitto W, Dumars KW. Potassium bromate poisoning. *J Pediatr.* 1949; 35:197–200.
4. Robertson HF, Flothow MW, Kissen MD. Potassium bromate poisoning. *J Pediatr.* 1950; 36:241–3.
5. Parker WA, Barr JR. Potassium bromate poisoning. *Br Med J.* 1951; 1:1363.
6. Benson GI. Potassium bromate poisoning. *Br Med J.* 1950; 1:1516.
7. Knappenberger RC. Potassium bromate poisoning. *J Pediatr.* 1952; 40:105–8.
8. Quick CA, Cole RA, Mauer SM. Deafness and renal failure due to potassium bromate poisoning. *Arch Otolaryngol.* 1975; 101:494–5.
9. Gradus D, Rhoads M, Bergstrom LB. Acute bromate poisoning associated with renal failure and deafness presenting as hemolytic uremic syndrome. *Am J Nephrol.* 1984; 4:188–91.
10. Warshaw BL, Carter MC. Bromate poisoning from hair permanent preparations. *Pediatrics.* 1985; 76:975–8.
11. Matsumoto I, Morizono T, Paparella MM. Hearing loss following potassium bromate: two case reports. *Otolaryngol Head Neck Surg.* 1980; 88:625–9.
12. Rumack BH, ed. Poisindex. 51st ed. Denver: Micromedix Inc.; 1987.
13. Sollman T, ed. A manual of pharmacology and its applications to pharmacology and toxicology. 2nd ed. Philadelphia: W. B. Saunders Company; 1922.
14. Santesson CG, Wickberg G. The action of sodium bromate. *Skandinav Arch Physiol.* 1913; 30:337.
15. Oh SH, Lee HY, Chung SH. Acute renal failure due to potassium bromate poisoning. *Ynsei Med J.* 1980; 21:106–9.
16. Shigematsu M, Hirata K. Acute renal failure due to bromate poisoning: report of 8 cases. *Nishinihon J Urol.* 1973; 35:280–90.
17. Kuwahara T, Ikehara Y, Kanatsu K. Two cases of potassium bromate poisoning requiring long-term hemodialysis therapy for irreversible tubular damage. *Nephron.* 1984; 37:278–80.
18. Niwa T, Ito T, Matsui E. Serial renal biopsy in potassium bromate intoxication. *Jpn Circ J.* 1974; 38:387–92.

Treatment of oral candidiasis with amphotericin B solution

Renée Brandell, Sandra L. Chase, and John R. Cohn

Clin Pharm. 1988; 7:70–2

Candida albicans, a fungus, is the most common cause of oral thrush or candidiasis.[1] Oral thrush occurs in a variety of patient populations, including infants, particularly newborns, the elderly, immunocompromised patients, and even healthy adults. Although considered a minor ailment, it is often distressing to the patient and if not properly treated may develop into a chronic condition. The condition may appear benign; therefore, oral thrush should be given prompt attention to prevent spread to adjacent tissues or progression to systemic candidiasis. Current therapeutic modalities for the treatment of oral candidiasis include nystatin suspension, troches, or vaginal tablets; clotrimazole troches; gentian violet; ketoconazole; and miconazole.[2] However, these products are not always effective. We describe the use of amphotericin B oral solution in a patient with oral candidiasis that was refractory to conventional treatment.

Case Report. The patient was a 66-year-old white woman with a three-year history of common variable agammaglobulinemia and cutaneous anergy. Since the time of diagnosis, the disease had been treated with intravenous immune globulin (Gammagard; Hyland Therapeutics Division, Travenol Laboratories, Inc., Glendale, CA) on an outpatient basis and during hospitalizations for treatment of various infections that developed secondary to her disease. She first developed symptomatic oral thrush in early 1985. Her medical history was notable for several years of chronic respiratory and urinary-tract infections, non-insulin-dependent diabetes mellitus, asthma, mitral valve prolapse, ventricular arrhythmias, peptic ulcer disease, and non-A, non-B hepatitis.

In October 1986 the patient was hospitalized for evaluation of abdominal pain and subsequently

Renée Brandell is Staff Pharmacist, Department of Pharmacy, Thomas Jefferson University Hospital, Philadelphia, PA. Sandra L. Chase, Pharm.D., is Cardiopulmonary Clinical Pharmacist, Department of Pharmacy, Thomas Jefferson University Hospital. John R. Cohn, M.D., is Clinical Assistant Professor of Medicine and Pediatrics, Jefferson Medical College, Philadelphia, PA.

Address reprint requests to Dr. Chase at the Department of Pharmacy, Thomas Jefferson University Hospital, 111 S. 11th Street, Philadelphia, PA 19107.

Presented at the 44th ASHP Annual Meeting, Washington, DC, June 3, 1987.

Copyright © 1988, American Society of Hospital Pharmacists, Inc. All rights reserved. 0278-2677/88/0101-0070$00.75.

received another course of immune globulin. She was a pleasant, thin white woman in no apparent distress. Physical examination was notable for multiple ulcers with raised white borders on the lateral edge of the tongue bilaterally and a sharp nonradiating abdominal pain. Medications on admission included quinidine sulfate 200 mg orally four times a day, verapamil hydrochloride 80 mg orally three times a day, sustained-release theophylline 200 mg orally twice a day, ranitidine 150 mg orally twice a day, furosemide 40 mg orally daily, nitrofurantoin 50 mg orally once a day, nystatin suspension 500,000 units orally four times a day, and triamcinolone acetonide oral inhaler, which she used episodically.

Many antifungal regimens had been tried in the past with varying degrees of success. The severity of the oral candidiasis could not be related to the immune globulin treatment schedule. Treatment of the patient's oral thrush began in early 1985 with the administration of nystatin suspension orally three times a day. Initially, treatment produced some improvement; however, the patient continued to experience some discomfort. The nystatin was discontinued, and ketoconazole orally once daily was initiated. This treatment was discontinued shortly thereafter due to patient complaints of severe headaches. Clotrimazole troches were started on an outpatient basis in May 1985. When the patient was last admitted for immune globulin therapy in July 1986, she complained that her oral thrush was not improving even though she had continued treatment with clotrimazole troches; therefore, the otolaryngology service was consulted. During this admission a throat swab was performed, and results showed no fungal elements present. Diagnosis was based on physical examination and previous improvement with antifungal therapy. One of the recommendations was administration of nystatin vaginal tablets orally three times a day. Nystatin tablets were not administered, and clotrimazole troches, one lozenge dissolved in the mouth five times a day, were started because of patient preference. Therapy was unsatisfactory, and the patient was restarted on nystatin suspension and discharged.

During the patient's hospital stay in October 1986, her oral candidiasis worsened, causing her much discomfort. An infectious-disease consultant suggested treatment with oral amphotericin B solution. The solution was prepared with 50 mg of amphotericin B injection (Fungizone; E. R. Squibb & Sons, Inc.) diluted in 500 mL of sterile water, resulting in a final concentration of 0.1 mg/mL. The dosage ordered was 15 mL to swish and expectorate four times a day. After four days of therapy, the number of white plaques present decreased. Subjectively, the patient believed that there had been substantial improvement. The patient was discharged with arrangements made for the amphotericin B solution to be prepared on an outpatient basis. The patient was advised to refrigerate the solution and to store it in the amber bottle in which it was dispensed.

Subsequent admissions and visits to her physician over the next six months revealed that therapy with amphotericin B solution continued to be successful. The patient also stated that the flavorless solution prevented the eruption of lesions. According to the patient, if she used the amphotericin B solution less frequently than prescribed, the lesions worsened. No adverse effects have yet been reported.

Discussion. In the United States, amphotericin B is commonly administered intravenously for the treatment of systemic fungal infections and topically for both cutaneous and mucocutaneous mycotic infections. Amphotericin B is a polyene antibiotic derived from a strain of *Streptomyces nodosus*. The drug is highly active in vitro against a wide variety of fungal species, among them *Candida*.[1] The antifungal spectrum of amphotericin B is broader than that of nystatin, but like the latter amphotericin B has no antibacterial activity.[1] When administered orally or topically the drug is nontoxic and nonirritating.[1] Amphotericin B can be readily prepared as a suspension without loss of potency. It is also manufactured commercially outside the United States (Funglin; Squibb, United Kingdom) as a 100-mg tablet, a 10-mg lozenge, a 50-mg pessary, a 100-mg/mL suspension, and a 2% adhesive base (Funglin in Orabase).

Various studies have been done using amphotericin B in a lozenge or tablet form. Ewing[1] studied the use of amphotericin B in a lozenge form for the treatment of candidiasis of the mouth, tongue, and lips. The study consisted of 81 patients from any age group and with any type of oral lesion that upon mycological swab or culture, or both, demonstrated the presence of *C. albicans*. The average number of lozenges administered was four daily for an average of seven days. Of the 81 patients, 71 (87%) were clinically cured; of those 71 patients, 52 (73%) were mycologically cured of *C. albicans*, and 19 (27%) still showed the presence of yeasts, but in reduced numbers.

A study conducted by Montes et al.[3] examined the treatment of chronic candidiasis in four patients over a six-month period. Two of the patients were young children with oral candidiasis as well as candidal granulomas and onchomycosis. Two subjects had oral candidiasis with systemic involvement. Dosages administered ranged from 1000 mg to 1800 mg per day in the form of an oral 200-mg tablet. At completion of the treatment period, two of the patients were free of all lesions. One subject showed clearing of oral lesions, whereas therapy was discontinued in another patient after three months because of lack of efficacy.

Because of earlier successful results with amphotericin B tablets, Montes et al.[4] studied 10 patients ranging in age from 4 to 61 years who had either long-standing chronic mucocutaneous candidiasis (five patients) or oral candidiasis alone (five patients). These patients were treated with 100-mg and 200-mg amphotericin B tablets. The patients dissolved the tablets slowly in the mouth three to four times daily. The total daily dosage ranged from 400 mg to 1600 mg. Therapy was evaluated after two weeks. All patients experienced excellent clinical and mycological response without adverse effects. Posttreatment cultures from the five patients with oral candidiasis alone were negative. Only very small numbers of colonies of *C. albicans* were obtained from the five patients with chronic mucocutaneous candidiasis.

Oral candidiasis has also been treated with amphotericin B in a topical preparation.[5] This preparation, containing 2% amphotericin B in an adhesive base (Orabase), was applied to oral candidal lesions after meals and at bedtime. Twenty-eight of 33 patients showed definite improvement, and four showed slight improvement.

A study conducted by Ching et al.[6] in 1983 reviewed the absorption of orally administered amphotericin B. Rather than the conventional microbiological methods previously used to determine serum concentrations of the drug, a more sensitive assay method, high-pressure liquid chromatography, was used. Fourteen patients with normal renal and hepatic function, suffering from various malignancies and receiving antineoplastic-drug therapy, were evaluated. The subjects received 10-mg lozenges either three or four times a day as prophylaxis against candidiasis. Duration of therapy ranged from two days to several months. Serum amphotericin B concentrations of up to 125 ng/mL and 165 ng/mL were found in patients receiving daily dosages of 30 and 40 mg, respectively. No apparent signs of toxicity were noted.

These results are in contrast to previous studies showing plasma concentrations of less than 3 ng/mL. Many of these earlier studies used daily dosages of amphotericin B of 2–10 g. Several factors may account for the absorption demonstrated by Ching and associates. In this study the 10-mg lozenges were retained in the mouth until dissolved, whereas previously they were swallowed. This fact suggests that the absorption across the buccal mucosa is superior to the gastrointestinal absorption of amphotericin B, which is unstable in acid and therefore in the stomach contents.[6] In addition, the more sensitive assay could have been responsible, at least in part, for the higher plasma concentrations recorded. These studies demonstrate the efficacy of various forms of amphotericin B such as tablets, lozenges, and an adhesive base. Adverse effects associated with the lozenges and tablets are minimal, but gastrointestinal upset has been reported when daily dosages exceeding 3 g were continued for several months.[7] This irritation was mild and readily cleared on cessation of treatment. In addition, amphotericin B is flavorless (in contrast to the unpleasant flavor of nystatin), which may enhance patient compliance. The antifungal spectrum of amphotericin is broader than that of nystatin, which may be beneficial in patients with oral candidiasis.

Conclusion. We have described the successful use of a 0.1-mg/mL oral solution of amphotericin B for the treatment of oral candidiasis refractory to other antifungal regimens. Although little information is available on the use of oral amphotericin B and comparative studies have not been performed, clinicians should be aware that this may be a therapeutic alternative if conventional treatment is not effective.

References

1. Ewing AE. Amphotericin B lozenges in the treatment of oral thrush. *Practitioner.* 1967; 199:62–7.
2. Petersdorf RG, Adams RD, Braunwald E et al., eds. Harrison's principles of internal medicine. New York: McGraw-Hill Book Co.; 1983:1060–1.
3. Montes LF, Cooper MD, Bradford LG et al. Treatment of chronic mucocutaneous candidiasis with amphotericin B. *Arch Dermatol.* 1971; 104:45–56.
4. Montes LF, Moore WJ, Soto TG et al. Amphotericin B tablets in oral candidiasis. *Cutis.* 1973; 11:146–8.
5. Martindale: the extra pharmacopoeia. 27th ed. Wade A, ed. London: The Pharmaceutical Press; 1977:719.
6. Ching MS, Raymond K, Bury RW et al. Absorption of orally administered amphotericin B lozenges. *Br J Clin Pharmacol.* 1983; 16:106–8.
7. APBI data sheet compendium, 1986–1987. London: Datapharm Publications Limited; 1986:1480.

ASHP Report

Procedure for submission of manuscripts to journals published by the American Society of Hospital Pharmacists

—Detach or copy these pages and mail with manuscript—

To expedite manuscript review, the American Society of Hospital Pharmacists requires that a copy of this form be completed and enclosed with each paper submitted for publication to the *American Journal of Hospital Pharmacy* or *Clinical Pharmacy*. Authors thereby certify that their papers comply with the major stylistic requirements of ASHP's journals, which are generally in conformance with the Uniform Requirements for Manuscripts Submitted to Biomedical Journals (*Am J Hosp Pharm*. 1982; 39:1538–43 and *Clin Pharm*. 1986; 5:33). ASHP exceptions to the Uniform Requirements are noted with an asterisk (*). Authors must comply with and check each point on the list (or mark "NA" for not applicable). If a manuscript is received without a completed form, the editor will mail a blank form to the author and not process the paper until the form has been completed. *The procedure applies to all manuscripts except letters, book reviews, therapy consultations, and management consultations.* (*For letters to the editor, see the first page of the Letters column in any issue.*)

Authors are requested to include with each manuscript a letter of transmittal, the minimum content of which is noted in the checklist below. Authors are encouraged to suggest appropriate reviewers for a manuscript. For exceptionally important work, the editors will consider requests by the authors for expedited ("fast track") review.

Unsolicited manuscripts are acknowledged within one week of their receipt with a letter from the editors. The letter includes a code number that should be cited in all communications regarding the manuscript.

Manuscripts should be submitted to the editor of the appropriate journal at the following address: 4630 Montgomery Avenue, Bethesda, MD 20814.

Letter of Transmittal

_____Summarizes in no more than two sentences the nature of the manuscript.
_____Includes information on prior or duplicate publication or submission elsewhere of any part of the work.
_____Includes a statement of financial or other relationships that might lead to a conflict of interests.

General

_____The corresponding author for this manuscript is

____

_____The preferred mailing address for the corresponding author is

____

____

____

____

_____The corresponding author can be reached during business hours at the following telephone number:

____

_____Six complete copies (including photostatic copies of all figures) of the manuscript are submitted. One set of camera-ready figures is submitted. The authors understand that the editors are not obligated to return any of this material.
_____Manuscript is typed double-spaced *throughout* (including tables, references, footnotes, figure captions, and author identification) on 21.6 × 27.9-cm white paper with margins of at least 2.5 cm all around.
_____Manuscript is not typed using all upper-case letters.
_____All pages are numbered consecutively (in the upper right-hand corner), beginning with the title page and including tables.
_____Each of the following elements begins on a separate page, in this sequence: title page, author identification page, abstract, text, footnotes, references, tables, figure captions, and figures.*
_____Abbreviations are in accordance with the *CBE Style Manual*, 5th ed. (pages 241–68). No drug or chemical names are abbreviated.
_____Pharmacokinetic abbreviations agree with those given in the following article: Rowland M, Tucker G. Symbols in pharmacokinetics. *J Pharmacokinet Biopharm*. 1980; 8:497–507.
_____If the manuscript reports the results of a survey, three copies of the survey instrument should be sent for use in the review process (not for publication).
_____Manuscript is accompanied by copies of any permission to reproduce published material, to use illustrations of identifiable persons, or to name persons for their contributions.

Title Page

_____Contains concise, informative title and no other information.

Author Identification Page

_____Lists as authors only those individuals who have participated sufficiently in the work to take public responsibility for the content. (Participation solely in the collection of data does not justify authorship. See *Clin Pharm*. 1986; 5:33 for elaboration.)
_____Lists the authors near the top of the page, giving first name, middle initial, and last name of each.
_____Identifies each author in the format used in the author identification section of papers published in the *American Journal of Hospital Pharmacy* and *Clinical Pharmacy*, giving highest academic degree, position, department, and institution.
_____Denotes address for reprint requests.
_____Identifies in one or more paragraphs, as appropriate, (a) contributions that need acknowledging but do not justify authorship, (b) acknowledgments of technical help, (c) acknowledgments of material and financial support (including grant numbers), and (d) financial relationships that may constitute a conflict of interest.
_____If the paper was presented in whole or in part at a meeting, include name of meeting, location, and date.

Abstract (not required for Letters, Notes, Research Notes, Drug Experience, Commentaries, or Reflections)

_____Is less than 200 words.
_____For research reports, concisely states objectives, methods (procedures), main results (including specific data and their statistical significance, if possible), and principal conclusions.
_____For *AJHP* descriptive reports, concisely states purpose of program, how the program works, and conclusions.
_____For review articles and primers, concisely identifies main topics covered in the review, summary of major points, and conclusion.

Text

_____When reporting experiments on humans, indicates whether the procedures followed were in accord with the ethical standards of the institution's committee on human experimentation or in accord with the Helsinki Declaration of 1975.
_____When reporting experiments on animals, indicates whether the institution's or the National Research Council's guide for the care and use of laboratory animals was followed.
_____Names of authors, institutions, or patients are not mentioned, except in descriptive reports where institution identification is essen-

tial to understanding the program.

_____For Drug Experience papers, patients' age, gender, race, weight, pertinent past medical history, and baseline laboratory values are included, as well as the generic names, manufacturers, trade names, formulations, and routes of administration of all drug products used.

_____Descriptive headings are used to identify major sections of the paper; subheadings also may be used.

_____For stability studies, includes documentation that the assay used is stability indicating (see *Am J Hosp Pharm.* 1983; 40:1159–60.)

_____Identifies in the Methods section all statistical tests used and the a priori level of significance; unusual or complex statistical methods are explained briefly or referenced.

_____If more than one statistical test is used, the data evaluated by each test are clearly identified in the Methods section.

_____Mean values for study results are accompanied by some measure of variability or precision (e.g., standard deviations); the use of confidence intervals, when appropriate, is encouraged.

_____Identifies precisely all drugs and chemicals used by generic name (with salt, if applicable). Trade names are used only to identify that a specific brand of drug was used.

_____Measurements are reported in the units in which they were made. Volume, distance, and weight measurements should be expressed in metric units.*

_____For commercial products important to the paper, denotes, in parentheses, the trade name or model number; the manufacturer's name, city, state, and zip code; and the lot number. If such designations are numerous, they are listed as footnotes at the end of the text.

_____Every reference, figure, table, and appendix is cited in the text in numerical order. (Order of mention in text determines the number given to each.)

_____Footnotes are identified consecutively in the text by superscript, lower-case letters.*

References

_____Are identified in text, tables, and legends by superscript* Arabic numbers.

_____Are typed double-spaced on sheets separate from the text and numbered consecutively as they appear in the text.

_____Do not include any "unpublished observations" and "personal communications." (References to written, not oral, communications may be inserted, in parentheses, in the text or included as footnotes.)

_____Have been verified by the author(s) against the original documents.

_____Abbreviations of journal titles conform to those used in *Index Medicus* (January issue).

_____Include inclusive page numbers.

_____Are in the style adopted by the U.S. National Library of Medicine and used in *Index Medicus* with the exception that only the first three authors (last name and two initials, if available) are ever listed. Examples of this style follow:

(a) Standard journal article—(list all authors when three or less; when four or more, list only first three and add et al.*):

1. Roberts LW, O'Donnell J, Matsuda T et al. Pharmacy-assisted burn unit skin bank program. Am J Hosp Pharm. 1977; 34:1353–4.

(b) Article from journal paginated by issue:

2. Goldschmidt L. Remodeling on a shoe-string improves pharmacy's efficiency. Hospitals. 1979; 53(May 1):115–6.

(c) Letter, editorial, or abstract:

3. Wightkin WT, Buckhammer CR. Simple method for intravenous-to-oral theophylline dose conversion. Clin Pharm. 1982; 1:300–1. Letter.
4. Zellmer WA. Prescribing pharmacists. Am J Hosp Pharm. 1982; 39:1481. Editorial.
5. Bartle WR, Walker SE, Shapero T. Effect of cimetidine on phenytoin metabolism. Clin Pharmacol Ther. 1982; 31:202. Abstract.

(d) Book—personal author(s):

6. Osler AG. Complement: mechanisms and functions. Englewood Cliffs, NJ: Prentice-Hall; 1976.

(e) Chapter or article in a book:

7. Weinstein L, Swartz MN. Pathogenic properties of invading microorganisms. In: Sodeman WA Jr, Sodeman WA, eds. Pathologic physiology: mechanisms of disease. Philadelphia: WB Saunders; 1974: 457–72.

(f) Editor, compiler, or chairman as author of book:

8. Wertheimer AI, Smith MC, eds. Pharmacy practice: social and behavioral aspects. 7th ed. Baltimore: University Park Press; 1981.

(g) Governmental agency publication:

9. National Center for Health Statistics. Acute conditions: incidence and associated disability, United States July 1968–June 1969. Rockville, MD: National Center for Health Statistics, 1972; DHEW publication no. (HSM) 72-1036. (Vital and health statistics; series 10: Data from the National Health Survey; no. 69.)

(h) Package insert:

10. Roche Laboratories. Accutane package insert. Nutley, NJ: 1982 May.

(i) Paper presented at a meeting:

11. Stern NB, Millburg WJ, Steckel SD. Managing proper disposal of antineoplastic agents. Paper presented to 17th Annual ASHP Midyear Clinical Meeting. Los Angeles, CA: 1982 Dec 7.

Tables

_____Are typed double-spaced, each (complete with title and footnotes) on a separate page (not submitted as photographs).

_____Are submitted in the original typed size, not photo-reduced.

_____Do not contain information duplicated in the text or figures.

_____Are in the style used in ASHP's journals.

_____Do not contain horizontal or vertical rules within the tabulated information.

_____Use superscript letters for footnote designations.*

_____If use data from another published or unpublished source, permission is obtained from the source (proof submitted with paper) and the source is acknowledged.

Figure Captions

_____Are typed double-spaced on a sheet separate from the text.

_____Are numbered consecutively as they are cited in the text.

_____All abbreviations and symbols used in the figure are defined; when appropriate, the measure of variability or precision represented is identified (e.g., do error bands represent standard deviation(s) or a confidence interval?).

Figures

_____Are professionally drawn and photographed. (Freehand or typewritten lettering is unacceptable.)

_____Are submitted as sharp, glossy, black-and-white photographic prints, usually 12.7 × 17.3 cm but no larger than 20.3 × 25.4 cm.

_____Are designed such that, when reduced to one-column width (8 cm), are legible and occupy no more than 10 cm of column length.

_____Axis labels appear outside the axes.

_____Titles and detailed explanations (including keys to symbols used) are in the captions, not the illustrations themselves.

_____If previously published, the original source is acknowledged, and written permission from the copyright holder to reproduce the material is submitted.

_____Each photographic print has a label pasted on its back indicating the figure number and title of the paper. (Do not note authors' names.* Do not write on the back.)

Copyright

_____The following copyright transferal statement is submitted on a separate sheet identified with the title of the paper and signed and dated by *each* author:

In consideration of the American Society of Hospital Pharmacists (ASHP) taking action in reviewing and editing my (our) submission, the author(s) undersigned hereby transfer(s), assign(s), or otherwise convey(s) all ownership rights in the submission and all copyright ownership to the American Society of Hospital Pharmacists. In the event that such work is not published by ASHP, all said rights shall be released.

_____If this paper has been presented at a meeting other than one sponsored by ASHP, a copy of a release from the sponsors of that meeting, permitting publication elsewhere, is enclosed.

Exclusive Publication Statement

I certify that none of the material in this manuscript has been previously published and none of this material is under consideration, or has been accepted for publication elsewhere. This includes journal articles, letters to the editor, symposia, editorials, proceedings, transactions, books, articles published by invitation, news reports, and preliminary publications of any kind except an abstract of 400 words or less.

____

(Signature of Corresponding Author) (Date)

_____If the item immediately above has not been obeyed, an explanation is included in the letter of transmittal.

Final Check

_____By signing below, I certify that this manuscript has been carefully checked for compliance with requirements stated in this checklist.

____

(Signature of Corresponding Author) (Date)

CP Continuing Education

The ASHP Continuing Education system gives readers a self-assessment mechanism for selected articles in Clinical Pharmacy *and the* American Journal of Hospital Pharmacy. *It also allows readers to obtain continuing-education credit for these articles.*

For the purpose of CE-credit enrollment a blank answer sheet is published at the end of each installment of the column for the CE articles in that issue. An enrollee accumulates these answer sheets until the enrollment is submitted, using the form that is published in the June and December issues of Clinical Pharmacy *and in the June and December issues of the* American Journal of Hospital Pharmacy. *Any combination of tests within a 18-month period, from both* Clinical Pharmacy *and* American Journal of Hospital Pharmacy, *may be included in an enrollment. More complete details about enrollment in the system will appear in the semiannual enrollment form.*

Article 680-204-8801 (see page 37)
Qualifies for 1.0 hour of CE Credit

Sulbactam: A β-lactamase inhibitor

Learning Objectives

After studying this article, the reader should be able to

1. Identify the reasons for adding sulbactam to a β-lactam antibiotic.
2. List seven properties of a good β-lactamase inhibitor.
3. Identify the spectrum and mechanism of β-lactamase inhibition by sulbactam.
4. Describe the chemistry and pharmacokinetics and list the adverse drug reactions and contraindications of sulbactam–ampicillin.
5. State the FDA-approved labeling indications for sulbactam–ampicillin and compare the uses of sulbactam–ampicillin with those of other antibiotic regimens.

Self-assessment Questions

For each question there is one best answer only.

1. The addition of sulbactam sodium to ampicillin sodium for injection
   a. Produces a stability profile similar to that of sulbactam alone.
   b. Increases the activity of ampicillin.
   c. Increases the storage life of ampicillin.
   d. Increases the solubility of ampicillin.

2. Sulbactam is a β-lactamase inhibitor that is
   a. Water insoluble.
   b. A naturally occurring compound.
   c. Extremely unstable in solution at 37 °C.
   d. Known also as penicillanic acid sulfone.

3. A property that is not desirable for β-lactamase inhibitors is
   a. Activity against a wide range of β-lactamase enzymes.
   b. Similarity between the inhibitor and its β-lactam antibiotic partner with respect to pharmacologic properties.
   c. Hydrolysis of the inhibitor by β lactamases.
   d. Lack of induction of β-lactamase enzyme production.

4. Which one of the following statements best describes the β-lactamase inhibitory activity of sulbactam?
   a. Binding at the active site of the β-lactamase enzyme is reversible.
   b. Binding at the active site of the β-lactamase enzyme is noncompetitive.
   c. Inactivation of β lactamase renders both the inhibitor and enzyme incapable of further action.
   d. Sulbactam is highly reactive in the native form.

5. Which one of the following statements concerning the pharmacokinetics of sulbactam is not correct?
   a. The primary route of elimination is renal.
   b. Sulbactam metabolites have not been described.
   c. Drug accumulation has not been reported after repetitive dosing in healthy volunteers, surgical patients, and premature newborns.
   d. Serum concentration–time data obtained after intravenous administration suggest a one-compartment model.

6. The major adverse effects of sulbactam–ampicillin include all of the following except
   a. Pain at the injection site.
   b. Bleeding disorders and nephrotoxicity.
   c. Hypersensitivity reactions.
   d. Overgrowth of resistant organisms.

7. Sulbactam and clavulanic acid are similar with respect to
   a. Hydrolysis by β-lactamase enzymes.
   b. Spectrum of β-lactamase inhibitory activity.

c. Activity on a weight basis.
d. Interaction with penicillin-binding proteins.

8. Which one of the following statements best describes the effects of probenecid on sulbactam?

a. Probenecid decreases the serum concentrations of sulbactam.
b. Probenecid enhances tubular secretion of sulbactam.
c. Probenecid prolongs the elimination of sulbactam.
d. Probenecid does not interact with sulbactam.

9. The recommended dosage of sulbactam sodium–ampicillin sodium in patients with normal renal function is

a. Ampicillin 1–2 g plus sulbactam 0.5–1 g every six hours; the daily dosage of sulbactam should not exceed 4 g.
b. Ampicillin 1–2 g plus sulbactam 2–4 g every six hours; the daily dosage of sulbactam should not exceed 8 g.
c. A total daily dosage of greater than 12 g (equivalent to ampicillin 8 g plus sulbactam 4 g) for serious infections.
d. Ampicillin 2 g plus sulbactam 2 g every eight hours; the dosage interval should be increased to 12 or 24 hours in patients with renal failure.

10. Sulbactam sodium–ampicillin sodium for injection has FDA-approved labeling indications for all of the following conditions except

a. Upper-respiratory-tract infections.
b. Intra-abdominal infections.
c. Skin and skin structure infections.
d. Gynecologic infections.

Answer sheet

January 1988 ***Clinical Pharmacy***

Note: An enrollment form for the ASHP Continuing-Education System appears in the June and December issues. Please accumulate all the answer sheets you wish to use in one enrollment and submit them at one time with a completed enrollment form.

Place an X in the box(es) at the top of the column(s) corresponding to the test(s) you are taking. Darken the boxes corresponding to the correct answers.

☐
680-204-8801
1.0 hour

	a b c d		a b c d
1.	☐☐☐☐	6.	☐☐☐☐
2.	☐☐☐☐	7.	☐☐☐☐
3.	☐☐☐☐	8.	☐☐☐☐
4.	☐☐☐☐	9.	☐☐☐☐
5.	☐☐☐☐	10.	☐☐☐☐

ASHP Use Only
(1.0)8801 _______ (3)

NOW . . .

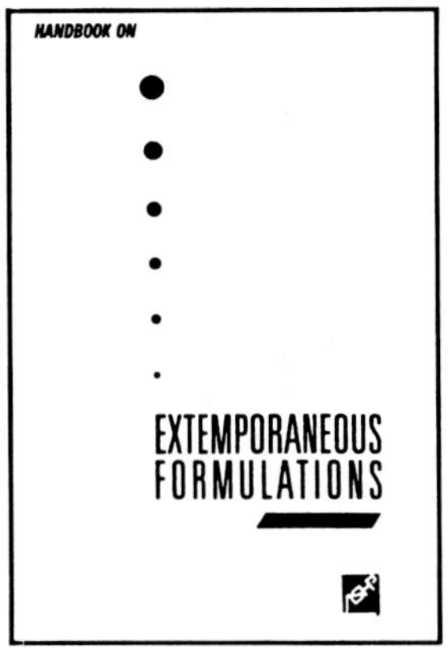

One comprehensive resource provides you 51 leading formulations for oral suspension.

The *Handbook on Extemporaneous Formulations*—new from ASHP—features those formulations most often requested for neonates, pediatric and geriatric patients, and others unable to take oral solids.

Concise instructions for each formulation provides:

- ingredients
- compounding instructions
- auxiliary labeling
- stability
- references (where available)

Spiralbound. Spill-resistant. Just $15.
Order this time saver today!

Prepared by the Committee on Extemporaneous Formulations, ASHP Special Interest Group (SIG) on Pediatric Pharmacy Practice.

ORDER FORM

YES! Please send me _______ copies of P254, the *Handbook on Extemporaneous Formulations*, at $15.00 each.

☐ Enclosed is my check for $ _______ .
(Checks must be drawn on a U.S. bank and payable to ASHP.)

☐ Enclosed is our purchase order # _______ ; please issue an invoice and add postage and handling.

OR

Charge $ _______ to my:
☐ MasterCard ☐ VISA

Acct. # _______ Exp. _______ month/year

Signature _______

Name _______

Institution _______

ASHP I.D.# _______

Address _______

City _______ State _______ Zip _______

Send to: ASHP Publication Records Dept., 4630 Montgomery Avenue, Bethesda, MD 20814

Current Literature

Drug Reaction Alerts

Drug Reaction Alerts focuses primarily on serious, unlabeled reactions to new chemical entities. The citations are compiled monthly from International Pharmaceutical Abstracts, *which covers over 800 pharmacy and health-related journals worldwide. An address for reprints (when available) follows the name of the corresponding author in each citation.*

Antifungals

Ormerod AD (Aberdeen Royal Infirmary, Aberdeen AB9 2ZB, Scotland), White MI. Cold urticaria triggered by **griseofulvin.** *Br Med J.* 1987; 295:612. Case. (14-year-old female atopy patient with *Trichophyton rubrum* infection; received griseofulvin 500 mg/day for six weeks; developed cold-induced urticaria; no resolution upon drug withdrawal)

Anti-infective Agents

Penmetcha M (Derbyshire Royal Infirmary, Derby DE1 2QY, England). **Trimethoprim**-induced erythema multiforme. *Br Med J.* 1987; 295:556. Case. (45-year-old woman with chronic sinusitis; received trimethoprim 200 mg twice daily for seven days; developed erythema multiforme; resolved upon drug withdrawal)

Anti-inflammatory Agents

Beun GD (Department of Nephrology and Immunology, University Hospital, Maastricht, Netherlands), Leunissen KM, Vriesman PJ et al. Isolated minimal change nephropathy associated with **diclofenac.** *Br Med J.* 1987; 295:182–3. Cases. (Two women; aged 56 and 70 years; received diclofenac 100 mg/day for three months or 150 mg/day for two periods of 13 and 20 days; developed lipoid nephrosis; one patient received atenolol, chlorthalidone, and hydralazine; kidney function returned to normal upon diclofenac withdrawal and therapy with a sodium-restricted diet, furosemide, and albumin by intravenous injection in one patient and with prednisone in the other)

Antivirals

Shea BF (New England Deaconess Hospital, 185 Pilgrim Road, Boston, MA 02215), Harbison MA, Sesin GP et al. **Acyclovir**-associated fever: a case report. *Pharmacotherapy.* 1987; 7:54–5. Case. (44-year-old woman with disseminated herpes simplex viral infection; received intravenous acyclovir 300 mg every 12 hours for 10 days; fever spike recorded two hours after first dose and again 24 hours after drug was discontinued)

Anxiolytics, Sedatives, and Hypnotics

Penfold NW (Addenbrooke's Hospital, Cambridge CB2 2QQ, England). Arrhythmias related to **propofol** infusion. *Br Med J.* 1987; 295:556. Case. (39-year-old man; received i.v. propofol [2,6-diisopropylphenol] 10 mg; developed ventricular tachycardia; resolved upon withdrawal of propofol and therapy with lidocaine)

Cardiac Drugs

Samlowski WE (Division of Hematology/Oncology, Department of Medicine, University of Utah, 1400 E. 2nd South Street, Salt Lake City, UT 84112), Frame RN, Logue GL. **Flecainide**-induced immune neutropenia: documentation of a hapten-mediated mechanism of cell destruction. *Arch Intern Med.* 1987; 147:383–4. Case. (66-year-old man; received flecainide acetate 100 mg three times daily; developed severe immune-mediated granulocytopenia; resolved upon drug withdrawal)

Central Nervous System Stimulants

Passmore AP (Queen's University of Belfast, Belfast BT9 7BL, Northern Ireland), Kondowe GB, Johnston GD. **Caffeine** and hypokalemia. *Ann Intern Med.* 1986; 105:468. Study. (Double-blind, crossover; 8 healthy men received single oral doses of caffeine 45, 90, 180, or 360 mg; serum potassium concentrations decreased with increased dosages of caffeine over time)

Corticosteroids

Lasser EC (Department of Radiology, M-032, University of California, La Jolla, CA 92093), Berry CC, Talner LB et al. Pretreatment with corticosteroids to alleviate reactions to intravenous contrast material. *N Engl J Med.* 1987; 317:845–9. Study. (Multicenter, randomized, placebo; 6763 patients; 2513 patients received a single dose of **methylprednisolone** 32 mg before administration of ionic contrast agent; 1759 patients received methylprednisolone 32 mg 12 hours and 2 hours before administration of ionic contrast agent; remaining patients received placebos in dosage schedules similar to single or multiple methylprednisolone regimens; incidence of adverse reactions of all types [except hives] significantly less with two-dose methylprednisolone regimen)

Drug Interactions

Budd JS (Princess Margaret Hospital, Swindon, Wiltshire SN1 4JU, England), Hoghton MA. Interaction of **captopril** and **Dyazide** causing hypotension and abdominal pain. *Br Med J.* 1987; 295:612. Case. (59-year-old male hypertensive patient; received captopril 25 mg 3 times daily for four months; developed hypotension and abdominal pain following a single oral dose of hydrochlorothiazide 25 mg with triamterene 50 mg; resolved after i.v. injection of colloids; continued therapy with hydrochlorothiazide 25 mg with triamterene 50 mg controlled hypertension without further effects)

Morris HH (Cleveland Clinic Foundation, Desk S 53, 9500 Euclid Avenue, Cleveland, OH 44106), Estes ML. Traveler's amnesia: transient global amnesia secondary to **triazolam.** *JAMA.* 1987; 258:945–6. Cases. (Three patients, aged 33–45 years; received triazolam 0.5 mg in a single dose for prevention of jet lag and **ethyl alcohol**; developed transient global amnesia lasting 8–11 hours)

Heavy Metal Antagonists

Miyagawa S (Department of Dermatology, Nara Medical University, Nara 634, Japan), Yoshioka A, Hatoko M et al. Systemic sclerosis-like lesions during long-term **penicillamine** therapy for Wilson's disease. *Br J Dermatol.* 1987; 116:95–100. Case. (14-year-old boy with Wilson's disease; received oral penicillamine 500 mg per day for 11 years; developed systemic sclerosis-like lesions)

Roentgenographic Agents

Evans JR (Loma Linda University School of Medicine, Loma Linda, CA 92350), Shankel SW, Cutler RE. Low osmolar contrast agents and nephrotoxicity. *Ann Intern Med.* 1987; 107:116. Cases. (Three patients, aged 36–65 years; received **iohexol** 70 mL or 83 mL or **iopamidol** 116 mL; developed decreased renal function; patients receiving iohexol recovered; patient receiving iopamidol required maintenance hemodialysis

Skeletal Muscle Relaxants

Nab HW (Institution of Neurology, Catholic University, 6525 GC Nijmegen, Netherlands), Hommes OR. Depression associated with **tizanidine.** *Br Med J.* 1987; 295:612. Case. (37-year-old man with multiple sclerosis; received oral tizanidine [5-chloro-4(2-imidazolin-2-yl-amino)-2,1,3-benzothiadiazole] 4 mg/day for nine days; developed depression; resolution upon drug withdrawal; positive rechallenge)

Sympatholytic Agents

Aron NB (Wolfson Hospital, Holon, 58100 Israel). **Phenoxybenzamine**-induced hyponatremia simulating the syndrome of inappropriate antidiuretic hormone secretion. *Ann Intern Med.* 1987; 107:119–20. Case. (73-year-old man; received phenoxybenzamine hydrochloride 10 mg daily for 10 days; developed hyponatremia mimicking syndrome of inappropriate antidiuretic hormone; symptoms improved rapidly upon treatment with furosemide and 3% sodium chloride injection)

Tranquilizers

Lobo AJ (Hinchingbrooke Hospital, Cambridgeshire PE18 INT, England), Dickinson RJ. Cricopharyngeal dyskinesia induced by **prochlorperazine.** *Br Med J.* 1987; 295:333. Case. (87-year-old woman receiving prochlorperazine 15 mg daily for two months; developed dysphagia resulting from esophageal dyskinesia; concomitant spironolactone, dichloralphenazone, acetaminophen–propoxyphene hydrochloride; symptoms resolved when drug withdrawn)

Vaccines

Fried M (Outpatient Clinic and Division of Gastroenterology, University Hospital, CH-4031 Basel, Switzerland), Conen D, Conzelmann M et al. Uveitis after hepatitis B vaccination. *Lancet.* 1987; 2:631–2. Case. (20-year-old female nurse; developed acute posterior uveitis after first and second booster doses of hepatitis B vaccine)

Xanthine Oxidase Inhibitors

Dykman D (Department of Medicine, Jewish Hospital of St. Louis, 216 S. Kingshighway Boulevard, St. Louis, MO 63178), Simon EE, Avioli LV. Hyperuricemia and uric acid nephropathy. *Arch Intern Med.* 1987; 147:1341–5. Case. (76-year-old woman; received allopurinol 300 mg/day; developed fever, stomatitis, skin rash, hypoxemia, and gastrointestinal symptoms; recovery upon treatment with high-dose steroids and antibiotics)

Book Review

Cancer Chemotherapy by Infusion

Edited by Jacob J. Lokich.

Published by Precept Press, Inc., 160 East Illinois St., Chicago, IL 60611, 1987. xxvii + 747 p. Price $99.

In recent years there has been a growing trend toward the delivery of cancer chemotherapy via continuous infusion. To date, the literature dealing with infusion chemotherapy is well dispersed throughout the medical oncology, pharmacy, and nursing literature, leaving the novice in the field with the formidable task of assembling up-to-date information. Therefore, it seems only appropriate that a focused text be developed regarding this modality of cancer therapy.

Dr. Jacob Lokich, the editor of this text and a prominent oncology researcher in the field of infusion therapy, has assembled an impressive group of medical oncologists, nurses, and pharmacists to review all aspects of injectable antineoplastic drug therapy. This book is divided into five sections: (1) rationale and technical aspects, (2) chemotherapeutic agents, (3) systemic infusion by tumor category, (4) regional infusion, and (5) special categories of infusion chemotherapy.

The first two sections will be of greatest value to hospital and home-care pharmacists who are involved in chemotherapy programs. The first three chapters of the text are devoted to outlining the experimental and theoretical rationale for chemotherapy by infusion. In the first chapter, the editor concisely reviews the rationale and historical development of the field. This chapter will be of interest to pharmacists who are unfamiliar with the concepts.

The chapters dealing with drug administration systems (chapter 4) and pharmaceutical issues (chapter 7) will be of the most use to hospital pharmacists who are involved in chemotherapy programs. Both chapters are well written and contain much practical information. The chapter on administration systems summarizes the technical aspects of the various types of infusion devices for ambulatory patients. The text is supplemented by several helpful schematic figures that aid the reader in understanding the mechanics and infusion patterns of these devices. A detailed table describing the characteristics of some of the available devices is also provided; the reader should be cautioned, however, that many available devices are not included in this table. This section also includes guidelines for selecting devices, which will be helpful to practitioners unfamiliar with the technology in this field, and it describes the technical and nursing aspects of long-term venous access.

The chapter on pharmaceutical aspects appropriately draws expertise from representatives of two institutions that have been innovators in injectable antineoplastic drug therapy (M. D. Anderson Hospital in Houston and New England Deaconess in Boston). This chapter explains to the reader stability and compatibility issues that must be dealt with when such therapy is being contemplated. Also contained in this chapter is probably the most extensive compilation of short-term and 30-day stability data available for many antineoplastic agents in various types of containers.

Continued on page 80

Editorial positions available at ASHP headquarters in Bethesda, Maryland, a progressive suburb of Washington, D.C.

Assistant Editor, Special Projects

An Assistant Editor position in the Special Projects Division is available beginning January 1, 1988. Responsibilities include identifying and producing new multimedia publications (primarily books) for practitioners in organized health care settings. The successful candidate will coordinate work of contributors and prepare and edit copy for publication projects.

Qualifications include pharmacy degree, exceptional writing skills, ASHP-accredited residency or equivalent hospital pharmacy practice experience, attention to detail, familiarity with pharmacy literature, and appreciation of the information needs of practitioners.

Assistant Editor, AJHP and CP

Join a professional team of ten editors and assistants in producing the *American Journal of Hospital Pharmacy* and *Clinical Pharmacy*.

Job content: planning future editorial content; reviewing manuscripts; working with reviewers and authors.

Minimum requirements: pharmacy degree, excellent command of the English language (including writing skills and ability to critically analyze the writing of others); keen perception of important issues of drug therapy and hospital pharmacy practice; interest in the pharmacy literature; attention to detail; ability to function well as a team member while executing independent assignments.

Drug Information Analyst, AHFS DI

This position offers a great opportunity to *begin* or *advance* your career potential and to utilize your clinical and drug information skills in serving national and international audiences. Your contribution for this highly respected and visible publication will be applied and appreciated by a broad-based audience of health professionals. Competence in the critical selection, evaluation, and use of drug information is essential. A Pharm.D. or equivalent background in therapeutics and the clinical use of drugs is preferred. Be a part of *AHFS Drug Information* and experience the professional recognition and satisfaction that this position can provide.

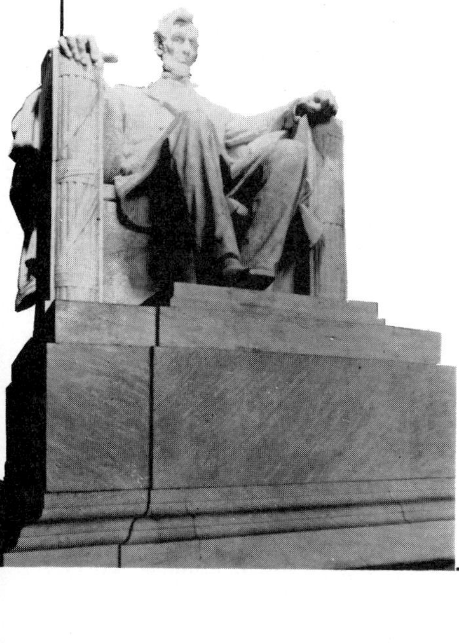

Salary negotiable; excellent benefits; assistance with moving expenses. Applicants should send resume, and salary requirements to: Thomas K. Somers, ASHP Director of Human Resources, Box 30068, Bethesda, MD 20814.

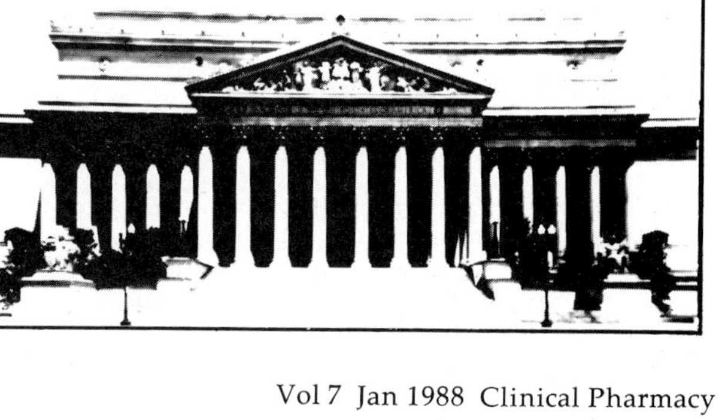

Continued from page 78

The next two sections provide in-depth summaries of injectable drug therapy according to individual drugs and to tumor types. This approach creates a certain amount of redundancy in the text, because many clinical studies and areas of interest are covered both by drug and by tumor type. The 11 chapters dealing with chemotherapeutic agents provide much information that will be helpful to hospital pharmacists; however, the content from chapter to chapter is inconsistent. For example, the chapters on bleomycin and the epipodophyllotoxins contain pertinent pharmaceutical information, while most others do not. Many investigational agents are also covered in these chapters.

The remaining two sections deal with regional infusions and other special categories of injectable antineoplastic drug therapy. Many of these chapters cover the technical aspects, clinical applications, and adverse consequences of novel routes and methods of infusion, including hepatic arterial; intra-arterial for head and neck and brain tumors; and intraperitoneal, intraventricular, and intravesical therapy.

In another chapter, which will interest both patient-oriented and administrative pharmacists, the editor addresses the issue of cost-effectiveness in cancer chemotherapy. This chapter brings to light many factors that should be considered when infusion programs are being planned.

One annoying feature of the text's format is that all references are grouped at the end of the book. For the reader who likes to refer to the references chapter by chapter, this arrangement necessitates much flipping back and forth.

Despite its being a comprehensive review of infusion chemotherapy, this text has the usual shortcomings of a work that addresses a still-developing and rapidly changing field. That is, the reader must recognize that a number of changes have occurred in the field since the various chapters were written. Overall, this text will be a valuable reference for hospital and home-health-care pharmacists who deal with active chemotherapy infusion programs. In view of the $99 price, institutions or individuals with limited budgets and minimal activity in infusion programs but wishing to purchase an oncology text would be better off to select one that is more comprehensive.

Reviewed by Rebecca S. Finley, Pharm.D., M.S., University of Maryland Cancer Center and School of Pharmacy, 22 South Greene Street, Baltimore, MD 21201.

Books Received

Books are listed as soon as received; selected books may be reviewed in Book Reviews in subsequent issues.

Cardiovascular Drug Therapy, edited by Stephen N. Hunyor. Published by Williams & Wilkins and Associates PTY Limited, 404 Sydney Road, Balgowlah, NSW 2093, Australia, 1987. Available from Williams & Wilkins, 428 E. Preston St., Baltimore, MD 21202. 309 p. Price $60.

Drug Treatment of the Rheumatic Diseases, Third Edition, edited by Frank Dudley Hart. Published by Williams & Wilkins and Associates PTY Limited, Balgowlah, Australia, 1987. Available through Williams & Wilkins, 428 East Preston St., Baltimore, MD 21202. x + 229 p. Price $48.

Immunology, Immunopathology, and Immunity, by Stewart Sell. Published by Elsevier Science Publishing Company, Inc., 52 Vanderbilt Ave., New York, NY 10017, 1987. xvii + 852 p. Price $55.00.

Neurobiology of Drug Abuse, edited by J. Marwah. Published by S. Karger AG, P.O. Box, CH-4009, Basel, Switzerland, 1987. 162 p. Price $98.00.

New Cardiovascular Drugs 1987, edited by Alexander Scriabine. Published by Raven Press, 1185 Avenue of the Americas, New York, NY 10036, 1987. xi + 271 p. Price $69.

Pharmacognosy, 9th edition, by Varro E. Tyler, Lynn R. Brady, and James E. Robbers. Published by Lea & Febiger, 600 Washington Square, Philadelphia, PA 19106-4198, 1988. viii+ 519 p. Price $39.50.

Side Effects of Drugs Annual 11—1987: A Worldwide Yearly Survey of New Data and Trends, edited by M.N.G. Dukes and L. Beeley. Published by Elsevier Science Publishers B.V., Amsterdam, the Netherlands, 1987. Available from Elsevier Science Publishing Co., Inc., 52 Vanderbilt Ave., New York, NY 10017. xviii + 516 p. Price $97.75, Dfl. 220.00.

USAN and the USP Dictionary of Drug Names. Published by the United States Pharmacopeial Convention, Inc., 12601 Twinbrook Parkway, Rockville, MD 20852, 1987. 708 p. Price $69.50 (1 to 24 copies), $55.60 (25 to 99 copies), additional discounts on larger quantities.

Advertising Index

American Society of Hospital Pharmacists
Clinical Pharmacy, 13
Handbook on Extemporaneous Formulations, 76
Pocket Guide to Injectable Drugs, 17
Positions Available, 79
Beecham Laboratories
Ticar, 20
Merieux Institute, Inc.
Multitest CMI, 19
Roxane Laboratories, A Boehringer Ingelheim Company
Intensols, inside front cover
Marinol, inside back cover, outside back cover
E. R. Squibb & Sons, Inc.
Azactam, 3–6
Stuart Pharmaceuticals, Division of ICI Americas, Inc.
Cefotan, 8–10
The Upjohn Company
Cleocin, 15–16

News

Recombinant tissue-plasminogen activator approved by FDA

Alteplase, recombinant (Activase, Genentech, Inc.), a recombinant-DNA tissue-plasminogen activator, was approved by FDA in November for use in the management of acute myocardial infarction. Alteplase has been reported to lyse coronary-artery thrombi, improve ventricular function, and reduce the incidence of congestive heart failure after myocardial infarction. The tissue-plasminogen activator product was reviewed in the May 1987 issue of *Clinical Pharmacy*.

Alteplase binds to fibrin contained in thrombi, converting entrapped plasminogen to plasmin and thereby initiating local fibrinolysis. Systemic fibrinolysis is limited. Approximately 80% of alteplase is cleared from the plasma within 10 minutes, primarily by the liver.

Clinical studies were begun in February 1984, and a new drug application was filed with FDA in April 1986. In controlled studies conducted by Genentech, reperfusion of obstructed coronary vessels was achieved within 90 minutes in approximately 70% of patients treated with alteplase. Following a May 1987 request by FDA's Cardio–Renal Advisory Committee for information on the effects of alteplase on myocardial function or survival, Genentech submitted data from two placebo-controlled studies demonstrating improvement in myocardial function.

A double-blind, placebo-controlled, randomized study of 138 patients with acute myocardial infarction showed improved left ventricular function 10 days after alteplase administration; compared with baseline values, the mean ejection fraction (measured by gated blood-pool scan) increased 3.6% in the alteplase group and decreased 4.7% in the placebo group. Alteplase treatment was associated with a lower incidence of congestive heart failure (14%, alteplase group; 33%, placebo group). A second double-blind, placebo-controlled, randomized study involving 136 patients also showed improvements in left ventricular function with treatment; alteplase recipients had higher ejection fractions at 21 days (mean follow-up) than did placebo recipients (62% versus 54%, ejection fraction measured by contrast ventriculogram; 54% versus 48%, ejection fraction measured by gated blood-pool scan). The benefit of anticoagulants after fibrinolytic therapy has not been proven definitively, but heparin has been administered to more than 90% of patients.

Bleeding is the most common complication of alteplase therapy. Thus, precautions and contraindications to therapy are similar to those for other forms of thrombolytic therapy. Arrhythmias may be associated with reperfusion. Substantial blood loss from the gastrointestinal or genitourinary tract has been reported in 4–5% of alteplase-treated patients. Intracranial hemorrhage is more common with higher doses; bleeding has occurred in 0.4% of patients treated with alteplase 100 mg and in 1.3% of those receiving a 150-mg dose.

A total dose of 100 mg infused intravenously over three hours is recommended; the first 60 mg should be administered over one hour, with the initial 6–10 mg given over one to two minutes. The remaining 40 mg should be administered over the second and third hours. Higher doses should be avoided because of the risk of intracranial hemorrhage. Patients weighing less than 65 kg should receive a total dose of 1.25 mg/kg. Alteplase is intended for intravenous use only.

Activase is supplied as a lyophilized powder in vials of 20 mg (biological potency of 11.6 million IU) and 50 mg (29 million IU). The cost of Activase per treatment course is approximately $2200.

Efficacy of intravenous streptokinase after myocardial infarction confirmed; labeled indications expanded

Labeling indications for streptokinase (Streptase, Hoechst-Roussel Pharmaceuticals Inc. and KabiKinase, KabiVitrum, Inc. and Smith Kline & French Laboratories) have been expanded to include intravenous administration in the management of acute myocardial infarction.

Recent studies have shown that intravenous administration of streptokinase soon after the onset of chest pain improves left ventricular function and short-term survival after myocardial infarction. The controlled, nonblinded multicenter trial of the Italian Group for the Study of Streptokinase in Myocardial Infarction involved 11,806 patients.[1] Overall mortality at 21 days was 18% lower in the streptokinase group than in the control group. Differences in mortality between the two groups were significant only when treatment was begun within six hours after the onset of symptoms; mortality was reduced 47% among patients treated within one hour, 23% among those treated within three hours, and 17% among those treated between three and six hours after the onset of symptoms. A follow-up report indicated that these early differences in mortality between the control group and the group of patients treated within six hours persisted for 12 months.[2]

In a double-blind, placebo-controlled study of 219 patients, the group receiving streptokinase 1.5 million units intravenously within four hours after the onset of chest pain had a higher mean left ventricular ejection fraction and lower mortality compared with the placebo group; reinfarction rates were similar for the two groups.[3] An earlier placebo-controlled study of 1741 patients showed a trend toward reduced mortality with intravenous streptokinase therapy.[4]

1. Gruppo Italiano per lo studio della Streptochinasi nell'Infarto Miocardico (GISSI). Effectiveness of intravenous thrombolytic treatment in acute myocardial infarction. *Lancet*. 1986; 1:397–402.
2. GISSI. Long-term effects of intravenous thrombolysis in acute myocardial infarction: final report of the GISSI study. *Lancet*. 1987; 2:871–4.
3. White HD, Norris RM, Brown MA et al. Effect of intravenous streptokinase on left ventricular function and early survival after acute myocardial infarction. *N Engl J Med*. 1987; 317:850–5.
4. The I.S.A.M. Study Group. A prospective trial of intravenous streptokinase in acute myocardial infarction (I.S.A.M.). *N Engl J Med*. 1986; 314:1465–71.

Study shows gemfibrozil reduces risk of coronary heart disease

Alterations in the lipoprotein profile produced by gemfibrozil lower the incidence of coronary heart disease (CHD) in men with primary dyslipidemia, according to results of the randomized, double-blind, placebo-controlled five-year Helsinki Heart Study.[1] Effects of treatment became evident during the second year of therapy.

A total of 18,966 men 40–55 years of age were screened for eligibility and willingness to participate in the study. Of these, 4081 were enrolled in the study; 2051 were assigned to treatment with gemfibrozil 600 mg twice daily, and 2030 were assigned to receive placebo. In all cases, the sum of the low-density lipoprotein (LDL) cholesterol and very-low-density (VLDL) lipoprotein cholesterol concentrations exceeded 200 mg/dL on two occasions. Patients with clinical findings of CHD, electrocardiographic abnormalities, congestive heart failure, or other diseases that could influence study results were excluded. Individuals with hypertension or "mild" non-insulin-dependent diabetes mellitus were allowed to participate.

The study was completed by 70% of the enrollees. For each of the five years of treatment, compliance was estimated to be within the range of 82–86%. Gemfibrozil raised high-density lipoprotein (HDL) cholesterol concentrations by more than 10% and lowered concentrations of total cholesterol by 11%, LDL cholesterol by 10%, non-HDL cholesterol by 14%, and triglycerides by 43%. HDL cholesterol concentrations declined slightly over time, HDL and non-HDL cholesterol values remained reasonably constant, and triglyceride concentrations increased slightly toward the end of the study. The placebo group had small, random variations and seasonal variations in lipid concentrations. The frequency of cardiac events (fatal or nonfatal myocardial infarction and cardiac death) was reduced 34% with gemfibrozil therapy; these cardiac events occurred at frequencies of 27.3 per 1000 in the gemfibrozil group and 41.4 per 1000 in the placebo group. The reduction in cardiac events was greatest (37%) for patients who had nonfatal myocardial infarctions. Mortality rates (21.9 per 1000, gemfibrozil; 20.7 per 1000, placebo) and causes of death were similar. Moderate to severe gastrointestinal symptoms were reported during the first year by 11.3% of gemfibrozil recipients and 7% of the placebo group. Thereafter, reported rates were 2.4% and 1.2%, respectively.

The reduction in CHD risk from pharmacologic modification of lipoprotein profiles in the Helsinki Heart Study is consistent with the findings of earlier studies of clofibrate and cholestyramine.

1. Frick MH, Elio O, Haapa K et al. Helsinki Heart Study: primary-prevention trial with gemfibrozil in middle-aged men with dyslipidemia. *N Engl J Med*. 1987; 317:1237–45.

Ganciclovir shows promise against cytomegalovirus, but data are insufficient for approval recommendation

FDA's Anti-Infective Drug Products Advisory Committee recommended against early approval of ganciclovir (formerly DHPG; Cytovene, Syntex Corporation), a congener of acyclovir, at its October 26 meeting; the drug is under review at FDA for the treatment of cytomegalovirus (CMV) retinitis in patients with AIDS. Effective treatments for this condition are not currently available. Clinical experience with ganciclovir suggests that the drug is potentially useful in the treatment of serious CMV infections, but controlled clinical trials of CMV retinitis have not been conducted. The lack of controlled studies on retinitis and the reported adverse effects of ganciclovir were important factors in the committee's decision.

The committee reviewed data obtained retrospectively from compassionate-use protocols; historical controls were used in data analysis. Treatment of 254 patients with ganciclovir led to improved vision in 56%, stabilization of vision in 26%, and deterioration in 18%; of 48 patients with retinitis who received no treatment, 45 had disease progression and 3 had stabilization.[1] Neutropenia developed during treatment in nearly 50% of the 716 patients who received ganciclovir for retinitis or other serious CMV infections.

Several uncontrolled studies suggesting that ganciclovir has beneficial effects in patients who have AIDS-associated serious CMV infections have been reported recently. Results of an open-label, compassionate-use multicenter study of ganciclovir in 97 patients with AIDS and serious CMV infections (retinitis, 56 patients; retinitis and pneumonia, 7; retinitis and gastrointestinal disease, 3; retinitis and multi-organ disease, 1; pneumonitis, 13; gastrointestinal disease, 12; central nervous system involvement, 2; other sites, 3) indicate that treatment suppresses disease activity; however, progression or recurrence of disease occurred after discontinuation of therapy in all patients for whom follow-up information was available.[2] Among the 60 patients with retinitis in whom response to ganciclovir could be evaluated, 30 improved and 22 had stabilization of disease activity. Dosages used in the study ranged from 3 to 15 mg/kg/day. The mean duration of therapy was 14 days. Neutropenia occurred in 55% of patients and frequently limited therapy. Results of a second study of 14 patients with AIDS and CMV infections were similar.[3] Ganciclovir 3–7.5 mg/kg/day for 5–24 days resulted in clinical improvement in 19 of 22 treatment courses, but most patients experienced relapses after discontinuation of therapy.

Continued on page 88

When it comes to taking their medicine, some patients need—

SPECIAL DELIVERY

INTENSOL™

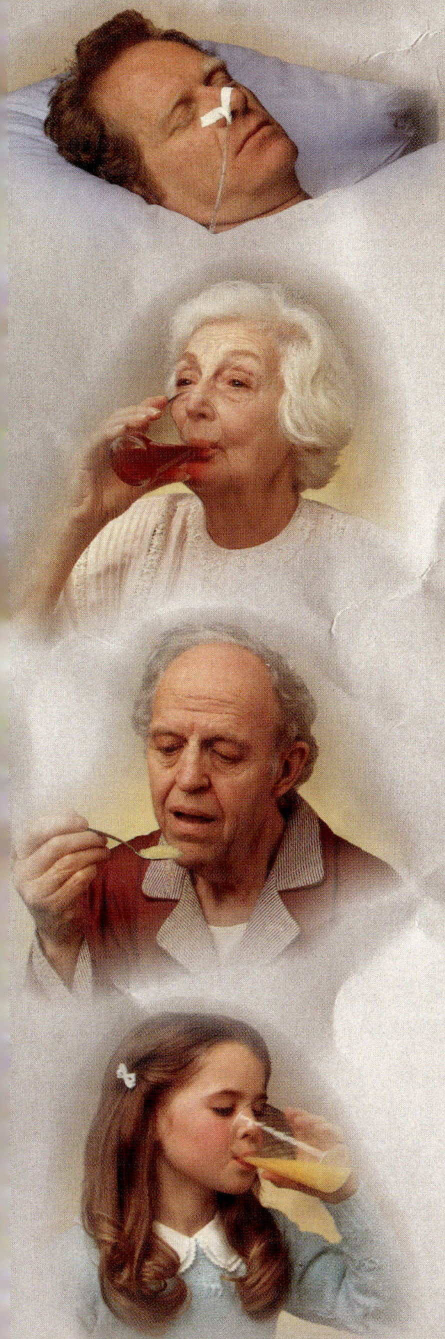

For patients who have difficulty with tablets

The nasogastric patient

The elderly or debilitated patient

The cancer patient on high or variable doses

The pediatric patient

Concentrated oral solutions

Intensols are highly concentrated medications—Chlorpromazine, Dexamethasone, DHT, Hydrochlorothiazide, Prednisone, Thioridazine, to name a few—in low volume solutions.

Easier than swallowing tablets

Intensols can be mixed with juice or semisolid foods, or even administered through nasogastric tubing.

Most Intensols have no flavor, so medications taste like the food or liquid they are mixed with. Each bottle comes with a calibrated dropper for easy dosage titration.

Easy to dispense

- Every dose is accurate.
- Ends the need to crush or break tablets—yielding inexact doses.
- Enhances patient compliance.
- Eliminates pharmacy compounding.

INTENSOLS...
A SPECIAL DELIVERY SYSTEM
for special patients.

Roxane
Laboratories, Inc.
Columbus, Ohio 43216

Intensols for your special patients

To find out more about INTENSOLS for your patients, fill out the following and mail to: Roxane Laboratories, Inc., PO Box 16532, Columbus, Ohio 43216.

Name ______

Address ______

Specialty ______

Continued from page 86

A third study, a prospective evaluation of ganciclovir 5 mg/kg intravenously every 12 hours for 14 days in 41 patients with AIDS and serious CMV gastrointestinal infections, showed clinical improvement in 30 patients and virologic response in 32.[4] Thirteen of the 33 patients who could be evaluated relapsed within nine weeks (median value) after the start of therapy. Moderate to severe leukopenia or neutropenia occurred in eight and six patients, respectively.

Ganciclovir has also been used to treat CMV infections in other immunocompromised patients, including transplant recipients.

1. Anon. FDA committee rules AIDS drug toxicity too uncertain to approve. *Med World News*. 1987; 28(22):38–39.
2. Laskin OL, Cederberg DM, Mills J et al. Ganciclovir for the treatment and suppression of serious infections caused by cytomegalovirus. *Am J Med*. 1987; 83:201–7.
3. Laskin OL, Stahl-Bayliss CM, Kalman CM et al. Use of ganciclovir to treat serious cytomegalovirus infections in patients with AIDS. *J Infect Dis*. 1987; 155:323–7.
4. Chachoua A, Dietrich D, Krasinski K et al. 9-(1,3-dihydroxy-2-propoxymethyl) guanine (ganciclovir) in the treatment of cytomegalovirus gastrointestinal disease with the acquired immunodeficiency syndrome. *Ann Intern Med*. 1987; 107:133–7.

Periodic dressing changes of peripheral venous catheter sites not indicated, study shows

Redressing of peripheral venous catheter sites at periodic intervals to prevent phlebitis or infection is not necessary for most hospitalized patients, according to a recent study of four dressing techniques.[1]

A total of 2088 peripheral venous catheters from 1259 patients were evaluated. All catheters were Teflon, had been inserted by a medical house officer or nurse, and had been in place at least 12 hours. Patients without neutropenia who were to have intravenous catheters inserted were randomly assigned to have one of the following types of dressings: sterile gauze and tape, replaced every 48 hours; gauze, left in place until catheter removal; a polyurethane transparent dressing, left in place until catheter removal; and a transparent dressing with iodophor antiseptic incorporated in the adhesive, left in place until catheter removal. The skin was cleansed with 10% povidone iodine before catheter insertion and during all subsequent dressing changes. Catheter sites were evaluated daily, and each patient was followed for three days after catheter removal.

Approximately 80% of the catheters were placed in surgical patients, and 25–30% were inserted while the patient was in an intensive-care unit. Among the four groups, catheters were used at similar frequencies in patients with high blood glucose concentrations (31–37% of the catheters evaluated), neoplastic disease (17–22%), urinary catheters (43–48%), and "active" unrelated infections (19–21%) and in patients receiving concurrent antibiotic therapy (74–77%). Approximately one half of catheter removals in each group were considered to be routine (i.e., intravenous access no longer needed or decision made to rotate sites). Catheters remained in place an average of 52 to 55 hours in the four groups.

The investigators concluded that all four dressing techniques were satisfactory. Moisture accumulated under the occlusive dressings more often than under the nonocclusive dressings. The iodophor-transparent dressing was somewhat less adherent than the other dressings. Inflammation, discomfort, and phlebitis occurred at similar frequencies in all four groups. At the time of catheter removal, the number of colonized catheter sites was significantly less with either the iodophor transparent dressing or the routinely changed gauze and tape dressing than with the unchanged gauze dressing. The incidence of local catheter-related infections was similar in the four groups; no cases of catheter-related bacteremia were reported. Colonization at the catheter insertion site, contamination of the catheter hub, moisture under the dressing, and duration of catheter placement were predictive of infection.

The authors concluded that most patients who have peripheral venous catheters do not need periodic dressing changes. In drawing this conclusion, they expressed support for current recommendations calling for rotation of access sites every 48–72 hours. The authors also cautioned that discontinuation of routine dressing changes should not lead to abandonment of at least daily inspection of catheter sites.

1. Maki DG, Ringer M. Evaluation of dressing regimens for prevention of infection with peripheral intravenous catheters: gauze, a transparent polyurethane dressing, and an iodophor-transparent dressing. *JAMA*. 1987; 258:2396–403.

CDC advises on detection and control of antibiotic-resistant *Neisseria gonorrhoeae*

Guidelines for the surveillance, control, detection, and treatment of antibiotic-resistant strains of *Neisseria gonorrhoeae* have been issued by the Centers for Disease Control (CDC).[1] The report focuses on the three most important forms of resistance, namely, penicillinase-producing strains of *N. gonorrhoeae* (PPNG), strains with chromosomally mediated resistance to penicillin (CMRNG), and strains with plasmid-mediated resistance to tetracycline (TRNG).

Although surveillance for all types of resistance is ideal, the primary focus of local surveillance programs should be detection of PPNG. According to CDC, all *N. gonorrhoeae* isolates should be tested for β-lactamase production. If all isolates cannot be tested for plasmid-mediated tetracycline resistance or chromosomally mediated penicillin resistance, selected isolates (i.e., positive post-treatment isolates, isolates from patients with disseminated gonococcal infections or gonococcal ophthalmia, and isolates from members of groups at high risk for infection with resistant strains) should be tested. The guidelines stress the need for surveillance systems to be representative and timely in reporting of results.

CDC outlined the elements of state and local control programs for endemic areas (areas in which PPNG accounts for <1% of all cases of gonorrhea over a two-month period), endemic areas (PPNG accounts for 1–3% of cases), and hyperendemic areas (PPNG accounts for >3% of cases). Recommendations pertained to manage-

Continued on page 92

Does so much for so much less than cefoxitin

In a study conducted in a 900-bed hospital, 100 patients were treated with CEFOTAN and retrospectively compared with 100 cefoxitin-treated patients with similar medical and surgical problems. CEFOTAN 1 to 2 g every 12 hours appeared equal to cefoxitin 1 to 2 g every 6 to 8 hours in terms of efficacy and safety.

Side effects were remarkably similar

Hematologic as well as nonhematologic side effects were infrequent in both groups.

"Abnormalities in hemostasis were similar; cefotetan-treated patients exhibited no apparent predisposition to overt bleeding or PT/PTT elevations."

$125,000

projected annual savings over cefoxitin

CLASSIFICATION OF CLINICAL OUTCOME FROM RETROSPECTIVE AUDIT

Outcome	CEFOTAN (n = 100*)	Cefoxitin (n = 100)
Empiric cure	88	80
Failure	0	1
Uncertain	1	1
Death	2†	5†
No data	1	13

*Eight patients who received CEFOTAN for prophylaxis were excluded.
†None was specifically related to infection.
—adapted from Quintiliani et al, p 278

By calculating drug costs and delivery for each regimen, investigators projected an annual savings of $125,000 for their institution.

In intra-abdominal and gynecologic infection due to indicated organisms

CEFOTAN® IM/IV
(cefotetan disodium)

Does so much for so much less than cefoxitin.

REFERENCE: Quintiliani R, Cooper BW, Briceland LL, et al: Formulary replacement policies: Cefotetan vs cefoxitin. *Infect Med,* July/August 1987, pp 275-279.

© 1988 ICI Americas Inc

Continued from page 88

ment information systems, *N. gonorrhoeae* culturing, testing for antimicrobial resistance, quality assurance of screening procedures, reporting of results, treatment, posttreatment testing, education, and activities of disease intervention specialists. Recommended methods of susceptibility testing were reviewed, and interpretive categories based on zone-size results and agar-dilution correlates were provided.

A treatment approach based on local PPNG prevalence was recommended by CDC. In nonendemic areas, if a regimen such as amoxicillin plus probenecid is used to treat gonorrhea, routine susceptibility testing and posttreatment evaluation of cure should be performed. Ceftriaxone was considered to be a desirable alternative. In endemic and hyperendemic areas, ceftriaxone is the drug of choice. A single intramuscular dose of ceftriaxone 250 mg (as the sodium salt) plus a seven-day regimen of doxycycline 100 mg orally twice daily or tetracycline hydrochloride 500 mg orally four times daily was recommended in endemic and hyperendemic areas for adults with uncomplicated urethral, endocervical, pharyngeal, or rectal gonorrhea. Erythromycin (erythromycin base or stearate 500 mg, erythromycin ethylsuccinate 800 mg, or equivalent doses of other erythromycin products four times daily for seven days) may be substituted for tetracycline for patients who should not take or cannot tolerate tetracyclines. Treatment recommendations for gonococcal infections at other anatomic sites are summarized in the table.

Treatment of Various Gonococcal Infections Diagnosed in PPNG-Endemic or PPNG-Hyperendemic Areas[a]

Indication	Treatment
Disseminated gonococcal infection	Ceftriaxone 1 g (as the sodium salt) i.m. daily for seven days[b]
Meningitis	A third-generation cephalosporin (high-dose) i.v. for 10–14 days
Endocarditis	A third-generation cephalosporin (high-dose) i.v. for at least one month
Ophthalmia	
Adults	Ceftriaxone 1 g (as the sodium salt) i.m. or i.v. daily for five days[b]
Neonates	Ceftriaxone 25–50 mg/kg/day (as the sodium salt) i.v. or i.m. for seven days[b]
Neonatal prophylaxis	1% silver nitrate solution, 1% tetracycline solution or ointment, or 0.5% erythromycin ointment applied topically to the eye within one hour after birth
	Ceftriaxone 125 mg (as the sodium salt) i.m. (25–50 mg/kg for low-birth-weight infants)[c]
Acute pelvic inflammatory disease	
Suspected primary pathogen is *Neisseria gonorrhoeae* or *Chlamydia trachomatis*	Doxycycline 100 mg i.v. twice daily plus cefoxitin 2 g (as the sodium salt) i.v. four times daily for at least four days and at least 48 hours after the patient improves, followed by doxycycline 100 mg orally twice daily to complete 10–14 days of therapy
Suspected primary pathogens are gram-negative bacilli or anaerobes	Clindamycin 900 mg (as the phosphate salt) i.v. three times daily mixed in the same infusion with gentamicin 2 mg/kg (as the sulfate salt) i.v. for the first dose, followed by 1.5 mg/kg/dose (adjusted based on renal function and serum concentrations) for at least four days and at least 48 hours after the patient improves; i.v. therapy should be followed by clindamycin 450 mg (as the hydrochloride salt) orally four times daily to complete 10–14 days of therapy

[a] PPNG = penicillinase-producing *Neisseria gonorrhoeae.*
[b] An equivalent third-generation cephalosporin may be used.
[c] Indicated for neonates born to mothers with peripartum gonococcal infections.

1. Centers for Disease Control. Antibiotic-resistant strains of *Neisseria gonorrhoeae:* policy guidelines for detection, management, and control. *MMWR.* 1987; 36(Suppl 5S):1S–18S.

Upcoming Specialty Meetings

American College of Cardiology . . . Atlanta, GA . . . March 27–31 . . . contact: W. D. Nelligan, CAE, 9111 Old Georgetown Road, Bethesda, MD 20814; 301-897-5400.

NIH Consensus Development Conference on Kidney Stones: Prevention and Treatment . . . Bethesda, MD . . . March 28–30 . . . contact: Conference Registrar, Prospect Associates, Suite 500, 1801 Rockville Pike, Rockville, MD 20852; 301-468-6338.

Sickle Cell Disease: The State of the Art . . . Bethesda, MD . . . April 11–13 . . . contact: Conference Department, New York Academy of Science, 2 E. 63rd Street, New York, NY 10021; 212-838-0280.

Arachidonic Acid Metabolism in the Nervous System: Physiological and Pathological Significance . . . Bethesda, MD . . . April 14–16 . . . contact: Conference Department, New York Academy of Science, 2 E. 63rd Street, New York, NY 10021; 212-838-0230.

American College of Preventive Medicine . . . Atlanta, GA . . . April 14–17 . . . contact: W. Kane, Ph.D., 1015 15th Street N.W., Washington, DC 20005; 202-789-0003.

International Symposium: Ethics and the Health Professional's Role in Communicating Health Risks . . . Washington, DC . . . April 18–19 . . . contact: J. Higginson, M.D., Institute for Health Policy Analysis, 2121 Wisconsin Ave. N.W., Suite 220, Washington, DC 20007.

American Trauma Society . . . Washington, DC . . . April 18–20 . . . contact: S. Bond-Lilicropp, P.O. Box 13526, Baltimore, MD 21203; 301-328-6304.

American Society for Clinical Nutrition . . . Washington, DC . . . April 28–30 . . . contact: S. Schiaffino, Ph.D., 9650 Rockville Pike, Bethesda, MD 20814; 301-530-7110.

American Society for Clinical Investigation . . . Washington, DC . . . April 29–May 5 . . . contact: I. H. Fox, M.D., A7119A University Hospital, Ann Arbor, MI 48109-0108; 313-936-8080.

Therapy Consultation

The Therapy Consultation *section provides brief advice, in question-and-answer format, on how to handle specific drug-therapy problems. Readers are invited to submit questions, which will be referred to a consultant for an answer. The problems should not be highly specialized or unusual, nor should they be mundane. Questions are answered briefly, based largely on the judgment and personal experience of the consultant, although selected references may be cited to substantiate the consultant's advice.*

Assistance in identifying Therapy Consultation *topics is provided by the drug information centers at the following institutions: Albert B. Chandler Medical Center and College of Pharmacy, University of Kentucky, Lexington; Arizona Health Sciences Center, Tucson; Medical College of Virginia Hospitals, Richmond; University of California Medical Center, San Diego; and University of Michigan Medical Center, Ann Arbor.*

Metronidazole for pseudomembranous colitis

Question: Is metronidazole effective for the treatment of pseudomembranous colitis that is unresponsive to oral vancomycin therapy? Should metronidazole be considered a first-line agent?

Answer: Oral vancomycin is the most recognized drug for the treatment of pseudomembranous colitis (PMC). Vancomycin is absorbed poorly from the gastrointestinal tract and is excreted primarily in the feces. After oral administration of vancomycin in recommended doses, fecal drug concentrations far exceed the minimum inhibitory concentration for *Clostridium difficile*. The optimum dosage and duration of vancomycin therapy for PMC is not yet established; a 10-day course with vancomycin 500–2000 mg/day orally (as the hydrochloride salt) in four divided doses is generally suggested.

Vancomycin therapy for PMC has several drawbacks. Treatment is expensive: Pharmacy acquisition cost at our hospital for a 10-day course of vancomycin 2 g/day is approximately $640. Furthermore, response to vancomycin is inadequate in approximately 6–9% of patients, and 3–5% of patients treated with vancomycin fail to respond.[1] Disease relapse has been reported in as many as 39% of patients receiving a full course of vancomycin, and relapses can be multiple.[2] Comparison of patients with and without relapses has shown no differences in the total daily dosage or duration of therapy. Variations in the regimen—use of high doses, low doses, tapered doses, or extended courses of treatment—have failed to prevent disease recurrence. Presumably, *C. difficile* persists in the colon as spores that are inherently resistant to vancomycin, returning to the vegetative form when the drug is discontinued. It has also been suggested that reinfection with viable spores from the patient's surrounding environment can lead to recolonization with *C. difficile*.

Metronidazole has been proposed as an effective alternative to vancomycin for PMC. In vitro tests have shown that most strains of *C. difficile* are highly susceptible to metronidazole at minimum inhibitory concentrations of 0.25–1.0 mg/L. Metronidazole has been used successfully to treat patients with PMC.[3-6] Several clinical trials have evaluated metronidazole in dosages of 1.0 to 2.0 g/day for 7 to 10 days. Symptomatic improvement with resolution of disease usually occurs within one to five days of starting therapy and is accompanied by eradication of *C. difficile* and its toxin.

In a large prospective, randomized trial of metronidazole versus vancomycin for PMC, Teasley et al.[6] randomly assigned 94 patients to receive a 10-day course of either metronidazole 250 mg orally four times a day or vancomycin 500 mg orally four times a day. Mean time to resolution of diarrhea was 2.8 ± 1.8 days for vancomycin and 2.4 ± 1.9 days for metronidazole; the difference was not statistically significant. Clinical response, treatment failure, and relapse rates were similar for both groups. It was concluded that metronidazole and vancomycin are equally effective for PMC.

In recent years, several concerns have been expressed regarding the use of metronidazole for PMC. Unlike oral vancomycin, metronidazole given orally is rapidly and completely absorbed from the gastrointestinal tract, raising doubt as to whether metronidazole can achieve bactericidal concentrations in the colon that are sufficient for the eradication of *C. difficile*. In a recent trial, Bolton et al.[5] measured fecal concentrations of metronidazole during oral and intravenous therapy for PMC. Findings from the trial showed that fecal drug concentrations after the administration of metronidazole 400 mg orally every eight hours or 500 mg intravenously every eight hours far exceeded the minimum inhibitory concentration for *C. difficile*. Fecal concentrations of metronidazole were bactericidal, and all patients responded satisfactorily to treatment. Clinical resolution of symptoms was accompanied by eradication of *C. difficile* and its toxin. Patients receiving metronidazole intravenously also showed a good response to therapy. In contrast, intravenously administered vancomycin has been reported to be ineffective for PMC. Systemic toxicity from the oral absorption of metronidazole was minimal or absent in the larger studies; thus, patients appear to tolerate metronidazole as well as oral vancomycin.

Disease relapse does occur following treatment with metronidazole. The frequency of relapse appears to be similar to that reported with vancomycin. If sporulation is the underlying mechanism for recurrence of disease, these results would be anticipated because spores are inherently resistant to all antibiotics including vancomycin and metronidazole. Patients with recurrent disease usually respond well to repeat courses of metronidazole. Occasional refractory cases may require a change to vancomycin.

Metronidazole appears to be effective for treating patients with PMC who fail to respond to or relapse after a course of vancomycin.[7-9] Eglington et al.[7] reported that a 59-year-old patient with PMC failed to respond to two courses of vancomycin 500 mg given orally every six hours but showed rapid clinical improvement and disease resolution after a change to oral metronidazole. The patient remained asymptomatic with no evidence of disease six months after the completion of metronidazole therapy. Other investigators have reported similar results.[8,9]

Pseudomembranous colitis may occasionally develop after treatment with metronidazole.[10] This should not preclude its use, however, because any antibiotic can cause the disorder; PMC after vancomycin has also been reported.

In conclusion, metronidazole may be used as an effective, first-line drug in a majority of patients with PMC. In an era of increasing cost consciousness and budget reductions in most hospitals, one cannot overlook the differences in the cost of treatment with metronidazole and vancomycin. Pharmacy acquisition cost at our hospital for a 10-day course of oral metronidazole 1.5 g/day amounts to approximately $6.60 as compared with $160 for the lowest recommended vancomycin dosage (125 mg orally four times daily). Metronidazole also offers the added advantage of intravenous use in situations where oral therapy is not possible. Vancomycin should be reserved for patients who are allergic or fail to respond to metronidazole.

1. Bartlett JG. Treatment of antibiotic-associated pseudomembranous colitis. *Rev Infect Dis*. 1984; 6(Suppl):S235–S241.
2. George WL, Rolfe RD, Harding GKM et al. *Clostridium difficile* and cytotoxin in feces of patients with antimicrobial agent-associated pseudomembranous colitis. *Infection*. 1982; 10:205–7.
3. Cherry RD, Portnoy D, Jabbari M et al. Metronidazole: an alternative therapy for antibiotic-associated colitis. *Gastroenterology*. 1982; 82:849–51.
4. Nicolopoulos NG, Stathapoulos EN, Douzinas EE et al. Pseudomembranous colitis. Treatment by metronidazole. *Hepatogastroenterology*. 1981; 28:120–2.
5. Bolton RP, Culshaw MA. Faecal metronidazole concentrations during oral and intravenous therapy for antibiotic associated colitis due to *Clostridium difficile*. *Gut*. 1986; 27:1169–72.
6. Teasley DG, Olson MM, Gerding DN et al. Prospective randomised trial of metronidazole versus vancomycin for *Clostridium-difficile*-associated diarrhea and colitis. *Lancet*. 1983; 2:1043–6.
7. Eglington GS, Mayes GR, Potts DW. Pseudomembranous colitis unresponsive to oral vancomycin therapy. *South Med J*. 1982; 75:1279–80.
8. Oldenberger D, Miller JA. Treatment of pseudomembranous colitis with oral metronidazole after relapse following vancomycin. *Am J Gastroenterol*. 1980; 74:359–60.
9. Mitchell SR, Gaver WR. Intermittent therapy with metronidazole for relapse of pseudomembranous colitis. *JAMA*. 1984; 251:3082. Letter.
10. Daly JJ, Chowdary KVS. Pseudomembranous colitis secondary to metronidazole. *Dig Dis Sci*. 1983; 28:573–4.

Ujjaini Khanderia, M.S., Pharm.D.
Clinical Assistant Professor, College of Pharmacy
Clinical Pharmacist–Internal Medicine, University of Michigan Medical Center
Ann Arbor, MI 48109-0008

The VA Medical Center, Syracuse, New York has an immediate opening for a clinical pharmacist interested in adult ambulatory care medicine. Responsibilities include evaluation of drug regimens, making dosage recommendations, providing drug information to professional staff, instructing resident staff concerning the concepts of effective prescribing and drug use evaluation. The Syracuse VA Medical Center is a 379-bed acute care facility which is affiliated with the SUNY College of Medicine and operates many ambulatory care clinics representing all major surgical and medical subspecialities.

A Pharm.D. or equivalent professional degree is required; residency experience preferred. Two or more years of work experience in a clinical capacity is desirable, but the major requirement is a motivated individual with strong professional and interpersonal skills. Salary is commensurate with qualifications and experience. Salary range $32,567 to $42,341 per year.

If you are interested in a challenging practice within a dynamic outpatient setting, we want to know more about you. Qualified candidates should send resumes to:

VA Medical Center
Personnel Service (05)
800 Irving Avenue
Syracuse, N.Y. 13210
(315) 476-7461, ext. 2311

Equal Opportunity Employer

Letters

The Letters *column is a forum for rapid exchange of ideas among readers of* CP. *Liberal criteria are applied in the review of submissions to encourage contributions to this column.*

The Letters *column includes the following types of contributions: (1) comments, addenda, and minor updates on previously published work, (2) alerts on potential problems related to drug therapy or clinical research, (3) observations or comments on trends in drug therapy or clinical research, and (4) brief expressions of opinion about controversies in drug therapy or clinical research.*

Letters need not be submitted with the journal's manuscript checklist. The following conditions, however, must be adhered to: (1) the body of the letter must be no longer than two typewritten pages, (2) the use of references, tables, and illustrations should be minimized, (3) the authors' names, affiliations, and mailing addresses must be typed at the end of the letter in the format used by CP, *and (4) the entire letter (including references, tables, and authors' names) must be typed double spaced on plain white paper (not letterhead). Following acceptance of a letter, the authors are required to sign an exclusive publication statement and a copyright-transferral form.*

Anabolic steroid use as an AIDS risk factor

The recent review by Kibble and Ross[1] concerning the adverse effects of anabolic steroids in athletes was a timely and comprehensive summary of the topic. We would like to point out another harmful, potentially life-threatening consequence of the use of injectable anabolic steroids—transmission of infectious agents, including the human immunodeficiency virus (HIV).

Sklarek et al.[2] reported a case of AIDS in a bodybuilder using anabolic steroids. The patient, a 37-year-old white man, had experienced progressive weight loss, fever, and shortness of breath over a six-month period; transbronchial biopsy revealed *Pneumocystis carinii* pneumonia. Although the patient denied any history of homosexual activity, he did admit to injecting anabolic steroids intramuscularly every week over the previous four years. Needles were often shared among bodybuilders from various gyms. The patient claimed to have discontinued this practice two years before admission after an episode of hepatitis B.

Shared needles are a known vector for transmission of HIV.[3] Educating athletes about the possibility of transmission of HIV may serve as a more persuasive deterrent to the use of anabolic steroids than educating them about other adverse effects, such as liver function abnormalities and hyperlipidemia. As pharmacists, we can convey this information to our patients and perhaps decrease the use of anabolic steroids by athletes.

1. Kibble MW, Ross MB. Adverse effects of anabolic steroids in athletes. *Clin Pharm.* 1987; 6:686–92.
2. Sklarek HM, Mantovani RP, Erens E et al. AIDS in a bodybuilder using anabolic steroids. *N Engl J Med.* 1984; 311:1701. Letter.
3. Castro KG, Hardy AH, Curran JW. The acquired immunodeficiency syndrome: epidemiology and risk factors for transmission. *Med Clin North Am.* 1986; 70:635–49.

WALTER J. MCCLAIN, PHARM.D., Clinical Pharmacist
Lenox Hill Hospital
100 East 77th Street
New York, NY 10021

KATHRYN K. BUCCI, PHARM.D., Family Medicine Fellow
Medical University of South Carolina
171 Ashley Avenue
Charleston, SC 29425

Wanted: Insightful authors of review articles

I would like to commend Zellmer[1] on his nicely outlined criteria for good journal review articles in the December 1987 issue of *CP*. I believe that an essential ingredient of a good review article is an author who is very aware of the area being reviewed, preferably one who is performing original research in the area. Sophisticated "clinician–educators" can prepare very insightful reviews. Unfortunately, the authors of review articles not uncommonly are young individuals who lack the perspective needed to write critically but fairly. The pressure to "publish or perish" often stimulates young faculty members to look at review articles as an easy avenue to getting published. I believe that journal editors can play an important role in limiting the number of superficial review articles by making sure that prospective authors have the necessary credentials.

I am not sure that we need *more* review articles, but we certainly need more *good* review articles.

1. Zellmer WA. Review articles. *Clin Pharm.* 1987; 6:969. Editorial.

JOHN H. RODMAN, PHARM.D., Acting Chairman
Pharmaceutical Division
St. Jude Children's Research Hospital
332 North Lauderdale
P.O. Box 318
Memphis, TN 38101-0318

"SURPRISE"!

Given a choice of having only one agent on their hospital formulary, the majority of respondents to a nationwide survey involving hospital specialists said they'd keep TICAR rather than another commonly used anti-pseudomonal penicillin.*

Ticar® (TICARCILLIN DISODIUM) plus an Aminoglycoside

Still preferred—when all is said and done.

* Data on file, BEECHAM Laboratories.

TICAR®
(Sterile Ticarcillin Disodium)

for Intramuscular or Intravenous Use

For complete prescribing information, consult official package insert.

ACTIONS: Ticarcillin is bactericidal; it is not absorbed orally, therefore, it must be administered intravenously or intramuscularly.

INDICATIONS: TICAR (Ticarcillin Disodium) is indicated for the treatment of the following infections:

Bacterial septicemia†
Skin and soft-tissue infections†
Acute and chronic respiratory tract infections†‡
†caused by susceptible strains of *Pseudomonas aeruginosa*, *Proteus* species (both indole-positive and indole-negative) and *Escherichia coli*.
‡(Though clinical improvement has been shown, bacteriological cures cannot be expected in patients with chronic respiratory disease or cystic fibrosis.)
Genitourinary tract infections (complicated and uncomplicated) due to susceptible strains of *Pseudomonas aeruginosa*, *Proteus* species (both indole-positive and indole-negative), *Escherichia coli*, *Enterobacter* and *Streptococcus faecalis* (enterococcus).

Ticarcillin is also indicated in the treatment of the following infections due to susceptible anaerobic bacteria:

(1) Bacterial septicemia.
(2) Lower respiratory tract infections such as empyema, anaerobic pneumonitis and lung abscess.
(3) Intra-abdominal infections such as peritonitis and intra-abdominal abscess (typically resulting from anaerobic organisms resident in the normal gastrointestinal tract).
(4) Infections of the female pelvis and genital tract such as endometritis, pelvic inflammatory disease, pelvic abscess and salpingitis.
(5) Skin and soft-tissue infections.

Although Ticarcillin is primarily indicated against Gram-negative infections, its *in vitro* activity against Gram-positive organisms should be considered in treating infections caused by both Gram-negative and Gram-positive organisms.

Based on the *in vitro* synergism between Ticarcillin and gentamicin sulfate or tobramycin sulfate against certain strains of *Pseudomonas aeruginosa*, combined therapy has been successful, using full therapeutic dosages.

Culturing and susceptibility testing should be performed initially and during treatment.

CONTRAINDICATIONS: A history of allergic reaction to any of the penicillins is a contraindication.

WARNINGS: Anaphylaxis may occur, especially in patients with an allergic diathesis. Check for a history of allergy to penicillins, cephalosporins or other allergens. If an allergic reaction occurs, the drug should be discontinued unless, in the opinion of the physician, the condition being treated is life-threatening and amenable only to Ticarcillin therapy. Serious anaphylactic reactions require immediate emergency treatment with epinephrine, oxygen, intravenous steroids and airway management.

Some patients receiving high doses of Ticarcillin may develop hemorrhagic manifestations associated with abnormalities of coagulation tests. Patients with renal impairment, in whom excretion of Ticarcillin is delayed, should be observed for bleeding manifestations. Such patients should be dosed strictly according to recommendations. If bleeding manifestations appear, Ticarcillin treatment should be discontinued and, if necessary, appropriate therapy instituted.

PRECAUTIONS: During prolonged treatment, periodic checking for organ system dysfunction (renal, hepatic and hematopoietic) is advisable. If overgrowth of resistant organisms occurs, the appropriate therapy should be initiated.

Since the theoretical sodium content is 5.2 milliequivalents (120 mg) per gram of Ticarcillin, electrolyte and cardiac status should be monitored carefully.

In a few patients receiving intravenous Ticarcillin, hypokalemia has been reported. Serum potassium should be measured periodically.

USAGE DURING PREGNANCY: Reproduction studies have been performed in mice and rats and have revealed no evidence of impaired fertility or harm to the fetus due to Ticarcillin. There are no well-controlled studies in pregnant women, but investigational experience does not include any positive evidence of adverse effects on the fetus. Although there is no clearly defined risk, such experience cannot exclude the possibility of infrequent or subtle damage to the fetus. Ticarcillin should be used in pregnant women only when clearly needed.

ADVERSE REACTIONS: The following adverse reactions may occur: skin rashes, pruritus, urticaria, drug fever, nausea, vomiting, anemia, thrombocytopenia, leukopenia, neutropenia, eosinophilia. SGOT and SGPT elevations have been reported. Patients, especially those with impaired renal function, may experience convulsions or neuromuscular excitability when very high doses of the drug are administered.

Local reactions at the site of injection have been reported. Vein irritation and phlebitis can occur, particularly when undiluted solution is directly injected into the vein.

DOSAGE AND ADMINISTRATION: Usual adult recommended dosage in bacterial septicemia, respiratory tract infections, skin and soft-tissue infections, intra-abdominal infections and infections of the female pelvis and genital tract, is 3 grams by intravenous infusion every 3, 4 or 6 hours depending on weight and severity of infection; in uncomplicated urinary tract infections, 1 gram I.M. or direct I.V. q.i.d.; in complicated urinary tract infections, 3 grams q.i.d. by I.V. infusion.

Please consult official package insert for details on dosages for patients with renal insufficiency, children, neonates and directions for use.

Supplied: 1 Gm, 3 Gm and 6 Gm Standard Vials; 3 Gm and 6 Gm Piggyback Bottles

7182BS1/86

TSM-1272

Beecham laboratories
Bristol, Tennessee 37620

Drug Review

Nicardipine, nitrendipine, and bepridil: New calcium antagonists for cardiovascular disorders

GUY R. HASEGAWA

Abstract: The chemistry, pharmacology, pharmacokinetics, clinical uses, and adverse effects of nicardipine, nitrendipine, and bepridil are reviewed.

Nicardipine, nitrendipine, and bepridil are calcium antagonists under investigation for the treatment of cardiovascular disorders. Nicardipine and nitrendipine share a common dihydropyridine nucleus with the calcium antagonist nifedipine; bepridil is unrelated to other known calcium antagonists. Like nifedipine, nicardipine and nitrendipine produce peripheral vasodilation as their predominant in vivo effect. Bepridil has vascular, sinoatrial and atrioventricular nodal, and myocardial effects qualitatively similar to those of the calcium antagonist verapamil; it also interferes with the fast sodium channel and prolongs refractoriness in atrial and ventricular tissue. Nicardipine and nitrendipine undergo extensive first-pass hepatic extraction after oral administration; oral bioavailability of bepridil is about 60%. All three drugs are highly protein bound and have been reported to increase plasma digoxin concentrations.

Both nicardipine and nitrendipine are effective antihypertensive agents used alone or combined with diuretics, β blockers, or angiotensin-converting enzyme inhibitors. Nicardipine and bepridil effectively control angina, and preliminary studies indicate that nitrendipine has antianginal properties. Bepridil may be useful in the treatment of various cardiac arrhythmias; however, its tendency to cause or worsen cardiac arrhythmias and its association with torsade de pointes may limit its usefulness. Nicardipine and nitrendipine have similar adverse effect profiles, with vasodilation-related complaints being most common.

Since nicardipine, nitrendipine, and nifedipine are similar in efficacy and safety, the eventual availability of sustained-release dosage forms may determine how these drugs are ultimately used. Bepridil is an effective antianginal drug, but, because of its proarrhythmic potential, it should probably not be used as a first-line agent.

Index terms: Angina pectoris; Angiotensin-converting enzyme inhibitors; Arrhythmia; Bepridil; Binding; Blood levels; Cardiac drugs; Combined therapy; Digoxin; Diuretics; Drug interactions; Drugs, availability; Excretion; Metabolism; Nicardipine; Nifedipine; Nitrendipine; Pharmacokinetics; Sustained-action medications; Sympatholytic agents; Toxicity
Clin Pharm. 1988; 7:97–108

Calcium antagonists have, in the past few years, become important components in the treatment of various cardiovascular disorders. The properties and uses of the agents currently available in the United States—nifedipine, diltiazem, and verapamil—have been summarized previously.[1,2] This article reviews three other calcium antagonists—nicardipine, nitrendipine, and bepridil—that are under investigation primarily for cardiovascular indications. Use of these drugs for other indications has not been well described and will not be discussed here. Other calcium antagonists are being developed for cardiovascular indications but are in earlier stages of investigation.

Chemistry

Although the calcium antagonists exhibit a vast diversity of structure, nicardipine and nitrendipine share a common dihydropyridine nucleus with nifedipine (Figure 1). Some structure–activity relationships for the dihydropyridines have been described.[3] Bepridil is chemically unrelated to other known calcium antagonists. Nicardipine, nitrendipine, and bepridil all have an asymmetric center and are used clinically as racemic mixtures. Enantiomers of calcium antagonists may differ in potency and pharmacologic properties[3]; whether such differences are important when nicardipine,

GUY R. HASEGAWA, PHARM.D., is Clinical Pharmacist, St. Joseph Mercy Hospital, Catherine McAuley Health Center, Ann Arbor, MI, and Clinical Assistant Professor, College of Pharmacy, The University of Michigan, Ann Arbor.

Address reprint requests to Dr. Hasegawa at the Department of Pharmacy, St. Joseph Mercy Hospital, P.O. Box 995, Ann Arbor, MI 48106.

This is **article 680-204-8802** in the **ASHP Continuing Education System;** it qualifies for 1.0 hour of continuing-education credit. See page 158 for learning objectives and test questions.

Copyright © 1988, American Society of Hospital Pharmacists, Inc. All rights reserved. 0278-2677/88/0201-0099$03.00.

Figure 1. Chemical structures of nicardipine, nitrendipine, nifedipine, and bepridil.

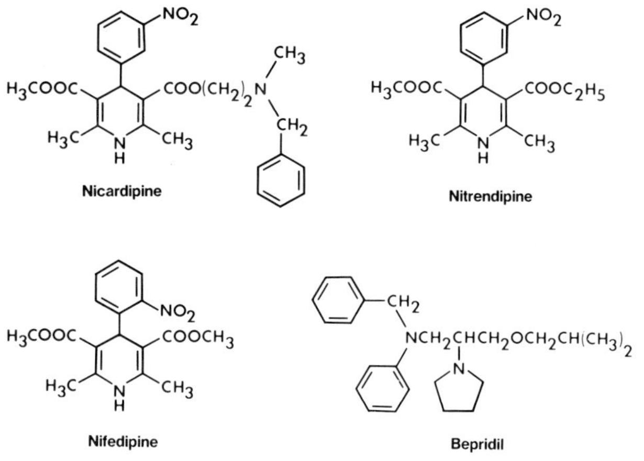

nitrendipine, and bepridil are used in humans as racemic mixtures is not known. Nicardipine and bepridil are used as hydrochloride salts.

Pharmacology

Calcium antagonists produce their various physiologic effects, at least in part, through inhibition of transmembrane calcium influx. In the sinoatrial (SA) and atrioventricular (AV) nodes of the heart, calcium is the major ion involved in depolarization. Thus, interference with calcium influx may cause sinus bradycardia or impair conduction through the AV node. In cardiac and smooth muscle, a decrease in calcium influx may inhibit excitation–contraction coupling, weakening the force of cardiac contraction and inducing vasodilation. The dissimilar effects elicited by calcium antagonists may result from differences in the site, affinity, and mode of interaction with calcium channels, as well as possible interactions with intracellular structures.[4,5]

Many classification schemes for the calcium antagonists have been proposed.[5-8] One system, developed by Singh et al.,[6] groups agents by pharmacologic profile. Type 1 drugs, including diltiazem and verapamil, slow AV nodal conduction and depress myocardial contractility in vivo while relaxing vascular smooth muscle. Type 2 drugs, the dihydropyridines such as nifedipine, nicardipine, and nitrendipine, inhibit SA and AV nodal function in vitro but not in vivo. Their potent vasodilatory effects may be accompanied in vivo by reflex increases in heart rate, AV nodal conduction, and contractility. Type 3 drugs, such as the investigational agents cinnarizine and flunarizine, are vasodilators with little direct cardiac effect. Finally, type 4 drugs, including bepridil, inhibit calcium influx into cardiac and vascular tissue but also have other complex electrophysiologic properties. Although the potential uses of an agent may be surmised from its type, differences within groups (e.g., selectivity for certain vascular beds) limit the usefulness of this scheme in further predicting a particular drug's therapeutic role.

Nicardipine[9] and nitrendipine[10] are qualitatively similar to nifedipine[11] in pharmacologic activity, producing peripheral vasodilation as their predominant in vivo effect. Reflex increases in heart rate occur initially with administration of the drugs but may not persist with long-term use. These agents generally do not impair cardiac impulse conduction or substantially depress myocardial contractility in vivo.

Bepridil has vascular, SA and AV nodal, and myocardial effects qualitatively similar to those of the type 1 calcium antagonist verapamil.[6,12] Bepridil also exerts quinidine-like effects, interfering with the fast sodium channel and prolonging refractoriness in atrial and ventricular tissue.[13,14]

Pharmacokinetics

Nicardipine. Single oral doses of nicardipine in healthy fasting volunteers are well absorbed and produce peak plasma drug concentrations in 20 minutes to two hours.[15] When doses are taken with or one hour after a meal, however, absorption is delayed, and both the peak plasma drug concentration and total bioavailability are reduced.[15,16] Nicardipine undergoes extensive presystemic, or first-pass, extraction, producing large intersubject and intrasubject variations in plasma concentration after single oral doses.[15] This variation is reduced, and bioavailability appears to increase, after continued dosing over three days, suggesting saturation or equilibration of first-pass processes.[15] In addition, bioavailability appears to increase as oral dosage increases, possibly a result of first-pass saturation. In one study, bioavailability increased from $6.5 \pm 1.1\%$ to $30.3 \pm 2.2\%$ (mean ± S.E.) as the single oral dose increased from 10 to 40 mg.[17] In another study, bioavailability increased from $10 \pm 6\%$ to $43 \pm 18\%$ (mean ± S.D.) as the oral dosage increased from 10 to 40 mg three times a day.[15] Nicardipine is at least 98% protein bound.[18,19]

Nicardipine is extensively metabolized in the liver,[17,20] with 60% of an oral dose excreted in the urine, primarily as glucuronide conjugates.[16] Compared with nicardipine, the metabolites have little or no cardiovascular activity.[21,22] About 35% of the radioactivity from administration of labeled oral nicardipine is recovered in the feces,[23] and elimination of unchanged drug in the urine is negligible.[23,24] Reported values for clearance vary widely. Administration of intravenous nicardipine has not demonstrated dose-dependent plasma clearance,[25] but clearance appears to decrease with increasingly larger oral doses.[17] Methods of reporting clearance data have been inconsistent, hindering comparison of study results. Reported elimination half-life values in healthy volunteers vary greatly, ranging from 35 minutes to 12 hours, with most values averaging about 1 hour.[15,17,18,23,26–28] Although the differing sensitivity of various assay methods may partly account for the extreme variability in reported half-lives, no particular assay has been consistently associated with either high or low values. Pharmacokinetic variables in elderly hypertensive patients are similar to those found in younger healthy volunteers.[23] Although some investigators[23,29] have found reduced nicardipine clearance values, increased peak drug concentrations in serum, and increased area under the plasma concentration–time curve (AUC) in patients with renal disease compared with healthy volunteers, others[30] have found no such differences and have concluded that dosage adjustments are unnecessary even for patients on hemodialysis. Silke et al.[25] reported reduced plasma nicardipine clearance in patients with coronary artery disease and attributed this change to diminished hepatic blood flow. Other conditions that compromise hepatic function might be expected to prolong nicardipine elimination half-life.

Few pharmacokinetic drug interactions have been reported involving nicardipine. In one study, 10 patients receiving maintenance digoxin therapy were given oral nicardipine hydrochloride 60 mg/day for two weeks.[31] Mean (± S.D.) plasma digoxin concentrations increased by about 20% ($p < 0.05$), from 1.08 ± 0.4 to 1.3 ± 0.6 ng/mL, exceeding 2 ng/mL in only one patient. Nicardipine has been reported to double trough cyclosporine concentrations in blood.[32] In dogs, isoflurane has decreased nicardipine volume of distribution and clearance.[33]

Nitrendipine. Like nicardipine, nitrendipine is also well absorbed after oral administration and undergoes first-pass hepatic extraction,[34,35] with peak plasma concentrations occurring one to two hours after a dose.[36–38] The oral bioavailability of a single 20-mg dose in six healthy subjects averaged about 23%.[35] AUC increases linearly as nitrendipine doses are increased from 5 to 20 mg[38]; AUC may also increase slightly with multiple dosing over several days.[39] Nitrendipine, like nicardipine, is about 98% protein bound.[10,35]

Nitrendipine is extensively metabolized in the liver, a process not saturated with clinically used dosages, to inactive pyridine analogs.[34,37,38] These metabolites eventually appear, primarily in the urine, as either the free pyridine forms or their glucuronide conjugates. Negligible amounts of unchanged nitrendipine appear in the urine.[37] Mean elimination half-life values vary widely, ranging from 2 to 31 hours in healthy volunteers,[36,37,39–41] patients with renal insufficiency,[36,40] and elderly patients.[42] As with nicardipine, neither high nor low half-life values have been consistently associated with any particular assay method. AUC and plasma half-life values are increased in patients with liver disease,[39,43] and AUC may be increased in elderly patients.[42,44] Reported values for clearance are variable, and study results have been reported in an inconsistent manner.

The pharmacokinetics of nitrendipine has been reported to be unaffected by concurrent administration of cimetidine, ranitidine, digoxin, digitoxin, atenolol, metoprolol, and acebutolol.[45] When given to eight patients receiving maintenance digoxin therapy, nitrendipine 20 mg/day increased peak plasma digoxin concentrations by 57% and digoxin AUC (from 0 to 12 hours) by 15% while decreasing digoxin clearance by 13% ($p < 0.05$ for all changes); renal digoxin clearance remained unchanged.[46] Effects on postdistribution concentrations of digoxin were not reported. Nitrendipine 10 mg/day did not alter digoxin pharmacokinetics. In another study, nitrendipine 20 mg twice daily had no effect on the pharmacokinetics of β-acetyldigoxin, another cardiac glycoside.[47]

Bepridil. Bepridil is well absorbed orally, with peak plasma concentrations occurring about two hours after drug administration.[48,49] When bepridil is given immediately after a meal, peak concentrations occur at about four hours, but the extent of absorption is not affected.[50] Although hepatic first-pass extraction reduces oral bioavailability to about 60%, plasma concentrations are linearly related to dose over the proposed dosage range.[49–51] Like nicardipine and nitrendipine, bepridil is highly protein bound (greater than 99%).[52]

Complete hepatic transformation of bepridil produces no fewer than 17 metabolites,[48] at least 1 of which may have cardiovascular activity.[50] Urinary excretion is the primary route of elimination for bepridil metabolites; little or no unchanged drug appears in the urine.[48] The terminal plasma half-life of bepridil averages 33 ± 15 hours (mean ± S.D.) after a single oral dose[50] but increases to 42 ± 12 hours with multiple dosing.[49] This prolongation of half-life is associated with decreased drug clearance and enhanced bioavailability.[50] Surprisingly, preliminary evidence suggests that hepatic disease does not affect bepridil pharmacokinetics to an important degree.[50] Bepridil clearance is apparently unchanged in patients with renal failure, and the drug is not removed by hemodialysis.[53]

Like nicardipine and nitrendipine, bepridil has also been reported to increase plasma digoxin concentrations. When given to patients receiving maintenance digoxin therapy, bepridil hydrochloride 300 mg/day for one week caused a 34% increase in trough digoxin concentrations ($p < 0.001$); plasma bepridil concentrations were unaffected by digoxin.[54] In another study, bepridil increased peak digoxin concentrations by 48%, digoxin AUC by 21%, and renal digoxin clearance by 30% while reducing plasma digoxin clearance by 16%.[55] Effects on postdistribution concentrations of digoxin were not described, and changes in individual subjects were not always reported. Propranolol and bepridil have been used together; neither drug influences the pharmacokinetics of the other.[56]

Treatment of Hypertension

Calcium antagonists have been studied extensively for the treatment of hypertension. Although vasodilation through calcium antagonism is the major antihypertensive property of these drugs, some may also act through α-adrenergic blockade[57] or myocardial depression.[58] Because long-term use of calcium antagonists apparently does not cause undesirable changes in glucose or lipid metabolism,[59] the renin–angiotensin–aldosterone system,[60] or renal function,[60] these drugs may assume a prominent, possibly first-step, role in the treatment of hypertension. Nifedipine, verapamil, and diltiazem have all been shown to be effective antihypertensive agents when used alone or in combination with other drugs.[59] Nicardipine and nitrendipine have been studied as well. Oral bepridil therapy, however, does not lower blood pressure in normotensive patients,[56,61–63] and the drug has received little attention as a possible antihypertensive agent.

Nicardipine is similar to nifedipine in its antihypertensive actions and efficacy. Both drugs decrease peripheral vascular resistance without dilating venous capacitance vessels.[64,65] Reflex tachycardia occurs initially with administration of either drug[65,66] but may lessen or abate completely with continued therapy.[67,68] In dosages of 30–120 mg/day in three doses, nicardipine hydrochloride has reduced systolic and diastolic blood pressure in patients with mild to moderate essential hypertension by about 10–20%, and it has produced satisfactory antihypertensive control (systolic blood pressure of <160 and diastolic blood pressure of <95 mm Hg) in about 60% of patients.[69–72] Antihypertensive effects have persisted for at least two years[69] and are apparent in patients with or without renal impairment.[29,30] Nicardipine has additive antihypertensive effects when used with β blockers,[72,73] enalapril,[74] or hydrochlorothiazide,[75] and it is as effective as propranolol,[76] verapamil,[77] or hydrochlorothiazide[75] as a first-step agent.

Like nifedipine and nicardipine, nitrendipine decreases vascular resistance, effectively reducing systolic and diastolic blood pressure in patients with essential hypertension and producing a reflex tachycardia that diminishes with long-term therapy.[78] When used in combination therapy or alone in dosages of 10–60 mg/day in one or two doses, nitrendipine has satisfactorily controlled blood pressure in the majority of patients for up to a year. Among patients who respond to nitrendipine, systolic and diastolic blood pressure decrease by about 10–20% in those with mild to moderate hypertension[79–84] and by about 25% in those with severe hypertension.[85–87] Nitrendipine is at least as effective as nifedipine,[82,88] verapamil,[82] captopril,[89] enalapril,[89] β blockers,[38,83,90,91] and hydralazine,[92,93] and it has been used successfully in combination with β blockers,[78,84,85] diuretics,[84,85,94,95] captopril,[96] and enalapril.[97] Nitrendipine is effective in elderly patients,[82,98] patients with low plasma renin activity,[82] and black as well as white patients.[81,87,90] Preliminary reports indicate that nitrendipine may also be useful in the treatment of renal[99,100] and pregnancy-induced hypertension,[101,102] as well as systolic hypertension in elderly patients.[103]

In the treatment of hypertension, the major clinical difference among the dihydropyridines—nifedipine, nicardipine, and nitrendipine—appears to be duration of action, with nifedipine and nicardipine therapy requiring three daily doses and nitrendipine one or two. Eventual introduction of sustained-release forms of nifedipine[59,104,105] and nicardipine[24] may make the current differences in duration unimportant. Though effective alone, all three drugs may be successfully combined with diuretics, angiotensin-converting enzyme inhibitors, or β blockers. Of the calcium antagonists, the dihydropyridines are probably the preferred agents in patients with cardiac conduction disturbances or severely diminished left ventricular function. The addition of nifedipine to β-blocker therapy may rarely worsen left ventricular function since reflex sympathetic activity may not compensate for nifedipine's intrinsic myocardial depressant properties.[106] Worsening of contractile function would be even more unusual if nicardipine or nitrendipine were added to β-blocker therapy since these dihydropyridines, unlike nifedipine, have no in vivo negative inotropic effects.[107–109]

Verapamil and diltiazem, although effective antihypertensive agents, may worsen pre-existing bradycardia, heart block, and congestive heart failure, and the combined use of verapamil and a β blocker would be even more likely to produce marked left ventricular dysfunction or symptomatic bradycardia.[58] Verapamil and diltiazem are logical choices for patients with normal cardiac conduction and contractility since these drugs generally elicit fewer complaints of unacceptable adverse effects than the dihydropyridines[2] (see Adverse Effects section).

Treatment of Angina Pectoris

Numerous investigators have studied nicardipine and bepridil for the treatment of angina pectoris. Although small, single-dose studies[110–112] have indicated that nitrendipine also has antianginal properties, the current long-term clinical data are insufficient for further discussion of the drug for this indication.

How nicardipine prevents angina pectoris is not

completely understood. Nicardipine is a potent coronary vasodilator and may, in some patients, enhance myocardial oxygen supply by increasing coronary blood flow.[64,113] The drug has minimal effects on preload in patients without congestive heart failure (CHF),[64,114] but a nicardipine-induced reduction in afterload may lower myocardial wall tension and lessen oxygen demand.[114,115] Nicardipine therapy allows patients with coronary artery disease to achieve more intense exercise levels before angina occurs. The heart rate–blood pressure product (an indicator of myocardial oxygen demand) when angina finally does occur is often the same or greater than the pretreatment value.[66,116-118] This suggests not only that nicardipine allows more work to be done with the same oxygen expenditure, but also that delivery or cellular use of oxygen may be enhanced.[66,116]

In patients with chronic stable angina pectoris, total daily nicardipine hydrochloride dosages of 90–120 mg have produced beneficial responses, increasing total exercise time or exercise time to onset of angina by about 10–40%[66,116-120] and decreasing anginal frequency and nitroglycerin consumption by about 50%.[66,118,120] Studies examining nicardipine's antianginal efficacy have lasted up to one year,[121] although most have been much shorter in duration. As an antianginal drug, nicardipine appears to be as effective as nifedipine,[116,122] propranolol,[118,123] and atenolol,[124] but in one study[119] was inferior to verapamil. Combination therapy using nicardipine and a β blocker should theoretically be safe and effective in the treatment of angina pectoris[109,125]; this presumption, however, is unsupported by adequate clinical data. Like nifedipine,[126] nicardipine may occasionally worsen symptoms of angina,[117] possibly by inducing reflex tachycardia or lowering coronary perfusion pressure. Preliminary evidence indicates that nicardipine may also be effective in preventing angina caused by coronary artery spasm.[67]

The precise mechanism of bepridil's antianginal effect is also unknown. By reducing afterload, the drug may lower myocardial oxygen requirements during exercise.[62] Bepridil may also improve coronary blood flow or favorably alter coronary blood distribution.[62] Despite bepridil's intrinsic negative inotropic properties,[127] left ventricular performance has been preserved or enhanced in patients treated with the drug.[62,128]

In daily dosages of 200–450 mg, bepridil hydrochloride produces definite clinical improvement in patients with chronic stable angina pectoris. Compared with placebo, bepridil therapy has reduced anginal frequency and nitroglycerin consumption by at least 50%[61,62,128-131] and increased total exercise time or exercise time to onset of angina by about 20–30%.[61,63,128,129,131,132] Beneficial effects have persisted for at least one to two years of therapy.[129,130] Bepridil appears to be as effective as propranolol,[63] and bepridil provides an additional antianginal effect for patients already receiving propranolol.[56] Because of its proarrhythmic potential (see Adverse Effects section), bepridil should probably be reserved for patients refractory to other, possibly safer, agents. Studies documenting bepridil's efficacy in refractory angina, however, are not currently available.[133]

The roles of nicardipine, nitrendipine, and bepridil in the treatment of angina pectoris are not clearly defined. Like the currently available calcium antagonists, nicardipine probably deserves consideration as a first-choice antianginal agent. Preliminary studies have demonstrated the antianginal properties of nitrendipine, but the drug cannot be recommended for this indication until more data are available. Bepridil effectively controls angina, but concern over its arrhythmogenicity may discourage clinicians from using it as a first-line drug.

Treatment of Arrhythmias

Nicardipine[134] and nitrendipine[135] do not have cardiac electrophysiologic properties in vivo that would be useful in the treatment of arrhythmias. Bepridil, on the other hand, prolongs refractoriness and slows conduction in the AV node,[13,136,137] much like verapamil.[138] In addition, bepridil has important electrophysiologic effects in other cardiac tissue. Although bepridil does not consistently slow atrial and ventricular conduction, it does prolong atrial, ventricular, and accessory pathway (antegrade and retrograde) refractoriness.[13,136,137] Thus, in addition to having possible antiarrhythmic effects in the ventricles, bepridil might also be useful in the treatment of supraventricular tachyarrhythmias, including those associated with pre-excitation syndromes.

Bepridil has been tested in patients with sustained AV re-entry tachycardia inducible by programmed electrical stimulation and associated with dual AV nodal or accessory pathways. In most patients, intravenous bepridil has caused prompt termination of induced arrhythmia whether given before or after induction. In a study by Rowland et al.,[136] the administration of intravenous bepridil stopped supraventricular tachycardia (SVT) within five minutes in 12 of 20 patients. Roy et al.[137] studied five patients with inducible sustained SVT. Although intravenous bepridil did not prevent reinduction of SVT in any patient, the drug stopped the arrhythmia within 10 beats in three of the patients. Therapy with oral bepridil hydrochloride 300–400 mg/day has either caused prompt termination of induced arrhythmia or prevented induction altogether in the majority of patients. Rowland et al.[136] and Roy et al.[137] studied the effects of oral bepridil in a total of 29 patients with inducible sustained SVT. After therapy, SVT was not inducible in 9 patients. Arrhythmia was still inducible in the remaining 20 patients, but in half of those it became nonsustained. Patients with inducible sustained arrhythmia after 7–10 days of oral therapy have tended to experience recurrences of arrhythmia during long-term treatment (up to 10 months) with bepridil hydrochloride 200–400 mg/day.[137]

Little is known about bepridil's effects on atrial fibrillation or flutter. In one study, intravenous bepridil caused a nonsignificant slowing of mean ventricular rate during induced atrial fibrillation in patients with accessory pathways.[137] Unlike intravenous verapamil,[139] bepridil prolongs refractoriness in accessory pathways.[137] Therefore, acceleration of the ventricular rate during atrial fibrillation in the Wolff–Parkinson–White syndrome, sometimes observed after verapamil administration,[139] should not occur with bepridil therapy. Clearly, further investigation is needed to define bepridil's properties and potential usefulness in the treatment of atrial fibrillation or flutter in patients with and without accessory pathways.

Intravenous bepridil has been tested in patients with ventricular tachycardia (VT) previously inducible by programmed electrical stimulation. Though not as effective as intravenous procainamide or quinidine,[140] bepridil has prevented reinduction of VT in about 50% of patients[140,141] and increased VT cycle length (by 30–105 milliseconds) in others.[141] Successful prevention by intravenous bepridil of VT induction appears to predict a successful outcome (i.e., absence of arrhythmia recurrence) with oral therapy lasting up to 13 months.[141] The frequency of premature ventricular complexes (PVCs) and nonsustained VT has been reduced by at least 70% and 95%, respectively, in about 50% of patients treated with oral bepridil hydrochloride 200–400 mg/day and evaluated by ambulatory electrocardiographic recording.[142]

Although bepridil appears to have a wider antiarrhythmic spectrum than verapamil or diltiazem, additional studies are needed to define its therapeutic role. Long-term efficacy and the potential for worsening arrhythmias are issues requiring clarification before bepridil can be recommended for use as an antiarrhythmic.

Treatment of Congestive Heart Failure

Because they produce vasodilation without marked myocardial depression, diltiazem[143] and the dihydropyridines may be beneficial as afterload reducers in the treatment of CHF. In addition, verapamil[144] and nifedipine[145] have improved left ventricular diastolic function in patients with hypertrophic cardiomyopathy. This suggests that calcium antagonists may theoretically be useful in patients without hypertrophic cardiomyopathy whose congestive symptoms may be due to diastolic rather than systolic dysfunction. The effects of nicardipine and nitrendipine on diastolic function, however, are not well described, and the following discussion is limited to the use of calcium antagonists in patients without hypertrophic cardiomyopathy. Nifedipine therapy has produced inconsistent results in such patients,[146,147] and only preliminary data are available for nicardipine and nitrendipine.

In patients with New York Heart Association (NYHA) class II–III CHF, intravenous nicardipine has increased left ventricular ejection fraction by 23% while significantly lowering blood pressure and raising heart rate.[148] Oral nicardipine hydrochloride, 30 mg every eight hours for a week, has caused significant increases in cardiac index and stroke volume index and decreases in mean arterial blood pressure, systemic vascular resistance, pulmonary artery pressure, and pulmonary artery wedge pressure in patients with NYHA class III–IV CHF during both rest and exercise.[108] Similarly, a single oral dose of nitrendipine 10–20 mg has raised cardiac index and stroke volume index, while reducing mean arterial pressure, systemic vascular resistance, right atrial pressure, pulmonary artery pressure, and pulmonary artery wedge pressure in patients with NYHA class III–IV CHF at rest.[107] Although nicardipine and nitrendipine appear to produce favorable hemodynamic responses, how the drugs would affect the symptoms and prognosis of CHF during long-term oral therapy is unknown and should be assessed with further studies.

Adverse Effects

Nicardipine. Although up to one half of patients receiving nicardipine may complain of adverse effects,[71] many of the effects occur with similar frequency in patients receiving placebo.[71,117] Most adverse effects are related to nicardipine's vasodilatory properties. Headache, palpitations, dizziness, flushing, or pedal or ankle edema occur in about 20% of patients.[66,72,117,121] According to one investigator,[73] some of these effects can be minimized by concurrent β-blocker therapy. Worsened angina pectoris is occasionally associated with nicardipine administration,[116,117,119] as are noncardiac effects such as nausea or epigastric discomfort,[66,73,118] weakness or fatigue,[72,73] and skin rash.[67] Adverse effects, though generally well tolerated, have forced discontinuation of drug administration in up to 10% of patients in some studies.[72,118,121] Nicardipine appears not to alter laboratory indicators of hematologic or biochemical status (e.g., electrolytes, cardiac enzymes, cholesterol or triglycerides, or renal, thyroid, or liver function tests),[66,72,116,118] and patients receiving nicardipine are notably free from adverse metabolic or endocrine effects.[149]

Nitrendipine. Nitrendipine is essentially indistinguishable from nicardipine in the types and frequency of adverse effects caused and the tolerance of these effects by patients. Although the majority of patients receiving nitrendipine in some studies have experienced adverse effects,[85,92] placebo administration has often been associated with the same complaints.[150] Complaints related to nitrendipine-induced vasodilation predominate, with gastrointestinal and central nervous system symptoms being less common and rash occurring rarely.[80,85,92,99,150] Many nitrendipine-induced adverse effects diminish with continued therapy[80,150] and may, according to some clinicians,[85] be controlled with concurrent β-blocker or diuretic therapy. Nitrendipine has been associated rarely with elevations in liver function test values without clinical evidence of liver disease.[93] Otherwise, nitrendipine does not appear to change serum biochemical, hematologic, or lipid values (including cholesterol, triglycerides, and lipoproteins).[38,85,150]

Bepridil. In some studies,[61,142] the majority of patients receiving bepridil have experienced adverse effects. Fortunately, bepridil's most worrisome adverse effect, its tendency to cause or worsen cardiac arrhythmias, appears to be uncommon. Bepridil does not consistently widen either the PR or QRS interval, but it can significantly prolong the QT (or corrected QT) interval,[61,131,132,142,151] sometimes causing concomitant flattening or notching of the T wave.[131,151] QT prolongation is a prerequisite for torsade de pointes,[152] a ventricular arrhythmia that has in fact occurred, though rarely, during bepridil therapy.[153,154] Bepridil-induced torsade de pointes has been reported most commonly in elderly women and has been associated with low serum potassium and high serum bepridil concentrations.[153,154] Bepridil has also caused new monomorphic VT and sped the rate of pre-existing VT. Levy et al.[141] studied the effects of oral bepridil in nine patients with inducible VT. One patient had previously inducible nonsustained VT (cycle length 470 milliseconds) that, after bepridil treatment, was still inducible, had a shorter cycle length (290 milliseconds), and required cardioversion. Nestico et al.[142] gave oral bepridil to 21 patients with benign or potentially lethal ventricular arrhythmias. One patient had an asymptomatic increase in PVC frequency, and another developed sustained VT that required cardioversion. Haerer et al.[155] gave oral bepridil to three patients with hypertrophic obstructive cardiomyopathy and reported that one patient developed new atrial flutter and another had new nonsustained VT. Bepridil does not appear to be more arrhythmogenic than other antiarrhythmic agents,[140] but sufficient comparative data are not available. In addition, more data are needed to clearly identify the patients most likely to experience bepridil's proarrhythmic effect. Bepridil apparently causes few other cardiovascular adverse effects, although it does tend to slow heart rate.[131,132,151]

The most common noncardiac adverse effects of bepridil involve the gastrointestinal and central nervous systems. Occurring in up to 20% of patients, gastrointestinal effects include diarrhea, constipation, dyspepsia, and nausea[56,131,132,136,142]; paralytic ileus has been reported in at least one patient.[141] Central nervous system effects, also occurring in about 20% of patients, include headache, dizziness, diplopia, tremor, nervousness, weakness, insomnia, drowsiness, anorexia, and poor memory.[56,131,132,136,137,142] Dry mouth also occurs,[132,142] and the intravenous drug preparation can cause thrombophlebitis.[136] Except for abnormal liver function tests in one patient,[132] bepridil has not been associated with biochemical, hematologic, lipid, or ophthalmologic changes.[61]

Comparison of Calcium Antagonists. Nicardipine, nitrendipine, and nifedipine cause similar adverse effects with similar frequency[9–11]; one agent cannot be identified as safer or more tolerable than the others. Vasodilation-related adverse effects are most common, although some may diminish with continued drug use or the addition of β-blocker or diuretic therapy. Slowing drug absorption by the use of sustained-release dosage forms or by giving the drugs with food may also reduce the severity of these effects.[59] In general, the dihydropyridines are safe drugs, causing bothersome, but rarely life-threatening, adverse effects. Verapamil and diltiazem appear to be better tolerated than the dihydropyridines,[2] and they are probably just as safe if used in patients without cardiac conduction abnormalities or severe left ventricular dysfunction.

Although bepridil causes different adverse effects than the other calcium antagonists, it is probably comparable to the dihydropyridines in patient tolerance. The major safety concern regarding bepridil is its proarrhythmic potential. Although its frequency and clinical importance are not fully known, this possibly life-threatening adverse effect might well be considered a notable hazard of bepridil therapy by some clinicians.

Dosage

A starting oral nicardipine hydrochloride dosage of 20 mg three times daily has been recommended for the treatment of hypertension or angina pectoris.[9] Because equilibration or saturation of first-pass processes may take three days, at least that interval should elapse between dosage adjustments; an interval of two weeks has been suggested.[9] Maximum dosage in most studies has been 40 mg three times daily. Dosage in patients with renal disease should probably not require adjustment, but a smaller-than-usual dosage should be used in the presence of hepatic disease. Taking the drug with food may prevent some vasodilation-related adverse effects, but doing this may also reduce drug bioavailability.

Antihypertensive therapy with oral nitrendipine has been effective at dosages of 10–60 mg/day in one or two doses. A daily morning dose of 10–20 mg would be a reasonable starting point, with dosage adjustments being made no more often than every week or so. Dosage reductions are advisable for patients with liver disease, but they are probably unnecessary for patients with renal dysfunction.

The usual dosage of oral bepridil hydrochloride for the treatment of angina pectoris or cardiac arrhythmias has been 200–400 mg once daily. Bepridil's long half-life indicates that dosage adjustments should probably not be made more often than every week. Some investigators[54,141,142] have used oral loading doses of 800–900 mg/day for one or two days; loading may have been related to a proarrhythmic effect in one patient.[142] Because they appear to be at highest risk to develop torsade de pointes,[154] elderly patients probably should receive conservatively low dosages of bepridil. Patients with liver disease may also require relatively low dosages, although preliminary evidence[50] suggests that dosage adjustment may be unnecessary. Dosage adjustments should not be necessary for patients with renal dysfunction.

Formulary Recommendations

Nicardipine and nitrendipine may have potential therapeutic advantages over nifedipine. Nitrendipine is a long-acting antihypertensive drug; its use, compared with use of either nifedipine or nicardipine, could enhance compliance with therapy. Nicardipine and nitrendipine lack myocardial depressant effects in vivo, but this apparent advantage may only have marginal clinical importance. Nifedipine rarely causes worsening of cardiac contractility, but it may do so in patients with preexisting left ventricular dysfunction[146,147] or when used in combination with a β blocker.[106] On the other hand, clinicians have considerable experience using nifedipine, and data regarding less common uses of the dihydropyridines (e.g., for coronary artery spasm, hypertensive crisis, Raynaud's phenomenon, esophageal spasm) are more plentiful for nifedipine than for nicardipine and nitrendipine.

It would be reasonable to have nifedipine and nitrendipine on the formulary simultaneously: nifedipine because it is versatile and widely used, and nitrendipine because it requires only one or two daily doses for treating hypertension. If proven effective for the treatment of angina pectoris, nitrendipine may become the dihydropyridine of choice for this indication. Nicardipine, in its present dosage form, might not be a useful formulary addition because it presents no important advantages over nifedipine. However, because of nicardipine's proven value in the treatment of angina as well as hypertension, it could replace nitrendipine if it becomes available in a once-daily dosage form. Should nifedipine become available in a once-daily dosage form that causes minimal adverse effects,[59] it might well be the only one of the three dihydropyridines needed.

Bepridil, too, would be a useful formulary item. Its long duration of action makes it an appealing antianginal drug, and it may also prove useful in the treatment of some cardiac arrhythmias. Although its potential for causing or worsening arrhythmias is not fully defined, clinicians may wish to reserve antianginal therapy with bepridil for those patients not responding satisfactorily to other drugs.

Verapamil and diltiazem are safe, effective, and versatile agents that are different enough from nicardipine, nitrendipine, and bepridil that they should not be displaced by the introduction of the latter drugs.

Conclusion

Nicardipine and nitrendipine are calcium antagonists much like nifedipine in action, uses, and safety. Nicardipine is an effective antianginal drug, and nitrendipine may prove effective as well; both are useful antihypertensive agents. Neither drug will replace nifedipine, but how any of the dihydropyridines—nifedipine, nicardipine, or nitrendipine—will eventually be used may depend on the availability of sustained-release dosage forms.

Bepridil is a long-acting calcium antagonist with verapamil-like effects on vascular and cardiac tissue, as well as other electrophysiologic properties that may make it a useful antiarrhythmic agent. Bepridil is an effective antianginal drug, but its role in the treatment of arrhythmias is not yet clear. Because of its proarrhythmic potential, clinicians may choose not to use bepridil as a first-line antianginal drug.

References

1. Leonard RG, Talbert RL. Calcium-channel blocking agents. *Clin Pharm.* 1982; 1:17–33.
2. Talbert RL, Bussey HI. Update on calcium-channel blocking agents. *Clin Pharm.* 1983; 2:403–16.
3. Triggle DJ. Antihypertensive mechanism of action and binding sites of nitrendipine. *Am J Cardiol.* 1986; 58:35D–38D.
4. Schwartz A, Matlib MA, Balwierczak J et al. Pharmacology of calcium antagonists. *Am J Cardiol.* 1985; 55:3C–7C.
5. Andersson K-E. Calcium-entry blockers. A heterogeneous family of compounds. *Acta Med Scand [Suppl].* 1984; 694:142–52.
6. Singh BN, Baky S, Nademanee K. Second-generation calcium antagonists: search for greater selectivity and versatility. *Am J Cardiol.* 1985; 55:214B–221B.

7. Godfraind T. Classification of calcium antagonists. *Am J Cardiol.* 1987; 59:11B–23B.
8. Vanhoutte PM. The expert committee of the World Health Organization on classification of calcium antagonists: the viewpoint of the raporteur. *Am J Cardiol.* 1987; 59:3A–8A.
9. Sorkin EM, Clissold SP. Nicardipine: a review of its pharmacodynamic and pharmacokinetic properties, and therapeutic efficacy, in the treatment of angina pectoris, hypertension and related cardiovascular disorders. *Drugs.* 1987; 33:296–345.
10. Goa KL, Sorkin EM. Nitrendipine: a review of its pharmacodynamic and pharmacokinetic properties, and therapeutic efficacy in the treatment of hypertension. *Drugs.* 1987; 33:123–55.
11. Sorkin EM, Clissold SP, Brogden RN. Nifedipine: a review of its pharmacodynamic and pharmacokinetic properties, and therapeutic efficacy, in ischaemic heart disease, hypertension and related cardiovascular disorders. *Drugs.* 1985; 30:182–274.
12. Alpert JS, Benotti JR, Brady PM et al. Hemodynamic effects of intravenous bepridil in patients with normal left ventricular function. *Am J Cardiol.* 1985; 55:20C–24C.
13. Singh BN, Nademanee K, Feld G et al. Comparative electrophysiologic profiles of calcium antagonists with particular reference to bepridil. *Am J Cardiol.* 1985; 55:14C–19C.
14. Prystowsky EN. Electrophysiologic and antiarrhythmic properties of bepridil. *Am J Cardiol.* 1985; 55:59C–62C.
15. Graham DJM, Dow RJ, Freedman D et al. Pharmacokinetics of nicardipine following oral and intravenous administration in man. *Postgrad Med J.* 1984; 60(Suppl 4):7–10.
16. Graham DJM, Dow RJ, Hall DJ et al. The metabolism and pharmacokinetics of nicardipine hydrochloride in man. *Br J Clin Pharmacol.* 1985; 20(Suppl 1):23S–28S.
17. Higuchi S, Shiobara Y. Comparative pharmacokinetics of nicardipine hydrochloride, a new vasodilator, in various species. *Xenobiotica.* 1980; 10:447–54.
18. Martinez JJ, Monkus EF, Ling T et al. Nicardipine pharmacokinetics in the elderly. *J Clin Pharmacol.* 1985; 25:468. Abstract.
19. Urien S, Albengres E, Comte A et al. Plasma protein binding and erythrocyte partitioning of nicardipine in vivo. *J Cardiovasc Pharmacol.* 1985; 7:891–8.
20. Higuchi S, Shiobara Y. Metabolic fate of nicardipine hydrochloride, a new vasodilator, by various species in vitro. *Xenobiotica.* 1980; 10:889–96.
21. Clarke B, Eglen RM, Patmore L et al. Cardioselective calcium entry blocking properties of a nicardipine metabolite. *Br J Pharmacol.* 1984; 83(Suppl):437P. Abstract.
22. Shibanuma T, Iwanami M, Fujimoto M et al. Synthesis of the metabolites of 2-(*N*-benzyl-*N*-methylamino)ethyl methyl 2,6-dimethyl-4-(*m*-nitrophenyl)-1,4-dihydropyridine-3,5-dicarboxylate hydrochloride (nicardipine hydrochloride, YC-93). *Chem Pharm Bull (Tokyo).* 1980; 28:2609–13.
23. Dow RJ, Graham DJM. A review of the human metabolism and pharmacokinetics of nicardipine hydrochloride. *Br J Clin Pharmacol.* 1986; 22(Suppl 3):195S–202S.
24. Thuillez C, Gueret M, Duhaze P et al. Nicardipine: pharmacokinetics and effects on carotid and brachial blood flows in normal volunteers. *Br J Clin Pharmacol.* 1984; 18:837–47.
25. Silke B, Graham DJM, Verma SP et al. Pharmacokinetic, haemodynamic and radionuclide studies with nicardipine in coronary artery disease. *Eur J Clin Pharmacol.* 1986; 29:651–7.
26. Jamieson MJ, Jeffers TA, Dow R et al. Nicardipine infusion: pharmacokinetics, haemodynamics and effects on the systolic time intervals. *Br J Clin Pharmacol.* 1985; 19:536P. Abstract.
27. Nelson GIC, Silke B, Verma SP et al. Pharmacokinetic and haemodynamic studies with nicardipine in coronary artery disease. *Br J Clin Pharmacol.* 1984; 17:635P. Abstract.
28. Campbell B, Kelman A, Sumner D et al. Non-invasive measurement of the acute haemodynamic effects of a new calcium channel blocker, nicardipine. *Br J Clin Pharmacol.* 1984; 17:188P–189P. Abstract.
29. Lee SM, Williams R, Warnock D et al. The effects of nicardipine in hypertensive subjects with impaired renal function. *Br J Clin Pharmacol.* 1986; 22(Suppl 3):297S–306S.
30. Clair F, Bellet M, Guerret M et al. Hypotensive effect and pharmacokinetics of nicardipine in patients with severe renal failure. *Curr Ther Res.* 1985; 38:74–82.
31. Lessem J, Bellinetto A. Interaction between digoxin and the calcium antagonists nicardipine and tiapamil. *Clin Ther.* 1983; 5:595–602.
32. Bourbigot B, Guiserix J, Airiau J et al. Nicardipine increases cyclosporin blood levels. *Lancet.* 1986; 1:1447. Letter.
33. Merin RG, Chelly JE, Hysing ES et al. Effect of isoflurane on nicardipine pharmacokinetics. *Clin Pharmacol Ther.* 1986; 39:210. Abstract.
34. Krol GJ, Lettieri JT, Yeh SC et al. Disposition and pharmacokinetics of ^{14}C-nitrendipine in healthy volunteers. *J Cardiovasc Pharmacol.* 1987; 9(Suppl 4):S122–S128.
35. Mikus G, Eichelbaum M. Pharmacokinetics, bioavailability, metabolism, and hemodynamic effects of the calcium channel antagonist nitrendipine. *J Cardiovasc Pharmacol.* 1987; 9(Suppl 4):S140–S141.
36. Aronoff GR. Pharmacokinetics of nitrendipine in patients with renal failure: comparison to normal subjects. *J Cardiovasc Pharmacol.* 1984; 6(Suppl 7):S974–S976.
37. Kann J, Krol GJ, Raemsch KD et al. Bioequivalence and metabolism of nitrendipine administered orally to healthy volunteers. *J Cardiovasc Pharmacol.* 1984; 6(Suppl 7):S968–S973.
38. Johnson BF, Romero L, Marwaha R. Hemodynamic and metabolic effects of the calcium channel blocking agent nitrendipine. *Clin Pharmacol Ther.* 1986; 39:389–94.
39. Lasseter KC, Cooper Shamblen E, Murdoch AA et al. Steady-state pharmacokinetics of nitrendipine in hepatic insufficiency. *J Cardiovasc Pharmacol.* 1984; 6(Suppl 7):S977–S981.
40. Aronoff GR, Sloan RS. Nitrendipine kinetics in normal and impaired renal function. *Clin Pharmacol Ther.* 1985; 38:212–8.
41. Krol GJ, Lettieri JT, Mazzu AL et al. Bioequivalence of different nitrendipine tablet dosage formulations. *J Cardiovasc Pharmacol.* 1987; 9(Suppl 4):S129–S135.
42. Lettieri J, Krol G, Yeh S et al. Pharmacokinetics of nitrendipine in elderly and young healthy volunteers. *J Cardiovasc Pharmacol.* 1987; 9(Suppl 4):S142–S147.
43. Kirch W, Dylewicz P, Hutt HJ et al. Pharmacokinetics of nitrendipine in liver disease. *J Clin Pharmacol.* 1985; 25:467. Abstract.
44. Kendall MJ, Lobo J, Jack DB et al. The influence of age on the pharmacokinetics of nitrendipine. *J Cardiovasc Pharmacol.* 1987; 9(Suppl 4):S96–S100.
45. Kirch W, Hutt HJ, Heidemann H et al. Drug interactions with nitrendipine. *J Cardiovasc Pharmacol.* 1984; 6(Suppl 7):S982–S985.
46. Kirch W, Logemann C, Heidemann H et al. Effect of two different doses of nitrendipine on steady-state digoxin level and systolic time intervals. *Eur J Clin Pharmacol.* 1986; 31:391–5.
47. Ziegler R, Wingender W, Boehme K et al. Study of pharmacokinetic and pharmacodynamic interaction between nitrendipine and digoxin. *J Cardiovasc Pharmacol.* 1987; 9(Suppl 4):S101–S106.
48. Ng KT, Hills JF, Wu WN. The absorption, excretion and biotransformation of bepridil HCl in man. *Fed Proc.* 1984; 43:655. Abstract.
49. Desiraju RK, Gemzik B, Nayak RK et al. Steady-state dose proportionality and pharmacokinetics of bepridil in healthy volunters. *Clin Pharmacol Ther.* 1984; 35:234. Abstract.
50. Benet LZ. Pharmacokinetics and metabolism of bepridil. *Am J Cardiol.* 1985; 55:8C–13C.

51. Lesko LJ, Benotti JR, Alpert JS et al. Pharmacokinetics of intravenous bepridil in patients with coronary disease. *J Pharm Sci*. 1986; 75:952–4.
52. Pritchard JF, McKown LA, O'Neill PJ. Comparative studies on the plasma protein binding of bepridil HCl. *Pharmacologist*. 1983; 25:112. Abstract.
53. Nayak RK, Halstenson CE, Opsahl JA et al. Pharmacokinetics of bepridil in hemodialysis patients. *Clin Pharmacol Ther*. 1987; 41:238. Abstract.
54. Belz GG, Wistuba S, Matthews JH. Digoxin and bepridil: pharmacokinetic and pharmacodynamic interactions. *Clin Pharmacol Ther*. 1986; 39:65–71.
55. Doose DR, Wallen S, Nayak RK et al. Pharmacokinetic interaction of bepridil and digoxin at steady-state. *Clin Pharmacol Ther*. 1987; 41:204. Abstract.
56. Frishman WH, Charlap S, Farnham J et al. Combination propranolol and bepridil therapy in stable angina pectoris. *Am J Cardiol*. 1985; 55:43C–49C.
57. Maisel AS, Motulsky HJ, Insel PA. Hypotension after quinidine plus verapamil: possible additive competition at alpha-adrenergic receptors. *N Engl J Med*. 1985; 312:167–70.
58. Soward AL, Vanhaleweyk GLJ, Serruys PW. The haemodynamic effects of nifedipine, verapamil and diltiazem in patients with coronary artery disease. *Drugs*. 1986; 32:66–101.
59. Frishman WH, Stroh JA, Greenberg SM et al. Calcium-channel blockers in systemic hypertension. *Curr Probl Cardiol*. 1987; 12:285–346.
60. Bauer JH, Reams G. Short- and long-term effects of calcium entry blockers on the kidney. *Am J Cardiol*. 1987; 59:66A–71A.
61. DiBianco R, Alpert J, Katz RJ et al. Bepridil for chronic stable angina pectoris: results of a prospective multicenter, placebo-controlled, dose-ranging study in 77 patients. *Am J Cardiol*. 1984; 53:35–41.
62. Narahara KA, Shapiro W, Weliky I et al. Hemodynamic actions of bepridil during treatment of stable angina pectoris. *Am J Cardiol*. 1985; 55:55C–58C.
63. Parker JO, Farrell B. Comparative antianginal effects of bepridil and propranolol in angina pectoris. *Am J Cardiol*. 1986; 58:449–52.
64. Lambert CR, Hill JA, Nichols WW et al. Coronary and systemic hemodynamic effects of nicardipine. *Am J Cardiol*. 1985; 55:652–6.
65. Guazzi M, Olivari MT, Polese A et al. Nifedipine, a new antihypertensive with rapid action. *Clin Pharmacol Ther*. 1977; 22:528–32.
66. Khurmi NS, Bowles MJ, Baba Subramanian V et al. Short- and long-term efficacy of nicardipine, assessed by placebo-controlled single- and double-blind crossover trials in patients with chronic stable angina. *J Am Coll Cardiol*. 1984; 4:908–17.
67. Gelman JS, Feldman RL, Scott E et al. Nicardipine for angina pectoris at rest and coronary arterial spasm. *Am J Cardiol*. 1985; 56:232–6.
68. Littler WA, Stallard TJ, Watson RDS et al. The effect of nifedipine on arterial pressure and reflex cardiac control. *Postgrad Med J*. 1983; 59(Suppl 2):109–13.
69. Murray TS, Langan J, Coxhead PF et al. Long-term effects of nicardipine in the treatment of essential hypertension. *Br J Clin Pharmacol*. 1986; 22(Suppl 3):249S–257S.
70. Littler WA, Young MA, Smith SA. The acute and chronic effects of nicardipine on blood pressure, heart rate, neurocirculatory reflexes and renal function in hypertensive patients. *Br J Clin Pharmacol*. 1986; 22(Suppl 3):239S–241S.
71. Brown ST III, Freedman D, DeVault GA et al. Safety, efficacy and pharmacokinetics of nicardipine in elderly hypertensive patients. *Br J Clin Pharmacol*. 1986; 22(Suppl 3):289S–295S.
72. Bellet M, Loria Y, Lallemand A. First-step treatment of mild to moderate uncomplicated essential hypertension by a new calcium antagonist: nicardipine. *J Cardiovasc Pharmacol*. 1985; 7:1149–53.
73. Kolloch R, Stumpe KO, Overlack A. Blood pressure, heart rate and A-V conduction responses to nicardipine in hypertensive patients receiving atenolol. *Br J Clin Pharmacol*. 1985; 20(Suppl 1):130S–134S.
74. Donnelly R, Elliott HL, Reid JL. Nicardipine combined with enalapril in patients with essential hypertension. *Br J Clin Pharmacol*. 1986; 22(Suppl 3):283S–287S.
75. Fagan TC, Conrad KA, Mar JH et al. Nicardipine and hydrochlorothiazide in essential hypertension. *Clin Pharmacol Ther*. 1986; 39:191. Abstract.
76. Murray TS, East BW, Robertson JIS. Nicardipine vs propranolol in the treatment of essential hypertension: effect on total body elemental composition. *Br J Clin Pharmacol*. 1986; 22(Suppl 3):259S–265S.
77. Al-Khawaja IM, Caruana MP, Lahiri A et al. Nicardipine and verapamil in essential hypertension. *Br J Clin Pharmacol*. 1986; 22(Suppl 3):273S–282S.
78. Nannan ME, Melin JA, Vanbutsele RJ et al. Acute and long-term effects of nitrendipine on resting and exercise hemodynamics in essential hypertension. *J Cardiovasc Pharmacol*. 1984; 6(Suppl 7):S1043–S1048.
79. Esper RJ, Esper RC, Baglivo HP et al. Long-term effectiveness of BAY e 5009-nitrendipine in the treatment of mild to moderate arterial hypertension. *J Cardiovasc Pharmacol*. 1984; 6(Suppl 7):S1096–S1099.
80. Tourkantonis A, Lasaridis A, Settas L. Clinical experience with long-term nitrendipine treatment in essential hypertension. *J Cardiovasc Pharmacol*. 1984; 6(Suppl 7):S1090–S1095.
81. Moser M, Lunn J, Nash DT et al. Nitrendipine in the treatment of mild to moderate hypertension. *J Cardiovasc Pharmacol*. 1984; 6(Suppl 7):S1085–S1089.
82. Müller FB, Bolli P, Erne P et al. Antihypertensive therapy with the long-acting calcium antagonist nitrendipine. *J Cardiovasc Pharmacol*. 1984; 6(Suppl 7):S1073–S1076.
83. Rüddel H, Schmieder R, Langewitz W et al. Efficacy of nitrendipine as baseline antihypertensive therapy. *J Cardiovasc Pharmacol*. 1984; 6(Suppl 7):S1049–S1052.
84. Weber MA, Drayer JIM. The calcium channel blocker nitrendipine in single- and multiple-agent antihypertensive regimens: preliminary report of a multicenter study. *J Cardiovasc Pharmacol*. 1984; 6(Suppl 7):S1077–S1084.
85. Jain AK, McMahon FG, Ryan JR et al. Efficacy and safety of nitrendipine in patients with severe hypertension: a multiclinic study. *J Cardiovasc Pharmacol*. 1984; 6(Suppl 7):S1053–S1059.
86. Burris JF, Mroczek WJ, Brobyn R et al. Long-term efficacy and safety of nitrendipine in severe hypertension. *J Cardiovasc Pharmacol*. 1987; 9(Suppl 4):S306–S310.
87. Jain AK, McMahon FG, Michael R et al. Nitrendipine, a new calcium channel blocker in the management of severe hypertension. *Clin Pharmacol Ther*. 1985; 37:203. Abstract.
88. Franz I-W, Wiewel D. Antihypertensive effects on blood pressure at rest and during exercise of calcium antagonists, beta-receptor blockers, and their combination in hypertensive patients. *J Cardiovasc Pharmacol*. 1984; 6(Suppl 7):S1037–S1042.
89. Gennari C, Nami R, Bianchini C et al. Nitrendipine and the angiotensin converting enzyme inhibitors in the treatment of hypertension. *J Cardiovasc Pharmacol*. 1987; 9(Suppl 4):S245–S251.
90. M'Buyamba-Kabangu JR, Fagard R, Lijnen P et al. Calcium entry blockade or beta-blockade in long-term management of hypertension in blacks. *Clin Pharmacol Ther*. 1987; 41:45–54.
91. Fritschka E, Distler A, Gotzen R et al. Crossover comparison of nitrendipine with propranolol in patients with essential hypertension. *J Cardiovasc Pharmacol*. 1984; 6(Suppl 7):S1100–S1104.
92. Fagan TC, Sternleib C, Vlachakis N et al. Efficacy and safety comparison of nitrendipine and hydralazine as antihypertensive monotherapy. *J Cardiovasc Pharmacol*. 1984; 6(Suppl 7):S1109–S1113.

93. Lopez LM, Mehta JL, Baz R et al. Effects of nitrendipine and hydralazine on plasma catecholamines in essential hypertension. *Clin Pharmacol Ther.* 1984; 36:444–50.
94. Massie BM, Tubau JF, Szlachcic J et al. Comparison and additivity of nitrendipine and hydrochlorothiazide in systemic hypertension. *Am J Cardiol.* 1986; 58:16D–19D.
95. Schoenberger JA, Glasser SP, Ram CVS et al. Comparison of nitrendipine combined with low-dose hydrochlorothiazide to hydrochlorothiazide alone in mild to moderate essential hypertension. *J Cardiovasc Pharmacol.* 1984; 6(Suppl 7):S1105–S1108.
96. Brouwer RML, Bolli P, Erné P et al. Antihypertensive treatment using calcium antagonists in combination with captopril rather than diuretics. *J Cardiovasc Pharmacol.* 1985; 7(Suppl 1):S88–S91.
97. Lang R, Degenhardt S, Ollenschläger G et al. Effect of a low-dose combination nitrendipine/enalapril in less-severe degrees of hypertension. *J Cardiovasc Pharmacol.* 1987; 9(Suppl 4):S254–S255.
98. Borzellino M, Homes G, Finizola A et al. Nitrendipine in elderly hypertensives. *J Cardiovasc Pharmacol.* 1987; 9(Suppl 4):S290–S294.
99. Höffler D, Stoepel K. Nitrendipine in hypertension that is difficult to control. *J Cardiovasc Pharmacol.* 1984; 6(Suppl 7):S1060–S1062.
100. Rosenthal J, Köhle W, Lehmann H. Nitrendipine in renal hypertension. Paper presented to Second International Nitrendipine Symposium. Lisbon, Portugal:1986 Apr 17–19.
101. Broughton Pipkin F, Lawrence MR. Preliminary studies on the cardiovascular effects of nitrendipine in human pregnancy. *J Cardiovasc Pharmacol.* 1987; 9(Suppl 4):S286–S289.
102. Allen J, Maigaard S, Forman A et al. Acute effects of nitrendipine in pregnancy-induced hypertension. *Br J Obstet Gynaecol.* 1987; 94:222–6.
103. Ferreira-Filho SR, Saragoça MA, Oliveira PC et al. Use of nitrendipine in the treatment of systolic hypertension in elderly patients. *J Cardiovasc Pharmacol.* 1987; 9(Suppl 4):S218–S220.
104. Landmark K, Dale J. Antihypertensive, haemodynamic and metabolic effects of nifedipine slow-release tablets in elderly patients. *Acta Med Scand.* 1985; 218:389–96.
105. Kleinbloesem CH, van Brummelen P, van de Linde JA et al. Nifedipine: kinetics and dynamics in healthy subjects. *Clin Pharmacol Ther.* 1984; 35:742–9.
106. Robson RH, Vishwanath MC. Nifedipine and beta-blockade as a cause of cardiac failure. *Br Med J.* 1982; 284:104.
107. Olivari MT, Levine TB, Cohn JN. Acute hemodynamic effects of nitrendipine in chronic congestive heart failure. *J Cardiovasc Pharmacol.* 1984; 6(Suppl 7):S1002–S1005.
108. Ryman KS, Kubo SH, Lystash J et al. Effect of nicardipine on rest and exercise hemodynamics in chronic congestive heart failure. *Am J Cardiol.* 1986; 58:583–8.
109. Pouleur H, Etienne J, Van Mechelen H et al. Effects of nicardipine or nifedipine added to propranolol in patients with coronary artery disease. *Postgrad Med J.* 1984; 60(Suppl 4):23–8.
110. Brügmann UE. Acute antihypertensive and anti-ischemic effects of nitrendipine: results of a double-blind, randomized, crossover, and placebo-controlled study. *J Cardiovasc Pharmacol.* 1987; 9(Suppl 4):S197–S200.
111. Rutsch W, Schmutzler H. Efficacy of nitrendipine in stable angina pectoris. *J Cardiovasc Pharmacol.* 1987; 9(Suppl 4):S214–S217.
112. Prager G, Varchmin G, Hönig E. Nitrendipine in coronary heart disease. *J Cardiovasc Pharmacol.* 1987; 9(Suppl 4):S208–S213.
113. Thomassen A, Bagger JP, Nielsen TT et al. Metabolic and hemodynamic effects of nicardipine during pacing-induced angina pectoris. *Am J Cardiol.* 1987; 59:219–24.
114. Lipkin D, Poole-Wilson PA. Effect of nicardipine on myocardial contractility and on angina induced by atrial pacing in patients with coronary artery disease. *Postgrad Med J.* 1984; 60(Suppl 4):21–2. Abstract.
115. Visser CA, Jaarsma W, Kan G et al. Immediate and longer-term effects of nicardipine, at rest and during exercise, in patients with coronary artery disease. *Postgrad Med J.* 1984; 60(Suppl 4):17–20.
116. Bowles MJ, Khurmi NS, O'Hara MJ et al. Randomized double-blind placebo-controlled comparison of nicardipine and nifedipine in patients with chronic stable angina pectoris. *Chest.* 1986; 89:260–5.
117. Scheidt S, LeWinter MM, Hermanovich J et al. Efficacy and safety of nicardipine for chronic, stable angina pectoris: a multicenter randomized trial. *Am J Cardiol.* 1986; 58:715–21.
118. McGill D, McKenzie W, McCredie M. Comparison of nicardipine and propranolol for chronic stable angina pectoris. *Am J Cardiol.* 1986; 57:39–43.
119. Rodrigues EA, Kohli RS, Lahiri A et al. Comparison of nicardipine and verapamil in the treatment of chronic stable angina. *Br J Clin Pharmacol.* 1986; 21:593P. Abstract.
120. Deedwania PC, Thao TP, Andrew HT et al. Nicardipine, a new calcium channel blocker in the treatment of chronic stable angina. *Clin Pharmacol Ther.* 1985; 37:190. Abstract.
121. Armstrong C, Garnham J, Blackwood R et al. Long-term safety and efficacy of nicardipine in the treatment of stable angina pectoris. *Br J Clin Pharmacol.* 1986; 22(Suppl 3):331S–337S.
122. Armstrong C, Garnham J, Blackwood R. Comparison of the efficacy of nicardipine and nifedipine in patients with chronic stable angina. *Br J Clin Pharmacol.* 1986; 22(Suppl 3):325S–330S.
123. Bjerle P, Olofsson BO, Glimvik O. Nicardipine and propranolol in angina pectoris: a comparative study with special reference to ergometer working capacity tests. *Br J Clin Pharmacol.* 1986; 22(Suppl 3):339S–343S.
124. Logan RL, Ikram H, Webster MW et al. Comparative efficacy of nicardipine hydrochloride and atenolol in the treatment of chronic stable angina. *Br J Clin Pharmacol.* 1986; 22(Suppl 3):345S–350S.
125. Silke B, Verma SP, Frais MA et al. Haemodynamic analysis of the effects of nicardipine and metoprolol alone and in combination in coronary artery disease. *Eur Heart J.* 1985; 6:930–8.
126. Jariwalla AG, Anderson EG. Production of ischaemic cardiac pain by nifedipine. *Br Med J.* 1978; 1:1181–2.
127. Tamari I, Borer JS, Moses JW et al. Hemodynamic assessment of intravenous bepridil administration in ischemic heart disease. *Am J Cardiol.* 1985; 55:25C–29C.
128. Zusman RM, Christensen DM, Kanarek DJ et al. Evaluation of bepridil for the treatment of angina pectoris: evidence for preservation of left ventricular function. *Am J Cardiol.* 1985; 55:30C–35C.
129. Sharma MK, Prasad R, Teague S et al. Monotherapy with bepridil in angina pectoris: long-term evaluation by serial exercise testing. *Clin Pharmacol Ther.* 1987; 41:197. Abstract.
130. DiBianco R, Katz RJ, Chesler E et al. Long-term efficacy of bepridil in patients with chronic stable angina pectoris: results of a multicenter, placebo-controlled study of extended bepridil use. *Am J Cardiol.* 1985; 55:50C–54C.
131. Shapiro W, DiBianco R, Thadani U et al. Comparative efficacy of 200, 300 and 400 mg of bepridil for chronic stable angina pectoris. *Am J Cardiol.* 1985; 55:36C–42C.
132. Hill JA, O'Brien JT, Scott E et al. Effects of bepridil on exercise tolerance in chronic stable angina: a double-blind, randomized, placebo-controlled, crossover trial. *Am J Cardiol.* 1984; 53:679–83.
133. Morganroth J, Horowitz LN. Are there unnecessary delays in the development of new cardiac drugs in the United States? *Am J Cardiol.* 1986; 58:1265–7. Editorial.
134. Matsui M, Nishiwaki H, Yoshino J et al. Effects of nicardipine hydrochloride on the conduction system of the heart in man. *Jpn Heart J.* 1982; 23(Suppl 1):243–5.
135. Rutsch W, Schmutzler H. Comparison of the acute hemodynamic effects of nifedipine with nitrendipine and a

study of the electrophysiological effects of nitrendipine in man. *J Cardiovasc Pharmacol.* 1984; 6(Suppl 7):S1011–S1015.
136. Rowland E, McKenna WJ, Krikler DM. Electrophysiologic and antiarrhythmic actions of bepridil: comparison with verapamil and ajmaline for atrioventricular reentrant tachycardia. *Am J Cardiol.* 1985; 55:1513–9.
137. Roy D, Montigny M, Klein GJ. Electrophysiologic effects and long-term efficacy of bepridil for recurrent supraventricular tachycardias. *Am J Cardiol.* 1987; 59:89–92.
138. Rinkenberger RL, Prystowsky EN, Heger JJ et al. Effects of intravenous and chronic oral verapamil administration in patients with supraventricular tachyarrhythmias. *Circulation.* 1980; 62:996–1010.
139. Gulamhusein S, Ko P, Carruthers SG et al. Acceleration of the ventricular response during atrial fibrillation in the Wolff–Parkinson–White syndrome after verapamil. *Circulation.* 1982; 65:348–54.
140. Somberg J, Torres V, Flowers D et al. Prolongation of QT interval and antiarrhythmic action of bepridil. *Am Heart J.* 1985; 109:19–27.
141. Levy S, Cointe R, Metge M et al. Bepridil for recurrent sustained ventricular tachycardias: assessment using electrophysiologic testing. *Am J Cardiol.* 1984; 54:579–81.
142. Nestico PF, Morganroth J, Horowitz LN et al. Bepridil hydrochloride for treatment of benign or potentially lethal ventricular arrhythmias. *Am J Cardiol.* 1986; 58:1001–4.
143. Walsh RW, Porter CB, Starling MR et al. Beneficial hemodynamic effects of intravenous and oral diltiazem in severe congestive heart failure. *J Am Coll Cardiol.* 1984; 3:1044–50.
144. Bonow RO, Rosing DR, Bacharach SL et al. Effects of verapamil on left ventricular systolic function and diastolic filling in patients with hypertrophic cardiomyopathy. *Circulation.* 1981; 64:787–96.
145. Lorell BH, Paulus WJ, Grossman W et al. Modification of abnormal left ventricular diastolic properties by nifedipine in patients with hypertrophic cardiomyopathy. *Circulation.* 1982; 65:499–507.
146. Elkayam U, Weber L, McKay C et al. Spectrum of acute hemodynamic effects of nifedipine in severe congestive heart failure. *Am J Cardiol.* 1985; 56:560–6.
147. Brooks N, Cattell M, Pidgeon J et al. Unpredictable response to nifedipine in severe cardiac failure. *Br Med J.* 1980; 281:1324.
148. Lahiri A, Robinson CW, Tovey J et al. Intravenous nicardipine in patients with chronic heart failure: a nuclear stethoscope study. *Postgrad Med J.* 1984; 60(Suppl 4):35–8.
149. Feely J, Cullen M, Collins W. Metabolic and endocrine consequences of calcium channel blockade. *Br J Clin Pharmacol.* 1986; 22(Suppl 3):231S–236S.
150. Stoepel K, Deck K, Corsing C et al. Safety aspects of long-term nitrendipine therapy. *J Cardiovasc Pharmacol.* 1984; 6(Suppl 7):S1063–S1066.
151. Duchêne-Marullaz P, Kantelip J-P, Trolèse J-F. Effects of bepridil, a new antianginal agent, on ambulatory electrocardiography in human volunteers. *J Cardiovasc Pharmacol.* 1983; 5:506–10.
152. Tzivoni D, Keren A, Stern S. Torsades de pointes versus polymorphic ventricular tachycardia. *Am J Cardiol.* 1983; 52:639–40. Editorial.
153. Leclercq JF, Kural S, Valère PE. Bépridil et torsades de pointes. *Arch Mal Coeur.* 1983; 76:341–8.
154. Manouvrier J, Sagot M, Caron C et al. Nine cases of torsade de pointes with bepridil administration. *Am Heart J.* 1986; 111:1005–7.
155. Haerer W, Weritz D, Stauch M. Bepridil in hypertrophic obstructive cardiomyopathy. *Am Heart J.* 1987; 113:1536. Letter.

"

Understanding the Immune System

It could be said that immunology is both the most ancient and the most modern of sciences, the most theoretical and the most practical. The basic concept of immunology was mentioned by Thucydides, writing during the time of the Peloponnesian Wars. He noted that the sick could be treated by those who had recovered since they were free of fear. The idea that survivors of infection were immune to a second infection thus appeared long ago. Edward Jenner's perception in regard to milk maids' smooth complexions—that is, with faces unscarred by smallpox—led to the idea that vaccination with cowpox might protect against smallpox. Louis Pasteur built on this concept of an attenuated virus to start the era of ever more extensive vaccination and immunities in the world today....

The importance of the immune system is indicated by the fact that the number of cells in our bodies devoted to the immune system is approximately equal to the number of cells in the brain. Only a few years ago, immunologists elicited derision from "hard scientists" by defining an antibody as "a molecule generated by an antigen" and an antigen as "a molecule which reacts with an antibody." That seemingly circuitous reasoning has revealed the most sophisticated molecular and practical applications of any biological system. This field has mysteries still unsolved but it is one in which every step along the path produces some benefit to mankind.

—Koshland DE Jr. Frontiers in immunology. *Science.* 1987; 238:1023. Editorial.

"

Therapy Reviews

Rocky Mountain spotted fever

CLAUDIA A. KAMPER, KATHERINE HAMMOND CHESSMAN, AND STEPHANIE J. PHELPS

Abstract: The epidemiology, pathogenesis, clinical features, and treatment of Rocky Mountain spotted fever are reviewed.

Rocky Mountain spotted fever is a severe infection caused by *Rickettsia rickettsii* transmitted to man by various species of ticks. High-incidence areas exist in the southeast and south central United States. Only 60–70% of patients with the disease report a history of tick bite or exposure to tick-infested areas. The disease is initially characterized by fever, headache, gastrointestinal complaints, myalgia, and a generalized rash. In several days generalized vasculitis may lead to periorbital edema and nonpitting edema of the face and extremities. Central nervous system involvement is common. Because signs and symptoms associated with the disease are nonspecific, the diagnosis is often delayed or missed. Traditionally diagnostic confirmation relied on serologic testing, but an indirect fluorescent antibody assay will soon be commercially available. Rocky Mountain spotted fever is usually treated with the rickettsiostatic agents chloramphenicol or tetracycline, but few comparative data on these agents in patients with the disease are available. For patients who cannot tolerate oral medications, intravenous chloramphenicol sodium succinate is the preferred treatment; chloramphenicol is also the drug of choice for children less than eight years of age. Otherwise, oral tetracycline hydrochloride is the drug of choice. Antibiotic therapy should be continued for 7–10 days or until the patient is afebrile for two to five days. All cases of Rocky Mountain spotted fever must be reported to the Centers for Disease Control.

The best ways to decrease the morbidity and mortality of the disease are to increase awareness of its signs and symptoms and to prevent exposure to ticks.

Index terms: Chloramphenicol; Chloramphenicols; Chloramphenicol sodium succinate; Pediatrics; Rocky Mountain spotted fever; Tetracycline; Tetracycline hydrochloride; Tetracyclines
Clin Pharm. 1988; 7:109–116

Rocky Mountain spotted fever was first recognized on the North American continent by American Indians. Tribes inhabiting the wooded Rocky Mountain region attributed the illness to "evil spirits," and braves avoided the disease by sending their squaws into especially "hazardous" areas.[1] In 1899, Rocky Mountain spotted fever was described as ". . . an acute, endemic, noncontagious but probably infectious, febrile disease, characterized by a continuous moderately high fever, severe arthritic and muscle pains, and a profuse petechial or purpuric eruption in the skin, appearing first on the ankles, wrists, and forehead, but rapidly spreading to all parts of the body."[2] In 1906, the etiologic agent, *Rickettsia rickettsii*, was identified by Howard Taylor Ricketts.[3]

Despite current understanding of the tick's role in transmitting Rocky Mountain spotted fever, the disease cannot yet be prevented. Figure 1 depicts the incidence of the disease since reporting began in 1920[4]; the number of reported cases rose dramatically during the 1970s after the Centers for Disease Control (CDC) initiated a surveillance program. Incidence peaked in 1981 with 1192 reported cases (0.51/100,000 population) and has since declined[5] with only 755 cases reported in 1986.[6] Although

CLAUDIA A. KAMPER, PHARM.D., is Assistant Professor, School of Pharmacy, Samford University, Birmingham, AL; KATHERINE HAMMOND CHESSMAN, PHARM.D., is Pediatric Clinical Pharmacist, Department of Hospital Pharmacy Practice and Administration, Medical University of South Carolina, Charleston; and STEPHANIE J. PHELPS, PHARM.D., is Assistant Professor, Department of Clinical Pharmacy, The Center for Pediatric Pharmacokinetics and Therapeutics, The University of Tennessee, Memphis, and Clinical Pharmacist, Le Bonheur Children's Medical Center, Memphis. At the time this manuscript was prepared, Dr. Kamper was a Research Fellow and Dr. Chessman was a Pediatric Pharmacy Resident, Department of Clinical Pharmacy, The University of Tennessee, Memphis.

Address reprint requests to Dr. Phelps at the Department of Clinical Pharmacy, The University of Tennessee, Memphis, 26 South Dunlap Street, Suite 307C, Memphis, TN 38163.

Supported in part by a Center of Excellence grant from the State of Tennessee.

Copyright © 1988, American Society of Hospital Pharmacists, Inc. All rights reserved. 0278-2677/88/0201-0109$02.00.

Figure 1. Incidence of Rocky Mountain spotted fever (number of cases per 100,000 population) in the United States from 1920 to 1984; the asterisk represents provisional data. (Reprinted from reference 4.)

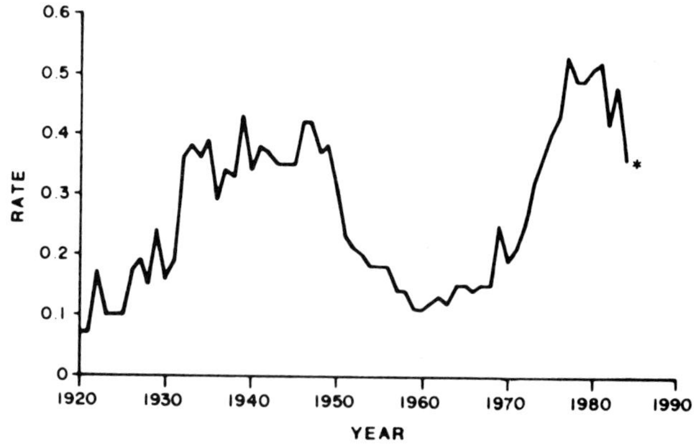

the number of deaths from Rocky Mountain spotted fever has decreased secondary to the decreasing incidence, the death-to-case ratio has remained at about 4% during the last five years.[6]

This article reviews the epidemiology, pathogenesis, clinical features, diagnosis, and pharmacologic management of Rocky Mountain spotted fever.

Epidemiology and Pathogenesis

Rickettsia rickettsii is the etiologic agent of Rocky Mountain spotted fever. It is one of five antigenically related rickettsial species known to cause human disease and accounts for more than 90% of rickettsial disease reported in the United States. Rocky Mountain spotted fever is the only rickettsiosis still associated with a substantial number of deaths.[7] *R. rickettsii* is a highly fastidious, rod-shaped, gram-negative, obligate intracellular parasite containing both RNA and DNA. In contrast to other rickettsial organisms, *R. rickettsii* is not confined to the cytoplasm but can invade the nucleus.

Although Rocky Mountain spotted fever was reported initially in the Rocky Mountain states, this region was responsible for less than 5% of all cases in the United States from 1964 through 1977.[8] The disease has been reported in every state except Maine, Hawaii, and Alaska. Because the disease is not geographically limited, the term "Rocky Mountain spotted fever" is a misnomer; the term "tick typhus" has been suggested as a more appropriate descriptor of the disease.[9] High-incidence regions exist in the Southeast and South Central States. While North Carolina reported the largest number of cases in 1985, Oklahoma had the highest incidence rate for 1982 through 1985.[5] Other states having high incidence rates include South Carolina, Arkansas, Tennessee, Montana, Kansas, Virginia, and Georgia.[4,5,10,11] The distribution of Rocky Mountain spotted fever for the United States in 1986 is shown in Figure 2.[6]

Early settlers first recognized the association between ticks and Rocky Mountain spotted fever.[1] Different tick species are responsible for transmitting the disease in different regions. Transmission to man is primarily via the wood tick (*Dermacentor andersoni*) in the West, the dog tick (*Dermacentor variabilis*) in the East, and the Lone-Star tick (*Amblyomma americanum*) in the Southwest.[12] Actual transmission of disease usually occurs via tick bite. A carrier tick changes from a hibernating state to an infective state with the first blood meal; consequently, attachment of an infected tick for several hours is required for transferral of rickettsiae to the host.[13] Transdermal transmission via infected tissue juices or tick feces through skin abrasions may occur upon crushing an infected tick, and this may be an important portal of entry for young children.[12] Needle[14] and aerosol transmission[14,15] have been reported rarely. Case reports of aerosol transmission have led to speculation that person-to-person respiratory transmission may occur.[15]

The reservoir, or continual source of infection, for Rocky Mountain spotted fever is maintained through transovarial passage of rickettsiae from the adult female tick to her offspring. An adult female can transmit the infection to 100% of her larvae for up to 12 generations.[16] Maturing of these infected offspring may explain the two peaks of illness during the active tick season.[17] Additionally, pathogenic rickettsiae in hibernating ticks do not lose virulence during the winter. They emerge from hibernation in the spring with diminished virulence but regain full virulence within weeks. Consequently, human illness occurs most frequently in April through September paralleling maximal tick activity. Additionally, intermittent animal carriers, including the ground squirrel, rabbit, chipmunk, wood rat, meadow mouse, and weasel, may provide temporary reservoirs for *R. rickettsii* while remaining disease free.

Prevalence of infected ticks varies from region to region. In general, woodland and uncultivated areas have a greater percentage of both infected and noninfected ticks. As many as 14,000 ticks per acre have been found in areas of Oklahoma.[18] An infectivity rate of 2–15% of the tick population has been reported in areas with frequent occurrence of Rocky Mountain spotted fever.[19]

Clinical Features

A history of tick bite or exposure to possible tick-infested areas may be reported in only 60–70% of patients with Rocky Mountain spotted fever;[4–6,10,11] therefore, if the clinical signs and symptoms suggest the disease, a high index of suspicion must be maintained even in the absence of a known tick exposure. The incubation period for Rocky Mountain spotted fever in humans ranges from 1 to 14

Figure 2. Incidence of Rocky Mountain spotted fever by state in 1986. (Reprinted from reference 6.)

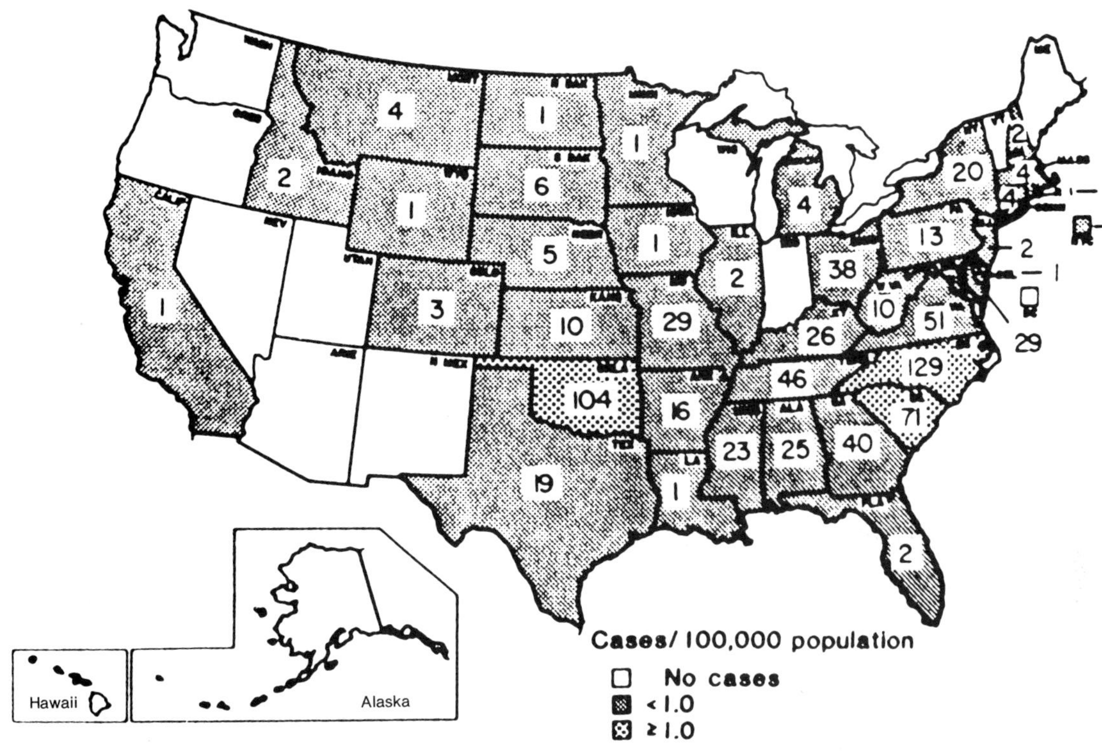

days with an average of four to eight days.[1,20] Studies in monkeys have suggested that the duration of the incubation period and the severity of disease may be related to the size of the inoculum.[21] Others have found no correlation between incubation period and severity of illness.[20]

Characteristics of Rocky Mountain spotted fever cases reported in 1986 are shown in Table 1.[6] Onset of symptoms is usually acute with early symptoms being nonspecific. Fever (39.4–40 °C) is nearly always present during the first two to three days of infection and may precede other signs by a week or more.[1] Fever is often unresponsive to either antipyretics or antibiotics.[22] Headache is reported in most cases. Pain associated with headache is often frontal in nature and can be unrelenting despite analgesic agents. Abdominal pain, nausea, anorexia, vomiting, and diarrhea occur frequently. In one series of patients, initial complaints in 32% of fatal cases were primarily gastrointestinal.[23] Chills, arthralgia, and myalgia may also be seen in the early phase of disease.

A characteristic rash is commonly associated with Rocky Mountain spotted fever. However, in 4–16% of laboratory-confirmed cases the rash is reportedly absent[17,24]; for these cases the term "Rocky Mountain spottless fever" has been coined.[25] Contrary to classic textbook descriptions, some exanthemata may be sparse and transient and

Table 1.
Characteristics of Cases of Rocky Mountain Spotted Fever Reported in 1986[a]

Characteristic	Percentage (*n* = 654)
Onset between April 1 and September 30	95
Male gender	62
Age less than 20 years	45
Caucasian race	92
Symptoms	
Fever	94
Headache	89
Myalgia	87
Rash	87
Rash including soles and palms	53
No known tick exposure	62

[a] Adapted from reference 6.

possibly overlooked on dark-skinned individuals.

When present, the rash usually occurs by the fifth day of illness but may occur as early as the first febrile day and as late as the eighth day.[26] Usually the rash is noted first on the ankles and feet but spreads within hours to the wrists and hands, including the palms and soles, and finally to the trunk and head. On initial appearance, the rash may be macular, maculopapular, or occasionally petechial. Lesions are approximately 2 to 6 mm in diameter and irregular.[27] Early in the disease, the rash blanches with applied pressure; however, in advanced stages of Rocky Mountain spotted fever, blanching no longer occurs as petechial and purpuric skin lesions coalesce into extensive areas of hemorrhage and necrosis. Skin lesion biopsy shows vasculitis secondary to rickettsial invasion of vascular endothelial cells. Resolution of the rash occurs with appropriate treatment; however, it may persist after other symptoms have abated.

Three to four days after the appearance of a rash, periorbital edema and nonpitting, nondependent edema of the face and extremities may develop.[22] Like the rash, edema occurs because of a generalized vasculitis and is not secondary to cardiac, renal, or endogenous serum protein abnormalities. Vasculitis may also lead to microthrombi, luminal occlusion, and microinfarction of virtually any organ.

Clinical evidence of central nervous system involvement is common and may be seen at any stage of illness. Nervous system abnormalities are attributed primarily to thrombovasculitis and range from headache and lethargy to coma. Some patients remain alert but are amnesic about the illness upon recovery.[28] Coma is a late consequence of severe disease. Stiff neck and other signs of meningeal irritation may be present. Encephalitis, seizures with electroencephalographic changes, and transient deafness have been observed. Other neurologic manifestations include tremor, paralysis, ataxia, opisthotonos, deafness, aphasia, or blindness. Permanent neurologic deficits have been reported rarely.[28]

Frequently noted ocular manifestations of Rocky Mountain spotted fever include conjunctivitis and photophobia; papilledema may be seen occasionally. Splenomegaly occurs in as many as 30–50% of patients.[1,29] Hepatomegaly with altered liver function is less common but may occur as the disease progresses. Similarly, renal function is rarely impaired in early disease, but oliguria and anuria may be present in critically ill patients. Myocardial involvement, including myocarditis, myocardial necrosis, and electrocardiogram changes, can occur. Arrhythmias have led occasionally to sudden death.[29] Lymphadenopathy is not associated with Rocky Mountain spotted fever.

Routine laboratory studies may be helpful in supporting a presumptive diagnosis of Rocky Mountain spotted fever. These laboratory findings may also be useful in monitoring the course of the disease.

Serum sodium and chloride concentrations are decreased frequently in the early stages of illness because of urinary losses. Further aberrations in electrolytes may be associated with neurologic involvement and inappropriate secretion of antidiuretic hormone.

Thrombocytopenia is common and may progress to disseminated intravascular coagulation with depressed fibrinogen concentrations and other coagulation abnormalities. Liver function test values are often normal early in the disease but are elevated in seriously ill patients. Serum albumin may be decreased secondary to decreased production, vascular leaks, and negative nitrogen balance.[8] Hematuria may occur because of widespread vasculitis. Serum creatinine and lactate dehydrogenase may increase progressively as a result of diffuse disease of skeletal and cardiac muscle and the lung.

White blood cell counts are usually normal early in the disease but may be elevated in more severe cases. Analysis of cerebrospinal fluid most frequently reveals a lymphocytic pleocytosis consistent with aseptic meningitis.[1]

Differential Diagnosis and Laboratory Confirmation

The nonspecific character of the initial signs and symptoms associated with Rocky Mountain spotted fever may lead to a missed or delayed diagnosis. Early treatment before irreversible tissue damage occurs is of primary importance in reducing both mortality and morbidity. Therefore, it is imperative that a thorough history regarding possible tick exposure be obtained in any patient with clinical features suggesting Rocky Mountain spotted fever.

While a variety of diseases may have signs and symptoms similar to Rocky Mountain spotted fever, those most frequently encountered are meningococcemia, rubeola, pneumonia, infectious mononucleosis, salmonellosis, and enterovirus infections. Table 2 compares and contrasts several of these diseases with Rocky Mountain spotted fever.

Allergic drug reactions are also frequently associated with skin rashes, as well as fever, and should be included in the differential diagnosis of Rocky Mountain spotted fever.

Traditionally diagnostic confirmation of Rocky Mountain spotted fever has relied on serologic testing. One of the more commonly used methods for rickettsial identification is the Weil–Felix agglutinins reaction. It has been suggested, however, that this method is "archaic and misleading."[30] Weil–Felix reactions depend on cross-reaction of *Proteus* antigens (*Proteus* OX-19, OX-2, OX-K) with antirickettsial antibodies. Rickettsial agglutinins appear 5–12 days after infection and peak by week three or four. Elevation of agglutinins may be delayed with early institution of appropriate antibiotic therapy. A single titer of 1:320 or a fourfold rise in convalescent over acute titer is considered presumptive evidence of Rocky Mountain spotted fever. The absence of agglutinins does not exclude rickettsial disease, however, because not all patients develop *Proteus* agglutinins. False-positive results occur with leptospirosis, severe liver disease, *Borrelia* infections, and *Proteus* infections.

Immunofluorescence studies performed on tis-

Table 2.
Characteristics of Rocky Mountain Spotted Fever and Other Infections with Similar Initial Features[a]

Feature	Rocky Mountain Spotted Fever	Meningococcemia	Enterovirus	Measles
History	Tick exposure; tick-infested area		Febrile illness in family or community	Exposure to measles or killed vaccine
Season	Late spring or summer	Late winter or early spring	Summer or fall	Winter or spring
Onset	Fever; rash in two or three days	Fever and rash within 24 hours	Fever and rash appear together	Severe prodrome; fever for three or four days before rash
Rash	Starts peripherally and spreads centrally; involves palms and soles; may progress from macular or maculopapular to petechial	May appear either as a few generalized, macular lesions or as extensive purpuric, ecchymotic, necrotic lesions with peripheral distribution that may involve palms and soles	Starts on face or trunk; may involve palms and soles; appears maculopapular; may be urticarial, petechial, or vesicular	Starts on head and spreads to trunk and extremities; atypically may start on extremities and involve palms and soles
Other features		Gram-negative diplococci in petechiae, buffy coat, or cerebrospinal fluid	May be associated with aseptic meningitis	Koplik spots during prodrome

[a] Adapted from reference 20.

sue obtained from a punch biopsy of an involved skin lesion may allow for a rapid and early diagnosis of Rocky Mountain spotted fever. In 1976, Woodward and colleagues[31] identified *R. rickettsii* in a specimen obtained from a skin biopsy. The presence of organisms in the skin sample was demonstrated on days four and eight of illness in two patients using an immunofluorescent technique. The biopsy can be taken from petechial, macular, or papular portions of the rash, not necessarily from the site of the tick bite. While this technique is available in many research centers, it may not be available routinely in all institutions. Previous treatment with antibiotics may cause negative immunofluorescence results.

Complement fixation is a more specific and sensitive method for identifying rickettsial infections, but this technique is more difficult and time consuming. Complement fixation titers tend to rise later (i.e., 10–14 days) and remain elevated longer. Serologic confirmation requires a single complement fixation titer ≥1:16 or a fourfold rise in convalescent over acute titer.

Newer, more sensitive and specific diagnostic tests allowing for early, accurate diagnosis will soon be commercially available. The microimmunofluorescent test, which is an indirect fluorescent antibody (IFA) assay, is now available on an investigational basis for detecting and quantifying the human humoral response to the spotted fever and typhus group rickettsiae. The IFA assay detects class-specific antibodies, such as IgG, IgM, and IgA, allowing separation of long-lived IgG response from short-lived acute-phase IgM antibody response. An IgG titer ≥1:16 is considered positive for infection but cannot distinguish past from present illness. An IgG titer ≥1:128 is considered a presumptive test for recent infection. Seroconversion or a fourfold or more increase in titer between acute and convalescent sera is considered strong evidence for recent infection. Detection of IgM antibody may help identify early infection and may reduce the need for convalescent sera to document rise in IgG titer. Antibodies of either type are variably absent for one to two weeks after onset of symptoms, and an initial negative titer should not exclude the diagnosis.[32]

Latex agglutination and enzyme-linked immunosorbent assay are two other laboratory procedures with increased sensitivity for rickettsial detection that are now investigational.

Treatment

In 1945, large doses of aminobenzoic acid were used to treat Rocky Mountain spotted fever.[33] Its use was associated with serious adverse effects and minimal effectiveness. Following the introduction of chloramphenicol and the tetracyclines, mortality from the disease decreased substantially from an average of 20–30% to less than 4% in 1986.[6] To our knowledge, however, no studies have compared the outcome of patients randomly treated with either chloramphenicol or tetracycline.

Both the tetracyclines and chloramphenicol are rickettsiostatic agents; they do not kill the organism but stop replication, allowing host defenses to develop and limit the course of disease. Both agents have been used successfully in the treatment of Rocky Mountain spotted fever, and no resistance has been reported.[34]

Chloramphenicol. Intravenous chloramphenicol sodium succinate in doses of 50–100 mg/kg/day (of chloramphenicol) is used frequently in the initial stages of disease when oral medications cannot be tolerated. Chloramphenicol may be preferred in this setting because the use of intravenous tetracycline is associated with pain and thrombophlebitis, especially with prolonged therapy or the use of a single vein for repeated infusions.[35] In addition, high daily doses of intravenous tetracycline have been linked to hepatic necrosis.[36,37] In children younger than eight years, chloramphenicol is preferred because the tetracyclines have been shown to mottle teeth and retard bone growth.

No published studies have evaluated various dosage regimens of chloramphenicol in patients with Rocky Mountain spotted fever. Serum chloramphenicol concentrations should be monitored routinely to avoid concentration-related toxicity, particularly in patients with hepatic or renal dysfunction secondary to the infection. Little published pharmacokinetic data exist for chloramphenicol given to patients with the disease. DuPont et al.[38] evaluated serum concentrations following intramuscular administration of chloramphenicol to nine adult volunteers infected with *R. rickettsii*. Approximately one third of the total plasma chloramphenicol remained as inactive unhydrolyzed succinate.

Chloramphenicol is hepatically metabolized and is an inhibitor of hepatic enzymes; therefore, it may interact with other drugs cleared by the liver that are used in patients with Rocky Mountain spotted fever. Phenytoin[39-43] and phenobarbital[41] metabolism may be inhibited by chloramphenicol. Conversely, because phenytoin, phenobarbital, and other drugs stimulate hepatic enzyme function, their concomitant administration with chloramphenicol may result in lower serum chloramphenicol concentrations.[44-46] Decreased chloramphenicol clearance in children treated with either phenobarbital or phenytoin before chloramphenicol has been attributed to competition for hepatic enzyme activity.[47] Krasinski et al.[46] reported five patients in whom concomitant chloramphenicol and phenytoin administrations resulted in elevated serum concentrations of chloramphenicol. Competition for protein binding sites at the microsomal level has been proposed as the mechanism of interaction between the two drugs. Decreased chloramphenicol elimination by acetaminophen has been reported in one patient[48] but has not been confirmed by other investigators.[49]

The adverse effects associated with chloramphenicol are discussed in detail in several review articles.[50-54] The hematologic abnormalities that can occur are of two types: dose-related bone marrow suppression and nondose-related idiosyncratic aplastic anemia. Dose-related hematological toxicities secondary to chloramphenicol have been shown to occur at peak serum chloramphenicol concentrations greater than 25 $\mu g/mL$[55]; however, bone marrow and mitochondrial changes have been reported at concentrations as low as 12 $\mu g/mL$.[56] Oski[57] recommended a hematological evaluation, including complete blood count, reticulocyte count, and platelet count, at the beginning of therapy, at the end of one week of therapy, and subsequently at three-day intervals if treatment continues. There is, however, no way of predicting the development of aplastic anemia; it has been reported to occur weeks to months after discontinuing the drug.[58]

Tetracycline. Tetracycline hydrochloride in doses of 20–50 mg/kg/day in children older than eight years of age and 500 mg four times daily in adults is the drug of choice for patients with Rocky Mountain spotted fever who can tolerate oral medications. Dosage adjustments for patients with renal failure are required for most commonly prescribed tetracycline derivatives, except doxycycline.[59,60] Doxycycline is the tetracycline of choice in patients with renal failure, since it does not induce changes in blood urea nitrogen or serum creatinine.[60]

Concomitant administration of tetracyclines and compounds containing divalent cations, such as antacids, milk, and vitamin and mineral supplements, decreases the absorption of certain tetracyclines and should be avoided. However, doxycycline is only minimally affected by these divalent cations.

As mentioned previously, tetracyclines can cause hepatic necrosis and vein irritation; they are also associated with diarrhea, rash, and hematologic abnormalities.[61]

Duration of Therapy. Antibiotic therapy should be continued for 7–10 days or until the patient is afebrile for two to five days. Appreciable response to treatment in the form of decreased fever and improved rash generally occurs 36–48 hours after beginning antibiotic therapy.[34] However, recovery may be delayed for several days in seriously ill patients; adjunctive treatment with intravenous fluids and blood products may be necessary. The use of short-term, high-dose corticosteroid therapy in critically ill patients with widespread vasculitis and encephalitis with cerebral edema is controversial but may be considered.[34]

Relapse is infrequent, and recurrence of Rocky Mountain spotted fever infection has not been reported.[34]

Prognosis. Age appears to affect both the clinical features and mortality of Rocky Mountain spotted fever. Mortality is higher in older patients. In 1986, infection in individuals 40 years of age or older was associated with a case-fatality rate of 5.8%, compared with 1.9% in younger individuals.[6] Analysis of 262 confirmed or highly probable cases from six states during a three-year period showed that children less than 15 years of age were more likely to display classic symptoms.[62] Patients older than 15 years had more atypical symptoms: less frequent history of rash and tick exposure, later onset of rash, and longer delays in seeking medical care.[56] The delayed treatment may increase the risk of death from the disease.

A difference in case-fatality rate has also been noted between races. Although the majority of patients (81%) were white, the case-fatality rate for blacks was 16% compared with 3% for Caucasians.[5] This difference may reflect difficulty in early recognition of rash on dark skin.

Prevention and Surveillance

The first killed vaccine for *R. rickettsii*, which was derived from infected ticks, was developed in 1925.[63] Subsequently, Cox developed a killed vaccine from infected embryonated chick eggs.[64] Neither agent was studied prospectively until 1973 when DuPont et al.[26] demonstrated no difference in attack rates in a group of volunteers given either vaccine. Based on this report, FDA withdrew the only commercially available vaccine, and no vaccine has since been marketed in the United States.

The best methods for preventing Rocky Mountain spotted fever are avoiding tick-infested areas when possible and wearing heavy clothing when walking in wooded areas. In addition, skin, hair, and clothing should be routinely inspected because tick bites often go unnoticed. If a tick is found and is not yet embedded in the skin, it can simply be brushed off.

Recommendations for tick removal have been published previously.[65] An embedded tick should be removed by grasping it with blunt forceps or tweezers as close to the point of attachment as possible and steadily pulling upward until removed. Fingers should not be used to remove ticks from animals or humans; a facial tissue, paper towel, or rubber gloves protecting the fingers may be used when tweezers are unavailable. Squeezing or crushing the tick should be avoided because of possible spread of disease through tick saliva, hemolymph, or gut contents. Skin contacting the tick during removal should be washed thoroughly.

Coating the tick with petroleum jelly or nail polish or bringing a heated object close to but not touching the tick have long been described as effective methods for inducing the tick to withdraw its feeding apparatus. These tactics should be avoided, however, because they are ineffective and may burn the patient.[65]

CDC currently operates two reporting systems for Rocky Mountain spotted fever.[60] One system involves a weekly telephone report of the number of cases for that week reported to each state health department. These statistics are then included in the *Morbidity and Mortality Weekly Report* (*MMWR*). A second system operated by the CDC's Division of Viral Disease uses brief surveillance forms completed for each case. This form includes epidemiologic, clinical, and laboratory information about each case.

Physicians and hospitals are required by state law to report cases of Rocky Mountain spotted fever to CDC through one of these two mechanisms. Annual summaries of all reported cases are published each spring in the *MMWR*.

Conclusion

Rocky Mountain spotted fever is a potentially fatal illness that can be successfully treated if diagnosed early and accurately. Prevention of the disease through vaccination is not possible, and eradication of either the rickettsiae or the tick vector is unlikely because of the large numbers found in endemic areas. To decrease the morbidity and mortality associated with Rocky Mountain spotted fever, the general public needs more information about preventing tick exposure and health professionals need an increased awareness of the signs and symptoms of the disease, especially in endemic areas.

References

1. Kelsey DS. Rocky Mountain spotted fever. *Pediatr Clin North Am*. 1979; 26:367–76.
2. Maxey EE. Some observations on the so-called spotted fever of Idaho. *Med Sentinel*. 1899; 7:433–8.
3. Ricketts HT. The study of "Rocky Mountain spotted fever" (tick fever?) by means of animal inoculations. *JAMA*. 1906; 47:33–6.
4. Centers for Disease Control. Rocky Mountain spotted fever—United States, 1984. *MMWR*. 1985; 34:195–7.
5. Centers for Disease Control. Rocky Mountain spotted fever—United States, 1985. *MMWR*. 1986; 35:247–9.
6. Centers for Disease Control. Rocky Mountain spotted fever—United States, 1986. *MMWR*. 1987; 36:314–5.
7. Hattwick MAW, Peters AH, Gregg MB et al. Surveillance of Rocky Mountain spotted fever. *JAMA*. 1973; 225:1338–43.
8. Woodward WE, Hornick RB. *Rickettsia rickettsii* (Rocky Mountain spotted fever). In: Mandell GL, Douglas RG, Bennett JE, eds. Principles and practice of infectious diseases. 2nd ed. New York: John Wiley & Sons Publishers; 1985: 1082–7.
9. Kelsey WM, Harrell GT. Management of tick typhus (Rocky Mountain spotted fever) in children. *JAMA*. 1948; 137:1356–61.
10. Centers for Disease Control. Rocky Mountain spotted fever—United States, 1982. *MMWR*. 1983; 32:229–32.
11. Centers for Disease Control. Rocky Mountain spotted fever—United States, 1983. *MMWR*. 1984; 33:188–95.
12. Feigin RD, Kissane JM, Eisenberg CS. Rocky Mountain spotted fever: successful application of new insights into physiologic changes during acute infections to successful management of a severely-ill patient. *Clin Pediatr*. 1969; 8:331–43.
13. Spencer RR, Parker RR. Studies on Rocky Mountain spotted fever: infectivity of fasting and recently fed ticks. *Public Health Rep*. 1923; 38:333–9.
14. Johnson JE, Kadull PJ. Rocky Mountain spotted fever acquired in a laboratory. *N Engl J Med*. 1967; 277:842–7.
15. Oster CN, Burke DS, Kenyon RH et al. Laboratory-acquired Rocky Mountain spotted fever: the hazard of aerosol transmission. *N Engl J Med*. 1977; 297:859–63.

16. Burgdorfer W, Brinton LP. Mechanisms of transovarial infection of spotted fever rickettsiae in ticks. *Ann NY Acad Sci.* 1976; 266:71–2.
17. Hattwick MAW, O'Brien RJ, Hanson BF. Rocky Mountain spotted fever: epidemiology of an increasing problem. *Ann Intern Med.* 1976; 84:732–9.
18. Sonenshine DE, Peters AH, Levy GF. Rocky Mountain spotted fever in relation to vegetation in the Eastern United States, 1951–1971. *Am J Epidemiol.* 1972; 96:59–69.
19. Loving SM, Smith AB, DiSalvo AF et al. Distribution and prevalence of spotted fever group rickettsiae in ticks from South Carolina, with an epidemiological survey of persons bitten by infected ticks. *Am J Trop Med Hyg.* 1978; 27:1255–60.
20. Linneman CC, Janson PJ. The clinical presentations of Rocky Mountain spotted fever. *Clin Pediatr.* 1978; 17:673–9.
21. Saslaw S, Carlisle HN, Wolf GL et al. Rocky Mountain spotted fever: clinical and laboratory observations of monkeys after respiratory exposure. *J Infect Dis.* 1966; 116:243–55.
22. Haynes RE, Sanders DY, Cramblett HG. Rocky Mountain spotted fever in children. *J Pediatr.* 1970; 76:685–93.
23. Hattwick MAW, Retailliau H, O'Brien RJ et al. Fatal Rocky Mountain spotted fever. *JAMA.* 1978; 240:1499–1503.
24. Wilfert CM, MacCormack JN, Kleeman K et al. Epidemiology of Rocky Mountain spotted fever as determined by active surveillance. *J Infect Dis.* 1984; 150:469–79.
25. Westerman EL. Rocky Mountain spotless fever: a dilemma for the clinician. *Arch Intern Med.* 1982; 142:1106–7.
26. DuPont HL, Hornick RB, Dawkins AT et al. Rocky Mountain spotted fever: a comparative study of the active immunity induced by inactivated and viable pathogenic *Rickettsia rickettsii*. *J Infect Dis.* 1973; 128:340–4.
27. MacCaughelty TC, Ernst G, Holtz AS. Rocky Mountain spotted fever from St. Louis County: implications for early diagnosis and treatment. *Crit Care Med.* 1982; 10:124–6.
28. Massey EW, Thames T, Coffey CE et al. Neurologic complications of Rocky Mountain spotted fever. *South Med J.* 1985; 78:1288–90.
29. Woodward TE. The rickettsioses. In: Harrison's principles of internal medicine. 10th ed. Petersdorf RG, Adams RD, Braunwald E et al., eds. New York: McGraw Hill Book Company; 1983:1069–78.
30. Newby JG. The Weil–Felix test is archaic and misleading. *JAMA.* 1986; 255:1022. Letter.
31. Woodward TE, Pedersen CE, Oster CN et al. Prompt confirmation of Rocky Mountain spotted fever: identification of rickettsiae in skin tissue. *J Infect Dis.* 1976; 134:297–301.
32. Hillcrest Biologicals, Inc. Rickettsial IFA kits product information. Cypress, CA; 1986 Feb.
33. Rose HM, Duane RB, Fischel EE. The treatment of spotted fever with para-aminobenzoic acid. *JAMA.* 1945; 129:1160–1.
34. Woodward TE. Rocky Mountain spotted fever: epidemiological and early clinical signs are keys to treatment and reduced mortality. *J Infect Dis.* 1984; 150:465–8.
35. American hospital formulary service—drug information 85. McEvoy GK, ed. Bethesda, MD: American Society of Hospital Pharmacists; 1985.
36. Dowling HF, Lepper MH. Hepatic reactions to tetracycline. *JAMA.* 1964; 188:307–9.
37. MacFarlane MD, McCarron MM. Fatty metamorphosis of the liver after i.v. tetracycline. *Drug Intell Clin Pharm.* 1972; 6:310–3.
38. DuPont HL, Hornick RB, Weiss CF et al. Evaluation of chloramphenicol acid succinate therapy of induced typhoid fever and Rocky Mountain spotted fever. *N Engl J Med.* 1970; 282:53–7.
39. Christensen LK, Skovsted L. Inhibition of drug metabolism by chloramphenicol. *Lancet.* 1969; 2:1397–9.
40. Ballek RD, Reidenberg MM, Orr L. Inhibition of diphenylhydantoin metabolism by chloramphenicol. *Lancet.* 1973; 1:150. Letter.
41. Vincent FM, Mills L, Sullivan JK. Chloramphenicol-induced phenytoin intoxication. *Ann Neurol.* 1978; 3:469. Letter.
42. Koup JR, Gibaldi M, McNamara P et al. Interaction of chloramphenicol with phenytoin and phenobarbital: case report. *Clin Pharmacol Ther.* 1978; 24:571–5.
43. Powell DA, Nahata MC, Durrell DC et al. Interaction among chloramphenicol, phenytoin, and phenobarbital in a pediatric patient. *J Pediatr.* 1981; 98:1001–3.
44. Bloxham RA, Durbin GM, Johnson T et al. Chloramphenicol and phenobarbitone—a drug interaction. *Arch Dis Child.* 1979; 54:76–7.
45. Sack CM, Koup JR, Smith AL. Chloramphenicol pharmacokinetics in infants and young children. *Pediatrics.* 1980; 66:579–84.
46. Krasinski K, Kusmiesz H, Nelson JD. Pharmacologic interactions among chloramphenicol, phenytoin, and phenobarbital. *Pediatr Infect Dis.* 1982; 1:232–5.
47. Rose JQ, Choi HK, Schentag JJ et al. Intoxication caused by interaction of chloramphenicol and phenytoin. *JAMA.* 1977; 237:2630–1.
48. Buchanan N, Moodley GP. Interaction between chloramphenicol and paracetamol. *Br Med J [Clin Res].* 1979; 2:307–8.
49. Kearns GL, Bocchini JA, Brown RD et al. Absence of a pharmacokinetic interaction between chloramphenicol and acetaminophen in children. *J Pediatr.* 1985; 107:134–9.
50. Smith AL, Weber A. Pharmacology of chloramphenicol. *Pediatr Clin North Am.* 1983; 30:209–36.
51. Laferriere CI, Marks MI. Chloramphenicol: properties and clinical use. *Pediatr Infect Dis.* 1982; 1:257–64.
52. Marks MI, Laferriere CI. Chloramphenicol: recent developments and clinical indications. *Clin Pharm.* 1982; 1:315–20.
53. Ambrose PJ. Clinical pharmacokinetics of chloramphenicol and chloramphenicol succinate. *Clin Pharmacokinet.* 1984; 9:222–38.
54. Messner HC, Smith AL. The current status of chloramphenicol. *Pediatrics.* 1979; 64:348–56.
55. Gussoff BD, Lee SL. Chloramphenicol-induced hematopoietic depression: a controlled trial with tetracycline. *Am J Med Sci.* 1966; 251:8–12.
56. Martello OJ, Manyan DR, Smith US. Chloramphenicol and bone marrow mitochondria. *J Lab Clin Med.* 1969; 74:927–30.
57. Oski FA. Hematologic consequences of chloramphenicol therapy. *J Pediatr.* 1979; 94:515–6.
58. Best WR. Chloramphenicol-associated blood dyscrasias. *JAMA.* 1967; 201:181–8.
59. Mahon WA, Johnson GE, Endrenyi L et al. The elimination of tritiated doxycycline in normal subjects and in patients with severely impaired renal function. *Scand J Infect Dis.* 1976; Suppl 9:24–31.
60. Alestig K. Studies on doxycycline during intravenous and oral treatment with reference to renal function. *Scand J Infect Dis.* 1973; 5:193–8.
61. Barza M, Schiefe RT. Antimicrobial spectrum, pharmacology, and therapeutic use of antibiotics: part 1. Tetracyclines. *Am J Hosp Pharm.* 1977; 34:49–57.
62. Helmick CG, Bernard KW, D'Angelo LJ. Rocky Mountain spotted fever: clinical, laboratory, and epidemiological features of 262 cases. *J Infect Dis.* 1984; 150:480–8.
63. Spencer RR, Parker RR. Rocky Mountain spotted fever: vaccination of monkeys and man. *Public Health Rep.* 1925; 40:2159–67.
64. Cox HR. Rocky Mountain spotted fever: protective value for guinea pigs of vaccine prepared from rickettsiae cultivated in embryonic chick tissues. *Public Health Rep.* 1939; 54:1070–7.
65. Needham GR. Evaluation of five popular methods for tick removal. *Pediatrics.* 1985; 75:997–1002.

Pathophysiology and treatment of the anemia of renal failure

CURTIS A. JOHNSON AND MICHAEL I. S. CHESTER

Abstract: The pathophysiology of anemia associated with renal failure and the major pharmacologic agents used in the treatment of this anemia are reviewed.

Patients with renal failure are often anemic primarily because of diminished circulating erythropoietin and suppressed erythropoiesis in the bone marrow. The anemia may cause malaise, fatiguability, aggravated angina, and decreased exercise tolerance. Many patients require frequent red blood cell transfusions.

Therapy has included anabolic androgen administration, iron and vitamin supplementation, and the administration of red blood cells. These approaches generally have not resulted in sustained improvement of the anemia. The recent development of recombinant human erythropoietin may represent a major therapeutic advance for the treatment of anemia associated with renal failure. Previously, erythropoietin therapy was not possible because of lack of sufficient quantities of the purified hormone. Clinical trials indicate, however, that recombinant human erythropoietin may improve erythropoiesis in most patients. Adverse effects have generally been mild and easily managed; however, increases in blood pressure and arteriovenous fistula clotting have been reported. Although initial reports are encouraging, larger and longer clinical trials are needed to determine proper dosing and to understand more completely the potential adverse effects of recombinant human erythropoietin.

Previous pharmacologic attempts to improve the anemia associated with renal failure have been largely unsatisfactory; initial reports on the use of recombinant human erythropoietin are promising.

Index terms: Androgens; Anemia; Blood; Erythropoietin; Iron; Iron preparations; Kidney failure; Toxicity; Vitamins
Clin Pharm. 1988; 7:117–22

Anemia is a common consequence of acute and chronic renal insufficiency and often leads to fatigue and general malaise.[1] In many patients, this anemia may be severe and may require repeated blood transfusions. Although it has many causes, the anemia is usually characterized by hypoproliferation of normocytic, normochromic red blood cells.[2] Most pharmacologic attempts to increase red blood cell production have proven to be unsatisfactory; however, the recent development of recombinant human erythropoietin shows promise for treating this disorder. Improved therapy of anemia is needed to avoid the risks associated with repeated blood transfusions—iron overload,[3] the transmission of infectious agents such as hepatitis and human immunodeficiency viruses,[4,5] and the development of transfusion reactions. This paper examines the factors that contribute to the anemia of renal failure and reviews the major pharmacologic agents other than blood administration that are used in its treatment.

Pathophysiology

Deficiency of Erythropoietin Production. A major cause of the anemia associated with renal failure is decreased production of erythropoietin by the kidneys.[6] Although extrarenal sites of production exist, probably in the liver, most patients with renal failure show evidence of erythropoietin deficiency, with concentrations in serum well below those of patients with comparable anemia without renal failure.[7] Some patients with renal failure who have anemia may have elevated concentrations of bioactive erythropoietin in serum.[8] However, it is believed that these patients may experience a relative erythropoietin deficiency in response to the increased demand for red blood cell production that occurs in these patients. In contrast to the anemia observed in most patients with renal failure, patients with polycystic kidney disease often have an elevated red blood cell count and hematocrit. It has been suggested that renal cysts present in this disease are capable of producing abnormal amounts of erythropoietin.[9] Individuals with polycystic kidney disease often do not become anemic or may develop only a mild reduction in hematocrit.

Interpretation of early investigations of erythropoietin production has been complicated by the imprecise and insensitive analytical methods for erythropoietin that have been used. Three types of assays have been used to measure erythropoietin and its activity.[10] An in vivo assay using polycythemic mice is reliable and specific; however, it lacks sensitivity and is a slow assay to perform. An in

CURTIS A. JOHNSON, PHARM.D., is Professor (Center for Health Sciences), School of Pharmacy, and Clinical Associate Professor, School of Medicine, University of Wisconsin, Madison. MICHAEL I. S. CHESTER is a graduate student and hospital pharmacy resident at the University of Wisconsin School of Pharmacy and the University of Wisconsin Hospital and Clinics.

Address reprint requests to Dr. Johnson at the School of Pharmacy, University of Wisconsin, 425 North Charter Street, Madison, WI 53706.

Copyright © 1988, American Society of Hospital Pharmacists, Inc. All rights reserved. 0278-2677/88/0201-0117$01.50.

vitro bioassay has improved sensitivity but diminished specificity. A radioimmunoassay is now considered the method of choice but is not yet widely available. A limitation of the radioimmunoassay is its cross-detection of biologically inactive forms of erythropoietin. The availability of improved analytical methods will lead to a more complete understanding of erythropoietin deficiency and the anemia of renal failure.

Inhibitors of Erythropoiesis. Several investigators have demonstrated that one or more substances in uremic serum suppress the proliferation of erythroid progenitor cells.[7,11–13] Studies using in vitro assays for colony-forming and blast-forming units have shown that uremic serum can inhibit the formation of red blood cells even in the presence of erythropoietin. Substances that may inhibit erythropoiesis include parathyroid hormone,[12] spermine,[14] and other low-molecular-weight polypeptides.[15] However, the contribution these compounds make to the development of anemia remains controversial.[16]

Both the presence and the inhibitory role of these substances are supported by the observation that patients with renal failure who have elevated concentrations of erythropoietin may still have suppressed erythropoiesis.[8] This implies the presence of one or more substances that diminish the bone marrow response to erythropoietin. In addition, it has been noted that the initiation of hemodialysis or peritoneal dialysis may lead to a rise in hematocrit without substantial changes in plasma erythropoietin concentrations.[1] This suggests that dialysis may remove the erythropoiesis-inhibiting substances found in uremic blood.

The inhibitory effect of parathyroid hormone has been challenged by Lutton and co-workers,[17] who failed to show any association between in vitro erythropoiesis and endogenous parathyroid hormone concentrations in human uremic serum. Other investigators also have failed to establish a correlation between parathyroid hormone concentrations and the anemia of renal failure.[18]

Although spermine has been shown to be a potent inhibitor of erythropoiesis in vitro,[14] Spragg et al.[19] have shown that concentrations of spermine and other low-molecular-weight polyamines are not elevated in uremic serum. This observation suggests that inhibitors of erythropoiesis may be compounds of larger molecular weight. Although uremic serum apparently contains one or more compounds that suppress red blood cell production, debate continues about the identity and specific activity of these compounds.

Altered Erythrocyte Survival. Another factor contributing to the anemia of renal failure is diminished red blood cell survival or hemolysis.[20,21] Hemolysis is thought to be caused by an extracorpuscular factor and not by any abnormality within the red blood cell.[6] Cell destruction is variable and may not be present at all. Altered red blood cell morphology with marked distortion and fragmentation of cells is often seen.

The factor(s) responsible for reduced cell survival is unknown. Giovannetti et al.[22] have suggested that guanidine derivatives present in uremic serum may cause hemolysis. Others have implicated parathyroid hormone as the cause of shortened red blood cell survival time in uremic patients.[23,24]

The contribution of altered erythrocyte survival time to the anemia of renal failure is probably secondary compared with erythropoietin deficiency and inhibitors of erythropoiesis. Adequate dialysis has been reported to return red blood cell survival time to normal.[25] Therefore, hemolysis in a well-dialyzed patient may be of minor clinical importance.

Iron Deficiency. The anemia of renal failure is usually characterized as a normocytic and normochromic type with normal marrow iron stores. Although iron transport in uremic patients is normal, iron deficiency may occur in some patients as a result of blood loss or reduced dietary iron intake. Occult gastrointestinal bleeding occurs in more than 20% of patients on dialysis.[26] Hemodialysis patients receive small amounts of heparin during dialysis and therefore may be at increased risk of bleeding. These patients also may experience the repetitive obligate loss of small amounts of blood in the dialysis machine. No blood loss is associated with peritoneal dialysis. Repeated venipuncture for laboratory tests also contributes to blood loss. Finally, iron deficiency may occur as a result of antacid-induced reduction of iron absorption across the intestinal mucosa. Antacids, often prescribed for the treatment of hyperphosphatemia, have been shown to decrease iron absorption.[27]

Vitamins. Because the water-soluble vitamins pyridoxine and folic acid are removed during dialysis, deficiencies of these vitamins may contribute to anemia. Vitamin B_{12} deficiency is rarely seen in patients with chronic renal failure. In the absence of impaired vitamin B_{12} absorption, large body stores of the vitamin prevent the rapid development of B_{12} deficiency.

Hypervitaminosis A also has been implicated as contributing to the anemia of renal failure.[28] Serum vitamin A concentrations are frequently elevated in cases of chronic renal failure, perhaps because of diminished metabolism of retinol to retinoic acid and an increased concentration of retinol-binding protein. The mechanism by which vitamin A may cause a reduction in hematocrit is unknown. Many clinicians now recommend avoiding vitamin A supplements in patients with chronic renal failure.

Aluminum Intoxication. A syndrome of aluminum intoxication in patients with renal failure has recently been described. One component of this syndrome has been the development of a microcytic anemia.[29] The precise method by which aluminum causes microcytosis is unclear; however, it has been suggested that aluminum may interfere with the incorporation of iron into erythroid cells.[1] Treatment with the chelating agent deferoxamine reverses the red blood cell microcytosis and improves the anemia. Because deferoxamine also chelates iron, patients receiving this drug should be observed for the possible development of iron deficiency.

Clinical Course

Anemia is seen in virtually all patients whose serum creatinine concentration is above 3.5 mg/dL.[9] However, hematocrits may vary widely among patients. With moderate renal failure, anemia is not severe and is unlikely to cause symptoms. As renal failure progresses, the anemia may worsen. Many patients tolerate the anemia well, perhaps because of compensatory lowering of hemoglobin–oxygen affinity leading to more effective delivery of oxygen to the tissues.[30] However, some patients develop symptoms that may lead to diminished exercise tolerance, myocardial ischemia, and reduced blood flow to the brain.

The severity of the anemia is not determined by the etiology of renal failure. It is impossible to predict the degree of anemia that will occur with end-stage renal disease. As mentioned previously, a wide variance in hematocrits can be seen in large groups of patients with chronic renal failure. With end-stage disease, however, the hematocrit for any individual will remain relatively constant. Some patients may develop a stable hematocrit as low as 18–20%. Any abrupt change in hematocrit may indicate the development of a complication.

Diagnosis

The anemia of renal failure is usually associated with certain laboratory findings.[9] Because of the varying degrees of severity of anemia, the diagnostic characteristics also vary. A common feature, however, is a normochromic, normocytic anemia with a diminished reticulocyte index. Bone marrow morphology is usually normal. Coexisting folate or iron deficiencies may alter the mean red cell volume.

Folic acid deficiency is best determined by measurement of serum folate concentrations and by the presence of red blood cell macrocytosis. Unfortunately, serum folate concentrations do not always correlate well with tissue stores of folate. In addition, several drugs (e.g., phenytoin, methotrexate, estrogens, phenobarbital, ampicillin, chloramphenicol) may interfere with the measurement of serum folate concentrations.

With no iron deficiency, the serum iron concentration is usually normal or high and the iron-binding capacity of serum is normal or low. A low serum ferritin concentration is consistent with iron deficiency; however, a normal or high value does not rule out iron deficiency because concomitant diseases, recent transfusions, and impaired incorporation of iron into hemoglobin may falsely raise the test results.[31] In spite of these limitations, however, measurement of the serum ferritin concentration remains the most useful diagnostic tool for the assessment of iron stores.

Examination of the peripheral blood smear may reveal morphologic abnormalities such as Burr cells, acanthocytes, target cells, and red cell inclusion bodies.

The total white blood cell count is usually normal; however, lymphocytopenia is often seen in uremic patients. The platelet count is normal, but abnormal platelet function (increased bleeding time) is usually seen.

Androgen Therapy

Androgen therapy has been advocated as a method to increase erythropoiesis in patients with renal failure.[32,33] The mechanism of improved erythropoiesis is androgenic stimulation of erythropoietin production.[34] The classes of anabolic androgenic steroids that have been used are testosterone esters, nortestosterone, and 17-methylated androgenic steroids.[9] The results of numerous therapeutic trials have been reviewed elsewhere.[35] Some patients demonstrate substantial improvement in erythropoiesis after androgen administration. Such a response may not develop for several months, however. It is also apparent that many patients experience little or no benefit from androgen therapy. Failure to respond within six months is an indication for discontinuing therapy. Patients who are anephric generally show no response to therapy.[26] Studies of anephric patients given androgens have failed to show a statistically significant improvement in erythropoiesis, but individual patients have shown an improvement in hematocrit. In general, androgen administration should be reserved for patients with native kidneys; however, a limited trial of androgens may be warranted in some anephric patients.

The choice of androgen remains controversial. Because of the adverse effects that have been observed, it has been suggested that males should be given either nandrolone decanoate or testosterone enanthate, whereas females should be given nandrolone decanoate, which has a high anabolic-to-androgenic ratio.[26] Both compounds are given intramuscularly: testosterone enanthate in a dosage of 4–7 mg/kg per week and nandrolone decanoate in a dosage of 1.5–2.5 mg/kg per week.

There has been great concern about the potential toxicities of long-term androgen therapy. Observed adverse effects include virilization, muscle soreness, abnormal hair growth, priapism, acne, and pain with injection. Orally administered 17-methylated androgenic steroids have been associated with hepatic dysfunction and hepatocellular carcinoma. As a result, use of the 17-methylated compounds is limited. The use of androgens has often resulted in weight gain and an increase in serum creatinine concentrations.[36] Blood urea nitrogen values usually remain unchanged. In a study of fluoxymesterone administration to a group of patients with chronic renal failure, the drug was associated with an increase in serum triglyceride concentrations.[37] Serum cholesterol levels were unaffected. Since hypertriglyceridemia is a common feature of chronic renal failure and since cardiovascular disease is a primary cause of death in uremic patients, androgens should be used cautiously in patients with lipid abnormalities.

Iron and Vitamin Supplementation

As described previously, the anemia of renal failure is usually not caused by iron deficiency. Therefore, administration of oral or injectable iron is generally not indicated. It is important, however, that the appropriate laboratory tests be performed periodically to detect the presence or development of iron deficiency. Stimulation of erythropoiesis by the administration of erythropoietin or androgens may cause increased use of iron stores with subsequent iron deficiency.

Prophylactic multivitamin preparations containing water-soluble vitamins, especially pyridoxine and folic acid, are usually prescribed for patients on dialysis. In particular, it is recommended that patients be given 10 mg of pyridoxine hydrochloride and 1 mg of folic acid daily.[38] Many inexpensive multivitamin formulations contain most of the water-soluble vitamins. However, many of these preparations contain inadequate amounts of pyridoxine and folic acid and contain unwanted fat-soluble vitamins. Dialysis patients receiving long-term vitamin A supplementation have developed hypervitaminosis A.[28] Likewise, the long-term use of multivitamin preparations containing the fat-soluble vitamin D may lead to vitamin D intoxication and hypercalcemia. This is particularly troublesome in those patients with pronounced hyperparathyroidism. To provide adequate amounts of water-soluble vitamins and to avoid excessive amounts of fat-soluble vitamins, several multivitamin preparations have been designed especially for patients with renal failure. Although these preparations may cost slightly more, their advantages support their use.

Recombinant Human Erythropoietin Therapy

In the past, administering erythropoietin was not possible because of a lack of sufficient quantities of the purified hormone. However, with the identification of the human gene for erythropoietin,[39] it has been possible to produce erythropoietin from recombinant sources. The potential value of erythropoietin administration has been demonstrated in uremic sheep given multiple infusions of plasma rich in sheep erythropoietin.[40] This nonpurified form of the hormone caused improved erythropoiesis as evidenced by increased reticulocyte formation, improved ferrokinetics, and hemoglobin C synthesis. These effects were maintained for several weeks after the infusions were discontinued.

Similar beneficial effects of erythropoietin have been observed after administration of rat plasma erythropoietin to uremic rats.[41] After 10 days of subcutaneous injection of the hormone, hemoglobin, hematocrit, and reticulocyte counts improved.

Clinical trials of therapy with recombinant human erythropoietin are now being conducted. Winearls and associates[42] studied 10 hemodialysis patients treated with recombinant human erythropoietin. Escalating doses of erythropoietin were administered intravenously three times a week at the end of each dialysis in a nonrandomized fashion. The dosage range was 3–192 units/kg/dose. The dosage was increased until the hemoglobin concentration increased at least 2 g/dL. Treatment was continued for up to 12 weeks. All patients had an increase in hemoglobin concentration and reticulocyte count. In nine patients treated for 12 weeks, the mean hemoglobin concentration after erythropoietin therapy was 10.3 g/dL compared with a mean pretherapy value of 6.2 g/dL. Transfusions were no longer required in those patients who were previously transfusion dependent. Nearly all patients reported subjective improvements in exercise tolerance and general well-being. Four patients noted transient aching in limbs and the pelvis two hours after erythropoietin injection. Two patients developed a clot in an arteriovenous fistula, and one patient developed hypertensive encephalopathy during treatment.

In a larger Phase I–II trial, Eschbach et al.[43] administered recombinant human erythropoietin to 25 patients on chronic hemodialysis. In this open-label study, patients received the hormone in intravenous dosages ranging from 1.5 to 500 units/kg body weight three times a week at the end of dialysis for three weeks. Response was assessed by transfusion requirements, hematocrit, use of iron and reticulocyte count.

Patients receiving 1.5 and 5.0 units/kg per dose failed to show improved erythropoiesis by the end of three weeks. Doses of 15 units/kg and greater produced favorable results in most patients in a dose-dependent fashion. Those patients receiving 150 or 500 units/kg per dose achieved mean hematocrit values of greater than 35% after three weeks, compared with baseline values of approximately

21%. Improved use of iron and increased reticulocyte counts also indicated enhanced erythropoiesis.

In a recently reported Phase III multicenter trial, Eschbach and coworkers[44] reported on 247 hemodialysis patients treated with recombinant human erythropoietin for up to four months. Patients were given 150–300 units/kg/dose intravenously three times a week. An increase in hematocrit was seen in all but six patients. The mean pretreatment hematocrit was 22.9% and rose to 33.5% after therapy. Before erythropoietin therapy, 127 patients were transfusion dependent; only 3 required transfusions after receiving erythropoietin.

In both studies by Eschbach et al., an increase in blood pressure was noted during therapy. In the multicenter trial, 32% of all patients experienced an increase in diastolic blood pressure of at least 10 mm Hg or required more antihypertensive medication. Two patients experienced seizures associated with the rise in blood pressure. Another consequence of erythropoietin therapy has been the development of iron deficiency. The suggested explanation for this observation is that increased hemoglobin synthesis exceeds the ability of the reticuloendothelial system to release iron. A decrease in serum ferritin concentration has been noted in some patients. Simultaneous intravenous or oral iron therapy was required to maintain improved erythropoiesis during erythropoietin treatment. Other adverse effects that have been seen following erythropoietin administration include a rise in predialysis concentrations of serum creatinine, urea nitrogen, and potassium.

The consequences of improved erythropoiesis leading to increased blood volume have been debated. Although normalization of the hematocrit is a desirable therapeutic goal,[45] a rising hematocrit with reduced plasma volume may adversely affect solute mass transfer, thus reducing the efficiency of the hemodialysis procedure.[46] Likewise, the possible relationship of increased red blood cell volume to thrombosis must be studied. Winearls et al.[42] reported that 2 of 10 patients developed a clot in an arteriovenous fistula. Eschbach and Adamson[47] noted that 2 of 21 patients with hematocrits greater than 30% had increased clotting of arteriovenous fistulae. Whether these occurrences are due to erythropoietin administration remains to be determined. Ahmad and Hand[48] have suggested that dialysis patients with near-normal levels of hemoglobin have increased clotting of arteriovenous fistulae. Further studies must be done to clarify how erythropoietin administration and normalization of the hematocrit affect blood coagulability in dialysis patients.

Although published data on the pharmacokinetics of erythropoietin in humans are limited, Mladenovic et al.[49] have studied the hormone's pharmacokinetics in a sheep model. Using a radioimmunoassay for erythropoietin, these investigators determined that the plasma half-life of this compound was 9 to 10 hours in both normal and uremic sheep. In the sheep model, it appears that the kidney plays a minor role in erythropoietin catabolism. The results of this study suggest that intermittent dosing of erythropoietin will adequately sustain a therapeutic effect.

Although the initial reports on the use of recombinant human erythropoietin indicate a favorable response in most patients, the results of larger and longer clinical trials are needed. Erythropoietic response has been shown to occur within three weeks in most patients receiving adequate doses. However, the metabolic adverse effects of this hormone must be better understood. In particular, the relationship between erythropoietin administration and the subsequent development of hypertension, iron deficiency, and access-site clotting needs to be determined. Should worsening of hypertension and hypercoagulability prove to be frequent adverse effects of erythropoietin, the need for increased antihypertensive therapy and antiplatelet drugs must be assessed.

Prostaglandin Therapy

Prostaglandin E_2 has been shown to stimulate erythropoiesis in mouse and dog models.[50] In a small clinical trial of four male, transfusion-dependent hemodialysis patients, prostaglandin E_2 was administered three times a week for eight weeks.[51] Although an increase in peripheral blood erythroid progenitor cells was noted, only one patient had a substantial rise in serum erythropoietin activity. The value of prostaglandin therapy for correcting the anemia of renal failure is unknown.

Conclusion

Anemia continues to be a frequent consequence of renal failure. Previous pharmacologic attempts to correct the anemia have been largely unsatisfactory. Repeated transfusions of red blood cells continue to present the risk of iron overload and the transmission of infectious agents. A major therapeutic breakthrough may result from the recent production of recombinant human erythropoietin. Clinical experience with this agent remains limited; however, initial reports are encouraging.

References

1. Eschbach JW, Adamson JW. Anemia of end-stage renal disease (ESRD). *Kidney Int*. 1985; 28:1–5.
2. Dodds A, Nicholls M. Haematological aspects of renal disease. *Anaesth Intensive Care*. 1983; 11:361–8.
3. Ali M, Fayemi AO, Rigolosi R et al. Hemosiderosis in hemodialysis patients. *JAMA*. 1980; 244:343–5.
4. Dienstag JL, Wands JR, Koff RS. Acute hepatitis. In: Petersdorf RG, Adams RD, Braunwald E et al., eds. Harrison's principles of internal medicine. 10th ed. New York:

McGraw-Hill; 1983:1789–1801.
5. Anon. Update: acquired immunodeficiency syndrome—United States. Leads from the *MMWR*. *JAMA*. 1986; 255:594–8.
6. Fisher JW. Mechanism of the anemia of chronic renal failure. *Nephron*. 1980; 25:106–11.
7. McGonigle RJS, Wallin JD, Shadduck RK et al. Erythropoietin deficiency and inhibition of erythropoiesis in renal insufficiency. *Kidney Int*. 1984; 25:437–44.
8. Caro J, Brown S, Miller O et al. Erythropoietin levels in uremic nephric and anephric patients. *J Lab Clin Med*. 1979; 93:449–58.
9. Anagnostou A, Kurtzman NA. Hematological consequences of renal failure. In: Brenner BM, Rector FC, eds. The kidney. Philadelphia: W. B. Saunders; 1986:1631–56.
10. Fried W, Morley C. Update on erythropoietin. *Int J Artif Organs*. 1985; 8:79–82.
11. Freedman MH, Cattran DC, Saunders EF. Anemia of chronic renal failure: inhibition of erythropoiesis by uremic serum. *Nephron*. 1983; 35:15–9.
12. Pierratos A, Toor P, Ayiomamitis A et al. Immunoreactive parathyroid hormone and in vitro inhibition of erythropoiesis by uremic serum in patients on continuous ambulatory peritoneal dialysis. *Am J Nephrol*. 1986; 6:465–8.
13. Fukushima Y, Fukuda M, Yoshida K et al. Serum erythropoietin levels and inhibitors of erythropoiesis in patients with chronic renal failure. *Tohoku J Exp Med*. 1986; 150:1–15.
14. Radtke HW, Rege AB, La Marche MB et al. Identification of spermine as an inhibitor of erythropoiesis in patients with chronic renal failure. *J Clin Invest*. 1981; 67:1623–9.
15. Gutman RA, Huang AT. Inhibitor of marrow thymidine incorporation from sera of patients with uremia. *Kidney Int*. 1980; 18:715–24.
16. Delwiche F, Segal GM, Eschbach JW et al. Hematopoietic inhibitors in chronic renal failure: lack of in vitro specificity. *Kidney Int*. 1986; 29:641–8.
17. Lutton JD, Solangi KB, Ibraham NG et al. Inhibition of erythropoiesis in chronic renal failure: the role of parathyroid hormone. *Am J Kidney Dis*. 1984; 3:380–4.
18. McGonigle RJS, Wallin JD, Husserl F et al. Potential role of parathyroid hormone as an inhibitor of erythropoiesis in the anemia of renal failure. *J Lab Clin Med*. 1984; 104:1016–26.
19. Spragg BP, Bentley DP, Coles GA. Anaemia of chronic renal failure. Polyamines are not raised in uraemic serum. *Nephron*. 1984; 38:65–6.
20. Hocken AG. Haemolysis in chronic renal failure. *Nephron*. 1982; 32:28–31.
21. Hefti JE, Blumberg A, Marti HR. Red cell survival and red cell enzymes in patients on continuous peritoneal dialysis (CAPD). *Clin Nephrol*. 1983; 19:232–5.
22. Giovannetti S, Cioni L, Balestri PL et al. Evidence that guanidines and some related compounds cause haemolysis in chronic uraemia. *Clin Sci*. 1968; 34:141–8.
23. Saltissi D, Carter GD. Association of secondary hyperparathyroidism with red cell survival in chronic haemodialysis patients. *Clin Sci*. 1985; 68:29–33.
24. Akmal M, Telfer N, Ansari A et al. Erythrocyte survival in chronic renal failure. Role of secondary hyperparathyroidism. *J Clin Invest*. 1985; 76:1695–8.
25. Von Hartitzsch B, Carr D, Kjellstrand CM et al. Normal red cell survival in well dialyzed patients. *Trans Am Soc Artif Intern Organs*. 1973; 19:471–4.
26. Neff MS, Goldberg J, Slifkin RF et al. Anemia in chronic renal failure. *Acta Endocrinol (Copenh)*. 1985; 271(Suppl):80–5.
27. Hall GJ, Davis AE. Inhibition of iron absorption by magnesium trisilicate. *Med J Aust*. 1969; 2:95–6.
28. Ono K, Waki Y, Takeda K. Hypervitaminosis A: a contributing factor to anemia in regular dialysis patients. *Nephron*. 1984; 38:44–7.
29. Wills MR, Savory J. Aluminum poisoning: dialysis encephalopathy, osteomalacia, and anemia. *Lancet*. 1983; 2:29–34.
30. Mitchell TR, Pegrum GD. The oxygen affinity of haemoglobin in chronic renal failure. *Br J Haematol*. 1971; 21:463–72.
31. Moreb J, Popovtzer MM, Friedlaender MM et al. Evaluation of iron status in patients on chronic hemodialysis: relative usefulness of bone marow hemosiderin, serum ferritin, transferrin saturation, mean corpuscular volume and red cell protoporphyrin. *Nephron*. 1983; 35:196–200.
32. Eschbach JW, Adamson JW. Improvement in the anemia of chronic renal failure with fluoxymesterone. *Ann Intern Med*. 1973; 78:527–32.
33. Williams JS, Stein JH, Ferris TF et al. Nandrolone decanoate therapy for patients receiving hemodialysis. *Arch Intern Med*. 1974; 134:289–92.
34. Alexanian R. Erythropoietin and erythropoiesis in anemic man following androgens. *Blood*. 1969; 33:564–72.
35. Alexander MR. Use of androgens in chronic renal failure patients on hemodialysis. *Am J Hosp Pharm*. 1976; 33:242–8.
36. Mirahmadi MK, Vaziri ND. Long-term nandrolone and testosterone administration in hemodialysis patients. *Drug Intell Clin Pharm*. 1980; 14:493–7.
37. Dombeck DH, Lindholm DD, Vieira JA. Lipid metabolism in uremia and the effects of dialysate glucose and oral androgen therapy. *Trans Am Soc Artif Intern Organs*. 1973; 19:150–3.
38. Kopple JD, Blumenkrantz MJ. Nutritional requirements for patients undergoing continuous ambulatory peritoneal dialysis. *Kidney Int*. 1983; 24(Suppl 16):S294–S302.
39. Jacobs K, Shoemaker C, Rudersdorf R et al. Isolation and characterization of genomic and cDNA clones of erythropoietin. *Nature*. 1985; 313:806–10.
40. Eschbach JW, Mladenovich J, Garcia JF et al. The anemia of chronic renal failure in sheep. Response to erythropoietin-rich plasma in vivo. *J Clin Invest*. 1984; 74:434–41.
41. Malgor LA, Barrios L, deAlbarenque ME et al. Erythropoietic effects of triiodothyronine on the anemia of renal failure in rats: comparative studies with testosterone and erythropoietin. *Exp Hematol*. 1986; 14:250–6.
42. Winerls CG, Oliver DO, Pippard MJ et al. Effect of human erythropoietin derived from recombinant DNA on the anaemia of patients maintained by chronic haemodialysis. *Lancet*. 1986; 2:1175–8.
43. Eschbach JW, Egrie JC, Downing MR et al. Correction of the anemia of end-stage renal disease with recombinant human erythropoietin. *N Engl J Med*. 1987; 316:73–8.
44. Eschbach JW, Adamson JW. Correction of the anemia of hemodialysis (HD) patients with recombinant human erythropoietin (rHuEpo): results of a multicenter study. Paper presented to 20th Annual American Society of Nephrology Meeting. Washington, DC: 1987 Dec 15.
45. Erslev AJ. Recombinant erythropoietin for the anemia of chronic renal failure. *N Engl J Med*. 1987; 317:169–70. Letter.
46. Walczyk MH, Golper TA. Correction of the anemia of end-stage renal disease with recombinant human erythropoietin. *N Engl J Med*. 1987; 317:249. Letter.
47. Eschbach JW, Adamson JW. Correction of the anemia of end-stage renal disease with recombinant human erythropoietin. *N Engl J Med*. 1987; 317:250–1. Letter.
48. Ahmad R, Hand M. Recombinant erythropoietin for the anemia of chronic renal failure. *N Engl J Med*. 1987; 317:169. Letter.
49. Mladenovic J, Eschbach JW, Koup JR et al. Erythropoietin kinetics in normal and uremic sheep. *J Lab Clin Med*. 1985; 105:659–63.
50. Gross DM, Brookins J, Fink GD et al. Effects of prostaglandin A_2, E_2 and $F_{2\alpha}$ on erythropoietin production. *J Pharmacol Exp Ther*. 1976; 198:489–96.
51. Ortega JA, Dukes PP, Ma A et al. A clinical trial of prostaglandin E_2 to increase erythropoiesis in anemia of end stage renal disease. *Prostaglandins Leukotrienes Med*. 1984; 14:411–6.

Management of hypophosphatemia

CHARLES W. LLOYD AND CARY E. JOHNSON

Abstract: The etiology, clinical presentation, and management of hypophosphatemia are reviewed.

Phosphorus is a major intracellular anion and plays an important role in many biochemical pathways relating to normal physiologic functions. Approximately 60 to 90% of the 1 to 1.5 g of daily dietary phosphorus intake is absorbed, and of that amount, about two thirds is excreted in the urine. The overall incidence of hypophosphatemia is about 2 to 3% of all hospitalized patients. Factors associated with hypophosphatemia include phosphate-binding antacid therapy, nasogastric suction, liver disease, sepsis, alcoholism, and acidosis associated with diabetic ketoacidosis. Patients receiving parenteral nutrient solutions were also at higher risk for hypophosphatemia before the routine supplementation of these formulations with phosphate. Patients with hypophosphatemia may be asymptomatic or may experience weakness, malaise, anorexia, bone pain, and respiratory arrest. The major systems involved include the neuromuscular, hematologic, and skeletal systems.

Phosphorus-containing products used to treat hypophosphatemia are a combination of monobasic and dibasic phosphate salts. Therefore, it is essential to calculate doses in millimoles rather than milligrams or milliequivalents to more accurately reflect the phosphorus concentration and to avoid potentially serious dosage errors. Normal daily requirements are readily maintained by dietary sources of phosphorus such as milk products or may be supplemented by phosphate-containing products administered orally or intravenously.

Since phosphorus is a key factor in many organ systems, it is essential to monitor serum phosphorus concentrations in patients at risk for hypophosphatemia.

Index terms: Calculations; Dosage; Drug administration routes; Hypophosphatemia; Minerals; Nutrition; Phosphates; Phosphorus
Clin Pharm. 1988; 7:123–128

Phosphorus, a major intracellular anion, is instrumental in metabolic and enzymatic reactions in normal body states. It is important in the formation of adenosine triphosphate (ATP) for the metabolism of cellular substrates. Total body content of phosphorus is approximately 700 g (23,000 mmol), 80% of which can be found in bone. The intracellular–extracellular soluble phosphate ratio is 100:1. The total body space of phosphorus is extremely difficult to calculate because phosphorus is primarily an intracellular solute.[1] Hypophosphatemia may result from decreased intake, increased renal losses, or transcellular ionic shifts.[2,3] Commonly occurring etiologies include alcoholism, phosphate-binding antacids, total parenteral nutrition (TPN) therapy without phosphorus, and diabetic ketoacidosis (DKA).[1] Since phosphorus is widely found in many food groups, decreased intake is less likely to be the primary cause of hypophosphatemia.[2]

The normal daily dietary intake of phosphorus is 1 to 1.5 g, of which 60–90% is absorbed, primarily in the jejunum of the small intestine.[3] Dietary sources that are high in phosphate include red meats, milk products, fish, and poultry. The kidneys are the most important regulator by which the body maintains phosphate homeostasis. Phosphorus is filtered at the glomerulus, and 80 to 90% is reabsorbed in the proximal renal tubules.[4] Two thirds (450 to 1020 mg or 15 to 33 mmol/day) of the amount of phosphorus ingested daily is excreted in urine.[2,4] Hormonal influences on serum phosphorus include parathyroid hormone and ergocalciferol (1,25-dihydroxyvitamin D_3), which have been shown to decrease renal phosphate reabsorption, and growth hormone and thyroxine, which are believed to increase phosphate reabsorption.[3] Recommended daily requirements of phosphorus are 0.4 to 1.2 mmol/kg for children and 0.14 to 0.4 mmol/kg for adults.[5] Normal blood concentrations of inorganic phosphorus and the ranges for moderate and severe hypophosphatemia are listed in Table 1. When the serum phosphorus concentration falls below 1 mg/dL, the clinical manifestations of hypophosphatemia are more commonly seen.[2–4]

The overall prevalence of hypophosphatemia

Table 1.
Serum Phosphorus Concentrations[a]

Normal	Moderate Hypophosphatemia	Severe Hypophosphatemia
3–4.5 (1–1.5)	1.0–2.0 (0.3–0.7)	<1.0 (<0.3)

[a] Concentrations given in milligrams per deciliter; numbers in parentheses are concentrations in millimoles per liter.

CHARLES W. LLOYD, PHARM.D., is Health Maintenance Facility Scientist, Krug International, NASA, Johnson Space Center, Houston, TX. At the time the paper was prepared he was Assistant Professor of Pharmacy, College of Pharmacy, The University of Michigan, and Clinical Pharmacist–Surgery, University of Michigan Hospitals, Ann Arbor. CARY E. JOHNSON, PHARM.D., is Associate Professor of Pharmacy, College of Pharmacy, The University of Michigan, and Clinical Pharmacist–Pediatrics, University of Michigan Hospitals.

Address reprint requests to Dr. Lloyd at Krug International, NASA, Johnson Space Center, SD—12, Houston, TX 77058.

Copyright © 1988, American Society of Hospital Pharmacists, Inc. All rights reserved. 0278-2677/88/0201-0125$01.50.

has been reported to be approximately 2 to 3% of all hospitalized patients.[6,7] Of these cases, 40% are believed to result from the use of TPN solutions without phosphorus supplementation, 12% are believed to be caused by vomiting, and 26% are due to unknown causes. Other factors such as phosphate-binding antacid therapy of greater than two weeks' duration, nasogastric suction, liver disease, gram-negative sepsis, familial hypophosphatemia, and insulin therapy accounted for 22% of the cases. The incidence of hypophosphatemia in patients with a diagnosis of acute alcoholism was determined to be approximately 10%.[8-11]

Parenteral nutrition can also induce hypophosphatemia by transcellular ionic shifts. When glucose is administered to cachectic or alcoholic patients, it stimulates the production of high-energy phosphate compounds as a result of glycolysis. A decrease in the serum phosphorus concentration normally occurs in the disposal of glucose, and this drop is accentuated in the fasting state. An ionic shift is seen with the administration of insulin, in which the serum phosphorus concentration falls with the cellular influx of glucose. Other substantial cellular shifts of phosphorus are seen with systemic alkalosis and with liver disease.[12-16]

Clinical Presentation

The clinical presentation of hypophosphatemia is more readily understood when the effects on selected major systems are described. The systems affected by hypophosphatemia—neuromuscular, hematologic, and skeletal—are summarized in Table 2.

Neuromuscular Effects. Neuromuscular manifestations associated with phosphorus concentrations of 2 mg/dL or less include weakness, malaise, anorexia, bone pain, and joint stiffness.[17] These signs and symptoms also occur with the more commonly considered diagnoses of hyperparathyroidism and abnormal calcium levels.[18] If the serum phosphorus concentrations fall below 1 mg/dL, the clinical presentation is more likely to include signs and symptoms such as anisocoria, ballismus, hyporeflexia, electroencephalographic changes, paresthesia, convulsions, and subsequently coma and death. Hypophosphatemia has been associated with depressed myocardial function and has been shown to be caused by ingestion of large quantities of phosphate-binding antacids in several cases.[19,20] The CNS presentation has been attributed to decreased brain-cell ATP production[21] and a reduction in delivery of oxygen to the brain as a result of decreased 2,3-diphosphoglycerate (2,3-DPG) in the red blood cells.[14,22-25] In most cases, the reduction in severity of symptoms correlated best with the correction of the serum phosphorus concentration to at least 2 mg/dL.[26]

Recently, concerns regarding severe hypophosphatemia in critically ill patients have addressed the problem of respiratory failure and ventilatory weaning.[27,28-31] In all cases the patients had chronic pulmonary disease, and after the administration of TPN therapy the patients were noted to have serum phosphate concentrations of less than 1 mg/dL. In a case report, Agusti et al.[29] were able to show a positive correlation between maximum inspiratory pressure (PImax) values ranging from 11 to 52 cm H_2O PImax and serum phosphorus concentrations of 0.4 to 3.0 mg/dL ($r = 0.97$; $p < 0.01$). This relationship highlights the importance of metabolic factors in the treatment of critically ill patients.

Hematologic Effects. Hematologic effects have involved erythrocytes, leukocytes, and platelets. Both the structure and function of red blood cells can be affected. A decreased serum phosphorus concentration will result in a reduction of erythrocyte ATP production and will affect the cell wall integrity and plasticity.[22,32,33] The red blood cell membranes become rigid with a decrease in cellular ATP, resulting in a shorter life span. Decreased serum phosphorus and 2,3-DPG concentrations result in a shift to the left in the oxyhemoglobin dissociation curve and decreased oxygen delivery to the tissue because of greater affinity between oxygen and hemoglobin.[25,33]

Leukocyte dysfunction is most commonly associated with serum phosphorus concentrations below 1 mg/dL.[34] The dysfunction is believed to be caused by decreased ATP production, resulting in

Table 2.
Systems Affected by Hypophosphatemia

Signs and Symptoms
Neuromuscular
Muscle weakness
Anorexia
Tremor
Paresthesia
Convulsions
Coma
Hyporeflexia
Irritability
Numbness
Abnormal EEG
Cardiomyopathy
Respiratory failure
Hematologic
Rhabdomyolysis
Hemolytic anemia
Decreased oxygen release
Decreased chemotaxis
Decreased phagocytosis
Decreased platelet survival
Myoglobinuria
Thrombocytopenia
Skeletal
Osteomalacia
Joint arthralgias
Pathologic fractures

decreased chemotactic, phagocytic, and bactericidal activity. The production of phagocytic vacuoles and ameboid movement involving actin and myosin depend on the availability of ATP.[35] The incidence of infection appears to be higher in patients receiving TPN therapy if they are also hypophosphatemic.[2,4] Other patients at risk for infection and leukocyte dysfunction include those with chronic alcoholism or diabetes and those receiving a combination of antacids and corticosteroids.[2]

Platelet dysfunction is believed to be caused by ATP deficiency and may result in an overall reduction in platelet survival, mucosal bleeding, epistaxis, and absence of clot retraction.[14] The thrombopathy of alcoholism or uremia can therefore be complicated by hypophosphatemia-associated platelet dysfunction.

Skeletal Effects. Skeletal manifestations of hypophosphatemia include large-joint arthralgias, inflammatory arthritis, or clinical and roentgenographic findings associated with sacroiliitis. These symptoms may be misdiagnosed as ankylosing spondylitis.[18] Pathologic fractures resulting from chronic hypophosphatemia have been reported in patients receiving phosphate-binding antacids.[36]

Patients with alcoholic liver disease are predisposed to hypophosphatemia. Several factors are believed to result in hypophosphatemia and hepatic hypoxemia in chronic alcoholic patients. These patients are commonly cachectic and are receiving intravenous glucose and large quantities of antacids. Alcoholic liver disease is also aggravated by hypophosphatemia, which causes a decrease in tissue respiration in the liver.[15] Patients with alcoholic liver disease are often hypokalemic or hypomagnesemic (or both), two factors known to induce renal tubular losses of phosphorus.[6,8,37]

Management

Since most products containing phosphorus are a combination of the monobasic and biphosphate salts (KH_2PO_4, formula weight [FW] = 136; NaH_2PO_4, FW = 120; $NaH_2PO_4 \cdot H_2O$, FW = 138) and the dibasic salts (K_2HPO_4, FW = 174; Na_2HPO_4, FW = 142; $Na_2HPO_4 \cdot 7H_2O$, FW = 268), it needs to be stressed that phosphorus is a polyvalent anion and should be discussed in terms of millimoles or milligrams versus milliequivalents. The use of milliequivalents does not reflect the concentration of the phosphorus preparation accurately and may lead to large dosage errors.[38,39] To convert between millimoles and milligrams of elemental phosphorus, use the following equivalencies: 1 mg = 0.032 mmol, 31 mg = 1 mmol.

Prevention of Hypophosphatemia Associated with TPN. The key to avoiding hypophosphatemia associated with TPN therapy is to monitor serum phosphorus concentrations and supplement with phosphorus in the standard TPN formulation. Phosphorus requirements per 24 hours in patients with normal serum concentrations of phosphorus and adequate renal function are 0.1 to 0.2 mmol/kg, plus an additional 10 mmol/L of nonprotein calories administered.[40] Therefore, the usual daily requirements are the same as if food were taken by mouth (30 to 90 mmol/day). Severe hypophosphatemia may occur if TPN therapy is instituted too aggressively.[27,41,42] This aggressive nutritional repletion creates a sudden demand for the production of phosphorylated compounds of glycolysis, resulting in a precipitous drop in the serum phosphorus concentration.[27,41,42] This phenomenon is termed the "refeeding syndrome" and is manifested by serious neurological and muscular disorders and eventually respiratory failure.[40-44] This complication occurs most frequently in patients being refed after severe weight loss.[4] Before initiation of TPN therapy, the serum phosphorus concentration is often normal, and the depletion syndrome does not become apparent until refeeding is started.[4] TPN therapy should be started slowly, and the daily amounts of both nonprotein and protein calories should be increased gradually.

Treatment of Moderate Hypophosphatemia. The available oral, rectal, and injectable phosphorus-containing products are outlined in Table 3. Milk has been added to the list as a dietary source. The dose and rate of administration depend on the patient's needs. Whenever possible, hypophosphatemia should be prevented by the supplementation of phosphorus by mouth or in TPN solutions.

Attempts should be made to supplement the diet with 30 to 90 mmol of phosphorus per day.[43-45] When the patient can tolerate oral feeding, milk can be used to deliver approximately 900 mg (29 mmol) of elemental phosphorus per liter.[43-45] If the patient is intolerant to milk products, Fleet Phospho-Soda, which contains 4.15 mmol of phosphorus per milliliter, can be used. A reasonable regimen would be to administer 5 mL, mixed with 120 mL of cold water or in at least 500 mL of tube feedings to avoid diarrhea, three to four times daily. The Fleet's enema can also be administered orally; however, it contains approximately one third the amount of phosphorus per milliliter (Table 3). If the use of a tablet or capsule formulation is preferred, these products contain between 4 and 8 mmol of phosphorus and should be given in a regimen of two to three tablets or capsules two to four times daily.[44]

The administration of phosphorus in diabetic ketoacidosis is controversial.[46] When hypophosphatemia is associated with hypokalemia, as occurs in diabetic ketoacidosis and alcohol withdrawal, it has been suggested that supplementation with a combination of phosphorus, potassium, and chloride is most appropriate.[43,47] A possible regimen would consist of the administration of half of the potassium deficit as the chloride salt and half as the

Table 3.
Phosphorus-Containing Products

Drug	Phosphorus (mmol)	Sodium (meq)	Potassium (meq)
Oral Agents			
Cow's milk	0.029/mL	0.025/mL	0.035/mL
Fleet's Oral Solution (Fleet)	4.15/mL	4.8/mL	None
Fleet's Enema (Fleet)	1.38/mL	1.6/mL	None
Neutra-Phos-K (Willen)	8.0/capsule	None	14.0/capsule
Neutra-Phos (Willen)	8.0/capsule	7.0/capsule	7.0/capsule
K-Phos Neutral Tab (Beach)	8.0/tablet	13.0/tablet	1.1/tablet
K-Phos Neutral Liq (Beach)	16.0/5 mL	None	28/5 mL
K-Phos Original (Beach)	3.7/tablet	None	3.7/tablet
K-Phos M. F. (Beach)	4.0/tablet	2.9/tablet	1.1/tablet
K-Phos No. 2 (Beach)	8.0/tablet	5.8/tablet	2.3/tablet
URO-KP-Neutral Tab (Star)	5.6/tablet	9.9/tablet	1.3/tablet
Injectable Agents			
Potassium phosphate injection (various manufacturers)	3.0/mL	None	4.4/mL[a]
	3.0/mL	None	4.5/mL[b]
Sodium phosphate injection (various manufacturers)	3.0/mL	4.0/mL	None

[a] Potassium phosphate, monobasic 224 mg/mL and potassium phosphate, dibasic 236 mg/mL (Abbott and LyphoMed).
[b] Potassium phosphate, monobasic 180 mg/mL and potassium phosphate, dibasic 292 mg/mL (Kendall McGaw).

phosphate salt. However, when an attempt is made to correct a metabolic imbalance of two predominantly intracellular ions such as potassium and phosphorus, it is important to monitor both serum concentrations to avoid serious toxicities.[42]

Treatment of Severe Hypophosphatemia. The amount of phosphorus necessary to correct hypophosphatemia remains unclear. The treatment of severe hypophosphatemia, in which the injectable form of phosphorus is indicated, has been addressed by several authors.[28,45,48] Dosage recommendations outlined by Lentz and coworkers[45] of 0.08 to 0.24 mmol/kg infused intravenously over six hours are based on the etiology of hypophosphatemia and the intensity and duration of the underlying process. They suggest an initial dose of phosphorus of 0.08 mmol/kg if hypophosphatemia is recent and uncomplicated and 0.16 mmol/kg of body weight if it is prolonged and has multiple causes. The initial dose should be increased by 25 to 50% if the patient is symptomatic and lowered by 25 to 50% if the patient is hypercalcemic. Kingston and Al-Siba'I[48] subdivided the group of severe hypophosphatemics into those with serum phosphorus concentrations less than 0.5 mg/dL and those who had an initial serum phosphorus concentration of 0.5 to 1.0 mg/dL. They recommended doses of 0.25 to 0.5 mmol/kg infused intravenously over four hours and determined that a dose of 0.25 mmol/kg of body weight raised the serum phosphorus concentration on the average by 1.2 mg/dL. No new complications or arrhythmias were noted with this therapy.[48] When injectable phosphorus therapy is used to correct the serum phosphorus concentration, the amounts of sodium and potassium contained in these preparations must be considered. Both studies excluded patients with renal insufficiency and based their dose on ideal body weight if the patient was obese. If the recommendations from these studies are converted into units of millimoles per kilogram per hour, then the range of doses can be more easily evaluated. However, the rate and duration of therapy remains unclear and appears to be primarily based on symptomatology and renal function (Table 4).

Concerns about dosage and rate of administration continue to be reported in the literature. Vannatta et al.[28] suggest a dose of 0.16 mmol/kg over six hours; however, they administered a fixed dose of 9 mmol infused intravenously over 12 hours.

Clinical Laboratory Monitoring. The recommended frequency for monitoring serum phosphorus concentrations depends on the severity of the hypophosphatemia. Serum phosphorus concentrations should probably be determined at the end of an infusion of potassium phosphate and at least weekly if the previous levels were within the normal range. Calcium, magnesium, sodium, and potassium levels should also be closely monitored when intravenous phosphate solutions are being administered.[3,43,45,48]

Potential Adverse Effects of Phosphorus Therapy. Adverse reactions to phosphorus therapy encompass the combined effects of both the phosphorus and the sodium or potassium salt used. The signs and symptoms include hypotension, cardiac arrhythmias and possible cardiac arrest, symptoms of hypocalcemic tetany, mental confusion, paresthesia of the extremities, metastatic calcification, hyperkalemia, hypernatremia, hypocalcemia, and hypomagnesemia.[2-4,46,49] The predominant adverse reaction to orally administered phosphorus is diarrhea. The incidence of adverse reactions is

Table 4.
Dosage Range of Phosphorus for Treatment of Severe Hypophosphatemia[a]

Regimen	Comments
Low Dose	
0.0125 mmol/kg/hr[b] for six hours	Based on the usual dose recommended by Lentz.[45] Recheck serum phosphorus concentration at the end of the infusion.
Intermediate Dose	
0.03–0.04 mmol/kg/hr[b] for six hours	The 0.03- and 0.04-mmol doses are recommended by Lentz[45] only to initiate therapy in patients who are symptomatic and have multiple underlying etiologies. Recheck the serum phosphorus concentration at the end of the infusion.
0.06 mmol/kg/hr[b] for four hours	Based on the recommended dose by Kingston[48] for patients with an initial serum phosphorus concentration of 0.5 to 1.0 mg/dL. Recheck the serum phosphorus concentration at the end of the infusion.
High Dose	
0.125 mmol/kg/hr[b] for four hours	Recommended only for patients noted to have an initial serum phosphorus concentration of <0.5 mg/dL.[44] Recheck the serum phosphorus concentration at the end of the infusion.

[a] This therapy is recommended only for patients with normal renal function.
[b] Weight should be based on ideal body weight for all patients, including those noted to be obese.

even greater if phosphorus is given in doses of 50 mmol or more over three hours or less.[50]

Conclusion

Phosphorus is a key factor in maintaining normal physiologic function of many organ systems, and it is imperative that serum phosphorus concentrations be monitored. If a normal diet is not possible or if the patient is critically ill, it becomes even more likely that phosphorus supplementation will be required. Phosphorus can be administered either orally or intravenously. However, if the intravenous route is selected, care must be used to avoid administering excessive amounts of the potassium or sodium salts. Also, phosphorus should be administered with caution in patients with renal insufficiency since phosphorus may accelerate deterioration of renal function. Whenever intravenous solutions of phosphorus are administered, follow-up serum phosphorus concentrations should be obtained immediately after completion of the dose.

References

1. Juan D, Elrazak MA. Hypophosphatemia in hospitalized patients. *JAMA.* 1979; 242:163–4.
2. Fitzgerald FT. Hypophosphatemia. *Adv Intern Med.* 1978; 23:137–57.
3. Stoff JS. Phosphate homeostasis and hypophosphatemia. *Am J Med.* 1982; 72:489–95.
4. Knochel JP. The pathophysiology and clinical characteristics of severe hypophosphatemia. *Arch Intern Med.* 1977; 137:203–20.
5. Nesbakken R, Reinlie S. Magnesium and phosphorus: the electrolytes of energy metabolism. *Acta Anaesthesiol Scand.* 1985; 29:60–4.
6. Betro MG, Pain RW. Hypophosphatemia and hyperphosphatemia in a hospital population. *Br Med J.* 1972; 1:273–6.
7. Larsson L, Rebel K, Sorbo B. Severe hypophosphatemia—a hospital survey. *Acta Med Scand.* 1983; 214:221–3.
8. Stein JH, Smith WO, Ginn HE. Hypophosphatemia in acute alcoholism. *Am J Med Sci.* 1966; 252:78–83.
9. Territo MC, Tanaka KR. Hypophosphatemia in chronic alcoholism. *Arch Intern Med.* 1974; 134:445–7.
10. Jacob HS, Ansdem T. Acute hemolytic anemia with rigid red cells in hypophosphatemia. *N Engl J Med.* 1971; 285:1446–50.
11. Klock JC, Williams HE, Mentzer WC. Hemolytic anemia and somatic cell dysfunction in severe hypophosphatemia. *Arch Intern Med.* 1974; 134:360–4.
12. Okel BB, Hurst JW. Prolonged hyperventilation in man: associated electrolyte changes and subjective symptoms. *Arch Intern Med.* 1961; 108:757–62.
13. Mostellar ME, Tuttle EP. The effects of alkalosis on plasma concentration and urinary excretion of inorganic phosphate in man. *J Clin Invest.* 1964; 43:138–49.
14. Jacob HS. Severe hypophosphatemia: a previously ignored cause of cellular dysfunction. *West J Med.* 1975; 122:501–2.
15. Rajan KS, Levinson R, Leevy CM. Hepatic hypoxia secondary to hypophosphatemia. *Clin Res.* 1973; 21:521. Abstract.
16. Keating JP, Karl IE, DeVivo DC et al. Hypophosphatemia in Reye's syndrome. *Lancet.* 1975; 2:39–40. Letter.
17. Lotz M, Zisman E, Bartter FC. Evidence for a phosphorus-depletion syndrome in man. *N Engl J Med.* 1968; 278:409–15.
18. Moser CR, Fessel WJ. Rheumatic manifestations of hypophosphatemia. *Arch Intern Med.* 1974; 134:674–8.
19. O'Connor LR, Wheeler WS, Bethune JE. Effect of hypophosphatemia on myocardial performance in man. *N Engl J Med.* 1977; 297:901–3.
20. Darsee JR, Nutter DO. Reversible severe congestive cardiomyopathy in three cases of hypophosphatemia. *Ann Intern Med.* 1978; 89:867–70.
21. Yawata Y, Craddock P, Habbel R et al. Hyperalimentation hypophosphatemia: hematologic-neurologic dysfunction due to ATP depletion. *Clin Res.* 1973; 21:729. Abstract.
22. Travis SF, Sugerman HJ, Ruberg RL et al. Alterations of red-cell glycolytic intermediates and oxygen transport as a consequence of venous hyperalimentation. *N Engl J Med.* 1971; 285:763–8.
23. Alberti KG, Darley JH, Emerson PM et al. 2,3-di-phosphoglycerate and tissue oxygenation in uncontrolled diabetes mellitus. *Lancet.* 1972; 2:391–5.
24. Oski FA, Marshall BE, Cohen PJ et al. The role of the left-shifted or right-shifted oxygen-hemoglobin equilibrium curve. *Ann Intern Med.* 1971; 74:44–6.
25. Thomas HM, Lefrak SS, Irwin RS et al. The oxyhemoglobin dissociation curve in health and disease. Role of 2,3-diphosphoglycerate. *Am J Med.* 1974; 57:331–48.
26. Boelens PA, Norweed W, Kjellstrand C et al. Hypophosphatemia with muscle weakness due to antacids and hemodialysis. *Am J Dis Child.* 1970; 120:350–3.
27. Takala J, Neuvonen P, Klossner J. Hypophosphatemia in hypercatabolic patients. *Acta Anaesthesiol Scand.* 1985; 29:65–7.
28. Vannatta JB, Whang R, Papper S. Efficacy of intravenous phosphorus therapy in the severely hypophosphatemic patient. *Arch Intern Med.* 1981; 141:885–7.
29. Agusti AG, Torres A, Estopa R et al. Hypophosphatemia as a cause of failed weaning: the importance of metabolic factors. *Crit Care Med.* 1984; 12:142–3.

30. Brown EL, Jenkins G. A case of respiratory failure complicated by acute hypophosphataemia. *Anaesthesia.* 1980; 35:42–5.
31. Varsano S, Shapiro M, Taragan R et al. Hypophosphatemia as a reversible cause of refractory ventilatory failure. *Crit Care Med.* 1983; 11:908–9.
32. Weed RI, LaCelle PL, Merrill EW. Metabolic dependence of red cell deformability. *J Clin Invest.* 1969; 48:795.
33. Klocke RA. Oxygen transport and 2,3-diphosphoglycerate (DPG). *Chest.* 1972; 62(Suppl part 2):79s–85s.
34. Craddock PR, Yawata Y, VanSanten L et al. Acquired phagocyte dysfunction: a complication of the hypophosphatemia of parenteral hyperalimentation. *N Engl J Med.* 1974; 290:1403–7.
35. Tatsumi N, Shibata N, Okamura Y et al. Actin and myosin-A from leucocytes. *Biochim Biophys Acta.* 1973; 305:433–44.
36. Abrams DE, Silcott RB, Terry R et al. Antacid induction of phosphate depletion syndrome in renal failure. *West J Med.* 1974; 120:157–60.
37. Vianna NJ. Severe hypophosphatemia due to hypokalemia. *JAMA.* 1971; 215:1497–8.
38. Turco SJ, Burke WA. Methods of ordering and use of intravenous phosphate (meq vs. mM). *Hosp Pharm.* 1975; 10:320–6.
39. Pestana C, ed. Fluids and electrolytes in the surgical patient. 3rd ed. Baltimore: Williams & Wilkins, 1985:24.
40. McSweeney GW. Parenteral nutrition. In: Katcher BS, Young LY, Koda-Kimble MA, eds. Applied therapeutics: the clinical use of drugs. San Francisco: Applied Therapeutics, Inc.; 1983:629–50.
41. Youssef HA. Hypophosphatemic respiratory failure complicating total parenteral nutrition—an iatrogenic potentially lethal hazard. *Anesthesiology.* 1982; 57:246. Letter.
42. Weinsier RL, Krumdieck CL. Death resulting from overzealous total parenteral nutrition: the refeeding syndrome revisited. *Am J Clin Nutr.* 1981; 34:393–9.
43. Berkelhammer C, Bear RA. A clinical approach to common electrolyte problems: 3. Hypophosphatemia. *Can Med Assoc J.* 1984; 130:17–23.
44. Dickerson RN. Treating hypophosphatemia. *Hosp Pharm.* 1985; 20:920–5.
45. Lentz RD, Brown DM, Kjellstrand CM. Treatment of severe hypophosphatemia. *Ann Intern Med.* 1978; 89:941–4.
46. Kebler R, McDonald FD, Cadnapaphornchai P. Dynamic changes in serum phosphorus levels in diabetic ketoacidosis. *Am J Med.* 1985; 79:571–6.
47. Winter RJ, Harris CJ, Phillips LS et al. Diabetic ketoacidosis: induction of hypocalcemia and hypomagnesemia by phosphate therapy. *Am J Med.* 1979; 67:897–900.
48. Kingston M, Al-Siba'I MB. Treatment of severe hypophosphatemia. *Crit Care Med.* 1985; 13:16–8.
49. Chernow B, Rainey TG, Georges LP et al. Iatrogenic hyperphosphatemia: a metabolic consideration in critical care medicine. *Crit Care Med.* 1981; 9:772–4.
50. Shackney S, Hasson J. Precipitous fall in serum calcium, hypotension, and acute renal failure after intravenous phosphate therapy of hypercalcemia. *Ann Intern Med.* 1967; 66:906–16.

"

Keeping Neonates Free of Pain

It has generally been assumed that the ability of a child to feel pain increases with age and that neonates may not perceive pain or may perceive it only minimally. Assumed by whom? Certainly not by those of us at the bedside of critically ill infants, who see them flinch from procedures, startle in response to loud noises, and turn from bright lights and various other forms of stimulation. Not by those who have heard infants' anguished cries and seen their vigorous withdrawals from painful stimuli. Not by those who have observed their increasing heart and respiratory rates and profuse sweating in response to heel sticks or circumcision. And finally, not by those who have seen babies gasp for every breath as they die from incurable chronic lung disease. . . .

The reason [that certain painful] procedures are done without anesthesia is not barbarism. One must remember that neonatology, and perhaps neonatal anesthesiology specifically, are relatively new fields. Many sick neonates who are surviving through intensive care and surgery today would not have lived 20 years ago. In our preoccupation with survival and improved outcome, relatively little attention has been paid to pain and its control. It was not indifference or lack of concern but a lack of awareness and a fixed but unfocused outlook that led to this situation. . . .

[T]he evidence that nociceptive activity constitutes a physiologic stress in newborns is so overwhelming that physicians can no longer act as if infants were indifferent to pain. Neonatologists, anesthesiologists, and surgeons must join with parents to guarantee that the best is done for newborns and to ensure that they are kept as free of pain as possible.

—Fletcher AB. Pain in the neonate. *N Engl J Med.* 1987; 317:1347–8. Editorial. "

Research

Comparison of equal-weight oral dosages of verapamil hydrochloride and diltiazem hydrochloride in patients with mild to moderate hypertension

JOHN W. HOLLIFIELD, JAMES J. HEUSNER, MARY DESCHAMPS, JAMES GRAY, DANIEL A. SPYKER, KARL E. PEACE, AND BRIAN DICKSON

Abstract: The clinical efficacy, safety, and tolerability of oral verapamil and diltiazem, at total daily dosages of equal weight, were evaluated in a placebo-controlled, double-blind crossover study.

Thirty-six ambulatory patients with chronic, stable, mild to moderate hypertension (supine diastolic blood pressure of 94–116 mm Hg) received a dosage of either verapamil or diltiazem 80 mg t.i.d. as the hydrochloride salt for one week after an antihypertensive-drug washout period. Each then received 120 mg of the same drug t.i.d. for one week. After another two-week washout period, the patients were crossed over to the other drug. Each patient had a 12-lead electrocardiogram and measurement of supine and standing blood pressure weekly.

In the 32 patients completing the study, low-dose verapamil reduced supine diastolic blood pressure (DBP) from a mean of 101.5 ± 5.2 to 95.3 ± 9.5 mm Hg; high dose verapamil reduced DBP to 90.9 ± 7.4 mm Hg. Standing DBP was reduced to a similar degree. Diltiazem showed an almost identical effect: Supine DBP was reduced from a mean of 101.7 ± 5.3 to 94.0 ± 10.1 mm Hg with the low dose and to 91.0 ± 8.6 mm Hg with the high dose, with similar effects on standing DBP. The high dose of both drugs significantly increased the QT_C interval, and both doses of diltiazem significantly increased the PR interval compared with baseline.

Both drugs exhibited consistent efficacy with minimal adverse effects. The electrophysiologic safety profile of verapamil was superior to that of diltiazem.

Index terms: Cardiac drugs; Diltiazem hydrochloride; Dosage; Hypertension; Toxicity; Verapamil hydrochloride
Clin Pharm. 1988; 7:129–34

The calcium-channel blockers verapamil and diltiazem have demonstrated efficacy in the treatment of angina pectoris[1] and hypertension. Since they are so well tolerated, they encourage compliance. In addition, verapamil has recently been approved in the United States for the treatment of hypertension. Because the comparative antihypertensive efficacy of equal doses of verapamil and diltiazem has not been evaluated previously, this study was undertaken to evaluate the clinical efficacy, safety, and tolerability of oral verapamil and diltiazem, at total daily dosages of equal weight in milligrams, in outpatients with chronic, stable, mild to moderate hypertension. The effects of both drugs on electrophysiologic measurements were also compared.

JOHN W. HOLLIFIELD, M.D., is Director, Center for Blood Pressure Control, and Clinical Instructor, Department of Medicine, University of Tennessee and Baptist Hospital, Nashville, TN. JAMES J. HEUSNER, PH.D., is Senior Clinical Research Scientist, Scientific Affairs, U.S. Region, Searle Laboratories. MARY DESCHAMPS is a nurse on the staff of Hypertension Research Associates, Inc., Nashville, TN. JAMES GRAY, M.D., is Associate Professor of Medicine, Department of Medicine, Baylor University, Waco, TX. DANIEL A. SPYKER, M.D., is Associate Professor of Medicine, University of Virginia School of Medicine, Charlottesville, VA. KARL E. PEACE, PH.D., is Senior Director, G.I. Clinical Studies, Clinical Data Information Management, Corporate Medical & Scientific Affairs, Searle Laboratories. BRIAN DICKSON, M.D., is Vice President, Scientific Affairs, U.S. Region, Searle Laboratories.

Address reprint requests to Dr. Hollifield at the Hypertension Center of Nashville, 1900 Patterson Street, Nashville, TN 37203.

Presented at the Clinical Research Forum, 22nd Annual ASHP Midyear Clinical Meeting, Atlanta, GA, December 9, 1987.

Copyright © 1988, American Society of Hospital Pharmacists, Inc. All rights reserved. 0278-2677/88/0201-0129$01.50.

Methods

Thirty-six ambulatory patients from two centers participated in this randomized, double-blind crossover study with a single-blind placebo washout period before the study and between treatments. Written informed consent was obtained after approval by appropriate institutional review boards. Inclusion criteria provided for men and women aged 45 to 80 years with mild to moderate hypertension and a resting supine diastolic blood pressure (DBP) between 94 and 116 mm Hg. Six patients, two of whom were 43 years old and four of whom were 44 years old, were included in the analysis as exceptions to the protocol. Exclusion criteria included severe cardiac disease (e.g., unstable angina, serious conduction abnormality, history of stroke, myocardial infarction, or coronary-artery bypass graft within the past three months), presence of substantial renal or liver dysfunction, pregnancy, noncompliance, or concomitant use of diuretics, antihypertensive drugs, or investigational agents.

Commercially available verapamil hydrochloride and diltiazem hydrochloride were used in this study. Tablets, broken along the scored lines, were inserted in opaque capsules for the purpose of blinding. All capsules (active and placebo) were identical in appearance.

The study design is described in Figure 1. All antihypertensive medications were discontinued for at least one week before visit 0; patients whose antihypertensive medications required gradual withdrawal were seen by the investigator once each week during the withdrawal period. At visit 0, an initial baseline blood pressure was taken and patients were evaluated through the results of a general medical and cardiovascular history, complete physical examination, and 12-lead electrocardiogram (ECG). After an additional one-week placebo washout period, eligible patients, as determined by a supine DBP of 94–116 mm Hg, were then randomized to one of two active treatments for a one-week course of therapy. Group A received 80 mg of verapamil hydrochloride three times daily (t.i.d.) and group B received 80 mg of diltiazem hydrochloride three times daily (t.i.d.) for one week. In both groups, the dose of each drug was increased after the first week of treatment to 120 mg t.i.d. (high dose); this dose was also given for a one-week period. At the end of the first two-week double-blind phase, patients entered a two-week placebo washout phase and were then crossed over to the second double-blind phase in which they were treated with the low dose of the other active treatment for one week, followed by the high dose for one week.

Figure 1. Design for comparative study of the calcium-channel blockers (CCBs) verapamil and diltiazem. The duration of the washout period was dependent on the type of previous antihypertensive medication.

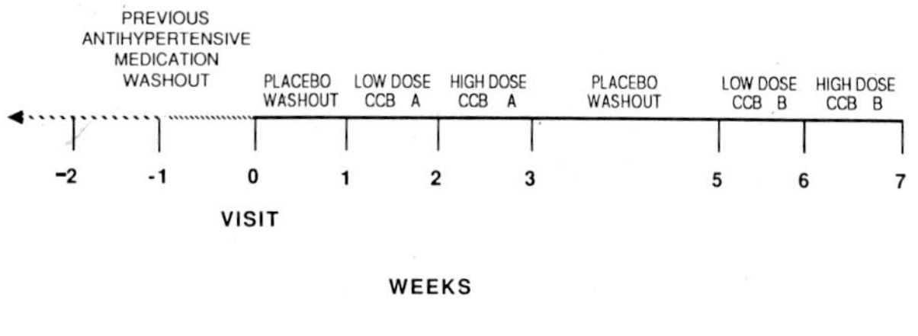

Blood pressure (BP) was measured and recorded weekly, preferably in the morning. Patients were instructed to hold their morning dose of medication on the day of each clinic visit. The patients were placed in the supine position for 10 minutes and, after this rest period, BP measurements were taken in the non-dominant arm every two minutes until two consecutive readings were within 4 mm Hg. The average of the last two readings was used to determine baseline values and drug response. Heart rate was measured in conjunction with each BP measurement. After completion of the supine measurements, the patients were asked to stand, and BP and pulse were measured immediately and after two minutes. Phases I and V of the Korotkoff sounds were used for systolic and diastolic measurements, respectively.

In addition to BP and heart rate measurements, 12-lead ECG readings and interim assessments (i.e., clinical changes in the physical examination results, with particular attention to the cardiovascular system, symptomatology, review of concomitant therapy and compliance check) were done weekly, beginning at baseline. Adverse effects were also evaluated weekly and graded subjectively by the investigators with respect to severity (mild, moderate, or severe) and relationship to study drug (remote, possible, or probable). A complete blood count with differential and platelet estimate and blood chemistry analysis and a urinalysis were done at the end of weeks 1, 3, and 7. Physical examinations were performed before and after the study.

Statistical Methods. All pairwise comparisons were carried out using within-patient differences. For comparisons between baseline and on-study response to each regimen, and for comparisons between responses to the two compounds, Student's t test with average differences and the associated patient-to-patient standard deviation was used, with an a priori p value ≤ 0.05 considered significant.

Results

Of the 36 patients initially enrolled, 32 completed the four treatment phases defined by the protocol. Three patients dropped out during the first active phase, for the following reasons: urinary tract infection, anxiety-related adverse effects, and supine DBP of 85 mm Hg. One patient was dropped because of adverse effects during the placebo washout (week 5) before entering the crossover active treatment. The characteristics of the 32 patients were as follows: 19 men and 13 women; 23 Caucasians and 9 blacks; mean age 55.3 years; mean height 67 inches; and mean weight 86.9 kilograms. The patients selected from each of the participating study centers differed only with respect to age; there was a mean difference between the two groups of 9.9 years. There were no significant demographic differences among the patients in the various treatment regimens.

Figure 2 summarizes the antihypertensive effects of both drugs. Table 1 presents the means ± standard deviations for blood pressure, heart rate, and electrophysiologic data with low-dose verapamil and diltiazem compared with baseline. The reduction in supine DBP (from 101.5 ± 5.2 to 95.3 ± 9.5 mm Hg) and in supine SBP (from 160.1 ± 18.4 to 154.3 ± 18.5 mm Hg) with low-dose verapamil was significant. Standing DBP and SBP were also significantly reduced. None of the other BP, heart rate, or ECG measurements showed significant variation.

Low-dose diltiazem showed an almost identical pattern, with significant reductions in supine DBP (from 101.7 ± 5.3 to 94.0 ± 10.1 mm Hg) and SBP (from 160.3 ± 15.6 to 151.4 ± 18.1 mm Hg), as well as in standing DBP and SBP. None of the other BP, heart rate, or ECG measurements showed significant variation, with the exception of the PR interval, which was prolonged to 104% of baseline.

Table 2 presents the mean BP, heart rate, and electrophysiologic data for high-dose verapamil and diltiazem compared with baseline. Supine DBP and SBP were significantly decreased with high dose verapamil (101.5 ± 5.2 to 90.9 ± 7.4 mm Hg and 160.1 ± 18.4 to 146.9 ± 17.2 mm Hg, respectively). Standing DBP and SBP were also significantly reduced. No other BP, heart rate, or ECG measurement showed a significant change except the QT_C interval, which increased to 103% of baseline.

High-dose diltiazem also significantly reduced supine DBP (from 101.7 ± 5.3 to 91.0 ± 8.6 mm Hg) and SBP (from 160.3 ± 15.6 to 149.6 ± 14.6 mm Hg), as well as standing DBP and SBP. There were no other significant changes in BP and heart rate mea-

Figure 2. Supine systolic and diastolic blood pressures (mean ± S.D.) for 32 study patients treated with equal low and high dosages of verapamil or diltiazem. Asterisk indicates significant difference from baseline.

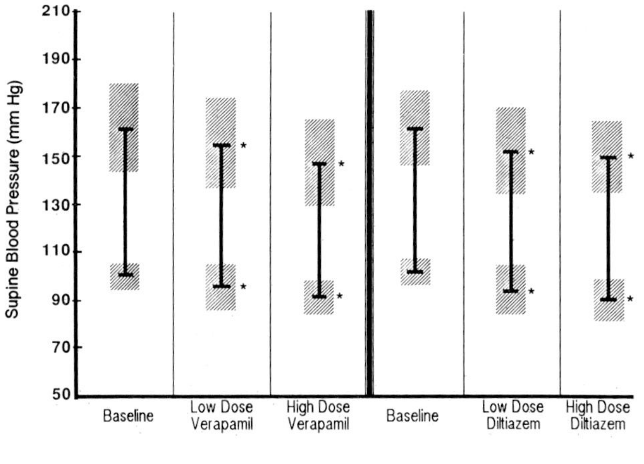

Table 1.
Mean (± S.D.) Blood Pressure and Electrocardiogram Readings of 32 Patients Receiving Low-Dose Verapamil or Diltiazem

Variable[a]	Low-Dose Drug Treatment	Baseline	Difference
Verapamil			
Supine			
Diastolic BP	95.3 ± 9.5	101.5 ± 5.2	−6.2 ± 8.2[b]
Systolic BP	154.3 ± 18.5	160.1 ± 18.4	−5.9 ± 13.1[b]
Heart rate	71.3 ± 8.4	71.7 ± 8.2	−0.4 ± 5.7
ECG interval			
PR	168.4 ± 24.5	166.6 ± 21.6	1.9 ± 15.1
QRS	73.1 ± 12.8	70.6 ± 12.7	2.5 ± 10.5
QT_C	384.1 ± 24.7	380.6 ± 20.8	3.4 ± 25.5
Standing			
Imm systolic BP	151.3 ± 19.0	158.5 ± 16.9	−7.2 ± 18.1[b]
Imm diastolic BP	97.1 ± 10.2	103.8 ± 6.4	−6.7 ± 9.2[b]
Imm heart rate	78.1 ± 8.8	77.0 ± 8.2	1.1 ± 7.5
2-Min systolic BP	151.8 ± 17.5	159.2 ± 16.9	−7.4 ± 18.1[b]
2-Min diastolic BP	98.3 ± 9.4	104.0 ± 6.5	−5.7 ± 8.2[b]
2-Min heart rate	76.3 ± 7.6	75.4 ± 7.5	0.8 ± 6.6
Diltiazem			
Supine			
Diastolic BP	94.0 ± 10.1	101.7 ± 5.3	−7.7 ± 7.8[b]
Systolic BP	151.4 ± 18.1	160.3 ± 15.6	−8.9 ± 12.4[b]
Heart rate	72.0 ± 8.8	73.6 ± 9.5	−1.7 ± 6.5
ECG interval			
PR	172.2 ± 28.4	165.0 ± 26.0	7.2 ± 16.7[b]
QRS	72.5 ± 12.4	72.8 ± 15.5	−0.3 ± 9.0
QT_C	377.5 ± 42.9	373.8 ± 26.2	3.7 ± 34.4
Standing			
Imm systolic BP	150.0 ± 18.5	163.0 ± 16.9	−13.0 ± 14.9[b]
Imm diastolic BP	97.1 ± 10.1	103.9 ± 8.4	−6.8 ± 7.9[b]
Imm heart rate	78.0 ± 10.3	80.8 ± 11.4	−2.8 ± 9.6
2-Min systolic BP	152.2 ± 16.1	163.2 ± 18.6	−10.9 ± 17.3[b]
2-Min diastolic BP	97.3 ± 10.2	105.2 ± 7.0	−7.8 ± 7.0[b]
2-Min heart rate	75.9 ± 9.2	77.1 ± 10.6	−1.3 ± 7.0

[a] Blood pressure in mm Hg, heart rate in beats/minute, ECG intervals in milliseconds; Imm = immediate, 2-Min = after two minutes.
[b] Significant difference.

Table 2.
Mean ± S.D. Blood Pressure and Electrocardiogram Readings of 32 Patients Receiving High-Dose Verapamil or Diltiazem

Variable[a]	High-Dose Drug Treatment	Baseline	Difference
Verapamil			
Supine			
Diastolic BP	90.9 ± 7.4	101.5 ± 5.2	−10.6 ± 6.7[b]
Systolic BP	146.9 ± 17.2	160.1 ± 18.4	−13.3 ± 11.7[b]
Heart rate	70.1 ± 7.8	71.7 ± 8.2	−1.7 ± 5.0
ECG interval			
PR	170.9 ± 24.9	166.6 ± 21.6	4.4 ± 15.0
QRS	73.4 ± 11.2	70.6 ± 12.7	2.8 ± 8.1
QT_C	393.1 ± 30.1	380.6 ± 20.8	12.5 ± 30.2[b]
Standing			
Imm systolic BP	144.2 ± 15.9	158.5 ± 16.9	−14.3 ± 16.5[b]
Imm diastolic BP	93.6 ± 8.6	103.8 ± 6.4	−10.2 ± 7.4[b]
Imm heart rate	76.3 ± 10.9	77.0 ± 8.2	−0.8 ± 10.3
2-Min systolic BP	146.7 ± 17.2	159.2 ± 16.9	−12.5 ± 14.6[b]
2-Min diastolic BP	95.1 ± 9.7	104.0 ± 6.5	−8.9 ± 8.2[b]
2-Min heart rate	74.6 ± 10.7	75.4 ± 7.5	−0.8 ± 9.3
Diltiazem			
Supine			
Diastolic BP	91.0 ± 8.6	101.7 ± 5.3	−10.7 ± 7.2[b]
Systolic BP	149.6 ± 14.6	160.3 ± 15.6	−10.7 ± 12.8[b]
Heart rate	72.0 ± 9.8	73.6 ± 9.5	−1.6 ± 6.9
ECG interval			
PR	172.8 ± 31.2	165.0 ± 26.0	7.8 ± 18.6[b]
QRS	72.5 ± 11.4	72.8 ± 15.5	−0.3 ± 10.0
QT_C	385.3 ± 32.3	373.8 ± 26.2	11.6 ± 24.9[b]
Standing			
Imm systolic BP	147.6 ± 16.6	163.0 ± 16.9	−15.4 ± 14.5[b]
Imm diastolic BP	93.9 ± 9.2	103.9 ± 8.4	−9.9 ± 7.0[b]
Imm heart rate	78.8 ± 11.4	80.8 ± 11.4	−1.9 ± 10.0
2-Min systolic BP	149.3 ± 17.4	163.2 ± 18.6	−13.8 ± 17.7[b]
2-Min diastolic BP	94.2 ± 10.3	105.2 ± 7.0	−11.0 ± 8.7[b]
2-Min heart rate	76.1 ± 10.5	77.1 ± 10.6	−1.1 ± 7.7

[a] Blood pressure in mm Hg, heart rate in beats/minute, ECG intervals in milliseconds; Imm = immediate, 2-Min = after two minutes.
[b] Significant difference.

Table 3.
Mean (± S.D.) Blood Pressure and Electrocardiogram Readings of 32 Patients Receiving Verpamil or Diltiazem

Variable[a]	Verapamil	Diltiazem	Difference
Low-Dose Verapamil versus Diltiazem			
Supine			
Diastolic BP	95.3 ± 9.5	94.0 ± 10.1	1.3 ± 8.2
Systolic BP	154.3 ± 18.5	151.4 ± 18.1	2.8 ± 13.2
Heart rate	71.3 ± 8.4	72.0 ± 8.8	−0.7 ± 7.4
ECG interval			
PR	168.4 ± 24.5	172.2 ± 28.4	−3.8 ± 13.4
QRS	73.1 ± 12.8	72.5 ± 12.4	0.6 ± 11.9
QT_C	384.1 ± 24.7	377.5 ± 42.9	6.6 ± 38.4
Standing			
Imm systolic	151.3 ± 19.0	150.0 ± 18.5	1.3 ± 18.1
Imm diastolic	97.1 ± 10.2	97.1 ± 10.1	−0.1 ± 8.6
Imm heart rate	78.1 ± 8.8	78.0 ± 10.3	0.1 ± 9.5
2-Min systolic	151.8 ± 17.5	152.2 ± 16.1	−0.5 ± 19.1
2-Min diastolic	98.3 ± 9.4	97.3 ± 10.2	1.0 ± 7.6
2-Min heart rate	76.3 ± 7.6	75.9 ± 9.2	0.4 ± 8.7
High-Dose Verapamil versus Diltiazem			
Supine			
Diastolic	90.9 ± 7.4	91.0 ± 8.6	−0.1 ± 6.5
Systolic	146.9 ± 17.2	149.6 ± 14.6	−2.7 ± 13.3
Heart rate	70.1 ± 7.8	72.0 ± 9.8	−2.0 ± 7.8
ECG interval			
PR	170.9 ± 24.9	172.8 ± 31.2	−1.9 ± 16.5
QRS	73.4 ± 11.2	72.5 ± 11.4	0.9 ± 7.8
QT_C	393.1 ± 30.1	385.3 ± 32.3	7.8 ± 30.0
Standing			
Imm systolic	144.2 ± 15.9	147.6 ± 16.6	−3.4 ± 13.6
Imm diastolic	93.6 ± 8.6	93.9 ± 9.2	−0.4 ± 7.4
Imm heart rate	76.3 ± 10.9	78.8 ± 11.4	−2.6 ± 8.4
2-MIn systolic	146.7 ± 17.2	149.3 ± 17.4	−2.7 ± 13.9
2-Min diastolic	95.1 ± 9.7	94.2 ± 10.3	0.9 ± 8.4
2-Min heart rate	74.6 ± 10.7	76.1 ± 10.5	−1.4 ± 9.4

[a] Blood pressure in mm Hg, heart rate in beats/minute, ECG intervals in milliseconds; Imm = immediate, 2-Min = after two minutes.
[b] Significant difference.

surements, but this dosage level significantly prolonged the PR interval (105% of baseline) and the QT_C interval (103% of baseline).

Table 3 compares the BP, heart rate, and electrophysiologic measurements for verapamil and diltiazem. There was no difference between the two drugs for either low or high doses in BP, heart rate, or ECG measurements. The ECGs of two patients exhibited asymptomatic nonspecific T-wave changes; one occurred with high-dose verapamil and one with high-dose diltiazem. Both resolved during the placebo washout period without sequelae.

Figures 3, 4, and 5 summarize the electrophysiologic effects of verapamil and diltiazem. Both drugs significantly increased the QT_C interval during high-dose treatment. Neither verapamil nor diltiazem significantly affected QRS duration, although there was a trend toward an increase from baseline with verapamil. Diltiazem significantly prolonged PR interval at both low-dose and high-dose levels.

The biochemical and hematologic variables examined for drug effect included glucose, aspartate aminotransferase, alanine aminotransferase, urea nitrogen, alkaline phosphatase, total protein, serum creatinine, total bilirubin, and eosinophil and lymphocyte percentages. No clinically important changes occurred in any of these measurements.

Forty-four adverse events were reported during the study; half occurred with active treatment and half with placebo. The number of incidents of each event is displayed in Table 4. The overall safety profiles for each of the two compounds were generally similar.

Figure 3. Measurements of QT_C interval (mean ± S.D.) for 32 study patients treated with equal low and high dosages of verapamil or diltiazem. Asterisk indicates significant difference from baseline.

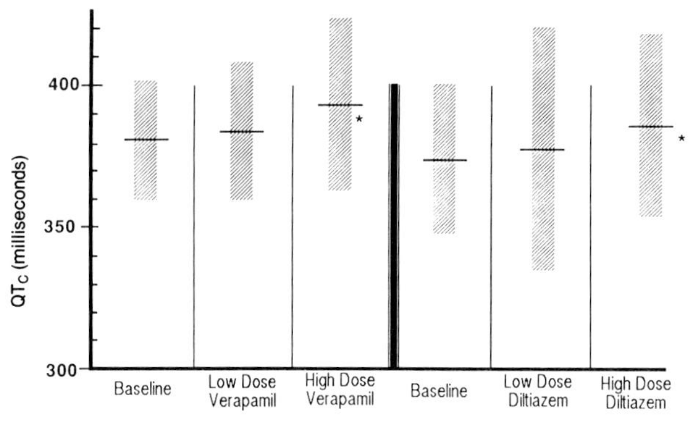

Figure 4. Measurements of QRS interval (mean ± S.D.) for 32 patients treated with equal low and high dosages of verapamil or diltiazem.

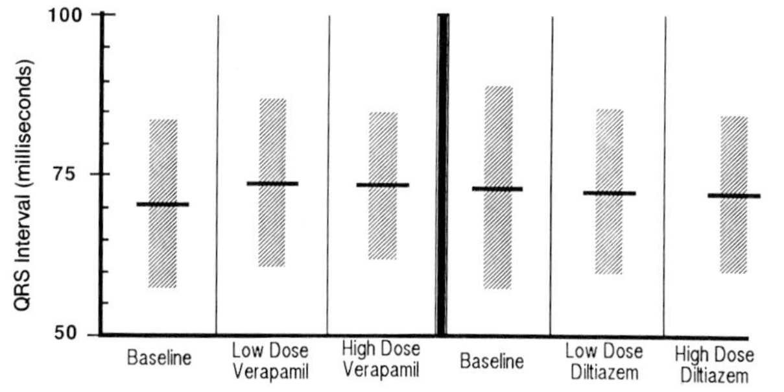

Figure 5. Measurements of PR interval (mean ± S.D.) for 32 patients treated with equal low and high dosages of verapamil or diltiazem. Asterisk indicates significant difference from baseline.

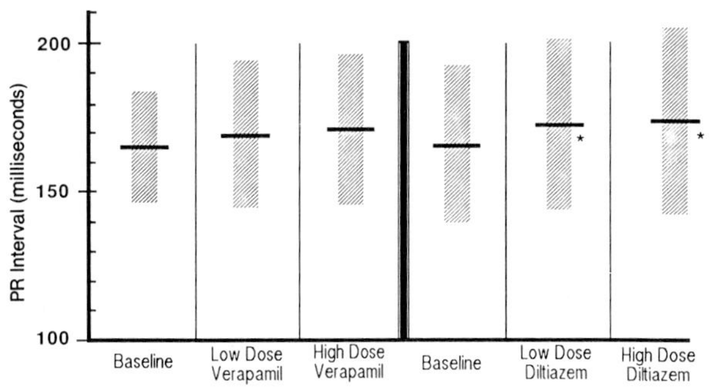

With the exception of two adverse events considered "probably" related to drug therapy, all the other adverse effects were considered to be either possibly or remotely related to study medication. One of the two "probably" related events was first degree (1%) A–V block, which developed during treatment with both agents at both low and high doses and was considered "mild"; no action was taken and the block resolved. The other adverse event was a rash occurring during diltiazem therapy, considered "moderate" in severity; it was treated with diphenhydramine hydrochloride 50 mg q.i.d., and the patient was withdrawn from the study. The rash resolved in nine days without any sequelae. This patient was not included in the efficacy analysis.

Table 4.
Adverse Events during Verapamil, Diltiazem, and Placebo Phases of Study

Adverse Event	No. of Incidents
Verapamil	
Headache	2
Dizziness	2
Leg cramps	2
Skin rash	2
Increased PR interval	1
Right ear "closed"	1
Sinus congestion	1
Back discomfort	1
Diltiazem	
Headache	2
Sinus congestion	2
Increased PR interval	1
Anxiety	1
Tinnitus	1
Rash	1
Low-grade fever	1
Cold or stuffy nose or cough	1
Urinary-tract infection	1
Placebo	
Headache	8
Dizziness	2
Sore throat	2
Tiredness	1
Weakness	1
Head congestion	1
Sinus congestion	1
Sleeplessness	1
Back discomfort	1
"Rapid heart beat"	1
Nervousness	1
"Cold"	1
Infected right ear	1

Discussion

Calcium flow and its regulation are thought to play a major role in the pathogenesis of hypertension.[2,3] It has been theorized that calcium antagonists reverse the increased entry of calcium into the smooth-muscle cell and appear to reverse the physiology of hypertension.[4] The Joint National Committee on the Detection, Evaluation and Treatment of Hypertension, in a 1984 reassessment of the "stepped-care" approach to the treatment of hypertension, suggested that antihypertensive agents such as calcium-channel blockers might play potentially useful roles as therapy for mild to moderate essential hypertension.

This drug class has been reported to be effective in a variety of cardiovascular disorders including angina and supraventricular arrhythmias[5,6] as well as in hypertension.[7–9] However, there are few studies directly comparing calcium-channel blockers as therapy for hypertension.

Conclusion

This study has demonstrated a reduction in blood pressure at equal oral doses of verapamil or diltiazem, which occurred without a reduction in heart rate. The primary distinction between these two agents was a significant prolongation of the PR interval during diltiazem treatment. Our results indicate that verapamil is a well-tolerated and efficacious alternative treatment in step one monotherapy of mild to moderate hypertension.

References

1. Frishman WH, Sonneblick EH. Calcium channel blockers. In: Hurst JW, Logue RB, Rackley CE et al., eds. The heart. New York: McGraw-Hill; 1986:1624–39.
2. Hulthen UL, Bolli P, Buhler FR. Calcium influx mediated vasoconstriction: studies in patients with mild and moderate essential hypertension. *J Hypertens.* 1983; 1 (Suppl 2):105–8.
3. Muller FB, Bolli P, Erne P et al. Use of calcium antagonists as monotherapy in the management of hypertension. *Am J Med.* 1984; 7:11–5.
4. Resnick L. Calcium metabolism in essential hypertension. In: Epstein S, ed. Current status of calcium channel blockers in hypertension. New York: Biomed Info Corp; 1986:19–26.
5. Winnifordd MD, Mauritson DR, Hillis LD. Verapamil therapy for paroxysmal supraventricular tachycardia. In: Packer M, Frishman WH, eds. Calcium channel antagonists in cardiovascular disease. Norwalk, CT: Appleton-Century-Crofts; 1984:245–56.
6. Opie LH. Calcium antagonists. Mechanism, therapeutic indications and reservations: a review. *Q J Med.* 1984; 53:1–16.
7. Anavekar SN, Christophidis N, Louis WJ et al. Verapamil in the treatment of hypertension. *J Cardiovasc Pharmacol.* 1981; 3:287–92.
8. Frishman WH, Weinberg P, Peled H et al. Calcium entry blockers for the treatment of severe hypertension and hypertensive crisis. *Am J Med.* 1984; 77(2b):35–45.
9. Halperin AK, Cubeddu LX. The role of calcium channel blockers in the treatment of hypertension. *Am Heart J.* 1986; 111:363–82.

“

Indications for Low-Osmolality Contrast Agents

. . . In most patients whose conditions are stable and uncomplicated, conventional [contrast] agents should be used. In patients with marked anxiety or those in whom pain, nausea, or vomiting might be hazardous because of underlying cardiac, pulmonary, or central nervous system disease or because of resultant inability to cooperate, one of the three low-osmolality agents should be used. Alternatively, digital subtraction arteriography may be substituted for certain studies, using a diluted conventional agent with lowered osmolality. In patients with a strong allergic diathesis or a history of a clear reaction following the administration of a contrast agent (i.e., other than pain, nausea, or a vasovagal response), pretreatment with a two-dose regimen of corticosteroids can be given. . . . In patients with renal dysfunction, an argument can be made for either conventional or lower-osmolality agents, and it is best to limit the dose of contrast and encourage diuresis. In patients with marked cardiac dysfunction, and probably in those with severe pulmonary disease and secondary right heart failure, it is advisable, mainly on the basis of experimental data, to use one of the three new agents.

—Bettmann MA. Radiographic contrast agents—a perspective. *N Engl J Med.* 1987; 317:891–3. Editorial.

”

Comparative bioavailability of two oral sustained-release procainamide products

Brian A. Baker, John R. Reynolds, Louis Gleckel, Edward A'Zary, and Monty M. Bodenheimer

Abstract: The bioavailability characteristics of two sustained-release oral procainamide preparations, Procan SR and Pronestyl-SR, were compared in 10 patients with arrhythmias.

Each patient was randomly assigned to receive either Procan SR 1 g or Pronestyl-SR 1 g, both administered orally every six hours. The initial drug was continued for 48 hours (eight doses), at which time the second drug, given at the same dosage and dosing interval, was substituted for a 48-hour period. Serum samples for procainamide determination were obtained hourly between 42 and 48 and between 90 and 96 hours after initiation of procainamide therapy. Values for area under the serum concentration–time curve (AUC) during the steady-state dosing interval, maximum serum drug concentration (C_{max}), minimum serum drug concentration (C_{min}), C_{max}:C_{min} ratio (representing fluctuations in serum drug concentrations within the dosing interval), and the time to maximum serum drug concentration (t_{max}) were determined.

Mean (± S.D.) t_{max} values for Procan SR and Pronestyl-SR were 2.2 ± 0.8 hours and 3.8 ± 1.1 hours, respectively. Only the differences between t_{max} values were statistically significant. The study had an 83% chance of detecting a 20% difference in AUC values. The chances of detecting a 20% difference in values for C_{max} and C_{min} were 62% and 71%, respectively.

These two preparations would probably possess similar therapeutic properties when given at the same dosage and dosing schedule; however, studies with larger subject populations are needed to project bioavailability data to the general population.

Index terms: Arrhythmia; Blood levels; Cardiac drugs; Drugs, availability; Equivalency, generic; Procainamide hydrochloride; Sustained-action medications
Clin Pharm. 1988; 7:135–138

Procainamide hydrochloride is used extensively in the prophylaxis and treatment of cardiac arrhythmias. Because of an average half-life of 2.5 to 3.5 hours,[1-3] non-sustained-release (conventional) formulations of procainamide must be administered every three to four hours in most patients to maintain therapeutic serum concentrations of drug throughout the dosing interval. A relationship between serum drug concentrations and therapeutic effects has been established.[2,4-8] When serum drug concentrations fluctuate substantially, peak concentrations may be excessive and result in toxic effects. Conversely, subtherapeutic serum drug concentrations occurring immediately before the next dose may increase the likelihood of "breakthrough" arrhythmias.[9]

With sustained-release procainamide formulations, these limitations are partly overcome because the drug concentrations throughout the dosing interval fluctuate less. Procan SR (Parke–Davis, Morris Plains, NJ) is formulated in a wax matrix that facilitates prolonged release of the drug throughout the gastrointestinal tract. Pronestyl-SR (E. R. Squibb & Sons Inc., Princeton, NJ) consists of a bilayer polymer that interacts with the environment of the gastrointestinal tract to form a gummy, nondisintegrating matrix core. It is this polymer matrix that controls drug release, a process that occurs by diffusion. In addition, a tablet coating controls drug release during the first 30 to 60 minutes after oral administration. The differences between these two formulations conceivably could result in dissimilar release characteristics. Studies have compared the pharmacokinetics of various sustained-release procainamide formulations[10,11]; however, to our knowledge Procan SR and Pronestyl-SR, the two most widely prescribed oral sustained-release procainamide preparations, have not been compared. The objective of our study was to compare the bioavailability characteristics of these two products in patients requiring procainamide for the treatment of arrhythmias.

Brian A. Baker, Pharm.D., is Assistant Clinical Professor, College of Pharmacy, St. John's University, Jamaica, NY, and Clinical Coordinator—Cardiology, Department of Pharmacy Services, Long Island Jewish Medical Center (LIJMC), New Hyde Park, NY. John R. Reynolds, Pharm.D., is Associate Clinical Professor, College of Pharmacy, St. John's University, and Clinical Pharmacokinetic Coordinator, Department of Pharmacy Services, LIJMC. Louis Gleckel, M.D., is Cardiology Fellow, Department of Cardiology, LIJMC. Edward A'Zary, Ph.D., is Director of Toxicology Laboratory, LIJMC. Monty Bodenheimer, M.D., is Chief of Adult Cardiology, LIJMC, and Professor of Medicine, State University of New York at Stony Brook.

Address reprint requests to Dr. Baker at the College of Pharmacy, St. John's University, Jamaica, NY 11439.

The assistance of the 7 South and coronary-care-unit nursing staff at Long Island Jewish Medical Center is acknowledged.

Presented at the Clinical Research Forum, 22nd Annual ASHP Midyear Clinical Meeting, Atlanta, GA, December 9, 1987.

Copyright © 1988, American Society of Hospital Pharmacists, Inc. All rights reserved. 0278-2677/88/0201-0137$01.00.

Methods

The study used a nonblinded, randomized, crossover design in which each patient served as his or her own control. The study protocol was approved by the institution's review board, and written informed consent was obtained from each patient.

Patients who were eligible for inclusion in the study included (1) those who were diagnosed as having acute myocardial infarction and who required continued antiarrhythmic therapy after discontinuance of lidocaine and (2) non-myocardial-infarction patients who were started on procainamide therapy for arrhythmia control. All patients were hospitalized at the time of the study. The following patients were excluded from the study: patients less than 21 years of age, patients with unstable renal function (greater than 25% change in serum creatinine or blood urea nitrogen during the blood sampling period or one week before) or with evidence of renal insufficiency (indicated by a serum creatinine concentration of greater than 2.0 mg/dL), patients with a history of procainamide allergy or adverse reactions such as lupus-like syndrome or blood dyscrasias, pregnant women, patients with malabsorption syndromes, and patients who were receiving cimetidine or ranitidine.

Seven men and three women participated in the study. The mean (± S.D.) patient weight was 75.1 ± 16.9 kg, and the mean (± S.D.) age was 65.2 ± 11.4 years. Patient characteristics are listed in Table 1. The procainamide dosage used in this study averaged 53.3 mg/kg/day; the therapeutic dosage generally is 50 mg/kg/day.[2,4]

Each patient was randomized to receive either Procan SR 1 g (two 500-mg tablets, lot 00616D) or Pronestyl-SR 1 g (two 500-mg tablets, lot 5A213) orally every six hours. The drug was continued for 48 hours (eight doses), at which time the second drug was substituted for a 48-hour period at the same dosage and dosing interval. Serum samples for procainamide determination were obtained via a heparin lock at 42 (trough concentration), 43, 44, 45, 46, 47, 48, 90 (trough concentration), 91, 92, 93, 94, 95, and 96 hours after initiation of procainamide therapy.

Procainamide was extracted from the serum at an alkaline pH into organic solvent. The organic extract was dried at room temperature, dissolved in mobile phase, and then analyzed by high-performance liquid chromatography on a C18 reverse-phase column.[12] The between-day coefficient of variation for the assay was less than 8% and the limit of detection was 0.2 mg/L.

Values for area under the serum concentration–time curve (AUC) during the steady-state dosing interval, maximum serum drug concentration (C_{max}), minimum serum drug concentration (C_{min}), C_{max}:C_{min} ratio (representing fluctuations in serum drug concentrations within the dosing interval), and time to maximum serum drug concentration (t_{max}) were determined from the serum concentration–time data. The AUC was calculated by the trapezoidal method.[13] Values for C_{max}, C_{min}, and t_{max} were determined by visual inspection of the concentration–time curves. All comparative data were evaluated by Student's t test for paired data. Statistical significance was determined at the p <0.05 level. The power of the statistical test was determined according to the method described by Bolton.[14]

Results and Discussion

Serum drug concentration-versus-time data are shown in Figure 1. Individual patient values and mean values for AUC, C_{max}, C_{min}, C_{max}:C_{min}, and

Table 1.
Patient Characteristics[a]

Patient No.	Age (yr)	Wt (kg)	Sex	Indication(s) for Procainamide Use	Concurrent Disease States	Concurrent Medications
1	65	74.5	F	MI	HTN, DM, hypothyroidism	Insulin, furosemide, levothyroxine, potassium chloride, dipyridamole, verapamil
2	47	90.5	M	VT	MI	Diazepam, aspirin
3	56	90.9	F	AF	RA, HTN	Warfarin, nadolol, hydrochlorothiazide, digoxin, potassium chloride
4	66	103.6	M	PVCs	MI, CHF	Furosemide, digoxin, nifedipine, transdermal nitroglycerin, potassium chloride
5	54	68.2	M	VT	None	Docusate, flurazepam
6	69	72.7	M	AF/PVCs	CHF, CVA	Digoxin
7	83	75.5	M	PVCs	MI	Diltiazem, transdermal nitroglycerin
8	63	56.4	M	PVCs	HTN, angina, MI	Nifedipine, furosemide, digoxin, captopril, potassium chloride, docusate, nitroglycerin ointment, flurazepam
9	67	72.7	M	AF	HTN	Nadolol, minoxidil, furosemide, digoxin, low-dose heparin
10	82	45.5	F	SVT/PVCs	None	Digoxin, triazolam, ferrous sulfate, folate

[a] MI = myocardial infarction, HTN = hypertension, DM = diabetes mellitus, VT = ventricular tachycardia, AF = atrial fibrillation, RA = rheumatoid arthritis, PVCs = premature ventricular contractions, CHF = congestive heart failure, CVA = cerebrovascular accident, SVT = supraventricular tachycardia.

t_{max} are reported in Table 2. Only the differences between t_{max} values were significant. The power analysis indicated that there was an 83%, 62%, and 71% chance of detecting 20% differences in AUC, C_{max}, and C_{min} values, respectively.

The characteristics of the plotted data for serum drug concentration versus time, which shape the AUC, are different between rapidly absorbed and slowly absorbed drugs. This difference is evidenced by differences in C_{max} and t_{max} values. Despite a significant difference in t_{max} values for the two sustained-release preparations in this study, there was no significant difference in the AUC values. Therefore, we can assume that the total amount of drug absorbed from each formulation throughout the dosing interval was the same.

In general, patients receiving Procan SR exhibited earlier C_{max} values (i.e., lower t_{max} values) than those receiving Pronestyl-SR; this was found to be statistically significant. The mean (± S.D.) t_{max} values for Procan SR and Pronestyl-SR were 2.2 ± 0.8 hours and 3.8 ± 1.1 hours, respectively. By comparison, peak serum drug concentrations generally occur within 0.75 to 2 hours after oral administration of non-sustained-release procainamide preparations.[2,4,5] This suggests that management of acute arrhythmias should be initiated with non-sustained-release preparations, or, if necessary, the injectable drug. Sustained-release preparations appear to be best suited either for long-term maintenance therapy or for initiating antiarrhythmic therapy in patients for whom therapy is not deemed urgent.

It is interesting to note that t_{max} values for patients 9 and 10 occurred at the end of the dosing interval after administration of Pronestyl-SR. It has been reported that gastrointestinal absorption of procainamide from non-sustained-release formulations is delayed in many patients compared with that in healthy volunteers.[3,4] The factors that are responsible for this delayed rate of absorption for orally administered procainamide are unknown, but they may include disease states such as congestive heart failure, acute myocardial infarction, delayed gastric emptying rates, and drug–drug interactions. Whether these factors also affect the absorption of sustained-release procainamide preparations is unclear. However, none of these conditions was evident in either of these patients.

Despite the differences between the t_{max} values of the two preparations, it is unlikely that a clinically important difference exists because the respective C_{max} and C_{max}:C_{min} values are similar. The C_{max}:C_{min} ratio represents fluctuations of serum drug concentrations within a specific dosing interval. Thus, this ratio indicates the likelihood that, relative to the defined therapeutic range, a patient will have either toxic or subtherapeutic drug concentrations at any time during the dosing interval. For example, a C_{max}:C_{min} ratio of 1.0 demonstrates that no fluctuation in serum drug concentration occurred during the dosing interval, a circumstance similar to that seen with a continuous intra-

Figure 1. Mean (± S.D.) serum procainamide concentrations after administration of Procan SR (▲) and Pronestyl-SR (●), 1 g every six hours.

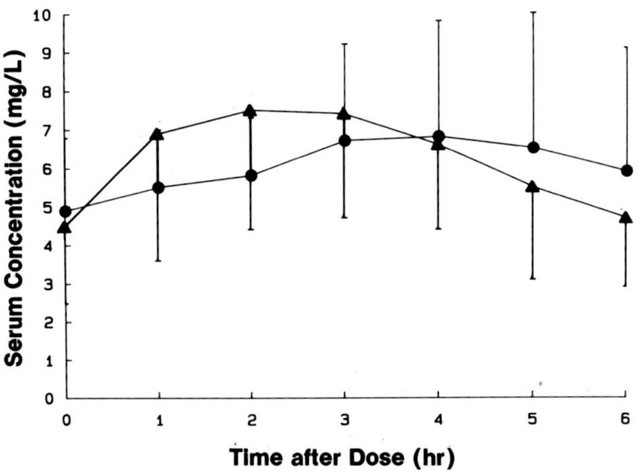

Table 2.
Pharmacokinetics of Procan SR and Pronestyl-SR in Study Patients

Patient No.	Procan SR AUC (mg/L · hr)	C_{max} (mg/L)	C_{min} (mg/L)	C_{max}: C_{min}	t_{max} (hr)	Pronestyl-SR AUC (mg/L · hr)	C_{max} (mg/L)	C_{min} (mg/L)	C_{max}: C_{min}	t_{max} (hr)
1	36.55	8.8	3.4	2.6	3	33.28	6.9	4.0	1.7	4
2	21.21	4.2	2.6	1.6	3	18.14	3.6	2.4	1.5	4
3	25.15	5.3	2.8	1.9	3	24.39	4.7	2.5	1.9	4
4	37.20	6.9	4.6	1.5	2	34.87	6.8	5.0	1.4	3
5	26.40	5.6	2.5	2.2	3	35.59	7.0	2.6	2.7	2
6	34.70	7.8	4.9	1.6	2	36.10	6.5	5.4	1.2	3
7	40.20	8.0	5.2	1.5	1	34.70	7.8	4.1	1.9	3
8	51.00	11.0	6.0	1.8	2	36.35	6.8	5.1	1.3	4
9	31.75	6.9	3.2	2.2	1	42.65	9.6	5.7	1.7	6
10	73.55	14.7	8.4	1.8	2	71.15	15.8	8.2	1.9	5
Mean ± S.D.	37.77 ± 15.17	7.9 ± 3.1	4.4 ± 1.9	1.9 ± 0.4	2.2 ± 0.8[a]	36.72 ± 13.90	7.6 ± 3.3	4.5 ± 1.8	1.7 ± 0.4	3.8 ± 1.1[a]

[a] Significant difference between values for Procan SR and Pronestyl-SR.

venous infusion under steady-state conditions. Conversely, a C_{max}:C_{min} ratio of 2.0 indicates a situation where the serum drug concentration varies twofold within the dosing interval. As compared with the first example (C_{max}:C_{min} ratio of 1.0), these fluctuations in serum drug concentrations are more likely to result in either toxic effects that correspond with excessive peak concentrations or subtherapeutic serum drug concentrations that could lead to the development of "breakthrough" arrhythmias.

Since this study involved administration of multiple doses of procainamide to patients with arrhythmias, there could be no drug washout period. To minimize the influence of a carryover effect from the first procainamide treatment to the second, drug concentration sampling was not performed until 42 hours after initiation of the second therapy. Assuming that steady-state conditions are achieved after approximately four elimination half-lives of fixed-dose, fixed-interval dosing and that the usual elimination half-life of procainamide in patients such as ours is approximately three to six hours, patients were considered to be at steady state after 12 to 24 hours. We delayed blood sampling until 42 hours to ensure that steady state was reached.

Because of the small number of patients studied, it may not be possible to extrapolate the study results to the general population. This study had an 83% chance of detecting a 20% difference in AUC values, indicating that an adequate sample size was used to detect differences in the AUC values. However, the chances of detecting a 20% difference in values for C_{max} and C_{min} were 62% and 71%, respectively.

Conclusion

In the patient population studied, there were no significant differences in the AUC, C_{max}, C_{min}, or C_{max}:C_{min} ratio between Procan SR and Pronestyl-SR. It is likely that these two preparations would possess similar therapeutic properties when given at the same dosage and dosing schedule. Studies with larger subject populations are needed to project comparative bioavailability data to the general population.

References

1. Dutcher JS, Strong JM, Lucas SV et al. Procainamide and *N*-acetylprocainamide kinetics investigated simultaneously with stable isotope methodology. *Clin Pharmacol Ther.* 1977; 22:447–57.
2. Koch-Weser J, Klein SW. Procainamide dosage schedules, plasma concentrations, and clinical effects. *JAMA.* 1971; 215:1454–60.
3. Lima JJ. Procainamide. In: Evans WE, Schentag JJ, Jusko WJ, eds. Applied pharmacokinetics—principles of therapeutic drug monitoring. San Francisco: Applied Therapeutics; 1980:404–35.
4. Giardina EGV, Fenster PE, Bigger JT Jr et al. Efficacy, plasma concentrations and adverse effects of a new sustained release procainamide preparation. *Am J Cardiol.* 1980; 46:855–62.
5. Koch-Weser J. Pharmacokinetics of procainamide in man. *Ann NY Acad Sci.* 1971; 179:370–82.
6. Shaw TRD, Kumana CR, Royds RB et al. Use of plasma levels in evaluation of procainamide dosage. *Br Heart J.* 1974; 36:265–70.
7. Koch-Weser J. Serum procainamide levels as therapeutic guides. *Clin Pharmacokinet.* 1977; 2:389–402.
8. Myerburg RJ, Kessler KM, Kiem I et al. Relationship between plasma levels of procainamide, suppression of premature ventricular complexes and prevention of recurrent ventricular tachycardia. *Circulation.* 1981; 64:280–90.
9. Arstila M, Katila M, Sundquist H et al. Dosage, plasma concentration and antiarrhythmic effect of procainamide in sustained-release tablets. *Acta Med Scand.* 1974; 195:217–22.
10. Ihlen H, Ditlefsen EML. Procainamide in acute myocardial infarction: a study on two different tablet preparations of sustained release type. *Curr Ther Res.* 1975; 18:720–6.
11. Hore P, Bones P, Rollinson T et al. A pharmacokinetic comparison of two sustained-release oral procainamide preparations. *Br J Clin Pharmacol.* 1979; 8:267–71.
12. Butterfield AG, Cooper JK, Midha KK. Simultaneous determination of procainamide and *N*-acetylprocainamide in plasma by high-performance liquid chromatography. *J Pharm Sci.* 1978; 67:839–42.
13. Ritschel WA, ed. Handbook of basic pharmacokinetics. 3rd ed. Hamilton, IL: Drug Intelligence Publications; 1986.
14. Bolton S. Pharmaceutical statistics—practical and clinical applications. New York: Marcel Dekker; 1984.

Indications for Gemfibrozil

"Until all the necessary data are available, it would seem appropriate to consider the use of gemfibrozil in patients with hypercholesterolemia (but without hypertriglyceridemia) that is insufficiently responsive to diet, weight control, and the resins or nicotinic acid or both, especially when HDL cholesterol levels are low. Its relative lack of side effects may ensure better compliance than is usual with the first-choice drugs. Gemfibrozil is also suitable for patients with hypertriglyceridemia, with or without hypercholesterolemia, but the effects of treatment should be carefully monitored to ensure that LDL cholesterol levels do not increase. Whatever the final place of gemfibrozil in the treatment scheme, it should be regarded as a welcome addition to that limited group of lipid-altering drugs that have been shown to reduce the incidence of coronary heart disease.

—Rifkind BM. Gemfibrozil, lipids, and coronary risk. *N Engl J Med.* 1987; 317:1279–81. Editorial."

Effect of diphenoxylate with atropine sulfate on the bioavailability of quinidine sulfate in healthy subjects

JOHN J. PONZILLO, JOSEPH M. SCAVONE, ROBERT P. PAONE, GEORGE P. LEWIS, CAROLYN M. RAYMENT, AND WILLIAM E. FITZSIMMONS

Clin Pharm. 1988; 7:139–42

Quinidine sulfate has been used for many years in the treatment of cardiac arrhythmias. Its usefulness has been limited, in part, by adverse effects such as nausea, vomiting, and diarrhea. Gastrointestinal intolerance may occur in as many as 30% of patients and may be severe enough to require discontinuation in as many as 10%.[1,2] These adverse effects may be caused by stimulation of the motor activity of the smooth muscle of the small intestine; they are not related to the dose of quinidine or to the concentration of quinidine in the blood.[3]

The management of quinidine-induced diarrhea has centered on the use of aluminum-containing antacids. This originated from the work of Romankiewicz et al.,[2] who studied the effect of aluminum hydroxide gel (Amphojel, Wyeth) on the absorption of quinidine sulfate. They used a randomized crossover design in four healthy volunteers and concluded that Amphojel had no significant effect on the absorption of quinidine sulfate.

Since the proposed mechanism of quinidine-induced diarrhea is increased smooth-muscle activity, it would seem reasonable to use a drug such as diphenoxylate with atropine sulfate (Lomotil) to decrease intestinal smooth-muscle activity. Before the use of Lomotil for the treatment of quinidine-induced diarrhea can be advocated, the effect of Lomotil on quinidine bioavailability should be studied. Thus, we examined the effect of Lomotil on the single-dose bioavailability of quinidine sulfate.

Methods. *Study Population.* The study group included eight healthy male volunteers. Subjects ranged in age from 20 to 27 years (mean, 22.8 years) and all were within 15% of ideal weight relative to height and frame size. Participants were selected on the basis of finding normal results in the physical examination, 12-lead electrocardiogram, and clinical laboratory tests including automated blood chemistry, complete blood-cell count, and urinalysis. None of the subjects included in the study had cardiac disease, renal or hepatic impairment, allergy to any of the study medications, or a history of a convulsive disorder. In addition, none of the subjects had taken prescription or nonprescription drugs within the last two weeks before the study or ingested alcoholic beverages during the week before the study. The protocol was reviewed and approved by the hospital's institutional review board. The purpose, hazards, and procedures were explained to each participant, and written informed consent was obtained.

Treatments. A randomized crossover design was used for the study. Subjects were assigned to either the control or the treatment group during the first phase of the study. After a washout period of one week, the groups were switched in accordance with the crossover design. Each subject served as his own control.

The control phase consisted of the ingestion of a single 300-mg dose of quinidine sulfate (Rugby Laboratories, lot 28464) on the morning of the study day. The treatment phase consisted of the ingestion of two tablets of diphenoxylate 2.5 mg with atropine sulfate 0.025 mg (Lomotil, Searle

JOHN J. PONZILLO, PHARM.D., is Clinical Pharmacy Specialist in Internal Medicine, The University of Connecticut Health Center, Farmington; at the time of this study, he was a graduate student, Massachusetts College of Pharmacy and Allied Health Sciences (MCP/AHS), Boston, MA. JOSEPH M. SCAVONE, M.S., PHARM.D., is Associate Professor of Clinical Pharmacy, MCP/AHS, and Clinical Research Coordinator, Division of Clinical Pharmacology, New England Medical Center, Boston, MA. ROBERT P. PAONE, PHARM.D., is Associate Professor of Clinical Pharmacy, MCP/AHS, and Associate Director, Division of Clinical Pharmacology, Lemuel Shattuck Hospital, Jamaica Plain, MA. GEORGE P. LEWIS, M.D., is Director, Division of Clinical Pharmacology, Lemuel Shattuck Hospital. CAROLYN M. RAYMENT, PHARM.D., is Director, New England Drug Information Consultation Service, Boston, MA. WILLIAM E. FITZSIMMONS, PHARM.D., is Clinical Pharmacokinetics Specialist, Department of Pharmacy, Rush-Presbyterian-St. Luke's Medical Center, Chicago, IL.

Address reprint requests to Dr. Ponzillo at the Department of Pharmacy, The University of Connecticut Health Center, Farmington, CT 06032.

The assistance of Nathan Lipsyc of Medic Drug, Inc., is acknowledged.

Submitted by Dr. Ponzillo to MCP/AHS in partial fulfillment of requirements for the Pharm.D. degree.

Presented at the Clinical Research Forum, 22nd Annual ASHP Midyear Clinical Meeting, Atlanta, GA, December 9, 1987.

Copyright © 1988, American Society of Hospital Pharmacists, Inc. All rights reserved. 0278-2677/88/0201-0139$01.00.

Pharmaceuticals, Inc., lot 1284-719) at midnight before the study day. On the morning of the study, an additional two tablets of Lomotil were taken approximately 60 minutes before a 300-mg tablet of quinidine sulfate. Subjects fasted for seven hours before and three hours after the ingestion of quinidine. All doses were administered with 120 mL of water.

Sampling. Blood samples (approximately 7 mL) were obtained from each subject either via a heparinized indwelling venous catheter or by direct venipuncture. For both trials, venous blood samples were drawn into heparinized tubes (Vacutainer, Becton-Dickinson, Rutherford, NJ). Samples were obtained at 0, 0.33, 0.66, 1, 1.5, 2, 4, 6, 8, 12, and 24 hours after the administration of the quinidine. The blood samples were centrifuged, and the plasma was separated and frozen at −4 °C until the time of assay.

Concentrations of quinidine in all samples were determined by high-performance liquid chromatography (HPLC),[4-6] with modifications only of the mobile phase to adjust for interlab variability and column age. One milliliter of each subject's plasma, to which 2.5 μg of bupivicaine was added as the internal standard, was alkalinized with 0.25 mL of 1.0 M sodium hyroxide and extracted with 3.0 mL of ethyl acetate. The samples were gently agitated in the upright position on a vortex-type mixer for 60 to 90 seconds. After centrifugation for 10 minutes at 400 *g*, an aliquot of the upper organic layer was transferred to a conical glass tube and evaporated to dryness under mildly reduced pressure at 45 °C. The residue was redissolved with 0.2 mL of the mobile phase. The mobile phase was 21.5% acetonitrile in a 30.1 mM phosphate buffer solution at pH 3.7 as previously described.[4] The buffer was prepared by dissolving 4.1 g of potassium phosphate in 1 L of distilled water containing 4.0 mL of tetrahydrofuran. The pH of the buffer was adjusted to 3.7 with 85% phosphoric acid.

Fifteen microliters of each reconstituted sample was autoinjected and analyzed by HPLC (Waters Associates, Milford, MA). The assay equipment consisted of a solvent-delivery system, ultraviolet absorbance detector (M440), data processor, and automatic sampling system (WHISP 710B). We used a 25-cm μC18 10-μm column (Analytical Sciences Inc., Santa Clara, CA) with a guard holder (Supelco, Bellefonte, PA) employing a LC-18-DB 5 μm cartridge. The column effluent was quantitated with the absorbance detector set at a wavelength of 214 nm with 0.05 absorbance units full scale. The flow rate was 1.5 mL/min, and analyses were performed at room temperature. Standard curves were prepared by similar extractions from drug-free plasma to which known concentrations of quinidine (0.05–10 μg/mL) were added. The sensitivity of this assay was 0.05 μg/mL and the coefficient of variation was less than 4% at all concentrations. In addition, the analytical recovery was 101% over the calibration range. All samples from a given subject's pair of trials were extracted and analyzed on the same day using the same calibration standard.

Pharmacokinetic and Statistical Analysis. Area under the concentration–time curve (AUC), elimination rate constant (k), time to peak concentration (t_{max}), and peak serum concentration (C_{max}) were determined for each treatment regimen. AUC was determined by applying the trapezoidal rule to the observed-plasma-concentration-versus-time data and extrapolating the terminal phase of the linear portion of the curve to infinity. The k value was determined from the slope of the log-linear portion of the concentration-versus-time curve using the BASIC computer program ESTRIP.[7] C_{max} and t_{max} are reported as observed values.

The two-tailed Student's t test for paired data was used to determine statistical difference. Differences were judged to be significant if the results of the test yielded a value for $p < 0.05$.

Results. A summary of the pharmacokinetic analysis is presented in Table 1. Plots of the mean serum concentrations versus time for all subjects during both phases of the study are shown in Figure 1.

Table 1.
Effect of Lomotil Pretreatment on Quinidine Pharmacokinetics[a]

Subject	t_{max} (hr)		C_{max} (μg/mL)		AUC (mg · hr/L)		k (hr^{-1})		$t_{1/2}$ (hr)	
	Control	Treatment	Control	Treatment	Control	Treatment	Control	Treatment	Control	Treatment
1	1.0	1.5	2.94	1.78	18.19	16.65	0.118	0.110	5.87	6.30
2	1.0	1.0	2.77	1.53	24.56	17.36	0.106	0.100	6.54	6.93
3	0.66	1.5	1.47	1.27	13.03	16.79	0.104	0.086	6.66	8.06
4	0.66	0.66	1.58	1.56	11.68	11.86	0.109	0.104	6.36	6.66
5	1.50	2.00	0.88	0.76	10.07	8.84	0.110	0.094	6.30	7.37
6	1.00	1.00	1.38	1.24	9.17	8.48	0.131	0.127	5.29	5.46
7	0.66	1.00	3.74	3.24	27.17	27.81	0.138	0.088	5.02	7.88
8	0.66	1.00	2.03	1.80	8.87	13.38	0.178	0.166	3.89	5.97
Mean ± S.D.	0.89 ± 0.30	1.21 ± 0.43	2.10 ± 0.97	1.65 ± 0.73	15.34 ± 7.17	15.15 ± 6.19	0.124 ± 0.025	0.103 ± 0.014	5.74 ± 0.96	6.83 ± 0.91

[a] Control = quinidine sulfate 300 mg; treatment = two tablets of Lomotil (diphenoxylate 2.5 mg with atropine sulfate 0.025 mg) before quinidine dose.

Figure 1. Mean (± one S.D.) serum quinidine concentration versus time for all subjects. Control phase (□) = quinidine alone; treatment phase (◇) = Lomotil pretreatment plus quinidine.

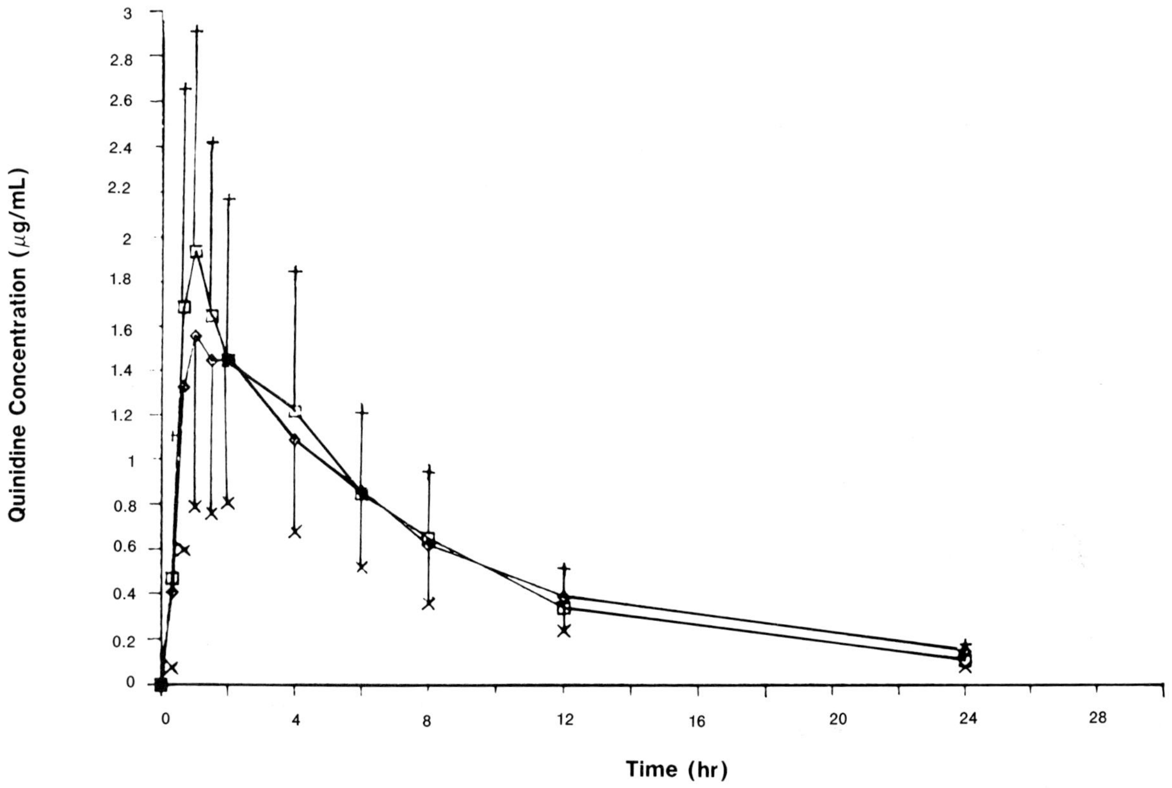

Analysis of t_{max} showed that the peak was reached later for the treatment group than for the control group. The mean t_{max} for the treatment group was 1.21 hr, versus 0.89 hr for the controls. This difference was statistically significant.

The mean C_{max} was lower in the treatment than in the control group (1.65 versus 2.10 μg/mL, respectively). This difference was also significant.

In comparing the data for AUC, we found no significant difference between the treatment and the control groups. In comparing the mean elimination rate constants, we found that the rate of elimination was significantly faster in the control group.

Discussion. The purpose of this study was not to look at the effect of pretreatment with Lomotil on decreasing diarrhea, but rather to study the effect of Lomotil pretreatment on the pharmacokinetics of quinidine sulfate. Many factors affect drug absorption, including changes in gastrointestinal motility. In general, drugs that reduce gastrointestinal motility and emptying rate tend to delay drug absorption.[8]

In this study, the rate of elimination of quinidine was decreased in the treatment group, but this may be due to changes in the rate of absorption. Koup and Gibaldi[9] point out that significant differences in half-life may result from changes in the rate of absorption. That is, treatments that cause a decrease in the rate of absorption may simultaneously affect the rate of decline of the drug concentration in the plasma. In general, the half-life of quinidine was still within the published range of 6.5 to 12 hr.[10-13] The AUC values did not differ significantly between the two groups; thus, the extent of absorption was not different.

In this study, we evaluated an immediate-release preparation of quinidine. Because this was a single-dose study, we did not measure any of the metabolites of quinidine. Thus, a multiple-dose study design would have been clinically more valid.

Conclusion. The coadministration of Lomotil with quinidine sulfate resulted in a significant decrease in C_{max} and k and an increase in t_{max}. There was no significant difference in the extent of absorption as measured by AUC. These data cannot be extrapolated to sustained-release preparations of quinidine because of their different release characteristics.

References

1. Selzer A. When quinidine is the right drug. *Drug Ther.* 1975; 9:115–21.
2. Romankiewicz JA, Reidenberg M, Drayder B. The noninter-

ference of aluminum hydroxide gel with quinidine sulfate: an approach to control quinidine-induced diarrhea. *Am Heart J*. 1978; 96:518–20.
3. Garrett JM, Schlegel JF, Code CF. Effect of quinidine on electrical and motor activity of canine small bowel. *Gut*. 1966; 7:362–5.
4. Dusci LJ, Hackett LP. Simultaneous determination of lidocaine, mexiletine, disopyramide, and quinidine in plasma by high performance liquid chromatography. *J Anal Toxicol*. 1985; 9:67–70.
5. Greenblatt DJ, Maltis R. Rapid high-performance liquid chromatographic analysis of oxaprozin, a non-steroidal anti-inflammatory agent. *J Chromatogr*. 1984; 310:445–9.
6. Greenblatt DJ, Locnistar A. Determination of ciramadol and dezocine, two new analgesics by high-performance liquid chromatography using electrochemical detection. *J Chromatogr*. 1986; 374:215–20.
7. Brown RD, Manno JE. ESTRIP, a BASIC computer program for obtaining initial polyexponential parameter estimates. *J Pharm Sci*. 1978; 67:1687–91.
8. Welling PG. Interactions affecting drug absorption. *Clin Pharmacokinet*. 1984; 9:404–34.
9. Koup JR, Gibaldi M. Some comments on the evaluation of bioavailability data. *Drug Intell Clin Pharm*. 1980; 14:327–30.
10. Ochs HR, Greenblatt DJ, Woo E. Clinical pharmacokinetics of quinidine. *Clin Pharmacokinet*. 1980; 5:150–68.
11. Brown JE, Shand DG. Therapeutic drug monitoring of antiarrhythmic agents. *Clin Pharmacokinet*. 1982; 7:125–48.
12. Greenblatt DJ, Pfeifer HJ, Ochs HR. Pharmacokinetics of quinidine in humans after intravenous, intramuscular, and oral administration. *J Pharmacol Exp Ther*. 1977; 202:365–78.
13. Ochs HR, Greenblatt DJ, Woo E. Single and multiple dose pharmacokinetics of oral quinidine sulfate and gluconate. *Am J Cardiol*. 1978; 41:770–7.

Effect of temperature on in vitro measurement of quinidine free fraction

CATHERINE N. VERME, THOMAS M. LUDDEN, AND STEVEN C. HARRIS

Clin Pharm. 1988; 7:142–6

Quinidine is a highly protein-bound drug frequently used for the treatment of both supraventricular and ventricular arrhythmias. Because of its narrow therapeutic index, monitoring of serum quinidine concentrations is often used to guide dosage adjustments. However, marked interindividual variability in the protein binding of quinidine has been reported. The mean quinidine free fraction reported in healthy volunteers has varied from 0.10[1] to 0.29.[2] Free drug concentrations in plasma or serum are believed to correlate with pharmacologic effects better than total drug concentrations.[3] Thus, the total serum quinidine concentration may not be a reliable indicator of arrhythmia suppression or potential toxicity, and measurement of serum concentration of free quinidine may be preferred.

Some of the discrepancies between studies examining quinidine protein binding may be caused by methodologic differences. Several factors are now known to influence quinidine binding in vitro, including blood-collection techniques[1,4,5] and conditions under which equilibrium dialysis or ultrafiltration is performed.[5] Although equilibrium dialysis followed by high-performance liquid chromatography (HPLC) has been the reference method for measurement of serum concentrations of free quinidine, these procedures are time consuming and are not suitable for routine clinical use. Recently, Ha et al.[6] described a rapid ultrafiltration assay for determination of serum concentration of free quinidine by the enzyme-multiplied immunoassay technique (EMIT). These authors demonstrated a good correlation ($r = 0.959$) between EMIT and HPLC and also between ultrafiltration and equilibrium dialysis when both methods were performed at the same temperature. The importance of adjusting the serum pH to physiologic values before measuring the serum concentration of free quinidine was also confirmed.[6]

Because it is now feasible to measure serum concentrations of free quinidine under clinical conditions by ultrafiltration, it is important to determine the extent to which temperature might influence the results of quinidine protein-binding studies. Woo and Greenblatt,[7] using blood-bank plasma from healthy volunteers supplemented in vitro with quinidine, evaluated the effect of temperature on quinidine binding using equilibrium dialysis. At 24 °C, quinidine unbound fraction was 0.25 ± 0.01 μg/mL, compared with 0.30 ± 0.01 μg/mL at 37 °C. Ha and colleagues[6] also observed temperature-dependent effects in patient samples when ultrafiltration at 25 °C resulted in lower quinidine free fraction values than when equilibrium dialysis at 37 °C was used. When these two methods were performed at the same temperature (25 °C), the quinidine free fraction values observed were similar. However, it is still unknown whether

CATHERINE N. VERME, PHARM.D., is Postgraduate Research Fellow, Research Service, Audie L. Murphy Memorial Veterans Hospital, San Antonio, TX, and The University of Texas Health Science Center at San Antonio. THOMAS M. LUDDEN, PH.D., is Consultant, Audie L. Murphy Memorial Veterans Hospital, and Professor, College of Pharmacy, University of Texas–Austin, and Department of Pharmacology, The University of Texas Health Science Center at San Antonio. STEVEN C. HARRIS, M.D., is Assistant Chief, Laboratory Service, and Chief, Therapeutic Drug Monitoring Laboratory, Audie L. Murphy Memorial Veterans Hospital; Associate Professor of Pathology and Pharmacology, The University of Texas Health Science Center at San Antonio; and Associate Professor of Pharmacy, University of Texas–Austin.

Address reprint requests to Dr. Harris at the University of Texas Health Science Center at San Antonio, 7703 Floyd Curl Drive, San Antonio, TX 78284.

This work was supported by the Veterans Administration.

The assistance of Ginny Wolfe, Duane Boyle, Pharm.D., Cindy Everitt, and Carolyn Mills is acknowledged.

there are intrasubject correlations among quinidine free fraction values obtained at various temperatures. Since ultrafiltration is often performed at room temperature, it is important to know whether free fractions of quinidine obtained at room temperature correlate with those at body temperature. The objective of this study was to compare serum concentrations of free quinidine and quinidine free fraction values obtained at three different temperatures in patient specimens using an enzyme immunoassay technique.

Methods. Serum samples were obtained from 20 men admitted to the Audie L. Murphy Memorial Veterans Hospital who were receiving quinidine and whose serum concentrations of free quinidine were determined for clinical purposes. Patient information is provided in Table 1. All samples were collected by venipuncture into anticoagulant-free Vacutainer-SST tubes (Becton-Dickinson, Rutherford, NJ, lot 6510-7H914). None of the patients was known to be receiving heparin. Our data indicate that the serum specimen from patient 13 was obtained before hemodialysis. However, since the specimen was drawn in the hemodialysis unit, it remains possible that heparin was administered before the serum sample was obtained.

After routine serum concentrations of total quinidine were determined in duplicate by enzyme immunoassay, samples were immediately frozen and stored at −20 °C until free serum quinidine concentrations were determined. All samples were frozen within approximately six hours after collection by venipuncture. The time period between sample collection and analysis of serum concentration of free quinidine varied between one and eight months. Since the same instrument and reagents were used to measure serum concentrations of both total and free quinidine, the measurement

Table 1.
Patient Characteristics

Patient No.	Diseases[a]	Concurrent Medications	Age (yr)	CL_{cr}[b] (mL/min)	Quinidine[c] Free Fraction (μg/mL) 4 °C	25 °C	37 °C
1	VTach, mild CHF	Amitriptyline, diltiazem, dipyridamole, nitroglycerin paste	60	67	0.07	0.13	0.13
2	VTach	Nifedipine, propranolol, furosemide, aspirin, dipyridamole	53	65	0.13	0.17	0.19
3	AFib, COPD, multiple myeloma	Doxepin, diltiazem, isosorbide dinitrate	54	106	0.09	0.15	0.17
4	VTach, mild CHF	Digoxin, warfarin, pentoxifylline	47	107	0.10	0.15	0.17
5	AFib, chronic ALD	Digoxin, nifedipine, ranitidine, ampicillin	61	102	0.13	0.20	0.18
6	AFib, mild CHF	Diltiazem, propranolol, cimetidine, aspirin, dipyridamole	61	70	0.06	0.12	0.13
7	AFib, VTach, COPD	Diltiazem, theophylline, prednisone	71	37	0.10	0.14	0.14
8	AFib, COPD, seizures	Digoxin, phenytoin, theophylline, metaproterenol	75	66	0.15	0.23	0.22
9	AFib, urosepsis	Ampicillin, amikacin	72	53	0.10	0.14	0.15
10	VTach, SVT	Ranitidine, warfarin, penicillin	74	30	0.06	0.11	0.12
11	PVCs, moderate CHF	Digoxin, nifedipine, nitroglycerin paste, ferrous sulfate	73	38	0.06	0.09	0.10
12	VTach, mild CHF, COPD	Thiothixene, lithium, diltiazem, theophylline, dexamethasone	66	79	0.09	0.14	0.16
13	AFib, ESRD (on HD)	Digoxin, nitroglycerin paste, metoclopramide, metronidazole, vancomycin	46	<10	0.19	0.26	0.27
14	AFib, mild CHF, chronic ALD	Digoxin, ampicillin, gentamicin	69	76	0.05	0.09	0.10
15	AFib, history of alcohol abuse	Digoxin, nitroglycerin paste, lorazepam, ranitidine, salsalate	59	85	0.14	0.18	0.21
16	AFib, severe CHF, MI	Digoxin, furosemide, aspirin, oxacillin, gentamicin	64	47	0.13	0.16	0.18
17	AFib	Digoxin, furosemide, aspirin, cefazolin	66	62	0.09	0.12	0.14
18	AFib, prostate CA, Parkinson's	Carbidopa–levodopa	86	38	0.15	0.17	0.19
19	VTach, mild CHF, small-bowel resection	Digoxin, ranitidine, ampicillin, gentamicin, metronidazole	81	32	0.11	0.12	0.13
20	SVT, mild CHF, MI, TB, COPD	Digoxin, verapamil, nitroglycerin paste, isoniazid, rifampin	77	57	0.10	0.11	0.13

[a] VTach = ventricular tachycardia, CHF = congestive heart failure, AFib = atrial fibrillation, COPD = chronic obstructive pulmonary disease, SVT = supraventricular tachycardia, MI = myocardial infarction, PVC = premature ventricular contraction, ESRD = end-stage renal disease, HD = hemodialysis, ALD = alcoholic liver disease, TB = tuberculosis, CA = cancer.

[b] CL_{cr} = creatinine clearance, which was determined by the following equation: (140 − age in years) × ideal body weight/(serum creatinine concentration × 72).

[c] Reported as the mean of duplicate determinations in 20 patients. Group mean ± S.D. at each temperature was as follows: 4 °C = 0.11 ± 0.035 μg/mL, 25 °C = 0.15 ± 0.043 μg/mL, and 37 °C = 0.16 ± 0.043 μg/mL.

of total serum quinidine concentrations was not repeated for this study. It had previously been shown that freezing and thawing of quinidine serum or plasma samples did not affect quinidine binding[7,8] and that samples were stable for at least two months at −20 °C.[8] After our samples were thawed to room temperature, the pH was adjusted to 7.4 with approximately 5–10 μL of 1 M phosphoric acid. Each sample was separated into three 0.75-mL portions and allowed to equilibrate at either 4, 25, or 37 °C. Ultrafiltration was then performed at each temperature, and the serum concentration of free quinidine was measured in duplicate by enzyme immunoassay.

Centrifree Micropartition System filters (Amicon, Danvers, MA, lot MU-0478-GAR) were used for ultrafiltration. Preliminary studies in this laboratory demonstrated that no substantial binding of quinidine to these filters occurred during ultrafiltration of solutions containing either 0.2 or 0.8 μg/mL quinidine base. A 0.75-mL aliquot of each sample was transferred by pipette into the reservoir, and the device was placed into a centrifuge equipped with a 35° fixed-angle head (M rotor, Sorvall-Du Pont Inst., Wilmington, DE). Samples were spun at 1700 g for 15 minutes at all temperatures.

Serum concentrations of both total and free quinidine were determined in duplicate by enzyme immunoassay using the COBAS-BIO Centrifugal Analyzer (Roche Analytical Instruments, Inc., Nutley, NJ) and EMIT quinidine reagents, serum calibrators, and controls (Syva Co., Palo Alto, CA). For measurement of serum concentration of free quinidine, the procedure was identical to that used for total concentrations, except that the sample volume was 15 μL instead of the usual 3 μL. Preliminary studies in this laboratory revealed that measurements in fresh serum samples supplemented with quinidine were approximately 15% higher than in quinidine-supplemented buffer samples. This is presumably due to a matrix effect. To eliminate this effect, calibrators containing 0.0, 0.1, 0.2, 0.4, 0.6, and 0.9 μg/mL quinidine base in tris(hydroxymethyl)aminomethane hydrochloride (Tris-hydrochloride) buffer (adjusted to pH 7.4 with concentrated hydrochloric acid) were prepared and assayed in duplicate. The serum equivalent values obtained by COBAS-BIO for the buffer-based calibrators were adjusted for differences in sample volume and then plotted against the known concentration of quinidine. A regression line was calculated using a weighted linear-regression analysis. From this equation, the serum concentration of free quinidine in each ultrafiltrate was calculated.

To ensure that buffer and ultrafiltrate samples produced similar results with this assay, three replicates each of drug-free ultrafiltrate and buffer were prepared at a concentration of 0.5 μg/mL quinidine base. All solutions were analyzed in triplicate using the procedure previously described. The ultrafiltrate-to-buffer concentration ratio was 1.02; therefore, it was concluded that buffer and ultrafiltrate samples produced similar results with this assay.

Assay performance was assessed by two methods. Previous studies using quinidine in Tris-hydrochloride buffer controls revealed coefficients of variation of 7.2% at 0.15 μg/mL (n = 5) and 3.3% at 0.75 μg/mL (n = 6). To control for the variability of the ultrafiltration process itself, drug-free serum was supplemented with quinidine to produce a total concentration of 3.0 μg/mL. After pH adjustment to 7.4, ultrafiltration was then performed (n = 8), and each ultrafiltrate was analyzed in duplicate for serum concentrations of free quinidine. The coefficient of variation for this procedure was 3.7%, with a mean serum concentration of free quinidine of 0.4 μg/mL.

Statistical analysis was performed using a two-way analysis of variance with a post hoc F test corrected for the number of comparisons.[9] Correlation coefficients were determined by both the Pearson (r) and Spearman Rank (Rs) methods. The a priori level of significance was $p \leq 0.05$.

Results. The mean (±S.D.) quinidine free fraction was 0.11 ± 0.035 at 4 °C, 0.15 ± 0.043 at 25 °C, and 0.16 ± 0.043 at 37 °C. Of 20 patients, 17 had an increase in free fraction as the ultrafiltration temperature increased. The remaining three patients had an increase in free fraction at 25 °C compared with 4 °C but a decrease in free fraction at 37 °C compared with 25 °C. Individual values for quinidine free fraction at different temperatures are included in Table 1 and are illustrated in Figure 1. The differences among the mean free fractions of quinidine at 4 and 25 °C, 25 and 37 °C, and 4 and 37 °C were all significant ($p \leq 0.001$). There was a strong correlation between mean free fraction at 4 and 25 °C (r = 0.893, Rs = 0.842), at 25 and 37 °C (r = 0.960, Rs = 0.964), and at 4 and 37 °C (r = 0.938, Rs = 0.893).

Serum concentrations of free quinidine ranged from 0.10 to 0.54 μg/mL at 4 °C, 0.12 to 0.95 μg/mL at 25 °C, and 0.13 to 1.0 μg/mL at 37 °C. Total serum quinidine concentrations ranged from 0.7 to 4.0 μg/mL. The range of quinidine free fraction was 0.05 to 0.19 at 4 °C, 0.09 to 0.26 at 25 °C, and 0.10 to 0.27 at 37 °C (Figure 1).

No correlation was found between quinidine free fraction and calculated creatinine clearance or age. There was also no correlation found between quinidine free fraction and the concurrent administration of tricyclic antidepressant agents, diltiazem, nifedipine, or enzyme-inducing agents (phenytoin, rifampin).

Discussion. The results of this study indicate there is a measurable change in free fraction of quinidine when ultrafiltration is performed at different temperatures. This is consistent with previ-

Figure 1. Temperature effects on quinidine free fraction. The free fraction of quinidine was calculated as the serum concentration of free quinidine divided by the total serum quinidine concentration. The temperature scale is discrete, and no implication about the shape of the free-fraction-versus-temperature relationship is intended.

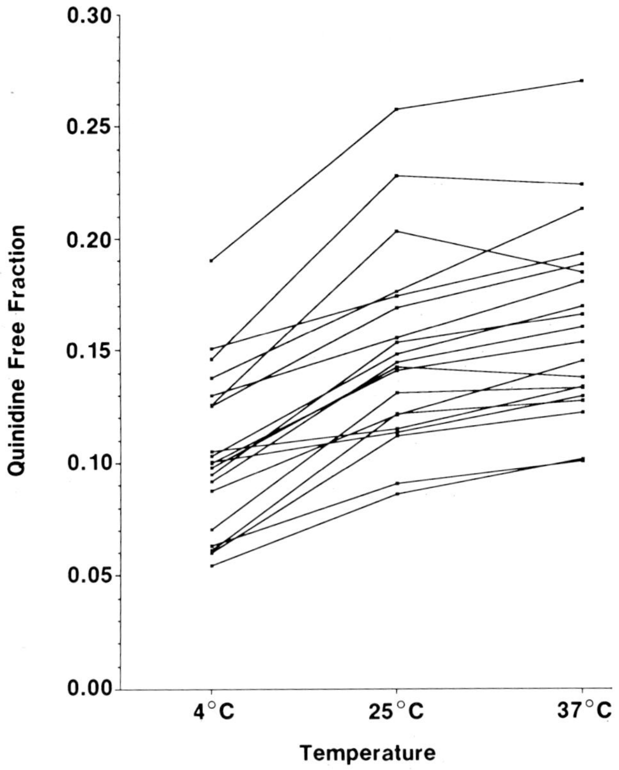

ous studies in which the free fraction of quinidine was determined by equilibrium dialysis.[6,7] The mean values for quinidine free fraction in this study were much lower than those reported by Woo and Greenblatt.[7] This is most likely attributable to the blood-bank plasma used in their study, since preservatives or anticoagulants, or both, added to these specimens may cause a dilutional or displacement effect.

The patient on hemodialysis (patient 13) had a much higher free fraction than the other 19 patients. Heparin administration could have contributed to this elevated free fraction.[1,4,5] Other possible explanations include accumulation of quinidine metabolites that have high free fractions[10] and that moderately cross-react with the assay used.[11] An elevated free fraction directly attributable to severe renal failure is also possible. However, this would not be expected since previous studies have shown that quinidine binding was not altered in renal disease[12,13] and since we found no correlation between calculated creatinine clearance and free fraction.

When ultrafiltration is performed at 37 °C, the mean values for quinidine free fraction are approximately 1.1 times higher than when ultrafiltration is performed at room temperature. When ultrafiltration is performed at 4 °C, the mean values for quinidine free fraction are approximately 60% of the values obtained at room temperature. Thus, our data suggest that values for serum concentrations of free quinidine that are determined in a clinical laboratory at room temperature adequately represent values at physiologic temperature. Although the serum concentrations of free quinidine and quinidine free fraction values obtained at room temperature were significantly different from those at body temperature, this difference is unlikely to be of clinical importance. In fact, the excellent rank correlation of free fraction among the three temperatures indicates that even 4 °C could be used if an appropriate adjustment in the desired free concentration range was made.

Measurement of α_1-acid glycoprotein and albumin concentrations is necessary to examine these results in more detail. Further studies are also necessary to demonstrate whether serum concentrations of free quinidine correlate better than total serum quinidine concentrations with efficacy or potential quinidine toxicity. Certainly, the wide interindividual variation that was observed in both serum concentrations of free quinidine and quinidine free fraction (Figure 1) supports the view that monitoring of serum concentrations of free quinidine rather than total serum quinidine concentrations may be clinically useful.

Conclusion. There is a significant intrapatient correlation in measured quinidine free fraction when ultrafiltration is performed at different temperatures. Serum concentrations of free quinidine determined after ultrafiltration at room temperature adequately reflect those at body temperature.

References

1. Kessler KM, Leech RC, Spann JF. Blood collection techniques, heparin and quinidine protein binding. *Clin Pharmacol Ther.* 1979; 25:204.
2. Kates RE, Sokoloski TD, Comstock TJ. Binding of quinidine to plasma proteins in normal subjects and patients with hyperlipoproteinemias. *Clin Pharmacol Ther.* 1978; 23:30.
3. MacKichan JJ. Pharmacokinetic consequences of drug displacement from blood and tissue proteins. *Clin Pharmacokinet.* 1984; 9(Suppl 1):32.
4. Naranjo CA, Sellers EM, Khouw V et al. Variability in heparin effect on serum drug binding. *Clin Pharmacol Ther.* 1980; 28:545.
5. Edwards DJ, Axelson JE, Slaughter RL et al. Factors affecting quinidine protein binding in humans. *J Pharm Sci.* 1984; 73:1264.
6. Ha HR, Vozeh S, Follath S. Evaluation of a rapid ultrafiltration technique for determination of quinidine protein binding and comparison with equilibrium dialysis. *Ther Drug Monit.* 1986; 8:331.
7. Woo E, Greenblatt DJ. Pharmacokinetic and clinical implications of quinidine protein binding. *J Pharm Sci.* 1979; 68:466.
8. Guentert TW, Oie S. Factors influencing the apparent protein binding of quinidine. *J Pharm Sci.* 1982; 71:325.
9. Winer BJ. Design and analysis of single-factor experiments. In: Statistical principles in experimental design. New York:

McGraw-Hill; 1962:69.
10. Drayer DE, Lowenthal DT, Restivo MS et al. Steady-state serum levels of quinidine and active metabolites in cardiac patients with varying degrees of renal function. *Clin Pharmacol Ther.* 1978; 24:31.
11. Lehmann CR, Boran KJ, Pierson WP et al. Quinidine assays: enzyme immunoassay versus high performance liquid chromatography. *Ther Drug Monit.* 1986; 8:336.
12. Skuterud B, Enger E et al. Serum protein binding of quinidine and diphenylhydantoin in healthy human volunteers and in patients with chronic renal failure. *Proc 5th Int Congr Pharmacol.* 1972:79.
13. Reidenberg MM, Affrime M. Influence of disease on binding of drugs to plasma proteins. *Ann NY Acad Sci.* 1973; 226:115.

Association between depression and propranolol use in ambulatory patients

DAVID BARTELS, MICHAEL GLASSER, ARTHUR WANG, AND PATRICK SWANSON

Clin Pharm. 1988; 7:146–50

Propranolol is a β-adrenergic-receptor-blocking agent that has well-documented central nervous system activity. The lipophilic nature of propranolol, allowing the achievement of high propranolol concentrations in the brain, probably accounts for this effect.[1-3] In a review of the literature on psychiatric and central nervous system adverse effects of antihypertensive medications, Paykel et al.[4] reported that the incidence of adverse effects caused by propranolol ranged from 1% to more than 20% in various studies. The reported symptoms included depression, sleep disorders, drowsiness, fatigue, and hallucinations.

Although depression is regularly mentioned as a possible adverse effect of propranolol therapy, clinical reports of depression have been infrequent,[5-9] with one author estimating that the risk of this adverse effect is less than 0.1%.[10] On the other hand, case reports using criteria from the *Diagnostic and Statistical Manual of Mental Disorders*, third edition (DSM-III) for the diagnosis of depression have noted a positive relationship between use of β-adrenergic-blocking agents and the appearance of depression. The debate over the effect of propranolol therapy on depression continues and is further complicated by the widely varying methodologies of different studies. The case reports tend to use the DSM-III criteria but they are applied only to selected patients, usually in a hospital setting. Large-scale studies, on the other hand, tend to use less reliable, often indirect measures of depression. For example, in looking at the records of 143,253 Medicaid patients, Avorn et al.[11] used the prescription of tricyclic antidepressants as the indicator for depression, assuming that all antidepressants were appropriately prescribed for depression and that all depressed patients were, in fact, prescribed tricyclic antidepressant agents. The confusion over the effect of propranolol use on depression is compounded by the fact that many of the symptoms of major depression are similar to some of the nonspecific pharmacological effects of propranolol, such as fatigue, reduced energy levels, and drowsiness, making it difficult to distinguish between the two in certain patients.

The present study compares the prevalance of depression in a group of ambulatory patients receiving propranolol therapy with that in a control group not receiving propranolol. In contrast to past studies, a number of instruments for the measurement of depression were used and the analysis involved more than case studies, as a control group was used for comparison of the prevalence of depression. This study presents additional data on the relationship between propranolol use and the appearance of depression.

Methods. Subjects participating in this study were recruited from the patient populations of three rural ambulatory-care teaching centers. Charts of patients who were diagnosed as having migraine headaches, hypertension, or angina pectoris were reviewed to determine if a patient was being treated with propranolol. Eligible patients were then contacted by telephone and asked to participate in the study. A control group of patients not using propranolol or any other β-blocking agent was recruited through one of three methods: (1) by letter, with the clinic patients whose names appeared on a computerized listing being sent a letter explaining the study and requesting their participation; (2) by bulletin or handout, with patients visiting the clinic being given a written description of the study requesting their participation; and (3) by personal contact, with patients visiting the clinic having the study explained to them by one of the project investigators while the patient waited to see the physician.

Written informed consent was obtained from all patients. The protocol and consent form had previ-

DAVID BARTELS, PHARM.D., is Assistant Professor of Clinical Pharmacy, MICHAEL GLASSER, PH.D., is Assistant Professor of Medical Sociology, and ARTHUR WANG and PATRICK SWANSON are Research Assistants, Department of Community Medicine, University of Illinois College of Medicine at Rockford.

Address reprint requests to Dr. Bartels at the Department of Community Medicine, University of Illinois College of Medicine at Rockford, 1601 Parkview Avenue, Rockford, IL 61107.

Presented at the 21st Annual ASHP Midyear Clinical Meeting, Las Vegas, NV, December 10, 1986.

Copyright © 1988, American Society of Hospital Pharmacists, Inc. All rights reserved. 0278-2677/88/0201-0146$01.25.

ously been approved by the local institutional review board. All patients agreeing to participate in the study were assessed for evidence of past or present depression using three different measurement strategies. First, the depression segment of the Diagnostic Interview Schedule (DIS) developed by the National Institute of Mental Health for epidemiological studies was administered to obtain a clinical diagnosis of depression.[12,13] The interviews, which were conducted by the project investigators, allowed for the determination of depression according to DSM-III criteria and thus distinguished grief reactions and symptoms of depression from single and recurrent episodes of depression. Second, a battery of self-rating scales for depression was administered to each patient, consisting of the Zung Depression Scale,[14-16] Beck's Depression Inventory,[17,18] the Carroll Rating Scale for Depression,[19] and the Demoralization Scale of the Psychiatric Epidemiology Research Inventory.[20,21] Also administered with these instruments was the Future Time Perspective or Hopelessness Scale.[22]

Finally, to obtain some potential indicator of the physiological basis for depression, the dexamethasone suppression test (DST) was used. Patients were given a 1-mg dose of dexamethasone to be taken at bedtime, with a visit to the health center scheduled for the next day between 1600 and 1700. At this time, a sample of 7 to 10 mL of blood was drawn for analysis of the cortisol concentration.[23-27] Patients were determined to be ineligible for study participation if they were using certain medications or were being treated for specific medical conditions that would interfere with a valid response on the DST.[23]

Analysis consisted of first determining whether there were significant differences in the backgrounds of the propranolol group and the control group. Characteristics that were examined included patients' sex, age, level of education, marital status, self-reported health status, and average number of visits to the physician in one year. Chi-square analysis was used to examine the relationship between the study groups and the following variables: whether or not the person had ever experienced two consecutive weeks of depression, as determined by the DIS; whether or not the individual had experienced a period of depression of two or more years as indicated by the DIS; the actual diagnosis of depression as derived from the DIS; and the Zung Index for depression, in which individuals' depression scores were standardized on a summary index for depression. Student's *t* test was used to compare the mean scores of the two study groups and their blood cortisol concentrations as measured by the DST; total current depressive symptoms, as derived from the DIS; total score on the Zung Self-Rating Scale; score on the Demoralization Scale of the Psychiatric Epidemiology Research Inventory; score on the Future Time Perspective Scale; total score on Beck's Depression Inventory; and overall score on the Carroll Rating Scale. The a priori level of significance for all comparisons was $p < 0.05$.

Results. A total of 127 patients participated in the study: 52 (40.9%) were undergoing propranolol therapy and 75 (59.1%) were control subjects. For the patients taking propranolol hydrochloride, the average dosage at the time of the study was 118 mg per day. The average maximum dosage anytime during their therapy with propranolol hydrochloride was 134 mg per day, with an average duration of 100 weeks. Of the 52 patients receiving propranolol, 31 were taking it for hypertension, 8 were taking it for migraine headaches, and 6 were taking it for angina pectoris. Five of the patients taking propranolol had both angina pectoris and hypertension, and two patients taking propranolol had both migraine headaches and hypertension. Of the 75 control subjects, 25 had no chronic medical problem and were being seen at the clinic only for an examination, 23 had hypertension, 7 had osteoporosis or degenerative joint disease, 5 had chronic headaches, 5 had diabetes mellitus, 5 had angina pectoris, and 5 had asthma or chronic obstructive lung disease.

Medication use was similar for those patients with hypertension, headaches, and angina pectoris in both the propranolol group and the control group. Most of the hypertensive patients in the propranolol group were treated with either propranolol alone or propranolol plus a diuretic, whereas in the control group, hypertensive patients were treated with a diuretic and a centrally acting α agonist or prazosin. Among those patients with headache, similar numbers in both groups were treated with ergot alkaloids, narcotic analgesics, and nonsteroidal anti-inflammatory agents, with the only difference between groups being whether they received propranolol. Patients with angina pectoris took the largest number of medications. Both the propranolol group and the control group had a large number of patients on nitrates, calcium-channel-blocking agents, digoxin, and diuretics. The use of these medications by both groups was similar; whether they were also receiving propranolol was the main difference.

The two study groups were similar with respect to sex, age, marital status, and level of education. Although there were more females in the propranolol group and this group tended to be somewhat younger than the control group, this difference was not significant. Furthermore, there were no significant differences between the groups relative to either self-reported health status or reported number of physician visits over a one-year period.

Tables 1 and 2 show the extent of the relationship between the study groups and the multiple measures of depression.

Table 1.
Chi-square Analysis of the Relationship between Study Group and Indicators of Depression

Indicator	No. (%) with Indicator[a] Propranolol Group (n = 52)	Control Group (n = 75)
Two consecutive weeks of depression in lifetime[b,c]		
Yes	25 (48.1)	47 (62.7)
No	27 (51.9)	28 (37.3)
Period of depression lasting for two years or more[b,d]		
Yes	3 (5.8)	19 (25.3)
Yes, but below critical	3 (5.8)	0 (0.0)
No	46 (88.4)	56 (74.7)
Clinical diagnosis[b,e]		
Depression absent	27 (51.9)	28 (37.3)
Depression but not severe	20 (38.5)	27 (36.0)
Depression—grief reaction	0 (0.0)	1 (1.3)
Depression—single episode	1 (1.9)	3 (4.0)
Depression—recurrent episodes	4 (7.7)	16 (21.3)
Zung Index[f,g]		
Within normal range	32 (72.7)	35 (57.4)
Mild to moderate depression	8 (18.2)	16 (26.2)
Moderate to marked depression	4 (9.1)	4 (6.6)
Severe to extreme depression	0 (0.0)	6 (9.8)

[a] Total number of subjects for both the propranolol and control groups may vary because of missing data.
[b] Based on Diagnostic Interview Schedule.
[c] $\chi^2 = 2.10$, d.f. = 1, $p = 0.147$.
[d] $\chi^2 = 11.84$, d.f. = 2, $p = 0.003$.
[e] $\chi^2 = 8.21$, d.f. = 4, $p = 0.145$.
[f] $\chi^2 = 6.21$, d.f. = 3, $p = 0.101$.
[g] Raw scores were standardized for comparison with national norms.

Table 2.
Mean ± S.D. Values for Selected Indicators of Depression for Propranolol and Control Groups

Indicator	Mean ± S.D. Values (No. of Subjects)[a] Propranolol Group (n = 52)	Control Group (n = 75)
Demoralization Scale (Psychiatric Epidemiology Research Inventory)	1.02 ± 0.53 (52)	1.43 ± 0.81[b] (75)
Beck's Depression Inventory	6.42 ± 5.15 (50)	9.75 ± 8.40[b] (71)
Carroll Rating Scale for Depression	7.98 ± 6.36 (43)	11.08 ± 8.38[b] (60)
Zung Self-Rating Depression Scale	34.11 ± 8.71 (44)	38.41 ± 10.50 (61)
Future Time Perspective Scale	2.50 ± 2.59 (48)	4.71 ± 5.16[b] (66)
No. of current depressive symptoms[c]	1.6 ± 1.92 (52)	3.29 ± 3.40[b] (75)
Blood cortisol concentration (μg/dL)	2.51 ± 2.80 (34)	2.33 ± 2.69 (69)

[a] Total number of subjects for both the propranolol and control groups may vary because of missing data.
[b] Significant at $p < 0.05$ (Student's t test).
[c] Based on Diagnostic Interview Schedule.

Discussion. The present study demonstrated that the prevalence of depression in patients receiving propranolol is no different from or is actually less than, by some measures, the prevalence of depression in a randomly selected group of patients not receiving propranolol. Patients in the propranolol group were less likely than the control-group patients to report depressive symptoms on the Demoralization Scale of the Psychiatric Epidemiology Research Inventory, Beck's Depression Inventory, the Carroll Rating Scale for Depression, the Future Time Perspective Scale, and the current depressive symptoms as derived from the DIS. However, with respect to the actual diagnosis of depression, as determined from the DIS, there was no difference in the appearance of depression between patients receiving propranolol and control subjects.

Limitations in study design may have contributed to the findings of this study. First, two of the three methods used to recruit the control group involved asking for volunteers, which may have resulted in a greater number of depressed people "volunteering" for the study. However, comparison of the three groups showed no difference in the frequency of depression among the three recruitment groups. Second, the control and propranolol groups were not matched for the type and severity of illness. Patients receiving propranolol all had one or more of the following illnesses: hypertension, migraine headaches, or angina pectoris. Similar numbers of patients in the control group had chronic disorders such as hypertension, headaches, and angina pectoris; however, this group had a large number of patients with no chronic illness who were not receiving any medications. The third possible limitation of the study design was that all the patients receiving propranolol had one of three diagnoses. The type of disease and the concomitant medications could have influenced their level of depression. If patients receiving propranolol are classified by diagnosis, the variables age, sex, and health status differ among the groups; however, the results of the depression interviews and scales administered to these patients are similar for each subgroup and for the propranolol group as a whole. Therefore, the potential limitations of study design apparently did not influence the results.

Whereas patients in this study were not directly assessed for anxiety using accepted scales or measures, many of the questions on the self-rating scales designed to measure depressive symptoms were actually assessing anxiety. Suzman,[28] in a study of propranolol in the treatment of anxiety, showed that of 513 anxious patients treated with propranolol, 271 were depressed before starting propranolol therapy. The high prevalence of depression in this group of patients was presumed to be because of the severity and chronicity of the anxiety caused by concomitant disease states and physical complaints. In 179 of these patients, the depression improved and anxiety was relieved after beginning propranolol, and only 92 patients needed to be treated with antidepressants. It appeared that when the majority of the patients were relieved of their chronic severe anxiety, their depression was also relieved.

The large number of depressed patients who benefited from the relief of anxiety in the Suzman study indicates that a high percentage of the patients probably had an adjustment disorder with depressed mood that was worsened by their anxiety. In the present study, the patients may have been experiencing a similar type of disorder, as shown by the results of the dexamethasone suppression test. Nonsuppressability on the DST has been shown to correlate with major depression,[29] which would not be affected by anxiety. In both groups in the present study, however, the patients did show suppression during the DST, and the serum cortisol concentrations did not correlate with the occurrence of depression, as previously reported for major forms of depression. This may indicate that the majority of these patients were suffering more from an adjustment disorder with depressed mood worsened by anxiety. This would have resulted in the lower frequency of depressive symptoms reported on the self-rating scales in the propranolol group compared with the control group but a similar frequency of major depression in the two groups as assessed by the DIS.

It has also been suggested by Oppenheim[5] that two types of depressive syndromes may actually be produced by propranolol therapy. The more common type is major depression resulting from biochemical abnormalities in the central nervous system, which is precipitated or exacerbated by propranolol and does not necessarily resolve when the propranolol is stopped. The other form of depression is a drug-dependent form that occurs when propranolol is started and reverses rapidly when it is stopped. This depressive syndrome may be the type of propranolol-induced depression reported relatively infrequently in case reports, whereas the other depressive syndrome described by Oppenheim may merely be a re-emergence of a major depressive illness in biologically predisposed individuals, occurring at a rate no greater than the incidence of depression in the general population. The lower rate at which depressive symptoms were reported on the self-rating scales by patients treated with propranolol in the present study may have been because of a beneficial effect on anxiety-induced depression, not because of either a positive or negative effect on either of the forms of depression described by Oppenheim.

The physiology of the relationship between propranolol and affective disorders needs to be explored in greater detail. Furthermore, replicating the present study using the same multiple instruments but a different comparison population and assessments of anxiety might be beneficial. Nevertheless, the present study using multiple, specific indicators for depression does call into question the contention that a relationship necessarily exists between propranolol therapy and the appearance of depression.

Conclusion. This study suggests that the prevalence of depression among propranolol-treated patients is not higher than that seen in a control group of patients not receiving propranolol. Propranolol may actually improve some of the anxiety-related depressive symptoms through its pharmacological effects on β-adrenergic receptors.

References

1. Cruickshank JM. The clinical importance of cardioselectivity and lipophilicity in beta blockers. *Am Heart J*. 1980; 100:160–78.
2. Taylor EA, Jefferson D, Carroll JD et al. Cerebrospinal fluid concentrations of propranolol, pindolol and atenolol in man: evidence for central actions of beta-adrenoceptor antagonists. *Br J Clin Pharmacol*. 1981; 12:549–59.
3. Neil-Dwyer G, Bartlett J, McAinsh J et al. Beta-adrenoceptor blockers and the blood brain barrier. *Br J Clin Pharmacol*. 1981; 11:549–53.
4. Paykel ES, Fleminger R, Watson JP. Psychiatric side effects of antihypertensive drugs other than reserpine. *J Clin Psychopharmacol*. 1982; 2:14–39.
5. Oppenheim G. Propranolol-induced depression: mechanism and management. *Aust NZ J Psychiatry*. 1983; 14:400–2.
6. Waal HJ. Propranolol-induced depression. *Br Med J*. 1967; 2:50.
7. McNeil GN, Shaw PK, Dock DS. Substitution of atenolol for propranolol in a case of propranolol-related depression. *Am J Psychiatry*. 1982; 139:1187–8.
8. Petrie WM, Maffucci RJ, Woosley RL. Propranolol and depression. *Am J Psychiatry*. 1982; 139:92–3.
9. Parker WA. Propranolol-induced depression and psychosis. *Clin Pharm*. 1985; 4:214–8.
10. Fitzgerald JD. Propranolol-induced depression. *Br Med J*. 1967; 11:372–3.
11. Avorn J, Everitt DE, Weiss S. Increased antidepressant use in patients prescribed beta-blockers. *JAMA*. 1986; 3:357–60.
12. Robins EN, Helzer JE, Croughan J et al. National Institute of Mental Health diagnostic interview schedule. *Arch Gen Psychiatry*. 1981; 38:381–9.
13. Eaton WW, Regier DA, Locke BZ et al. The epidemologic catchment area program of the National Institute of Mental Health. *Public Health Rep*. 1981; 96:319–25.
14. Zung WWK. A self-rating depression scale. *Arch Gen Psychiatry*. 1965; 12:63–70.
15. Zung WWK, Richards CB, Short MJ. Self-rating depression scale in an outpatient clinic. *Arch Gen Psychiatry*. 1965; 13:508–15.
16. Zung WWK. Factors influencing the self-rating depression scale. *Arch Gen Psychiatry*. 1967; 16:543–7.
17. Beck AT, Ward CH, Mendelson M et al. An inventory for measuring depression. *Arch Gen Psychiatry*. 1961; 4:53–63.
18. Beck AT, Beck RW. Screening depressed patients in family practice: a rapid technique. *Postgrad Med J*. 1972; 48:81–5.
19. Carroll BJ, Feinberg M, Smouse PE et al. The Carroll rating scale for depression. *Br J Psychiatry* 1981; 138:194–200.
20. Dohrenwend BP, Shrout PE, Egri G et al. Nonspecific psychological distress and other dimensions of psychopathology. *Arch Gen Psychiatry*. 1980; 37:1229–36.
21. Roberts RE, Vernon SW. Usefulness of the PERI demoralization scale to screen for psychiatric disorder in a community

sample. *Psychol Res.* 1981; 5:183–93.
22. Beck AT, Weissman A, Lester A et al. The measurement of pessimism: the hopelessness scale. *J Consult Clin Psychol.* 1974; 42:861–5.
23. Feiger AD. Biological testing in psychiatry. Kalamazoo, MI: The Upjohn Company; 1983. Monograph.
24. Asnis GM, Sechar EJ, Malbreich V et al. Cortisol secretion and dexamethasone response in depression. *Am J Psychiatry.* 1981; 138:1218–21.
25. Carroll BJ. Dexamethasone suppression test for melancholia. *Br J Psychiatry.* 1982; 140:292–304.
26. Carroll BJ. Use of the dexamethasone test in depression. *J Clin Psychol.* 1982; 42:44–50.
27. Schatzberg AF, Rothschild AJ, Stahl JB et al. The dexamethasone suppression test: identification of subtypes of depression. *Am J Psychiatry.* 1983; 140:88–91.
28. Suzman MM. Propranolol in the treatment of anxiety. *Postgrad Med J.* 1976; 52:168–74.
29. Ostrow DG, Okonek A, Gibbons R et al. Biologic markers and antidepressant response. *J Clin Psychol.* 1983; 44:10–3.

Comparison of 16-meq and 20-meq daily potassium supplement regimens

BONITA L. ROOHK, FRED L. MEISTER, MARY K. HEWETT, AND JOHN A. RUMSFELD

Clin Pharm. 1988; 7:150–2

Many patients taking postassium-depleting medications such as diuretics tend to develop an abnormally low serum potassium concentration.[1-4] Although some individuals can avoid hypokalemia with dietary supplementation, most are unable to consistently eat foods high in potassium, and other high-risk patients (i.e., those with severe liver disease or life-threatening arrhythmias) generally require potassium supplements.[5-7] A case can also be made for potassium supplementation in edematous patients, since they generally have some degree of secondary hyperaldosteronism.[6,8]

BONITA L. ROOHK, M.S., is Instructor, Golden West College, Huntington Beach, CA. FRED L. MEISTER, PHARM. D.,is Clinical Pharmacologist, Hoag Memorial Hospital Presbyterian, Newport Beach, CA, and Assistant Clinical Professor, School of Pharmacy, University of California, San Francisco. MARY K. HEWETT, M.S., is Head Nurse, Emergency Services, Hoag Memorial Hospital Presbyterian. JOHN A. RUMSFELD, M.D., practices pulmonary medicine in Newport Beach, CA.

Address reprint requests to Dr. Meister at Hoag Memorial Hospital Presbyterian, 301 Newport Boulevard, Box Y, Newport Beach, CA 92663.

Support in the form of drugs, clinical assessments, and laboratory testing was obtained from Ciba-Geigy.

Presented at the Clinical Research Forum, 22nd Annual ASHP Midyear Clinical Meeting, Atlanta, GA, December 9, 1987.

Copyright © 1988, American Society of Hospital Pharmacists, Inc. All rights reserved. 0278-2677/88/0201-0150$00.75.

The usual dosage for prevention of hypokalemia is from 16 to 24 meq of potassium daily.[5,9] This amount is usually adequate despite wide variations in dietary intake (i.e., 40 to 120 meq daily).[9,10] Because of the unpleasant taste of liquid potassium supplements, tablet formulations of potassium have been developed and are widely used,[5,6] with wax-matrix formulations being the most frequently prescribed oral potassium supplements.[11] The convenience and lack of unpleasant taste may improve patient compliance.[5,6,12] Several studies have shown that tablets are generally as effective as liquid potassium at maintaining potassium balance.[13-20] Hyperkalemia is rarely a problem with this degree of supplementation because of the kidneys' capacity to greatly increase sodium-potassium adenosine triphosphatase (ATPase) activity and increase potassium-ion secretion.[21,22] The purpose of this study was to determine if 16 meq of daily potassium supplement is clinically equivalent to 20 meq of daily potassium supplement in the average patient who requires potassium supplementation.

Methods. Twenty hypertensive subjects or subjects with compromised pulmonary function were selected. All were taking diuretics or glucocorticoids, or both, on a regular basis and had at one time been hypokalemic (serum potassium below 3.5 meq/L). All currently had normal serum potassium values (3.5–5.0 meq/L) maintained through the use of 20-meq daily doses of solid or liquid oral dosage forms of supplemental potassium. Subjects taking more than 20 meq of potassium supplement per day to maintain acceptable serum potassium levels were excluded from the study, as were patients whose prescribed medications were in a state of flux. In order to better approximate clinical conditions, patients on other drugs affecting potassium metabolism, such as β-adrenergic blocking agents and nonsteroidal anti-inflammatory drugs, were not excluded as long as their therapy was consistent throughout the duration of the study.

Eight men aged 56–82 years and 12 women aged 55–79 years were randomly assigned to one of two groups and evaluated over a nine-week period. During the first week, subjects were instructed to take their current potassium therapy twice daily, after breakfast and dinner. The remaining eight weeks were divided into two four-week segments. Group A received one 8-meq wax-matrix tablet (Slow-K, Ciba) twice daily, after breakfast and dinner. Group B received one 10-meq wax-matrix tablet (Klotrix, Mead Johnson) twice daily, after breakfast and dinner. After four weeks of therapy, crossover occurred, with group A receiving Klotrix and group B receiving Slow-K.

At every office visit, each patient was interviewed and serum potassium concentration was measured. The subjects were asked to describe their general well-being and the presence or absence of common hypokalemic symptoms and adverse reactions most commonly attributed to potassium supplements. All were asked to report any changes in their diet or medications during the previous week.

To standardize the blood tests as much as possible, subjects reported to the clinical unit in a fasting state and without taking their morning potassium supplement. Visits were scheduled at a fixed time of day (within one hour). Serum potassium was measured with a Beckman Astra analyzer, which uses an ion-selective electrode. Results were compared using Student's t test for paired data, $p < 0.05$ being considered significant.

In addition to the tests performed at each visit, each patient was physically evaluated three times during the study: at the beginning, crossover point, and end of the study (visits 2, 5, and 8). This assessment focused on evaluation of the neuromuscular and cardiovascular systems and included an ECG and arterial blood gas evaluation, when indicated. The ECGs were used as an additional indicator of potential hypokalemia, and the arterial blood gases were used to eliminate alkalosis as a cause for drops in plasma potassium that are not indicative of total body potassium loss.

Results and Discussion. Of the 20 patients beginning the study, 18 completed the entire nine weeks. One patient was removed from the study when his serum potassium concentration fell from 3.9 meq/L to 3.1 meq/L in one week. This patient was in the Slow-K group. Coincidentally, his medication before starting the study was also Slow-K. At the time of his removal from the study, this patient was in severe respiratory distress and his physician had given him a 2-mL injection of betamethasone sodium phosphate–betamethasone acetate suspension (Celestone Soluspan, Schering). This change in medication caused his removal from this study and could have contributed to the decrease in serum potassium concentration. A second patient, in the Klotrix group, chose to withdraw from the study for personal reasons. Data from these two patients are excluded from the final results.

In the 18 patients that remained, the two therapy regimens were compared with respect to alterations in both subjective and objective variables. At 19 of 135 visits, patients reported having not felt well; most reports were of asthma, respiratory distress, or fatigue. One patient reported two days of gastrointestinal disturbance, but since her spouse had the same symptoms a day later it was presumed that this gastrointestinal distress was not drug related. The bouts of fatigue and ill health seem unrelated to serum potassium. In 7 of these bouts, the serum potassium concentration increased, in 10 bouts it decreased, and in the other 2 it remained the same. In addition, one patient reported dark stools three days in a row; there was no gastrointestinal distress at the time, and the stool color subsequently returned to normal. This patients's hemoglobin concentration was high for a female (16.0 g/dL), so the attending physician elected to do no further tests unless the sign recurred.

No significant difference in serum potassium concentrations at visits 2, 5, and 8 was found between the regimens. All three of these data points were verified with arterial blood gas measurements that would identify serum potassium changes secondary to intracellular–extracellular shifts rather than changes in total body potassium. This is an important consideration, since a change of 0.1 unit in plasma pH can be accompanied by a change of 0.6 meq/L in plasma potassium ion concentration.[23,24] No recognizable shifts occurred.

Significance of changes in serum potassium concentrations must also be determined by relating the absolute value of the change to instrument accuracy and concentration changes expected from the dosage difference between the two regimens. The Beckman Astra, which we used to measure serum potassium values, has a coefficient of variation of 1.3% for serum potassium values in the midrange.[25] This exceeds the manufacturer's specifications for the instrument. At this level of accuracy, the instrument would measure a serum potassium of 4.3 meq/L within 0.056 meq. Using this instrument, any two values must differ more than 0.112 meq to exceed instrument variation. In addition, a 1-meq/L drop in plasma potassium requires approximately 100–200 meq loss of potassium from body stores,[9] although the exact amount varies with absolute serum potassium value as well as other factors.[4] At the 4-meq dose difference per day, a patient would require 25–50 days to show a 1-meq/L drop in plasma potassium. Each phase of the study was continued for four weeks (28 days). Therefore, a 0.5–1.0 meq/L drop in all patients at the lower dose would be expected should this difference in dosage be critical. Considering both the dosage difference and instrument variation, the patients should show a 0.6- to 1.1-meq/L change in serum potassium concentration for the difference in regimens to be clinically important.

Arguably, the second phase of the study in each group has fewer variables than the first because of the four weeks of potassium supplement stabilization that occurred in the patients during the first four weeks of the study. Group A patients took Klotrix (20 meq daily) during the second phase of the study. Their mean serum potassium concentration changed from 3.83 meq/L to 3.94 meq/L from visit 5 to visit 8, but this change did not exceed instrument variation. During this time, serum potassium concentrations in four of nine patients increased (+ 0.2, 0.2, 0.3, and 0.9 meq/L), in three others it decreased (− 0.1, 0.2, and 0.3 meq/L), and no change occurred in the remaining two patients. The differences in potassium concentrations were not significant. Group B patients took Slow-K (16 meq daily) during the second phase of the study. Their mean serum potassium changed from 4.31 meq/L to 4.08 meq/L from visit 5 to visit 8. During this time, one patient demonstrated an increase in serum potassium concentration (+ 0.7 meq/L), five showed a decrease (− 0.4, 0.4, 0.5, 0.6, and 0.9 meq/L), and three had no significant change. Again, the mean difference was not significant. Only two of the individual losses were of the magnitude predicted from the dosage differences, and the one increase is unexplained.

These minimal differences assume strict compliance with the prescribed regimen and no dietary change that would alter potassium intake. Compliance was virtually 100%, as judged by medication that remained after each phase of the study. Although no patients reported any dietary alterations, their diets were not closely regulated. This was not a major flaw in experimental design, since it more closely approximates clinical reality and since most patients reported habitual dietary preferences. However, the possibility exists that dietary intake might introduce some variation in the serum potassium values recorded.

A second question of interest in the study is whether the initiation of a wax-matrix form of potassium will change the potassium maintenance dose. Three patients in group A who started on Slow-K and one patient in group B who started on Klotrix were already on a wax-matrix type of supplement, so their values were not included in this comparison. All others were taking a liquid, powder, effervescent tablet, or capsular (Micro K Extencaps, Robins) form of supplement. A comparison of values from visits 2 and 5 showed no significant difference between the values for either group. Three patients in group A receiving Slow-K (16 meq daily) demonstrated an increase of 0.2 meq/L in serum potassium, one showed a decrease of 1.3 meq/L, and two showed no change. Three patients in group B receiving Klotrix (20 meq daily) demonstrated an increase in serum potassium (+ 0.2, 0.4, and 0.5 meq/L), three demonstrated a decrease (− 0.1, 0.2, and 0.5 meq/L), and two showed no change. The lack of change in serum potassium when patients changed drug forms to a wax-matrix supplement is not surprising in view of the literature supporting therapeutic equivalency of the various drug forms.[13-20]

Conclusion. Based on the results of this eight-week study, it would appear that a 16-meq dosage of potassium supplement per day is as effective as a 20-meq dosage of potassium supplement per day at maintaining potassium balance in patients requiring 20 meq or less per day. Also, wax-matrix tablets are equivalent to other dosage forms for maintaining serum potassium levels.

References

1. Anon. Drugs for hypertension. *Med Lett Drugs Ther.* 1981; 23:45–8.
2. Lawson D, Henry D, Lowe J et al. Severe hypokalemia in hospitalized patients. *Arch Intern Med.* 1979; 139:978–80.
3. Lindeman R. Hypokalemia: causes, consequences and correction. *Am J Med Sci.* 1976; 272:5–17.
4. Nardone D, McDonald W, Girard D. Mechanisms in hypokalemia: clinical correlation. *Medicine.* 1978; 57:435–46.
5. Anon. Klotrix and other slow-release potassium tablets. *Med Lett Drugs Ther.* 1981; 23:3–4.
6. Stanaszek WF, Romankiewicz JA. Current approaches to management of potassium deficiency. *Drug Intell Clin Pharm.* 1985; 19:176–83.
7. Sherlock P. Cardiovascular and renal drugs and gastrointestinal drugs advisory committee meeting. Bethesda, MD: Food and Drug Administration. 1983: 1–273.
8. Knochel JP. Role of glucoregulatory hormones in potassium homeostasis. *Kidney Int.* 1977; 11:443–52.
9. Boyd JR, ed. Facts and comparisons. St. Louis: J. B. Lippincott Company; 1986: 15–15b.
10. Mudge GH. Agents affecting volume and composition of body fluids. In: Goodman and Gilman's the pharmacological basis of therapeutics. 7th ed. Gilman AG, Goodman LS, Rall TW et al., eds. New York: Macmillan Publishing Company; 1985: 866–74.
11. McMahon FG, Rayan JR, Akdamar K et al. Effect of potassium chloride supplements on upper gastrointestinal mucosa. *Clin Pharmacol Ther.* 1984; 35:852–5.
12. Skoutakis VA, Carter CA, Acchiardo SR. Therapeutic assessment of Slow-K and K-Tab potassium chloride formulations in hypertensive patients treated with thiazide diuretics. *Drug Intell Clin Pharm.* 1987; 21:445–50.
13. Ben-Ishay D, Engleman K. Bioavailability of potassium from a slow-release tablet. *Clin Pharmacol Ther.* 1973; 14:250–3.
14. Cordano A, Vitale J, Hamby R et al. A new controlled release oral potassium supplement. *Clin Ther.* 1979; 2:263.
15. Dickerson J, Bressler R, Gelderman G. Bioavailability, efficacy, safety, and acceptance of Klotrix—a slow release potassium chloride supplement. *Curr Ther Res.* 1980; 28:340.
16. Ryan JR, Elliot BW. A multicenter trial of microencapsulated potassium chloride. *Curr Ther Res.* 1981; 29:838.
17. Skoutakis V, Acchiardo S, Hudgins L et al. Liquid and controlled release potassium chloride supplement. *Curr Ther Res.* 1980; 28:754.
18. Skoutakis VA, Acchiardo SR, Wojciechowski NJ et al. Liquid and solid potassium chloride: bioavailability and safety. *Pharmacotherapy.* 1984; 4:392–7.
19. Tannen R, Cordano A. Pharmacokinetics and effects on fecal blood loss of a controlled release potassium chloride tablet. *J Pharmacol Exp Ther.* 1978; 204:240–6.
20. Weintraub M, Wardell W. Slow release potassium. *Drug Ther.* 1975; 5:63–8.
21. Hayslett JP, Binder HJ. Mechanism of potassium adaption. *Am J Physiol.* 1982; 243:F103–F112.
22. Young DB. Relationship between plasma potassium concentration and renal potassium excretion. *Am J Physiol.* 1982; 242:F599–F603.
23. Adler S, Fraley DS. Potassium and intracellular pH. *Kidney Int.* 1977; 11:433–42.
24. Giebisch G, Thier S. Potassium: physiological and clinical importance. In: Siegel L, ed. Directions in cardiovascular medicine. Somerville, NJ: Hoechst-Roussel Pharmaceuticals, Inc.; 1977: 48.
25. Anon. Clinical laboratory internal quality control program. Newport Beach, CA: Hoag Memorial Hospital Presbyterian; 1986.

Drug Experience

Straightforward reports of unusual drug experiences are included in this section. These may be confirmations of previously reported drug experiences or brief apparent first reports. While selected references may be cited, the purpose of a Drug Experience report is not to present an extensive review of the literature.

A related section, Grand Rounds, includes papers that are well-documented patient case reports with a thorough review of the important literature to help put the case in perspective.

Phenytoin-induced pseudolymphoma with mycosis fungoides manifestations

L. EVANS COOKE, THOMAS C. HARDIN, AND DAN J. HENDRICKSON

Clin Pharm. 1988; 7:153–7

Pseudolymphoma is a well-defined, seldom reported, and often unrecognized adverse reaction to phenytoin. This syndrome can be clinically indistinguishable from malignant lymphoma, and it commonly involves local or generalized lymphadenopathy, fever, dermatologic disorders, and eosinophilia. Lymph nodal tissues show histologic changes that mimic malignant processes, and these may be morphologically indistinguishable from true malignancy. In all cases of pseudolymphoma, the syndrome completely resolves clinically and histologically when the offending agent is withdrawn.[1-8] Therefore, recognition of the drug-induced syndrome is important to ensure withdrawal of the drug and to avoid unnecessary therapy with antineoplastic agents.

The malignant processes most commonly simulated histologically are Hodgkin's lymphoma, non-Hodgkin's lymphoma, and lymphosarcoma. However, a small number of phenytoin-induced syndromes mimicking other malignant lymphomas have been reported over the years. Mycosis fungoides is a malignant, cutaneous T-cell lymphoma. Five cases of phenytoin-induced pseudolymphoma simulating this malignancy have been reported in the literature.[7,9,10] The following is an additional account of a patient who had phenytoin-induced pseudolymphoma with mycosis fungoides manifestations, and we present histological evidence to support this diagnosis.

Case Report. A 40-year-old Latin American man was hospitalized with new-onset seizures considered secondary to ethanol withdrawal, severe hyponatremia (serum sodium concentration, 117 meq/L), or an old small basal ganglial hemorrhagic infarct noted on computed tomography (CT) scan of the head. The patient was started on phenytoin 300 mg orally at bedtime and ultimately discharged with scheduled follow-up for further neurological evaluation.

Approximately one month after discharge, the patient was hospitalized again with malaise, low-grade fever (38.1 °C), 4.5-kg weight loss, severe facial and labial swelling and hyperpigmentation of the face, marked ulceration of the tongue and lips, and a scaly, pruritic, maculopapular erythematous rash on the trunk and extremities. No other remarkable physical abnormalities were found at this time. A complete blood count (CBC) revealed a white blood cell (WBC) count of 11,100/cu mm (65% segmented neutrophils, 2% band forms, 6% lymphocytes, 6% monocytes, 17% eosinophils, 2% basophils, and 2% atypical lymphocytes), hemoglobin (Hb) 9.3 g/dL, hematocrit (Hct) 27.3%, and mean corpuscular volume (MCV) of 91 cu μm. Total bilirubin, serum aspartate aminotransferase (AST, formerly SGOT), and serum alanine aminotransferase (ALT, formerly SGPT) were abnormally ele-

L. EVANS COOKE, PHARM.D., is Clinical Pharmacy Coordinator, Veterans Administration Medical Center, Amarillo, TX; at the time of this report, she was Clinical Pharmacy Specialty Practice Resident in Adult Medicine, Pharmacy Service, Audie L. Murphy Memorial Veterans Hospital (ALMMVH), San Antonio, TX. THOMAS C. HARDIN, PHARM.D., is Clinical Coordinator, Pharmacy Service, ALMMVH, and Clinical Assistant Professor, Department of Pharmacology, The University of Texas Health Science Center at San Antonio and College of Pharmacy, The University of Texas at Austin. DAN J. HENDRICKSON, M.D., is Internal Medicine Resident, Department of Medicine, The University of Texas Health Science Center at San Antonio.

Address reprint requests to Dr. Cooke at the Pharmacy Service (119), Veterans Administration Medical Center, 6010 Amarillo Blvd. West, Amarillo, TX 79106.

The assistance of Nanette Clare, M.D., in preparing the photographs and presenting the pathology of this case is acknowledged.

Copyright © 1988, American Society of Hospital Pharmacists, Inc. All rights reserved. 0278-2677/88/0201-0153$01.25.

vated (1.8 mg/dL, 40 U/L, and 114 U/L, respectively). The patient's condition was considered a hypersensitivity reaction to phenytoin, and the drug was discontinued. Dexamethasone phosphate 10 mg was given intravenously every eight hours for four doses. Within 24 hours the swelling and rash had greatly improved, and one week after admission the patient was discharged with complete resolution of symptoms.

Approximately one month later the patient again was hospitalized with facial and labial swelling, hyperpigmentation of the face, mucositis of the oral cavity, further weight loss (3.2 kg) secondary to dysphagia and anorexia, a maculopapular morbilliform rash on the trunk and arms, and generalized lymphadenopathy that was not present before. Because of an apparent miscommunication, the patient had resumed taking phenytoin when he returned home (positive rechallenge). Physical examination revealed cervical, periclavicular, axillary, epitrochlear, and inguinal lymphadenopathy, as well as hepatosplenomegaly. Results of urinalysis, blood chemistries, and CBC were normal except for eosinophilia (not quantified) and anemia (Hb 10.8 g/dL and Hct 31.2%).

The differential diagnosis at this time included phenytoin hypersensitivity reaction, phenytoin-induced pseudolymphoma, malignant lymphoma, and other less likely possibilities. Phenytoin was discontinued again, and the patient was treated with diphenhydramine hydrochloride 25 mg orally every six hours as needed for itching, codeine phosphate 30–60 mg orally as needed for mouth pain, and a 1:1:1 suspension of antacid–diphenhydramine hydrochloride–lidocaine hydrochloride swished and swallowed when needed for mouth pain.

A punch biopsy of the skin (Figure 1) revealed dermal–epidermal interface vacuolar changes where mononuclear cells were seen infiltrating and destroying the basal layer of the epidermis. A superficial, perivascular lymphohistiocytic infiltrate was also present. The rash quickly spread to the lower extremities, face, and neck with only the palms of his hands and the soles of his feet spared, and a fever of 39.2 °C was recorded. Five days after admission the rash began exfoliating and was extremely pruritic. Fever, adenopathy, and oral lesions persisted. Trace pedal edema was observed, and laboratory values indicated evidence of liver involvement (lactate dehydrogenase 263 U/L and alkaline phosphatase 286 U/L). The WBC count was also elevated (11,100/cu mm with 13% eosinophils).

Ten days after admission the oral pain and facial swelling had improved, but bilateral inguinal lymph nodes had increased in size and a new swollen cervical lymph node was found, with no improvement in other nodes. Bilateral nonpitting pedal edema was now 4+ and resembled lymphedema.

Figure 1. Biopsy specimen of skin showing lymphocytic infiltrate of upper dermis with lymphocytic epidermotropism. Upper photo is a paraffin section, hemotoxylin-eosin stained (original magnification × 40); lower photo is an electron micrograph showing lymphocyte in epidermis with convoluted nucleus (× 7560).

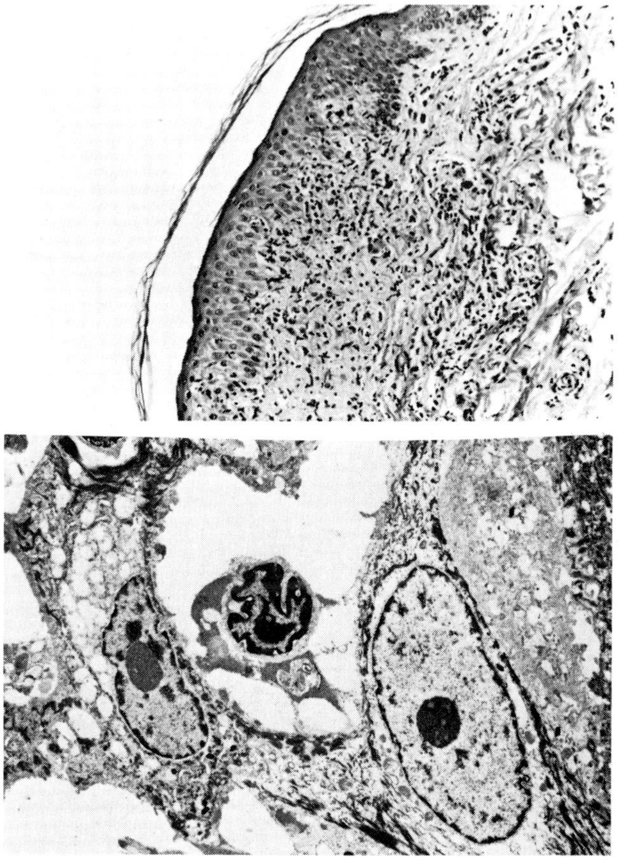

A CT scan of the abdomen and pelvis and an excisional cervical lymph node biopsy were performed to rule out frank lymphoma. The CT scan showed hepatosplenomegaly; cholelithiasis; normal pancreas, kidney, and adrenals; and multiple enlarged periaortic and inguinal lymph nodes. Examination of frozen and permanent sections of the lymph node (Figure 2) showed a lymphoproliferative process with dermatopathic hyperplasia. There was diffuse proliferation of the nodal architecture with histiocytes and small lymphocytes having convoluted nuclei. Electron microscopy confirmed these findings, which were consistent with mycosis fungoides.

Follow-up examination of a cell suspension from the lymphoid tissue showed an abnormally increased population of total T lymphocytes (89%, normal 72 ± 7%), a markedly elevated T-helper lymphocyte population of the total T lymphocytes (78%, normal 45 ± 11%), a decreased population of T-suppressor lymphocytes (12%, normal 28 ± 9%), and an excessively high T-helper/T-suppressor ra-

Figure 2. Lymph node section showing diffuse infiltrate of small lymphocytes with irregular nuclei and occasional histiocytes. Upper photo is a paraffin section, hemotoxylin-eosin stained (original magnification × 250); lower photo is an electron micrograph showing lymphocytes with convoluted nuclei (× 7560).

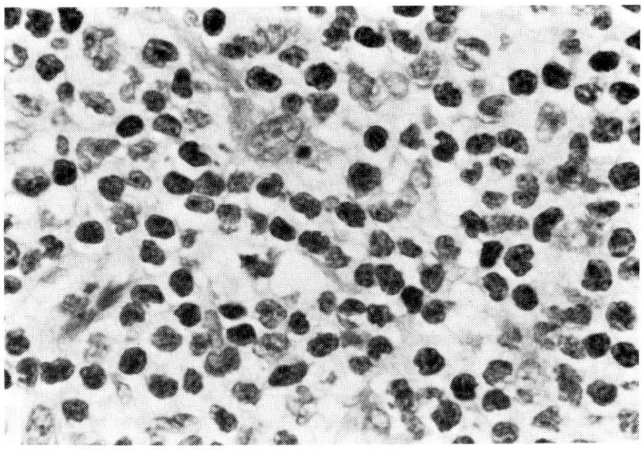

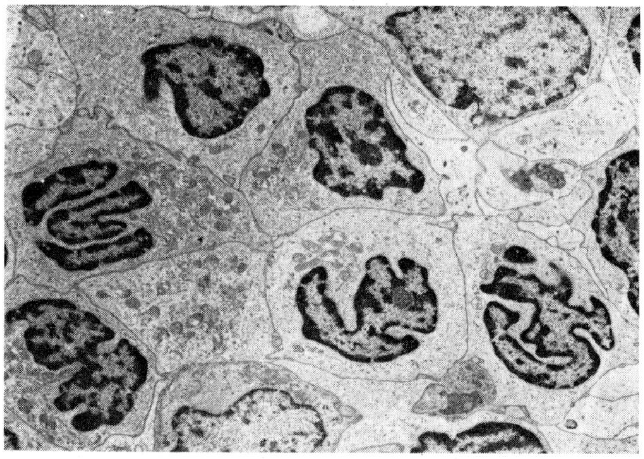

tio of 6.5. Concomitant microscopic examination of the peripheral blood (Figure 3) revealed circulating Sézary cells, which are neoplastic lymphocytes often found in patients with mycosis fungoides. A subsequent bone marrow aspirate was normal.

Despite the pathology reports, suspicion was high for phenytoin hypersensitivity, and the patient was observed.

By day 17 of hospitalization, the facial swelling and oral lesions were almost resolved. Lymphadenopathy remained, and the patient's palms and soles were now desquamating in thick, tough plaques. Skin tests to assess immunocompetency were nonreactive, consistent with anergy.

At day 24 of hospitalization, all oral lesions had cleared, and no appreciable facial or mucosal swelling remained. The rash continued to flake, but itching had decreased. Generalized lymphadenopathy persisted, but the pedal edema had decreased to 2+ and changed to pitting edema.

Overall signs and symptoms continued to improve until day 35, when only enlargement of cervical, axillary, and inguinal lymph nodes remained, although the nodes had decreased in size. The patient was markedly improved, and he was discharged for outpatient follow-up. Within two months of discontinuing phenytoin all lymph nodes had returned to normal, and all other signs and symptoms remained absent.

Figure 3. Electron micrograph of peripheral blood buffy coat preparation showing abnormal lymphocyte with convoluted nucleus (× 8820).

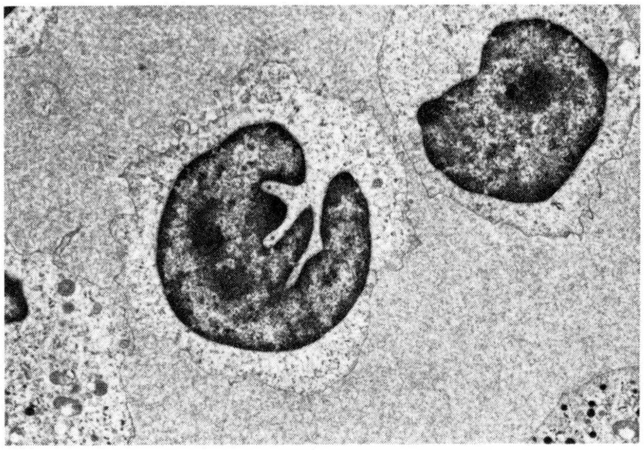

Discussion. Phenytoin-induced pseudolymphoma is an uncommon syndrome, considering that fewer than 200 cases have been reported despite phenytoin's use in millions of people since being marketed in 1938.[1-8] Coope and Burrows[1] reported the first case of phenytoin-induced lymphadenopathy in 1940. In 1959 Saltzstein and Ackerman[2] reviewed 75 previously reported cases of anticonvulsant-induced lymphadenopathy and reported seven new cases. All patients had clinical and histological evidence of malignant lymphoma. Most cases involved the use of mephenytoin, while other drugs implicated less often were trimethadione, thyphenyltoin, phensuximide, and ethotoin. Phenytoin was implicated in 11 cases.

Recognition of the drug-induced syndrome, initiation of proper treatment, and avoidance of unnecessary antineoplastic-drug therapy are important. Table 1 lists the most commonly encountered features of pseudolymphoma. Onset of signs and symptoms can occur from one week to two years after phenytoin therapy is begun; the majority of cases occur within four months. Lymphadenopathy and other features usually resolve within one to four weeks of phenytoin withdrawal, although some problems have persisted longer, as was the experience with our patient.[1-8]

Phenytoin-induced pseudolymphoma is considered a delayed hypersensitivity reaction because of the length of time required to develop the syndrome, regression when phenytoin is withdrawn, and recurrence when therapy is reinstituted. The histology of lymph nodal tissue is similar to that found in malignant processes and could be mistak-

Table 1.
Clinical Manifestations of Pseudolymphoma Syndrome

Most Common Features
- Lymphadenopathy: cervical nodes most common, but frequently generalized
- Fever
- Skin disorders: morbilliform or scarlatiniform rashes, urticaria, exfoliative dermatitis, and abnormal pigmentation
- Eosinophilia

Frequent Features
- Hepatosplenomegaly
- Malaise
- Weight loss
- Leukocytosis or leukopenia
- Elevated levels of hepatic enzymes: AST (SGOT), ALT (SGPT), lactate dehydrogenase, or alkaline phosphatase

Less Frequent Features
- Joint swelling: primarily lower extremities
- Arthralgias
- Oral mucositis
- Facial and labial swelling
- Conjunctivitis

en for such, but the tissue normalizes as clinical features disappear. Definitive treatment involves withdrawal of the drug and symptomatic relief. Steroids and antihistamines have been used to speed recovery, but they are not necessary for remission of the syndrome.[1-8]

In 1966 Hyman and Sommers[11] used the term pseudolymphoma to refer to this syndrome, which recedes with cessation of drug therapy. They also reported seven cases of malignant lymphoma associated with phenytoin use. Six patients were diagnosed initially as having frank lymphoma, and the seventh patient's diagnosis was confirmed by lymph node biopsy three years later. Phenytoin was implicated as a possible inducing factor of neoplastic transformation.

In 1968 Gams and coworkers[12] coined the phrase pseudo-pseudolymphoma to describe a case of phenytoin-induced lymphadenopathy that resolved after cessation of therapy; however, 20 months after phenytoin withdrawal, fatal malignant lymphoma developed. Table 2 summarizes the proposed classification system of hydantoin-induced lymphadenopathy based on the clinical syndrome and lymph node tissue histology. Our patient continues to be followed as an outpatient and one year later remains free of any signs or symptoms of a malignant process.

Reports of lymphoma and of pseudolymphoma followed by malignant lymphoma in patients receiving phenytoin have prompted several investigators to explore the drug's possible carcinogenic properties.[13-26] Phenytoin is known to cause immunosuppression involving a decline in suppressor T lymphocytes.[24] Gershwin and Steinberg[25] suggested that an antigenic stimulus like phenytoin could overcome compromised T-suppressor

Table 2.
Classification of Hydantoin-Induced Lymphadenopathy[12]

Diagnosis	Clinical Syndrome	Lymphoid Tissue
Lymphoid hyperplasia	Regularly regresses with cessation of therapy	Normal architecture with a pleomorphic cellular response or lymphadenitis (not to be confused with lymphoma)
Pseudolymphoma	Indistinguishable from the hyperplasia group	Alteration and effacement of nodal architecture with reticular cell hyperplasia (may appear frankly malignant)
Pseudo-pseudolymphoma	Regresses upon drug withdrawal; after a quiescent period symptoms reappear (without further drug treatment)	Consistent with hyperplasia or pseudolymphoma at first, later shows true malignant process
Lymphoma	Does not regress upon drug withdrawal	Diagnostic for malignancy

function, leading to pronounced lymphoid proliferation and ultimately a malignant state.

Rosenthal and colleagues[9] have proposed the name "pseudo-mycosis fungoides syndrome" for a subtype of the pseudolymphoma syndrome. They characterized this condition as the triad of exfoliative erythrodermic dermatitis, Pautrier's microabscesses of the epidermis, and generalized lymphadenopathy, along with various other features of pseudolymphoma. Five cases consistent with this description have been reported in the literature,[7,9,10] including three by Rosenthal.

We believe that our patient represents another such case, and we offer histological evidence not previously reported to support this diagnosis. Our patient had the following characteristics:

- Exfoliative erythrodermic dermatitis;
- A skin biopsy similar to those previously reported;
- Generalized lymphadenopathy;
- Histological evidence of mycosis fungoides in lymphoid tissue;
- Characteristically abnormal lymphocyte populations of lymphoid tissue;
- Circulating Sézary cells;
- Clinical manifestations of pseudolymphoma; and
- Complete regression of all physical, laboratory, and histologic abnormalities upon withdrawal of phenytoin.

Our patient's skin biopsy was not considered classic for Pautrier's microabscesses, which are collections of hyperchromatic mononuclear cells within the epidermis characterizing malignant lymphoma of the skin, particularly mycosis fungoides. Nevertheless, histologic findings were similar to other associated changes found in at least three of the previously reported subjects.[9,10]

Lymph node biopsies were performed in only three of the previously reported cases of pseudomycosis fungoides syndrome; all specimens were histologically abnormal and consistent with abnormalities found in pseudolymphoma.[7,9,10] However, histological examination of lymphoid tissue from our patient revealed convoluted lymphocytes and cerebriform nuclei characteristic of mycosis fungoides.[27] These findings were not reported in the five original cases. A cell suspension from our patient's lymphoid tissue contained an abnormal lymphocyte population that was consistent with true mycosis fungoides.[27] These findings were similar to the composition of cells that Rosenthal et al.[9] reported in the peripheral blood of their patients. In addition, circulating Sézary cells were found in the peripheral blood of our patient, as was reported by Rosenthal. This is another common finding in true mycosis fungoides.[27]

Bone marrow aspirates were performed on our patient and in two other previously reported cases.[7,10] All findings were normal. All reported cases, including our own, involved clinical manifestations of pseudolymphoma.

Conclusion. Recognition of phenytoin-induced pseudolymphoma is important for the initiation of proper treatment and avoidance of unnecessary therapy with antineoplastic agents. The patient described here had the characteristics of pseudo-mycosis fungoides syndrome, a rare subtype of pseudolymphoma. This is the sixth reported case of phenytoin-induced pseudolymphoma with mycosis fungoides manifestations; it is the first report containing histologic evidence to support the diagnosis.

References

1. Coope R, Burrows RGR. Treatment of epilepsy with sodium diphenyl hydantoinate. *Lancet*. 1940; 1:490–2.
2. Saltzstein SL, Ackerman LV. Lymphadenopathy induced by anticonvulsant drugs and mimicking clinically and pathologically malignant lymphomas. *Cancer*. 1959; 12:164–82.
3. Schwinghammer TL, Howrie DL. Phenytoin-induced lymphadenopathy. *Drug Intell Clin Pharm*. 1983; 17:460–2.
4. Oates RK, Tonge RE. Phenytoin and the pseudolymphoma syndrome. *Med J Aust*. 1971; 2:371–3.
5. Choovivathanavanich P, Wallace EM, Scaglione PR. Pseudolymphoma induced by diphenylhydantoin. *J Pediatr*. 1970; 76:621–3.
6. Rosenfeld S, Swiller AI, Shenoy MV et al. Syndrome simulating lymphosarcoma induced by diphenylhydantoin sodium. *JAMA*. 1961; 176:491–3.
7. Schreiber MM, McGregor JG. Pseudolymphoma syndrome. *Arch Dermatol*. 1968; 97:297–300.
8. Treyve EL, Duckert LG. Phenytoin-induced lymphadenopathy appearing as a nasopharyngeal malignant neoplasm. *Arch Otolaryngol*. 1981; 107:382–4.
9. Rosenthal CJ, Noguera CA, Coppola A et al. Pseudolymphoma with mycosis fungoides manifestations, hyperresponsiveness to diphenylhydantoin, and lymphocyte dysregulation. *Cancer*. 1982; 49:2305–14.
10. Wolf R, Kahane E, Sandbank M. Mycosis fungoides-like lesions associated with phenytoin therapy. *Arch Dermatol*. 1985; 121:1181–2.
11. Hyman GA, Sommers SC. The development of Hodgkin's disease and lymphoma during anticonvulsant therapy. *Blood*. 1966; 28:416–27.
12. Gams RA, Neal JA, Conrad FG. Hydantoin-induced pseudo-pseudolymphoma. *Ann Intern Med*. 1968; 69:557–68.
13. Matzner Y, Polliack A. Lymphoproliferative disorders in four patients receiving chronic diphenylhydantoin therapy: etiologic correlation or chance association? *Isr J Med Sci*. 1978; 14:865–9.
14. Anthony JJ. Malignant lymphoma associated with hydantoin drugs. *Arch Neurol*. 1970; 22:450–4.
15. Charlton MH, Lunsford D. Se sestanze di idantonia come possibili cause del linfoma maligno. *Minerva Med*. 1971; 62:2185. Abstract.
16. Li FP, Willard DR, Goodman R et al. Malignant lymphoma after diphenylhydantoin (Dilantin) therapy. *Cancer*. 1975; 36:1359–62.
17. Clemmesen J. Are anticonvulsants oncogenic? *Lancet*. 1974; 1:705–7.
18. Anon. Is phenytoin carcinogenic? *Lancet*. 1971; 2:1071–2. Editorial.
19. Lillie MA, Yang LC, Honig PJ et al. Erythroderma, hypogammaglobulinemia, and T-cell lymphocytosis—occurrence following therapy with phenytoin. *Arch Dermatol*. 1983; 119:415–8.
20. Sorrell TC, Forbes IJ, Burness FR et al. Depression of immunological function in patients treated with phenytoin sodium (sodium diphenylhydantoin). *Lancet*. 1971; 2:1233–5.
21. Bluming A, Homer S, Khiroya R. Selective diphenylhydantoin-induced suppression of lymphocyte reactivity in vitro. *J Lab Clin Med*. 1976; 88:417–21.
22. Sorrell TC, Forbes IJ. Depression of immune competence by phenytoin and carbamazepine—studies in vivo and in vitro. *Clin Exp Immunol*. 1975; 20:273–85.
23. Charlesworth EN. Phenytoin-induced pseudolymphoma syndrome—an immunologic study. *Arch Dermatol*. 1977; 113:477–80.
24. Duggan MAK, Court JB. A proposed mechanism of production of the autoimmune and lymphoproliferative side effects of beta-adrenergic-site-blocking drugs and hydantoin anticonvulsants. *Ann Clin Res*. 1981; 13:406–18.
25. Gershwin ME, Steinberg AD. Loss of suppressor function as a cause of lymphoid malignancy. *Lancet*. 1973; 2:1174–6.
26. Kruger GRF, Harris D. Is phenytoin carcinogenic? *Lancet*. 1972; 1:323. Letter.
27. Broder S, Bunn PA. Cutaneous T-cell lymphomas. *Semin Oncol*. 1980; 7:310–31.

CP Continuing Education

The ASHP Continuing Education system gives readers a self-assessment mechanism for selected articles in Clinical Pharmacy *and the* American Journal of Hospital Pharmacy. *It also allows readers to obtain continuing-education credit for these articles.*

For the purpose of CE-credit enrollment a blank answer sheet is published at the end of each installment of the column for the CE articles in that issue. An enrollee accumulates these answer sheets until the enrollment is submitted, using the form that is published in the June and December issues of Clinical Pharmacy *and in the June and December issues of the* American Journal of Hospital Pharmacy. *Any combination of tests within a 18-month period, from both* Clinical Pharmacy *and* American Journal of Hospital Pharmacy, *may be included in an enrollment. More complete details about enrollment in the system will appear in the semiannual enrollment form.*

Article 680-204-8802 (see page 97)
Qualifies for 1.0 hour of CE credit

Nicardipine, nitrendipine, and bepridil: New calcium antagonists for cardiovascular disorders

Learning Objectives

After studying this article, the reader should be able to

1. Describe the major pharmacologic properties of nicardipine, nitrendipine, and bepridil.
2. Describe the major pharmacokinetic properties of nicardipine, nitrendipine, and bepridil.
3. Identify the major adverse effects of nicardipine, nitrendipine, and bepridil.
4. List the cardiovascular disorders for which nicardipine, nitrendipine, and bepridil have been shown to be effective.

Self-assessment Questions

For each question there is one best answer only.

1. Actions of nicardipine, nitrendipine, and bepridil that may be useful in the treatment of cardiovascular disorders include

   a. Direct (in vitro) enhancement of myocardial contractility.
   b. Relaxation of vascular smooth muscle.
   c. Facilitation of atrioventricular nodal conduction.
   d. Lowering of serum calcium concentration.

2. Nicardipine, nitrendipine, and bepridil share a pharmacokinetic property in that all three drugs

   a. Form metabolites that have greater activity than the parent drug.
   b. Are highly protein bound.
   c. Undergo substantial first-pass metabolism.
   d. All of the above alternatives are correct.
   e. Alternatives b and c only are correct.

3. Serum digoxin concentrations have been reported to be increased by administration of

   a. Nicardipine.
   b. Nitrendipine.
   c. Bepridil.
   d. All of the above alternatives are correct.
   e. Alternatives a and b only are correct.

4. Multiple clinical trials have demonstrated the antihypertensive efficacy of

   a. Nicardipine and nitrendipine, but not bepridil.
   b. Nitrendipine and bepridil, but not nicardipine.
   c. Nicardipine and bepridil, but not nitrendipine.
   d. Nicardipine, nitrendipine, and bepridil.

5. Antianginal effects have been demonstrated in studies using long-term administration of

   a. Nicardipine and nitrendipine, but not bepridil.
   b. Nitrendipine and bepridil, but not nicardipine.
   c. Nicardipine and bepridil, but not nitrendipine.
   d. Nicardipine, nitrendipine, and bepridil.

6. Bepridil has cardiac electrophysiologic properties that may make it useful in the treatment of

   a. Symptomatic bradycardia.
   b. Complete heart block.
   c. Supraventricular tachyarrhythmias.
   d. Monomorphic ventricular tachycardia.
   e. Alternatives c and d only are correct.

7. When studied in patients with congestive heart failure, nicardipine and nitrendipine have caused

   a. A definite prolongation of survival.
   b. Increases in mean blood pressure.
   c. Increases in left ventricular ejection fraction or cardiac index.
   d. All of the above alternatives are correct.
   e. Alternatives b and c only are correct.

8. The tachycardia that occurs with the dihydropyridines
   a. Often lessens or abates with long-term therapy.
   b. Is a result of direct stimulation by the drugs of the sinoatrial node.
   c. Eliminates these drugs as useful antianginal agents.
   d. Makes these agents useful in the treatment of symptomatic bradycardia.

9. The reported proarrhythmic effects of bepridil have included the development of
   a. Torsade de pointes.
   b. New monomorphic ventricular tachycardia.
   c. New atrial flutter.
   d. All of the above alternatives are correct.
   e. Alternatives a and b only are correct.

10. The most commonly reported noncardiac adverse effects of bepridil include
   a. Gastrointestinal and central nervous system complaints.
   b. Flushing and peripheral edema.
   c. Thrombocytopenia.
   d. Photosensitivity.

Answer sheet

February 1988 ***Clinical Pharmacy***

Note: An enrollment form for the ASHP Continuing-Education System appears in the June and December issues. Please accumulate all the answer sheets you wish to use in one enrollment and submit them at one time with a completed enrollment form.

Place an X in the box(es) at the top of the column(s) corresponding to the test(s) you are taking. Darken the boxes corresponding to the correct answers.

□
680-204-8802
1.0 hour

	a	b	c	d	e
1.	□	□	□	□	
2.	□	□	□	□	□
3.	□	□	□	□	□
4.	□	□	□	□	
5.	□	□	□	□	
6.	□	□	□	□	□
7.	□	□	□	□	□
8.	□	□	□	□	
9.	□	□	□	□	□
10.	□	□	□	□	

ASHP Use Only
(1.0)8802________(3)

Ad Council

WHEN THERE
WILL BE
NO LONELINESS,
NO DESTITUTION,
NO SICKNESS,
NO WAR,
ONLY THEN
WILL THERE
BE NO NEED
FOR THE
AMERICAN
RED CROSS.

Contact your local chapter.

American Red Cross

Current Literature

Drug Reaction Alerts

Drug Reaction Alerts focuses primarily on serious, unlabeled reactions to new chemical entities. The citations are compiled monthly from International Pharmaceutical Abstracts, *which covers over 800 pharmacy and health-related journals worldwide. An address for reprints (when available) follows the name of the corresponding author in each citation.*

Anti-infective Agents

Alfaham M (University Hospital of Wales, Heath Park, Cardiff CF4 4XW, Wales), Holt ME, Goodchild MC. Arthropathy in a patient with cystic fibrosis taking **ciprofloxacin**. *Br Med J.* 1987; 295:699. Case. (16-year-old girl with cystic fibrosis and advanced lung disease; received ciprofloxacin 750 mg twice daily for 22 days; developed arthritis in the knees; concomitant floxacillin, stanozolol, gentamicin, carbenicillin, vitamins, and pancreatic enzyme supplements; resolution of all symptoms within two weeks after withdrawal of ciprofloxacin)

Antiprotozoals

Wharton JM (Division of Cardiology, Duke University Medical Center, P.O. Box 3371, Durham, NC 27710), Demopulos, PA, Goldschlager N. Torsade de pointes during administration of **pentamidine isethionate**. *Am J Med.* 1987; 83:571–6. Cases. (two men, ages 26 and 36 years; received pentamidine isethionate 4 mg/kg/day by i.v. or i.m. injection for 13 or 20 days; both patients developed QT-interval prolongation, precordial T-wave abnormalities, and ST-segment changes; electrocardiographic abnormalities resolved over several days to weeks corresponding to the elimination characteristics of pentamidine)

Antivirals

Melamed AJ (Memorial Sloan-Kettering Cancer Center, New York, NY), Muller RJ, Gold JW et al. Possible **zidovudine**-induced hepatotoxicity. *JAMA.* 1987; 258:2063. Cases. (three men with acquired immunodeficiency syndrome, aged 33–43 years; received zidovudine [AZT] 1200 mg/day for 2–3 weeks; developed alterations in several liver function tests; tests returned to normal upon drug withdrawal; negative rechallenge in two patients)

Richman DD (no reprints available), Fischl MA, Grieco MH et al. Toxicity of **azidothymidine** (AZT) in the treatment of patients with AIDS and AIDS-related complex: double-blind, placebo-controlled trial. *N Engl J Med.* 1987; 317:192–7. Study. (multicenter, placebo-controlled, double-blind; 282 patients with acquired immunodeficiency syndrome or AIDS-related complex; study patients received zidovudine 250 mg every four hours; anemia requiring multiple red cell transfusions, neutropenia, nausea, myalgia, insomnia, and severe headaches more common in patients receiving AZT)

Antituberculars

Mac-Moune Lai F (Chinese University of Hong Kong, Prince of Wales Hospital, Shatin, Hong Kong), Lai KN, Chong YW. Papillary necrosis associated with **rifampicin** therapy. *Aust N Z J Med.* 1987; 17:68–70. Case. (32-year-old woman with renal tuberculosis; received rifampin 450 mg/day for 14 months; concomitant pyridoxine; developed papillary necrosis, glomerulosclerosis, and granulomatous interstitial nephritis; renal failure progressed upon drug withdrawal and patient died)

Cardiac Drugs

Manolis AS (New England Medical Center, P.O. Box 98, 750 Washington St., Boston, MA 02111), Tordjman T, Mack KD et al. Atypical pulmonary and neurologic complications of **amiodarone** in the same patient: report of a case and review of the literature. *Arch Intern Med.* 1987; 147:1805–9. Case. (67-year-old woman with arrhythmia; received amiodarone 18 g over 10 days as a loading dose, then 400 mg/day for six months; developed pulmonary and hepatic nodules masquerading as metastatic carcinoma, later developed focal infiltrates and a large left pleural effusion mimicking infection, malignant neoplasm, or collagen vascular disease; incapacitating orthostatic hypotension persisted for six weeks after drug withdrawal; pleuropulmonary toxic effects resolved upon discontinuation of amiodarone; resolution hastened by therapy with prednisone tapered and discontinued over 10 days)

Drug Interactions

Edwards DJ (College of Pharmacy, Wayne State University, Detroit, MI 46202), Lavoie R, Beckman H et al. Effect of coadministration of **verapamil** on the pharmacokinetics and metabolism of **quinidine**. *Clin Pharmacol Ther.* 1987; 41:68–73. Study. (six healthy nonsmoking volunteers, aged 23–34 years; received single oral dose of quinidine sulfate 400 mg after pretreatment with oral verapamil 80 mg or 120 mg every eight hours for three days; half-life prolonged and oral clearance of quinidine decreased from 17 L/hr to 11.6 L/hr after 80-mg dose or 11.3 L/hr after 120-mg dose; clearance of (3S)-3-hydroxyquinidine reduced 61.2% and 70.6% after 80-mg and 120-mg doses, respectively; renal clearance of unchanged quinidine not affected)

Lucena MI (Department of Clinical Pharmacology, School of Medicine, Granada, Spain), Moreno A, Fernandez MC et al. **Digitoxin** elimination in healthy subjects taking **ampicillin**. *Int J Clin Pharmacol Res.* 1987; 7:33–7. Study. (six healthy subjects; received single dose of digitoxin 1 mg followed three days later by ampicillin 500 mg 4 times daily for five days; mean elimination half-life of digitoxin increased from 162 ± 12.9 hours to 181.3 ± 10.1 hours after ampicillin administration)

Ng HW (Department of Dermatology, Royal Liverpool Hospital, Liverpool L7 8XP, England), McFarlane AW, Graham RM et al. Near fatal drug interactions with **methotrexate** given for psoriasis. *Br Med J.* 1987; 295:752-3. Case. (80-year-old patient with psoriasis; received methotrexate 25 mg i.m. and oral **trimethoprim** 200 mg twice daily for 10 days; developed severe skin ulceration and leukopenia; received methotrexate previously without incident; skin healed within 7 days after beginning of folinic acid treatment and white cell count normalized within 10 days)

Novakova I (Department of Internal Medicine, University Hospital Nijmegen, 6500 HB Nijmegen, Netherlands), Donnelly P, Witte T et al. **Itraconazole** and **cyclosporin** nephrotoxicity. *Lancet.* 1987; 2:920–1. Study. (14 allogenic bone-marrow transplant recipients; received itraconazole 100 mg twice daily one week before transplantation; received cyclosporine 3 mg/kg/day i.v. one day before transplantation; cyclosporine blood concentrations not significantly higher in patients treated with both drugs than in those given cyclosporine alone, and no significant differences in serum creatinine concentrations when drugs taken concomitantly)

Reeves RA (Hypertension Unit, Edith Cavell Wing, Toronto Western Hospital, 399 Bathurst St., Toronto, Ontario, Canada M5T 2S8), Smith DL, Leenen FH. Hemodynamic interaction of nonselective vs beta-1-selective beta blockade with **hydralazine** in normal humans. *Clin Pharmacol Ther.* 1987; 41:326–35. Study. (randomized, double-blind, placebo-controlled, crossover; 8 healthy volunteers, aged 18–28 years; received pretreatment with **propranolol** 20 mg and 40 mg or **atenolol** 25 mg and 50 mg before receiving hydralazine 100 mg; both propranolol and atenolol blunted hydralazine-induced increases in heart rate, cardiac output, and venous return similarly, although heart rate and cardiac output were not completely normalized; atenolol did not affect hydralazine-induced decrease in afterload, whereas propranolol significantly opposed this change)

Hemorheologic Agents

Mass RD (University of California, San Francisco, CA 94143), Venook AP, Linker CA et al. **Pentoxifylline** and aplastic anemia. *Ann Intern Med.* 1987; 107:427–8. Cases. (two women, ages 70 and 80 years; received pentoxifylline 400 mg 2 or 3 times daily for 3 or 10 weeks; concomitant hydrochlorothiazide–triamterene, furosemide, prazosin, and chlorpropamide; blood cell counts remained depressed upon drug withdrawal; both patients developed septicemia and died despite antibiotic therapy)

Hypotensive Agents

Richter WO (no reprints available), Schwandt P. Serious side effect of **nifedipine**. *Arch Intern Med.* 1987; 147:1852. Case. (69-year-old hypertensive woman; received nifedipine 30–120 mg/day for six months; concomitant digitoxin, furosemide, prazosin hydrochloride, and allopurinol; developed cholestasis evidenced by elevated liver function test values; resolution upon drug withdrawal; positive rechallenge)

Book Reviews

Avery's Drug Treatment: Principles and Practice of Clinical Pharmacology and Therapeutics, Third Edition

Edited by Trevor M. Speight.

Published by ADIS Press Limited, Auckland, New Zealand, and Williams & Wilkins, 428 East Preston St., Baltimore, MD 21202, 1987. xvi + 1507 p. Price $60.00.

The third edition of Avery's text continues the trend set by the second edition, which was a major improvement over the original, published in 1976.

The structure and organization have not changed since the inception of the text—it makes use of a disease-oriented approach to the selection of the most appropriate drug and dosage regimen for a particular patient. It does so under the general headings of (1) the clinical pharmacologic basis of therapeutics, with a welcome emphasis on the importance of pharmacokinetics in drug selection and use, (2) the selection and rational use of drugs for a particular disease, (3) the influence of associated or intercurrent illness on drug pharmacokinetics and response, and (4) diseases that may be caused or exacerbated by drugs.

The text has undergone major revision. Fifteen of the previous edition's 30 chapters have been rewritten by new authors, and two entirely new chapters have been added, Therapeutic Drug Monitoring and Drug Use in the Critically Ill. In addition, the appendices have been updated to include (1) an extremely useful and exhaustive compilation of the population pharmacokinetic characteristics of literally hundreds of drug products, including data covering values for half-life, clearance, and volume of distribution, (2) the Bennett table for drug dosing in renal failure, (3) a newly added guide to drug dosing in hepatic failure, and (4) information concerning antibiotic selection and adverse drug reactions. The widely criticized Dettli nomogram for drug dosage estimation in renal failure is included as an appendix but is of questionable value, especially in view of the standard set by Bennett.

The text does have some limitations—distractions, really—that may be attributed more to language differences and writing-style idiosyncracies than to any inadequacies in the quality of information presented. For example, the terminology of disease states and even drug products (lignocaine as opposed to lidocaine) and the use of the British style of writing (wherewithal, amongst, whilst) may require some getting used to. More problematic, however, is the use of the standardized international units of measure—a blood glucose concentration of 10 mmol/L, for example. More than a distraction, the variation from the system used commonly in the United States makes it almost impossible to correlate the laboratory information to the discussions of drugs and disease states. The final limitation, which may actually be an advantage, is that many drugs not currently approved for use in the United States are discussed in the book. Because many of the drugs that are used overseas do eventually make it into the American marketplace, this coverage may provide us with drug information that, instead of becoming outdated, will be useful well into the future.

The book contains chapters on all of the major disease states, and it devotes entire chapters to drug use in premature infants, neonates, and pediatric and geriatric patients. It is a complete, well-referenced text that is written from a pharmacologic perspective. The pharmacist and the pharmacy student, along with other health-care providers, should find this reference a highly valuable addition to their holdings. I am pleased to recommend it strongly.

Reviewed by Michael J. Melby, M.S., Department of Pharmacy, New England Medical Center Hospitals, 171 Harrison Avenue, Boston, MA 02111.

Guide to Planning and Managing Multiple Clinical Studies

By Bert Spilker.

Published by Raven Press, 1185 Avenue of the Americas, New York, NY 10036, 1987. xxii + 410 p. Price $36.50.

Dr. Spilker, the head of the Department of Project Coordination at Burroughs Wellcome Company, offers this book as a follow-up to *Guide to Clinical Studies and Developing Protocols* and *Guide to the Clinical Interpretation of Data*. He refers frequently to the first two volumes for further discussion of particular issues. Nonetheless, this volume is complete enough to offer an encyclopedic overview of planning and undertaking multiple clinical studies. The author's stated purpose in this volume is to discuss the issues involved in designing and undertaking multiple studies that evaluate the clinical efficacy of drugs or devices. The author attempts to provide this information in a practical "nuts and bolts" style and aims his book toward readers with industrial, academic, and government affiliations.

The text is divided into three main sections. The first, "Planning and Conducting Multiple Clinical Studies," begins by describing how an organization (usually a pharmaceutical company) chooses drugs or devices and their applications for clinical development. Chapters on establishing project strategies and designs follow. Although these chapters assume that the reader is knowledgeable about Food and Drug Administration regulations and procedures, they do provide even the casual reader with a fascinating glimpse into the workings of a pharmaceutical firm and the interaction between individual investigators and the institution, as told from the institutional point of view. Subsequent chapters deal with collecting and integrating data from multiple studies, and they range from a general discussion of often self-evident points to suggested specific data-collection forms with limited general applicability. The chapter on safety data does contain an interesting discussion on the need for complete information about adverse reactions and much practical advice concerning the tabulation and interpretation of data collected from multiple studies by different investigators. The concluding chapter in the first section, "Potential Ethical Issues in Single and Multiple Studies," disappointingly limits its discussion to the premise that an unethical study is one that does not provide usable, meaningful data.

The second section of the book concerns planning clinical studies for special situations; it includes surgical studies, studies of devices, drugs for rare diseases, and special populations (e.g., elderly). The use of tables and flow charts with occasionally interesting discussions (e.g., the difficulties in truly randomizing surgical treatments) continues as in the earlier section of the book. The point of view is most definitely that of a pharmaceutical firm and how it decides which drugs, devices, or studies to pursue for the long-term benefit of the firm.

The third section concerns management of multiple clinical studies. Topics including coordination, allocation of resources, and monitoring are discussed from industry's point of view.

On the whole, the book is uneven in its presentation. While the general use of graphs and tables allows each chapter to be easily summarized, the discussion of many pertinent topics is superficial. The overall point of view is thoroughly from the industrial perspective and makes this book most useful for the person planning to work with or within the pharmaceutical industry.

Reviewed by Mark C. Norris, M.D., and Ghassem E. Larijani, Pharm.D., Department of Anesthesiology, Jefferson Medical College, Philadelphia, PA 19107.

Books Received

Books are listed as soon as received; selected books may be reviewed in Book Reviews in subsequent issues.

Drug Use in Respiratory Disease, edited by J. Douglas Wilson. Published by Williams & Wilkins and Associates PTY Limited, 43 Herbert Street, Artarmon, N.S.W. 2064, Australia, 1987. Available from Williams & Wilkins, 428 E. Preston St., Baltimore, MD 21202. 319 p. Price $60.

Essentials of General Pathology, by John R. Warren, Dante G. Scarpelli, Janardan K. Reddy et al. Published by Macmillan Publishing Company, 866 Third Ave., New York, NY 10022, 1987. vii + 259 p. Price $29.95.

Therapeutics in the Elderly, edited by Jeffrey C. Delafuente and Ronald B. Stewart. Published by Williams & Wilkins, 428 East Preston St., Baltimore, MD 21202, 1988. xii + 357 p. Price $33.95.

Advertising Index

American Red Cross
Institutional, 159
Beecham Laboratories
Ticar, 96
Roxane Laboratories, A Boehringer Ingelheim Company
Intensols, 87
Stuart Pharmaceuticals, Division of ICI Americas, Inc.
Cefotan, 89–91, inside back cover, outside back cover
The Upjohn Company
Cleocin, 83–84
Veterans Administration Medical Center (Syracuse)
Position Available, 94
Wyeth Laboratories
Tubex, inside front cover

When it comes to taking their medicine,
some patients need—

SPECIAL DELIVERY

INTENSOL™

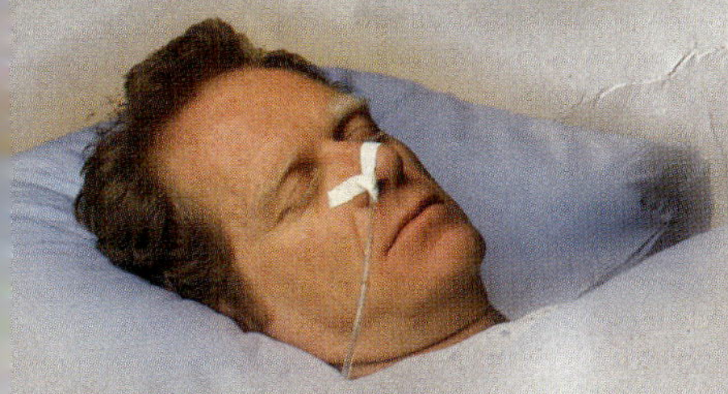

For patients who have difficulty with tablets

The nasogastric patient
The elderly or debilitated patient
The cancer patient on high or variable doses
The pediatric patient

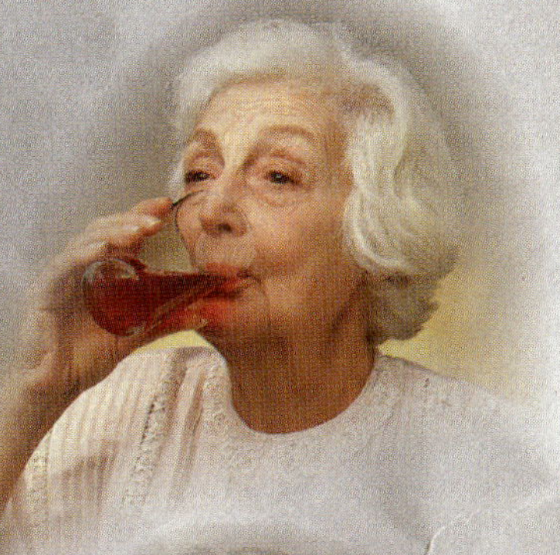

Concentrated oral solutions

Intensols are highly concentrated medications—Chlorpromazine, Dexamethasone, DHT, Hydrochlorothiazide, Prednisone, Thioridazine, to name a few—in low volume solutions.

Easier than swallowing tablets

Intensols can be mixed with juice or semisolid foods, or even administered through nasogastric tubing.

Most Intensols have no flavor, so medications taste like the food or liquid they are mixed with. Each bottle comes with a calibrated dropper for easy dosage titration.

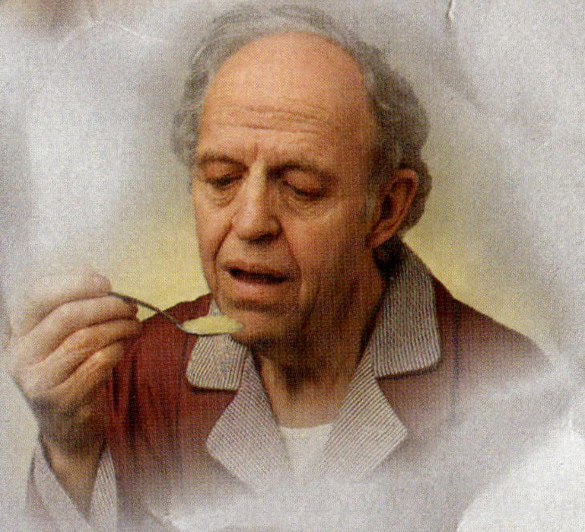

Easy to dispense

- Every dose is accurate.
- Ends the need to crush or break tablets—yielding inexact doses.
- Enhances patient compliance.
- Eliminates pharmacy compounding.

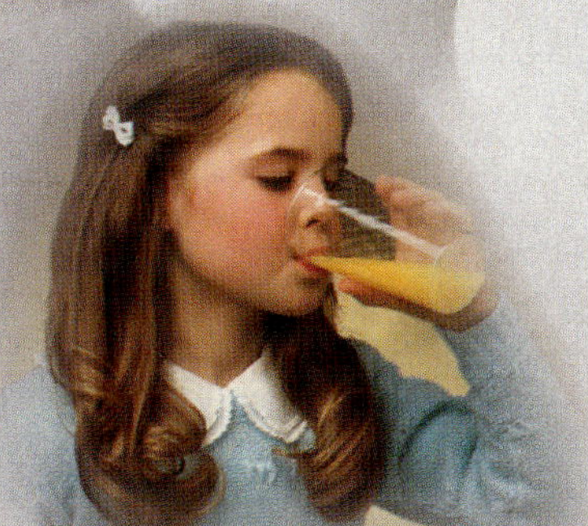

INTENSOLS...

A SPECIAL DELIVERY SYSTEM
for special patients.

Roxane Laboratories, Inc.
Columbus, Ohio 43216

Intensols for your special patients

To find out more about INTENSOLS for your patients, fill out the following and mail to: Roxane Laboratories, Inc., PO Box 16532, Columbus, Ohio 43216.

Name
Address
Specialty

News

FDA's drug review process is focus of attention in 1987; agency approves 27 new products

1987 was marked by intense scrutiny of FDA's drug approval process, best exemplified by the attention focused on the approval of alteplase, recombinant and decisions regarding agents under evaluation for the treatment of AIDS. During the year changes were made in drug regulations and FDA's organizational structure that will affect the drug approval process in the future: The treatment IND rule permitting broader use of investigational drugs in the treatment of certain serious or life-threatening conditions went into effect and, in response to pressures generated by AIDS and the drug review process, FDA's biologic and drug evaluation unit was divided into two units.

A total of 21 new drugs and 6 biologicals were approved by FDA during 1987. Six of the 21 drugs were considered by FDA to be modest therapeutic advances (indicated by a 1B rating) and two, lovastatin and zidovudine, were designated as important therapeutic advances (1A rating). The year was average in terms of the number of drug approvals. The approval of eight orphan drugs in 1987 was the highest yearly total since enactment of the Orphan Drug Act. Fifty-eight products were granted orphan status, raising the total number to 183.

Twenty-two of the 27 approvals were announced during the last quarter of the year; approval dates for 15 agents came during the final two weeks of December. The mean drug approval time decreased from 34.2 months in 1986 to 32.3 months in 1987. For drugs with 1A or 1B ratings, the mean approval time decreased from 32.1 to 22.7 months. Zidovudine, aplonidine, and lovastin were approved 3, 3.5, and 9.5 months, respectively, after NDA submission; review times for other drugs ranged from 18 to 87 months.

Two products were produced using recombinant-DNA technology. Results of a survey commissioned by the Pharmaceutical Manufacturers Association suggest that the number of biotechnology-based products will increase in the future. According to the survey, much of the corporate biotechnology research being conducted in the United States is directed toward pharmaceutical products. Of 1476 biotechnology patents issued in 1987, 845 (57%) were health-care related.

The following products were approved by FDA during 1987:

- Alteplase, recombinant (Activase, Genentech, Inc.), a tissue plasminogen activator for the treatment of acute myocardial infarction;
- Antihemophilic factor, human (Monoclate Factor VIII:c, Armour Pharmaceutical Company), the first human antihemophilic factor product to be purified using monoclonal antibody technology;
- Aplonidine hydrochloride (Iopidine, Alcon Laboratories, Inc.) an α adrenergic agonist for controlling postsurgical increases in intraocular pressure;
- Carprofen (Rimadyl, Hoffmann-La Roche, Inc.), a nonsteroidal anti-inflammatory agent;
- Cefmenoxime hydrochloride (Cefmax, TAP Pharmaceuticals), a cephalosporin indicated for the treatment of lower-respiratory-tract and urinary-tract infections;
- Ciprofloxacin hydrochloride (Cipro, Miles Inc.), an oral quinolone antimicrobial agent;
- Fluoxetine hydrochloride (Prozac, Dista Products Company), a serotonin-uptake inhibitor for the treatment of depression;
- Haemophilus b conjugate vaccine (ProHIBiT, Connaught Laboratories, Inc.), effective in preventing *H. influenzae* type b disease in children as young as 18 months of age;
- Iofetamine hydrochloride I 123 injection (Spectamine, Medi-Physics, Inc.), a lipid-soluble brain-imaging agent for use in the evaluation of strokes;
- Lisinopril (Prinivil, Merck Sharp & Dohme; Zestril, Stuart Pharmaceuticals), a once-a-day angiotensin-converting enzyme inhibitor indicated for the treatment of hypertension;
- Lovastatin (Mevacor, Merck Sharp & Dohme), a cholesterol-lowering agent that acts by inhibiting 3-hydroxy-3-methylglutaryl coenzyme A (HMG-CoA) reductase;
- Mesalamine, or 5-aminosalicylic acid (Rowasa, Reid-Rowell, Inc.), a rectal suspension enema for the treatment of ulcerative colitis, ulcerative proctitis, or ulcerative proctosigmoiditis;
- Milrinone (Sterling Drug Inc.), a phosphodiesterase inhibitor for intravenous administration in the treatment of congestive heart failure;
- Mitoxantrone (Novatrone, Lederle Laboratories), an anthracenedione indicated for the treatment of acute nonlymphocytic leukemia;
- Mometasone furoate 0.1% (Elocon, Schering Corporation), a topical synthetic corticosteroid;
- Mupirocin 2% (Bactroban, Beecham Laboratories), a topical antibacterial agent for the treatment of impetigo;
- Penbutolol sulfate (Levatol, Eli Lilly and Company), a β blocker for use in the treatment of hypertension;
- α_1-Proteinase inhibitor, human (Prolastin, Cutter Biological), for the treatment of emphysema resulting from α_1-antitrypsin deficiency;
- Poliovirus vaccine, inactivated (Connaught Laboratories, Inc.), a new inactivated poliovirus vaccine with more consistent potency and immunogenicity;
- Sodium benzoate with sodium phenylacetate (Ucephan, Kendall McGaw Laboratories) for the prevention and treatment of hyperammonemia caused by urea-cycle enzyme abnormalities;
- Technetium Tc 99m mebrofenin (Choletec, Squibb Diagnostics), a radiopharmaceutical for use in hepatobiliary system visualization;
- Terazosin (Hytrin, Abbott Health Care Products, Inc.), a once-a-day α_1-adrenergic blocker for the treatment of hypertension;
- Terconazole (Terazol 7, Ortho Pharmaceutical Corporation) for the treatment of vulvovaginal candidiasis;

Continued on page 169

Continued from page 166

- Teriparatide acetate (Parathar, Rorer Group, Inc.), a diagnostic agent for distinguishing between hypoparathyroidism and pseudohypoparathyroidism in patients with hypocalcemia;
- Ursodiol (Deursil, Gipharmex S.P.A./Ciba-Geigy Corporation) for the dissolution of gallstones;
- Zidovudine (Retrovir, Burroughs Wellcome Co.) for the treatment of certain patients with symptomatic human immunodeficiency virus (HIV) infection; and
- HIV Western blot test kit (Du Pont Company and Biotech Research Laboratories) for detection of antibodies to HIV.

Editor's note: This article also appears in the News column of the March issue of the *American Journal of Hospital Pharmacy*.

Immunization of younger children possible with new *Haemophilus influenzae* vaccine

A conjugate vaccine that will permit immunization against *Haemophilus influenzae* type b disease in children as young as 18 months of age was among the products approved at the end of 1987; the previously marketed polysaccharide vaccines are not indicated for use in children less than 24 months of age. Haemophilus b conjugate vaccine (diphtheria toxoid-conjugate), available from Connaught Laboratories, Inc. as ProHIBiT, is the first successful clinical application of conjugate vaccine technology. Covalent bonding of the capsular polysaccharide of *H. influenzae* type b to diphtheria toxoid enhances antibody response and immunologic memory in young children. Connaught has announced plans to discontinue distribution of its polysaccharide vaccine HibVAX after the conjugate vaccine is introduced. In children 18–20 months of age, mean antibody levels after immunization are about 30 times higher with the conjugate vaccine than with the polysaccharide vaccine. Clinical studies assessing the safety and efficacy of the conjugate vaccine in children as young as two months are ongoing. Although some immunologic response to the diphtheria toxoid component may occur, Haemophilus b conjugate vaccine does not eliminate the need for routine immunization against diphtheria. Administration of the conjugate vaccine with diphtheria–tetanus–pertussis (DTP) vaccine and inactivated poliovirus vaccine is not associated with a higher incidence of adverse reactions than with administration of the DTP vaccine alone.

A single intramuscular injection of 0.5 mL of the vaccine is recommended for immunization of children 18 months to 5 years of age. Each 0.5-mL dose contains 25 μg of purified capsular polysaccharide and 18 μg of conjugated diphtheria toxoid protein.

More potent inactivated poliovirus vaccine approved by FDA; CDC to review vaccination policies in 1988

The inactivated poliovirus vaccine (Poliovirus vaccine inactivated, Connaught Laboratories Ltd.) approved by FDA in December is a more potent version of the conventional inactivated (Salk) vaccine. The new vaccine is prepared using human cell cultures and requires only three primary immunizations, whereas the conventional inactivated vaccine is manufactured in monkey kidney cells and requires four primary immunizations.

Poliovirus vaccination policies will be reviewed by the Immunization Practices Advisory Committee of the Centers for Disease Control (CDC) later this year. Current immunization strategies rely primarily on use of the live, attenuated oral vaccine. Recognized indications for use of inactivated vaccines are (1) immunization of unvaccinated adults at increased risk of exposure to poliovirus and (2) immunization, if indicated, of individuals at increased risk of paralysis from oral poliovirus vaccine and their household members and other close contacts. Included in the second group are persons with congenital or acquired immune deficiency diseases or impairment of immune function as a result of other diseases or immunosuppressive therapy. Children with asymptomatic human immunodeficiency virus infection do not appear to be at increased risk of adverse reactions to the oral vaccine, but use of inactivated vaccine is recommended because other family members may be immunocompromised and at risk from contact with oral vaccine virus.

The recommended primary immunization schedule with the enhanced-potency vaccine consists of three 0.5-mL doses of vaccine administered subcutaneously. The second dose should be administered eight weeks after the first dose; an interval of 12 months between the second and third doses is recommended. The first dose can be given as early as six weeks of age, but administration at two months is preferred. A booster dose is indicated before school enrollment unless the primary immunization schedule is completed on or after the child's fourth birthday. The enhanced-potency inactivated vaccine can also be used to complete primary immunization begun with the conventional inactivated product.

The vaccine may contain trace quantities of streptomycin or neomycin. Individuals who have developed anaphylactic reactions to either of these drugs should not be immunized with the enhanced-potency product.

Serotonin-uptake inhibition accounts for activity of new antidepressant

The activity of fluoxetine hydrochloride (Prozac, Dista Products Company), an antidepressant approved by FDA at the end of 1987, is related to the drug's ability to inhibit the uptake of serotonin in the central nervous system. Inhibition of histamine, muscarinic, and α-adrenergic receptors is less with fluoxetine than with the tricyclic antidepressants. Fluoxetine is structurally unrelated to other antidepressant agents that are currently available.

Approximately 94.5% of fluoxetine binds in vitro to serum proteins, including albumin and α_1-glycoprotein. Fluoxetine is metabolized in the liver to a number of compounds; to date, the only active metabolite that has been identified is norfluoxetine. Fluoxetine and norfluoxetine are comparable in terms of serotonin-uptake inhibition. Norfluoxetine appears to be eliminated pri-

Continued on page 172

B fragilis group activity...

THE UNSURPASSED β-LACTAM CHOICE

TIMENTIN® ticarcillin disodium/ clavulanate potassium

B fragilis group coverage superior to cephalosporins and penicillins

Susceptibility Pattern (%) of 531 *B fragilis* Group Isolates in a Nationwide *in vitro Study[1]**

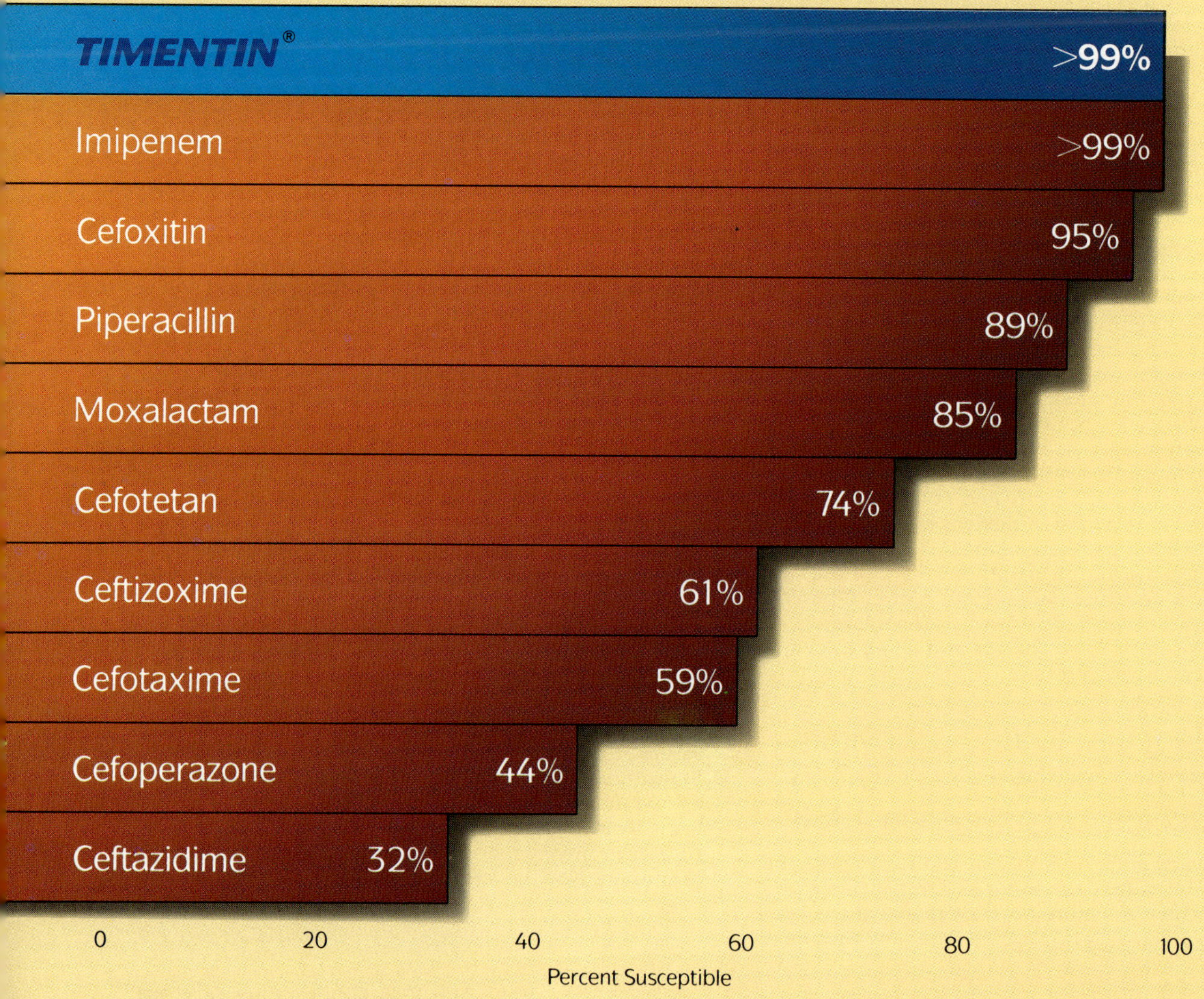

**In vitro* activity does not necessarily imply *in vivo* efficacy.

More active *in vitro** than traditional antianaerobic agents

Activity Against Clinical Isolates of *B fragilis* Group[2]		
Antibiotic	MIC_{50} (μg/mL)	MIC_{90} (μg/mL)
TIMENTIN†	≤1	4
Cefoxitin	8	32
Cefoperazone	32	128
Chloramphenicol	8	8
Clindamycin	0.5	8
Metronidazole	1	2

**In vitro* activity does not necessarily imply *in vivo* efficacy.
†Ticarcillin in the presence of a constant 2 μg/mL clavulanic acid.

More active *in vitro** than cefoxitin

Activity Against *B fragilis* Group[3]		
Organism (No. strains)	MIC_{90} (μg/mL) TIMENTIN†	Cefoxitin
B fragilis (32)	0.5	16
B vulgatus (21)	1	16
B thetaiotaomicron (19)	2	32
B ovatus (16)	1	32
B distasonis (13)	8	64

**In vitro* activity does not necessarily imply *in vivo* efficacy.
†Ticarcillin in the presence of a constant 1 μg/mL clavulanic acid.

Destroys β-lactamases that limit the usefulness of other β-lactam choices

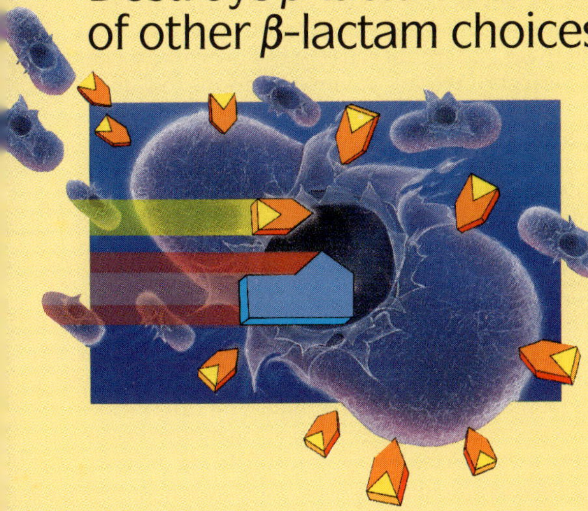

- "Most (90 percent) strains of B. fragilis produce constitutive beta-lactamases, which are primarily cephalosporinases. All other Bacteroides species probably produce beta-lactamases, but controversy exists concerning whether the enzymes are predominantly penicillinases or cephalosporinases."[4]
- "[Clavulanate potassium] inhibits the beta-lactamases of most Bacteroides species."[4]

△ Clavulanate potassium destroys ▶ most β-lactamases produced by Gram-positive and Gram-negative aerobes and anaerobes.
TIMENTIN destroys a broad range of aerobic and anaerobic bacteria regardless of β-lactamase production.

FOR ANAEROBIC CERTAINTY

TIMENTIN®

ticarcillin disodium/ clavulanate potassium

The unsurpassed β-lactam choice

Usual Dosage: 3.1 g every 4 to 6 hours.

Please see next page for brief summary of prescribing information.

THE CLAVULANATES Beecham laboratories BRISTOL, TENNESSEE 37620

© 1988, Beecham Laboratories.

BRIEF SUMMARY OF PRESCRIBING INFORMATION

TIMENTIN®

sterile ticarcillin disodium and clavulanate potassium

for Intravenous Administration

INDICATIONS AND USAGE: TIMENTIN® is indicated in the treatment of infections caused by susceptible strains of the designated organisms in the conditions listed below:

Bacterial Septicemia: including bacteremia, caused by β-lactamase producing strains of *Klebsiella* spp., *E. coli, Staphylococcus aureus* and *Pseudomonas aeruginosa* (and other *Pseudomonas* species).

Lower Respiratory Infections: caused by β-lactamase producing strains of *Staphylococcus aureus, Hemophilus influenzae* and *Klebsiella* spp.

Bone and Joint Infections: caused by β-lactamase producing strains of *Staphylococcus aureus.*

Skin and Skin Structure Infections: caused by β-lactamase producing strains of *Staphylococcus aureus, Klebsiella* spp., and *E. coli.*

Urinary Tract Infections (complicated and uncomplicated): caused by β-lactamase producing strains of *E. coli, Klebsiella* spp., *Pseudomonas aeruginosa* (and other *Pseudomonas* species), *Citrobacter* spp., *Enterobacter cloacae, Serratia marcescens,* and *Staphylococcus aureus.* While TIMENTIN is indicated only for the conditions listed above, infections caused by ticarcillin susceptible organisms are also amenable to TIMENTIN treatment due to its ticarcillin content. Therefore, mixed infections caused by ticarcillin susceptible organisms and β-lactamase producing organisms susceptible to TIMENTIN should not require the addition of another antibiotic.

Appropriate culture and susceptibility tests should be performed before treatment in order to isolate and identify organisms causing infection and to determine their susceptibility to TIMENTIN. Because of its broad spectrum of bactericidal activity against Gram-positive and Gram-negative bacteria, TIMENTIN is particularly useful for the treatment of mixed infections and for presumptive therapy prior to the identification of the causative organisms. TIMENTIN has been shown to be effective as single drug therapy in the treatment of some serious infections where normally combination antibiotic therapy might be employed. Therapy with TIMENTIN may be initiated before results of such tests are known when there is reason to believe the infection may involve any of the β-lactamase producing organisms listed above; however, once these results become available, appropriate therapy should be continued.

Based on the *in vitro* synergism between TIMENTIN and aminoglycosides against certain strains of *Pseudomonas aeruginosa,* combined therapy has been successful, especially in patients with impaired host defenses. Both drugs should be used in full therapeutic doses. As soon as results of culture and susceptibility tests become available, antimicrobial therapy should be adjusted as indicated.

CONTRAINDICATIONS: TIMENTIN is contraindicated in patients with a history of hypersensitivity reactions to any of the penicillins.

WARNINGS: SERIOUS AND OCCASIONALLY FATAL HYPERSENSITIVITY (ANAPHYLACTOID) REACTIONS HAVE BEEN REPORTED IN PATIENTS ON PENICILLIN THERAPY. THESE REACTIONS ARE MORE LIKELY TO OCCUR IN INDIVIDUALS WITH A HISTORY OF PENICILLIN HYPERSENSITIVITY AND/OR A HISTORY OF SENSITIVITY TO MULTIPLE ALLERGENS. THERE HAVE BEEN REPORTS OF INDIVIDUALS WITH A HISTORY OF PENICILLIN HYPERSENSITIVITY WHO HAVE EXPERIENCED SEVERE REACTIONS WHEN TREATED WITH CEPHALOSPORINS. BEFORE INITIATING THERAPY WITH TIMENTIN, CAREFUL INQUIRY SHOULD BE MADE CONCERNING PREVIOUS HYPERSENSITIVITY REACTIONS TO PENICILLINS, CEPHALOSPORINS, OR OTHER DRUGS. IF AN ALLERGIC REACTION OCCURS, TIMENTIN SHOULD BE DISCONTINUED AND THE APPROPRIATE THERAPY INSTITUTED. **SERIOUS ANAPHYLACTOID REACTIONS REQUIRE IMMEDIATE EMERGENCY TREATMENT WITH EPINEPHRINE. OXYGEN, INTRAVENOUS STEROIDS, AND AIRWAY MANAGEMENT, INCLUDING INTUBATION, SHOULD ALSO BE PROVIDED AS INDICATED.**

PRECAUTIONS: While TIMENTIN possesses the characteristic low toxicity of the penicillin group of antibiotics, organ system functions should be assessed periodically during therapy.

Bleeding manifestations have occurred in some patients receiving β-lactam antibiotics. These reactions have been associated with abnormalities of coagulation tests such as clotting time, platelet aggregation and prothrombin time and are more likely to occur in patients with renal impairment. If bleeding manifestations appear, TIMENTIN treatment should be discontinued and appropriate therapy instituted.

TIMENTIN has only rarely been reported to cause hypokalemia. Periodic monitoring of serum potassium may be advisable in patients receiving prolonged therapy.

Pregnancy (Category B): Reproduction studies have been performed in rats given doses up to 1050 mg/kg/day and have revealed no evidence of impaired fertility or harm to the fetus due to TIMENTIN. There are, however, no adequate and well-controlled studies in pregnant women. Because animal reproduction studies are not always predictive of human response, this drug should be used during pregnancy only if clearly needed.

DOSAGE AND ADMINISTRATION: TIMENTIN should be administered by intravenous infusion (30 min.). Usual recommended dose for systemic and urinary tract infections for average (60 kg) adults is 3.1 Gm TIMENTIN (3.1 Gm vial containing 3 Gm ticarcillin and 100 mg clavulanic acid) given every 4 to 6 hours. In urinary tract infections, a dosage of 3.2 Gm TIMENTIN (3.2 Gm vial containing 3 Gm ticarcillin and 200 mg clavulanic acid) given every 8 hours is adequate. Please see official package insert for details on dosages for other patients, including those with renal insufficiency, and directions for use.

SUPPLIED: 3.1 Gm and 3.2 Gm Standard Vials; 3.1 Gm and 3.2 Gm Piggyback Bottles: 31 Gm Bulk Pharmacy Package: 3.1 Gm ADD-Vantage™ Antibiotic Vial.

7548/E-BS

References

1. Cuchural GJ, Tally FP, Jacobus NV, et al: Susceptibility of Bacteroides fragilis group clinical isolates to newer beta-lactam drugs, abstract No. 1B8. Presented to the 3rd Panamerican Congress of Infectious Diseases and Chemotherapy, San Juan, Puerto Rico, Dec 9-13, 1986.
2. Barry AL, Jones RN, Packer RR: *In vitro* susceptibility of the *Bacteroides fragilis* group to cefoperazone, ampicillin, ticarcillin, and amoxycillin combined with β-lactamase inhibitors. *J Antimicrob Chemother* 1986;17:125-127.
3. Bourgault AM, Lamothe F, Parent M: *In vitro* activity of ticarcillin and amoxycillin in combination with clavulanic acid against species of the *Bacteroides fragilis* group, abstract No. 43. Program and abstracts of the 23rd Interscience Conference on Antimicrobial Agents and Chemotherapy, Las Vegas, Oct 24-26, 1983.
4. Neu HC: Contribution of beta-lactamases to bacterial resistance and mechanisms to inhibit beta-lactamases. *Am J Med* 1985;79(suppl 5B):2-12.

Beecham laboratories

BRISTOL, TENNESSEE 37620

© 1988, Beecham Laboratories.

News *Continued from page 169*

marily by metabolism to inactive compounds. The elimination half-lives of fluoxetine and norfluoxetine are two to three days and seven to nine days, respectively. Studies of patients treated with fluoxetine for up to three years suggest that steady-state plasma concentrations are reached within four to five weeks. Hepatic disease can impair elimination of fluoxetine. The effects of age and renal disease on the pharmacokinetics of fluoxetine and norfluoxetine have not been adequately evaluated in multidose studies.

The efficacy of fluoxetine was established in clinical trials of five to six weeks' duration; patients enrolled in the studies were outpatients with a diagnosis of major depression.

In these studies, the most frequently reported adverse reactions to fluoxetine were nervous system complaints (including nervousness, insomnia, anxiety, tremor, fatigue, and dizziness) and gastrointestinal complaints (including anorexia, nausea, and vomiting). Approximately 4% of patients developed a rash or urticaria, or both, during treatment. The drug was discontinued in almost one third of these patients because of the rash or associated systemic effects. Overall, adverse reactions to fluoxetine led to drug discontinuation in 15% of patients participating in clinical trials.

Nausea and vomiting are prominent features of overdoses involving high doses of fluoxetine. Central nervous system stimulation may also be important. Of the 38 reported overdoses, two cases, both involving ingestion of multiple drugs, resulted in death.

The recommended initial dosage of fluoxetine is 20 mg/day, administered in the morning. If clinical improvement is not apparent after several weeks of therapy, the dosage may be increased (using a twice-daily schedule) to a maximum of 80 mg/day. The full antidepressant effect may not be evident for at least four weeks.

Prozac is available as tablets containing 20 mg of fluoxetine as the hydrochloride salt.

Studies suggest possible role for sucralfate in critically ill patients

Two recent studies suggest that sucralfate may have a role in the prevention of upper gastrointestinal tract bleeding in critically ill, mechanically ventilated patients.

The results of a randomized study reported in the *Archives of Internal Medicine* suggest that sucralfate 1 g every six hours is as effective as antacids or cimetidine in the prevention of stress-related upper gastrointestinal tract bleeding in critically ill, mechanically ventilated patients.[1] The study involved 62 patients with respiratory failure of less than 48 hours' duration. Exclusion criteria included known active gastrointestinal tract bleeding, guaiac-positive stools, known bleeding diathesis, gastrointestinal tract surgery within the preceding 48 hours, and a requirement for dialysis. The study regimens consisted of sucralfate 1 g administered every six hours via a nasogastric tube, cimetidine 300 mg (as the hydrochloride salt) given intravenously every six hours

Continued on page 176

Does so much for so much less than cefoxitin

A retrospective chart review of four antibiotic regimens was conducted in an 800-bed hospital on a total of 141 patients. CEFOTAN was compared with cefoxitin as well as combination antibiotic therapy. The clinical success rate and incidence of adverse reactions were similar with CEFOTAN and cefoxitin.

Equally as effective as combination antibiotic therapy with a cost advantage

When CEFOTAN was compared with the ampicillin/aminoglycoside/clindamycin combination and the ampicillin/aminoglycoside/metronidazole combination, results were comparable.

40%

savings over cefoxitin

Clinical efficacy

Infection	CEFOTAN Success/Total	(%)	Cefoxitin Success/Total	(%)
OB/GYN	10/11	(91)	24/26	(92)
Abdominal	10/11	(91)	3/4	(75)
Miscellaneous	6/8	(75)	4/5	(80)
Prophylaxis	2/2	(100)	3/3	(100)
Total	28/32	(88)	34/38	(89)

—adapted from Sochalski et al

However, using CEFOTAN costs approximately 40% less than cefoxitin.

Clinical efficacy

Infections	CEFOTAN Success/ Total	(%)	Amp/Ag/Clin Success/ Total	(%)	Amp/Ag/Met Success/ Total	(%)
OB/GYN, abdominal, miscellaneous, and prophylaxis	19/21	(90)	27/29	(93)	17/21	(81)

—adapted from Sochalski et al

Cost comparisons showed that CEFOTAN was more cost-effective than the clindamycin- or metronidazole-containing regimens.

In intra-abdominal and gynecologic infection due to indicated organisms

CEFOTAN® IM/IV
(cefotetan disodium)

Does so much for so much less than cefoxitin.

REFERENCE: Sochalski A, Sullman S, Andriole VT: Cost effectiveness study of cefotetan versus cefoxitin and cefotetan versus combination antibiotic regimens. *Am J Surg*, submitted for publication.

© 1988 ICI Americas Inc

Continued from page 172

(dosage adjusted for renal dysfunction), and liquid antacids administered via a nasogastric tube in doses adequate to maintain the gastric pH at 4 or higher.

Efficacy could be evaluated in 59 of 62 patients. Four of 19 patients in the antacid group, 1 of 21 patients receiving cimetidine, and none of 19 sucralfate-treated patients had bright red blood in the nasogastric tube aspirate. Correction for a higher incidence of acute renal failure among antacid recipients did not alter the finding of a significant difference in bleeding between the antacid and sucralfate groups. The three treatment groups were similar with respect to other risk factors for bleeding. Coffee-ground heme-positive nasogastric aspirates were reported in 11 patients in the cimetidine group, 7 in the antacid group, and 4 in the sucralfate group. There were no differences in the incidence of guaiac-positive stools.

The average cost of therapy per patient, based solely on pharmacy charges, was $2.40/day for sucralfate, $6.60/day for antacids, and $78.40/day for cimetidine.

According to the second study, use of an agent such as sucralfate that does not raise gastric pH may be beneficial by protecting against bacterial overgrowth.[2] The study was based on the premise that when gastric pH is relatively high, gram-negative nosocomial pneumonia may be more likely to occur as a result of retrograde colonization of the pharynx with stomach flora.

Rates of gastric colonization and nosocomial pneumonia were evaluated in 130 mechanically ventilated patients who were randomly assigned to receive either sucralfate 1 g administered via a nasogastric tube every six hours or conventional treatment with a histamine H_2 antagonist or antacids, or both. Patients receiving sucralfate had a significantly higher proportion of gastric aspirates with a pH of 4 or less and significantly less colonization of the stomach, pharynx, and trachea with gram-negative organisms than did patients in the conventional treatment group. Pneumonia was diagnosed in 11.5% of patients treated with sucralfate and 23.2% of those receiving conventional therapy; the difference between the two groups was not significant. Mortality rates were 1.6 times higher with conventional therapy.

The two studies support further evaluation of the effects of sucralfate in critically ill patients.

1. Cannon LA, Heiselman D, Gardner W et al. Prophylaxis of upper gastrointestinal tract bleeding in mechanically ventilated patients: a randomized study comparing the efficacy of sucralfate, cimetidine, and antacids. *Arch Intern Med.* 1987; 147:2101–6.
2. Driks MR, Craven DE, Celli BR et al. Nosocomial pneumonia in intubated patients given sucralfate as compared with antacids or histamine type 2 blockers: the role of gastric colonization. *N Engl J Med.* 1987; 317:1376–82.

Rule on nonprescription first-aid antibiotics finalized by FDA

FDA has issued a final monograph on nonprescription first-aid antibiotic products intended for topical administration; the regulation arose from FDA's ongoing review of nonprescription drug products. The monograph lists active ingredients and drug concentrations that are permitted, defines the wording that may be used to describe the indications and directions for use, and lists the warning statements that must be included on product labels. Products may contain any of the following ingredients, either alone or in the combinations specified by FDA: bacitracin, bacitracin zinc, chlortetracycline hydrochloride, neomycin sulfate, and tetracycline hydrochloride. Inclusion of polymyxin B sulfate, oxytetracycline hydrochloride, and local anesthetics in certain combination products is permitted. Gramicidin, which was judged to have unproven efficacy, must be removed from first-aid antibiotic products or replaced by an effective ingredient. The regulations were published in the December 11, 1987, issue of the *Federal Register*.

News Brief

• A boxed warning concerning the use of **midazolam hydrochloride** (Versed, Roche Laboratories) for conscious sedation has been added to the product labeling; the statement warns of the potential for respiratory depression or arrest and the need for individualized dosing and continuous monitoring.

Upcoming Specialty Meetings

American College of Obstetricians and Gynecologists . . . Boston, MA . . . May 1–5 . . . contact: W. H. Pearse, M.D., ACOG, 600 Maryland Avenue S.W., Suite 300, Washington, DC 20024; 202-638-5577.

American Association of Immunologists . . . Las Vegas, NV . . . May 1–6 . . . contact: J. F. Saunders, M.D., 9650 Rockville Pke, Bethesda, MD 20814; 801-530-7178.

American Society of Pharmacology and Experimental Therapeutics . . . Las Vegas, NV . . . May 2–6 . . . K. A. Croker, ASPET, 9650 Rockville Pike, Bethesda, MD 20814; 301-530-7060.

Association for Research in Vision and Ophthalmology . . . Sarasota, FL . . . May 2–6 . . . contact: H. Quigley, M.D., The John Hopkins Hospital, Wilmer Eye Institute, Maumenee Building 1100, Baltimore, MD 21205; 301-571-1844.

American Lung Association . . . Las Vegas, NV . . . May 8–11 . . . contact: J. A. Swomley, 1740 Broadway, New York, NY 10019-4374; 212-645-4470.

American Thoracic Society . . . Las Vegas, NV . . . May 8–11 . . . contact: S. R. Iannotta, 1740 Broadway, New York, NY 10019; 212-315-8700.

American Gastroenterological Association . . . New Orleans, LA . . . May 14–20 . . . C. B. Slack, 6900 Grove Road, Thorofare, NJ 08086; 609-848-1000.

American Geriatrics Society . . . Anaheim, CA . . . May 19–22 . . . L. H. Barondess, American Geriatric Society, 770 Lexington Avenue, Suite 400, New York, NY 10021; 212-308-1414.

16th International Congress of Chemotherapy . . . Jerusalem, Israel . . . June 11–16 . . . contact: Professor E. Rubinstein, P.O. Box 983, Jerusalem 91009, Israel; 972-2-527335.

People count on you for the latest drug therapy information. You can count on linical Pharmacy to provide it.

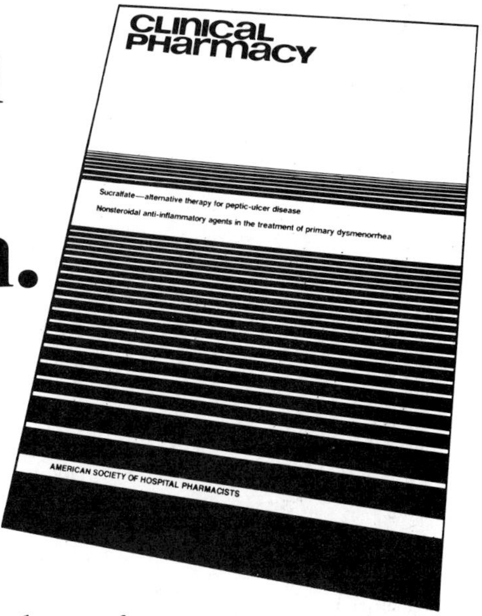

Clinical Pharmacy . . . the monthly journal that brings you the most current drug therapy information available.

here aren't enough hours in your day to uncover all the information available n new drugs, current therapies, the latest research results. That's why there's *linical Pharmacy*.

ach month, *Clinical Pharmacy* rovides you—

- an analysis of new drugs and new drug therapy
- current perspectives on existing drug therapies
- reviews of the latest drug literature
- reports on clinical research
- news from FDA and clinical centers around the country

or as little as $40 a year!*
linical Pharmacy keeps you current n the drugs and research you want o know about.

lew drugs recently featured iclude:

- mupirocin
- flecainide and encainide
- midazolam hydrochloride
- quinolone antimicrobials

This low annual fee applies to ASHP members only! Foreign, ASHP Student and Nonmember rates vary.

Original research recently featured . . .

- accuracy of four dosing methods for vancomycin
- minimum urine collection periods for accurate determination of creatinine clearance

Subscribing to *Clinical Pharmacy* is money and time well spent! Here are *just* three reasons why:

1. CP's Drug Tracking System. The *CP* staff identifies important new drugs and follows them through FDA approval. The result—articles on new drugs even before they reach the market.

2. CP's Editorial Expertise. Twenty-five clinical practitioners, researchers and educators advise the *CP* editorial staff on trends, developments and findings making an impact on drug therapy. The result—well-written, accurate reviews that analyze the appropriate therapy for major diseases.

3. CP's Continuing Education Opportunities. *CP* offers selected articles for continuing education (CE) credit. The American Society of Hospital Pharmacists is accredited by the American Council on Pharmaceutical Education as a CE provider. You can test your grasp of the material whether or not you're seeking CE credits.

Many turn to you for answers on the best drug therapies . . . latest research results . . . potential side effects.

Clinical Pharmacy can help you meet that challenge.

rder Form ☐ Please enter by subscription to *Clinical Pharmacy* at the rate I've noted below.
☐ Enclosed is my check for $ ______ . (Checks must be drawn on a U.S. bank and payable to ASHP.)
harge $ ______ to my: ☐ MasterCard ☐ VISA Acct. # ______________ Exp. __________ month/year

Signature ______________________

☐ My purchase order # ______________ is attached; please issue an invoice and add postage and handling.

lame ______________________

nstitution ______________________

SHP I.D. # ______________

ddress ______________________

ity ______ State ______ Zip ______

CP Rates

ASHP Member	$40/year
ASHP Student/Resident	$30/year
Nonmember	$63/year

(Outside the USA, please add $5)

Send to:
ASHP Publication Record Dept.
4630 Montgomery Ave
Bethesda, MD 20814

Therapy Consultation

Management of vancomycin-induced "red-man syndrome"

Question: A patient with bacteremia caused by a methicillin-resistant strain of *Staphylococcus aureus* developed "red-man syndrome" during treatment with vancomycin 1 g (as the hydrochloride salt) every 12 hours. Increasing the infusion time from one hour to two hours did not prevent the reaction from recurring. Are there other strategies that might alleviate the reaction?

Answer: The following additional maneuvers can be tried in an attempt to successfully complete therapy; unfortunately, most of these have not been evaluated prospectively.

1. If the reaction began during the second hour of the two-hour infusion, change the dosage to 500 mg (administered as a one-hour infusion) every six hours.
2. Increase the infusion time of the 1000-mg dose to three to four hours, and then gradually return to a shorter infusion time as tolerated by the patient.
3. Pretreat with either a histamine H_1 or H_2 blocker, or both.
4. Use ciprofloxacin if it is appropriate for this case.
5. Consider using trimethoprim–sulfamethoxazole if the organism is susceptible to this drug.
6. Obtain teicoplanin, an investigational glycopeptide antibiotic, for compassionate use.

The first three suggestions are based on the mechanism of the "red man (or red neck) syndrome," the most common adverse reaction to vancomycin. The reaction involves a spectrum of infusion-related effects, including one or more of the following events: pruritus (usually starting on the scalp and progressing to the upper torso and extremities), erythema over the same area, and angioedema.[1] Profound hypotension has been reported after very rapid infusions of vancomycin, such as administration of 1000 mg over 30 minutes or less.[2] Presumably these effects occur from the same underlying mechanism, namely, vancomycin-induced release of histamine and possibly other vasoactive substances. Since this nonallergic reaction occurs during infusion of the first dose, it is called an anaphylactoid reaction, to be distinguished from an anaphylactic reaction, which requires preformed antibodies.

My colleagues and I recently demonstrated that plasma histamine concentrations increase significantly in most healthy volunteers who receive vancomycin 1 g intravenously over one hour.[3] Although none of the 11 volunteers in our study experienced hypotension, the amount of released histamine correlated with the severity of the reaction. The incidence and severity of the reaction decreased with subsequent doses. In contrast, no infusion-related events occurred after administration of 500-mg doses over one hour, and histamine concentrations showed only minor changes. This evidence is the basis for the first two recommendations. Our study showed no relationship between serum vancomycin concentrations and reaction severity when 1000-mg doses were given. Thus, a major determinant of the reaction (aside from dose and infusion rate) is probably individual "sensitivity" of the receptors for histamine release. The patient described appears to be unusually sensitive to vancomycin.

Other drugs, such as narcotics given during anesthesia, have been reported to release histamine and cause anaphylactoid reactions. Investigations in the area of narcotic anesthesia have found that pretreatment with both H_1 and H_2 blockers provides greater protection against hypotension than treatment with either agent alone.[4] Whether H_1 and H_2 blockers provide similar protection against the cutaneous reactions induced by vancomycin is unknown, but use of these agents may be worthwhile if the first two suggestions are not successful.

If attempts to minimize the reaction fail, use of another antimicrobial agent may be indicated. Ciprofloxacin and trimethoprim–sulfamethoxazole have good in vitro activity against many methicillin-resistant strains of *Staphylococcus aureus*.[5,6] However, experience in treating bacteremia with either of these drugs is limited. Teicoplanin is similar in structure and in vitro activity to vancomycin.[7] To date, infusion-related reactions have been reported in only one patient (Barbara Fant, Merrell Dow Pharmaceuticals, Inc., personal communication, 1988 Jan 28), but histamine studies have not been undertaken.

1. Rothenberg HJ. Anaphylactoid reaction to vancomycin. *JAMA*. 1959; 171:1101–2.
2. Southorn PA, Plevak DJ, Wright AAJ et al. Adverse effects of vancomycin administered in the perioperative period. *Mayo Clin Proc*. 1986; 61:721–4.
3. Polk RE, Healy DP, Schwartz LB et al. Vancomycin and the "red man" syndrome: pharmacodynamics of histamine release. *J Infect Dis*. 1988; 157:502–7.
4. Philbin DM, Moss J, Akins CW et al. The use of H1 and H2 histamine antagonists with morphine anesthesia: a double-blind study. *Anesthesiology*. 1981; 55:292–6.
5. Nix DE, DeVito JM. Ciprofloxacin and norfloxacin, two fluoroquinolone antimicrobials. *Clin Pharm*. 1987; 6:105–17.
6. Neu HC. Treatment of methicillin-resistant *Staphylococcus* infections. *Antimicrob Newsl*. 1984; 1:47–8.
7. Williams AH, Gruneberg RN. Teicoplanin. *J Antimicrob Chemother*. 1984; 14:441–5.

Ron E. Polk, Pharm.D.
Associate Professor, Department of Pharmacy and Pharmaceutics
Instructor, Department of Medicine
Medical College of Virginia–Virginia Commonwealth University
Richmond, VA 23298

Drug Review

Guanfacine hydrochloride: A centrally acting antihypertensive agent

LAURA A. CORNISH

Abstract: The pharmacology, pharmacokinetics, clinical efficacy, adverse effects, and dosage of guanfacine hydrochloride are reviewed.

Guanfacine lowers blood pressure by activating CNS α adrenoreceptors, which results in sympathetic ouflow leading to reduced vascular tone. However, initial hypotensive response to guanfacine may be caused by stimulation of peripheral presynaptic receptors that inhibit sympathetic nerve function. Guanfacine is rapidly and completely absorbed from the gastrointestinal tract and apparently undergoes extensive distribution to all tissues. Steady-state plasma concentrations may be reached in four days. About 30% is excreted renally; the rest is metabolized hepatically. Its long duration of action is related to a slow elimination half-life.

In the few controlled clinical trials of guanfacine versus placebo, systolic and diastolic blood pressures were reduced in patients treated with guanfacine; daily dosages of guanfacine 1, 2, and 3 mg (as the hydrochloride salt) were comparable in efficacy. Several large open trials of guanfacine showed blood pressure reductions of about 16% after one year; some patients received other antihypertensive therapy concomitantly. Guanfacine and clonidine appear to have comparable effects in reducing both systolic and diastolic blood pressure when given as monotherapy and as step-2 therapy; data on the comparative blood-pressure-lowering effects of guanfacine and methyldopa are less consistent. Guanfacine's adverse reactions include dry mouth, sedation, and constipation. Adverse effects and reaction to sudden withdrawal of the drug may be less severe with guanfacine than with clonidine. A daily dose of guanfacine 1 mg (as the hydrochloride salt) at bedtime is recommended; 2 or 3 mg, or divided doses, may be given if needed.

Once-daily administration and fewer adverse effects may give guanfacine some advantage over other centrally acting antihypertensive agents. Further study is needed to determine whether it will be adequate as first-line therapy.

Index terms: Absorption; Blood levels; Clonidine; Dosage; Drugs, body distribution; Excretion; Guanfacine hydrochloride; Hypertension; Hypotensive agents; Mechanism of action; Metabolism; Methyldopa; Pharmacokinetics; Toxicity
Clin Pharm. 1988; 7:187–97

Guanfacine is a phenylacetyl-guanidine derivative with the chemical formula *N*-amidino-2-(2,6-dichlorophenyl) acetamide monohydrochloride. Guanfacine hydrochloride is marketed as an antihypertensive agent by A. H. Robins (as Tenex) in the United States and by Sandoz, Ltd. (as Estulic) in other countries.

This article reviews the pharmacology, pharmacokinetics, clinical efficacy, adverse effects, and dosage of guanfacine. In addition, formulary recommendations are made.

Pharmacology

The blood-pressure-lowering effects of guanfacine are mediated by α-adrenoreceptor activation within the central nervous system. Central stimulation of α receptors results in decreased sympathetic outflow. This reduction in outflow results in a reduced vascular tone. Peripheral effects may also contribute to the overall blood-pressure-lowering effects.

Evidence to support the central action of guanfa-

LAURA A. CORNISH, PHARM.D., is Clinical Assistant Professor of Pharmacy, College of Pharmacy, The University of Michigan, and Clinical Pharmacist, The University of Michigan Medical Center, Ann Arbor.

Address reprint requests to Dr. Cornish at The University of Michigan Hospitals, 1500 E. Medical Center Drive, B2D301 Box 0008, Ann Arbor, MI 48109.

This is **article 680-204-8803** in the **ASHP Continuing Education System.** See page 241 for learning objectives and test questions.

Copyright © 1988, American Society of Hospital Pharmacists, Inc. All rights reserved. 0278-2677/88/0301-0187$02.75.

cine comes from the animal model. In anesthetized dogs, guanfacine decreased blood pressure and heart rate after administration into the vertebral artery, but not after intravenous administration, of 1 μg/kg/min.[1] Similar findings have been noted in anesthetized cats.[1] Administration of guanfacine into the cerebral ventricles produced little effect on heart rate or blood pressure in cats pretreated with the α-adrenoreceptor-blocking agent phentolamine.[1] Other experiments in anesthetized cats have shown a reduction in the preganglionic sympathetic nerve activity. This reduction in spontaneous preganglionic nerve activity can be attributed to central inhibition of the sympathetic tone. This information strongly suggests a central α-adrenoreceptor-agonist mechanism of guanfacine.

Biochemical studies offer additional support for the central α-adrenoreceptor-agonist activity of guanfacine. In the rat model, guanfacine has been shown to decrease the cerebral norepinephrine turnover after blockade of norepinephrine synthesis by diethyldithiocarbamate.[1] Both guanfacine and clonidine significantly inhibited the diethyldithiocarbamate-induced disappearance of norepinephrine. This decrease in norepinephrine turnover in the CNS results from central α-adrenoreceptor stimulation.[2] Binding studies indicate that guanfacine is more selective for α_2 rather than α_1 adrenoreceptors and that its selectivity for this receptor is equal to or greater than that of clonidine.[3-5] In addition, the two drugs may have different central sites of action. This was demonstrated by the topical application of the two drugs to the exposed ventral surface of the medulla oblongata in the cat.[1] Application of clonidine 2 μg/kg induced a drop in mean arterial blood pressure by more than 50 mm Hg and in heart rate by more than 30 beats per minute. No changes were noted when guanfacine 20 μg/kg was applied in a similar fashion. Thus, although the two drugs are both central α agonists, they may work at different sites within the CNS.

Other receptor-binding studies have noted minimal or no effect of guanfacine on dopamine-, serotonin-, histamine H_1- and H_2-, and β_1- or β_2-adrenoreceptor sites.[5,6] This is in contrast to clonidine, which has been shown to stimulate central histamine H_2 receptors as well as to decrease dopamine turnover in the rat brain.[1,6]

In addition to its central site of action, guanfacine also stimulates peripheral α adrenoreceptors. An initial brief increase in blood pressure followed by a prolonged decrease in blood pressure has been reported in both animals[7,8] and humans.[9] Guanfacine's direct vascular α-adrenoreceptor-stimulant activity is the most likely explanation for this observation, as this response is prevented by α blockade with phentolamine but not by pretreatment with reserpine.[8] Since this pressor effect has not been noted with intracisternal administration of guanfacine, it has been proposed that the pressor effect seen after intravenous administration may be due to postsynaptic α-receptor stimulation in the vasculature.[7] The overall blood-pressure-lowering effects may be a summation of the peripheral and central effects, with the central effects predominating.[7]

Murphy and Brown[10] reported that in healthy volunteers given intravenous guanfacine a decrease in norepinephrine concentrations occurred before any evidence of central effects was seen. Thus, the initial hypotensive response may be due to peripheral adrenoreceptor activation. Brown et al.[11] further substantiated these findings in a group of healthy volunteers given intravenous guanfacine; they exhibited decreased blood pressure and plasma norepinephrine concentrations (an index of peripheral sympathetic nervous system activity) 20 minutes before an increase in growth hormone (an index of central α-adrenoreceptor stimulation) was observed. From these experiments, it seems likely that guanfacine stimulates peripheral presynaptic receptors that inhibit sympathetic nerve function. This peripheral sympathetic nervous system inhibition may contribute to guanfacine's overall antihypertensive effect.

Effects on Neuroendocrine System. Guanfacine has been shown to significantly reduce plasma renin activity (PRA) in both short-term and long-term studies[9,12]; this effect may occur because of decreased central and peripheral sympathetic activity[13] or because of direct actions on the α_2 receptors in the juxtaglomerular apparatus.[14] The magnitude of blood pressure reductions produced by guanfacine does not correlate with the effects of the drug on plasma renin activity nor with pretreatment basal PRA levels. Thus the antihypertensive effect of guanfacine may be independent of the renin–angiotensin system.

Both plasma norepinephrine and urinary catecholamine excretion decrease after guanfacine administration. Schoeppe and Brecht[12] reported no significant correlation between the simultaneous reductions in plasma norepinephrine concentrations or pretreatment basal plasma norepinephrine concentrations and the magnitude of blood pressure reduction. This is in contrast to the findings of others[15-17] who have reported a direct correlation. Lancranjan[18] reported that oral administration of guanfacine 3–6 mg/day for 7 to 10 days had no effect on plasma concentrations of prolactin, adrenocorticotrophic hormone, follicle-stimulating hormone, or luteinizing hormone. Growth hormone increased after single oral doses of 1–2 mg. Seven-day treatment with guanfacine 3 mg/day showed that the drug did not have a sustained stimulatory effect on growth hormone. Hypertensive patients with elevated prolactin levels experienced a reduction in serum prolactin. Hauger–Klevene and colleagues[19,20] reported that the reduction in serum prolactin concentration was maintained throughout a two- to seven-year period.

Pharmacokinetics

The available pharmacokinetic data for guanfacine are derived from studies in healthy volunteers and from single-dose and multidose trials in hypertensive patients, including those with renal insufficiency and those undergoing hemodialysis. All of these studies indicate that the pharmacokinetics of guanfacine is markedly different from that of other centrally acting antihypertensives. Many of the studies have used gas–liquid chromatography with electron capture[21] or gas chromatography–mass spectrometry[22] to measure plasma concentrations of the parent compound. High-pressure liquid chromatography has been used to identify radioactively labeled guanfacine metabolites in the urine.[23]

Guanfacine is rapidly and completely absorbed from the gastrointestinal tract, with nearly 100% bioavailability. This is probably because the drug exists predominantly (67%) in its free, lipid-soluble base form at physiologic pH.[23] Peak plasma concentrations occur approximately one to four hours after an oral dose.[23] There is a linear relationship between plasma concentration and guanfacine dosage.[23,24]

Animal studies indicate that guanfacine is widely distributed and produces its highest concentrations in highly perfused organs such as the kidney and liver; lower concentrations of the drug are found in the brain, testis, and plasma.[23] In humans the apparent volume of distribution is approximately 6 L/kg.[24] This large volume of distribution suggests that the drug is extensively distributed throughout the body tissues and fluids in humans as well as in animals. In human plasma approximately 20–30% of total guanfacine is bound to plasma proteins and 60%, to erythrocytes.[23] It is not known whether the drug is excreted in human breast milk. Animal studies indicate that placental transfer does occur.[23]

Approximately 80% of a given dose of guanfacine is excreted within four days. About 30% of the drug is excreted from the kidneys unchanged.[23] The remainder is metabolized in the liver.[23] The major metabolite in man is the inactive 3-hydroxy derivative, which is conjugated and excreted as the glucuronide (30–40%) or sulfate (8%) form.[23,25] Small amounts of oxidized mercapturic acid derivatives are also excreted in human urine.[23]

Guanfacine best fits a two-compartment open model with first-order absorption and elimination.[24] In a study by Weiss et al.[24] in hypertensive patients, the distribution (α) half-life ranged from 1.4 to 2.1 hours. The elimination (β) half-life has been reported in both healthy subjects and in hypertensive patients to range from 15.8 to 22.8 hours.[23,24] This long elimination half-life of guanfacine explains its long duration of action and allows once-daily administration. The total body clearance ranges from 15.4 to 21.6 L/hour.[26]

In a study of 18 hypertensive patients with various degrees of renal function, the elimination half-life did not differ significantly between patients with normal and impaired renal function, with a mean elimination half-life of 14 hours.[26] In addition, when compared with the patients with normal renal function, the patients with severe renal dysfunction showed no significant differences in the plasma concentration–time curves, total clearances, or serum guanfacine concentrations. However, the renal clearance of unchanged guanfacine is lower in patients with renal failure than in healthy subjects. Therefore, since the total drug clearance is unchanged in renal failure patients, there appears to be an increase in nonrenal elimination. A five-hour hemodialysis session removes approximately 15% of the drug from the circulation.[27] Thus, replacement doses are not required after hemodialysis.

Disposition of guanfacine differs between older and younger individuals; in older persons, somewhat more rapid absorption, slightly longer β half-life, decreased excretion of parent drug and renal clearance, and slightly higher plasma concentrations are seen.[22] In addition, a larger percentage of guanfacine metabolites (compared with parent drug) is seen in the urine of older patients. The explanation for these observations is thought to be the age-related decrease in renal function and subsequent increase in nonrenal metabolism. This prevents the usual dose of the drug from producing substantially higher blood levels at steady state than are seen in healthy volunteers.[22]

Depending on the elimination half-life of the drug in the individual, steady-state plasma concentrations of guanfacine may be reached in four days.[24] In one study in patients with essential hypertension, treatment with a mean daily oral dose of guanfacine 2 mg for one year produced a steady-state concentration of 4.1 μg/L.[28]

Hemodynamic Effects

Administration of guanfacine 4 mg intravenously over five minutes to five patients with essential hypertension resulted in increases in blood pressure, pulmonary artery pressure, and peripheral resistance immediately after the infusion; these effects were most likely due to the α-sympathomimetic effect of the drug.[29] Blood pressure began to decrease to values lower than initial readings approximately five minutes after the end of the infusion. This decrease corresponded to a decrease in cardiac output, as peripheral resistance was not changed. Reductions in blood pressure noted after three hours were due to decreases in peripheral resistance; these continued throughout the 20-hour observation period. Investigations using guanfacine 0.02 mg/kg intravenously report similar findings.[30]

The hemodynamic effects of guanfacine after moderate-term therapy in essential hypertension are different from the results of the single-dose studies. Treatment of 12 patients diagnosed as having essential hypertension with approximately 4 mg of guanfacine daily for six weeks reduced systemic vascular resistance (SVR) in both resting and exercising conditions by 20% and 15%, respectively; the effects on SVR most likely accounted for the antihypertensive response noted.[31] Irmer and Just,[30] using larger doses (4–7 mg/day) for longer periods of time (12 weeks), reported significant decreases in mean arterial pressure under both resting and exercise conditions, with concomitant reductions in SVR. Cardiac output was shown to decrease with exercise but not at rest; pulmonary capillary wedge pressure decreased under both resting and exercising conditions. Others have reported significant decreases in SVR with no changes in cardiac index.[28,32]

Placebo-Controlled Studies

Few studies have compared guanfacine with placebo. Most of these studies report a significant reduction in blood pressure with 0.5–3 mg of guanfacine while placebo-treated patients show no effect (Table 1). Decreases in systolic and diastolic blood pressure (BP) range from 17 to 57 mm Hg and 14 to 28 mm Hg, respectively.[33-38] The antihypertensive effect may be greater in the standing position than in the supine position.[34]

In one of the larger placebo-controlled, double-blind studies, 362 patients with essential hypertension (seated diastolic BP 95–114 mm Hg) were randomized to receive chlorthalidone 25 mg/day plus either placebo or guanfacine 0.5, 1, 2, or 3 mg for 12 weeks; 307 patients were included in the final analysis of efficacy.[38] Dosages of 1, 2, and 3 mg/day were comparable when efficacy was defined as the percentage of patients who achieved a diastolic blood pressure of less than 90 mm Hg. Blood pressure reductions with these three dosage levels were significantly different from that with placebo. Blood pressure reductions in the placebo and guanfacine 0.5 mg/day treatment groups were not significantly different; these reductions were probably due to the chlorthalidone. All blood pressure reductions occurred at two weeks and were near maximal after four weeks of therapy. In a double-blind, placebo-controlled, parallel trial, 68 patients with mild essential hypertension (diastolic blood pressure 90–100 mm Hg) were randomized to receive either guanfacine 1 mg daily at bedtime or placebo for eight weeks.[39] All patients treated with guanfacine had significant decreases in diastolic blood pressure, with average reductions of 13 mm Hg. Mean diastolic blood pressure for the placebo group was decreased by 1.6 mm Hg.

Open Clinical Trials

Unlike the placebo-controlled trials, open trials have studied large patient populations with mild, moderate, and severe hypertension for prolonged durations of therapy (Table 1). One multicenter trial assessed the antihypertensive efficacy of guanfacine in 580 hypertensive patients with blood pressures of 160/95 mm Hg or higher.[40] Guanfacine was begun at a dosage of 0.5 mg orally twice daily and increased until a satisfactory therapeutic effect was obtained. Diuretics, β-adrenergic-blocking drugs, or vasodilators were added if necessary. All patients were monitored for one year. Mean arterial blood pressure and diastolic blood pressure were reduced by 16%, while systolic blood pressure was reduced by 17%. Of the patients who were receiving guanfacine alone, 64% had a good therapeutic response (defined as a blood pressure equal to 50% of the difference between the pretreatment and the normal values). The rate of normalization of blood pressure for the group of patients as a whole was 54%. Normal blood pressure was defined as ≤145/90 mm Hg in patients younger than 40 years and ≤160/95 mm Hg in older patients. Once-daily and twice-daily dosing schedules produced the same antihypertensive effect as did three-times-daily administration, but the rate of blood pressure normalization was higher with once-daily or twice-daily administration (78%) than with three-times-daily administration (58%). In patients with mild to moderate hypertension (<200/110 mm Hg) guanfacine was effective as monotherapy at a mean dose of 3 mg/day; however, patients with moderate to severe hypertension (>200/110 mm Hg) usually required higher daily doses of guanfacine (mean 6 mg) combined with either a β-adrenergic antagonist and a diuretic or a vasodilator and a diuretic. These observations were confirmed in 169 patients who were followed for an additional year.[40,41] Patients who received guanfacine three times daily did not achieve normalized blood pressure as often as those who received the drug once or twice daily.

Another large, multicenter study used low single daily doses (1–2 mg) of guanfacine to treat patients with mild to severe hypertension (mean systolic blood pressure ≥180 mm Hg, diastolic ≥103 mm Hg).[41,42] The study involved 1234 patients followed for two months and 3504 patients followed for three months. Between 10% and 28% were on other antihypertensive therapy. A reduction in blood pressure by 50% of the difference between the pretreatment value and the normal value was achieved in 80% of patients. Blood pressure normalized (≤145/90 mm Hg in patients under 40

Table 1.
Clinical Trials of Guanfacine in the Treatment of Hypertension

Reference	Study Design[a]	Dosage Regimen[b]	Effect on Blood Pressure[c]	Comments
Jaattela[33]	PC,SB, CO	PB for 2 weeks, G 3 mg/day for 6 weeks (*n* = 24)	PB: 181 ± 4/109 ± 2 sitting[d] G: 149 ± 4/95 ± 2 sitting	
Lochaya et al.[34]	PC,DB,R	G 4–12 mg/day for 7 weeks (*n* = 19) PB for 1 week (*n* = 17)	G: 129 ± 15/96 ± 8 standing PB: 161 ± 22/111 ± 10 standing[d]	Similar reductions were reported for both sitting and supine blood pressure. Some patients were also receiving small doses of diuretics.
Heidbreder et al.[35]	PC,DB,R	G 2 mg/day for 2 weeks (*n* = 10) PB for 2 weeks (*n* = 10)	PT: 157 ± 7/115 ± 6 G: 135 ± 9/100 ± 7[e]	Blood pressure in the placebo group did not differ significantly before and after 2 weeks of placebo treatment.
Szam and Hollo[36]	PC,CO	G 0.5–5 mg/day for 24 weeks, PB for 2 weeks before and after G (*n* = 14)	PT: 207/117 sitting[d] G: 150/91 sitting	
Wever and VanBrummelen[37]	PC,SB, CO	G 0.5–3 mg/day for 4 weeks, PB for 2 weeks (*n* = 10)	G: 162 ± 19/95 ± 11 PB: 179 ± 17/107 ± 5[e]	6 of 10 patients also received a thiazide diuretic throughout the study.
Materson et al.[38]	PC,DB,R	G 0.5–3 mg/day for 12 weeks (*n* = 289) PB for 12 weeks (*n* = 73)	G: 14/13 mm Hg reduction in sitting BP PB: 5/7 mm Hg reduction in sitting BP	All patients were also receiving chlorthalidone 25 mg/day. Only patients receiving G ≥1 mg/day had a significant reduction in baseline BP.
Fillingim et al.[39]	PC,DB, P,R	G 1 mg/day for 8 weeks (*n* = 17) PB for 8 weeks (*n* = 9)	G: 13 mm Hg reduction in mean DBP PB: 1.6 mm Hg reduction in mean DBP[d,e]	
Jerie[40]	O	First year (*n* = 580) G 3.4 mg/day (mean dose, monotherapy) or 6 mg/day (mean dose, combination therapy) Second year (*n* = 169) G 3.2 mg/day (mean dose, monotherapy) or 5 mg/day (mean dose, combination therapy)	16% reduction in MAP 54% normalization of sitting BP[f] 17% reduction in MAP 60% normalization of sitting BP[f]	A 3-week period preceded and followed the 12-month treatment period. Some patients were also receiving other antihypertensive medications.
Jerie[41]	O	G 1–2 mg/day for 6 weeks (*n* = 4267) G 1–2 mg/day for 8 weeks (*n* = 1234) G 1–2 mg/day for 12 weeks (*n* = 3504)	15.6% reduction in SBP 14.5% reduction in DBP 61% normalization of supine BP[f] 16.6% reduction in SBP 16% reduction in DBP 70.5% normalization of supine BP[f] 16.4% reduction in SBP 17.4% reduction in DBP 58% normalization of supine BP[f]	Some patients were also receiving other antihypertensive medications.
Jerie and Lasance[42]	O	G 2.2 mg/day (mean dose, monotherapy, *n* = 22) or 5.7 mg/day (mean dose, combination therapy, *n* = 32) for 5–7 years	PT: 186 ± 22/112 ± 11[d] G: 149 ± 14/93 ± 19[e]	
Westelinck and Michotte[43]	O	G 2 mg/day (mean dose) for 6 weeks (*n* = 46)	PT: 176 ± 14/107 ± 9 sitting[d] G: 149 ± 11/92 ± 8 sitting	A two-week washout period preceded treatment.

[a] PC = placebo-controlled, SB = single-blind, DB = double-blind, CO = crossover, R = randomized, O = open, P = parallel.
[b] G = guanfacine, PB = placebo.
[c] Reported as mean ± S.D., absolute blood pressure (in mm Hg), or percentage absolute reduction in blood pressure; PT = pretreatment, MAP = mean arterial pressure, DBP = diastolic blood pressure, SBP = systolic blood pressure, BP = blood pressure.
[d] Significantly different from blood pressure values reported for guanfacine.
[e] Patient position (sitting, standing, supine) during blood pressure measurement not reported.
[f] Normal value defined as ≤145/90 mm Hg for patients <40 years old and ≤160/95 for older patients.

years, ≤160/95 mm Hg in patients over 40 years of age) in approximately 60% of all patients. The reduction in systolic and diastolic blood pressure was 16%, which is consistent with other reports.[40,43,44]

A few reports are available indicating that tolerance to guanfacine may develop, as evidenced by increasing blood pressures during treatment.[16,43,45] The mechanism of this tolerance is unclear; it may be a true drug tolerance or a worsening of the underlying condition. Should tolerance occur, it may be overcome by the addition of diuretics or other antihypertensive agents.[16,45] Increasing the guanfacine dose may not be advantageous; Jerie and Lasance[46] have suggested that higher doses (>3 mg/day) and frequent administration may actually lead to direct stimulation of peripheral α adrenoreceptors, which may result in a diminution of the antihypertensive effect.

Guanfacine may be useful in the treatment of hypertension due to preeclampsia. Phillipp[47] reported the use of guanfacine 2–6 mg daily for 16 to 68 days in 30 pregnant women with preeclampsia. Both statistically significant and clinically important reductions in blood pressure were noted during the first week of therapy, with blood pressures falling almost to normal levels before parturition in 24 of the women. Although six of the infants were "small-for-date," no other fetal abnormalities were reported.

Comparisons of Guanfacine with Other Drugs

Diuretics. No studies have compared the effectiveness of guanfacine with that of diuretics, each as monotherapy. However, a few studies have compared the effectiveness of diuretics alone with that of a combination of diuretic plus guanfacine. These studies are not in agreement as to the additive effect of combination therapy on lowering blood pressure. In one study of 18 patients with moderate to severe hypertension (blood pressure >160/95 mm Hg), guanfacine 2–15 mg/day (mean, 5.7 mg) was added to cyclopenthiazide 0.5 mg or hydrochlorothiazide 50 mg daily. With combination therapy, mean systolic and diastolic blood pressures decreased by 26% and 27%, respectively, over 12 months.[48] Murakami et al.,[49,50] in an eight-week trial involving 221 hypertensive patients, reported that the addition of a diuretic to guanfacine therapy resulted in lower dosage requirements of guanfacine (1.34 mg) in these patients than in patients receiving guanfacine as monotherapy (1.63 mg). In addition, guanfacine as monotherapy or in combination with a diuretic produced comparable decreases in systolic and diastolic blood pressures (14.6% and 10.1%, respectively, with guanfacine alone; 13.8% and 8.7%, respectively, with combination therapy).

Keenan et al.[51] suggest that guanfacine is an effective step-2 antihypertensive drug. Their 12-week, multicenter, double-blind, placebo-controlled study used 249 patients with mild to moderate essential hypertension (diastolic BP 95–114 mm Hg). All patients were stabilized on chlorthalidone 25 mg daily before the study. One hundred-twenty-six patients received guanfacine (1–3 mg daily) as step-2 therapy, while 123 received placebo. Both groups were further subdivided so that blood pressure measurements were determined at 12 or 24 hours after dosing. The addition of guanfacine to the chlorthalidone regimen significantly decreased sitting diastolic and systolic blood pressures and mean arterial pressure, as compared to placebo. These reductions occurred during the first week of the study with guanfacine doses of 1 mg/day and were maintained for the 12-week duration of the study. Dosages of guanfacine in excess of 3 mg/day did little to further reduce blood pressure. In addition, guanfacine's antihypertensive effects were similar at 12 and 24 hours after a once-daily dose, with decreases in diastolic blood pressure of 11 and 12 mm Hg, respectively.

Clonidine. Several controlled trials indicate that guanfacine and clonidine have comparable effects in reducing both systolic and diastolic blood pressure when given as monotherapy and as step-2 therapy.[52–55] Distler et al.,[52] in a double-blind, placebo-controlled, crossover trial, studied 16 patients with essential hypertension (diastolic blood pressure ≥105 mm Hg). All antihypertensive medications were withdrawn two weeks before the study; then, either guanfacine 1 mg two or three times daily or clonidine hydrochloride 0.15 mg two or three times daily was administered for five weeks. After another two-week placebo period, the crossover to the other agent occurred. Final daily doses of guanfacine and clonidine hydrochloride were 2 to 6 mg and 0.3 to 0.9 mg, respectively. There were no significant differences in the antihypertensive effect of guanfacine or clonidine. In fact, eight of nine patients receiving guanfacine and six of seven patients receiving clonidine achieved normalization of blood pressure (defined as diastolic blood pressure <95 mm Hg).

Guanfacine has been compared with clonidine as step-2 antihypertensive therapy in a few well-controlled studies. One of the largest of these trials was a double-blind, parallel study of 546 patients with essential hypertension (diastolic BP 95–114 mm Hg).[53] In addition to chlorthalidone 25 mg daily, patients received either guanfacine 1–3 mg at bedtime (n = 270) or clonidine hydrochloride 0.2–0.6 mg in two divided doses (n = 276) for 24 weeks. Diastolic blood pressure reduction occurred by the fourth week of therapy in all patients. Both guanfacine and clonidine exhibited equal antihypertensive efficacy; 149 of 275 (55%) guanfacine-treated and 164 of 276 (59%) clonidine-treated patients achieved a diastolic blood pressure of less than 90 mm Hg. Blood pressure reduction was maintained for the two treatment groups in both the sitting and standing positions for the duration of the study.

Methyldopa. Data concerning the comparable blood-pressure-lowering effects of guanfacine and methyldopa are less consistent than data on the effects of guanfacine and clonidine. Reports are somewhat conflicting as to whether there is a difference in the overall blood-pressure-lowering effects of the two drugs. Most of the studies have been small in patient numbers and not as well controlled as the guanfacine versus clonidine studies. Farooki et al.,[56] in a double-blind, parallel-group design study, compared once-daily guanfacine and twice-daily methyldopa administration in 40 patients with mild to moderate hypertension (BP >150/100 mm Hg). All antihypertensive medications except hydrochlorothiazide were withdrawn two weeks before the patients were randomized to receive either guanfacine 1 to 6 mg/day given once daily (mean dose 2.5 mg/day) or methyldopa 500 to 2000 mg/day given twice daily (mean dose 763 mg/day) for 16 weeks. All patients in both treatment groups achieved blood pressure reductions to at least 160/90 mm Hg, with blood pressure control usually being achieved within the first four to six weeks of treatment. Standing systolic blood pressure was significantly lower in the methyldopa-treated patients at weeks 8–16. This difference was not considered clinically important. Statistics for standing diastolic or supine systolic or diastolic blood pressure were not mentioned.

In a group of 22 hypertensive patients (diastolic blood pressure of 105 mm Hg or higher), methyldopa (mean dosage 1790 mg/day given in two divided doses) significantly reduced postexercise systolic and diastolic blood pressures.[57] However, patients receiving guanfacine (mean dose 4.6 mg given once daily) showed significant reductions in postexercise diastolic blood pressure only. Both drugs decreased supine and standing blood pressures taken at rest.

A few studies have reported guanfacine to produce greater reductions in diastolic and systolic BP than methyldopa.[58,59] In one placebo-controlled, crossover, randomized study of 20 patients with essential hypertension (diastolic blood pressure 100–120 mm Hg), 5 of 10 patients taking guanfacine (mean dose 3.5 mg once daily) achieved normalization of blood pressure (BP <145/95 mm Hg) and 18 had a good response (systolic BP 145–160; diastolic BP 95–110 mm Hg).[58] Normalization of blood pressure occurred in only three of the methyldopa-treated patients (mean dose 1.2 g daily) and a "good response" in nine of the patients.

It has been suggested that 1 mg of guanfacine is equivalent to 125 mg of methyldopa in terms of antihypertensive potency.[60] However, the fact that this estimation is based on the results of nine hypertensive patients treated with either guanfacine or methyldopa for an eight-week period makes the estimation less convincing. Based on the results of larger studies of longer duration, a potency ratio of greater than 250 to 1 is likely.[56–58]

Other Drugs. Few published studies have evaluted the comparative or additive effects of guanfacine with other centrally acting antihypertensives, β-adrenergic antagonists, or vasodilators. One recent study suggests that there is no difference between guanfacine and guanabenz in their antihypertensive effects but that guanfacine may be less sedating.[39]

Clement et al.[60] reported that the effect of metoprolol (200-mg sustained-release tablet once daily) and guanfacine (2 mg daily) on 12-hour ambulatory blood pressure was comparable. Both drugs significantly reduced blood pressure, but the effect of guanfacine was less pronounced than that of metoprolol.

The combination of guanfacine (2 to 6 mg/day) plus hydralazine hydrochloride (50 to 300 mg/day) has been shown to have a greater blood-pressure-lowering effect than guanfacine as a single agent.[61] Guanfacine was able to counteract hydralazine-induced increases in sympathetic nervous tone and thus may be an alternative to β-adrenergic antagonists for this purpose.

Adverse Effects

The adverse reactions to guanfacine are generally dose or dose-frequency dependent and are more frequent during the first year of therapy (Table 2). Because of guanfacine's central mechanism of action, the most common adverse reactions are dry mouth and sedation.

Jerie[62] has summarized the adverse reactions to guanfacine in a multicenter trial involving 580 hypertensive patients treated with guanfacine (mean

Table 2.
Incidence of Adverse Reactions during Guanfacine Therapy[a]

Reaction	Percent of Patients: Year 1 (*n* = 580)	Percent of Patients: Year 2 (*n* = 169)
Dry mouth	60	26
Constipation	14	4
Gastric pain	2.4	...[b]
Tiredness, sedation	33	8
Dizziness	15	7
Nausea, vomiting, diarrhea	2.8	1.2
Bitter taste	1.2	...
Insomnia	5.3	...
Palpitations	1.2	...
Impotence	4.0	...

[a] Adapted from reference 41.
[b] Not reported.

dose 3.4 mg) for one year; 169 patients were followed for an additional year (mean guanfacine dose 3.2 mg/day). Dry mouth and sedation occurred in 60% and 33% of the patients, respectively, during the first year of therapy and in 26% and 8% of the patients, respectively, during the second year. Of interest is the fact that the patients were taking smaller doses of guanfacine during the second year of therapy. Administration of guanfacine once daily and twice daily at low doses (2 mg or less) was associated with fewer adverse reactions than administration three times daily at higher doses. Only 52 of the original 580 patients studied dropped out during the first year because of adverse reactions, the most common being dry mouth (20 patients), sedation (12 patients), and constipation (7 patients). Patients receiving guanfacine as part of combination therapy experienced more adverse reactions than did those receiving the drug as monotherapy. This may be due in part to the fact that they were receiving higher guanfacine doses (mean dose after the first year, 6 mg/day; after the second year, 4.9 mg/day). Among 54 patients who were followed for five to seven years (mean dose 2.2 mg/day as monotherapy, 5.7 mg/day as combination therapy) dry mouth and sedation occurred in six and two, respectively.[41]

Dry mouth and sedation may occur less frequently with guanfacine than with clonidine. In a 24-week, double-blind, randomized, parallel evaluation of the safety and efficacy of clonidine and guanfacine, dry mouth was reported in 30% of guanfacine-treated patients (n = 270) and 37% of the clonidine-treated patients (n = 276).[53] There was a significant difference between the two drugs in the incidence of somnolence, occurring in 21% and 35% of the patients treated with guanfacine and clonidine, respectively. Similar findings have been reported by others.[63,64] Additionally, guanfacine may produce a lower incidence of orthostatic hypotension than guanethidine[66] or clonidine.[63]

Withdrawal of Guanfacine. The sudden cessation of centrally acting antihypertensives, clonidine in particular, may cause a withdrawal syndrome that is characterized by a rapid increase in blood pressure, headaches, tremor, restlessness, and nausea.[66] The withdrawal syndrome of clonidine may occur in as many as 50–80% of patients treated with doses over 1.2 mg/day. The withdrawal syndrome may begin 18 to 20 hours after cessation of therapy.[63,66,67] Blood pressure rises to pretreatment levels or higher within 24–48 hours and is often accompanied by insomnia, headache, flushing, sweating, and apprehension.[66] Additionally, both plasma and urinary catecholamine concentrations increase over 24–72 hours after cessation of therapy.[66]

In contrast to clonidine, this withdrawal syndrome is rarely seen on discontinuation of guanfacine therapy. One investigator suggests that the incidence may be 3%.[64] Some authors have reported catecholamine concentrations after guanfacine discontinuation that were significantly greater than pretreatment values, but these increased concentrations were not accompanied by the severe symptoms that have been observed with clonidine withdrawal.[13,68] A gradual recovery of pretreatment blood pressure occurs over two to four days after guanfacine withdrawal.[63,68] One group of authors reported that in two patients blood pressure surpassed pretreatment levels (30 mm Hg systolic and 10 mm Hg diastolic above initial values); however, the patients were asymptomatic.[36] Reid et al.[66] reported similar findings in five hypertensive patients.

Jain et al.[54] compared the efficacy and adverse reactions of guanfacine 1-3 mg/day and clonidine hydrochloride 0.1–0.3 mg twice daily in a 24-week, double-blind, randomized, parallel study of 42 hypertensive patients. In clonidine-treated patients, significant increases in blood pressure were noted from day 2 onward after abrupt drug withdrawal, and a maximum mean rise of 12/7 mm Hg from pretreatment baseline blood pressure was noted on day 3. In guanfacine-treated patients, significant increases in blood pressure were noted from day 3 onward after drug withdrawal, with a maximum mean rise of 9/5 mm Hg from pretreatment blood pressure on day 4. Increases in systolic blood pressure of at least 10 mm Hg occurred in 55% of the guanfacine-treated patients (n = 20) and in 86% of the clonidine-treated patients (n = 22). Likewise, 40% of guanfacine-treated patients and 64% of clonidine-treated patients experienced increases in diastolic blood pressure of at least 10 mm Hg. During this withdrawal phase, most subjects taking either guanfacine or clonidine remained asymptomatic despite blood pressure elevations.

Most authors suggest that the apparently less-severe withdrawal syndrome associated with guanfacine, as compared with clonidine, is related to its longer plasma half-life and time to recovery of pretreatment blood pressure.[13,36,54,68]

Other Effects. The short-term effects of guanfacine may be quite different from its long-term effects on glucose tolerence. Pagani et al.[69] report that after short-term use (three days) glucose tolerance was reduced and was associated with significant reductions in insulin concentrations. However, no hyperglycemic episodes have been reported when guanfacine was given to patients with glucose intolerance or healthy volunteers for periods up to two years.[70,71] One study in hypertensive patients with adult-onset, non-insulin-dependent diabetes mellitus noted an improvement in the glucose tolerance test with no significant effect on insulin secretion.[72]

Administration of guanfacine 2 mg/day for two years to 30 patients with essential hypertension led to significant reductions in both serum cholesterol and triglyceride concentrations.[73] A seven-year follow-up study of 22 of the original 30 patients reported a 7% incidence of cardiovascular complications in the guanfacine-treated patients and a 20% incidence in the nontreated patients.[20]

Drug Interactions

Thus far the only published drug interaction is between phenobarbital and guanfacine. The administration of phenobarbital 100 mg with guanfacine 4 mg to a hypertensive patient with chronic renal failure[74] resulted in a marked shortening of the elimination half-life (5 hr) as compared to guanfacine therapy alone (approximately 14 hr in renal failure patients). A withdrawal reaction was observed following cessation of guanfacine therapy. The authors suggest that the reaction was likely explained by an increase in the rate of elimination of guanfacine as a result of enzyme induction by phenobarbital.

FDA-Approved Labeling

The FDA has approved guanfacine for the management of hypertension. Since dosing information has been established in the presence of thiazide-type diuretics, the manufacturer recommends that guanfacine should be used in hypertensive patients who are already receiving a thiazide-type diuretic.

Dosage and Availability

The recommended dosage of guanfacine is 1 mg (as the hydrochloride salt) daily given at bedtime to minimize somnolence. Patients should already be receiving a thiazide-type diuretic. If after three to fours weeks of therapy 1 mg does not give a satisfactory result, doses of 2 and then subsequently 3 mg may be given. If the patient develops a rise in blood pressure near the end of the dosing interval, a divided dosing regimen may be used.[73]

If guanfacine is used as monotherapy and the desired reduction in blood pressure is not achieved with 2 to 3 mg daily given as a single dose, a diuretic should be added in the smallest recommended dose.

Use of guanfacine doses higher than 3 mg daily is not recommended because the incidence of adverse reactions increases substantially and there is no evidence of increased efficacy.[40]

Guanfacine hydrochloride is available as tablets containing 1 mg of guanfacine, supplied in bottles of 100 and 500 and in unit dose packs of 100, for oral administration. The average cost to the pharmacist for one month of therapy of guanfacine 1 mg/day is approximately $9; one month's costs for generic clonidine hydrochloride 0.1 mg twice daily and methyldopa 250 mg twice daily are approximately $10 and $9, respectively. Guanabenz acetate (Wytensin, Wyeth Laboratories) 4 mg twice daily costs approximately $16 per month of therapy.

Patient Instructions

Patients should be informed that the common adverse effects of guanfacine are dry mouth and somnolence. Patients who receive guanfacine should be cautioned against operating dangerous machinery or driving motor vehicles until they see how the drug affects them. In addition, they should be warned that their tolerance for alcohol and other CNS depressants may be diminished. Because of the potential for a withdrawal reaction, patients should be advised not to discontinue therapy abruptly.

Formulary Considerations

Guanfacine is a centrally acting antihypertensive with clinical efficacy similar to that of clonidine and methyldopa. Guanfacine offers some advantages over other centrally acting antihypertensives in that it has a longer elimination half-life, which allows once-daily administration. This may be advantageous for patients whose compliance is hindered by frequent medication administration times. The longer half-life of guanfacine may also account for a less severe withdrawal reaction than that seen with clonidine when the drug is discontinued abruptly. Additionally, guanfacine may cause less dry mouth and sedation than clonidine. For these reasons, guanfacine should be considered for formulary addition.

Conclusion

Guanfacine is a centrally acting antihypertensive medication. Its effects on peripheral α_2 adrenoreceptors may provide an additional mechanism of action. Most of the clinical trials that have evaluated guanfacine efficacy have used the drug in combination with a diuretic. Thus, it is difficult to assess whether guanfacine will be adequate as first-line therapy or as an alternative second-line therapy. Further study in this area is necessary.

The pharmacokinetic profile of guanfacine is considerably different from those of the other available centrally acting antihypertensive medications. Guanfacine has a long half-life, which allows once-daily administration and may account for a less severe withdrawal reaction when the drug is discontinued abruptly. Guanfacine appears to be associated with less dry mouth and sedation than clonidine. Thus, guanfacine may offer some advantages over other centrally acting antihypertensive medications in the areas of administration and adverse effects.

References

1. Scholtysik G, Lauener H, Eichenberger E et al. Pharmacological actions of the antihypertensive agent *N*-amidino-2-(2,6-dichlorophenyl) acetamide hydrochloride (BS 100-141). *Arzneimittelforschung*. 1975; 25:1483–91.
2. Zigun JR, Bannon MJ, Roth RH. Comparison of two alpha-noradrenergic agonists (clonidine and guanfacine) on norepinephrine turnover in the cortex of rats during morphine abstinence. *J Pharmacol*. 1981; 70:565–70.
3. Timmermans PBMWM, Schoop AMC, vanZwieten PA. Binding characteristics of [^{3}H]-guanfacine to rat brain alpha-adrenoreceptors: comparison with [^{3}H]-clonidine. *Biochem Pharmacol*. 1982; 31:899–905.
4. Louis WJ, Papanicolaou J, Summers RJ et al. Relationship between alpha-adrenoceptor selectivity and anticonvulsant activity after chronic clonidine like drugs in rats. *Br J Pharmacol*. 1982; 76:299P. Abstract.
5. Dausse JP, Cardot A, Meyer P. Specific binding of ^{3}H-guanfacine to alpha-two-adrenoceptors in rat brain. Comparison with clonidine. *J Pharmacol*. 1983; 14:35–46.
6. Medgett IC, McCulloch MW. Effects of clonidine, guanfacine and three imidazoline derivatives related to clonidine on blood pressure, heart rate and gastric acid secretion in the anesthetized rat. *Arch Int Pharmacodyn Ther*. 1979; 240:158–68.
7. Barber ND, Reid JL. Comparisons of the actions of centrally and peripherally administered clonidine and guanfacine in the rabbit: investigation of the differences. *Br J Pharmacol*. 1982; 77:641–7.
8. Saameli K, Scholtysik G, Waite R. Pharmacology of BS100-141, a centrally acting antihypertensive drug. *Clin Exp Pharmacol Physiol*. 1975; 2 (Suppl 2):207–12.
9. Rosenthal J. Effect of guanfacine on blood pressure and renin activity in hypertensive patients. *Br J Clin Pharmacol*. 1980; 10(Suppl 1):91–6.
10. Murphy MB, Brown MJ. Peripheral alpha-receptor activation by centrally acting drugs? *Pharmacologist*. 1983; 25:196. Abstract.
11. Brown MJ, Harland D, Murphy MB et al. Effect of centrally acting alpha-adrenergic agonists on sympathetic nervous system function in humans. *Hypertension*. 1984; 6(Suppl II):57–62.
12. Schoeppe W, Brecht HM. Guanfacine in essential hypertension: effect on blood pressure, plasma noradrenaline concentration and plasma renin activity. *Br J Clin Pharmacol*. 1980; 10(Suppl 1):97–101.
13. Reid JL, Zamboulis C, Hamilton CA. Guanfacine: effects on long-term treatment and withdrawal. *Br J Clin Pharmacol*. 1980; 10(Suppl 1):183–8.
14. Lefkowitz RJ, Caron MG, Stiles ML. Mechanism of membrane-receptor regulation. Biochemical, physiological and clinical insights derived from studies of the adrenergic receptors. *N Engl J Med*. 1984; 310:1570–9.
15. Collart F, Staroukine M, Verniory A. Relationships between blood pressure, heart rate and plasma epinephrine, norepinephrine, angiotensin II concentrations, plasma renin activity during chronic guanfacine therapy in patients with essential arterial hypertension. *Acta Cardiol*. 1985; 40:269–76.
16. Higuchi M, Overlack A, Stumpe KO. Evaluation of long-term treatment of essential hypertension with guanfacine. *Br J Clin Pharmacol*. 1980; 10(Suppl 1):61–4.
17. Manhem P, Hokfelt B. Blood pressure, heart rate, catecholamines and plasma renin activity following institution and withdrawal of guanfacine treatment in moderate hypertension. *Br J Clin Pharmacol*. 1980; 10(Suppl 1):109–14.
18. Lancranjan I. Effect of guanfacine on pituitary hormones in man. *Br J Clin Pharmacol*. 1980; 10(Suppl 1):151–6.
19. Hauger-Klevene JH, Pinkas MB, Gerber S. Blood pressure and prolactin: effects of guanfacine. Three year follow-up study. *Hypertension*. 1981; 3(Suppl II):222–5.
20. Hauger-Klevene JH, Balossi EC, Scornavacchi JC. Effects of guanfacine on growth hormone, prolactin, renin, lipoproteins and glucose in essential hypertension. *Am J Cardiol*. 1986; 27:27E–31E.
21. Guerret M, Julien-Larose C, Kiechel JR et al. Determination of 3-hydroxy-guanfacine in biological fluids by electron-capture gas-liquid chromatography. *J Chromatogr*. 1982; 233:181–92.
22. Kiechel JR. Pharmacokinetics of guanfacine in patients with impaired renal function and in some elderly patients. *Am J Cardiol*. 1986; 57:18E–21E.
23. Kiechel JR. Pharmacokinetics and metabolism of guanfacine in man: a review. *Br J Clin Pharmacol*. 1980; 10(Suppl 1):25–32.
24. Weiss YA, Lavene DL, Safar ME et al. Guanfacine kinetics in patients with hypertension. *Clin Pharmacol Ther*. 1979; 25:283–93.
25. Scholtysik G, Jerie P, Picard CW. Guanfacine. In: Scriabine A, ed. Pharmacology of antihypertensive drugs. New York: Raven Press; 1980:79–98.
26. Kirch W, Kohler H, Braun W. Elimination of guanfacine in patients with normal and impaired renal function. *Br J Clin Pharmacol*. 1980; 10(Suppl 1):33–5.
27. Kirch W, Kohler H, Axthelm T. Pharmacokinetics of guanfacine in patients undergoing hemodialysis. *Eur J Drug Metab Pharmacokinet*. 1982; 7:277–80.
28. Hedner F, Nyberg G, Mellstrand T. Guanfacine in essential hypertension: effects during rest and isometric exercise. *Clin Pharmacol Ther*. 1984; 35:604–9.
29. Magometschnigg G, Hitzenberger G, Bonelli J. Hemodynamic effects of guanfacine. *Br J Clin Pharmacol*. 1980; 10(Suppl 1):125–31.
30. Irmer M, Just H. Acute and long term effects of guanfacine. *Eur Heart J*. 1981; 2(Suppl A):59.
31. Schafer N, Rauh J, Rosenthal J. Hemodynamics in hypertensive patients before and during guanfacine treatment. *Br J Clin Pharmacol*. 1980; 10(Suppl 1):133–5.
32. Farsang C, Varga K, Vajda L et al. Effects of clonidine and guanfacine in essential hypertension. *Clin Pharmacol Ther*. 1984; 36:588–594.
33. Jaattela A. Clinical efficacy of BS 100-141 in essential hypertension. *Eur J Clin Pharmacol*. 1976; 10:69–72.
34. Lochaya S, Thongmitr V, Suvachittanont O. Antihypertensive effect of BS 100-141, a new central acting hypertensive agent. *Am Heart J*. 1980; 99:58–63.
35. Heidbreder E, Pagel G, Roeckel A et al. Effect of guanfacine on vigilance. *Br J Clin Pharmacol*. 1980; 10(Suppl 1):169–72.
36. Szam I, Hollo J. Long-term antihypertensive therapy with guanfacine. *Int J Clin Pharmacol Ther Toxicol*. 1982; 20:388–92.
37. Wever AMJ, VanBrummelen P. The influence of guanfacine on blood pressure and lung function in hypertensive patients with chronic obstructive lung disease. *Br J Clin Pharmacol*. 1983; 15(Suppl 4):521–3.
38. Materson BJ, Kessler WB, Alderman MH et al. A multicenter, randomized, double-blind dose-response evaluation of step-2 guanfacine versus placebo in mild to moderate hypertension. *Am J Cardiol*. 1986; 57:32E–37E.
39. Fillingim JM, Blackshear JL, Strauss A et al. Guanfacine as monotherapy for systemic hypertension. *Am J Cardiol*. 1986; 57:50E–54E.
40. Jerie P. Clinical experience with guanfacine in long-term treatment of hypertension. *Br J Clin Pharmacol*. 1980; 10(Suppl 1):37–47.
41. Jerie P. Long-term evaluation of therapeutic efficacy and safety of guanfacine. *Am J Cardiol*. 1986; 57:55E–59E.
42. Jerie P, Lasance A. Long-term efficacy and tolerance of the antihypertensive agent guanfacine. *Int J Clin Pharmacol Ther Toxicol*. 1984; 22:170–4.
43. Westelinck K, Michotte Y. Low dose guanfacine once-a-day for the treatment of hypertension in general practice: a multi-centre pilot study. *Curr Med Res Opin*. 1982; 7:631–8.
44. Jerie P. Low, single daily doses of guanfacine in the ambulatory treatment of hypertension. *Br J Clin Pharmacol*. 1983; 15(Suppl 4):479–83.

45. Hauger-Klevene JH, Pinkas MB. Long term treatment of essential hypertension with guanfacine: effect on cardiovascular complications, renin and prolactin. *Curr Med Res Opin*. 1982; 7:569–79.
46. Jerie P, Lasance A. Guanfacine in the treatment of hypertension: two years experience with low dose monotherapy. *Int J Clin Pharmacol Ther Toxicol*. 1981; 19:279–87.
47. Phillipp E. Guanfacine in the treatment of hypertension due to pre-eclamptic toxaemia in thirty women. *Br J Clin Pharmacol*. 1980; 10(Suppl 1):137–40.
48. Seedat YK. Long-term treatment of hypertension with guanfacine (BS 100-141) alone and in combination therapy. *Curr Ther Res*. 1978; 24:288–98.
49. Murakami M, Ikeda M, Miyahara M. Clinical pilot study with guanfacine alone or in combination with a diuretic. *Br J Clin Pharmacol*. 1980; 10(Suppl 1):89. Abstract.
50. Sorkin EM, Heel RC. Guanfacine: a review of its pharmacodynamic and pharmacokinetic properties, and therapeutic efficacy in the treatment of hypertension. *Drugs*. 1986; 31:301–36.
51. Keenan RE, Black PL, Freudenburg JC et al. Usefulness of low dose guanfacine, once a day, for 24 hour control of hypertension. *Am J Cardiol*. 1986; 57:38E–42E.
52. Distler A, Kirch W, Luth B. Antihypertensive effect of guanfacine: a double-blind cross-over trial compared with clonidine. *Br J Clin Pharmacol*. 1980; 10(Suppl 1):49–53.
53. Wilson MF, Haring O, Lewin A et al. Comparison of guanfacine versus clonidine for efficacy, safety and occurrence of withdrawal syndrome in step-two treatment of mild to moderate essential hypertension. *Am J Cardiol*. 1986; 57:43E–49E.
54. Jain AK, Hiremath A, Michael R et al. Clonidine and guanfacine in hypertension. *Clin Pharmacol Ther*. 1985; 37:271–6.
55. Lauro R, Reda G, Spalline L et al. Hypotensive effect of guanfacine in essential hypertension: a comparison with clonidine. *Br J Clin Pharmacol*. 1980; 10(Suppl 1):81–2.
56. Farooki MS, Farsky K, Bouchard S et al. Comparison of once-daily guanfacine and twice-a-day methyldopa in the treatment of mild to moderate hypertension. *Clin Ther*. 1985; 7:199–204.
57. Joshi RC, De A, Cameron EGM. Comparative study of a new alpha-adrenoceptor agonist, guanfacine and alpha-methyldopa in the treatment of hypertension. *Br J Clin Pract*. 1984; 38:66–71.
58. Roeckel A, Heidland A. Comparative studies of guanfacine and methyldopa. *Br J Clin Pharmacol*. 1980; 10(Suppl 1):55–9.
59. Bune AJ, Chalmers JP, Graham JR et al. Double-blind trial comparing guanfacine and methyldopa in patients with essential hypertension. *Eur J Clin Pharmacol*. 1981; 19:309–15.
60. Clement DL, Castro CM, DePue N et al. Effect of metoprolol and guanfacine on ambulatory blood pressure and its variations. *Br J Clin Pharmacol*. 1983; 15(Suppl 4):4715–85.
61. Velasco M, Urbina-Quintana A, Morillo J et al. Systemic and cardiac hemodynamic interactions between guanfacine and hydralazine in hypertensive patients. *Eur J Clin Pharmacol*. 1984; 27:393–6.
62. Jerie P. Clinical experience with guanfacine in long-term treatment of hypertension. Part II: adverse reactions to guanfacine. *Br J Clin Pharmacol*. 1980; 10(Suppl 1):1575–645.
63. Kirch W, Distler A. Antihypertensive effect of *N*-amidino-2-(2,6-diclorophenyl) acetamide hydrochloride: a double-blind cross-over trial versus clonidine. *Int J Clin Pharmacol*. 1978; 16:132–5.
64. Spiegel R, Devos JE. Central effects of guanfacine and clonidine during wakefulness and sleep in healthy subjects. *Br J Clin Pharmacol*. 1980; 10(Suppl 1):165–8.
65. Szam I, Kallay K. Comparative study of two antihypertensive agents: guanfacine and guanethidine. *Br J Clin Pharmacol*. 1980; 10(Suppl 1):85–7.
66. Reid JL, Wing LMH, Dargie HJ et al. Clonidine withdrawal in hypertension: changes in blood pressure and plasma and urinary noradrenaline. *Lancet*. 1977; 1:1171–4.
67. Hoobler SW, Kashima T. Central nervous system actions of clonidine in hypertension. *Mayo Clin Proc*. 1977; 52:395–8.
68. Zamboulis C, Reid JL. Withdrawal of guanfacine after long-term treatment in essential hypertension. Observations on blood pressure and plasma and urinary noradrenaline. *Eur J Clin Pharmacol*. 1981; 19:19–24.
69. Pagani G, Fiorella G, Benco R et al. Comparison of the effects of short term treatment with guanfacine and clonidine on glucose metabolism, plasma renin activity and some anterior pituitary hormones. *Curr Ther Res*. 1984; 36:155–62.
70. Sailer S, Lisch HJ, Patsch W. Guanfacine and glucose metabolism. *Br J Clin Pharmacol*. 1980; 10(Suppl 1):123–4.
71. Lancranjan I, del Pozo E, Marbach P et al. The effect of a new central alpha-adrenoceptor agonist on pituitary function in man. *Acta Endocrinol*. 1977; 85(Suppl 212):80. Abstract.
72. Hauger-Klevene JH, Scornavacchi JC. Improvement of glucose tolerance in hypertensive diabetic patients treated with guanfacine for one year. *Eur J Clin Pharmacol*. 1985; 29:391–3.
73. Hauger-Klevene JH. Hypolipemic effect of guanfacine: 2 year follow-up study. *Drugs Exp Clin Res*. 1984; 2:127.
74. Kiechel JR, Lavene D, Guerret M et al. Pharmacokinetic aspects of guanfacine withdrawal syndrome in a hypertensive patient with chronic renal failure. *Eur J Clin Pharmacol*. 1983; 25:463–6.
75. A. H. Robins Co. Tenex package insert. Richmond, VA; 1986 Oct.

“

Peripheral Intravenous Infusions and Infection Control

To summarize, the following infection control practices are appropriate for most peripheral intravenous infusions: fluid containers should be changed every 24 hours; administration sets and catheters may be changed together every 72 hours; and dressings need be applied only once, at the time of catheter insertion. We have introduced this protocol in our institution and already have received delighted comments from ward nurses and members of the infusion team. We suggest that all members of hospital infection control committees review these data and consider revising their own policies.

—Decker MD, Schaffner W. Intravenous therapy: expanding the bounds of safety. *JAMA*. 1987; 258:2418–9. Editorial.

”

Therapy Review

Drug dosing during continuous arteriovenous hemofiltration

SUSAN K. BICKLEY

Abstract: An overview of continuous arteriovenous hemofiltration (CAVH), which is an alternative to hemodialysis and peritoneal dialysis in the management of acute renal failure, is provided, and literature concerning drug clearance via hemofiltration is reviewed.

CAVH is a slow, continuous process that removes, by convective mass transport, non-protein-bound solutes smaller than 10,000 daltons from blood diverted through an extracorporeal filter. The system provides a creatinine clearance of approximately 10 mL/min. The sieving coefficient of a particular compound reflects its ability to permeate the filter membrane and is primarily influenced by protein binding. Clearance of a compound depends on its sieving coefficient and the ultrafiltration rate. Methods for estimating drug clearance, the amount of drug removed per time interval, and appropriate drug dosages are discussed. Many drugs commonly used in an intensive-care setting, including aminoglycosides, cephalosporins, acyclovir, vancomycin, phenobarbital, ranitidine, and theophylline, can be expected to have a limited but clinically important clearance during CAVH.

CAVH substantially enhances the current treatment of acute renal failure; although limited data for specific drugs are available in the literature, drug dosages may be adjusted based on the methods outlined in this review.

Index terms: Acyclovir; Aminoglycosides; Antibiotics; Anticonvulsants; Antivirals; Calculations; Cephalosporins; Dosage; Excretion; Filtration; Gastrointestinal drugs; Kidney failure; Phenobarbital; Ranitidine; Respiratory smooth-muscle relaxants; Theophylline; Vancomycin

Clin Pharm. 1988; 7:198–206

Continuous arteriovenous hemofiltration (CAVH) is a relatively new technique that is being used with increasing frequency in patients with acute renal failure. Described by Kramer et al.[1] in 1977, CAVH is an extracorporeal process by which fluid and electrolytes, as well as low- and mid-molecular-weight substances, are removed from the blood by means of low-pressure flow through hollow artificial fiber or flat plate membranes. The system simulates the function of the human glomerulus but is much less efficient, producing creatinine clearances of approximately 10 mL/min. CAVH candidates, who are usually found in the intensive-care-unit setting, include patients in whom massive fluid overload restricts adequate parenteral nutrition, patients unable to tolerate hemodialysis because of hemodynamic instability, and patients in whom peritoneal dialysis is not feasible.[2–8]

The use of CAVH is expected to increase because of its relative safety, simplicity, and cost-effectiveness.[9,10] This expected increase in use will create a greater need for clinicians to modify drug dosing. Drug clearance in this dialysis system is different from that in hemodialysis, which depends on the type and size of the dialyzer, pore size of the membrane, and blood flow. It is also different from peritoneal dialysis, during which drug clearance depends on the number and type of exchanges, dwell times, concurrent use of vasoactive drugs, presence of peritonitis, and protein losses.[11–13] Thus, it will be important for the clinician to exam-

SUSAN K. BICKLEY, PHARM.D., is Clinical Pharmacist, Surgery, University of Michigan Hospitals, Ann Arbor, MI, and Clinical Assistant Professor, University of Michigan, College of Pharmacy, Ann Arbor.

Address reprint requests to Dr. Bickley at the Department of Pharmacy Services, University of Michigan Medical Center, 1500 E. Medical Center Drive B2D301/0008, Ann Arbor, MI 48109

Adapted from an article that appeared in the May 1987 issue of the *Michigan Drug Letter*, a publication of the Department of Pharmacy Services, University of Michigan Medical Center, Ann Arbor.

Copyright © 1988, American Society of Hospital Pharmacists, Inc. All rights reserved. 0278-2677/88/0301-0198$02.25.

Figure 1. Typical hemodialysis blood circuit. Reprinted with permission from reference 14.

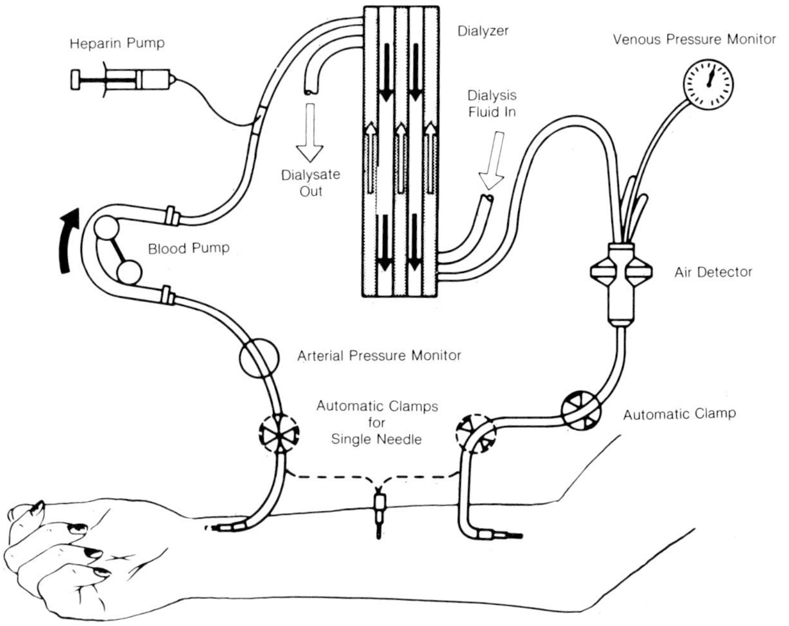

ine clearance data for drugs to determine doses or dose modifications in patients undergoing CAVH.

System Design

Since hemofiltration was developed as an alternative to hemodialysis, it would be appropriate to review the basic concepts of hemodialysis for comparison. Figure 1 depicts a typical hemodialysis setup, in which a patient's heparin-treated arterial blood is pumped at rates of 150–250 mL/min through a dialyzer and back into the venous circulation. A dialyzing membrane separates blood from the countercurrent flow (500 mL/min) of a dialysate solution. The dialysate contains sodium, chloride, calcium, magnesium, and bicarbonate or acetate in physiologic concentrations. The creatinine clearance during hemodialysis is roughly 150–160 mL/min. Patients are typically maintained on two to three four-hour dialysis sessions weekly. Solute clearance in hemodialysis is primarily caused by a diffusion process that is enhanced by blood and dialysate flow. In general, hemodialysis inadequately removes mid-molecular-weight (500- to 2000-dalton) solutes, while solutes weighing less than 500 daltons are preferentially cleared.[14] This is in contrast to CAVH, which has the capacity to slowly and continuously filter solutes weighing up to 5000 daltons.

In the CAVH procedure, the CAVH filter is placed extracorporeally, usually at the femoral site, creating an arteriovenous loop (Figure 2). The tubing contains arterial (prefilter) ports for heparin and fluid administration, an ultrafiltrate port for ultrafiltrate collection, and a venous (postfilter) port for administration of filtration replacement fluid. The filters have a pore size of 10,000 daltons. Filters containing 5000 hollow fibers are manufactured with either of two substances, polysulfone (Amicon, Amicon Division of W. R. Grace & Co., Danvers, MA 01923) or cellulose triacetate (Sartorius, Sartorius Filters Incorporated, Hayward, CA 94544).[10] Alternatively, flat plate filters (Hospal,

Figure 2. Extracorporeal circuit for continuous arteriovenous hemofiltration. Reprinted with permission from the Amicon Division, W. R. Grace & Co., Danvers, MA.

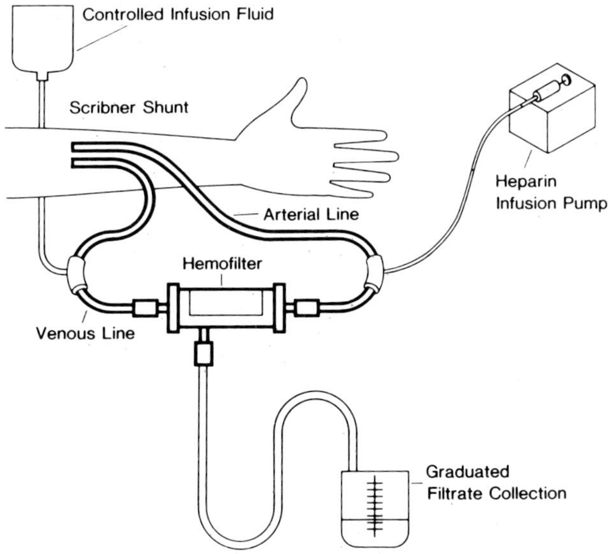

Hospal Medical Corporation, Edison, NJ 08837) are used in some centers. In this filter design, blood flows through multiple (2–20) parallel membranes. These membranes are flexible, prevent negative transmembrane pressure, and are thought to have a lower incidence of filter clotting. Unlike hemodialysis, in which the major mode of solute removal is diffusion into a dialysate solution, these devices freely filter water and non-protein-bound molecules weighing less than inulin (5200 daltons) by the process of convective mass transfer, as expressed in the following equation:

$$C_{pw} \simeq (C_{wp})(\alpha) \quad (1)$$

where C_{pw} is the concentration of drug in the plasma water, C_{wp} is the concentration of the drug in whole plasma, and α is the unbound fraction of the drug. Fluid and solutes that pass through the hollow fiber pores are collected as ultrafiltrate when hydrostatic pressure (the pressure of a liquid that is dependent on systolic blood pressure, blood flow, access site, ultrafiltrate column height, and ultrafiltrate suction) is greater than oncotic pressure (the osmotic pressure exerted by colloids in solution). Thus, non-protein-bound molecules should be found at identical concentrations in simultaneous arterial and ultrafiltrate samples.

The ultrafiltration rate (UFR) is generally maintained at 400 to 600 mL/hr, although the rate is never constant. A systolic blood pressure of at least 50 to 70 mm Hg is necessary to produce ultrafiltrate. Blood pumps are usually not required unless the access site is an arteriovenous fistula. However, many investigators have chosen to use blood pumps to increase the blood flow, the UFR, and, consequently, the solute removal rate.[15-19]

Because such large volumes (10 to 16 L) are collected as ultrafiltrate daily, filtration replacement fluid containing calcium, chloride, magnesium, sodium, and bicarbonate must be administered at a rate of approximately 400 mL/hr. Filtration replacement fluid is composed of the following solutions: (1) 10.35 meq of calcium chloride in 1000 mL of 0.9% sodium chloride injection, (2) 6.4 meq of magnesium (as magnesium sulfate) in 1000 mL of 0.9% sodium chloride injection, (3) 1000 mL of 0.9% sodium chloride injection, and (4) 150 meq of sodium bicarbonate in 1000 mL of 5% dextrose in water. All four solutions are infused simultaneously at equal rates, which results in the following mixed concentrations: sodium 150 meq/L, chloride 110 meq/L, bicarbonate 35 meq/L, calcium 2.5 meq/L, and magnesium 1.6 meq/L. The composition of the solutions may vary, depending on electrolyte requirements. Potassium may be added if necessary. This filtration replacement fluid is infused either pre- or postfilter.[7,20] Many centers prefer prefilter infusion of replacement fluid for several reasons. Prefilter infusion results in dilution of the blood entering the filter, thereby reducing oncotic pressure and decreasing the diffusion of intracellular ions and urea into the extracellular space. Together, these factors contribute to enhancement of solute clearance via ultrafiltration. In addition, predilution results in a local decrease in the hematocrit, which is thought to lead to a lower incidence of filter clotting.

Hemofilters are primed before use with a solution of heparin and albumin in 0.9% sodium chloride injection. A major problem with these filters is the formation of blood clots within the hollow fibers. The priming procedure is thought to extend the life of the filter. The patient's blood should be anticoagulated before placement of a new filter. A loading dose of heparin sodium 20 units/kg is administered 20 minutes before the filter is to be used, followed by a continuous prefilter heparin sodium infusion of 500 units/hr or 10 units/kg/hr.[7,10,20] The dose is titrated by monitoring the activated clotting time (ACT), which should be 200 ± 50 seconds (not to exceed 300 seconds) or 20 to 30 seconds above that of control.[10,15] Although the actual heparin clearance through the hemofilter has not been reported, patients may experience some degree of systemic anticoagulation. Bleeding as a result of heparin treatment or tubing disconnection should be regarded as serious complications of CAVH. In cases of pre-existing coagulopathies, heparin administration is not mandatory.[10,20]

Principles of Drug Removal

Solute clearances during CAVH were published initially by Dodd and coworkers.[5] This study of 25 oliguric renal failure patients reported the clearance of many endogenous solutes. In accordance with the previously described theory of convective mass transfer, urea, creatinine, inulin (molecular weight, 5200), and vitamin B_{12} (molecular weight, 1400) were all found to have identical concentrations in plasma and ultrafiltrate samples.[21-23] Albumin is not filtered; however, it should be noted that free amino acids are filtered. It was also reported that only ionized calcium is filtered and, as expected, only non-protein-bound conjugated bilirubin is filtered.

To estimate the clearance of other endogenous and exogenous solutes (drugs) through the hemofilter, it is necessary to review the factors affecting removal. Several variables must be examined, including the UFR, the delivery of drug to the filter, and the ultrafiltration properties of the drug.[24]

The UFR is increased by increases in hydrostatic pressure and filter surface area, while increases in oncotic pressure and blood viscosity will decrease the UFR. Drug delivery to the filter is obviously crucial in assessing drug clearance. Blood flow should be maximized in the macrocirculation and microcirculation within the hemofilter. The phenomenon of protein concentration polarization, wherein protein build-up on the filter membrane causes an increase in oncotic pressure at the membrane and hydrodynamic resistance, with a subsequent decrease in the ultrafiltration flux, may influence drug delivery, but its clinical importance is questionable.[24] Another theoretical concern is presented by solutes involved in the Gibbs–Donan effect. In this process, negatively charged proteins (e.g., albumin) will bind cations (e.g., calcium) and thereby retard transmembrane movement.[10] Again, the clinical importance of this observation is unknown. Perhaps the most important factor in delivery of drug to the filter is the volume of distribution of the solute. Drugs with large degrees of protein binding or sequestration into fat or other body tissues will have relatively large volumes of distribution (e.g., digoxin, amphotericin B) and will not be substantially cleared by hemofiltration.

Lastly, the clearance of drugs is affected by their ultrafiltration properties: drug–protein binding, molecular size, steric hindrance, drug–membrane interactions, and sieving coefficients. The sieving coefficient is a constant for any particular membrane and solute and represents the proportion of solute that will cross the hemofilter membrane, much like a partition coefficient. In general, all drugs have molecular weights less than that of inulin and should therefore be potentially hemofilterable.

At any one point along the hemofilter, a drug's ability to permeate the membrane can be mathematically described by the following relationship:

$$S = C_{uf}/C_{pw} \quad (2)$$

where S represents the sieving coefficient and C_{uf} represents the concentration of the drug in the ultrafiltrate. When integrated to incorporate the total length of the hemofilter, equation 2 becomes

$$S = 2C_{uf}/(C_{arterial} + C_{venous}) \quad (3)$$

where $C_{arterial}$ is the arterial drug concentration and C_{venous} is the venous drug concentration. Colton et al.[21] and Henderson et al.[22] have found an excellent correlation ($r = 0.98$) between the sieving coefficient determined by equation 3 and that determined by equation 4, as follows:

$$S = C_{uf}/C_{arterial} \quad (4)$$

Thus, equation 4 is routinely used in determining the sieving coefficient for a particular solute. As stated previously, S should be constant. However, sudden changes in solute binding (i.e., drug displacement or enhanced binding), assay inaccuracy, or small numbers of observations could account for variations in reported coefficients. Variations of 0.1 or less in sieving coefficients are considered unimportant.

The amount of drug removed by the hemofilter system can be calculated simply, as follows:

$$A = (C_{arterial})(\alpha)(UFR_{avg})(t) \quad (5)$$

where A is the amount of drug removed and UFR_{avg} is the average ultrafiltration rate over the collection time (t). This can be simplified according to equation 1 to

$$A = (C_{uf})(V_{uf}) \quad (6)$$

where V_{uf} is the volume of the ultrafiltrate. Again, it should be emphasized that the rate of drug removal by CAVH is very low.

Although this method of dosing may seem logical, several drawbacks are evident. First, in the clinical setting, it is not always possible to obtain an assay for a particular drug. If an assay is available, it may not be practical to wait for assay results before calculating and giving the next dose. In addition, clinicians should not overlook concomitant routes of drug elimination (hepatic, biliary, renal) when calculating dosages. If equation 5 is used, it should be noted that literature values for the unbound fraction are generally determined in healthy individuals.[25] The protein binding of many drugs will change under various conditions, including uremia.[26,27]

An alternative to this dosing method is to calculate the hemofilter clearance of individual drugs, as follows:

$$CL_{uf} = (S)\ UFR_{avg} \quad (7)$$

This clearance may be substituted for the drug's renal clearance in pharmacokinetic dosing equations if the patient is anuric. For instance, for drugs cleared solely by the renal route the following equation can be used:

$$\text{Dose} = (C_{ss})(CL_{uf})(\tau)/(S_a)(F) \quad (8)$$

where C_{ss} is the steady-state drug concentration desired, τ is the dosing interval, S_a is the factor for conversion of the salt form of the drug, and F is the bioavailability of the drug. If the patient has some residual renal function, this clearance should be added to the drug's estimated renal clearance before it is substituted in these dosing equations. In addition, for drugs cleared by renal and nonrenal routes, the following equation can be used:

$$\text{Dose} = (C_{ss})(CL_{uf} + CL_{nr})(\tau)/(S_a)(F) \quad (9)$$

where CL_{nr} is the nonrenal clearance, which can usually be obtained from the literature.

Investigations of Drug Removal

Several investigators have determined the hemofilter's ability to clear endogenous solutes.[5-7]

Average sieving coefficients for most electrolytes, creatinine, urea nitrogen, and glucose are between 0.9 and 1.05. Exceptions to this are calcium (S = 0.64), albumin (S = 0.01), total protein (S = 0.02), and total bilirubin (S = 0.03).[7] Relatively few studies in the literature address the quantification of drug removal in CAVH. In fact, drug elimination during hemofiltration was first observed in patients on intermittent hemofiltration. Intermittent hemofiltration is based on the same general principles as CAVH; however, blood flow rates are increased to 200 to 400 mL/min by the use of a pump producing UFRs of 10 to 80 mL/min. Without a pump, blood flow into the filter is usually less than 90 mL/min. UFRs are approximately 25% of plasma flow rates, although this percentage can vary, with UFRs of less than 90 mL/min or greater than 250 mL/min. Drug clearance values obtained from studies of intermittent hemofiltration cannot be applied to the CAVH situation because of differences in ultrafiltration rates and transmembrane pressures. However, sieving coefficients obtained from intermittent hemofiltration data can be used in CAVH. This is because S is theoretically a constant for a given solvent wherein the hemofilter membrane and protein binding are unchanged, and it should not vary with fluctuating ultrafiltration rates. Therefore, it is worthwhile to evaluate studies of drug elimination in intermittent hemofiltration as well as CAVH. Sieving coefficients reported in various studies are shown in Table 1.

One of the first studies of drug clearance during hemofiltration was reported by Rumpf in 1977.[15] During single-dose studies, a linear relationship between clearance and S, as calculated by equations 4 and 7, was established for ampicillin, sulfamethoxazole, and clofibrate, but not for gentamicin or doxycycline. For the two latter drugs, linear relationships were found between S and filtration time. This means that S was not found to be constant at different ultrafiltration rates for gentamicin and doxycycline. These unexpected findings were postulated to be due to a membrane polarization effect that caused a rapid deposition of protein on the membrane at the beginning of hemofiltration. With time, protein deposition becomes saturated, allowing greater proportions of drug to be filtered. This theory remains unproven. Because the methodology in this study is substantially different from that in current use, the data presented cannot be extrapolated with certainty to the clinical setting.

Several investigations of cephalosporin clearance during hemofiltration have been reported. Garcia et al.[16] developed dosing guidelines for intermittent hemofiltration patients receiving cefoxitin. During a four-hour session, 61.96 ± 10.65% of a 30-mg/kg dose of cefoxitin (as the sodium salt) was eliminated, a significant increase from the 44% elimination for the same period with conventional hemodialysis. Ceftazidime elimination was investigated by Gravert and coworkers.[17] During intermittent hemofiltration times of 3.5 to 5 hours, 38 to 78% of an initial 0.5-g dose was recovered in the ultrafiltrate. As expected with this low-molecular-weight (637 daltons), minimally protein-bound (10%) molecule, ultrafiltrate concentrations were found to be almost the same as serum concentrations.

Aminoglycosides have received more attention in the hemofiltration literature than other agents, perhaps because of their frequent use and readily available assays.[a,6,8,15,24,28,30–32] Kennedy reported aminoglycoside levels obtained from ultrafiltrate, venous, and arterial samples to be identical in patients on continuous hemofiltration.[32] This was not an unexpected finding since aminoglycosides have a relatively large free fraction (α = 0.95). Ossenkoppele et al.[8] examined aminoglycoside elimination during CAVH with the Amicon 20 hemofilter and found similar results. A more detailed pharmacokinetic analysis of gentamicin elimination during CAVH was presented in a case by Lehman and Kolb.[28] In this study, ultrafiltration rates were enhanced by connecting the ultrafiltrate port to a wall suction unit. After a gentamicin loading dose, ultrafiltrate and serum concentrations were measured five times within a 30-hour period. A CAVH elimination rate constant of 0.01 hr^{-1} was calculated (r = 0.997), and a linear relationship was confirmed between clearance and UFR (r = 0.998). Akahoshi et al.[30] measured aminoglycoside concentrations in four CAVH patients. S was found to be similar to that reported by other investigators, and a correlation coefficient of 0.7 was demonstrated between UFR and clearance.

Vancomycin dosing was assessed in a recent investigation by Matzke and coworkers.[18] In addition to an analysis using an in vitro model, vancomycin clearance was determined in five patients undergoing intermittent hemofiltration. During the in vitro phase, vancomycin-spiked uremic blood was pumped through a hemofilter, while the in vivo phase used two Gambro hemofilters (Gambro Inc., Lincolnshire, IL 60069) in series. Patients were given 18 mg/kg of vancomycin (as the hydrochloride salt). Pharmacokinetic analysis revealed a vancomycin half-life of 136 hours when the patient was not undergoing hemofiltration and 4.1 hours during hemofiltration. Interestingly, significant rebound increases in vancomycin concentration (52.4 ± 15.6%) were observed within 2.8 to 45.8 hours after the completion of hemofiltration. An average of 32% of the vancomycin body stores were cleared during an average 172-minute treatment. Cumulative in vitro and in vivo data yielded the following linear relationship (r = 0.9914) between vancomycin hemofiltration clearance (CL_{hf}) and UFR (all units are in milliliters per minute):

$$CL_{hf} = 0.78(UFR) - 8.16 \qquad (10)$$

Table 1.
Measured Drug Sieving Coefficients in Continuous Arteriovenous Hemofiltration

Drug	Reference or Footnote	n[a]	α[b]	S[c]	Comments[d]
Amikacin	24	8	0.95	0.88 ± 0.03	
Amphotericin B	24	1	0.10	0.40	
Ampicillin	24	4	0.80	0.69 ± 0.21	
	15	10		0.60	IHF, UFR 10–70 mL/min, RP-G dialyzer (Rhône–Poulenc, France)
Cefoperazone	24	1	0.10	0.27	
Cefotaxime	24	2	0.62	0.51 ± 0.01	
Cefoxitin	16	7	0.25	N.R.[e]	IHF, blood flow 200 mL/min, Sartorius S.M. 40003 hemofilter (Sartorius Filters Incorporated, Hayward, CA)
Ceftazidime	17	N.R.	0.90	Reported as near 1.0	IHF, blood flow 300 mL/min, UFR 70 mL/min, Gambro hemofilter (Gambro Inc., Lincolnshire, IL)
Ceftriaxone	24	1	0.10	0.71	
Cephapirin	24	2	0.55	1.70 ± 0.49	
Clindamycin	24	1	0.75	0.98	
Clofibrate	15	7	0.04	0.06	IHF, UFR 10–70 mL/min, RP-G dialyzer
Digoxin	24	12	0.75	0.96 ± 0.06	
	6	N.R.		0.31	
	19	5		0.62	IHF, UFR 30–80 mL/min, RP 6 filters (Rhône–Poulenc)
	29	N.R.		0.5	
Doxycycline	15	N.R.	0.10	0.4–1.0	IHF, UFR 10–70 mL/min, RP-G dialyzer
Erythromycin	24	1	0.25	0.37	
Gentamicin	24	13	0.95	0.81 ± 0.02	
	30	5		0.88	UFR 100–900 mL/hr, Amicon 30 hemofilter (Amicon Division, W.R. Grace & Co., Danvers, MA)
	8	N.R.		0.87 ± 0.02	
	15	N.R.		0.1–0.4	IHF, UFR 10–70 mL/min, RP-G dialyzer
	a	9		0.85 ± 0.07	In vitro, Amicon minifilter
	31	3		0.75 ± 0.17	
Lidocaine	33,b	1	0.40	>20.0	Unexplained result
Metronidazole	24	4	0.80	0.86 ± 0.03	
Mezlocillin	24	4	0.68	0.68 ± 0.11	
N-acetylprocainamide	24	9	0.80	0.92 ± 0.02	
	6	N.R.		0.89	
Nafcillin	24	4	0.15	0.54 ± 0.12	
	6	N.R.		0.19	
Oxacillin	24	1	0.05	0.02	
Phenobarbital	24	2	0.06	0.86 ± 0.01	
Phenytoin	24	14	0.10	0.45 ± 0.06	
	a	9		0.1 ± 0.03	In vitro, Amicon minifilter
Procainamide	24	9	0.80	0.86 ± 0.02	
	6	N.R.		0.88	
Streptomycin	22	1	0.65	0.30	
Sulfamethoxazole	15	8	0.50	0.9	IHF, UFR 10–70 mL/min, RP-G dialyzer
Theophylline	24	2	0.47	0.85 ± 0.01	
Tobramycin	6	N.R.	0.95	0.89	
	24	6		0.78 ± 0.06	
	8	N.R.		0.87 ± 0.02	
	30	9		0.73 ± 0.18	
Vancomycin	24	11	0.90	0.69 ± 0.06	
	18	5		0.79 ± 0.07[f]	IHF, mean UFR 205 mL/min, two Gambro hemofilters in series
		5		0.66 ± 0.13[g]	IHF, mean UFR 205 mL/min, two Gambro hemofilters in series
		6		0.66 ± 0.031	In vitro, UFR 20–120 mL/min, Gambro FH202 hemofilter

[a] Number of observations.
[b] Unbound fractions obtained from reference 24.
[c] Average sieving coefficient with standard error of the mean if available.
[d] IHF = intermittent hemofiltration, UFR = ultrafiltration rate.
[e] N.R. = not reported.
[f] Determined one-half hour after start of hemofiltration.
[g] Determined at end of hemofiltration treatment.

Thus, vancomycin elimination may be important during hemofiltration, especially if very high ultrafiltration rates are used.

Clearance of cardiac glycosides has also been the subject of several hemofiltration studies.[6,19,24,29] In a series of five patients, Kramer et al.[19] measured elimination of strophanthin, digoxin, and digitoxin after single doses of each. During the six-hour intermittent hemofiltration treatment period, digoxin had an S of 0.62, with a clearance of 36.7 ± 6.6

mL/min, which is significantly greater than its hemodialysis clearance (25 ± 6 mL/min). The potential clinical use of this finding was tested in a report of digoxin toxicity by Lai and coworkers.[29] The Amicon 20 hemofilter was used with blood flow rates of 65 to 76 mL/min on a patient with a serum digoxin concentration of 3.3 ng/mL. The authors concluded that hemofiltration substantially enhanced digoxin clearance in this patient (creatinine clearance, 27 mL/min). The authors suggested that drug clearance can be increased with the use of a pump, although it was not demonstrated in this study, and that hemofiltration should be considered in treating patients who have very high digoxin levels, because the rate of digoxin removal is increased with higher plasma concentrations.

Several authors have reported *S* values for an array of drugs. Paganini et al.[6] used equation 3 to calculate *S* for tobramycin, procainamide, *N*-acetylprocainamide, nafcillin, and digoxin in a study of 23 oliguric renal failure patients. Unfortunately, dosing recommendations cannot be confidently derived from these values because of insufficient data points. Golper et al.[24,33] have contributed to the scant available literature concerning drug elimination in CAVH. Again, using the Amicon 20 hemofilter, these investigators collected data for 24 drugs administered in a series of patients. *S* values, which were calculated according to equation 4, are reported in Table 1. The *S* values were all based on random simultaneous plasma and ultrafiltrate levels. Pharmacokinetic variables were not calculated, and no attempt was made to correlate clearance with UFR. Many of the measured *S* values reported by Golper et al. do not correspond to the predicted value. This may be due to assay sensitivity, a low number of observations, or unknown changes in protein binding. The data for lidocaine are admittedly peculiar, because they imply that ultrafiltrate concentration greatly exceeds plasma concentration. The authors note that this sample was assayed twice with identical results, leaving this irrational *S* value unexplained.

One final study by Golper and Saad[a] is of interest since it investigates protein binding and protein membrane interactions in more detail. In this in vitro experiment, a closed-circuit, pump-driven system was constructed to analyze drug sieving coefficients through the Amicon Minifilter. In a series of tests, phenytoin was analyzed because of its relatively high level of protein binding. Drug concentrations were measured in ultrafiltrate and arterial samples in three solvents (uremic plasma water, uremic whole plasma, and uremic whole blood) at various concentrations. *S* values for plasma are reported in Table 2. Whole blood was not recommended for assay because of an artificial decrease in *S* in the arterial sample, which results because many drugs exhibit a substantial level of binding to red blood cells. In addition, Golper and Saad found that *S* may increase with increasing concentrations of drug, which may be related to saturation of membrane protein binding sites. Interestingly, this study also showed a 100% increase in *S* for phenytoin after the addition of free fatty acid to the solvent. Lastly, protein membrane polarization was confirmed, in accordance with previous studies, by the observation of a slow release of membrane-bound phenytoin.[34,35] The clinical importance of the above findings is not known but is thought to be minimal.

Dosage Adjustment during CAVH

The elimination of many drugs by CAVH can be theoretically predicted. Unfortunately, extensive data on this subject are not yet available. The method for estimating a given drug's potential for filtration is based primarily on protein-binding data. It has been illustrated that this information does not always correlate well with the actual measured sieving coefficients. When attempting to modify drug dosing for the CAVH patient, the method described in the appendix may be used.

Conclusion

CAVH is clearly a therapeutic modality that substantially enhances the current treatment of acute renal failure. Although limited data for the clearance of specific drugs are available in the literature, drug dosages may be adjusted based on the methods outlined in this review.

---

[a] Golper TA, Saad AA. Gentamicin and phenytoin in vitro sieving characteristics through hollow fiber polysulfone hemofilters. Submitted for review. Information on file. Danvers, MA: Amicon Division of W. R. Grace & Co.; 1985 Aug 8.

[b] Golper TA, Pulliam J, Bennett WM. Removal of cefotaxime, metronidazole and gentamicin by continuous arteriovenous hemofiltration. Information on file. Danvers, MA: Amicon Division of W. R. Grace & Co.; 1983.

References

1. Kramer P, Wigger W, Rieger J et al. Arteriovenous haemofiltration. A new and simple method for treatment of overhydrated patients resistant to diuretics. *Klin Wochenschr.* 1977; 55:1121–2.
2. Silverstein ME, Ford CA, Lysaght MJ et al. Treatment of severe fluid overload by ultrafiltration. *N Engl J Med.* 1974; 291:747–51.
3. Kramer P, Kaufhold G, Grone HJ et al. Management of anuric intensive care patients with arteriovenous hemofiltration. *Int J Artif Organs.* 1980; 3:225–30.
4. Lauer A, Saccaggi A, Ronco C et al. Continuous arteriovenous hemofiltration in the critically ill patient. Clinical use and operational characteristics. *Ann Intern Med.* 1983; 99:455–60.
5. Dodd NJ, O'Donovan RM, Bennett-Jones DN et al. Arteriovenous hemofiltration: a recent advance in the management of renal failure. *Br Med J.* 1983; 287:1008–10.
6. Paganini EP, O'Hara P, Nakamoto S. Slow continuous ultrafiltration in hemodialysis resistant oliguric acute renal failure patients. *Trans Am Soc Artif Intern Organs.* 1984; 30:173–8.
7. Kaplan AA, Longnecker RE, Folkert VW. Continuous arte-

Table 2.
Pharmacokinetic Data for Various Drugs in Adults[a]

Drug	Route of Elimination[b]	V(L/kg)[c]	α[d]	S[e]
Anti-infectives				
Aminoglycosides				
Amikacin	R	0.22–0.29	0.95	0.88
Gentamicin	R	0.23–0.26	0.95	0.75–0.88
Tobramycin	R	0.22–0.25	0.95	0.73–0.89
Penicillins				
Ampicillin	R(H)	0.17–0.31	0.80	0.65–0.69
Mezlocillin	R(H)	0.17–0.20	0.68	0.68
Nafcillin	H(R)	0.31–0.38	0.19	0.19–0.54
Oxacillin	R(H)	0.12–0.4	0.05	0.02
Penicillin G	R(H)	0.3–0.42	0.40–0.60	. . .[f]
Piperacillin	R(H)	0.18–0.30	0.78–0.84	. . .
Ticarcillin	R	0.14–0.21	0.55	. . .
Cephalosporins				
Cefazolin	R	0.13	0.20	. . .
Cefonocid	R	0.11–0.13	0.02–0.1	. . .
Cefotaxime	R(H)	0.15	0.62	0.51
Cefoxitin	R	0.13	0.25	. . .
Ceftazidime	R	0.18–0.31	0.90	1.0
Ceftriaxone	R(NR)	0.08–0.19[g]	0.10[g]	0.71
Cefuroxime	R	0.13–0.22	0.5–0.66	. . .
Other Antimicrobial Agents				
Acyclovir	R	0.6–0.8	0.70–0.85	. . .
Amphotericin B	NR	4.0	0.10	0.40
Clindamycin	H	0.6–1.2	0.75	0.98
Sulfamethoxazole–trimethoprim				
Sulfamethoxazole	H(R)	0.28–0.38	0.40–0.60	0.9
Trimethoprim	R(H)	1–2.2	0.30–0.7	. . .
Erythromycin	H	0.5	0.25	0.37
Imipenem	R(NR)	. . .	0.80	. . .
Metronidazole	H(R)	0.6–0.8	0.80	0.86
Vancomycin	R	0.47–0.84	0.9	0.66–0.79
Cardiovascular Agents				
Digoxin	R(NR)	7.5	0.75	0.31–0.96
Dopamine	NR	. . .	. . .	. . .
Dobutamine	NR	. . .	. . .	. . .
Hydralazine	H(NR)	0.5–0.9	0.13	. . .
Isoproterenol	NR	. . .	. . .	. . .
Labetalol	H(R)	3.2–15.7	0.5	. . .
Lidocaine	H(R)	1.3–2.2	0.4	>20
Methyldopa	R(H)	0.69	0.85	. . .
Nitroprusside	NR	. . .	. . .	. . .
Norepinephrine	NR	. . .	. . .	. . .
Phentolamine	NR	. . .	. . .	. . .
Procainamide	R(H)	1.4–2.5	0.8	0.86–0.88
Miscellaneous Agents				
Chlorpromazine	H	7–9	0.01–0.09	. . .
Cimetidine	R	0.8	0.8	. . .
Diazepam	H	0.7–2.6	1.0	. . .
Metoclopramide	R(H)	4.4	0.7–8	. . .
Phenobarbital	H(R)	0.7–1.0	0.6	0.86
Phenytoin	H	0.64	0.10	0.1–0.45
Ranitidine	H(R)	1.2–1.4	0.81–0.9	. . .
Theophylline	H	0.28–0.47	0.47	0.85

[a] Compiled from references 6, 8, 15, 17–19, 24, 25, 28, 30, 36, 37 and footnote a.
[b] R = renal elimination, H = hepatic elimination, NR = other nonrenal routes of elimination. Secondary routes are indicated in parentheses.
[c] V = volume of distribution.
[d] α = unbound fraction.
[e] S = sieving coefficient.
[f] Not determined.
[g] Dose dependent.

riovenous hemofiltration. A report of six months experience. *Ann Intern Med.* 1984; 100:358–67.
8. Ossenkoppele GJ, Van Der Meulen J, Bronsveld W et al. Continuous arteriovenous hemofiltration as an adjunctive therapy for septic shock. *Crit Care Med.* 1985; 13:102–4.
9. Anon. Continuous arteriovenous hemofiltration. *JAMA.* 1985; 253:1325–6.
10. Golper TA. Continuous arteriovenous hemofiltration in acute renal failure. *Am J Kidney Dis.* 1985; 6:373–86.
11. Henderson LW. Peritoneal ultrafiltration dialysis: enhanced urea transfer using hypertonic peritoneal dialysis fluid. *J Clin Invest.* 1966; 45:950–5.
12. Nolph KD, Ghods AJ, Brown PA et al. Effects of intraperitoneal nitroprusside on peritoneal clearances in man with variations of dose, frequency of administration and dwell times. *Nephron.* 1979; 24:114–20.
13. Hirszel P, Lasrich M, Maher JF. Augmentation of peritoneal mass transport by dopamine: comparison with norepinephrine and evaluation of pharmacologic mechanisms. *J Lab Clin Med.* 1979; 94:747–54.
14. Keshaviah PR, Shaldon S. Haemodialysis monitors and monitoring. In: Drukker W, Parsons FM, Maher JF, eds. Replacement of renal function by dialysis. Boston: Martinus Nijhoff; 1983:224.
15. Rumpf KW, Rieger J, Doht B et al. Drug elimination by hemofiltration. *J Dial.* 1977; 1:677–88.
16. Garcia JM, Dominguez-Gil A, Taberno JM et al. Pharmacokinetics of cefoxitin during hemofiltration. *Eur J Clin Pharmacol.* 1983; 25:395–8.
17. Gravert C, Schulz E, Sack K. Ceftazidime in intensive care medicine and hemofiltration. *J Antimicrob Chemother.* 1983; 12(Suppl A):177–80.
18. Matzke GR, O'Connell MB, Collins AJ et al. Disposition of vancomycin during hemofiltration. *Clin Pharmacol Ther.* 1986; 40:425–30.
19. Kramer P, Matthias C, Matthaei D et al. Elimination of cardiac glycosides through hemofiltration. *J Dial.* 1977; 1:689–95.
20. Mault JR. Continuous arterio-venous hemofiltration clinical protocol. 4th ed. Ann Arbor: University of Michigan Department of Surgery; 1985.
21. Colton CK, Henderson LW, Ford CA et al. Kinetics of hemodiafiltration. I. In vitro transport characteristics of a hollow fiber blood ultrafilter. *J Lab Clin Med.* 1975; 85:355–71.
22. Henderson LW, Colton CK, Ford CA. Kinetics of hemodiafiltration. II. Clinical characterization of a new blood cleansing modality. *J Lab Clin Med.* 1975; 85:572–91.
23. Henderson LW. Solute kinetics and fluid removal in hemofiltration. *Int J Artif Organs.* 1983; 6:5–8.
24. Golper TA, Wedel SK, Kaplan AS et al. Drug removal during continuous arteriovenous hemofiltration: theory and clinical observations. *Int J Artif Organs.* 1985; 8:307–12.
25. Bennett WM, Aronnoff GR, Morrison G et al. Drug prescribing in renal failure. Dosing guidelines for adults. *Am J Kidney Dis.* 1983; 3:155–93.
26. Tillement JP, Lhoste F, Guidicelli JF. Diseases and drug protein binding. *Clin Pharmacokinet.* 1978; 3:144–54.
27. Schulz P, Giacomini KM, Luttrell S et al. Effect of low doses of heparin on the plasma binding of phenytoin and prazosin in normal man. *Eur J Clin Pharmcol.* 1983; 25:211–4.
28. Lehman ME, Kolb KW. Gentamicin elimination in a patient undergoing continuous ultrafiltration. *Clin Pharm.* 1985; 4:327–30.
29. Lai KN, Ramasamyiyer S, Pun CO, Vallence-Owen J. Hemofiltration in digoxin overdose. *Arch Intern Med.* 1986; 146: 1219–20.
30. Akahoshi SK, Bollish SJ, Kerr LE. Clearance of aminoglycosides by continuous arteriovenous hemofiltration. Paper presented to 19th Annual ASHP Midyear Clinical Meeting. Dallas, TX: 1984 Dec 6.
31. Kaplan AA, Longnecker RE, Folkert VW. Continuous hemofiltration: in response. *Ann Intern Med.* 1984; 101:145–6. Letter.
32. Kennedy DJ, Greenberg RN, Miller LW. Continuous hemofiltration. *Ann Intern Med.* 1984; 101:145. Letter.
33. Golper TA, Pulliam J, Bennett WM. Removal of therapeutic drugs by continuous arteriovenous hemofiltration. *Arch Intern Med.* 1985; 145:1651–2.
34. Jaffrin MY, Vantard G, Granger A. A concentration polarization model of hemofiltration with highly permeable membranes. *ASAIO J.* 1979; 2:73–85.
35. Calderaro V, Memoli B, Andreucci VE et al. Influence of concentration polarization in post-dilutional hemofiltration of human plasma. *Artif Organs.* 1980; 4:317–21.
36. American hospital formulary service—drug information 86. McEvoy GK, ed. Bethesda, MD: American Society of Hospital Pharmacists; 1986.
37. Mandell GL, Douglas RG, Bennett JE, eds. Principles and practice of infectious diseases. 2nd ed. New York: John Wiley & Sons, Inc.; 1985.

Appendix—Dosage Adjustment during CAVH

The following method may be used to adjust drug dosages during CAVH. Units must be consistent in all equations.

1. S or α should be obtained from references.
2. If S or α is unknown, S should be measured. This is accomplished by measuring the drug concentration in simultaneous ultrafiltrate, arterial, and venous samples. These values are then used in equation 3 to compute S:

$$S = 2C_{uf}/(C_{arterial} + C_{venous}) \qquad (3)$$

   This equation should be used in preference to equation 4, especially if the drug concentration has not reached steady state, as is common in renal failure. If the drug concentration is thought to be near steady state, equation 4 may be substituted, eliminating the need for assay of a venous blood sample. In using equation 4, $C_{arterial}$ should be measured at the midpoint of the ultrafiltrate collection interval.
3. Clearance of the drug by the hemofilter is calculated using equation 7:

$$CL_{uf} = (S)\ UFR_{avg} \qquad (7)$$

4. The dose of the drug is estimated as follows:
   a. For drugs cleared solely by the renal route:

$$Dose = (C_{ss})(CL_{uf})(\tau)/(S_a)(F) \qquad (8)$$

   b. For drugs cleared by renal and nonrenal routes:

$$Dose = (C_{ss})(CL_{uf} + CL_{nr})(\tau)/(S_a)(F) \qquad (9)$$

Pharmacokinetic data for many agents that may be administered to the CAVH patient are summarized in Table 2. This information can be used to calculate appropriate dosage adjustments. Calculations of supplemental dosages that would be administered in addition to baseline dosages for severe renal failure are illustrated in the following examples:

1. Digoxin: Replacement doses are probably unnecessary because of a large volume of distribution.
2. Vancomycin: Daily supplemental dose

$$= (C_{ss})(CL)(\tau)/(S_a)(F)$$
$$= 15\ \mu g/mL\ (0.7 \times 500\ mL/hr \times 24\ hr/day)\ (1\ day)/1 \times 1$$
$$= 125\ mg/day$$

3. Gentamicin: Total daily dose is calculated via standard pharmacokinetic equations wherein (S) UFR is substituted for clearance.
4. Phenytoin: Replacement doses are probably unnecessary because of primary hepatic metabolism.

The values in Table 2 serve only as a general guide since they may not reflect actual values in the critically ill CAVH population. Until more-consistent data are available for individualizing drug dosing, the clinician should monitor levels as described above to determine patient-specific values for S and clearance for every possible drug.

Research

Intrapatient variation of aminoglycoside pharmacokinetics in critically ill surgery patients

DAVID W. FUHS, HENRY J. MANN, CAROL ANN M. KUBAJAK, AND FRANK B. CERRA

Abstract: Intrapatient variation in aminoglycoside pharmacokinetics was studied in 100 critically ill surgery patients, and the relationships between aminoglycoside pharmacokinetics and physiological variables were evaluated.

A one-compartment model and the DataMed Clinical Support Service System were used to calculate pharmacokinetic values from serum concentration–time data and to provide individualized dosage regimens.

A total of 323 pharmacokinetic analyses (2 to 9 per patient) were performed. There were significant intrapatient differences in clearance (CL) between analyses, and there was a downward trend in elimination rate constant (k) and an upward trend in half-life ($t_{1/2}$) with time. There were no significant differences in mean volume of distribution (V) between analyses and no strong correlations of V, k, and CL between analyses. The total daily dosage necessary to provide the desired serum aminoglycoside concentration decreased with time, while the dosing interval increased. The mean absolute changes in $t_{1/2}$, V, and CL between analyses were 3.2 hr, 7.1 L, and 15.7 mL/min, respectively. Dosing regimen changes were required in 90% of the patients, regardless of the time between analyses, including 75% (24/32) of the patients with analyses on consecutive days. There were weak correlations between changes in serum creatinine concentration and changes in dosing interval and between changes in weight and changes in V. Changes in calculated creatinine clearance, BUN, pulmonary capillary wedge pressure, central venous pressure, systemic vascular resistance, cardiac index, input minus output, and maximum temperature did not result in strong correlations with k, $t_{1/2}$, V, and CL by univariate or multivariate regression analyses.

The frequent and often large apparent changes in aminoglycoside pharmacokinetics in critically ill surgery patients cannot be reliably predicted by monitoring common physiological variables. In these patients, aminoglycoside pharmacokinetics must be frequently assessed so that dosages can be adjusted in a timely manner.

Index terms: Aminoglycosides; Blood levels; Dosage; Drugs, body distribution; Excretion; Half-life; Pharmacokinetics
Clin Pharm. 1988; 7:207–13

Aminoglycoside pharmacokinetics has been studied in a large number of disease states and patient groups, and serum concentrations have been related to both efficacy and toxicity.[1-11] Individualized dosing methods using a one-compartment model have been shown to be accurate and produce fewer potentially toxic serum concentrations than do various nomograms.[12,13] The high frequency of aminoglycoside use in critically ill patients and the almost exclusively renal route of elimination make the aminoglycosides a good model for demonstrating pharmacokinetic varia-

DAVID W. FUHS, PHARM.D., M.S., is Clinical Research Supervisor, United Hospital, St. Paul, MN; at the time of this study, he was Clinical Pharmacy Fellow in Critical Care, University of Minnesota Hospital and College of Pharmacy, University of Minnesota, Minneapolis. HENRY J. MANN, PHARM.D., is Associate Professor of Pharmacy Practice, College of Pharmacy, University of Minnesota, and Critical Care Pharmacist, University of Minnesota Hospital. CAROL ANN M. KUBAJAK, M.S., is Clinical Pharmacy Fellow in Critical Care, University of Minnesota Hospital and College of Pharmacy, University of Minnesota. FRANK B. CERRA, M.D., is Professor of Surgery, University of Minnesota, and Director, Surgical Critical Care, Nutrition, and Metabolism, University of Minnesota Hospital.

Address reprint requests to Dr. Fuhs at United Hospital, Department of Pharmacy, 333 North Smith Avenue, St. Paul, MN 55102.

Statistical analysis supported by a grant (RR-400) from the General Clinical Research Center Program of the Division of Research Resources, National Institutes of Health.

Presented at the Clinical Research Forum, 22nd Annual ASHP Midyear Clinical Meeting, Atlanta, GA, December 9, 1987.

Copyright © 1988, American Society of Hospital Pharmacists, Inc. All rights reserved. 0278-2677/88/0301-0207$01.75.

tion. Interpatient differences in aminoglycoside pharmacokinetics have been documented, and several variables (age, sex, hematocrit, weight, altered renal function, and body temperature) have been shown to correlate with aminoglycoside clearance.[1,2,14,15] Intrapatient variation has only recently been described,[3,4,16] and explanations for the variation, such as change in fluid status or organ function, have been suggested but not studied.[2]

Critically ill patients with sepsis have markedly altered physiological characteristics that make the dosing of drugs a clinical challenge. Heart rate, cardiac output, temperature, and white blood cell count are often elevated, while the systemic vascular resistance may be increased or decreased. The plasma protein profile changes rapidly in response to stress, and the patient is often hypermetabolic.[17,18] Septic and postsurgical patients often require fluid resuscitation and have alterations in the concentrations of hormones and vasoactive substances that may affect blood flow and organ function. Cardiac, respiratory, renal, and hepatic failure are common, alone and in combination, which complicates drug dosing and influences patient survival.[19]

In a previous study, we described altered aminoglycoside pharmacokinetics in critically ill surgery patients and the need to individualize dosage regimens because of significant differences compared with a population-based dosing method.[3] We also documented the need to adjust the dosage regimen from the first to the second pharmacokinetic analysis. The present study includes 62 patients from the previous report along with 38 additional critically ill patients and examines intrapatient variation through as many as four consecutive pharmacokinetic analyses. Because determining a relationship between changing physiological variables and pharmacokinetic variables in critically ill patients may allow more timely dosage adjustments, we also attempted to define indicators of intrapatient variation. This study was designed to (1) describe intrapatient variation of aminoglycoside pharmacokinetics in critically ill patients and (2) evaluate the relationships between changes in physiological variables and the intrapatient changes in the pharmacokinetics of aminoglycosides.

Methods

The study population consisted of 100 consecutive critically ill patients age 18 or older in the surgical intensive-care unit (SICU); each had two or more pharmacokinetic analyses (sets of two to four serum concentration determinations) while receiving gentamicin or tobramycin for known or suspected gram-negative sepsis. The study period began in November 1984 and continued through November 1986. The selection of an aminoglycoside was empiric until the results of bacteriological and sensitivity tests were available. To be considered for the study, patients were required to have pulmonary artery and urinary catheters in place. Patients requiring dialysis or an intra-aortic balloon pump were excluded from the study. This work was done in accord with the ethical standards of the committee on the use of human subjects in research.

Age, height, and sex were recorded with the initial pharmacokinetic analysis. Actual body weight (ABW), maximum temperature (T_{max}), blood urea nitrogen (BUN), and serum creatinine concentration (SCr) were recorded with each pharmacokinetic analysis. The body temperature recorded was the core temperature measured via the pulmonary artery catheter. Ideal body weight (IBW), determined by the method of Dubois,[20] was used for all weight-normalized terms unless ABW was less than IBW. Body surface area was calculated from body height and weight, and creatinine clearance (CL_{cr}) was estimated from the Cockcroft and Gault equation.[21] Each patient's fluid input minus output (I − O) was calculated as the difference between the total fluid input and the total fluid output, including urine, wound drainage, and nasogastric-tube losses, but excluding insensible losses.

The initial dosage regimen was not standardized, but 2 mg/kg was routinely used, with the frequency determined by an estimate of the elimination rate. Study doses of the aminoglycosides were administered using a volumetric chamber and pump-assisted constant intravenous infusion over approximately one hour. The start and finish of the aminoglycoside infusion and the exact time the serum concentrations were obtained for each analysis were recorded by the nurse who administered the drug. Each analysis was reviewed daily, and if the infusion or sampling times were missing, the data were not included in the study. If a patient's concentrations were estimated to be at steady state (defined as 4.5 times the estimated half-life), a minimum of one preinfusion and one postinfusion serum concentration were obtained. A minimum of two postinfusion serum concentrations were collected after the first dose. A preinfusion and at least two postinfusion concentrations were obtained if the patient had already received one or more doses but had not reached steady state. The first postinfusion concentration was routinely obtained one hour after the one-hour infusion. When more than one postinfusion concentration was obtained, the sampling interval was extended to include as least one estimated half-life ($t_{1/2}$) of the drug.

Blood samples were immediately transported to the hospital laboratory, where they were centrifuged and the serum was collected. If analysis was delayed, the serum was frozen at −20 °C until analysis. All serum aminoglycoside concentrations were analyzed in duplicate with a fluorescence polarization immunoassay method (TDx, Abbott Laboratories, Irving, TX) by the hospital laboratory. The coefficient of variation of this assay at our institution is 3.9% at a concentration of 1.94 μg/mL and 2.8% at a concentration of 4.95 μg/mL for both intrabatch and interbatch samples. Values for peak, trough, elimination rate constant (k), $t_{1/2}$, volume of distribution (V), and total body clearance (CL) were calculated from the concentration–time data with the DataMed Clinical Support Services system (DataMed, Inc., Minneapolis, MN), which uses least-squares linear regression analysis, a one-compartment model, and the Sawchuk–Zaske method.[12] The DataMed system is a flexible pharmacokinetic program that can be used for either a priori or individualized pharmacokinetic analysis of 23 drugs, including the aminoglycosides. Peak and trough concentrations were extrapolated to the end and the beginning of infusion, respectively. The dosage regimens were adjusted to achieve peak and trough concentrations of 8.0 and less than 2.0 μg/mL, respectively. Only the adjusted dosage regimens were then compared between analyses.

The hemodynamic variables heart rate (HR), stroke volume (SV), central venous pressure (CVP), pulmonary capillary wedge pressure (PCWP), cardiac output (CO), cardiac index (CI), and systemic vascular resistance (SVR) were determined by a cardiorespiratory technician during the time the aminoglycoside serum concentrations were obtained. PCWP was measured by one of the physicians responsible for the patient. The CO was measured in triplicate by the thermodilution technique and reported as the mean of the three observations. The CLINFO software system (BBN Software Products Corporation, Cambridge, MA) was used to calculate the descriptive statistics. The BMDP Statistical Software (University of California, Berkeley, CA) two-way analysis of variance (ANOVA) was used for the multiple paired comparisons of intrapatient variation, which eliminated any bias due to differences in the number of pharmacokinetic analyses per patient. Because of the correlations between pharmacokinetic variables and CL_{cr}, SCr, BUN, ABW, I − O, and T_{max} reported by others in studies of interpatient variation,[1,12,14,15] changes in these variables were correlated with changes in the aminoglycoside pharmacokinetic variables in an attempt to explain some of the intrapatient variation. In addition, the hemodynamic variables (CI, PCWP, CVP, and SVR) were also correlated with the pharmacokinetic changes. The univariate and multivariate analyses were carried out using the CLINFO database system and statistical package. After these univariate analyses, each of the physiological variables was added in a stepwise fashion to the regression model that best explained the intrapatient change in the pharmacokinetic variables to determine if a multivariate model would explain more of the intrapatient pharmacokinetic variation. The predetermined level of significance was set at $p < 0.05$ for all statistical tests.

Results

The 100 critically ill patients (61 men, 39 women) had 323 pharmacokinetic analyses (range, 2 to 9 per patient). The mean demographic and physiological data are displayed in Table 1. Most of the critically ill patients received ventilator support, ranitidine, blood replacement, and diuretics. Some of the patients also received one or more hemodynamically active drugs, such as dopamine, dobutamine, nitroglycerin, or nitroprusside during the course of the study. The aminoglycoside was often accompanied by clindamycin or metronidazole, a cephalosporin or vancomycin, and occasionally a penicillin. The first pharmacokinetic analysis generally occurred within 48 hours of beginning aminoglycoside therapy.

Of the 323 analyses, 17 (5.2%) consisted of two serum concentrations after the loading dose, 21 (6.5%) consisted of three serum samples after the loading dose, 48 (14.9%) consisted of one preinfusion and one postinfusion sample, 147 (45.5%) consisted of one preinfusion and two postinfusion samples, and 90 (27.9%) consisted of one preinfusion and three postinfusion samples. The mean pharmacokinetic values for the 323 analyses exhibited large standard deviations and wide ranges. The mean (± S.D.) k for the 323 pharmacokinetic analyses was 0.12 ± 0.076 hours^{-1} (range, 0.014 to 0.463 hours^{-1}) and the mean $t_{1/2}$ overall was 8.7 ± 6.7 hours (range, 1.5 to 49.5 hours). The mean V overall was 21.8 ± 8.3 L (range, 7.0 to 66.0 L), the mean V normalized to actual body weight (V_{ABW}) was 0.30 ± 0.10 L/kg (range, 0.10 to 0.73 L/kg) and

Table 1.
Demographic and Physiological Description of 100 Critically Ill Patients at Time of First Pharmacokinetic Analysis

Variable[a]	Mean ± S.D.	Range
Age (yr)	59.0 ± 16.3	19.0–89.0
Height (cm)	170.2 ± 10.8	145–193
TBW (kg)	75.0 ± 18.8	40.5–144.6
IBW (kg)	63.3 ± 11.5	38.1–86.8
SCr (mg/dL)	1.9 ± 1.2	0.6–6.8
CL_{cr} (mL/min)	45.7 ± 24.8	5.5–131.8
PCWP (mm Hg)	17.9 ± 5.7	5–36
CVP (mm Hg)	10.5 ± 5.0	1–27
CI (L/min/sq m)	4.5 ± 1.4	1.9–7.2
SVR (dynes·sec/cm^5)	781 ± 288	219–1580
T_{max} (°C)	38.3 ± 0.9	36.2–40.0

[a] TBW = total body weight; IBW = ideal body weight; SCr = serum creatinine concentration; CL_{cr} = calculated creatinine clearance; PCWP = pulmonary capillary wedge pressure; CVP = central venous pressure; CI = cardiac index; SVR = systemic vascular resistance; T_{max} = maximum temperature per 24 hours.

the mean V normalized to ideal body weight (V_{IBW}) was 0.36 ± 0.12 L/kg (range, 0.14 to 0.88 L/kg). The CL overall was 42.1 ± 28.2 mL/min (range, 6.4 to 183.6 mL/min) and the CL normalized to actual body weight was 0.58 ± 0.36 mL/min/kg. The mean extrapolated peak concentration was 7.8 ± 2.8 μg/mL (range, 2.4 to 16.8 μg/mL), and the mean extrapolated trough concentration was 1.6 ± 0.9 μg/mL (range 0 to 5.5 μg/mL).

The multiple, paired comparisons (two-way ANOVA) of the pharmacokinetic values by analysis number are displayed in Table 2. There were 295 analyses evaluated (195 comparisons) in patients having two to four analyses. Because of the small number of patients having more than four analyses, these data were excluded from further analysis. There were no statistically significant differences in the intrapatient k and $t_{1/2}$ between each of the successive analyses, but there was a downward trend in k and an upward trend in $t_{1/2}$ with time. The differences between k and $t_{1/2}$ for analyses 2, 3, and 4 were significant when compared with analysis 1. There were no significant differences in the V, V_{ABW}, and V_{IBW} between analyses by pairwise comparison. There were significant differences in the intrapatient CL between analyses. The total daily dosage (mg/day and mg/kg/day) necessary to provide the desired concentrations decreased with time, while the dosing interval increased.

To determine whether there was a relationship for each pharmacokinetic variable with time, the correlations of the pharmacokinetic variables on successive analyses were determined. The pharmacokinetic variables k, V, and CL for the earlier analysis were plotted on the x-axis (independent variable) and the variables for the subsequent analysis on the y-axis (dependent variable). The correlation coefficient, slope, and y-intercept for each analysis pair are displayed in Table 3. The slope of the regression equation was less than 1 in each case, and the majority of the data points were below the line of identity, which indicates that each of the variables tended to decrease with time; however, the correlations were not strong.

Table 2.
Comparison of Pharmacokinetic and Dosing Variables by Analysis Number[a]

Variable[b]	Analysis 1 (n = 100)	Analysis 2 (n = 100)	Analysis 3 (n = 64)	Analysis 4 (n = 31)
k (hr^{-1})	0.14 ± 0.08	0.12 ± 0.07[c]	0.12 ± 0.07[c]	0.11 ± 0.06[c,d]
$t_{1/2}$ (hr)	7.1 ± 5.4	8.1 ± 7.4[c]	8.4 ± 5.1[c]	8.5 ± 5.2[c]
V (L)	21.7 ± 8.7	22.7 ± 8.7	21.2 ± 7.3	20.4 ± 7.0
V_{ABW} (L/kg)	0.29 ± 0.09	0.31 ± 0.11	0.29 ± 0.11	0.29 ± 0.07
V_{IBW} (L/kg)	0.35 ± 0.12	0.37 ± 0.14	0.35 ± 0.13	0.34 ± 0.10
CL (mL/min)	49.3 ± 31.3	43.4 ± 29.0[c]	40.4 ± 26.5[c,d]	34.3 ± 17.2[c,d,e]
Dosage in mg/day	256 ± 158	229 ± 157[c]	218 ± 143[c,d]	179 ± 85[c,d]
Dosage in mg/kg/day	3.40 ± 2.0	2.98 ± 1.9[c]	2.83 ± 1.7[c,d]	2.65 ± 1.2[c,d]
Dosing interval (hr)[f]	12	12	18	18
Day of therapy	1.7 ± 1.2	5.2 ± 2.7	8.0 ± 3.6	10.0 ± 4.1

[a] Values expressed as mean ± S.D. except where noted otherwise.
[b] k = elimination rate constant; $t_{1/2}$ = half-life; V = volume of distribution; V_{ABW} = V based on actual body weight; V_{IBW} = V based on ideal body weight; CL = clearance.
[c] Significantly different from analysis 1 (two-way ANOVA for multiple paired comparisons).
[d] Significantly different from analysis 2 (two-way ANOVA for multiple paired comparisons).
[e] Significantly different from analysis 3 (two-way ANOVA for multiple paired comparisons).
[f] Median.

Table 3.
Correlation of Pharmacokinetic Variables between Analyses[a]

Variable[b]	1 vs. 2 (n = 100)	2 vs. 3 (n = 64)	3 vs. 4 (n = 31)
k	$y = 0.64x + 0.03$, $r = 0.66$	$y = 0.68x + 0.03$, $r = 0.76$	$y = 0.65x + 0.03$, $r = 0.70$
V	$y = 0.26x + 17.2$, $r = 0.26$	$y = 0.16x + 17.6$, $r = 0.21$	$y = 0.32x + 13.7$, $r = 0.34$
CL	$y = 0.62x + 12.5$, $r = 0.67$	$y = 0.67x + 8.8$, $r = 0.77$	$y = 0.39x + 18.6$, $r = 0.53$

[a] The pharmacokinetic variables for the first analysis of each pair of analyses were plotted on the x-axis (independent variable); the subsequent analysis was on the y-axis (dependent variable). Results expressed as regression equation (correlation coefficient, r).
[b] k = elimination rate constant; V = volume of distribution; CL = clearance.

Large intrapatient changes in the $t_{1/2}$, V, and CL were evident when the absolute intrapatient change in each of the variables was evaluated (Table 4). The V changed more than 1 L (range, 1 to 36.8 L) in 83% (162/195) and more than 5 L in 48% (93/195) of the intrapatient comparisons. The CL changed by 10 mL/min or more (range, 10 to 108 mL/min) in 51% (99/195) of the intrapatient comparisons. These within-patient differences were not evident in the analysis of the mean intrapatient differences because the pharmacokinetic variables both increased and decreased, which minimized the mean differences.

The impact of this intrapatient pharmacokinetic variation is illustrated by the number of dosage regimen changes necessary to maintain the desired aminoglycoside concentrations. A comparison of the recommended dosage regimens from analyses 1 and 2 revealed that it was necessary to change either the dose, the dosing interval, or both in 77 of the 100 patients. A clinically important change in the dose was defined as 30 mg or more, because this translates into a 1- to 2-μg/mL change in the serum concentration. Of the 23 patients who did not have a marked regimen change between analyses 1 and 2, 9 patients did not have a third analysis, but 13 of the 14 remaining patients had clinically important regimen changes between analyses 2 and 3. The net result was that 90 of the 100 patients required a significant regimen change by the third analysis. When successive analyses were performed on consecutive days, it was necessary to change the dose, the dosing interval, or both in 75% (24/32) of the patients.

The SCr is frequently monitored as an indicator of changing renal function and, therefore, changing aminoglycoside elimination. A change in the SCr of 0.3 mg/dL or more was considered clinically important, given the laboratory duplicate range of 0.2 mg/dL (alkaline picrate method). However, there was an inconsistent relationship between changes in the SCr and the changes in the dosing interval (Table 5). The intrapatient change in dosing interval ranged from an increase of 72 hours to a decrease of 48 hours, and the change in SCr ranged from an increase of 2.9 mg/dL to a decrease of 2.8 mg/dL between analyses.

Table 4.
Absolute Intrapatient Changes in Pharmacokinetic Variables between Analyses

Variable[a]	1 vs. 2 (n = 100)	2 vs. 3 (n = 64)	3 vs. 4 (n = 31)
$t_{1/2}$ (hr)	3.7 ± 6.1	2.8 ± 4.1	2.4 ± 3.5
V (L)	7.1 ± 7.8	7.8 ± 10.9	6.0 ± 8.3
CL (mL/min)	16.8 ± 18.8	14.5 ± 15.2	14.6 ± 15.1

[a] Expressed as mean ± S.D.; $t_{1/2}$ = half-life; V = volume of distribution; CL = clearance.

A change in the ABW is often used as an indicator of a patient's fluid balance. However, there was not an apparent relationship between changes in ABW and changes in V (Table 6).

The univariate correlation of the intrapatient changes in the physiological variables with the intrapatient changes in the pharmacokinetic variables is shown in Table 7. The best univariate correlations were for changes in CL_{cr} with the change in

Table 5.
Intrapatient Changes in Serum Creatinine Concentration (SCr) versus Changes in Dosing Interval

SCr Change[a]	Dosing Interval Change[b] Increase	Decrease	Unchanged
Increased (n = 59)	42 (71.2)	4 (6.8)	13 (22.0)
Decreased (n = 49)	9 (18.4)	16 (32.7)	24 (48.9)
Unchanged (n = 87)	23 (26.4)	11 (12.6)	53 (61.0)

[a] Change defined as ≥0.3 mg/dL.
[b] No. (%) of analyses.

Table 6.
Intrapatient Changes in the Actual Body Weight (ABW) versus Changes in Volume of Distribution (V)

ABW Change[a]	V Change[b,c] Increased	Decreased	Unchanged
Increased (n = 67)	33 (49.3)	21 (31.3)	13 (19.4)
Decreased (n = 80)	26 (32.5)	41 (51.3)	13 (16.2)
Unchanged (n = 48)	23 (47.9)	18 (37.5)	7 (14.6)

[a] Change defined as ≥1 kg.
[b] Change defined as ≥1 L.
[c] No. (%) of analyses.

Table 7.
Univariate Correlation (r) of Change in Physiological Variables with Change in Pharmacokinetic Variables (n = 195)

Physiological Variables[a]	Pharmacokinetic Variables[b] k	$t_{1/2}$	V	CL
CL_{cr} (mL/min)	0.43	−0.26	0.03	0.36
SCr (mg/dL)	−0.29	0.31	−0.03	−0.25
BUN (mg/dL)	−0.25	0.20	0.06	−0.11
ABW (kg)	−0.22	0.17	0.15	0.02
PCWP (mm Hg)	−0.14	0.11	0.09	0.01
CVP (mm Hg)	−0.29	0.13	0.05	−0.14
SVR (dynes · sec/cm^5)	0.06	0.02	0.10	0.12
CI (L/min/sq m)	0.05	0.003	−0.02	0.03
I − O (mL)	0.12	−0.04	−0.18	−0.15
T_{max} (°C)	−0.08	0.03	0.01	−0.10

[a] CL_{cr} = calculated creatinine clearance; SCr = serum creatinine concentration; BUN = blood urea nitrogen; ABW = actual body weight; PCWP = pulmonary capillary wedge pressure; CVP = central venous pressure; SVR = systemic vascular resistance; CI = cardiac index; I − O = total input minus output; T_{max} = maximum temperature on the day of analysis.
[b] k = elimination rate constant; $t_{1/2}$ = half-life; V = volume of distribution; CL = clearance.

k (r = 0.43) and in CL (r = 0.36). Changes in SCr correlated best with changes in $t_{1/2}$ (r = 0.31). The intrapatient change in ABW showed the best correlation with changes in V (r = 0.15). Overall, the univariate correlations of the physiological variables did not reveal any strong relationships with the pharmacokinetic variables. In addition, there were no apparent relationships between any of the hemodynamically active drugs and the pharmacokinetic variables.

When the physiological variables were added in a stepwise fashion to even the best univariate relationships, the resulting multivariate analyses showed no significant improvement in the predictability of change in the pharmacokinetic variables. The multivariate correlation of changes in k versus changes in CL_{cr}, I − O, CI, PCWP, and BUN was r = 0.45. The multivariate correlation of V versus changes in ABW, PCWP, CL_{cr}, I − O, and T_{max} was r = 0.21, and the multivariate correlation of changes in CL versus changes in CL_{cr}, ABW, CI, I − O, and T_{max} was r = 0.36.

Discussion

This study documents wide intrapatient variation in the pharmacokinetics of aminoglycosides in critically ill surgery patients. These pharmacokinetic changes resulted in the need to alter the dosage regimen by a clinically important amount at least once during the treatment course in 90% of the patients. Large changes in the pharmacokinetic values occurred even when the analyses were performed on consecutive days and continued through four analyses. Unfortunately, there were no physiological variables that reliably identified the direction, frequency, or magnitude of these pharmacokinetic changes. The data presented here indicate for the first time that critically ill patients with no identifiable changes in commonly monitored physiological variables often have dramatic variations in pharmacokinetic values and, consequently, changes in dosage requirements. These previously unreported variations in pharmacokinetics may subject the patient to either subtherapeutic or potentially toxic serum concentrations.

There is a degree of error in the measurement and calculation of the pharmacokinetic and physiological variables. However the Sawchuk–Zaske method has been shown to accurately predict the concentrations observed after dosage adjustment in stable patients.[12] The intrapatient pharmacokinetic variability described here may be due in part to variations in drug delivery, flushing of the intravenous line, the assay method, sampling strategies, and the inability of a one-compartment model to account for two-compartment accumulation. Because of these possible errors, the variation may represent apparent rather than actual changes in the intrapatient pharmacokinetic variables. In order to quantify the true intrapatient pharmacokinetic variation, a larger number of standardized serum samples and a more controlled drug delivery process would be necessary. The optimal number of serum concentrations for characterizing the intrapatient pharmacokinetic variation is not known. The majority of the patients in this study had two or more postinfusion concentration determinations. Because of the magnitude of the apparent pharmacokinetic changes reported in this study, we believe that the variation was primarily due to changes in the patient rather than error in the method. Regardless of whether the variation is true or apparent, we believe clinicians are often obligated to make corresponding changes in the dosage regimens in critically ill patients.

Intrapatient variation of aminoglycoside pharmacokinetics has also been demonstrated in three studies of cystic fibrosis patients.[4,16,22] There was a significant decrease in the $t_{1/2}$ between day 1 and day 6 or beyond in the study by Bosso et al.[16] and between week 1 and week 2 in the study by Munzenberger et al.[22] There are also two preliminary reports of the intrapatient variation of aminoglycoside pharmacokinetics in surgical intensive-care patients.[8,23] The large volumes of distribution reported in the present study are similar to our previous report and are consistent with data published by several others.[3,6–8,23] Our finding of a lack of significant difference in V between analyses is supported by several of these reports.[16,22,23] However, large ranges and standard deviations for each of the pharmacokinetic variables were reported. Frequent monitoring and dosage adjustment were recommended in all of these studies.

The correlations previously found between physiological variables (SCr, ABW, T_{max}),[1,12,14,15] which were based on interpatient variation, did not hold true in this study population. The Cockcroft–Gault method[21] is a common method of estimating CL_{cr} and was used for comparison with pharmacokinetic variables as in previous reports.[1,12,14,15] It is possible that using a method of calculating CL_{cr} that considers changing renal function (e.g., Jeliffe and Jeliffe[24]) may improve the relationship to changes in pharmacokinetic variables. In our critically ill patients, variables such as SCr and ABW are not reliable indicators of pharmacokinetic changes and are often misleading. In addition, changes in I − O, CVP, and PCWP, which are often used to guide fluid replacement therapy, were not at all related to changes in the aminoglycoside CL or V. Dasta and Armstrong[23] also have reported that fluid excess (I − O) does not correlate with V. Therefore, the decision about when to reanalyze aminoglycoside pharmacokinetics in a critically ill patient cannot be based on whether there are changes in the commonly monitored physiological variables. Rather, the decision must be based on the amount of risk the clinician is willing to assume if the pharmacokinetic variables are different from what is expected.

One of the problems in describing relationships between changes in physiological and pharmacokinetic variables is the multifactorial nature of these changes. We tried to include as many of the physiological variables as possible in the multivariate analysis, but we were unable to improve the correlations. It is frustrating that we are unable to predict changes in V or clearance, especially since we know that the patient population studied undergoes large fluid shifts because of surgery, sepsis, hypovolemia, and drug therapy, all of which may affect serum concentrations. It is possible that future research may identify other markers of organ function or fluid balance that will correlate with changes in pharmacokinetic variables in critically ill patients. However, at present we are left with the need to measure the aminoglycoside pharmacokinetic values frequently to detect such changes. Our current standard of practice is to repeat a pharmacokinetic analysis at least every three days in critically ill patients with aminoglycoside dosing intervals less than 48 hours and at least every other dose when the dosing interval is longer than 48 hours.

Conclusion

Critically ill surgery patients have frequent and often large apparent changes in aminoglycoside pharmacokinetics that require substantial dosage adjustments. There is a downward trend in clearance with time, but the intrapatient variation in the pharmacokinetic variables is not reliably predicted by common physiological variables. Aminoglycoside pharmacokinetics in critically ill patients must be assessed frequently so that dosages can be adjusted in a timely manner and the number of subtherapeutic or potentially toxic serum concentrations can be minimized.

References

1. Zaske DE, Cipolle RJ, Rotschafer JC et al. Gentamicin pharmacokinetics in 1640 patients: method for control of serum concentrations. *Antimicrob Agents Chemother.* 1982; 21:407–11.
2. Zaske DE, Cipolle RJ, Strate RJ. Gentamicin dosage requirements: wide interpatient variations in 242 surgery patients with normal renal function. *Surgery.* 1980; 87:64–9.
3. Mann HJ, Fuhs DW, Awang R et al. Altered aminoglycoside pharmacokinetics in critically ill patients with sepsis. *Clin Pharm.* 1987; 6:154–9.
4. Mann HJ, Canafax DM, Cipolle RJ et al. Increased dosage requirements of tobramycin and gentamicin for treating pseudomonas pneumonia in patients with cystic fibrosis. *Pediatr Pulmonol.* 1985; 1:238–43.
5. Zaske DE, Irvin P, Strand LM et al. Wide interpatient variations in gentamicin dose requirements for geriatric patients. *JAMA.* 1982; 248:3122–6.
6. Kloth DD, Tegtmeier BR, Kong C et al. Altered gentamicin pharmacokinetics during the perioperative period. *Clin Pharm.* 1985; 4:182–5.
7. Summer WR, Michael JR, Lipsky JJ. Initial aminoglycoside levels in the critically ill. *Crit Care Med.* 1983; 11:948–50.
8. Niemiec PW, Allo MD, Miller CF. Effect of altered volume of distribution on aminoglycoside levels in patients in surgical intensive care. *Arch Surg.* 1987; 122:207–12.
9. Moore RD, Smith CR, Lietman PS. The association of aminoglycoside plasma levels with mortality in patients with gram-negative bacteremia. *J Infect Dis.* 1984; 149:443–8.
10. Moore RD, Smith CR, Lipsky JJ et al. Risk factors for nephrotoxicity in patients treated with aminoglycosides. *Ann Intern Med.* 1984; 100:352–7.
11. Zaske DE, Bootman SL, Solem LD et al. Increased burn patient survival with individualized doses of gentamicin. *Surgery.* 1982; 91:142–9.
12. Sawchuck RJ, Zaske DE, Cipolle RJ et al. Kinetic model for gentamicin dosing with the use of individual patient parameters. *Clin Pharmacol Ther.* 1977; 21:362–7.
13. Lesar TS, Rotschafer JC, Strand LM et al. Gentamicin dosing errors with four commonly used nomograms. *JAMA.* 1982; 248:1190–3.
14. Barza M, Brown RB, Shen D et al. Predictability of blood levels of gentamicin in man. *J Infect Dis.* 1975; 132:165–74.
15. Pennington JE, Dale DC, Reynolds HY et al. Gentamicin sulfate pharmacokinetics: lower levels of gentamicin in blood during fever. *J Infect Dis.* 1975; 132:270–5.
16. Bosso JA, Relling MV, Townsend PL et al. Intrapatient variation in aminoglycoside disposition in cystic fibrosis. *Clin Pharm.* 1987; 6:54–8.
17. Cerra FB, Seigel JH, Border JR et al. Correlations between metabolic and cardiopulmonary measurements in patients after trauma, general surgery, and sepsis. *J Trauma.* 1979; 19:621–9.
18. Moyer ED, Border JR, McMenamy RH et al. Multiple systems organ failure: V. Alterations in the plasma protein profile in septic trauma—effects of intravenous amino acids. *J Trauma.* 1981; 21:645–9.
19. Knaus WA, Draper EA, Wagner DP et al. Prognosis in acute organ-system failure. *Ann Surg.* 1985; 202:685–93.
20. DuBois D, DuBois EF. The measurement of the surface area of man. *Arch Intern Med.* 1916; 17:868–43.
21. Cockcroft DW, Gault MH. Prediction of creatinine clearance from serum creatinine. *Nephron.* 1976; 16:31–41.
22. Munzenberger PJ, Commissaris RL, Massoud N et al. Variability of tobramycin pharmacokinetics in cystic fibrosis. *Pediatr Infect Dis.* 1987; 6:739–43.
23. Dasta JF, Armstrong DK. More on variability in aminoglycoside volume of distribution. *Clin Pharm.* 1986; 6:193. Letter.
24. Jelliffe RW, Jelliffe SM. A computer program for estimation of creatinine clearance from unstable serum creatinine levels, age, sex, and weight. *Math Biosci.* 1972; 14:17–24.

Effect of infusion pump fill-stroke flow interruption on response to sodium nitroprusside in surgical patients

HENRY J. MANN, DAVID W. FUHS, AND FRANK B. CERRA

Abstract: The influence of the piston-cassette pump fill stroke on the pharmacodynamic response to sodium nitroprusside was evaluated prospectively in 10 adult patients in the surgical intensive-care unit.

Simultaneous analog recordings of blood pressure and fill stroke were made over three complete pump fill cycles in each patient. Sodium nitroprusside flow rates and concentrations were recorded throughout the data-collection period. Analysis was based on the maximum pressure obtained during the two-minute baseline period before a fill stroke (Pmax baseline), the pressure at the initiation of the fill stroke (P initial), and the maximum pressure obtained during the two-minute period after the fill stroke (Pmax postfill).

The maximum systolic blood pressure (SBP), diastolic blood pressure (DBP), and mean blood pressure (MBP) during the baseline and post-fill-stroke periods were significantly different. The mean (± S.D.) variability in pressure between the time periods Pmax baseline and Pmax postfill was 3.9 ± 5.8 mm Hg for SBP (range, −8 to +16), 3.5 ± 5.7 mm Hg for DBP (range, −7 to +13), and 3.6 ± 5.6 mm Hg for MBP (range, −7 to +14). The likelihood of a pharmacodynamic change was inconsistent both between and within patients. Within patients the difference between cycles for the variability between time periods ranged from a minimum of 2 mm Hg to a maximum of 16 mm Hg for SBP, 2 mm Hg to 17 mm Hg for DBP, and 1 mm Hg to 17 mm Hg for MBP. The variability within the baseline period (Pmax baseline − P initial) in SBP was significantly greater than the variability between the time periods, while the differences for DBP and MBP were not significant.

In adult surgical intensive-care-unit patients receiving sodium nitroprusside for blood pressure control, there is a small, detectable pharmacodynamic effect that may be associated with the fill stroke of a piston-cassette pump. The pharmacodynamic effect is inconsistent both between and within patients and is not greater than the variation in blood pressure observed during a baseline period preceding the fill stroke, and it is unlikely that a more pronounced effect would be demonstrated with other commonly used agents in the surgical intensive-care unit.

Index terms: Devices; Drug administration; Flow; Hypertension; Hypotensive agents; Sodium nitroprusside
Clin Pharm. 1988; 7:214–9

The continuous infusion of short-acting drugs such as dopamine, dobutamine, sodium nitroprusside, and nitroglycerin is a frequently used therapeutic modality in the critical-care unit. The general availability and use of electronic infusion-control devices have aided the proliferation of these therapies by allowing clinicians to safely and accurately control the rate of infusion of these potent medications. Two studies have raised questions concerning the effect that mechanical design and flow characteristics of infusion devices may have on the delivery of short-acting drugs.[1,2]

In the first study reported, Floyd[1] used a pharmacokinetic model to develop computer simulations of serum concentrations for various agents with short half-lives infused with a piston-valve infusion pump. The objective of the study was to determine if the brief period of no flow associated with the fill stroke of piston-valve infusion pumps could affect serum drug concentrations in a clinically important way. The author concluded that decrements in serum concentration associated with the fill stroke do occur, but in adults they "are unlikely to be clinically important when drug half-life exceeds two minutes." However, two drugs were noted to have half-lives shorter than two minutes: nitroglycerin (1.7 minutes) and nitroprusside (0.4 minutes). The implication based on this pharmacokinetic model is that large swings in the pharmacodynamic effects of these two agents might be attributable to infusion pumps that interrupt flow for short periods during a fill stroke.

The second study by Leff et al.[2] was designed to assess the ability of a novel gravimetric technique

HENRY J. MANN, PHARM.D., is Associate Professor of Pharmacy Practice, College of Pharmacy, University of Minnesota, and Critical Care Pharmacist, University of Minnesota Hospital and Clinic (UMHC), Minneapolis. DAVID W. FUHS, PHARM.D., M.S., is Clinical Research Supervisor, Department of Pharmacy Services, United Hospital, St. Paul, MN; at the time of this study, he was Clinical Pharmacy Fellow in Critical Care at UMHC. FRANK B. CERRA, M.D., is Professor of Surgery, University of Minnesota, and Director, Surgical Critical Care, Nutrition, and Metabolism, UMHC.

Address reprint requests to Dr. Mann at the College of Pharmacy, University of Minnesota, HSUF-7-109, 308 Harvard Street, S.E., Minneapolis, MN 55455.

This research was supported by a grant from IMED Corporation.

Presented at the Clinical Research Forum, 22nd Annual ASHP Midyear Clinical Meeting, Atlanta, GA, December 9, 1987.

Copyright © 1988, American Society of Hospital Pharmacists, Inc. All rights reserved. 0278-2677/88/0301-0214$01.50.

to determine the flow properties of a peristaltic infusion pump and a piston-valve infusion pump. This in vitro technique demonstrated differences in the effusion profiles for the two devices tested. Although there was not a significant difference in the actual delivery of fluid during 10-second intervals of effusion, the fill stroke had a clearly visible effect on flow continuity with the piston-valve infusion device. During this period, the actual effused weight decreased to approximately 25% of the desired effusion rate. The authors believed that the technique might simulate effects on clinical response to an infused drug that are attributable to pump-operating mechanisms. It was further postulated that the lack of adverse effects reported from flow-rate alterations are "likely the result of a failure to recognize the occurrence of variations in flow continuity; as a result, adverse effects are attributed to other factors." The authors called for further studies to identify the degree of flow continuity that is clinically acceptable for infusion devices.

To date, there are no published clinical studies that have evaluated the effect of flow continuity on the pharmacodynamic effect of short-acting drugs. This prospective study was designed to evaluate the influence of the piston-cassette pump fill stroke on the pharmacodynamic response to sodium nitroprusside in adult patients in a surgical intensive-care unit (SICU).

Methods

This study was conducted in accord with the ethical standards of the institution's committee on the use of human subjects in research. Ten adult surgery patients admitted to the SICU and requiring sodium nitroprusside to control postoperative hypertension were prospectively enrolled in the study. The decision to administer sodium nitroprusside and the guidelines for blood pressure control were made by the physicians caring for the patient. To be included in the study, patients had to receive sodium nitroprusside for at least two hours before the initiation of the study and have adequate blood pressure control as determined by the investigators. All patients had a functioning arterial blood pressure line connected to a bedside monitor for continuous assessment of arterial blood pressure.

The experimental setup consisted of a specially adapted piston-cassette infusion pump (IMED model 980, IMED Corporation, San Diego, CA 92131). The pump was connected to one channel of a two-channel FM tape recorder (Bruel and Kjaer model 7006, Bruel and Kjaer, Marlborough, MA 01752). The other channel of the tape recorder was connected to the output signal of the patient's bedside arterial blood pressure monitor. The pump was adapted to give an electrical impulse to the tape recorder at the same time and for the same duration as the 5.5-second fill stroke of the pump. In all other respects, the pump was a standard production version. Thus, an analog record of the patient's arterial blood pressure measurements was simultaneously recorded along with the analog signal indicating the precise times and duration of the pump fill stroke.

Demographic characteristics of the patient population and details of the sodium nitroprusside flow rates and concentrations were recorded throughout the data-collection period. Patients were switched from the hospital's standard infusion pump to the experimental setup at identical flow rates. After a five-minute stabilization period, data from the blood pressure monitor were recorded on the FM tape recorder for a total of three complete fill cycles in each patient. The occurrence of cassette fill strokes was simultaneously recorded on the other channel. Since each cassette holds approximately 3.5 mL of fluid, a minimum of 10.5 mL of sodium nitroprusside solution was administered by the experimental setup over the time course of three complete fill cycles. The time course for data collection thus varied with the infusion rate and ranged from 30 minutes to 2.5 hours. At the completion of data collection, the patient was switched back to the hospital's standard infusion device.

The analog blood pressure and fill-stroke data were plotted for each patient on a two-channel strip chart recorder. The maximum pressure during the two-minute period immediately preceding a fill stroke (Pmax baseline) and the two-minute period immediately after each fill stroke (Pmax postfill) were determined (Figure 1). Systolic blood pressure (SBP) and diastolic blood pressure (DBP) determinations were made graphically from the strip chart recording. Mean blood pressure (MBP) was calculated as $MBP = [(2 \times DBP) + SBP] \times 0.33$. For each time period, the maximum SBP and its corresponding DBP were identified and the MBP calculated. The initial pressure (P initial) at the start of the cassette fill stroke was also recorded.

The maximum SBP, DBP, and MBP for Pmax baseline, Pmax postfill, and P initial were compared by two-way analysis of variance (ANOVA). If a difference at an a priori level of significance of $p < 0.05$ was found by two-way ANOVA, multiple two-tailed Student's t tests for paired data were then performed to isolate the difference. Correlations between pressures and flow rates were made using a simple linear-regression model.

Results

A total of 30 complete fill cycles were recorded in 10 patients (5 men, 5 women). Because of technical problems with the recorder, all three fill cycles for patient number one were excluded from the analysis. One fill cycle in patient number seven was excluded from the analysis because of a gain change in the strip chart recorder occurring within the baseline two-minute period; therefore, all data analysis is based on 26 fill cycles. Demographic data for the patients and details of the SNP administration for each cycle are shown in Table 1. The median pump flow rate was 15 mL/hr (range, 5 to 30), and both the median and mean doses of SNP were 2.6 μg/kg/min (range, 0.69 to 5.13).

The SBP, DBP, and MBP at the initiation of the fill stroke and the maximum SBP, DBP, and MBP values during the two-minute baseline period and

Figure 1. Diagram of the experimental setup, illustrating the relationships between fill cycles A and B (C is not shown), the experimental periods (baseline, fill stroke, and postfill), and the pressure tracing from which the maximum pressure obtained in the two-minute period preceding a fill stroke (Pmax baseline), the pressure when the fill stroke was initiated (P initial), and the maximum pressure obtained in the two-minute period after a fill stroke (Pmax postfill) were derived.

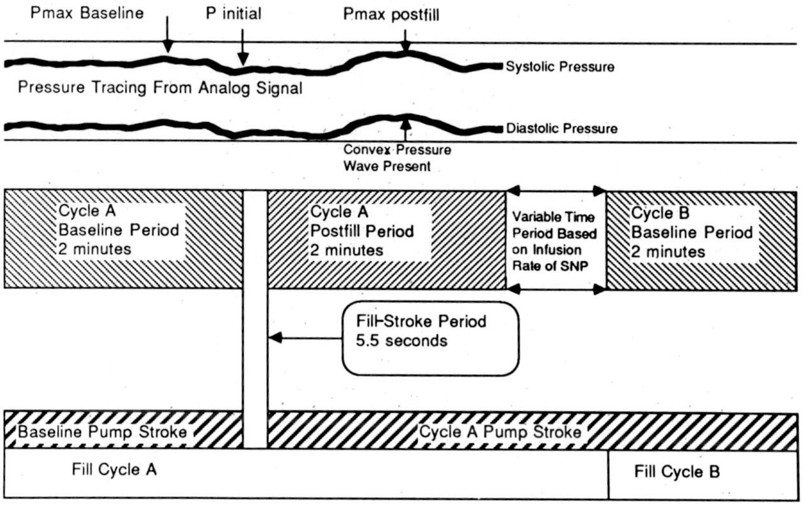

Table 1.
Demographic and Infusion Data for SICU Patients Treated with Sodium Nitroprusside (SNP)[a]

Patient Cycle	Sex	Age (yr)	Weight (kg)	SNP Concentration (μg/mL)	Flow Rate (mL/hr)	Flow Rate (μg/kg/min)
2a	F	53	91.4	800	15	2.19
2b				800	10	1.46
2c				800	5	0.73
3a	F	65	61.2	800	10	2.18
3b				800	10	2.18
3c				800	10	2.18
4a	M	35	74.8	400	15	1.34
4b				400	15	1.34
4c				400	15	1.34
5a	M	73	70	800	30	5.13
5b				800	30	5.13
5c				800	30	5.13
6a	M	50	78	800	18	3.12
6b				800	18	3.12
6c				800	18	3.12
7b	M	71	77	800	15	2.6
7c				800	15	2.6
8a	M	60	96.5	800	5	0.69
8b				800	10	1.38
8c				800	10	1.38
9a	F	44	67.1	800	15	2.98
9b				800	15	2.98
9c				800	15	2.98
10a	F	55	60	400	11	3.64
10b				400	10	3.31
10c				400	10	3.31

[a] SICU = surgical intensive-care unit.

the two-minute post-fill-stroke period for each patient are shown in Table 2. The maximum SBP, DBP, and MBP during the baseline and post-fill-stroke periods were significantly different. The mean (± S.D.) change from Pmax baseline to Pmax postfill was 3.9 ± 5.8 mm Hg for SBP, 3.5 ± 5.7 mm Hg for DBP, and 3.6 ± 5.6 mm Hg for MBP. The change from Pmax baseline to Pmax postfill ranged from a decrease of 8 mm Hg to an increase of 16 mm Hg for SBP, a decrease of 7 mm Hg to an increase of 13 mm Hg for DBP, and a decrease of 7 mm Hg to an increase of 14 mm Hg for MBP. The change from Pmax baseline to Pmax postfill for DBP was strongly correlated with the same change in SBP in both direction and magnitude ($r = 0.90$).

In 16 of 26 (62%) cycles there was a recognizable convex wave in the pressure tracing after a fill stroke (Table 1 and Figure 1). In 8 of 26 (31%) cycles, the Pmax postfill SBP and DBP exceeded the Pmax baseline SBP and DBP by 5 mm Hg or more, and in each case a visible convex wave in the pressure tracing was present. Four patients consistently demonstrated a convex wave in the pressure tracing, three were inconsistent, and two failed to demonstrate a convex wave in the pressure tracing.

The likelihood of a pharmacodynamic change appears to be inconsistent both between and within patients. The Pmax postfill increased by more than 5 mm Hg over the Pmax baseline for SBP in 8 of 26 (31%) cycles, for DBP in 10 of 26 (38%) cycles, and for MBP in 9 of 26 (35%) cycles. In four of the nine patients, the Pmax postfill did not increase by more than 5 mm Hg over Pmax baseline during all 12 fill cycles for SBP, DBP, or MBP. In one of these patients, the Pmax postfill was actually less than the Pmax baseline by more than 5 mm Hg for SBP, DBP, and MBP during one fill cycle. Within patients, the difference between cycles for the variability between time periods (Pmax postfill − Pmax baseline) ranged from a minimum of 2 mm

Table 2.
Individual Pharmacodynamic Responses of SICU Patients to 26 Fill-Stroke Cycles of a Piston-Cassette Infusion Pump[a]

Patient Cycle	P initial[b] (mm Hg)			Pmax Baseline[c] (mm Hg)			Pmax Postfill[d] (mm Hg)			Convex Wave Present[e]
	SBP[f]	DBP[g]	MBP[h]	SBP	DBP	MBP	SBP	DBP	MBP	
2a	123	65	84	135	65	88	146	75	99	Yes
2b	104	62	77	121	75	90	124	73	90	Yes
2c	140	65	90	151	67	95	164	78	106	Yes
3a	115	55	75	120	55	77	136	68	91	Yes
3b	123	59	80	140	67	92	144	69	94	Yes
3c	136	67	90	146	70	95	148	75	99	Yes
4a	106	56	73	105	60	75	105	58	74	No
4b	105	55	72	115	57	76	107	50	69	No
4c	106	59	75	112	59	77	113	58	76	No
5a	105	60	75	140	65	90	146	71	96	Yes
5b	105	60	75	140	63	89	144	71	95	Yes
5c	102	58	73	133	59	84	144	71	95	Yes
6a	101	55	70	109	55	73	125	68	87	Yes
6b	103	57	72	121	66	84	121	61	81	Yes
6c	84	50	61	97	51	66	101	59	73	Yes
7b	109	55	73	113	56	74	117	60	79	Yes
7c	118	56	77	135	64	87	131	62	85	No
8a	123	70	88	126	75	92	128	73	91	No
8b	119	64	82	127	64	85	136	75	95	Yes
8c	139	76	97	149	84	106	155	87	110	Yes
9a	103	67	79	108	67	81	106	69	81	No
9b	103	69	80	102	69	80	105	71	82	No
9c	100	68	79	106	75	85	106	75	85	No
10a	104	54	71	102	46	66	104	48	67	Yes
10b	126	65	85	126	65	85	126	65	85	No
10c	120	64	83	126	70	89	126	70	89	No
Mean ± S.D.	112 ± 13	61 ± 6	78 ± 8	123[g] ± 16	64[g] ± 8	84[g] ± 9	127[i,j] ± 18	68[i,j] ± 9	88[i,j] ± 11	

[a] SICU = surgical intensive-care unit.
[b] P initial = pressure when the fill stroke was initiated.
[c] Pmax baseline = maximum pressure obtained in the two-minute period preceding a fill stroke.
[d] Pmax postfill = maximum pressure obtained in the two-minute period after a fill stroke.
[e] A visible convex wave is present in the pressure tracing after a fill stroke.
[f] SBP = systolic blood pressure.
[g] DBP = diastolic blood pressure.
[h] MBP = mean blood pressure.
[i] Significantly different ($p < 0.05$) from P initial.
[j] Significantly different ($p < 0.05$) from Pmax baseline.

Hg to a maximum of 16 mm Hg for SBP, 2 mm Hg to 17 mm Hg for DBP, and 1 mm Hg to 17 mm Hg for MBP. Thus, the hemodynamic changes between sample periods approximated or exceeded the changes within sample periods in many instances.

A greater appreciation for the variability in pressure changes is obtained when the Pmax baseline and the Pmax postfill are examined relative to the pressure obtained at the start of the fill stroke (P initial). Systolic, diastolic, and mean blood pressures for both Pmax baseline and Pmax postfill were significantly greater than the corresponding P initial value. The mean (± S.D.) pressure change after a fill stroke (Pmax postfill − P initial) was 15 ± 12 mm Hg for SBP, 7 ± 6 mm Hg for DBP, and 9 ± 7 mm Hg for MBP. The corresponding pressure changes within a baseline sample period (Pmax baseline − P initial) were 11 ± 10 mm Hg for SBP, 3 ± 4 mm Hg for DBP, and 6 ± 5 mm Hg for MBP.

There was a strong correlation in variability of pressure changes within patients between the post-fill-stroke period and the baseline period, represented as Pmax postfill − P initial versus Pmax baseline − P initial, for SBP (r = 0.89) and a relatively weaker correlation for DBP (r = 0.35) and MBP (r = 0.66) using simple linear regression. The variability within the baseline period, represented as Pmax baseline − P initial, in SBP was significantly greater than the variability between the time periods, represented as Pmax baseline − Pmax postfill, while the differences for DBP and MBP were not significant.

The mean (± S.D.) time from P initial to Pmax postfill was 47 ± 14 seconds (range, 27 to 81 seconds). During all cycles in which an obvious convex wave in the pressure tracing occurred after a fill stroke, the pressure tracing returned to baseline within three minutes. Simple linear regression showed a very weak correlation between time to Pmax postfill and flow rate of sodium nitroprusside in milliliters per hour (r = 0.31) and in micrograms per kilogram per minute (r = 0.24). Flow rate of sodium nitroprusside in milliliters per hour and in micrograms per kilogram per minute failed to correlate with the change in the time period represented as Pmax postfill − Pmax baseline for SBP (r = 0.07), DBP (r = 0.25), and MBP (r = 0.19).

Discussion

The results of this study support the implication that interruptions in flow caused by a fill stroke in infusion pumps may have an effect on the pharmacodynamic response to a very short acting drug such as nitroprusside. The increase in mean blood pressure during the post-fill-stroke period was significant as compared with the baseline period. This effect was not consistent between or within patients, however, and appeared to have little clinical importance in the model tested. To be clinically important, in our opinion, the blood pressure effect should be consistent within patients and exceed normal variation to a degree that would necessitate a change in therapy. In this study, the pharmacodynamic alteration that could be associated with the lack of flow continuity was not consistent either between or within patients. In addition, the degree of variability in pressure observed during the baseline period was greater than the degree of change in maximum SBP between the baseline and the post-fill-stroke period. There was no difference in variability within and between the two time periods for DBP and MBP. A change in therapy because of fluctuations in pressure surrounding a fill stroke was not required during the study, which is consistent with clinical practice, wherein piston-cassette pumps are in widespread use without noticeable problems in regulation of drug infusions. Two patients in this study did have dosage adjustments of sodium nitroprusside to maintain blood pressure guidelines established by their physicians; however, this was not related to the fill stroke of the infusion device.

The results do not support the ability of an in vitro effusion profile to simulate the effects on clinical response of an infused drug that are attributable to pump-operating mechanisms. The pump used in this study would generate an effusion profile very similar to that described for the IMED model 960 in the study by Leff et al.[2] The use of sodium nitroprusside, which has a direct pharmacologic effect and an extremely short half-life, as the infused agent in combination with continuous analog monitoring of arterial pressure represents one of the most likely situations in which an effect of the pump mechanism on a pharmacodynamic response would be detected. As the half-life of the infused agent gets longer in relation to the time for the fill stroke in which flow continuity is stopped, the expected change in serum concentration from steady state decreases. Similarly, the less directly related the serum concentration is to the mechanism of response, the less likely a short interruption in flow continuity is to result in a detectable change in the measured response. Therefore, it would seem very unlikely that the results obtained with other agents commonly infused in the critical-care unit, such as dopamine or dobutamine, would demonstrate a consistent pharmacodynamic response to a fill stroke when sodium nitroprusside did not. It further seems likely that the reported lack of adverse effects from flow-rate alterations is a result of these alterations having little clinical importance, rather than a lack of recognition of variations in flow continuity, as suggested by Leff et al.[2]

Conclusion

In adult surgical intensive-care patients receiving sodium nitroprusside for blood pressure control, there is a small, detectable pharmacodynamic effect that may be associated with the fill stroke of a piston-cassette pump. The pharmacodynamic effect is inconsistent both between and within patients and is not greater than the variation in blood pressure observed during a baseline period preceding the fill stroke. It is unlikely that a more pronounced effect would be demonstrated with other commonly used agents in a surgical intensive-care unit. If agents with shorter half lives and direct pharmacodynamic effects become available, or if infusion devices with longer flow interruptions relative to the half-life of the infused agent are used, the likelihood of observing an effect from the flow interruption will increase. Further clinical studies with well-defined pharmacodynamic endpoints will be required to verify our conclusions. Data from other infusion devices, drugs, and patient populations may provide different results, since our conclusions are based on assumptions that may vary for both the pharmacokinetic and pharmacodynamic models, including the use of a one-compartment model and a direct pharmacologic effect of the drug.

References

1. Floyd RA. Effect of infusion pump fill-stroke flow interruptions on simulated serum concentrations of short half-life drugs. *Am J Hosp Pharm*. 1984; 41:2399–400.
2. Leff RD, True WR, Roberts RJ. A gravimetric technique for evaluating flow continuity from two infusion devices. *Am J Hosp Pharm*. 1987; 44:1388–91.

Efficacy of individualized phenytoin sodium loading doses administered by intravenous infusion

FRANCINE G. DELA CRUZ, MICHELE Z. KANTER, JAMES H. FISCHER, JERROLD B. LEIKIN

Abstract: The safety and efficacy of administering individualized phenytoin sodium loading doses by intravenous infusion were studied on 40 occasions in 37 adult patients having seizures.

Doses were calculated based on an average volume of distribution (0.75 L/kg) and desired plasma phenytoin concentration. Total and free phenytoin concentrations were determined before and after the infusion. Phenytoin sodium doses of 225–1300 mg were administered by intravenous infusion at a rate of 40 mg/min after dilution in 0.9% sodium chloride injection to concentrations ranging from 4.5 to 13.5 mg/mL. Infusion rates were reduced if adverse effects occurred.

The dosing method accurately achieved desired phenytoin concentrations (predicted mean ± S.D. concentration, 18.3 ± 1.6 μg/mL; observed mean concentration, 17.4 ± 2.5 μg/mL). Postinfusion concentrations of free phenytoin ranged from 0.8 to 3.6 μg/mL (mean ± S.D., 1.7 ± 0.6 μg/mL). Of 21 patients evaluated for efficacy, 16 responded. A total of 45% of patients experienced pain at the infusion site, which diminished when the infusion rate was reduced. No serious cardiovascular or neurological toxicities occurred.

The intravenous infusion method of administration is safe and effective and is useful for rapid achievement of therapeutic phenytoin concentrations in the emergency room setting.

Index terms: Additives; Anticonvulsants; Blood levels; Dosage; Drug administration; Phenytoin; Phenytoin sodium; Seizures; Sodium chloride; Toxicity
Clin Pharm. 1988; 7:219–24

Efforts to develop guidelines for the safe and effective administration of large intravenous loading doses of phenytoin have been hindered by differences in patient characteristics, administration methods, and dosages among published studies. Intravenous loading doses of phenytoin have been administered by two different methods: direct manual i.v. injection and i.v. infusion of dilute phenytoin solutions. In early studies, phenytoin sodium loading doses were administered by manual i.v. injection to patients with status epilepticus or acute repetitive seizures at rates of 50–100 mg/

FRANCINE G. DELA CRUZ, PHARM.D., is Clinical Assistant Professor, Department of Pharmacy Practice, College of Pharmacy, University of Illinois at Chicago (UIC); at the time of this study she was a clinical pharmacy resident in emergency medicine/critical care. MICHELE Z. KANTER, PHARM.D., is Clinical Assistant Professor, Department of Pharmacy Practice, and JAMES H. FISCHER, PHARM.D., is Associate Professor, Department of Pharmacy Practice, and Assistant Director, Clinical Pharmacokinetics Laboratory, College of Pharmacy, UIC. JERROLD B. LEIKIN, M.D., is Physician-in-Charge, Emergency Services Department, University of Illinois Hospital, and Assistant Professor in Medicine, Department of Medicine, College of Medicine, UIC.

Address reprint requests to Dr. Dela Cruz at the Department of Pharmacy Practice, College of Pharmacy, University of Illinois at Chicago, 833 S. Wood St., Room 244, Chicago, IL 60612.

Presented at the 21st Annual ASHP Midyear Clinical Meeting, Las Vegas, NV, December 10, 1986.

Copyright © 1988, American Society of Hospital Pharmacists, Inc. All rights reserved. 0278-2677/88/0301-0219$01.50.

min.[1-4] These rapid rates of administration were associated with relatively high incidences of phlebitis and cardiovascular toxicity, most likely caused by too rapid administration of propylene glycol, the diluent in phenytoin injection solutions.[1,3,5] Manual i.v. administration poses additional difficulties, including variable administration rates that may result in small bolus doses of highly concentrated phenytoin solution being delivered to the patient. Manual administration also represents inefficient use of physician or nursing staff time for drug administration.

Studies have demonstrated that an acceptable margin of safety and convenience can be achieved when dilute phenytoin sodium solutions are administered by i.v. infusion at rates of 40 mg/min or less.[6-8] In these studies, phenytoin sodium dosages were determined by two different methods: administration of a fixed number of milligrams (500–1500 mg), or a dosage predicated on body weight (15–18 mg/kg).[4,6,8] The use of large fixed dosages may cause plasma concentrations greater than 20 μg/mL, which may be higher than necessary to control non-life-threatening seizure exacerbations and may increase the potential for adverse reactions. The use of these set doses is complicated by the fact that some patients have substantial preinfusion serum phenytoin concentrations. Curtis et al.[9] found that 13.7% of patients with acute seizures had phenytoin concentrations exceeding 15 μg/mL. Administration of set doses may cause plasma concentrations to exceed the desired therapeutic range, potentially inducing toxicity.

Individualizing phenytoin loading doses to achieve desired plasma concentrations has been made possible by the availability of assays that rapidly measure baseline plasma phenytoin concentrations.[9] The ability to accurately and rapidly attain therapeutic plasma concentrations with individualized phenytoin doses minimizes the potential for toxicity from i.v. administration. Decreasing the risk of toxicity may also reduce the need for hospital admission or extended patient observation. Therapeutic concentrations could be achieved rapidly in noncompliant patients or postictal patients with subtherapeutic concentrations, facilitating their timely discharge from outpatient acute-treatment settings.

The purpose of this study was to determine the safety and efficacy of administering loading doses of phenytoin by intravenous infusion to achieve desired phenytoin concentrations in patients treated for seizures in an emergency room.

Methods

Patients 16 years of age or older who were seen in the emergency room and whose physicians ordered an intravenous loading dose of phenytoin for management of seizures were eligible to enter the study. Evaluation of patients included a history, physical examination, clinically indicated laboratory studies (including determining serum concentrations of electrolytes, calcium, magnesium, phosphorus, and antiepileptic drugs, as well as a complete blood count with differential), and an electrocardiogram. Patients were excluded if any of the following were noted: a total plasma phenytoin concentration of 15 μg/mL or greater before the infusion, hypotension (systolic blood pressure less than 80 mm Hg), atrial or ventricular cardiac dysrhythmia, severe conduction disturbances such as second- or third-degree heart block, bradycardia (heart rate less than 50 beats per minute), severe congestive heart failure, absence or minor motor seizures, or history of hydantoin hypersensitivity. The protocol for this study was approved by the institutional review board.

Patients were entered into the study during a 12-month period. The phenytoin dose required for each patient was calculated by one of three clinical pharmacists present in the emergency room using the following equation:

$$\text{Loading dose} = V \times \text{TBW} \times (C_{\text{desired}} - C_{\text{observed}})/0.92$$

where V is the mean apparent volume of distribution of phenytoin, 0.75 L/kg,[3] TBW is total body weight in kilograms, C_{desired} is the desired plasma phenytoin concentration, C_{observed} is the observed preinfusion plasma phenytoin concentration, and 0.92 is the fraction of phenytoin sodium present as phenytoin. The volume of distribution was calculated in each patient by rearranging the equation in terms of V, in which case C_{desired} became the observed postinfusion serum phenytoin concentration.

Admixtures of phenytoin for i.v. administration were prepared by pharmacy personnel in the emergency room by diluting phenytoin injection (Parenteral Dilantin, Parke-Davis, Morris Plains, NJ 07950) with 0.9% sodium chloride injection (Travenol Laboratories Inc., Deerfield, IL 60015). The total volume of the admixture depended on the dose. Doses of 799 mg or less were prepared in 50 mL of 0.9% sodium chloride injection; doses of 800–1199 mg were prepared in 100 mL; and doses of 1200–1999 mg were prepared in 150 mL. The admixtures were administered by volumetric infusion pump (IMED Corporation, Model 927, San Diego, CA 92131) at a rate of 40 mg/min. An inline filter was not used. The infusion rate was reduced in increments of 25% if patients developed intolerable pain at the i.v. site, hypotension, bradycardia, cardiac dysrhythmias, or conduction abnormalities. The primary i.v. fluid (0.9% sodium chloride injection) was administered at a constant rate of approximately 126 mL/hr (21 drops/min) during the phenytoin infusion.

Patients were monitored for adverse effects including hypotension (defined as a symptomatic decrease in blood pressure by more than 20%), irregular pulse, bradycardia, phlebitis, pain at the i.v. site, dizziness, nausea, vomiting, headache, lethargy, respiratory depression, and ataxia. An electrocardiogram was ordered if an irregular pulse or severe hypotension was noted. Vital signs were monitored before the infusion and every 5 to 15 minutes during the infusion until the infusion was complete.

The clinical pharmacist in the emergency room analyzed the plasma phenytoin concentrations before the infusion and 30 to 60 minutes after the infusion using an enzyme-mediated immunoassay technique (EMIT QST phenytoin assay, Syva Co., Palo Alto, CA). The intraday and interday precision values, as represented by the coefficient of variation for replicate samples, were 3.5% and 6%, respectively, over the concentration range of 2.5 to 40 μg/mL. Preinfusion and postinfusion concentrations of free phenytoin were measured using the EMIT FreeLevel System at 25 °C (Syva Co., Palo Alto, CA). The intraday and interday coefficients of variation for replicate samples were 4.2 and 7.5%, respectively.

Seizure frequency was classified according to the following categories:

1. Status epilepticus: seizure activity (generalized, complex partial, or simple partial) continued for 30 minutes or longer, or repetitive seizures occurred without the patient regaining consciousness between events;
2. Recurrent seizures: three or more seizures occurred in a 24-hour period;
3. Isolated seizures: one or more seizures occurred in a 24-hour period.

Seizure type was determined from the patient's clinical history or by observation in conjunction with the patient's electroencephalogram (EEG) and classified using the International Classification of Epileptic Seizures.[10]

Response to treatment was classified as successful if no further seizures occurred for 24 hours after the infusion. If seizures were reduced in frequency, extent, or severity, the treatment was considered partially successful. If there was no improvement or if seizure activity recurred within 24 hours, treatment was considered unsuccessful. Diazepam, additional phenytoin, or phenobarbital was administered as needed to control additional seizures.

The ability of this method of determining a loading dose to predict postinfusion serum phenytoin concentrations was assessed from the mean prediction error (bias) and root mean squared prediction error (precision), which were calculated by comparing observed and predicted postinfusion serum phenytoin concentrations.[11] Differences between observed and predicted phenytoin concentrations were also compared using a paired Student's *t* test.

Differences in serum concentrations of total or free phenytoin for patients in the successful and unsuccessful treatment groups were assessed by Student's *t* test for independent samples. Fisher's Exact Test was used to evaluate the relationship between a patient's age and the occurrence of pain at the infusion site. The a priori level of significance was set at $p < 0.05$.

Results

A total of 40 i.v. infusions of phenytoin were administered to 25 men and 12 women. The patients ranged in age from 17 to 72 years (mean, 33 years). The patients' total body weights ranged from 38.6 to 99.5 kg. Sixteen patients were taking concomitant antiepileptic drugs. Preinfusion serum concentrations of total and free phenytoin ranged from 0 to 13.9 μg/mL (mean ± S.D., 3.1 ± 4.2 μg/mL) and from 0 to 1.0 μg/mL (mean ± S.D., 0.3 ± 0.3 μg/mL), respectively. Characteristics of the patients' seizures are shown in Table 1. Of the three patients with status epilepticus, one patient's seizure was classified as generalized, one was classified as complex partial, and one was classified as simple partial (epilepsia partialis continua). Of the 37 patients, 82% had experienced at least one seizure less than 10 hours before the phenytoin infusion. Four patients with alcohol-related seizures were later found to have epileptogenic foci on their EEGs. Fifty-six percent of the patients on long-term phenytoin therapy had nondetectable concentrations.

The use of the above equation resulted in the administration of loading doses of phenytoin sodi-

Table 1.
History, Type, Frequency, and Etiology of Seizures

Seizure Characteristic	No. of Patients[a] (*n* = 40)
History	
New onset	10
Chronic epilepsy	29
Unknown	1
Type	
Generalized tonic–clonic	15
Complex partial with generalization	23
Complex partial without generalization	1
Simple partial with generalization	1
Frequency	
Status epilepticus	3
Recurrent	5
Isolated	32
Etiology	
Subtherapeutic plasma concentration	21
Anticonvulsant withdrawal	2
Brain tumor or metastasis	3
Alcohol or sedative withdrawal	7
Cerebrovascular accident	2
Undetermined	5

[a] One of the 37 patients had two episodes of seizures during the study period, and one patient had three episodes.

um of 225–1300 mg, which were administered at a mean rate of 30 mg/min (range, 5.6–40 mg/min). These doses were calculated to achieve plasma concentrations of 15–23 μg/mL (mean 18.3 ± 1.6 μg/mL); the actual postinfusion plasma concentrations that resulted from these doses ranged from 12.2 to 22.4 μg/mL (mean, 17.4 ± 2.5 μg/mL) (Table 2). The dosing method was successful in achieving desired plasma phenytoin concentrations, as demonstrated by the mean prediction error (bias) of 0.9 μg/mL (95% confidence interval, 0.1–1.7 μg/mL) and root mean squared prediction error (precision) of 2.6 (95% confidence interval, 2.1–3.1). Predicted and observed postinfusion plasma concentrations were not significantly different. The small number of patients whose total body weight was more than 40% greater than their ideal body weight (i.e., the ratio of total body weight to ideal body weight was greater than 1.4) did not allow us to evaluate the accuracy of the dosing method in obese patients. The mean apparent volume of distribution for phenytoin in the patients was 0.83 ± 0.20 L/kg; this supports the use of the literature value of 0.75 L/kg in the calculation of the loading doses.

Postinfusion serum concentrations of free phenytoin varied from 0.8 to 3.6 μg/mL (mean 1.7 ± 0.6 μg/mL), and the mean free fraction was 9.8 ± 3.8%. There was a significant correlation between free fraction and serum albumin concentration ($r = -0.45$). Thirteen samples were noted to have phenytoin free fractions greater than 10%. Two of these samples were obtained from a pregnant patient who received two infusions at 19 weeks' gestation (free fractions on the separate occasions were 14.7% and 23%). Her serum albumin concentration was normal. An elevated free fraction (13.4%) in a patient with chronic alcoholism could be explained by hypoalbuminemia (2.4 mg/dL; normal range, 3.8–5.1 mg/dL). There was no obvious cause for elevated free fractions in the remainder of the cases, including concomitant drugs.

Data concerning the efficacy of the phenytoin loading dose during the 24 hours after the infusion was available in 21 cases. Treatment was successful in 16 (76%) of these cases. One infusion was partially successful, and four were unsuccessful. Of the five instances of partially successful and unsuccessful treatment, four seizures were of the complex partial type with secondary generalization, and one was generalized tonic–clonic. There were no significant differences between the successful and unsuccessful treatment groups for postinfusion mean concentrations of total phenytoin (17.1 ± 2.7 μg/mL and 16.4 ± 3.0 μg/mL, respectively) or postinfusion mean concentrations of free phenytoin (1.8 ± 0.8 μg/mL and 1.9 ± 0.6 μg/mL, respectively). One patient with a total phenytoin concentration greater than 20 μg/mL continued to have complex partial secondarily generalized seizures after the loading dose. Three failures occurred with peak concentrations of free phenytoin greater than 2.0 μg/mL.

No clinically important changes were observed in heart rate or systolic or diastolic blood pressure. The mean maximum change in systolic blood pressure was −5.2% from baseline; the mean maximum change in diastolic blood pressure was −1.8%; and the mean maximum change in heart rate was 0.8%. The maximum change in blood pressure and heart rate occurred at variable times during the infusion.

The most common complication was pain at the i.v. site. Forty-five percent of the patients experienced intolerable pain, necessitating a reduction in

Table 2.
Serum Phenytoin Concentrations Desired and Achieved after Administration of Individualized Loading Doses

Patient No.	Total:Ideal Body Weight Ratio	Serum Phenytoin Concentration (μg/mL) Desired	Observed	% Error[a]
1	1.77	20	20.7	(3.5)[b]
2	1.01	18	17.9	0.6
3	1.03	16	16.2	(1.2)
4[c]	1.34	18	14.2	21.1
5	0.96	15	15.6	(4.0)
6	0.92	18	19.2	(6.7)
7	1.35	18	12.2	32.2
8	1.06	20	16.0	20.0
9	1.16	16	16.2	(1.2)
10	0.92	20	17.8	11.0
11[c]	1.02	19	21.2	(11.6)
12	1.00	18	19.8	(10.0)
13	1.02	18	22.2	(23.3)
14	0.97	18	14.6	18.9
15[d]	1.22	18	14.1	21.7
16[d]	1.22	20	15.5	22.5
17	0.96	17	14.2	16.5
18	0.84	18	14.6	18.9
19	0.83	20	15.0	25.0
20	1.40	15	13.7	8.7
21	1.00	18	17.4	3.3
22	1.05	18	15.6	13.3
23	1.05	19	18.0	5.3
24	1.33	18	18.9	(5.0)
25	1.24	20	21.0	(5.0)
26	1.21	19	16.3	14.2
27	0.82	19	16.4	13.7
28	1.50	17	18.7	(10.0)
29	1.13	19	19.3	(1.6)
30	1.75	17	18.8	(10.6)
31	1.56	18	17.6	2.2
32	1.00	23	17.8	22.6
33[d]	1.24	20	22.4	(12.0)
34	1.15	20	18.2	9.0
35	1.10	18	16.3	9.4
36	1.01	15	16.9	(12.7)
37	1.09	18	16.1	10.6
38	1.65	18	21.4	(18.9)
39	0.93	18	20.7	(15.0)
40	0.84	20	17.9	10.5

[a] Calculated as product of ($C_{desired} - C_{observed}/C_{desired}$) (100).
[b] Parentheses denote negative variance.
[c] Same patient had two separate visits.
[d] Same patient had three separate visits.

the infusion rate. Thirty-five percent of the patients experienced little or no pain, and 20% of the patients could not be evaluated for pain because of postictal central nervous system depression. Examination of data revealed that patients older than 50 years of age tended to better tolerate pain during infusion than did younger patients, but this relationship was not significant. The concentrations of phenytoin in the admixtures were similar for patients with and without pain (range, 4.5–13.2 mg/mL and 8.0–13.5 mg/mL, respectively).

Neurological adverse effects, consisting of dizziness, headache, tinnitus, mild drowsiness, and difficulty in walking, were observed in only three patients and resolved shortly after the infusion.

Discussion

To our knowledge this is the first study that implemented an individualized dosing method for calculating intravenous loading doses of phenytoin. This method takes into account the patient's preinfusion phenytoin concentration and estimated volume of distribution. Set milligram doses of phenytoin have been shown to yield highly variable plasma concentrations.[1-3,7] Cranford et al.[3] found that uniform doses of 1000 mg of phenytoin produced two-hour postinfusion concentrations varying from 10.0 to 35.2 μg/mL in patients with preinfusion concentrations less than 1 μg/mL. Wallis et al.[1] noted values of 11–33 μg/mL 15 minutes after administration of phenytoin sodium 1000 mg by i.v. push, followed by 500 mg administered intramuscularly.[1]

Doses based on body weight result in a narrower and more predictable range of plasma phenytoin concentrations. However, this dosing method may result in supratherapeutic values in patients with detectable preinfusion phenytoin concentrations. Carducci et al.[8] administered phenytoin sodium 18 mg/kg to 38 seizure patients with preinfusion plasma concentrations less than 6 μg/mL.[8] Four patients had preinfusion concentrations ranging from 2.5 to 5.5 μg/mL. Fifty-one percent of the patients had four-hour postinfusion concentrations greater than 20 μg/mL, which may potentially induce acute adverse effects, such as nystagmus, ataxia, nausea, and vomiting.[3]

The apparent volume of distribution for phenytoin is relatively constant and can be used to calculate doses for attaining desired phenytoin concentrations.[3] Our results and those of Cranford et al.[3] suggest that the volume of distribution for phenytoin is approximately 0.75–0.8 L/kg total body weight. The availability of assays capable of rapidly determining phenytoin concentrations allows for measurement of preinfusion phenytoin concentrations, and doses can be calculated on a patient-specific basis. Our results show that this prospective dosing method can safely and accurately achieve desired phenytoin concentrations.

Pain at the infusion site was the most common complication noted in this study. In all cases the irritation was relieved by slowing the infusion rate. The relatively high prevalence of pain may be related to crystallization of phenytoin in intravenous fluids. Crystallization in 0.9% sodium chloride injection has been detectable after four to nine hours at concentrations of 1 mg/mL,[12] and shortly after admixture at concentrations of 4.6–18.4 mg/mL.[13] Crystals in filtered dextrose solutions of phenytoin have been previously identified by melting point determination.[14] The clinical importance of these crystals, which range in diameter from 5 to 200 μm, is unknown. Cloyd et al.[13] suggested the use of a 0.22- or 0.45-μm filter with phenytoin admixtures. Prefiltration and postfiltration phenytoin concentrations have been reported to be similar.[12,13] The use of inline filters has not been clinically evaluated. However, the low prevalence of pain (10%) in a previous study using an inline 0.22 μm filter suggests that filters may be beneficial.[8]

Although there were no clinically important changes in blood pressure or heart rate, the maximum change occurred at highly variable times. The unpredictable occurrence of these changes, and the potential for severe hypotension occurring shortly after completion of the infusion, suggests the need for regular monitoring of vital signs during and after the infusion.[3,7]

The development of guidelines for safely and effectively infusing intravenous phenytoin has been difficult. The published literature contains few studies, and these differ in population size, patient characteristics, solution concentrations, infusion rates, methods of infusion control, and dosing methods. Administration of standard doses to patients with subtherapeutic phenytoin concentrations may result in supratherapeutic concentrations and increase the risk of adverse effects. Our dosing technique may help to minimize dose- or concentration-related adverse effects associated with rapid infusion of phenytoin loading doses.

Conclusion

The administration of individualized loading doses of phenytoin by constant intravenous infusion is a reasonable approach to the acute management of seizures. Dosage calculations incorporating preinfusion plasma phenytoin concentration and the apparent volume of distribution of the drug permit the accurate attainment of desired increases in plasma concentrations. We recommend this method when preinfusion measurement of phenytoin concentrations can be accomplished and rapid attainment of a therapeutic plasma concentration is a primary goal of therapy.

References

1. Wallis W, Kutt H, McDowell F. Intravenous diphenylhydantoin in treatment of acute repetitive seizures. *Neurology.* 1968; 18:513–25.
2. Wilder BJ, Ramsay RE, Willmore J et al. Efficacy of intravenous phenytoin in the treatment of status epilepticus: kinetics of central nervous system penetration. *Ann Neurol.* 1977; 1:511–8.
3. Cranford RE, Leppik IE, Patrick B et al. Intravenous phenytoin: clinical and pharmacokinetic aspects. *Neurology.* 1978; 28:874–80.
4. Cranford RE, Leppik IE, Patrick B et al. Intravenous phenytoin in acute treatment of seizures. *Neurology.* 1979; 29:1474–9.
5. Louis S, Kutt H, McDowell F. The cardiocirculatory changes caused by intravenous Dilantin and its solvent. *Am Heart J.* 1967; 74:523–9.
6. Salem RB, Wilder BJ, Yost RL et al. Rapid infusion of phenytoin sodium loading doses. *Am J Hosp Pharm.* 1981; 38:354–7.
7. Earnest MP, Marx JA, Drury LR. Complications of intravenous phenytoin for acute treatment of seizures. *JAMA.* 1983; 249:762–5.
8. Carducci B, Hedges JR, Beal JC et al. Emergency phenytoin loading by constant intravenous infusion. *Ann Emerg Med.* 1984; 13:1027–31.
9. Curtis RA, Hutchinson RA, Bederka J et al. Effect of empiric dosing on blood levels of theophylline and phenytoin. *Ann Emerg. Med.* 1985; 14:213–7.
10. Commission on Classification and Terminology of the International League Against Epilepsy. Proposal for revised clinical and electroencephalographic classification of epileptic seizures. *Epilepsia.* 1981; 2:489–501.
11. Scheiner LB, Beal SL. Some suggestions for measuring predictive performance. *J Pharmacokinet Biopharm.* 1981; 9:503–12.
12. Bauman JL, Siepler JK, Fitzloff J. Phenytoin crystallization in intravenous fluids. *Drug Intell Clin Pharm.* 1977; 11:646–9.
13. Cloyd JC, Bosch DE, Sawchuk RJ. Concentration–time profile of phenytoin after admixture with small volumes of intravenous fluids. *Am J Hosp Pharm.* 1978; 35:45–8.
14. Bauman JL, Siepler JK. Intravenous phenytoin (concluded). *N Engl J Med.* 1977; 296:111. Letter.

Glipizide pharmacokinetics in young and elderly volunteers

KELLY A. KOBAYASHI, LARRY A. BAUER, JOHN R. HORN, KENT OPHEIM, FRANCIS WOOD, JR., AND WAYNE A. KRADJAN

Abstract: The effects of aging on the pharmacokinetics of glipizide were studied.

Ten healthy young men (24.9 ± 1.9 years of age) and 10 healthy older men (74.4 ± 7.9 years of age) each ingested a single 5-mg tablet of glipizide after an overnight fast. Blood samples were obtained immediately before drug ingestion and at 10, 20, 30, 45, 60, 90, and 120 minutes and at 3, 4, 6, 8, 10, 12, and 24 hours after drug ingestion. Serum samples were assayed for glipizide content by a modified high-pressure liquid chromatographic method. Clearance, volume of distribution at steady state, and half-life were estimated from the serum concentration–time curve data. Area under the concentration–time curve and area under the moments curve were calculated using the trapezoidal rule.

The mean values for young and older subjects for time to peak concentration (2.1 versus 2.5 hours), peak concentrations (465 versus 399 μg/mL), elimination half-life (4.2 versus 4.0 hours), clearance (38.8 versus 38.1 mL/min), and distribution volume at steady state (12.5 versus 14.3 L) were not significant. However, two older individuals had a markedly prolonged time to peak concentration (six to eight hours). For 8 of the 20 subjects a more prolonged terminal half-life may have existed.

Further study is required to determine whether significant pharmacokinetic differences between young and elderly subjects appear with multiple dosing of glipizide.

Index terms: Age; Antidiabetic agents; Blood levels; Drugs, body distribution; Excretion; Geriatrics; Glipizide; Half-life; Pharmacokinetics

Clin Pharm. 1988; 7:224–8

The physiologic changes that occur with advancing age have been known for some time[1]; however, only recently has much attention focused on their influence on pharmacokinetics. It is now recognized that elderly adults have altered pharmacokinetic values for certain drugs.[2–4] Although reduced

KELLY A. KOBAYASHI is a Pharm.D. candidate and Pharmacy Resident, School of Pharmacy and Department of Pharmacy, University of Washington, Seattle. LARRY A. BAUER, PHARM.D., and JOHN R. HORN, PHARM.D., are Associate Professors, Department of Pharmacy Practice, University of Washington. KENT OPHEIM, PH.D., is Associate Professor, Department of Laboratory Medicine, University of Washington, and Children's Orthopedic Hospital Medical Center, Seattle. FRANCIS WOOD, JR., M.D., is Associate Professor, Department of Medicine, Division of Endocrinology, and WAYNE A. KRADJAN, PHARM.D., is Associate Professor, Department of Pharmacy Practice, University of Washington.

Address reprint requests to Dr. Kradjan at the School of Pharmacy, SC-69, University of Washington, Seattle, WA 98195.

The assistance of Vern Ainardi in performing the glipizide assays is acknowledged.

This project was supported by a contract with Pfizer Pharmaceuticals. A portion of this work was conducted through the Clinical Research Center of the University of Washington and the Diabetes–Endocrinology Research Center and was supported by grant Nos. RR-37 and AM17047 from the National Institutes of Health.

Presented in the Clinical Research Forum, 22nd Annual ASHP Midyear Clinical Meeting, Atlanta, GA, December 9, 1987.

Copyright © 1988, American Society of Hospital Pharmacists, Inc. All rights reserved. 0278–2677/88/0301-0224$01.25.

renal function and associated impairment in excretion of drugs or their metabolites in the elderly often necessitates dosage reduction, the effects of age on hepatic metabolism and excretion of various drugs are highly variable and unpredictable. Because aging can affect many physiologic factors, very few generalities can be made regarding the effects of aging on the pharmacokinetics of specific drugs, and it is often difficult to establish specific dosing guidelines for geriatric patients. Therefore, it is desirable to study the effects of aging on all drugs that may be used in an older population.

Oral hypoglycemic agents are often used in treating the elderly, and the risk of prolonged hypoglycemia is potentially dangerous in this population. Glipizide, a sulfonylurea compound with hypoglycemic activity, has been marketed in the United States since 1983 and is indicated for use in patients with non-insulin-dependent diabetes mellitus (NIDDM), many of whom are over the age of 65. Although this drug has undergone extensive premarketing research and evaluation, most of the data regarding its pharmacokinetics and pharmacodynamics were obtained in studies of either healthy young volunteers[5] or mixed populations of diabetics with ages ranging from 30 to more than 65 years.[6,7] Ages are not identified in other studies.[8,9] In a recent paper, Arrigoni et al.[10] described a decrease in the clearance of chlorpropamide, another oral hypoglycemic agent, in elderly diabetic patients compared with young healthy adults. Some of this difference may be explained by the long half-life of chlorpropamide and a high percentage of renal clearance for both chlorpropamide and its active metabolites. In contrast, glipizide is primarily metabolized by the liver to inactive metabolites, and no studies to date have examined the effects of aging on glipizide pharmacokinetics. This study was undertaken to compare the pharmacokinetics of glipizide in young healthy adults and older healthy adults.

Methods

Ten healthy young men (24.9 ± 1.9 years of age, mean ± S.D.) and ten healthy older men (74.4 ± 7.9 years of age) participated in the investigation. A complete medical history, a physical examination, and an electrocardiogram were performed at the time of study entry, and screening laboratory data included a complete blood count, urinalysis, 12-panel serum chemistry determination (SMA-12) and liver-function tests (aspartate aminotransferase, bilirubin, alkaline phosphatase). All values, including serum albumin, were within normal limits for all subjects. The subjects did not smoke tobacco-containing products or take any other medications throughout the study period. Criteria for exclusion were allergy to sulfa drugs; a history of diabetes, congestive heart failure, pulmonary disease, renal insufficiency (serum creatinine concentration > 1.5 mg/dL or creatinine clearance < 60 mL/min) or hepatic dysfunction (results of liver-function tests reveal values greater than two times normal values); or taking any medication that may affect serum glucose concentrations or insulin release or act as an inducer or inhibitor of hepatic enzymes. The study was approved by the institution's review board, and informed consent was obtained from all study participants.

The subjects were admitted to the clinical research center after an overnight fast. At approximately 0800, a single 5-mg tablet of glipizide (Glucotrol, Roerig Pharmaceuticals, lot no. 6813A) was administered orally with 8 oz of water. Standardized meals (providing 2065 kcal: 86.8 g of protein, 69.9 g of fat, and 275 g of carbohydrate) were provided 30 minutes, 4 hours, and 10 hours after tablet ingestion. Subjects remained seated either on a bed or in a chair for four hours after the dose. Blood samples (5 mL each) were collected immediately before tablet ingestion and at 10, 20, 30, 45, 60, 90, and 120 minutes and at 3, 4, 6, 8, 10, 12, and 24 hours after drug ingestion for measurement of glipizide concentrations.

Subjects were observed for signs and symptoms of hypoglycemia, as well as for other possible adverse effects of the drug. No such reactions were observed in either group of subjects. Blood glucose concentrations were not routinely measured; these measurements were to be done only if the subject exhibited a suspected hypoglycemic reaction. After 12 hours of observation, subjects were allowed to return home for the night. All subjects returned the next morning for the 24-hour blood sample.

Blood samples were allowed to clot, and serum was separated and stored at −20 °C. Serum samples of glipizide were assayed using a modification of the high-pressure liquid chromatographic method with ultraviolet-light detection as originally reported by Wahlin-Boll et al.[11] The coefficient of variation (CV) of the modified assay was 10.8% at a serum glipizide concentration of 60 μg/L and 6.4% at a serum concentration of 521 μg/L. The detection limit of glipizide is 10 ng/mL, using an injection volume of 40 μL. Two serum controls were run with each set of patient samples.

Time to peak concentration and peak concentration were determined for all subjects by inspecting the serum concentration–time data. The area under the concentration–time curve (AUC) and the area under the moments curve (AUMC) were calculated using the trapezoidal rule. Volume of distribution at steady state (V_{ss}) was calculated as follows:

$$V_{ss} = [(F)\,(\text{Dose})\,(\text{AUMC})/\text{AUC}^2)] - [(F)\,(\text{Dose})/(k_a)\,(\text{AUC})]$$

where k_a is the absorption rate constant and bioavailability (F) was assumed to equal one.[5,6] Clearance was estimated from the glipizide concentration–time curve using model-independent equations.[12] PCNONLIN, a nonlinear least-squares regression program, was used to fit the individual serum data to the appropriate exponential equation.[13] Equal weighting and $1/C^2_{observed}$ weighting were used. The best fit was determined by inspection of the residual plots. Half-life ($t_{1/2}$) was calculated from the terminal elimination rate constant.

Statistical analysis was performed using the two-tailed Student's t test. A p value of < 0.01 was considered significant.

Results

The important pharmacokinetic values for glipizide in young and old healthy subjects are summarized in Table 1. Absorption was rapid in both young and old subjects, with no difference in peak concentrations (465 ± 139 versus 399 ± 96 μg/L) or times to peak concentration (2.1 ± 0.9 versus 2.5 ± 2.3 hours). However, two of the older subjects displayed delayed and erratic absorption, with times to peak concentration in the range of six to eight hours. These two subjects displayed no unusual laboratory values or other abnormalities that would explain this difference. Values of area under the concentration–time curve extrapolated to infinity, volume of distribution at steady state, clearance, and elimination half-life were not significantly different between the young and older subjects. Subject 10 in the younger group displayed unusual elimination characteristics, with a markedly prolonged elimination half-life of 11.4 hours. Even if the results of this subject are excluded from analysis, the differences between the two groups are still not significant with respect to clearance (41.5 ± 14.2 versus 38.1 ± 8.9 mL/min; $p = 0.57$) or elimination half-life (3.4 ± 0.7 versus 4.0 ± 0.9 hours; $p = 0.09$).

Discussion

For most subjects in both age groups, concentrations of glipizide were not detectable until 20 minutes after tablet ingestion. All but one younger subject attained detectable levels by 45 minutes after tablet ingestion; glipizide levels were detectable in this individual by one hour. Prior studies in healthy volunteers and type II diabetics indicate that the absorption of glipizide is delayed 30–60 minutes when the drug is given with meals. However, the area under the concentration–time curve remains unchanged.[14] In our study the dose was given 30 minutes before breakfast, which has been shown to more closely mimic the normal pattern of insulin release in response to increases in blood glucose.[15] Therefore, it appears that it generally takes about 20–30 minutes before detectable levels of glipizide appear in the serum after the drug is

Table 1.
Patient Demographic and Pharmacokinetic Data[a]

Subject	Age (yr)	Weight (kg)	t_{max} (hr)	C_{max} (μg/L)	$t_{1/2}$ (hr)	$AUC_{0-\infty}$ (μg/L/hr)	CL (mL/min)	V_{ss} (L)
Young Men								
1	23	86	1.0	539	5.0	2468.6	33.8	12.4
2	25	67	4.0	543	3.5	3505.8	23.8	9.5
3	27	93	2.0	290	2.6	1214.5	68.8	15.8
4	28	100	1.5	351	3.2	1421.7	58.6	15.4
5	28	80	2.0	404	3.0	2012.1	41.4	10.7
6	24	75	1.0	755	3.7	2615.8	31.9	8.2
7	24	71	3.0	374	3.9	2936.8	28.4	13.2
8	23	74	2.0	304	2.6	1610.9	51.7	12.0
9	23	61	3.0	581	2.9	2345.6	35.5	13.0
10	24	70	1.3	509	11.4	5709.2	14.6	13.7
Mean ± S.D.	24.9 ± 1.9	77.8 ± 11.4	2.1 ± 0.9	465 ± 139	4.2 ± 2.6	2584.1 ± 1237.5	38.8 ± 15.7	12.5 ± 2.3
Older Men								
1	97	65	1.5	517	5.3	3567.0	23.4	11.5
2	73	84	1.5	316	4.1	1763.8	47.3	16.7
3	71	93	1.0	365	3.3	1736.6	48.0	14.4
4	74	69	1.5	527	3.2	2680.8	31.1	10.2
5	66	79	6.0	235	5.0	2119.1	39.3	21.3
6	70	75	1.0	491	3.7	2074.8	40.2	13.2
7	73	83	1.5	455	2.8	1611.9	51.7	11.1
8	75	89	1.0	444	4.3	2437.6	34.2	14.1
9	72	84	1.5	323	5.3	2124.3	39.2	14.8
10	73	91	8.0	312	3.5	3138.0	26.6	15.6
Mean ± SD	74.4 ± 7.9	81.2 ± 8.8	2.5 ± 2.3	399 ± 96	4.0 ± 0.9	2325.4 ± 604.8	38.1 ± 8.9	14.3 ± 3.1
p		0.48	0.66	0.26	0.88	0.58	0.90	0.17

[a] t_{max} = time to maximum concentration, C_{max} = peak concentration, $t_{1/2}$ = half-life, $AUC_{0-\infty}$ = area under the concentration–time curve from time zero to infinity, CL = total plasma drug clearance, V_{ss} = volume of distribution at steady state.

taken on an empty stomach.

Other investigators have shown that glipizide, like other sulfonylureas, is well absorbed after oral administration, with bioavailability being essentially 100%.[5,6] After a 5-mg oral dose, glipizide is rapidly absorbed, with peak serum concentrations attained at one to three hours and mean peak serum concentrations reported to range from 450 to 550 μg/L.[5-8] Our results are in close agreement with those of these investigations, with the time to peak concentration being 2.1 and 2.5 hours for young and older subjects, respectively. Similarly, peak concentrations were 465 and 399 μg/L. Of note is the greater variability in the times to achieve peak concentration in the older subjects (range, one to eight hours) versus the younger subjects (range, one to four hours). In particular, two older subjects exhibited markedly delayed times to reach peak concentration (six and eight hours).

The mean elimination half-life of glipizide has been reported to range from two to seven hours.[5-8] In our study, terminal elimination half-lives of 4.2 hours for the younger subjects and 4.0 hours for the older subjects confirm the findings of previous studies. Although no single pharmacokinetic model could be used to describe the disposition of the drug in all 20 subjects, most fit a two-compartment model. After rapid absorption and a short alpha distribution phase, most subjects entered into the beta elimination phase by four to six hours after drug ingestion. Two subjects in each group did not clearly demonstrate an alpha phase and were best described using a one-compartment model. Because of the drug's short half-life, 11 of 20 subjects had serum levels below the limits of assay detection at 24 hours.

An interesting observation was made regarding serum concentrations in the terminal phase. For eight of the nine subjects with detectable serum levels at 24 hours, it appeared that a more prolonged terminal half-life may have existed. Since no samples were drawn between 12 and 24 hours and because the 24-hour concentrations were near the lower limits of the assay, this terminal phase cannot be accurately described. Additionally, as noted in the results, one of the younger subjects clearly demonstrated a prolonged half-life of 11.4 hours. This subject reached a peak concentration of 509 μg/L at 1.3 hours and had a slow elimination over the next 16 hours, with the concentration still being 78 μg/L at 24 hours. This phenomenon has been previously described with glipizide by other authors.[6] Balant et al.[9] suggested the possibility of a slowly equilibrating deep compartment. Further research is needed to investigate whether glipizide accumulates with multiple dosing.

The apparent volume of distribution for the central compartment of glipizide has been reported to range from 6 to 13 L.[16] We calculated the volume of distribution at steady state because it better reflects drug distribution in the body. The volume of distribution at steady state described in our study (12.5 versus 14.3 L) reflects the high degree of serum protein binding of glipizide (98–99%).[17] The clearance values attained in our study of 38.8 mL/min for the young subjects and 38.1 mL/min for the older subjects are similar to, but slightly slower than, those reported by Wahlin-Boll et al. (51.6 mL/min).[6] Overall, the rapid clearance, small volume of distribution, and short elimination half-life of glipizide in our subjects support previous observations that glipizide is rapidly eliminated. Since glipizide is primarily metabolized, it appears to be less affected by aging than chlorpropamide, which has a greater dependence on renal elimination.[10]

One recognized limitation of our study, being a single-dose study, is that it does not address the possibility of diurnal variation in the pharmacokinetic variables for glipizide or accumulation of metabolites that may occur with multiple dosing. Few data are available regarding these issues. However, based on glipizide's short elimination half-life and rapid elimination, clinically important accumulation would probably not occur with long-term dosing. In addition, since serum glucose and insulin concentrations were not measured, no conclusions can be made regarding any differences in pharmacodynamic response to glipizide between the two groups.

Conclusion

Special attention should be given in prescribing drugs for the elderly. However, in our study, none of the pharmacokinetic values were significantly different in the older subjects compared with the younger subjects. The clinical importance of the greater variability in the time to peak concentration in the older population with respect to insulin release and blood glucose concentrations remains to be assessed. Similarly, further investigation with multiple dosing of glipizide is needed.

References

1. Shand DG. Biological determinants of altered pharmacokinetics in the elderly. *Gerontology*. 1982; 28(Suppl):8–17.
2. Plein JB, Plein EM. Aging and drug therapy. In: Eisdorfer C, ed. Annual review of gerontology and geriatrics. New York: Springer Publishing Company; 1981:211–54.
3. Geokas M. Clinics in geriatric medicine: symposium on the aging process. Philadelphia: W. B. Saunders and Company; 1986.
4. Vestal R, ed. Drug treatment in the elderly. Sydney, Australia: ADIS Health Science Press; 1984.
5. Schmidt HAE, Schoog M, Schweer KW. Pharmacokinetics and pharmacodynamics as well as metabolism following orally and intravenously administered ^{14}C-glipizide, a new antidiabetic. *Diabetologia*. 1973; 9(Suppl):320–30.
6. Wahlin-Boll E, Almer LO, Melander A. Bioavailability, pharmacokinetics and effects of glipizide in type 2 diabetics. *Clin Pharmacokinet*. 1982; 7:363–72.
7. Ostmann J, Christenson I, Jansson B et al. The antidiabetic effect and pharmacokinetic properties of glipizide. *Acta*

Med Scand. 1981; 210:173–80.
8. Balant L, Zahnd GR, Gorgia A et al. Pharmacokinetics of glipizide in man: influence of renal insufficiency. *Diabetologia.* 1973; 9(Suppl):331–8.
9. Balant L, Fabre J, Zahnd GR. The pharmacokinetics of glipizide and glibenclamide in man. *Eur J Clin Pharmacol.* 1975; 8:63–9.
10. Arrigoni L, Fundak G, Horn J et al. Chlorpropamide pharmacokinetics in young healthy adults and older diabetic patients. *Clin Pharm.* 1987; 6:162–4.
11. Wahlin-Boll E, Melander A, Sartor G. High-performance liquid chromatographic determination of glipizide and some other sulphonylurea drugs in serum. *J Chromatogr.* 1979; 164:541–6.
12. Gibaldi M, Perrier D. Pharmacokinetics. New York: Marcel Dekker; 1982.
13. Statistical Consultants, Inc. PCNONLIN and NONLIN84: software for the statistical analysis of nonlinear models. *Am Stat.* 1986; 40:52–6.
14. Sartor G, Schersten B, Melander A. Effects of glipizide and food intake on the blood levels of glucose and insulin in diabetic patients. *Acta Med Scand.* 1978; 203:211–4.
15. Wahlin-Boll E, Melander A, Sartor G et al. Influence of food intake on the absorption and effect of glipizide in diabetics and in healthy subjects. *Eur J Clin Pharmacol.* 1980; 18:279–83.
16. Brogden RN, Heel RC, Pakes GE et al. Glipizide: a review of its pharmacological properties and therapeutic use. *Drugs.* 1979; 18:329–53.
17. Crookes MJ, Brown KF. Interaction of glipizide with human serum albumin. *Biochem Pharmacol.* 1975; 24:298–9.

Effect of food and gastric acidity on absorption of orally administered ketoconazole

PARICHAT LELAWONGS, JOSEPH A. BARONE, JOHN L. COLAIZZI, ALICE T. M. HSUAN, WITOLD MECHLINSKI, ROBERT LEGENDRE, AND JOSEPH GUARNIERI

Abstract: Effects of food and gastric acidity on the bioavailability of ketoconazole tablets were investigated in 12 volunteers using a six-treatment, randomized, Latin-square crossover design.

All volunteers received all treatments, as follows: (A) ketoconazole 200 mg administered after a fast; (B) ketoconazole 200 mg with a standardized high-fat meal; (C) ketoconazole 200 mg with a standardized high-carbohydrate meal; (D) ketoconazole 200 mg after pretreatment with glutamic acid hydrochloride 680 mg as capsules; (E) ketoconazole 200 mg in a simulated achlorhydric state induced with cimetidine and sodium bicarbonate; and (F) ketoconazole 200 mg administered with glutamic acid hydrochloride in a simulated achlorhydric state. Ketoconazole concentrations were measured by high-performance liquid chromatography in plasma samples drawn immediately before and at various times over 24 hours after drug administration. Bioavailability variables, including natural logarithm transformation for area under the concentration–time curve (AUC), were subjected to analysis of variance followed by Duncan's Multiple Range testing.

Treatments B and C significantly prolonged the times required to achieve the peak plasma ketoconazole concentration, and treatment C also significantly reduced the peak plasma ketoconazole concentration (C_{max}) compared with treatment A. There was a trend toward increased AUC values with treatment B and decreased AUC values with treatment C. Treatment D produced a higher C_{max} compared with treatment A, and treatment E produced large, significant reductions in C_{max} and AUC values compared with treatment A. Treatment F significantly increased AUC values and C_{max} compared with treatment E.

Food appears to diminish the rate of ketoconazole absorption, and the effect on extent of absorption may be related to food composition. Glutamic acid hydrochloride capsules may provide an effective, convenient method of enhancing ketoconazole absorption in patients with reduced gastric acidity.

Index terms: Absorption; Achlorhydria; Antifungals; Blood levels; Drugs, availability; Drug interactions; Food; Glutamic acid hydrochloride; Hydrogen ion concentration; Ketoconazole
Clin Pharm. 1988; 7:228–35

PARICHAT LELAWONGS, M.S., is a graduate student, College of Pharmacy, Rutgers–The State University of New Jersey, Piscataway. JOSEPH A. BARONE, PHARM. D., is Assistant Professor of Clinical Pharmacy, and Director of Clinical Programs, College of Pharmacy, Rutgers, and Assistant Director for Academic Affairs, Robert Wood Johnson University Hospital, New Brunswick, NJ. JOHN L. COLAIZZI, PH.D., is Dean and Professor of Pharmacy, College of Pharmacy, Rutgers. ALICE T. M. HSUAN, PH.D., is Director, Biostatistics and Clinical Data Processing; WITOLD MECHLINSKI, PH.D., is Director, Analytical Laboratories; ROBERT LEGENDRE, M.S., is Project Director, Infectious Diseases; and JOSEPH GUARNIERI, PH.D., is a biostatistician, Janssen Pharmaceutica, Piscataway, NJ.

Address reprint requests to Dr. Barone at Rutgers–The State University of New Jersey, College of Pharmacy, Piscataway, NJ 08854.

The secretarial assistance of Margaret Snyder and Ellen Held is acknowledged.

Presented at the Clinical Research Forum, 21st Annual ASHP Midyear Clinical Meeting, Las Vegas, NV, December 10, 1986.

Copyright © 1988, American Society of Hospital Pharmacists, Inc. All rights reserved. 0278-2677/88/0301-0228$02.00.

Ketoconazole (Nizoral, Janssen Pharmaceutica) is a potent, orally active imidazole piperazine compound with broad-spectrum antifungal activity and systemic efficacy against a wide variety of yeast, dimorphic fungal, and dermatophytic infections.[1-3] Because the drug is often used to treat critically ill and immunocompromised patients, adequate absorption after oral administration is important.

There have been conflicting statements regarding the effects of food on ketoconazole absorption, with reports indicating both enhancement and reduction of absorption by food.[4-8] The manufacturer has indicated that food increases the absorption of ketoconazole and causes a greater consistency in blood levels achieved,[9] and *USP Dispensing Information* indicates that ketoconazole "may be taken with a meal or snack to minimize nausea and vomiting and to promote absorption."[10] The bioavailability of ketoconazole also has been shown to be affected by the pH of gastric contents, since an acidic pH is needed for adequate tablet dissolution.[11] Increased gastric pH results in decreased drug absorption.[9] Therefore, it is recommended that ketoconazole not be given concomitantly with drugs that increase gastrointestinal pH and that for achlorhydric patients the drug be dissolved in diluted hydrochloric acid solution and administered via a plastic or glass straw to avoid staining of the teeth or erosion of dental enamel.[11] It is also recommended that additional water be administered after the acidic solution to prevent oropharyngeal irritation.[9] The obvious inconvenience of using the acidic solution warrants investigation of alternative methods of acidifying gastrointestinal contents.

The effects of food and altered gastric pH on ketoconazole absorption have not been studied in the same group of subjects. The purpose of this study was to characterize the effects of food, gastric acidification, and drug-induced achlorhydria on the absorption of ketoconazole in humans and to evaluate the use of glutamic acid hydrochloride capsules as an alternative to the use of diluted hydrochloric acid as a gastric acidifying agent.

Methods

Subjects. Twelve healthy, nonsmoking volunteers (eight men and four women) aged 23 to 42 years and ranging in weight from 51.8 to 73.6 kg (mean ± S.D., 64.3 ± 7.4 kg) and in height from 156.2 to 177.2 cm (mean ± S.D., 169.8 ± 7.3 cm) were entered in the study. All subjects completed the study. None of the subjects was taking concurrent medications, and none had a history of drug abuse or any acute or chronic cardiovascular, gastrointestinal, hepatic, renal, endocrine, or metabolic disease.

Each subject was determined to be in good health based on prestudy physical examinations and clinical laboratory tests. These tests included complete blood, platelet, and differential counts and determinations of hematocrit and serum concentrations of hemoglobin, creatinine, urea nitrogen, alkaline phosphatase, total bilirubin, aspartate aminotransferase (AST, also called SGOT), alanine aminotransferase (ALT, also called SGPT), total protein, total cholesterol, calcium, and uric acid. Urine was also collected and checked for glucose, casts, albumin, red blood cells, and white blood cells. Before each study period, temperature, blood pressure, pulse, and respiratory rate were determined and recorded.

Informed consent was obtained from each subject before admission into the study. The research protocol was approved by the institutional review board.

Treatments. Subjects were randomly assigned to treatment sequences according to a Latin-square crossover design. Patient numbers were assigned post hoc. Specific treatments were as follows: treatment A: ketoconazole 200 mg as one tablet (Nizoral, Janssen Pharmaceutica, Inc., Piscataway, NJ 08854, control number 24C062) administered to fasting subjects; treatment B: ketoconazole 200 mg as one tablet administered immediately after a standard high-fat meal consisting of egg, bologna, whole milk, toast with butter, and canned peaches; treatment C: ketoconazole 200 mg as one tablet administered immediately after a standard high-carbohydrate meal consisting of egg, bologna, chocolate milk, toast with jam, and fresh banana; treatment D: ketoconazole 200 mg as one tablet preceded by pretreatment with glutamic acid hydrochloride 680 mg as two capsules (Acidulin, Eli Lilly & Co., Indianapolis, IN 46285, control number 8FD27A) given five minutes before ketoconazole, all to fasting subjects; treatment E: ketoconazole 200 mg as one tablet preceded by pretreatment with cimetidine 300 mg as one tablet (Tagamet, Smith Kline & French Laboratories, Philadelphia, PA 19101, control number 365T13) given two hours before ketoconazole and sodium bicarbonate 2 g as three 650-mg tablets (Purepac Pharmaceutical Co., Division of Kalipharma, Inc., Elizabeth, NJ 07202, lot number 45766) given one hour before ketoconazole, all to fasting subjects; and treatment F: ketoconazole 200 mg as one tablet preceded by pretreatment with cimetidine 300 mg as one tablet given two hours before ketoconazole, sodium bicarbonate 2 g as three 650-mg tablets given one hour before ketoconazole, and glutamic acid hydrochloride 680 mg as two capsules given 15 minutes before ketoconazole, all to fasting subjects.

Standardized Diets. The components of the standardized high-fat and high-carbohydrate meals are described in Tables 1 and 2. The diets are designed to contain approximately the same caloric content, caloric density, weight, and percentage of

Table 1.
Standardized High-Fat Meal

Food Item	Amount	Weight (g)	Water (g)	Energy (kcal)	Protein[a] (g)	Fat[b] (g)	Carbohydrate[c] (g)
Whole milk	1 cup	244	212.3	160	9	9	12
Egg (large), scrambled	1	50	37.0	80	6	6	...
With butter	1 tbsp	14	2.2	100	...	12	...
With butter and cream	1 tbsp	15	12.0	20	1	2	1
Bologna	2 slices	26	14.6	80	3	7	...
White bread, toasted	2 slices	44	11.0	152	4.8	1.8	28.2
Butter	1 tbsp	14	2.2	100	...	12	...
Peach, water packed	1/2 cup	122.5	123.41	37.5	0.5	...	10

[a] Total food energy from protein was 97.2 kcal (13.0% of total food energy).
[b] Total food energy from fat was 448.2 kcal (59.7% of total food energy).
[c] Total food energy from carbohydrate was 204.8 kcal (27.3% of total food energy).

Table 2.
Standardized High-Carbohydrate Meal

Food Item	Amount	Weight (g)	Water (g)	Energy (kcal)	Protein[a] (g)	Fat[b] (g)	Carbohydrate[c] (g)
Skim milk	1 cup	245	220.5	90	9	...	12
With chocolate syrup	2 tbsp	40	9.6	98	1	0.4	23.4
Egg (large), boiled	1	50	37.0	80	6	6	...
Bologna	1 slice	13	7.3	40	1.5	3.5	...
White bread, toasted	2 slices	44	15.4	152	4.8	1.8	28.2
Jam	3 tbsp	60	17.4	165	...	...	42
Banana	1	175	110.0	100	1	...	26

[a] Total food energy from protein was 93.2 kcal (12.9% of total food energy).
[b] Total food energy from fat was 105.3 kcal (14.5% of total food energy).
[c] Total food energy from carbohydrate was 526.4 kcal (72.6% of total food energy).

water. A major consideration in the selection of these meals was to control gastric emptying time, based on the concept that isocaloric contents and equal meal weights of food will produce similar effects on the gastric emptying rate.[12,13]

Achlorhydria Model. To simulate an achlorhydric state using healthy subjects, gastric acid secretion had to be inhibited, and the acid produced in the stomach overnight had to be neutralized. Cimetidine 300 mg was administered to inhibit gastric acid secretion; investigators have shown that varied doses of cimetidine given to patients cause decreased gastric acid secretion compared with either basal secretion or acid secretion after placebo.[14] A 300-mg dose was found to decrease mean basal acid secretion to almost zero for at least five hours after ingestion, and the onset of effect occurred within one hour after cimetidine ingestion. In addition, the inhibitory effect of cimetidine administration on gastric secretion also occurs in healthy subjects.[15]

In fasting, healthy, young adults, the acidity of gastric juice is 40–60 meq/L with a pH of 0.9–1.2; the average volume secreted overnight is about 400 mL, or 16–24 meq.[16] Since 1 g of sodium bicarbonate neutralizes 12 meq of acid, 2 g of sodium bicarbonate would be required to neutralize the gastric acid produced overnight.[17]

In this study, one 300-mg cimetidine tablet was administered two hours before the dose of ketoconazole, and three 650-mg sodium bicarbonate tablets were administered one hour before ketoconazole to simulate an achlorhydric state in healthy subjects. Treatment F, in which 680 mg of the acidifying agent glutamic acid hydrochloride was administered, was necessary to investigate whether it would be possible to reverse the effect of a drug-induced achlorhydric state on the absorption of ketoconazole.

Study Design. Subjects were admitted to the clinical research unit at 1700 on the day before each treatment period. Vital signs (temperature, blood pressure, pulse, and respiratory rate) were monitored at the time of check-in. Subjects were provided with a standard dinner and underwent a supervised fast of at least 12 hours' duration begun after the completion of dinner and continuing until the time of dosing the next morning.

According to a randomized, crossover design, ketoconazole was administered to each subject in the fasting state or with meals, alone or concomitantly with other medications, depending on the treatment. Eleven 10-mL blood samples were collected from the antecubital vein into heparin-treated Vacutainer tubes using standard venipuncture technique immediately before drug administration and at 0.5, 1, 1.5, 2, 3, 4, 6, 8, 12, and 24 hours after the administration of ketoconazole. Plasma was separated immediately by centrifugation, harvested into plasma collection tubes, and stored frozen at −20 °C until analyzed. A standard lunch was served four hours after ketoconazole dosing. Subjects were allowed to leave the clinical research unit after the 12-hour blood sample but were required to return to the testing facility for the 24-hour blood sample the next morning. A washout period of one week separated each treatment period. This was considered adequate since the terminal elimination half-life of ketoconazole is approximately eight hours.[18]

Analytical Procedure. The determination of ketoconazole in human plasma was based on a high-performance liquid chromatographic (HPLC) method developed by Janssen Pharmaceutica. The method involves extraction of ketoconazole and an internal standard into an alkalinized heptane–isoamyl alcohol (95:5) mixture, followed by acidification and a back-extraction procedure and analysis by HPLC using a reverse-phase column with ultraviolet detection at 240 nm. Quantitation was accomplished by measuring the peak height ratio of ketoconazole relative to the internal standard, terconazole (Janssen-R42 470), (+)-cis-1-[4-[[(2,4-dichlorophenyl)-2-(1H-1,2,4-triazol-1-ylmethyl)-1,3-dioxolan-4-y1]methoxy]phenyl]-4-(1-methylethyl) piperazine. The calibration curves were found to be linear to well over 10 μg/mL. The detection limit of the procedure was 0.005 μg/mL, and the coefficient of variation at the limit of detection was 21%. The mean (± S.D.) maximum extraction recovery for ketoconazole was 80.5 ± 6.0%. The mean maximum extraction recovery for terconazole was 94.5 ± 1.7%.

Statistical Analysis. The following variables were compared to assess the absorption profiles of ketoconazole under the influence of food composition and acidity as provided by the six different treatments: the geometric mean (the antilogarithm of the mean logarithm to the base e) of the area under the plasma concentration–time curve (AUC), the peak plasma concentration (C_{max}), and the time to peak plasma concentration (t_{max}).

Values for AUC from time zero to 24 hours were calculated by the trapezoidal rule.[19] A logarithmic transformation (using the natural logarithm (ln) or logarithm to the base e) was applied to the AUC data to minimize the variability among treatments. (Since the values of p that resulted from comparisons of t_{max} and C_{max} data all were less than 0.002, and since these variables are usually not transformed, the transformation was only applied to AUC data.[20])

The null hypothesis was that the mean values of AUC, C_{max}, and t_{max} for each of the six treatments would be equal. Mean data were subjected to analysis of variance for Latin-square crossover design[21]; the statistical model accounted for variation arising from sequence, volunteers within sequences, weeks, and treatments. Each study variable (i.e., AUC, C_{max}, and t_{max}) was analyzed separately. The a priori level of significance was set at $p < 0.05$. Duncan's Multiple Range Test[22] was used for multiple comparisons when the overall treatment comparison was significant.

Results

The mean plasma ketoconazole concentrations at each sampling time for the 12 subjects for each treatment are depicted in Figure 1. Values for the C_{max}, t_{max}, and AUC_{0-24} for each subject and each treatment are summarized in Table 3. Table 3 also shows the mean values for each subject's C_{max}, t_{max}, and AUC. Table 4 summarizes significant differences for the 12 subjects' AUC (geometric mean), C_{max}, and t_{max} values, which are the important bioavailability variables for comparing the six treatments.

After a single 200-mg ketoconazole tablet was administered orally to the fasting control subjects, a mean peak plasma ketoconazole concentration of 4.37 μg/mL was achieved at 1.21 hours. Both high-fat and high-carbohydrate meals significantly prolonged the times required to achieve the peak plasma ketoconazole concentration. The high-carbohydrate meal also significantly reduced the peak plasma ketoconazole concentration as compared with values for the control model. As shown in Table 4, mean peak plasma ketoconazole concentrations of 4.42 and 3.01 μg/mL were reached at mean peak times of 2.33 and 2.38 hours after administration of the drug with high-fat and high-carbohydrate meals, respectively. As shown in Table 4, significant differences in peak plasma ketoconazole concentrations were observed between high-fat-meal and high-carbohydrate-meal conditions. No significant differences in peak plasma ketoconazole concentrations were observed between the high-fat meal and the fasting condition.

As is shown in Table 4, the geometric mean (antilogarithm of mean logarithm to the base e) of AUC for the fasting state was 15.25 μg·hr/mL. The high-fat-meal treatment increased this mean value to 20.47 μg·hr/mL, while the high-carbohydrate-meal treatment resulted in a decrease of the mean value to 12.74 μg·hr/mL. However, there were no significant differences among treatment groups A, B, and C.

The mean peak plasma concentration was significantly higher for the glutamic acid hydrochloride treatment compared with values for the fasting subjects (5.47 versus 4.37 μg/mL). However, the times to peak plasma concentration were not significantly different when ketoconazole was ad-

Figure 1. Mean plasma ketoconazole concentration at each sampling time after oral administration of a 200-mg tablet in treatment groups A (□), B (■), C (△), D (▲), E (×), and F (+).

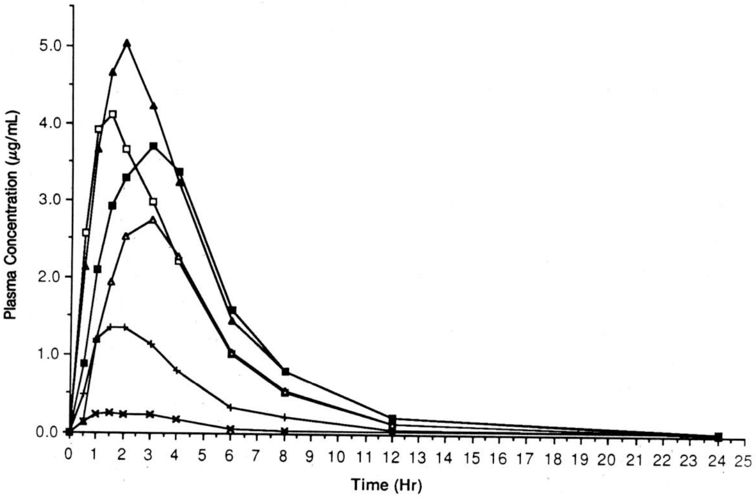

Table 3.
Values for C_{max} (µg/mL), t_{max} (hr) and AUC (µg·hr/mL) for 12 Subjects after Oral Administration of a 200-mg Ketoconazole Tablet[a]

Subject	Treatment A			Treatment B			Treatment C			Treatment D			Treatment E			Treatment F		
	C_{max}	t_{max}	AUC	C_{max}	t_{max}	AUC	C_{max}	t_{max}	AUC	C_{max}	t_{max}	AUC	C_{max}	t_{max}	AUC	C_{max}	t_{max}	AUC
1	0.590	1.00	1.75	5.050	4.00	20.55	1.380	3.00	5.89	1.530	1.00	5.29	0.240	1.50	1.10	0.230	2.00	1.23
2	4.120	0.50	13.00	4.610	3.00	23.95	4.260	3.00	20.15	7.310	2.00	32.54	0.160	1.50	1.84	6.120	2.00	30.42
3	4.680	1.59	21.12	3.880	4.00	18.69	2.850	2.00	13.44	5.100	1.50	22.62	0.190	3.00	1.19	0.075	1.00	.85
4	3.980	1.00	19.88	4.560	1.00	24.81	4.160	2.00	27.03	7.390	2.00	35.89	1.250	1.50	5.46	1.840	1.50	8.37
5	2.440	1.00	7.62	3.540	2.00	20.63	2.070	1.50	6.87	6.360	2.00	27.27	0.087	2.00	.90	4.000	2.00	17.08
6	5.290	1.50	21.18	4.500	2.00	18.58	2.000	1.50	7.89	4.490	1.50	22.08	0.055	3.00	.52	0.110	3.00	1.13
7	6.960	1.00	26.61	5.580	1.50	25.40	4.540	2.00	20.24	6.240	1.00	23.01	0.760	3.00	2.81	0.110	3.00	1.05
8	5.780	1.50	32.53	4.320	2.00	21.25	3.990	3.00	19.11	5.420	2.00	28.00	0.180	1.00	.99	0.310	1.50	1.53
9	2.490	1.00	7.74	3.550	0.50	12.00	1.830	1.50	7.78	2.920	3.00	12.85	0.054	1.00	.54	0.230	1.50	.91
10	6.410	1.50	37.92	6.960	2.00	42.69	4.570	3.00	28.57	8.890	1.50	53.00	0.170	3.00	1.97	1.870	1.00	7.19
11	3.590	1.50	15.83	2.820	3.00	13.72	2.090	3.00	8.63	3.870	2.00	14.70	0.140	2.00	.58	0.490	2.00	3.47
12	6.080	1.50	25.47	3.720	3.00	16.27	2.370	3.00	10.56	6.080	2.00	26.15	0.520	2.00	2.09	2.100	1.00	9.01

[a] C_{max} = peak concentration, t_{max} = time to peak concentration, AUC = area under the concentration–time curve.

Table 4.
Summary of Significant Differences among Treatment Groups for Bioavailability Variables

Variable[a]	Treatment						Comparisons between Treatments[b]														
	A	B	C	D	E	F	A & B	A & C	A & D	A & E	A & F	B & C	B & D	B & E	B & F	C & D	C & E	C & F	D & E	D & F	E & F
AUC_{0-24}[c] (µg·hr/mL)	15.25	20.47	12.74	22.18	1.29	3.30	–	–	–	+	+	–	–	+	+	+	+	+	+	+	+
C_{max} (µg/mL)	4.37	4.42	3.01	5.47	0.32	1.46	–	+	+	+	+	+	+	+	+	+	+	+	+	+	+
t_{max} (hr)	1.21	2.33	2.38	1.71	2.04	1.79	+	+	–	+	–	–	–	–	–	+	–	–	–	–	...

[a] AUC_{0-24} = area under the concentration–time curve from time zero to 24 hours.
[b] + = treatments that are significantly different ($p < 0.05$); – = treatments that are not significantly different ($p > 0.05$).
[c] Geometric mean (antilogarithm of mean LOGAREA [base e]).

ministered with the gastric acidifying agent. The mean values for t_{max} were 1.21 hours for ketoconazole alone and 1.71 hours for ketoconazole with glutamic acid hydrochloride. There was no significant difference in the geometric mean of AUC between the glutamic acid hydrochloride group and the fasting group, with values of 22.18 and 15.25 μg·hr/mL, respectively.

The mean peak plasma concentration dropped from 4.37 μg/mL in the fasting state to 0.32 μg/mL in the achlorhydria model, and the difference was significant. The geometric mean of AUC for the achlorhydria model was 1.29 μg·hr/mL compared with 15.25 μg·hr/mL for the fasting state, with the difference being significant. The mean peak time was also significantly prolonged when the drug was given in the achlorhydric state, and the peak plasma ketoconazole concentration was reached at 2.04 hours, compared with 1.21 hours in the fasting state.

In treatment group F, the geometric mean of AUC was significantly increased with the administration of glutamic acid hydrochloride in the simulated achlorhydria model as compared with values for the achlorhydric state alone (3.30 versus 1.29 μg·hr/mL). The mean peak plasma ketoconazole concentration was also significantly increased (1.46 versus 0.32 μg/mL). Glutamic acid hydrochloride treatment appeared to increase the mean plasma concentrations of ketoconazole in subjects with induced achlorhydria at different sampling times, but none of these differences was significant. There was also no significant difference in t_{max} between these two treatments.

Discussion

Some clinicians recommend that ketoconazole be given with food to improve absorption, based on observations of higher and more consistent plasma concentrations when the drug was given with food.[4,5] However, Brass et al.[6] found a reduction in mean AUC and peak concentration when ketoconazole was given with food to seven subjects, although the reductions were not significant. Mannisto et al.[7] demonstrated a significant reduction in ketoconazole absorption when the drug was coadministered with food in 10 subjects. Daneshmend et al.[8] studied ketoconazole in eight subjects and showed that food did not reduce the absorption of ketoconazole at either 200-, 400-, 600-, or 800-mg doses and had a tendency to enhance the absorption of 400- and 600-mg doses.

Such conflicting reports are difficult to interpret. Our study evaluated the effects of different diets and levels of stomach acidity in the same 12 subjects. Although we did not perform a power analysis to determine sample size, we found that both high-carbohydrate and high-fat meals significantly increased the time required to achieve peak serum ketoconazole concentrations, implying a decrease in the absorption rate of ketoconazole. There was an increase in the mean peak ketoconazole concentration with the high-fat meal compared with the fasting state, but the difference was not significant. There was a significant decrease (31.1%) in the peak plasma ketoconazole concentration with the high-carbohydrate meal. There was a 16.5% decrease in the geometric mean of AUC with the high-carbohydrate meal and a 34.2% increase in AUC with the high-fat meal. However, these differences were not significant.

These effects may be caused by a number of factors. For example, increased viscosity of gastrointestinal contents by food may inhibit dissolution of ketoconazole. Possible complexation or adsorption of ketoconazole by food components could diminish absorption. Since the pH of stomach contents is known to become briefly elevated after a meal,[23,24] such an elevation in gastric pH could diminish the extent or rate of dissolution of ketoconazole. Fatty meals may increase the absorption of lipophilic drugs such as ketoconazole by increasing their rates of dissolution or by increasing the flow of bile into the intestinal tract.[25] High-fat meals also result in more-delayed gastric emptying compared with other types of meals.[26] Such prolonged residence time in the stomach in the case of ketoconazole would provide longer exposure to the acidic environment, thus ensuring more extensive dissolution.[25-27]

The results also suggest a trend toward increased extent of absorption with the high-fat-meal treatment, especially when compared with results from the high-carbohydrate-meal treatment. Of the 12 subjects, 11 had a higher value for AUC for the high-fat-meal treatment compared with the high-carbohydrate-meal treatment in the same subject.

Achlorhydria is a failure of the stomach to produce gastric juice with a pH less than 6, after stimulation by either pentagastrin or histamine.[28] In the elderly, gastric pH rises slightly, and gastric acid secretion decreases to 25 to 35% of that of a 20-year-old person.[29] Pernicious anemia, gastric carcinoma, tropical sprue, hypothyroidism, gastrojejunotomy, and complete and partial gastrectomy have been shown to be associated with achlorhydria.[30-33] Achlorhydria may influence drug absorption by affecting pH or the gastric-emptying rate. Ketoconazole is a poorly soluble, weakly basic drug, and its dissolution is favored in an acidic solution; an increased gastric pH may be expected to substantially impair absorption.[6,34,35] Subjects in the simulated-achlorhydria group showed significant decreases in mean peak plasma ketoconazole concentration, as well as in geometric mean of AUC. The mean time to peak plasma concentration was also significantly delayed, indicating a decrease in the rate of absorption of the drug in the achlorhydria model compared with the control. Since one can assume that the achlorhydria model created a less acidic gastric pH, the dissolution of ketoconazole in the stomach would have been affected, resulting in the observed decrease in the rate and extent of drug absorption. It is also possible that an increased gastric-emptying rate resulting from an alkaline gastric medium could have rapidly transported undissolved drug to the relatively alkaline environment of the intestine, where drug dissolution would be impaired.

Baxter et al.[36] have shown that there is a significant increase in the extent of absorption when ketoconazole is given orally to humans as an acidified solution compared with oral administration in tablet form. Disadvantages to the use of acidified solutions of ketoconazole, as recommended in the package insert,[11] include problems of palatability, damage to dental enamel, and irritation to the oropharyngeal mucous membranes. Also, since an oral liquid dosage form is not commerically available, an acidified solution must be extemporaneously prepared using crushed tablets.

Glutamic acid hydrochloride is easy to administer in capsule form and releases hydrochloric acid upon reacting with aqueous stomach contents. The mean peak plasma ketoconazole concentration was significantly higher for the glutamic acid hydrochloride group when compared with values for the control fasted subjects. The geometric mean of AUC for the group treated with glutamic acid hydrochloride was also increased by 45%, but the difference was not significant. Because glutamic acid hydrochloride was administered 15 minutes before ketoconazole, it is probable that the acid content of the gastric medium was sufficiently increased to provide a more favorable environment for the dissolution and subsequent absorption of ketoconazole compared with that in fasted control subjects.

When ketoconazole was administered with glutamic acid hydrochloride to subjects in the achlorhydric group, the geometric mean of AUC was significantly increased by a factor of 2.6 compared with values for the achlorhydric subjects who received only ketoconazole. The peak plasma ketoconazole concentration was also significantly increased by a factor of 4.6. The dose of glutamic acid hydrochloride was not enough to achieve the same absorption pattern as was seen in the fasting state. The dose of glutamic acid hydrochloride used in this study was based on work by Shay and Cohen,[37] who reported that by giving two capsules of glutamic acid hydrochloride with a meal in achlorhydric patients, the pH of gastric fluid was decreased from pH 7 to 8 to pH 2 to 3 for approximately one hour and then rose to pH 3 to 4 during the second hour. They also showed that gastric pH was decreased from pH 7 to 8 to pH 2 to 3 for a longer period when three or four capsules of glutamic acid hydrochloride were administered. To further increase ketoconazole absorption so that blood levels approach those seen in the fasting state, a larger dose of glutamic acid hydrochloride would probably have to be administered.

Conclusion

Coadministration of ketoconazole with food may diminish the rate of drug absorption, and coadministration of the drug with a high-carbohydrate meal may decrease the peak plasma concentration of ketoconazole. The use of two or more glutamic acid hydrochloride capsules may provide an effective and convenient method of enhancing the absorption of ketoconazole tablets in patients with reduced gastric acidity.

References

1. Heeres J, Backx LJJ, Mostmans JH et al. Antimycotic imidazoles. Part 4. Synthesis and antifungal activity of ketoconazole, a new potent orally active broad spectrum antifungal agent. *J Med Chem.* 1979; 22:1003–5.
2. Levine HB, Borelli D, Fuentes J et al. Ketoconazole, an oral antifungal: laboratory and clinical assessment of imidazole drugs. *Postgrad Med J.* 1979; 55:657–61.
3. Levine HB. Ketoconazole in the management of fungal disease. 1st ed. Australia: ADIS Press; 1982.
4. Dismukes WE, Stamm AM, Graybill JR et al. Treatment of systemic mycoses with ketoconazole: emphasis on toxicity and clinical response in 52 patients. *Ann Intern Med.* 1983; 98:13–20.
5. Daneshmend TK, Warnock DW, Turner A et al. Pharmacokinetics of ketoconazole in normal subjects. *J Antimicrob Chemother.* 1981; 8:299–304.
6. Brass C, Galgiani JN, Blaschke TF et al. Disposition of ketoconazole, an oral antifungal, in humans. *Antimicrob Agents Chemother.* 1982; 21:151–8.
7. Mannisto PT, Mantyla R, Nyanen S et al. Impairing effect of food on ketoconazole absorption. *Antimicrob Agents Chemother.* 1982; 21:730–3.
8. Daneshmend TK, Warnock DW, Ene MD et al. Influence of food on the pharmacokinetics of ketoconazole. *Antimicrob Agents Chemother.* 1984; 25:1–3.
9. American hospital formulary service–drug information 85. McEvoy G, ed. Bethesda, MD: American Society of Hospital Pharmacists; 1985:65–8.
10. Heller WM, ed. USP dispensing information. 5th ed. Volume 1. Drug information for the health care provider. Rockville, MD: The United States Pharmacopeial Convention, Inc.; 1984:729–31.
11. Janssen Pharmaceutica. Nizoral package insert. Piscataway, NJ: Sep 1984.
12. Guthrie HA. Introductory nutrition. 3rd ed. St. Louis: The C.V. Mosby Co.; 1975:503–32.
13. Robinson CH. Fundamentals of normal nutrition. 3rd ed. New York: Macmillan Publishing Co., Inc.; 1978:490–512.
14. Henn RM, Isenberg JI, Maxwell V et al. Inhibition of gastric acid secretion by cimetidine in patients with duodenal ulcer. *N Engl J Med.* 1975; 293:371–5.
15. Domschke W, Domschke S, Reim E et al. Human gastric mucosal blood flow during cimetidine inhibition of acid secretion. In: Greutzfeldt W, ed. Cimetidine. Amsterdam: Excerpta Medica; 1978:81–5.
16. Brooks FP. Gastrointestinal system secretion. In: West JB, ed. Best and Taylor's physiological basis of medical practice. 11th ed. Baltimore: Williams & Wilkins; 1985:698–9.
17. Harvey SC. Gastric antacids, miscellaneous drugs for the treatment of peptic ulcers, digestants, and bile acids. In: Goodman and Gilman's the pharmacological basis of therapeutics. 7th ed. Gilman AG, Goodman LS, Rall TW et al., eds.

New York: Macmillan Publishing Co., Inc.; 1985:980–6.
18. Hume AL, Kerkering TM. Ketoconazole. *Drug Intell Clin Pharm.* 1983; 17:169–74.
19. Gibaldi M, Perrier D. Pharmacokinetics. 2nd ed. New York: Marcel Dekker, Inc.; 1982:445–9.
20. Bolton S. Pharmaceutical statistics, practical and clinical applications. New York: Marcel Dekker, Inc.; 1984:282.
21. Grizzle JE. The two period changeover design and its use in clinical trials. *Biometrics.* 1965; 21:467–80.
22. Scheffe H. The analysis of variance. New York: John Wiley and Sons, Inc.; 1959:78–83.
23. Gibaldi M. Gastrointestinal absorption—biologic considerations. In: Gibaldi M. Biopharmaceutics and clinical pharmacokinetics. 3rd ed. Philadelphia: Lea & Febiger; 1984:34–40.
24. Fordtran JS, Walsh JH. Gastric acid secretion rate and buffer content of the stomach content after eating. *J Clin Invest.* 1973; 52:645–57.
25. Welling PG. How food and fluid affect drug absorption. *Postgrad Med.* 1977; 62:73–82.
26. Welling PG. Influence of food and diet on gastrointestinal drug absorption. *J Pharmacokinet Biopharm.* 1977; 5:291–34.
27. Welling PG. Effect of food on bioavailability of drugs. *Pharm Int.* 1980; Jan:14–8.
28. Brooks FP. Tests related to the stomach. In: Berk JE, ed. Gastroenterology. 4th ed. Philadelphia: W. B. Saunders Company; 1985:367–77.
29. Benet LZ. Pharmacokinetic basis for drug treatment. 1st ed. New York: Raven Press; 1984:32–3.
30. Hurst AF. The clinical importance of achlorhydria. *Br Med J.* 1934; Oct:664–9.
31. Saeed-uz-Zafar M. The thyroid. In: Berk JE, ed. Gastroenterology. 4th ed. Philadelphia: W. B. Saunders Company; 1985:4624–8.
32. Sheehy TW. Tropical sprue. In: Berk JE, ed. Gastroenterology. 4th ed. Philadelphia: W. B. Saunders Company; 1985:1758–80.
33. Kalser MH. Absorption of cobalamin (vitamin B_{12}), folate, and other water-soluble vitamins. In: Berk JE, ed. Gastroenterology. 4th ed. Philadelphia: W. B. Saunders Company; 1985:1553–66.
34. van der Meer JWM, Keuning JJ, Schiejgrong HW et al. The influence of gastric acidity on the bioavailability of ketoconazole. *J Antimicrob Chemother.* 1980; 6:552–4.
35. Carlson JA, Mann HJ, Canafax DM. Effect of pH on disintegration and dissolution of ketoconazole tablets. *Am J Hosp Pharm.* 1983; 40:1334–6.
36. Baxter JG, Brass C, Schentag JJ et al. Pharmacokinetics of ketoconazole administered intravenously to dogs and orally as tablet and solution to humans and dogs. *J Pharm Sci.* 1986; 75:443–7.
37. Shay H, Cohen JG. A comparison of the effectiveness of glutamic acid hydrochloride and diluted hydrochloric acid as the replacement therapy in anacidity measured by fractional gastric acid titration and hydrogen-ion concentration curves. *Ann Intern Med.* 1936; 9:1628–37.

Research Note

Effects of diltiazem hydrochloride on glucose tolerance in persons at risk for diabetes mellitus

BARBARA J. JONES, JAMES M. MCKENNEY, JACKSON T. WRIGHT, JR., AND ROBERT P. GOODMAN

Clin Pharm. 1988; 7:235–8

Diltiazem hydrochloride (Cardizem, Marion Laboratories) is a calcium-channel-blocking agent used clinically in the treatment of angina pectoris. Data from recent studies suggest that diltiazem is also effective for the treatment of mild to moderate hypertension.[1-4] Like other calcium-channel-blocking agents, diltiazem inhibits transmembrane calcium influx. It appears to cause coronary and peripheral vasodilation by inhibiting calcium-mediated smooth muscle contraction in blood vessels.[5]

In vitro, the secretion of a number of hormones, including insulin, depends on calcium ion influx.[6] Calcium is known to play a critical role in insulin release, the secretory process apparently being triggered by an accumulation of this cation in the cytosol.[7-9] In vitro studies with verapamil suggest that calcium-channel blockade reduces insulin secretion.[10-12] However, most of the studies of verapamil and nifedipine in patients have not shown adverse changes in insulin levels or tolerance to a glucose load.[13-17] The three studies that showed modest changes in insulin levels or glucose tolerance—one with intravenous verapamil[18] and two

BARBARA J. JONES, PHARM.D., is Coordinator, Home Health Care Pharmacy Services, Medical College of Virginia Hospitals, Virginia Commonwealth University, Richmond. JAMES M. MCKENNEY, PHARM.D., is Professor, School of Pharmacy, Medical College of Virginia, Virginia Commonwealth University (MCV–VCU). JACKSON T. WRIGHT, JR., M.D., PH.D., is Associate Professor, School of Medicine, (MCV–VCU). ROBERT P. GOODMAN, M.D., is Assistant Professor, School of Medicine, (MCV–VCU).

Address reprint requests to Dr. Jones at Box 42, MCV Station, Richmond, VA 23298.

Presented at the meeting of The American Federation for Clinical Research, Washington, DC, May 3, 1986.

Copyright © 1988, American Society of Hospital Pharmacists, Inc. All rights reserved. 0278-2677/88/0301-0235$01.00.

with oral nifedipine[19,20]—suggest that the effect may be related to dose or concentration.

Little is known about the effect of diltiazem on glucose tolerance and insulin levels. Segrestaa et al.[21] reported that oral diltiazem produced no significant change in basal glucose levels, glucose tolerance, or insulin secretion in 12 healthy male volunteers. Its effect in patients with diabetes mellitus or persons at risk for diabetes mellitus is unknown. One subgroup that may be at particular risk of this adverse effect is obese persons with family history of diabetes mellitus, a subgroup known to be predisposed to both cardiovascular disease and diabetes mellitus. Since hypertension and diabetes are particularly common to this subgroup and often occur simultaneously,[22] it is essential to examine diabetogenic potential of these agents in this subgroup.

We investigated the effect of therapeutic doses of diltiazem on glucose tolerance in obese, nondiabetic women with family history of diabetes mellitus. We hypothesized that diltiazem, compared with placebo, would produce a statistically significant increase in these subjects' serum glucose levels and area under the glucose tolerance curve in response to a standard glucose load.

Methods. We recruited 11 obese black women with family history of type II diabetes mellitus but no history of hypertension and no other serious medical problems (as determined by history, physical examination, complete blood count, and automated chemistry panel). The study had been approved by the institutional review board. Obese black women with family history of type II diabetes mellitus were chosen as our study population because they possessed several risk factors that are thought to contribute to the development of diabetes.[23, 24] The subjects were not taking any medications before the study and took no medications during the study period that might have affected blood glucose or interacted with diltiazem. All gave informed written consent. The mean age was 30 years (range, 19 to 43 years), mean height was 147.2 cm (range, 140.3 to 154.1 cm), and mean weight was 92.3 kg (range, 71.8 to 150.9 kg). None of the subjects was more than 20% heavier than the standard weight for her age and height, as specified by the Metropolitan Life Insurance Company weight tables.[25] Seven of the subjects had family history of diabetes in their grandparents only, two in their parents only, and two in both grandparents and parents.

The study used a randomized crossover design consisting of two nine-day double-blind drug periods separated by a five-day washout period. Diltiazem hydrochloride 60 mg or an identical-appearing placebo was ingested every six hours during study weeks, with the last capsule taken in the morning of day 9 of each study week.

Subjects' compliance was monitored by capsule counts. Before each glucose tolerance test, adverse effects were evaluated by interviewing the subject, checking blood pressure and heart rate, and obtaining an ECG rhythm strip.

A standard oral glucose tolerance test (75 g glucose) was administered on the second and ninth day of each double-blind period immediately after ingestion of the morning dose of diltiazem or placebo. After an overnight 12-hour fast, blood samples were collected at time 0 (fasting) and 30, 60, 120, and 240 minutes after glucose ingestion and analyzed for glucose and C-peptide concentrations. In addition, the fasting time 0 sample was used for measurement of insulin.

Glucose concentrations were determined by a standard glucose analyzer. Plasma C-peptide and insulin concentrations were measured by radioimmunoassay.

Mean values and standard error were calculated for each treatment group, at each time point for glucose and C-peptide concentrations. The area under the plasma glucose and C-peptide concentration–time curves above the baseline levels was calculated using the trapezoidal rule.[26] Mean values and standard error were also calculated for fasting insulin concentrations. Statistical evaluation was performed using analysis of variance, looking at the effects of the four different treatment groups (placebo day 2, placebo day 9, diltiazem day 2, and diltiazem day 9) on glucose and C-peptide concentrations at each time point and on baseline insulin levels. A Student's t test was performed comparing mean baseline glucose, insulin, and C-peptide concentrations on day 2 of each double-blind period to evaluate an order effect. An alpha value of $p < 0.05$ was chosen as our level of significance.

Results. Of the 11 study subjects, 6 received placebo first. There were no significant differences caused by the order of the dosing.

Compliance with study regimens was documented by capsule counts and adverse-effect profile. The mean percentage of capsules taken by the study subjects during the first and second treatment periods was 99.5. Headache, a commonly known adverse effect of diltiazem, was noted in 10 of 11 subjects (91%) in the active drug phase and in 1 of 11 in the placebo phase.

Mean plasma glucose concentrations were normal at baseline. Mean plasma glucose concentrations at baseline and 30, 60, 120, and 240 minutes after the oral glucose load were not significantly different with diltiazem than with placebo (Figure 1). Mean plasma glucose concentration 30 minutes after the glucose load was 13% higher after one week of diltiazem therapy than after one week of placebo, but this difference was not significant. None of the concentrations after two days of diltiazem was significantly different from the corresponding concentration after nine days, indicating

Figure 1. Plasma glucose concentration over time after an oral glucose load in subjects receiving diltiazem and placebo.

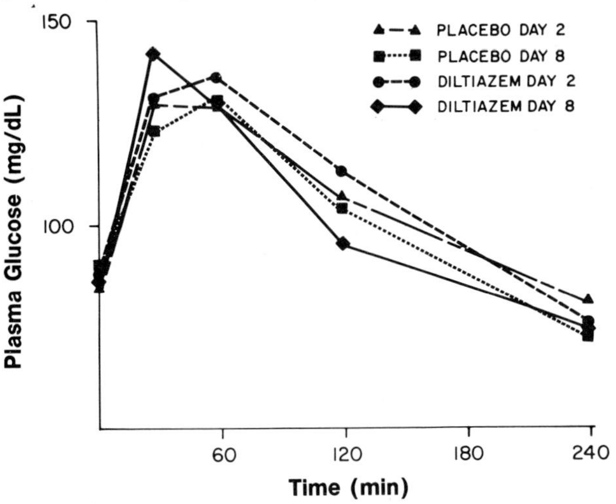

Figure 2. Plasma C-peptide concentration over time after an oral glucose load in subjects receiving diltiazem and placebo.

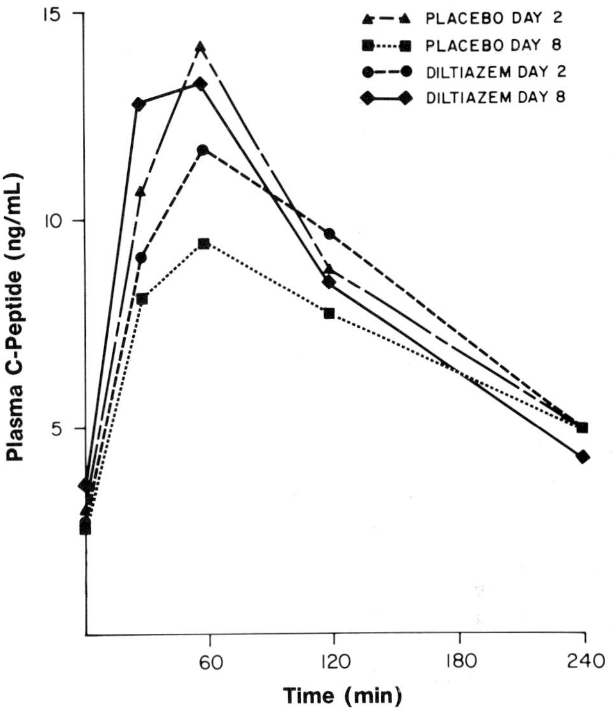

no difference in glucose tolerance in initial versus long-term treatment.

Mean C-peptide levels at baseline and 30, 60, 120, and 240 minutes after an oral glucose load were not significantly different with diltiazem than with placebo (Figure 2). The measurements of C-peptide responses gave no indication of appreciable inhibition of β-cell function in the pancreas at any time during the study.

Plasma insulin concentrations on days 2 and 8 of placebo and days 2 and 8 of diltiazem (mean ± S.E.) were 29.64 ± 4.49, 33.09 ± 4.76, 29.01 ± 4.15, and 28.73 ± 3.96 μg/mL, respectively. The values during diltiazem treatment were not significantly different from those for placebo.

The mean areas under the plasma glucose and C-peptide concentration–time curves were not significantly different with diltiazem than with placebo (Table 1).

Table 1.
Area Under the Curve for Plasma Glucose and C-Peptide Concentrations in 11 Subjects Receiving Diltiazem and Placebo

Therapy	Plasma Glucose (mean ± S.E.)	Plasma C-Peptide (mean ± S.E.)
Placebo day 2	424 ± 19	35 ± 6
Placebo day 9	411 ± 23	29 ± 6
Diltiazem day 2	436 ± 20	34 ± 5
Diltiazem day 9	407 ± 23	34 ± 5

Discussion. No significant changes in mean concentrations of plasma glucose and C-peptide were found at any time period in subjects receiving diltiazem, nor were clinically important changes in these measurements seen in any individual. This indicates that diltiazem hydrochloride 240 mg daily for up to one week does not cause substantial glucose intolerance. In addition, diltiazem does not appear to affect fasting baseline glucose, insulin, or C-peptide.

The lack of significant differences in glucose concentrations between the diltiazem and placebo treatment periods support the findings of Segrestaa et al.[21] They found no significant difference in plasma glucose, insulin, or glucagon levels after an oral glucose load during treatment for eight days with diltiazem hydrochloride 180 mg daily in 12 healthy volunteers.

Conclusion. The results of our study indicate that diltiazem hydrochloride at a daily dosage of 240 mg may be given for up to one week to obese black women with family history of diabetes without precipitating clinically important glucose intolerance.

References

1. McAuley BJ, Schroeder MD. The use of diltiazem hydrochloride in cardiovascular disorder. *Pharmacotherapy*. 1982; 2:121–33.
2. Safer ME, Simon AC, Levenson JA et al. Hemodynamic effects of diltiazem in hypertension. *Circ Res*. 1983; 52:1169–73.
3. Smith MS, Verghese CP, Shand DG et al. Pharmacokinetic and pharmacodynamic effects of diltiazem. *Am J Cardiol*. 1983; 51:1369–74.
4. Maeda K, Takasugi T, Tsukano Y et al. Clinical study on the hypotensive effect of diltiazem hydrochloride. *Int J Clin*

Pharmacol Ther Toxicol. 1981; 19:47–55.

5. Sawaii K. Effects of long-term administration of diltiazem hydrochloride in hypertensive patients. *Clin Ther.* 1983; 5:422–35.
6. Shamoon H, Baylor P, Kambosos D et al. Influence of oral verapamil on glucoregulatory hormones in man. *J Clin Endocrinol Metab.* 1985; 60:536–41.
7. Malaisse WJ, Herchuelz A, Devis G et al. Regulation of calcium fluxes and their regulatory roles in pancreatic islets. *Ann NY Acad Sci.* 1978; 307:562–81.
8. Malaisse WJ, Hutton JC, Sever A et al. Calcium antagonist and islet function. VII. Effect of calcium deprivation. *J Membr Biol.* 1978; 38:193–208.
9. Lebron P, Malaisse WJ, Herchuelz A. Evidence for two distinct modalities of Ca^{+2} influx into pancreatic B cell. *Am J Physiol.* 1982; 242:E59–66.
10. Malaisse WJ, Pipeleers DG, Malaisse-Lagae F et al. Effect of a verapamil derivative (D 600) on calcium uptake and insulin release by isolated islets. *Diabetologia.* 1973; 9:80.
11. Devis G, Somer G, Van Obberghen E et al. Calcium antagonists and islet function I. Inhibition of insulin release by verapamil. *Diabetes.* 1975; 24:547–51.
12. Malaisse WJ, Herchuelz A, Levy J et al. Calcium antagonists and islet function. III. The possible site of action of verapamil. *Biochem Pharmacol.* 1977; 26:735–40.
13. Dante A. Nifedipine and fasting glycemia. *Ann Intern Med.* 1986; 104(1):125–6. Letter.
14. Donnelly T, Harrower ADB. Effect of nifedipine on glucose tolerance and insulin secretion in diabetic and non-diabetic patients. *Curr Med Res Opin.* 1980; 6:690–3.
15. Greenwood RH. Hyperglycemic effect of nifedipine. *Br Med J.* 1982; 284:50.
16. Andersson DEH, Rojdmark S. Improvement of glucose tolerance by verapamil in patients with non insulin dependent diabetes mellitus. *Acta Med Scand.* 1981; 2210:27–33.
17. Rojdmark S, Andersson DEH. Influence of verapamil on glucose tolerance *Acta Med Scand.* [Suppl] 1984; 681:37–42.
18. Rojdmark S, Andersson DEH, Hed R et al. Effect of verapamil on glucose response to intravenous injection of glucagon and insulin in healthy subjects. *Horm Metab Res.* 1980; 12:285–90.
19. Charles S, Ketelslegers JM. Guyschaert M et al. Hyperglycemic effect of nifedipine. *Br Med J.* 1980; 283:19–20.
20. Gingliano D, Torella R, Cacciapuoti F et al. Impairment of insulin secretion in man by nifedipine. *Eur J Clin Pharmacol.* 1980; 18:395–8.
21. Segrestaa JM, Caulin C, Dahan R et al. Effect of diltiazem on plasma glucose, insulin and glucagon during an oral glucose tolerance test in healthy volunteers. *Eur J Clin Pharmacol.* 1984; 26:481–3.
22. McKenney JM, Goodman RP, Wright JT. Use of antihypertensive agents in patients with glucose intolerance. *Clin Pharm.* 1985; 4:649–56.
23. Bennett PH, Harris M, Murphy RS. Geographic and ethnic differences in diabetes frequency in the Americas. In: Mngola EN, ed. Diabetes 1982. New York: Elsevier Science; 1983: 131–6.
24. Born DM. Diabetes in the family. Bowie, MD: Prentice-Hall; 1982; 10, 117–8.
25. Anon. Weights of insured persons in the United States associated with the lowest mortality. *Stat Bull Metropol Life Insur Co.* 1959; (Nov-Dec): 40.
26. Gibaldi M, Perrier D, eds. Pharmacokinetics. 2nd ed. New York: Marcel Dekker, Inc.; 1982:445–9.

“

Understanding Immunoregulation

The key reason for the booming interest in immunology in current biomedical science is its appeal at many levels. From a public health viewpoint, vaccines have proved to be history's most cost-effective tool, and the search for new and improved vaccines is on in earnest. For the physician interested in chronic diseases, it is clear that disordered immune processes form at least part of the etiologic and pathogenetic spectrum in many disorders. For the oncologist, even though the concept of tumor-specific antigens has lost some of its shine, the possibilities for prophylaxis, diagnosis, and therapy through immunologic approaches remain tantalizing. For the transplantation surgeon, regulation of the immune response represents the rate-limiting step for further triumphs. For the basic scientist, the system as a whole, with its capacity for recognition and learning, is fascinating, and its cellular and molecular components yield useful models for analysis at all levels from biophysics to physiology.

The basic components of the immune system are now understood in reasonable detail. We have a conceptual atlas and many detailed analyses about which consensus has been reached or is near. Yet, in many immunopathologic situations, our capacity for therapeutic intervention falls far short of the ideal because our knowledge of regulation and control is still relatively primitive. Despite this period of heady growth, we must not shirk the patient task of understanding immunoregulation much more deeply.

—Nossal GJV. Current concepts: immunology—the basic components of the immune system. *N Engl J Med.* 1987; 316:1320–5.

”

Commentary

Selection of a human growth hormone product

KELLY J. BURCH AND
MARIELA ALVARADO-HUGHES

Clin Pharm. 1988; 7:239–40

Before the introduction of biosynthetic human growth hormone in 1985, growth hormone was obtained by extraction from human cadaver pituitary glands. The clinical use of pituitary human growth hormone was restricted because it was scarce and expensive. In 1985, the National Institutes of Health halted distribution of its pituitary growth hormone product after reports of Creutzfeldt–Jakob disease in patients treated with pituitary human growth hormone.[1,2]

Currently, two biosynthetic hormones are available in the United States. Both hormones are synthesized by a strain of *Escherichia coli* that has been modified by the addition of a gene for human growth hormone. Somatrem, or methionyl human growth hormone (Protropin, Genentech, Inc.), introduced in 1985, was the first polypeptide hormone of recombinant-DNA origin, followed by somatropin (Humatrope, Eli Lilly and Company), marketed early last year. In the future r-DNA somatropin may be available from other manufacturers, including Genentech. Somatrem and somatropin contain 192 and 191 amino acids, respectively, and have a molecular weight of approximately 22,000.[3,4] The amino acid sequence of somatrem and somatropin is identical to that of pituitary human growth hormone except that somatrem differs by an additional amino acid, methionine, at the *N*-terminal end of the molecule.

Formation of Antibodies to Human Growth Hormone. Potential differences in antigenicity between the r-DNA growth hormone products are of interest because the products differ by one amino acid. Formation of antibodies to growth hormone is of concern because of the potential for attenuation of the growth effect of growth hormone therapy. Early studies showed that the formation of antibodies to pituitary-derived and methionyl growth hormone depended on the quality of the product. As a more purified product has become available, antibody formation has decreased. Immunogenicity of the two growth hormone molecules has been evaluated in clinical trials sponsored by Lilly Research Laboratories using both Humatrope and the methionyl human growth hormone developed by Lilly.[5] Measurable binding capacity was detected in 3.3% of the patients treated with Humatrope, as opposed to 50% of the patients receiving the methionyl human growth hormone.

Clinical research has confirmed the minimal antibody formation seen with r-DNA somatropin. A multicenter clinical trial evaluated 69 patients treated with r-DNA somatropin for six months to one year and detected no anti-human-growth-hormone antibodies in these patients.[6] In contrast to the Lilly study, one long-term multicenter study compared the antibody formation in 84 patients treated for 6 to 30 months with two Protropin products of different quality.[7] In patients receiving the more purified injection, the percentage developing antibodies against growth hormone was smaller than that in patients receiving an earlier, less purified preparation. In patients who developed antibodies, the antibodies had very low binding capacity, and levels needed to depress the growth-promoting action of human growth hormone

KELLY J. BURCH, PHARM.D., is Clinical Consultant for Nutritional Support Services, Le Bonheur Children's Medical Center, Memphis, TN, and Assistant Professor of Clinical Pharmacy, College of Pharmacy, University of Tennessee, Memphis. MARIELA ALVARADO-HUGHES, PHARM.D., is Resident in Pediatric Pharmacy Practice, Le Bonheur Children's Medical Center.

Address reprint requests to Dr. Burch at the Department of Pharmacy Services, Le Bonheur Children's Medical Center, One Children's Plaza, Memphis, TN 38103.

Copyright © 1988, American Society of Hospital Pharmacists, Inc. All rights reserved. 0278-2677/88/0301-0239$00.50.

(>1 mg/dL) were reached in only one patient.

Although patients treated with somatrem may have a higher degree of antibody formation than patients receiving r-DNA somatropin, the antibodies do not usually reach the levels of binding capacity needed to decrease growth velocity; hence, we believe that the differences in antigenicity between these two hormones are not clinically important and should not influence product selection. Should attenuation of growth velocity occur in a specific patient, drug inactivation by antibody binding may be an etiology. Switching to the alternative product may be indicated.

Indications and Dosage Recommendations. Somatrem and somatropin are indicated for long-term treatment of children with growth failure resulting from inadequate secretion of endogenous growth hormone.[3,4] The recommended dosage for Protropin is 0.1 mg (0.26 IU) per kg i.m. three times per week. The recommended dosage for patients receiving Humatrope is 0.066 mg (0.16 IU) per kg i.m. three times per week. The milligram-to-International-Unit conversion is the same for both hormones. In 1986, the World Health Organization reevaluated the international standards for human growth hormone. The first standards, established in 1982, state that 1 mg is equal to 2 IU. The revised standards state that 1 mg is equal to 2.6 IU.[8] Protropin labeling is being updated. The recommended dosage for Humatrope is lower than that for Protropin because the recommendations are based on the dosage levels used in manufacturer-sponsored premarketing studies.

Eli Lilly and Company evaluated Humatrope and methionyl human growth hormone in two 12-month trials. The dosage regimen was standard for both products (0.06 mg/kg intramuscularly three times per week), and therapeutic results were equivalent.[5] Genentech has not evaluated Protropin at the lower dosage regimen, and thus the package insert recommends the studied dosage of 0.1 mg/kg three times per week. Based on currently available information, we believe both hormones are equipotent and dosage requirements should be the same.

Availability and Cost. Both biosynthetic hormones are supplied as sterile, white, lyophilized powder for intramuscular injection. Each Protropin vial contains somatrem 5 mg (13 IU), mannitol 40 mg, and sodium phosphate 1.7 mg. Two 5-mg vials are supplied in a package with one 10-mL vial of diluent. The diluent is Bacteriostatic Water for Injection, USP, preserved with 0.9% benzyl alcohol.[3] Each Humatrope vial contains somatropin 5 mg (13 IU), mannitol 25 mg, glycine 5 mg, and sodium phosphate 1.3 mg. Each vial of its diluent contains water for injection preserved with 0.3% *m*-cresol and 1.7% glycine.[4] One Humatrope vial is packaged with one 5-mL vial of diluent. Humatrope is also available in Lilly's Redi-vial packaging. Both products should be refrigerated before and after reconstitution and should be discarded seven days after reconstitution. Thus, neither product offers any real advantage with respect to packaging, storage condition, or expiration; however, Humatrope is available in a single 5-mg package, whereas the Protropin package contains two 5-mg vials.

Known hypersensitivity to the specific diluent or preservative may influence product selection. The Protropin diluent contains benzyl alcohol; however, the small dose of the alcohol, administered only three times weekly, should pose no danger even to the infant patient.

List prices of the two products are comparable but, because of the wholesaler distribution system used by Eli Lilly and Company, wholesaler markups may add to overall cost to pharmacies and to patients receiving Humatrope.

Conclusion. Differences between the two r-DNA growth hormone products are of minimal clinical importance. Differences in antibody formation are not clinically important and should not influence product selection. However, Protropin and Humatrope are not generic equivalents. The issue of generic equivalency is particularly pertinent in light of the high cost of this therapy (at least $7500/year), which is usually borne, at least in part, by third-party payers. Interchange may be considered if the two drugs are judged by the practitioner to be therapeutically equivalent. If patients are changed from one product to the other, the issue of third-party coverage of the alternate product should be explored.

References

1. Howrie DL. Growth hormone for the treatment of growth failure in children. *Clin Pharm*. 1987; 6:283–91.
2. Schaff-Blass E, Burstein S, Rosenfield RL. Advances in diagnosis and treatment of short stature, with special reference to the role of growth hormone. *J Pediatr*. 1984; 104:801–13.
3. Genentech Incorporated. Protropin package insert. San Francisco, CA; 1985 Oct.
4. Eli Lilly Corporation. Humatrope package insert. Indianapolis, IN; 1987 Feb.
5. Sportsman JR, Heisserman JA, Frank B et al. Methionyl-human growth hormone provokes elevated levels of antibodies to human growth hormone relative to natural sequence human growth hormone. Paper presented to the 69th Annual Meeting of the Endocrine Society. Indianapolis, IN: 1987 Jun 10.
6. Banke MB, Bierich JR. Clinical experience with authentic recombinant somatropin—German Collaborative Study. *Acta Pediatr Scand*. 1987; 331(Suppl): 9–17.
7. Kaplan SL, Underwood LE, August GP et al. Clinical studies with recombinant-DNA derived methionyl human growth hormone in growth hormone deficient children. *Lancet*. 1986; 1:697–700.
8. National Institute for Biological Standards and Control. The international standard for growth hormone, human, for bioassay. London: The National Institute for Biological Standards and Control; 1987.

CP Continuing Education

The ASHP Continuing Education system gives readers a self-assessment mechanism for selected articles in Clinical Pharmacy *and the* American Journal of Hospital Pharmacy. *It also allows readers to obtain continuing-education credit for these articles.*

For the purpose of CE-credit enrollment a blank answer sheet is published at the end of each installment of the column for the CE articles in that issue. An enrollee accumulates these answer sheets until the enrollment is submitted, using the form that is published in the June and December issues of Clinical Pharmacy *and in the June and December issues of the* American Journal of Hospital Pharmacy. *Any combination of tests within a 18-month period, from both* Clinical Pharmacy *and* American Journal of Hospital Pharmacy, *may be included in an enrollment. More complete details about enrollment in the system will appear in the semiannual enrollment form.*

Article 680-204-8803 (see page 187)
Qualifies for 1.0 hour of CE credit

Guanfacine hydrochloride: A centrally acting antihypertensive agent

Learning Objectives

After studying this article, the reader should be able to

1. List the potential mechanisms by which guanfacine exerts its antihypertensive effect.
2. Explain the pharmacokinetic profile of guanfacine.
3. Compare and contrast the antihypertensive efficacy of guanfacine, clonidine, and methyldopa.
4. Identify common adverse effects of guanfacine.
5. Recommend a dosage regimen of guanfacine for a given patient.

Self-assessment Questions

For each question there is one best answer only.

1. The major mechanism of action of guanfacine is
   a. Peripheral α_2-adrenoreceptor stimulation.
   b. Central stimulation of α adrenoreceptors.
   c. Competitive inhibition of β adrenoreceptors.
   d. Stimulation of peripheral α_1 adrenoreceptors.

2. What percentage of guanfacine is protein bound?
   a. 30%.
   b. 50%.
   c. 60%.
   d. 90%.

3. Which one of the following statements best describes the pharmacokinetic profile of guanfacine?
   a. Guanfacine has a rapid onset of action and a short half-life.
   b. Guanfacine has a rapid onset of action and a long half-life.
   c. Guanfacine has a delayed onset of action and a long half-life.
   d. Guanfacine has a delayed onset of action and a short half-life.

4. Which one of the following statements best describes the effects of aging on the pharmacokinetics of guanfacine?
   a. The elimination half-life is shorter in older individuals.
   b. Drug absorption is somewhat slower in older individuals.
   c. Total drug clearance is decreased in older individuals.
   d. Plasma concentrations of guanfacine are substantially higher in older individuals.

5. How many days are required for guanfacine to reach steady-state plasma concentrations?
   a. One.
   b. Two.
   c. Three.
   d. Four.

6. Which one of the following statements best describes the development of tolerance to guanfacine therapy?
   a. Tolerance to guanfacine's blood-pressure-lowering effects has not been reported.
   b. The guanfacine dose should always be increased to overcome tolerance.

c. Should tolerance occur it may be overcome by the addition of a diuretic or other antihypertensive agent.
d. Tolerance should be minimized by more frequent drug administration.

7. The withdrawal reaction associated with abrupt discontinuation of therapy

a. Occurs at a higher frequency with guanfacine than with clonidine.
b. Is less severe with guanfacine than with clonidine; this difference may be related to the longer half-life of guanfacine.
c. Is followed by a gradual recovery of pretreatment blood pressure; with guanfacine recovery occurs over a six- to eight-day period.
d. Is similar in severity and frequency of occurrence with guanfacine and clonidine.

8. Administration of guanfacine for several years to patients with essential hypertension has been associated with

a. Reductions in serum cholesterol and triglyceride concentrations.
b. Increases in serum cholesterol and triglyceride concentrations.
c. No change in serum cholesterol or triglyceride concentrations.
d. Reductions in serum triglyceride concentrations but no effect on cholesterol concentrations.

9. The only drug that has been reported to interact with guanfacine is

a. Cimetidine.
b. Phenobarbital.
c. Rifampin.
d. Diazepam.

10. An appropriate starting dose of guanfacine is

a. 3 mg b.i.d.
b. 1 mg daily at bedtime.
c. 2 mg b.i.d.
d. 3 mg daily at bedtime.

FACULTY POSITION
ASSISTANT/ASSOCIATE PROFESSOR
SCHOOL OF PHARMACY
DIVISION OF PHARMACY PRACTICE
UNIVERSITY OF NORTH CAROLINA
AT CHAPEL HILL

The University of North Carolina School of Pharmacy invites applications and nominations for a tenure track faculty position in the Division of Pharmacy Practice. Individuals must possess recognized clinical and research expertise in psychopharmacy. Experience in analytical research methodology will be considered of benefit in evaluation of candidates.

The individual selected will be expected to participate in both undergraduate, graduate, and Pharm.D. student instruction, clinical service at the North Carolina Memorial Hospital, and to conduct scholarly research. The selected individual will also be expected to fulfill certain administrative duties, such as committee participation, with the School of Pharmacy, Department of Psychiatry, and Department of Pharmacy.

Salary and rank will be commensurate with experience and qualifications. Applications will be received until May 1, 1988. Interested candidates shall submit a letter of application, curriculum vitae, and the names and addresses of three references to:

Ralph H. Raasch, Pharm.D.
Associate Professor
School of Pharmacy
CB# 7360, Beard Hall
University of North Carolina
Chapel Hill, NC 27599-7360
(919) 962-0071

Equal Opportunity Employer

Answer sheet

March 1988 ***Clinical Pharmacy***

Note: An enrollment form for the ASHP Continuing Education System appears in the June and December issues. Please accumulate all the answer sheets you wish to use in one enrollment and submit them at one time with a completed enrollment form.

Place an X in the box(es) at the top of the column(s) corresponding to the test(s) you are taking. Darken the boxes corresponding to the correct answers.

☐
680-204-8803
1.0 hour

	a	b	c	d
1.	☐	☐	☐	☐
2.	☐	☐	☐	☐
3.	☐	☐	☐	☐
4.	☐	☐	☐	☐
5.	☐	☐	☐	☐
6.	☐	☐	☐	☐
7.	☐	☐	☐	☐
8.	☐	☐	☐	☐
9.	☐	☐	☐	☐
10.	☐	☐	☐	☐

ASHP Use Only
(1.0)8803________(3)

Current Literature

Drug Reaction Alerts

Drug Reaction Alerts focuses primarily on serious, unlabeled reactions to new chemical entities. The citations are compiled monthly from International Pharmaceutical Abstracts, *which covers over 800 pharmacy and health-related journals worldwide. An address for reprints (when available) follows the name of the corresponding author in each citation.*

Antidiabetic Agents

Goodman RC (Division of Endocrinology and Metabolism, Department of Medicine, Department of Pathology, and Clinical Research Center, University of Tennessee, Memphis, TN 38163), Dean PJ, Radparvar A et al. **Glyburide** induced hepatitis. *Ann Intern Med.* 1987; 106:837–9. Cases. (two women, aged 61 and 63 years; received glyburide 10 mg twice daily for one to four weeks; developed hepatitis-like syndrome; no serologic evidence of viral infection, liver biopsy consistent with drug-induced hepatitis; rapid recovery upon drug withdrawal)

Anti-Infective Agents

Temperley D (Dr. Steevens' Hospital and Trinity College Medical School, Dublin 8, Ireland), Casey E, Connolly R et al. **Vancomycin**-associated lacrimation. *Lancet.* 1987; 2:1337. Case. (49-year-old man with rheumatoid arthritis; received vancomycin 750 mg twice daily for septic arthritis in second right metatarsophalangeal joint; developed profuse tearing within two days of starting vancomyin therapy; patient also developed conjunctivitis but no rash and blood pressure was not altered; patient-blinded placebo administration did not lead to lacrimation; lacrimation ceased when vancomycin was discontinued; positive rechallenge)

Antineoplastic Agents

Weinstein A (New York Medical College, Westchester Medical Center, Valhalla, NY), Bujak D, Mittelman A et al. Erythema nodosum in a patient with renal cell carcinoma treated with **interleukin 2** and lymphokine-activated killer cells. *JAMA.* 1987; 258:3120–1. Case. (26-year-old woman with kidney neoplasm; received interleukin 2 and lymphokine-activated killer cell therapy; concomitant methadone, diazepam, aluminum hydroxide and magnesium hydroxide, merperidine hydrochloride, diphenhydramine hydrochloride, scopolamine, and docusate sodium; developed erythema nodosum; symptoms resolved upon therapy with prednisone 20 mg/day initially and tapered over three weeks; positive rechallenge)

Antiviral agents

Furth PA (University of Maryland Medical School, Box 243, 22 S. Greene Street, Baltimore, MD 21201), Kazakis AM. Nail pigmentation changes associated with azidothymidine **(zidovudine).** *Ann Intern Med.* 1987; 107:350. Cases. (36-year-old black woman and 38-year-old black man with human immunodeficiency viral infection; received zidovudine 20 mg every four hours for two to four weeks for treatment of *Pneumocystis carinii* pneumonia; developed increased pigmentation of toenails and fingernails)

Gill PS (University of Southern California, Norris Cancer Hospital and Research Institute, 1441 Eastlake Avenue, Los Angeles, CA 90003), Rarick M, Brynes RK et al. Azidothymidine associated with bone marrow failure in the acquired immunodeficiency syndrome (AIDS). *Ann Intern Med.* 1987; 107:502–5. Cases. (four men with acquired immunodeficiency syndrome, aged 36–53 years; received **zidovudine** 100–400 mg four times daily for various periods of time; developed severe pancytopenia and bone marrow aplasia; partial bone marrow recovery in three patients within four to five weeks and no recovery in one patient six months after drug withdrawal)

Anti-Inflammatory Agents

Ballesteros JA (Internal Medicine Department, Hospital del Insalud "Son Dureta," 07014 Palma de Mallorca, Spain), Badosa AM, Usandizaga I et al. Hepatotoxicity due to **bendazac.** *Lancet.* 1987; 2:1030–1. Cases. (two women, aged 67 and 76 years; received bendazac 500 mg every eight hours for several months and bendazac 500 mg/day for last three months [reduced from 1.5 g/day], respectively; developed hepatotoxicity; symptoms disappeared and laboratory values returned to normal by three months after drug withdrawal; positive rechallenge in one patient)

Drugs, Adverse Reactions

Barucha C (Belfast City Hospital, Belfast BT9 7AD, Northern Ireland) McMillan JC. Eczema after intravenous infusion of **immunoglobulin.** *Br Med J.* 1987; 295:1141. Case. (75-year-old woman with idiopathic thrombocytopenic purpura; received globulin immune 1 g/kg i.v. every six or seven weeks for three doses; developed eczema; patient treated with systemic hydrocortisone, chlorpheniramine, and topical corticosteroids; eruption faded between first and second doses and between second and third doses of globulin immune; eczema became permanent after third dose of globulin immune)

Drug Interactions

Isley WL (University of Missouri, School of Medicine [Gold 5], 2411 Holmes, Kansas City, MO 61408). Effect of **rifampin** therapy on thyroid function tests in a hypothyroid patient on replacement **L-thyroxine.** *Ann Intern Med.* 1987; 107:517–8. Case. (31-year-old hypothyroid woman; received levothyroxine 0.1 mg/day and rifampin 200 mg every 12 hours for septicemia; concomitant propranolol, hydrochlorothiazide, calcitriol, heparin, and warfarin; developed asymptomatic biochemical hypothyroidism; biochemical parameters improved upon withdrawal of rifampin; positive rechallenge)

Lodwick R (Dudley Road Hospital, Birmingham B18 7QH, England), McConkey B, Brown AM et al. Life-threatening interaction between **tamoxifen** and **warfarin**. *Br Med J.* 1987; 295:1141. Case. (65-year-old woman; received warfarin 27–

28.5 mg/wk for 11 years and tamoxifen 10 mg twice daily for an infiltrating duct carcinoma; developed hemorrhage; prothrombin times returned to normal upon withdrawal of warfarin and therapy with fresh frozen plasma)

Prolactin Inhibitors

Lopez JM (University Catolica de Chile, Casilla 114-D, Santiago, Chile), Fardella CB. **Bromocriptine** therapy and hyperprolactinemia. *Ann Intern Med.* 1987; 106:909–10. Case. (55-year-old man with prolactinoma; received bromocriptine 1.25 mg/day initially; reduction of bromocriptine to 3 mg/day led to 87% reduction in serum prolactin concentration to 600 ng/mL; increase in bromocriptine dosage to 1.25 mg/day decreased serum prolactin concentration to 90 ng/mL)

Book Reviews

Cardiovascular Drug Therapy

Edited by Stephen N. Hunyor.

Published by Williams & Wilkins and Associates PTY Limited, 404 Sydney Road, Balgowlah, NSW 2093, Australia, 1987. Available from Williams & Wilkins, 428 East Preston St., Baltimore, MD 21202. 309 p. Price $60.

This book contains an exhaustive 33 separate chapters on a variety of cardiovascular topics. A number of the chapters focus on topics not usually covered in a traditional therapeutics or pharmacology text. The flavor of this book is truly international, with only 3 of 42 authors affiliated with institutions in the United States. Most of the authors are from the United Kingdom and Australia. In addition, this book is directed solely at the clinical use of cardiac drugs.

The initial entries in the book include the common topics of how to manage angina pectoris, acute myocardial infarction, cardiac failure, cardiac arrhythmias, peripheral vascular disease, valvular heart disease, cardiomyopathies, hypertension, hypotension, and hyperlipidemias. Following these chapters are discussions of the major classes of cardiac drugs, such as acetylcholinesterase inhibitors, digitalis and other positive inotropics, diuretics, β blockers, α blockers, anticoagulants, and calcium antagonists. Interspersed among these chapters are less traditional reviews on the use of drugs in circulatory arrest, drugs after myocardial infarction, coronary artery spasm, adjunctive medical therapy to percutaneous transluminal coronary angioplasty, drug therapy during and after cardiac surgery, cardiac pacing, when to stop cardiac drugs, and cardiovascular iatrogenic disease and drug interactions.

The major advantage of this book lies in the large variety of topics covered in addition to those nontraditional ones already mentioned; also, the topics are covered succinctly, with most chapters being less than 10 pages.

The major disadvantage of the text is the fact that specific recommendations are not referenced. At the end of each chapter, three to five general references are listed as suggested reading; hence, the reader is left with the sense that recommendations of the authors reflect personal opinion rather than literature-based facts.

I see this book as having its greatest utility for individuals with some background or training in cardiovascular diseases who are looking for texts to help update their knowledge of cardiac drug therapy. Physicians, pharmacists, nurses, and other allied health professionals with some understanding of cardiac drugs will appreciate this disease-state-based overview of cardiovascular therapy. This is a clinically oriented text. Those looking for detailed pharmacologic information would be better advised to look elsewhere.

Reviewed by Daniel E. Hilleman, Pharm.D., Creighton Cardiac Center, 601 North 30th Street, Omaha, NE 68131

Drug Treatment of the Rheumatic Diseases, Third Edition

Edited by Frank Dudley Hart.

Published by Williams & Wilkins and Associates PTY Limited, Balgowlah, Australia, 1987. Available from Williams & Wilkins, 428 East Preston St., Baltimore, MD 21202. x + 229 p. Price $48.

This edition of *Drug Treatment of the Rheumatic Diseases* retains the same format and authors as the previous edition. The first portion of this book discusses the pharmacologic properties, indications, adverse effects, and drug interactions of antirheumatic drugs, including a number of drugs not currently approved in the United States such as flurbiprofen, fenbufen, tiaprofenic acid, flufenamic acid, diclofenac, isoxicam, tenoxicam, orgotein, and levamisole. The second portion reviews management considerations of the more common rheumatic disorders, such as rheumatoid arthritis, osteoarthritis, gouty arthritis, seronegative spondylarthritides, polymyalgia rheumatica/giant cell arteritis, systemic lupus erythematosus, vasculitic syndromes, dermatomyositis/polymyositis, progressive systemic sclerosis, infective arthropathies, rheumatic fever, and juvenile rheumatoid arthritis. As an overview, this book succeeds in concisely summarizing a vast amount of information.

The stated goal of this textbook, "helping the clinician in the decision-making process of which drug to use," is laudable but not realized. The very scope of the subject matter reviewed preordains failure when the text limits the discussion of any one disease state to less than 10 pages. By necessity, only a selective overview of therapeutic strategies is possible, and application to individual patients is limited. For the practitioner lacking an extensive background in the pathophysiology of these disorders, an appropriate awareness of the empiric nature of drug treatment, and the controversy associated with the use of some treatments, this book is insufficient as a sole source of information on drug therapy of rheumatic disease.

Perhaps this text's greatest asset lies in its contributing authors who, for the most part, were trained in and who practice in the United Kingdom. The content of the textbook reflects the collective experiences and perceptions of practitioners from a different economic climate and health-care system. For the practitioner trained in the United States, this book reveals a number of differences in the approach to treatment of rheumatic diseases. For example, in this country, aspirin is still considered the nonsteroidal drug of choice for initiating treatment in rheumatoid arthritis. In the United Kingdom, the "modern nonsteroidal anti-inflammatory drugs naproxen, piroxicam, and diclofenac" are considered the anti-inflammatory drugs of choice. Penicillamine enjoys the status of being the preferred second-line agent for rheumatoid arthritis in the United Kingdom, whereas most rheumatologists in the United States prefer gold therapy. There appears to be much less enthusiasm for methotrexate in the United Kingdom compared with its rather broad-based acceptance in the United States.

Although the information contained in this book is available in standard rheumatology, pharmacology, and drug information texts that are readily available in most libraries and drug information centers, practitioners wishing to compare and contrast their experiences in managing rheumatic disorders with their United Kingdom counterparts may find this book to be a useful supplement to these standard references.

Reviewed by Stephen L. Dahl, Pharm.D., University of Missouri–Kansas City Schools of Medicine and Pharmacy, UMKC School of Medicine, 2411 Holmes Street, Kansas City, MO 64108-2792.

Pharmacokinetics and Pharmacodynamics: Research and Analysis

Edited by Randall B. Smith, Patricia D. Kroboth, and Randy P. Juhl.

Published by Harvey Whitney Books, 4906 Cooper Road, P.O. Box 42696, Cincinnati, OH 45242, 1986. viii + 103 p. Price $8.

This book is a presentation of a symposium held at the University of Pittsburgh May 16–17, 1985. The presenters providing chapters to this text are well-known researchers in the areas that they discuss. In general, the text is well written and concise.

Each topic covered in this book is supported both by theoretical considerations and by practical examples from the literature. Designs of clinical trials intended to establish the link between pharmacokinetics and pharmacodynamics are presented with an acceptable balance of idealism and practicality. Examples of difficult clinical study designs, patient-recruitment problems, and practical equations are provided. Particularly broad-reaching examples are provided for the researcher who has ever had to "justify" a study designed to examine the association between pharmacokinetics and pharmacodynamics. Some hard-core analytical presentations, such as the equation required for modeling and NONMEM application, are also included.

By the time most individuals receive this text, almost three years will have elapsed since the symposium was held. This is an unfortunate reality regarding textbook information as opposed to periodical literature. Also on the negative side is an obvious editorial blunder in a figure, on page 44, in which numerical labels of EC50 have been inadvertently misplaced. (This is the only such error that I found.)

Although none of the information provided in this book is truly new, the book's most positive attribute is that it is one of the most complete compilations of such specialized knowledge of which I am aware. Until more consistent pharmacologic measures are available for all drugs, analysts in this field must learn from other researchers' experiences. This book is replete with important examples, along with excellent supporting theories. For these reasons, it is a useful addition to a pharmacokineticist's library.

Reviewed by David A. Graves, Pharm.D., Clinical Pharmacology Department, Pennwalt Corporation, 755 Jefferson Road, Rochester, NY 14623.

Pharmacology in Medicine: Principles and Practice

Edited by Sachin N. Pradhan, Roger P. Maickel, and Samar N. Dutta.

Published by SP Press International Inc., 7806 Honeybee Court, Bethesda, MD 20817, 1986. xii + 1087 p. Price $55 (U.S.), $71.50 (Canada).

This book covers the principles of pharmacology in 121 chapters that are divided among seven sections. Each chapter begins with a brief outline to give the reader a sense of the major points that will be addressed by the chapter authors. There are 60 coauthors, so any attempt to standardize the format of the chapters would have been largely impossible.

The 75-page introductory section includes a history of pharmacology and related federal drug regulations and general principles of pharmacokinetics, pharmacodynamics, and toxicology. However, discussion of pharmacokinetic parameters is divided between this introductory portion and the only appendix in the textbook. It might have been more appropriate to include the narrative portion of the five-page appendix within the introductory section to facilitate the reader's understanding of this important area of pharmacology.

The third chapter, entitled "Pharmacodynamic Aspects of Drug Action," presents an excellent discussion of dose–response relationships and theories of drug action and antagonism. In this chapter, as well as in many others throughout the textbook, the principles are well illustrated with bold, legible figures and tables. Differences in the responsiveness of individuals to drugs are addressed in a short special chapter, entitled "Pharmacogenetics and Toxicogenetics." One small point that is disturbing to me in this chapter is the discussion of the differences in tissue cholinesterase. The dibucaine test for the evaluation of patients with atypical forms of serum cholinesterase is mentioned here and in another chapter (in section two on depolarizing neuromuscular blocking agents), but a concise description of the test or a literature reference to the procedure is never offered anywhere in the text. This omission, although troublesome, is not surprising because most pharmacology textbooks fail to mention the dibucaine test.

In section two, drug actions on both peripheral and central neuronal systems are thoroughly described, beginning with the fundamentals of autonomic and neuromuscular pharmacology and ending with therapy of central nervous system disorders and the problems associated with substance abuse. Section three is devoted to the actions of drugs on the hormone systems, kinins, the immune system, and vitamins.

Section four continues the organ-system approach to pharmacology initiated in the previous section, starting with the circulatory system, progressing to respiratory and alimentary systems, and concluding with chapters on the special sensory systems—the ocular, auditory and vestibular, and olfactory senses. In some chapters there is no mention of investigational drugs. For example, experimental antihypertensive agents such as the serotonin-2 receptor blockers currently in clinical trials do not appear in this section, although investigational drugs are included in the discussion of hypolipidemic and antiarrhythmic agents. The physiology and pharmacology of the kidney are reasonably clear; however, it is unfortunate that the diuretic agents are classified as major and minor in terms of their clinical usefulness since this classification might be confused with the concept of diuretic efficacy (in other words, there are clinically useful—i.e., major—diuretics with relatively low diuretic efficacy).

Section five is devoted to all forms of chemotherapy and contains a comprehensive review of various categories, including therapies for sexually transmitted diseases. However, the discussion of viral venereal diseases does not provide any information on the acquired immunodeficiency syndrome (AIDS).

The chapters on chemotherapy of neoplastic diseases and interactive effects of radiation and drugs provide a comprehensive review of the state of knowledge in these areas. The chapters on environmental pollutants review the risks associated with inappropriate exposure to chemicals found in a home environment and list appropriate treatments for acute poisonings. Industrial and agricultural chemicals and their toxicities after accidental exposure are documented.

In the final section of the textbook the authors deal with what is referred to as special areas of pharmacology, e.g., pediatric and geriatric pharmacology, adverse drug reactions, and treatment of acute poisoning. The first two chapters in this section would be helpful in selecting the proper dosages for patients at the upper and lower ends of the age spectrum. These are areas in which more information is needed for the practice of pharmacy, and the authors have provided some specific examples. On the other hand, the chapter on adverse drug reactions gives the impression of being too superficial. Less prose and more presentation of examples would help the reader to quickly digest the practical information that should be included in this chapter.

Overall, the authors have done a good job in assembling the principles and practices of pharmacology in a 1087-page textbook.

Reviewed by Jon W. Banning, Ph.D., Department of Pharmaceutical Sciences, College of Pharmacy and Allied Health Professions, Wayne State University, 105 Shapiro Hall, Detroit, MI 48202.

Problems in Pediatric Drug Therapy, Second Edition

Edited by Louis A. Pagliaro and Ann M. Pagliaro.

Published by Drug Intelligence Publications, Inc., 1241 Broadway, Hamilton, IL 62341, 1987. xii + 674 p. Price $38.50.

Problems in Pediatric Drug Therapy is a well-referenced compilation of data concerning the use and effects of drugs in the fetus, infant, and child. It is useful for health-care professionals who specialize in pediatrics and for those who do not have extensive backgrounds in pediatrics and only occasionally need pediatric drug information. The book's editors, contributing authors, and Pediatric Advisory Committee are multidisciplinary, a fact that has increased the book's practicality for nurses and physicians as well as for pharmacists.

A major change in this edition is the expansion of the handbook from 6 to 10 chapters to include material on drug administration, drug interactions, intravenous medications, and immunizations. Chapters updated and expanded from the first edition cover human teratogens, drugs excreted in human milk, pediatric poisoning, adverse drug reactions, drug dosing in neonates, and drug dosing in infants and children. The drug dosing tables are comprehensive and include information about many recently marketed drugs, such as the newer cephalosporins. A useful addition to the book is the table entitled "Intravenous Medication Guidelines," which lists drug name, pH, initial reconstituting diluent and dilution, methods of administration, further dilution, recommended rate of infusion, compatible infusion solutions, cautions, and incompatibilities. The index is detailed, and the reader can rapidly and easily find needed information.

This book has no information on resuscitation, such as a table on emergency drug doses, nor does it include pediatric neonatal pharmacokinetic data or information about extemporaneous formulation of oral liquids from solid dosage forms. However, it might cease to be a "handbook" if it were all-inclusive. It should be used in conjunction with other frequently used resources on pediatric drug therapy, such as *The Harriet Lane Handbook*, *The Pediatric Drug Handbook*, *The Pocketbook of Pediatric Antimicrobial Therapy*, *Drug Therapy in Infants*, and *The Handbook on Extemporaneous Formulations*.

Reviewed by Karin E. Zenk, Pharm.D., Department of Pharmacy, University of California Irvine Medical Center, 101 City Drive South, Orange, CA 92668.

Books Received

Books are listed as received; selected books may be reviewed in Book Reviews in subsequent issues.

The Merck Manual, Fifteenth Edition, Robert Berkow, Editor-in-Chief. Published by Merck Sharp & Dohme Research Laboratories, Rahway, NJ 07065-0900, 1987. xxvii + 2696 p. Price $21.50.

Tropical Diseases: A Therapeutic Update, edited by P. F. D'Arcy and D.W.G. Harron. Published by F.I.P. Publications, Alexanderstraat 11, 2514 JL The Hague, The Netherlands, 1987. 82 p. Price $10, Dutch fl.20, U.K. £5.00, plus postage.

Advertising Index

American Society of Hospital Pharmacists
Clinical Pharmacy, 183
Beecham Laboratories
Ticar, 186
Timentin, 170–172
Eli Lilly and Company
Tazidime, 167–168
Merieux Institute, Inc.
Multitest CMI, 185
Roxane Laboratories, A Boehringer Ingelheim Company
Intensols, 165
Marinol, inside back cover, outside back cover
E. R. Squibb & Sons, Inc.
Azactam, 177–180
Stuart Pharmaceuticals, Division of ICI Americas, Inc.
Cefotan, 173–175
University of North Carolina-Chapel Hill
Positions Available, 242
The Upjohn Company
Cleocin, 181–182
Wyeth Laboratories
Tubex, inside front cover

News

Record number of orphan drug designations granted in 1987

Designation of 58 biologicals and drugs as orphan drug products during 1987 brought to 183 the total number of orphan designations. Last year's total was the highest annual total since the Orphan Drug Act was passed in 1983. Product names, sponsors, and designated uses of the 1987 orphan drug products are listed in the following table. The list of products is updated quarterly and a cumulative list is published annually in the *Federal Register*.

Primary prevention study finds cardiovascular benefit with aspirin therapy

A report from the Physicians' Health Study Research Group provides preliminary evidence that aspirin, given at a dose of 325 mg on alternate days, may reduce the incidence of fatal and nonfatal myocardial infarctions in men.[1] Significant differences between the aspirin and placebo groups led to early termination of the component of the study evaluating aspirin for primary preven-

1987 Orphan Drug Designations[a]

Agent (Sponsor)	Designated Use
Biologicals	
Anti-TAP-72 immunotoxin (XOMA Corporation, San Francisco, CA)	Treatment of metastatic colorectal cancer (adenocarcinoma)
Benzylpenicillin, benzylpenicilloic acid, and benzylpenilloic acid (Kremers-Urban Co.)	Penicillin allergy testing (major and minor determinants)
CD5 T-lymphocyte immunotoxin (XOMA Corporation)	Treatment of graft-versus-host disease or rejection in bone-marrow transplant recipients
Cytomegalovirus immune globulin, human (Massachusetts Public Health Biologic Laboratories)	Prevention or attenuation of primary cytomegalovirus disease in immunosuppressed organ-transplant recipients
Erythropoietin, human, recombinant (McDonnell Douglas Corporation, St. Louis, MO; Ortho Pharmaceutical; Chugai Pharmaceutical Co., Ltd., Japan; and Organon Teknika Corporation, Durham, NC)	Treatment of anemia associated with end-stage renal disease
Interferon alfa-n1 (Burroughs Wellcome Co.)	Treatment of human papillomavirus in patients with severe or recurrent respiratory (laryngeal) papillomatosis
Interferon alfa-2a, recombinant (Hoffmann-La Roche, Inc.)	Treatment of AIDS-related Kaposi's sarcoma
Interferon alfa-2b, recombinant (Schering Corporation)	Treatment of chronic myelogenous leukemia, metastatic renal cell carcinoma, AIDS-related Kaposi's sarcoma, and ovarian carcinoma
Iodine I 131 Lym-1 monoclonal antibody (Lederle Laboratories)	Treatment of B cell lymphoma
ST1-RTA immunotoxin (Sanofi, Inc., New York, NY)	Use in the prevention of acute graft-versus-host disease in allogenic bone-marrow transplantation Treatment of B chronic lymphocytic leukemia
Technetium Tc 99m antimelanoma antibody kit (NeoRx Corporation, Seattle, WA)	Use in detection (by imaging) of metastases of malignant melanoma
Trisaccharides A and B (Chembiomed Ltd., Edmonton, Alberta, Canada)	Treatment of moderate to severe forms of neonatal hemolytic disease caused by placental transfer of antibodies against blood group substances A and B Use in ABO-incompatible organ transplantation Treatment of moderate to very severe transfusion reactions caused by transfusion of ABO incompatible blood, blood products, or blood derivatives
Drugs	
Acetylcysteine, i.v. (Bristol-Myers Company)	Management of moderate to severe acetaminophen overdoses
Allopurinol (Burroughs Wellcome Co.)	Use in ex vivo preservation of cadaveric kidneys for transplantation
AS 101 (Scientific Testing, Inc., New Brunswick, NJ)	Treatment of AIDS
Baclofen, intrathecal (Medtronics, Inc., Minneapolis, MN)	Treatment of intractable spasticity caused by spinal cord injury or multiple sclerosis

Continued

1987 Orphan Drug Designations *(continued)*

Agent (Sponsor)	Designated Use
BW 12C (Burroughs Wellcome)	Treatment of sickle cell disease crisis
Calcitonin, human (Ciba-Geigy Corp.)	Treatment of symptomatic Paget's disease of bone
Copolymer 1 (TAG Pharmaceuticals, Sellersville, PA)	Treatment of multiple sclerosis
Dantrolene sodium (Norwich Eaton Pharmaceuticals)	Treatment of neuroleptic malignant syndrome
Dextran sulfate sodium (Ueno Fine Chemicals Industry, Ltd., Japan)	Treatment of AIDS
Epidermal growth factor, human (Ethicon, Inc., Somerville, NJ)	Promotion of cutaneous wound healing in extreme burns
Ifosfamide (Bristol-Myers)	Treatment of testicular cancer
Luteinizing hormone releasing hormone (LHRH), (Roberts Laboratories, Inc., Eatontown, NJ)	Treatment of central precocious puberty
LHRH (Ortho Pharmaceutical)	Use in the induction of ovulation in women with hypothalamic amenorrhea caused by deficient or abnormal secretion of LHRH
Mefloquine (Mephra AG, Switzerland)	Treatment and prevention of chloroquine-resistant falciparum malaria
Mesna (Adria Laboratories Inc.)	Inhibition of urotoxic effects of oxazaphosphorine compounds (e.g., cyclophosphamide)
Metronidazole, topical	
(Curatek Pharmaceuticals, Inc.)	Treatment of acne rosacea
(G.D. Searle & Company)	Treatment of grade III and IV anaerobically infected decubitus ulcers
Morphine sulfate concentrate, preservative free (Elkins-Sinn, Inc.)	For administration via microinfusion devices in repeated doses or by constant infusion, for epidural use when systemic analgesic therapy is ineffective or epidural therapy is considered preferable, and for intrathecal use in patients with refractory cancer pain
Pentamidine isethionate, by inhalation (Fisons Corporation)	Prevention of *Pneumocystis carinii* pneumonia in patients at high risk
Pentostatin (Warner-Lambert Company)	Treatment of hairy cell leukemia
Piracetam (U.S.B., Secteur Pharmaceutique, Belgium)	Treatment of myoclonus
Sodium oxybate (Biocraft Laboratories, Inc., Elmwood Park, NJ)	Treatment of narcolepsy and the auxiliary symptoms of cataplexy, sleep paralysis, hypnagogic hallucinations, and autonomic behavior
Somatropin	
(Saizen, Serno Laboratories Inc., Randolph, MA)	Treatment of idiopathic or organic growth hormone deficiency in children with growth failure
(Protropin II, Genentech, Inc.)	Long-term treatment of children who have growth failure due to inadequate growth hormone secretion
(Norditropin, Nordisk-USA)	Treatment of growth failure in children due to inadequate growth hormone secretion
	For adjunctive use in the induction of ovulation in women with infertility due to (1) hypogonadotropic hypogonadism and (2) bilateral tubal occlusion or unexplained infertility, who are undergoing in vivo fertilization procedures or in vitro fertilization with embryo transfer procedures, respectively, who fail to ovulate in response to gonadotropic therapy alone
	For use in the treatment of short stature associated with Turner's syndrome
Surfactant, human, amniotic-fluid derived (T. Allen Merritt, UCSD Medical Center)	Prevention and treatment of neonatal respiratory distress syndrome
Teriparatide (Rorer Group, Inc.)	Use in establishing a diagnosis in patients with clinical and laboratory evidence of hypocalcemia caused by either hypoparathyroidism or pseudohypoparathyroidism
Thymoxamine hydrochloride (C.Y.C. Pak, M.D., University of Texas Health Science Center, Dallas)	Use in the prevention of cystine nephrolithiasis in patients with homozygous cystinuria
Tranexamic acid (Kabi Vitrum, Inc.)	Treatment of patients undergoing prostatectomy complicated by hemorrhage or risk of hemorrhage as a result of increased fibrinolysis or fibrinogenolysis
Urofollitropin (Serono Laboratories, Inc.)	For use in induction of ovulation in patients with polycystic ovarian disease who have an elevated LH-to-FSH ratio and have not responded to clomiphene
4-Aminopyridine (Rush–Presbyterian–St. Luke's Medical Center, Chicago, IL)	Relief of symptoms of multiple sclerosis
5-Aza-2′-deoxycytidine (Pharmachemie B.V., Holland)	Treatment of acute leukemia
2′,3′-Dideoxyadenosine (National Cancer Institute)	Treatment of AIDS
24,25-Dihydroxycholecalciferol (Lemmon Company–TAG Pharmaceuticals)	Treatment of uremic osteodystrophy

[a] Adapted from *Fed Regist.* 1988; 53:2680–8.

Continued on page 260

More active *in vitro** than traditional antianaerobic agents

Activity Against Clinical Isolates of *B fragilis* Group[2]		
Antibiotic	MIC_{50} (μg/mL)	MIC_{90} (μg/mL)
TIMENTIN†	≤1	4
Cefoxitin	8	32
Cefoperazone	32	128
Chloramphenicol	8	8
Clindamycin	0.5	8
Metronidazole	1	2

**In vitro* activity does not necessarily imply *in vivo* efficacy.
†Ticarcillin in the presence of a constant 2 μg/mL clavulanic acid.

More active *in vitro** than cefoxitin

Activity Against *B fragilis* Group[3]		
Organism (No. strains)	MIC_{90} (μg/mL) TIMENTIN†	Cefoxitin
B fragilis (32)	0.5	16
B vulgatus (21)	1	16
B thetaiotaomicron (19)	2	32
B ovatus (16)	1	32
B distasonis (13)	8	64

**In vitro* activity does not necessarily imply *in vivo* efficacy.
†Ticarcillin in the presence of a constant 1 μg/mL clavulanic acid.

Destroys β-lactamases that limit the usefulness of other β-lactam choices

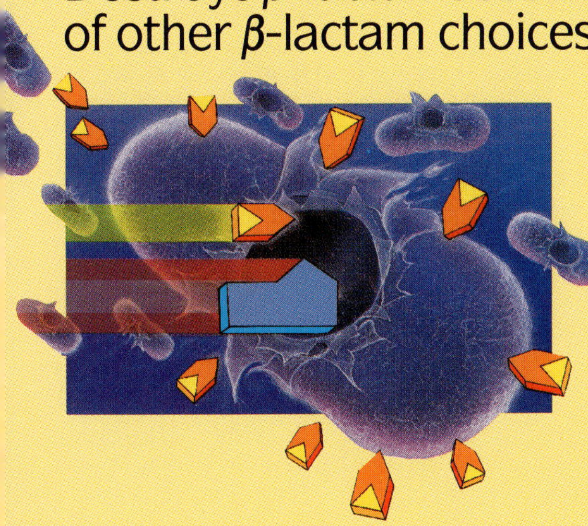

- "Most (90 percent) strains of B. fragilis produce constitutive beta-lactamases, which are primarily cephalosporinases. All other Bacteroides species probably produce beta-lactamases, but controversy exists concerning whether the enzymes are predominantly penicillinases or cephalosporinases."[4]
- "[Clavulanate potassium] inhibits the beta-lactamases of most Bacteroides species."[4]

△ Clavulanate potassium destroys ▶ most β-lactamases produced by Gram-positive and Gram-negative aerobes and anaerobes.
TIMENTIN destroys a broad range of aerobic and anaerobic bacteria regardless of β-lactamase production.

FOR ANAEROBIC CERTAINTY

TIMENTIN®

ticarcillin disodium/ clavulanate potassium

The unsurpassed β-lactam choice

Usual Dosage: 3.1 g every 4 to 6 hours.

Please see next page for brief summary of prescribing information.

THE CLAVULANATES Beecham laboratories
BRISTOL, TENNESSEE 37620

© 1988, Beecham Laboratories.

BRIEF SUMMARY OF PRESCRIBING INFORMATION

TIMENTIN®

sterile ticarcillin disodium and clavulanate potassium
for Intravenous Administration

INDICATIONS AND USAGE: TIMENTIN® is indicated in the treatment of infections caused by susceptible strains of the designated organisms in the conditions listed below:

Bacterial Septicemia: including bacteremia, caused by β-lactamase producing strains of *Klebsiella* spp., *E. coli, Staphylococcus aureus* and *Pseudomonas aeruginosa* (and other *Pseudomonas* species).

Lower Respiratory Infections: caused by β-lactamase producing strains of *Staphylococcus aureus, Hemophilus influenzae* and *Klebsiella* spp.

Bone and Joint Infections: caused by β-lactamase producing strains of *Staphylococcus aureus*.

Skin and Skin Structure Infections: caused by β-lactamase producing strains of *Staphylococcus aureus, Klebsiella* spp., and *E. coli*.

Urinary Tract Infections (complicated and uncomplicated): caused by β-lactamase producing strains of *E. coli, Klebsiella* spp., *Pseudomonas aeruginosa* (and other *Pseudomonas* species), *Citrobacter* spp., *Enterobacter cloacae, Serratia marcescens*, and *Staphylococcus aureus*. While TIMENTIN is indicated only for the conditions listed above, infections caused by ticarcillin susceptible organisms are also amenable to TIMENTIN treatment due to its ticarcillin content. Therefore, mixed infections caused by ticarcillin susceptible organisms and β-lactamase producing organisms susceptible to TIMENTIN should not require the addition of another antibiotic.

Appropriate culture and susceptibility tests should be performed before treatment in order to isolate and identify organisms causing infection and to determine their susceptibility to TIMENTIN. Because of its broad spectrum of bactericidal activity against Gram-positive and Gram-negative bacteria, TIMENTIN is particularly useful for the treatment of mixed infections and for presumptive therapy prior to the identification of the causative organisms. TIMENTIN has been shown to be effective as single drug therapy in the treatment of some serious infections where normally combination antibiotic therapy might be employed. Therapy with TIMENTIN may be initiated before results of such tests are known when there is reason to believe the infection may involve any of the β-lactamase producing organisms listed above; however, once these results become available, appropriate therapy should be continued.

Based on the *in vitro* synergism between TIMENTIN and aminoglycosides against certain strains of *Pseudomonas aeruginosa*, combined therapy has been successful, especially in patients with impaired host defenses. Both drugs should be used in full therapeutic doses. As soon as results of culture and susceptibility tests become available, antimicrobial therapy should be adjusted as indicated.

CONTRAINDICATIONS: TIMENTIN is contraindicated in patients with a history of hypersensitivity reactions to any of the penicillins.

WARNINGS: SERIOUS AND OCCASIONALLY FATAL HYPERSENSITIVITY (ANAPHYLACTOID) REACTIONS HAVE BEEN REPORTED IN PATIENTS ON PENICILLIN THERAPY. THESE REACTIONS ARE MORE LIKELY TO OCCUR IN INDIVIDUALS WITH A HISTORY OF PENICILLIN HYPERSENSITIVITY AND/OR A HISTORY OF SENSITIVITY TO MULTIPLE ALLERGENS. THERE HAVE BEEN REPORTS OF INDIVIDUALS WITH A HISTORY OF PENICILLIN HYPERSENSITIVITY WHO HAVE EXPERIENCED SEVERE REACTIONS WHEN TREATED WITH CEPHALOSPORINS. BEFORE INITIATING THERAPY WITH TIMENTIN, CAREFUL INQUIRY SHOULD BE MADE CONCERNING PREVIOUS HYPERSENSITIVITY REACTIONS TO PENICILLINS, CEPHALOSPORINS, OR OTHER DRUGS. IF AN ALLERGIC REACTION OCCURS, TIMENTIN SHOULD BE DISCONTINUED AND THE APPROPRIATE THERAPY INSTITUTED. **SERIOUS ANAPHYLACTOID REACTIONS REQUIRE IMMEDIATE EMERGENCY TREATMENT WITH EPINEPHRINE. OXYGEN, INTRAVENOUS STEROIDS, AND AIRWAY MANAGEMENT, INCLUDING INTUBATION, SHOULD ALSO BE PROVIDED AS INDICATED.**

PRECAUTIONS: While TIMENTIN possesses the characteristic low toxicity of the penicillin group of antibiotics, organ system functions should be assessed periodically during therapy.

Bleeding manifestations have occurred in some patients receiving β-lactam antibiotics. These reactions have been associated with abnormalities of coagulation tests such as clotting time, platelet aggregation and prothrombin time and are more likely to occur in patients with renal impairment. If bleeding manifestations appear, TIMENTIN treatment should be discontinued and appropriate therapy instituted.

TIMENTIN has only rarely been reported to cause hypokalemia. Periodic monitoring of serum potassium may be advisable in patients receiving prolonged therapy.

Pregnancy (Category B): Reproduction studies have been performed in rats given doses up to 1050 mg/kg/day and have revealed no evidence of impaired fertility or harm to the fetus due to TIMENTIN. There are, however, no adequate and well-controlled studies in pregnant women. Because animal reproduction studies are not always predictive of human response, this drug should be used during pregnancy only if clearly needed.

DOSAGE AND ADMINISTRATION: TIMENTIN should be administered by intravenous infusion (30 min.). Usual recommended dose for systemic and urinary tract infections for average (60 kg) adults is 3.1 Gm TIMENTIN (3.1 Gm vial containing 3 Gm ticarcillin and 100 mg clavulanic acid) given every 4 to 6 hours. In urinary tract infections, a dosage of 3.2 Gm TIMENTIN (3.2 Gm vial containing 3 Gm ticarcillin and 200 mg clavulanic acid) given every 8 hours is adequate. Please see official package insert for details on dosages for other patients, including those with renal insufficiency, and directions for use.

SUPPLIED: 3.1 Gm and 3.2 Gm Standard Vials; 3.1 Gm and 3.2 Gm Piggyback Bottles: 31 Gm Bulk Pharmacy Package: 3.1 Gm ADD-Vantage™ Antibiotic Vial.

7548/E-BS

References

1. Cuchural GJ, Tally FP, Jacobus NV, et al: Susceptibility of Bacteroides fragilis group clinical isolates to newer beta-lactam drugs, abstract No. 1B8. Presented to the 3rd Panamerican Congress of Infectious Diseases and Chemotherapy, San Juan, Puerto Rico, Dec 9-13, 1986.
2. Barry AL, Jones RN, Packer RR: *In vitro* susceptibility of the *Bacteroides fragilis* group to cefoperazone, ampicillin, ticarcillin, and amoxycillin combined with β-lactamase inhibitors. *J Antimicrob Chemother* 1986;17:125-127.
3. Bourgault AM, Lamothe F: In-vitro activity of amoxycillin and ticarcillin in combination with clavulanic acid compared with that of new β-lactam agents against species of the *Bacteroides fragilis* group. *J Antimicrob Chemother* 1986;17:593-603.
4. Neu HC: Contribution of beta-lactamases to bacterial resistance and mechanisms to inhibit beta-lactamases. *Am J Med* 1985;79(suppl 5B):2-12.

Beecham laboratories
BRISTOL, TENNESSEE 37620
© 1988, Beecham Laboratories.

News *Continued from page 254*

tion of myocardial infarction; the good cardiovascular health of the study participants (cardiovascular mortality rate approximately 12% of the expected rate) also meant that obtaining definitive data on cardiovascular mortality by the scheduled close of the trial was unlikely. The ongoing portion of the study tests whether administration of β carotene decreases the incidence of cancer.

The study group consisted of 22,071 male physicians 40 to 84 years of age in 1982 who had no personal history of myocardial infarction, stroke, transient ischemic attacks, or cancer; no current liver or renal disease, peptic ulcer disease, or gout; no contraindications to the use of aspirin; and no current use of aspirin, nonsteroidal anti-inflammatory agents, other platelet-active drugs, or vitamin A supplements.

The risk of myocardial infarction was 47% lower with aspirin therapy after an average follow-up time of 57 months. The risk of stroke was 15% higher (nonsignificant increase) among aspirin recipients. Inclusion of nonfatal myocardial infarctions and strokes and cardiovascular deaths in the risk-to-benefit analysis showed that risk was 23% lower with aspirin therapy. The difference in the incidences of gastrointestinal distress for the two study groups was 0.6%. A prerandomization run-in phase helped exclude individuals who would not comply with or tolerate aspirin therapy. The investigators concluded that decisions on the use of aspirin for primary prevention of cardiovascular disease must be individualized, taking into account the demonstrated benefits and well-recognized risks of aspirin therapy.

The study provides important preliminary information on a new role for aspirin. In the precisely defined study population, clear benefits were evident. However, questions remain as to the relative benefits and safety of therapy in the general population.

1. The Steering Committee of the Physicians' Health Study Research Group. Preliminary report: findings from the aspirin component of the ongoing Physicians' Health Study. *N Engl J Med*. 1988; 318:262–4.

Panel cites deficiencies in cholesterol testing, urges national laboratory standardization

Considerable improvement in the reliability of blood cholesterol determinations performed by clinical laboratories is needed if efforts to identify and treat individuals at high risk of coronary heart disease are to be successful; this was the conclusion of the Laboratory Standardization Panel of the National Cholesterol Education Program, sponsored by the National Heart, Lung, and Blood Institute. The report, issued in January 1988, identifies the levels of precision and accuracy deemed by the panel to be acceptable and provides general recommendations for standardization of cholesterol measurements.

The panel urged adoption of the concentration-defined categories of risk proposed in the October 1987 report of the Expert Panel on Detection, Evaluation, and

Continued on page 263

News *Continued from page 260*

Treatment of High Blood Cholesterol in Adults. Acceptance of this recommendation would require national standardization of cholesterol measurements and use of reliable analytical methods.

A survey cited in the panel's report found that approximately one half of cholesterol values reported by clinical laboratories participating in the survey deviated from the true concentration value by more than 5%. Deviation by 5% is currently recommended by the panel, with reduction to 3% within five years. Precision (reproducibility) appears to be less of a problem. A degree of precision consistent with a coefficient of variation of 5% was also recommended by the panel; a level of 3% or less is the eventual goal.

Although preliminary studies indicate that some of the new portable analyzers are comparable in accuracy and precision to analyzers used in large clinical laboratories, further evaluation of these instruments was deemed necessary before they could be recommended for routine use in clinical practice.

The panel members stated that, in an effort to standardize cholesterol measurements by clinical laboratories throughout the United States, cholesterol values should be traceable to the reference method of the Centers for Disease Control or the definitive method of the National Bureau of Standards. Specific changes in analytical techniques will be addressed in a second report.

Study shows photoaged skin improves with topical tretinoin

Short-term topical application of tretinoin can improve skin color and the wrinkling and roughness associated with chronic sun exposure, according to results of a 16-week randomized, double-blind, vehicle-controlled study of 30 caucasian subjects 35 to 70 years of age.[1] Phase III studies of the effects of topical tretinoin on photodamaged skin are under way at six medical centers in the United States.

All study participants had a clinical diagnosis of dermatoheliosis of the face and forearms. Subjects applied either 0.1% tretinoin cream or placebo vehicle cream once nightly to the face and left forearm; the alternate treatment was applied to the right forearm.

All tretinoin-treated forearms, but none of the vehicle-treated forearms, showed improvement in fine wrinkling and increased pinkness. Roughness and coarse wrinkling were significantly different between the two treatments; however, the extent of improvement in these two variables generally was less, and improvements were noted in fewer patients. Facial skin also improved, but the extent of change was less than that with forearm skin. Histologic changes were noted in tretinoin-treated areas only. Almost all patients experienced some degree of dermatitis with treatment, but clinical improvements could not be attributed to edematous changes. Longer studies will be needed to determine whether the histologic changes and clinical improvements persist.

1. Weiss JS, Ellis CN, Headington JT et al. Topical tretinoin improves photoaged skin: a double-blind vehicle-controlled study. *JAMA*. 1988; 259:527–32.

Continued on page 264

ANNOUNCING

A Decision Model for the Treatment of Cancer Pain

A Software Diskette and Continuing Education Program to Help in Assessment and Management of Cancer Pain

Developed by: Charles S. Cleeland, PhD, and Armando Rotondi, MS, Pain Research Group, University of Wisconsin-Madison. Based on research conducted under Grant CA-26582 of the National Cancer Institute.

Medical Consultants: Russell Portenoy, MD, Department of Neurology, Albert Einstein College of Medicine, Bronx, New York; Theresa Brechner, MD,Department of Anesthesiology, University of California-Los Angeles.

Sponsored by: Roxane Laboratories, Inc., Columbus, Ohio.

To Order: A check for $17.50 should be made payable to the University of Wisconsin—133K613. Wisconsin residents add 5% sales tax. Send the check to:

Charles S. Cleeland, PhD
Department of Neurology
Pain Research Group
H6/530 Clinical Science Center
600 Highland Avenue
Madison, WI 53792

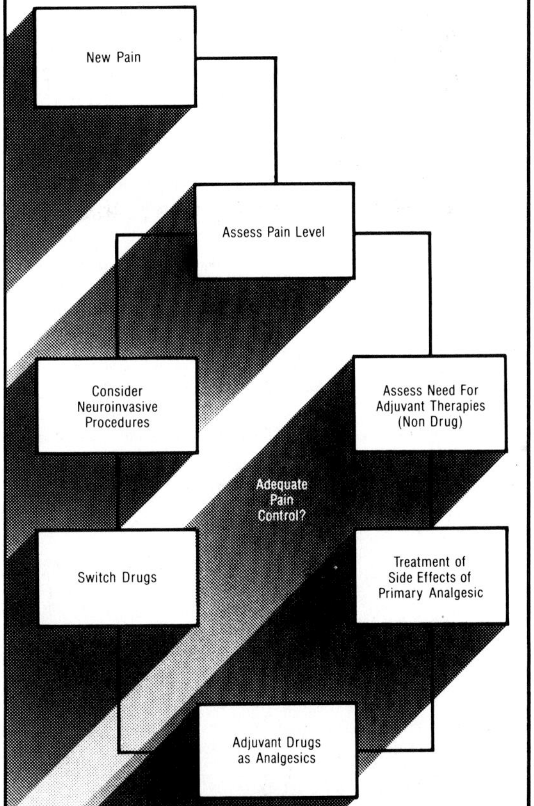

Experimental antineoplastic regimen granted treatment IND status

Under the guidelines of the 1987 treatment IND regulations, FDA has approved an experimental antineoplastic therapy for use in patients with germ cell carcinoma of the testes, ovary, or extragonadal sites that has not responded to conventional therapy. The regimen consists of cisplatin and either vinblastine or etoposide in combination with the experimental agents ifosfamide and mesna. Ifosfamide is a structural analogue of cyclophosphamide. Mesna is used to prevent severe hemorrhagic cystitis, a major adverse effect of ifosfamide.

An estimated 250 patients may be eligible to receive this treatment annually. Preliminary study data released by FDA show that approximately one third of more than 50 patients who have been treated with this regimen in the ongoing study have achieved complete remission, and 15–20% of all patients in the study have remained in complete remission for more than one year.

Second AIDS vaccine enters clinical trials

Bristol-Myers has received approval from FDA to conduct clinical tests of an experimental vaccine intended to prevent infection with human immunodeficiency virus (HIV). The vaccine, the second to enter clinical trials in the United States, is prepared using recombinant-DNA technology. Genes that code for HIV envelope proteins are inserted into vaccinia virus. The study approved by FDA is designed to assess the safety of the vaccine and its ability to induce antibody production. The vaccine will be tested in 30 to 60 homosexual volunteers not infected with HIV. A similar group of volunteers serving as the control group will receive smallpox vaccine.

News Briefs

- Results of a Phase I study of **2′,3′-dideoxycytidine** alone or alternating with zidovudine in 20 patients with AIDS or AIDS-related complex were reported in the January 16, 1988, issue of *The Lancet*. The study suggests that the antiviral agent has activity against the human immunodeficiency virus and has a toxicity profile different from that of zidovudine.

- FDA recently approved a **radioimmunoassay for the measurement of cyclosporine concentrations** (Sandimmune Radioimmunoassay Kit, Sandoz Pharmaceuticals Inc.). Measurements made using the radioimmunoassay and high-performance liquid chromatography are not interchangeable because of differences in specificity. The radioimmunoassay antibody crossreacts with several cyclosporine metabolites. Thus, therapeutic ranges established for the two assay techniques are not interchangeable.

Assistant Director

Accreditation Services Department

This position will be responsible for assisting in the direction of the department, conducting residency and technician training program accreditation surveys, and assisting with general matters related to accreditation. Requirements: Active pharmacist license, completion of an ASHP-accredited residency program, post-residency practice experience, experience as a preceptor of residents, and exceptional organizational and oral and written communication skills. Extensive travel will be required. Submit curriculum vitae (with list of references and publications), approximate date of availability, and compensation expectations to:

Thomas K. Somers, Director
Human Resources Division
American Society of Hospital Pharmacists
P.O. Box 30068
Bethesda, MD 20814
Phone: 301-657-3000

Equal Opportunity Employer

Upcoming Specialty Meetings

The Expanding Role of Folates and Fluoropyrimidines in Cancer Chemotherapy . . . Buffalo, NY . . . April 28–29 . . . contact: Gayle Bersani, Education Office, Roswell Park Memorial Institute, 666 Elm Street, Buffalo, NY 14263; 716-845-2339.

Biomedical Advances in Aging: Molecular and Immunological Mechanisms, Intervention and Clinical Approaches to Treatment . . . Washington, DC . . . May 9–13 . . . Allan L. Goldstein, Department of Biochemistry, The George Washington University School of Medicine and Health Sciences, 2300 Eye Street N.W., Washington, DC 20037; 202-994-3517 or 3709.

American Cancer Society . . . Cleveland, OH . . . June 7–10 . . . contact: G. R. Gadberry, 90 Park Avenue, New York, NY 10016; 212-736-3030.

Endocrine Society . . . New Orleans, LA . . . June 8–10 . . . contact: N. C. Karpin, 9650 Rockville Pike, Bethesda, MD 20814; 301-571-1802.

American Diabetes Association . . . New Orleans, LA . . . June 11–14 . . . contact: R. S. Boan, 1660 Duke Street, Alexandria, VA 22314; 703-549-1500.

Conference on Management of Psychiatric and Substance Abuse Services . . . San Diego, CA . . . June 15–17 . . . contact: N. Gordon, American Hospital Association, 840 North Lake Shore Drive, Chicago, IL 60611; 312-280-6650.

Therapy Consultation

The Therapy Consultation *section provides brief advice, in question-and-answer format, on how to handle specific drug-therapy problems. Readers are invited to submit questions, which will be referred to a consultant for an answer. The problems should not be highly specialized or unusual, nor should they be mundane. Questions are answered briefly, based largely on the judgment and personal experience of the consultant, although selected references may be cited to substantiate the consultant's advice.*

Assistance in identifying Therapy Consultation *topics is provided by the drug information centers at the following institutions: Albert B. Chandler Medical Center and College of Pharmacy, University of Kentucky, Lexington; Arizona Health Sciences Center, Tucson; Medical College of Virginia Hospitals, Richmond; University of California Medical Center, San Diego; and University of Michigan Medical Center, Ann Arbor.*

Choice of diluents for intrathecal drug administration

Question: What is the diluent of choice for drugs that will be administered intrathecally? Preservative-free 0.9% sodium chloride injection is preferred by some because it is available in small containers. However, some clinicians prefer lactated Ringer's injection, claiming it is more physiologic. Others prefer Elliott's B solution, although it is not available commercially and must be compounded or obtained from the National Cancer Institute.

Answer: The diluent of choice for intrathecal administration of drugs continues to be a controversial problem for oncology pharmacists. The appropriate choice is important because some acute CNS toxicities observed after intrathecal injection of antineoplastic agents may be due to the type of diluent used. Acute toxicities reported after administration of intrathecal agents include vomiting, fever, headache, and paraplegia.

Currently, the diluents considered to be acceptable for intrathecal administration are preservative-free 0.9% sodium chloride injection, lactated Ringer's injection, sterile water, and Elliott's B solution. These diluents differ in ionic composition, pH, and osmolarity. Ideally, we would like a diluent that has characteristics as close to those of cerebrospinal fluid (CSF) as possible. CSF is essentially an electrolyte solution containing bicarbonate as a buffer. CSF may be withdrawn from patients and used as a drug vehicle, although this is not done routinely because of practical considerations. Of the vehicles currently available, Elliott's B solution most closely resembles CSF. Concentrations of ions and glucose in Elliott's B solution are within the normal range of CSF values. Sodium, potassium, and calcium concentrations in CSF, Elliott's B solution, and lactated Ringer's injection are very similar, but lactated Ringer's injection does not contain magnesium, phosphate, bicarbonate, or sulfate. The formulation of Elliott's B solution available from the National Cancer Institute (NCI) contains sodium chloride 7.3 mg, potassium chloride 0.3 mg, calcium chloride 0.2 mg, magnesium sulfate 0.3 mg, sodium phosphate, dibasic 0.2 mg, dextrose hydrous 0.3 mg, sodium bicarbonate 1.9 mg, and phenolsulfonphthalein 0.1 μg per milliliter; the pH of the solution is adjusted to 6–7.5 with carbon dioxide.

The differences among these solutions may be clinically important. Investigators have suggested that because of the relatively small CSF volume and poor CSF buffering capacity, injections into the CSF should closely match the CSF in pH and osmolarity. Geiser et al.[1] reported that the incidence of major adverse effects (vomiting, headache, and fever lasting two to five days) after intrathecal methotrexate administration varied with the diluent used. In a retrospective review of 71 courses of methotrexate prophylaxis, the incidence of these adverse effects was 12.5% when Elliott's B solution was used as the diluent and 61% when 0.9% sodium chloride injection was used as the diluent. No prospective studies have been conducted to verify these findings. Other investigators have demonstrated increased neurotoxicity in animals given intrathecal cytarabine under nonphysiologic conditions.[2] Pharmaceutical research evaluating the stability, osmolarity, and buffering capacity of methotrexate, cytarabine, and hydrocortisone diluted in Elliott's B solution, lactated Ringer's injection, and 0.9% sodium chloride injection in various concentrations showed Elliott's B solution to be superior to the other diluents with respect to buffering capacity.[3]

Although there is no conclusive evidence that Elliott's B solution is the diluent of choice for intrathecal administration of drugs, the available data indicate that it should be used whenever possible. Unfortunately, Elliott's B solution is still an investigational agent. It may be obtained from the NCI, but supplies may be used with NCI protocols only. Furthermore, methotrexate is the only drug for which the NCI has an approved investigational new drug (IND) application for use with Elliott's B solution. However, Elliott's B solution may be compounded at your institution. The Johns Hopkins Hospital compounds its own Elliott's B solution, and we use it as a diluent for most intrathecal antineoplastic drugs. One exception is thiotepa. Because of the high osmolarity of thiotepa, sterile water is used as the diluent so the osmolarity of the final solution will be closer to that of CSF. If Elliott's B solution is not available at your hospital, either 0.9% sodium chloride injection or lactated Ringer's injection may be used. Lactated Ringer's injection has a slightly higher buffering capacity than 0.9% sodium chloride.

In conclusion, no prospective clinical comparison has proven that one diluent is better than another. One ret-

Continued on page 266

9th Annual Meeting AMERICAN COLLEGE OF CLINICAL PHARMACY

July 24–27, 1988
Wyndham Franklin Plaza Hotel
Philadelphia

Sunday, July 24
5:00 pm – 7:00 pm
Annual Business Meeting
7:00 pm – 9:00 pm
Opening Reception

Monday, July 25
8:30 am – 9:45 am
Therapeutic Frontiers Lecture:
"Monoclonal Antibodies in the Treatment of Cancer"
Paul A. Bunn, Jr., M.D.
10:15 am – 11:45 am
Therapeutic Symposium:
"Treatment of Hyperlipidemia: Which Drugs and Why"
11:45 am – 1:45 pm
Pharmacy Industry Forum Exhibits
2:00 pm – 3:30 pm
Therapeutic Symposium:
"New Methodologies for Clinical Pharmacy Research: Beyond Kinetics"
3:45 pm – 5:30 pm
Joint Symposium:
ACCP and the European Society of Clinical Pharmacy

Tuesday, July 26
8:00 am – 10:30 am
Poster Presentations
10:30 am – 12:30 pm
Research Institute Program
12:30 pm – 2:30 pm
Pharmacy Industry Forum Exhibits
2:30 pm – 5:30 pm
Contributed Scientific Papers I, II, III
4:00 pm – 5:30 pm
Innovative Clinical Pharmacy Practice Forum

Wednesday, July 27
8:30 am – 11:30 am
Therapeutic Symposium:
"Biotechnology: The Future of New Drug Therapy"
11:30 am – 1:00 pm
Residency and Fellowship Forum
Committee Meetings
1:00 pm – 2:30 pm
Therapeutic Symposium:
"Promoting Clinical Pharmacy Services: Issues in Cost Effectiveness"
2:45 pm – 5:30 pm
Contributed Scientific Papers IV, V, VI
6:00 pm – 7:00 pm
President's Reception
7:00 pm – 9:00 pm
Banquet

For Information:
American College of Clinical Pharmacy
3101 Broadway, Suite 350
Kansas City, Missouri 64111
(816) 531-2177

accp
American College of Clinical Pharmacy

Therapy Consultation *Continued from page 265*

rospective study in humans and animal and pharmaceutical research indicate that Elliott's B solution may be superior because of its superior buffering capacity. Elliott's B solution should be used as the diluent for intrathecal administration of drugs if it is available. Otherwise, preservative-free 0.9% sodium chloride injection and lactated Ringer's solution are appropriate alternatives.

1. Geiser CF, Bishop Y, Jaffee N et al. Adverse effects of intrathecal methotrexate in children with acute leukemia in remission. *Blood*. 1975; 45:189–95.
2. Duttera MH, Gallelli JF, Kleinman LM et al. Intrathecal methotrexate. *Lancet*. 1972; 1:540.
3. Cradock JC, Kleinman LM, Rahman A. Evaluation of some pharmaceutical aspects of intrathecal methotrexate sodium, cytarabine and hydrocortisone. *Am J Hosp Pharm*. 1978; 35:402–5.

LAURENCE GREEN, PHARM.D.
Assistant Director of Pharmacy
The Johns Hopkins Hospital
Baltimore, MD 21205

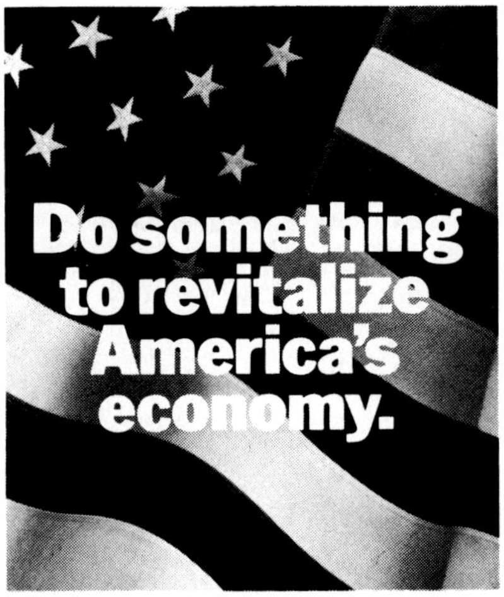

Support America's colleges. Because college is more than a place where young people are preparing for their future. It's where *America* — and American business — is preparing for *its* future.

Give to the college of your choice.

Ad Council A Public Service of This Publication
COUNCIL FOR AID TO EDUCATION CFAE

Letters

The Letters *column is a forum for rapid exchange of ideas among readers of* CP. *Liberal criteria are applied in the review of submissions to encourage contributions to this column.*

The Letters *column includes the following types of contributions: (1) comments, addenda, and minor updates on previously published work, (2) alerts on potential problems related to drug therapy or clinical research, (3) observations or comments on trends in drug therapy or clinical research, and (4) brief expressions of opinion about controversies in drug therapy or clinical research.*

Suspected gentamicin allergy could be sulfite sensitivity

A 58-year-old man with a history of spinal astrocytoma, spastic quadriparesis, and neurogenic bladder was admitted to our hospital for surgical treatment of nonhealing sacral decubitus ulcers and drug therapy of a urinary-tract infection caused by *Pseudomonas aeruginosa*. The patient had no known allergies. During an initial infusion of gentamicin injection (Elkins–Sinn, Inc.) the patient developed cyanosis, wheezing, dyspnea, tachypnea, tachycardia, and hypoxemia, with a P_{O_2} value of 48. Intravenous administration of epinephrine and diphenhydramine hydrochloride and discontinuation of the gentamicin infusion resulted in an immediate improvement in the patient's condition.

The patient's bronchospastic reaction initially was attributed to a gentamicin allergy. However, anaphylactic reactions to gentamicin are quite rare; only one case has been reported in the literature.[1] It is more likely that this patient's reaction was the result of a sensitivity to sodium bisulfite, the preservative in gentamicin injection. Skin testing is of limited value in the diagnosis of sulfite sensitivity, so the diagnosis must be established by a cautious provocative challenge. No such rechallenge was conducted with this patient, since another antimicrobial agent was used to treat his urinary-tract infection.

Reactions to sulfites are common; although they occur more frequently in patients with asthma,[2] they occur in nonasthmatic individuals as well.[3] Bronchospasm is the most frequently reported reaction to sulfites,[2] but life-threatening loss of consciousness and anaphylactic shock can occur. Health-care practitioners should be aware that sulfiting agents are used as antioxidants in a variety of drug products, including antimicrobial agents such as gentamicin.[4] Reactions such as the one experienced by the patient we describe should not automatically be attributed to the drug. Doing so could prevent the patient from receiving sulfite-free formulations of that or similar drugs in the future.

1. Hall JF. Anaphylaxis after gentamicin. *Lancet*. 1977; 2:455. Letter.
2. Stevenson DD, Simon RA. Sensitivity to ingested metabisulfites in asthmatic subjects. *J Allergy Clin Immunol*. 1981; 68:26–32.
3. Clayton DE, Busse W. Anaphylaxis to wine. *Clin Allergy*. 1980; 10:341–3.
4. Dalton–Bunnow MF. Sulfite content of drug products. *Am J Hosp Pharm*. 1985; 42:2196–2201.

DENNIS J. MIKOLICH, M.D., Chief
Division of Infectious Disease

WILLIAM W. MCCLOSKEY, PHARM.D., Clinical Pharmacist
Department of Medicine

Veterans Administration Medical Center
Davis Park
Providence, RI 02908

Magnesium gluconate can be used as oral supplement

In the Therapy Consultation column about treatment of magnesium deficiency, which appeared in the November 1987 issue of *Clinical Pharmacy*, Montgomery[1] neglected to mention magnesium gluconate in her discussion of agents that can be administered orally to patients with hypomagnesemia. Magnesium gluconate contains 4.4 meq of magnesium per 1000 mg of salt.[2]

1. Montgomery P. Treatment of magnesium deficiency. *Clin Pharm*. 1987; 6:834–5. Therapy Consultation.
2. Martindale: The extra pharmacopoeia. 28th ed. Wade A, ed. London: The Pharmaceutical Press; 1982;626.

HARRY WONG, PHARM.D.
Pharmacy Department
Kaiser Permanente of Sacramento
6600 Bruceville Road
Sacramento, CA 95831

Corrections

Effect of two cimetidine regimens on prothrombin time and warfarin pharmacokinetics during long-term warfarin therapy (June 1987, Research Note). In the last sentence of the Results section on page 494, the 0.221 value reported in parentheses is that of the coefficient of determination R^2, not the correlation coefficient r.

Encainide and flecainide: Two class 1c antiarrhythmic agents (November 1987, Continuing Education). Because of an error in the wording of question 10 of continuing-education article number 680-204-8717 on page 901, there is no correct answer. Responses to question 10 will be excluded from calculations of test scores for continuing-education credit.

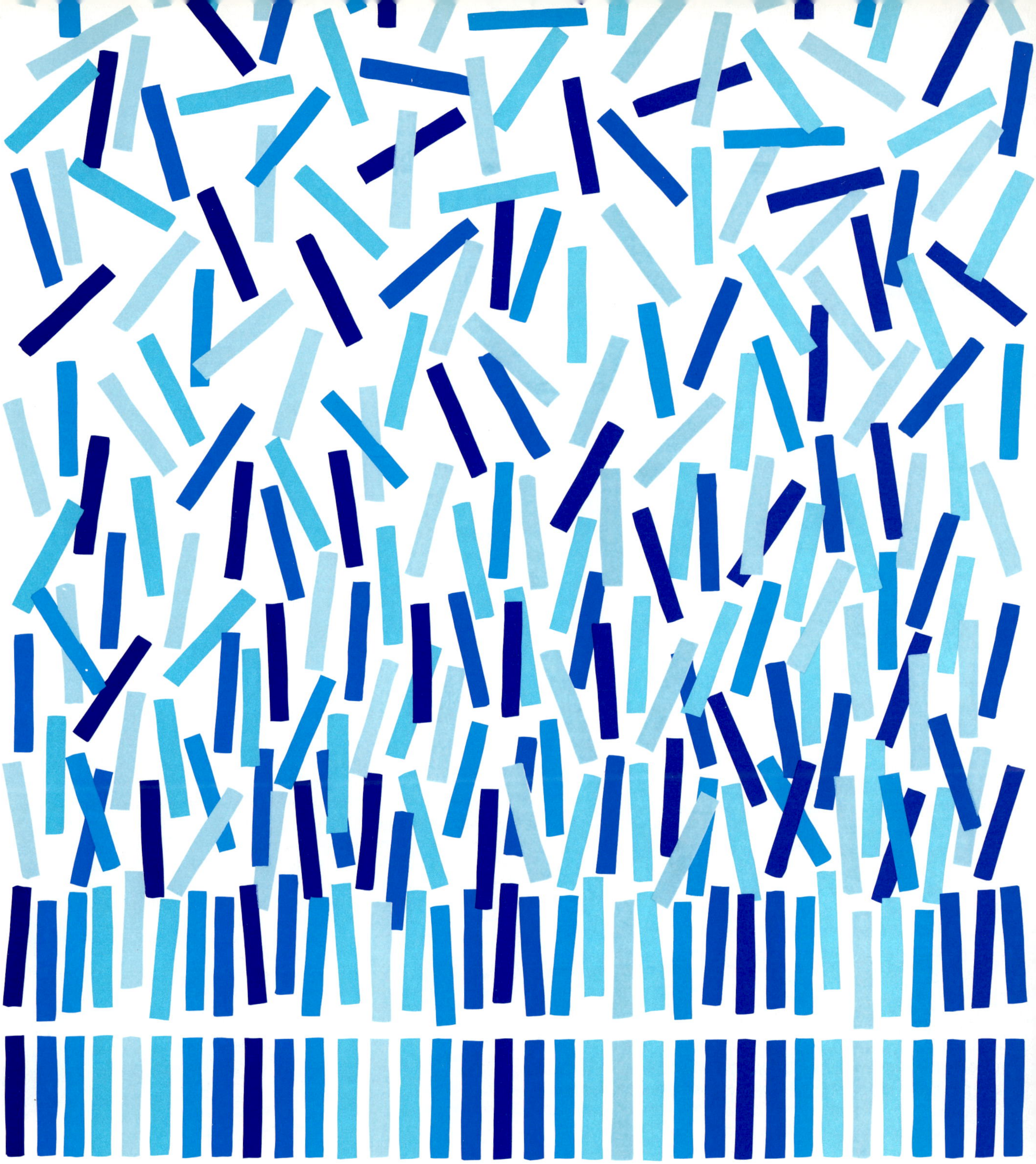

Coming Soon

Rythmol™
propafenone HCl

from Knoll Pharmaceuticals

Knoll Pharmaceuticals
A Unit of BASF K&F Corporation
Whippany, New Jersey 07981

© 1988 BASF K&F Corporation

BASF Group

knoll®

4826/12-87

Printed in U.S.A.

Drug Reviews

Comparison of famotidine with cimetidine and ranitidine

ROSEMARY R. BERARDI, ROBERTA M. TANKANOW, AND TIMOTHY T. NOSTRANT

Abstract: The pharmacodynamic, therapeutic, and toxicologic properties of famotidine are evaluated and compared with those of cimetidine and ranitidine.

Famotidine, an H_2-receptor antagonist with a thiazole nucleus, is approximately 7.5 times more potent than ranitidine and 20 times more potent than cimetidine on an equimolar basis. Therapeutic trials indicate that famotidine 20 mg b.i.d. or 40 mg at bedtime is as effective as standard doses of cimetidine and ranitidine for healing duodenal ulcers. A dose of 40 mg at bedtime appears to heal benign gastric ulcers. A single nocturnal dose of 20 mg is effective in preventing duodenal ulcer relapse. Further studies are required that compare the efficacy of famotidine with cimetidine and ranitidine in the treatment of gastric ulcers and in the prevention of recurrent duodenal ulcers. The overall incidence of adverse effects observed with famotidine appears to be similar to that reported for cimetidine and ranitidine. Like ranitidine, famotidine does not have antiandrogenic effects or substantially inhibit the hepatic metabolism of drugs. Because of its increased antisecretory potency and lack of antiandrogenic effects at higher doses, famotidine may be the H_2-receptor antagonist of choice in treating Zollinger–Ellison syndrome.

Additional clinical experience, as well as cost and safety factors, will determine the place of famotidine in treating and preventing acid-peptic disorders.

Index terms: Cimetidine; Dosage; Drug interactions; Famotidine; Gastrointestinal drugs; Ranitidine; Toxicity; Ulcers
Clin Pharm. 1988; 7:271–284

Famotidine (Pepcid, Merck Sharp & Dohme) is the latest histamine H_2-receptor antagonist to be approved by the Food and Drug Administration (FDA) for the treatment of acid-peptic disorders. The drug was developed in an attempt to increase antisecretory potency and to decrease the incidence and types of adverse effects and drug interactions reported with the previously approved H_2-receptor antagonists, cimetidine (Tagamet, Smith Kline & French) and ranitidine (Zantac, Glaxo).

This article evaluates the pharmacodynamic, therapeutic, and toxicologic properties of famotidine and compares these and other factors with what is known regarding cimetidine and ranitidine.

Chemistry

Famotidine differs structurally from the earlier H_2-receptor antagonists in that it contains a thiazole ring nucleus rather than the imidazole ring of cimetidine or the furan ring of ranitidine (Figure 1). With the development of ranitidine, it became evident that inhibition of histamine at the H_2 receptors was not determined exclusively by compounds containing the imidazole group. In general, molecular manipulations have resulted in H_2-receptor antagonists with increased potency and enhanced specificity. Some structural modifications have produced agents such as tiotidine that have been associated with potential toxicities.[1]

ROSEMARY R. BERARDI, PHARM.D., is Associate Professor of Pharmacy, College of Pharmacy, The University of Michigan, and Clinical Pharmacist–Gastroenterology, The University of Michigan Hospitals (UMH), Ann Arbor, MI; ROBERTA M. TANKANOW, M.S., is Investigational Drug Service Clinical Pharmacist, UMH, and Clinical Assistant Professor of Pharmacy, College of Pharmacy, The University of Michigan; TIMOTHY T. NOSTRANT, M.D., is Associate Professor of Medicine, School of Medicine, The University of Michigan, and Gastroenterologist, Department of Internal Medicine, UMH.

Address reprint requests to Dr. Berardi at the College of Pharmacy, The University of Michigan, Ann Arbor, MI 48109-1065.

This is **article 680-204-8804** in the **ASHP Continuing Education System;** it qualifies for 1.0 hour of continuing-education credit. See page 326 for learning objectives and test questions.

Copyright © 1988, American Society of Hospital Pharmacists, Inc. All rights reserved. 0278-2677/88/0401-0271$03.50.

Figure 1. Chemical structures of the H_2-receptor antagonists (from top to bottom) famotidine, ranitidine, and cimetidine.

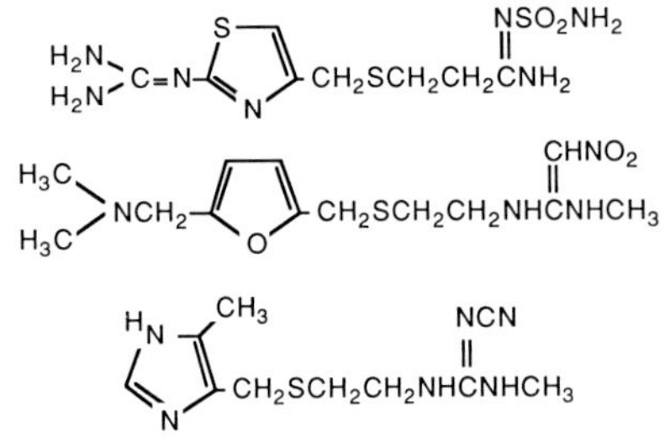

Pharmacology

Famotidine acts as a reversible competitive inhibitor of histamine at the H_2 receptors without producing discernible effects on muscarinic, nicotinic, histamine H_1, or sympathetic α and β receptors.[2] The binding specificity of the drug appears to resemble that of ranitidine and probably accounts for its similar adverse-effects profile. On an equimolar basis, it is reported to be about 7.5 times more potent than ranitidine and about 20 times more potent than cimetidine in inhibiting basal and pentagastrin-stimulated gastric acid secretion in humans.[3] However, other reports in humans have suggested an antisecretory potency of 12 to 15 times that of ranitidine and 40 to 60 times that of cimetidine.[4] Increased potency does not necessarily confer a therapeutic advantage, since increasing the dose of a less potent agent usually provides a similar quantitative response.

Gastric Antisecretory Effects. The effect of famotidine on gastric acid secretion has been evaluated in healthy subjects, in patients with duodenal ulcer disease, and in patients with Zollinger–Ellison syndrome after basal and nocturnal acid secretion and after pentagastrin-, histamine-, and meal-stimulated acid secretion.[4–8]

McCallum et al.[5] compared single oral doses of famotidine 5 mg, 10 mg, and 20 mg with cimetidine 300 mg in a five-way, double-blind, placebo-controlled trial in 10 healthy volunteers. Plasma concentrations of famotidine and cimetidine were monitored over a seven-hour period. All doses of famotidine and cimetidine inhibited pentagastrin-stimulated gastric acid secretion and volume in the initial two to four hours ($p < 0.05$); however, the 10- and 20-mg doses of famotidine were more potent than cimetidine ($p < 0.05$). The 5-mg famotidine dose resulted in acid suppression similar to that of 300 mg of cimetidine. In the five- to seven-hour period, all doses of famotidine continued to suppress acid secretion, while the effect of cimetidine 300 mg did not differ from that of placebo. The 20-mg famotidine dose resulted in higher gastric pH levels compared with all other treatments throughout the duration of the study ($p < 0.05$).

The plasma concentrations of famotidine appeared to be dose related, while the cimetidine concentrations were consistent with those previously reported.[9] However, the frequency and duration of blood sampling did not permit pharmacokinetic characterization of the plasma concentration–time curve and precise correlations between plasma concentrations and gastric antisecretory activity. Additional reports suggest that after pentagastrin stimulation the duration of the antisecretory response to an oral dose of famotidine 20 mg lasts 10 to 12 hours and that measurable reductions in basal and nocturnal acid secretion occur at 18 hours after the oral administration of a 40-mg dose.[4,6]

In a double-blind, placebo-controlled trial of eight subjects (basal gastric acid output > 5 meq/hr), Ryan et al.[7] compared the antisecretory effects of single oral (20 mg) and intravenous (10 and 20 mg) doses of famotidine on the inhibition of nocturnal acid secretion. All famotidine treatments decreased gastric acid secretion for up to 12 hours after drug administration when compared with placebo ($p < 0.01$). Maximal suppression occurred two and four hours after treatment and was 97.4%, 99.7%, and 99.4% after the 10-mg intravenous, 20-mg intravenous, and 20-mg oral doses, respectively. At 12 hours, 73.8%, 77.2%, and 83.3% of gastric secretion was inhibited for the respective treatments. Seven of eight subjects had pH values > 3.0 for up to seven hours after each treatment. All seven responders maintained this pH for up to 12 hours after the 20-mg intravenous dose. The area under the concentration–time curve for the 20-mg oral dose was similar to that of the 10-mg intravenous dose and was approximately one half that of the 20-mg intravenous dose, suggesting an oral bioavailability of 50%. There was no clear association between the plasma famotidine concentration and the magnitude of the antisecretory effect, although inadequate blood sampling and assay insensitivity limited the investigators' ability to make a pharmacokinetic and pharmacodynamic association.

Howard et al.[8] compared the antisecretory effects of famotidine with cimetidine and ranitidine in nine patients with Zollinger–Ellison syndrome. Equally potent doses of the three drugs were established by determining the minimum dose required (when given every six hours) to inhibit acid secretion to < 10 meq/hr during the hour immediately preceding the next dose. To compare the duration of each drug's antisecretory effects, gastric acid secretion was measured from 5 to 12 hours after equipotent doses of each drug were discontinued. The average minimum daily requirement of each drug to control gastric acid hypersecretion was 0.24 g (range, 0.08–0.48 g) of famotidine, 2.1 g (range 0.6–3.6 g) of ranitidine, and 7.8 g (range 1.2–13.2 g) of cimetidine. Gastric acid secretion could not be suppressed to < 10 meq/hr in one patient with famotidine 0.64 g/day, ranitidine 6.0 g/day, or cimetidine

14.4 g/day; administration of isopropramide 5 mg (as the iodide salt) every six hours was required. Although equally potent doses of the three H_2-receptor antagonists had a similar onset of action, the antisecretory duration of famotidine was 30% longer than that of either cimetidine or ranitidine ($p < 0.05$). However, this study did not establish whether famotidine's longer duration of action resulted in a less frequent dosing interval compared with those of cimetidine and ranitidine in treating patients with Zollinger–Ellison syndrome.[10]

Results of these gastric secretory studies suggest that famotidine effectively suppresses basal, nocturnal, and stimulated acid secretion and that the duration of its antisecretory action may be dose related. Famotidine differs from cimetidine in its increased potency and prolonged duration of acid inhibition. Although famotidine is more potent than ranitidine, the duration of its antisecretory effects, when equipotent doses are given, appears to be similar to that of ranitidine in healthy subjects and prolonged in patients with Zollinger–Ellison syndrome.[3,8] The longer famotidine elimination half-life (Table 1) probably does not account for the difference in duration of antisecretory activity, since variations in the elimination half-life of cimetidine and ranitidine are reported to range from one to three hours.[9,11] Increased potency and duration of acid inhibition may not result in clinically important differences for most patients, since equipotent doses of cimetidine or ranitidine may be administered.

Other Pharmacologic Actions. Famotidine, like cimetidine and ranitidine, does not appear to alter gastric emptying, exocrine pancreatic function, and the basal tone of the lower esophageal sphincter.[4,6] Pepsin output is decreased and is comparable to the magnitude observed with oral 200- to 300-mg doses of cimetidine.[12] Serum gastrin concentrations are not significantly altered in patients with gastric or duodenal ulcers.[13,14] However, oral administration of single antisecretory doses of famotidine in healthy subjects resulted in small increases (within normal limits) of serum gastrin levels, similar to those observed with cimetidine and ranitidine.[4,6,14–17]

Small decreases in serum prolactin concentrations have been observed after oral and intravenous administration of famotidine, but concentrations remained within the range of normal physiological variation.[13,14] In contrast, dose-related increases of prolactin have been reported after intravenous bolus injections of cimetidine and ranitidine.[15–17] Famotidine is similar to ranitidine in that it does not appear to possess antiandrogenic activity.[14,16] Unlike cimetidine, it does not displace dihydrotestosterone from androgen binding sites.[14,17]

Single doses of famotidine 40 mg (oral) and 20 mg (intravenous) did not have a significant effect on blood pressure, heart rate, or electrocardiographic patterns in healthy volunteers.[6] In patients with various degrees of renal impairment, inulin and endogenous creatinine clearances were not affected by single 10-mg intravenous doses of famotidine.[18] In contrast to cimetidine, therapeutic doses of famotidine do not appear to inhibit the hepatic cytochrome P-450 mixed-function oxidase system.[19,20] Ranitidine has less of an effect on cytochrome P-450 than does cimetidine.[16] Studies are needed to determine the immunological effects of famotidine in humans.

Table 1.
Pharmacokinetics of Famotidine, Ranitidine, and Cimetidine[a]

Variable	Famotidine	Ranitidine	Cimetidine
Oral bioavailability (%)	37–45	39–87	63–78
Protein binding (%)	15–20	15–20	15–20
Volume of distribution (L/kg)	1.1–1.4	1.2–1.9	0.8–1.2
Time of peak effect after oral dose (hr)	1–3	1–3	1–2
Elimination half-life (hr)	3.5	2.5	2.0
% Excreted unchanged in urine 24 hr after i.v. dose	70	70	75
Renal clearance (L/hr)	15–27	24–32	24–36
Mean plasma concentration resulting in 50% inhibition of stimulated acid secretion (ng/mL)	13	100	750

[a] Data compiled from references 9, 11, 12, 14, and 21–25.

Pharmacokinetics

The pharmacokinetics of famotidine has been studied in healthy subjects, in patients with renal insufficiency, and in patients with liver disease.[12,21–27] Table 1 compares some of the more important pharmacokinetic variables of famotidine, ranitidine, and cimetidine.

The bioavailability of famotidine after oral administration ranges from 37% to 45% and is consistent with an antisecretory potency of approximately one half that of the intravenous dose.[7,21] The reported mean peak plasma concentrations for a 5-mg, 10-mg, 20-mg, and 40-mg oral dose are 17–22 ng/mL, 29–33 ng/mL, 50–60 ng/mL, and 78 ng/mL, respectively.[12,14,21–23] The plasma concentrations required to inhibit 50% of pentagastrin-stimulated acid are shown in Table 1. These concentrations do not correlate directly with dose or therapeutic response.

Famotidine is eliminated primarily in the urine, the remaining portion being metabolized to a sulfoxide metabolite of unknown activity.[21-23] The mean total plasma clearance after intravenous administration ranges from 25 to 29 L/hr, with the mean renal clearance reported to be 15 to 27 L/hr, indicating active tubular secretion of the drug.[21,23,24]

Takabatake et al.[24] studied the pharmacokinetics of famotidine in 24 patients with various degrees of renal function and in seven subjects with normal renal function. The elimination half-life was 2.59 hours in patients with normal renal function (creatinine clearance [CL_{cr}] >90 mL/min) or mild renal impairment (CL_{cr} 60–90 mL/min), and increased to 4.72 hours in moderate renal failure (CL_{cr} 30–60 mL/min) and to 12.07 hours in patients with severe renal failure (CL_{cr} <30 mL/min). Total body clearance and renal clearance were correspondingly reduced in patients with severely impaired renal function; nonrenal clearance remained unchanged in patients with moderate renal insufficiency but decreased in patients with severe failure. Volume of distribution was unchanged. Others have confirmed the prolonged half-life of famotidine in severe renal failure and the need for a possible reduction in famotidine dosage.[25] The elimination half-life of famotidine is reported to be 13.71 hours in patients undergoing hemodialysis.[26] No significant differences in famotidine disposition were observed in patients with compensated or decompensated cirrhosis after administration of single intravenous doses.[27]

Overview of Clinical Trials

The treatment of peptic ulcer disease with H_2-receptor antagonists is well established for cimetidine and ranitidine.[16,28] Famotidine, a more potent antisecretory agent, is equally effective as cimetidine and ranitidine in healing duodenal ulcers and appears to be as effective in healing gastric ulcers and in preventing recurrence of duodenal ulcers. Controlled clinical trials that assess the efficacy of famotidine in other acid-peptic disorders are in progress in the United States. Of the few reports that have been published, most are abstracts. Currently, FDA labeling for famotidine, ranitidine, and cimetidine includes the indications listed in Table 2.

Numerous uncontrolled open studies evaluating the efficacy of famotidine in the treatment of active gastric or duodenal ulcer have been conducted throughout Japan and Europe. A few of these studies using endoscopy to verify ulcer presence and confirm ulcer healing are summarized and published elsewhere.[14] In addition, famotidine has been compared with gefarnate (geranyl farnesyl acetate), an agent used primarily in Japan and Europe that is associated with duodenal and gastric ulcer healing rates similar to those achieved by placebo. These studies will not be discussed in this review, since it is unlikely that gefarnate will be available in the United States as an alternative to placebo. A summary of the more important studies comparing famotidine with gefarnate are reported elsewhere.[14,29] In general, ulcer healing rates for gastric and duodenal ulcers and adverse effects reported in the open trials and studies using gefarnate are similar to those observed in the larger, controlled, double-blind studies discussed in this review.

Treatment of Active Duodenal Ulcer

The methods, design, and results of the double-blind controlled clinical trials comparing the efficacy of various oral dosage regimens of famotidine with placebo or ranitidine in the treatment of active duodenal ulcer are summarized in Table 3.[30-36] Compliance with drug therapy was verified in three of the seven studies.[30,31,36] In all of the studies except for that of Dobrilla et al.,[36] various amounts of liquid or tablet antacids were used when necessary, enabling patients to obtain relief from occasional ulcer pain. It is possible that antacids, when used in smaller doses than originally recommended, may contribute to successful ulcer healing.[37,38] Antiulcer medications (other than p.r.n. antacids) were discontinued before the start of each study, and patients receiving ulcerogenic medications

Table 2.
FDA-Approved Labeling and Dosages for Famotidine, Ranitidine, and Cimetidine

Indication	Dosages		
	Famotidine	Ranitidine[a]	Cimetidine
Active duodenal ulcer			
Short-term treatment	20 mg p.o. b.i.d. 40 mg p.o. h.s	150 mg p.o. b.i.d. 300 mg p.o. h.s	300 mg p.o. q.i.d. 400 mg p.o. b.i.d. 800 mg p.o. h.s
Maintenance therapy	20 mg p.o. h.s	150 mg p.o. h.s	400 mg p.o. h.s
Active benign gastric ulcer (short-term treatment)		150 mg p.o. b.i.d.	300 mg p.o. q.i.d.
Gastroesophageal reflux disease		150 mg p.o. b.i.d.	
Pathological hypersecretory states[b]	20 mg p.o. q6h	150 mg p.o. b.i.d.	300 mg p.o. q.i.d.
Intravenous therapy[c]	20 mg q12h	50 mg q6–8h	300 mg q6–8h[c]

[a] Given as the hydrochloride salt.
[b] Doses should be adjusted to meet the needs of individual patients.
[c] In hospitalized patients with pathological hypersecretory states or in patients who are unable to take oral medication.

(aspirin and nonsteroidal anti-inflammatory agents) were excluded from participation.

In a multicenter, randomized, placebo-controlled study in the United States, Gitlin et al.[30] evaluated the efficacy of three dosage regimens of famotidine. The patient characteristics for the four treatment subgroups showed a similar distribution for single versus multiple ulcers, duration of ulcer history, sex, age, cigarette smoking, and alcohol and caffeine ingestion. Both ulcer healing and ulcer pain frequency with famotidine therapy were significantly superior to placebo at two, four, and eight weeks. The 95% confidence interval for ulcer healing was similar among the famotidine treatment groups, indicating that the daily dose of 40 mg/day was equivalent to 80 mg/day and that the 40-mg dose at bedtime was equivalent to the 20-mg b.i.d. regimen. Antacid use was decreased at two, four, and eight weeks in the famotidine groups compared with placebo, except for the group receiving famotidine 40 mg at bedtime ($p < 0.01$). No significant differences in ulcer healing rates were shown for smokers compared with nonsmokers, but nonsmokers tended to heal better in both the famotidine treatment groups and the placebo control group.

McCullough[31] summarized the results of a large international multicenter study that included 68 investigators from 19 countries. A total of 1031 patients were enrolled in the trial, which compared three famotidine treatment regimens with a twice-daily regimen of ranitidine. Protocol violations prevented the evaluation of healing rates in 51 patients, the number of which was similar for all groups. Age, sex, smoking, alcohol consumption, single versus multiple ulcers, and the duration of ulcer history were similar among the treatment groups. The difference in antacid consumption between the famotidine groups and those receiving ranitidine was not significant at any time during the study. The authors reported that ulcer-healing rates were not significantly different among any of the famotidine groups at two, four, and eight weeks and between any famotidine group and ranitidine. Ulcer pain improved and antacid use decreased in all groups equally. This large study emphasizes the importance of inhibiting nocturnal acid secretion in healing duodenal ulcers and con-

Table 3.
Double-Blind Controlled Trials Comparing Famotidine with Placebo or Ranitidine in the Treatment of Active Duodenal Ulcer

Reference	Drug and Dose (mg)[a]	Defined Ulcer Healing	Frequency of Scheduled Endoscopy[b]	No. of Evaluable Patients	% Healed at Indicated Time		
					2 weeks	4 weeks	8 weeks
30	P b.i.d.	Yes	2, 4, 8 weeks	97	17[c]	31[c]	45[c]
	F 40 h.s.			89	32	70	83
	F 20 b.i.d.			84	38	67	82
	F 40 b.i.d.			93	34	75	82
31	F 40 h.s.	Yes	2, 4, 8 weeks	240	34[d]	67[d]	87
	F 20 b.i.d.			247	N.D.[e]	N.D.	92
	F 40 b.i.d.			247	N.D.	N.D.	92
	R 150 b.i.d.			246	38[d]	75[d]	90
32	F 40 h.s.	Yes	2, 4, 8 weeks	51	46	75	92
	F 20 b.i.d.			55	42	83	97
	F 40 b.i.d.			55	47	81	93
	R 150 b.i.d.			49	46	78	90
33	F 40 h.s.	Yes	2, 4, 8 weeks	42	67	91	98
	F 20 b.i.d.			42	57	83	95
	F 40 b.i.d.			41	63	90	100
	R 150 b.i.d.			43	65	93	93
34	F 40 h.s.	No	2, 4, 8 weeks	15	40	73	87
	F 20 b.i.d.			18	44	83	94
	F 40 b.i.d.			15	47	100	100
	R 150 b.i.d.			17	53	88	94
35	F 40 h.s.	No	2, 4 weeks	48	64	94	...
	R 300 h.s.			50	46	90	...
36	F 40 h.s.	Yes	4, 6 weeks	116	...	76[f]	...
	R 300 h.s.			112	...	76[g]	...

[a] P = placebo, F = famotidine, R = ranitidine given as the hydrochloride salt.
[b] Baseline endoscopies were performed in all cases.
[c] $p \leq 0.05$ when placebo was compared with each famotidine dosage regimen.
[d] Estimates obtained from figures; numerical data not reported.
[e] Data not reported.
[f] By six weeks, 91% of patients were healed.
[g] By six weeks, 87% of patients were healed.

firms that famotidine, in a dosage of 40 mg/day, is as effective as ranitidine 150 mg (as the hydrochloride salt) b.i.d. in the treatment of active duodenal ulcer. As shown in Table 3, two similar European multicenter studies comparing famotidine 40 mg at bedtime, 20 mg b.i.d., and 40 mg b.i.d. with ranitidine 150 mg (as the hydrochloride salt) b.i.d. confirm the results previously described.[32,33]

In a multicenter trial, Rohner and Gugler[35] compared single oral nocturnal doses of famotidine 40 mg with ranitidine 300 mg (as the hydrochloride salt).[35] There were no significant differences between treatment groups with regard to age, sex, and smoking; however, patients in the ranitidine group tended to have larger or multiple ulcers, consumed more alcohol, and had a longer history of duodenal ulcer. Antacid consumption in both groups was low during the first week and lower throughout the remainder of the study. Before entry into the study, all patients reported ulcer-related pain during the day, but only 77 (famotidine, 35; ranitidine, 42) patients had pain during the night. Symptomatic response was similar in both treatment groups, with two thirds of the patients being free of daytime ulcer-related pain after one week of treatment. A tendency toward increased pain relief during the day in the famotidine group was not significant. Differences in nighttime pain were obscured because the initial night pain distribution was uneven for both groups. The results of this study indicate that single nocturnal doses of famotidine 40 mg and ranitidine 300 mg (as the hydrochloride salt) are equally effective in healing duodenal ulcers and in providing relief from ulcer pain. Another study comparing nocturnal oral doses of famotidine 40 mg and ranitidine 300 mg (as the hydrochloride salt) has found similar ulcer healing rates and pain control.[36]

Equivalent healing rates for famotidine, ranitidine, and cimetidine should be expected when equipotent doses of each drug are administered at the same time of day, since they have similar effects on basal and stimulated gastric acid secretion. In addition, the duration of acid secretory inhibition and the pharmacokinetics of famotidine and ranitidine are similar (Table 1). However, differences in antisecretory duration between cimetidine and ranitidine have failed to translate into differences in efficacy when equipotent doses of each drug are used to treat duodenal ulcers.[16] Possibly only nocturnal acid suppression is required for healing duodenal ulcers or, once the amount and duration of acid suppression is achieved, additional suppression does not significantly increase ulcer healing. Alternatively, the lack of a significant difference between treatment groups may indicate that an insufficient number of patients was studied to permit detection of a difference between drugs or drug regimens that are expected to exert a high rate of efficacy (beta error).

The healing rates obtained in the famotidine multicenter studies included in this review are similar to those reported in the literature for the numerous trials conducted to determine the efficacy of cimetidine and ranitidine in the treatment of active duodenal ulcers.[16,28] These similarities in efficacy are supported by additional trials comparing single nocturnal doses of H_2 antagonists with multiple daily doses.[39,40] Therefore, it is reasonable to conclude that famotidine in a dose of 20 mg orally b.i.d. or 40 mg at bedtime is equally effective; that both dosage regimens accelerate duodenal ulcer healing to the same extent as recommended daily doses of ranitidine or cimetidine; and that a single daily dose of 40 mg of famotidine is as effective as ranitidine 300 mg (as the hydrochloride salt) or cimetidine 800 mg orally at bedtime (Table 2). Patient compliance with the three H_2-receptor antagonists should be similar if the frequency of the daily dosing regimen is the same for each drug.

Treatment of Active Benign Gastric Ulcer

Four similar controlled trials have been conducted to determine the efficacy of famotidine in healing active benign gastric ulcer.[41–44] One additional trial compared a bedtime dose of famotidine 40 mg orally with ranitidine 150 mg (as the hydrochloride salt) twice daily.[45] The methods, design, and results of these double-blind studies are summarized in Table 4. In all trials, patients receiving ulcerogenic medications were excluded, and previous antiulcer regimens were withheld. Compliance with drug therapy was verified in three of the studies.[41–43] Occasional antacid use was reported in four of the five trials.[41,43–45]

It is important to note that only two of the controlled gastric ulcer trials have been conducted in the United States,[44,45] although approximately 4% of participants in the worldwide study reported by Lyon[41] were North Americans. Worldwide studies provide valuable information regarding the efficacy of H_2-receptor antagonists in healing gastric and duodenal ulcers; however, differences in placebo and ulcer healing rates may vary depending on geographical location.[46] Additional clinical trials evaluating the efficacy of famotidine in healing gastric ulcers are in progress in the United States.

Lyon[41] reported the results of a worldwide study involving 14 countries that compared famotidine 40 mg orally at bedtime with placebo. The two treatment groups were comparable with regard to age, sex, country of residence, previous peptic ulcer history, cigarette smoking, and median ulcer size; however, the placebo group had a greater proportion of patients who regularly used alcohol. Antacid consumption and the frequency and severity of ulcer pain were quantitated daily. At four, six, and eight weeks, the famotidine group showed a significant increase in gastric ulcer healing.

Table 4.
Double-Blind Controlled Trials Comparing Famotidine with Placebo or Ranitidine in the Treatment of Active Benign Gastric Ulcer[a]

Reference	Drug and Dose (mg)[a]	Defined Ulcer Healing	Frequency of Scheduled Endoscopy[b]	No. of Evaluable Patients	% Healed at Indicated Time		
					4 weeks	6 weeks	8 weeks
41	P h.s.	No	4, 6, 8 weeks	169[c]	31[e]	46[e]	54[e]
	F 40 h.s.			167[c]	47	65	80
42	P h.s.	No	4, 6, 8 weeks	39	45	64[f]	70[e]
	F 40 h.s.			34	56	84	94
43	P h.s.	Yes	4, 6, 8 weeks	29	31	45	66[e]
	F 40 h.s.			33	42	61	97
44	P h.s.	No	4, 6, 8 weeks	149[d]	39	44[e]	64[e]
	F 40 h.s.				45	66	78
45	F 40 h.s.	No	4, 6, 8 weeks	175[d]	49	70	82
	R 150 b.i.d.				48	69	81

[a] P =placebo, F = famotidine, R = ranitidine given as the hydrochloride salt.
[b] Baseline endoscopies were performed in all cases.
[c] Represents number of patients entered into study.
[d] Represents total number of evaluable patients; specific numbers of patients in drug treatment or placebo groups were not identified.
[e] $p < 0.01$ when placebo was compared with each famotidine dosage.
[f] $p < 0.05$ when placebo was compared with each famotidine dosage.

Country of residence did not appear to influence the response to famotidine, since 13 of the 14 countries had higher healing rates with famotidine than with placebo. Among patients with a high level of alcohol ingestion, 78% of the group treated with famotidine and 56% of the placebo group had healed gastric ulcers by the eighth week. The median time for complete relief of daytime pain was shorter for patients in the famotidine group (14 days versus 35 days for the placebo group, $p < 0.01$). A total of 22% of patients receiving famotidine and 34% of patients receiving placebo continued to have some residual pain at the end of the study. The difference in time required to abolish nocturnal pain was of borderline significance ($0.05 < p < 0.055$). A total of 16% of patients in the famotidine group and 21% in the control group failed to achieve complete relief of nighttime pain. Antacid use was less for the famotidine group during the first week ($p < 0.05$ except for day 3) and during weeks four, six, and eight, although these later differences were not significant. This study indicates that gastric ulcer healing and the relief of ulcer pain are enhanced by famotidine 40 mg at bedtime.

Dammann et al.[42] conducted a randomized, placebo-controlled multicenter trial in Austria and Germany. The proportion of patients whose ulcers healed was higher in the famotidine group throughout the study period, with significance reached by weeks 6 and 8. Reduction of daytime and nocturnal pain was similar in both groups, with no significant difference between treatments. However, approximately 70% in each group were asymptomatic by the fourth week. Although 13 patients were asymptomatic at the end of the study, an unhealed gastric ulcer was evident upon endoscopy.

Two additional multicenter studies have compared single nocturnal doses of famotidine with placebo and have reported similar results.[43,44] When once-daily famotidine was compared with twice-daily ranitidine in a community-based multicenter trial, both treatment regimens were equivalent in accelerating gastric ulcer healing and in relieving associated symptoms.[45]

The placebo healing rates for gastric ulcers tend to be higher and more variable than those observed with duodenal ulcers. In addition, the response to drug therapy appears to be lower, and longer treatment periods are required.[46] Thus, establishing a significant difference in ulcer healing rates (especially during a four- to eight-week period) may be difficult in gastric ulcer trials. Although studies comparing famotidine, ranitidine, and cimetidine with placebo indicate that they are effective in healing duodenal ulcers, the efficacy of these agents in healing gastric ulcers is less convincing.[15,16,41–44,46] The comparative efficacy of oral regimens of ranitidine 150 mg (as the hydrochloride salt) b.i.d. and cimetidine 1000 mg (in divided daily doses of 200 mg, 200 mg, 200 mg, and 400 mg) or 1200 mg (300 mg q.i.d.) has been evaluated in controlled trials, and, in most instances, they are associated with similar gastric ulcer healing rates.[16,46] It appears that a single bedtime dose of famotidine 40 mg orally is significantly more effective than placebo in healing gastric ulcers and may be as effective as ranitidine administered two times per day and cimetidine administered four times per day. However, additional efficacy trials comparing single versus multiple dosing per day with the three H_2-receptor antagonists are required to confirm this supposition. Only cimetidine and ranitidine are approved by the FDA for the treatment of gastric ulcers (Table 2).

Maintenance Therapy

Texter et al.[47] reported the results from a 12-month, double-blind, placebo-controlled, multicenter trial conducted in the United States that evaluated 303 patients receiving maintenance therapy for up to one year with oral famotidine 20 mg at bedtime, 40 mg at bedtime, or placebo. Endoscopies were performed before entry into the study and repeated at 3, 6, and 12 months and if symptoms suggested a relapse. The treatment groups were comparable as to age, sex, race, level of cigarette smoking and alcohol consumption, initial ulcer size, and type of medical treatments used to heal the initial ulcer. During the study period, patients were excluded if they were noncompliant with treatment medication or if they used prohibited medications such as aspirin. Antacid use was not discussed by the investigators.

Relapse rates were calculated using the life-table analysis method, a rigorous statistical evaluation that adjusts for dropouts in each assessment period by assuming that they were at risk for half the period and that the risk was the same for those patients who did not drop out.[48] Values for the cumulative relapses at the end of 12 months are reported in Table 5. Relapse rates at all time points were significantly lower in patients receiving either famotidine 20 mg or 40 mg orally at bedtime compared with placebo ($p < 0.01$). However, no significant difference between the two famotidine groups was observed during the study. Because of similar efficacy, the 20-mg bedtime dose of famotidine is recommended. Fewer relapses occurred in women and in nonsmokers, while more relapses were reported for patients under 40 years of age and in those with a long history of ulcer disease.

In most instances, the rate of ulcer recurrence with famotidine 20 mg at bedtime appears to be similar to rates reported for ranitidine 150 mg (as the hydrochloride salt) at bedtime and cimetidine 400 mg at bedtime when the life-table analysis method is used to calculate cumulative recurrence rates in duodenal ulcer maintenance trials.[48] This finding is not surprising in light of the importance of effective nocturnal acid suppression in preventing duodenal ulcer relapse. However, an oral famotidine dose of 20 mg appears to be equipotent to ranitidine 150 mg and cimetidine 800 mg. Comparative clinical trials of the three H_2-receptor antagonists are required to determine the superiority of any one agent in preventing recurrent duodenal ulcers.

Although the efficacy of the H_2-receptor antagonists in preventing duodenal ulcer recurrence is established, their effectiveness in preventing gastric ulcer recurrence is not as conclusive. Studies with cimetidine suggest that the prevention of gastric ulcer relapse may require higher doses than those used for duodenal ulcer maintenance.[48] Ranitidine 150 mg (as the hydrochloride salt) orally at bedtime appears to be effective, but the number of patients studied is insufficient to provide a definitive answer.[48] Controlled, double-blind studies that evaluate the efficacy of famotidine maintenance therapy in treating gastric ulcers have not yet been published in the United States. There are no H_2-receptor antagonists approved by the FDA for the prevention of gastric ulcer relapse.

Treatment of Zollinger–Ellison Syndrome

A study comparing the potency, onset, and duration of antisecretory action of famotidine, ranitidine, and cimetidine in patients with Zollinger–Ellison syndrome was summarized above.[8] After completion of the initial phase of the study, the investigators evaluated the efficacy of famotidine in eight of the same patients by using each patient's minimal dosage requirement (one fourth of the total daily dosage given every six hours), established in the earlier phase of the study.[8] If a famotidine dose of 0.64 g (0.16 g every six hours) did not suppress gastric acid secretion to <10 meq/hr in the hour tested, then isopropamide 5 mg (as the iodide salt) every six hours was added to the regimen. Patients were treated for up to nine months (mean, six months) with famotidine and evaluated initially at two weeks and at two-month intervals thereafter. A single increase in famotidine dosage was required in three patients, and two additional patients required two dosage increases. Of these five patients, two required the addition of isopropamide to maintain the desired level of gastric acid

Table 5.
Results of Duodenal Ulcer Maintenance Trial Comparing Famotidine with Placebo

Reference	No. of Patients	Drug and Dose (mg)[a]	Recurrence Rate (%)[b] 3 months	6 months	12 months
47	99	P h.s.	39[c]	52[c]	57[c]
	97	F 20 h.s.	14	16	23
	107	F 40 h.s.	9	21	25

[a] P = placebo, F = famotidine.
[b] Recurrence rates were calculated by the life-table analysis method.
[c] $p < 0.01$ when placebo was compared with each famotidine dosage regimen.

output. Famotidine remained effective in controlling acid hypersecretion for up to nine months. The frequency of dosage adjustments was approximately the same as those reported for cimetidine and ranitidine, suggesting that rapid tolerance did not develop with famotidine.[10,49]

Vinayek et al.[50] studied 33 patients with gastric hypersecretory states (32 with Zollinger–Ellison syndrome), five of whom were initially treated in the second phase of the study conducted by Howard et al.[8] Before famotidine therapy, 27 patients required an average ranitidine maintenance dose of 2.3 g/day (as the hydrochloride salt, range 0.6 to 5.4 g/day), and 6 patients required an average cimetidine dose of 4.6 g/day (range 1.2 to 9.0 g/day). Fourteen patients required an additional anticholinergic agent. Thirty-two patients received long-term famotidine treatment for up to 34 months (mean, 10 months); 21 patients were studied for at least 6 months, 9 for at least 12 months, and 6 for at least 24 months. The mean daily maintenance dose of famotidine required was 0.33 g/day (range 0.05 to 0.8 g/day), while five patients needed the addition of an anticholinergic agent. Hypersecretion of gastric acid was controlled in seven patients using less frequent dosing with famotidine (every six to eight hours) than what they were previously receiving with cimetidine or ranitidine (every four to six hours). However, this study was not originally designed to assess the antisecretory duration and effective dosing interval of famotidine. No toxicities or adverse effects were reported in any of the patients treated with famotidine for as long as 34 months.

The results of these two studies demonstrate that famotidine, like ranitidine and cimetidine, is effective in the long-term treatment of hypersecretory states and that its action is potentiated by anticholinergic agents. As is true for cimetidine and ranitidine, higher doses of famotidine are required in patients who have documented gastric acid hypersecretion. In addition, patients requiring a high dose of either of the two H_2 antagonists will probably require a high dose of famotidine. The frequency of dosage increments is approximately the same for all three drugs, although it appears that in some patients the dosing interval may be less frequent with famotidine. Because the requirements of H_2-receptor antagonists may increase with time, even with potent agents such as famotidine, newer antisecretory agents such as omeprazole may be more effective in patients with Zollinger–Ellison syndrome.[51,52]

Treatment of Other Acid–Peptic Disorders

There are only a few published clinical trials that have evaluated the efficacy of famotidine in the treatment of acid–peptic disorders such as gastroesophageal reflux disease or gastritis, prevention of stress-related mucosal lesions, treatment of active acute upper gastrointestinal hemorrhage, or prevention of the pulmonary acid-aspiration syndrome associated with anesthesia.[53–56] Many of these published reports are open trials conducted in locations other than the United States. Of the three H_2-receptor antagonists, only ranitidine is approved by the FDA for the treatment of reflux esophagitis (Table 2); however, neither cimetidine nor ranitidine has FDA approval for the other acid–peptic disorders for which they are commonly used. Although it is likely that famotidine is at least as effective as cimetidine and ranitidine in the prevention and treatment of these disorders, comparative, double-blind clinical trials conducted in the United States are required before such assumptions can be confirmed.

Adverse Reactions

Extensive preclinical safety studies were performed with famotidine before the drug was administered to humans. To date, the overall incidence of adverse effects reported in patients receiving famotidine is low.[6,7,13,23,29–36,41–45,47,50,57–59] The drug has been well tolerated by patients in both the short-term controlled trials for the treatment of peptic ulcer disease and in the long-term studies for the prevention of ulcer relapse and Zollinger–Ellison syndrome. In short-term trials comparing famotidine with cimetidine or ranitidine, the incidence of adverse clinical effects was similar, and no significant differences were reported.

Miyoshi et al.[59] summarized the results of open and controlled trials in Japan in which 2001 patients received 20 to 60 mg of famotidine per day over eight weeks. Patients received famotidine therapy for various peptic disorders including gastric and duodenal ulcer, anastomotic ulcer, and reflux esophagitis. The overall incidence of adverse effects was 2.8%, or 57 patients of whom 8 had severe reactions that necessitated discontinuation of therapy. Other reported adverse effects included constipation, diarrhea, and skin rash, which occurred in 1.3%, 0.4%, and 0.2% of the patients, respectively.

The safety of famotidine in patients receiving 40 mg/day for the treatment of gastric ulcer was examined in a worldwide study and in Japan.[41] In the worldwide study, 44 (13%) of the 336 patients experienced an adverse reaction, with no difference observed between the famotidine-treated patients and the placebo group with regard to number of incidents. The frequency and severity of the reported reactions were similar for individuals over 65 years of age and younger patients. Headache occurred in 4.7% of the famotidine-treated patients. Other infrequent (incidence $< 1.0\%$) reactions in the famotidine group included muscle cramps, skin rash, impotence, and mild disorientation. Eleven patients were withdrawn from the study because of an adverse experience (six in the famotidine group and five in the placebo group). Results from the Japanese study indicated that 8.3% of patients receiving famotidine and 18.8% of those taking gefarnate reported at least one adverse experience. Among the famotidine-treated patients, the only adverse effects occurring in more than 2.0% of the patients were constipation (4.2%) and nausea (2.1%). A causal relation was unlikely since the identical incidences were reported in the gefarnate group.

In the worldwide study, laboratory abnormalities were observed in 11 patients (famotidine, 5; placebo, 6) and included leukocytosis; prolonged erythrocyte sedimentation rate; elevated concentrations of blood urea nitrogen, serum alkaline phosphatase, and serum aminotransferase; and proteinuria. No patients were withdrawn from the study because of these effects. Similar abnormalities were reported in 15% of the Japanese study patients and were evenly distributed between the famotidine and placebo groups.

McCullough[31] evaluated the efficacy and safety of famotidine 40 to 80 mg/day and ranitidine 300 mg/day (as the hydrochloride salt) in 1031 patients with active duodenal ulcer disease during an eight-week treatment period. The type and frequency of adverse reactions reported in the famotidine-treated patients included headache (3.1%–3.9%), diarrhea (1.2%–1.6%), dizziness (0.4%–1.2%), somnolence (0.4%–0.8%), and asthenia (0.0%–1.2%), with the incidences of each being equally distributed among the different famotidine dosages. Both the type and frequency of adverse experiences reported with ranitidine were similar to those reported with famotidine. Of the 872 patients receiving famotidine, nine withdrew from the study because of adverse experiences including abdominal pain, generalized pain, headache, and anorexia. Of 259 ranitidine-treated patients, three withdrew because of diarrhea and depression. There were no reported changes in laboratory values in either drug group.

When famotidine was studied in 33 patients with hypersecretory states (doses ranging from 0.05 g/day to 0.8 g/day), no hematologic or biochemical evidence of toxicity was detected.[50] No neurologic or antiandrogenic (breast tenderness, gynecomastia, impotence) effects occurred in the famotidine-treated male patients; however, one patient who had been receiving cimetidine before entry into the study reported gynecomastia and impotence while taking cimetidine. In the eight cases in which famotidine therapy had to be stopped, none had to be discontinued because of adverse effects attributable to the drug.

It appears that the overall incidence of adverse effects observed with famotidine is similar to that reported with cimetidine and ranitidine.[15-17] All three H_2-receptor antagonists have an excellent safety profile, although it is probable that ranitidine and cimetidine have been used in more patients for a longer time. Famotidine differs from cimetidine but resembles ranitidine in that long-term treatment using high doses in men is not associated with antiandrogenic adverse effects.[16,17,50,60] This appears to favor the use of either ranitidine or famotidine in patients with hypersecretory states that require high doses of H_2-receptor antagonists.

Cimetidine and ranitidine, like famotidine, have also been associated with gastrointestinal adverse effects and headache, but these adverse experiences usually resolve with continued treatment. Substantial increases in aminotransferase concentrations have been reported with intravenous doses of ranitidine 100 mg (as the hydrochloride salt) q.i.d.[61] Although the CNS effects that are reported to occur with cimetidine (primarily in the elderly and those with severe renal impairment) have been reported in fewer patients receiving ranitidine, it is difficult to conclude that there is a difference in incidence between the two drugs. In contrast to cimetidine and ranitidine, intravenous famotidine does not significantly affect serum prolactin levels.[13,14] Famotidine appears to be a safe and valuable agent for patients requiring treatment with H_2 antagonists and may be well tolerated by the elderly.[62] However, early predictions of adverse effects and safety have been revised with the continued use of cimetidine and ranitidine.

Drug Interactions

Famotidine appears to be similar to ranitidine in that usual therapeutic doses do not significantly affect the elimination of drugs that are metabolized by the cytochrome P-450 mixed-function oxidase system.[19,20,63,67] In contrast, cimetidine has been reported to decrease the hepatic clearance of theophylline, warfarin, phenytoin, lidocaine, chlordiazepoxide, and other drugs metabolized by hepatic microsomal enzymes.[68] The dissolution of drugs and the disintegration of oral dosage forms that are pH-dependent could be affected by increased gastric pH resulting from the administration of H_2-receptor antagonists.[69]

Theophylline pharmacokinetics (single intravenous dose of 5 mg/kg) was studied in 10 healthy volunteers after the oral administration of famotidine 40 mg b.i.d. and cimetidine 300 mg every six hours for five days. Cimetidine significantly decreased plasma clearance of theophylline and prolonged the elimination half-life, whereas famotidine had no effect on the metabolic elimination of theophylline.[64] Sambol et al.[65] examined the effect of famotidine and cimetidine on phenytoin pharmacokinetics and indocyanine green clearance. The plasma clearance of phenytoin remained unchanged after famotidine administration but was significantly decreased with cimetidine.

In a study by Locniskar et al.[66] therapeutic doses of cimetidine significantly increased the elimination half-life and the area under the concentration–time curve and decreased the total clearance of diazepam in 12 healthy subjects, while famotidine did not significantly affect the disposition of the drug.[66] Klotz et al.[67] studied the effect of famotidine on the pharmacokinetics of diazepam and procainamide to determine changes in hepatic metabolism (for diazepam) and tubular secretion (for procainamide). Famotidine did not intensify the sedative and muscle-relaxing action of diazepam, nor did it affect the pharmacodynamics of procainamide. The elimination half-life and the total plasma clearance of both drugs were not significantly altered. This is in contrast to the documented effects of cimetidine on hepatic microsomal enzymes and the renal tubular secretion of procainamide and *N*-acetyl procainamide.[68]

Thus, it appears that famotidine, like ranitidine, does not interact in a clinically important manner with drugs that are metabolized by the cytochrome P-450 system. Alternatively, hepatic enzyme interactions with cimetidine appear to be dose related within its therapeutic range.[70,71] The lower cimetidine daily doses (800 mg for duodenal ulcer treatment and 400 mg for duodenal ulcer prevention), as well as the once-daily dosing regimen, may reduce the magnitude of potential cimetidine drug interactions. Cimetidine, and to a lesser extent ranitidine, may inhibit the renal clearance of drugs that undergo tubular secretion. All H_2-receptor antagonists may alter drug absorption through their effects on gastric pH. Because a wide range of interpatient and intrapatient factors appears to affect the degree of cimetidine and ranitidine drug interactions, caution should be exercised until additional clinical experience is gained with famotidine.

Dosage

The recommended oral dosage regimens of famotidine for the treatment of active duodenal ulcer are shown in Table 2. Famotidine 40 mg orally at bedtime appears to heal benign gastric ulcers, although FDA labeling does not include this indication. As with all H_2-receptor antagonists, treatment should be continued for four to eight weeks or until ulcer healing is confirmed by endoscopy. Since the efficacy of divided daily doses appears to be the same as for a single nocturnal dose, once-daily dosing for cimetidine, ranitidine, and famotidine is usually recommended in an attempt to enhance patient compliance. Lower nocturnal doses of famotidine, like cimetidine and ranitidine, are recommended for the prevention of recurrent duodenal ulcer.

The manufacturer recommends that the dose of famotidine be decreased to 20 mg or that the dosing interval be lengthened (36–48 hours) when the creatinine clearance falls below 10 mL/min.[72] Takabatake et al.[25] recommend that the dosage in renal failure be adjusted according to the following guidelines: $CL_{cr} > 60$ mL/min, give usual dose; $CL_{cr} = 30–60$ mL/min, reduce dose by 50%; $CL_{cr} <$ 30 mL/min, give 25% of recommended dose. Dosage reductions in renal failure are also recommended for cimetidine and ranitidine.[9,11] As with cimetidine and ranitidine, the famotidine dosage schedule should be adjusted to coincide with the end of hemodialysis.[9,11,26] The pharmacokinetics of famotidine in patients on continuous ambulatory peritoneal dialysis has not been reported.

Patients with pathological hypersecretory conditions such as Zollinger–Ellison syndrome should initially receive famotidine 20 mg every six hours. The dosage should be increased depending on the severity of the patient's condition or the dose of the previous H_2-receptor antagonist. Doses as high as 0.2 g every six hours have been used in patients with severe disease.[50]

The intravenous route of administration is intended for patients who are unable to take oral medication or who have severe hypersecretory conditions or intractable ulcers. The recommended intravenous dose of famotidine is 20 mg every 12 hours versus the more frequent dosing regimens recommended for cimetidine and ranitidine.

Availability and Cost

Famotidine is available as 20- and 40-mg oral tablets, a 10-mg/mL injection (with or without preservatives), and a 40-mg/5 mL oral suspension. The oral suspension requires reconstitution and is stable for 30 days upon refrigeration. The undiluted intravenous preparation must be stored at 2–8 °C. Both cimetidine and ranitidine are available as oral tablets and as injections; although there is an oral liquid solution (does not require reconstitution) of cimetidine, there is no commercially available oral liquid formulation of ranitidine. Neither of the undiluted injectable forms of cimetidine or ranitidine requires refrigeration. The costs associated with various H_2-antagonist treatments are shown in Table 6. These costs will vary in the hospital setting depending on competitive bidding by the manufacturer of each drug.

Place in Therapy

Famotidine 20 mg b.i.d. or 40 mg at bedtime is as effective as standard doses of cimetidine and ranitidine in healing duodenal ulcers. A single bedtime dose of 40 mg appears to be effective in the treatment of active benign gastric ulcer. The results of a well-controlled maintenance trial indicate that a famotidine dose of 20 mg at bedtime is effective in preventing duodenal ulcer recurrence. Although comparisons have not been made with cimetidine and ranitidine, it is likely that a single nocturnal dose of famotidine 20 mg will prove to be equally effective in preventing duodenal ulcers.

Famotidine appears to be as effective as cimetidine and ranitidine when equipotent doses are used to treat patients with Zollinger–Ellison syndrome. Like ranitidine, high antisecretory doses appear to be devoid of antiandrogenic effects. It is possible that its prolonged antisecretory action may permit less frequent dosing in the treatment of patients with hypersecretory diseases. Treatment failures have been associated with all three H_2-receptor antagonists. The value of famotidine in "cimetidine-resistant" or "ranitidine-resistant" ulcers remains to be demonstrated.

Large multicenter placebo-controlled clinical trials for short-term ulcer treatment and long-term maintenance therapy have shown that most patients tolerate therapeutic doses very well. The adverse effects and safety profile resemble those of ranitidine. Therapeutic doses of famotidine do not appear to affect the pharmacokinetics of drugs that undergo hepatic elimination and renal tubular secretion. As with the other H_2-receptor antagonists, renal elimination is decreased in patients with renal impairment, and a reduction in dose may be indicated. Famotidine, like cimetidine, is available in an oral liquid dosage form for patients unable to take oral tablets; thus, there is a less expensive alternative to the injectable form of the drug. Because the three drugs are similar in efficacy, cost and safety will be important considerations in drug selection and formulary decisions.

Conclusion

Famotidine, ranitidine, and cimetidine appear to be equally effective in treating gastric and duodenal ulcers when adequate doses are administered. A single nocturnal dose of famotidine, like cimetidine and ranitidine, is effective in healing duodenal ulcers and may enhance patient compliance. The efficacy of famotidine, ranitidine, and cimetidine in preventing duodenal ulcer recurrence may also be similar. Famotidine, because of its increased potency and lack of antiandrogenic adverse effects at higher doses, may be the drug of choice for treating hypersecretory conditions such as Zollinger–Ellison syndrome. Famotidine and ranitidine do not significantly inhibit the hepatic clearance of drugs metabolized by cytochrome P-450 mixed-function oxidase, although lower daily doses of cimetidine appear to decrease the magnitude of this drug interaction.

Additional clinical experience and controlled trials are necessary to determine the safety and comparative efficacy of famotidine in treating acid–peptic disorders. However, safety and cost, rather than increased potency and efficacy, will probably be the deciding factors in selecting the most appropriate H_2-receptor antagonist for treating acid–peptic disorders.

Table 6.
Cost Comparison of Famotidine, Ranitidine, and Cimetidine

Drug	Dosage Form	Dose (mg)	Cost/Day ($)[a]	Cost/Month ($)[a]
Famotidine (Pepcid)	20-mg tablet	20 h.s.	1.02	30.60
		20 b.i.d.	2.04	61.20
	40-mg tablet	40 h.s.	1.97	59.10
	40-mg/5-mL liquid, 50-mL bottle	20 h.s.	2.71	81.30
		20 b.i.d.	5.42	162.60
	20-mg/2-mL injection, 2-mL vial	20 q12h	11.88	...
	20-mg/2-mL injection, 4-mL vial	20 q12h	9.20	...
Ranitidine (Zantac)	150-mg tablet	150 h.s.	1.09	32.70
		150 b.i.d.	2.18	65.40
	300-mg tablet[b]	300 h.s.	1.98	59.40
	50-mg/2-mL injection, 2-mL vial[b]	50 q8h	11.97	...
		50 q6h	15.96	...
	50-mg/2-mL injection, 10-mL vial[b]	50 q8h	9.26	...
		50 q6h	12.36	...
Cimetidine (Tagamet)	200-mg tablet	400 h.s.	0.88	26.40
	300-mg tablet	300 q.i.d.	1.84	55.20
	400-mg tablet	400 h.s.	0.87	26.10
		400 b.i.d.	1.74	52.20
	800-mg tablet	800 h.s.	1.68	50.40
	300-mg/5-mL liquid, 240-mL bottle[b]	300 q6h	4.26	127.80
	300-mg/2-mL injection, 2-mL vial (packages of 30)[b]	300 q8h	11.18	...
		300 q6h	14.92	...
	300-mg/2-mL injection, 8-mL vial (packages of 25)[b]	300 q8h	8.65	...
		300 q6h	11.53	...

[a] Average wholesale price based on *Drug Topics Redbook Annual Pharmacist's Reference*, Update 1988.
[b] As the hydrochloride salt.

References

1. Streett CS, Cimprich RE, Robertson JL. Pathologic findings in the stomachs of rats treated with the H2-receptor antagonist tiodidine. *Scand J Gastroenterol.* 1984; 19(Suppl 101):109–17.
2. Takagi T, Takeda M, Fujihara A et al. General pharmacological properties of a new potent H2-blocker, famotidine (YM-11170). *Pharmacometrics.* 1983; 26:599–611.
3. Dammann HG, Muller P, Simon B. 24 hour intragastric acidity and single night-time dose of three H2-blockers. *Lancet.* 1983; 2:1078. Letter.
4. Smith JL. Clinical pharmacology of famotidine. *Digestion.* 1985; 32(Suppl 1):15–23.
5. McCallum RW, Chremos AN, Kuljian B et al. MK-208, a novel histamine H2-receptor inhibitor with prolonged antisecretory effect. *Dig Dis Sci.* 1985; 12:1139–44.
6. Chremos AN. Pharmacodynamics of famotidine in humans. *Am J Med.* 1986; 81(Suppl 4B):3–7.
7. Ryan JR, Vargas R, McMahon FG et al. Comparison of effects of oral and intravenous famotidine on inhibition of nocturnal gastric acid secretion. *Am J Med.* 1986; 81(Suppl 4B):60–4.
8. Howard JM, Chremos AN, Collen MJ et al. Famotidine, a new, potent, long-acting histamine H2-receptor antagonist; comparison with cimetidine and ranitidine in the treatment of Zollinger–Ellison syndrome. *Gastroenterology.* 1985; 88:1026–33.
9. Somogyi A, Gugler R. Clinical pharmacokinetics of cimetidine. *Clin Pharmacokinet.* 1983; 8:463–95.
10. Jensen RT, Collen MJ, McArthur KE et al. Comparison of the effectiveness of ranitidine and cimetidine in inhibiting acid secretion in patients with gastric hypersecretory states. *Am J Med.* 1984; 77:(Suppl 5B):90–105.
11. Roberts CJC. Clinical pharmacokinetics of ranitidine. *Clin Pharmacokinet.* 1984; 9:211–21.
12. Miwa M, Tani N, Miwa T. Inhibition of gastric secretion by a new H2-antagonist, YM-11170, in healthy subjects. *Int J Clin Pharmacol Ther Toxicol.* 1984; 22:214–7.
13. Hayakawa A, Ohe K, Miyoshi A et al. Properties of famotidine in relation to safety. *Ital J Gastroenterol.* 1984; 16:174–6.
14. Campoli-Richards DM, Clissold SP. Famotidine: pharmacodynamic and pharmacokinetic properties and a preliminary review of its therapeutic use in peptic ulcer disease and Zollinger–Ellison syndrome. *Drugs.* 1986; 32:197–221.
15. Freston JW. Cimetidine II. Adverse reactions and patterns of use. *Ann Intern Med.* 1982; 97:728–34.
16. Brogden RN, Carmine AA, Heel RC et al. Ranitidine: a review of its pharmacology and therapeutic use in peptic ulcer disease and other allied diseases. *Drugs.* 1982; 24:267–303.
17. McGuigan JE. A consideration of the adverse effects of cimetidine. *Gastroenterology.* 1981; 80:181–92.
18. Opsahl JA, Abrahams PA, Halstenson CE et al. Renal function after famotidine administration. *Clin Pharmacol Ther.* 1986; 39:218. Abstract.
19. Staiger C, Korodnay B, Devries JX et al. Comparative effects of famotidine and cimetidine on antipyrine kinetics in healthy volunteers. *Br J Clin Pharmacol.* 1984; 18:105–6. Letter.
20. Somerville KW, Kitchingman GA, Langman MJS. Effect of famotidine on oxidative drug metabolism. *Eur J Clin Pharmacol.* 1986; 30:279–81.
21. Kawai R, Yamada S, Kawamura S et al. Metabolic fate of famotidine (YM-11170), a new potent H2-receptor antagonist: absorption and excretion in dogs and humans. *Pharmacometrics.* 1984; 27:73–7.
22. Hucker HB, Hutt JE, Chremos AN et al. Disposition and metabolism of famotidine, a potent H2-receptor blocker, in man. *Fed Proc.* 1984; 43:655. Abstract.
23. Ryan R. Clinical pharmacology of famotidine: summary of data from the United States. *Ital J Gastroenterol.* 1984; 16:171–4.
24. Takabatake T, Ohta H, Maekawa M et al. Pharmacokinetics of famotidine, a new H2-receptor antagonist, in relation to renal function. *Eur J Clin Pharmacol.* 1985; 28:327–31.
25. Halstenson CE, Abrahams PA, Opsahl JA et al. Disposition of famotidine in renal insufficiency. *Clin Pharmacol Ther.* 1986; 39:197. Abstract.
26. Takabatake T, Ohta H, Maekawa M et al. Pharmacokinetics of famotidine in patients with renal insufficiency. *Shinryo to Shinyaki.* 1983; 20:2061–8.
27. Morgan MY, Stambuk D. Famotidine pharmacokinetics following oral and intravenous administration in patients with liver disease: results of a preliminary study. *Postgrad Med J.* 1986; 62:(Suppl 2):29–37.
28. Freston JW. Cimetidine I. Developments, pharmacology, and efficacy. *Ann Intern Med.* 1982; 97:573–80.
29. Bianchi Porro G. Famotidine in the treatment of gastric and duodenal ulceration: overview of clinical experience. *Digestion.* 1985; 32(Suppl 1):62–9.
30. Gitlin N, McCullough AJ, Smith JL et al. A multicenter, double-blind, randomized, placebo-controlled comparison of nocturnal and twice-a-day famotidine in the treatment of active duodenal ulcer disease. *Gastroenterology.* 1987; 92:48–53.
31. McCullough AJ. A multicenter, randomized, double-blind study comparing famotidine with ranitidine in the treatment of active duodenal ulcer disease. *Am J Med.* 1986; 81(Suppl 4B):17–24.
32. Barbara L, Corinaldesi R, Bianchi Porro G et al. Famotidine in the management of duodenal ulcer: experience in Italy. *Digestion.* 1985; 32(Suppl 1):24–31.
33. Simon B, Dammann HG, Jakob G et al. Famotidine versus ranitidine for the short-term treatment of duodenal ulcer. *Digestion.* 1985; 32(Suppl 1):32–7.
34. Hetzel DJ, Shearman DJC, Korman MG et al. Famotidine (MK 208) in the treatment of duodenal ulcer: short term multicentre studies and a maintenance trial. *Aust NZ J Med.* 1985; 15(Suppl 2):547. Abstract.
35. Rohner HG, Gugler R. Treatment of active duodenal ulcers with famotidine. *Am J Med.* 1986; 81(Suppl 4B):13–6.
36. Dobrillo G, De Pretis G, Piazzi L et al. Comparison of once-daily bedtime administration of famotidine and ranitidine in the short-term treatment of duodenal ulcer: a multicenter, double-blind, controlled study. *Scand J Gastroenterol.* 1987; 22(Suppl 143):21–8.
37. Weberg R, Berstad A, Loange O et al. Duodenal ulcer healing with four antacid tablets daily. *Scand J Gastroenterol.* 1985; 20:1041–5.
38. Bianchi Porro G, Parente F, Lazzaroni M et al. Medium-dose antacids versus cimetidine in the short-term treatment of duodenal ulcer. *J Clin Gastroenterol.* 1986; 8:141–5.
39. Valenzuela JE, Dickson B, Dixon W et al. Efficacy of a single nocturnal dose of cimetidine in active duodenal ulcer: results of a United States multicenter trial. *Postgrad Med.* 1985; Nov:35–41.
40. Conlin-Jones DG, Ireland A, Gear P et al. Reducing overnight secretion of acid to heal duodenal ulcers: comparison of standard divided dose of ranitidine with a single dose administered at night. *Am J Med.* 1984; 77(Suppl 5B):116–22.
41. Lyon DT. Efficacy and safety of famotidine in the management of benign gastric ulcers. *Am J Med.* 1986; 81(Suppl 4B):33–41.
42. Dammann HG, Walter TA, Hentschel E et al. Famotidine: nocturnal dosing for gastric ulcer healing. *Digestion.* 1985; 32(Suppl 1):45–50.
43. Paoluzi P, Tarsoli A, Bianchi Porro G et al. Famotidine (MK-208) in the treatment of gastric ulcer: results of a multicenter double-blind controlled study. *Digestion.* 1985; 32(Suppl 1):38–44.
44. McCullough A, Petrozza J, Roufail WM et al. Famotidine 40 mg once daily in the treatment of acute gastric ulcer: a U.S. multicenter placebo-controlled trial. *Gastroenterology.* 1987; 92:1525. Abstract.
45. Brazer R, Pancotto FS, Brice RS et al. A comparison of famotidine 40 mg once daily with ranitidine 150 mg twice daily

in the treatment of benign gastric ulcer: a community-based U.S. multicenter trial. *Gastroenterology*. 1987; 92:1327. Abstract.

46. Legerton CW. Duodenal and gastric ulcer healing rates: a review. *Am J Med*. 1984; 77(Suppl 5B):2–6.
47. Texter EC, Navab F, Mantell G et al. Maintenance therapy of duodenal ulcer with famotidine: a multicenter United States study. *Am J Med*. 1986; 81(Suppl 4B):25–32.
48. Berardi RR, Savitsky ME, Nostrant TT. Maintenance therapy for prevention of recurrent peptic ulcers. *Drug Intell Clin Pharm*. 1987; 21:493–501.
49. Collen MJ, Howard JM, McArthur KE et al. Comparison of ranitidine and cimetidine in the treatment of gastric hypersecretion. *Ann Intern Med*. 1984; 100:52–8.
50. Vinayek R, Howard JM, Maton PN et al. Famotidine in the therapy of gastric hypersecretory states. *Am J Med*. 1986; 81(Suppl 4B):49–59.
51. Jensen RT. Basis for failure of cimetidine in patients with Zollinger-Ellison syndrome. *Dig Dis Sci*. 1984; 29:363–6.
52. Delchier JC, Soule JC, Mignon M et al. Effectiveness of omeprazole in seven patients with Zollinger-Ellison syndrome resistant to histamine H2-receptor antagonists. *Dig Dis Sci*. 1986; 31:693–9.
53. Orr WC, Robinson MG, Humphries TJ et al. Dose response effects of famotidine on gastroesophageal reflux (GER). *Gastroenterology*. 1987; 92:1562. Abstract.
54. Sekiguchi T, Nishioka T, Kogure M et al. Once-daily administration of famotidine for reflux esophagitis. *Scand J Gastroenterol*. 1987; 22(Suppl 134):51–4.
55. Miwa T, Miyoshi A. Famotidine in the treatment of gastritis. *Scand J Gastroenterol*. 1987; 22(Suppl 134):46–50.
56. Aoki T. Clinical benefits of intravenously administered famotidine in the treatment of upper gastrointestinal hemorrhage caused by peptic ulcer and stress ulcer disease. *Scand J Gastroenterol*. 1987; 22(Suppl 134):41–5.
57. Berlin RG, Clineschmidt BV, Majka JA. Famotidine: an appraisal of its mode of action and safety. *Am J Med*. 1986; 81(Suppl 4B):8–12.
58. Burek JD, Majka JA, Bokelman DL. Famotidine: summary of preclinical safety assessment. *Digestion*. 1985; 32(Suppl 1):7–14.
59. Miyoshi A, Muto V, Miwa T et al. Famotidine: summary of overall safety from Japanese clinical studies. *Ital J Gastroenterol*. 1984; 16:177–8.
60. Jensen RT, Collen MJ, Pandol SJ et al. Cimetidine-induced impotence and breast changes in patients with gastric hypersecretory states. *N Engl J Med*. 1983; 303:833–7.
61. Cohen A, Fabre L. Tolerance to repeated intravenous doses of ranitidine HCl and cimetidine HCl in normal volunteers. *Curr Ther Res*. 1983; 34:475–82.
62. Dickinson RJ, Royston CMS, Sutton DR. A comparison of famotidine and ranitidine in an elderly population: a multicentre study. *Postgrad Med J*. 1986; 62(Suppl 2):63–5.
63. Kirch W, Hoensch H, Janish HD. Interactions and noninteractions with ranitidine. *Clin Pharmacokinet*. 1984; 9:493–510.
64. Chremos AN, Lin JH, Yeh KC et al. Famotidine does not interfere with the disposition of theophylline in man: comparison to cimetidine. *Clin Pharmacol Ther*. 1986; 39:187. Abstract.
65. Sambol NC, Upton RA, Chremos AN et al. Influence of famotidine and cimetidine on the disposition of phenytoin and indocyanine green. *Clin Pharmacol Ther*. 1986; 39:225. Abstract.
66. Locniskar A, Greenblatt DJ, Harmatz JS et al. Interaction of diazepam with famotidine and cimetidine, two H2-receptor antagonists. *J Clin Pharmacol*. 1986; 26:299–303.
67. Klotz U, Arvela P, Rosenkranz B. Famotidine, a new H2-receptor antagonist, does not affect hepatic elimination of diazepam or tubular secretion of procainamide. *Eur J Clin Pharmacol*. 1985; 28:671–5.
68. Nazario M. The hepatic and renal mechanisms of drug interactions with cimetidine. *Drug Intell Clin Pharm*. 1986; 20:342–8.
69. Powell JR, Donn KH. Histamine H2-antagonist drug interactions in perspective: mechanistic concepts and clinical implications. *Am J Med*. 1984; 77(Suppl 5B):57–84.
70. Cohen IA, Johnson CJ, Berardi RR et al. Cimetidine–theophylline interaction: effects of age and cimetidine dose. *Ther Drug Monit*. 1985; 7:426–34.
71. Bartle WR, Walker SE, Shapero T. Dose-dependent effect of cimetidine on phenytoin kinetics. *Clin Pharmacol Ther*. 1983; 33:649–55.
72. Merck Sharp & Dohme Laboratories. Pepcid prescribing information. West Point, PA; 1986 Oct.

Advances in Immunosuppressive Therapy

“Greater potency and specificity and less toxicity have been the objectives in developing immunosuppressive therapies. Nevertheless, the standard immunosuppressants used in renal allotransplantation still have substantial nonspecificity. The major advances in their use have been to administer them in lower doses, to use them as combination therapy (also in low doses), to give high-dose antirejection therapy for shorter periods, and to treat rejection only when there is a low-risk/high-benefit potential. The more prudent management of immunosuppressants, the use of prophylactic antibiotics, improvements in surgical techniques, and the prompt recognition and treatment of complications resulted first in an improvement in patient survival and subsequently an improvement in allograft survival. The introduction of a more potent form of antilymphocyte globulin, liberal and innovative transfusion policies, as well as the availability of cyclosporine have accelerated the improvement in allograft success rates.

—American Medical Association Council on Scientific Affairs. Introduction to the management of immunosuppression. *JAMA*. 1987; 257:1781–5.”

Use of cephalosporins with enhanced antianaerobic activity for treatment and prevention of anaerobic and mixed infections

JOSEPH T. DIPIRO AND J. RUSSELL MAY

Abstract: The microbiology, adverse-effect profiles, pharmacokinetics, published results of comparative clinical trials, and costs of cephalosporins with enhanced antianaerobic activity are reviewed.

Cefoxitin, ceftizoxime, cefotetan, and moxalactam have been used as single agents in the treatment or prophylaxis of anaerobic or mixed aerobic and anaerobic infections, including intra-abdominal, female genital tract, and soft-tissue infections. None of these agents is as active against *Bacteroides* species as is clindamycin or metronidazole, but differences among the four cephalosporins do not appear to be clinically important. These agents differ somewhat in their activity against gram-positive and gram-negative bacteria. The majority of adverse reactions to these agents are immunological; disulfiram-like reactions and alterations in normal hemostasis have also been observed with cefotetan and moxalactam. All of these agents are well absorbed after intramuscular injection and produce serum concentrations adequate to treat most infections. Only ceftizoxime and moxalactam produce cerebrospinal fluid concentrations adequate for treatment of gram-negative meningitis. The primary route of elimination is renal, and each agent requires dosage adjustments in patients with renal impairment. Major differences exist among the elimination half-lives of the agents in patients with normal renal function.

The decision to use a cephalosporin for treatment of anaerobic infections should be based on the results of clinical trials that have demonstrated the efficacy of the agent. Data are available to support the use of cefoxitin, ceftizoxime, and moxalactam in the treatment of intra-abdominal infections; cefoxitin and moxalactam to prevent infection of traumatic injury to the abdomen; all four agents in the treatment of female genital tract infections; and all four agents for prophylactic use in surgical procedures that may involve enteric anaerobes, especially *B. fragilis*.

Cephalosporins with enhanced antianaerobic activity appear to have similar in vitro microbiological activity and have efficacy similar to that of combination regimens for the treatment and prophylaxis of intra-abdominal infections, abdominal contamination, obstetric and gynecological infections, and soft-tissue infections.

Index terms: Antibiotics; Cefotetan; Cefoxitin; Ceftizoxime; Cephalosporins; Costs; Drugs; Equivalency, therapeutic; Moxalactam; Pharmacokinetics; Surgical wound infection; Toxicity
Clin Pharm. 1988; 7:285–302

Over the past 20 years anaerobic bacteria have been increasingly recognized as pathogens in many infectious processes. Anaerobic bacteria are likely to be involved in intra-abdominal infections, female genital tract infections, some respiratory-tract infections (such as aspiration pneumonia, lung abscess, and empyema), some soft-tissue infections (such as foot infections in diabetic patients), and brain abscesses. The approach to treating these infections has changed over the past decade, but it focuses on surgical intervention (i.e., drainage of abscesses or excision of devitalized tissue) and antimicrobial regimens. Although surgical intervention is accepted as an important component of therapy, the choice of antimicrobial agents continues to be debated.

Traditionally, antimicrobial treatments for anaerobic or mixed infections have included penicillins for clostridial infections and clindamycin, chloramphenicol, or metronidazole for infections potentially involving *Bacteroides fragilis*. When other organisms, such as aerobic gram-negative bacilli, are present, these agents must be combined with other antimicrobial agents (such as aminoglycosides). Since the introduction of cefoxitin in 1978, clinicians have used cephalosporins for treatment of anaerobic or mixed anaerobic and aerobic bacterial infections. Although certain cephalosporins are commonly used to treat or prevent mixed or anaerobic infections, two key questions remain: (1) Is treatment with cephalosporins justified for anaerobic or mixed infections (i.e., are they as effec-

JOSEPH T. DIPIRO, PHARM.D., is Associate Professor of Pharmacy Practice, University of Georgia College of Pharmacy, and Associate Clinical Professor of Surgery, Medical College of Georgia, Augusta, GA. J. RUSSELL MAY, PHARM.D., is Assistant Director of Pharmacy, Medical College of Georgia Hospital and Clinics, and Adjunct Associate Professor of Pharmacy Practice, University of Georgia College of Pharmacy.

Address reprint requests to Dr. DiPiro at the Medical College of Georgia, Room CN-137, 1459 Laney Walker Blvd., Augusta, GA 30912.

This is **article 680-204-8805** in the **ASHP Continuing Education System.** See page 327 for learning objectives and test questions.

Copyright © 1988, American Society of Hospital Pharmacists, Inc. All rights reserved. 0278-2677/88/0401-0285$04.50.

tive as combination regimens)? (2) If so, which cephalosporins should be chosen for treatment or prevention of anaerobic infections?

A number of cephalosporins are available with qualities similar to those of cefoxitin. Whether these agents should serve as alternatives to cefoxitin for treatment or prevention of anaerobic infections is a question currently being posed by many pharmacy and therapeutics (P&T) committees. The purpose of this review is to examine the situations in which cephalosporins have been considered for therapy of anaerobic or mixed aerobic and anaerobic infections and to discuss the in vitro and clinical information on cephalosporins that have been proposed as alternatives to cefoxitin. The discussion concentrates on those agents with enhanced antianaerobic activity: cefoxitin, ceftizoxime, cefotetan, and moxalactam. Other agents, such as piperacillin, mezlocillin, imipenem–cilastatin, ampicillin–sulbactam, and ticarcillin–clavulanate have antianaerobic activity and may be alternatives to traditional antianaerobic agents or cephalosporins; however, those agents are not the focus of this review.

Common Infections Involving Anaerobes

Cephalosporins with enhanced activity against common anaerobic pathogens are used for various infections, including intra-abdominal, female genital tract, and soft-tissue infections. The aerobic and anaerobic character of these infections has been clearly established to include various *Bacteroides* species, *Fusobacteria*, gram-positive anaerobic cocci (such as peptococci and peptostreptococci), gram-positive bacilli (such as *Eubacterium* and *Bifidobacterium*), and *Clostridia*, in addition to enteric gram-negative bacilli or aerobic gram-positive cocci.

Intra-abdominal Infections. Intra-abdominal infections (secondary bacterial peritonitis or abscess) typically are caused by the usual bacterial flora of the gastrointestinal tract.[1] In the distal ileum and colon, numerous anaerobes can be isolated, and concentrations of anaerobes can be as high as 10^{10}–10^{11} per milliliter of intestinal contents.[2] The predominant anaerobes include *Bacteroides* spp., peptostreptococci, and *Clostridia*. High concentrations of aerobes also can be isolated; therefore, abdominal infections generally involve mixtures of aerobes and anaerobes. Infected intra-abdominal sites yield an average of 2.5–5 types of organisms, with 1.4–2 aerobes and 2.4–3 anaerobes.[3,4]

The importance of aerobic and anaerobic bacteria in intra-abdominal infections has been demonstrated in animal studies with defined bacterial contamination of the abdomen.[5–7] In these experiments gram-negative bacilli such as *Escherichia coli* were responsible for the peritonitis phase of intra-abdominal contamination and resulted in early mortality. Anaerobic bacteria (*B. fragilis*) did not cause peritonitis and early mortality, but they were associated with the formation of intra-abdominal abscesses. The combination of gram-negative bacilli and anaerobes is believed to result in synergistic antimicrobial virulence.[8,9]

Female Genital Tract Infections. Infections of the female genital tract often involve anaerobic bacteria. Common types of infections involving anaerobic bacteria include postoperative pelvic or wound infection (e.g., after hysterectomies), postpartum endomyometritis (particularly in association with cesarean section), septic abortions, tubo-ovarian abscesses, and salpingitis. Usually these tend to be mixed infections, with anaerobic bacteria found along with other organisms (e.g., gram-negative bacilli and gram-positive cocci). Of the anaerobic bacteria, *Bacteroides* species (other than *B. fragilis*) are isolated most frequently from female genital tract infections.[10]

Postpartum endomyometritis classically has been associated with β-hemolytic streptococci, but since the advent of aseptic techniques and antibiotic therapies, the predominant pathogens have changed. Enteric anaerobes along with facultative organisms are isolated most commonly. The greatest risk for postpartum endomyometritis is after cesarean section. Other potential risk factors include the use of invasive fetal monitoring devices, long labor, premature rupture of membranes, and low socioeconomic status.[11]

Postoperative infections are a common problem after gynecological operations, since there is a contaminated field (i.e., the operation extends into the vagina). Gynecological surgery may result in vaginal cuff infections, wound infections (e.g., when there is an abdominal incision), and pelvic abscesses. Vaginal hysterectomies have a generally higher rate of postoperative infection than other types of hysterectomies. Risk factors for hysterectomies as described by Shapiro[12] include a longer duration of operation, failure to administer antimicrobial agents prophylactically, a young age, being a clinic patient, and the use of an abdominal approach. As with other female genital tract infections, postoperative gynecological infections are most often caused by a mixture of anaerobic bacteria (particularly *Bacteroides* species) and facultative bacteria (particularly gram-negative bacilli such as *E. coli*).[11]

Septic abortions occur as a result of retained products of conception or from traumatic injury or perforation of the uterus. Clearly, these infections were more common in the era before the legal availability of medical abortions. About two thirds to three fourths of these infections involve anaerobic bacteria (particularly *B. fragilis*).[10,13] These infections may also involve gram-negative bacilli and less frequently *Staphylococcus aureus, Neisseria gonorrhea*, group A β-hemolytic streptococci, or *Clostridia*.

Community-acquired female genital tract infections may also involve anaerobic bacteria. Salpingitis may be caused initially by *N. gonorrhea* or *Chlamydia trachomatis* and may progress to involve other pathogens. In up to one half of patients, *B. fragilis* can be isolated.[10,14] Tubo-ovarian abscesses typically involve a mixture of anaerobic and aerobic bacteria, and *Bacteroides* species are the most common anaerobes.[15]

Pulmonary Infections. Anaerobic bacteria are involved in various pulmonary infections, including empyema, lung abscess, and aspiration or necrotizing pneumonia. Anaerobic bacteria are introduced into the lung by one of four possible mechanisms: aspiration of oropharyngeal or gastric contents, bacterial implantation from penetrating trauma or surgery, through the bloodstream from a distant site of infection, or extension from an adjacent infected focus. Of these, the most common mechanism is aspiration of oropharyngeal or gastric contents.

Aspiration pneumonia usually occurs because of compromised consciousness or dysphagia. The former may be associated with alcoholism, cerebrovascular accident, general anesthesia, seizure disorders, or sedative drug ingestion. The latter may be the result of neurological disorders or esophageal stricture. Aspiration pneumonia commonly involves anaerobic bacteria; however, community-acquired infections and hospital-acquired infections involve different pathogens. With community-acquired infections, the causative bacteria are more likely to be anaerobic (oropharyngeal anaerobes such as *Bacteroides* species and *Fusobacteria*). Hospital-acquired infections are more likely to involve a mixture of bacteria, such as anaerobes with *S. aureus* or gram-negative bacilli (*Klebsiella, Enterobacter, Serratia,* or *Pseudomonas*). *B. fragilis* can be isolated in up to 15% of aspiration pneumonias.[16]

Lung abscess may result from anaerobic lung infections such as aspiration pneumonia, and up to 100% of lung abscesses may involve anaerobes. Finegold[17] reported that anaerobes alone were isolated from 58% of lung abscesses and a combination of anaerobes and aerobes was isolated from 42%. The most frequently isolated anaerobes included *Bacteroides* species, *Fusobacteria,* and anaerobic streptococci. In most of these infections antimicrobial agents alone will provide sufficient treatment.

Empyema is a purulent collection in the pleural cavity and may be the result of parenchymal disease (such as necrotizing pneumonia or ruptured lung abscess) or a complication of abdominal or genitourinary infection. Finegold[17] reported anaerobic isolates from 76% of patients with empyemas, and anaerobes alone were isolated in 35%. In contrast to lung abscesses, empyemas require surgical drainage for adequate treatment and are associated with a mortality rate of 10% to 20%.

Soft-Tissue Infections. Infections of the skin and soft tissues may be caused by various bacterial and nonbacterial microorganisms and may involve any or all of the soft-tissue components. Soft-tissue infections may be classified as cellulitis (clostridial or nonclostridial) if they involve the skin and subcutaneous tissues, as fascitis if they involve superficial fascia, or as myonecrosis if they cause destruction of muscle tissue. These infections may be related to traumatic injury or ulcers (decubitus ulcers or foot ulcers in diabetic patients), or they may occur after bites.

Many soft-tissue infections involve anaerobic organisms. Classically anaerobic soft-tissue infections have been associated with *Clostridia,* for example, clostridial cellulitis, gas gangrene, and clostridial myonecrosis. However, over the past two decades the anaerobic character of many other soft-tissue infections has been recognized. Necrotizing fascitis is usually a serious infection and frequently involves the trunk, perineum, perirectal area, buttock, or thigh. These infections characteristically are caused by a mixture of aerobic and anaerobic bacteria (including *Bacteroides* species and anaerobic gram-positive cocci).[18] Foot ulcers in diabetic patients and decubitus ulcers are also frequently infected with mixtures of aerobic and anaerobic bacteria. Wheat and associates[19] reported that staphylococci and enterococci and other streptococci were the most common aerobic isolates from diabetic foot infections and that *Peptostreptococcus* species and *Bacteroides* species (including *B. fragilis, B. thetaiotamicron,* and *B. melaninogenicus*) were the most frequently isolated anaerobes. Fierer and associates[20] also reported that *B. fragilis* and *Peptostreptococcus* species were isolated most frequently from infected feet of diabetics. These investigators observed that anaerobic bacteria were involved in more than 50% of diabetic foot infections and that infections involving anaerobes were generally more serious than those not involving anaerobes. Infected decubitus ulcers also frequently involve a mixture of aerobic and anaerobic bacteria.[18]

Cephalosporins in the Treatment of Anaerobic Infections

Cephalosporins often are used to treat anaerobic or mixed infections; however, debate continues as to which antimicrobial regimens should be chosen. The antimicrobial options usually considered include aminoglycosides used with clindamycin, metronidazole, or extended-spectrum penicillins; imipenem–cilastatin alone; extended-spectrum penicillins alone; ampicillin–sulbactam; or cephalosporins. In some cases, the choice of a cephalosporin alone is appropriate.

Traditionally, cephalosporins have been classified into "generations." This system is useful in that it indicates which agents have the greatest activity against aerobic gram-positive bacilli (first-generation) and which are most active against aerobic gram-negative bacilli (third-generation) and gives some idea of the relative cost of the agent (first-generation agents generally are least expensive). However, the classification system is impractical for many recently introduced cephalosporins since some of these new agents do not clearly fit in any one generation. It would be preferable to describe cephalosporins by some notable aspect of their antimicrobial activity (e.g., antipseudomonal, antistaphylococcal, or enhanced antianaerobic activity). Applying this latter approach to the subject of this review makes it necessary to discuss agents that are traditionally classified as either second- or third-generation cephalosporins, since agents with enhanced antianaerobic activity are not limited to any one generation. We believe that it is inappropriate to choose a cephalosporin based on its generation alone; a number of other factors should be considered.

To address the issues involved in cephalosporin use for anaerobic or mixed infections, the pertinent in vitro and clinical data must be reviewed. In the following sections we address the microbiology, adverse-effect profiles, pharmacokinetics, published results of clinical trials, and costs of these agents. In the section on clinical use we discuss studies that compare two or more cephalosporins or that compare cephalosporin efficacy with that of other regimens. The microbiology, adverse-effect, pharmacokinetics, and cost sections focus on comparisons among the enhanced antianaerobic cephalosporins.

Susceptibility Testing of Anaerobic Bacteria

Competitive marketing of cephalosporins with enhanced antianaerobic activity has been intense. If pharmacists are to be able to sift through the many various promotional claims, they must appreciate the differences among these agents' activity against anaerobic and aerobic bacteria and understand the controversies and variability associated with anaerobic susceptibility testing methods.

Antimicrobial susceptibility testing of anaerobic bacteria has become more important recently because of recognition of the clinical importance of anaerobes, less predictable susceptibility patterns, and introduction of new antimicrobial agents.[21] To adequately compare the relative activities of cefoxitin, ceftizoxime, cefotetan, moxalactam, and other agents, the variability of susceptibility testing methods, geographical differences, and advances in the identification of organisms must be understood. Antimicrobial susceptibility information for anaerobes generally is not available to clinicians for individual patients; therefore, they must rely on published susceptibility data.

The technology of anaerobic culture techniques and identification has progressed remarkably in the past two decades. Major advances include the availability of a standardized reference method and development of practical methods of anaerobic susceptibility testing. The National Committee for Clinical Laboratory Standards (NCCLS) recognized the need for standardization and formed a subcommittee to develop a reference method for the performance of susceptibility tests for anaerobes.[22] The agar dilution method that was chosen, although not well suited to routine use in a clinical laboratory because of time, complexity, and cost, serves as the standard from which the accuracy of other, more practical tests can be determined. Laboratories are encouraged to select a method verified as providing results similar to those of the NCCLS reference method. Such verification has been provided for the limited agar dilution, broth microdilution, and the broth disk elution methods.[22]

Problems with Susceptibility Testing. A recent comparison of a microbroth panel with the agar dilution method yielded some interesting results.[23] For the nine drugs tested, 35% of the minimum inhibitory concentration (MIC) results differed by one or more dilutions and 17% differed by two or more dilutions. Although the microbroth panel method was considered by the authors to be an acceptable alternative to the standard, potential exists for conflicting information in published reports on in vitro sensitivities. To further complicate the comparison of in vitro anaerobic susceptibility data, geographical differences may exist, resistance may develop, or differences in the broth may cause conflicting results. One multicenter study clearly demonstrated that susceptibilities to antimicrobial agents vary among medical institutions.[24] Resistance of *B. fragilis* to clindamycin ranged from 0% to 27% of isolates. Also, patterns of susceptibility may change over time, as observed in a study that detected a trend of increasing cefoxitin resistance from 8% in 1981 to 16% in 1983.[24] Resistance rates for moxalactam remained stable or declined over the same time period. Culture media or broth may also influence in vitro results.[25] The MIC_{90} of ceftizoxime against *Bacteroides* changed from 0.25 μg/mL to 8 μg/mL with a change of culture media using the agar dilution method.

The *Bacteroides* group represents important anaerobic pathogens in humans. Those organisms, formerly classified as subspecies of *B. fragilis*, are now recognized to be separate species: *B. fragilis, B. distasonis, B. vulgatus, B. ovatus*, and *B. thetaiotamicron*. When comparing in vitro data, one must recognize that in many studies, several of these species are grouped together as the *B. fragilis* group. As will be discussed, susceptibility to antimicrobials varies among these species.

In Vitro Comparisons of Cephalosporin Activity

Anaerobes. Table 1 shows the susceptibilities of

Table 1.
Comparative Susceptibilities of *Bacteroides* Species

Study	Ref. No.	MIC$_{90}$ (μg/mL) Cefoxitin	Cefotetan	Ceftizoxime	Moxalactam	Cefotaxime
B. fragilis						
Kamimura et al., 1979	101	6.25	...	6.25	...	6.25
Fu and Neu, 1980	108	25	...	...	25	100
Greenwood et al., 1980	112	...	...	4	...	16
Drulak and Chow, 1981	103	16	...	52	...	...
Yu and Washington, 1983	104	8	...	...	1	16
Garzone et al., 1983	32	16	...	54	32	>128
Fass, 1983	105	...	...	8	1	16
Kesado et al., 1984	109	8	4	32	8	64
Aldridge et al., 1984	110	16	16	8	...	...
Bansal et al., 1984	111	...	...	32	8	32
La Mothe et al., 1984	113	16	...	16	1	64
Del Bene et al., 1985	27	32	32	...	8	256
Watt and Brown, 1985	28	16	16	...	...	...
Thornsberry, 1985	33	16	...	16	32	16
Neu et al., 1985	106	8	...	...	4	128
Souza Dias et al., 1985	107	16	...	...	8	64
Bourgault and La Mothe, 1986	102	16	...	16	8	...
B. distasonis						
Kamimura et al., 1979	101	12.5	...	6.25	...	12.5
Drulak and Chow, 1981	103	32	...	16	...	...
Aldridge et al., 1984	110	32	64	8	...	...
La Mothe et al., 1984	113	64	...	2	128	4
Watt and Brown, 1985	28	32	32	...	...	...
Souza Dias et al., 1985	107	32	...	...	256	128
Bourgault and La Mothe, 1986	102	64	...	64	>128	...
B. ovatus						
Kamimura et al., 1979	101	12.5	...	6.25	...	12.5
Aldridge et al., 1984	110	64	128	16	...	...
La Mothe et al., 1984	113	32	...	16	32	128
Watt and Brown, 1985	28	16	32	...	...	...
Bourgault and La Mothe, 1986	102	32	...	32	32	...
B. thetaiotamicron						
Drulak and Chow, 1981	103	52	...	46	...	...
Yu and Washington, 1983	104	32	...	...	8	64
Aldridge et al., 1984	110	32	128	64	...	...
La Mothe et al., 1984	113	64	...	64	128	128
Watt and Brown, 1985	28	32	32	...	...	...
Bourgault and La Mothe, 1986	102	32	...	32	16	...
B. vulgatus						
Kamimura et al., 1979	101	6.25	...	3.13	...	6.25
La Mothe et al., 1984	113	8	...	1	2	4
Aldridge et al., 1984	110	16	64	8	...	...
Souza Dias et al., 1985	107	32	...	...	128	64
Bourgault and La Mothe, 1986	102	16	...	8	4	...
B. fragilis group[a]						
Fu and Neu, 1980	108	50	...	50	...	100
Yu and Washington, 1983	104	16	...	...	32	16
Garzone et al., 1983	32	...	...	>32	>32	>32
Aldridge et al., 1984	110	32	128	16	...	...
Thornsberry, 1985	33	16	...	8	16	16
Neu et al., 1985	106	16	...	...	32	>128
Souza Dias et al., 1985	107	32	...	...	64	128
Cuchural and Tally, 1986	24	32	...	...	32	128
Aldridge and Sanders, 1986	114	32	...	16	...	64

[a] Study does not separate *B. distasonis, B. ovatus, B. thetaiotamicron,* or *B. vulgatus.*

Bacteroides species to cephalosporins with enhanced antianaerobic activity. Because cefotaxime is often included in third-generation comparisons, it is also included in the table. A possible synergistic effect of cefotaxime and its desacetyl metabolite against *B. fragilis* strains is being investigated, but the clinical importance of this potential interaction is not known. A recent report concluded that discrepancies in in vitro susceptibility reports on cefotaxime may result from degradation of the drug.[26]

Although the references cited in Table 1 are not all-inclusive, they are representative and show the trend of susceptibility patterns. None of these cephalosporins is as active against *Bacteroides* as is clindamycin or metronidazole.[24,27,28] For most *Bacteroides* species, the MIC_{90} ranges from 1 to 4 μg/mL for clindamycin and from 1 to 2 μg/mL for metronidazole. Cefotaxime appears to be the least active. In addition, various species have different susceptibilities. Although these cephalosporins appear to vary in their activity against specific *Bacteroides* species, the clinical relevance of these differences is not apparent. Comparative in vitro data for cefotetan relative to the other agents are lacking, especially for the species formerly combined as the *B. fragilis* group. Because in vitro activity does not necessarily imply in vivo effectiveness, available clinical data must be carefully evaluated.

Other Clinically Important Pathogens. Results of in vitro studies of these agents' activity against gram-positive and gram-negative organisms have been more consistent.[29-33] For gram-positive bacteria, only minor differences exist among these agents. All of the agents are active against *S. aureus* (except methicillin-resistant strains) and streptococci (except enterococci), although none is considered first-line therapy for documented gram-positive infections. Activity against *Staphylococcus epidermidis* should be considered intermediate, at best, for all of these agents. In fact, many *S. epidermidis* strains may be resistant.

Ceftizoxime and moxalactam are clearly more active than cefoxitin is against several gram-negative organisms (Table 2). In general, cefotetan's activity falls somewhere between that of cefoxitin and the other agents. These cephalosporins should not be used alone for treating serious infections caused by *Ps. aeruginosa*.

A potentially important characteristic of some cephalosporins is the ability to interact with certain gram-negative bacteria, causing the bacteria to produce more β-lactamases (β-lactamase induction)

Table 2.
Comparative Susceptibilities of Gram-Negative Bacteria

Study	Ref. No.	MIC_{90} (μg/mL)			
		Cefoxitin	Cefotetan	Ceftizoxime	Moxalactam
Escherichia coli					
Garzone et al., 1983	32	8.2	...	0.25	0.5
Richards and Heel, 1985	30	...	...	0.03–0.5	0.08–0.5
Ward and Richards, 1985	29	3.8–100	0.13–3.12	...	0.125–2
Thornsberry, 1985	33	8	...	0.12	0.25
Enterobacter cloacae					
Richards and Heel, 1985	30	...	...	0.25–32	0.1–12.5
Ward and Richards, 1985	29	32–128	2–160	...	0.25–50
Thornsberry, 1985	33	64	...	16	8
Haemophilus influenzae					
Garzone et al., 1983	32	5.9	...	0.03	0.08
Richards and Heel, 1985	30	12.5–16	...	0.0015–0.25	0.02–0.25
Ward and Richards, 1985	29	...	1–4	...	...
Thornsberry, 1985	33	4	...	0.01–0.03	0.06–0.12
Klebsiella pneumoniae					
Garzone et al., 1983	32	5.1	...	0.1	0.5
Richards and Heel, 1985	30	...	...	0.03–0.1	0.1–0.8
Ward and Richards, 1985	29	2–8	0.12–4	...	0.12–4
Thornsberry, 1985	33	8	...	0.03	0.25
Neisseria gonorrheae					
Garzone et al., 1983	32	1.6	...	0.12	0.25
Richards and Heel, 1985	30	1–2	...	0.002–0.125	0.06–0.25
Ward and Richards, 1985	29	...	1–4	...	...
Thornsberry, 1985	33	2–4	...	0.01–0.03	0.06–0.12
Proteus mirabilis					
Richards and Heel, 1985	30	...	...	0.006–0.5	0.1–0.5
Ward and Richards, 1985	29	2–64	0.06–1	...	0.07–0.5
Thornsberry, 1985	33	8	...	0.01	0.25
Serratia marcescens					
Garzone et al., 1983	32	64	...	3.7	9.3
Richards and Heel, 1985	30	...	...	0.06–32	0.25–16
Ward and Richards, 1985	29	64–256	3.2–32	...	2–6.25
Thornsberry, 1985	33	64	...	2	4

and to select mutants that are stably derepressed to β-lactamase production. Bacteria that are likely to possess these inducible enzymes include *Enterobacter, Citrobacter, Serratia,* and *Pseudomonas*.[34] The importance of this ability is that bacteria exposed to these cephalosporins may become resistant to a wide range of other β-lactam antimicrobial agents including β-lactamase-stable agents. Among the most potent inducers of β-lactamase production are cefoxitin and moxalactam.[35] The clinical importance of this interaction is not yet fully understood.

Adverse Effects

When first introduced, broad-spectrum cephalosporins were proposed as replacements for combination therapy.[36] It was thought that using cephalosporins might be safer. As these agents were administered to more patients, their toxicity profiles became clearer, and potentially dangerous adverse effects were recognized with some cephalosporins. Fortunately, serious reactions are rare.

The majority of adverse reactions seen with cephalosporins are immunological. Urticaria, rash, and pruritus are reported most commonly, but the overall incidence of skin reactions is approximately 3% or less.[37] Severe skin reactions are extremely rare. Only two cases of exfoliative dermatitis have been reported, both complications of cefoxitin therapy.[38,39] Cross-sensitivity among the penicillins and cephalosporins has been reported to be about 8%.[40] However, in a more recent study with moxalactam, only 14 of 344 (4.1%) patients with a documented allergy to penicillin experienced a reaction to moxalactam.[41] The frequency of febrile reactions is probably lower with cephalosporins than with the penicillins.[37] There is no information to suggest that any one of the cephalosporins under discussion poses a greater risk of hypersensitivity reactions.

As the chemical structures of cephalosporins were modified in search of broader-spectrum and longer-acting agents, some undesirable toxicological properties were recognized, most notably adverse effects similar to those of the disulfiram-alcohol reaction and alterations in normal hemostasis. These two reactions have been associated with a methylthiotetrazole (MTT) side chain at the 3 position of the cephem nucleus. Cefotetan and moxalactam possess this side chain; cefoxitin and ceftizoxime do not.

Only cephalosporins that contain the MTT side chain have been reported to cause a disulfiram-like reaction in patients or healthy subjects after ingestion of alcohol.[37] Symptoms of a disulfiram-like reaction include flushing, headache, respiratory difficulty, nausea, vomiting, hyperventilation, tachycardia, hypotension, syncope, vertigo, blurred vision, and confusion.

Several potential mechanisms exist for the bleeding problems reported with cephalosporins involving hypoprothrombinemia and impaired platelet function. Some authors suggest that the hypoprothrombinemia occurs secondary to inhibition or destruction of the natural gastrointestinal flora that produce vitamin K.[42,43] This theory is supported by the observation that in many patients, the hypoprothrombinemia is rapidly reversed by the administration of phytonadione. Also, poor nutritional status is a common finding in patients with this adverse effect. Several studies suggest that the mechanism may be much more complex, involving an alteration in vitamin K metabolism.[44,45] Moxalactam, in addition to causing hypoprothrombinemia, may also interfere with platelet function.[46,47] The clinical importance of these theories has been demonstrated in recent studies.[48,49]

In patients at risk for developing bleeding problems or in patients with coagulopathies associated with underlying disease or age, cephalosporins with the MTT side chain, particularly moxalactam, probably should be avoided. The risk of using cefotetan in these patients has not been well defined.

Pharmacokinetics

A factor to consider in choosing one cephalosporin over another is the pharmacokinetic profile. An agent's pharmacokinetics can affect cost, ease of administration, and efficacy in some specific situations. In this section, the pertinent pharmacokinetic characteristics of cefoxitin, cefotetan, ceftizoxime, and moxalactam are compared.

Serum Concentrations. These cephalosporins are well absorbed after intramuscular administration and produce serum concentrations adequate to treat most infections. After a 1-g i.m. dose the highest serum concentration is achieved by cefotetan (52–79 μg/mL),[29] followed by moxalactam given as the disodium salt (27–52 μg/mL),[50] ceftizoxime given as the sodium salt (35–41 μg/mL),[30] and cefoxitin (22 μg/mL).[31]

Schumacher[51] recently calculated values for the maximum ($C_{ss_{max}}$) and minimum ($C_{ss_{min}}$) steady-state plasma concentrations achieved during recommended dosing intervals of various agents. These values are reported, along with a summary of published pharmacokinetic data, in Table 3. After 2-g doses, ceftizoxime (given as the sodium salt) had the highest $C_{ss_{max}}$, 123 μg/mL, with an eight-hour dosing interval. Cefotetan given every 12 hours had the lowest $C_{ss_{max}}$, 34 μg/mL. All agents except cefoxitin had a $C_{ss_{max}}$ above 2 μg/mL at the end of the dosing interval. Given every six hours, cefoxitin had a $C_{ss_{min}}$ of 0.3 μg/mL. In an earlier study using similar methods, cefoxitin when administered every four hours produced a $C_{ss_{max}}$ of 107 μg/mL and a $C_{ss_{min}}$ of 3.1 μg/mL,[52] similar to values produced by ceftizoxime and moxalactam when given every eight hours.

Distribution. Discussion of cephalosporin distribution sometimes centers around issues of documented importance, such as the concentrations achieved in cerebrospinal fluid (CSF), or issues of questionable importance, such as the degree of serum protein binding. Neither of these examples is relevant to the treatment of most anaerobic infections. The agents clearly differ in the extent to which they bind to serum proteins (Table 3); however, the clinical importance is debatable and this factor should not affect cephalosporin selection.

Of the four agents, only ceftizoxime and moxalactam produce CSF concentrations adequate for treatment of meningitis caused by gram-negative bacilli.[53] Documentation of cefotetan's penetration into CSF is currently insufficient to adequately compare it with the other cephalosporins.

Elimination. The primary route of elimination for these cephalosporins is renal, and each agent requires dosage adjustments in patients with renal impairment. Major differences exist among the elimination half-lives of the agents in patients with normal renal function. Cefotetan has the longest half-life, at 4.2 hours,[54] which justifies its recommended 12-hour dosing interval. Moxalactam and ceftizoxime have half-lives of 2.0 hours and 1.9 hours, respectively.[53] Both can be given every 8 to 12 hours for most infections. Cefoxitin has the shortest half-life, ranging from 38 to 58 minutes.[31] As mentioned earlier, when cefoxitin is given every six hours, serum concentrations may fall well below 1 μg/mL at the end of the dosing interval. Therefore, cefoxitin should be given every six hours, and in serious or life-threatening infections, a four-hour dosing interval should be considered.

Clinical Use of Cephalosporins for Mixed Infections

The decision to use a cephalosporin for treatment of anaerobic infections should be based primarily on clinical trials demonstrating efficacy of the agent. In this section, we present only information on clinical trials done in situations where common enteric anaerobic bacteria (such as *Bacteroides* species) are likely pathogens. Other infections, such as clostridial infections of soft tissues, will not be discussed here. The major areas for discussion include intra-abdominal infections, obstetric and gynecological infections, some soft-tissue infections, and prevention of postoperative polymicrobic infections (such as after gastrointestinal or obstetric and gynecological operations).

The majority of studies fall into one of two categories: comparisons of cephalosporins with combination regimens (such as an aminoglycoside with clindamycin or metronidazole) or comparisons of two or more cephalosporins. The former may be used to assess the relative benefit of cephalosporins in the treatment of anaerobic infections, and the latter may be used to support the choice of a specific cephalosporin. Many of the studies discussed are flawed in some way; however, the most serious and consistent fault is that usually too few patients were studied for there to have been a high probability of detecting a significant difference among regimens even if one did exist. Therefore, a Type II error is probable.[55] Because of this problem, the conclusion that no significant difference exists among regimens is often suspect. The more important studies relating to these topics are presented below.

Intra-abdominal Infection. Treatment of intra-abdominal infections has been a focus of study for many new antimicrobial agents, including the cephalosporins under discussion (Table 4). In a relatively large number of trials, cephalosporins were compared with clindamycin–aminoglycoside combinations. Cefoxitin,[56,57] ceftizoxime,[58,59] and moxalactam[60,61] seemed comparable to the combination regimens in terms of infectious outcome. Since some of these trials included relatively few patients,[56,58,59] the ability to discriminate among treatments is limited. The trial by Schentag et al.[60] is particularly important because it included older patients with established intra-abdominal infec-

Table 3.
Comparative Pharmacokinetic Parameters

Drug	Dosage	Serum Concentration[a] Maximum (μg/mL)	Serum Concentration[a] Minimum (μg/mL)	Half-Life (hr)	Protein Binding (%)
Cefoxitin[31,51,52]	2 g every 6 hr	56	0.3	0.63–0.97	65
	2 g every 4 hr	107	3.1		
Cefotetan[29,51,54]	2 g every 12 hr	34	2.0	4.2	78–91
Ceftizoxime[51,53] (as the sodium salt)	2 g every 8 hr	123	2.2	1.9	30
Moxalactam[51,53] (as the disodium salt)	2 g every 8 hr	101	6.8	2.0	51

[a] Mean steady-state peak and trough levels as calculated by Schumacher.[51,52]

tions—the patients about whom most clinicians would have concerns if single-agent regimens were used. The results of the trial demonstrated that moxalactam was as effective as the clindamycin–tobramycin combination.

A large number of patients were studied in a series of trials by Stone et al.[61,62] In these trials, moxalactam, cefotaxime, and cefoperazone were demonstrated to be equivalent in efficacy to clindamycin–gentamicin. One criticism of some of the early trials by Stone et al. was that the relatively low doses of clindamycin used (5 mg/kg) may have affected outcomes from the combination therapy. In another comparative trial of cephalosporins, ceftizoxime, and cefoxitin were judged to be equally efficacious.[63]

The trials that included cephalosporins that are not very active against *B. fragilis* have provided inconsistent results. Cefotaxime, cefoperazone, and cefamandole have demonstrated efficacy equivalent to that of clindamycin–gentamicin combinations in some trials.[61,62,64] However, two reports of patients with perforated or gangrenous appendices suggest that the clindamycin–gentamicin combination may be superior to cefoperazone and cefamandole.[65,66] In a relatively large trial of patients with perforated or gangrenous appendices, cefotaxime and cefoperazone were determined to be less effective than moxalactam.[67]

For established intra-abdominal infections, the information available on cefoxitin, ceftizoxime, and moxalactam appears to support their use; however, clinical trials with larger numbers of patients are needed. Results of comparative trials with cefotetan have not yet been published. For agents that are relatively inactive against *B. fragilis* (e.g., cefoperazone, cefotaxime, and cefamandole), the published information is inconsistent; therefore, these agents cannot be recommended for routine use for anaerobic infections.

Abdominal Trauma. A common setting for the study of new antimicrobials has been cases of traumatic injury involving the abdomen (Table 5). These trials usually included patients who sustained a penetrating abdominal injury with risk of intra-abdominal infection. Abdominal trauma is frequently studied because this type of injury is commonly seen in urban medical centers. These

Table 4.
Comparative Studies of Cephalosporin Use in Intra-abdominal Infections

Study	Ref. No.	Agent(s)	No. (%) of Patients Cured
Stone et al., 1982	62	Cefotaxime	101/125 (81)
		Clindamycin and gentamicin	100/124 (81)
Drusano et al., 1982	56	Cefoxitin	16/26 (62)
		Clindamycin and an aminoglycoside	11/21 (52)
Berne et al., 1982[a]	65	Cefamandole	37/48 (77)[b]
		Cefoperazone	41/48 (85)[b]
		Clindamycin and gentamicin	48/49 (98)[b]
Heseltine et al., 1983[a]	66	Cefoperazone	40/47 (85)[b]
		Cefamandole	37/48 (77)[b]
		Clindamycin and gentamicin	51/52 (98)[b]
Schentag et al., 1983	60	Moxalactam	37/49 (76)
		Clindamycin and tobramycin	36/49 (73)
Stone et al., 1983	61	Moxalactam	65/77 (84)
		Cefotaxime	65/78 (83)
		Cefoperazone	68/78 (87)
		Clindamycin and gentamicin	159/227 (70)
Busuttil et al., 1984	64	Cefamandole	24/31 (77)
		Clindamycin and gentamicin	29/34 (85)
Harding et al., 1984	58	Ceftizoxime	21/24 (88)
		Clindamycin and tobramycin	13/15 (87)
Solomkin and Lentnek, 1984	59	Ceftizoxime	26/29 (90)
		Clindamycin and tobramycin	27/30 (90)
Lou et al., 1985	63	Ceftizoxime	46/46 (100)
		Cefoxitin	58/59 (98)
Malangoni et al., 1985	57	Cefoxitin	49/59 (83)
		Clindamycin and tobramycin	42/53 (79)
Lau et al., 1985[a]	67	Cefotaxime	59/77 (77)[c]
		Cefoperazone	62/78 (79)[c]
		Moxalactam	69/75 (92)[c]
Tally et al., (1981)	100	Cefoxitin (with or without amikacin)	29/33 (88)
		Moxalactam	26/33 (79)

[a] Study included patients with perforated and gangrenous appendices only.
[b] Cure rates with clindamycin and gentamicin were significantly higher than were cure rates with either cefamandole or cefoperazone sodium.
[c] Moxalactam was associated with a significantly better cure rate than was either cefotaxime or cefoperazone.

studies should be clearly differentiated from studies of established intra-abdominal infection because relatively few patients with abdominal trauma develop established peritonitis or abscess. Finally, these trials should not be interpreted to support the use of these agents for treatment of established intra-abdominal infection but rather for the situations of relatively low infectious risk under which they were studied.

In the majority of published studies, cephalosporins have been compared with combinations of an aminoglycoside and clindamycin. Cefoxitin has been shown to be as effective as the combinations of clindamycin–gentamicin,[68,69] clindamycin–tobramycin,[70,71] ticarcillin–tobramycin,[72] and aminoglycoside–ampicillin–clindamycin.[73] In two other trials, moxalactam has demonstrated efficacy equivalent to that of combinations of clindamycin and tobramycin.[70,74]

In two trials, patients who received cefamandole had significantly higher infection rates than did patients who received cefoxitin,[71,72] whereas in two other trials, cefamandole was as effective as cefoxitin alone[70] or tobramycin–cephalothin.[75] In a relatively large trial of more than 400 patients, Feliciano and associates[76] found that cefoxitin was equivalent in efficacy to moxalactam but superior to cefotaxime.

In summary, for abdominal trauma, adequate support exists for the use of some cephalosporins, particularly cefoxitin and moxalactam, but not for others known to be relatively inactive against *B. fragilis*. Published information in this area is not yet available for ceftizoxime and cefotetan, but it is likely that these agents would be as effective as cefoxitin or moxalactam.

Female Genital Tract Infections. Female genital tract infections may be diverse, including endomyometritis, salpingitis, and tubo-ovarian abscesses, among others. Unfortunately, most studies of female genital tract infections included mixed types of infections, making comparison of studies difficult. In addition, most of the published studies are based on relatively few patients, with the largest study group less than 200 patients.

A variety of cephalosporins have been evaluated for the treatment of female genital tract infections, many in comparison with aminoglycoside–clindamycin combinations (Table 6). Cefoxitin has demonstrated efficacy equivalent to that of clindamycin combined with gentamicin[77,78] or other aminoglycosides[56] in three studies. However, Apuzzio and associates[79] found both cefoxitin and ceftizoxime to be less effective than clindamycin–gentamicin. The difference in efficacy was significant for cefoxitin but not for ceftizoxime. Moxalactam,[80,81] cefoperazone,[82] and cefotaxime[83] all have demonstrated efficacy similar to that of clindamycin–aminoglycoside combinations.

In the only trials that compared cephalosporins,

Table 5.
Comparative Studies of Cephalosporin Use in Abdominal Trauma

Study	Ref. No.	Agent(s)	No. (%) of Patients Who Became Infected
Crenshaw et al., 1983	75	Cefamandole	3/49 (6)
		Tobramycin and cephalothin	5/40 (11)
Hofstetter et al., 1984	73	Cefoxitin	10/69 (15)
		Aminoglycoside, ampicillin, and clindamycin	9/50 (18)
Gentry et al., 1984	72	Cefamandole	9/51 (18)[a]
		Cefoxitin	3/50 (6)[a]
		Ticarcillin and tobramycin	5/51 (10)
Nichols et al., 1984	69	Cefoxitin	14/70 (20)
		Clindamycin and gentamicin	17/75 (23)
Rowlands and Ericsson, 1984	70	Cefamandole	10/51 (20)[b]
		Cefoxitin	11/54 (20)[b]
		Clindamycin and tobramycin	5/46 (11)[b]
		Moxalactam	1/47 (2)
		Clindamycin and tobramycin	4/45 (9)
Jones et al., 1985	71	Cefamandole	23/78 (29)[a]
		Cefoxitin	12/94 (13)[a]
		Clindamycin and tobramycin	17/85 (20)
Nelson et al., 1986	74	Moxalactam	10/78 (13)
		Clindamycin and tobramycin	8/85 (9)
Heseltine et al., 1986	68	Cefoxitin	3/34 (9)
		Clindamycin and gentamicin	3/41 (7)
Feliciano et al., 1986	76	Cefoxitin	4/149 (3)
		Cefotaxime	19/124 (15)
		Moxalactam	11/153 (7)

[a] Cefamandole had a significantly higher infection rate than did cefoxitin.
[b] Cefamandole and cefoxitin had significantly higher infection rates than did clindamycin and tobramycin for wound infections only.

cefotetan and cefoxitin were found to have similar efficacy,[84] and cefoxitin and ceftizoxime were equally efficacious.[79] The majority of studies support the use of cephalosporins for female genital tract infections. Cephalosporins that do not have substantial activity against *B. fragilis* (such as cefoperazone, cefamandole, and cefotaxime) appear to be effective.

Anaerobic Soft-Tissue Infections. Few comparative studies of the effectiveness of antimicrobial therapy for anaerobic soft-tissue infections have been conducted (Table 7). Patients with soft-tissue infections were included in a large series of trials conducted by Stone and associates.[61] In these trials, cefotaxime, cefoperazone, and moxalactam were equivalent in effectiveness to the combination of clindamycin and gentamicin. Hughes and associates[85] compared ceftizoxime with cefoxitin in patients with lower-extremity infections associated with diabetes mellitus or peripheral vascular disease. More than 80% of the infections were polymicrobic, and the outcomes of the treatments were similar. It is difficult to provide recommendations based on the available published literature. Although these studies are favorable, in many soft-tissue infections the major therapeutic measures are surgery and proper wound management. Antimicrobial therapy is a secondary measure, and the value of secondary therapies is usually more difficult to establish.

Anaerobic Pulmonary Infections. Although there are numerous trials of cephalosporins for the

Table 6.
Comparative Studies of Cephalosporin Use in Female Genital Tract Infections

Study	Ref. No.	Agent(s)	No. (%) of Patients Cured
Post-Cesarean-Section Endomyometritis			
Gibbs et al., 1982	115	Cefamandole	93/106 (88)
		Clindamycin and gentamicin	76/92 (83)
Hemsell et al., 1983	83	Cefotaxime	79/81 (98)
		Clindamycin and gentamicin	37/39 (95)
Gibbs et al., 1983	81	Moxalactam	52/56 (93)
		Clindamycin and gentamicin	55/57 (96)
Apuzzio et al., 1985	79	Ceftizoxime	49/68 (72)
		Cefoxitin	15/24 (62)[a]
		Clindamycin and gentamicin	28/32 (88)[a]
Herman et al., 1986	78	Cefoxitin	36/48 (75)
		Clindamycin and gentamicin	38/50 (76)
Faro et al., 1987	116	Cefoxitin	40/49 (82)
		Mezlocillin	46/53 (87)
		Clindamycin and gentamicin	44/50 (92)
Miscellaneous Female Genital Tract Infections			
Drusano et al., 1982	56	Cefoxitin	20/20 (100)
		Clindamycin and an aminoglycoside	22/23 (96)
Sweet et al., 1985	80	Moxalactam	29/30 (97)
		Clindamycin and tobramycin	29/30 (97)
O'Bryan et al., 1986	84	Cefotetan	26/26 (100)
		Cefoxitin	10/11 (91)
Gilstrap et al., 1986	82	Cefoperazone	47/51 (92)
		Clindamycin and gentamicin	48/51 (94)
Larsen et al., 1986	77	Cefoxitin	37/41 (90)
		Clindamycin and gentamicin	42/50 (84)
Poindexter et al., 1986	117	Cefotetan	34/34 (100)
		Moxalactam	8/8 (100)
		Cefoxitin	5/5 (100)

[a] Clindamycin and gentamicin had a significantly better cure rate than did cefoxitin.

Table 7.
Comparative Studies of Cephalosporin Use in Anaerobic Soft-Tissue Infections

Study	Ref. No.	Agent(s)	No. (%) of Patients Cured
Stone et al., 1983	61	Moxalactam	58/62 (94)
		Cefotaxime	33/41 (80)
		Cefoperazone	46/51 (90)
		Clindamycin and gentamicin	125/145 (86)
Hughes et al., 1985	81	Ceftizoxime	23/28 (82)
		Cefoxitin	17/25 (68)

treatment of lower respiratory infections, information that specifically applies to anaerobic lung infections is scarce. At present, these infections should be treated with a penicillin or clindamycin. If pulmonary infections are believed to be caused by a mixture of organisms that include gram-negative bacilli as well as anaerobes, then cephalosporins may be considered for treatment.

Prevention of Anaerobic Infections

The agents discussed here—cefoxitin, ceftizoxime, moxalactam, and cefotetan—have been studied for prophylactic use in surgical procedures for which anaerobic bacteria are common postoperative pathogens. The main procedures of this type are colorectal operations, hysterectomies, and cesarean sections (Table 8). For these procedures, infection rates in the absence of antimicrobial prophylaxis are relatively high, and antimicrobial use has lowered infection rates in placebo-controlled trials. However, a major question remains: What is the most effective antimicrobial agent for prophylactic use in these procedures?

Oral and injectable antimicrobial agents have been recommended for prophylaxis of colorectal operations. The oral antimicrobial agents of choice have been neomycin sulfate and erythromycin. There is controversy about the injectable agents; some published recommendations suggest using agents with activity against *B. fragilis*, whereas others indicate that first-generation cephalosporins such as cefazolin are suitable. In trials in which cephalosporins were directly compared, ceftizoxime, cefoxitin, and cefazolin were judged to be equivalent in efficacy,[86] as were cefazolin and moxalactam.[87] When combined with oral neomycin sulfate and erythromycin, cefazolin was judged to be as effective as cefoxitin alone and more effective for operations lasting more than four hours.[88] In a variety of trials, cefoxitin and moxalactam were compared with various combination regimens (usually including metronidazole) and were found to be as effective as those regimens in preventing postoperative infection.[89-91]

Cephalosporins have frequently been used for obstetric and gynecological operations. In direct comparisons of cephalosporins, cefonicid, cefotaxime, and cefazolin (which do not have good activity against *B. fragilis*) did not differ significantly in effectiveness from cefoxitin and moxalactam (Table 8). Most of the first-, second-, and third-generation cephalosporins studied have had equivalent efficacy. The available information suggests that ceftizoxime and cefotetan also are effective for prophylaxis of obstetric and gynecological operations.

Two approaches can be taken to choosing injectable cephalosporins for prophylaxis of surgical procedures that may involve enteric anaerobes. If the available information suggests that activity against *B. fragilis* is not required, then a relatively inexpensive agent such as cefazolin can be selected. If activity against *B. fragilis* is necessary, then the choice should come from among the available cephalosporins with enhanced antianaerobic activity (i.e., cefoxitin, ceftizoxime, cefotetan, and moxalactam).

Cost

Providng cost-effective antimicrobial therapy has been a goal of P&T committees for many years. With the introduction of prospective pricing according to diagnosis-related groups, the pursuit of this goal has intensified. Numerous studies of the costs of antimicrobial therapy have appeared in the pharmacy and medical literature.[92-96] A comparative study of cefoxitin versus the combination of clindamycin and an aminoglycoside pointed out the potential cost benefit of using a cephalosporin alone when treating mixed aerobic and anaerobic infections.[92]

Several factors must be considered when comparing the costs of antianaerobic cephalosporins. These factors include acquisition costs, supply costs, intravenous drug delivery system costs, and the pharmacokinetic and toxicity profiles of the agents. Because of differences among institutions, any cost comparisons should be highly individualized. Acquisition costs should be calculated for antimicrobial agents in the dosage ranges commonly employed in the institution. Table 9 gives this information for the Medical College of Georgia Hospital and Clinics. Daily supply costs (the cost of materials associated with drug administration) are institution-specific and relate to the type of intravenous drug delivery system used (e.g., minibags, infusion pumps). The sum of these costs represents the total daily cost. Some studies include personnel time as a cost item[93,97]; however, the actual usefulness of this information has been questioned.[96]

Individualized cost comparisons can be conducted more easily since the advent of computer programs that incorporate institution-specific costs.[97] The computer program described by Parr and associates[97] factors in laboratory costs, primarily for assays of serum drug concentration needed for therapeutic monitoring. The cost of tests to monitor for specific drug toxicities, such as coagulopathies, should also be considered when comparing cephalosporins. As shown in Table 9, a longer half-life offers potential savings in daily drug costs. These savings increase when drug administration costs are added. Cefoxitin, although less expensive than other agents on a per-gram basis, may actually be more expensive when large doses are required.

Formulary Considerations

Cephalosporins are promoted for the treatment

Table 8.
Comparative Studies of Cephalosporin Use for Prophylaxis of Infections in Which Anaerobes Are Common Pathogens

Study	Ref. No.	Agent(s)	No. (%) of Patients Who Became Infected
Colorectal Operations			
Slama et al., 1979	118	Cephalothin	5/16 (31)
		Cefamandole	6/18 (30)
Hoffman et al., 1981	119	Cefoxitin[a]	1/32 (3)[b]
		Placebo[a]	9/33 (27)[b]
Lewis et al., 1981	120	Cephradine	25/70 (36)[c]
		Metronidazole and erythromycin	6/60 (10)[c]
Maki and Aughey, 1982	86	Cefazolin	4/31 (13)
		Cefoxitin	1/32 (3)
		Ceftizoxime	2/30 (7)
McDonald and Karran, 1983	90	Cefoxitin	8/52 (15)
		Gentamicin and metronidazole	7/48 (15)
Kaiser et al., 1983	88	Cefazolin, neomycin and erythromycin	2/63 (3)
		Cefoxitin	7/56 (13)
Plouffe et al., 1985[d]	87	Moxalactam	10/83 (12)
		Cefazolin	6/98 (6)
McCulloch et al., 1986	91	Moxalactam	6/41 (15)
		Gentamicin and metronidazole	7/45 (16)
Jones et al., 1987	121	Cefazolin	1/35 (3)
		Cefoxitin	1/36 (3)
		Cefotaxime	4/29 (14)
Hinchey et al., 1987	89	Moxalactam	5/64 (8)
		Neomycin and metronidazole	3/67 (4)
Vaginal Hysterectomy			
Hemsell et al., 1983	122	Cefazolin	5/100 (5)
		Moxalactam	6/93 (6)
Maki et al., 1984	123	Cefonicid	4/29 (14)
		Cefoxitin	2/31 (6)
Littlejohn et al., 1985	124	Cefonicid	0/40 (0)
		Cefoxitin	0/39 (0)
Benigno et al., 1986	125	Cefoxitin	3/60 (5)
		Cephalothin	5/87 (6)
		Piperacillin	8/151 (5)
Abdominal Hysterectomy			
Maki et al., 1984	123	Cefonicid	0/37 (0)
		Cefoxitin	3/49 (6)
Hemsell et al., 1984	126	Cefoperazone	6/50 (12)
		Cefoxitin	2/51 (4)
Periti et al., 1984	127	Cefotaxime	1/112 (1)
		Ceftriaxone	2/97 (2)
Hemsell et al., 1985	128	Cefazolin	4/54 (7)
		Ceftriaxone	4/54 (7)
Tuomala et al., 1985	129	Cefazolin	6/108 (6)
		Moxalactam	6/100 (6)
Abdominal and Vaginal Hysterectomy			
Orr et al., 1986	130	Cefotetan	2/47 (4)
		Cefoxitin	1/23 (4)
Jones et al., 1987	121	Cefazolin	2/50 (4)
		Cefoxitin	4/45 (9)
		Cefotaxime	2/43 (5)
Cesarean Sections			
Stiver et al., 1983	131	Cefazolin	8/119 (7)
		Cefoxitin	7/124 (6)
Parsons et al., 1985	132	Cefonicid	9/90 (10)
		Cefoxitin	9/62 (15)
Saltzman et al., 1985	133	Ceftizoxime	4/50 (8)[e]
		Placebo	14/49 (29)[e]
Varner et al., 1986	134	Cefotetan	2/20 (10)
		Cefoxitin	0/9 (0)
Periti et al., 1984	127	Cefotaxime	2/46 (4)
		Ceftriaxone	0/30 (0)
McGregor et al., 1986	135	Cefotetan	7/46 (15)
		Cefoxitin	2/24 (8)

[a] Patients in both groups received oral kanamycin preoperatively.
[b] Patients who received placebo had a significantly higher infection rate than did patients who received cefoxitin.
[c] Patients who received cephradine had a significantly higher infection rate than did patients who received metronidazole and erythromycin.
[d] Mixed gastrointestinal operations.
[e] Patients who received placebo had a significantly higher infection rate than did patients who received ceftizoxime.

Table 9.
Comparative Costs of Cephalosporins with Enhanced Antianaerobic Activity

Drug	Unit Cost ($)[a]	Dosage	Cost ($) of One Day's Therapy[b]
Cefoxitin (as the sodium salt)	6.82/1-g vial 13.59/2-g vial	1 g every 4–6 hr 2 g every 4–6 hr	27.28–81.54
Cefotetan (as the sodium salt)	7.95/1-g vial 15.60/2-g vial	1–2 g every 12 hr	15.90–31.20
Ceftizoxime (as the sodium salt)	7.94/1-g vial 15.17/2-g vial	1–2 g every 8–12 hr	15.88–45.41
Moxalactam (as the disodium salt)	10.28/1-g vial 20.54/2-g vial	1–2 g every 8–12 hr	20.56–61.62

[a] Acquisition cost at the Medical College of Georgia Hospital and Clinics.
[b] Includes drug costs only.

of many types of infections, including those caused by anaerobes or combinations of aerobic microorganisms. There are two major issues associated with the use of cephalosporins for anaerobic or mixed infections: (1) Are cephalosporins as effective as combination regimens (such as an aminoglycoside and clindamycin or metronidazole? (2) Which cephalosporins are most effective in treating these infections? To address these issues, clinical, laboratory, and financial information should be considered. P&T committees should also consider that a number of agents may be used to treat anaerobic or mixed infections (including clindamycin, metronidazole, chloramphenicol, mezlocillin, piperacillin, ticarcillin–clavulanate, imipenem–cilastatin, and ampicillin–sulbactam); these are additional alternatives to the use of cephalosporins.

The question of whether cephalosporins have efficacy equivalent to that of combination regimens is primarily addressed by comparative clinical trials. The majority of published trials suggest that those cephalosporins with enhanced antianaerobic activity are as effective as combination regimens for treatment of intra-abdominal infections and intra-abdominal contamination from traumatic injury, female genital tract infections, and soft-tissue infections. However, some investigators have indicated that aminoglycosides should be included in the regimens until antimicrobial susceptibilities are determined.[56,98–100] Determining which cephalosporin is best for anaerobic or mixed infections should be based on results of clinical trials, as well as other pertinent information. The available clinical trials suggest that cephalosporins with enhanced activity against anaerobes, such as *B. fragilis*, are more effective than other cephalosporins for treatment of some anaerobic and mixed infections. For prophylaxis of infection associated with colorectal operations, hysterectomies, and cesarean sections, the advantage of cephalosporins with activity against *B. fragilis* is not clearly demonstrated, although many clinicians believe that antianaerobic activity is necessary.

Microbiological factors, safety factors, and costs are important considerations when selecting from among cephalosporins with enhanced antianaerobic activity. The four available agents with enhanced antianaerobic activity appear to have relatively minor differences in anaerobic activity. However, ceftizoxime, moxalactam, and cefotetan are considerably more active against gram-negative bacilli than cefoxitin is. For P&T committees to evaluate available microbiological data, susceptibility trends reported by several in vitro studies should be reviewed; decisions should not be made on the basis of individual studies. If possible, institutional susceptibility patterns should be considered. The issue of β-lactamase induction (or selection of derepressed mutants) should not influence the cephalosporin selection process until the clinical relevance of this issue is defined. The cephalosporins have fairly similar adverse effects, although those cephalosporins with the MTT side chain pose a greater risk of adverse hematological effects. This risk is well established for moxalactam but not for cefotetan. P&T committees may want to reserve judgment on cefotetan until more data are available. Finally, there are important pharmacokinetic factors (such as half-life) that relate to the required dosing frequency and cost. Cefoxitin has the shortest half-life, requiring dosing every 4 to 6 hours, whereas the alternative agents may be given at 8- to 12-hour intervals. The number of daily doses required and the cost per dose determine the overall cost of the cephalosporin regimens. There may be substantial differences in the total regimen cost mainly because of differences in the number of required daily doses. If the P&T committee wants to select one agent to meet a variety of needs, (e.g., for treatment of meningitis), CSF penetration may be important.

After considering the above factors, a cephalosporin can be chosen for treatment of anaerobic and mixed infections. Selection should be based on information demonstrating that an agent has efficacy equivalent to that of established regimens. If an agent is less effective than those regimens, the other factors are not important. If agents have equivalent efficacy, then other factors may be considered. The risk of adverse effects (e.g., hematological effects with moxalactam) should be considered. In many institutions, clinicians have preferred to avoid using moxalactam because of the greater risk of adverse effects. Finally, the cost of the regimen may determine which cephalosporin is selected. In choosing an agent with enhanced antianaerobic activity, the so-called generation of the cephalosporin should not be considered, since this system does not relate to clinical application. The specific choice of agent will depend on an institution's priorities. If clinical experience with an agent is more important, cefoxitin would be the best choice. If cost savings is a high priority, ceftizoxime or cefotetan should be chosen.

Conclusion

Cephalosporins with enhanced antianaerobic activity (cefoxitin, ceftizoxime, cefotetan, and moxalactam) appear to have similar in vitro microbiological activity, with cefotetan and moxalactam possibly less active against some anaerobic species and cefoxitin less active against some aerobic gram-negative bacilli. Clinical trials of these agents for the treatment of intra-abdominal infections, abdominal contamination, obstetric and gynecological infections, and soft-tissue infections have demonstrated that these cephalosporins have efficacy similar to that of combination regimens (most trials involved cefoxitin). Decisions to use antianaerobic cephalosporins should be based on consideration of alternative regimens (e.g., clindamycin, metronidazole, chloramphenicol, mezlocillin, piperacillin, ticarcillin–clavulanate, imipenem–cilastatin, and ampicillin–sulbactam), clinical experience, and cost of therapy. Selection of an antianaerobic cephalosporin should not be constrained by considerations of cephalosporin generation.

References

1. Wilson SE. Secondary bacterial peritonitis. In: Wilson SE, Finegold SM, Williams RA, eds. Intra-abdominal infections. New York: McGraw-Hill Book Co.; 1982:62–8.
2. Finegold SM. Microflora of the gastrointestinal tract. In: Wilson SE, Finegold SM, Williams RA, eds. Intra-abdominal infection. New York: McGraw-Hill Book Co.; 1982:1–21.
3. Lorber B, Swenson RM. The bacteriology of intra-abdominal infections. *Surg Clin North Am.* 1975; 55:1249–355.
4. Nichols RL. Empiric antibiotic therapy of intra-abdominal infections. *Rev Infect Dis.* 1983; 5(Suppl):590–7.
5. Onderdonk AB, Weinstein WM, Sullivan NM et al. Experimental intra-abdominal abscesses in rats: quantitative bacteriology of infected animals. *Infect Immun.* 1974; 10:1256–9.
6. Weinstein WM, Onderdonk AB, Bartlett JG et al. Antimicrobial therapy of experimental intra-abdominal sepsis. *J Infect Dis.* 1975; 132:282–6.
7. Onderdonk AB, Bartlett JG, Louie T et al. Microbial synergism in experimental intra-abdominal abscess. *Infect Immun.* 1976; 13:22–6.
8. Mackowiak PA. Microbial synergism in human infections. *N Engl J Med.* 1978; 298:21–5, 83–7.
9. Rotstein OD, Pruett TL, Simmons RL. Lethal microbial synergism in intra-abdominal infections. *Arch Surg.* 1985; 120:146–51.
10. Bartlett JG. Anaerobic infection of the pelvis. *Clin Obstet Gynecol.* 1979; 21:351–60.
11. Ledger WJ. Infection in the female. 2nd ed. Philadelphia: Lea and Febiger; 1986: 169–95, 249–78.
12. Shapiro M, Munoz A, Tager I et al. Risk factors for infection at the operative site after abdominal or vaginal hysterectomy. *N Engl J Med.* 1982; 307:1661–6.
13. Rotteram ER Jr, Schick SF. Nonclostridial anaerobic bacteria in septic abortion. *Am J Med.* 1969; 46:80–9.
14. Eschenbach DA, Buchanan TM, Pollock HM et al. Polymicrobial etiology of acute pelvic inflammatory disease. *N Engl J Med.* 1975; 293:166–71.
15. Landers DV, Sweet RL. Tubo-ovarian abscess: contemporary approach to management. *Rev Infect Dis.* 1983; 5:876–84.
16. Johanson WG, Harris GD. Aspiration pneumonia, anaerobic infections, and lung abscess. *Med Clin North Am.* 1980; 3:385–94.
17. Finegold SM. Anaerobic bacteria in human disease. New York: Academic Press; 1977.
18. Simmons RL, Ahrenholz DH. Infections of the skin and soft tissues. In: Simmons RL, Howard RJ, eds. Surgical infectious diseases. New York: Appleton-Century-Crofts; 1982:507–84.
19. Wheat LJ, Allen SD, Henry M et al. Diabetic foot infections. Bacteriologic analysis. *Arch Intern Med.* 1986; 146:1935–40.
20. Fierer J, Daniel D, Davis C. The fetid foot: lower-extremity infections in patients with diabetes mellitus. *Rev Infect Dis.* 1979; 1:210–7.
21. Rosenblatt JE. Antimicrobial susceptibility testing of anaerobic bacteria. *Rev Infect Dis.* 1984; 6(Suppl 1):S242–S248.
22. National Committee for Clinical Laboratory Standards. Reference agar dilution procedure for antimicrobial susceptibility testing of anaerobic bacteria; approved standard. Villanova, PA: National Committee for Clinical Laboratory Standards; 1985. NCCLS publication no. M11-A.
23. Baron EJ, Bruckner DA. Comparison of susceptibilities of anaerobic bacteria determined by agar dilution and by a microbroth method. *Rev Infect Dis.* 1984; 6(Suppl 1):S249–S253.
24. Cuchural GJ, Tally FP. *Bacteroides fragilis:* current susceptibilities, mechanisms of drug resistance and principles of antimicrobial therapy. *Drug Intell Clin Pharm.* 1986; 20:567–73.
25. Borobio MV, Pascual A, Cominguez MC et al. Effect of medium, pH, and inoculum size on activity of ceftizoxime and Sch-34343 against anaerobic bacteria. *Antimicrob Agents Chemother.* 1986; 30:626–7.
26. Marchbanks C, Yost R, White R. Cefotaxime stability during in vitro microbiologic testing. *Antimicrob Agents Chemother.* 1987; 31:1375–8.
27. Del Bene VE, Carek PJ, Twitty JA et al. In vitro activity of cefbuperazone compared with that of other β-lactam agents against anaerobic gram bacilli and contribution of β-lactamase to resistance. *Antimicrob Agents Chemother.* 1985; 27:817–20.
28. Watt B, Brown FV. The comparative in vitro activity of cefotetan against anaerobic bacteria. *J Antimicrob Chemother.* 1985; 15:671–7.
29. Ward A, Richards DM. Cefotetan. A review of its antibacterial activity, pharmacokinetic properties and therapeutic use. *Drugs.* 1985; 30:382–426.
30. Richards DM, Heel RC. Ceftizoxime. A review of its antibacterial activity, pharmacokinetic properties and therapeutic use. *Drugs.* 1985; 29:281–329.
31. Brogden RN, Heel RC, Speight TM et al. Cefoxitin. A

review of antibacterial activity, pharmacological properties and therapeutic use. *Drugs.* 1979; 17:1–37.
32. Garzone P, Lyon J, Yu VL. Third generation and investigational cephalosporins: II. Microbiological review and clinical summaries. *Drug Intell Clin Pharm.* 1983; 17:615–22.
33. Thornsberry C. Review of in vitro activity of third generation cephalosporins and other newer β-lactam antibiotics against clinically important bacteria. *Am J Med.* 1985; 79(Suppl 2A):14–20.
34. Sanders CC. Novel resistance selected by the new expanded-spectrum cephalosporins: a concern. *J Infect Dis.* 1983; 147:585–9.
35. Hemsell DL. Induction of β-lactamase enzymes: clinical applications for the obstetric-gynecologic patient. *Am J Obstet Gynecol.* 1987; 156:504–6.
36. Barza M. Three generations of cephalosporins. *Clin Pharm.* 1982; 1:165–7.
37. Norrby SR. Adverse reactions and interactions with newer cephalosporin and cephamycin antibiotics. *Medical Toxicology.* 1986; 1:32–46.
38. Kannangara DW, Smith B, Cohen K. Exfoliative dermatitis during cefoxitin therapy. *Arch Intern Med.* 1982; 142:1031–2.
39. Tietze KJ, Gaska JA. Cefoxitin-associated exfoliative dermatitis. *Clin Pharm.* 1983; 2:582–4.
40. Petz LD. Immunologic cross reactivity between penicillins and cephalosporins: a review. *J Infect Dis.* 1978; 137(Suppl):S74–S79.
41. Kammer RB. Moxalactam: clinical summary of efficacy and safety. *Rev Infect Dis.* 1982; 4(Suppl):S712–S719.
42. Bang NU, Kammer RB. Hematologic complications associated with β-lactam antibiotics. *Rev Infect Dis.* 1983; 5(Suppl 2):S380–S393.
43. Rotomar K, Conly JM, Chubb H et al. Production of menaquinolones by intestinal anaerobes. *J Infect Dis.* 1984; 158:213–8.
44. Lipsky JJ, Lewis JC, Novick WJ. Production of hypoprothrombinemia by moxalactam and 1-methyl-5-thiotetrazole in rats. *Antimicrob Agents Chemother.* 1984; 25:380–1.
45. Barza M, Furie B, Brown AE et al. Defects in vitamin K-dependent carboxylation associated with moxalactam treatment. *J Infect Dis.* 1986; 153:1166–9.
46. Bang NU, Tessler SS, Heindenreich RO et al. Effects of moxalactam on blood coagulation and platelet function. *Rev Infect Dis.* 1982; 4(Suppl)S546–S545.
47. Weitekamp MR, Aber RC. Prolonged bleeding time and bleeding diathesis associated with moxalactam administration. *JAMA.* 1982; 249:69–71.
48. Brown RB, Klar J, Lemeshaw S et al. Enhanced bleeding with cefoxitin or moxalactam. Statistical analysis within a defined population of 1493 patients. *Arch Intern Med.* 1986; 146:2159–64.
49. Nichols RL, Wikler MA, McDevitt JT et al. Coagulopathy associated with extended-spectrum cephalosporins in patients with serious infections. *Antimicrob Agents Chemother.* 1987; 31:281–5.
50. Balant L, Dayer P, Auckenthaler R. Clinical pharmacokinetics of the third generation cephalosporins. *Clin Pharmacokinet.* 1985; 10:101–43.
51. Schumacher GE. Comparison of antibiotic dosage regimens using pharmacokinetic and microbiologic factors. *Clin Pharm.* 1987; 6:59–68.
52. Schumacher GE. Pharmacokinetic and microbiologic evaluation of dosage regimens for newer cephalosporins and penicillins. *Clin Pharm.* 1983; 2:448–57.
53. Neu HC. Ceftizoxime: a β-lactamase-stable, broad spectrum cephalosporin. Pharmacokinetics, adverse effects, and clinical use. *Pharmacotherapy.* 1984; 4:47–60.
54. Smith BR, LeFrock JL, Thyrum PT et al. Cefotetan pharmacokinetics in volunteers with various degrees of renal function. *Antimicrob Agents Chemother.* 1986; 29:887–93.
55. Polk RE, Hepler CD. Controversies in antimicrobial therapy: critical analysis of clinical trials. *Am J Hosp Pharm.* 1986; 43:630–40.
56. Drusano GL, Warren JW, Saah AJ et al. A prospective randomized controlled trial of cefoxitin versus clindamycin-aminoglycoside in mixed anaerobic-aerobic infections. *Surg Gynecol Obstet.* 1982; 154:715–20.
57. Malangoni MA, Condon RE, Spiegel CA. Treatment of intra-abdominal infections is appropriate with single-agent or combination antibiotic therapy. *Surgery.* 1985; 98:648–55.
58. Harding GKM, Nicolle LE, Haase DA et al. Prospective, randomized, comparative trials in the therapy for intra-abdominal and female genital tract infections. *Rev Infect Dis.* 1984; 6:S283–S292.
59. Solomkin JS, Lentnek AL. A randomized trial of ceftizoxime vs. tobramycin/clindamycin for intra-abdominal infection. Proceedings of the 24th International Conference on Antimicrobial Agents and Chemotherapy. Washington, DC: American Society of Microbiology; 1984:957. Abstract 957.
60. Schentag JJ, Wel PB, Reitberg DP et al. A randomized clinical trial of moxalactam alone versus tobramycin plus clindamycin in abdominal sepsis. *Ann Surg.* 1983; 198:35–41.
61. Stone HH, Strom PR, Fabian TC et al. Third-generation cephalosporins for polymicrobial surgical sepsis. *Arch Surg.* 1983; 118:193–200.
62. Stone HH, Geheber CE, Kolb LD et al. Clinical comparison of cefotaxime versus the combination of gentamicin plus clindamycin in the treatment of peritonitis and similar polymicrobial soft-tissue surgical sepsis. *Clin Ther.* 1982; 4:67–80.
63. Lou MA, Valdepenas E, Mackabee J et al. A comparative evaluation of ceftizoxime and cefoxitin in the treatment of intra-abdominal infections. Proceedings of the 14th International Congress of Chemotherapy. Kyoto, Japan: 1985. Abstract S-25-5, p 2, 3, 7–9.
64. Busuttil RW, McGratten MA, Freischlag J. A comparative study of cefamandole versus gentamicin plus clindamycin in the treatment of documented or suspected bacterial peritonitis. *Surg Gynecol Obstet.* 1984; 158:1–8.
65. Berne TV, Yellin AW, Appleman MD, Heseltine PNR. Antibiotic management of surgically treated gangrenous or perforated appendicitis. *Am J Surg.* 1982; 144:8–13.
66. Heseltine PNR, Yellin AE, Appleman MD et al. Perforated and gangrenous appendicitis: an analysis of antibiotic failures. *J Infect Dis.* 1983; 148:322–9.
67. Lau WY, Fan ST, Chu KW et al. Randomized, prospective, and double-blind trial of new β-lactams in the treatment of appendicitis. *Antimicrob Agents Chemother.* 1985; 28:639–42.
68. Heseltine PNR, Berne TV, Yellin AE et al. The efficacy of cefoxitin versus clindamycin/gentamicin in surgically treated stab wounds of the bowel. *J Trauma.* 1986. 26:241–5.
69. Nichols RL, Smith JW, Klein DB et al. Risk of infection after penetrating abdominal trauma. *N Engl J Med.* 1984; 311:1065–70.
70. Rowlands BJ, Ericsson CD. Comparative studies of antibiotic therapy after penetrating abdominal trauma. *Am J Surg.* 1984; 148:791–5.
71. Jones RC, Thal ER, Johnson NA et al. Evaluation of antibiotic therapy following penetrating abdominal trauma. *Ann Surg.* 1985; 201:576–85.
72. Gentry LO, Feliciano DV, Lea AS et al. Perioperative antibiotic therapy for penetrating injuries of the abdomen. *Ann Surg.* 1984; 200:561–6.
73. Hofstetter SR, Pachter HL, Bailey AA et al. A prospective comparison of two regimens of prophylactic antibodies in abdominal trauma: cefoxitin versus triple drug. *J Trauma.* 1984; 24:307–10.
74. Nelson RM, Benitex PR, Newell MA et al. Single-antibiotic use for penetrating abdominal trauma. *Arch Surg.* 1986; 121:153–6.
75. Crenshaw C, Glanges E, Webber C et al. A prospective random study of a single agent versus combination antibiotics as therapy in penetrating injuries of the abdomen.

Surg Gynecol Obstet. 1983; 156:289–94.
76. Feliciano DV, Gentry LO, Bitondo CG et al. Single-agent cephalosporins prophylaxis for penetrating abdominal trauma. *Am J Surg*. 1986; 152:674–81.
77. Larsen JW, Voise CT, Grossman JH. Comparison of cefoxitin and clindamycin-gentamicin for pelvic infections. *Clin Ther*. 1986; 9:77–83.
78. Herman G, Cohen AW, Talbot GH et al. Cefoxitin versus clindamycin and gentamicin in the treatment of postcesarean section infections. *Obstet Gynecol*. 1986; 67:371–6.
79. Apuzzio JJ, Ganesh V, Pelosi MA et al. Comparative clinical evaluation of ceftizoxime with clindamycin and gentamicin and cefoxitin in the treatment of postcesarean endomyometritis. *Surg Gynecol Obstet*. 1985; 161:518–22.
80. Sweet RL, Ohm-Smith M, Landers DV et al. Moxalactam versus clindamycin plus tobramycin in the treatment of obstetric and gynecologic infections. *Am J Obstet Gynecol*. 1985; 152:808–17.
81. Gibbs RS, Blanco JD, Duff P et al. A double-blind, randomized comparison of moxalactam versus clindamycin-gentamicin in treatment of endomyometritis after cesarean section delivery. *Am J Obstet Gynecol*. 1983; 146:769–72.
82. Gilstrap LC, St. Clair PJ, Gibbs RS et al. Cefoperazone versus clindamycin plus gentamicin for obstetric and gynecologic infections. *Antimicrob Agents Chemother*. 1986; 30:808–9.
83. Hemsell DL, Cunningham FG, DePalma RT et al. Cefotaxime sodium therapy for endomyometritis following cesarean section: dose-finding and comparative studies. *Obstet Gynecol*. 1983; 62:489–96.
84. O'Bryan D, Knuppel R, Lake M. Cefotetan: comparative and noncomparative studies in obstetric and gynecologic infections. *South Med J*. 1986; 79:35. Abstract.
85. Hughes CE, Johnson CC, Bamberger DM et al. Treatment and long-term follow-up of foot infections in patients with diabetes or ischemia: a randomized, prospective, double-blind comparison of cefoxitin and ceftizoxime. *Clin Ther*. 1987; 10(Suppl A):36–49.
86. Maki DG, Aughey DR. Comparative study of cefazolin, cefoxitin, and ceftizoxime for surgical prophylaxis in colorectal surgery. *J Antimicrob Chemother*. 1982; 10(Suppl C):281–7.
87. Plouffe JF, Perkins RL, Fass RJ et al. Comparison of the effectiveness of moxalactam and cefazolin in the prevention of infection in patients undergoing abdominal operations. *Diagn Microbiol Infect Dis*. 1985; 3:25–31.
88. Kaiser AB, Herrington JL, Jacobs JK et al. Cefoxitin versus erythromycin, neomycin, and cefazolin in colorectal operations. *Ann Surg*. 1983; 198:525–30.
89. Hinchey EJ, Richards GK, Lewis R et al. Moxalactam as single-agent prophylaxis in the prevention of wound infection following colon surgery. *Surgery*. 1987; 101:15–9.
90. McDonald PJ, Karran SJ. A comparison of intravenous cefoxitin and a combination of gentamicin and metronidazole as prophylaxis in colorectal surgery. *Dis Colon Rectum*. 1983; 26:661–4.
91. McCulloch PG, Blamey SL, Finlay IG et al. A prospective comparison of gentamicin and metronidazole and moxalactam in the prevention of septic complications associated with elective operations of the colon and rectum. *Surg Gynecol Obstet*. 1986; 162:521–4.
92. Scheife RT, Tally FP, McGowan K et al. Cost comparison of two antimicrobial regimens for treating mixed aerobic-anaerobic infections. *Am J Hosp Pharm*. 1981; 38:1466–9.
93. Rapp RP, Bannon CL, Bivins BA. The influence of dose frequency and agent toxicity on the cost of parenteral antibiotic therapy. *Drug Intell Clin Pharm*. 1982; 16:935–8.
94. Brooks GF, Barriere SL. Clinical use of the new β-lactam antimicrobial drugs. *Ann Intern Med*. 1983; 98:530–5.
95. Gleckman R, Gantz NM. Cost-effective antibiotic prescribing. *Pharmacotherapy*. 1983; 3:239–48.
96. Scalley RD, Stuart CC. Is there cost reduction potential for extended half-life cephalosporins? *Drug Intell Clin Pharm*. 1986; 20:975–80.
97. Parr MD, Hansen LA, Waite WW et al. Computer program for comparing total costs of intravenous antibiotic regimens. *Am J Hosp Pharm*. 1986; 43:2189–93.
98. Ho J, Barza M. Role of aminoglycoside antibiotics in the treatment of intra-abdominal infections. *Antimicrob Agents Chemother*. 1987; 31:485–91.
99. Nicolle L, Harding G, Louie T et al. Cefoxitin plus tobramycin and clindamycin plus tobramycin. *Arch Surg*. 1986; 121:891–986.
100. Tally FP, McGowan K, Kellum JM et al. A randomized comparison of cefoxitin with or without amikacin and clindamycin plus amikacin in surgical sepsis. *Ann Surg*. 1981; 193:318–23.
101. Kamimura T, Matsomoto Y, Okada N et al. Ceftizoxime (FK 749), a new parenteral cephalosporin: in vitro and in vivo antibacterial activities. *Antimicrob Agents Chemother*. 1979; 16:540–8.
102. Bourgault AM, La Mothe F. In vitro activity of amoxicillin and ticarcillin in combination with clavulanic acid compared with that of new β-lactam agents against species of the *Bacteroides fragilis* group. *J Antimicrob Chemother*. 1986; 17:593–603.
103. Drulak MW, Chow AW. Comparative in vitro activity of ceftizoxime, cefoperazone, and cefoxitin against anaerobic bacteria. *Antimicrob Agents Chemother*. 1981; 20:683–5.
104. Yu PK, Washington JA. Bactericidal activities of new β-lactam antibiotics against *Bacteroides fragilis*. *Antimicrob Agents Chemother*. 1983; 24:1–4.
105. Fass RJ. Comparative in vitro activities of third generation cephalosporins. *Arch Intern Med*. 1983; 143:1743–5.
106. Neu HC, Chin NX, Labthavikul P. The in vitro activity of a novel penem FCE 22101 compared to other β-lactam antibiotics. *J Antimicrob Chemother*. 1985; 16:305–13.
107. Souza Dias BM, Jacobus NV, Gorbach SL et al. In vitro activity of cefbuperazone against *Bacteroides* spp. *Antimicrob Agents Chemother*. 1985; 27:968–70.
108. Fu KP, Neu HC. Antibacterial activity of ceftizoxime, a β-lactamase-stable cephalosporin. *Antimicrob Agents and Chemother*. 1980; 17:583–90.
109. Kesado T, Watanabe K, Asahi Y et al. Comparative antibacterial activities of 7-methoxy cephalosporins and 7-methoxyiminoacetamido cephalosporins against *Bacteroides fragilis*. *Antimicrob Agents Chemother*. 1984; 26:131–3.
110. Aldridge KE, Sanders CV, Janney A et al. Comparison of the activities of penicillin G and new β-lactam antibiotics against clinical isolates of *Bacteroides* species. *Antimicrob Agents Chemother*. 1984; 26:410–3.
111. Bansal MB, Chuah SK, Thadepalli H. Susceptibility of intestinal anaerobes to new β-lactam antibiotics. *Chemotherapy*. 1984; 30:237–43.
112. Greenwood D, Pearson N, Eley A et al. Comparative in vitro activities of cefotaxime and ceftizoxime (FK749): new cephalosporins with exceptional potency. *Antimicrob Agents Chemother*. 1980; 17:397–401.
113. La Mothe F, Auger F, Lacroix JM. Effects of clavulanic acid on the activities of ten β-lactam agents against members of the *Bacteroides fragilis* group. *Antimicrob Agents Chemother*. 1984; 25:662–5.
114. Aldridge KE, Sanders CV. Comparison of the activity of Carumonam (RO 17-2301) with other broad-spectrum antibiotics: in vitro antibacterial spectrum, inoculum effect, and synergy studies. *Curr Ther Res*. 1986; 40:515–27.
115. Gibbs RS, Blanco JD, Castaneda YS, St. Clair PJ. A double-blind, randomized comparison of clindamycin-gentamicin versus cefamandole for treatment of postcesarean section endomyometritis. *Am J Obstet Gynecol*. 1982; 144:261–7.
116. Faro S, Phillips LE, Baker JL et al. Comparative efficacy and safety of mezlocillin, cefoxitin, and clindamycin plus gentamicin in postpartum endometritis. *Obstet Gynecol*. 1987; 69:760–6.

117. Poindexter AN, Sweet R, Ritter M. Cefotetan in the treatment of obstetric and gynecologic infections. *Am J Obstet Gynecol.* 1986; 154:946–50.
118. Slama TG, Carey LC, Fass RJ. Comparative efficacy of prophylactic cephalothin and cefamandole for elective colon surgery: results of a prospective, randomized, double-blind study. *Am J Surg.* 1979; 137:593–6.
119. Hoffman CEJ, McDonald PJ, Watts JM. Use of perioperative cefoxitin to prevent infection after colonic and rectal surgery. *Ann Surg.* 1981; 193:353–6.
120. Lewis RT, Allan CM, Goodall RG et al. Preventing anaerobic infection in surgery of the colon. *Can J Surg.* 1981; 24:139–41.
121. Jones RN, Wojeski W, Bakke J et al. Antibiotic prophylaxis of 1036 patients undergoing elective surgical procedures. *Am J Surg.* 1987; 153:341–6.
122. Hemsell DL, Hemsell P, Nobles B et al. Moxalactam versus cefazolin prophylaxis for vaginal hysterectomy. *Am J Obstet Gynecol.* 1983; 147:379–85.
123. Maki DG, Lammers JL, Aughey DR. Comparative studies of multiple-dose cefoxitin vs. single dose cefonicid for surgical prophylaxis in patients undergoing biliary tract operations or hysterectomy. *Rev Infect Dis.* 1984; 6(Suppl):887–95.
124. Littlejohn TW, Evrard HM, Moonsammy G. Comparison of cefonicid and cefoxitin for prevention of infection following vaginal hysterectomy. *Adv Ther.* 1985; 2:240–9.
125. Benigno BB, Evrard J, Faro S et al. A comparison of piperacillin, cephalothin and cefoxitin in the prevention of postoperative infections in patients undergoing vaginal hysterectomy. *Surg Gynecol Obstet.* 1986; 163:421–7.
126. Hemsell DL, Johnson ER, Bawdon RE et al. Cefoperazone and cefoxitin prophylaxis for abdominal hysterectomy. *Obstet Gynecol.* 1984; 63:467–72.
127. Periti P, Mazzei T, Lamanna S et al. Single dose ceftriaxone versus multiple-dose cefotaxime antimicrobial prophylaxis in gynecologic and obstetric surgery. *Chemotherapia.* 1984; 3:299–304.
128. Hemsell DL, Johnson ER, Bawdon RE et al. Ceftriaxone and cefazolin prophylaxis for hysterectomy. *Surg Gynecol Obstet.* 1985; 161:197–203.
129. Tuomala RE, Fisher SG, Munoz A et al. A comparative trial of cefazolin and moxalactam as prophylaxis for preventing infection after abdominal hysterectomy. *Obstet Gynecol.* 1985; 66:372–6.
130. Orr JW, Varner RE, Kilgore LC et al. Cefotetan versus cefoxitin as prophylaxis in hysterectomy. *Am J Obstet Gynecol.* 1986; 154:960–3.
131. Stiver HG, Forward KR, Livingstone RA et al. Multicenter comparison of cefoxitin versus cefazolin for prevention of infectious morbidity after non-elective cesarean section. *Am J Obstet Gynecol.* 1983; 145:158–63.
132. Parsons MT, Gibson R, Rimando RJ et al. Comparison of single-dose cefonicid and multiple-dose cefoxitin for surgical prophylaxis in women undergoing cesarean section. *Adv Ther.* 1985; 2:233–9.
133. Saltzman DH, Eron LJ, Kay HH et al. Single-dose antibiotic prophylaxis in high risk patients undergoing cesarean section. *Obstet Gynecol.* 1985; 65:655–7.
134. Varner MW, Weiner CP, Petzold CR et al. Comparison of cefotetan and cefoxitin as prophylaxis in cesarean section. *Am J Obstet Gynecol.* 1986; 154:951–4.
135. McGregor JA, French JI, Makowski E. Single-dose cefotetan versus multi-dose cefoxitin for prophylaxis in cesarean section in high-risk patients. *Am J Obstet Gynecol.* 1986; 154:955–60.

“

Research in Monoclonal Antibodies

[T]he moderate successes of monoclonal antibody therapy are extremely encouraging. However, they include therapies that work in a very limited set of circumstances. The therapy must be exogenous, as in bone marrow transplantation, or administered once, as in the treatment of blood poisoning and transplant rejection. To overcome these limitations it is clear that more basic research is required before antibody therapy can be used safely. In particular, further research in immunology will be critical for learning how to control tolerance to the immunogenic effects of antibodies and how to avoid uptake of antibodies by the reticuloendothelial system. Both of these goals will be assisted by genetic engineering on antibody molecules which might make them less immunogenic and remove their recognition sequences for reticuloendothelial cell uptake. For example, several research groups have developed the technology for producing "chimeric" antibodies. These are composed of the antigen combining site and variable region of a mouse monoclonal antibody, genetically engineered to be attached to a human immunoglobulin constant region. In addition, more basic research is needed to understand the cell biology of receptor internalization and signaling. The effects of monoclonal antibodies do not stop at surface receptors. Their binding can trigger or block activity within the cell and their uptake can alter the metabolism of conjugated drugs and toxins. Fortunately, research in both immunology and receptor biology has entered a revolutionary age and it is likely that new insights applicable to antibody therapy will soon be discovered.

—Brodsky FM. Monoclonal antibodies as magic bullets. *Pharm Res.* 1988; 5:1–9.

”

Research

Delivery of gentamicin by a controlled-release infusion system versus a minibag system

DEE MARIE MUNOZ, ELAINE R. GREEN, MARGARET M. CHRYMKO, JOSEPH M. MYLOTTE, AND JACK G. KITRENOS

Abstract: Delivery of gentamicin via a new controlled-release intravenous infusion system was compared with conventional delivery via small-volume injections in minibags by measuring serum drug concentrations in 10 healthy men.

Each volunteer received gentamicin (as the sulfate salt) 2 mg/kg. In phase 1, subjects randomly received the drug either as a 50-mL admixture in 5% dextrose injection (D5W) or from the controlled-release system (CRIS, IVAC Corporation), in which drug was diluted in a vial with 10 mL of sterile water for injection (density of drug solution, approximately 1.5% w/v) and was delivered when the primary solution (D5W; density, 5% w/v) displaced drug from the vial and infused it into the subject over 30 min; subjects were then crossed over. In phase 2, nine of the subjects received the drug via CRIS with the diluent changed to 10 mL of 5% dextrose and 0.9% sodium chloride injection (D5NS; density of drug solution, approximately 5.9% w/v). In phase 3, 10 men (seven of the original subjects) received the gentamicin dose via CRIS with 20 mL of D5NS as the diluent or via minibags in a crossover design. The amount of drug remaining in each vial used with the CRIS system was determined.

Drug administration via CRIS with 10 mL of sterile water diluent resulted in serum concentrations approximately 35% of those obtained with the minibag system, and a substantial portion (71 ± 8%) of the dose to be administered remained in the vials. With D5NS 10 mL as the diluent, less than 1% of the dose remained in the vials and postdistribution serum gentamicin concentrations were comparable to those for minibag doses. Approximately 4% of the dose prepared in 20 mL of D5NS remained in the CRIS vials.

If the manufacturer's recommendations for use are followed, CRIS may be satisfactory for delivery of small doses of potent drugs. The diluent should be chosen so that the drug solution will be more dense than the primary solution being infused.

Index terms: Aminoglycosides; Blood levels; Density; Devices; Dextrose; Diluents; Drug administration; Drugs; Gentamicin; Gentamicin sulfate; Injections; Sodium chloride; Volume; Water for injection
Clin Pharm. 1988; 7:303–7

Administration methods for intravenous fluids and drugs have been an area of advancing technology over the last decade. Several drug and device manufacturers have developed systems that attempt to improve efficiency, safety, and cost-effectiveness of drug delivery.[1–6] At the same time, success of these systems has required that they also be easily integrated into the patient-care setting.

DEE MARIE MUNOZ, PHARM.D., is Assistant Chief Pharmacist, Kaiser Foundation Health Plan Pharmacy, San Francisco, CA; at the time of this study, she was Clinical Resident, Department of Pharmaceutical Services, Erie County Medical Center (ECMC), Buffalo, NY. ELAINE R. GREEN, PHARM.D., is Clinical Assistant Professor of Pharmacy, School of Pharmacy, State University of New York at Buffalo (SUNYAB) and Clinical Faculty, ECMC. MARGARET M. CHRYMKO, PHARM.D., is Assistant Director for Clinical Pharmacy Services and Research, ECMC, and Clinical Assistant Professor of Pharmacy, School of Pharmacy, and Clinical Instructor, School of Medicine, SUNYAB. JOSEPH M. MYLOTTE, M.D., is Attending Physician, Infectious Disease Service, Veterans Administration Medical Center, Buffalo, NY, and ECMC, and Assistant Professor of Medicine, School of Medicine, SUNYAB. JACK G. KITRENOS, PHARM.D., is Director, Department of Pharmaceutical Services, ECMC, and Clinical Associate Professor of Pharmacy, School of Pharmacy, and Clinical Assistant Professor of Medicine, School of Medicine, SUNYAB.

Address reprint requests to Dr. Kitrenos at the Department of Pharmaceutical Services, Erie County Medical Center, 462 Grider Street, Buffalo, NY 14215.

The assistance of Mary Ellen Gliosca in typing this manuscript and of Carolyn Kalinka, Kathy Catanzaro, and Robert Vinti is acknowledged.

Supported by the IVAC Corporation.

Presented at the 21st Annual ASHP Midyear Clinical Meeting, Las Vegas, NV, December 10, 1986.

Copyright © 1988, American Society of Hospital Pharmacists, Inc. All rights reserved. 0278-2677/88/0401-0303$01.25.

In 1986, the IVAC Corporation marketed the CRIS controlled-release infusion system, a novel means by which intermittent drug doses can be administered directly from the vial in which the drug dose is prepared. The CRIS system functions by allowing flow from the primary fluid container into the vial containing the drug. The primary fluid displaces the drug from the vial and infuses it into the patient. This mechanism of action suggests that drug delivery from the CRIS device may be affected by relative densities of the primary solution and the contents of the vial.

During product development, the IVAC Corporation and Eli Lilly and Company characterized the performance of this system by establishing drug output patterns in in vitro tests and by predicting drug concentrations in blood by using computer-generated pharmacokinetic models.[7]

The purpose of our study was to compare profiles of in vivo serum concentrations when gentamicin was administered in identical doses through the CRIS device and standard minibag systems and to determine effect on drug delivery caused by varying the densities and volumes of the CRIS vial contents.

Methods

Thirteen healthy male volunteers participated in this randomized, crossover investigation. The following selection criteria were used: age between 21 and 50 years, weight within 20% of ideal body weight, normal results of complete blood count, and serum creatinine concentration between 0.5 and 1.3 mg/dL. Exclusion criteria included history of hepatic, renal, cardiac, hematologic, or gastrointestinal disease, or serious adverse reaction to gentamicin or other aminoglycoside antibiotics.

The protocol for this investigation was approved by the joint hospital and university investigational review board. In all cases, informed consent was obtained after the details of the study were explained to the participants. One physician conducted medical histories and physical examinations and reviewed laboratory data on all subjects admitted to the study.

The crossover study was conducted in three phases, separated in all cases by at least 14 days. Each subject had a peripheral i.v. line placed in one arm for the infusion of primary fluid and drug and an indwelling venous catheter (heparin lock) in the opposite arm to facilitate blood sample collection.

Phase 1. In phase 1, 10 subjects were randomly selected for either the traditional minibag administration system (Baxter Healthcare Corporation, Deerfield, IL) or the controlled-release infusion system (CRIS, IVAC Corporation, San Diego, CA). A gentamicin dose of 2 mg/kg (rounded off to the nearest 10 mg) was used for all subjects, independent of method of administration. In all cases, standard intravenous admixture procedures were used for drug preparation.

The minibag system contained 50 mL of 5% dextrose injection (D5W) to which the calculated dose of gentamicin (as the sulfate salt) had been added. An infusion rate was established to allow for administration of the drug and solution over approximately 30 minutes. This rate and method are consistent with hospital intravenous administration guidelines. The rate was set at 120 mL/hr and controlled by an IVAC 230 rate controller. In all cases, fluid and drug administration simulated routine nursing-unit drug administration. After drug administration, the secondary infusion lines were flushed with the primary solution to ensure complete drug delivery.

The CRIS system delivered the gentamicin in 10 mL of sterile water for injection (SWI); the primary i.v. fluid was D5W. The infusion rate was established at 120 mL/hr, controlled by an IVAC 230 rate controller. The density of the drug dose prepared in SWI (mean, 1.5% w/v) was much less than the density of the D5W primary solution (5% w/v). After 30 minutes, the CRIS infusion was stopped and the line was flushed with the primary fluid.

Blood samples (5 mL) were collected at 0, 5, 10, 15, 30, 45, 60, 120, and 240 minutes after the start of the infusion. Heparin lock flush (heparin sodium 10 units/mL) was used to maintain heparin lock patency. Samples were centrifuged and the serum was separated. All samples were frozen until assay. The volume remaining in the CRIS vial was measured and a sample was assayed for remaining drug contents. All serum gentamicin assays were performed, in duplicate, within one week of sample collection, using a fluorescence polarization immunoassay (TDx Analyzer, Abbott Laboratories, Irvine, TX). The lower limit of assay sensitivity was 0.3 μg/mL. Controls were performed across the concentration range of 1–8 μg/mL with a coefficient of variation of less than 10%.

All subjects were then crossed over to the opposite drug administration system. Data were collected as described above.

Phase 2. In phase 2, nine of the subjects from phase 1 received gentamicin 2 mg/kg infused through the CRIS adapter; 5% dextrose and 0.9% sodium chloride injection (D5NS) 10 mL was used as the diluent; the primary i.v. fluid was D5W. In phase 2, the density of the gentamicin prepared in D5NS (approximately 5.9% w/v) was greater than that of the D5W primary solution (5% w/v).

Phase 3. The methods used in phase 3 were similar to those in phases 1 and 2. Ten subjects (seven from phases 1 and 2) received the CRIS and minibag doses of gentamicin (2 mg/kg) in a crossover design. The volume of the diluent in the CRIS vial was increased to D5NS 20 mL for phase 3. The relative densities of the solutions were unchanged from phase 2.

Statistical Analysis. Serum gentamicin concentrations achieved with the two delivery systems were compared using the Student's *t* test for paired data (phase 3) and analysis of variance (ANOVA) (phases 1 and 2). A significant difference was defined by $p < 0.05$.

Results

Thirteen volunteers participated in the three phases of this study. Seven of these completed all three phases over a six-month period. The only reason that a subject did not complete all phases was relocation. The mean age of the volunteers was 28 years (range, 24 to 39 years). The mean gentamicin dose was 150 mg (range, 120–180 mg).

The mean serum gentamicin concentrations for doses administered in phases 1 and 2 are outlined in Table 1 and shown graphically in Figure 1. Serum concentrations achieved using CRIS and SWI 10 mL were significantly different from those for minibag administration at 30, 45, 60, 120, and 240 minutes. For CRIS and D5NS 10 mL, significant differences from minibag administration occurred at 10, 15, 30, 60, 120, and 240 minutes. Gentamicin serum concentrations when the drug was administered via CRIS and D5NS 20 mL were significantly different from those achieved with minibag administration at 15 and 30 minutes (Table 2 and Figure 2).

Administration of gentamicin via CRIS using 10 mL of sterile water as the diluent resulted in serum gentamicin concentrations approximately 35% of those obtained with the minibag system. A substantial portion (71 ± 8%) of the dose to be administered remained in the CRIS vials with this diluent. When the diluent was changed to 10 mL of D5NS, less than 1% of the dose remained in the CRIS vials, and postdistribution serum gentamicin concentrations were comparable to those of the minibag doses. Approximately 4% of the dose prepared in 20 mL of D5NS was recovered in the CRIS vials. Minibags were not analyzed for remaining drug contents.

Discussion

The results of this study show that the CRIS system is apparently sensitive to differences in density between primary and secondary solutions and that these differences can affect drug delivery. Because the CRIS drug delivery depends, in large part, on displacement of the drug solution from the vial by the primary solution, a requirement for reliable delivery seems to be that the secondary solution remains at the bottom of the inverted vial and is displaced as the lighter primary solution enters at the bottom and rises to the top of the vial.

The discovery that gentamicin was not adequately delivered by the CRIS system and SWI led to the manufacturer's current statement that the density within the CRIS vial should be equal to or greater than 6% w/v. Most primary solutions have densities less than 6% on a weight/volume (w/v) basis. D5W is 5% w/v, 0.9% sodium chloride injection is 0.9% w/v, and D5NS is 5.9% w/v. Therefore, if the concentration of the drug in the vial will be less than 60 mg/mL (6% w/v), the diluent for the dose should be chosen to contribute the needed density so that the drug solution will be more dense than the primary solution that is being infused.

Table 1.
Mean (± S.D.) Serum Gentamicin Concentrations (μg/mL) in Phases 1 and 2[a]

Time (min)	Phase 1: Minibag (*n* = 10)	Phase 1: CRIS–SWI 10 mL (*n* = 10)	Phase 2: CRIS–D5NS 10 mL (*n* = 9)
0	<0.3	<0.3	<0.3
5	<0.3	<0.3	<0.3
10	2.5 ± 1.31	2.67 ± 1.58	9.41 ± 6.19[b]
15	4.92 ± 1.75	3.34 ± 1.28	14.98 ± 4.84[b]
30	9.36 ± 1.78	3.19 ± 0.60[c]	11.37 ± 0.88[b]
45	8.43 ± 0.83	2.88 ± 0.78[c]	8.96 ± 0.55[d]
60	6.8 ± 0.59	2.37 ± 0.54[c]	7.46 ± 0.41[b]
120	4.12 ± 0.41	1.44 ± 0.28[c]	4.69 ± 0.37[b]
240	1.85 ± 0.28	0.83 ± 0.14[c]	2.23 ± 0.32[b]

[a] Phase 1: minibag contained 5% dextrose injection (D5W), CRIS (controlled-release infusion system) diluent was sterile water for injection (SWI), and CRIS was used with D5W primary infusion; phase 2: CRIS diluent was 5% dextrose and 0.9% sodium chloride injection and CRIS was used with D5W primary infusion.

[b] Significantly different from minibag and CRIS–SWI 10 mL.

[c] Significantly different from minibag and CRIS–D5NS 10 mL.

[d] Significantly different from CRIS–SWI 10 mL.

Figure 1. Mean serum gentamicin concentrations in phases 1 and 2. ● = minibag containing drug diluted in 5% dextrose injection (D5W); ◇ = controlled-release infusion system (CRIS) with drug diluted in 10 mL of 5% dextrose and 0.9% sodium chloride injection; ◆ = CRIS with drug diluted in 10 mL of sterile water. For CRIS with both diluents, primary infusion was D5W.

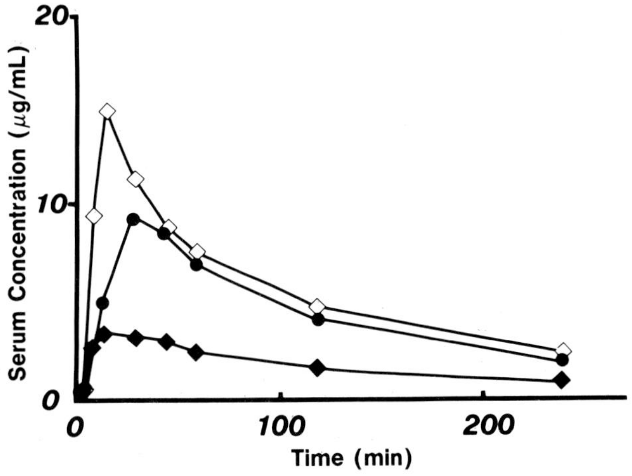

For simplicity, choice of 10 mL of D5NS as the diluent for all drug doses less than 600 mg ensures that the secondary solution will possess density characteristics such that it will be delivered predictably by the CRIS device. Doses larger than 600 mg/10 mL of solution, e.g., doses for many antibiotics, will be heavier than the 6% w/v limit because of the drug alone and therefore will need no special choice of diluent.

The volume of diluent in the CRIS vial also appears to affect drug delivery. The 20-mL volume resulted in lower serum concentrations during the distributive phase than did the CRIS 10-mL infusion, and the 20-mL volume produced a serum gentamicin profile more similar to that achieved with traditional minibag administration. Postdistributive peak concentrations 60 minutes after initiation of infusion were comparable for the minibag, CRIS–10 mL D5NS, and CRIS–20 mL D5NS infusions.

The postdistributive serum gentamicin concentrations were similar for the minibag, the CRIS–D5NS 10 mL, and the CRIS–D5NS 20 mL infusions. The postdistributive gentamicin concentrations at 60 minutes would be comparable to peak concentrations measured in clinical practice. The peaks achieved for the minibag, the CRIS–D5NS 10 mL, and the CRIS–D5NS 20 mL systems were within the generally accepted therapeutic peaks of 6–8 μg/mL for serious infections. Gentamicin concentrations during infusions and during drug distribution may consistently achieve concentrations above the defined therapeutic range. In this study, the gentamicin concentrations of 8–15 μg/mL may be initially disturbing to the clinician. However, the reason for waiting 60 minutes to obtain the true peak is to avoid measuring the higher concentrations that occur during the distribution phase. The 60-minute concentration is the standard for which our therapeutic definitions have been established. No toxicity was associated with the brief periods of gentamicin concentrations greater than 8 μg/mL.

When comparing CRIS drug administration with the traditional minibag infusion system, we observed several other differences. First, the CRIS vial maintains its original volume throughout the infusion period, as the primary solution displaces the contents of the drug vial. We speculate that nurses may potentially be concerned that they cannot visually confirm that drug infusion is completed or in progress. This concern can be partially alleviated by drop chamber inspection, by use of an electronic infusion instrument to control the infusion, and by inservice education regarding the principles of the CRIS system. Since IVAC recommends that expended vials should be left in place until the next scheduled dose,[8] nurses should be instructed to mark vials to indicate when the drug infusion was initiated.

Some drugs may require dilution to volumes greater than 20 mL. In these cases, adjustment may be necessary to ensure drug delivery by the CRIS system in accordance with the manufacturer's recommendation.

Once the allotted time for drug infusion has elapsed, the primary solution is infusing at the rate set for drug delivery. This rate may not be desirable or acceptable in some clinical situations. An infustion instrument that delivers a specific volume and then sounds an alarm when that infusion is complete will call the nurse back to the bedside. The nurse can then program the infusion device for continuation of the primary fluid at the appropriate rate. Some infusion instruments can be programmed to run at the secondary rate for a specific volume and then automatically switch back to the primary rate.

Table 2.
Mean (± S.D.) Serum Gentamicin Concentrations (μg/mL) in Phase 3[a]

Time (min)	Minibag (n = 10)	CRIS–D5NS 20 mL (n = 10)
0	<0.3	<0.3
5	1.2 ± 2.6	<0.3
10	3.4 ± 2.1	3.3 ± 4.0
15	5.6 ± 1.6	11.6 ± 3.7[b]
30	10.4 ± 3.5	12.0 ± 1.5[b]
45	8.8 ± 1.7	8.7 ± 0.7
60	7.3 ± 1.1	7.6 ± 0.6
120	4.5 ± 1.2	5.4 ± 0.6
240	1.9 ± 0.5	2.4 ± 0.5

[a] Phase 3: minibag contained 5% dextrose injection (D5W); CRIS (controlled-release infusion system) diluent was 5% dextrose and 0.9% sodium chloride injection, and CRIS was used with D5W primary infusion.
[b] Significantly different.

Figure 2. Mean serum gentamicin concentrations in phase 3. ◇ = minibag containing drug diluted in 5% dextrose injection (D5W); ◆ = controlled-release infusion system with drug diluted in 20 mL of 5% dextrose and 0.9% sodium chloride injection; D5W used as primary infusion.

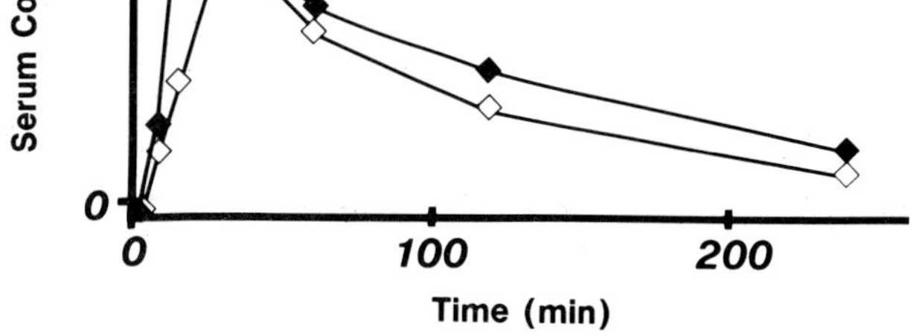

The CRIS device in effect becomes part of the primary set. A secondary set and a minibag are no longer necessary for doses that can be administered through the CRIS adapter. This is most advantageous for drugs that are available in 10- or 20-mL vials ready for reconstitution in standardized doses. The CRIS system may enable the institution to save on preparation, auxiliary equipment, and inventory costs.

The CRIS device is recommended primarily for drugs with direct "i.v. push" administration indications.[8] Further studies are warranted to ensure appropriate administration of other drugs that, like gentamicin, have no specific i.v. push instructions in their approved labeling. Additional compatibility studies may also be necessary.

Conclusion

The IVAC controlled release infusion system (CRIS) appears to possess characteristics that make it satisfactory for delivery of small doses of potent drugs such as gentamicin when IVAC recommendations regarding secondary solution density are observed. To ensure complete delivery of the dose, a diluent that will make the drug solution more dense than the primary solution must be selected.

References

1. Markowsky SJ, Kitrenos JG. Comparison of six methods for preparing cefazolin sodium for intermittent injection. *Am J Hosp Pharm.* 1983; 40:1653–8.
2. Tribble DA, Fotis M, McDonald DE. Unit of use versus traditional intravenous piggyback drug administration systems. *Am J Hosp Pharm.* 1979; 36:739–42.
3. Fraterrigo CC, Jorgenson JA. Accuracy and efficiency of three methods of preparing piggyback admixtures. *Am J Hosp Pharm.* 1982; 39:1920–3.
4. Dreiman RK. Comparison of six methods of preparing piggyback doses of cephalothin sodium. *Am J Hosp Pharm.* 1980; 37:1342–6.
5. Pohorylo EM, Lewis FM, Anderson ER Jr. Time and cost comparison of four methods of filling piggyback bottles. *Am J Hosp Pharm.* 1983; 40:87–90.
6. Smith TS, Kitrenos JG. Comparison of seven methods of preparing and administering cefazolin sodium small volume injections. *Am J Hosp Pharm.* 1986; 43:1930–5.
7. Kirsch LE, Ragozzino JL. Drug delivery with the IVAC CRIS controlled release infusion system. *Pharm Pract News.* 1986; 13(Jul):1–4.
8. IVAC Corporation. CRIS package insert. San Diego, CA; 1986.

Simulated effect of gentamicin assay errors on calculated pharmacokinetic values

ERIC G. BOYCE AND CAROL B. PUGH

Abstract: The effects of errors in gentamicin concentrations were assessed using computer simulation.

Steady-state concentrations at the end of a one-hour infusion (C_{max}) and at the end of the dosing interval (C_{min}) were calculated for four simulated patients with three dosing schemes each. Errors from −80% to +80% were systematically induced in C_{max} or C_{min}, or both. Pharmacokinetic values were calculated from the error concentrations and then used to determine new dosing regimens given specific desired concentrations. True C_{max} and C_{min} values were calculated using the new dosing regimens and original pharmacokinetic values.

As the absolute value of the induced error increased, increases were generally seen in the absolute value of the resultant error and in the deviation of the true C_{max} and C_{min} from desired values. Resultant error was more evident with induced error less than zero, when error was induced into C_{max}, and with shorter dosing intervals. Resultant error in pharmacokinetic variables was greater than induced error at induced errors as low as ±5%. Toxic and suboptimal values for the true C_{max} and C_{min} rarely occurred with induced errors of −20% to +20%.

Errors in serum gentamicin concentration measurements are more likely to cause larger resultant errors as the errors in concentration values (1) increase in magnitude, (2) result in underreporting of the concentration values, or (3) affect peak concentration values. Shorter dosing intervals may also increase the influence of assay errors.

Index terms: Aminoglycosides; Blood levels; Calculations; Computers; Dosage schedules; Errors, medication; Gentamicin; Methodology; Models; Pharmacokinetics: Time
Clin Pharm. 1988; 7:307–13

ERIC G. BOYCE, PHARM.D., and CAROL B. PUGH, PHARM.D., are Assistant Professors of Clinical Pharmacy, Department of Pharmacy Practice and Pharmacy Administration, Philadelphia College of Pharmacy and Science, Philadelphia, PA.

Address reprint requests to Dr. Boyce at the Philadelphia College of Pharmacy and Science, Woodland Avenue at 43rd Street, Philadelphia, PA 19104-4495.

Presented at the Clinical Research Forum, 22nd Annual ASHP Midyear Clinical Meeting, Atlanta, GA, December 9, 1987.

Copyright © 1988, American Society of Hospital Pharmacists, Inc. All rights reserved. 0278-2677/88/0401-0307$01.75.

Precise, accurate measurement of serum drug concentrations is one crucial aspect of a successful pharmacokinetics service. In most clinical laboratories, serum aminoglycoside concentrations are measured using immunoassay methods with intra-assay coefficients of variation of 10% or less. However, studies have revealed interassay differences in concentration measurement ranging from 18 to 115%.[1,2] Results from immunoassays can also be influenced by patient or sample factors such as hyperbilirubinemia,[3] presence of ticarcillin,[4] and presence of heparin.[5] However, each assay is not similarly affected by each factor.[6] Differences in assay results can cause potentially serious consequences by leading to the use of toxic or subtherapeutic dosage regimens. Thus, an understanding of the impact of assay errors on the calculation of pharmacokinetic values and subsequent dosing regimens is of clinical importance.

We used computer simulation to assess the effects of errors in serum gentamicin concentration values on the calculation of pharmacokinetic values and dosing regimens and their resultant concentration values. The resulting errors and concentration values were examined to determine the presence of general trends and the effects of patient characteristics (elimination rate constant and volume of distribution); induction of error in the peaks or troughs, or both; and changes in dosing (dose and dosing interval). We also attempted to determine the induced errors that would produce toxic or suboptimal concentrations and higher-than-expected resultant errors.

Methods

Study Design. A spreadsheet program (Symphony, Lotus Corporation) was used on a personal computer to determine serum gentamicin concentrations in simulated "patients." A one-compartment model was used to calculate steady-state concentrations resulting from simulated doses administered by zero-order intermittent intravenous infusion over one hour. The methods used to induce error in the concentration values were developed to assess potential interassay errors and intra-assay differences. A systematic approach was used to provide reproducible results.

The creation of four "patients" allowed the simulation of some commonly encountered clinical situations, as well as the analysis of trends for each set. The variables used for each patient simulation are listed in Table 1. Patient A represents a lean patient with mild renal dysfunction, and patient B simulates a lean patient with moderate renal dysfunction. The obese patient with mild renal dysfunction is represented by patient C, and the obese patient with moderate renal dysfunction is portrayed by patient D.

Calculations. Doses and dosing intervals that would yield concentrations at the end of a one-hour infusion (C_{max}) of 6.5 mg/mL and at the end of a dosing interval (C_{min}) of 1.0 mg/L were calculated for each "patient" using the pharmacokinetic values listed in Table 1 and the following equations:

$$\tau = t_{inf} + [\ln (C_{max}/C_{min})/k] \quad (1)$$

$$D = C_{max}(k)(t_{inf})(V)(1 - e^{-k\tau})/(1 - e^{-kt_{inf}}) \quad (2)$$

where τ is the dosing interval in hours, t_{inf} is the duration of the infusion in hours, C_{max} is the concentration at the end of the infusion in milligrams per liter, C_{min} is the concentration at the end of the dosing interval in milligrams per liter, k is the elimination rate constant in inverse hours, D is the dose in milligrams, and V is the volume of distribution in liters. The values calculated for each simulation are listed in Table 1.

Error was then introduced into (1) C_{max} only, (2) C_{min} only, (3) both C_{max} and C_{min} of the same magnitude and in the same direction, and (4) both C_{max} and C_{min} of the same magnitude but in opposite directions. The induced errors used for each scenario were ±80, ±60, ±40, ±30, ±20, ±15, ±10, and ±5%. The resulting concentration values were termed $C_{max\ error}$ and $C_{min\ error}$. Throughout this report, the direction of induced error for the fourth error pattern (C_{max} and C_{min} in opposite directions) is expressed in terms of C_{max}. For example, an error of −15% represents −15% error in C_{max} and +15% error in C_{min}.

The elimination rate constant (k_{error}), volume of distribution (V_{error}), and clearance (CL_{error}) were determined from each pair of $C_{max\ error}$ and $C_{min\ error}$ values for each of the four error patterns. The following equations were used:

Table 1.
Patient Simulations and Initial Dosage Regimens

Simulated Patient	Elimination Rate Constant (hr^{-1})	Volume of Distribution (L)	Clearance (L/hr)	Dose (mg)	Dosing Interval (hr)
A	0.267	12.2	3.27	80	8
B	0.110	12.7	1.39	75	18
C	0.267	18.4	4.91	120	8
D	0.110	18.6	2.01	110	18

$$k_{error} = [\ln (C_{max\ error}/C_{min\ error})]/(\tau - t_{inf}) \quad (3)$$

$$V_{error} = D\,(1 - e^{-k_{error}t_{inf}}) / k_{error}t_{inf}\,[C_{max\ error} - (C_{min\ error}\,e^{-k_{error}t_{inf}})] \quad (4)$$

$$CL_{error} = (k_{error})(V_{error}) \quad (5)$$

If the $C_{max\ error}$ or $C_{min\ error}$ values were not within the desired ranges (6.0 to 7.0 mg/L for $C_{max\ error}$, 0.8 to 1.2 mg/L for $C_{min\ error}$), the dose or the dosing interval, or both, were modified. Desired concentrations were set for C_{max} (6.5 mg/L) and C_{min} (1.0 mg/L). The new interval (τ*) was initially determined by substituting k_{error} and desired C_{max} and C_{min} values into equation 1. The new interval was then rounded to the nearest of the following dosing intervals: 3, 4, 6, 8, 12, 18, 24, 36, and 48 hours. Increments of 24 hours were used for intervals greater than 48 hours.

The new dose (D*) was then determined by substituting the desired C_{max} value, τ*, k_{error}, and V_{error} in equation 2. The resulting dose was rounded to the nearest 5 mg. The new maximum concentration (C_{max}*) and minimum concentration (C_{min}*) were then calculated by substituting k_{error}, V_{error}, τ*, and D* into equations 6 and 7, as follows:

$$C_{max}^* = D^*\,(1 - e^{-k_{error}t_{inf}}) / (V_{error})(k_{error})\,(t_{inf})(1 - e^{-k_{error}\tau^*}) \quad (6)$$

$$C_{min}^* = C_{max}^*\,e^{-k_{error}(\tau^* - t_{inf})} \quad (7)$$

Dose and interval were adjusted to keep both C_{max}* and C_{min}* within the desired ranges of 6.0 to 7.0 mg/L and 0.8 to 1.2 mg/L, respectively. If this was not possible, the dose or dosing interval was adjusted to keep C_{max}* within the desired range and to allow C_{min}* to drop into the range of 0.5 to 0.8 mg/L. Changes in dose were attempted before changes in dosing interval. Adjustments were made to minimize the differences between the new concentrations and the desired ranges of 6.0 to 7.0 mg/L for C_{max}* and 0.8 to 1.2 mg/L for C_{min}*.

The true C_{max} ($C_{max\ true}$) and C_{min} ($C_{min\ true}$) values were determined for each simulated patient by substituting the new dose (D*) and interval (τ*) and the original values for k and V into equations 6 and 7.

In addition to the initial dosing, two other dosing schemes were evaluated in each of the simulated patients. In the second dosing scheme, the dose was increased to 120 (patient A), 100 (patient B), 155 (patient C), and 150 (patient D) mg, but the dosing intervals were unchanged from initial values. These increases in dose resulted in C_{max} and C_{min} values that ranged from 8.4 to 9.8 mg/L and from 1.3 to 1.5 mg/L, respectively. In the third dosing scheme, the initial dose used for each simulated patient was unchanged, but the dosing intervals were lengthened to 12 hours for patients A and C and to 24 hours for patients B and D. C_{max} was 6.0 mg/L, and C_{min} ranged from 0.3 to 0.5 mg/L for this third dosing scheme. These simulations were carried out as outlined above and were also examined for trends based on changes in dose and dosing interval.

Analysis of Data. The difference between true and error values was determined for the elimination rate constant, volume of distribution, clearance, dosing interval, dose, and total daily dose. Any difference (taken as the absolute value of the percentage of the true value) greater than the absolute value of the induced error was considered to be unexpectedly high. Any $C_{max\ true}$ values greater than 10.0 mg/L or $C_{min\ true}$ values greater than 2.0 mg/L were considered to be toxic. Any $C_{max\ true}$ values less than 4.0 mg/L and $C_{min\ true}$ values less than 0.5 mg/L were considered to be suboptimal.

Each pharmacokinetic variable, dosing variable, and concentration value was examined for general trends in the resultant errors. The data were further evaluated to determine trends based on the pattern of induced error in C_{max} or C_{min}, or both, and simulated patient (changes in pharmacokinetic values).

Results

General Trends. Several general trends were evident in the data generated. As the absolute value of the induced percentage error increased, corresponding increases were noted in the absolute value of the resultant error and in the deviation of $C_{max\ true}$ and $C_{min\ true}$ from the desired values. Error induced in the negative direction (less than zero) generally caused larger absolute values of resultant errors and more toxic and suboptimal concentrations compared with error induced in the positive direction (greater than zero).

Overall, there were few differences among the "patients" in the resultant errors in pharmacokinetic variables and dosing regimens and in the resultant concentrations that were toxic and suboptimal (Table 2). Resultant errors were usually within 1 or 2%, and true concentrations were within 0.2 mg/L for C_{min} and 0.4 mg/L for C_{max} among "patients" for the same pattern of induced error and dosing scheme; however, as discussed below, exceptions existed. A consistent grouping of patients A and C versus patients B and D was noted (Table 2). Patients B and D simulated patients with moderate renal dysfunction, as evidenced by gentamicin elimination rate constants of 0.11 hours^{-1} and clearances of 1.39 and 2.01 L/hr, respectively, compared with patients A and C, who had mild renal dysfunction, as demonstrated by elimination rate constants of 0.267 hours^{-1} and clearances of 3.27 and 4.91 L/hour, respectively.

Trends were also observed among the error patterns and dosing schemes. Error induced in C_{max} only or both C_{max} and C_{min} (same or opposite direction) caused the greatest resultant error, while error induced in C_{min} only caused the least. A slight trend was noted among the dosing schemes. The dosing scheme involving the lengthening of the dosing interval was associated with equal or lower resultant errors or problem concentrations (toxic or suboptimal) for all error calculations except for errors in clearance and daily doses when error was induced in C_{max} only and in both C_{max} and C_{min} in opposite directions.

Errors in Individual Pharmacokinetic Variables. The resultant errors in the elimination rate constant were influenced by the pattern of induced errors (Table 2). Errors induced in both C_{max} and C_{min} in opposite directions caused the most problems in the elimination rate constant. Error induced in C_{max} only or C_{min} only caused unexpectedly high resultant errors when the induced error was −80%, but errors of equal magnitude and direction induced in both C_{max} and C_{min} caused no error in the elimination rate constant. When the dosing interval was lengthened, patients B and D had larger errors in the elimination rate constant than patients A and C for all patterns of error except the one in which errors were induced in both C_{max} and C_{min} in the same direction.

Unexpectedly high errors in the volume of distribution data were seen over a wide range when errors were induced in C_{max} and C_{min} in opposite directions, in C_{max} only, and in C_{max} and C_{min} in the same direction (Table 2). Error induced in C_{min} alone affected the volume of distribution the least.

Unexpectedly high error values for clearance were most evident when errors were induced in C_{max} and C_{min} in the same direction or in C_{max} only (Figure 1 and Table 2). Error induced in C_{min} only and in C_{max} and C_{min} in opposite directions caused the least amount of resultant error in clearance. For the dosing schemes in which the dose was increased and the interval was lengthened, patients B and D had larger errors in clearance than patients A and C when errors were induced in C_{min} only. Conversely, in all dosing schemes patients A and C had larger errors in clearance than patients B and D when errors were induced in C_{max} only or in both C_{max} and C_{min} in opposite directions.

Resultant errors in dosing interval, dose, and daily dose generally followed the distribution of errors in the elimination rate constant, volume of distribution, and clearance, respectively (data not shown).

Resultant True Concentrations. $C_{max\,true}$ and $C_{min\,true}$ values were calculated using the original values for k and V and the dosing interval (τ^*) and dose (D^*) derived from the erroneous pharmacokinetic values. The $C_{max\,true}$ was defined as toxic when greater than 10.0 mg/L and suboptimal when less than 4.0 mg/L. Error induced in C_{min} only did not cause toxic or suboptimal true C_{max} concentrations (Figure 2 and Table 2). Toxic $C_{max\,true}$ values were seen at induced errors as low as 30% (absolute value) and suboptimal values at errors of 60% or greater (absolute value).

Toxic $C_{min\,true}$ values, defined as concentrations greater than 2.0 mg/L, were noted for all "patients" when errors of 60% or greater (absolute value) were induced in C_{max} and C_{min} in the same

Table 2.
Range of Induced Errors (%) Yielding Unexpectedly High Errors in Pharmacokinetic Variables[a] or Toxic or Suboptimal Gentamicin Concentrations[b]

Pattern of Induced Error	Simulation	Pharmacokinetic Variable[c]			True Concentration (mg/mL)[d]			
					C_{max}		C_{min}	
		k	V	CL	Toxic	Suboptimal	Toxic	Suboptimal
C_{max} only	A and C	−80	−80 to +15	−80 to −40	−80 to −30	+60 to +80[e]	. . .	−80 to −60
	B and D	−80	−80 to +15	−80 to −50	−80 to −40	+80	. . .	−80 to −50
C_{min} only	A and C	−80	. . .	. . .	. . .	. . .	. . .	+30 to +80
	B and D	−80	. . .	. . .	. . .	. . .	−80 to −60	. . .
C_{max} and C_{min} in same direction	A and C	. . .	−80 to −5	−80 to −5	−80 to −40	+80	−80 to −60	. . .
	B and D	. . .	−80 to −5	−80 to −5	−80 to −40	+60 to +80[f]	−80 to −60	. . .
C_{max} and C_{min} in opposite directions[h]	A and C	−80 to +80	−80 to +30	−80	−80 to −30[g]	. . .	. . .	−80 to −40, −15
	B and D	−80 to +80	−80 to +20	−80	−80 to −40	. . .	. . .	−80 to −40

[a] The absolute value of the induced percentage error in the pharmacokinetic variable was greater than the absolute value of the percentage error induced in the initial concentration values.

[b] Toxic gentamicin concentrations were defined as peak concentrations >10.0 mg/L or trough concentrations >2.0 mg/L. Suboptimal concentrations were defined as peak concentrations <4.0 mg/L or trough concentrations <0.5 mg/L.

[c] k = elimination rate constant, V = volume of distribution, CL = clearance.

[d] C_{max} = concentration at the end of a one-hour infusion, C_{min} = concentration at the end of a dosing interval.

[e] Simulated patient A demonstrated suboptimal true C_{max} at +80% induced error only.

[f] Simulated patient D demonstrated suboptimal true C_{max} at +80% induced error only.

[g] Simulated patient C demonstrated toxic true C_{max} at −80% to −40% induced error.

[h] Values given are those for the error induced in C_{max}. Errors in C_{min} are of equal magnitude but in the opposite direction.

Figure 1. Resultant errors in gentamicin clearance versus errors induced in simulated gentamicin concentrations for patient A. Error was induced in the following: □ = C_{max} only; + = C_{min} only; ◇ = C_{max} and C_{min} in the same magnitude and direction; △ = C_{max} and C_{min} in the same magnitude but opposite directions (using the error in C_{max} for graphing purposes).

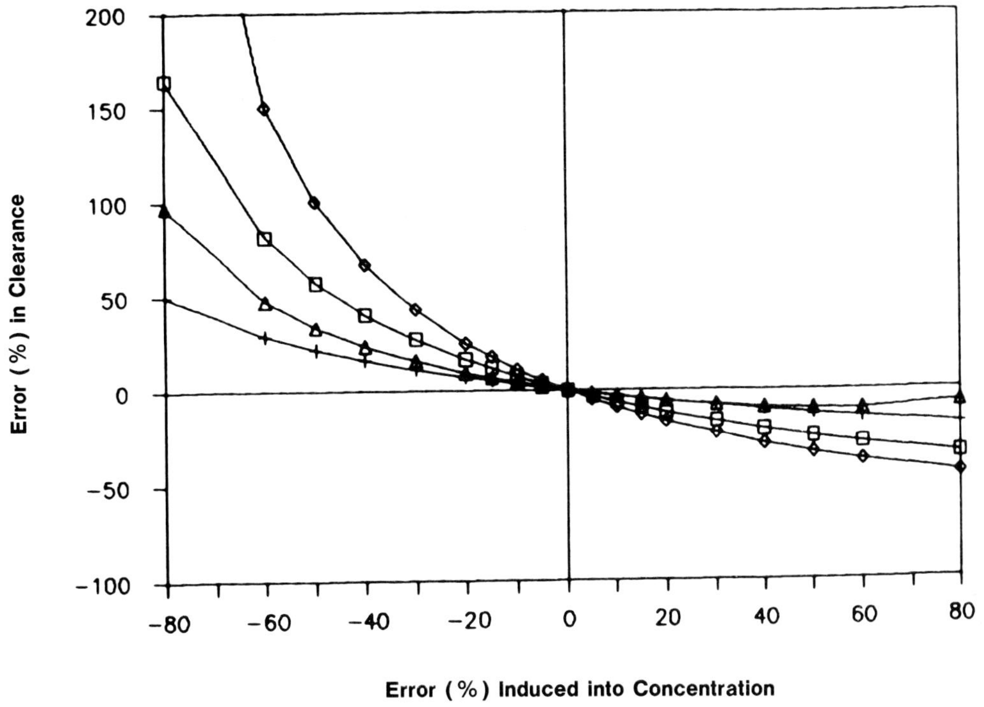

Figure 2. Resulting maximum steady-state concentrations ($C_{max\ true}$, or true maximum concentrations) versus the errors induced in simulated serum gentamicin concentrations for patient A. Error was induced in the following: □ = C_{max} only; + = C_{min} only; ◇ = C_{max} and C_{min} in the same magnitude and direction; △ = C_{max} and C_{min} in the same magnitude but opposite directions (using the error in C_{max} for graphing purposes).

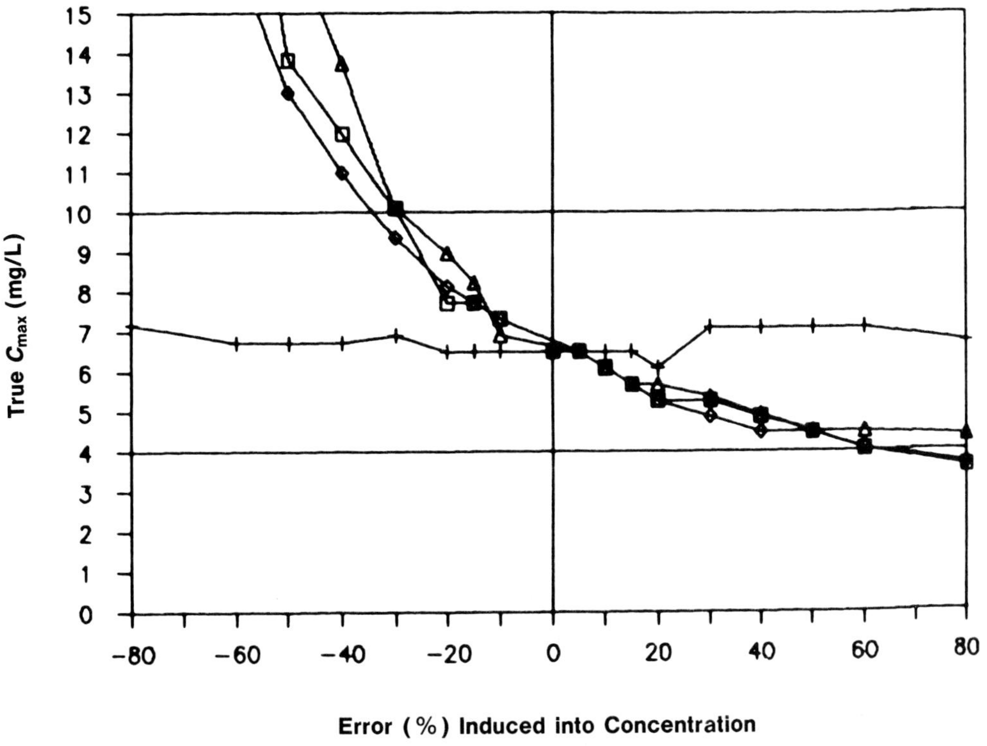

direction and for "patients" B and D when errors of 60% or greater were induced in C_{min} alone (Figure 3 and Table 2). Suboptimal $C_{min\ true}$ values, defined as concentrations less than 0.5 mg/L, were associated with induced errors in C_{max} only, C_{min} only, and both C_{max} and C_{min} (opposite directions). Suboptimal $C_{min\ true}$ values were consistently observed at induced errors as low as 30% (absolute value); however, isolated suboptimal $C_{min\ true}$ values occurred at induced error rates of −15% or −20%, depending on the dosing scheme, when errors were induced in C_{max} and C_{min} in opposite directions.

Discussion

Several trends were noted in this computer simulation of errors in serum gentamicin concentrations. As expected, increases in the absolute value of induced error led to increases in the absolute value of resultant error. The direction, but not the magnitude, of the resultant errors in the elimination rate constant, volume of distribution, $C_{max\ true}$, and $C_{min\ true}$ could be predicted from the equations used. However, the nonlinearity of the resultant errors in some cases and the greater amount of resultant errors associated with negative induced errors were not expected. The resultant errors in clearance were more difficult to predict since clearance was calculated as the product of the elimination rate constant and the volume of distribution. An unexpectedly high amount of error in pharmacokinetic values did not necessarily result in true concentration values that were toxic or suboptimal.

The approach used in this study was very systematic and rigid. In one sense, this provided reproducible results with little left to judgment or interpretation. The definitions of toxic and suboptimal concentrations used were somewhat arbitrary and could be open to criticism. We believed the rigid dosing methods used in this simulation were a reasonable approach to the situations studied. However, those dosing methods may not apply to all patients and would need to be modified to reflect the clinical status of the patient. The methods used to induce error in C_{max} or C_{min}, or both, were developed to assess potential intra-assay errors and interassay differences. Although the induction of error in C_{max} and C_{min} in opposite directions may be the least likely scenario to be encountered, this scenario was included to cause the largest possible resultant error. Additional credence for the inclusion of the fourth error pattern (error induced in both C_{max} and C_{min} in opposite directions) is provided by Witebsky et al.,[7] who demonstrated that enzyme-multiplied immunoassay measured higher at low concentrations and lower at high concentrations than fluorescence-polarization immunoassay. Additionally, we did not induce error randomly in this study because it would not have provided the systematic, rigid approach we deemed necessary.

Several clinical applications of the results of this

Figure 3. Resulting minimum steady-state concentrations ($C_{min\ true}$, or true minimum concentrations) versus the errors induced in simulated gentamicin concentrations for patient A. Error was induced in the following: □ = C_{max} only; + = C_{min} only; ◇ = C_{max} and C_{min} in the same magnitude and direction; △ = C_{max} and C_{min} in the same magnitude but opposite directions (using the error in C_{max} for graphing purposes).

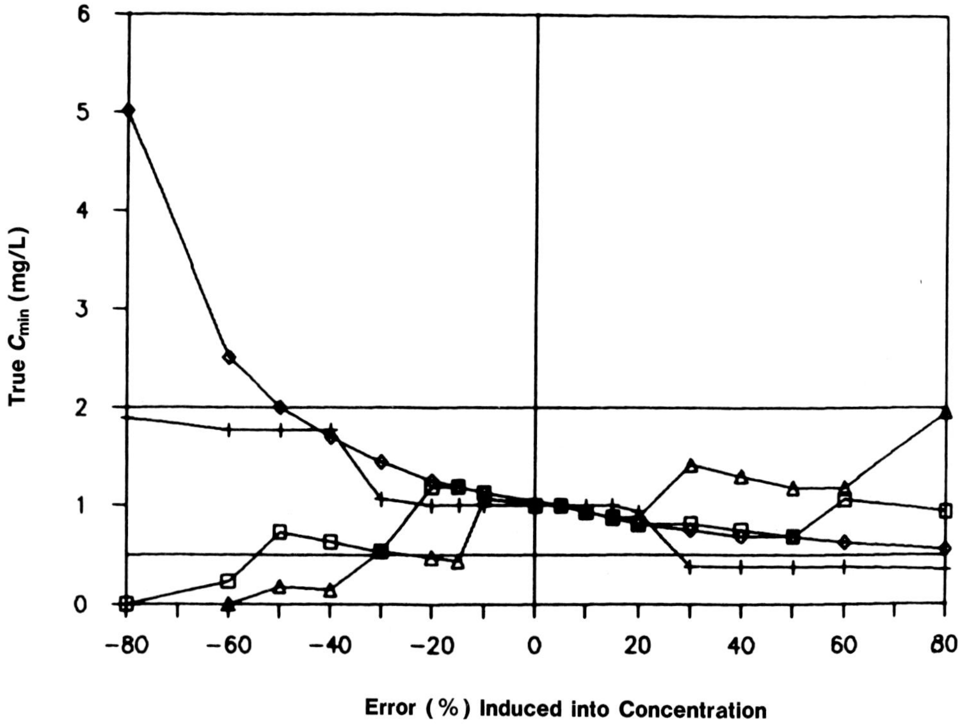

study may be possible. Negative induced error, which would correlate with an underreporting of concentration values, caused the largest amount of resultant error in nearly every error pattern. The possible clinical importance of this is demonstrated by the in vitro drug–drug interaction between aminoglycosides and the antipseudomonal penicillins that leads to falsely lowered aminoglycoside concentrations for some patients.[8] Errors in C_{max} caused more resultant error than errors in C_{min}, particularly in the calculation of the volume of distribution. Thus, errors in peak concentration values may be of greater clinical importance than errors in trough concentration values. Additionally, patients with shorter dosing intervals may be at increased risk if errors in concentration values occur.

The results from this simulation might also be used to determine acceptable limits for errors in serum gentamicin concentration measurements. At induced errors as small as ±5%, the absolute values of the resultant errors in pharmacokinetic variable and dosing calculations were greater than the absolute values of the induced errors. Therefore, the error in concentrations may not be useful in predicting the potential maximum of resultant errors in variables and dosing. A second, potentially more useful definition of acceptable error might include only those induced errors that do not cause toxic or suboptimal concentrations. Using this second definition, an acceptable limit of induced error would be ±20% given the methodology we used.

Errors in other factors may also cause resultant errors in pharmacokinetic values and doses or dosing intervals that could result in toxic or suboptimal concentrations. Such errors could occur in the amount of drug actually administered, in recording when a dose was given or when blood samples were obtained, in estimating the length of the infusion, and in obtaining blood samples before steady-state concentrations are reached. Errors in calculations or in making incorrect assumptions are also possible. Although errors in concentrations were the only aspect we attempted to evaluate, other errors may be equally important.

Attempts should be made to diminish errors in all components of pharmacokinetic monitoring, including concentration measurements. Since interrun variability is less than intrarun variability, it would be best to have samples for peak and trough determinations analyzed in the same batch. Changes in assay methodology could lead to different results and place patients at risk for toxicity or loss of efficacy. Although consistency of assay methodology would seem to be desirable, improvements in clinical assays occur constantly. Clinical laboratories should evaluate the consistency of assay results when assay systems are replaced and when different lots of assay reagents are used. Clinicians and pharmacokineticists who use the assay results should be informed of any differences in results. Differences between assays should also be considered when population values for pharmacokinetic parameters are applied to individual patients.

Conclusion

Since errors or differences in concentration measurements cannot be completely eliminated, it is important to understand the impact of the remaining errors. If safety and efficacy are the major considerations, errors of ±20% in serum gentamicin concentration measurements may be clinically acceptable. Errors in serum gentamicin concentration measurements are more likely to cause larger resultant errors as the errors in concentration values (1) increase in magnitude, (2) result in underreporting of the concentration values, or (3) affect peak concentration values. Shorter dosing intervals may also increase the influence of assay errors or differences.

References

1. Fukuchi H, Yoshida M, Tsukiai S et al. Comparison of enzyme immunoassay, radioimmunoassay, and microbiologic assay for amikacin in plasma. *Am J Hosp Pharm*. 1984; 41:690–3.
2. Matzke GR, Hunt S, Gwizdala C et al. Accuracy of gentamicin assays. *Am J Hosp Pharm*. 1980; 37:1049–50. Letter.
3. Munro AJ, Smith DS, Shaw EJ. A simplified quenching fluoroimmunoassay for gentamicin and the effects of some potential interfering factors. *J Antimicrob Chemother*. 1982; 9:47–51.
4. Dalmady-Israel C, Green PJ, Sloskey GE et al. Ticarcillin and assay of tobramycin. *Ann Intern Med*. 1984; 100:460–1. Letter.
5. Walters MI, Roberts WH. Gentamicin/heparin interactions: effects on two immunoassays and on protein binding. *Ther Drug Monit*. 1984; 6:199–202.
6. Witebsky FG, Selepak ST. Feasibility of gentamicin measurement in icteric sera by the Syva EMIT system. *Antimicrob Agents Chemother*. 1983; 23:172–4.
7. Witebsky FG, Sliva CA, Selepak ST et al. Evaluation of four gentamicin and tobramycin assay procedures for clinical laboratories. *J Clin Microbiol*. 1983; 18:890–4.
8. Pickering LK, Rutherford I. Effect of concentration and time upon inactivation of tobramycin, gentamicin, netilmicin and amikacin by azlocillin, carbenicillin, mecillinam, mezlocillin and piperacillin. *J Pharmacol Exp Ther*. 1981; 217:345–9.

Research Notes

Evaluation of lithium–tetracycline interaction

MARTHA P. FANKHAUSER, JAMES L. LINDON, BRIGID CONNOLLY, AND WALTER J. HEALEY

Clin Pharm. 1988; 7:314–7

Lithium is the drug of choice for treating acute mania and for preventing recurrences of bipolar disorder.[1] The recommended serum lithium concentrations are 0.8 to 1.2 meq/L for acute mania and 0.6 to 1.0 meq/L for long-term maintenance therapy.[2] Blood samples for determination of serum lithium concentration should be drawn 12 hours ± 30 minutes after the last dose. Samples obtained outside this 12-hour interval may result in unreliable and misleading results. Lithium has an elimination half-life of approximately 24 hours in adults (it may exceed 36 hours in geriatric patients) and thus takes five to seven days to reach steady-state serum concentrations.[2]

Lithium is excreted primarily by the kidneys, and its elimination is dependent upon the glomerular filtration rate. Approximately 80% of lithium is reabsorbed in the proximal renal tubules.[3] Lithium is in competition with sodium for proximal renal tubular reabsorption, and reabsorption of lithium may be affected by sodium loading or depletion. Any condition or medication that increases renal excretion of sodium or decreases serum sodium concentration (e.g., dehydration, fever, vomiting, diarrhea, low sodium diets, thiazide diuretics) can reduce lithium clearance. Nonsteroidal anti-inflammatory drugs such as indomethacin, phenylbutazone, naproxen, and ibuprofen have been shown to reduce renal lithium clearance and increase lithium concentrations.[4-6] Interactions between lithium and other medications have also been reported.[7,8]

Several cases of lithium toxicity or adverse reactions have been reported when antibiotics are added to lithium therapy. Metronidazole, spectinomycin, and tetracycline have been reported to increase serum lithium concentrations.[9] A possible interaction between lithium carbonate and tetracycline in a 30-year-old woman with bipolar disorder was reported in 1978.[10] Lithium and tetracycline, however, have been used concomitantly without serious problems in many patients.[9,11] Tetracycline is frequently used to treat acneform eruptions caused by lithium.[12]

Since the initial case report in 1978 of a possible lithium–tetracycline interaction, there have been no other published reports or studies investigating the importance of the interaction. The purpose of this study was to determine the effect of tetracycline on steady-state serum lithium concentrations in healthy volunteers and to compare the frequency and severity of adverse effects in the lithium and the lithium–tetracycline treatment phases.

Methods. Fourteen healthy volunteers (eight women and six men) aged 21–35 years (mean ± S.D., 27.5 ± 4.0 years) participated in the study. The protocol was approved by the university's human-subject committee, and written informed consent was obtained from the participants. All subjects were screened by a physician for medical illnesses. A complete physical examination, blood chemistry tests, complete blood counts, and urinalyses were performed at baseline. Subjects were excluded if they had an upper gastrointestinal tract disease, renal or hepatic impairment, epilepsy, mental illness, or hypersensitivity to lithium or tetracycline, or if they were pregnant. During the study, women were required to use a birth control method acceptable to the investigators.

For a week before the study and during the study, subjects were not allowed to ingest any medication, caffeine-containing beverages, alcohol, or nicotine. Subjects were instructed to maintain a constant daily intake of sodium and fluids and to not make any dietary or exercise changes during the study. When subjects were taking tetracycline, they were instructed not to drink milk or ingest other dairy products within one hour of taking tetracycline.

The study had a parallel design, with each sub-

MARTHA P. FANKHAUSER, M.S., is Clinical Assistant Professor, Department of Pharmacy Practice, College of Pharmacy, and Department of Psychiatry, College of Medicine, University of Arizona, Tucson. JAMES L. LINDON, PHARM.D., is a graduate student in Pharmacy Administration, College of Pharmacy, University of Arizona. BRIGID CONNOLLY, M.D., is a psychiatry resident, Department of Psychiatry, College of Medicine, University of Arizona. WALTER J. HEALEY, M.D., is Staff Psychiatrist, Community Health and Counseling Services, Machias, ME.

Address reprint requests to Ms. Fankhauser at the Department of Pharmacy Practice, College of Pharmacy, University of Arizona, Tucson, AZ 85721.

Presented at the Clinical Research Forum, 22nd Annual ASHP Midyear Clinical Meeting, Atlanta, GA, December 9, 1987.

Copyright © 1988, American Society of Hospital Pharmacists, Inc. All rights reserved. 0278-2677/88/0401-0314$01.00.

ject serving as his or her own control. During each day of the 14-day study, subjects received controlled-release lithium carbonate 450-mg tablets (Eskalith-CR, Smith Kline & French, lot 236J10) twice daily at 0700 and 1900. During the treatment phase (days 8–14), subjects also received tetracycline hydrochloride 500-mg capsules (Cyclopar 500, Parke-Davis, lot 34366D) twice daily at 0700 and 1900. Two of the men received 450-mg controlled-release lithium carbonate tablets once daily at 1900: Subject 1 weighed 126 pounds and had attained a steady-state serum lithium concentration of 1.0 meq/L on 900 mg a day (when participating in a previous lithium pharmacokinetic study); subject 7 weighed 137 pounds, and the investigators wanted to be sure that his lithium concentrations would be low.

The first seven days of the study served as the control phase, and the last seven days of the study served as the treatment phase. Steady-state serum concentration was defined as a lithium concentration not varying by more than 15% for three consecutive days (i.e., days 6, 7, and 8 for the control phase and days 13, 14, and 15 for the treatment phase). Subjects were excluded from the study if any serum lithium concentration was greater than 1 meq/L or if a steady-state concentration was not achieved by day 8.

On days 6, 7, 8, 13, 14, and 15, a 12-hour blood sample was drawn between 0700 and 0730. The blood sample was collected in two red-top tubes and allowed to clot. The samples were centrifuged for five minutes, and the serum was transferred to two plastic transport tubes. One serum sample was frozen at −20 °C and stored as an extra sample. The other serum sample was refrigerated and analyzed within 24 hours of collection by flame-emission photometry at National Health Laboratories in Phoenix, Arizona (sensitivity = 0.1 meq/L; precision = 0.02 meq/L; accuracy = 0.03 meq/L).

Adverse effects were recorded daily throughout the study using a 14-item rating scale. The severity of each adverse effect was rated as 1 = none, 2 = mild, 3 = moderate, 4 = severe, and 5 = extreme. Subjects were weighed at baseline and on day 15.

A two-tailed Student's t test for paired data was used to analyze the data.[13] Steady-state lithium concentrations in the control phase (mean of days 6, 7, and 8) were compared with those in the treatment phase (mean of days 13, 14, and 15). The severity of adverse effects on days 1–7 (control phase) was compared with that for days 8–14 (treatment phase). A p value of less than 0.05 was considered significant.

Results. Thirteen of the subjects completed the study. Subject 7 was dropped from the study on day 6 because of increased difficulty in concentrating and impaired cognition. The subject received controlled-release lithium carbonate 450 mg daily, and the first steady-state serum concentration drawn on day 6 was 0.37 meq/L. All other subjects attained steady-state concentrations on day 6 (control phase) and on day 13 (treatment phase). Data for the mean steady-state serum concentrations are reported in Table 1. The overall mean (± S.D.) steady-state lithium concentrations for the 13 subjects were 0.51 ± 0.13 meq/L in the control phase and 0.47 ± 0.12 meq/L in the treatment phase, a mean difference of 0.04 ± 0.05, which was significant (p = 0.01). Calculation of a 95% confidence interval for the mean difference indicated that the mean steady-state lithium concentration would decrease by 0.03 to 0.06 meq/L when tetracycline was added to lithium therapy.

Adverse effects as determined by the mean daily ratings for subjects on days 1–7 and on days 8–14 are compared in Table 2. The mean severity rating for each adverse effect was not significantly different between the control phase and the treatment phase. Body weights obtained at baseline were not significantly different from those on day 15.

Discussion. The significant decrease in steady-state lithium concentrations when tetracycline was added to the lithium regimen does not support the earlier case report in which tetracycline significantly increased steady-state serum lithium concentrations. Despite the lowering of steady-state lithium concentrations in our study population, the clinical importance of the lithium–tetracycline interaction may be minimal. The decrease in lithi-

Table 1.
Serum Lithium Concentrations (meq/L) during Control (Lithium Alone) and Treatment (Lithium plus Tetracycline) Phases

Subject No.	Sex	Lithium Concentration[a,b] Control	Treatment
1[c]	M	0.35 ± 0.06	0.34 ± 0.03
2	F	0.49 ± 0.02	0.48 ± 0.02
3	F	0.45 ± 0.01	0.49 ± 0.04
4	F	0.56 ± 0.05	0.47 ± 0.04
5	F	0.39 ± 0.01	0.39 ± 0.01
6	M	0.54 ± 0.03	0.50 ± 0.01
7[c,d]	M	0.37[e]	. . .
8	F	0.38 ± 0.05	0.28 ± 0.03
9	F	0.75 ± 0.06	0.63 ± 0.03
10	F	0.70 ± 0.04	0.70 ± 0.04
11	M	0.49 ± 0.03	0.47 ± 0.04
12	M	0.41 ± 0.03	0.35 ± 0.02
13	F	0.65 ± 0.02	0.60 ± 0.04
14	M	0.50 ± 0.02	0.46 ± 0.06
Mean ± S.D.		0.51 ± 0.13	0.47 ± 0.12

[a] Mean ± S.D. (n = 3) for days 6–8 in control phase and for days 13–15 in treatment phase.

[b] Except as noted, subjects received lithium carbonate 450 mg twice daily.

[c] Received lithium carbonate 450 mg once daily.

[d] Subject dropped from the study on day 6.

[e] Steady-state serum lithium concentration obtained on day 6 only; subject not included in statistical analysis.

um concentrations by 0.03 to 0.06 meq/L is slightly greater than the 0.02-meq/L precision of the laboratory test and is probably not clinically important in most patients. Whether the interaction varies with different steady-state serum lithium concentrations could not be determined by this study, since lithium concentrations in all of our subjects were maintained between 0.3 and 0.8 meq/L.

The mean ratings of adverse effects reported for the control phase (days 1–7) and those reported for the treatment phase (days 8–14) by each subject were not significantly different. It should be noted that the gastrointestinal adverse effects (e.g., diarrhea and nausea) and some central nervous system adverse effects (e.g., dizziness, fatigue, headache, and weakness) were rated slightly higher during the treatment phase. Whether the increase in severity of adverse effects was in response to lithium, tetracycline, or the combination therapy could not be determined. Because both lithium and tetracycline cause gastrointestinal adverse effects (e.g., nausea, vomiting, diarrhea, abdominal discomfort), it would be expected that the combination therapy might increase the incidence and severity of these adverse effects.

Although there was no significant difference in weight measured at baseline and day 15, subject 8 gained 7 pounds during the two-week study (161 to 168 pounds). The increase in weight may have caused the subject's mean steady-state serum lithium concentration to decrease from 0.38 to 0.28 meq/L. The paired *t* test analysis was repeated excluding subject 8, and the mean (± S.D.) differences for the 12 remaining subjects were still significant (0.03 ± 0.04, p = 0.02). Thus, it does not appear that the weight gain in subject 8 accounted for the significant lowering of steady-state lithium concentrations.

Table 2.
Adverse Effects in 13 Subjects Receiving Lithium Alone (Control) and Lithium plus Tetracycline (Treatment)

Adverse Effect	Rating[a,b] Control	Treatment	*p*
Appetite increase	1.31 ± 0.53	1.49 ± 0.76	0.26
Confusion	1.02 ± 0.08	1.02 ± 0.08	1.00
Diarrhea	1.01 ± 0.04	1.08 ± 0.21	0.29
Dizziness	1.07 ± 0.24	1.17 ± 0.35	0.17
Drowsiness	1.10 ± 0.18	1.09 ± 0.19	0.89
Dry mouth	1.12 ± 0.25	1.14 ± 0.30	0.79
Fatigue	1.13 ± 0.39	1.21 ± 0.34	0.33
Headache	1.08 ± 0.17	1.12 ± 0.28	0.58
Nausea	1.08 ± 0.14	1.23 ± 0.46	0.19
Thirst increase	1.64 ± 0.65	1.50 ± 0.51	0.17
Tremor	1.06 ± 0.20	1.08 ± 0.17	0.76
Increased frequency of urination	1.69 ± 0.70	1.64 ± 0.78	0.47
Vomiting	1.02 ± 0.08	1.00 ± 0.00	0.34
Weakness	1.00 ± 0.00	1.10 ± 0.28	0.33

[a] Adverse effect severity scale: 1 = none; 2 = mild; 3 = moderate; 4 = severe; 5 = extreme.

[b] Adverse effect score expressed as mean ± S.D. for days 1–7 (control) and for days 8–14 (treatment).

The overall mean (± S.D.) steady-state serum lithium concentration (0.49 ± 0.12 meq/L) was below the standard therapeutic range of 0.6 to 1.2 meq/L. Only three subjects attained serum lithium concentrations greater than 0.6 meq/L. Whether higher serum lithium concentrations may predispose a patient to an increased risk of a drug interaction with tetracycline could not be determined by this study. The dose of tetracycline hydrochloride (500 mg twice daily) was on the lower end of the 1–3 g/day dosage range used to treat some infections. It is possible that a higher daily dose of tetracycline (or a single initial dose of 1.5 g) may affect the absorption or clearance of lithium. To determine the importance of the lithium–tetracycline interaction, further studies are needed at higher serum lithium concentrations and with higher tetracycline doses.

Tetracycline therapy may rarely increase the excretion of nitrogen and increase serum creatinine and urea nitrogen concentrations.[14] Patients with renal dysfunction may develop azotemia, hyperphosphatemia, and acidosis with usual doses of tetracycline. Patients with compromised renal function may be at greater risk for decreases in renal clearance and changes in serum lithium concentrations if tetracycline therapy is initiated. Because our subjects had normal renal function, this possible effect could not be determined. A reversible Fanconi-like syndrome has also been reported in patients taking outdated or deteriorated tetracycline.[14] The syndrome is characterized by nausea, vomiting, lethargy, polydipsia, polyuria, glycosuria, aminoaciduria, phosphaturia, proteinuria, acidosis, and hypokalemia. This reaction is unlikely to occur with currently marketed tetracycline preparations since citric acid (which accelerates the deterioration of tetracycline) is no longer used as an excipient.[14]

Patients with higher serum lithium concentrations or those on long-term lithium therapy may have an increased risk of renal impairment.[15] Elderly patients may have decreased glomerular filtration secondary to age-related histological changes and should be closely monitored if tetracycline is added to lithium therapy.[16] The combination therapy may increase the gastrointestinal adverse effects when lithium and tetracycline are coadministered. Patients should be instructed to separate the doses if this adverse effect occurs.

Conclusion. In these healthy volunteers, serum lithium concentrations were significantly lower during concurrent tetracycline administration. The decrease in lithium concentrations may not be clinically important, and further study of this interaction in patients with higher serum lithium concentrations is needed.

References

1. Consensus Development Panel. Mood disorder: pharmacologic prevention of recurrences. *Am J Psychiatry.* 1985; 142:469–76.
2. Jefferson JW, Greist JH, Ackerman DL et al., eds. Lithium: an overview. In: Lithium encyclopedia for clinical practice. 2nd ed. Washington, DC: American Psychiatric Press; 1987:1–31.
3. Ereshefsky L, Jann MW. Lithium. In: Mungall DR, ed. Applied clinical pharmacokinetics. 2nd ed. New York: Raven Press; 1983:245–70.
4. Kristoff CA, Hayes PE, Barr WH et al. Effect of ibuprofen on lithium plasma and red blood cell concentrations. *Clin Pharm.* 1986; 5:51–5.
5. Ragheb MA, Powell AL. Lithium interaction with sulindac and naproxen. *J Clin Psychopharmacol.* 1986; 6:150–4.
6. Ragheb M. Ibuprofen can increase serum levels in lithium-treated patients. *J Clin Psychiatry.* 1987; 48:161–3.
7. Amdisen A. Lithium and drug interactions. *Drugs.* 1982; 24:133–9.
8. Jefferson JW, Greist JH, Baudhuin M. Lithium: interactions with other drugs. *J Clin Psychopharmacol.* 1981; 1:124–34.
9. Jefferson JW. Greist JH, Ackerman DL et al., eds. Antibiotics. In: Lithium encyclopedia for clinical practice. 2nd ed. Washington DC: American Psychiatric Press; 1987:69–71.
10. McGennis AJ. Lithium carbonate and tetracycline interaction. *Br Med J.* 1978; 1:1183.
11. Jefferson JW. Lithium and tetracycline. *Br J Dermatol.* 1982; 107:370. Letter.
12. Deandrea D, Walker N, Mehlmauer M et al. Dermatological reactions to lithium: a critical review of the literature. *J Clin Psychopharmacol.* 1982; 2:199–204.
13. Snedecor GW, Cochran WG, eds. Statistical methods. 6th ed. Ames, IA; The Iowa State University Press; 1967.
14. American hospital formulary service—drug information 87. McEvoy GK, McQuarrie GM, eds. Tetracycline. Bethesda, MD: American Society of Hospital Pharmacists; 1987:296–303.
15. Norman TR, Walker RG, Burrows GD. Renal function related changes in lithium kinetics. *Clin Pharmacokinet.* 1984; 9:349–53.
16. Hardy BG, Shulman KI, MacKenzie SE et al. Pharmacokinetics of lithium in the elderly. *J Clin Psychopharmacol.* 1987; 7:153–8.

Effect of ranitidine and cimetidine on ibuprofen pharmacokinetics

DAVID W. STEPHENSON, RALPH E. SMALL, JOHN H. WOOD, HAYES E. WILLIS, STEVEN M. JOHNSON, H. THOMAS KARNES, AND KUSUMA RAJASEKHARAIAH

Clin Pharm. 1988; 7:317–21

Ibuprofen (Motrin, The Upjohn Company) was the first of the propionic acid derivative nonsteroidal anti-inflammatory drugs (NSAIDs) to be introduced in the United States.[1] The use of ibuprofen as an analgesic, antipyretic, and anti-inflammatory agent is well established. Unfortunately, ibuprofen can cause gastric mucosal damage and bleeding in humans. Administration of NSAIDs results in inhibition of gastric prostaglandin E_2 synthesis.[2] Prostaglandin E_2 protects the lining of the stomach from acid production by supporting the gastrointestinal mucosal barrier. Ulcerations may be healed by decreasing intragastric acidity via administration of antacids, sucralfate, or histamine H_2-receptor antagonists.[3,4] Ranitidine (Zantac, Glaxo, Inc.) and cimetidine (Tagamet, Smith Kline & French Laboratories) are competitive antagonists of histamine at H_2-receptor sites in the stomach. Ranitidine and cimetidine have been shown in placebo-controlled trials to increase the rate of healing of duodenal and gastric ulcers over a four- to six-week period.[4] These drugs vary in their ability to inhibit hepatic oxidative metabolism of other drugs. Rani-

DAVID W. STEPHENSON, PHARM.D., is Director of Education and Clinical Service Coordinator, Comp-U-Dose Pharmacies, Chesapeake, VA, and Adjunct Professor, School of Nursing, Old Dominion University, Norfolk, VA; at the time of this study, he was a Pharm.D. candidate at Medical College of Virginia–Virginia Commonwealth University (MCV–VCU), Richmond. RALPH E. SMALL, PHARM.D., is Associate Professor of Pharmacy and Pharmaceutics, and Associate Professor of Medicine (Division of Rheumatology, Allergy, and Immunology); JOHN H. WOOD, PH.D., is Professor of Pharmacy and Pharmaceutics; and HAYES E. WILLIS, M.D., is Assistant Professor of Medicine (Division of Rheumatology, Allergy, and Immunology), MCV–VCU. STEVEN M. JOHNSON, PHARM.D., is Clinical Research Assistant, Marion Laboratories, Kansas City, MO; at the time of this study, he was Clinical Pharmacy Fellow in Immunology and Rheumatology, MCV–VCU. H. THOMAS KARNES, PH.D., is Assistant Professor of Pharmacy and Pharmaceutics, and KUSUMA RAJASEKHARAIAH, M.PHARM., is a Doctor of Philosophy candidate, Department of Pharmacy and Pharmaceutics, MCV–VCU.

Address reprint requests to Dr. Small at the Department of Pharmacy and Pharmaceutics, Medical College of Virginia–Virginia Commonwealth University, Box 581, MCV Station, Richmond, VA 23298-0581.

Supported by a grant from Glaxo, Inc., Research Triangle Park, NC 27709.

Presented at the Clinical Research Forum, 22nd Annual ASHP Midyear Clinical Meeting, Atlanta, GA, December 9, 1987.

Copyright © 1988, American Society of Hospital Pharmacists, Inc. All rights reserved. 0278-2677/88/0401-0317$01.25.

tidine has a 10-fold-lower binding affinity for cytochrome P-450 and P-448 than does cimetidine.[5] Ibuprofen is metabolized via this oxidative pathway to form two inactive metabolites. Since ranitidine has fewer clinically important drug interactions than cimetidine and since either could be used to treat ibuprofen-induced ulceration, a comparison of the effect of these drugs on the pharmacokinetics of ibuprofen would be valuable.

The purpose of this study was to determine whether ranitidine or cimetidine can affect the pharmacokinetics of ibuprofen at steady-state conditions.

Methods. Twelve healthy volunteers between 18 and 55 years of age with normal results from a complete physical examination, an automated blood chemistry analysis, a complete blood count, and a urinalysis were selected for the study. Exclusion criteria included a history of upper gastrointestinal, renal, or hepatic disease; blood dyscrasias; hypersensitivity to ibuprofen, other nonsteroidal anti-inflammatory agents, ranitidine, or cimetidine; pregnancy or missed menstrual period; and ingestion of an alcoholic beverage or any medications within two weeks before the beginning of the study. The protocol was approved by the committee on the conduct of human research of the Medical College of Virginia–Virginia Commonwealth University. Informed consent was obtained from all participants.

The subjects were randomized to one of three treatment groups using a random number table. Each group participated in three treatment phases. In phase 1, the subjects received ibuprofen 600 mg (The Upjohn Co., Kalamazoo, MI, lot 341WC) four times a day (with meals and at bedtime) for three days. On day 4, one 600-mg dose of ibuprofen was given in the morning at 0800. In phase 2, the subjects received 600 mg of ibuprofen four times a day (with meals and at bedtime) and ranitidine hydrochloride 300 mg (Glaxo, Inc., Research Triangle Park, NC, lot Z0336BP) at breakfast for three days. On day 4, one 300-mg dose of ranitidine hydrochloride was given two hours before the 0800 dose of ibuprofen to permit evaluation of the effect of pH on ibuprofen absorption. In phase 3, the subjects received ibuprofen 600 mg four times a day (with meals and at bedtime) and cimetidine 800 mg (Smith Kline & French Laboratories, Philadelphia, PA, lot X8076T27) at breakfast for three days. On day 4, one 800-mg dose of cimetidine was given two hours before the 0800 ibuprofen dose. Morning doses of ranitidine and cimetidine were selected over evening doses to eliminate the necessity of collecting blood samples during the earliest hours of the morning. All medicines were given with 240 mL of water. On day 4 of drug administration, subjects fasted for eight hours before and three hours after ingestion of the last ibuprofen dose in each phase. A washout period of one week separated each phase.

Serum samples were collected one and two hours before and at times 0, 0.25, 0.5, 0.75, 1, 1.25, 1.5, 1.75, 2, 3, 4, 5, 6, 8, 12, and 16 hours after the last ibuprofen dose in each phase. Samples were transferred to labeled vials and frozen at −20 °C until time of assay. Concentrations of ibuprofen were determined using high-performance liquid chromatography (HPLC).[6]

Pharmacokinetic values were determined from plots of serum concentration-versus-time and log serum concentration-versus-time. The elimination rate constant (k) was determined as the slope of the least-squares regression line of the terminal elimination phase. Area under the concentration–time curve from time zero to the last measured serum concentration (AUC_{0-16}) was calculated using the trapezoidal rule.[7] Extrapolated area under the curve from 16 hours to infinity ($AUC_{16-\infty}$) was calculated from the following equation: $AUC_{16-\infty} = C_{16}/k$, where C_{16} is the serum concentration at the 16-hour sample and k is the elimination rate constant. Total area under the curve ($AUC_{0-\infty}$) was the sum of these areas. Since the data reported here are from the last administration of a multiple-dose study, concentration values at time 0 were finite. Consequently, the $AUC_{0-\infty}$ had to be adjusted to make valid comparisons. Adjusted area under the curve ($AUC_{0-\infty adjusted}$) was calculated in the following manner: $AUC_{0-\infty} = AUC_{0-\infty adjusted} - C_0/k$ where C_0 is the serum ibuprofen concentration at time zero. The time to peak serum concentration (t_{max}) and actual peak serum concentration (C_{max}) were determined by inspection of the serum concentration-versus-time curve. Clearance (CL) was calculated from the following equation: $CL = dose/AUC_{0-\infty adjusted}$. Multivariate repeated measure analysis of variance (ANOVA) was used to analyze all data for significance.[8] The a priori level of significance was set at $p < 0.05$. All subjects were monitored for possible adverse effects.

Results. Demographic data describing the study group are summarized in Table 1. All 12 subjects completed the study.

Figure 1 illustrates the mean serum ibuprofen concentrations from all three phases of the study. Values for $AUC_{0-\infty adjusted}$, C_{max}, t_{max}, CL, k, and $t_{1/2}$ for ibuprofen for the three phases of the study were not significantly different (Table 2). The power of this study to detect a 50% difference between control and active treatment was greater than 99% for $AUC_{0-\infty adjusted}$, C_{max}, CL, k, and $t_{1/2}$. The power was 82% for t_{max}.

The semilogarithmic plot of serum ibuprofen concentration–time profiles for the three treatment phases is shown in Figure 2. Ibuprofen elimination rates are represented by the negative slopes of the terminal segment of each curve and are virtually identical. No differences were seen in any of the three treatment groups with respect to elimination half-life.

Headache and nausea were the only adverse effects reported. Two subjects reported these adverse effects during the cimetidine treatment phase, and one other subject noted headache and nausea during all three treatment phases. None of the subjects required treatment for these conditions.

Discussion. This study indicates that ranitidine hydrochloride 300 mg or cimetidine 800 mg in a once-daily, morning dosing schedule does not significantly affect ibuprofen pharmacokinetics. A once-daily dosing schedule for the H_2 antagonists was chosen on the assumption that this regimen will become popular. The efficacy of once-daily dosing in acute treatment of duodenal ulcers has been confirmed in controlled clinical trials.[9] This is the first study to evaluate ibuprofen pharmacokinetics after multiple doses; many patients with arthritis require long-term ibuprofen therapy to control pain and inflammation.

The subjects received the H_2-antagonist dose two hours before ibuprofen administration on the sampling day to allow for maximum effect on gastric pH. Cimetidine and ranitidine achieve plasma concentrations necessary to cause a 50% maximum inhibitory effect within 30 minutes; these levels are maintained for 2.5 hours (cimetidine) and 6 hours (ranitidine).[10] Oral administration of H_2 antagonists will achieve maximum effect on gastric pH between 1 and 2 hours after dosing. This has the potential to increase the bioavailability of weak acids. Ibuprofen is a weak acid, and the higher gastric pH could enhance dissolution of the tablet by increasing ionization.

Ochs et al.[11] evaluated the effect of ranitidine and cimetidine on ibuprofen in a single-dose, crossover design. Ibuprofen 600 mg was taken concurrently with cimetidine 400 mg or ranitidine hydrochloride 150 mg. Cimetidine was administered every eight hours for two additional doses, and administration of ranitidine was repeated once in 12 hours. Significant increases in ibuprofen area under the curve and peak serum concentrations

Table 1.
Demographic Data of the Study Population

Subject	Sex	Race[a]	Age (yr)	Weight (kg)	Height (cm)
1	F	W	25	56.8	170
2	F	W	21	52.2	173
3	F	W	27	61.4	170
4	M	W	25	81.8	180
5	F	B	27	55.0	170
6	M	W	24	68.2	173
7	F	B	29	59.0	168
8	F	B	23	56.8	180
9	M	W	26	100	185
10	M	B	26	76.8	180
11	M	B	24	64.5	173
12	M	B	24	68.6	170
Mean ± S.D.			25 ± 2	66.8 ± 13.2	174 ± 5

[a] W = white, B = black.

Figure 1. Mean serum ibuprofen concentration versus time (□ = control, + = ranitidine, ◇ = cimetidine).

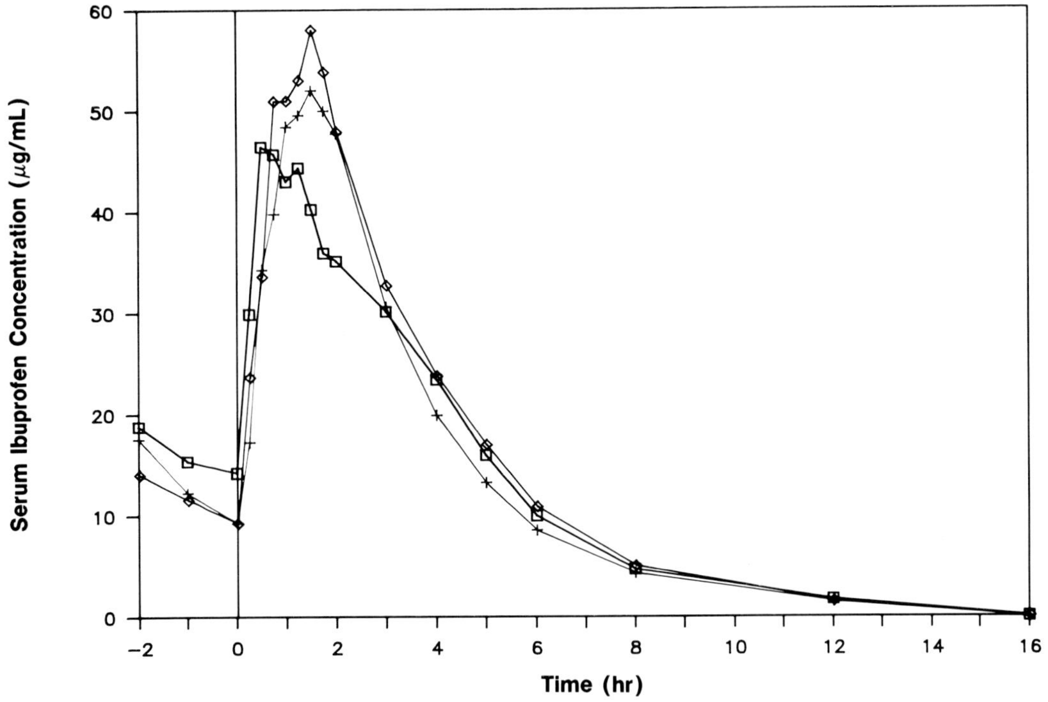

were demonstrated during the cimetidine treatment phase. Pharmacokinetic values during the ranitidine treatment phase did not differ significantly from those during the ibuprofen phase.

A study by Conrad et al.[12] was unable to show any difference in ibuprofen pharmacokinetics with the administration of a single 400-mg ibuprofen dose after one week of administration of cimetidine 300 mg every six hours. This study evaluated six healthy volunteers who were randomly assigned to one week with cimetidine and crossed over to one week without cimetidine. Values for AUC and $t_{1/2}$ for these two groups were not significantly different.

Mailhot et al.[13] evaluated the effect of cimetidine on the pharmacokinetics of another nonsteroidal anti-inflammatory agent, piroxicam. The main metabolic pathway for piroxicam is hydroxylation; it is potentially susceptible to the same interference from cimetidine as ibuprofen. Serum piroxicam concentrations were determined in 10 healthy volunteers after a single 20-mg dose on day 1 and then on day 15 after 7 days of administration of cimetidine 300 mg four times a day. A significant difference in AUC was observed, with a mean 15% increase after cimetidine administration.

Headache and nausea were anticipated based on previous reports on the administration of high once-daily doses of cimetidine.[9] Ibuprofen was administered with meals to decrease the incidence of nausea, but one subject still experienced nausea during treatment. The headaches experienced by

Table 2.
Ibuprofen Pharmacokinetic Values (Mean ± S.D.) after Concomitant Administration of Ranitidine or Cimetidine

Variable[a]	Control (n = 12)	Ranitidine (n = 12)	Cimetidine (n = 12)
$AUC_{0-\infty adjusted}$ (μg·hr/min)	166.71 ± 34.78	175.36 ± 36.36	200.25 ± 69.37
C_{max} (μg/mL)	63.36 ± 23.63	71.34 ± 12.54	66.76 ± 18.79
t_{max} (hr)	1.65 ± 1.29	1.08 ± 0.55	1.27 ± 0.42
CL (mL/min)	62.05 ± 11.01	58.81 ± 9.70	53.96 ± 13.57
k (hr^{-1})	0.41 ± 0.08	0.38 ± 0.10	0.39 ± 0.08
$t_{1/2}$ (hr)	1.75 ± 0.26	1.92 ± 0.46	1.85 ± 0.37

[a] $AUC_{0-\infty adjusted}$ = adjusted area under the curve, C_{max} = peak serum concentration, t_{max} = time to peak serum concentration, CL = clearance, k = elimination rate constant, $t_{1/2}$ = elimination half-life.

Figure 2. Logarithmic mean serum ibuprofen concentration versus time (□ = control, + = ranitidine, ◇ = cimetidine).

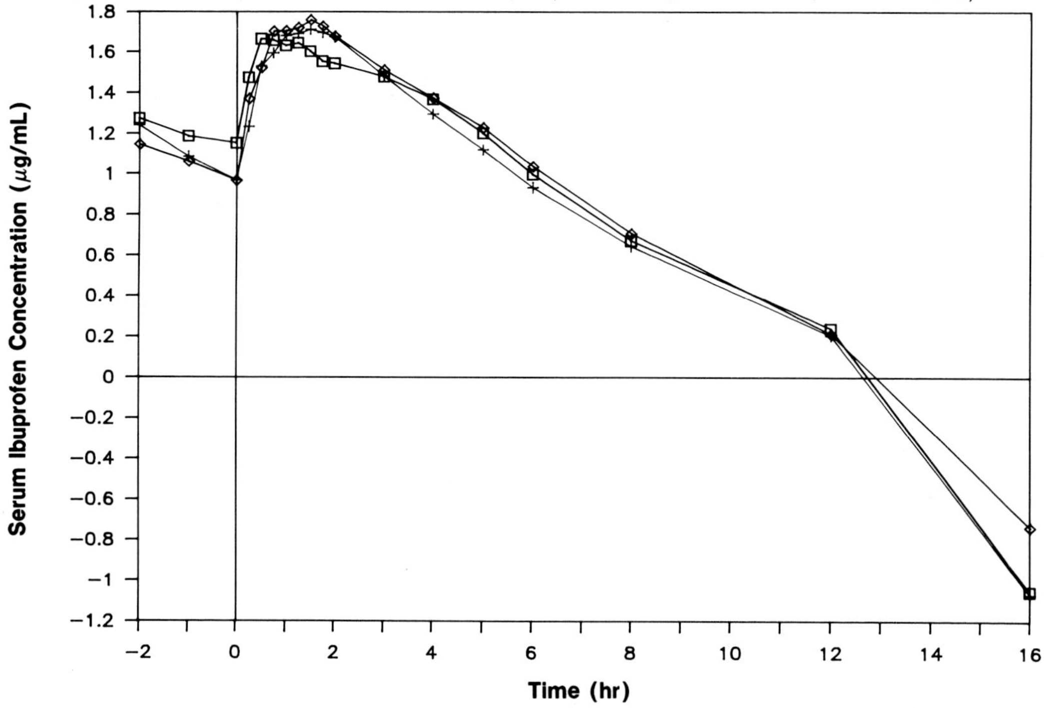

two other subjects may be related to cimetidine administration, since the effect was not observed in these subjects during the control or ranitidine treatment phases.

Based on the serum concentrations that were achieved in this study and the pharmacokinetic values that were calculated, the coadministration of ranitidine or cimetidine with ibuprofen does not significantly decrease clearance or prolong the half-life of ibuprofen. The small decrease in ibuprofen clearance caused by cimetidine is of little clinical importance considering the wide therapeutic range of ibuprofen. However, these results do not necessarily apply to patients such as the elderly, who may have diminished hepatic function or concomitant disease states. The administration of the H_2 antagonists two hours before ibuprofen dosing on the sampling day did not contribute to enhanced absorption as anticipated.

Conclusion. In young, healthy adults, neither cimetidine nor ranitidine administered at the dosages studied significantly alters the pharmacokinetics of ibuprofen.

References

1. Flower RJ, Moncada S, Vane JR. Analgesic-antipyretics and anti-inflammatory agents: drugs employed in the treatment of gout. In: Goodman LS, Gilman A, eds. The pharmacological basis of therapeutics. New York: MacMillan Publishing Co., Inc., 1985:674–715.
2. Cohen MM. Mucosal cytoprotection by prostaglandin E2. *Lancet*. 1978; 2:1253–4.
3. Konturek SJ, Obtulowitz W, Kwiecien N et al. Comparison of ranitidine and cimetidine in inhibition of histamine, sham feeding and meal-induced gastric secretion in duodenal ulcer patients. *Gut*. 1980; 21:181–6.
4. Ashton MG, Holdsworth CD, Ryan FP et al. Healing of gastric ulcers after one, two, and three months of ranitidine. *Br Med J*. 1982; 284:467–8.
5. Speeg KV, Patwardhan RV, Avant GR et al. Inhibition of microsomal drug metabolism by histamine H_2-receptor antagonism in vitro and in vivo in rodents. *Gastroenterology*. 1982; 82:89–96.
6. Lockwood GF, Wagner JG. High-performance liquid chromatographic determination of ibuprofen and its major metabolites in biological fluids. *J Chromatogr*. 1982; 232:335–43.
7. Niazi S. Textbook of biopharmaceutics and clinical pharmacokinetics. New York: Appleton-Century-Crofts; 1979:61.
8. Wilkinson L. REGM: a multivariate general linear hypothesis program for least squares analysis of multivariate data. *Behav Res Methods Instrum*. 1975; 7:485–6.
9. Valenzuela JE, Dickson B, Dixon W. Efficiency of a single nocturnal dose of cimetidine in active duodenal ulcer. *Postgrad Med*. 1985; 32:35–41.
10. Richards DA. Comparative pharmacodynamics and pharmacokinetics of cimetidine and ranitidine. *J Clin Gastroenterol*. 1983; 5(Suppl):81–90.
11. Ochs HR, Greenblatt DJ, Matlis R et al. Interaction of ibuprofen with the H-2 receptor antagonists ranitidine and cimetidine. *Clin Pharmacol Ther*. 1985; 38:648–51.
12. Conrad KA, Mayersohn M, Bliss M. Cimetidine does not alter ibuprofen kinetics after a single dose. *Br J Clin Pharmacol*. 1984; 18:624–6.
13. Mailhot C, Dahl SL, Ward JR. The effect of cimetidine on serum concentrations of piroxicam. *Pharmacotherapy*. 1986; 6:112–7.

"

Gentamicin-Resistant Enterococci

Although it is unclear how gentamicin-resistant enterococci will figure in the hospital environment of the future, their increasing prevalence is clearly cause for concern. Rigorous infection control, more careful selection of antimicrobial agents, and systematic screening for isolates with high-level resistance to gentamicin are all likely to be important in limiting the spread of these organisms. The first step, however, is to recognize their existence and probable epidemiology.

—Hoffman SA, Moellering RC Jr. The enterococcus: "putting the bug in our ears." *Ann Intern Med*. 1987; 106:757–61.

"

Drug Experience

Straightforward reports of unusual drug experiences are included in this section. These may be confirmations of previously reported drug experiences or brief apparent first reports. While selected references may be cited, the purpose of a Drug Experience report is not to present an extensive review of the literature.

A related section, Grand Rounds, includes papers that are well-documented patient case reports with a thorough review of the important literature to help put the case in perspective.

Continuous infusion of midazolam hydrochloride to control status epilepticus

CATHERINE B. CRISP, RICHARD GANNON, AND FREDERIC KNAUFT

Clin Pharm. 1988; 7:322–4

Like all benzodiazepines, midazolam has anxiolytic, hypnotic, anticonvulsant, muscle relaxant, and antegrade amnestic effects.[1] There have been only two published reports of midazolam being successfully used to treat seizures in humans. In one report, intramuscular midazolam 0.15–0.30 mg/kg (as the hydrochloride salt) terminated seizures in 12 of 15 patients. Four of these successfully treated patients had status epilepticus.[2] In another report, status epilepticus was terminated in a 14-year-old with a single intravenous dose of midazolam 15 mg.[3] We describe a case in which midazolam was given as a continuous intravenous infusion for the treatment of life-threatening status epilepticus in a hemodynamically unstable patient. The seizures in this patient probably had multiple etiologies, including hypoxia, renal failure, central nervous system bleeding secondary to disseminated intravascular coagulation, hypocalcemia, and potentially high nafcillin concentrations.

Case Report. A 68-year-old, 40-kg woman was admitted because of worsening respiratory status with hypoxemia, fever (37.8–38.3 °C), dehydration, obtundation, and staphylococcal facial cellulitis. The patient had a six-month history of persistent cough, dyspnea, and weight loss and a two-month history of recurrent right-sided herpes zoster involving the head, face, eye, and upper torso. Four months before admission an abdominal computed tomography scan had shown an enlarged head of the pancreas, presumed malignant. The patient had refused permission for biopsy of the mass at that time. During this admission a chest roentgenogram revealed patchy, nodular, and streaking infiltrates in both the right and left upper lobes of the lungs.

Results of laboratory studies were as follows: urea nitrogen (BUN) 34 mg/L; serum creatinine 0.4 mg/dL; ionized calcium 1.88 meq/L; aspartate aminotransferase (AST, formerly called SGOT) 63 U/L; alanine aminotransferase (ALT, formerly called SGPT) 72 U/L; lactate dehydrogenase (LDH) 252 U/L; total bilirubin 0.9 mg/dL; white blood cell (WBC) count 10,900 with a differential of 78% neutrophils, 13% bands, 5% lymphocytes, and 4% monocytes. Spinal fluid was abnormal: protein 94 g/dL; glucose 80 mg/dL (serum glucose 107 mg/dL); red blood cell count 400/cu mm; WBC count 100/cu mm (57% neutrophils, 36% lymphocytes, 7% monocytes); no bacteria seen on Gram's stain; and cultures negative.

Empirically, treatment with intravenous cefotaxime and acyclovir was started. Two days later nafcillin was added because admission blood cultures grew *Staphylococcus aureus*. Despite these antibiotics the patient continued to have fever spikes. Tobramycin 80 mg (as the sulfate salt) every 12 hours was added for synergy against *Staph. aureus*. She continued to deteriorate, and on the third hospital day she was intubated and transferred to the medical intensive-care unit (ICU) because of increased

CATHERINE B. CRISP, PHARM.D., is Critical Care Pharmacy Fellow and Assistant Clinical Professor, School of Pharmacy, University of Connecticut, Storrs, CT. RICHARD GANNON, PHARM.D., is Clinical Pharmacist, Medical Intensive Care Unit, Department of Pharmacy, Hartford Hospital, Hartford, CT, and Assistant Clinical Professor, School of Pharmacy, University of Connecticut. FREDERIC KNAUFT, M.D., is Clinical Assistant Professor for Respiratory Therapy, University of Hartford, Hartford, CT; Clinical Instructor, School of Medicine, University of Connecticut, Farmington; and Associate Director, Department of Respiratory Therapy, Hartford Hospital.

Address reprint requests to Dr. Gannon at the Pharmacy Department, Hartford Hospital, 80 Seymour Street, Hartford, CT 06115.

Copyright © 1988, American Society of Hospital Pharmacists, Inc. All rights reserved. 0278-2677/88/0401-0322$00.75.

respiratory distress (respiratory rate 40/min; pH 7.43; Po_2 39; Pco_2 27; 54% oxygen saturation), low blood pressure (80/40 mm Hg), and persistent fever.

The next morning she had a 10-second generalized tonic-clonic seizure, which resolved spontaneously. Early that afternoon she required continuous infusions of norepinephrine 37 μg/min (as the bitartrate salt) and dopamine hydrochloride 13–20 μg/kg/min to maintain her systolic blood pressure above 90 mm Hg. About eight hours after the first seizure, a second generalized seizure occurred, which again resolved spontaneously. At this time she had acute renal and liver failure with disseminated intravascular coagulation. Laboratory test values were as follows: prothrombin time 16 sec; partial thromboplastin time 47 sec; thrombin time 48 sec; fibrinogen 0.8 g/L; fibrinogen split products 80 μg/mL; platelets 75,000; BUN 71 mg/L, serum creatinine 1.8 mg/dL; AST 76 U/L; ALT 25 U/L; LDH 242 U/L; and total bilirubin 5.2 mg/dL (59% conjugated).

The nafcillin dosage was decreased from 2 g (as the sodium salt) every four hours to 1 g every four hours. An attempt was made to measure the nafcillin concentration; however, only a bioassay (*Micrococcus* species) was available. Since both cefotaxime and tobramycin interfere with the assay, the result would have been inaccurate.

The patient experienced additional seizure activity overnight, and the next morning (ICU day 2) she was given an intravenous loading dose of phenytoin sodium 800 mg (20 mg/kg) and started on 300 mg/day (7.5 mg/kg) intravenously. Her first phenytoin maintenance dose was given eight hours after the loading dose. A pulmonary lavage was done, with a preliminary Gram's stain showing *Pneumocystis carinii*. Subsequently the antibiotics were stopped, and sulfamethoxazole–trimethoprim (400 mg–80 mg) intravenously every eight hours was started.

That night, starting at 2300 (approximately 36 hours after first seizure), the patient began to have four to six generalized seizures every hour. Each seizure lasted about 10 seconds and was accompanied by a drop in blood pressure, heart rate, and arterial oxygen saturation. During this period she received one 150-mg intravenous dose of phenobarbital sodium without effect on the seizures. Her systolic blood pressure dropped transiently to 85 mm Hg; therefore, administration of a full loading dose (20 mg/kg) of phenobarbital sodium was thought to be inappropriate. She required dopamine hydrochloride 5.3 μg/kg/min and norepinephrine 15 μg/min (as the bitartrate salt) to maintain a systolic blood pressure of 90 mm Hg and a urine output of 20 mL/hr. During the night, seizures were not treated with bolus doses of diazepam for fear of increasing hypotension. At this time a do-not-resuscitate order was issued, and no further laboratory tests were ordered.

In the morning it was decided that a midazolam hydrochloride infusion would be used. An intravenous loading dose of midazolam 5 mg (0.125 mg/kg) was given, followed by a continuous intravenous infusion of 3 mg/hr. A continuous infusion was used because it was thought that bolus dosing of any benzodiazepine might cause more severe hypotension. Once the midazolam was given, the patient had no more witnessed seizures. Four hours later her systolic blood pressure decreased to 82–88 mm Hg. Norepinephrine was increased to a maximum of 24 μg/min. The midazolam infusion was subsequently decreased to 2 mg/hr, which allowed the norepinephrine dosage to be titrated back down to 15 μg/min (which it had been before midazolam was added). The infusion of midazolam was continued for a total of 30 hours, until the patient died the next day after all vasopressors were stopped. Results of an enzyme-linked immunosorbent assay (ELISA) and a Western blot test were subsequently reported to be positive for antibody to the human immunodeficiency virus.

Discussion. No anticonvulsant serum concentrations were obtained because the family did not want the patient to have any more blood tests. Most likely the phenobarbital concentration was subtherapeutic because of the low dose used. As for phenytoin sodium, the patient received 27.5 mg/kg within an eight-hour period. Because of the patient's high loading dose, impaired liver function, and sulfamethoxazole therapy, a subtherapeutic phenytoin concentration was highly unlikely.

An EEG was not done, at the family's request. The patient may have been having subclinical seizures during the midazolam infusion; however, her previous seizures had been manifested clinically.

At this institution and others, patients in the ICU have been sedated with constant infusions of midazolam.[4–6]

We use midazolam (as the hydrochloride salt) 100 mg/100 mL of 5% dextrose injection or 0.9% sodium chloride injection prepared in a polyvinyl chloride minibag. A loading dose of 0.1–0.5 mg/kg is followed by the continuous infusion of 0.5–5.0 μg/kg/min. We have not seen adverse effects on blood pressure or respiratory rate that could not be controlled by decreasing the infusion rate. Because midazolam is highly lipophilic at physiologic pH and is compatible with common intravenous fluids, we postulate that it could be an effective anticonvulsant in treating status epilepticus. We have described one case in which continuous infusion of midazolam controlled life-threatening seizures in a hemodynamically unstable patient.

Benzodiazepines administered by continuous intravenous infusion are considered by some to be the drugs of choice for treatment of status epilepticus after phenytoin has failed.[7,8] If phenytoin therapy fails, a decision must be made whether to use phenobarbital or continuous-infusion benzodiazepines. In this instance, since phenobarbital caused hypotension the most likely choice was a benzodiazepine infusion.

Diazepam has been administered by continuous intravenous infusion for treatment of status epilepticus.[9,10] Since diazepam requires suspension in a lipoid substance, there is a high incidence of thrombophlebitis with intravenous administration and problems with compatibility.[4,9-11] Also, because of the long elimination half-life of diazepam and its metabolites, prolonged sedation may occur after the continuous infusion is stopped.

Midazolam is one of the newest benzodiazepines to be marketed in the United States. This drug exhibits different pharmacologic and pharmacokinetic properties than other benzodiazepines.[1] In acidic media, such as 5% dextrose injection, 0.9% sodium chloride injection, and lactated Ringer's injection, midazolam is highly water soluble. It is compatible with other intravenous solutions, and administration causes little local irritation. At physiologic pH the drug is highly lipophilic, resulting in a rapid onset of action after administration. The drug is rapidly hydroxylated by hepatic enzymes (elimination half-life of one to four hours).[1] The half-life of midazolam is much shorter than that of other benzodiazepines.

Conclusion. Based on the known mechanism of action and the ease by which this drug can be administered intravenously, we propose that it may be an alternative therapy for treating status epilepticus, even in hemodynamically unstable patients. However, further experience with this drug, administered as a continuous infusion, is necessary before conclusions about its usefulness in treating status epilepticus can be made.

References

1. Reves JG, Fragen RJ, Vinik R et al. Midazolam: pharmacology and uses. *Anesthesiology*. 1985; 62:310–24.
2. Egli M, Albani C. Relief of status epilepticus after IM administration of the new short-acting benzodiazepine midazolam (Dormicum). In: Program and abstracts of 12th World Congress of Neurology. Princeton, NJ: Excerpta Medica; 1981:44. Abstract 137.
3. Kaneko S, Kurahashi K, Fujita S et al. Potentiation of GABA by midazolam and its therapeutic effect against status epilepticus. *Folia Psychiatr Neurol Jpn*. 1983; 37:307–9.
4. Dirksen MSC, Vree TB, Oriessen JJ. Midazolam in the intensive care unit. *Drug Intell Clin Pharm*. 1986; 20:805–6.
5. Michalle S, Moncorge C, Fichelle A et al. Long term midazolam infusion for basal sedation in intensive care. A clinical and pharmacokinetic study. *Anesthesiology*. 1986; 65:A66.
6. Cheng EY, Westphal LM, White PF et al. Use of a midazolam infusion for sedation following aortocoronary bypass surgery. *Anesthesiology*. 1986; 65:A67.
7. Rawal K, D'Souza BJ. Status epilepticus. *Crit Care Clin*. 1985; 1:339–53.
8. Delgado-Escueta AV, Wasterlain C, Treiman DM et al. Management of status epilepticus. *New Engl J Med*. 1982; 306:1337–40.
9. Prensky AL, Raff MC, Moore MJ et al. Intravenous diazepam in the treatment of prolonged seizure activity. *N Engl J Med*. 1967; 276:779–84.
10. Bell HE, Bertino JS. Constant diazepam infusion in the treatment of continuous seizure activity. *Drug Intell Clin Pharm*. 1984; 18:965–70.
11. Michael KA, Lehman ME, Amersosn AB. Diazepam infusions. *Drug Intell Clin Pharm*. 1984; 18:214–5.

"

Refocusing on Constipation

[P]rimary caregivers as well as researchers need to refocus their attention and attitude toward the problem of constipation. From early adulthood on, the problem should be actively sought and proper management instituted. This requires education in good bowel habits, dietary management, and the need to *avoid* irritant laxatives unless specific indications are present, i.e., weakened abdominal or perineal muscles, a necessary constipating medication, loss of rectal reflex, or anorexia and weight loss secondary to constipation. This requires taking the necessary time to educate patients but should be done instead of quickly writing a prescription for the "dynamite" of choice. Chronically constipated patients will benefit from this approach as well but will require a more involved, individualized, and persistent approach. Developing a framework for management and treatment (similar to the step-care approach for hypertension) may help stimulate physician interest and understanding. . . . Much of the cause of chronic constipation may be reversible if proper management and education are instituted early in the course of disease. . . . As the population ages and medical care shifts away from acute (infectious) care toward care of chronic disease, treatment of problems such as constipation will be important in improving quality of life for our patients.

—Castle SC. Constipation: a pressing issue. *Arch Intern Med*. 1987; 147:1702–3. Editorial.

"

"SURPRISE"!

Given a choice of having only one agent on their hospital formulary, the majority of respondents to a nationwide survey involving hospital specialists said they'd keep TICAR rather than another commonly used anti-pseudomonal penicillin.*

Ticar® (TICARCILLIN DISODIUM)
plus an Aminoglycoside

Still preferred—when all is said and done.

*Data on file, BEECHAM Laboratories.

TICAR®
(Sterile Ticarcillin Disodium)

For Intramuscular or Intravenous Use

For complete prescribing information, consult official package insert.

ACTIONS: Ticarcillin is bactericidal; it is not absorbed orally, therefore, it must be administered intravenously or intramuscularly.

INDICATIONS: TICAR (Ticarcillin Disodium) is indicated for the treatment of the following infections:

Bacterial septicemia†
Skin and soft-tissue infections†
Acute and chronic respiratory tract infections†‡
†caused by susceptible strains of *Pseudomonas aeruginosa, Proteus* species (both indole-positive and indole-negative) and *Escherichia coli*.
‡(Though clinical improvement has been shown, bacteriological cures cannot be expected in patients with chronic respiratory disease or cystic fibrosis.)
Genitourinary tract infections (complicated and uncomplicated) due to susceptible strains of *Pseudomonas aeruginosa, Proteus* species (both indole-positive and indole-negative), *Escherichia coli, Enterobacter* and *Streptococcus faecalis* (enterococcus).

Ticarcillin is also indicated in the treatment of the following infections due to susceptible anaerobic bacteria:

1) Bacterial septicemia.
2) Lower respiratory tract infections such as empyema, anaerobic pneumonitis and lung abscess.
3) Intra-abdominal infections such as peritonitis and intra-abdominal abscess (typically resulting from anaerobic organisms resident in the normal gastrointestinal tract).
4) Infections of the female pelvis and genital tract such as endometritis, pelvic inflammatory disease, pelvic abscess and salpingitis.
5) Skin and soft-tissue infections.

Although Ticarcillin is primarily indicated against Gram-negative infections, its *in vitro* activity against Gram-positive organisms should be considered in treating infections caused by both Gram-negative and Gram-positive organisms.

Based on the *in vitro* synergism between Ticarcillin and gentamicin sulfate or tobramycin sulfate against certain strains of *Pseudomonas aeruginosa*, combined therapy has been successful, using full therapeutic dosages.

Culturing and susceptibility testing should be performed initially and during treatment.

CONTRAINDICATIONS: A history of allergic reaction to any of the penicillins is a contraindication.

WARNINGS: Anaphylaxis may occur, especially in patients with an allergic diathesis. Check for a history of allergy to penicillins, cephalosporins or other allergens. If an allergic reaction occurs, the drug should be discontinued unless, in the opinion of the physician, the condition being treated is life-threatening and amenable only to Ticarcillin therapy. Serious anaphylactic reactions require immediate emergency treatment with epinephrine, oxygen, intravenous steroids and airway management.

Some patients receiving high doses of Ticarcillin may develop hemorrhagic manifestations associated with abnormalities of coagulation tests. Patients with renal impairment, in whom excretion of Ticarcillin is delayed, should be observed for bleeding manifestations. Such patients should be dosed strictly according to recommendations. If bleeding manifestations appear, Ticarcillin treatment should be discontinued and, if necessary, appropriate therapy instituted.

PRECAUTIONS: During prolonged treatment, periodic checking for organ system dysfunction (renal, hepatic and hematopoietic) is advisable. If overgrowth of resistant organisms occurs, the appropriate therapy should be initiated.

Since the theoretical sodium content is 5.2 milliequivalents (120 mg) per gram of Ticarcillin, electrolyte and cardiac status should be monitored carefully.

In a few patients receiving intravenous Ticarcillin, hypokalemia has been reported. Serum potassium should be measured periodically.

USAGE DURING PREGNANCY: Reproduction studies have been performed in mice and rats and have revealed no evidence of impaired fertility or harm to the fetus due to Ticarcillin. There are no well-controlled studies in pregnant women, but investigational experience does not include any positive evidence of adverse effects on the fetus. Although there is no clearly defined risk, such experience cannot exclude the possibility of infrequent or subtle damage to the fetus. Ticarcillin should be used in pregnant women only when clearly needed.

ADVERSE REACTIONS: The following adverse reactions may occur: skin rashes, pruritus, urticaria, drug fever, nausea, vomiting, anemia, thrombocytopenia, leukopenia, neutropenia, eosinophilia. SGOT and SGPT elevations have been reported. Patients, especially those with impaired renal function, may experience convulsions or neuromuscular excitability when very high doses of the drug are administered.

Local reactions at the site of injection have been reported. Vein irritation and phlebitis can occur, particularly when undiluted solution is directly injected into the vein.

DOSAGE AND ADMINISTRATION: Usual adult recommended dosage in bacterial septicemia, respiratory tract infections, skin and soft-tissue infections, intra-abdominal infections and infections of the female pelvis and genital tract, is 3 grams by intravenous infusion every 3, 4 or 6 hours depending on weight and severity of infection; in uncomplicated urinary tract infections, 1 gram I.M. or direct I.V. q.i.d.; in complicated urinary tract infections, 3 grams q.i.d. by I.V. infusion.

Please consult official package insert for details on dosages for patients with renal insufficiency, children, neonates and directions for use.

Supplied: 1 Gm, 3 Gm and 6 Gm Standard Vials; 3 Gm and 6 Gm Piggyback Bottles

7182BS1/86

TSM-1272

Beecham
laboratories
Bristol, Tennessee 37620

CP Continuing Education

The ASHP Continuing Education system gives readers a self-assessment mechanism for selected articles in Clinical Pharmacy *and the* American Journal of Hospital Pharmacy. *It also allows readers to obtain continuing-education credit for these articles.*

For the purpose of CE-credit enrollment a blank answer sheet is published at the end of each installment of the column for the CE articles in that issue. An enrollee accumulates these answer sheets until the enrollment is submitted, using the form that is published in the June and December issues of Clinical Pharmacy *and in the June and December issues of the* American Journal of Hospital Pharmacy. *Any combination of tests within a 18-month period, from both* Clinical Pharmacy *and* American Journal of Hospital Pharmacy, *may be included in an enrollment. More complete details about enrollment in the system will appear in the semiannual enrollment form.*

Article 680-204-8804 (see page 271)
Qualifies for 1.0 hour of CE credit

Comparison of famotidine with cimetidine and ranitidine

Learning Objectives

After studying this article, the reader should be able to

1. Compare the chemical structure, potency, antisecretory effects, and pharmacokinetics of famotidine with those of cimetidine and ranitidine.
2. Compare the clinical efficacy and dosage regimens of famotidine with those of cimetidine and ranitidine in the treatment of active duodenal ulcer, active benign gastric ulcer, prevention of ulcer recurrence, and Zollinger–Ellison syndrome.
3. State two of the most frequent adverse effects reported with famotidine therapy.
4. Compare the drug interaction profile of famotidine with that of cimetidine and ranitidine.
5. Compare the availability and cost of famotidine, cimetidine, and ranitidine dosage forms.

Self-assessment Questions

For each question there is one best answer only.

1. Which one of the following is true with regard to the chemical ring structures of famotidine, cimetidine, and ranitidine?

   a. Famotidine = imidazole, cimetidine = furan, ranitidine = thiazole.
   b. Famotidine = benzimidazole, cimetidine = imidazole, ranitidine = furan.
   c. Famotidine = thiazole, cimetidine = imidazole, ranitidine = furan.
   d. Famotidine = thiazole, cimetidine = imidazole, ranitidine = benzimidazole.

2. On an equimolar basis, famotidine is

   a. Less potent than cimetidine and ranitidine.
   b. More potent than cimetidine but less potent than ranitidine.
   c. Equipotent to cimetidine and ranitidine.
   d. More potent than cimetidine and ranitidine.

3. When used to heal active duodenal ulcers, famotidine given for six to eight weeks at full doses appears to be

   a. More effective than cimetidine and ranitidine.
   b. Approximately equal to cimetidine and ranitidine.
   c. More effective than cimetidine but less effective than ranitidine.
   d. Less effective than cimetidine and ranitidine.

4. The recommended oral famotidine dosage regimen(s) for healing uncomplicated duodenal ulcers is (are)

   a. 10 mg b.i.d., 20 mg at bedtime.
   b. 20 mg b.i.d., 40 mg at bedtime.
   c. 40 mg b.i.d., 80 mg at bedtime.
   d. 20 mg every six hours.

5. When used to prevent duodenal ulcer recurrence, famotidine therapy after one year appears to be

   a. Less effective than cimetidine and ranitidine.
   b. More effective than cimetidine and less effective

than ranitidine.
c. Approximately equal to cimetidine and ranitidine.
d. More effective than cimetidine and ranitidine.

6. The recommended dosage of oral famotidine for preventing duodenal ulcer recurrence is

a. 5 mg at bedtime.
b. 10 mg at bedtime.
c. 20 mg at bedtime.
d. 40 mg at bedtime.

7. Antiandrogenic adverse effects in men have been primarily associated with the long-term use of high doses of

a. Cimetidine.
b. Ranitidine.
c. Cimetidine and famotidine.
d. Ranitidine and famotidine.

8. Two of the most frequent adverse effects reported with famotidine are

a. Elevated levels of liver enzymes and headache.
b. Mental-status changes and constipation.
c. Skin rash and diarrhea.
d. Headache and constipation.

9. Which of the following H_2-receptor antagonists appear to substantially affect the eliminination of drugs that are metabolized by hepatic microsomal enzymes?

a. Cimetidine.
b. Cimetidine and ranitidine.
c. Cimetidine and famotidine.
d. Cimetidine, ranitidine, and famotidine.

10. Which one of the following statements is true with regard to famotidine dosage formulations?

a. There is no commercially available oral liquid.
b. The oral liquid does not require reconstitution.
c. There is no commercially available injectable dosage form.
d. The undiluted injectable dosage form requires refrigeration.

Article 680-204-8805 (see page 285)
Qualifies for 1.0 hour of CE credit

Use of cephalosporins with enhanced antianaerobic activity for treatment and prevention of anaerobic and mixed infections

Learning Objectives

After studying this article the reader should be able to

1. List four major loci of infections for which cephalosporins with enhanced antianaerobic activity have been demonstrated to be useful.
2. Contrast the spectra of activity of cefoxitin, cefotetan, ceftizoxime, and moxalactam.
3. Identify important adverse reactions associated with cephalosporins with enhanced antianaerobic activity.
4. Contrast the absorption, distribution, and elimination of cefoxitin, cefotetan, ceftizoxime, and moxalactam.
5. Discuss important considerations for pharmacy and therapeutics committees in regard to selecting from among cephalosporins with enhanced antianaerobic activity.

Self-assessment Questions

For each question there is one best answer only.

1. Antimicrobial susceptibility testing of anaerobic bacteria has assumed greater importance in recent years because

a. Organisms formerly thought to be subspecies of *Bacteroides fragilis* have been recognized to be separate species.
b. A practical agar dilution testing method has become available for routine use in clinical laboratories.
c. Bacterial susceptibilities to antimicrobial agents vary among institutions.
d. Both a and c are correct.
e. All of the above answers are correct.

2. Which one of the following statements best describes the in vitro activity of cefoxitin, cefotetan, ceftizoxime, and moxalactam against *Bacteroides* species?

a. All four agents are as active against *Bacteroides* species as clindamycin and metronidazole.
b. None of the four agents is as active against *Bacteroides* species as clindamycin or gentamicin.
c. The four agents vary in their activity in slight but clinically important ways.
d. Moxalactam is most active and cefoxitin is least active; insufficient data are available for cefotetan.

3. Which one of the following statements best describes the activity of cefoxitin, cefotetan, ceftizoxime, and moxalactam against gram-positive and gram-negative organisms?

a. No clear differences exist in their activity against these organisms.
b. Any of the four agents could be used as first-line therapy for documented gram-positive infections.
c. Ceftizoxime and moxalactam are clearly more active than cefoxitin against several gram-negative organisms.
d. Cefoxitin and moxalactam can interact with certain gram-negative bacteria to inhibit β-lactamase production.

4. Disulfiram-like reactions and hematologic abnormalities have been associated with

a. Cefotetan and moxalactam.
b. Cefoxitin and ceftizoxime.
c. Cefotetan and cefoxitin.
d. All four of these agents.

5. Following a 1-g intramuscular injection, the highest serum concentrations are achieved by

   a. Cefotetan.
   b. Cefoxitin.
   c. Ceftizoxime.
   d. Moxalactam.

6. Of the four cephalosporins with enhanced antianaerobic activity, which two could achieve cerebrospinal fluid concentrations adequate for the treatment of gram-negative meningitis?

   a. Cefotetan and moxalactam.
   b. Cefoxitin and ceftizoxime.
   c. Cefotetan and cefoxitin.
   d. Ceftizoxime and moxalactam.

7. In patients with normal renal function, which of the four cephalosporins with enhanced antianaerobic activity could be administered every 12 hours?

   a. Cefotetan only.
   b. Cefotetan and cefoxitin.
   c. Cefotetan, ceftizoxime, and moxalactam.
   d. Cefotetan, cefoxitin, and moxalactam.

8. Which one of the following statements is true regarding the treatment of intra-abdominal infections?

   a. All four of the cephalosporins with enhanced antianaerobic activity are as effective as the combination of clindamycin and an aminoglycoside.
   b. Sufficient information exists to support the use of cefoxitin, ceftizoxime, and moxalactam.
   c. Sufficient information exists to support the use of cefoxitin, cefotetan, and moxalactam.
   d. Insufficient information exists to clearly support the use of the cephalosporins.

9. The most important consideration in choosing an injectable cephalosporin for prophylaxis of postsurgical infection is

   a. Whether *Bacteroides fragilis* is a likely pathogen.
   b. Whether the cephalosporin is first, second, or third generation.
   c. The cost of the agent.
   d. The agent's onset of action.

10. When comparing the costs associated with cefoxitin, cefotetan, ceftizoxime, and moxalactam, which of the following factors should be considered?

    a. Drug acquisition and administration costs.
    b. Associated laboratory costs.
    c. Pharmacokinetic profiles of the drugs.
    d. Both a and b are correct.
    e. All of the above answers are correct.

Clinical Pharmacists

CLINICAL PHARMACIST ONCOLOGY

Opportunities exist for career advancement in VA Health Care System. Complete benefits package available. 40-hour week, no weekends or holidays. Responsibilities include the institution and development of antineoplastic drug program (i.e., patient drug monitoring, pharmacokinetic monitoring, inservice lectures, and general staff development). Time allotted for research.

CLINICAL PHARMACIST INFECTIOUS DISEASES

Opportunities exist for career advancement in VA Health Care System. Complete benefits package available. 40-hour week, no weekends or holidays. Responsibilities include development of an existing antibiotic drug program (i.e., patient drug monitoring, pharmacokinetic monitoring, In-Service lectures and general staff development). Time allotted for research.

May be licensed in any state. Two years clinical experience required (Pharm.D. or equivalent preferred).

Both positions are affiliated with Rutgers University College of Pharmacy. Salary commensurate with qualifications, starting at $35,825.00 per annum.

Contact **Louis E. Cobuzzi, Chief of Pharmacy Service, Veterans Administration Medical Center, Bronx, New York 10468. 212-579-1611.**

Equal Opportunity Employer.

Answer sheet

April 1988 *Clinical Pharmacy*

Note: An enrollment form for the ASHP Continuing-Education System appears in the June and December issues. Please accumulate all the answer sheets you wish to use in one enrollment and submit them at one time with a completed enrollment form.

Place an X in the box(es) at the top of the column(s) corresponding to the test(s) you are taking. Darken the boxes corresponding to the correct answers.

	□ 680-204-8804 1.0 hour a b c d		□ 680-204-8805 1.0 hour a b c d e
1.	□□□□	1.	□□□□□
2.	□□□□	2.	□□□□
3.	□□□□	3.	□□□□
4.	□□□□	4.	□□□□
5.	□□□□	5.	□□□□
6.	□□□□	6.	□□□□
7.	□□□□	7.	□□□□
8.	□□□□	8.	□□□□
9.	□□□□	9.	□□□□
10.	□□□□	10.	□□□□□

ASHP Use Only
(1.0)8804 ________ (3)
(1.0)8805 ________ (3)

Current Literature

Drug Reaction Alerts

Drug Reaction Alerts focuses primarily on serious, unlabeled reactions to new chemical entities. The citations are compiled monthly from International Pharmaceutical Abstracts, *which covers over 800 pharmacy and health-related journals worldwide. An address for reprints (when available) follows the name of the corresponding author in each citation.*

Antibiotics

Lacouture PG (Slone Epidemiology Unit, 1371 Beacon Street, Brookline, MA 02146), Epstein MF, Mitchell AA. **Vancomycin** associated shock and rash in newborn infants. *J Pediatr.* 1987; 111:615–6. Cases. (two neonates; received vancomycin hydrochloride 15 mg/kg every 12 hours via i.v. infusion over 20 minutes; developed shock and rash; symptoms resolved within five minutes in first neonate and second neonate received albumin and diphenhydramine, which resulted in immediate increase in blood pressure and increased responsiveness; received subsequent dosages of vancomycin over one hour with no reaction)

Antineoplastic Agents

Harrison PV (Department of Dermatology, Beaumont Hospital, Slyne Road, Lancaster LA1 2JF, England). **Methotrexate**-induced epidermal necrosis. *Br J Dermatol.* 1987; 116:867–9. Case. (86-year-old woman with erythrodermic psoriasis and borderline renal failure; received i.v. infusion of methotrexate 7.5 mg over 48 hours; concomitant aspirin; developed epidermal necrosis and elevated plasma methotrexate concentration 36 hours after drug administration)

Antituberculars

Goldin HM (Department of Medicine, Cook County Hospital, Chicago, IL 60612-9989), Schweitzer WJ, Bronson DM. **Rifampin** and exfoliative dermatitis. *Ann Intern Med.* 1987; 107:789. Case. (63-year-old man with tuberculosis; received rifampin 600 mg/day for six months; developed exfoliative dermatitis; skin healed slowly upon drug withdrawal)

Cathartics and Laxatives

Bowyer RC (St. Richards Hospital, Chichester PO19 4SE, England), Urquhart J. Fecal peritonitis induced by **Picolax:** response. *Br Med J.* 1987; 295:1413. Case. (75-year-old woman; received oral sachet of citric acid, magnesium oxide, and sodium picosulfate; developed large-bowel infarction; infarction corrected surgically; patient developed myocardial infarction 18 days later and died)

Drug Interactions

Anderson DJ (VA Medical Center, Minneapolis, MN 55417), Janoff EN. Herpes zoster infection in a patient on **methotrexate** given **prednisone** to prevent postherpetic neuralgia. *Ann Intern Med.* 1987; 107:783. Case. (66-year-old woman with rheumatoid arthritis; received methotrexate 2.5 mg every other day; prednisone 30 mg/day added to drug regimen; developed disseminated herpes zoster infection; prednisone and methotrexate discontinued and patient received i.v. acyclovir 30 mg/kg daily)

Cook B (Ninewells Hospital and Medical School, Dundee DD1 9SY, Scotland). Angiotensin converting enzyme inhibitors and diuretics. *Br Med J.* 1987; 295:1351–2. Case. (85-year-old man with heart failure; received **captopril** 25 mg/day and combination of **furosemide** 40 mg and **triamterene** 50 mg three times daily for two weeks; developed dehydration and hyperkalemia; electrolyte imbalance resolved upon withdrawal of hypotensive drugs and therapy with insulin, dextrose, and calcium polystyrene sulfonate)

Leor J (Tel-Aviv University, Tel-Hashomer, Israel), Levartowsky D, Sharon C. *Ann Intern Med.* 1987; 107:601. Case. (61-year-old woman; received **warfarin** 2.5–5 mg/day for six years and **nalidixic acid** 1 g three times daily for 10 days for treatment of urinary-tract infection; prothrombin time became excessively prolonged; prothrombin time normalized upon withdrawal of warfarin for six days and substitution of ampicillin and gentamicin for nalidixic acid; warfarin therapy reintroduced without incident)

Mesmer RE. Don't mix miso with MAOIs. *JAMA.* 1987; 258:3515. Case. (41-year-old woman with depression; received therapy with **phenelzine sulfate** 60 mg/day; concomitant alprazolam and triazolam; interaction between **tyramine** in miso soup and phenelzine resulted in hypertensive crisis; patient recovered spontaneously)

Heavy Metal Antagonists

Windus DW (Box 8129, 4949 Barnes Hospital Plaza, St. Louis, MO 63110), Stokes TJ, Julian BA et al. Fatal rhizopus infections in hemodialysis patients receiving **deferoxamine.** *Ann Intern Med.* 1987; 107:678–80. Cases. (four hemodialysis patients with chronic renal failure, aged 36–49 years; received deferoxamine 1.5–6 g/wk for nine weeks to one year; became infected with *Rhizopus* species infections and developed cerebral micromycosis; all patients died)

Hypotensive Agents

Stricker BH (Netherlands Center for Monitoring of Adverse Reactions to Drugs, P.O. Box 5406, 2280 HJ Rijswijk, Netherlands). Skin reactions and fever with **indapamide**. *Br Med J.* 1987; 295:1313–4. Cases. (16 hypertensive patients, aged 42–80 years; received indapamide 2.5 mg/day for 1–12 days; developed skin reactions sometimes accompanied by fever; rashes resolved upon withdrawal of indapamide and three patients received antihistamines)

Continued on page 330

NOW . . .

One comprehensive resource provides you 51 leading formulations for oral suspension.

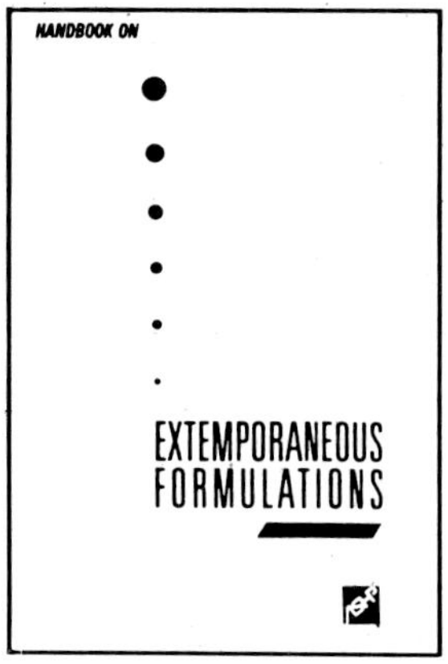

The *Handbook on Extemporaneous Formulations*—new from ASHP—features those formulations most often requested for neonates, pediatric and geriatric patients, and others unable to take oral solids.

Concise instructions for each formulation provides:

- ingredients
- compounding instructions
- auxiliary labeling
- stability
- references (where available)

Spiralbound. Spill-resistant. Just $15.
Order this time saver today!

Prepared by the Committee on Extemporaneous Formulations, ASHP Special Interest Group (SIG) on Pediatric Pharmacy Practice.

YES! Please send me __________ copies of P254, the *Handbook on Extemporaneous Formulations*, at $15.00 each.

☐ Enclosed is my check for $ __________ .
(Checks must be drawn on a U.S. bank and payable to ASHP.)

☐ Enclosed is our purchase order # ______________ ; please issue an invoice and add postage and handling.

OR

Charge $ ______________ to my:
☐ MasterCard ☐ VISA

Acct. # ______________________ Exp. __________ month/year

Signature ______________________

Name ______________________

Institution ______________________

ASHP I.D.# ______________________

Address ______________________

City __________ State __________ Zip __________

Send to: ASHP Publication Records Dept., 4630 Montgomery Avenue, Bethesda, MD 20814

Payments to ASHP are not deductible as charitable contributions for Federal Income Tax purposes. However, they may be deductible under other provisions of the Internal Revenue Code.

Current Literature *Continued from page 329*

Parasympathomimetic Agents

Nadal J (Hospital de St. Pau, Avda S, Antoni M. Claret 167, Barcelona, Spain), De La Fuente V, Abadias M et al. Toxic coma induced by anticholinergic eye drops. *Br Med J.* 1987; 295:1352. Case. (6-year-old boy; received two drops in each eye of ophthalmic solution containing **atropine sulfate** 2%, **scopolamine bromhidrate** 0.5%, and **phenylephrine hydrochloride** 4%; approximately 3 mg atropine sulfate, 0.75 mg scopolamine bromhidrate, and 6 mg phenylephrine hydrochloride instilled; patient became comatose because of atropine intoxication; recovery upon therapy with two doses of physostigmine salicylate 9.5 mg i.v. 10 minutes apart)

Books Received

Books are listed as soon as received; selected books may be reviewed in Book Reviews in subsequent issues.

The Acetylator Genes and Drug Response, by Wendell W. Weber. Published by Oxford University Press, 200 Madison Ave., New York, NY 10016, 1987. xiii + 248 p. Price $49.95.

Modern Nutrition in Health and Disease, Seventh Edition, edited by Maurice E. Shils and Vernon R. Young. Published by Lea & Febiger, 600 Washington Square, Philadelphia, PA 19106-4198, 1988. xx + 1694 p. Price $75.

Therapeutic Drug Monitoring: A Guide to Clinical Application, by Mary H. Diers Caviness, Janis J. MacKichan, Michael B. Bottorff et al. Published by Abbott Laboratories, Diagnostic Division, 1921 Hurd St., P.O. Box 152020, Irving, TX 75015-2020, 1987. xiv + 438 p. Price $25; $20/copy for quantities of 14 or more.

Advertising Index

Aid to Higher Education Campaign
Institutional, 266
American College of Clinical Pharmacy
9th Annual Meeting, 266
American Society of Hospital Pharmacists
Handbook on Extemporaneous Formulations, 330
Position Available, 264
Beecham Laboratories
Ticar, 325
Timentin, 258–260
Knoll Pharmaceuticals
Rythmol, 270
Eli Lilly and Company
Nebcin, 261–262
Tazidime, 255–256
Partnership for a Drug-Free America
Institutional, 257
Roxane Laboratories, A Boehringer Ingelheim Company
Computer Program, 263
E. R. Squibb & Sons, Inc.
Azactam, 249–252
Stuart Pharmaceuticals, Division of ICI Americas, Inc.
Cefotan, inside back cover, outside back cover
The Upjohn Company
Cleocin, 267–268
Veterans Administration Medical Center (Bronx)
Positions Available, 328
Wyeth Laboratories
Tubex, inside front cover

When it comes to taking their medicine, some patients need—

SPECIAL DELIVERY

INTENSOL™

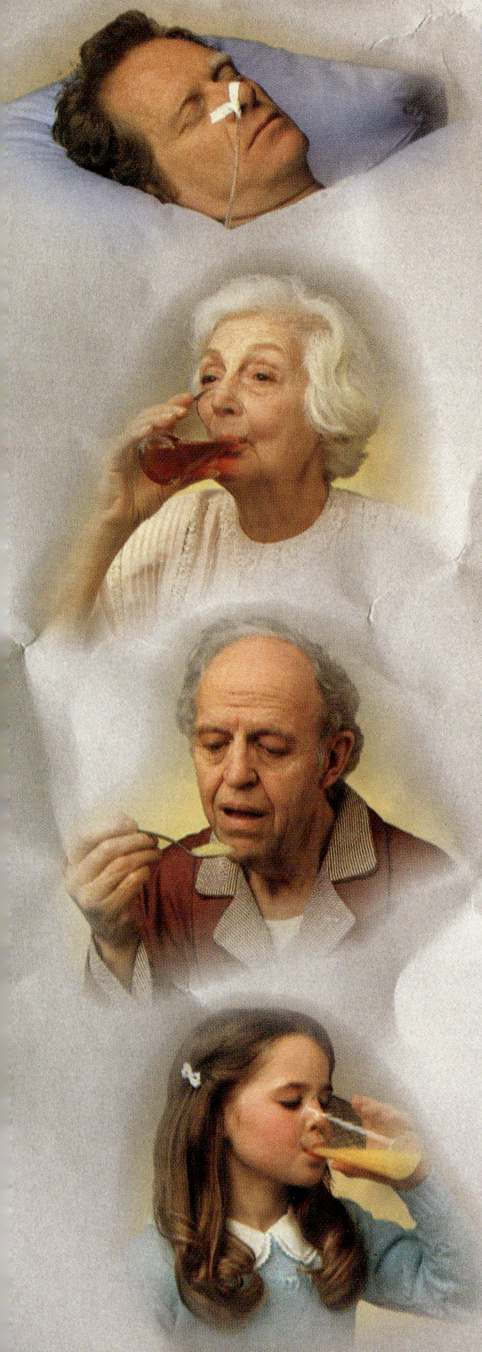

For patients who have difficulty with tablets

The nasogastric patient
The elderly or debilitated patient
The cancer patient on high or variable doses
The pediatric patient

Concentrated oral solutions

Intensols are highly concentrated medications—Chlorpromazine, Dexamethasone, DHT, Hydrochlorothiazide, Prednisone, Thioridazine, to name a few—in low volume solutions.

Easier than swallowing tablets

Intensols can be mixed with juice or semisolid foods, or even administered through nasogastric tubing.

Most Intensols have no flavor, so medications taste like the food or liquid they are mixed with. Each bottle comes with a calibrated dropper for easy dosage titration.

Easy to dispense

- Every dose is accurate.
- Ends the need to crush or break tablets—yielding inexact doses.
- Enhances patient compliance.
- Eliminates pharmacy compounding.

INTENSOLS...
A SPECIAL DELIVERY SYSTEM
for special patients.

Roxane Laboratories, Inc.
Columbus, Ohio 43216

Intensols for your special patients

To find out more about INTENSOLS for your patients, fill out the following and mail to: Roxane Laboratories, Inc., PO Box 16532, Columbus, Ohio 43216.

Name

Address

Specialty

News

Report supports FDA's bioequivalence evaluation criteria, advocates more stringent statistical testing

Major changes are not needed in FDA's process for approving generic drug products, according to a report issued on February 11 by the Bioequivalence Task Force assembled by FDA. The task force was formed to review issues raised at a hearing on the bioequivalence of immediate-release solid oral dosage forms held September 29–October 1, 1986. More than 800 representatives of academia, the pharmaceutical industry, the medical profession, and government attended the hearing. The task force concluded that FDA's guiding principle that "drug products delivering comparable blood levels of a therapeutic substance yield comparable therapeutic results" is scientifically sound. Moreover, the report supports FDA's assertion that if a product is deemed by FDA to be therapeutically equivalent, a physician "can feel secure that authorizing substitution of that product for any other therapeutically equivalent drug will provide the same intended effect."

Criteria for Bioequivalence Decisions. The task force recommended that bioequivalence decisions should be made using a 90% confidence interval based on the two one-sided *t* test method rather than the 75/75 rule. According to the 75/75 rule, a generic product is bioequivalent if at least 75% of subjects achieve drug concentrations in blood that are 75% to 125% of those achieved with the original (reference) product. The task force also concluded that for some drugs or drug classes, clinical evidence may indicate a need for requirements that are more stringent than the generally applied rule requiring mean values to be within ±20% of the values determined for the reference product. The report stated that FDA should consider using as an "additional nonstatistical criterion" a mean difference in area-under-the-curve of ±10%; however, the task force concluded that this additional criterion is not essential to ensuring generic drug bioequivalence. As reported by the task force, the mean difference in bioavailability between generic and innovator products approved during a two-year period (since 1962, under the Waxman–Hatch bill) was 3.5%; 80% of the values for generic drugs approved since 1984 are within 5% of the reference value. Although current requirements were considered adequate for ensuring quality and uniformity of drug products, variability among products and the treatment of outliers were deemed to deserve further study by FDA's Division of Biometrics.

Regulatory Aspects. According to the task force, FDA's criteria for bioequivalence decisions, including exceptions for which standards are either more or less stringent, should be made widely available. Publication of a formal guideline or a supplement to *Approved Drug Products with Therapeutic Equivalence Evaluations* (FDA's list of therapeutic equivalents, commonly known as the Orange Book) was suggested as a means for providing full information on evaluation procedures and decision criteria. The task force stated that the Orange Book format should be modified so the basis of drug ratings (in vivo bioequivalence studies or in vitro dissolution testing) could be determined. The task force also recommended that the Orange Book be advertised more widely to pharmacists.

According to the report, FDA should encourage marketing of fully bioavailable products when the innovator product is poorly bioavailable and the generic product "matches the bioavailability of a more fully bioavailable formulation and produces blood levels equivalent to those of the innovator product when given at a lower dose." However, such products would not be considered to be bioequivalent to the innovator product. According to the report, the number of poorly bioavailable products currently on the market is small.

Development of a detailed method for identifying and investigating clusters of reports of therapeutic failures with a given product was urged by the task force. The goal of such a program would be distinguishing consistent patterns of poor product performance from isolated cases of therapeutic failure.

Design of Bioequivalence Studies. The task force concluded that single-dose studies are adequate for most drugs and that use of both a solution and the innovator product as reference standards is generally not required. Use of a solution is necessary only when the relative bioavailability of a product is unknown or the bioavailability is known to be poor. Metabolite concentrations should be determined if the metabolite's pharmacologic effects are clinically important. According to the report, it is preferable to perform bioequivalence tests on healthy volunteers, but FDA should be prepared to act on "any credible leads" indicating that patient-specific factors not accounted for in current testing methods may affect bioequivalence results. The use of an alternate study design to determine intrasubject variability is being considered.

As stated in the report, in vitro dissolution testing is important in ensuring lot-to-lot uniformity and in supporting the acceptability of minor changes in drug products, but no particular dissolution pattern has been shown to ensure bioequivalence. Dissolution testing can be used for drugs that have established in vivo–in vitro relationships. It is also used for drugs approved before 1962 if bioavailability problems are not suspected or are

Continued on page 337

Continued from page 334

considered to be unlikely. In vivo bioequivalence testing is required for at least one strength of all other solid oral drugs. The task force reaffirmed the soundness of FDA's policy on in vivo testing, which applies to both generic and innovator products: "If a product meets in vivo bioequivalence study requirements at one strength, and the formulations of additional strengths are proportional to the strength tested in the in vivo bioequivalence study, and the additional strengths meet dissolution requirements, then further in vivo equivalence studies are not required for the additional strengths unless there is evidence of safety or efficacy problems."

Regulatory Issues. The report recommended further discussion of the need for bioequivalence studies of reformulated products. In general, FDA waives the requirement for in vivo evidence of bioequivalence for "minor" changes in formulation (e.g., color). However, there is no clear distinction between major and minor reformulations, and a series of minor reformulations could mimic the effect of a major reformulation.

With respect to the effect of excipients on bioavailability, the task force stated that the effects of excipients is assessed by current bioequivalence studies and that voluntary labeling guidelines will alert patients to the drug's allergenic potential.

Copies of the Report by the Bioequivalence Task Force on Recommendations from the Bioequivalence Hearing Conducted by the Food and Drug Administration can be obtained by writing to the Dockets Management Branch (HFA-305), Room 4-62, 5600 Fishers Lane, Rockville, MD 20857. Two self-addressed adhesive labels should be submitted with the written request.

FDA approves treatment IND protocol for trimetrexate

An approved treatment investigational new drug (IND) protocol for trimetrexate will allow more widespread use of the drug by AIDS patients with *Pneumocystis carinii* pneumonia who develop severe or life-threatening adverse reactions to pentamidine and trimethoprim-sulfamethoxazole; the approval was announced by FDA on February 19. The drug will be available from the National Institute of Allergy and Infectious Diseases (NIAID) to patients who meet the protocol criteria. Details of the distribution program can be obtained by contacting the NIAID hotline at 1-800-426-7527 (or 1-800-833-0014 in Michigan).

Trimetrexate, a quinazolone analogue of methotrexate, was synthesized in 1969 by scientists at Warner-Lambert Company and was developed as an antineoplastic agent. The potential for use of trimetrexate in the treatment of *P. carinii* pneumonia was proposed by NIAID scientists in 1985. Trimetrexate inhibits both mammalian and protozoan dihydrofolate reductase. Leucovorin is given with trimetrexate to protect mammalian cells. Both drugs will be supplied by the NIAID.

The treatment IND regulations permitting broader use of investigational drugs in certain circumstances became effective in June 1987. The trimetrexate treatment protocol is the third to be approved under these regulations. Two requests were approved in the fourth quarter of 1987. One permits use of cytomegalovirus immune globulin to prevent cytomegalovirus infection in renal transplant recipients; the other permits use of certain four-drug regimens containing ifosfamide and mesna in the treatment of refractory germ cell carcinoma. According to FDA Commissioner Frank E. Young, 12 applications for treatment IND status have been submitted to FDA. Of these, three have been approved, two did not meet the criteria for FDA review, one is under discussion with the sponsor, and six are on "clinical hold" because of insufficient data on efficacy or safety.

Focus of new FDA division is AIDS, opportunistic infections

A new division, the Division of Anti-Viral Drug Products, will be created within FDA's Center for Drug Evaluation and Research. The unit will be responsible for reviewing all antiviral drugs and all other antimicrobial agents that are potential treatments for AIDS-related opportunistic infections. Other antimicrobial agents will remain under the purview of FDA's Division of Anti-Infective Drug Products. Establishment of a division within the Center for Biologic Evaluation and Research for reviewing AIDS-related biological products is under consideration.

FDA challenges Alzheimer's disease study findings

FDA has challenged the findings of a preliminary study[1] examining the efficacy of tetrahydroaminoacridine (THA) in patients with Alzheimer's disease. An audit conducted by the agency failed to locate all data supporting the researchers' reported findings of symptomatic improvement with THA and raised questions as to the adequacy of the double-blinding procedures. Letters published in the June 18, 1987, issue of the *New England Journal of Medicine* also were critical of the methodology and the analysis and reporting of data. All issues raised by FDA investigators have not yet been resolved.

This preliminary study was an impetus for a multicenter study begun in September 1987. The larger clinical trial was halted by FDA after two months because of evidence of hepatotoxicity in 20% of patients. Since that time FDA has approved resumption of the study at a lower dose. Theoretical support for a possible beneficial effect of THA on Alzheimer's disease is provided by the drug's ability to enhance cholinergic activity.

1. Summers WK, Majovski LV, Marsh GM et al. Oral tetrahydroaminoacridine in long-term treatment of senile dementia, Alzheimer type. *N Engl J Med*. 1986; 312:1241–5.

Study suggests limited role for comprehensive toxicology testing in drug overdoses

Discordance between clinical impression and toxicology test results is relatively frequent, according to results

Continued on page 340

B fragilis group activity...

THE UNSURPASSED β-LACTAM CHOICE

TIMENTIN® ticarcillin disodium/ clavulanate potassium

B fragilis group coverage superior to cephalosporins and penicillins

Susceptibility Pattern (%) of 531 *B fragilis* Group Isolates in a Nationwide *in vitro Study[1]**

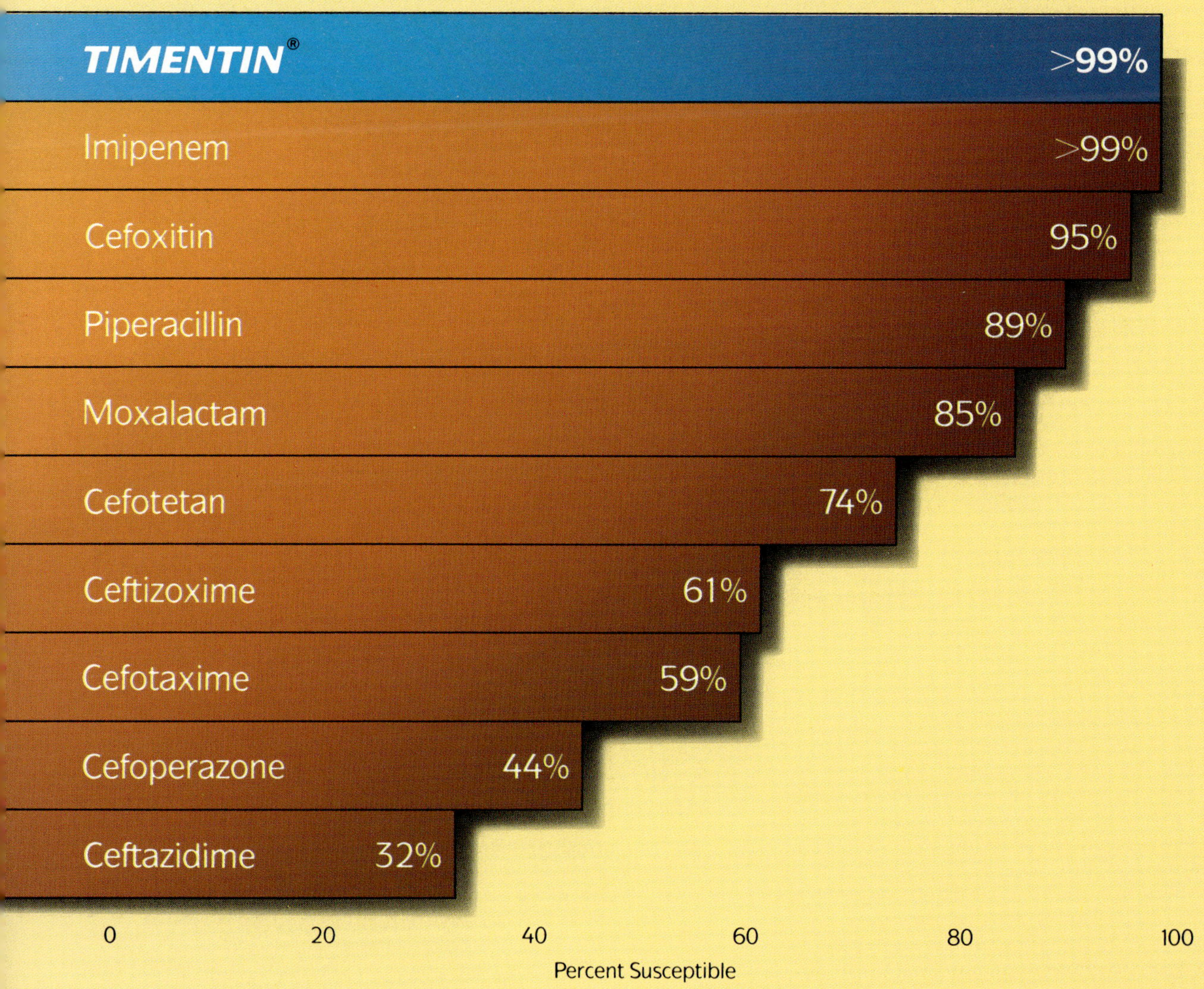

**In vitro* activity does not necessarily imply *in vivo* efficacy.

More active *in vitro** than traditional antianaerobic agents

Activity Against Clinical Isolates of *B fragilis* Group[2]		
Antibiotic	MIC_{50} (μg/mL)	MIC_{90} (μg/mL)
TIMENTIN†	≤1	4
Cefoxitin	8	32
Cefoperazone	32	128
Chloramphenicol	8	8
Clindamycin	0.5	8
Metronidazole	1	2

**In vitro* activity does not necessarily imply *in vivo* efficacy.
†Ticarcillin in the presence of a constant 2 μg/mL clavulanic acid.

More active *in vitro** than cefoxitin

Activity Against *B fragilis* Group[3]		
Organism (No. strains)	MIC_{90} (μg/mL) TIMENTIN†	Cefoxitin
B fragilis (32)	0.5	16
B vulgatus (21)	1	16
B thetaiotaomicron (19)	2	32
B ovatus (16)	1	32
B distasonis (13)	8	64

**In vitro* activity does not necessarily imply *in vivo* efficacy.
†Ticarcillin in the presence of a constant 1 μg/mL clavulanic acid.

Destroys β-lactamases that limit the usefulness of other β-lactam choices

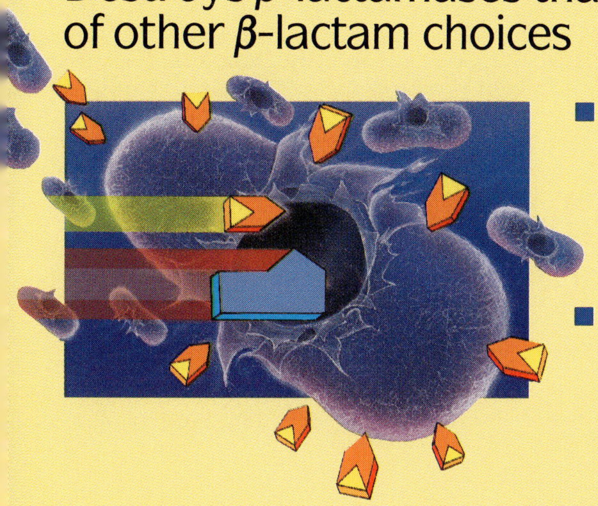

- "Most (90 percent) strains of B. fragilis produce constitutive beta-lactamases, which are primarily cephalosporinases. All other Bacteroides species probably produce beta-lactamases, but controversy exists concerning whether the enzymes are predominantly penicillinases or cephalosporinases."[4]
- "[Clavulanate potassium] inhibits the beta-lactamases of most Bacteroides species."[4]

△ Clavulanate potassium destroys most β-lactamases produced by Gram-positive and Gram-negative aerobes and anaerobes.
TIMENTIN destroys a broad range of aerobic and anaerobic bacteria regardless of β-lactamase production.

FOR ANAEROBIC CERTAINTY

TIMENTIN®

ticarcillin disodium/ clavulanate potassium

The unsurpassed β-lactam choice

Usual Dosage: 3.1 g every 4 to 6 hours.

Please see next page for brief summary of prescribing information.

THE CLAVULANATES Beecham laboratories BRISTOL, TENNESSEE 37620

© 1988, Beecham Laboratories.

BRIEF SUMMARY OF PRESCRIBING INFORMATION

TIMENTIN®

sterile ticarcillin disodium and clavulanate potassium

for Intravenous Administration

INDICATIONS AND USAGE: TIMENTIN® is indicated in the treatment of infections caused by susceptible strains of the designated organisms in the conditions listed below:

Bacterial Septicemia: including bacteremia, caused by β-lactamase producing strains of *Klebsiella* spp., *E. coli, Staphylococcus aureus* and *Pseudomonas aeruginosa* (and other *Pseudomonas* species).

Lower Respiratory Infections: caused by β-lactamase producing strains of *Staphylococcus aureus, Hemophilus influenzae* and *Klebsiella* spp.

Bone and Joint Infections: caused by β-lactamase producing strains of *Staphylococcus aureus*.

Skin and Skin Structure Infections: caused by β-lactamase producing strains of *Staphylococcus aureus, Klebsiella* spp., and *E. coli*.

Urinary Tract Infections (complicated and uncomplicated): caused by β-lactamase-producing strains of *E. coli, Klebsiella* spp., *Pseudomonas aeruginosa* (and other *Pseudomonas* species), *Citrobacter* spp., *Enterobacter cloacae, Serratia marcescens*, and *Staphylococcus aureus*. While TIMENTIN is indicated only for the conditions listed above, infections caused by ticarcillin susceptible organisms are also amenable to TIMENTIN treatment due to its ticarcillin content. Therefore, mixed infections caused by ticarcillin susceptible organisms and β-lactamase producing organisms susceptible to TIMENTIN should not require the addition of another antibiotic.

Appropriate culture and susceptibility tests should be performed before treatment in order to isolate and identify organisms causing infection and to determine their susceptibility to TIMENTIN. Because of its broad spectrum of bactericidal activity against Gram-positive and Gram-negative bacteria, TIMENTIN is particularly useful for the treatment of mixed infections and for presumptive therapy prior to the identification of the causative organisms. TIMENTIN has been shown to be effective as single drug therapy in the treatment of some serious infections where normally combination antibiotic therapy might be employed. Therapy with TIMENTIN may be initiated before results of such tests are known when there is reason to believe the infection may involve any of the β-lactamase producing organisms listed above; however, once these results become available, appropriate therapy should be continued.

Based on the *in vitro* synergism between TIMENTIN and aminoglycosides against certain strains of *Pseudomonas aeruginosa*, combined therapy has been successful, especially in patients with impaired host defenses. Both drugs should be used in full therapeutic doses. As soon as results of culture and susceptibility tests become available, antimicrobial therapy should be adjusted as indicated.

CONTRAINDICATIONS: TIMENTIN is contraindicated in patients with a history of hypersensitivity reactions to any of the penicillins.

WARNINGS: SERIOUS AND OCCASIONALLY FATAL HYPERSENSITIVITY (ANAPHYLACTOID) REACTIONS HAVE BEEN REPORTED IN PATIENTS ON PENICILLIN THERAPY. THESE REACTIONS ARE MORE LIKELY TO OCCUR IN INDIVIDUALS WITH A HISTORY OF PENICILLIN HYPERSENSITIVITY AND/OR A HISTORY OF SENSITIVITY TO MULTIPLE ALLERGENS. THERE HAVE BEEN REPORTS OF INDIVIDUALS WITH A HISTORY OF PENICILLIN HYPERSENSITIVITY WHO HAVE EXPERIENCED SEVERE REACTIONS WHEN TREATED WITH CEPHALOSPORINS. BEFORE INITIATING THERAPY WITH TIMENTIN, CAREFUL INQUIRY SHOULD BE MADE CONCERNING PREVIOUS HYPERSENSITIVITY REACTIONS TO PENICILLINS, CEPHALOSPORINS, OR OTHER DRUGS. IF AN ALLERGIC REACTION OCCURS, TIMENTIN SHOULD BE DISCONTINUED AND THE APPROPRIATE THERAPY INSTITUTED. **SERIOUS ANAPHYLACTOID REACTIONS REQUIRE IMMEDIATE EMERGENCY TREATMENT WITH EPINEPHRINE. OXYGEN, INTRAVENOUS STEROIDS, AND AIRWAY MANAGEMENT, INCLUDING INTUBATION, SHOULD ALSO BE PROVIDED AS INDICATED.**

PRECAUTIONS: While TIMENTIN possesses the characteristic low toxicity of the penicillin group of antibiotics, organ system functions should be assessed periodically during therapy.

Bleeding manifestations have occurred in some patients receiving β-lactam antibiotics. These reactions have been associated with abnormalities of coagulation tests such as clotting time, platelet aggregation and prothrombin time and are more likely to occur in patients with renal impairment. If bleeding manifestations appear, TIMENTIN treatment should be discontinued and appropriate therapy instituted.

TIMENTIN has only rarely been reported to cause hypokalemia. Periodic monitoring of serum potassium may be advisable in patients receiving prolonged therapy.

Pregnancy (Category B): Reproduction studies have been performed in rats given doses up to 1050 mg/kg/day and have revealed no evidence of impaired fertility or harm to the fetus due to TIMENTIN. There are, however, no adequate and well-controlled studies in pregnant women. Because animal reproduction studies are not always predictive of human response, this drug should be used during pregnancy only if clearly needed.

DOSAGE AND ADMINISTRATION: TIMENTIN should be administered by intravenous infusion (30 min.). Usual recommended dose for systemic and urinary tract infections for average (60 kg) adults is 3.1 Gm TIMENTIN (3.1 Gm vial containing 3 Gm ticarcillin and 100 mg clavulanic acid) given every 4 to 6 hours. In urinary tract infections, a dosage of 3.2 Gm TIMENTIN (3.2 Gm vial containing 3 Gm ticarcillin and 200 mg clavulanic acid) given every 8 hours is adequate. Please see official package insert for details on dosages for other patients, including those with renal insufficiency, and directions for use.

SUPPLIED: 3.1 Gm and 3.2 Gm Standard Vials; 3.1 Gm and 3.2 Gm Piggyback Bottles: 31 Gm Bulk Pharmacy Package: 3.1 Gm ADD-Vantage™ Antibiotic Vial.

7548/E-BS

References

1. Cuchural GJ, Tally FP, Jacobus NV, et al: Susceptibility of Bacteroides fragilis group clinical isolates to newer beta-lactam drugs, abstract No. 1B8. Presented to the 3rd Panamerican Congress of Infectious Diseases and Chemotherapy, San Juan, Puerto Rico, Dec 9-13, 1986.
2. Barry AL, Jones RN, Packer RR: *In vitro* susceptibility of the *Bacteroides fragilis* group to cefoperazone, ampicillin, ticarcillin, and amoxycillin combined with β-lactamase inhibitors. *J Antimicrob Chemother* 1986;17:125-127.
3. Bourgault AM, Lamothe F: In-vitro activity of amoxycillin and ticarcillin in combination with clavulanic acid compared with that of new β-lactam agents against species of the *Bacteroides fragilis* group. *J Antimicrob Chemother* 1986;17:593-603.
4. Neu HC: Contribution of beta-lactamases to bacterial resistance and mechanisms to inhibit beta-lactamases. *Am J Med* 1985;79(suppl 5B):2-12.

Beecham laboratories

BRISTOL, TENNESSEE 37620

© 1988, Beecham Laboratories.

News *Continued from page 337*

of a retrospective review of 209 cases of intentional drug overdose.[1] The investigator suggested that laboratory tests could be used more selectively without compromising patient care.

Medical records of patients who took overdoses of drugs having the potential to cause acute deterioration of respiratory, cardiovascular, or neurologic function or multiple-drug overdoses involving acetaminophen were reviewed. Toxicology tests were performed in 198 of 209 overdoses. Laboratory results and clinical impression of the ingested drug were in accordance in 47% of cases, at least one clinically suspected drug was not confirmed in 25% of cases, at least one drug not suspected clinically was reported by the laboratory in 14% of cases, and both types of discordance were present in 14% of cases. A clinically unsuspected drug was found in 54 of 198 cases. In eight of these cases, the unsuspected drug was the only laboratory finding. The investigator detected a change in patient management because of an unexpected laboratory result in only three cases; all three involved alkalinization or forced diuresis for barbiturate overdoses. Institution of therapy specific for the ingested drug did not appear to substantially affect patient outcome. These findings prompted Brett to conclude that comprehensive toxicology analysis has a limited role in many overdoses. According to Brett, general toxicology screens are useful in determining the cause of unexplained alterations in mental status and also are valuable in seriously ill patients who have taken overdoses, but the overall focus of toxicology testing should be drugs for which specific therapies are available.

1. Brett AS. Implications of discordance between clinical impression and toxicology analysis in drug overdose. *Arch Intern Med.* 1988; 148:437–41.

News Brief

• FDA has withdrawn marketing approval for certain combinations of **amphotericin B and tetracycline** (Mysteclin F capsules and syrup, E. R. Squibb & Sons, Inc.); evidence of efficacy for the labeled indication, prevention of candidal disease attributable to antibiotic therapy, was lacking. Approval of 14 antifungal–antibiotic combination products was withdrawn in 1985.

Upcoming Specialty Meetings

International Convocation on Immunology (11th) . . . June 12–16 . . . Buffalo, NY . . . contact: J. F. Mohn, Ernest Witebsky Center for Immunology, 240 Sherman Hall, State University of New York at Buffalo, Buffalo, NY 14214; 716-831-2848.

The Johns Hopkins Graduate Summer Program in Epidemiology—1988 . . . June 20–July 8 . . . Baltimore, MD . . . contact: Helen Walters, Program Coordinator, Graduate Summer Program in Epidemiology, 615 North Wolfe Street, Baltimore, MD 21205; 301-955-7158.

Second International Congress on Cancer Pain . . . July 14–17 . . . Rye, NY . . . contact: Mary Callaway, Executive Director, Second International Congress on Cancer Pain, 1275 York Avenue, Box 52, Room C799, New York, NY 10021; 212-794-7456.

Does so much for so much less than cefoxitin

In a 900-bed hospital, CEFOTAN 1 or 2 g every 12 hours replaced cefoxitin 1 or 2 g every 6 to 8 hours. During the course of the year that CEFOTAN was added to formulary, patients were prospectively monitored for efficacy and side effects. Two retrospective audits were also conducted. Results indicated comparable efficacy and incidence of coagulopathies in CEFOTAN- and cefoxitin-treated groups.

Cost advantages also seen over other antibiotics

One retrospective audit reviewed patients treated with CEFOTAN or an aminoglycoside administered with clindamycin or mezlocillin.

Clinical outcomes were similar; however, analysis showed that CEFOTAN was the least costly antibiotic regimen.

$124,961

actual annual savings over cefoxitin

After one year of cefoxitin formulary replacement with CEFOTAN, the savings realized at this hospital amounted to $124,961.

Substantial savings with CEFOTAN

Cefoxitin CEFOTAN

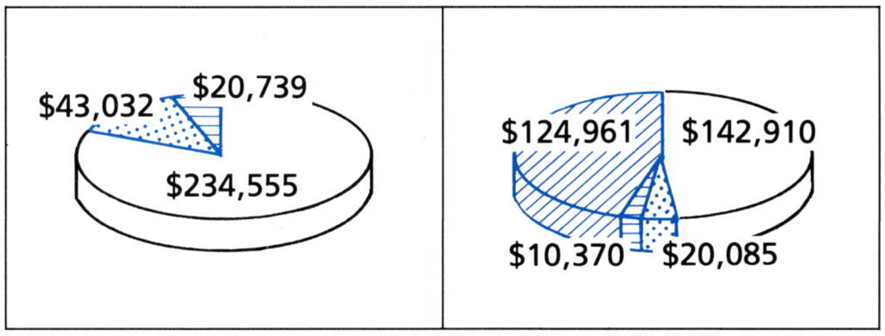

TOTAL COST = $298,326 TOTAL COST = $173,365

DRUG COST SUPPLY COST LABOR COST SAVINGS

—adapted from Nightingale et al, Figure 1

In intra-abdominal and gynecologic infection due to indicated organisms

CEFOTAN® IM/IV
(cefotetan disodium)

Does so much for so much less than cefoxitin.

REFERENCE: Nightingale CH, Smith KS, Quintiliani R, et al: The conversion of cefoxitin usage to cefotetan: An interdisciplinary approach. *Am J Surg*, submitted for publication.

© 1988 ICI Americas Inc

Therapy Consultation

The Therapy Consultation *section provides brief advice, in question-and-answer format, on how to handle specific drug-therapy problems. Readers are invited to submit questions, which will be referred to a consultant for an answer. The problems should not be highly specialized or unusual, nor should they be mundane. Questions are answered briefly, based largely on the judgment and personal experience of the consultant, although selected references may be cited to substantiate the consultant's advice.*

Assistance in identifying Therapy Consultation *topics is provided by the drug information centers at the following institutions: Albert B. Chandler Medical Center and College of Pharmacy, University of Kentucky, Lexington; Arizona Health Sciences Center, Tucson; Medical College of Virginia Hospitals, Richmond; University of California Medical Center, San Diego; and University of Michigan Medical Center, Ann Arbor.*

Topical cromolyn sodium for recurrent aphthous ulcers

Question: Is the topical use of cromolyn sodium an alternative to topical administration of tetracycline or corticosteroids in patients with recurrent aphthous ulcers?

Answer: Most reports of topical cromolyn sodium use in dermatology are anecdotal cases. A few controlled evaluations with inconclusive results have been reported. In practice, cromolyn sodium is rarely used and is considered only when other modalities have failed.

Although multiple local and systemic factors have been identified in triggering aphthous ulcer formation, the etiology is not well understood. Patients often note a painful area of erythema, either flat or indurated, for one to three days before ulceration. Lesions are most painful for the first two to three days after ulcer formation. Discomfort typically persists for 15 days thereafter. Various microorganisms have been isolated from lesions; *Streptococcus sanguis* has been noted most frequently and has been hypothesized to produce a delayed hypersensitivity response in patients with recurrent aphthae. The initial ulceration is thought to result from a cell-mediated immune reaction but is apparently not influenced by cromolyn sodium.[1] Mast cells appear in large numbers in the early stages of ulcer formation and decrease, presumably via degranulation, during the most painful phase.[1,2] Cromolyn sodium is hypothesized to reduce pain from ulcers by inhibiting release of histamine, slow-reacting substance of anaphylaxis (SRS-A), and other mediators from mast cells.[1,2]

Two randomized double-blind, placebo-controlled, crossover trials have evaluated lozenge formulations of cromolyn in patients with recurrent aphthous ulcers.[1,2] Kowolik et al.[2] compared disodium cromoglycate as a 20-mg lozenge given four times a day with placebo in 21 patients. Patients were randomly assigned to receive either disodium cromoglycate or placebo for six weeks and then were crossed over to the alternate treatment for six weeks. No significant difference in relief of pain or number of new lesions was noted between the placebo and disodium cromoglycate treatment periods. However the group receiving placebo followed by disodium cromoglycate showed more ulcer-free days ($p < 0.05$). Rash and a tight feeling in the chest were noted in two patients on active medication. No other adverse effects were reported. Further investigation with higher doses of disodium cromoglycate is indicated.

Lozenges containing 200 mg of cromoglycic acid (the acid form of disodium cromoglycate) given four times a day were compared with a calcium phosphate placebo in a study reported by Dolby and Walker.[1] Fifteen patients received either active or placebo lozenges for 30 days; after a 14-day washout period the alternate lozenge was given for 30 days. The number of very painful days was reduced significantly by cromoglycic acid, although the total number of ulcer-free days was not significantly different between the two groups. One patient experienced nausea from the taste of cromoglycic acid and withdrew from the trial. The authors stated that cromoglycic acid would be of considerable value in symptomatic treatment of recurrent aphthous ulcers in view of the adverse effects associated with topical corticosteroid therapy.

Other case reports note improvement in 91 of 154 patients with recurrent aphthous ulcers after using 2.5% cromolyn sodium (Intal, Fisons Corporation) incorporated into toothpaste three times a day.[3,4] Treatment failures and variable results in these reports may be attributed to the various salts and formulations used. Frost[4] noted improvement in 17 of 31 nonresponders when patients rinsed with a soap mouthwash before using cromolyn toothpaste. Presumably, this maintained the cromolyn in an acid form for better absorption.[4] Effectiveness of cromolyn may also be limited by the poor rate of absorption through the oral mucosa.[1] The phase of ulceration in which the patient initiates treatment may also influence the results. This factor was not addressed by any of the investigators.

Continued on page 346

OW AVAILABLE IN
UNIT DOSE PACKAGING.

EPITOL™

CARBAMAZEPINE TABLETS, USP 200MG

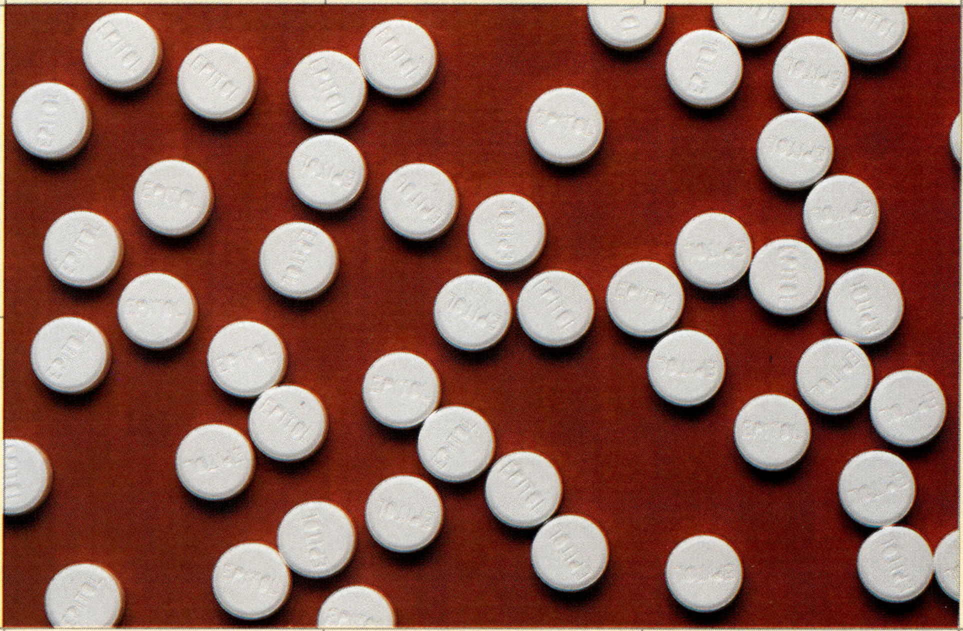

- Available for immediate delivery through your local wholesaler or direct from LEMMON.
- Available in both Unit Dose and bulk packaging.
- Full bioequivalency data available upon request.

Epitol Tablets
200mg
NDC 0093-0090-01
100's

Epitol Tablets
200mg
NDC 0093-0090-05
500's

Epitol Tablets
200mg
NDC 0093-0090-10
1000's

Epitol Tablets
200mg
NDC 0093-0090-93
U/D 100's

QUALITY • PURITY • SERVICE
LEMMON

LEMMON COMPANY
Sellersville, PA 18960
CALL TOLL FREE 800-523-6542
IN PENNSYLVANIA 215-723-5544

CLINICAL PHARMACISTS
SAUDI ARABIA

EXCELLENT TAX FREE SALARIES, plus free accommodation and flights, generous vacation, good recreational facilities and other substantial benefits in accordance with international company practice are offered.

REZAYAT MEDICAL SERVICES have been awarded a prestigious hospital contract for a new 380 bed referral hospital in Saudi Arabia, constructed and equipped to the highest international standards. Your skills are urgently required to contribute to these high standards in care and expertise.

Send your résumé and copy of your qualification certificate(s) to **Janet Grieve, c/o Rezayat America Inc., 5177 Richmond Avenue, Suite 780, Houston, Texas 77056.**

An Equal Opportunity Employer

Therapy Consultation *Continued from page 344*

Numerous other therapies for aphthous ulcers, such as topical tetracycline, chlorhexidine, or corticosteroids, have been explored.[5] These agents are not curative, but they are considered standards of therapy and are widely used. Despite somewhat positive results seen with cromolyn sodium, cost–benefit comparison to other regimens for recurrent aphthous ulcers precludes routine use.

1. Dolby AE, Walker DM. A trial of cromoglycic acid in recurrent aphthous ulceration. *Br J Oral Surg*. 1975; 12:292–5.
2. Kwolik MJ, Muir KF, MacPhee IT. Di-sodium cromoglycate in the treatment of recurrent aphthous ulceration. *Br Dent J*. 1978; 144:384–6.
3. Frost M. Cromoglycate in aphthous stomatitis. *Lancet*. 1973; 2:389. Letter.
4. Frost M. Cromoglycate in aphthous stomatitis. *Br Dent J*. 1978; 144:269. Letter.
5. Rennie JS, Reade PC, Scully C. Recurrent aphthous stomatitis. *Br Dent J*. 1985; 159:361–8.

JEAN RUMSFIELD, PHARM.D.

Clinical Assistant Professor
Department of Dermatology
College of Medicine
University of Illinois
Chicago, IL 60680

Medical Information Scientist
GenDerm Corporation
Northbrook, IL 60062

ARE YOU READY TO BE CHALLENGED?

The U.S. Public Health Service has just the pharmacy opportunities you're looking for...

- ☐ Prescriptive authority.
- ☐ Diversity of assignments.
- ☐ Patient counseling.
- ☐ Team partnership on clinical rounds.
- ☐ Advice on drug regimens.
- ☐ Opportunities for advancement.

If you're an entry-level pharmacist who wants to be on the leading edge, practicing high-tech pharmacy at its best, call us.

We need you in many areas: INDIAN HEALTH SERVICE, FOOD & DRUG ADMINISTRATION AND NATIONAL INSTITUTES OF HEALTH. And we have clinical, regulatory, administrative and research positions available nationwide.

Call or write Pharmacist Recruitment Officer
RM 7A-39 Parklawn Building
5600 Fishers Lane
Rockville, Maryland 20857
(301) 443-5740
U.S. Public Health Service

Therapy Review

Parenteral nutrition in pediatric patients

EMILY B. COCHRAN, STEPHANIE J. PHELPS, AND RICHARD A. HELMS

Abstract: Protein, calorie, fluid, fat, and micronutrient requirements of pediatric patients are reviewed, as are methods of nutritional assessment and complications associated with the use of parenteral nutrition in these patients.

In general, preterm infants and neonates require greater per-kilogram amounts of protein, calories, fluid, and micronutrients than older children. In addition, preterm infants and neonates have deficiencies in enzymes that metabolize certain amino acids, making otherwise nonessential amino acids essential. These unique protein needs have been addressed in amino acid formulations designed specifically for this group of patients. Supplying the neonate with the calcium and phosphorus needed for bone growth can be difficult because of solubility limitations in parenteral nutrient solutions. The use of intravenous fat emulsion in infants with hyperbilirubinemia or pulmonary complications is controversial. However, only rarely does fat emulsion have to be completely withheld. Complications associated with parenteral nutrition in pediatric patients include infection, metabolic disorders (cholestasis, bone demineralization), and mechanical problems. Cholestasis induced by parenteral nutrition has been shown to be more common in low-birth-weight infants; however, the precise etiology is unknown and may be multifactorial.

Basic requirements necessary to promote growth while pediatric patients are receiving parenteral nutrition have been determined. However, current studies are challenging what were thought to be standards of pediatric parenteral nutrition therapy.

Index terms: Age; Amino acids; Caloric agents; Contraindications; Fat emulsions; Hyperbilirubinemia; Nutrition; Pediatrics; Proteins; Toxicity; Weight
Clin Pharm. 1988; 7:351–66

The first report of the successful use of total parenteral nutrition in an infant appeared in 1944.[1] Since that time, recommendations for the amount of calories, protein, and micronutrients to be provided to pediatric patients have been developed, allowing practitioners to individualize parenteral nutrition based on age, weight, nutritional status, and disease. Essential macronutrient and micronutrient needs of pediatric patients continue to be studied and have resulted in the development of new products and the recognition of the essentiality of nutrients previously thought to be nonessential. The development of laboratory techniques using small sample volumes allows the practitioner to monitor the efficacy and toxicity of parenteral nutrition routinely and enables the researcher to develop and study new products. This article will discuss current methods of nutritional assessment, determination of parenteral nutrient formulation, management and monitoring of pediatric patients receiving parenteral nutrition, and complications that may result from the use of parenteral nutrition.

EMILY B. COCHRAN, PHARM.D., is ASHP Research and Education Foundation Pediatric Pharmacotherapy Fellow, Department of Clinical Pharmacy, The University of Tennessee, Memphis, and Le Bonheur Children's Medical Center, Memphis. STEPHANIE J. PHELPS, PHARM.D., is Assistant Professor, Department of Clinical Pharmacy, The Center for Pediatric Pharmacokinetics and Therapeutics, The University of Tennessee, and Clinical Pharmacist, Le Bonheur Children's Medical Center. RICHARD A. HELMS, PHARM.D., is Associate Professor, Department of Clinical Pharmacy, The Center for Pediatric Pharmacokinetics and Therapeutics, and Director, Nutritional Support Services, Le Bonheur Children's Medical Center.

Address reprint requests to Dr. Helms at the Department of Clinical Pharmacy, 26 South Dunlap Street, Memphis, TN 39163.

Supported in part by a grant from the American Society of Hospital Pharmacists Research and Education Foundation, sponsored by McNeil Consumer Products, and a Center of Excellence grant from the state of Tennessee.

This is **article 680-204-8806** in the **ASHP Continuing Education System;** it qualifies for 1.0 hour of continuing-education credit. See page 402 for learning objectives and test questions.

Copyright © 1988, American Society of Hospital Pharmacists, Inc. All rights reserved. 0278-2677/88/0501-0351$04.00.

Nutritional Assessment

Nutritional status is assessed by evaluating weight, height, somatic and visceral proteins, and the body's ability to mount an immune response.[2–4] The initial physical examination can reveal important information about the nutritional status of a patient. For example, muscle wasting, edema, scaly skin, and dry or brittle hair may suggest protein-calorie malnutrition.[4] Changes in the oral mucosa, pale conjunctiva, pallor, growth retardation, and skin lesions may indicate vitamin or trace element deficiencies.[3–6]

Intake and Output. Weight and intake and output should be measured daily for all pediatric patients receiving parenteral nutrition. Infants should be weighed with the same amount of clothing and using the same scales each day. Addition or deletion of wound dressings or arm boards can alter the apparent weight of the small infant and may make interpretation of the change in weight difficult.

Intake consists of all fluids given to a patient, including maintenance fluids, replacement fluids, and medications. Output includes urine, stool, nasogastric tube or gastrostomy tube drainage, emesis, ventriculostomy drainage, and wound drainage. Urine and stool output can be measured by weighing diapers before and after elimination. Whenever possible, stool and urine amount should be recorded separately. Evaluation of daily weight and daily monitoring of total intake and output aid in assessing fluid balance and reflect the adequacy of nutritional support.

Growth Curves. Standards for height, weight, and head circumference derived from large populations of pediatric patients in the United States have been compiled in chart form, allowing data for an individual patient to be compared graphically to age-related population standards.[7] Information obtained from growth charts can be used for preliminary assessment of nutritional status and can aid in discriminating between acute and chronic malnutrition.[8] Weights below population standards are usually indicative of acute malnutrition, whereas chronic malnutrition is manifested by decreasing weight and height for age.[8] Growth charts are useful for longitudinal assessment of growth and response to parenteral nutrition.[9] Because frequent plotting of weight on growth charts can be cumbersome, average daily weight gains for a given age can be extrapolated from the growth chart. It is often necessary to evaluate weight change over several days, particularly in the neonate, because weights can fluctuate widely from day to day.

Anthropometric Measurements. Anthropometric measurements including subscapular skinfold thickness, triceps skinfold thickness, and midarm muscle circumference allow estimation of body fat and muscle mass. Like growth charts, these measurements have been compiled in population standards. An age-related nomogram was developed for arm circumference and triceps skinfold thickness from the United States Ten-State Nutrition Survey of 1968–70.[10] Using arm muscle area and triceps skinfold values determined from the nomogram, Frisancho[11] calculated age-related percentiles for arm muscle area, arm muscle diameter, and arm muscle circumference that can be used for a general assessment of nutritional status. Subscapular skinfold standards have also been developed based on data obtained for British children.[12] To ensure accuracy and minimize variability in consecutive measurements, the measurement site should be consistent, the appropriate caliper should be used, and the same person should measure an individual patient whenever possible. Because anthropometric measurements are not done routinely on all patients receiving parenteral nutrition, these standards are used less frequently than the standards for height and weight. However, when measurements are made appropriately, anthropometrics can be an effective means of monitoring response to parenteral nutrition.[9]

Visceral Proteins. Visceral protein markers include serum albumin, transferrin, transthyretin (prealbumin), and retinol-binding protein.[13] Although albumin and transferrin are used to assess nutritional status, they do not increase early in nutritional repletion because of the relatively long half-lives of 20 days[14] and 8 days,[15] respectively. On the other hand, transthyretin and retinol-binding protein have half-lives of 2 days[16] and 10 hours,[17] respectively, and therefore increase in response to nutritional support earlier. Transthyretin and retinol-binding protein increased after institution of nutritional supplementation in otherwise healthy appropriate-for-gestational-age infants[18] and premature infants,[19] as well as in critically ill malnourished infants receiving parenteral nutrition.[20] In the past, transthyretin was not used as a routine monitoring marker because the assay methodology was not readily available. Recently, a simplified, less expensive nephelometric prealbumin kit (PAB, Beckman Instruments, Inc., Brea, CA) was introduced that may increase the use of transthyretin as a monitoring marker in pediatric patients. If transthyretin levels are to be used to monitor response to nutritional repletion, measurements should be done upon initiation of parenteral nutrition and weekly until values are normal. Somatomedin-C[21] and fibronectin[22] levels have also been used to monitor response to nutritional repletion in adults, but their use has not been evaluated in children.

Urine Studies. Although a 24-hour urine collection for nitrogen balance is used routinely to assess response to nutritional support in adults,[23] problems exist when similar studies are attempted in neonates and infants.[24] To collect urine for 24 hours in uncatheterized infants, a urine collection bag must be placed around the infant's genital area with an adhesive and must remain in place for 24 hours. Problems with this procedure include collection bags that are too large for the infant, adhesives that do not stick properly, skin breakdown under the adhesive, and stool contamination of collected urine. During collections, a substantial amount of urine may be lost onto the preweighed diaper, which can be quantified by reweighing the wet diaper. In this case, determination of total urine nitrogen output must be extrapolated to the total volume of urine excreted. When 24-hour urine collections are difficult, a six-hour urine collection for urea nitrogen can be used to estimate nitrogen balance.[25] In spite of difficulties encountered with urine collections in infants, skilled nursing care and accurate record keeping allow these collections to be made and nitrogen balance to be calculated reliably.

Another method of determining adequacy of nutritional intake is the creatinine height index (CHI), which was designed to estimate relative muscle mass and reflect protein status. CHI is calculated as follows:[26]

CHI = 24-hour creatinine excretion (patient) / 24-hour creatinine excretion (normal for height)

Normal values for CHI approach 1 in children who are not malnourished and are less than 1 in children with protein–calorie malnutrition.[27] The CHI is not done routinely in infants because of the aforementioned difficulty with urine collections.

3-Methylhistidine, a byproduct of skeletal muscle catabolism, is excreted unchanged in the urine. Seashore et al.[28] studied healthy and stressed premature infants and found that a milligram ratio of 3-methylhistidine to creatinine excreted in 24 hours of 0.2 or less generally indicated normal metabolic status. Ratios greater than 0.2 were seen only in stressed patients or patients receiving inadequate calories.[28] The same problems with 24-hour urine collections that were discussed for nitrogen excretion also exist in the determination of 3-methylhistidine and creatinine excretion.

Immune Function. Total lymphocyte count and intradermal skin testing can partially assess the body's ability to mount an immune response and are used as indicators of nutritional status.[2,3] Helms and coworkers[29] reported improved lymphocyte function and enhanced expression of T-cell populations in malnourished infants less than three months of age who received parenteral nutrition. Because developmental and environmental factors determine immune function, lack of response to immunologic challenges may not indicate malnutrition but may be attributable to immaturity of the immune system.[30,31] For example, only 12% of normal infants up to seven months of age experienced a delayed hypersensitivity response to the *Candida* intradermal skin test, whereas 80% of infants 7–12 months old had a positive response.[31]

Role of Assessment Techniques. Many nutritional-status assessment techniques have been evaluated, but their overall usefulness in the pediatric population is limited. Thus, monitoring daily weight, daily fluid balance, and routine metabolic markers adequately assesses response to parenteral nutrition in an infant that appears normal and has an appropriate weight and height for age. Patients with clinical or laboratory signs of malnutrition may benefit from more in-depth nutritional assessment techniques. Weekly anthropometric measurements used in conjunction with laboratory values, such as levels of transthyretin or retinol-binding protein, can result in a relatively sensitive and specific assessment of response to nutritional support. Neonates and small infants have relatively low total blood volumes of approximately 75–100 mL/kg; it is therefore important to be selective in the blood tests that are performed.

Fluid Requirements

Fluid requirements depend on hydration status, size, environmental factors (i.e., radiant warmers, ultraviolet light therapy), and disease.[6,24,32–39] A common method of approximating requirements for maintenance fluids in pediatric patients has been developed and is found in Table 1.[36] Maintaining desired fluid balance is essential because dehydration, hypernatremia, and hyperosmolarity may occur with inadequate administration of fluids, and peripheral edema, pulmonary edema, and congestive heart failure can result from fluid overload.[6,34–36] Daily evaluation of weight and assessment of intake and output are effective methods of estimating hydration status.

Neonates and infants, with relatively large body surface areas for body weight and greater insensible losses from skin, require proportionally more fluids to maintain adequate hydration.[33,34] Fluids must be managed cautiously in the premature infant, who is at increased risk for the development of a variety of diseases or exacerbation of existing disease when excessive fluids are administered. Studies have shown a relationship between patent ductus arteriosus,[40] bronchopulmonary dyspla-

Table 1.
Daily Maintenance Fluid Requirements

Body Weight (kg)	Amount of Fluid per Day
1–10	100 mL/kg
11–20	1000 mL plus 50 mL/kg for each kilogram above 10 kg
>20	1500 mL plus 20 mL/kg for each kilogram above 20 kg

sia,[41] necrotizing enterocolitis,[42] and intraventricular hemorrhage[43] in low-birth-weight neonates receiving excessive fluid volumes. Patients with underlying cardiac defects, head trauma, or renal compromise may require fluid restriction to facilitate recovery or prevent exacerbation of underlying disease. On the other hand, patients with high urinary output, increased ostomy output, diarrhea, and vomiting should be given replacement fluid for these excessive losses in addition to maintenance fluid requirements. Fever and the use of radiant warmers or ultraviolet lights increase fluid losses, thus increasing fluid needs by approximately 20–25%.[34,37–39] Occasionally, an infant with high urine output who receives phototherapy may require maintenance fluid amounts of 200 mL/kg/day or more.[37,38]

Electrolyte and Mineral Requirements

Daily electrolyte, mineral, and trace element requirements are shown in Table 2.[6,24,32,34,36,44] In addition to daily maintenance requirements, all patients with excessive body fluid losses should receive replacement fluid with comparable electrolytes (Table 3).[45] Serum electrolytes should be assessed daily for the first two to three days of parenteral nutrition, then every other day for about four days. After a week or more of therapy when the infant is stable and the electrolyte content of the parenteral nutrient solution is not being changed, electrolytes can be assessed weekly or every two weeks. If the electrolyte content of the parenteral nutrient solution is changing or if the infant is not stable, serum electrolytes should be monitored more frequently.

The premature neonate often has increased fluid and electrolyte requirements because the immature kidney is unable to effectively regulate urinary water and electrolyte losses.[6,34,46] Neonates may also have glycosuria, which may increase fluid and electrolyte losses.[47] In addition, diuretics such as furosemide are frequently used in neonates and infants and may result in preferential excretion of considerable amounts of potassium and calcium along with mobilization of fluids.

Electrolytes may also be provided from sources that are overlooked. For example, patients receiving TrophAmine (Kendall McGaw, Irvine, CA) or Aminosyn-PF (Abbott Laboratories, North Chicago, IL) with L-cysteine hydrochloride supplementation (40 mg of L-cysteine hydrochloride/g of protein) receive an additional 0.5 to 1 meq/kg/day of chloride.[48] Premature neonates with arterial lines infusing 0.9% sodium chloride injection can receive their total daily sodium needs from the arterial line infusion. Medications with high electrolyte content (e.g., carbenicillin) may be used. Conversely, discontinuation of arterial lines or medications with increased electrolyte content may result in a need to alter electrolyte content of the parenteral nutrient solution. Therefore, close monitoring of changes in serum electrolyte concentrations, followed by adjustments in the parenteral nutrient solution, is mandatory.

Potassium. Premature neonates may require increased concentrations of potassium salts in parenteral nutrient solutions to replenish potassium losses incurred by immature renal function or through diuretic use. When infused peripherally in high concentrations, potassium is irritating to veins.[49,50] Infiltration of concentrated potassium can result in severe sequelae, including skin sloughing and tissue necrosis.[51,52] Up to 80 meq/L of potassium salts has been used peripherally for short periods of time; however, peripheral-vein solutions containing 40 meq/L or less of potassium are recommended to minimize the possibility of phlebitis.[49] Higher concentrations of potassium can be infused through a central venous catheter. Regardless of the route of administration, the cumulative rate of potassium administration should not exceed 0.5 meq/kg/hr because of potential induction of cardiac arrhythmias.[50,53]

Calcium and Phosphorus. Pediatric patients may require increased concentrations of calcium in parenteral nutrient solutions. The premature neonate may require up to 150 mg/kg/day (7.5 meq/kg/day) of elemental calcium to maintain in utero calcium, primarily bone, accretion rates.[44] In addition, neonates may receive diuretics, which can increase calcium needs by increasing excretion of calcium. Because parathyroid hormone stimulates mobilization of calcium from bone, serum calcium can be normal even though intake is inadequate.[54]

Table 2.
Daily Electrolyte and Mineral Requirements

Element	Amount	
	Neonates	Infants and Children
Sodium	1.6–9 meq/kg	2–4 meq/kg
Potassium	1.4–10 meq/kg	2–3 meq/kg
Chloride	1.1–4.5 meq/kg	2–3 meq/kg
Phosphorus	1–2 mmol/kg	1–2 mmol/kg
Magnesium	80 mg/kg	30–60 mg/kg
Calcium (Elemental)	150 mg/kg	400–1200 mg/day

Table 3.
Electrolyte Content of Body Fluids

Fluid	Electrolyte		
	Sodium (meq/L)	Potassium (meq/L)	Chloride (meq/L)
Gastric	10–115	5–35	10–155
Pancreatic	115–150	5–10	55–95
Ileal	105–145	5–30	90–135
Cecal	50	10	40
Bile	130–165	5–15	90–120
Saliva	35	10	35

Thus, serum calcium concentrations may not accurately reflect actual calcium needs for bone growth.[54] The adequacy of calcium intake can be assessed by reviewing and comparing bone density on sequential routine chest roentgenograms obtained for other clinical purposes. Maintenance of normal serum calcium concentration is partly dependent on normal magnesium concentrations; therefore, magnesium and calcium concentrations should be assessed simultaneously. Like potassium, calcium can produce severe tissue necrosis if concentrated solutions infiltrate peripherally.[51,52] We routinely use 0.5 to 0.8 meq of calcium per kg in parenteral nutrient solutions administered through a peripheral vein without serious infiltration sequelae. Solutions containing higher concentrations of calcium can be infused through a central venous catheter.

Providing sufficient quantities of calcium to the neonatal patient is difficult because of calcium and phosphorus solubility limitations in parenteral nutrient solutions. Precipitation of calcium phosphate can occur with increasing temperature, pH, or concentration of calcium and phosphorus.[55-58] Placing an infant in an isolette or administering ultraviolet light therapy results in a warmer temperature close to the infant. If solutions containing calcium and phosphorus in concentrations near the limits of solubility become warmed, calcium phosphate may precipitate in the intravenous line.

Early attempts to deliver required amounts of calcium and phosphorus resulted in preparation of two parenteral nutrient solutions a day, one with calcium alone and one with phosphorus alone.[59] One solution was infused for 12 hours and was followed by infusion of the alternate solution for 12 hours.[59] This method of calcium and phosphorus administration resulted in alternating periods of high and low serum concentrations of calcium and phosphorus depending on which solution was being infused.[59] Infusion of solutions containing both calcium and phosphorus resulted in stable calcium and phosphorus concentrations.[59]

Other methods of increasing calcium and phosphorus solubility in parenteral nutrient solutions have been examined. L-Cysteine hydrochloride, addition of which is required for specialty pediatric amino acid formulations, decreases solution pH. Use of L-cysteine hydrochloride with FreAmine III (Kendall McGaw) to increase solubility of calcium and phosphorus was less expensive than the daily administration of calcium and phosphorus in separate solutions.[60] Concentrations of calcium 50 meq/L and phosphate 20 mmol/L were compatible in solutions containing 2% TrophAmine, 10% dextrose, and 0.08% L-cysteine.[57] A subsequent study compared the results of calcium-phosphate solubility previously found with TrophAmine solutions to results for similar Aminosyn-PF solutions and showed that calcium phosphate solubility was less with Aminosyn-PF.[58] These findings suggest that calcium and phosphate solubility must be evaluated separately for each amino acid product.

Protein Requirements

Early intravenous amino acid solutions were composed of protein hydrolysates that were contaminated with various minerals and ammonia.[61-64] Problems with hyperammonemia and poor nitrogen use commonly seen with protein hydrolysates have been alleviated by the introduction of purer, crystalline amino acid formulations. Because hydrochloride salt forms of amino acids were used almost exclusively in early crystalline amino acid products, metabolic acidosis often resulted from their use.[62,63] Products now contain the acetate salt form of amino acids whenever possible. In addition to decreased toxicity, crystalline amino acids promote greater rates of nitrogen retention than protein hydrolysates.[65] All amino acid formulations currently marketed consist of crystalline amino acids.

Protein needs must be determined on an individual basis because requirements vary according to patient age, development, and disease. Premature neonates should receive sufficient protein and calories to achieve intrauterine growth rates, whereas older children need to be maintained in respective growth percentiles for age.[66] Enteral protein given at 4 to 6 g/kg/day was shown to promote nitrogen retention and growth in premature neonates.[67-69] Parenteral protein needs are less than enteral requirements, and generally, 2.5 to 3.0 g/kg/day of protein promotes nitrogen retention in premature neonates and infants.[6,24,32,65,66,70-73] Protein requirements slowly decrease to 1.5 to 2.0 g/kg/day after about one year of age,[66] and by adolescence adult requirements of 1.0 to 1.5 g/kg/day are achieved.[66] Routine assessments of response to therapy, such as nitrogen balance and visceral protein status, will ensure adequate provision of protein for pediatric patients with above-average requirements and avoid overuse of expensive, potentially harmful protein solutions in a patient who requires less protein.

Several investigators examined the amount of protein as crystalline amino acids required to produce nitrogen accretion in neonates[71-73]; they found that as protein and calorie intake increases, nitrogen accretion rates increase. Otherwise healthy, postsurgical neonates of 35–40 weeks' gestation receiving as little as 1.7 to 1.8 g/kg/day of protein achieved positive nitrogen balance (mean, approximately 200 mg/kg/day) when 40–50 cal/kg/day of lipid or dextrose was concurrently provided.[71] Provision of 2.5 g/kg/day of protein and 60 cal/kg/day resulted in a mean positive nitrogen balance of 178 mg/kg/day in preterm neonates.[72] Preterm neonates given 2.5 to 3.5 g/kg/day of protein and 81 cal/kg/day achieved mean intrauterine nitrogen accretion rates of 320 mg/kg/day.[73]

Special Amino Acid Formulations. Standard crystalline amino acid products (Travasol, Baxter Healthcare Corporation, Deerfield, IL; FreAmine III, Kendall McGaw; Aminosyn, Abbott Laboratories) are composed of essential and nonessential amino acids and were developed based on adult requirements. Aberrant steady-state plasma amino acid patterns were noted in premature neonates and infants receiving these crystalline amino acid products, suggesting different amino acid needs for pediatric patients.[62,74,75] Because certain enzymes are poorly developed in neonates, cysteine,[75-78] taurine,[67] tyrosine,[67] and histidine[79] may be essential amino acids in neonates. In neonates, hepatic cystathionase insufficiency results in impaired conversion of methionine to cysteine (Figure 1), and since cysteine is converted to taurine, there is also a deficiency of taurine.[76]

Two crystalline amino acid products (TrophAmine, Aminosyn-PF) that claim to meet the specific amino acid needs of infants have been marketed. The amino acid contents of these products are compared in Table 4. Both products contain less methionine, phenylalanine, and glycine than the products developed for adults. In addition, both products contain taurine and the dicarboxylic amino acids (glutamate and aspartate) and require the addition of L-cysteine hydrochloride, which is unstable in solution for prolonged periods of time, before infusion. TrophAmine has *N*-acetyl-L-tyrosine added as a water-soluble source of tyrosine.

Newborn animals developed neurotoxicity when given large doses of dicarboxylic amino acids; this raised questions about the safety of these amino acids in newborn human infants.[80] To investigate this potential problem, Bell et al.[81] compared plasma and erythrocyte aspartate concentrations and erythrocyte glutamate concentrations in infants receiving Neopham (Cutter Laboratories, Berkeley, CA; not currently marketed) with aspartate 107 mg/dL and glutamate 186 mg/dL to those concentrations in infants receiving Travasol with no added dicarboxylic amino acids. Although plasma glutamate concentrations were higher in infants receiving Neopham, erythrocyte aspartate and glutamate concentrations in the two groups were similar; this led to the conclusion that dicarboxylic amino acids could be used safely in infants.[81]

Figure 1. Transsulfuration pathway for conversion of methionine to cysteine and taurine.

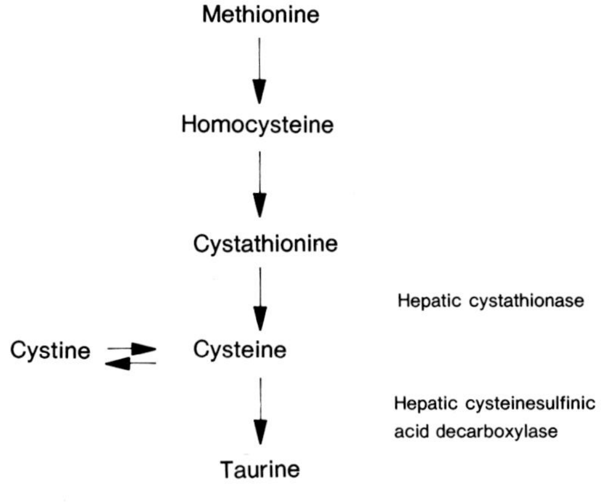

Assuming that postprandial plasma amino acid patterns are important in enhancing protein synthesis, duplicating normal (enterally fed) values may result in better weight gain and nitrogen retention.[62,74,82-87] Plasma amino acid patterns have been determined in healthy primarily human-milk-fed[82-85] and formula-fed[86,87] infants. Plasma amino acid concentrations from human-milk-fed infants[82] have been compared with those of infants receiving TrophAmine[88,89] or FreAmine III.[88] Neonates receiving TrophAmine had plasma amino acid patterns similar to those of infants fed human milk, whereas neonates receiving FreAmine III had elevated plasma concentrations of methionine, phenylalanine, and glycine and low concentrations of tyrosine.[88] Neonates who received TrophAmine also had significantly greater weight gain and nitrogen balance when compared with neonates who received FreAmine III.[88]

Little clinical experience has been documented for the Aminosyn-PF formulation.[90,91] Table 5 compares mean plasma amino acid concentrations in 11 infants 1 to 13 weeks of age who received an average of 2.7 g/kg/day of Aminosyn-PF and 100 cal/kg/day with plasma amino acid concentrations reported in infants primarily fed human milk.[82-85]

Table 4.
Comparison of Pediatric Amino Acid Products

Amino Acid	Composition (mol %)	
	TrophAmine 6%	Aminosyn-PF 7%
L-Isoleucine	8.11	7.42
L-Leucine	13.89	11.55
L-Lysine	7.27	5.92
L-Methionine	2.91	1.53
L-Phenylalanine	3.82	3.31
L-Tryptophan	1.28	1.12
L-Threonine	4.56	5.51
L-Valine	8.70	7.03
L-Arginine	9.09	9.01
L-Histidine	4.06	2.59
L-Alanine	7.79	10.03
L-Proline	7.72	9.03
Glycine	6.36	6.56
L-Serine	4.75	6.02
L-Tyrosine	0.48	0.44
N-Acetyl-L-tyrosine (tyrosine equivalents)	1.17	0.00
L-Glutamic acid	4.43	7.14
L-Aspartic acid	3.10	5.07
L-Cysteine	0.24	0.00
Taurine	0.26	0.73
Total	99.99	100.01

Plasma concentrations for 1/2 cystine, histidine, tyrosine, and glutamine were low compared with standards for infants.[82-85] Results of a multicenter trial comparing clinical outcome of neonates receiving Aminosyn-PF or TrophAmine will be available soon.

Specific amino acid formulations may ultimately allow adequate growth to be maintained while protein and calorie intake is reduced.[65,92] Helms et al.[92] reported positive nitrogen balance and weight gain (>200 mg/kg/day and >10 g/kg/day, respectively) with low doses of TrophAmine (2 g/kg/day) and calories (50 cal/kg/day) in preterm infants receiving parenteral nutrition. In the past, these results were achievable only with high-calorie and standard protein intakes.

Caloric Requirements

Sufficient nonprotein calories must be provided as carbohydrate or fat to meet basal metabolic energy demands, to ensure growth and development, and to prevent use of protein from the parenteral nutrient solution, muscle, or visceral protein merely as an energy source. Infants generally require more enteral than parenteral calories.[93] Enterally fed low-birth-weight infants had global energy requirements of 150 cal/kg/day.[94] About 12% of daily calories were lost primarily in stool as fat. Of the remaining 132 cal/kg/day ingested, maintenance of normal metabolism required 63 cal/kg/day, daily activities used 4 cal/kg/day, and the balance of 65 cal/kg/day produced growth rates of 16 g/kg/day.[94]

Table 5.
Mean (± S.E.) Amino Acid Concentrations in Infants Receiving Aminosyn-PF Compared with Concentration Ranges in Enterally Fed Infants[a]

Amino Acid	Concentration (μmol/L) Aminosyn-PF	Enteral Feedings[b]
Threonine	137.0 ± 7.1	65–338
Valine	83.0 ± 3.9	78–270
Leucine	59.3 ± 2.4	46–199
Isoleucine	39.0 ± 2.0	26–98
Lysine	82.6 ± 3.6	71–304
Methionine	11.6 ± 0.6	6–53
1/2 Cystine	5.3 ± 0.5[c]	26–92
Histidine	41.7 ± 1.3[c]	44–254
Phenylalanine	27.5 ± 1.0	16–110
Tyrosine	9.0 ± 1.0[c]	32–200
Tryptophan	19.9 ± 1.0	18–101
Aspartic acid	30.3 ± 1.9	0.1–191
Serine	115.9 ± 4.9	94–476
Glutamic acid	189.3 ± 15.5	18–243
Glutamine	129.3 ± 9.1[c]	142–959
Proline	135.9 ± 7.4	82–329
Glycine	188.0 ± 7.0	62–577
Alanine	173.3 ± 10.3	125–702
Arginine	44.4 ± 3.0	17–148

[a] Feedings consisted primarily of human milk.
[b] Lowest and highest reported values from references 82–85.
[c] Mean values below the target range.

Parenteral calorie needs of the preterm infant have been estimated to be 85–130 cal/kg/day.[6,32,61,73,95,96] Studies have shown that premature infants receiving as few as 50 cal/kg/day and 2.5 to 3 g/kg/day of protein can achieve positive nitrogen balance.[73] To produce weight gains of 9–15 g/kg/day in the low-birth-weight infant, 80–100 cal/kg/day may be needed.[61,73,95] Current evidence suggests that with amino acid formulations designed specifically for neonates (TrophAmine), adequate weight gain can be achieved with lower calorie intake.[92] During the first year of life, caloric requirements begin to decrease, and usually 75–90 cal/kg/day is sufficient for children one to seven years of age.[96] Caloric requirements continue to decrease to 60–75 cal/kg/day from 7 to 12 years of age and reach adult needs of 30–60 cal/kg/day by about 18 years of age.[96] These recommendations are only guidelines, and actual measurements of growth and development should be used to individualize the number of calories provided.

Carbohydrates

In the past, ethanol,[6,97,98] fructose,[99] and galactose[6] were used as calorie sources for parenteral nutrition. One current product designed for peripheral use in the postsurgical adult, ProcalAmine (Kendall McGaw), uses 3% glycerol to provide calories because the transport of glycerol across the cell membrane does not depend on insulin.[100] However, dextrose is used almost exclusively in parenteral nutrient solutions as the source of carbohydrate calories.

Nutritional support solutions infused peripherally are usually limited to 10% to 12.5% dextrose[95,101] because infusion of more hypertonic solutions into peripheral veins can result in phlebitis or severe infiltration sequelae. With dextrose concentrations of 10% to 12.5%, adequate calories for preterm neonates can be provided peripherally if the patient can tolerate large fluid loads and maximum doses of fat emulsion.[95,102] Patients who require parenteral nutrition for long periods of time usually have central venous catheters placed to allow for the infusion of hypertonic solutions of dextrose and amino acids. Therapy should be initiated with approximately 10 g/kg/day of dextrose in older infants and children. Increases of 5 g/kg every 12 to 24 hours up to 30 g/kg/day can be made if the patient has central venous access and normal glucose tolerance. Neonates, particularly premature neonates, may not tolerate large amounts of glucose initially and are at risk for hyperosmolar coma and intraventricular hemorrhage as a result of hyperglycemia.[6,103] Thus neonates should be started on about 5 g/kg/day of dextrose, which is slowly increased by 3 g/kg/day with close monitoring of serum glucose. Children receiving corticosteroids may become hyperglycemic with infusion of more than 15 to 20 g/kg/day of dextrose. These individuals should have dextrose concentrations increased slowly as tolerated and may need to receive maximal calories from fat emulsion to avoid insulin therapy.

Patients receiving parenteral nutrition should have glucose tolerance assessed through monitoring of serum glucose every 8 to 12 hours using Chemstrip bG (Bio-Dynamics, Indianapolis, IN) or Dextrostix (Ames Division, Miles Laboratories, Inc., Elkhart, IN). Errors in technique or interfering substances can produce erroneously high or low results with these rapid assessments of serum glucose. Patients with unexplained hyperglycemia or hypoglycemia as determined by these methods should have serum glucose measured from blood drawn via venipuncture for verification of results.

Glucose intolerance in patients who require parenteral nutrition can be managed with insulin to normalize serum glucose. Although insulin is compatible with parenteral nutrient solutions, it does adsorb to glass, polyvinyl chloride, and filters, resulting in decreased insulin delivery to the patient.[104] Albumin has been added to bind insulin and presumably decrease the binding of insulin to solution containers.[55,104] Pediatric patients frequently have changing insulin requirements that preclude the direct addition of insulin (with albumin) to parenteral nutrient solutions. In this case, a separate continuous infusion of regular insulin (beginning dose 0.1 U/kg/hr[105]) is titrated to serum glucose concentration, offering a practical solution and minimizing waste of the parenteral nutrient solution.[106]

Because glycosuria can result in osmotic diuresis with excessive fluid and electrolyte loss (see earlier discussion regarding fluid requirements), urine should be assessed for glucose (Chemstrip, Bio-Dynamics; Keto-Diastix, Clinitest, Ames Division, Miles Laboratories, Inc.) and ketones (Keto-Diastix, Clinitest, Ames Division, Miles Laboratories, Inc.). Neonates have a lower renal threshold for glucose and may excrete glucose in their urine even when euglycemic.[47] In this case, increasing the dextrose concentration in parenteral nutrient solutions to meet caloric requirements is acceptable provided fluid losses are manageable.

Fat

Indications and Clinical Use. Fat emulsions (Liposyn and Liposyn II, Abbott Laboratories; Intralipid, KabiVitrum, Alameda, CA; Travamulsion, Baxter Heathcare Corporation; Soyacal, Alpha Therapeutics, Los Angeles, CA) prevent or reverse essential fatty acid deficiency and provide a concentrated, isotonic source of calories (Table 6). Biochemical evidence of essential fatty acid deficiency is demonstrated by a triene:tetraene ratio greater than 0.4 and is primarily a result of linoleic acid deficiency.[107,108] Previously it was thought that linoleic acid was the only essential fatty acid, but current evidence suggests that linolenic acid may also be essential.[109] Because Liposyn contained less than 0.1% linolenic acid, Abbott Laboratories introduced a second-generation Liposyn product (Liposyn II) containing 4.2% linolenic acid. Recently, medium-chain triglycerides (MCT Oil, Mead Johnson, Evansville, IN) have been used as a calorically dense product; however, this product does not prevent essential fatty acid deficiency, and parenteral use in pediatric patients has not been evaluated.

The premature neonate with limited fat stores may develop biochemical evidence of essential fatty acid deficiency in one to two days, ultimately resulting in reduced growth, dry skin and hair, decreased platelets, and impaired wound healing.[110-112] Friedman et al.[112] reported that topically applied sunflower seed oil reversed biochemical and clinical evidence of essential fatty acid deficiency in two neonates on fat-free parenteral nutrition. However, a later study conducted in 15 neonates showed that cutaneous administration of safflower oil did not uniformly reverse or prevent

Table 6.
Composition of Fat Emulsions

Ingredient or Characteristic	Liposyn II	Travamulsion	Soyacal	Intralipid
Source				
Soybean oil (%)	50	100	100	100
Safflower oil (%)	50	...	...	...
Ingredient				
Linoleic acid (%)	65.8	56	49–60	50
Oleic acid (%)	17.7	23	21–26	26
Palmitic acid (%)	8.8	11	9–13	10
Linolenic acid (%)	4.2	6	6–9	9
Stearic acid (%)	3.4	4	3–5	3.5
Egg yolk phospholipids (%)	1.2	1.2	1.2	1.2
Glycerin (%)	2.5	2.25	2.21	2.25
Calories (per milliliter)				
10% Emulsion	1.1	1.1	1.1	1.1
20% Emulsion	2.0	2.0	2.0	2.0

essential fatty acid deficiency.[113] Provision of 2–4% of the required total daily calories as intravenous fat emulsion (1–2% linoleic acid) will prevent the clinical signs of essential fatty acid deficiency.[108]

Metabolism of fat emulsion results in lipid peroxidation and free radical formation, which can damage cell membranes if vitamin E, a scavenger of free radicals, is deficient.[114,115] Although lipid emulsions contain small amounts of vitamin E, supplementation with a multiple-vitamin preparation is required.[115] The vitamin E:PUFA (polyunsaturated fatty acids) ratio is a crude measure of the adequacy of vitamin E intake and is useful only when ratios are maintained at a fixed level for weeks. Maintaining a vitamin E:PUFA ratio greater than 0.6 mg/g is usually sufficient to prevent peroxidative injury.[114,115]

Fat therapy should be started at a dose of 0.5 g/kg/day in premature neonates, whereas term infants and infants older than one month can usually be started on 1 g/kg/day. Ideally, lipid emulsion should be given continuously over 24 hours to promote clearance from circulation.[108] Visual inspection of plasma for turbidity does not correlate well with measured serum triglyceride or free fatty acid concentrations.[116] Therefore, fat tolerance should be assessed by measuring serum triglycerides and free fatty acids. If serum triglycerides or free fatty acids are within normal limits, fat emulsion can be increased by 0.25 g/kg/day to a maximum of 3 g/kg/day in preterm neonates and by 0.5 to 1 g/kg/day up to 4 g/kg/day in term and older infants.[70] At our institution, patients who have triglyceride concentrations of up to 200 mg/dL are maintained on their current dose of fat emulsion, and serum triglyceride concentrations are monitored to be sure that enzymatic clearance is not exceeded. Because egg phospholipids are used to emulsify fat emulsions, patients beginning fat therapy should be monitored for hypersensitivity, which may consist of allergic reactions, fever, chills, dyspnea, cyanosis, nausea, headache, dizziness, or chest and back pain.[117,118]

The use of fat emulsion with parenteral nutrition has distinct advantages. Essential fatty acid deficiency can be prevented or reversed. Patients who cannot tolerate large glucose loads can receive sufficient calories if fat emulsion is added to a dextrose and amino acid regimen. The inclusion of fat with parenteral nutrient solutions infused through a peripheral vein can provide enough calories for growth in preterm neonates and infants who can tolerate fluid loads of 140 mL/kg/day.[92,96,102] Also, continuous coadministration of fat emulsion with a parenteral nutrient regimen prolongs viability of peripheral intravenous lines in infants who may have limited venous access.[119]

Neonates and infants are able to effectively use fat as an energy source in the first day of life.[120,121] However, infants who are small for their gestational age and who receive fat emulsion may have a limited ability to metabolize fat, as demonstrated by elevated serum triglyceride concentrations.[121–123] A study in low-birth-weight infants showed that Liposyn, a safflower oil-based fat emulsion with 0.1% linolenic acid, was cleared less efficiently than Intralipid, a soybean oil-based product with 8–9% linolenic acid.[123] Differences in particle size between the two solutions were postulated to account for the difference in triglyceride clearance.[123] Low-birth-weight infants with sepsis may have a decreased clearance of fat emulsion.[124,125] Septic low-birth-weight infants receiving 3 g/kg/day of fat emulsion had higher triglyceride and free fatty acid concentrations than nonseptic low-birth-weight infants.[124,125]

Carnitine facilitates the transport of fatty acids across mitochondrial membranes to the site of fat oxidation.[126] Premature neonates and newborn infants have limited carnitine stores and immature enzyme systems that synthesize carnitine.[127,128] Thus, carnitine insufficiency may explain poor lipid use in these patients. Intravenous L-carnitine supplementation of 10 mg/kg/day in preterm neonates[129] and 10 mg/kg/day orally in infants receiving long-term parenteral nutrition[130] increased ketogenesis, suggesting improved use of fat emulsion.[129,130] An oral L-carnitine product (Kendall McGaw) is available for use in patients with a genetic carnitine deficiency, and the intravenous product is available investigationally.

Heparin, which augments lipoprotein lipase activity, was postulated to be effective in reducing serum triglyceride concentrations in neonates receiving fat emulsion.[131–133] Bolus doses of heparin (10 U/kg) stimulated lipolytic activity and temporarily improved lipid clearance.[131] Neonates receiving bolus doses of heparin (10 U/kg) in addition to heparin (1 U/mL) mixed with the parenteral nutrient solution had significantly lower triglyceride concentrations than patients receiving bolus doses of heparin (10 U/kg) only.[132,133] These studies were conducted over a four-hour time period; thus, long-term effects of heparin therapy in neonates and infants are unknown.

Controversies in the Use of Fat Emulsion. The use of fat emulsion in patients with hyperbilirubinemia is controversial. When serum bilirubin concentrations exceed 18–20 mg/dL, kernicterus, deposition of unconjugated bilirubin in brain cells, can occur. The resulting neurologic syndrome can range in severity from mild neuromuscular incoordination to more severe symptoms including mental retardation, ataxia, and seizures.[134] Neonates, particularly premature neonates, frequently develop physiologic jaundice and hyperbilirubinemia because of immature hepatic enzymes that conjugate bilirubin. Because fatty acids and bilirubin competitively bind to albumin, bilirubin can be displaced from high-affinity albumin-binding sites by free fatty acids, resulting in increased unconjugated bilirubin concentrations and increased risk of kernicterus. Andrew et al.[135] found that molar ratios of serum free fatty acid to albumin must be greater than 6 to displace bilirubin from albumin. Further, an in vitro study found that Intralipid and Liposyn enhanced reserve capacity for binding of bilirubin to albumin.[136] Therefore, hyperbilirubinemia alone does not absolutely restrict the use of intravenous fat emulsion; providing 2–4% of the total daily calorie needs as fat emulsion to prevent essential fatty acid deficiency should not present a problem.[70]

In septic adults receiving 20% Intralipid at rates of 50, 100, and 200 mL/hr, impaired immunologic function correlated with hypertriglyceridemia and partially impaired leukocyte function.[137] On the other hand, neither functional nor numerical studies of cell-mediated immunity were adversely affected by Intralipid infusion in 15 infants receiving clinically used Intralipid doses of 1.1 to 3.2 g/kg/day.[29] No infant had hypertriglyceridemia in the latter study.[29]

The use of lipids in patients with pulmonary compromise is also controversial. Because fat emboli were found in pulmonary capillaries during postmortem examinations of neonates who received Intralipid, the infusion of fat emulsion in neonates with respiratory compromise was postulated to further alter pulmonary function.[138-140] Schroder et al.[141] found no pulmonary fat accumulation in 22 infants, 13 of whom received Intralipid, when lungs were fixed in situ immediately after death; they attributed the previous findings to artifact secondary to delayed fixation of the lungs. Pereira et al.,[122] in a study of pulmonary function in premature neonates, found that appropriate-for-gestational-age neonates who were less than one week of age, had respiratory-distress syndrome, and received Intralipid 1 g/kg over four hours ($n = 4$) had lower PO_2 values than age-related neonates receiving no Intralipid ($n = 4$). No other changes in pulmonary function were demonstrated, and the lower PO_2 did not correlate with elevations in serum triglycerides.[122] Brans and coworkers[142] found that oxygen diffusion in the lungs of premature neonates was not affected by infusion of up to 4 g/kg/day of Intralipid over 24 hours. Therefore, to avoid excessive fat concentrations in circulation and potential changes in pulmonary microcirculation that may result in a lowering of PO_2, the total daily dose of fat emulsion should be infused over 24 hours whenever possible.[108,142]

Vitamin and Trace Element Requirements

Vitamins. In general, intravenous vitamin requirements, particularly for water-soluble vitamins, are more than the Recommended Dietary Allowances (RDA) for oral vitamins for several reasons. Vitamins in solution may interact with each other or with the plastic intravenous tubing, and certain B vitamins (cyanocobalamin, folic acid, pyridoxine, riboflavin, thiamine) and ascorbic acid degrade when exposed to light.[55,143] These interactions result in smaller amounts of vitamins actually being delivered to the patient.[55,143] In an attempt to minimize these interactions, vitamins are added just before infusion. In addition to problems with interactions, intravenous vitamins are presented to the kidney soon after infusion, resulting in early urinary clearance of the water-soluble vitamins.

In 1975, the American Medical Association Nutrition Advisory Group (AMA–NAG) published guidelines for the use of intravenous vitamins in the pediatric population.[144] MVI Pediatric (Armour Pharmaceutical Co., Kankakee, IL), containing the currently recommended total daily requirements for children weighing more than 10 kg, was subsequently marketed as a powder for reconstitution in 5-mL vials. Infants weighing less than 10 kg were to be given 10% per kilogram of the recommended vitamin formulation (the equivalent of 0.5 mL/kg of MVI Pediatric) to fulfill their daily vitamin needs.[144] FDA currently recommends that 30% of a diluted vial be given to infants weighing less than 1 kg, 65% be given to infants weighing between 1 and 3 kg, and the entire 5 mL of the diluted vial be given to infants weighing more than 3 kg and to children up to 11 years of age.[145] Investigators measured serum vitamin concentrations in infants and children who received 5 mL of MVI Pediatric and in premature neonates who received 3.5 mL (65% of a vial).[146,147] These doses prevented vitamin deficiency states; however, serum concentrations of certain vitamins (cyanocobalamin, pantothenate, biotin) were above the normal ranges in all patients and ascorbic acid concentrations were increased in preterm infants.[146] Serum vitamin concentrations do not necessarily reflect concentrations in tissue, which is the site of activity.

Because vitamins accumulate during the third trimester of pregnancy, premature neonates have minimal vitamin stores at birth, and vitamin deficiency can develop soon after birth if no supplementation is provided.[148] Vitamin E, a free radical scavenger that protects cell membranes against lipid peroxidation, may confer protection against retinopathy of prematurity and anemia that may occur shortly after birth.[115] Premature infants weighing less than 1 kg given 30% of a vial of MVI Pediatric had mean serum vitamin E concentrations of 0.79 to 1.28 mg/dL.[149] However, 44% of those infants had vitamin E concentrations of ≤ 1 mg/dL, which is below the therapeutic range.[150] Currently, maintenance of serum concentrations of α-tocopherol (vitamin E) between 1 and 2 mg/dL is recommended,[151] which requires a vitamin E dose of 2.1 to 4.6 mg/dL or 30% to 65% of a vial of MVI Pediatric.[150]

Infants and children with specific diseases such

as cystic fibrosis may require more fat-soluble vitamins than recommened by the AMA-NAG,[152] whereas children with renal impairment may require lower amounts of water-soluble vitamins since the ability to excrete vitamins in the urine may be compromised.[153]

Trace Elements. The major trace elements known to be essential to normal growth and development are copper, zinc, chromium, manganese, selenium, iodine, and iron. Copper, zinc, chromium, and manganese are available together as PedTE-PAK-4 (SoloPak Laboratories, Franklin Park, IL), PTE-4 (LyphoMed, Inc., Melrose Park, IL), and Multitrace Pediatric (Armour Pharmaceutical Co.). When solutions were used at a dosage of 0.4 mL/kg/day in preterm infants, in utero retention rates for zinc and copper were achieved.[154] Preterm neonates should receive trace element supplementation upon institution of parenteral nutrition. It is recommnended that neonates and infants be given 0.3 mL/kg/day of a trace element product.[155] Older children are generally given 0.1 mL/kg/day with a maximum dose of 5 mL of the aforementioned trace element products. Term neonates and infants who are going to receive parenteral nutrition for two weeks or less do not require trace element supplementation. Selenium deficiency results in decreased glutathione peroxidase activity[156]; therefore, selenium should be added at 3 μg/kg/day to a maximum of 40 μg/day,[157] particularly in infants receiving substantive lipid doses (>2.0 g/kg/day). Topical povidone iodine solution or ointment used to cleanse the catheter insertion site usually results in sufficient iodine absorption to prevent deficiency.[158] Thyroid profile monitoring is recommended for pediatric patients receiving long-term parenteral therapy. Patients receiving parenteral nutrition longer than one month who are older than two months of age and do not receive enteral iron may need to be given intravenous iron dextran. Preterm infants less than two months of age who are given iron may experience hemolysis due to oxidative destruction of the erythrocyte lipid membrane and are not candidates for exogenous supplementation.[159] Factors to be considered before iron supplementation include red blood cell indices and a history of blood transfusions. Microcytic red blood cells and low hemoglobin values may suggest a need for intravenous iron supplementation. A patient with normocytic red blood cells who has received a blood transfusion may not need intravenous iron even if enteral intake is inadequate. Iron needs can be calculated from the following formula:

Body weight (pounds) × (100 − % Hgb) × 0.3
= milligrams of iron[160]

where % Hgb is expressed as a percentage of the normal age-related hemoglobin. The calculated elemental iron dose is administered over three days; the daily dose should not exceed 25 mg. This procedure can be done on a monthly basis in those individuals receiving all their nutritional needs by vein. Iron can be provided daily in parenteral nutrient solutions[66]; however, it is time consuming and expensive to add iron every day when monthly replacements are adequate. Usual precautions for anaphylaxis should be observed with the first exposure to parenteral iron.

Complications

Patients receiving parenteral nutrition are at risk of developing technical, metabolic, and infectious complications.[24,32,63,64,161-177]

Technical Complications. Technical complications that occur at the time of catheter insertion in pediatric patients are similar to those in adults and include pneumothorax, hemothorax, injury to arteries and veins, air embolism, and cardiac perforation. After catheter placement, thrombus formation, dislodgment of the catheter, fibrin clots on the catheter tip, and precipitates in the catheter may occur. Central venous catheters are inserted through an incision in the neck and are tunneled under the skin to an exit site on the chest. This procedure can result in scarring that may be embarrassing as the child grows up. Therefore, placement of catheter exit sites should be made with sensitivity to the future.

Infection. Sepsis is a potentially life-threatening complication associated with central venous access, with a reported incidence of up to 45% in neonates and children[161,162] and 3–27% in adults.[163,164] Because the catheter provides direct access to the central circulation, the line must be kept clean to avoid infections. Infused solutions should be changed carefully, a sterilizing ointment or solution should be applied around all connections, and the insertion site dressing should be changed every two or three days.[165] Infants receiving parenteral nutrition should be supervised closely because playing with or chewing on intravenous lines can damage the tubing or disconnect taped connections and contaminate the intravenous line. If the line is contaminated for any reason, the patient should be monitored closely for impending infection. Any signs of infection such as fever, hyperglycemia or hypoglycemia, increased irritability, or redness at the insertion site with or without constitutional symptoms should be responded to immediately. Protocols have been established that provide a systematic approach to the patient with suspected central venous line infection. These include obtaining peripheral and central blood cultures before institution of antibiotic therapy and determination of the specific antibiotics and dosages to be used before final culture and sensitivity reports. In addition to catheter care, other methods to minimize infection are being investigated. For example, catheters with bonded antibiotics prevented colonization of catheter tips in animals inoculated with *Staphylococcus aureus.*[166]

After positive cultures have been obtained, a systematic treatment plan should follow. If the catheter is to be removed, the catheter tip should be cultured on removal to document the infecting organism, and appropriate antibiotic therapy should be instituted. After central and peripheral blood cultures, patients requiring continued central venous access may have the catheter changed over a guidewire[167] or a new catheter placed at a different site. Antibiotics are infused through the newly placed catheter to treat the sepsis and to prevent seeding of the newly placed catheter. Pediatric patients have limited sites for central venous catheter placement; therefore, the decision to remove the catheter and place a new catheter in a different site must be made judiciously. The pediatric patient with presumed central venous catheter infection who needs to have central venous access preserved can be treated by infusions of antibiotics through the infected catheter. A study in 17 pediatric patients with documented central venous catheter bacteremia showed that 65% of patients were successfully treated without removal of the catheter.[168] Central and peripheral blood cultures should be repeated every three days until all culture results are negative to ensure eradication of the infecting organism.

A thrombus on the catheter tip can occlude the catheter or become a nidus for central venous line infection. Urokinase (Abbokinase, Abbott Laboratories; Breokinase, Breon Laboratories, Inc., New York, NY), an enzyme that will lyse thrombi, used in conjunction with antibiotics resulted in successful resolution of central-line infections in 20 adults.[169] Although no comparable studies have been conducted in pediatric patients, urokinase has been used successfully in pediatric patients to clear central venous lines occluded by thrombi.[170]

Metabolic Complications. Metabolic complications can occur and some can be very difficult to manage. Casein and fibrin hydrolysates were commonly associated with hyperammonemia in neonates, resulting from preformed ammonium ion content in these products.[62] With the currently available crystalline amino acid products, hyperammonemia is an infrequent problem in infants and children without liver disease. The early crystalline amino acid solutions (primarily as hydrochloride salts) were frequently responsible for metabolic acidosis.[63] Crystalline amino acids are now provided as a mixture of hydrochloride and acetate salts resulting in a less frequent occurrence of metabolic acidosis. Administration of excessive amino acids can result in azotemia, as evidenced by an elevated blood urea nitrogen (BUN), and must be differentiated from increases in BUN caused by dehydration.[6,24]

Most electrolyte-, mineral-, and trace element-related problems are iatrogenic and can be prevented through appropriate supplementation and monitoring. Rickets has been noted in neonates receiving long-term parenteral nutrition, probably because of an inability to provide sufficient calcium for bone growth.[171] The addition of L-cysteine hydrochloride to parenteral nutrient solutions can improve solubility of greater concentrations of calcium and phosphorus and minimizes problems with osteoporosis secondary to inadequate calcium intake. However, metabolic bone disease in parenterally fed infants may not simply be the result of inadequate calcium intake. Alterations in vitamin D metabolism, the production of antimetabolites, and end-organ resistance all may play a part in this complex picture of demineralization.[172]

Cholestasis can be a serious complication of parenteral nutrition. Should it occur, cholestasis usually becomes evident after about two weeks of parenteral nutrition.[173] Because sepsis, hepatitis, and other physiologic and anatomical factors can also induce cholestasis, these should be ruled out as the cause of abnormal liver function tests in any patient on parenteral nutrition. Black et al.[174] evaluated indicators of hepatocellular sinusoidal membrane function and integrity (serum aminotransferases and bile salts) and measures of canalicular membrane function (γ-glutamyl transpeptidase, 5′-nucleotidase, and conjugated bilirubin) in 21 infants receiving parenteral nutrition or glucose and electrolyte solutions. After one week, infants receiving parenteral nutrition had significantly higher concentrations of γ-glutamyl transpeptidase, 5′-nucleotidase, and conjugated bilirubin than did the infants receiving glucose and electrolyte solutions, indicating canalicular membrane damage.[174]

Bell et al.[175] retrospectively evaluated 624 infants less than 30 days old who received parenteral nutrition and found that infants with intracranial hemorrhage, patent ductus arteriosus, sepsis, or gastrointestinal surgery were more likely to develop cholestasis. Other investigators have shown that cholestasis induced by parenteral nutrition is more common in low-birth-weight infants, with the incidence increasing from 14–38% in infants weighing less than 2000 g[176–178] to 50% in those weighing less than 1000 g.[179] Amino acids, calorie overload, and fasting have been proposed as etiologies in the development of liver disease induced by parenteral nutrition; however, the precise etiology remains unknown and may be multifactorial.[173] If feasible, withdrawal of parenteral nutrition will usually reverse the liver dysfunction, but fibrosis and death have been reported when the liver disease progressed to cirrhosis.[176] Management of the patient with cholestasis induced by parenteral nutrition who cannot be taken off parenteral nutrition includes (1) cycling the patient off parenteral nutrition for part of the day, (2) providing adequate, not excessive, calories to maintain normal metabolism and growth, (3) administering appropriate types and amounts of amino acids, and (4) initiating minimal enteral feedings for gut stimulation when possible.[173] Although phenobarbital has been used effectively in other types of cholestasis, it has not proven to be beneficial in cholestasis induced by parenteral nutrition.[180]

Conclusion

Basic requirements necessary to promote growth while pediatric patients are receiving parenteral nutrition have been determined. However, considerable research continues, particularly in the area of complications associated with parenteral nutrition and the attainment of normal development. Amino acid solutions specific for pediatric patients have been designed, and investigators are only beginning to understand the therapeutic implications of their use. Micronutrient deficiencies are being reported and require the practitioner's attention in creating an appropriate nutritional solution. Thus, current studies are challenging what were thought to be standards of pediatric parenteral nutrition therapy, requiring clinicians to continue evaluating current literature to ensure provision of optimal nutritional support to pediatric patients.

References

1. Helfrick FW, Abelson NM. Intravenous feeding of a complete diet in a child: report of a case. *J Pediatr*. 1944; 25:400–4.
2. Costa G. Determination of nutritional needs. *Cancer Res*. 1977; 37:2419–24.
3. Merritt RJ, Blackburn GL. Nutritional assessment and metabolic response to illness of the hospitalized child. In: Suskind RM, ed. Textbook of pediatric nutrition. New York: Raven Press; 1981:285–307.
4. Grant JP, Custer PG, Thurlow J. Current techniques of nutritional assessment. *Surg Clin North Am*. 1981; 61:437–63.
5. Morriss FH. Trace minerals. *Semin Perinatol*. 1979; 3:369–79.
6. Kerner JA, Sunshine P. Parenteral alimentation. *Semin Perinatol*. 1979; 3:417–34.
7. Hamill PVV, Drizd TA, Johnson CL et al. Physical growth: National Center for Health Statistics percentiles. *Am J Clin Nutr*. 1979; 32:607–29.
8. Waterlow JC. Some aspects of childhood malnutrition as a public health problem. *Br Med J*. 1974; 4:88–90.
9. Helms RA, Miller JL, Burckart GL et al. Clinical outcome as assessed by anthropometric parameters, albumin and cellular immune function in high-risk infants receiving total parenteral nutrition. *J Pediatr Surg*. 1983; 18:564–9.
10. Gurney JM, Jelliffe DB. Arm anthropometry in nutritional assessment: nomogram for rapid calculation of muscle circumference and cross-sectional muscle and fat areas. *Am J Clin Nutr*. 1973; 26:912–5.
11. Frisancho AR. Triceps skin fold and upper arm muscle size norms for assessment of nutritional status. *Am J Clin Nutr*. 1974; 27:1052–8.
12. Tanner JM. Whitehouse RH. Revised standards for triceps and subscapular skinfolds in British children. *Arch Dis Child*. 1975; 50:142–5.
13. Ingenbleek Y, van den Schrieck H, de Nayer P et al. Albumin, transferrin, and the thyroxine-binding prealbumin/retinol binding protein (TBPA-RBP) complex in assessment of malnutrition. *Clin Chim Acta*. 1975; 63:61–7.
14. Rothschild MA, Oratz M, Schreiber SS. Albumin synthesis. *N Engl J Med*. 1972; 286:748–57.
15. Awai M, Brown EB. Studies of the metabolism of I^{131}-labeled human transferrin. *J Lab Clin Med*. 1963; 61:363–96.
16. Oppenheimer JH, Surks MI, Bernstein G et al. Metabolism of I-131 labeled thyroxine binding prealbumin in man. *Science*. 1965; 149:748–51.
17. Peterson PA. Demonstration in serum of two physiological forms of the human retinol-binding protein. *Eur J Clin Invest*. 1971; 1:437–44.
18. Giacoia GP, Watson S, West K. Rapid turnover transport proteins, plasma albumin, and growth in low birth weight infants. *J Parenter Enter Nutr*. 1984; 8:367–70.
19. Moskowitz SR, Pereira G, Spitzer A et al. Prealbumin as a biochemical marker of nutritional adequacy in premature infants. *J Pediatr*. 1983; 102:749–53.
20. Helms RA, Dickerson RN, Ebbert ML et al. Retinol-binding protein and prealbumin: useful measures of protein repletion in critically ill, malnourished infants. *J Pediatr Gastroenterol Nutr*. 1986; 5:586–92.
21. Clemmons DR, Underwood LE, Dickerson RN et al. Use of somatomedin-C/insulin-like growth factor I measurements to monitor the response to nutritional repletion in malnourished patients. *Am J Clin Nutr*. 1985; 41:191–8.
22. Kirby DF, Marder RJ, Craig RM et al. The clinical evaluation of plasma fibronectin as a marker for nutritional depletion and repletion and as a measure of nitrogen balance. *J Parenter Enter Nutr*. 1985; 9:705–8.
23. Forbes GB, Bruining GJ. Urinary creatinine excretion and lean body mass. *Am J Clin Nutr*. 1976; 29:1359–66.
24. Heird WC, Winters RW. Total parenteral nutrition. *J Pediatr*. 1975; 86:2–16.
25. Lopez AM, Wolfsdorf J, Raszynski A et al. Estimation of nitrogen balance based on a six-hour urine collection in infants. *J Parenter Enter Nutr*. 1986; 10:517–8.
26. Bistrian BR, Blackburn GL, Sherman M et al. Therapeutic index of nutritional depletion in hospitalized patients. *Surg Gynecol Obstet*. 1975; 141:512–6.
27. Viteri FE, Alvarado J. The creatinine height index: its use in the estimation of the degree of protein depletion and repletion in protein calorie malnourished children. *Pediatrics*. 1970; 46:696–706.
28. Seashore JH, Huszar GB, Davis EM. Urinary 3-methylhistidine excretion and nitrogen balance in healthy and stressed premature infants. *J Pediatr Surg*. 1980; 15:400–4.
29. Helms RA, Herrod HG, Burckart GJ et al. E-Rosette formation, total T-cells and lymphocyte transformation in infants receiving intravenous safflower oil emulsion. *J Parenter Enter Nutr*. 1983; 7:541–5.
30. Lawton AR, Cooper MD. Ontogeny of immunity. In: Stiehm ER, Bulginiti VA, eds. Immunologic disorders in infants and children. Philadelphia: W. B. Saunders Company; 1980:36–51.
31. Shannon DC, Johnson G, Rosen FS et al. Cellular reactivity to *Candida albicans* antigen. *N Engl J Med*. 1966; 275:690–3.
32. Shaw JCL. Parenteral nutrition in the management of sick low birthweight infants. *Pediatr Clin North Am*. 1973; 20:333–58.
33. Dreszer M. Fluid and electrolyte requirements in the newborn infant. *Pediatr Clin North Am*. 1977; 24:537–46.
34. Bell EF, Oh W. Fluid and electrolyte balance in very low birth weight infants. *Clin Perinatol*. 1979; 6:139–50.
35. Oh W. Disorders of fluid and electrolytes in newborn infants. *Pediatr Clin North Am*. 1976; 23:601–9.
36. Perkins RM, Levin DL. Common fluid and electrolyte problems in the pediatric intensive care unit. *Pediatr Clin North Am*. 1980; 27:567–86.
37. Oh W, Karecki H. Phototherapy and insensible water loss in the newborn infant. *Am J Dis Child*. 1972; 124:230–2.

38. Bell EF, Weinstein MR, Oh W. Heat balance in premature infants: comparative effects of convectively heated incubator and radiant warmer, with and without plastic heat shield. *J Pediatr.* 1980; 96:460–5.
39. Baumgart S. Partitioning of heat losses and gains in premature newborn infants under radiant warmers. *Pediatrics.* 1985; 75:89–99.
40. Bell EF, Warburton D, Stonestreet BS et al. Effect of fluid administration on the development of symptomatic patent ductus arteriosus and congestive heart failure in premature infants. *N Engl J Med.* 1980; 302:598–604.
41. Brown ER, Start A, Sosenko I et al. Bronchopulmonary dysplasia: possible relationship to pulmonary edema. *J Pediatr.* 1978; 92:982–4.
42. Goldman HI. Feeding and necrotizing enterocolitis. *Am J Dis Child.* 1980; 134:553–5.
43. Goldberg RN, Chung D, Goldman SL et al. The association of rapid volume expansion and intraventricular hemorrhage in the preterm infant. *J Pediatr.* 1980; 96:1060–3.
44. Knight PJ, Buchanan S, Clatworthy H. Calcium and phosphate requirements of preterm infants who require prolonged hyperalimentation. *JAMA.* 1980; 243:1244–6.
45. Edelman IS, Leibman J. Anatomy of body water and electrolytes. *Am J Med.* 1959; 27:256–77.
46. Siegel SR, Oh W. Renal function as a marker of human fetal maturation. *Acta Paediatr Scand.* 1976; 65:481–5.
47. Cowett RM, Oh W, Pollak A et al. Glucose disposal of low birth weight infants: steady state hyperglycemia produced by constant intravenous glucose infusion. *Pediatrics.* 1979; 63:389–96.
48. Abbott Hospital Products. L-Cysteine hydrochloride product information. Irvine, CA; 1987 Feb.
49. Lawson DH. Clinical use of potassium supplements. *Am J Hosp Pharm.* 1975; 32:708–11.
50. Ash SR. The perils of IV potassium: are they exaggerated? *Parenterals.* Dec 1986/Jan 1987:1–8.
51. Upton J, Mulliken JB, Murray JE. Major intravenous extravasation injuries. *Am J Surg.* 1979; 137:497–506.
52. Yosowitz P, Ekland DA, Shaw RC. Peripheral intravenous infiltration necrosis. *Ann Surg.* 1975; 182:553–6.
53. Surawicz B. Relationship between electrocardiogram and electrolytes. *Am Heart J.* 1967; 73:814–34.
54. Popovtzer MM, Knochel JP. Disorders of calcium, phosphorus, vitamin D, and parathyroid hormone activity. In: Schrier RW, ed. Renal and electrolyte disorders. Boston: Little, Brown and Company; 1986:251–329.
55. Niemiec PW, Vanderveen TW. Compatibility considerations in parenteral nutrient solutions. *Am J Hosp Pharm.* 1984; 41:893–911.
56. Eggert LD, Rusho WJ, MacKay MW et al. Calcium and phosphorus compatibility in parenteral nutrition solutions for neonates. *Am J Hosp Pharm.* 1982; 39:49–53.
57. Fitzgerald KA, MacKay MW. Calcium and phosphate solubility in neonatal parenteral nutrient solutions containing TrophAmine. *Am J Hosp Pharm.* 1986; 43:88–93.
58. Fitzgerald KA, MacKay MW. Calcium and phosphate solubility in neonatal parenteral nutrient solutions containing Aminosyn PF. *Am J Hosp Pharm.* 1987; 44:1396–1400.
59. Kimura S, Nose O, Seino Y. Effects of alternate and simultaneous administrations of calcium and phosphorus on calcium metabolism in children receiving total parenteral nutrition. *J Parenter Enter Nutr.* 1986; 10:513–6.
60. Schmidt GL, Baumgartner TG, Fischlschweiger W et al. Cost containment using cysteine HCl acidification to increase calcium/phosphate solubility in hyperalimentation solutions. *J Parenter Enter Nutr.* 1986; 10:203–7.
61. Driscol JM, Heird WC, Schullinger JN et al. Total intravenous alimentation in low-birth weight infants: a preliminary report. *J Pediatr.* 1972; 81:145–53.
62. Ghadimi H, Abaci F, Kumar S et al. Biochemical aspects of intravenous alimentation. *Pediatrics.* 1971; 48:955–65.
63. Heird WC, Dell RB, Driscoll JM et al. Metabolic acidosis resulting from intravenous alimentation mixtures containing synthetic amino acids. *N Engl J Med.* 1972; 287:943–8.
64. Johnson JD, Albritton WL, Sunshine P. Hyperammonemia accompanying parenteral nutrition in newborn infants. *J Pediatr.* 1972; 81:154–61.
65. Duffy B, Gunn T, Collinge J et al. The effect of varying protein quality and energy intake on the nitrogen metabolism of parenterally fed very low birthweight (<1600 g) infants. *Pediatr Res.* 1981; 15:1040–4.
66. Zlotkin SH, Stallings VA, Penchary PB. Total parenteral nutrition in children. *Pediatr Clin North Am.* 1985; 32:381–400.
67. Malloy MH, Gaull GE. Enteral protein and amino acid nutrition in preterm infants. *Semin Perinatol.* 1979; 3:315–20.
68. Davidson M, Levine SZ, Bauer CH et al. Feeding studies in low-birth-weight infants. *J Pediatr.* 1967; 70:695–713.
69. Goldman HI, Freudenthal R, Holland B et al. Clinical effects of two different levels of protein intake on low-birth-weight infants. *J Pediatr.* 1969; 74:881–9.
70. Committee on Nutrition, American Academy of Pediatrics. Commentary on parenteral nutrition. *Pediatrics.* 1983; 71:547–52.
71. Rubecz I, Mestyan J, Varga P et al. Energy metabolism, substrate utilization, and nitrogen balance in parenterally fed postoperative neonates and infants. *J Pediatr.* 1981; 98:42–6.
72. Anderson TL, Muttart CR, Bilber MA et al. A controlled trial of glucose versus glucose and amino acids in premature infants. *J Pediatr.* 1979; 94:947–51.
73. Zlotkin SH, Bryan MH, Anderson GH. Intravenous nitrogen and energy intakes required to duplicate in utero nitrogen accretion in prematurely born human infants. *J Pediatr.* 1981; 99:115–20.
74. Stegink LD, Baker GL. Infusion of protein hydrolysates in the newborn infant: plasma amino acid concentrations. *J Pediatr.* 1971; 78:595–602.
75. Das JB, Filler RM. Amino acid utilization during total parenteral nutrition in the surgical neonate. *J Pediatr Surg.* 1973; 8:793–9.
76. Gaull G, Sturman JA, Raiha NCR. Development of mammalian sulfur metabolism: absence of cystathionase in human fetal tissues. *Pediatr Res.* 1972; 6:538–47.
77. Malloy MH, Rassin DK, Richardson CJ. Total parenteral nutrition in sick preterm infants: effects of cysteine supplementation with nitrogen intakes of 240 and 400 mg/kg/day. *J Pediatr Gastroenterol Nutr.* 1984; 3:239–44.
78. Zlotkin SH, Bryan MH, Anderson GH. Cysteine supplementation to cysteine-free intravenous feeding regimens in newborn infants. *Am J Clin Nutr.* 1981; 34:914–23.
79. Snyderman SE, Boyer A, Roitman E et al. The histidine requirement of the infant. *Pediatrics.* 1963; 31:786–801.
80. Olney JW, Ho OL. Brain damage in infant mice following oral intake of glutamate, aspartate, and cysteine. *Nature.* 1970; 227:609–11.
81. Bell EF, Filer LJ, Wong AP et al. Effects of a parenteral nutrition regimen containing dicarboxylic amino acids on plasma, erythrocyte, and urinary amino acid concentrations of young infants. *Am J Clin Nutr.* 1983; 37:99–107.
82. Wu PYK, Edwards NB, Storm MC. Plasma amino acid pattern in normal term breast-fed infants. *J Pediatr.* 1986; 109:347–9.
83. Andersen GE, Bucher D, Friis-Hansen B et al. Plasma amino acid concentrations in newborn infants during parenteral nutrition. *J Parenter Enter Nutr.* 1983; 7:369–73.
84. Pohlandt F. Plasma amino acid concentrations in newborn infants breast-fed ad libitum. *J Pediatr.* 1979; 92:614–6.
85. Thom JC, Victor T, Pichanick AME et al. The effect of intravenous amino acids on plasma amino acid concentration during total parenteral nutrition in infants with necrotizing enterocolitis. *S Afr Med J.* 1981; 59:946–9.
86. Ghadimi H, Pecora P. Plasma amino acids after birth. *Pediatrics.* 1964; 34:182–91.

87. Filer LJ, Stegink LD, Chandramouli B. Effect of diet on plasma aminograms of low birth weight infants. *Am J Clin Nutr.* 1977; 30:1036–43.
88. Helms RA, Christensen ML, Mauer EC et al. Comparison of a pediatric versus standard amino acid formulation in preterm neonates requiring parenteral nutrition. *J Pediatr.* 1987; 110:466–70.
89. Heird WC, Dell RB, Helms RA et al. Evaluation of an amino acid mixture designed to maintain normal plasma amino acid patterns in infants and children receiving parenteral nutrition. *Pediatrics.* 1987; 80:401–8.
90. Helms RA, Johnson MR, Christensen ML et al. Evaluation of two pediatric amino acid formulations. *J Parenter Enter Nutr.* 1988; 12 (Suppl):45. Abstract.
91. Adamkin DH, Sims A, Radmacher P. Plasma amino acids in premature (PT) neonates receiving a pediatric amino acid formulation (PA) containing taurine, glutamate, and aspartate. *Clin Res.* 1984; 32:898A. Abstract.
92. Helms RA, Johnson MR, Christensen ML et al. Altered caloric and protein requirement in neonates receiving a pediatric amino acid formulation. *Pediatr Res.* 1987; 21:429A. Abstract.
93. Reichman B, Chessex P, Putet G et al. Diet, fat accretion, and growth in premature infants. *N Engl J Med.* 1981; 305:1495–1500.
94. Reichman BL, Chessex P, Putet G et al. Partition of energy metabolism and energy cost of growth in the very low-birth-weight infant. *Pediatrics.* 1982; 69:446–51.
95. Coran AG. The long-term total intravenous feeding of infants using peripheral veins. *J Pediatr Surg.* 1973; 8:801–7.
96. Kerner JA Jr. Caloric requirements. In: Kerner JA Jr, ed. Manual of pediatric parenteral nutrition. New York: John Wiley & Sons; 1983:63-7.
97. Benda GIM, Babson SG. Peripheral intravenous alimentation of the small premature infant. *J Pediatr.* 1971; 79:494–8.
98. Peden VH, Sammon TJ, Downey DA. Intravenously induced infantile intoxication with ethanol. *J Pediatr.* 1973; 88:490–3.
99. Hessov I. Which carbohydrates should we recommend for intravenous nutrition? *Acta Anaesthesiol Scand.* 1985; 29:30–1.
100. Freeman JB, Fairfull-Smith R, Rodman GH Jr et al. Safety and efficacy of a new peripheral intravenously administered amino acid solution containing glycerol and electrolytes. *Surg Gynecol Obstet.* 1983; 156:625–31.
101. Coran AG. Parenteral nutrition in infants and children. *Surg Clin North Am.* 1981; 61:1089–1100.
102. Cashore WJ, Sedaghatian MR, Usher RH. Nutritional supplements with IV administered lipid protein hydrolysates and glucose in small premature neonates. *Pediatrics.* 1975; 56:8–16.
103. Thomas DB. Hyperosmolality and intraventricular haemorrhage in premature babies. *Acta Paediatr Scand.* 1976; 65:429–32.
104. Weber SS, Wood WA, Jackson EA. Availability of insulin from parenteral nutrient solutions. *Am J Hosp Pharm.* 1977; 34:353–7.
105. Fort P, Waters SM, Lifshitz F. Low-dose insulin infusion in the treatment of diabetic ketoacidosis: bolus versus no bolus. *J Pediatr.* 1980; 96:36–40.
106. Sajbel TA, Dutro MP, Radway PR. Use of separate insulin infusions with total parenteral nutrition. *J Parenter Enter Nutr.* 1987; 11:97–9.
107. Press M, Kikuchi H, Shimoyama T et al. Diagnosis and treatment of essential fatty acid deficiency in man. *Br Med J.* 1974; 2:247–50.
108. Committee on Nutrition, American Academy of Pediatrics. Use of intravenous fat emulsions in pediatric patients. *Pediatrics.* 1981; 68:738–43.
109. Bivins BA, Bell RM, Rapp RP et al. Linoleic acid versus linolenic acid: what is essential? *J Parenter Enter Nutr.* 1983; 7:473–8.
110. Friedman Z, Danon A, Stahlman MT et al. Rapid onset of essential fatty acid deficiency in the newborn. *Pediatrics.* 1976; 58:640–9.
111. Paulsrud JR, Pensler L, Witten CF et al. Essential fatty acid deficiency in infants induced by fat free intravenous feedings. *Am J Clin Nutr.* 1972; 25:897–904.
112. Friedman Z, Shochat SJ, Maisels MJ et al. Correction of essential fatty acid deficiency in newborn infants by cutaneous application of sunflower-seed oil. *Pediatrics.* 1976; 58:650–4.
113. Hunt CE, Engel RR, Modler S et al. Essential fatty acid deficiency in neonates: inability to reverse deficiency by topical applications of EFA-rich oils. *J Pediatr.* 1978; 92:603–7.
114. Committee on Nutrition, American Academy of Pediatrics. Nutritional needs of low-birth-weight infants. *Pediatrics.* 1977; 50:519–30.
115. Bell EF, Filer LJ Jr. The role of vitamin E in the nutrition of premature infants. *Am J Clin Nutr.* 1981; 34:414–22.
116. Schreiner RL, Glick MR, Nordschow CD et al. An evaluation of methods to monitor infants receiving intravenous lipids. *J Pediatr.* 1979; 94:197–200.
117. Kerner JA Jr. Fat requirements. In: Kerner JA Jr, ed. Manual of pediatric parenteral nutrition. New York: John Wiley & Sons; 1983:103–27.
118. Pelham LD. Rational use of intravenous fat emulsions. *Am J Hosp Pharm.* 1981; 38:198–208.
119. Phelps SJ, Cochran EC, Kamper CA. Peripheral venous line infiltration in infants receiving 10% dextrose, 10% dextrose/amino acids, 10% dextrose/amino acids/fat emulsion. *Pediatr Res.* 1987; 21:67A. Abstract.
120. Paust H, Schroder H, Park W et al. Fat elimination in parenterally fed low birth weight infants during the first two weeks of life. *J Parenter Enter Nutr.* 1983; 7:557–9.
121. Andrew F, Chan G, Schiff D. Lipid metabolism in the neonate. *J Pediatr.* 1976; 88:273–8.
122. Pereira GR, Fox WW, Stanley CA et al. Decreased oxygenation and hyperlipemia during intravenous fat infusions in premature infants. *Pediatrics.* 1980; 66:26–30.
123. Cooke RJ, Burckart GJ. Hypertriglyceridemia during the intravenous infusion of a safflower oil-based fat emulsion. *J Pediatr.* 1983; 103:959–61.
124. Park W, Paust H, Brosicke H et al. Impaired fat utilization in parenterally fed low-birth-weight infants suffering from sepsis. *J Parenter Enter Nutr.* 1986; 10:627–30.
125. Park W, Paust H, Schroder H. Lipid infusion in premature infants suffering from sepsis. *J Parenter Enter Nutr.* 1984; 8:290–2.
126. Bremer J. Carnitine metabolism and functions. *Physiol Rev.* 1983;63:1420–80.
127. Schmidt-Sommerfeld E, Penn D, Wolf H. Carnitine blood concentrations and fat utilization in parenterally alimented premature newborn infants. *J Pediatr.* 1982; 100:260–4.
128. Yeh Y, Cooke RJ, Zee P. Impairment of lipid emulsion metabolism associated with carnitine insufficiency in premature infants. *J Pediatr Gastroenterol Nutr.* 1985; 4:795–8.
129. Schmidt-Sommerfeld E, Penn D, Wolf H. Carnitine deficiency in premature infants receiving total parenteral nutrition: effect of L-carnitine supplementation. *J Pediatr.* 1983; 102:931–5.
130. Helms RA, Whitington PF, Mauer EC et al. Enhanced lipid utilization in infants receiving oral L-carnitine during long-term parenteral nutrition. *J Pediatr.* 1986; 109:984–8.
131. Dhanireddy R, Hamosh M, Sivasubramanian KN et al. Post heparin lipolytic activity and Intralipid clearance in very low-birth-weight infants. *J Pediatr.* 1981; 98:617–22.
132. Zaidan H, Dhanireddy R, Hamosh M et al. Effect of continuous heparin administrtion on Intralipid clearing in very low-birth-weight infants. *J Pediatr.* 1982; 101:599–602.
133. Zaidan H, Dhanireddy R, Hamosh M et al. Lipid clearing in premature infants during continuous heparin infusion: role of circulating lipases. *Pediatr Res.* 1985; 19:23–5.
134. Overall JC Jr. Jaundice and hyperbilirubinemia in the newborn infant. In: Nelson WE, ed. Nelson textbook of

pediatrics. Philadelphia: W. B. Saunders Company; 1987:405–7.
135. Andrew G, Chan G, Schiff D. The effect of Intralipid on bilirubin binding in vitro and in vivo. *J Pediatr.* 1976; 88:279–84.
136. Burckart GJ, Whitington PF, Helms RA. The effect of two intravenous fat emulsions and their components on bilirubin binding to albumin. *Am J Clin Nutr.* 1982; 36:521–6.
137. Nordenstrom J, Jarstrand C, Wiernik A. Decreased chemotactic and random migration of leukocytes during Intralipid infusion. *Am J Clin Nutr.* 1979; 32:2416–22.
138. Friedman Z, Marks KH, Maisels J et al. Effect of parenteral fat emulsion on the pulmonary and reticulo-endothelial systems in the newborn infant. *Pediatrics.* 1978; 61:694–8.
139. Barson AJ, Chiswick ML, Doig MC. Fat embolism in infancy after intravenous fat infusions. *Arch Dis Child.* 1978; 53:218–3.
140. Hertel J, Tystrup I, Andersen GE. Intravascular fat accumulation after Intralipid infusion in the very low-birth-weight infant. *J Pediatr.* 1982; 100:975–6.
141. Schroder H, Paust H, Schmidt R. Pulmonary fat embolism after Intralipid therapy—a post-mortem artefact? *Acta Paediatr Scand.* 1984; 73:461–4.
142. Brans YW, Dutton EB, Andrew DS et al. Fat emulsion tolerance in very low birth weight neonates: effect on diffusion of oxygen in the lungs and on blood pH. *Pediatrics.* 1986; 78:79–84.
143. Greene HL. Vitamins in total parenteral nutrition. *Drug Intell Clin Pharmacol.* 1972; 6:355–60.
144. Multivitamin preparations for parenteral use—a statement by the Nutrition Advisory Group (AMA, Dept. of Foods and Nutrition). *J Parenter Enter Nutr.* 1979; 3:258–62.
145. Armour Pharmaceutical Company. M.V.I. Pediatric product information. Kankakee, IL; 1986 May.
146. Moore MC, Greene HL, Phillips B et al. Evaluation of a pediatric multiple vitamin preparation for total parenteral nutrition in infants and children. *Pediatrics.* 1986; 77:530–8.
147. Greene HL, Moore MEC, Phillips B et al. Evaluation of a pediatric multiple vitamin preparation for total parenteral nutrition. *Pediatrics.* 1986; 77:539–47.
148. Mock DM. Water-soluble vitamin requirements of the preterm infant. *J Pediatr Gastroenterol Nutr.* 1987; 6:323–5.
149. Franck LS, Greene HL, Phillips BL. Alpha tocopherol (E) levels in premature infants during and after intravenous multivitamin supplementation. *Clin Res.* 1986; 34:115A. Abstract.
150. Greene HL, Phillips BL. Vitamin dosages in premature infants. *Pediatrics.* 1987; 79:655. Letter.
151. Polland RL. Vitamin E: what should we do? *Pediatrics.* 1986; 77:788. Letter.
152. Blanc WA, Reid JD, Andersen DH. Avitaminosis E in cystic fibrosis of the pancreas. *Pediatrics.* 1958; 22:494–505.
153. DeBari VA, Frank O, Baker H et al. Water soluble vitamins in granulocytes, erythrocytes, and plasma obtained from chronic hemodialysis patients. *Am J Clin Nutr.* 1984; 39:410–5.
154. Zlotkin SH, Buchanan BE. Meeting zinc and copper intake requirements in the parenterally fed preterm and full-term infant. *J Pediatr.* 1983; 103:441–6.
155. American Medical Association. Guidelines for essential trace element preparations for parenteral use. *JAMA.* 1979; 241:2051–4.
156. Rotruck JT, Pope AL, Ganther HE et al. Selenium: biochemical role as a component of glutathione peroxidase. *Science.* 1973; 179:588–90.
157. SoloPak Laboratories. Sele-Pak product information. Franklin Park, IL; 1986 Apr.
158. Pyati SP, Ramamurthy RS, Krauss MT et al. Absorption of iodine in the neonate following topical use of povidone iodine. *J Pediatr.* 1977; 91:825–8.
159. Melhorn DK, Gross S. Vitamin E dependent anemia in the premature infant: I. Effects of large doses of medicinal iron. *J Pediatr.* 1971; 79:569–80.
160. American hospital formulary service—drug information 86. McEvoy GK, ed. Iron preparations. Bethesda, MD: American Society of Hospital Pharmacists; 1986:638–40.
161. Johnson DG. Total intravenous nutrition in newborn surgical patients: a 3 year perspective. *J Pediatr Surg.* 1970; 5:601–5.
162. Eichelberger MR, Rous PG, Hoelzer D et al. Percutaneous subclavian venous catheters in neonates and children. *Pediatr Surg.* 1981; 16:547–52.
163. Pinilla JC, Ross DF, Martin T et al. Study of the incidence of intravascular catheter infection and associated septicemia in critically ill patients. *Crit Care Med.* 1983; 11:21–5.
164. Goldman DA, Maki DG. Infection control in total parenteral nutrition. *JAMA.* 1973; 223:1360–4.
165. Murphy LM, Lipman TO. Central venous catheter care in parenteral nutrition: a review. *J Parenter Enter Nutr.* 1987; 11:190–201.
166. Trooskin SZ, Donetz AP, Harvey RA et al. Prevention of catheter sepsis by antibiotic bonding. *Surgery.* 1985; 97:547–51.
167. Bozzetti F, Terno G, Bonfanti G et al. Prevention and treatment of central venous catheter sepsis by exchange via a guidewire. *Ann Surg.* 1983; 198:48–52.
168. Flynn PM, Shenep JL, Stokes DC et al. In situ management of confirmed central venous catheter-related bacteremia. *Pediatr Infect Dis.* 1987; 6:729–34.
169. Glynn MFX, Langer B, Jeejeebhoy KN. Therapy for thrombotic occlusion of long-term intravenous alimentation catheters. *J Parenter Enter Nutr.* 1980; 4:387–90.
170. Winthrop AL, Wesson DE. Urokinase in the treatment of occluded central venous catheters in children. *J Pediatr Surg.* 1984; 19:536–8.
171. Leape LL, Valaes T. Rickets in low birth weight infants receiving total parenteral nutrition. *J Pediatr Surg.* 1976; 11:665–74.
172. Venkataraman PS, Tsang RC, Stichen JJ et al. Early neonatal hypocalcemia in extremely preterm infants. *Am J Dis Child.* 1986; 140:1004–8.
173. Merritt RJ. Cholestasis associated with total parenteral nutrition. *J Pediatr Gastroenterol Nutr.* 1986; 5:9–22.
174. Black DD, Suttle EA, Whitington PF et al. The effect of short-term total parenteral nutrition on hepatic function in the human neonate: a prospective randomized study demonstrating alteration of hepatic canalicular function. *J Pediatr.* 1981; 99:445–9.
175. Bell RL, Ferry GD, Smith EO et al. Total parenteral nutrition-related cholestasis in infants. *J Parenter Enter Nutr.* 1986; 10:356–9.
176. Sondheimer JM, Bryan H, Andrews W et al. Cholestatic tendencies in premature infants on and off parenteral nutrition. *Pediatrics.* 1978; 62:984–9.
177. Beale EF, Nelson RM, Bucciarelli RL et al. Intrahepatic cholestasis associated with parenteral nutrition in premature infants. *Pediatrics.* 1979; 64:342–7.
178. Pereira GR, Sherman MS, DiGiacomo J et al. Hyperalimentation-induced cholestasis. Increased incidence and severity of premature infants. *Am J Dis Child.* 1981; 135:842–5.
179. Postuma R, Trevenen CL. Liver disease in infants receiving total parenteral nutrition. *Pediatrics.* 1979; 63:110–5.
180. Gleghorn EE, Merritt RJ, Subramanian N et al. Phenobarbital does not prevent total parenteral nutrition-associated cholestasis in noninfected neonates. *J Parenter Enter Nutr.* 1986; 10:282–3.

Research

Accuracy of tobramycin delivery by four i.v. infusion methods

ROY A. PLEASANTS, WILLIAM T. SAWYER, DENNIS M. WILLIAMS, WILLIAM R. MCKENNA, JOHN M. BROWN, AND J. ROBERT POWELL

Abstract: The accuracy of tobramycin delivery by four methods of intermittent intravenous infusion was studied in 11 healthy male volunteers.

Subjects received intravenous tobramycin (as the sulfate salt) 1.5 mg/kg by each of four infusion methods in a nonblinded, randomized, four-way crossover design. The methods used for intravenous infusion were (1) minibag via gravity flow (MG), (2) minibag with the secondary infusion tubing inserted below a volumetric infusion pump (MP), (3) metered chamber via volumetric infusion pump (MC), and (4) syringe pump (SP). Doses were diluted to a volume of 50 mL, except for the two minibag methods, for which the dilution was necessarily greater because of manufacturer overfill. Intravenous flow rates for both primary fluid and drug administration were set at 100 mL/hr, and the duration of drug infusion was documented by observation for each administered dose. The fluid volume of 12 minibags was measured to assess manufacturer overfill. Fluid remaining in the secondary i.v. tubing for the minibag methods was collected after the infusion. Seventeen blood samples were obtained before and at various time intervals after each dose and analyzed in duplicate for tobramycin content by fluorescence polarization immunoassay.

A mean of 10% of each dose remained in the secondary i.v. tubing at the completion of the infusion for the minibag methods, whereas less than 1% of each dose remained in the secondary tubing for the SP method. Since the proportion of the dose administered was lower with minibag administration than with the syringe-pump or metered-chamber methods, the values for the area under the concentration–time curve from time zero to infinity for the subjects receiving the drug via the minibag methods were significantly lower than those for the subjects using the other methods. The duration of infusion was significantly longer for both minibag methods than for either the metered-chamber or the syringe-pump method.

In comparison with the metered-chamber and syringe-pump methods, the two minibag methods used in this investigation were associated with prolonged and incomplete delivery of tobramycin.

Index terms: Aminoglycosides; Blood levels; Devices; Drug administration systems; Injections; Surgical supplies; Tobramycin; Tobramycin sulfate

Clin Pharm. 1988; 7:367–73

The relative influence of different intravenous infusion methods on drug delivery is particularly important to clinicians because of patient-care implications. In pediatric patients, use of conventional methods for intermittent i.v. infusion, such as metered (volumetric) chambers alone, has been shown to result in untimely and incomplete drug delivery.[1–3] To improve the efficiency of drug administration by i.v. infusion in this patient population, techniques such as retrograde administration

ROY A. PLEASANTS, PHARM.D., is Senior Clinical Specialist in Infectious Diseases, North Carolina Memorial Hospital, Chapel Hill, NC, and Clinical Assistant Professor, School of Pharmacy, University of North Carolina at Chapel Hill (UNCCH). WILLIAM T. SAWYER, M.S., is Assistant Director of Clinical Services, Department of Pharmacy, North Carolina Memorial Hospital, and Associate Professor, School of Pharmacy, UNCCH. DENNIS M. WILLIAMS, PHARM.D., is Clinical Assistant Professor, School of Pharmacy; WILLIAM R. MCKENNA, M.D., is Fellow, Division of Infectious Diseases, School of Medicine; and JOHN M. BROWN, M.D., is Resident in Internal Medicine, School of Medicine, UNCCH. J. ROBERT POWELL, PHARM.D., is Head, Clinical Pharmacokinetics, Glaxo Inc., Research Triangle Park, NC; at the time of this study, he was Associate Professor, School of Pharmacy, UNCCH.

Address reprint requests to Dr. Pleasants at the Department of Pharmacy, North Carolina Memorial Hospital, Manning Dr., Chapel Hill, NC 27514.

Supported in part by Becton Dickinson and Company, Infusion Systems, Lincoln Park, NJ 07006; IMED Corporation, San Diego, CA 92131; and Clinical Research Unit, School of Medicine, UNCCH (NIH grant RR46).

Presented at the 21st Annual ASHP Midyear Clinical Meeting, Las Vegas, NV, December 11, 1986.

Copyright © 1988, American Society of Hospital Pharmacists, Inc. All rights reserved. 0278-2677/88/0501-0367$01.75.

and syringe pumps have become more widely employed.

Previous in vitro investigations of representative methods used for adults, gravity-flow minibag[4] and volumetric chamber,[5] have been documented to be associated with prolonged tobramycin delivery. A recent report has indicated that drug delivery by minibags may result in altered serum drug concentration data in adults.[6] Therefore, we conducted this investigation to evaluate the effect of four i.v. infusion methods on the timeliness and completeness of tobramycin administration in healthy adult volunteers.

Methods

Twelve healthy male volunteers, ≥18 years of age and within 20% of ideal body weight, were selected for a nonblinded, randomized, four-way crossover study. Subjects were chosen based on normal results of a medical history and physical examination, measurement of vital signs, and laboratory tests including blood chemistries and urinalysis. Healthy adult volunteers were chosen instead of patients to minimize intersubject and intrasubject variation in tobramycin pharmacokinetic disposition. The study protocol was approved by the institution's committee on the protection of the rights of human subjects, and all subjects gave their written informed consent before initiation of the study. Subjects were instructed to abstain from other medications, alcohol, and caffeine at least 24 hours before and during each study day.

Each subject received four single doses of intravenous tobramycin (as the sulfate salt) 1.5 mg/kg of total body weight, on different occasions, each separated by a one-week washout period. Once randomization had been established, doses were administered to the subjects in an identical sequence on each study day. A single lot of tobramycin (Nebcin, Eli Lilly and Company, Indianapolis, IN, lot 9NP77B) was used, and samples from this lot were assayed for drug concentration to determine the actual dose administered. Doses were prepared within 24 hours of administration, refrigerated at 8 °C, and allowed to reach room temperature before administration. Doses were diluted with 0.9% sodium chloride injection to a volume of 50 mL; however, this dilution was necessarily greater with minibags because of manufacturer overfill. On each study day, an indwelling venous catheter (Flash-Cath, Travenol Laboratories, Deerfield, IL 60015 and PRN Adapter, Deseret Med., Inc., Sandy, UT 64070) was inserted in each subject's arm for blood sampling, and a second venous catheter was inserted in the opposite arm for drug administration.

Infusion Methods. Tobramycin was delivered to subjects by each of the following intravenous infusion systems: (1) minibag via gravity flow (MG), (2) minibag with the secondary infusion tubing inserted below a volumetric pump (MP), (3) metered chamber via volumetric pump (MC), and (4) syringe pump (SP). These systems are shown in Figures 1–4. The first three methods were selected to simulate the methods, i.v. tubing, and techniques used most frequently at this institution. Fifty-milliliter minibags were selected to allow comparison among the methods in which similar fluid volumes and flow rates were used. Although both minibag methods employed gravity flow for actual drug administration, the technique of primary i.v. fluid administration differed between the two methods. For the MG method, primary fluid was administered by gravity flow, whereas a volumetric infusion pump was used for primary fluid administration for the MP method. The sequence of infusion methods was randomly selected for each subject before initiation of the study. Subjects remained

Figure 1. Diagram of the minibag gravity intravenous infusion method. LVI = large-volume injection.

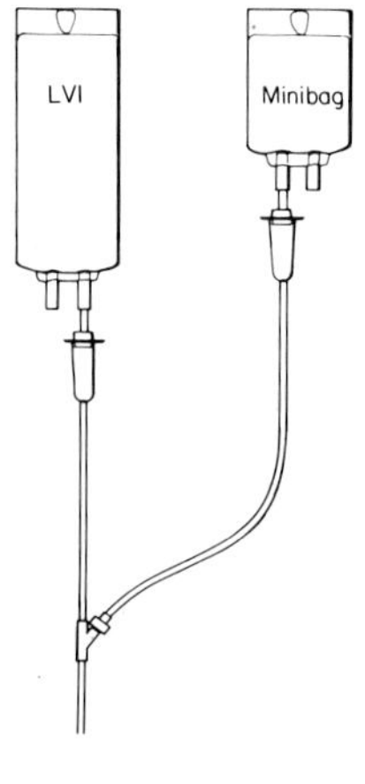

Figure 2. Diagram of the minibag pump intravenous infusion method. LVI = large-volume injection.

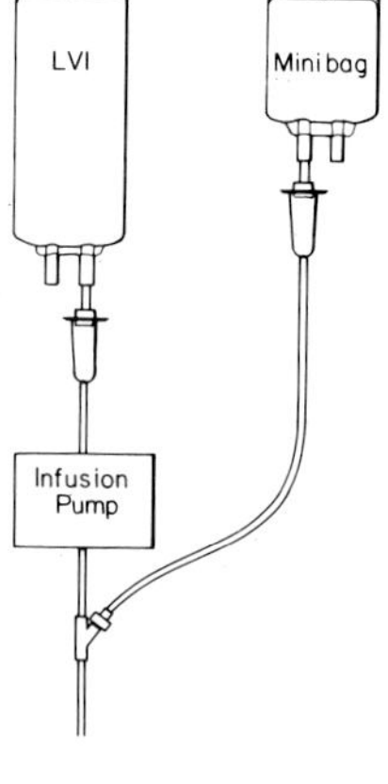

Figure 3. Diagram of the metered-chamber intravenous infusion method. LVI = large-volume injection.

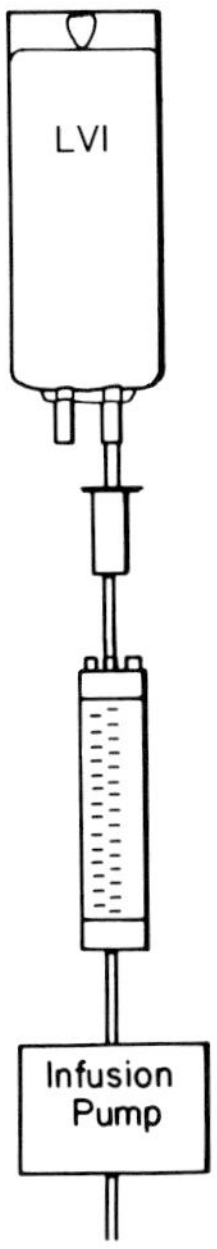

Figure 4. Diagram of the syringe-pump intravenous infusion method. LVI = large-volume injection.

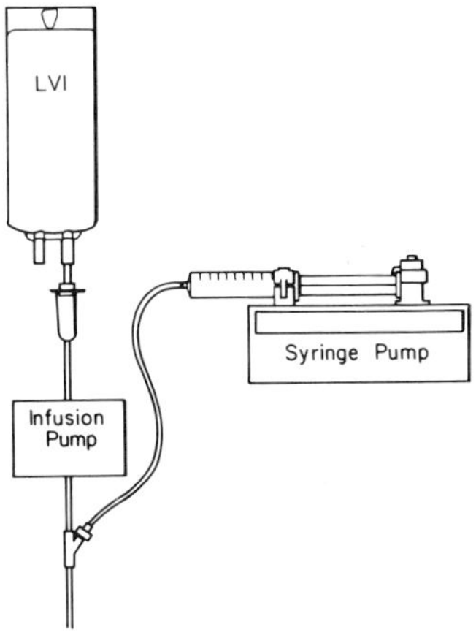

seated during the infusion of fluids to minimize alterations in flow rates related to postural changes.

Flow rates for drug and fluid administration were initially set to theoretically administer each dose over 30 minutes based on measured (MC and SP) or reported (MG and MP) volumes of diluent; no additional changes were made afterward to compensate for possible alterations in flow rates. An electronic drop-rate counter (IMED 340, IMED Corp., San Diego, CA 92131) was used to establish drip rates for gravity-flow i.v. fluid and drug administration for the MG and MP methods. Flow rates for pump-assisted drug and fluid delivery were set by the appropriate devices on the volumetric and syringe pumps. Intravenous fluid was allowed to empty from the minibags and become stationary in the secondary tubing. Secondary i.v. sets for the MG, MP, and SP methods remained attached to the primary tubing until primary fluid administration was complete. Primary fluid administration was maintained for 90 minutes after initiation of the tobramycin infusion for each method. A single lot of minibags was used for this study (Viaflex, Travenol Laboratories, lot ZP001347), and overfill was determined by measuring the volume of i.v. fluid contained in 12 minibags.

The observed infusion time, defined as the time required for i.v. fluid flow to stop in the secondary tubing for the minibag methods and the time required for the syringe or metered chamber to empty, was documented for each dose in each subject. Actual (adjusted) duration of infusion (t') was determined from the observed infusion time plus the estimated time required for the volume of fluid containing drug to completely cease delivery from the infusion systems (e.g., calculated time required for drug remaining in primary line to be infused after cessation of flow from minibag set plus observed infusion time). Predicted infusion time was calculated from the initial flow rate, the volume of fluid containing tobramycin, and the estimated time required for the drug to begin entering the systemic circulation, depending on where the drug was introduced into the i.v. set. Details of each infusion method are described below.

Minibag Gravity. The minibag gravity (MG) method included one large-volume injection (LVI), 500 mL of 0.9% sodium chloride injection (Viaflex, lot C007278, Travenol Laboratories), one primary i.v. tubing set (Saftiset, code 811-91, 60 drops/mL, 80 inch, i.d. = 0.105 inch, nonvented set with check valve, lot NJ5477, Cutter Biologicals, Berkeley, CA 94710), one secondary i.v. tubing set (Saftiset, code 811-90, 10 drops/mL, 70 inch, i.d. = 0.105 inch, nonvented set, lot NJ5860, Cutter), and one 50-mL minibag containing 0.9% sodium chloride injection and tobramycin. The primary i.v. tubing was primed and set at a flow rate of 100 mL/hr. The secondary i.v. set was primed and piggybacked into the primary line at the Y-site proximal to the subject, and a flow rate of 100 mL/hr was established at the onset of the infusion.

Minibag Pump. The minibag pump (MP) method included one LVI, 500 mL of 0.9% sodium chloride injection (Viaflex, Travenol Laboratories), one primary i.v. tubing and cassette (Accuset, code 9215, i.d. above cassette = 0.118 inch, i.d. below cassette = 0.060 inch, lot 86I09632, IMED Corp.), one secondary i.v. tubing set (Saftiset, code 811-90, Cutter), a volumetric infusion pump (model 960, IMED Corp.), and one 50-mL minibag containing 0.9%

sodium chloride injection and tobramycin. The primary i.v. tubing was primed, and the infusion pump was set at a flow rate of 100 mL/hr. The secondary set inclusive of the minibag was primed and piggybacked into the Y-site proximal to the subject (below the infusion pump), and a flow rate of 100 mL/hr was established at the onset of the infusion.

Metered Chamber. The metered-chamber (MC) method included one LVI, 500 mL of 0.9% sodium chloride injection (Viaflex, Travenol Laboratories), one metered chamber, i.v. tubing, and cassette (Accuset, code 9225, lot 6A04203, IMED Corp.), and a volumetric infusion pump (model 960, IMED Corp.). The i.v. set was primed with primary fluid, and then undiluted tobramycin, previously drawn into a syringe, was injected into the metered chamber and diluted with the primary fluid to yield a total volume of 50 mL. The flow rate was set at 100 mL/hr. At the end of the drug infusion, the infusion pump was stopped, and 100 mL of primary i.v. fluid was added into the metered chamber. The infusion pump was restarted and allowed to run for an additional 60 minutes at the same flow rate.

Syringe Pump. The syringe-pump (SP) method included one LVI, 500 mL of 0.9% sodium chloride injection (Viaflex, Travenol Laboratories), one primary i.v. tubing and cassette (Accuset, code 9215, lot 86I09632, IMED Corp.), a volumetric infusion pump (model 960, IMED Corp.), a syringe pump (model 360, Becton Dickinson and Co., Lincoln Park, NJ 07006), one i.v. extension tubing (Microbore Extension Set, code 2804, 60 inch, i.d. = 0.02 inch, lot 54401, Becton Dickinson), and one 60-mL syringe containing tobramycin diluted with 0.9% sodium chloride injection to a volume of 50 mL. The extension set was attached to the syringe, primed, and piggybacked into the lower Y-site (below the infusion pump). The primary i.v. line was primed, and both the volumetric and syringe pumps were set at a flow rate of 100 mL/hr.

Specimen Collection and Analysis. Serum samples for creatinine determination were obtained before the study and on each study day to monitor potential changes in renal function. Blood samples were obtained just before and 10, 20, 30, 35, 40, 45, 60, 75, 90, 105, 120, 150, 180, 240, 360, and 480 minutes after initiation of the drug infusion. At each sampling time, an initial aliquot of blood was obtained through the appropriate intravenous catheter and discarded, and a second aliquot of blood was then drawn into a separate syringe. Intravenous catheters were kept patent after blood samples were obtained by flushing them with a minimum of 3.0 mL of 0.9% sodium chloride injection. Each sample was transferred to a non-heparin-treated blood collection tube (Venoject, lot 8605223E1, Terumo Medical Corp., Elkton, MD 21921), allowed to clot, and centrifuged for 10 minutes. Serum was harvested, stored at −20 °C, and batch analyzed within 30 days. Fluid remaining in the secondary tubing for both minibag methods was also collected for analysis to quantitate the amount of drug remaining in the intravenous tubing.

Each sample was analyzed in duplicate for tobramycin content by fluorescence polarization immunoassay using reagent of a single lot (92-135-AZ, TDx, Abbott Diagnostics, Irving, TX 75015). The lower limit of detection of this method is 0.18 μg/mL. Intrabatch and interbatch assay precision (coefficient of variation) is 1.8% and 3.9%, respectively, at a concentration of 1.0 μg/mL. Triplicate analyses of drug remaining in secondary i.v. sets for the MP and MG methods were performed after the drug containing i.v. fluid was diluted with buffer solution as recommended by the manufacturer to a predicted concentration of approximately 4 μg/mL. A similar technique was used to quantitate the concentration of tobramycin from the manufacturer's lot.

Pharmacokinetic and Data Analysis. Serum tobramycin concentration–time data for each dose were fitted to a biexponential decay model with zero-order input and first-order disposition using a nonlinear least-squares regression program.[7] The area under the serum concentration–time curve from time zero to infinity ($AUC_{0\rightarrow\infty}$) was calculated by the trapezoidal rule from 0 to 8 hours plus the ratio of the measured eight-hour concentration and the terminal elimination rate constant (β).[8] The time interval from initiation of the infusion to occurrence of the maximum serum concentration (t_{max}) was determined directly from the serum concentration–time data. Estimated creatinine clearance was calculated from baseline serum creatinine values by the method of Cockcroft and Gault.[9]

Data were compared statistically using nonparametric, one-way analysis of variance (Kruskal–Wallis), with Duncan's Multiple range test used to detect differences between individual infusion methods.[10] An a priori level of significance was set at $p < 0.05$.

Results

Eleven subjects completed the study; one subject was terminated from the study after the first week because of inadequate vascular access. The following were the mean ± S.D. (range) values for the subjects: age, 26 ± 3.0 years (21–31 years); weight, 78.8 ± 11.4 kg (62–93.4 kg); and estimated creatinine clearance, 110 ± 21.3 mL/min/72 kg (94.2–162.9 mL/min/72 kg). No adverse reactions as a result of tobramycin administration, as evidenced by either changes in serum creatinine concentration greater than 0.3 mg/100 mL or subjective symptomatology, occurred during the study. Values for $AUC_{0\rightarrow\infty}$, t_{max}, actual t', and predicted t' are shown in Table 1.

Table 1.
Differences in Infusion Times and Pharmacokinetic Variables among the Infusion Methods[a]

Variable	Minibag Gravity	Minibag Pump	Metered Chamber	Syringe Pump
Duration of infusion (min)				
Predicted	37	37	38	31
Actual	51 ± 8.0[b,c] (36–60)	48 ± 11.5[c] (35–70)	37 ± 4.0[d] (30–42)	32 ± 5.0[d] (30–45)
t_{max} (min)	46 ± 7.5[e] (35–62)	41 ± 9.0[e] (30–60)	37 ± 4.0[f] (30–41)	32 ± 5.5[f] (30–46)
$AUC_{0\to\infty}$ (μg · hr/mL)	16.7 ± 2.0[g] (13.5–19.8)	17.0 ± 2.9[g,h] (13.2–20.2)	19.9 ± 2.0[i] (15.5–21.9)	18.7 ± 1.9[h,i] (15.4–20.7)

[a] Values expressed as mean ± S.D. (range) for 11 subjects.
[b] All mean values were significantly different from all other mean values for a given variable unless otherwise indicated.
[c–i] No significant differences between pairs of data that are indicated by matching footnote letters, according to Duncan's Multiple range test (e.g., for actual duration of infusion, 51 minutes[c] [minibag gravity] is not significantly different from 48 minutes[c] [minibag pump]).

Completeness of Administration. The mean measured tobramycin concentration from the manufacturer's lot used for this study was determined to be 102.5% (41 mg/mL) of the stated concentration (40 mg/mL). The mean measured fluid volume for the lot of minibags used in this investigation was 57.3 ± 0.78 mL), indicating a 14.6% overfill. Addition of the dosages of tobramycin used in this study would have yielded a volume of approximately 60 mL. For both minibag methods, a mean of 6.0 mL remained in the secondary i.v. tubing after completion of the infusion period and, as a result, a mean of 10% of each dose was not administered (range 2.5–19.7%). Less than 1% (0.3 mL) of drug remained in the extension tubing for the syringe-pump method. Because the intravenous tubing was flushed as a result of continued fluid administration after the end of the tobramycin infusion, drug delivery was assumed to be 100% for the MC method.

The minibag infusion methods (MG, MP) delivered approximately 15% less drug according to $AUC_{0\to\infty}$ values than the MC method ($p < 0.05$), while the SP method was not significantly different from the MC method (MC > MG, MP; SP > MG; $p < 0.05$). When $AUC_{0\to\infty}$ values for the MG and MP methods were corrected to account for the mean drug loss of 10% in the secondary i.v. tubing, the differences in $AUC_{0\to\infty}$ observed among the methods were not significant ($p = 0.293$).

Timeliness of Delivery. The actual duration of tobramycin infusion varied substantially among the infusion methods (Figure 5). The mean t' values were significantly greater than predicted for both minibag methods ($p < 0.05$), and both were significantly longer than t' for the MC and SP methods. For the SP method, t' was 30 minutes for all but two subjects in whom tobramycin delivery was delayed after the syringe pump shut off in response to an occlusion alarm. In each case, the alarm apparently resulted from incorrect placement of the extension set needle against the intraluminal wall of the primary i.v. tubing. After the needle tip was directed away from the tubing wall, the remaining volume was infused without further interruption. There was a lag time in the actual initiation of intravascular tobramycin delivery of eight minutes with the MC method, reflecting the time required for the i.v. tubing to be primed with the diluted tobramycin after the infusion began. This delay was equivalent to the product of the flow rate and the volume of i.v. fluid between the metered chamber and the subject. The greatest variability in the duration of infusion within methods occurred with the minibag methods. Of the 11 subjects, the duration of infusion was as predicted for only 1 subject for the MG method and only 2 subjects for the MP method.

Figure 5. Distributions of the duration of infusion for each infusion method. MG = minibag gravity flow, MP = minibag pump, MC = metered chamber, and SP = syringe pump. Vertical lines represent mean ± S.D.

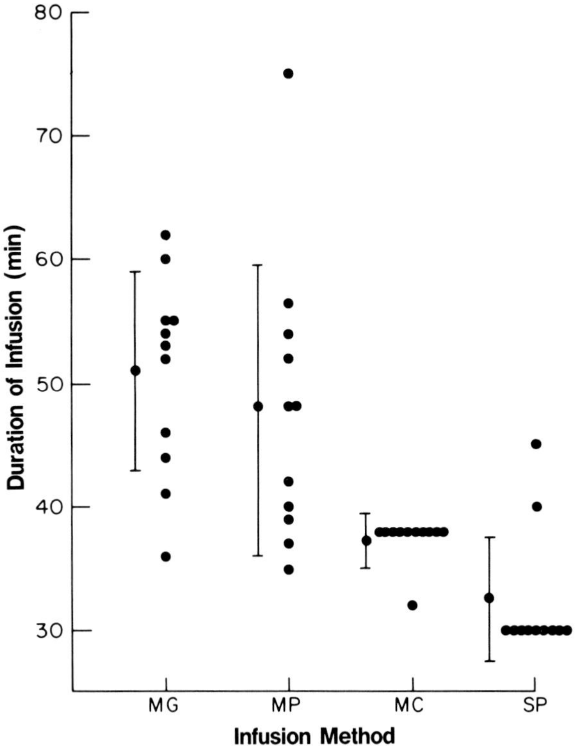

In contrast, the duration of infusion was as predicted in 9 subjects (of 11) for the SP method. When the lag time was considered for the MC method, t' was as predicted in 10 of 11 subjects. The variability in actual t' for the MP method (CV = 24.0%) was twofold greater than observed with the MC method (CV = 10.8%). Variability for the SP (CV = 15.6%) and MG (CV = 15.7%) methods was similar.

The differences in the observed t_{max} values among the methods were significant (Table 1). For the MC and SP methods t_{max} occurred at the end of the infusion, whereas for the minibag methods t_{max} occurred at approximately five minutes before the end of the infusion.

Discussion

When interpreting serum drug concentrations in adults, practitioners frequently assume that intravenous drug administration by intermittent infusion is associated with complete and timely drug delivery. This study clearly documents significant differences in the relative performance of four intermittent i.v. infusion methods used to administer tobramycin in adults. The two minibag methods used in this investigation, which are similar to those used at the study institution, provided incomplete and prolonged delivery of tobramycin. In contrast, the use of a metered chamber or a syringe pump with a volumetric infusion pump was associated with more consistent, complete, and timely drug delivery.

The incomplete delivery of tobramycin observed with both minibag methods was the result of several factors. After emptying from the minibags, the i.v. admixture fluid became stationary in the secondary tubing at a level approximately horizontal to the drip chamber on the primary set and thus was not administered. This resulted in a reduction in the proportion of the dose administered and subsequently in significantly lower $AUC_{0\rightarrow\infty}$ values for the minibag methods compared with the syringe-pump or metered-chamber systems. In an in vitro study evaluating tobramycin delivery by two methods,[4] minibag via gravity flow or dual-rate infusion controller, a greater proportion of the dose (≥95%) was delivered than we observed in this investigation. This difference is primarily attributable to differences in the volume of i.v. fluid remaining in the tubing after completion of the infusion and the concentration of drug in the fluid remaining in the tubing. The secondary i.v. tubing used in an in vitro study[4] was reported to contain 4.6 mL of fluid, whereas the secondary tubing used in this study contained approximately 8.5 mL, excluding the drip chamber. At the same time, the concentration of drug remaining in the tubing was lower in the in vitro investigation (0.8–1.6 mg/mL) than in this study (1.8–2.6 mg/mL). Thus, use of smaller i.v. secondary tubing or a larger small-volume injection would result in more complete drug delivery. Drug loss could also be decreased by flushing the fluid remaining in the secondary tubing. We did not evaluate flushing techniques since they are rarely employed in drug administration at our institution. However, such manipulations do not eliminate the problem of prolonged administration of tobramycin with gravity-flow systems.

The durations of infusion for the minibag methods were prolonged because of overfill of the minibags and the influence of gravity-flow administration. Manufacturer overfill for large- and small-volume injections has previously been reported.[11-13] Minibag overfill (approximately 10 mL including tobramycin) resulted in infusion periods longer than the desired interval of 30 minutes because drip rates were calculated on the basis of a theoretical 50-mL volume. At the same time, decreased infusion rates after the onset of the infusion occurred. Previous studies have demonstrated prolonged in vitro delivery of tobramycin when administered from minibags[4] or a volumetric chamber[5] by gravity flow. Intravenous flow rates for the gravity-flow minibag method were reported to decrease from the initial rate five minutes after initiation of the infusion and were approximately 40% less than the initial rate of 120 mL/hr at the end of the infusion.[4] This resulted in a net prolongation of drug delivery of approximately 30 minutes beyond the predicted time interval. In contrast, the use of the dual-rate infusion controller was associated with timely tobramycin administration. Similar results were observed with tobramycin delivery by a volumetric-chamber method.[5] In our study, the actual mean infusion time was 14 (range, 0–25 minutes) and 11 (range, −2–38 minutes) minutes longer than predicted for the MG and MP methods, respectively.

Substantial intramethod variability was also observed with the MG and MP infusion methods. In addition, for these two methods, the actual t' was as predicted in only a few instances. This variability prevents an accurate prediction of t' based on i.v. fluid volume and flow rate. Loss of tobramycin in the secondary i.v. tubing also varied widely, ranging from 2.5 to 19.7%. Thus, no assumptions can be made about usual drug loss or typical duration of infusion to compensate for these deficiencies.

Decreased i.v. flow rate over time has also been documented for large-volume injections when a gravity-flow technique is used.[11] Inability to maintain a constant primary i.v. fluid flow rate could influence secondary drug administration. We chose to evaluate both minibag methods because of this potential factor and because both methods are used at our institution. In this investigation, the use of a volumetric infusion pump on the primary i.v. line did result in a slight but not significantly shorter duration of infusion for the MP method as compared with the MG method (Table 1). Attachment of the secondary i.v. tubing to the primary i.v. set above the volumetric pump for the MP method may have resulted in more timely delivery. However, because this method is not used at our institution, we did not evaluate it. In contrast to minibag delivery, both the MC and SP methods were associated with a more predictable onset and completion of drug delivery. The delay observed in this study for the MC method (eight minutes) can be minimized by priming the i.v. tubing with drug solution or by considering the delay when choosing peak sampling times for measuring serum aminoglycoside concentrations.

The method of intravenous infusion also significantly influenced t_{max} values (Table 1). In contrast to the use of minibag methods, where t_{max} occurred approximately five minutes before the end of the infusion, mean t_{max} values occurred at the end of the infusion period for the MC and SP methods. This is consistent with the previously noted decrease in the i.v. flow rate for the minibag methods over the course of the infusion compared with the initial rate selected. The i.v. flow rate for the minibags apparently decreases to the extent that the amount of drug entering the systemic circulation is less than the amount being removed during the latter portion of the infusion period.

This study was conducted in a controlled research environment, and differences among the infusion methods may be greater in the actual patient-care setting. In a previous clinical study evaluating gentamicin delivery by minibags in patients, a number of factors were identified that influence serum concentration data.[12] In particular, drug delivery was both incomplete and prolonged with minibag administration. In that report, drug loss accounted for a portion of observed differences between predicted and measured peak serum gentamicin concentrations.

In a related study,[14] we examined the effect of the four infusion methods on tobramycin pharmacokinetic variables and predicted dosages in healthy volunteers.

Conclusion

In this investigation, use of either a syringe-pump or a metered-chamber infusion system that incorporated a volumetric infusion pump resulted in more accurate, consistent, and predictable tobramycin delivery than observed with two minibag methods. Based on these results, the method of intravenous administration can significantly influence the completeness and timeliness of drug administration in adults.

References

1. Nahata MC, Powell DA, Durrell D et al. Delivery of tobramycin by three infusion methods. *Chemotherapy.* 1984; 30:84–7.
2. Gould T, Roberts RJ. Therapeutic problems arising from the use of the intravenous route for drug administration. *J Pediatr.* 1979; 465–71.
3. Rajchgot P, Radde IC, MacLeod SM. Influence of specific gravity on intravenous drug delivery. *J Pediatr.* 1981; 99:658–61.
4. Nahata MC, Durrell DE, Miller MA. Accuracy of tobramycin piggyback delivery using gravity flow versus a controller. *Am J Hosp Pharm.* 1986; 43:947–9.
5. Nahata MC, Durrell DE, Miller MA. Accuracy of tobramycin delivery with a controller and a volumetric chamber or syringe. *Am J Hosp Pharm.* 1986; 43:2239–41.
6. Pleasants RA, Sawyer WT, Dupuis RE et al. Patient-location-specific alterations in aminoglycoside volume of distribution. *Clin Pharm.* 1986; 5:872–3. Letter.
7. Gibaldi M, Perrier D. Pharmacokinetics. 2nd ed. New York: Marcel Dekker; 1982.
8. Metzler CM. NONLIN. Kalamazoo, MI: The Upjohn Company; 1985.
9. Cockcroft DW, Gault MH. Prediction of creatinine clearance from serum creatinine. *Nephron.* 1976; 16:31–41.
10. Wilkinson L. SYSTAT user's guide. Evanston, IL: SYSTAT, Inc.; 1985.
11. Flack FC, Whyte TD. Behavior of standard gravity-fed administration sets used for intravenous infusion. *Br Med J.* 1974; 3:439–43.
12. Armistead JA, Nahata MC. Effect of variables associated with intermittent gentamicin infusion on pharmacokinetic predictions. *Clin Pharm.* 1983; 2:153–6.
13. Kleinberg ML, Chang P. Overfill of common piggyback admixture solutions. *Hosp Pharm.* 1984; 19:657–8.
14. Pleasants RA, Sawyer WT, Williams DM et al. Effect of four intravenous infusion methods on tobramycin pharmacokinetics. *Clin Pharm.* 1988; 7:374–9.

“

Clinical Evaluation of Ganciclovir

Unlike the studies for all other antivirals, ganciclovir studies to date have not used placebo controls in the evaluation of targeted patients. This is surprising in spite of the life- and sight-threatening nature of the disease. Whether the lack of placebo-controlled trials for chorioretinitis [is] a result of perceived differences in "orphan drug" development, public pressure from the AIDS community, or such "dramatic improvement" compared to historic controls is debatable. It is likely that the Food and Drug Administration will have to weigh the value of ganciclovir without the benefit of a placebo-controlled trial, as many clinical investigators and patients now would not allow a placebo arm for therapy of cytomegalovirus chorioretinitis on ethical grounds.

—Whitley RJ. Ganciclovir—have we established clinical value in the treatment of cytomegalovirus infections? *Ann Intern Med.* 1988; 108:452–4. Editorial.

”

Effect of four intravenous infusion methods on tobramycin pharmacokinetics

ROY A. PLEASANTS, WILLIAM T. SAWYER, DENNIS M. WILLIAMS, WILLIAM R. MCKENNA, AND J. ROBERT POWELL

Abstract: The influence of four intermittent intravenous infusion methods on the determination of tobramycin pharmacokinetic values and predicted doses was evaluated in 11 healthy adult volunteers.

Each subject received tobramycin (as the sulfate salt) 1.5 mg/kg by each of four i.v. infusion methods: (1) minibag via gravity flow (MG), (2) minibag with the secondary infusion tubing inserted below a volumetric pump (MP), (3) metered chamber via volumetric pump (MC), and (4) syringe pump (SP). Infusion rates were initially set to administer each dose over a 30-minute period. Sixteen blood samples were obtained over an eight-hour period before and at various time intervals after each dose and were analyzed for tobramycin content by fluorescence polarization immunoassay. Area under the serum concentration–time curve from time zero to infinity ($AUC_{0-\infty}$) was calculated by the trapezoidal rule. Serum tobramycin concentration data for each subject were fitted to a biexponential decay model with zero-order input. β and V_β were calculated from fitted data. One-compartment pharmacokinetic values, elimination rate constant (k), apparent volume of distribution (V), and predicted doses to achieve steady-state peak concentrations of 6 μg/mL were calculated by the method of Sawchuk and Zaske.

There were no significant differences in either β or k among the infusion methods. V_β values (mean ± S.D.) for the methods were 0.240 ± 0.025 (MG), 0.257 ± 0.025 (MP), 0.221 ± 0.027 (MC), and 0.231 ± 0.032 (SP) L/kg. Values for the methods for V were 0.244 ± 0.041 (MG), 0.258 ± 0.036 (MP), 0.205 ± 0.021 (MC), and 0.225 ± 0.037 (SP) L/kg (V_β and V; SP > MP, MC > MG, MP, $p < 0.05$). Predicted dosages (mean ± S.D.) were 4.88 ± 0.83 (MG), 5.01 ± 0.83 (MP), 3.84 ± 0.40 (MC), and 4.24 ± 0.51 (SP) mg/kg/day (MB, MP > MC, SP, $p < 0.05$). Observed maximum serum concentrations were 5.45 ± 0.77 (MG), 5.50 ± 1.04 (MP), 8.20 ± 0.83 (MC), and 8.21 ± 0.97 (SP) μg/mL (MC, SP > MG, MP, $p < 0.05$). Serum concentrations measured 60 minutes after the initiation of the infusion were significantly different only for the MC method. Predicted serum concentrations 30 minutes after the initiation of the infusion were higher than measured concentrations for only the minibag methods ($p < 0.05$).

In this investigation the two minibag methods were associated with larger volume of distribution values and predicted doses compared with pump-assisted metered-chamber and syringe-pump methods.

Index terms: Aminoglycosides; Blood levels; Devices; Dosage; Drug administration systems; Drugs, body distribution; Injections; Pharmacokinetics; Tobramycin; Tobramycin sulfate
Clin Pharm. 1988; 7:374–9

The appropriate application of clinical pharmacokinetic principles to the individualization and optimization of drug therapy involves consideration of all variables that may affect the relationship among the dose, the concentration, and patient response. In particular, the method of drug administration may represent an important influence. In pediatric patients, conventional intravenous infusion methods have been shown to result in altered serum aminoglycoside concentrations and calculated pharmacokinetic values as a result of delayed, prolonged, and incomplete drug delivery, usually associated with the use of large-bore infusion tubing and relatively slow rates of infusion.[1-3] However, the influence of i.v. infusion techniques or methods on serum drug concentration data has not been fully characterized in adult patients.

In another study, the influence of four different intravenous infusion methods on the completeness and timeliness of tobramycin delivery was examined in adult volunteers.[4] The objective of this investigation was to evaluate the effect of these observed differences on the determination of

ROY A. PLEASANTS, PHARM.D., is Senior Clinical Specialist in Infectious Diseases, North Carolina Memorial Hospital, Chapel Hill, NC, and Clinical Assistant Professor, School of Pharmacy, University of North Carolina at Chapel Hill (UNCCH). WILLIAM T. SAWYER, M.S., is Assistant Director of Clinical Services, Department of Pharmacy, North Carolina Memorial Hospital, and Associate Professor, School of Pharmacy, UNCCH. DENNIS M. WILLIAMS, PHARM.D., is Clinical Assistant Professor, School of Pharmacy, and WILLIAM R. MCKENNA, M.D., is Fellow, Division of Infectious Diseases, School of Medicine, UNCCH. J. ROBERT POWELL, PHARM.D., is Head, Clinical Pharmacokinetics, Glaxo Inc., Research Triangle Park, NC; at the time of this study, he was Associate Professor, School of Pharmacy, UNCCH.

Address reprint requests to Dr. Pleasants at the Department of Pharmacy, North Carolina Memorial Hospital, Manning Drive, Chapel Hill, NC 27514.

Supported in part by Becton Dickinson and Company, Infusion Systems, Lincoln Park, NJ 07006; IMED Corporation, San Diego, CA 92131; and Clinical Research Unit, School of Medicine, UNCCH (NIH grant RR46).

Presented at the 21st Annual Midyear Clinical Meeting, Las Vegas, NV, December 11, 1986.

Copyright © 1988, American Society of Hospital Pharmacists, Inc. All rights reserved. 0278-2677/88/0501-0374$01.50.

pharmacokinetic values and predicted dosages. Pharmacokinetic values were calculated after multicompartment analysis to accurately assess the impact of the infusion method and also by a standard one-compartment approach to delineate the influence on pharmacokinetic calculations in the patient-care setting.

Methods

The study was conducted in 11 healthy men.[4] Each volunteer received tobramycin (as the sulfate salt) 1.5 mg/kg by each of four methods of intermittent i.v. infusion, with doses administered one week apart to allow for adequate washout of residual drug. Three infusion methods, minibag via gravity flow (MG), minibag with the secondary infusion tubing inserted below a volumetric infusion pump (MP), and metered chamber via volumetric infusion pump (MC), were used to simulate routine i.v. aminoglycoside administration at the study institution. A fourth method, syringe pump (SP), was also included in the investigation.

The observed serum drug concentration–time data for each subject and infusion method were analyzed using both one- and two-compartment pharmacokinetic models. To estimate the terminal elimination rate constant, β (hr^{-1}), serum tobramycin concentration–time data were fitted to a biexponential decay model with zero-order input using a computerized nonlinear regression-analysis program (NONLIN).[5] Area under the serum concentration–time curve from time zero to infinity ($AUC_{0-\infty}$) was calculated by the trapezoidal method for the zero- to eight-hour interval, with the remaining area determined from the ratio of the measured eight-hour serum concentration to the terminal elimination rate constant.[6] For purposes of comparing a multicompartment volume term, V_β was determined. V_β (L), normalized to total body weight (TBW), was calculated from the following equation:

$$V_\beta = D/(AUC_{0-\infty})(\beta)TBW \quad (1)$$

where D = dose (mg).

To simulate the use of serum drug concentration–time data under routine clinical conditions, one-compartment, first-order pharmacokinetic values were calculated by the method of Sawchuk and Zaske.[7] The terminal elimination rate constant, k (hr^{-1}), was calculated by linear regression using three postinfusion serum concentrations obtained over approximately three half-lives at 60, 180, and 360 minutes after the initiation of the infusion. The apparent volume of distribution, V (L), was calculated by the following equation:

$$V = (k_o/k)(1 - e^{-kT})/(C_{60}/e^{-kt}) \quad (2)$$

where k_o = dose (mg/hr), C_{60} = serum tobramycin concentration (μg/mL) measured at 60 minutes after initiation of the infusion, T = actual duration of infusion (hr), and t = time interval between the occurrence of the observed C_{60} and the end of the infusion period (hr). The concentration before the dose was not included in the determination of V because this value was zero. A value of V normalized to total body weight (L/kg) was also calculated. Based on these variables, a predicted dose was calculated to achieve a steady-state peak serum concentration of 6 μg/mL, at the end of the infusion, using a dosage interval of eight hours. Doses were based on the actual T and calculated V for each individual subject and infusion method. To assess the effect of incomplete or prolonged drug delivery observed with the minibag methods, dosage was also calculated for each individual subject and infusion method by (1) adjustment of V to compensate for the mean 10% of each dose not administered by the minibag methods and using the actual T and (2) use of the calculated V and an optimal T of 30 minutes.

Measured and predicted serum tobramycin concentrations for each infusion method were compared. The maximum observed concentration (C_{max}) was determined directly from serum concentration–time data. Measured serum concentrations 60 minutes after the infusion began (C_{60}) were compared among the infusion methods. In addition, serum tobramycin concentrations predicted to occur 30 minutes after the initiation of the infusion (C_{30}) were calculated from the following equation:

$$C_{30} = C_{60}/e^{-kt} \quad (3)$$

Nonparametric, one-way analysis of variance (Kruskal–Wallis) was used to compare differences in serum concentrations (measured C_{max}, predicted versus measured C_{30}, and measured C_{60}), pharmacokinetic variables, and predicted dosage requirements among infusion methods. Duncan's Multiple range test was used to determine differences between infusion methods.[8] An a priori level of significance was set at $p < 0.05$.

Results

The mean serum tobramycin concentration–time profiles for the 11 subjects and each infusion method are shown in Figure 1. Mean calculated values for β, k, V_β, V, C_{max}, C_{60}, and C_{30} are summarized in Table 1. Predicted doses, based on actual and adjusted pharmacokinetic values, are shown in Table 2.

Statistical differences in V_β and V were observed among the infusion methods ($p < 0.05$, Table 1). Values for V_β and V were significantly lower for the MC method than for either minibag infusion method. V_β and V values for the SP method were significantly different from only the MP method ($p < 0.05$). No significant differences in either β or k were noted among the infusion methods.

Significant differences in predicted doses among methods were observed (Table 2). Within individual subjects, differences of as much as 97 mg per dose were observed between the infusion methods (Figure 2). However, if an adjusted V was used or the dose was infused over an optimal time interval (30 minutes) for the minibag methods, the difference in predicted doses among the infusion methods was smaller (Table 2).

C_{max} values for the MC and SP methods were significantly greater than those observed for the minibag methods. Values of C_{60} observed with the MC method were significantly different from those noted with the other three methods ($p < 0.05$). The predicted C_{30} value was higher than the measured C_{30} value for 9 of the 11 subjects with the MG method and 7 of the subjects for the MP method. In addition, the predicted C_{30} was greater than C_{max} in 6 of the subjects for the MG method and 3 of the subjects for the MP method. In contrast, predicted C_{30} values were less than measured C_{30} and C_{max} values in all instances for the MC and SP methods.

Figure 1. Mean serum concentration–time profile for each intravenous infusion method and all subjects (n = 11). □ —•— □ = syringe pump, ■ •••• ■ = metered chamber, O – – – O = minibag gravity, ●—● = minibag pump.

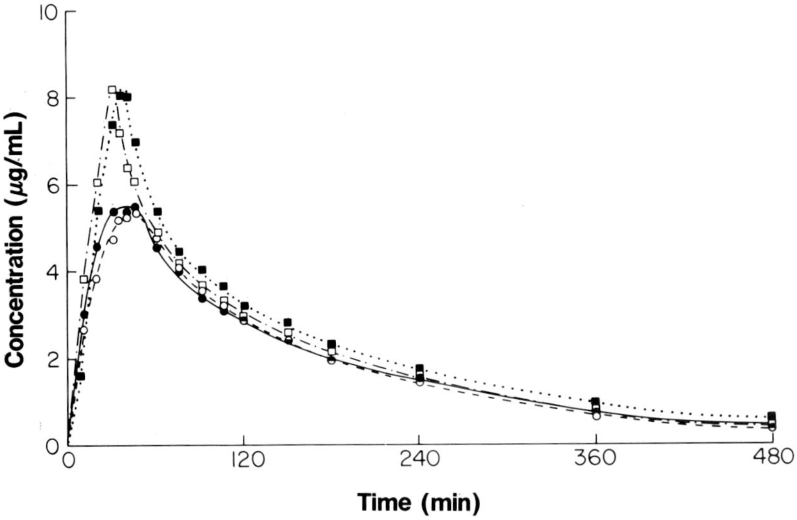

Table 1.
Pharmacokinetic and Serum Concentration Data for the Four Infusion Methods

Variable	Infusion Method[a,b] MG	MP	MC	SP
Observed C_{max} (µg/mL)	5.45 ± 0.77[c,d] (4.95–7.85)	5.50 ± 1.04[d] (4.35–7.40)	8.20 ± 0.83[e] (7.25–9.50)	8.21 ± 0.97[e] (7.30–9.95)
Measured C_{60} (µg/mL)	4.78 ± 0.58[f] (3.99–5.59)	4.58 ± 0.56[f] (3.67–5.50)	5.42 ± 0.48 (4.91–6.36)	4.88 ± 0.55[f] (4.03–5.89)
Measured C_{30} (µg/mL)	4.70 ± 0.74[g] (3.83–6.63)	5.37 ± 1.25[g] (3.18–7.38)	7.62 ± 1.11[h] (6.27–9.48)	8.18 ± 1.32[h] (5.55–9.95)
Predicted C_{30} (µg/mL)	5.65 ± 0.68 (4.64–6.54)	5.45 ± 0.65 (4.40–6.94)	6.42 ± 0.54 (5.79–7.01)	5.73 ± 0.60 (4.81–6.70)
β (hr^{-1})[q]	0.3430 ± 0.033[i] (0.2885–0.3957)	0.3439 ± 0.037[i] (0.2838–0.4030)	0.3303 ± 0.047[i] (0.2557–0.4102)	0.3269 ± 0.036[i] (0.2575–0.3726)
k (hr^{-1})[r]	0.3726 ± 0.044[j] (0.2948–0.4512)	0.3510 ± 0.042[j] (0.2816–0.4180)	0.3639 ± 0.040[j] (0.3019–0.4296)	0.3674 ± 0.033[j] (0.3086–0.4331)
V_β (L/kg)	0.240 ± 0.025[k,l] (0.220–0.302)	0.257 ± 0.025[k] (0.191–0.285)	0.221 ± 0.027[m] (0.191–0.238)	0.231 ± 0.032[l,m] (0.185–0.266)
V (L/kg)	0.244 ± 0.041[n,o] (0.205–0.317)	0.258 ± 0.036[n] (0.210–0.334)	0.205 ± 0.021[p] (0.170–0.229)	0.225 ± 0.037[o,p] (0.181–0.311)

[a] MG = minibag gravity, MP = minibag pump, MC = metered chamber, and SP = syringe pump.
[b] Values expressed as mean ± S.D. (range).
[c] All mean values were significantly different from all other mean values for a given variable unless otherwise indicated.
[d–p] Each pair (i.e., data with matching footnote letters) not significantly different according to Duncan's Multiple range test (e.g., for observed C_{max}, 8.20 µg/mL[e] [MC] is not significantly different from 8.21 µg/mL[e] [SP].
[q] Terminal elimination rate constant calculated using two-compartment model.
[r] Terminal elimination rate constant calculated using one-compartment model.

Discussion

A number of factors can contribute to altered serum drug concentration–time profiles in adult patients. In particular, certain disease states have been clearly shown to influence the pharmacokinetic disposition of aminoglycosides.[9] However, as evidenced by the results of this investigation, inefficient drug administration methods may also influence considerably the perceived relationship between the administered drug dose and resulting serum concentrations. More important, differences in i.v. drug administration methods may be associated with substantial variation in calculated pharmacokinetic values and doses predicted to achieve equivalent peak serum concentrations during maintenance therapy. Differences in the efficiency of the method of i.v. drug delivery, which result in significant alterations in the duration of the infusion and completeness of tobramycin delivery, therefore represent a clinically important variable in interpreting serum drug concentrations and designing drug dosage regimens.

Figure 2. Predicted doses (milligrams per kilogram, every eight hours) for individual subjects and infusion methods, where MG = minibag gravity, MP = minibag pump, MC = metered chamber, and SP = syringe pump. Vertical bars represent mean ± S.D.

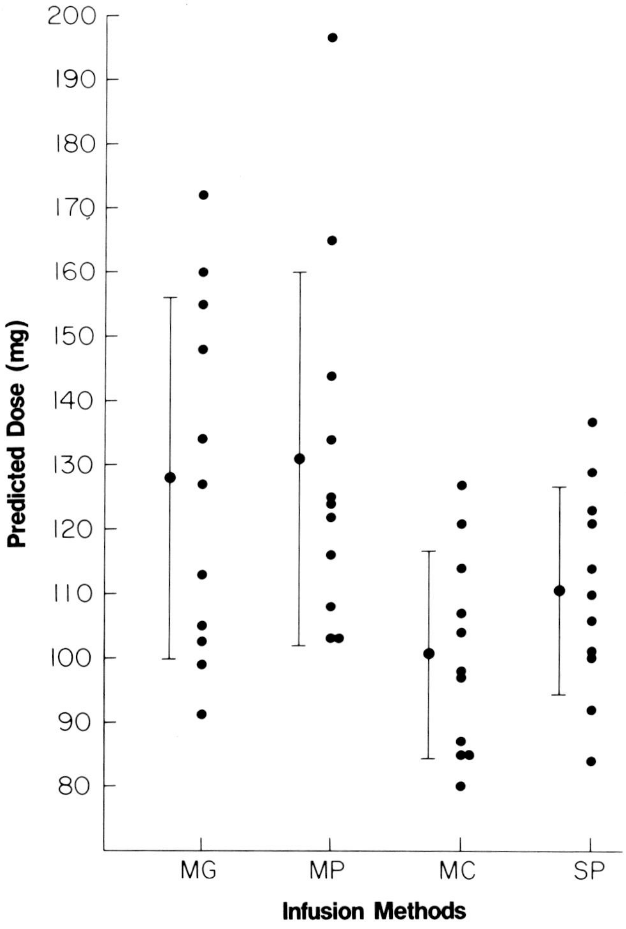

In this study, the method of drug delivery affected select pharmacokinetic values. No significant differences in either β or k were noted among the infusion methods. However, aminoglycosides do not exhibit dose-dependent elimination, and differences in either variable would not be expected to be associated with incomplete drug administration. Delayed initiation of intravascular delivery observed with the MC method could potentially influence calculation of the elimination rate constant through an increased influence of the initial rapid distribution (α) phase on peak serum drug concentrations, resulting in excessively large elimination rate constants. Nonetheless, β and k values for the MC method were similar to or less than those observed with the other three infusion methods (Table 1) and were not appreciably altered as a consequence of delayed tobramycin delivery. In contrast, however, the method of drug delivery significantly influenced the calculated volume of distribution and maintenance dose estimates.

Larger calculated values for both volume of distribution variables, V_β and V, were observed for the minibag methods. These observations are most likely the result of incomplete tobramycin delivery associated with drug remaining in the secondary

Table 2.
Doses (mg/kg/day) Predicted To Achieve Steady-State Peak Concentrations of 6 μg/mL Using Actual and Assumed Volume (*V*) and Infusion Time (*T*) Estimates

Variable	Infusion Method[a,b]			
	MG	MP	MC	SP
Calculated *V*, actual *T*	4.88 ± 0.83[c,d] (3.60–5.91)	5.01 ± 0.83[d] (4.10–6.77)	3.84 ± 0.40[e] (3.13–4.42)	4.24 ± 0.51[e] (3.56–5.11)
Adjusted *V*, actual *T*	4.43 ± 0.74[f,g] (3.24–5.77)	4.50 ± 0.74[f] (3.68–6.09)	3.84 ± 0.40[h] (3.13–4.42)	4.24 ± 0.51[g,h] (3.56–5.11)
Calculated *V*, optimal *T*	4.55 ± 0.74[i,j] (3.42–5.56)	4.85 ± 0.72[i] (3.89–6.25)	3.84 ± 0.40[k] (3.13–4.42)	4.24 ± 0.51[j,k] (3.56–5.11)

[a] MG = minibag gravity, MP = minibag pump, MC = metered chamber, SP = syringe pump.
[b] Values expressed as mean ± S.D. (range).
[c] All mean values were significantly different from all other mean values for a given variable unless otherwise indicated.
[d–k] Each pair (i.e., data with matching footnote letters) not significantly different according to Duncan's Multiple range test (e.g., for calculated *V*, actual *T*, 3.84 mg/kg/day[e] [MC] is not significantly different from 4.24 mg/kg/day[e] [SP]).

i.v. tubing after the infusion. Calculated volume of distribution values were not significantly different among the infusion methods when this drug loss was considered in the calculation. However, volume estimates were significantly elevated for both minibag methods when 100% drug administration was assumed in the calculation.

The results of the current study in healthy volunteers are similar to clinical observations of larger mean *V* values noted in patients receiving aminoglycosides by gravity-flow minibag methods (0.33 L/kg) compared with those in patients receiving aminoglycosides by a pump-assisted metered-chamber method (0.27 L/kg).[10] It is notable that, while the mean volume value is increased modestly, the range of observed alterations may be quite wide. We have recently noted that some relatively healthy adult patients hospitalized in the study facility have improbable calculated *V* values, ranging from 0.6 to 1.2 L/kg. It is therefore possible that drug delivery may be even more variable in the patient-care setting than in a controlled research setting using healthy volunteers. Of particular clinical relevance is the fact that in a substantial number of these adult patients in whom large *V* values were observed, therapeutic peak serum aminoglycoside concentrations were not achieved during therapy when doses were determined on the basis of population *V* values (0.25 L/kg).

Higher estimated *V* values and predicted doses occurred with the minibag methods because (1) the actual duration of drug infusion observed in the current study was significantly longer than predicted for both minibag methods and (2) a greater amount of drug was consequently eliminated during the infusion period. Because of the differences in the duration of infusion, higher doses are required with the MG and MP methods to attain peaks similar to those achieved with the MC and SP methods. Second, incomplete delivery also results in a calculated *V* that is falsely elevated because 100% drug delivery is assumed in calculating the volume term. Therefore, incomplete delivery also contributes to a proportionally higher predicted dose necessary to achieve similar peak serum concentrations. These influences of drug delivery on calculated *V* and predicted dose are clearly reflected in the marked differences in the maximum observed serum concentrations (C_{max}) noted among infusion methods. Although the serum tobramycin concentration–time profiles of the four methods begin converging 60 minutes after the initiation of the infusion (Figure 1), it is common practice to estimate peak concentrations at the end of the infusion period when using a one-compartment model.[11-14] In addition, without precise documentation, *T* is frequently assumed to be the recommended infusion time. Therefore, by assuming that the actual infusion duration is the same as the recommended time of infusion (30 minutes at our institution and also for the current study), peak serum concentrations at the end of the infusion period are predicted to be higher than the actual measured values for the minibag infusion methods used in this study.

Additionally, in a substantial number of study subjects, tobramycin delivery by the minibag methods was associated with predicted concentrations at the end of the infusion that were higher than the maximum observed serum concentration at any time. Thus, with infusion methods that are associated with a prolonged duration of infusion, the "predicted" peak concentrations may never be achieved.

The clinical impact of the differences in peak serum tobramycin concentrations observed among the infusion methods was not evaluated in this study. In a previously reported simulation of the effect of different infusion durations on tissue concentrations of drugs exhibiting biexponential elimination, no differences in predicted tissue drug concentrations were noted.[15] Nonetheless, the implications of the results of this study and others are of concern. Although the simulation study failed to show differences in predicted tissue concentrations, obvious differences in blood concentrations would occur. Also, while in vivo data describing the effect of different infusion durations on tissue aminoglycoside concentrations have not been published, changes have been observed in animals. In a report describing the penetration of tobramycin into interstitial fluid in a rabbit model, significantly higher interstitial fluid concentrations of gentamicin were measured at 30 and 60 minutes after drug administration when the drug was given by a 5-minute bolus dose compared with a 30-minute infusion.[16] At two hours after drug administration, tissue concentrations were still higher with bolus delivery than with the slower infusion (1.8 versus 1.3 μg/mL); however, the difference between the two administration methods was not significant.

Differences in the timeliness and consistency of tobramycin delivery among the infusion methods could influence a clinician's ability to make accurate and appropriate dosage adjustments. With a gravity-flow system, the duration of infusion may vary from dose to dose, thus influencing serum concentrations and associated pharmacokinetic calculations. Also, differences in the completeness of drug delivery will influence not only the serum concentrations achieved but also the dose required to achieve therapeutic serum concentrations. Further, in an institution where more than one method for secondary i.v. drug administration is used, patients could potentially be overdosed or underdosed if the infusion method were changed (e.g., as a result of the patient's being transferred to an area that uses a different infusion method).

The mean differences observed among the infusion methods in the current study in predicted daily dosage could also result in differences in drug expenditures. This does not even consider the potential for increased costs that may be associated with more frequent serum sampling undertaken to make dosage adjustments in situations in which secondary drug administration occurs by an inconsistent and inefficient i.v. infusion method. Thus, we propose that differences in efficiency of drug delivery should be included in the overall cost evaluation of i.v. infusion systems.

In addition to the impact on patient care, these observations may have implications for interpretation of previous studies that have demonstrated enlarged aminoglycoside volume of distribution values in specific patient populations where completeness and timeliness of drug delivery were not controlled. Few clinical studies of aminoglycoside pharmacokinetics have described in detail the specific methods of i.v. drug infusion. Interpatient[17] and intrapatient[18] variability in aminoglycoside pharmacokinetic values could be partially attributed to inconsistency in drug administration. We recommend that an infusion method that provides for complete and timely delivery be used for administration of i.v. aminoglycosides. In this study, the pump-assisted metered-chamber and syringe-pump methods were more efficient in this regard than either minibag method. Other minibag methods of aminoglycoside delivery not used at the study institution were not evaluated; thus, we cannot conclude that gravity-flow minibag methods are necessarily associated with inefficient drug delivery in all circumstances. However, the two methods used in this investigation clearly were suboptimal.

Conclusion

Based on the results of this study and other reports, the method of intravenous infusion should constitute a major consideration in the interpretation of serum aminoglycoside concentrations in adults. The two minibag methods used in this investigation were associated with larger volume of distribution values and predicted doses compared with pump-assisted metered-chamber and syringe-pump methods. We strongly encourage each institution to evaluate its own techniques of drug administration, particularly in regard to the timeliness, consistency, and completeness of drug administration, especially those with a narrow therapeutic range, such as aminoglycosides.

References

1. Nahata MC, Powell DA, Durrell DE et al. Effect of infusion methods on tobramycin serum concentrations in newborn infants. *J Pediatr.* 1984; 104:136–8.
2. Nahata MC, Powell DA, Glazer JP et al. Effect of intravenous flow rate and injection site on in vitro delivery of chloramphenicol succinate and in vivo kinetics. *J Pediatr.* 1981; 99:463–7.
3. Leff RD, Roberts RJ. Methods of intravenous drug administration in the pediatric patient. *J Pediatr.* 1981; 98:631–5.
4. Pleasants RA, Sawyer WT, Williams DM et al. Accuracy of tobramycin delivery by four i.v. infusion methods. *Clin Pharm.* 1988; 7:367–73.
5. Metzler CM. NONLIN. Kalamazoo, MI: The Upjohn Company; 1985.
6. Gibaldi M, Perrier D. Pharmacokinetics. 2nd ed. New York: Marcel Dekker; 1982.
7. Sawchuk RJ, Zaske DE. Pharmacokinetics of dosing regimens that utilize multiple intravenous infusions: gentamicin in burn patients. *J Pharmacokinet Biopharm.* 1976; 4:183–95.
8. Wilkinson L. SYSTAT user's guide. Evanston, IL: SYSTAT, Inc.; 1985.
9. Evans WE, Schentag JJ, Jusko WJ. Applied pharmacokinetics. 2nd ed. Spokane, WA: Applied Therapeutics, Inc.; 1986.
10. Pleasants RA, Sawyer WT, Dupuis RE et al. Patient-location-specific alterations in aminoglycoside volume of distribution. *Clin Pharm.* 1986; 5:872–3. Letter.
11. Kloth DD, Tegtmeier BR, Kong C et al. Altered gentamicin pharmacokinetics during the perioperative period. *Clin Pharm.* 1985; 4:182–5.
12. Evans WE, Taylor RH, Feldman S et al. A model for dosing gentamicin in children and adolescents that adjusts for tissue accumulation with continuous dosing. *Clin Pharmacokinet.* 1980; 5:295–306.
13. Gardner D, Schneider PJ. Gentamicin dosage requirements in postpartum patients. *Clin Pharm.* 1984; 3:416–8.
14. Deziel-Evans LM, Murphy JE, Job JL. Correlation of pharmacokinetic indices with therapeutic outcomes in patients receiving aminoglycosides. *Clin Pharm.* 1986; 5:319–24.
15. Morgan DJ, Raymond K. The effect of duration of intravenous infusion on maximum and threshold blood concentrations for drugs exhibiting biexponential elimination kinetics. *J Pharmacokinet Biopharm.* 1982; 10:93–107.
16. Kozok AJ, Gerding DN, Peterson LR et al. Effect of gentamicin intravenous infusion rate on interstitial fluid concentration. *Antimicrob Agents Chemother.* 1977; 12:606–8.
17. Hendeles L, Iafrate RP, Stillwell PC et al. Individualizing gentamicin dosage in cystic fibrosis: limitations to pharmacokinetic approach. *J Pediatr.* 1987; 110:303–10.
18. Hoppe M, Hill M, Schnapf B et al. Small variability in tobramycin pharmacokinetics in cystic fibrosis. *Drug Intell Clin Pharm.* 1987; 21:13A. Abstract.

Research Note

Pharmacokinetic and pharmacodynamic comparison of mezlocillin and ticarcillin

ROBERT G. DEETER, STEVEN L. BARRIERE, AND ROBERT FEKETY

Clin Pharm. 1988; 7:380–4

Mezlocillin and ticarcillin are used interchangeably in the treatment of serious gram-negative infections. The two drugs are similar with regard to in vitro activity[1-4] and appear to produce equivalent clinical results.[4-7] The pharmacokinetic disposition of the new penicillins, azlocillin, mezlocillin, and piperacillin, are well defined.[8-11] Mezlocillin, azlocillin, and piperacillin exhibit dose-dependent elimination, which is supported by the prolonged half-life, increased area under the curve per gram, and decreased total and renal clearances observed as the dosage is increased. There are three pharmacokinetic studies wherein successively larger doses of ticarcillin were administered.[12-14] These studies suggested that ticarcillin does not undergo dose-dependent elimination. No studies have compared the dose dependency of ticarcillin with that of the newer penicillins.

The pharmacodynamics of antipseudomonal penicillins have largely been unexplored. In one study, the serum bactericidal activity of mezlocillin, azlocillin, and ticarcillin against clinical isolates of *Pseudomonas aeruginosa* was determined.[15] However, the dose-dependent elimination of these agents and resultant pharmacodynamic effects has not been assessed. Therefore, the purposes of this study were to (1) compare the pharmacokinetic disposition of mezlocillin and ticarcillin, (2) determine whether ticarcillin exhibits dose-dependent pharmacokinetics, and (3) ascertain whether this phenomenon might be clinically relevant.

Methods. *Experimental Procedures.* Six healthy male nonsmoking volunteers (mean ± S.D. values: weight, 75.1 ± 10.0 kg; height, 180.1 ± 6.3 cm; body surface area, 1.82 ± 0.18 sq m; and creatinine clearance, 134.2 ± 22.7 mL/min/1.73 sq m) participated in this study. Each subject was informed of the nature and risk of the investigation, and consent was obtained before participation. A panel of laboratory tests, consisting of serum chemistries (SMA-12), complete blood cell and platelet counts, urinalysis, and creatinine clearance, was performed, and a complete medical history was taken. Physical examinations were performed before and after the study. All results were normal. The subjects did not ingest any medication for one week before the study and abstained from alcohol and beverages containing caffeine for 24 hours before and after each drug administration.

Each subject received, on separate occasions in randomized fashion at weekly or greater intervals, single intravenous doses of mezlocillin 80 mg/kg and 50 mg/kg (as the sodium salt) and ticarcillin 80 mg/kg and 50 mg/kg (as the disodium salt). Mezlocillin sodium (Mezlin, Miles Pharmaceuticals, lot B1A5), 3-g vial, was reconstituted with 30 mL of sterile water for injection so that each milliliter of solution contained 100 mg of mezlocillin. The appropriate dose was then diluted to 50–100 mL with Sterile Water for Injection, USP, before infusion. Ticarcillin disodium (Ticar, Beecham Laboratories, lot BK3784), 6-g vial, was reconstituted with 24 mL of Sterile Water for Injection, USP, so that each milliliter of solution contained 200 mg of ticarcillin. The appropriate dose was then diluted to 50 mL as described. Each dose was infused over 25 minutes into a peripheral vein in the arm with a constant-rate infusion pump. Mezlocillin vials were assayed and determined to contain 96.8% of the labeled amount. Ticarcillin vials were assayed and determined to contain 98.7% of the labeled amount.

Blood samples (10 mL each) for assay were collected before the drug was administered (time zero) and at 0.5, 0.75, 1.0, 1.25, 1.5, 2.0, 3.0, 4.0, 5.0, 6.0, and 8.0 hours after administration. Samples were immediately placed on ice and centrifuged,

---

ROBERT G. DEETER, PHARM.D., is Assistant Professor, College of Pharmacy, Rutgers University, Piscataway, NJ, and Clinical Pharmacist, Robert Wood Johnson University Hospital, New Brunswick, NJ; at the time of this study, he was Clinical Pharmacy Resident, University of Michigan Hospitals and College of Pharmacy, Ann Arbor. STEVEN L. BARRIERE, PHARM.D., is Specialist in Infectious Diseases, Department of Pharmaceutical Services, and Adjunct Associate Professor, Departments of Medicine and Pharmacology, School of Medicine, UCLA Medical Center, Los Angeles, CA; at the time of this study, he was Associate Professor of Pharmacy and Internal Medicine, University of Michigan. ROBERT FEKETY, M.D., is Professor of Internal Medicine and Chief, Division of Infectious Diseases, University of Michigan.

Address reprint requests to Dr. Deeter at the Department of Pharmacy Practice and Administration, College of Pharmacy, Rutgers University, Piscataway, NJ 08855-0789.

Presented in part at the 25th Interscience Conference on Antimicrobial Agents and Chemotherapy, Minneapolis, MN, September 30, 1985.

Copyright © 1988, American Society of Hospital Pharmacists, Inc. All rights reserved. 0278-2677/88/0501-0380$01.25.

and serum was harvested. Blood samples (10 mL each) for serum bactericidal titer determinations were collected at 0, 0.5, 4.0, 6.0, and 8.0 hours and were handled similarly. Urine samples were collected before drug administration, hourly up to 2 hours, and every 2 hours up to 8 hours and then pooled from 8 hours to 12 hours and 12 hours to 24 hours. After collection, initial urine samples were placed on ice, and pooled samples were refrigerated during the collection period. All serum and urine samples were kept frozen at −20 °C until analyzed; all samples were assayed within 60 days of collection.

Analytical Methods. Serum and urine samples were analyzed for mezlocillin and ticarcillin content using high-performance liquid chromatography. In the mezlocillin assay, serum samples (0.2 mL) were deproteinized with 0.5 mL of acetonitrile containing the internal standard furosemide. After the samples were mixed in a Vortex mixer and centrifuged, the supernatant was injected directly onto the column. Urine samples were diluted and injected directly onto the column after the addition of furosemide. A Waters Chromatography System with a model 481 variable-wavelength spectrophotometer set at 220 nm was used. The assay was carried out on a μ-Bondapak phenyl column (Waters Associates, Milford, MA) with a solvent system of 30% acetonitrile, 9% tetrahydrofuran, and phosphate buffer titrated with sodium hydroxide to a pH of 3. The solvent flow rate was 1 mL/min. The lowest limit of detection was 0.5 μg/mL for serum and 5 μg/mL for urine. The coefficient of variation for this assay was 3.9%. No interference from serum or urine was noted.

The following changes were made in the above procedure for the ticarcillin assay: the internal standard for the serum and urine samples was cefoperazone, the variable-wavelength spectrophotometer had a detector setting of 205 nm, and the solvent system consisted of 30% acetonitrile, 0.03% tetramethylammonium chloride, and phosphate buffer. The assay was run as described above. The lowest limit of detection was 0.5 μg/mL for serum and 5 μg/mL for urine. The coefficient of variation for this assay was 8.1%. No interference from serum or urine was noted.

Serum Bactericidal Titers. The bactericidal titers from mezlocillin and ticarcillin against a resistant clinical (serum) isolate of *Escherichia coli* were determined. The microorganism had a minimum inhibitory concentration and minimum bactericidal concentration of 4 μg/mL for ticarcillin and mezlocillin as determined by macrodilution techniques.[16] Serum bactericidal activity was assessed via the standard methodology.[17]

Pharmacokinetic and Pharmacodynamic Analysis. Pharmacokinetic values for each drug were determined using compartment-independent methods.[18] Elimination half-life was calculated by dividing 0.693 by the elimination rate constant (λ_z) estimated from the terminal portion of the serum concentration–time curve. The area under the plasma concentration–time curve (AUC) was calculated by the log trapezoidal rule. AUC beyond the last measured point was estimated by dividing the value of the last point by λ_z. The area under the bactericidal titer–time curve (AUBC) was determined by plotting the inverse of the serum bactericidal titer versus time and calculating the area by the trapezoidal rule.[19]

Estimates of plasma clearance (CL) and volume of distribution at steady state (V_{ss}) were calculated using the following noncompartmental equations:

$$\mathrm{CL} = \mathrm{Dose}/\mathrm{AUC} \quad (1)$$

$$V_{ss} = (\mathrm{Dose})(\mathrm{AUMC})/(\mathrm{AUC})^2 - (\mathrm{Dose})(T)/2(\mathrm{AUC}) \quad (2)$$

AUMC is the area under the first moment of the plasma drug concentration–time curve calculated using the log trapezoidal rule, and T is the infusion time.[20]

Renal clearance (CL_R) and nonrenal clearance (CL_{NR}) were calculated using the following noncompartmental equations:

$$CL_R = Ae_{t_1-t_2}/AUC_{t_1-t_2} \quad (3)$$

$$CL_{NR} = CL - CL_R \quad (4)$$

where $AUC_{t_1-t_2}$ is the area under the plasma concentration–time curve over the time interval t_1 to t_2. $Ae_{t_1-t_2}$ is the total amount of drug excreted in the urine over the time interval t_1 to t_2.

Statistical Analysis. Pharmacokinetic values for the high and low doses for each drug were compared using Student's t test for paired data. The Wilcoxon Rank Sum test was used to evaluate pharmacodynamic values. A significant difference was defined as $p < 0.05$, and results are reported as mean ± S.D.

Results. *Pharmacokinetics.* All subjects completed the study. Pharmacokinetic values for mezlocillin and ticarcillin in the six subjects after single 80-mg/kg (high) and 50-mg/kg (low) doses are listed in Table 1. Mean plasma concentration–time curves for high- and low-dose mezlocillin and ticarcillin are shown in Figures 1 and 2.

The total, renal, and nonrenal clearances were significantly lower at the 80-mg/kg dose of mezlocillin compared with the 50-mg/kg dose. Also, the peak concentration, elimination half-life, and area under the curve per gram of drug (AUC/g) were greater for high-dose mezlocillin compared with low-dose mezlocillin. The mezlocillin fraction excreted unchanged and steady-state volume of distribution did not change with a dose increase. In contrast to the significant changes observed with mezlocillin, the clearances, elimination half-life, and AUC/g for ticarcillin did not change significantly between the high and low doses.

Table 1.
Pharmacokinetic Variables for Mezlocillin and Ticarcillin[a]

Pharmacokinetic Variable[b]	Mezlocillin Dose (mg/kg) 50	Mezlocillin Dose (mg/kg) 80	Ticarcillin Dose (mg/kg) 50	Ticarcillin Dose (mg/kg) 80
C_{max} (μg/mL)	152.1 ± 28.0	282.4 ± 49.5	181.5 ± 56.5	215.9 ± 42.6
$t_{1/2}$ (min)	67.5 ± 3.9	89.8 ± 11.8[c]	83.5 ± 19.6	84.3 ± 24.8
V_{ss} (L/1.73 sq m)	24.9 ± 2.3	21.1 ± 1.9	25.0 ± 2.8	29.3 ± 3.2
fe (%)	43.9 ± 5.6	46.2 ± 6.4	87.5 ± 12.5	89.2 ± 12.4
CL (mL/min/1.73 sq m)	376.6 ± 31.3	284.4 ± 53.1[c]	297.2 ± 82.2	285.2 ± 46.0
CL_R (mL/min/1.73 sq m)	165.6 ± 27.1	126.0 ± 18.9[c]	265.7 ± 92.5	266.3 ± 72.8
CL_{NR} (mL/min/1.73 sq m)	211.1 ± 24.5	158.2 ± 45.4[c]	31.2 ± 22.7	27.2 ± 29.7
AUC (μg·hr/mL/1.73 sq m)	151.1 ± 9.4	337.2 ± 56.4	205.0 ± 61.0	327.3 ± 65.7
AUC/g (μg·hr/mL/1.73 sq m)	42.5 ± 3.2	59.5 ± 12.0[c]	58.0 ± 18.8	57.6 ± 12.8

[a] Data expressed as mean ± S.D.

[b] C_{max} = peak concentration after 25-minute infusion, $t_{1/2}$ = elimination half-life, V_{ss} = steady-state volume of distribution, *fe* = percentage of drug excreted unchanged in urine in 24 hours, CL = total clearance, CL_R = renal clearance, CL_{NR} = nonrenal clearance, AUC = area under the serum concentration–time curve, and AUC/g = area under the concentration–time curve per gram of drug.

[c] Significantly different from value for lower dose of same drug.

Figure 1. Serum mezlocillin concentrations (mean ± S.D.) after the 80-mg/kg dose (upper curve) and the 50-mg/kg dose (lower curve).

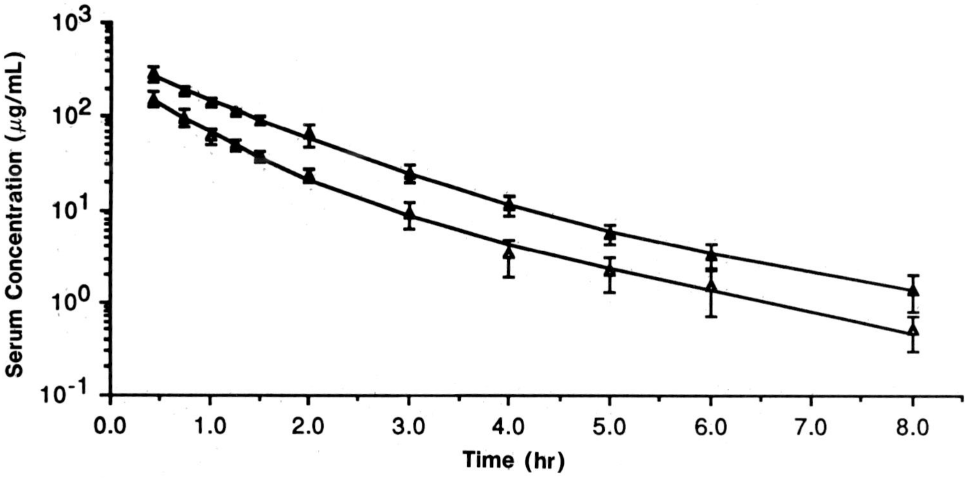

Figure 2. Serum ticarcillin concentrations (mean ± S.D.) after the 80-mg/kg dose (upper curve) and the 50-mg/kg dose (lower curve).

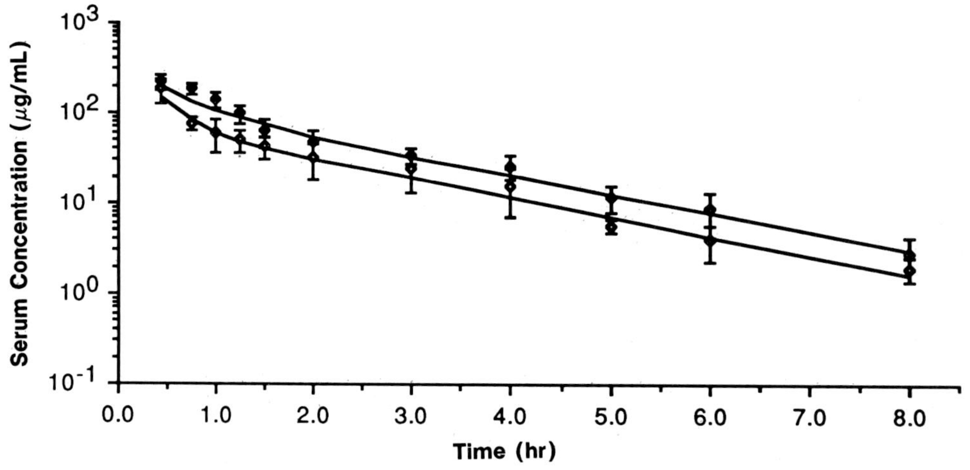

Pharmacodynamics. The pharmacodynamic variables for mezlocillin and ticarcillin in the six subjects after single 80-mg/kg and 50-mg/kg doses are listed in Table 2. The area under the bactericidal titer–time curves (AUBCs) for the 80-mg/kg dose were significantly greater than those for the 50-mg/kg dose for both mezlocillin and ticarcillin. However, when these AUBC values were normalized for dose administered (AUBC/g), the values for ticarcillin were not significantly different. The normalized AUBC/g of mezlocillin at the 80-mg/kg dose was significantly greater than that for the 50-mg/kg dose. The increase in peak serum bactericidal titers for mezlocillin between the low and high doses was significantly greater than that observed for ticarcillin.

Discussion. The results of this investigation support previous findings that mezlocillin is subject to dose-dependent pharmacokinetics. This dose dependency, better termed capacity-limited elimination, is probably due to saturation of elimination pathways. The renal clearance and nonrenal clearance of mezlocillin were significantly reduced with a dose increase. Our data also suggest that ticarcillin is not subject to dose-dependent disposition. The total clearance of ticarcillin did not change. The possibility that ticarcillin undergoes dose-dependent elimination with decreased kidney function needs to be explored.

Serum clearances for mezlocillin have ranged from 171.7 to 417.9 mL/min[8–11] and for ticarcillin, from 95.9 to 154.0 mL/min.[12–14] The pharmacokinetics of mezlocillin has been well studied, and our clearance values are similar to those reported. In contrast, the pharmacokinetics of ticarcillin has not been so extensively studied. Our values are higher than those previously reported. The large range of clearance values for a particular antipseudomonal penicillin is probably due to differences in study designs, concentration detection methods, pharmacokinetic calculation methodologies, and stability of these agents during storage. These factors account for the discrepancy between our clearance values and those previously reported. This discrepancy illustrates the importance of crossover, comparative studies; in studies of this design, comparisons can be made because methodologic differences are not a problem and the clinical utility of the data is not biased.

The clinical implication of capacity-limited elimination for ureidopenicillins is that larger doses can be given less frequently with potentially equivalent clinical efficacy. This is supported by calculating total daily AUC of mezlocillin for each dose. The 50-mg/kg dose is generally given every four hours for the treatment of serious infections. Multiplication of the individual mezlocillin AUC for the 50-mg/kg dose by six results in a mean value of 907 μg·hr/mL. A comparable value is obtained by multiplication of the AUC for the 80-mg/kg dose by three (1012 μg·hr/mL). Hence, the 80-mg/kg dose for mezlocillin could potentially be given every eight hours (three doses/day) and provide an equal or larger total AUC compared to the 50-mg/kg dose administered every four hours (six doses/day). In contrast, multiplication of the mean ticarcillin AUC for the 50-mg/kg dose times six results in daily AUCs of 1230 μg·hr/mL, and multiplication of the AUC for the 80-mg/kg dose times three results in daily AUCs of 982 μg·hr/mL. The daily AUC for the high dose of ticarcillin is smaller than that for the low dose. Administration of ticarcillin 80 mg/kg every eight hours (high dose) does not provide the same daily AUC and amount of available drug per 24 hours compared with the 50-mg/kg dose administered every four hours (low dose).

Further support for this concept is provided by analyzing the AUBC. The dose dependency of mezlocillin is evident by the significant increase in AUBC per gram of administered drug. The total daily AUBCs for mezlocillin (calculated as above)

Table 2.
Bactericidal Activity of Mezlocillin and Ticarcillin[a]

Variable[b]	Mezlocillin Dose (mg/kg)		Ticarcillin Dose (mg/kg)	
	50	80	50	80
Reciprocal of SBT at indicated time after drug administration (hr)				
0.5	69.3 ± 31.5[c]	234.7 ± 52.3	64.0 ± 0.0	117.3 ± 26.1
4.0	3.7 ± 0.8	7.3 ± 1.6	8.7 ± 3.9	12.0 ± 4.4
6.0	2.0 ± 0.0	4.0 ± 0.0	3.7 ± 0.8	6.0 ± 2.2
8.0	0.0 ± 0.0	1.8 ± 0.4	0.7 ± 0.5	3.2 ± 1.3
AUBC				
Total	153.0 ± 61.0[d]	499.0 ± 104.0	160.0 ± 11.0[d]	283.0 ± 57.0
Per gram of drug	41.1 ± 15.8[d]	85.7 ± 24.3	43.2 ± 7.2	47.2 ± 8.6

[a] Data expressed as mean ± S.D.
[b] SBT = serum bactericidal titer, AUBC = area under the bactericidal titer–time curve.
[c] Change in titers from low dose to high dose was significantly different from that for ticarcillin.
[d] Significantly different from value for lower dose of same drug.

at the low and high doses were 918 and 1497 μg·hr/mL ($p < 0.05$), respectively. This difference may be primarily due to enhanced peak titers with high-dose mezlocillin. There was essentially no change in the AUBC for ticarcillin with a dose increase. The total daily AUBCs for ticarcillin at low and high doses were 960 and 849 μg·hr/mL ($p > 0.05$), respectively. Thus, the dose increase for mezlocillin provides significantly enhanced bactericidal activity, whereas the bactericidal activity for ticarcillin 80 mg/kg given every eight hours is not significantly different from that provided by 50 mg/kg given every four hours.

The duration of antibacterial activity is also important. Both drugs produced adequate bactericidal activity for six hours at the 50-mg/kg dose against the *E. coli* isolate. Additionally, both drugs produced minimal but detectable bactericidal activity at eight hours after the 80-mg/kg dose. This suggests that the higher-dose, longer-dosing-interval schedule may be effective for ticarcillin since bactericidal activity persists throughout an eight-hour dosing interval. Multiple-dose studies comparing high- and low-dose regimens that allow for drug accumulation need to be performed.

These alternative dosage regimens may be cost-effective. If the clinical efficacy of administering 80 mg/kg every eight hours (240 mg/kg/day) proves to be comparable to administering 50 mg/kg every four hours (300 mg/kg/day), cost savings can be realized since 20% less drug is administered in half as many doses.

Conclusion. Mezlocillin exhibited dose dependency that resulted in significantly enhanced serum bactericidal activity against the *E. coli* isolate used for this study. The AUBC for ticarcillin at a higher dose was no greater than that for the lower dose, although activity was present in serum eight hours after administration. Further pharmacokinetic–pharmacodynamic studies with ticarcillin are needed. Clinical trials with mezlocillin comparing a regimen using 80 mg/kg every eight hours with a regimen using 50 mg/kg every four hours should be initiated.

References

1. White GS, Malow JB, Zimelis VM et al. Comparative in-vitro activity of azlocillin, ampicillin, mezlocillin, piperacillin, and ticarcillin, alone and in combination with an aminoglycoside. *Antimicrob Agents Chemother.* 1979; 15:540–3.
2. Fass RJ. Statistical comparison of the antibacterial activities of broad-spectrum penicillins against gram-negative bacilli. *Antimicrob Agents Chemother.* 1983; 24:156–62.
3. Thadepalli H, Roy I, Bach VT et al. In-vitro activity of mezlocillin and its related compounds against aerobic and anaerobic bacteria. *Antimicrob Agents Chemother.* 1979; 15:487–90.
4. Drusano GL, Schimpff SC, Hewitt WL. The acylampicillins: mezlocillin, piperacillin, and azlocillin. *Rev Infect Dis.* 1984; 6:13–32.
5. Gonzalez MA. Comparison of the efficacy and safety of mezlocillin and ticarcillin in the treatment of patients with serious systemic infections. *J Antimicrob Chemother.* 1982; 9(Suppl. C):1–16.
6. Leal del Rosal P. Mezlocillin and ticarcillin in the treatment of patients with serious systemic infections. *J Antimicrob Chemother.* 1982; 9(Suppl A):227–8.
7. McCloskey RV, Killebrew D, Tutlane V et al. A randomized, double blinded comparison of mezlocillin and ticarcillin for the treatment of patients with respiratory infections. *J Antimicrob Chemother.* 1982; 9(Suppl A):209–13.
8. Viollier A, Standiford HC, Drusano GL et al. Comparative pharmacokinetics and serum bactericidal activity of mezlocillin, ticarcillin, and piperacillin, with and without gentamicin. *J Antimicrob Chemother.* 1985; 15:597–606.
9. Bergan T. Overview of acylureidopenicillin pharmacokinetics. *Scand J Infect Dis.* 1981; 29(Suppl):33–48.
10. Bergan T. Overview of the pharmacokinetics of mezlocillin. *J Antimicrob Chemother.* 1983; 11(Suppl C):1–16.
11. Flaherty JF, Barriere SL, Mordenti J et al. Effect of dose on the pharmacokinetics and serum activity of mezlocillin. *Antimicrob Agents Chemother.* 1987; 31:895–8.
12. Dalhoff A, Hoffler D, Wulfing JA. Ticarcillin pharmacokinetics in man according to different administration schedules. *J Int Med Res.* 1977; 5:308–12.
13. Libke RD, Clark JT, Ralph ED et al. Ticarcillin vs carbenicillin: clinical pharmacokinetics. *Clin Pharmacol Ther.* 1975; 17:441–6.
14. Guglielmo BJ, Flaherty JF, Batman R et al. Comparative pharmacokinetics of low and high-dose ticarcillin. *Antimicrob Agents and Chemother.* 1986; 30:359–60.
15. Coppens L, Klastersky J. Comparative study of anti-pseudomonas activity of azlocillin, mezlocillin and ticarcillin. *Antimicrob Agents Chemother.* 1979; 15:396–9.
16. National Committee for Clinical Laboratory Standards. Standard methods for dilution antimicrobial susceptibility tests for bacteria which grow aerobically: tentative standards. NCCLS document M7-T. Villanova, PA: National Committee for Laboratory Standards; 1983.
17. National Committee for Clinical Laboratory Standards. Methodology for the serum bactericidal test: proposed guidelines. NCCLS document M21-P. Villanova, PA: National Committee for Laboratory Standards; 1987.
18. Jusko WJ. Guidelines for collection and pharmacokinetic analysis of drug disposition data. In: Evans WE, Schentag JJ, Jusko WJ, eds. Applied pharmacokinetics. San Francisco: Applied Therapeutics; 1980:639–80.
19. Barriere SL, Kapusnik JE, Ely E et al. Analysis of a new method to determine antibacterial synergy; area under bactericidal time curve. *J Antimicrob Chemother.* 1985; 16:49–60.
20. Benet LZ, Galeazzi RL. Noncompartmental determination of the steady-state volume of distribution. *J Pharm Sci.* 1979; 68:1071–4.

Commentary

Aminoglycosides: A reassessment of their therapeutic role

STEVEN L. BARRIERE

Clin Pharm. 1988; 7:385–90

Over the last 20 years, aminoglycosides have become standard therapy for the treatment of gram-negative bacillary infection, either alone or in combination with β-lactam compounds. Additionally, in combination with either penicillins or vancomycin, aminoglycosides are agents of choice for various forms of streptococcal and staphylococcal endocarditis.[1] This widespread use has occurred because of their broad, potent gram-negative spectrum, their rapid bactericidal action, and their ability to exert a synergistic effect when combined with β lactams or other compounds.

However, the introduction of the third-generation cephalosporins and more recently imipenem, aztreonam, and the fluoroquinolones has led to a substantial decrease in the use of aminoglycosides.[2,3] These new agents are potent, have a broad spectrum, and are bactericidal. Moreover, they penetrate well into deeper sites of infection (e.g., the CNS) and do not require serum concentration monitoring for toxicity.

What then is the current role for aminoglycosides? Should they be regarded as relics, only to be remembered rather than applied? The purpose of this paper is to attempt to answer these questions. Advantages and disadvantages of aminoglycosides compared with other compounds will be assessed, and their comparative efficacy will be reviewed in an attempt to define the established clinical role of aminoglycosides.

STEVEN L. BARRIERE, Pharm.D., is Specialist in Infectious Diseases, Department of Pharmaceutical Services, and Adjunct Associate Professor, Division of Infectious Diseases, Department of Medicine, UCLA Center for the Health Sciences, Los Angeles, CA.

Address reprint requests to Dr. Barriere at Room A4-215 CHS, UCLA Medical Center, 10833 LeConte Avenue, Los Angeles, CA 90024.

Presented at the 21st Annual ASHP Midyear Clinical Meeting, Las Vegas, NV, December 11, 1986.

Copyright © 1988, American Society of Hospital Pharmacists, Inc. All rights reserved. 0278-2677/0501-0385$01.50.

Disadvantages of Aminoglycosides

There are several real, and apparent, disadvantages to aminoglycosides. First, their spectrum is limited to aerobic bacteria because the mechanism of aminoglycoside uptake by bacterial cells is oxygen dependent.[4] Thus, anaerobic bacteria are resistant to aminoglycosides. This necessitates the inclusion of a drug active against anaerobes in the treatment of mixed infections such as those found in the abdomen and female pelvis.[5] Newer β lactams such as cefoxitin, cefotetan, ceftizoxime, and especially imipenem are active against both aerobic and anaerobic organisms. These latter compounds seldom require the addition of a second agent for mixed infection.[5]

Second, aminoglycosides penetrate poorly into certain sites of infection.[6] This is due, in part, to limitation in dose and achievable serum concentrations because the relative penetration of these drugs into extracellular fluid spaces is comparable to that of β lactams. However, penetration into the CNS is limited because of the drugs' polarity and water solubility. Therefore, CNS infection attributable to gram-negative bacilli usually requires direct injection of aminoglycosides into the subarachnoid space.[7] A frequent result of prolonged treatment in this fashion is irritation of the local tissues or arachnoiditis.[8] In contrast, third-generation cephalosporins such as cefotaxime or ceftazidime are widely regarded as the drugs of choice for meningitis caused by gram-negative bacilli, and need only be given intravenously.[9]

None of the newer β lactams or fluoroquinolones are associated with dose-related toxicity such as renal damage, hearing loss, and vestibular damage. Aminoglycosides produce these effects at various frequencies depending on many risk factors; these adverse effects appear to occur in at least 5–10% of patients treated with the drugs.[10] Toxicity is generally believed to occur at drug concentrations that are only slightly higher than therapeutic levels. Therefore, the therapeutic index of aminoglycosides is quite low. This requires that serum concentrations of the drugs be monitored in most patients, which adds to the expense of aminoglycoside therapy.[11] Moreover, toxicity may occur even in carefully monitored patients.[12] Therefore, there has been an increasing tendency to eliminate the use of aminoglycosides in favor of less toxic β-lactam compounds. This has been especially true in patients receiving other nephrotoxins such as amphotericin B or cyclosporine.

Finally, unlike β lactams the activity of aminoglycosides is diminished in the presence of low pH, such as is found in cases of abscess. The presence of purulence and necrotic tissue also inactivates aminoglycosides.[4]

Advantages of Aminoglycosides

Some recent investigations have shed new light on the potential clinical utility of aminoglycosides. These data, in combination with prior knowledge about the bactericidal potency of these drugs, have raised new interest in the use of aminoglycosides.

Aminoglycosides are consistently bactericidal. Unlike many other commonly used compounds, their activity is not diminished in the presence of large inocula of bacteria ($>10^5$/mL).[4] Additionally, synergistic killing is obtained by combining a β-lactam compound with an aminoglycoside.[13] This is found for both gram-positive and gram-negative aerobic bacteria. In contrast, synergy is infrequently observed when combinations of β-lactam compounds are tested.[14] These observations have been extended to in vivo situations involving experimental infection. Johnson et al.[15] compared the efficacy of piperacillin, amikacin, and ceftazidime alone or in combination in the treatment of experimental infection caused by *Pseudomonas aeruginosa*. The results are illustrated in Table 1. Seven groups of 20 animals each were infected and then treated with various regimens. The aminoglycoside (amikacin) alone was more effective than either β lactam. Moreover, the aminoglycoside–β-lactam combinations were clearly more effective than the double β-lactam regimen in all respects. Finally, the amikacin–β-lactam combinations were slightly more effective than amikacin given alone.

Again, unlike β lactams, as the ratio of the concentration of aminoglycoside to minimum inhibitory concentration (MIC) is increased, the rate of killing is increased. In other words, the higher the concentration of aminoglycoside in a testing system, the more rapid and completely the inoculum of bacteria is killed.[16]

As with most other antimicrobials that affect protein, DNA, or RNA synthesis, a postantibiotic effect (PAE) is found in vitro when aminoglycosides are tested against gram-positive and, especially, gram-negative bacteria.[17] This phenomenon is persistent suppression of bacterial growth beyond the time that the organisms are exposed to inhibitory concentrations of the antimicrobial agent. Cell-wall-active agents such as penicillins and cephalosporins exert only a minimal PAE against gram-positive bacteria and none against gram-negative bacteria.[16,17] Only imipenem (a carbapenem) exerts a modest PAE against gram-negative bacteria. In general, the greater the concentration-to-MIC ratio, the longer the PAE. The clinical implication of this is that dosing intervals for drugs with pronounced PAEs can be extended longer than would be apparent from their elimination half-life.

These characteristics of aminoglycosides have generated interest in assessing the efficacy and tolerance of dosage regimens that take advantage of these phenomena. For example, combining the entire daily dose of a drug such as gentamicin or tobramycin and administering it as a single daily injection has been tested. In an in vitro model of infection, Blaser et al.[18] assessed the effects of identical total daily doses of netilmicin, administered as continuous or intermittent infusions in various dosage schedules, against several strains of bacteria including *Ps. aeruginosa*. They found that once-daily administration of the aminoglycoside provided the best response overall in terms of rapidity of bacterial killing and eradication of the organisms from the infection site. Additionally, they noted that no bacterial killing occurred after the first dose unless the ratio of peak drug concentration to MIC was >6. In a similar study using the same model, these authors noted that bacterial regrowth occurred within 24 hours unless the peak concentration-to-MIC ratio exceeded 8:1.[19]

Kapusnik et al.[20] compared the efficacy of 4-hour versus 24-hour dosing intervals of tobramycin in a guinea-pig model of *Ps. aeruginosa* pneumonia.[20] The half-life of the drug in the guinea pig was 0.5 hours. The dose given produced serum concentra-

Table 1.
Comparative Efficacy of Various Regimens in the Treatment of Experimental *Pseudomonas aeruginosa* Infection[a]

Regimen[b]	Survival (%)	Positive Blood Cultures (%)	Emergence of Resistance (%)
Control	5	95	0
Piperacillin	45	75	40
Ceftazidime	50	65	15
Amikacin	95	10	10
Piperacillin plus amikacin	100	5	0/5[c]
Ceftazidime plus amikacin	100	0	0/0
Piperacillin plus ceftazidime	75	55	25/35

[a] Adapted from reference 15.
[b] Each treatment group consisted of 20 animals.
[c] Percentage for first agent/percentage for second agent.

tions similar to those observed in humans. In this model of pneumonia, the efficacy of the once-daily dosing of the aminoglycoside was the same as the every-four-hours regimen. The average peak concentrations of tobramycin in the once-daily regimen were approximately seven times higher than in the every-four-hours regimen.

In another study, tobramycin was given once daily or continuously to 52 patients with cystic fibrosis who, after 10 days of therapy, had no change in creatinine clearance or hearing despite the presence of peak serum concentrations of 40 μg/mL.[21] In terms of clinical response, the two regimens were equally effective. In the same study, these authors also found that acute pneumonia caused by *Ps. aeruginosa* in guinea pigs responded better to once-daily than more frequent dosing of tobramycin. Chronic pneumonia in rats and endocarditis in rabbits responded equally to both regimens.[21] In contrast, Pechere et al.[22] found that, in a study of the efficacy of tobramycin in murine *Klebsiella* bronchopneumonia, eight-hour dosing of the drug was significantly more effective than 24-hour dosing. However, it was also noted that eight-hour intervals were equivalent to 16 half-lives of tobramycin in the mouse species used.

Petty et al.[23] administered tobramycin sulfate to healthy volunteers in doses of 5 mg/kg (of tobramycin) once daily or 1.7 mg/kg three times daily. They assessed urinary enzyme excretion (alanine aminopeptidase and *N*-acetylglucosaminodase), serum creatinine, and creatinine clearance before and after nine days of treatment. There was no difference observed between the two regimens for any variable, except for a slight (5 mL/min) decrease in creatinine clearance in the group given divided doses of tobramycin compared with a slight (4 mL/min) increase in clearance among those receiving single daily doses.

In another study, 28 women (17–40 years of age) with pelvic inflammatory disease were randomly assigned to receive daily or three-times-daily doses of netilmicin sulfate in a total daily dosage of 6.6 mg/kg (of netilmicin).[24] The duration of therapy was seven days for both groups. All patients also received ampicillin and tinidazole. Despite peak concentrations of netilmicin in excess of 20 μg/mL with the daily regimen, results of audiometric testing before, during, and after treatment revealed no differences between the two groups. Additionally, urinary phospholipid excretion, a marker of kidney cellular damage, was actually less in the patients receiving daily doses. These reports suggest that an aminoglycoside dosing regimen using fewer doses per day may be as effective and no more toxic than standard regimens.

In a retrospective analysis, Moore et al.[25] assessed the importance of the peak concentration-to-MIC ratio in clinical response to aminoglycoside therapy.[25] These investigators found strong associations between this ratio and clinical response, even after adjustment for underlying severity of illness and other factors correlated with response. Response rates increased from <70% with peak concentration-to-MIC ratios of <6 to >80% with ratios >6. In three separate investigations of the efficacy of amikacin in the treatment of gram-negative infections, a peak concentration-to-MIC ratio of 8–10:1 was associated with clinical cure.[26]

Aminoglycosides administered as a single daily dose should achieve peak concentration-to-MIC ratios of at least 5 to 6 for susceptible organisms (MIC ≤4 μg/mL, gentamicin or tobramycin; MIC ≤16 μg/mL, amikacin). Thus, the response to aminoglycosides is enhanced by the achievement of higher concentrations. Single-daily-dose therapy may be advantageous from an efficacy standpoint and may be less toxic.

Comparative Efficacy of Aminoglycosides versus Other Antimicrobials

The list of agents that are competing to replace aminoglycosides is growing. Currently, the third-generation cephalosporins, imipenem, and aztreonam have been demonstrated to be as effective as aminoglycosides in the treatment of most gram-negative bacillary infections. Exceptions include serious infection caused by *Ps. aeruginosa,* wherein a combination of drugs is probably more effective,[27] and the treatment of enterococcal infection, wherein an aminoglycoside is required for synergistic bactericidal activity. The new fluorinated quinolone derivatives have been shown to be effective in the treatment of many infections attributable to *Ps. aeruginosa,* but the development of resistance has been problematic.[28] The combination of a quinolone and an antipseudomonal penicillin appears promising in this regard.[29]

In an attempt to avoid the nephrotoxicity of aminoglycosides yet provide broad-spectrum coverage for seriously ill patients, combinations of β-lactam compounds are being used more frequently. Unlike aminoglycoside–β-lactam combinations, the "double β-lactam" regimens are seldom synergistic in vitro and occasionally behave antagonistically.[14] Although these combinations have been shown to be as effective as aminoglycoside regimens in seriously ill patients, some words of caution are in order. The evidence that the double β-lactam combinations are as effective as aminoglycoside regimens in the treatment of infection caused by *Ps. aeruginosa* is sparse. As was found in experimental infections, some investigators have noted a poorer response rate in patients treated without an aminoglycoside. Moreover, in profoundly granulocytopenic patients, some studies have found that β-lactam combinations are less effective.[14,30]

For example, Winston et al.[30] compared the efficacy of moxalactam plus piperacillin versus moxalactam plus amikacin in the treatment of febrile granulocytopenic patients. They found that the response rates for patients whose granulocyte counts remained less than 100/cu mm were 48% for the double β-lactam group versus 77% for the aminoglycoside regimen.

Several studies have compared the efficacy of various new β lactams to aminoglycosides in nongranulocytopenic patients. In general, the new β lactams appear to be as effective as aminoglycosides, except in infection caused by *Ps. aeruginosa*, and are less toxic.[3] For example, Smith et al.[31] compared the effectiveness of cefotaxime sodium, in a dose of 12 g per day (of cefotaxime), to a combination of nafcillin plus tobramycin in a randomized, double-blind study. The patients treated had serious bacterial infections. The overall response rates were 90% for cefotaxime and only 60% for the aminoglycoside regimen. Moreover, adverse effects (diarrhea and nephrotoxicity) were seen more frequently in the aminoglycoside group. These differences held true even after confounding factors were analyzed. However, the dosage of cefotaxime that was used is 1.5 to 2 times larger than those most frequently used for infection outside of the central nervous system. Use of more commonly employed dosages may result in somewhat lower efficacy. Regardless, the efficacy of the β lactam in a "safe" dosage was at least equivalent to that of the aminoglycoside.

In an experimental study, neutropenic rats were challenged with multiple lethal doses of *Ps. aeruginosa*.[32] Imipenem, moxalactam, and amikacin alone and in combinations were compared in terms of protective efficacy (Table 2). After the largest inoculum of organisms (250 times the 50% lethal dose) was administered, all animals given saline died. Most of the animals given either moxalactam or amikacin died. Imipenem alone and the combination of moxalactam plus amikacin protected about half of the animals. The most effective regimen was the combination of amikacin plus imipenem. These data support the long-held tenet that infection caused by *Ps. aeruginosa* requires combination therapy. Even the newest, most active β lactams such as ceftazidime, imipenem, and aztreonam are not adequate as sole agents for serious infection caused by this organism. Soft-tissue, bone and joint, and urinary-tract infection may respond adequately, but infection of the central nervous system, pneumonia, endovascular infection, and other deep-seated infections caused by *Ps. aeruginosa* should be treated with aminoglycoside-containing combinations.[27,33]

Table 2.
Mortality of Neutropenic Rats at 72 Hours after Challenge with 250 Times the 50% Lethal Dose of *Pseudomonas aeruginosa*[a]

Therapy	Dead/Challenged
Saline	20/20
Moxalactam	17/20
Amikacin	18/20
Imipenem	8/20[b]
Moxalactam plus amikacin	10/20[b]
Imipenem plus amikacin	1/20[b]

[a] Adapted from reference 32.
[b] $p < 0.05$.

In two recent comparative studies, aztreonam has been compared with aminoglycoside therapy. Gudiol et al.[34] conducted an open, randomized comparison of aztreonam versus an aminoglycoside in 57 adult, nongranulocytopenic patients who had aerobic gram-negative septicemia.[34] Thirty-one patients received aztreonam (1 g every eight hours), and 26 received an aminoglycoside (1.5 mg/kg every eight hours) (13 received gentamicin, and 13 received tobramycin). No other drugs with gram-negative activity were given. The overall cure rate was 84% for aztreonam and 77% for aminoglycosides. Only one of the failures was attributable to *Ps. aeruginosa* (gentamicin). The only therapeutic difference between the groups was a significantly higher incidence of colonization and superinfection in the aztreonam group. Nearly all of these episodes were caused by enterococci.

In the other study, the efficacy of aztreonam alone or in combination with amikacin was compared with a double β-lactam regimen (moxalactam–ticarcillin) in the treatment of febrile granulocytopenic patients.[35] The regimens were equally effective overall, with the only evident difference being a somewhat lower response rate in *Pseudomonas* infections to aztreonam alone versus aztreonam plus amikacin (four of seven versus seven of seven).

The new fluorinated quinolones, such as ciprofloxacin, show promise in treating gram-negative infections, especially since they can be given orally. To date, there have been no published studies comparing them directly with aminoglycosides. However, the results of treatment both in open studies and in trials comparing them with third-generation cephalosporins are encouraging.[28] Again, the treatment of deep-seated, serious infection caused by *Ps. aeruginosa* remains problematic. Resistance has emerged during therapy in a substantial proportion of patients.[36]

The quinolones, however, have been shown to act synergistically with both β lactams and aminoglycosides. Experimental work with drugs such as azlocillin in combination with ciprofloxacin suggests that the emergence of resistant subpopulations of organisms is suppressed.[37] More work in this area is necessary to determine the true effectiveness of quinolones, either alone or in combination.

Established Clinical Roles for Aminoglycosides

Given the above information, and other evidence beyond the scope of this paper, aminoglycosides will likely remain as standards of therapy for selected situations.[38] Infection caused by *Ps. aeruginosa* may frequently be effectively treated with β lactams or quinolones given alone. However, aminoglycoside combinations currently remain the most effective regimens, especially for serious infection in sites such as the central nervous system and lower respiratory tract.

The treatment of serious enterococcal infection (endocarditis, meningitis) requires bactericidal activity, which is not provided unless an aminoglycoside is added to a cell-wall-active agent.[1]

Listeria monocytogenes is killed more effectively and rapidly by a combination of penicillin or ampicillin plus an aminoglycoside, and some authorities recommend the combination for the treatment of life-threatening infection.[39] Aminoglycosides are often listed as drugs of choice for the treatment of infrequently encountered organisms such as *Francisella tularensis* and certain atypical mycobacteria.[40]

Finally, most authorities recommend that empiric therapy for febrile granulocytopenic patients should contain an aminoglycoside.[41]

Conclusion

Aminoglycosides have important in vitro advantages over β lactams. Moreover, they are consistently more effective in experimental infection caused by *Ps. aeruginosa*, especially in combination with an active β lactam. Clinical trials seldom treat enough patients with infection attributable to *Ps. aeruginosa* to generate meaningful results. However, there is a general trend towards superior efficacy with aminoglycoside regimens.

Even in 1988 there are clearly established roles for aminoglycosides. Therefore, they are not relics. With further exploration of new dosage regimens that maximize efficacy and minimize toxicity, we may even see a resurgence in their use.

References

1. Sande MA, Scheld WM. Combination antibiotic therapy of bacterial endocarditis. *Ann Intern Med*. 1980; 92:390–5.
2. Levin S, Karakusis PH. Future trends in aminoglycoside therapy. *Am J Med*. 1986; 80(Suppl 6B):190–4.
3. Moellering RC. Have the new beta-lactams rendered the aminoglycosides obsolete for the treatment of serious nosocomial infections? *Am J Med*. 1986; 80(Suppl 6B):44–7.
4. Siegenthaler WE, Bonetti A, Luthy R. Aminoglycoside antibiotics in infectious diseases—an overview. *Am J Med*. 1986; 80(Suppl 6B):2–14.
5. DiPiro JT, Mansberger JA, Davis JB. Current concepts in clinical therapeutics: intra-abdominal infections. *Clin Pharm*. 1986; 5:34–50.
6. Edson RS, Keys TF. The aminoglycosides. *Mayo Clin Proc*. 1983; 58:99–102.
7. Kaiser AB, McGee ZA. Aminoglycoside therapy of gram-negative bacillary meningitis. *N Engl J Med*. 1975; 293:1215–20.
8. Buckley RM, Watters W, MacGregor RR. Persistent meningeal inflammation associated with intrathecal gentamicin. *Am J Med Sci*. 1977; 274:207–9.
9. Landesman SH, Cherubin CE, Corrado ML. Gram-negative bacillary meningitis. New therapy and changing concepts. *Arch Intern Med*. 1982; 142:439–40.
10. Whelton A. Therapeutic initiatives for the avoidance of aminoglycoside toxicity. *J Clin Pharmacol*. 1985; 25:67–81.
11. Gladen HE. Cost-effective aminoglycoside therapy in surgical patients. *Am J Med*. 1986; 80(Suppl 6B):228–33.
12. Flint LM, Gott J, Short L et al. Serum level monitoring of aminoglycoside antibiotics. *Arch Surg*. 1985; 120:99–103.
13. Lyon MD, Smith KR, Saag MS et al. In vitro activity of piperacillin, ticarcillin, and mezlocillin alone and in combination with aminoglycoside against *Pseudomonas aeruginosa*. *Antimicrob Agents Chemother*. 1986; 30:25–30.
14. Barriere SL. Therapeutic considerations in using combinations of newer β-lactam antibiotics. *Clin Pharm*. 1986; 5:24–33.
15. Johnson DE, Thompson B, Calia FM. Comparative activities of piperacillin, ceftazidime, and amikacin, alone and in all possible combinations, against experimental *Pseudomonas aeruginosa* infection in neutropenic rats. *Antimicrob Agents Chemother*. 1985; 27:735–9.
16. Vogelman BS, Craig WA. Kinetics of antimicrobial activity. *J Pediatr*. 1986; 108:835–40.
17. Vogelman BS, Craig WA. Postantibiotic effects. *J Antimicrob Chemother*. 1985; 15(Suppl A):37–46.
18. Blaser J, Stone BB, Zinner SH. Efficacy of intermittent versus continuous administration of netilmicin in a two-compartment in vitro model. *Antimicrob Agents Chemother*. 1985; 27:343–9.
19. Blaser J, Stone BB, Groner MC et al. Comparative study with enoxacin and netilmicin in a pharmacodynamic model to determine importance of ratio of antibiotic peak concentration to MIC for bactericidal activity and emergence of resistance. *Antimicrob Agents Chemother*. 1987; 31:1054–60.
20. Kapusnik JE, Gordin F, Scott K et al. Efficacy of once daily vs conventional aminoglycoside therapy for experimental pseudomonas pneumonia. *Clin Res*. 1985; 33:57A.
21. Powell SH, Thompson WL, Luthe MA et al. Once-daily vs continuous aminoglycoside dosing: efficacy and toxicity in animal and clinical studies of gentamicin, netilmicin, and tobramycin. *J Infect Dis*. 1983; 147:918–32.
22. Pechere M, Letarte R, Pechere JC. Efficacy of different dosing schedules of tobramycin for treating a murine *Klebsiella pneumoniae* bronchopneumonia. *J Antimicrob Chemother*. 1987; 19:487–91.
23. Petty BG, Baumgardner JY, Lietman PS. Comparison of the renal effects of single vs thrice daily dosing of tobramycin in healthy volunteers. *Proc 26th Intersci Conf Antimicrob Agents Chemother*. 1986:101.
24. Clerckx-Braun F, Donnez J, Ibrahim S et al. Study of the tolerance of netilmicin once a day vs thrice a day in 28 cases of pelvic inflammatory disease. *Proc 27th Intersci Conf Antimicrob Agents Chemother*. 1987:101.
25. Moore RD, Lietman PS, Smith CR. Clinical response to aminoglycoside therapy: importance of the ratio of peak concentration to minimal inhibitory concentration. *J Infect Dis*. 1987; 155:93–9.
26. Williams PJ, Hull JH, Sarubbi FA et al. Factors associated with nephrotoxicity and clinical outcome in patients receiving amikacin. *J Clin Pharmacol*. 1986; 26:79–86.
27. Bodey GP, Bolivar R, Fainstein V et al. Infections caused by *Pseudomonas aeruginosa*. *Rev Infect Dis*. 1983; 5:279–313.
28. Nix DE, DeVito JM. Ciprofloxacin and norfloxacin, two fluoroquinolone antimicrobials. *Clin Pharm*. 1987; 6:105–17.
29. Zinner SH, Dudley MN. Bactericidal activity of ciprofloxacin alone and in combination with azlocillin in an in-vitro

capillary model. *J Antimicrob Chemother.* 1986; 18(Suppl D):49–54.
30. Winston DJ, Barnes RC, Ho WG et al. Moxalactam plus piperacillin versus moxalactam plus amikacin in febrile, granulocytopenic patients. *Am J Med.* 1984; 77:442–50.
31. Smith CR, Ambinder R, Lipsky JJ et al. Cefotaxime compared with nafcillin plus tobramycin for serious bacterial infections. *Ann Intern Med.* 1984; 101:469–77.
32. Wade JC, Standiford HL, Drusano GL et al. Potential of imipenem as single-agent empiric antibiotic therapy of febrile neutropenic patients with cancer. *Am J Med.* 1985; 78(Suppl 6A):62–72.
33. Fong IW, Tomkins KB. Review of *Pseudomonas aeruginosa* meningitis with special emphasis on treatment with ceftazidime. *Rev Infect Dis.* 1985; 7:604–12.
34. Gudiol F, Pallares CR, Ariza X et al. Comparative clinical evaluation of aztreonam vs. aminoglycosides in gram-negative septicemia. *J Antimicrob Chemother.* 1986; 17:661–72.
35. Jones PG, Rolston KVI, Fainstein V et al. Aztreonam therapy in neutropenic patients with cancer. *Am J Med.* 1986; 81:243–8.
36. Scully BE, Parry MF, Neu HC et al. Oral ciprofloxacin therapy of infections due to *Pseudomonas aeruginosa. Lancet.* 1986; 1:819–22.
37. Dudley MN, Mandler HD, Gilbert D et al. Pharmacokinetics and serum bactericidal activity of intravenous ciprofloxacin: studies in vitro and in an in vitro dynamic model. *Am J Med.* 1987; 82(Suppl 4A):363–8.
38. Neu HC. Antibiotics in the second half of the 1980's. Areas of future development and the effect of new agents on aminoglycoside use. *Am J Med.* 1986; 80(6B):195–203.
39. Scheld WM, Fletcher DD, Fink FN et al. Response to therapy in an experimental rabbit model of meningitis due to *Listeria monocytogenes. J Infect Dis.* 1979; 140:287–94.
40. Anon. The choice of antimicrobial drugs. *Med Lett Drugs Ther.* 1986; 28:33–40.
41. Young LS. Empirical antimicrobial therapy in the neutropenic host. *N Engl J Med.* 1986; 315:580–1.

“

Cathartics as an Adjunct in Clinical Toxicology

Because of their ability to accelerate gastrointestinal transit, cathartics have become a useful adjunct in clinical toxicology, where they are used as facilitators of gastrointestinal decontamination. Typically, when an acute toxic ingestion occurs, gastric evacuation is carried out by lavage or emesis followed by administration of activated charcoal with a cathartic added to expedite expulsion of the reversible drug–charcoal complex. With ingestions of drugs including phenobarbital, theophylline and tricyclic antidepressants, activated charcoal and a cathartic are given repetitively to provide continued drug binding and removal, respectively.

The use of cathartics in toxicology has, however, been questioned. Clearly guidelines are needed for their rational use based on the literature and the known pharmacology of these agents. . . .

Continued use of cathartics in the management of acute poisoning appears, in our view, to be appropriate. The availability of a number of agents offers options based on the patient and the drug ingested. Whole bowel irrigation is appearing as another potentially useful means of catharsis. Further research is clearly needed to define efficacy, particularly in the face of abnormalities of bowel function, a very common situation in toxic ingestions. These offer exciting avenues for further investigation.

—Shannon M, Fish SS, Lovejoy FH Jr. Cathartics and laxatives: do they still have a place in management of the poisoned patient? *Med Toxicol.* 1986; 1:247–52.

”

Grand Rounds

Death of a child associated with multiple overdoses of acetaminophen

KATHRYN V. BLAKE, DAVID BAILEY, GARY M. ZIENTEK, AND LESLIE HENDELES

Abstract: A case of long-term acetaminophen overdosage in a six-year-old child, which contributed to her death despite optimal medical management including oral acetylcysteine therapy, is reported.

Acetaminophen 325 mg every six hours was prescribed for fever associated with measles. Believing that acetaminophen was nontoxic, the child's mother progressively increased the dose over three days, first in response to fever and subsequently for abdominal pain probably secondary to unrecognized acetaminophen toxicity. On admission to the hospital, the patient's serum acetaminophen concentration was 163 μg/mL (11 hours after the last dose); subsequently, the acetaminophen half-life was determined to be 15 hours. A course of oral acetylcysteine therapy (a loading dose of 140 mg/kg as the sodium salt followed by 70 mg/kg every four hours for 17 doses) was begun. Hepatic and renal failure developed within two days, followed by the onset of seizures, and brain death occurred on the 11th day. Autopsy findings consistent with acetaminophen toxicity included centrilobular hepatic and renal tubular necrosis. *Aspergillis fumigatus* and *Cryptococcus neoformans* isolates from pulmonary abscesses and bronchopulmonary lymph nodes, respectively, were an unexpected finding. However, in the absence of acetaminophen overdosage, death would have been unlikely. Cryptococcal lymphadenitis was believed to have been the initial febrile illness that was treated with supratherapeutic doses of acetaminophen.

Fatalities in children from a single overdose of acetaminophen have been rare, and there is only one previous report of a fatality after long-term administration of multiple excessive doses. The lethal outcome in this case illustrates the need to educate the public on the potential toxicity of nonprescription medications.

Index terms: Acetaminophen; Acetylcysteine sodium; Analgesics and antipyretics; Antidotes; Blood levels; Dosage; Dosage schedules; Drug administration; Errors, medication; Half-life; Pediatrics; Toxicity
Clin Pharm. 1988; 7:391–7

Fatalities in children after a single acute overdose of acetaminophen have been reported but are extremely rare even in patients with serum concentrations that would be hepatotoxic in adults.[1–3] Although adults and children metabolize acetaminophen through similar pathways, albeit in differing proportions, it is not yet clear why children are less susceptible to acetaminophen hepatotoxicity.[4]

We report a case of long-term acetaminophen overdosing that contributed to the death of a child and review acetaminophen metabolism and mechanisms of toxicity.

There have been only a few reports of hepatotoxicity in children after repeated overdoses of acetaminophen.[3,5–9] This case is unusual as there is only one previous report of a fatality in a child resulting from administration of excessive doses of

KATHRYN V. BLAKE, PHARM.D., is Fellow, College of Pharmacy and Division of Pediatric Pharmacology/Toxicology, College of Medicine, University of Florida, Gainesville. DAVID BAILEY, M.D., is Major, U.S. Army, and Chief of Pediatric Gastroenterology, Tripler Army Medical Center, Honolulu, HI; at the time of this report, he was a fellow in the Division of Pediatric Gastroenterology, Department of Pediatrics, The University of Florida. GARY M. ZIENTEK, M.D., is Resident, Department of Pathology, University of Florida. LESLIE HENDELES, PHARM.D., is Professor, College of Pharmacy and Department of Pediatrics, University of Florida.

Address reprint requests to Dr. Blake at the University of Florida, J. Hillis Miller Health Center, Box J-486, Gainesville, FL 32610-0486.

The assistance of William H. Donnelly, Jr., M.D., Professor of Pathology, University of Florida, is acknowledged.

The opinions or assertions presented here are those of the authors and are not to be construed as official or as reflecting the views of the Department of the Army.

This is **article 680-204-8807** in the **ASHP Continuing Education System;** it qualifies for 1.0 hour of continuing-education credit. See page 403 for learning objectives and test questions.

Copyright © 1988, American Society of Hospital Pharmacists, Inc. All rights reserved. 0278-2677/88/0501-0391$01.75.

Papers in the Grand Rounds section are patient case reports and literature review combined in a way that gives them high educational value. The papers lead off with a well-documented case report of an unusual drug experience (e.g., adverse drug reaction or other unexpected drug response, experimental use of a drug). The case generally deals with a difficult therapeutic problem or dilemma that is commonly encountered but may be overlooked or misunderstood. (Esoteric or rare occurrences of minor importance do not make good Grand Rounds material.) A literature review puts the case in perspective with previously reported similar cases and alternative treatments. The review is integrated with related discussion of the case being reported.

CP *readers are encouraged to use Grand Rounds for educational group discussions. For this purpose, discussion questions are printed at the end of Grand Rounds papers.*

acetaminophen over several days[3]; all other reports are of fatalities that occurred after a single overdose.

Case Report

Two months before admission, this white, six-year-old, 21-kg girl had chickenpox. For the subsequent two months, she had brief recurrent bouts of fever and vomiting of unknown origin. It is unknown whether she received treatment for these episodes.

Three days before admission, the patient was taken to a local emergency room with a temperature of 40.6 °C of 12 hours' duration, a maculopapular rash of 24 hours' duration, vomiting, conjunctivitis, and bilateral anterior cervical lymphadenopathy. A diagnosis of measles was made. The child was sent home, and the mother was instructed by the physician to give one regular-strength Tylenol (325 mg of acetaminophen, McNeil Consumer Products Company) every six hours as needed for fever.

The child reportedly was given Extra-Strength Tylenol (500 mg of acetaminophen) every 4 hours during the next 48 hours (143 mg/kg/day). Then, because of sustained fever and abdominal pain, the dose was increased to 500 mg every 2 to 3 hours for the next 12 hours. The total dose was estimated to be 7 g over the three-day period (330 mg/kg).

On the day of admission the child was taken back to the same emergency room in an incoherent state. Important physical findings included a blood pressure of 64/40 mm Hg, a pulse rate of 80 beats per minute, a respiratory rate of 30 breaths per minute, a generalized purplish rash, and hepatomegaly, with the liver extending below the umbilicus. The initial laboratory findings included a serum acetaminophen concentration of 163 μg/mL (11 hours after the last dose); serum glucose, 17 mg/dL; prothrombin time (PT), 37.5 seconds; partial thromboplastin time (PTT), 43.2 seconds; blood ammonia, 191 μg/dL; total bilirubin, 3.8 mg/dL; direct bilirubin, 2.7 mg/dL; white blood cells (WBC), 15,400/cu mm; platelets, 424,000/cu mm; aspartate aminotransferase (AST, formerly called SGOT), 5000 IU/L; lactate dehydrogenase (LDH), 6000 IU/L; and serum bicarbonate, 6 meq/L. Hypoglycemia was corrected with administration of 25 g of dextrose followed by a solution of 50% dextrose in 0.9% sodium chloride injection infused at a rate of 20 mL/hr for one hour and then 10 mL/hr. Blood glucose was 259 mg/dL measured eight hours after admission. Dopamine hydrochloride was begun at a rate of 5 μg/kg/min, which increased blood pressure to 110/60 mm Hg during the next two hours. The patient was given sodium bicarbonate, lactulose, an oral loading dose of 140 mg/kg of acetylcysteine (as the sodium salt), fresh-frozen plasma, 400 mL of 5% albumin, ampicillin (100 mg/kg, then 75 mg/kg as the sodium salt for two doses) and chloramphenicol (30 mg/kg, then 20 mg/kg as the sodium succinate salt for two doses) for possible sepsis, and was transferred to the University of Florida's pediatric intensive-care unit.

On admission, approximately 12 hours after being taken to the local emergency room, the patient had stable vital signs, a generalized rash, and hepatomegaly and responded only to painful stimuli. She had no focal neurological deficit. Laboratory values at that time included a serum acetaminophen concentration of 101 μg/mL; blood urea nitrogen (BUN), 34 mg/dL; creatinine, 1.9 mg/dL; total bilirubin, 5.2 mg/dL; direct bilirubin, 2.9 mg/dL; AST, 10,440 IU/L; alanine aminotransferase (ALT, formerly called SGPT), 5,140 IU/L; LDH, 15,800 IU/L; albumin, 3.2 g/dL; total protein, 5.2 g/dL; bicarbonate, 12.7 meq/L; platelets, 183,000/cu mm; and WBC, 10,900/cu mm with a differential of 65% neutrophils, 26% lymphocytes, 4% monocytes, 3% eosinophils, and 5% bands. Serological tests for hepatitis B surface antigen, Epstein–Barr virus antibody, and cytomegalovirus antibody were negative. Rubella antibody and antihepatitis B surface antigen serological tests were positive. Urinary output was negligible. Medications begun included nafcillin 700 mg i.v. every four hours (200 mg/kg/day as the sodium salt); a single 50-mg dose of gentamicin (2.4 mg/kg as the sulfate salt); lactulose 50 mL every six hours as a retention enema; phytonadione 10 mg i.v. daily; and two doses of intravenous furosemide of 20 mg (1 mg/kg) and 50 mg (2.4 mg/kg). The ampicillin and chloramphenicol were discontinued. A standard course of acetylcysteine (a 70-mg/kg oral dose given at four-hour intervals for 17 doses) was given after the loading dose.

On the second hospital day, the patient had hepatic and renal failure: creatinine was 3.2 mg/dL; BUN, 48 mg/dL; PT, 20.0 seconds; PTT, 37.0 seconds; blood ammonia, 196 μg/dL; creatine phosphokinase, >80,000 IU/L; platelets, 95,000/cu mm; and a serum acetaminophen concentration of 25.5 μg/mL. Her urine output was 0.02 mL/kg/hr. No organisms were cultured from cerebrospinal fluid or blood. Dexamethasone therapy was initiated with 5 mg i.v. and continued at the rate of 2 mg i.v. every six hours because of increased intracranial pressure confirmed by computed axial tomography (CAT) scan. No other therapy was used to manage the increased intracranial pressure.

By the third hospital day the full course of acetylcysteine had been completed, and hemodialysis was initiated for increasing uremia. The serum acetaminophen concentration was estimated to be 8.4 μg/mL (Figure 1). Spontaneous movements were rare and seizures developed, which were treated with phenobarbital sodium and then with phenytoin sodium.

Although the patient's liver size had decreased considerably by the fourth day, blood ammonia, total bilirubin, and direct bilirubin concentrations peaked at 258 μg/dL, 13.1 mg/dL, and 10.5 mg/dL, respectively. Declining AST and ALT concentrations were 1200 IU/L and

2220 IU/L (Figure 2), and the serum acetaminophen concentration was 2.4 μg/mL (Figure 1). The acetaminophen half-life was 15 hours using all data points. Blood cultures remained sterile. Intubation was required to manage decreasing respiratory function. By the sixth day after admission, cranial and peripheral nerve reflexes were absent. Over the next four days the anticonvulsants, nafcillin, lactulose, and dexamethasone were discontinued. On the 11th hospital day, after an angiogram documented the absence of cerebral blood flow, the patient was pronounced brain dead, and life support was discontinued.

Autopsy Findings. The autopsy revealed several pathological changes consistent with acetaminophen toxicity. The liver had centrilobular necrosis and severe acute passive congestion; there was no evidence of hepatitis or other viral infection. Postmortem viral antibody titers were not obtained. Both kidneys had uniform acute tubular necrosis with evidence of regeneration. These changes appeared to have occurred over a 10- to 12-day period. Unexplainable venous renal infarctions, old and recent, were also present.

The lungs had five small peripheral abscesses from which *Aspergillus fumigatus* was cultured. In addition, *Cryptococcus neoformans* was demonstrated histologically in multiple bronchopulmonary lymph nodes. Diffuse acute pancreatitis with considerable fibrosis was an unexpected finding. Examination of the heart revealed no pathological changes, which was consistent with the apparent lack of cardiac involvement during the course of the illness. The immediate cause of death was brainstem herniation due to diffuse cerebral edema.

Figure 1. Serial measurements of serum acetaminophen concentrations in a six-year-old child after multiple overdoses over several days. The first data point is 11 hours after the last dose. The half-life was 15 hours.

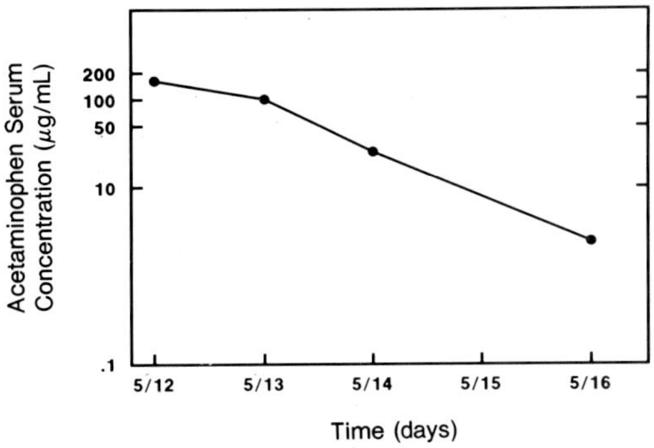

Figure 2. Serial measurements of aspartate aminotransferase (AST, formerly called SGOT) (IU/dL) (●- - -●), alanine aminotransferase (ALT, formerly called SGPT) (IU/dL) (O—O), direct bilirubin (mg/dL) (Δ—Δ), and serum ammonia (μg/dL) (▲- - -▲) over time in a six-year-old child after multiple overdoses of acetaminophen.

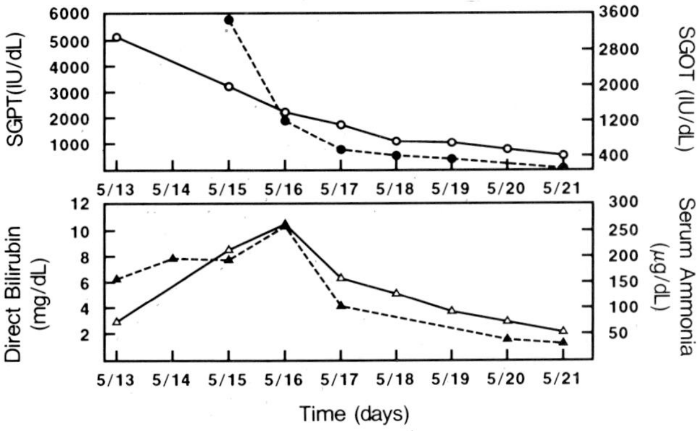

Discussion

Recent media advertisements emphasizing a possible link between aspirin and Reye's syndrome have encouraged many parents to switch from aspirin to acetaminophen for the treatment of fever, pain, and symptoms of the common cold in children. However, as in this case, some parents believe that acetaminophen lacks toxicity and can be used ad libitum. Fortunately, children appear to be remarkably resistant to acetaminophen-induced hepatotoxicity.[1,10]

The evidence in this case suggests that cryptococcal lymphadenitis was the primary febrile illness but that overdosage with acetaminophen contributed to this child's death. There was no indication of immunosuppression by history, immunizations were up-to-date, and neither cryptococcus nor granulomas were found in the brain, liver, or other organ systems. Cryptococcal lymphadenitis is generally a benign infection when confined to the lungs.[11] The *Aspergillus* infection may have developed secondary to intubation, as organisms were demonstrated only in the lungs and were not believed to be present in sufficient quantity to cause death.

The liver damage appeared to be of acute onset as the AST and ALT levels were extremely elevated on admission but the albumin level was slightly below normal. There was no evidence of recent or past inflammation in the liver to indicate a viral infection as the initiating illness. Currently, there is no proof that acetylcysteine administration more than 10 hours after acetaminophen ingestion potentiates hepatic toxicity or renal impairment[12]; therefore, this therapy is unlikely to have contributed to failure of these organs. In addition, the unusually long acetaminophen half-life of 15 hours indicates that substantial hepatotoxicity had occurred by the time of admission.

The diffuse renal tubular damage also appeared to be caused by the acetaminophen toxicity. Had the tubular necrosis been due to a severe ischemic event, more patchy necrosis would have been observed. The liver and kidney contain the cytochrome P-450 enzyme system, which oxidizes acetaminophen, and glutathione, which detoxifies the metabolite.[13] The toxic intermediate produced by the cytochrome P-450 metabolism of acetaminophen in the kidney may have caused the observed tubular necrosis.[13]

The pancreatic fibrosis was older than the 14-day history of the acute illness and may have resulted from the varicella infection. Serum amylase concentrations were not determined during the hospital stay. The patient had no history of mumps, eliminating it as the cause of the fibrosis. Pancreatitis has been reported in adults after acetaminophen overdose.[14,15]

This patient's history has many of the signs and symptoms found in Reye's syndrome, Kawasaki's disease (mucocutaneous lymph node syndrome), toxic shock syndrome, and non-A, non-B hepatitis. Although the clinical course was strikingly similar to Reye's syndrome, a patient with Reye's syndrome has fatty infiltration of the liver, heart, kidney, and pancreas, whereas no such changes were found at the autopsy of this patient. Lack of palmar or plantar erythema and desquamation eliminated both Kawasaki's disease and toxic shock syndrome. Lastly, there was no histological or serological evidence of hepatitis.

In summary, excessive doses of acetaminophen were given unknowingly to treat cryptococcal lymphadenitis, which is usually a benign disease. The resulting medical problems included hepatic failure, renal failure, seizures, respiratory dysfunction, and increased intracranial pressure with subsequent herniation and death. The patient also had had a varicella infection two months earlier. Multiple factors contributed to this child's death; however, it appears that if she had not been given an overdosage of acetaminophen, death would have been unlikely. Thus, the lethal outcome in this case illustrates the need to educate the public about the adverse effects of nonprescription drugs and the need to follow dosage instructions on the container. In addition, claims of safety in the media need to be tempered with sufficient information to make certain the public understands that many nonprescription drugs are potential poisons when used incorrectly.

Summary of Previously Reported Cases. Little information is available in the literature on long-term excessive acetaminophen dosing in children. Among the seven previously reported cases, there was only one fatal outcome (Table 1). In all cases (possibly excepting that of the seven-week-old child[5]) the duration of overdosing was longer than 24 hours and the amount administered was in excess of the recommended dosage for children of 40 to 60 mg/kg/day given in divided doses every four to six hours. The seven-week-old child also had the mildest liver dysfunction, with no elevation in PT, PTT, or bilirubin. Results of liver function tests were abnormally high in all cases, but severity of abnormality did not appear to predict outcome. Although in each case (excepting that of the 15-month-old child[8]) the serum acetaminophen concentration was in the "probable hepatic toxicity" range of the Rumack–Matthew nomogram,[16] this nomogram is not appropriate for predicting toxicity in cases of long-term overdosing since it was derived from data obtained from patients ingesting a single acute overdose. There have been reports of long-term excessive use over several weeks to years causing hepatic injury in adults,[17–21] but liver dysfunction was mild and coexisting alcohol abuse,[17] cancer,[17] and infectious mononucleosis[20] could

Table 1.
Reported Cases of Multiple Excessive Doses of Acetaminophen in Children

Ref	Age	Duration of Excessive Dosing	Dose	Conc; Time[a]	PT; PTT[b,c]	AST[b,d] (IU/L)	ALT[b,e] (IU/L)	Bilirubin[b] Total/Direct (mg/dL)	Outcome
5	6 wk	48 hr	30 mg every 4 hr plus additional unknown amount	119; 12	26; 53	2,350	825	1.1/. . .	Survived
5	7 wk	6–8 days	30 mg every 4–5 hr	10.7; 54	10; 26	1,180	480	0.6/. . .	Survived
9	7 mo	3 days	38 mg/kg/dose every 6 hr	72; 4	50.3; 80.3	7,120	6,600	2.2/1.5	Survived
6	11 mo	32 hr	70 mg/kg/dose every 4 hr	240; 11	29.6; 52.4	1,170	880	2.8/. . .	Survived
8	15 mo	2 wk	75–150 mg/kg/day plus an additional unknown amount	0; 30	24.1; 52.7	10,230	10,274	3.2/2.4	Survived
7	18 mo	2 days	12.3 mg/kg/dose every 2 hr	14; 36	68; 66	1,576	1,392	7.5/3.0	Survived
3	2 yr	70 hr	650 mg every 4 hr	25.8; >24	47.5; 46.5	26,840	10,000	3.4/2.6	Died
Present case	6 yr	3 days	23.8 mg/kg/dose every 2–4 hr	163; 11	37.5; 43.2	10,000	5,140	13.1/10.5	Died

[a] Serum concentration (μg/mL); time (hr) after last known dose.
[b] Maximum laboratory value.
[c] Prothrombin time; partial thromboplastin time.
[d] Aspartate aminotransferase (formerly called SGOT).
[e] Alanine aminotransferase (formerly called SGPT).

have predisposed patients to toxicity in several of the cases.

Metabolism. In adults and children, approximately 80% to 90% of an acetaminophen dose is sulfated or glucuronidated in the liver, and 5% is excreted unchanged in the kidney. Children excrete a larger proportion of a dose as the sulfate conjugate than adults, but adult patterns of metabolism are reached between 10 and 12 years of age (Table 2). Neither acetaminophen nor its sulfated or glucuronidated metabolites produce centrilobular necrosis. Several elegant studies in animals[26,27] demonstrated that a reactive intermediate of acetaminophen, *N*-acetyl-*p*-benzoquinoneimine,[28] covalently binds to hepatic proteins to cause necrosis. Only 5% to 25% of a nontoxic acetaminophen dose in adults is metabolized to *N*-acetyl-*p*-benzoquinoneimine, which is sulfated by glutathione to form the nontoxic metabolite mercapturic acid and excreted in the urine.[24,25] When single large doses of acetaminophen are ingested, the sulfation and glucuronidation pathways are believed to become saturated and a larger proportion of the dose is excreted as the mercapturic acid conjugate.[24,29] An early rise in unconjugated bilirubin levels, within 12 hours of acute ingestion, may indicate saturation of the sulfate and glucuronide conjugation pathways before clinical manifestations of toxicity are evident.[30] When the glutathione stores of the liver become depleted after an overdose in animals, the reactive intermediate metabolite binds to hepatic proteins and induces injury.[31] The amount bound to hepatic proteins is directly proportional to the severity of the necrosis.[27] Binding to hepatic proteins occurs when tissue stores of hepatic glutathione are depleted by 70% or more.[31,32]

Although a larger proportion of an acetaminophen dose is sulfated in children, that fact does not appear to be a sufficient explanation of why children are relatively resistant to hepatotoxicity after an acute overdose. The combined percentage of a dose excreted as the sulfate and glucuronide metabolites is the same in children as in adults, and neither of these metabolites is responsible for causing necrosis. The percentage of a nontoxic dose excreted as the mercapturic acid conjugate has not been studied in children, but it is reasonable to assume that the percentage is similar to that of adults because the total percentage of a dose recovered in the urine is approximately the same at all ages. Glutathione turnover was studied in rats by Lauterburg et al.[33] They observed that the rate of synthesis of glutathione declined linearly with increasing body weight, which correlated with animal age. In addition, the rate of synthesis after depletion of glutathione by diethylmaleate was much greater in the younger animals. These investigators concluded that children may have a more rapid rate of synthesis and a greater capacity to stimulate glutathione production after depletion of stores by acetaminophen overdose, and this probably protects them from hepatic necrosis. Hart and Timbrell[34] observed that younger mice developed less hepatotoxicity than adult mice when given the same acetaminophen dose. It was observed that although glutathione stores and hepatic cytochrome P-450 levels were much lower in neonatal mice than in adult mice, hepatic glutathione stores increased more rapidly than cytochrome P-450 levels with increasing age. Thus, perhaps in children, as in mice, the hepatoprotective effect of glutathione develops earlier than the enzyme producing the hepatotoxic metabolite.

Therapeutic Management. Treatment of acute acetaminophen overdose involves repletion of a sulfhydryl source for detoxification of the reactive intermediate. Exogenously administered intravenous glutathione is taken up into hepatocytes in animals only at large doses and is not used to treat overdosage in humans.[35,36] Glutathione precursors such as intravenous cysteamine, intravenous methionine, and intravenous and oral acetylcysteine are readily taken up into hepatocytes and protect

Table 2.
Relationship of Age to Excretion of Acetaminophen Metabolites after a Single Therapeutic Dose

	Percentage of Dose Excreted				
Age	Glucuronide Conjugate	Sulfate Conjugate	Mercapturic Acid Conjugate	Unchanged Drug	Reference
2–3 days	12.8	47.6	. . .	2.43	22
1–20 days	10–20	50–60	. . .	<4	4
3–9 yr	30–40	40–50	. . .	<4	4
7–10 yr	30–40	40–50	. . .	<10	23
12 yr	40–50	30	. . .	<4	4
Adult	50	30	. . .	<4	4
Adult	50	20–30	. . .	<10	23
Adult	45–55	20–30	15–25	2	24
Adult	. . .	. . .	4		25

against hepatic injury after acute overdosage in humans.[37-39] Prescott et al.[37] demonstrated protection from hepatic injury when intravenous methionine or cysteamine was given within 10 hours of the overdose. However, patients given methionine or cysteamine after 10 hours developed severe hepatic damage. It was thought that administration after 10 hours may have worsened outcome since the amino acid compounds could not be metabolized by the damaged liver and thus may have precipitated hepatic coma. Currently, orally administered acetylcysteine is the treatment of choice since it is equally effective and is associated with fewer adverse effects.[39] No adverse outcomes have been noted with its administration 10 hours or longer after an overdose.[12]

Assessment. The symptoms of chronic acetaminophen overdosage in children are nonspecific, including lethargy, disorientation, vomiting, and increased temperature. Laboratory findings of elevated AST, ALT, total bilirubin, PT, and PTT should alert the clinician to possible acetaminophen toxicity since acetaminophen is commonly given to children with and without a physician's prescription. For neonates, the recommended dosage is 5 to 10 mg/kg every four to six hours and for children it is 40 to 60 mg/kg/day given in divided doses every four to six hours.[40] In early reports of acute acetaminophen overdosage, Prescott et al.[41] suggested calculation of acetaminophen half-life to determine risk of hepatotoxicity. However, these authors also noted that acetaminophen was metabolized very rapidly (normal half-life) early after drug ingestion, even in patients who subsequently developed hepatic damage. Thus, half-life determination early after an acute overdosage may not be predictive of hepatotoxicity, but a prolonged half-life may be indicative of hepatotoxicity that has already occurred. The half-life after therapeutic doses of acetaminophen is similar at all ages and is 3.5 hours in newborns,[4,22] 4.0 hours in children 3 to 9 years,[4] and 3.6 to 3.8 hours in children 12 years to adult.[4]

Prescott et al.[41] also observed that all the patients in their study with a serum acetaminophen concentration greater than 300 μg/mL at four hours after acute overdosage developed hepatic damage. In no case did hepatic injury occur if the serum concentration was less than 120 μg/mL at 4 hours or less than 50 μg/mL at 12 hours after ingestion. These data, along with additional reports, were used to construct the Rumack–Matthew nomogram, which currently assists in assessing the need for acetylcysteine therapy in acutely poisoned patients.[16]

Treatment. Treatment of acetaminophen toxicity in cases of acute overdosage is well established. Even though acetaminophen is rapidly absorbed, attempts at preventing absorption with oral activated charcoal should be continued for at least 24 hours after ingestion since the reported time of ingestion is frequently inaccurate. Assessment of potential hepatotoxicity with the Rumack–Matthew nomogram currently is the standard of care after acute overdosage. The nomogram provides an assessment of hepatic injury based on a single serum acetaminophen concentration drawn at least four hours after the ingestion. If the serum concentration is within the toxic range, acetylcysteine therapy should be started with an oral loading dose of 140 mg/kg and then continued at 70 mg/kg for 17 additional doses. Acetylcysteine should also be started if the serum concentration is above 10 μg/mL and the time of ingestion is estimated to have been between 4 and 24 hours earlier.

There is no defined treatment in cases of long-term acetaminophen overdosage. Gastric emptying procedures and activated charcoal administration are of little value in cases of long-term ingestion of excessive doses. The protective value of giving acetylcysteine is questionable since it is usually the symptoms resulting from hepatic damage that bring the child in for medical care. Hemodialysis[42] and charcoal hemoperfusion[43] have not been found to improve outcome in acute overdose situations and similarly are not expected to be beneficial in cases of long-term overdosage. Although there is no literature to support the use of oral acetylcysteine in cases of long-term overdosage, there is little risk associated with administration. If the serum half-life of acetaminophen is prolonged after long-term overdosing, indicating that hepatic injury has occurred, oral acetylcysteine may be administered safely. Clearly, if the patient is in fulminant hepatic failure and the acetaminophen half-life is in excess of 12 hours, confirming severe damage,[41] acetylcysteine therapy is unlikely to provide any benefit. Intravenous acetylcysteine is being investigated in a multicenter trial in the United States and has been used successfully in Europe.[44,45] If proven safe and effective, intravenous acetylcysteine would replace oral therapy since it can be given to patients who are vomiting and it can be given concurrently with oral activated charcoal.

Conclusion

There is no defined treatment for long-term acetaminophen toxicity. Although not documented in the literature, oral acetylcysteine may be given in cases of long-term overdosage since little risk is associated with its administration. If the acetaminophen half-life is more than 12 hours and severe hepatic injury is evident, the patient should be managed with appropriate supportive care alone.

Discussion Questions

1. Discuss the proposed mechanism of hepatotoxicity caused by acetaminophen. What laboratory tests

can be used in patient assessment?

2. Explain the different routes of acetaminophen metabolism and the changes that occur in children as they reach 12 years of age.
3. Why is half-life determination not as accurate in predicting hepatotoxicity as the four-hour serum concentration used in the Rumack–Matthew nomogram for acute overdoses?
4. Is there a role for acetylcysteine in the treatment of chronic acetaminophen poisoning?

References

1. Rumack BH. Acetaminophen overdose in young children. *Am J Dis Child*. 1984; 138:428–33.
2. Nogen AG, Bremmer JE. Fatal acetaminophen overdosage in a young child. *J Pediatr*. 1978; 92:832–3.
3. Clark JH, Russell GJ, Fitzgerald JF. Fatal acetaminophen toxicity in a 2 year old. *J Indiana State Med Assoc*. 1983; 76:832–5.
4. Miller RP, Roberts RJ, Fischer LJ. Acetaminophen kinetics in neonates, children and adults. *Clin Pharmacol Ther*. 1976; 19:284–94.
5. Greene JW, Craft L, Ghishan F. Acetaminophen poisoning in infancy. *Am J Dis Child*. 1983; 137:386–7.
6. Henretig FM, Orel H, Werners S et al. Pediatric acetaminophen (APAP) hepatotoxicity after 36 hours of repeated overdosing. *Vet Hum Toxicol*. 1986; 28:489. Abstract.
7. Swetnam SM, Florman AL. Probable acetaminophen toxicity in an 18-month-old infant due to repeated overdosing. *Clin Pediatr*. 1984; 23:104–5.
8. Agran PF, Zenk KE, Romansky SG. Acute liver failure and encephalopathy in a 15-month-old infant. *Am J Dis Child*. 1983; 137:1107–14.
9. Smith DW, Isakson G, Frankel LR et al. Hepatic failure following ingestion of multiple doses of acetaminophen in a young child. *J Pediatr Gastroenterol Nutr*. 1986; 5:822–5.
10. Peterson RG, Rumack BH. Age as a variable in acetaminophen overdose. *Arch Intern Med*. 1981; 141:390–3.
11. Hammerman KJ, Powell KE, Christianson CS et al. Pulmonary cryptococcosis: clinical forms and treatment. *Am Rev Respir Dis*. 1973; 108:1116–23.
12. Vale JA, Meredith TJ, Goulding R. Treatment of acetaminophen poisoning. *Arch Intern Med*. 1981; 141:394–6.
13. Mitchell JR, McMurtry RJ, Statham CN et al. Molecular basis for several drug-induced nephropathies. *Am J Med*. 1977; 62:518–26.
14. Gilmore IT, Tourvas E. Paracetamol-induced acute pancreatitis. *Br Med J*. 1977; 1:753–4.
15. Timperley WR. Paracetamol-induced acute pancreatitis. *Br Med J*. 1977; 1:1086.
16. Rumack BH, Matthew H. Acetaminophen poisoning and toxicity. *Pediatrics*. 1975; 55:871–6.
17. Barker JD, de Carle DJ, Anuras S. Chronic excessive acetaminophen use and liver damage. *Ann Intern Med*. 1977; 87:299–301.
18. Johnson GK, Tolman KG. Chronic liver disease and acetaminophen. *Ann Intern Med*. 1977; 87:302–4.
19. Ware AJ, Upchurch KS, Eigenbrodt EH et al. Acetaminophen and the liver. *Ann Intern Med*. 1978; 88:267–8. Letter.
20. Rosenberg DM, Neelon FA. Acetaminophen and liver disease. *Ann Intern Med*. 1978; 88:129. Letter.
21. Bonkowsky HL, Mudge GH, McMurty RJ. Chronic hepatic inflammation and fibrosis due to low doses of paracetamol. *Lancet*. 1978; 1:1016–8.
22. Levy G, Khanna NK, Soda DM et al. Pharmacokinetics of acetaminophen in the human neonate: formation of acetaminophen glucuronide and sulfate in relation to plasma bilirubin concentration and D-glucaric acid excretion. *Pediatrics*. 1975; 55:818–25.
23. Alam SN, Roberts RJ, Fischer LJ. Age-related differences in salicylamide and acetaminophen conjugation in man. *J Pediatr*. 1977; 90:130–5.
24. Davis M, Simmons CJ, Harrison NG et al. Paracetamol overdose in man: relationship between pattern of urinary metabolites and severity of liver damage. *Q J Med*. 1976; 45:181–91.
25. Mitchell JR, Thorgeirsson SS, Potter WZ et al. Acetaminophen-induced hepatic injury: protective role of glutathione in man and rationale for therapy. *Clin Pharmacol Ther*. 1974; 16:676–84.
26. Jollow DJ, Mitchell JR, Potter WZ et al. Acetaminophen-induced hepatic necrosis: II. Role of covalent binding in vivo. *J Pharmacol Exp Ther*. 1973; 187:195–202.
27. Potter WZ, Davis DC, Mitchell JR et al. Acetaminophen-induced hepatic necrosis: III. Cytochrome P-450-mediated covalent binding in vitro. *J Pharmacol Exp Ther*. 1973; 187:203–10.
28. Miner DJ, Kissinger PT. Evidence for the involvement of *N*-acetyl-*p*-quinoneimine in acetaminophen metabolism. *Biochem Pharmacol*. 1979; 28:3285–90.
29. Slattery JT, Wilson JM, Kalhorn TF et al. Dose-dependent pharmacokinetics of acetaminophen: evidence of glutathione depletion in humans. *Clin Pharmacol Ther*. 1987; 41:413–8.
30. Davidson AR, Rojas-Bueno A, Thompson RPH et al. Unconjugated hyperbilirubinemia in paracetamol liver damage: clinical and experimental studies. *Digestion*. 1973; 8:444–5.
31. Mitchell JR, Jollow DJ, Potter WZ et al. Acetaminophen-induced hepatic necrosis: IV. Protective role of glutathione. *J Pharmacol Exp Ther*. 1973; 187:211–7.
32. Jollow DJ, Thorgiersson SS, Potter WZ et al. Acetaminophen-induced hepatic necrosis: VI. Metabolic disposition of toxic and nontoxic doses of acetaminophen. *Pharmacology*. 1974; 12:251–71.
33. Lauterburg BH, Vaishnav Y, Stillwell WG et al. The effects of age and glutathione depletion on hepatic glutathione turnover in vivo determined by acetaminophen probe analysis. *J Pharmacol Exp Ther*. 1980; 213:54–8.
34. Hart JG, Timbrell JA. The effect of hepatotoxicity on paracetamol hepatotoxicity in mice. *Biochem Pharmacol*. 1979; 28:3015–7.
35. Gazzard BG, Hughes RD, Portmann B et al. Protection of rats against the hepatotoxic effect of paracetamol. *Br J Exp Pathol*. 1974; 55:601–5.
36. Benedetti MS, Louis A, Malnoe A. Prevention of paracetamol-induced liver damage in mice with glutathione. *J Pharm Pharmacol*. 1975; 27:629–32.
37. Prescott LF, Park J, Sutherland GR et al. Cysteamine, methionine, and penicillamine in the treatment of paracetamol poisoning. *Lancet*. 1976; 2:109–13.
38. Prescott LF, Newton RW, Swainson CP et al. Successful treatment of several paracetamol overdosages with cysteamine. *Lancet*. 1974; 1:588–92.
39. Rumack BH, Peterson RC, Kock GG et al. Acetaminophen overdose. 662 cases with evaluation of oral acetylcysteine treatment. *Arch Intern Med*. 1981; 141:380–5.
40. Temple AR. Pediatric dosing of acetaminophen. *Pediatr Pharmacol*. 1983; 3:321–7.
41. Prescott LF, Wright N, Roscoe P et al. Plasma paracetamol half-life and hepatic necrosis in patients with paracetamol overdosage. *Lancet*. 1971; 1:519–22.
42. Farid NR, Glynn JP, Kerr DNS. Haemodialysis in paracetamol self poisoning. *Lancet*. 1972; 2:396–8.
43. Gazzard BG, Willson RA, Weston MJ et al. Charcoal haemoperfusion for paracetamol overdose. *Br J Clin Pharmacol*. 1974; 1:271–5.
44. Prescott L. Treatment of severe acetaminophen poisoning with intravenous acetylcysteine. *Arch Intern Med*. 1981; 141:386–9.
45. Prescott L, Illingworth RN, Critchley JAJH et al. Intravenous N-acetylcysteine: the treatment of choice for paracetamol poisoning. *Br Med J*. 1979; 2:1097–1100.

Drug Experience

Straightforward reports of unusual drug experiences are included in this section. These may be confirmations of previously reported drug experiences or brief apparent first reports. While selected references may be cited, the purpose of a Drug Experience report is not to present an extensive review of the literature.

A related section, Grand Rounds, includes papers that are well-documented patient case reports with a thorough review of the important literature to help put the case in perspective.

Neutropenia associated with oral acyclovir and multiple antibacterial agents in a patient with acquired immunodeficiency syndrome

MARY LYNN MCPHERSON AND
KAREN I. PLAISANCE

Clin Pharm. 1988; 7:398–401

Patients with the acquired immunodeficiency syndrome (AIDS) appear to be at an increased risk for experiencing adverse drug reactions. The greater incidence of multisystem reactions to trimethoprim–sulfamethoxazole in this group of patients has been well documented.[1] Patients with AIDS are more likely to develop neutropenia and thrombocytopenia when treated with trimethoprim–sulfamethoxazole,[1–3] although the mechanism behind the pancytopenia and the contribution of concomitant cytomegalovirus (CMV) infection are unclear.[4] Adverse reactions, including those involving the bone marrow, have been reported frequently with pentamidine,[2,5] pyrimethamine–sulfadoxine,[6] dapsone–trimethoprim,[7] flucytosine,[8,9] and danazol.[10]

We describe a patient with AIDS who developed neutropenia related to multiple antimicrobial agents and recovered upon discontinuation of drug therapy. This report also describes the first case of neutropenia associated with oral acyclovir therapy.

Case Report. The patient, a 32-year-old white man, was admitted to the psychiatric ward at our institution in September 1985 for treatment of depression. He was transferred to the medical service one day later for further evaluation and more intensive nursing care. The patient had a history of homosexuality, intravenous drug abuse, a 50- to 60-pound weight loss over the past eight months, and a positive antibody test for human immunodeficiency virus since July 1985.

In July 1985, the patient had been admitted and treated for shigellosis with intravenous trimethoprim–sulfamethoxazole 125 mg–500 mg every six hours. Over the eight days preceding exposure to antimicrobial agents, the patient's white blood cell (WBC) count and neutrophil count were stable (4250 ± 770 and 2806 ± 393 cells/cu mm, respectively). After exposure to trimethoprim–sulfamethoxazole, his neutrophil count fell from 2856 to 882 cells/cu mm (Figure 1). He completed his antibiotic course without other adverse reactions noted and was discharged on July 29, 1985.

One month later (August 25, 1985) he was seen as an outpatient. His WBC count was 3000 cells/cu mm with 50% segmented forms, 16% bands, and 22% lymphocytes. Perianal herpes simplex virus infection was diagnosed, and oral acyclovir 200 mg four times daily was started.

One week later, he was admitted to our institution. His only medication at that time was acyclovir, which, according to the patient's history, he had taken for only two days before admission. On admission he was found to have occasional urinary and fecal incontinence, weakness, lethargy, and diarrhea. Culture of perianal lesions was negative for herpes simplex virus. Renal function was normal; the WBC count was 3200 cells/cu mm with 58% segmented forms, 4% band forms, and 20% lymphocytes.

Oral acyclovir 200 mg four times daily was con-

MARY LYNN MCPHERSON, PHARM.D., is Clinical Pharmacist, Pharmacy Department, The Union Memorial Hospital, Baltimore, MD. KAREN I. PLAISANCE, PHARM.D., is Assistant Professor, Department of Clinical Pharmacy, School of Pharmacy, University of Maryland, Baltimore, MD.

Address reprint requests to Dr. Plaisance at the School of Pharmacy, University of Maryland, 20 N. Pine Street, Baltimore, MD 21201.

The contribution of Frank M. Calia, M.D., and the house staff and fellows of the University of Maryland Medical Systems in the care of this patient and the assistance of James C. Wade in the review of this manuscript are acknowledged.

Presented at the 22nd Annual ASHP Midyear Clinical Meeting, Atlanta, GA, December 9, 1987.

Copyright © 1988, American Society of Hospital Pharmacists, Inc. All rights reserved. 0278-2677/88/0501-0398$01.00.

Figure 1. Temporal relationship of neutrophil count to antimicrobial therapy. Abbreviations: tmp–smx = trimethoprim–sulfamethoxazole; a = acyclovir; gent = gentamicin; lac = β lactam; clinda = clindamycin.

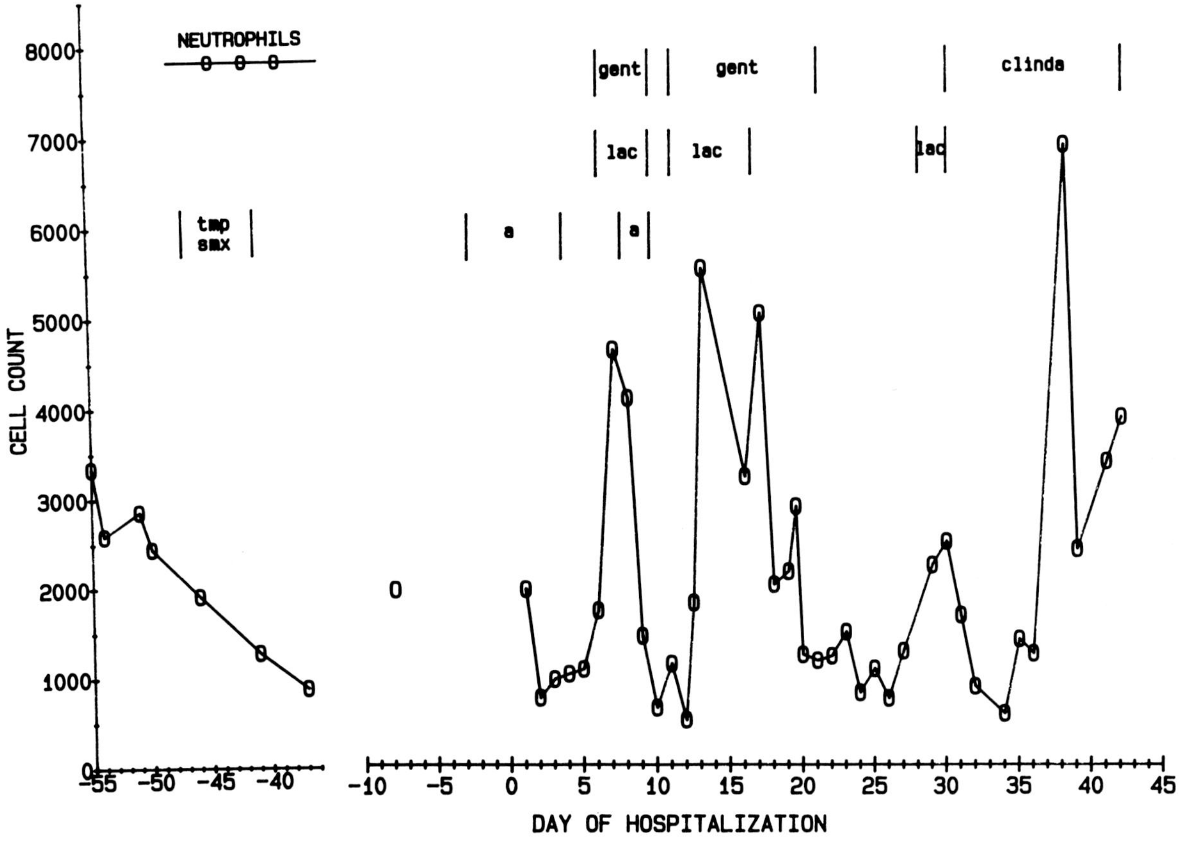

tinued as the only systemic medication. One day after admission, the WBC count fell to 1800 cells/cu mm with 38% segmented forms, 2% band forms, and 46% lymphocytes. His WBC count remained in this range over the next two days (Figure 1); on day 3 of hospitalization, acyclovir was discontinued because of concern that the neutropenia might be associated with the acyclovir therapy. The patient's WBC count rose on day 5 (two days after discontinuation of acyclovir) and continued to rise over the next two days to a peak neutrophil count of 4131 cells/cu mm (Figure 1).

On day 6, the patient developed a temperature of 41.1 °C and was empirically begun on intravenous nafcillin, sodium (1.5 g of nafcillin every six hours), ticarcillin sodium (3 g of ticarcillin every four hours), and gentamicin sulfate (loading dose of 100 mg of gentamicin, followed by 75 mg every eight hours). On day 7, the patient's primary physician was contacted, and a history of chronic leukopenia before acyclovir exposure was elicited. The patient was restarted on acyclovir 200 mg orally four times per day. One day later (day 8), the patient's WBC count was 2200/cu mm with 63% segmented forms, 3% band forms, and 24% lymphocytes. By day 9, the WBC count had declined to 1400/cu mm with a similar differential. Acyclovir and the antibacterial agents were discontinued. The reappearance of fever on day 11 led to reinitiation of the same antibacterial therapy. Over the next four days, the patient's neutrophil count rose from 1140 to 5580/cu mm (Figure 1).

Blood cultures obtained on day 11 were positive for *Klebsiella pneumoniae,* and on day 14 the antimicrobial therapy was changed to cefotaxime sodium (2 g of cefotaxime i.v.every six hours). Cefotaxime was discontinued within 48 hours, after the patient developed bronchospasm and rash. The patient finished a 14-day course of intravenous gentamicin therapy with his neutrophil count gradually decreasing to a nadir of 748 cells/cu mm over the next week. Again, when antimicrobial therapy was discontinued, the neutrophil count recovered to 2546 cells/cu mm. On day 28, the patient developed a superficial cellulitis and was begun on nafcillin. Over the next eight hours the patient developed a rash, fever, and peripheral eosinophilia. His neutrophil count declined to a nadir of 736/cu mm. Clindamycin phosphate (600 mg of clindamycin i.v. every eight hours) was substituted for nafcillin, and his neutrophil count subsequently rose over the next 48 hours.

The patient remained hospitalized, and over the next three weeks, he became progressively encephalopathic and died of respiratory failure on hospital day 65.

Discussion. Figure 1 demonstrates a reduction in neutrophil count on exposure to trimethoprim–sulfamethoxazole, oral acyclovir, and β-lactam agents. This decline occurred in association with a parallel decline in total white blood cells. In each case, removal of the antimicrobial agent was followed by recovery of the neutrophil count.

Immune-mediated leukopenia is usually manifested by rapid destruction of peripheral cells after an initial sensitization period. On re-exposure to drug, this leukopenia occurs rapidly and is often associated with fever, rash, pruritus, and eosinophilia.[11,12] This time course appears consistent with that observed in our patient.

Trimethoprim–sulfamethoxazole has been associated with the occurrence of hematologic adverse effects in AIDS and non-AIDS patients.[2,13] Additionally, the relative incidence of adverse effects with pentamidine and trimethoprim–sulfamethoxazole in patients with AIDS has been investigated. While a retrospective survey[1] suggested that there was a higher incidence of adverse effects with trimethoprim–sulfamethoxazole than with pentamidine, a prospective study[2] concluded that the incidence of adverse effects in AIDS patients receiving trimethoprim–sulfamethoxazole was similar to that in AIDS patients receiving pentamidine. Patients with AIDS appear to be at increased risk of developing adverse reactions to both of these agents compared with patients who have other immunodeficiencies.[2,3]

Our patient received a dose of trimethoprim–sulfamethoxazole much lower than that usually used to treat *Pneumocystis carinii* pneumonia. Yet he developed mild leukopenia during his week-long course, which appeared to resolve after drug removal.

Acyclovir represents an important advance in the therapy[14,15] and prophylaxis[16,17] of mucocutaneous herpes simplex infections in immunosuppressed patients. Minimal acyclovir-related adverse reactions have been reported with both the intravenous[18] and oral[19] formulations. Intravenous administration of acyclovir sodium has been associated with neutropenia in a small number of reported cases.[20–22]. Of 11 patients who developed neutropenia while receiving acyclovir, 5 were also receiving interferon alfa, which may have contributed to the neutropenia observed.[21] Three of the remaining six patients who received only acyclovir sodium were given high-dosage therapy (≥ 1500 mg/sq m/day) for the treatment of CMV pneumonia.[20] The highest peak and trough concentrations reported in these patients were 310 and 105 μM, respectively. The remaining three patients were being treated for resistant herpes simplex (72 mg/kg/day), herpes zoster, and CMV infections (30 mg/kg/day).[22] In vitro, acyclovir concentrations of 440 μM are required to induce a 50% decrease in granulocyte–monocyte colony-forming activity in cell culture.[23] These concentrations have not been achieved in vivo.

Dose-related bone marrow toxicity is not unexpected with agents that interfere with DNA metabolism, even for relatively viral-specific agents. However, our patient was receiving 800 mg of oral acyclovir daily. Oral acyclovir is poorly absorbed, with bioavailability ranging from 15% to 30%.[24] Therefore, mean steady-state peak acyclovir concentrations would be expected to be far lower (2.5 μM/L) than those previously associated with acyclovir-induced bone marrow suppression. Thus, it is unlikely that the bone marrow suppression observed in our patient was dose related.

Beta-lactam antibiotics are among the agents most commonly implicated as causing bone marrow suppression in non-AIDS patients. Our patient was receiving ticarcillin and nafcillin, both of which have been associated with neutropenia.[11,12] The development of neutropenia in our patient was consistent with an initial sensitization period, with re-exposure resulting in a rapid decline in WBC count along with rash, fever, and eosinophilia and subsequent recovery when therapy was discontinued.

The contribution of infections caused by the Herpetoviridae family of viruses to the development of neutropenia in patients with AIDS is unclear. Marrow suppression has been previously described in patients infected with CMV,[4] which is commonly implicated as a pathogen in patients with AIDS.[25]

Cultures for herpetoviruses were obtained from our patient on two occasions. On admission, culture of his perianal lesions was negative for herpes simplex. On day 48 of hospitalization, our patient underwent bronchoscopy, and washings from this procedure were obtained for CMV culture. Unfortunately, these specimens were contaminated, not allowing for isolation of CMV. Marrow suppression secondary to CMV may manifest as a waxing and waning process. We cannot exclude the contribution of active CMV disease to the production or aggravation of the bone marrow suppression in our patient. However, the temporal relationship of neutropenia on drug exposure and resolution on drug removal is striking.

Conclusion. We present a case of possible immune-mediated neutropenia developing in a patient with AIDS who was receiving multiple antimicrobial agents. Whether AIDS patients are at greater risk than other populations for drug-induced bone marrow toxicity in unclear. Further experience with these antimicrobial agents in AIDS patients may help to clarify this relationship.

References

1. Gordin FM, Simon GL, Wofsy CB et al. Adverse reactions to trimethoprim–sulfamethoxazole in patients with the acquired immunodeficiency syndrome. *Ann Intern Med.* 1984; 100:495–9.
2. Wharton JM, Coleman DL, Wofsy CB et al. Trimethoprim–sulfamethoxazole or pentamidine for *Pneumocystis carinii* pneumonia in the acquired immunodeficiency syndrome. *Ann Intern Med.* 1986; 105:37–44.
3. Kovacs JA, Hiemenz JW, Macher et al. *Pneumocystis carinii* pneumonia: a comparison between patients with the acquired immunodeficiency syndrome and patients with other immunodeficiencies. *Ann Intern Med.* 1984; 100:663–71.
4. Simmons RL, Lopez C, Balfour H Jr et al. Cytomegalovirus: Clinical virological correlations in renal transplant recipients. *Ann Surg.* 1974; 180:623–34.
5. Polsky B, Dryjanski J, Whimbey E et al. Severe neutropenia during pentamidine treatment of *Pneumocystis carinii* pneumonia in patients with AIDS. *JAMA.* 1984; 251:1253–4.
6. Navin TR, Miller KD, Satriale RD et al. Adverse reactions associated with pyrimethamine–sulfadoxine prophylaxis for *Pneumocystis carinii* infection in AIDS. *Lancet.* 1985; 1:1332.
7. Leoung GS, Mills J, Hopewell PC et al. Dapsone–trimethoprim for *Pneumocystis carinii* pneumonia in the acquired immunodeficiency syndrome. *Ann Intern Med.* 1986; 105:45–8.
8. Kovacs JA, Kovacs AA, Polis M et al. Cryptococcosis in the acquired immunodeficiency syndrome. *Ann Intern Med.* 1985; 103:533–8.
9. Zuger A, Louis E, Holzman RS et al. Cryptococcal disease in patients with the acquired immunodeficiency syndrome. *Ann Intern Med.* 1986; 104:234–40.
10. Metroka CE, Moore A, Sonnabend JA. Risks with danazol in the acquired immunodeficiency syndrome. *Ann Intern Med.* 1984; 101:564–5.
11. Kirkwood GR, Smith LL, Rustagi PK et al. Neutropenia associated with beta-lactam antibiotics. *Clin Pharm.* 1983; 2:569–78.
12. Bang NU, Kammer RB. Hematologic complications associated with beta-lactam antibiotics. *Rev Infect Dis.* 1983; 5(Suppl 2):380–93.
13. Hughes WT, Feldman S, Chaudhary SC et al. Comparison of pentamidine isethionate and trimethoprim–sulfamethoxazole in the treatment of *Pneumocystis carinii* pneumonia. *J. Pediatr.* 1978; 92:285–91.
14. Straus SE, Smith HA, Brickman C et al. Acyclovir for chronic mucocutaneous simplex virus infection in immunosuppressed patients. *Ann Intern Med.* 1982; 96:270–7.
15. Shepp DH, Newton BA, Dandliker PS et al. Oral acyclovir therapy for mucocutaneous herpes simplex virus infections in immunocompromised marrow transplant recipients. *Ann Intern Med.* 1985; 102:783–5.
16. Saral R, Ambinder RF, Burns WH et al. Acyclovir prophylaxis against herpes simplex virus infection in patients with leukemia. *Ann Intern Med.* 1983; 99:773–6.
17. Straus SE, Seidlin M, Takiff H et al. Oral acyclovir to suppress recurring herpes simplex virus infections in immunodeficient patients. *Ann Intern Med.* 1984; 100:522–4.
18. Laskin OL, Saral R, Burns WH et al. Acyclovir concentrations and tolerance during repetitive administration for 18 days. *Am J Med.* 1982; 73(Suppl):221–4.
19. Fiddian AP, Halsos AM, Kinge BR et al. Oral acyclovir in the treatment of genital herpes. *Am J Med.* 1982; 73(Suppl):335–7.
20. Wade JC, Hintz M, McGuffin RW et al. Treatment of cytomegalovirus pneumonia with high-dose acyclovir. *Am J Med.* 1982; 73(Suppl):249–56.
21. Wade JC, McGuffin RW, Springmeyer SC et al. Treatment of cytomegaloviral pneumonia with high-dose acyclovir and human leukocyte interferon. *J Infect Dis.* 1983; 148:557–62.
22. Bean B, Fletcher C. Neutropenia in immunocompromised patients receiving intravenous acyclovir. In: Program and Abstracts of the 25th Interscience Conference on Antimicrobial Agents and Chemotherapy. Washington, DC: American Society for Microbiology; 1985:237. Abstract 786.
23. McGuffin RW, Shiota FM, Meyers JD. Lack of toxicity of acyclovir to granulocyte progenitor cells in vitro. *Antimicrob Agents Chemother.* 1980; 18:471–3.
24. Laskin OL. Clinical pharmacokinetics of acyclovir. *Clin Pharmacokinet.* 1983; 8:187–201.
25. Masur H, Lane HC. The acquired immunodeficiency syndrome. In: Remington JS, Swartz MN, eds. Current clinical topics in infectious diseases. Vol. 6. New York: McGraw-Hill; 1985:1–39.

"

Indications for Antiarrhythmic Therapy

Few situations in medicine are comparable to that involving antiarrhythmic drugs, in which so many potentially toxic agents are given to so many patients without proof of benefit. . . . To date, the FDA has not required pharmaceutical sponsors to evaluate the effects of their drugs on mortality, but has accepted instead evidence that the new drugs can prevent induction of ventricular tachycardia by programmed electrical stimulation. Since induced ventricular tachycardia is usually associated with symptoms and predicts a high risk of mortality, the FDA has approved drug therapy for the indication, symptomatic ventricular arrhythmia—a reasonable compromise.

Until myocardial infarction can be prevented, ventricular arrhythmias and sudden death will continue to be major concerns for the practicing physician. Broader use of antiarrhythmic drugs in an open trial will be justified only when their use has been shown to be beneficial in patients with asymptomatic arrhythmias.

—Woosley RL. Indications for antiarrhythmic therapy: a wealth of controversy, a dearth of data. *Ann Intern Med.* 1988; 108:450–2. Editorial.

"

CP Continuing Education

Article 680-204-8806 (see page 351)
Qualifies for 1.0 hour of CE credit

Parenteral nutrition in pediatric patients

Learning Objectives

After studying this article, the reader should be able to

1. Describe the protein, calorie, fat, fluid, and micronutrient requirements of the neonate, infant, and child.
2. List the nutritional assessment techniques most useful in monitoring the adequacy of parenteral nutrition support in pediatric patients.
3. Identify the differences in metabolic pathways for amino acid metabolism in neonates compared with older children and adults.
4. Identify complications associated with the use of parenteral nutrient solutions in pediatric patients.
5. List variables that can be monitored to assess complications of parenteral nutrition in pediatric patients.

Self-assessment Questions

For each question there is one best answer only.

1. Protein requirements of the neonate
   a. Are generally greater on a per kilogram basis than are requirements of the older child.
   b. Are qualitatively similar to those of adults.
   c. Are less for enteral than for parenteral nutrition.
   d. All of the above alternatives are correct.
   e. Alternatives a and c only are correct.

2. Amino acid products designed for use in the neonate
   a. Result in normalization of plasma amino acid patterns in neonates.
   b. Have higher concentrations of phenylalanine and other amino acids identified as essential in the neonate.
   c. Have resulted in enhanced nitrogen retention and greater weight gain than products designed for use in adults.
   d. All of the above alternatives are correct.
   e. Alternatives a and c only are correct.

3. Which one of the following statements best explains why fluid or electrolyte requirements may be altered in neonates?
   a. Fluid requirements can be increased by ultraviolet light therapy or diuretic use.
   b. Calcium requirements are decreased because calcium needs are met in utero.
   c. Potassium requirements are low because neonates have a limited ability to excrete potassium in the urine.
   d. Cysteine requirements are decreased because neonates are unable to use cysteine.
   e. Alternatives a and c are both correct.

4. Which of the following statements best describes the usefulness of nutritional assessment techniques in the pediatric population?
   a. A 24-hour urine collection for creatinine is easy to perform in neonates and infants and is a reliable indicator of nutritional status.
   b. Growth curves provide an effective means of assessing nutritional status in infants and children.
   c. Use of daily weight alone may be a good indicator of the adequacy of nutritional intake in the neonate.
   d. All of the above alternatives are correct.
   e. Alternatives a and c only are correct.

5. Essential fatty acid deficiency in neonates
   a. Can be reversed by daily topical application of safflower oil.
   b. Does not occur before two weeks or more of fat-free parenteral nutrition.
   c. Is manifested biochemically as a triene:tetraene ratio of less than 0.4.
   d. Occurs when 30–50% of the total daily caloric requirements are not provided as fat emulsion.
   e. Is clinically evident as dry hair and skin, decreased growth, and impaired wound healing.

6. Which one of the following statements best describes the indications for use and administration of fat emulsion?
   a. Fat emulsion may be used as a concentrated, isotonic source of calories.
   b. Fat emulsion should be given as quickly as possible to avoid excessive exposure to lipid particles.
   c. Fat emulsion should not be used with peripheral nutritient solutions because its use has been shown to result in early infiltration.
   d. Fat emulsion should be withheld from small-for-gestational-age neonates because they have a limited ability to metabolize fat.

7. Controversial issues relating to the use of fat emulsions include
   a. Administration of fat emulsion to patients with hyperbilirubinemia.
   b. Administration of fat emulsion to patients with pulmonary disease.
   c. The role of concomitant heparin infusion in enhancing lipid clearance.
   d. All of the above alternatives are correct.
   e. Alternatives a and c only are correct.

8. In general, neonatal requirements for intravenously administered vitamins are

   a. Independent of age and pre-existing disease.
   b. Lower than the RDA for oral vitamins because they are administered directly into the circulation.
   c. Met when vitamins are administered at the dosages currently recommended by FDA.
   d. Similar for full-term and premature neonates because vitamin stores are similar at birth.

9. Which one of the following statements best describes the occurrence and management of complications of parenteral nutrition therapy?

   a. Complications are usually self-limiting and require no modification of therapy.
   b. Central venous catheter infections may be treated successfully in situ.
   c. Electrolyte imbalances are difficult to manage because of solubility considerations.
   d. Currently available amino acid solutions are composed of hydrochloride salt forms, resulting in a frequent occurrence of metabolic acidosis.
   e. Problems with rickets and bone demineralization have been totally eliminated since calcium requirements can be provided in nutrient solutions using amino acid products designed for neonates.

10. Cholestasis associated with parenteral nutrition

   a. Is more common in older infants with fully developed metabolic pathways.
   b. Usually occurs in the first few days of therapy and is first noted by an increase in serum aminotransferases.
   c. Occurs after about two weeks of parenteral nutrition and is transient and self-limiting.
   d. Can be treated by a cycling regimen wherein appropriate types and amounts of amino acids and appropriate amounts of calories are provided.
   e. Has been shown to respond to treatment with phenobarbital.

Article 680-204-8807 (see page 391)
Qualifies for 1.0 hour of CE credit

Death of a child associated with multiple overdoses of acetaminophen

Learning Objectives

After studying this article, the reader should be able to

1. Describe the signs and symptoms of chronic acetaminophen toxicity.
2. Compare the percentages of an acetaminophen dose conjugated with sulfate, glucuronide, or glutathione and excreted unchanged in the urine in children and adults.
3. List the appropriate therapeutic doses of acetaminophen in neonates and children.
4. Give the appropriate oral acetylcysteine dose used to treat acute acetaminophen overdosage.

Self-assessment Questions

For each question there is one best answer only.

1. Acute and chronic acetaminophen toxicity is commonly associated with elevations of

   a. Aspartate aminotransferase (AST, formerly called SGOT) and alanine aminotransferase (ALT, formerly called SGPT).
   b. Blood urea nitrogen and serum creatinine.
   c. Amylase.
   d. Prothrombin time, thromboplastin time, and bilirubin.
   e. Alternatives a and d only are correct.

2. Children up to 10 to 12 years of age excrete an acetaminophen dose largely

   a. As the sulfate conjugate.
   b. As the glucuronide conjugate.
   c. As the mercapturic acid conjugate.
   d. As unchanged drug.
   e. None of the above alternatives is correct.

3. The proposed mechanism for acetaminophen-induced hepatotoxicity includes all of the following except

   a. Depletion of glutathione stores.
   b. Binding of an intermediate metabolite to hepatocytes.
   c. Saturation of the glucuronidation pathway.
   d. Saturation of the *N*-demethylation pathway.
   e. Saturation of the sulfation pathway.

4. The treatment of choice in cases of acute overdose is

   a. Methionine.
   b. Cysteine.
   c. Cysteamine.
   d. Acetylcysteine.
   e. Glutathione.

5. The therapeutic dose for acetaminophen in children is

   a. 40 mg/kg/dose every four hours.
   b. 60 mg/kg/day every six hours.
   c. 60 mg/kg/dose every six hours.
   d. 10 mg/kg/dose every four hours.
   e. Alternatives b and d only are correct.

6. What percentage of a nontoxic acetaminophen dose may be excreted as the mercapturic acid conjugate?

   a. 100%.
   b. 75%.
   c. 50%.
   d. 25%.
   e. None of the above alternatives is correct.

7. The oral acetylcysteine dose (as the sodium salt) used to treat acute acetaminophen toxicity is a

   a. 140-mg loading dose, then 70 mg for 17 doses.
   b. 140 mg/kg loading dose, then 70 mg/kg for 17 doses.
   c. 14 mg/kg loading dose, then 7 mg/kg for 17 doses.
   d. 140 g/kg loading dose, then 70 g/kg for 17 doses.
   e. None of the above alternatives is correct.

9th Annual Meeting
AMERICAN COLLEGE OF CLINICAL PHARMACY

July 24–27, 1988
Wyndham Franklin Plaza Hotel
Philadelphia

Sunday, July 24

5:00 pm – 7:00 pm
Annual Business Meeting

7:00 pm – 9:00 pm
Opening Reception

Monday, July 25

8:30 am – 9:45 am
Therapeutic Frontiers Lecture:
"Monoclonal Antibodies in the Treatment of Cancer"
Paul A. Bunn, Jr., M.D.

10:15 am – 11:45 am
Therapeutic Symposium:
"Treatment of Hyperlipidemia: Which Drugs and Why"

11:45 am – 1:45 pm
Pharmacy Industry Forum Exhibits

2:00 pm – 3:30 pm
Therapeutic Symposium:
"New Methodologies for Clinical Pharmacy Research: Beyond Kinetics"

3:45 pm – 5:30 pm
Joint Symposium:
ACCP and the European Society of Clinical Pharmacy

Tuesday, July 26

8:00 am – 10:30 am
Poster Presentations

10:30 am – 12:30 pm
Research Institute Program

12:30 pm – 2:30 pm
Pharmacy Industry Forum Exhibits

2:30 pm – 5:30 pm
Contributed Scientific Papers I, II, III

4:00 pm – 5:30 pm
Innovative Clinical Pharmacy Practice Forum

Wednesday, July 27

8:30 am – 11:30 am
Therapeutic Symposium:
"Biotechnology: The Future of New Drug Therapy"

11:30 am – 1:00 pm
Residency and Fellowship Forum
Committee Meetings

1:00 pm – 2:30 pm
Therapeutic Symposium:
"Promoting Clinical Pharmacy Services: Issues in Cost Effectiveness"

2:45 pm – 5:30 pm
Contributed Scientific Papers IV, V, VI

6:00 pm – 7:00 pm
President's Reception

7:00 pm – 9:00 pm
Banquet

For Information:

American College of Clinical Pharmacy
3101 Broadway, Suite 350
Kansas City, Missouri 64111
(816) 531-2177

accp
American College of Clinical Pharmacy

CP Continuing Education *Continued from page 403*

8. The normal acetaminophen half-life for all age groups is
   a. 2–4 hours.
   b. 4–8 hours.
   c. 8–12 hours.
   d. 12–24 hours.
   e. Dose dependent.
9. Which one of the following statements best describes the treatment of acetaminophen overdoses?
   a. Hemodialysis and charcoal hemoperfusion have not been shown to improve outcome after acute overdoses and are not expected to be beneficial after chronic overdosage.
   b. Acetylcysteine has been shown to worsen hepatic encephalopathy if given more than 10 hours after an acute overdose.
   c. Acetylcysteine has been proven beneficial for treatment of chronic acetaminophen overdosing.
   d. None of the above alternatives is correct.
   e. Alternatives a and b only are correct.
10. Clinical manifestations of chronic acetaminophen toxicity may include
   a. Lethargy.
   b. Vomiting.
   c. Fever.
   d. Disorientation.
   e. All of the above alternatives are correct.

Answer sheet

May 1988 ***Clinical Pharmacy***

Note: An enrollment form for the ASHP Continuing Education System appears in the June and December issues. Please accumulate all the answer sheets you wish to use in one enrollment and submit them at one time with a completed enrollment form.

Place an X in the box(es) at the top of the column(s) corresponding to the test(s) you are taking. Darken the boxes corresponding to the correct answers.

	□ 680-204-8806 1.0 hour a b c d e		□ 680-204-8807 1.0 hour a b c d e
1.	□□□□□	1.	□□□□□
2.	□□□□□	2.	□□□□□
3.	□□□□□	3.	□□□□□
4.	□□□□□	4.	□□□□□
5.	□□□□□	5.	□□□□□
6.	□□□□	6.	□□□□□
7.	□□□□□	7.	□□□□□
8.	□□□□	8.	□□□□□
9.	□□□□□	9.	□□□□□
10.	□□□□□	10.	□□□□□

ASHP Use Only
(1.0)8806 ______(3)
(1.0)8807 ______(3)

Current Literature

Drug Reaction Alerts

Drug Reaction Alerts focuses primarily on serious, unlabeled reactions to new chemical entities. The citations are compiled monthly from International Pharmaceutical Abstracts, *which covers over 800 pharmacy and health-related journals worldwide. An address for reprints (when available) follows the name of the corresponding author in each citation.*

Antibiotics

Galland MC (Center Regional de Pharmacovigilance, Hopital Salvator, 249, Blvd. de Ste. Marguerite, 13009 Marseille, France), Rodor F, Jouglard J. **Spiramycin** and allergic toxidermy vasculitis. *Thérapie.* 1987; 42:227–9. Case. (34-year-old woman; received two doses of spiramycin 1 g; developed allergic vasculitis)

Anticoagulants

Mayou SC (Dowling Skin Unit, St. Thomas' Hospital, Lambeth Palace Road, London SE1 7EH, England), Kelly SE, McGibbon DH. Local cutaneous sensitivity to subcutaneous **heparin.** *Br J Dermatol.* 1987; 117:664–5. Case. (35-year-old pregnant woman with cardiomyopathy; received heparin 5000 U twice daily for five weeks; developed local cutaneous hypersensitivity reaction at injection site 7–36 hours after injection; reaction occurred with both bovine and porcine preparations)

Anticonvulsants

Cooke LE (Pharmacy Service [119], VA Medical Center, 6010 Amarillo Blvd. W., Amarillo, TX 79106), Hardin TC, Hendrickson DJ. **Phenytoin**-induced pseudolymphoma with mycosis fungoides manifestations. *Clin Pharm.* 1988; 7:153–7. Case. (40-year-old man; received phenytoin 300 mg at bedtime for seizures; developed pseudolymphoma with manifestations of mycosis fungoides; positive rechallenge after one month; facial and labial swelling, hyperpigmentation of face, mucositis of oral cavity, weight loss, maculopapular morbilliform rash on the trunk and arms, generalized lymphadenopathy and hepatosplenomegaly improved until day 35 and all physical, laboratory, and histologic abnormalities resolved within 60 days of discontinuation of phenytoin)

Antidepressants

Fisch RZ (Department of Psychiatry, Shaare Zedek Medical Center, Jerusalem 91000, Israel), Alexandrowitz A. Delirium in a patient treated with **mianserin.** *Br Med J.* 1988; 296:137. Case. (70-year-old woman with depression; received mianserin 30 mg/day for 14 days; developed delirium; recovery upon drug withdrawal)

Cardiac Drugs

Rayner HC (Leicester General Hospital, Leicester LE5 4PW, England), May S, Walls J. Penile erection due to **nifedipine.** *Br Med J.* 1988; 296:137. Case. (70-year-old man with angina pectoris; received nifedipine 10 or 20 mg as regular or slow-release preparation; concomitant digoxin, furosemide, allopurinol, warfarin, and quinine sulfate; developed penile erection; rechallenge in double-blind trial in same patient demonstrated that reaction was dose dependent)

Drug Interactions

Flessner MF (University of Virginia School of Medicine, Charlottesville, VA), Knight H. Prolongation of prothrombin time and severe gastrointestinal bleeding associated with combined use of **warfarin** and **ketoprofen.** *JAMA.* 1988; 259:353. Case. (62-year-old man; received long-term therapy with warfarin sodium 5 mg/day and ketoprofen 25 mg three times daily for seven days; concomitant digoxin, furosemide, captopril, verapamil, potassium chloride, and allopurinol; developed prolonged prothrombin time and gastrointestinal hemmorrhage; hemorrhage resolved upon withdrawal of ketoprofen and therapy with plasma and red blood cells)

Huang SM (Research Laboratory, Ortho Pharmaceutical Corp., Raritan, NJ 08869), Weintraub HS, Marriott TB et al. **Etintidine-theophylline** interaction study in humans. *Biopharm Drug Dispos.* 1987; 8:561–9. Study. (Double-blind, two-way cross-over; 10 men, aged 21–41 years; received etintidine hydrochloride 400 mg twice daily and oral dose of theophylline elixir 5 mg/kg; rapid absorption of etintidine in both placebo and theophylline-treated groups; etintidine had no significant effect on maximum concentration and time to maximum concentration of theophylline; etintidine prolonged elimination half-life and extended elimination of theophylline)

Lee K (University of Colorado Health Science Center, Denver, CO 80262), Mize R, Lowenstein SR. **Glyburide** induced hypoglycemia and **ranitidine.** *Ann Intern Med.* 1987; 107:261–2. Case. (72-year-old man; received glyburide 5 mg/day for six months; developed erosive esophagitis and received ranitidine 150 mg twice daily; glucose concentration 178 mg/dL upon discharge from hospital; patient developed hypoglycemia four days later with glucose concentrations of 20–40 mg/dL for which hospitalization and treatment with dextrose was necessary)

Lowenthal DT (Pharmacy Research Department, Du Pont Critical Care, 1600 Waukegan Road, Waukegan, IL 60085), Porter RS, Achari R et al. **Esmolol-digoxin** drug interaction. *J Clin Pharmacol.* 1987; 27:561–6. Study. (Open-label, baseline controlled; 11 healthy men, aged 22–33 years; received esmolol hydrochloride 50–300 mg i.v. and digoxin 0.2 mg orally twice daily; steady state concentration, elimination half-life, and total body clearance of esmolol did not change; peak concentration and time to reach peak concentration of digoxin not affected by esmolol; AUC of digoxin increased from 2.60 ± 0.59 to 2.88 ± 0.75 ng/hr/mL during the six-hour esmolol infusion)

Lutz M (Gastroenterology Unit, INTA, University of Chile, Santiago 11, Chile), Espinoza J, Arancibia A et al. Effect of **structured dietary fiber** on bioavailability of **amoxicillin.** *Clin Pharmacol Ther.* 1987; 42:220–4. Study. (10 healthy volunteers, aged 18–32 years; received either 7.8 g or 36.3 g of dietary fiber per day and tablets containing amoxicillin 500 mg; amoxicillin absorption slower with diet containing 7.8 g dietary fiber and bioavailability higher in those who received less fiber)

Shackleford EJ (Eagle Ridge Hospital and Health Care Center, 475 Guildford Way, Port Moody, British Columbia, Canada V3H 3W9), Watson FT. **Amiodarone-phenytoin** interaction. *Drug Intell Clin Pharm.* 1987;21:921. Case. (73-year-old woman; received amiodarone 200 mg three times daily initially and maintenance dose of 400 mg daily; concomitant therapy with phenytoin 400 mg/day; developed unsteady gait and drowsiness after 14 days of therapy with amiodarone; serum amiodarone concentrations on day 26 were elevated at 122 mmol/L; reduction of dosage of phenytoin to 200 mg/day resulted in prompt resolution of all symptoms)

Drugs, Adverse Reactions

Williams NR (Anon). Erythromycin: case of nightmares. *Br Med J.* 1988; 296:214. Case. (25-year-old woman with oropharyngeal sepsis; received **erythromycin** 250 mg four times daily for three days; experienced nightmares; nightmares subsided when drug withdrawn)

Steroids, cortico-

Dziewulski P (Department of Plastic Surgery, St. Thomas Hospital, London SE1 7EH, England), Gault DT, Davis PK. Systemic response to intralesional steroid therapy. *Br Med J.* 1988; 296:137. Case. (24-year-old man; received **triamcinolone acetonide** 5 mg by injection into keloid scar; developed rhinitis, bronchospasm, and angioedema; symptoms resolved spontaneously)

Book Review

Drug Use in Respiratory Disease

Edited by J. Douglas Wilson.

Published by William & Wilkins and Associates PTY Limited, 43 Herbert Street, Artarmon, N.S.W. 2064, Australia, 1987. Available from Williams & Wilkins, 428 E. Preston St., Baltimore, MD 21202. 319 p. Price $60.

Advances in the pharmacotherapy of respiratory diseases have led to the development and release of many new drugs in recent years. Changes in dosage forms, routes of administration, and treatment regimens with established drugs have also occurred. Presenting an overview of these new developments and evaluative clinical studies is the primary objective of *Drug Use in Respiratory Disease*.

The text consists of 20 chapters individually authored by an international group of physicians, primarily from Australia, England, New Zealand, Scotland, and the United States. The first 8 chapters review the pharmacology, pharmacokinetics, and modes of delivery of the most common respiratory drugs. Chapter titles include "Drug Delivery to the Lungs," "Oxygen Therapy and Toxicity," "Bronchodilators," and "Corticosteroid Therapy." The next 11 chapters present a review of the primary respiratory diseases, including pneumonia, chronic bronchitis and emphysema, respiratory failure, tuberculosis, cystic fibrosis, and asthma; diseases of the upper respiratory tract are not included. These chapters are subdivided into sections that review diagnostic features, natural history and prognosis, goals of treatment, drugs and regimens, and patient education.

The primary emphasis of each chapter is on drug treatment, and each drug is reviewed according to indications, dosage, delivery systems, and adverse effects. The final chapter presents an excellent review of adverse effects of drugs on the lungs.

The text is well referenced and provides many useful tables, summarizing both the disease state and drug information. An adequate index is also provided, making the book useful as a reference guide. The primarily international authorship of the text provides a beneficially different emphasis and perspective on treatment, including drug products, dosages, and delivery systems not currently available in the United States. The variation in authorship has also led to differences in the depth of drug information provided in some chapters; however, the overall quality of the text is very good.

This book would serve as a valuable reference for the clinical pharmacist with a background or interest in respiratory diseases and would be a reasonable addition to the drug information reference collection of most pharmacy libraries. The major problem with the book is the poor quality of the binding, which will not stand up to the wear and tear expected of a reference book.

Reviewed by Cary E. Johnson, Pharm.D., College of Pharmacy, University of Michigan, Ann Arbor, MI 48109.

Advertising Index

American College of Clinical Pharmacy
9th Annual Meeting, 404
Beecham Laboratories
Ticar, 350
Timentin, 338–340
Lemmon Company
Epitol Unit Dose, 345
Eli Lilly and Company
Nebcin, 335–336
Merieux Institute, Inc.
Multitest CMI, 349
Razayat Medical Services
Positions Available, 346
Roxane Laboratories, A Boehringer Ingelheim Company
Intensols, 333
Marinol, inside back cover, outside back cover
Stuart Pharmaceuticals, Division of ICI Americas, Inc.
Cefotan, 341–343
U.S. Public Health Service
Positions Available, 346
The Upjohn Company
Cleocin, 347–348
Wyeth Laboratories
Tubex, inside front cover

News

Guidelines for authors of biomedical journal articles revised

The recently released third edition of the *Uniform Requirements for Manuscripts Submitted to Biomedical Journals* addresses several problems in biomedical publishing that were not covered by earlier versions of the document.[1] These issues include minimum requirements for statistical reporting, qualifications for authorship, and policies for repetitive publication of a paper in different languages. The *American Journal of Hospital Pharmacy* and *Clinical Pharmacy* are among more than 300 biomedical journals that have agreed to consider for publication manuscripts prepared in the style specified by the *Uniform Requirements*. The checklist for ASHP's journals conforms to the *Uniform Requirements* in most respects; however, authors are encouraged to comply with the checklist requirements since papers that adhere to these specifications can be handled more expeditiously.[2]

Statistical Reporting. The guidelines for statistical reporting set forth in the *Uniform Requirements* are based on the view that an average reader who has a general knowledge of the topic should be able to comprehend a scientific report on the first reading. An accompanying statement explains the reasoning for the 15 points that constitute the minimum requirements for reporting statistical aspects of research.[3] These requirements are stated as follows:

1. Describe statistical methods with enough detail to enable a knowledgeable reader with access to the original data to verify the reported results.
2. When possible, quantify findings and present them with appropriate indicators of measurement error or uncertainty (such as confidence intervals).
3. Avoid sole reliance on statistical hypothesis testing, such as the use of *p* values, which fails to convey important quantitative information.
4. Discuss eligibility of experimental subjects.
5. Give details about randomization.
6. Describe the methods for, and success of, any blinding of observations.
7. Report treatment complications.
8. Give numbers of observations.
9. Report losses to observation (such as dropouts from a clinical trial).
10. References for study design and statistical methods should be to standard works (with pages stated) when possible rather than to papers where designs or methods were originally reported.
11. Specify any general-use computer programs used.
12. Put general descriptions of statistical methods in the Methods section. When data are summarized in the Results section, specify the statistical methods used to analyze them.
13. Restrict tables and figures to those needed to explain the argument of the paper and to assess its support. Use graphs as an alternative to tables with many entries; do not duplicate data in graphs and tables.
14. Avoid nontechnical uses of technical terms in statistics, such as "random" (which implies a randomizing device), "normal," "significant," "correlation," and "sample."
15. Define statistical terms, abbreviations, and most symbols.

Authorship. Persons designated as authors should have "participated sufficiently in the work to take public responsibility for the content." As stated in the guidelines, authorship is justified if an individual has made substantial contributions in *each* of the following three areas: (1) conception and design, or analysis and interpretation of data, (2) drafting the article or revising it critically for important intellectual content, and (3) final approval of the version to be published. Examples of activities that do not justify authorship include general supervision of the research group and participation that is limited to funding acquisition or data collection. Editors may require authors to defend authorship assignments.

Multiple Publication. Publication of study results in more than one journal is rarely acceptable. One possible exception is publication in another language, if the following five conditions, as stated in the *Uniform Requirements* document, are met:

1. The editors of both journals concerned are fully informed; the editor concerned with secondary publication should have a photocopy, reprint, or manuscript of the primary version.
2. The priority of the primary publication is respected by a publication interval of at least two weeks.
3. The paper for secondary publication is written for a different group of readers and is not simply a translated version of the primary paper; an abbreviated version will often be sufficient.
4. The secondary version reflects faithfully the data and interpretations of the primary version.
5. A footnote on the title page of the secondary version informs readers, peers, and documenting agencies that the paper was edited, and is being published, for a national audience in parallel with a primary version based on the same data and interpretations.

1. International Committee of Medical Journal Editors. Uniform requirements for manuscripts submitted to biomedical journals. *Ann Intern Med*. 1988; 108:258–65.
2. Knapp CA. Manuscript checklist for ASHP journals. *Am J Hosp Pharm*. 1988; 45:511. Questions and answers.
3. Bailear JC III, Mosteller F. Guidelines for statistical reporting in articles for medical journals: amplifications and explanations. *Ann Intern Med*. 1988; 108:266–73.

Continued on page 416

B fragilis group activity...

THE UNSURPASSED β-LACTAM CHOICE

TIMENTIN® *ticarcillin disodium/ clavulanate potassium*

B fragilis group coverage superior to cephalosporins and penicillins

Susceptibility Pattern (%) of 531 *B fragilis* Group Isolates in a Nationwide *in vitro Study[1]**

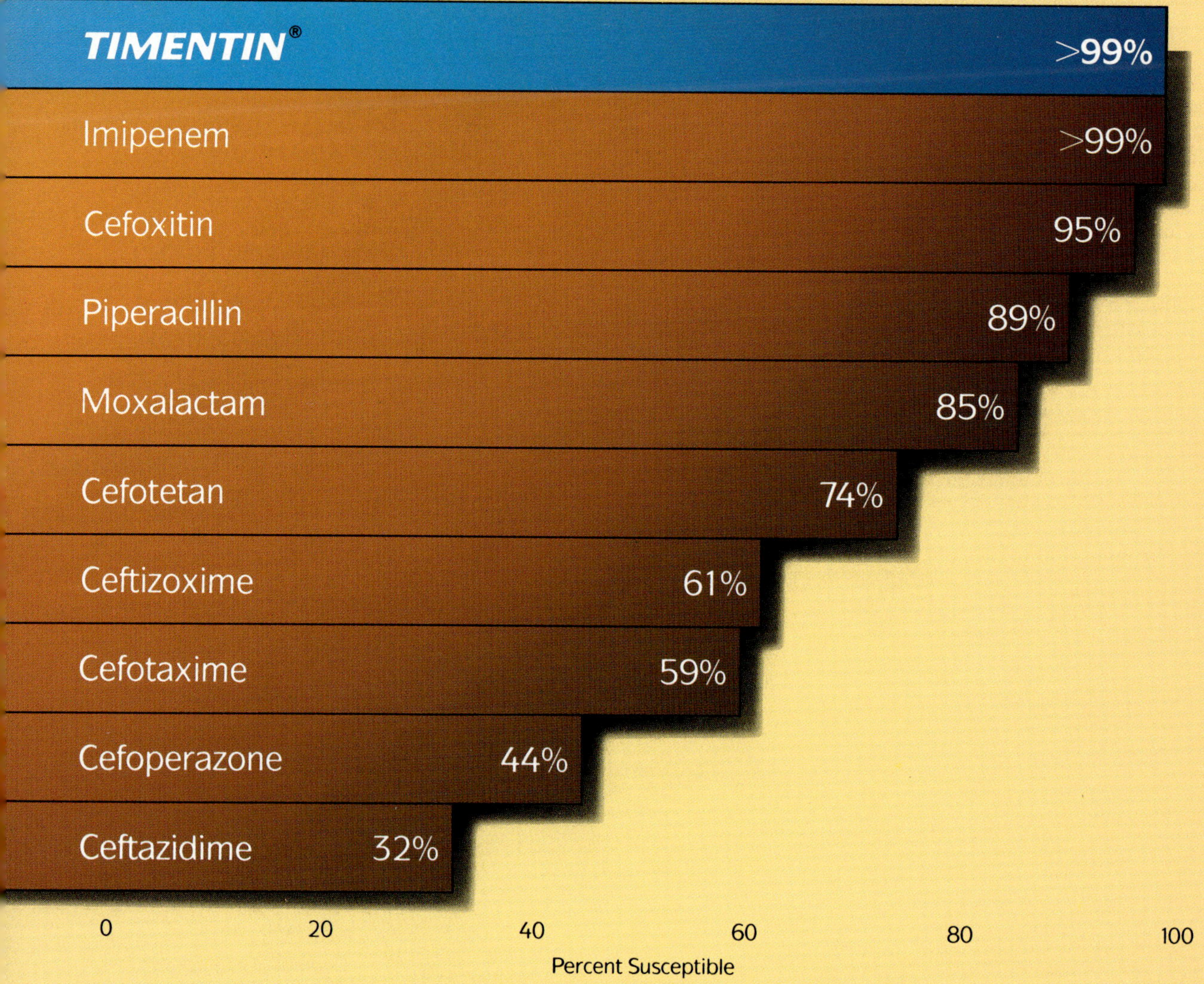

**In vitro* activity does not necessarily imply *in vivo* efficacy.

More active *in vitro** than traditional antianaerobic agents

Activity Against Clinical Isolates of *B fragilis* Group[2]		
Antibiotic	MIC50 (μg/mL)	MIC90 (μg/mL)
TIMENTIN†	≤1	4
Cefoxitin	8	32
Cefoperazone	32	128
Chloramphenicol	8	8
Clindamycin	0.5	8
Metronidazole	1	2

**In vitro* activity does not necessarily imply *in vivo* efficacy.
†Ticarcillin in the presence of a constant 2 μg/mL clavulanic acid.

More active *in vitro** than cefoxitin

Activity Against *B fragilis* Group[3]		
Organism (No. strains)	MIC90 (μg/mL) TIMENTIN†	MIC90 (μg/mL) Cefoxitin
B fragilis (32)	0.5	16
B vulgatus (21)	1	16
B thetaiotaomicron (19)	2	32
B ovatus (16)	1	32
B distasonis (13)	8	64

**In vitro* activity does not necessarily imply *in vivo* efficacy.
†Ticarcillin in the presence of a constant 1 μg/mL clavulanic acid.

Destroys β-lactamases that limit the usefulness of other β-lactam choices

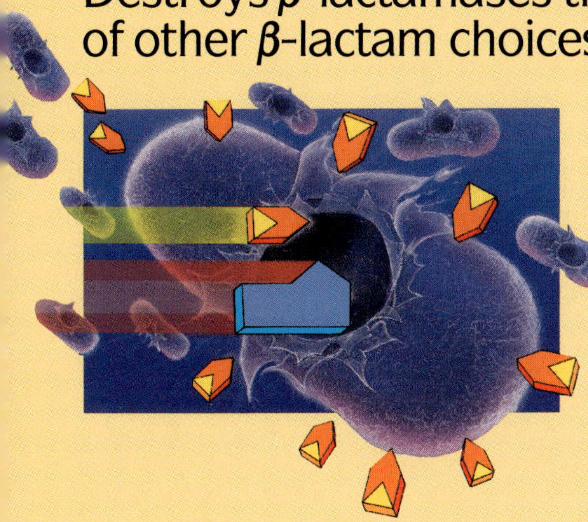

- "Most (90 percent) strains of B. fragilis produce constitutive beta-lactamases, which are primarily cephalosporinases. All other Bacteroides species probably produce beta-lactamases, but controversy exists concerning whether the enzymes are predominantly penicillinases or cephalosporinases."[4]
- "[Clavulanate potassium] inhibits the beta-lactamases of most Bacteroides species."[4]

△ Clavulanate potassium destroys most β-lactamases produced by Gram-positive and Gram-negative aerobes and anaerobes.
TIMENTIN destroys a broad range of aerobic and anaerobic bacteria regardless of β-lactamase production.

FOR ANAEROBIC CERTAINTY

TIMENTIN®

ticarcillin disodium/ clavulanate potassium

The unsurpassed β-lactam choice

Usual Dosage: 3.1 g every 4 to 6 hours.

Please see next page for brief summary of prescribing information.

THE CLAVULANATES Beecham laboratories BRISTOL, TENNESSEE 37620

© 1988, Beecham Laboratories.

BRIEF SUMMARY OF PRESCRIBING INFORMATION

TIMENTIN®

sterile ticarcillin disodium and clavulanate potassium

for Intravenous Administration

INDICATIONS AND USAGE: TIMENTIN® is indicated in the treatment of infections caused by susceptible strains of the designated organisms in the conditions listed below:

Bacterial Septicemia: including bacteremia, caused by β-lactamase producing strains of *Klebsiella* spp., *E. coli*, *Staphylococcus aureus* and *Pseudomonas aeruginosa* (and other *Pseudomonas* species).

Lower Respiratory Infections: caused by β-lactamase producing strains of *Staphylococcus aureus*, *Hemophilus influenzae* and *Klebsiella* spp.

Bone and Joint Infections: caused by β-lactamase producing strains of *Staphylococcus aureus*.

Skin and Skin Structure Infections: caused by β-lactamase producing strains of *Staphylococcus aureus*, *Klebsiella* spp., and *E. coli*.

Urinary Tract Infections (complicated and uncomplicated): caused by β-lactamase-producing strains of *E. coli*, *Klebsiella* spp., *Pseudomonas aeruginosa* (and other *Pseudomonas* species), *Citrobacter* spp., *Enterobacter cloacae*, *Serratia marcescens*, and *Staphylococcus aureus*. While TIMENTIN is indicated only for the conditions listed above, infections caused by ticarcillin susceptible organisms are also amenable to TIMENTIN treatment due to its ticarcillin content. Therefore, mixed infections caused by ticarcillin susceptible organisms and β-lactamase producing organisms susceptible to TIMENTIN should not require the addition of another antibiotic.

Appropriate culture and susceptibility tests should be performed before treatment in order to isolate and identify organisms causing infection and to determine their susceptibility to TIMENTIN. Because of its broad spectrum of bactericidal activity against Gram-positive and Gram-negative bacteria, TIMENTIN is particularly useful for the treatment of mixed infections and for presumptive therapy prior to the identification of the causative organisms. TIMENTIN has been shown to be effective as single drug therapy in the treatment of some serious infections where normally combination antibiotic therapy might be employed. Therapy with TIMENTIN may be initiated before results of such tests are known when there is reason to believe the infection may involve any of the β-lactamase producing organisms listed above; however, once these results become available, appropriate therapy should be continued.

Based on the *in vitro* synergism between TIMENTIN and aminoglycosides against certain strains of *Pseudomonas aeruginosa*, combined therapy has been successful, especially in patients with impaired host defenses. Both drugs should be used in full therapeutic doses. As soon as results of culture and susceptibility tests become available, antimicrobial therapy should be adjusted as indicated.

CONTRAINDICATIONS: TIMENTIN is contraindicated in patients with a history of hypersensitivity reactions to any of the penicillins.

WARNINGS: SERIOUS AND OCCASIONALLY FATAL HYPERSENSITIVITY (ANAPHYLACTOID) REACTIONS HAVE BEEN REPORTED IN PATIENTS ON PENICILLIN THERAPY. THESE REACTIONS ARE MORE LIKELY TO OCCUR IN INDIVIDUALS WITH A HISTORY OF PENICILLIN HYPERSENSITIVITY AND/OR A HISTORY OF SENSITIVITY TO MULTIPLE ALLERGENS. THERE HAVE BEEN REPORTS OF INDIVIDUALS WITH A HISTORY OF PENICILLIN HYPERSENSITIVITY WHO HAVE EXPERIENCED SEVERE REACTIONS WHEN TREATED WITH CEPHALOSPORINS. BEFORE INITIATING THERAPY WITH TIMENTIN, CAREFUL INQUIRY SHOULD BE MADE CONCERNING PREVIOUS HYPERSENSITIVITY REACTIONS TO PENICILLINS, CEPHALOSPORINS, OR OTHER DRUGS. IF AN ALLERGIC REACTION OCCURS, TIMENTIN SHOULD BE DISCONTINUED AND THE APPROPRIATE THERAPY INSTITUTED. **SERIOUS ANAPHYLACTOID REACTIONS REQUIRE IMMEDIATE EMERGENCY TREATMENT WITH EPINEPHRINE. OXYGEN, INTRAVENOUS STEROIDS, AND AIRWAY MANAGEMENT, INCLUDING INTUBATION, SHOULD ALSO BE PROVIDED AS INDICATED.**

PRECAUTIONS: While TIMENTIN possesses the characteristic low toxicity of the penicillin group of antibiotics, organ system functions should be assessed periodically during therapy.

Bleeding manifestations have occurred in some patients receiving β-lactam antibiotics. These reactions have been associated with abnormalities of coagulation tests such as clotting time, platelet aggregation and prothrombin time and are more likely to occur in patients with renal impairment. If bleeding manifestations appear, TIMENTIN treatment should be discontinued and appropriate therapy instituted.

TIMENTIN has only rarely been reported to cause hypokalemia. Periodic monitoring of serum potassium may be advisable in patients receiving prolonged therapy.

Pregnancy (Category B): Reproduction studies have been performed in rats given doses up to 1050 mg/kg/day and have revealed no evidence of impaired fertility or harm to the fetus due to TIMENTIN. There are, however, no adequate and well-controlled studies in pregnant women. Because animal reproduction studies are not always predictive of human response, this drug should be used during pregnancy only if clearly needed.

DOSAGE AND ADMINISTRATION: TIMENTIN should be administered by intravenous infusion (30 min.). Usual recommended dose for systemic and urinary tract infections for average (60 kg) adults is 3.1 Gm TIMENTIN (3.1 Gm vial containing 3 Gm ticarcillin and 100 mg clavulanic acid) given every 4 to 6 hours. In urinary tract infections, a dosage of 3.2 Gm TIMENTIN (3.2 Gm vial containing 3 Gm ticarcillin and 200 mg clavulanic acid) given every 8 hours is adequate. Please see official package insert for details on dosages for other patients, including those with renal insufficiency, and directions for use.

SUPPLIED: 3.1 Gm and 3.2 Gm Standard Vials; 3.1 Gm and 3.2 Gm Piggyback Bottles; 31 Gm Bulk Pharmacy Package; 3.1 Gm ADD-Vantage™ Antibiotic Vial.

7548/E-BS

References

1. Cuchural GJ, Tally FP, Jacobus NV, et al: Susceptibility of Bacteroides fragilis group clinical isolates to newer beta-lactam drugs, abstract No. 1B8. Presented to the 3rd Panamerican Congress of Infectious Diseases and Chemotherapy, San Juan, Puerto Rico, Dec 9-13, 1986.
2. Barry AL, Jones RN, Packer RR: *In vitro* susceptibility of the *Bacteroides fragilis* group to cefoperazone, ampicillin, ticarcillin, and amoxycillin combined with β-lactamase inhibitors. *J Antimicrob Chemother* 1986;17:125-127.
3. Bourgault AM, Lamothe F: In-vitro activity of amoxycillin and ticarcillin in combination with clavulanic acid compared with that of new β-lactam agents against species of the *Bacteroides fragilis* group. *J Antimicrob Chemother* 1986;17:593-603.
4. Neu HC: Contribution of beta-lactamases to bacterial resistance and mechanisms to inhibit beta-lactamases. *Am J Med* 1985;79(suppl 5B):2-12.

Beecham laboratories

BRISTOL, TENNESSEE 37620

© 1988, Beecham Laboratories.

News *Continued from page 413*

Marketing of intravenous enalaprilat approved by FDA

Approval for marketing of enalaprilat (Vasotec I.V., Merck Sharp & Dohme) was granted recently by FDA; the drug is the first injectable angiotensin-converting enzyme inhibitor to be made available in the United States. Enalaprilat is the active metabolite of the orally administered prodrug enalapril. Enalaprilat is labeled for use in the treatment of hypertension when oral therapy is not practical.

Single intravenous doses of enalaprilat produce a polyexponential serum concentration profile with a prolonged terminal elimination phase. Studies with oral enalapril indicate that the half-life of enalaprilat is approximately 11 hours. More than 90% of a dose of enalaprilat is excreted unchanged in the urine within 24 hours. Drug accumulation may occur when renal function is impaired (creatinine clearance less than 30 mL/min).

Enalaprilat reduces supine and standing systolic and diastolic blood pressure. Furosemide and enalaprilat have additive antihypertensive effects. Symptomatic orthostatic hypotension is uncommon but may occur, particularly in volume-depleted patients. Abrupt withdrawal of enalaprilat has not been reported to cause a rapid increase in blood pressure. In clinical trials involving 349 patients, the most common adverse reactions were hypotension (3.4%), headache (2.9%), and nausea (1.1%).

The recommended dosage of enalaprilat is 1.25 mg administered intravenously over five minutes every six hours. A clinical response usually occurs within 15 minutes, but peak effects may be delayed for up to four hours after the first dose. Peak effects after subsequent doses may be greater. If patients receiving enalaprilat are begun on oral enalapril maleate, an initial dose of 5 mg given orally once daily is recommended. Patients treated with diuretics and patients with renal impairment should receive lower doses of enalaprilat and enalapril.

Vasotec I.V. is supplied as a 1.25 mg/mL solution in 2-mL vials. The cost to the pharmacist is $16 per 2-mL vial.

Preliminary findings suggest APSAC reduces mortality after myocardial infarction

Anisoylated plasminogen streptokinase activator complex (APSAC, Eminase, Beecham Laboratories), an investigational thrombolytic agent, significantly reduces mortality 30 days after acute myocardial infarction, according to preliminary results of a randomized double-blind, placebo-controlled multicenter trial.[1] The preliminary report was based on the trial's second planned interim analysis and included data on 1004 of the first 1007 patients enrolled in the study; in accordance with predetermined statistical criteria, patient enrollment was halted after the interim analysis.

Eligibility requirements included age of 70 years or

Continued on page 419

less, ECG findings consistent with myocardial infarction, and onset of symptoms within the previous six hours. APSAC 30 units or placebo was given intravenously over five minutes; intravenous administration of heparin was begun six hours later, followed by warfarin for at least three months. Beta-blocker therapy was started during hospitalization if treatment was not contraindicated and was continued for up to one year. Data on survival and adverse events were collected for up to one year. Reperfusion was not assessed.

APSAC reduced 30-day mortality an estimated 47.5% (95% confidence interval, 21.0% to 65.2%); 32 of 502 (6.4%) APSAC-treated patients died within 30 days after myocardial infarction, compared with 61 of 502 (12.2%) patients in the placebo group. Mortality was lower among APSAC recipients in each of the following subgroups: age $\geq$ 65 years, age $<$ 65 years, randomization to treatment within four hours of the onset of symptoms, and randomization to treatment four to six hours after the onset of symptoms. Mortality was higher if randomization to treatment occurred at four hours or later. One-year follow-up was available for only 29% of patients. Data on baseline comparability of study groups and frequency of adverse events were incomplete.

One-year survival, frequency of adverse events, and a more detailed comparison of the treatment groups will be covered in a follow-up report.

1. AIMS Trial Study Group. Effect of intravenous APSAC on mortality after acute myocardial infarction: preliminary report of a placebo-controlled clinical trial. *Lancet*. 1988; 1:545–9.

Information sheets for institutional review boards available from FDA

New information sheets outlining the responsibilities of institutional review boards (IRBs) when research subjects will be paid or will be recruited through advertising are available from FDA; the sheets are entitled "Payment to Research Subjects" and "Advertising for Study Subjects." Other IRB information sheets are being revised to conform to the IND Rewrite Regulations (published in the March 19, 1987, issue of the *Federal Register*) and the regulations on treatment use and sale of investigational agents (May 22, 1987, issue of the *Federal Register*). FDA is also preparing a series of clinical investigator information sheets.

Conference for health-statistics data users set

The National Center for Health Statistics (NCHS), the federal government's principal vital and health statistics agency, will hold a conference for current and potential users of NCHS public-use data files in Bethesda, Maryland, July 27–29. There is no registration fee for conference attendees. More information can be obtained by writing to the National Center for Health Statistics, Sci-

Continued on page 420

ANNOUNCING

A Decision Model for the Treatment of Cancer Pain

A Software Diskette and Continuing Education Program to Help in Assessment and Management of Cancer Pain

Developed by: Charles S. Cleeland, PhD, and Armando Rotondi, MS, Pain Research Group, University of Wisconsin-Madison. Based on research conducted under Grant CA-26582 of the National Cancer Institute.

Medical Consultants: Russell Portenoy, MD, Department of Neurology, Albert Einstein College of Medicine, Bronx, New York; Theresa Brechner, MD,Department of Anesthesiology, University of California-Los Angeles.

Sponsored by: Roxane Laboratories, Inc., Columbus, Ohio.

To Order: A check for $17.50 should be made payable to the University of Wisconsin—133K613. Wisconsin residents add 5% sales tax. Send the check to:

Charles S. Cleeland, PhD
Department of Neurology
Pain Research Group
H6/530 Clinical Science Center
600 Highland Avenue
Madison, WI 53792

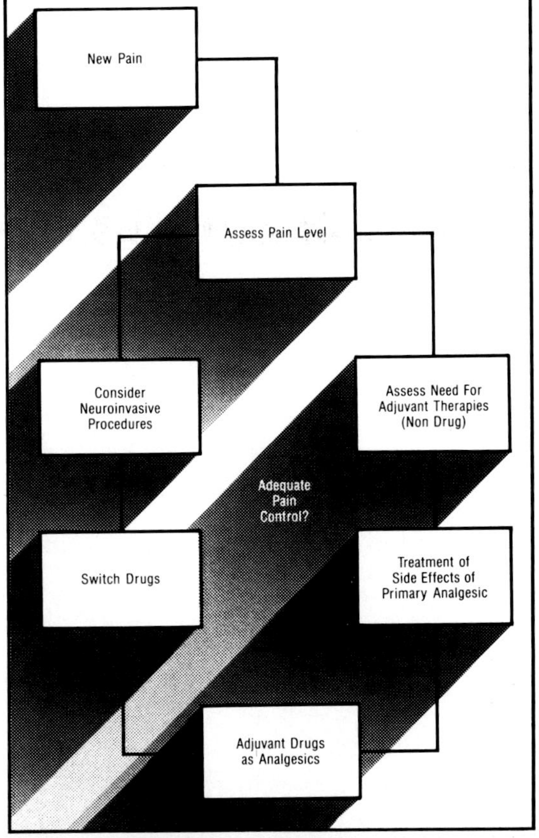

NOW AVAILABLE

The Handbook on Injectable Drugs Fifth Edition

by Lawrence A. Trissel
Published by the American Society of Hospital Pharmacists

This popular reference covers a wide scope of injectable drugs used in admixtures. The fifth edition features completely revised monographs on 240 commercial drug products, plus information on investigational drugs. New dosage sections have been greatly expanded.

Monographs cover information on:

- products
- stability
- dosage
- compatibility

New drugs in this edition include:

- Aztreonam
- Imipenem-Cilastatin Sodium
- Ceftazidime
- Pentamidine Isethionate

Order your copy today.

ORDER FORM:

Handbook on Injectable Drugs, 5th Edition; 758 pp.

Please send me _____ copies of the *Handbook* (P276) @ $60.00.

☐ Enclosed is my check for $ _________ (Checks must be drawn on a U.S. bank.)

☐ Enclosed is our purchase order # _________ ; please issue an invoice and add postage and handling.

Charge $ _________ to my: ☐ MasterCard ☐ Visa

Acct. # _______________ Exp. _________ month/year

Signature _______________

Name _______________

Address _______________

City _______________ State _____ Zip _________

ASHP I.D.# _______________

Send to: **ASHP Publications Records Department**
4630 Montgomery Avenue
Bethesda, Maryland 20814

ASHP is a trademark of the American Society of Hospital Pharmacists, Inc.; Registered in the U.S. Patent and Trademark Office.

Payments to ASHP are not deductible as charitable contributions for Federal Income Tax purposes. However, they may be deductible under other provisions of the Internal Revenue Code.

News *Continued from page 419*

entific and Technical Information Branch, 3700 East-West Highway, Room 1-57, Hyattsville, MD 20782 or by calling Debora Freeman at 301-436-8500.

News Briefs

• FDA has approved marketing of a liquid formulation of **loperamide hydrochloride** (Imodium A-D, McNeil Consumer Products Company) as a nonprescription product. The maximum recommended dose for nonprescription use in the treatment of acute nonspecific diarrhea is 8 mg/day for two days. The drug will be supplied as a 1 mg/5 mL solution in 2-, 3-, and 4-ounce bottles.

• A final rule identifying conditions under which **nonprescription ophthalmic drug products** are recognized by FDA as being safe and effective and not misbranded was published in the March 4, 1988, issue of the *Federal Register*. Ophthalmic anti-infective agents are not addressed in the monograph because of unresolved scientific issues. The monograph defines eyewashes and ophthalmic astringents, demulcents, emollients, hypertonicity agents, and vasoconstrictors; establishes the active ingredients in each of these categories that may be used; and sets standards for product labeling.

• FDA has withdrawn approval of the New Drug Application (NDA) for **hydrocodone with phenyltoloxamine** (Tussionex Suspension and Tablets, Pennwalt Corporation) because of lack of evidence of efficacy for the labeled indication; the regulation covers any identical or similar product that was not marketed under a separate approved NDA. FDA has approved Pennwalt's application for marketing a reformulated suspension containing **hydrocodone with chlorpheniramine.**

Upcoming Specialty Meetings

International Conference on Preventive Cardiology (2nd) . . . Washington, DC. . . June 18–22 . . . contact: International Conference on Preventive Cardiology, 9650 Rockville Pike, Bethesda, MD 20814.

American Society of Hypertension (3rd). . . New York, NY . . . June 22–26 . . . contact: C. Verneuil, CPC Communications, Box 4010, Greenwich, CT 06830; 203-661-0600.

Prenatal Abuse of Licit and Illicit Drugs . . . Bethesda, MD . . . September 7–9 . . . contact: New York Academy of Science, 2 East 63rd Street, New York, NY 10021; 212-838-0230.

American College of Nuclear Medicine . . . Lake Tahoe, NV . . . September 15–18 . . . contact: J. D. Watson, Jr., M.D., P.O. Box 5887, Columbus, GA 31906; 404-322-8049.

American College of Emergency Physicians . . . New Orleans, LA . . . September 26–29 . . . contact: C. C. Rorrie, Jr., Ph.D., P.O. Box 619911, Dallas, TX 75261-9911; 214-550-0911.

CU trouble spot: G drug administration

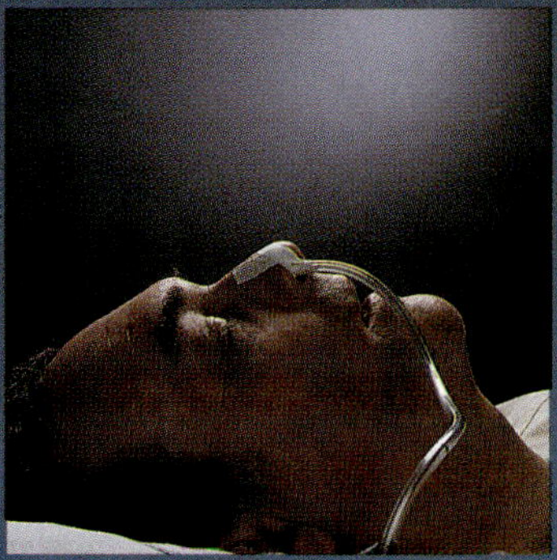

e solution is INTENSOLS™ oncentrated Oral Solutions

DEXAMETHASONE . . . . . . 1 mg/mL
PROPRANOLOL . . . . . . 80 mg/mL
PREDNISONE . . . . 5 mg/mL
DIAZEPAM . . . . 5 mg/mL

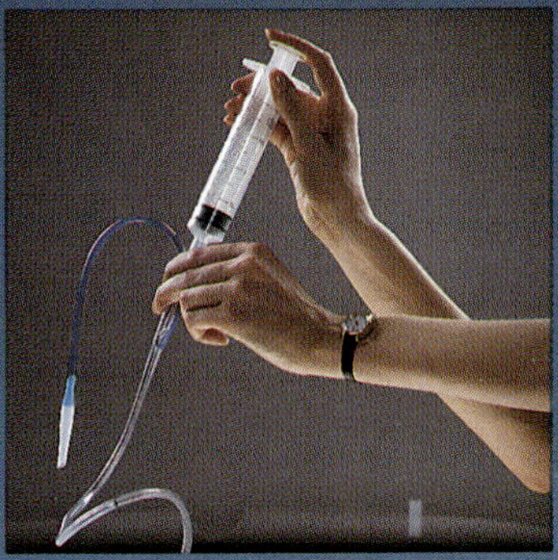

PALLIATIVE CARE AND CANCER PAIN PRODUCTS

Roxane Laboratories, Inc.
Columbus, Ohio 43216

nplifies drug ministration to sogastric patients

rsing benefits

- minates crushing tablets or dissolving apsules
- ore accurate and consistent dose
- on't clog NG tubes
- ves nursing time for more productive atient care activities

armacy benefits

- orrect dose is administered and osorbed by the patient
- ushing of sustained-release, sublingual, enteric-coated tablets is minimized
- ug/drug and acid/base interactions in ortar are avoided

y to dispense

ch bottle comes with a calibrated opper for accurate dosing and ation. Administering directly into NG oe is possible.

Ideal for patients who have difficulty swallowing tablets

- Geriatric, pediatric, and cancer patients on high or variable doses
- Mixable with soft foods or liquids; most Intensols are tasteless so they won't alter the flavor
- Easy to swallow for improved compliance

Many Intensol-formulated drugs are available

- Prednisone, dexamethasone, diazepam, propranolol, and more
- Easy to switch from injectables to orals

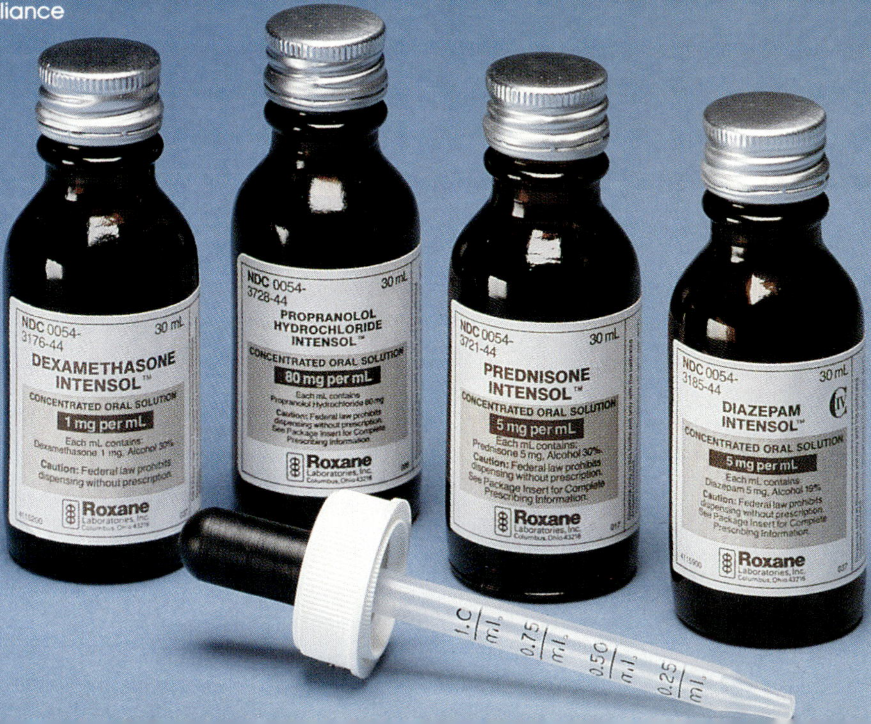

NTENSOLS™

olutions to tablet-taking problems

Therapy Consultation

The Therapy Consultation *section provides brief advice, in question-and-answer format, on how to handle specific drug-therapy problems. Readers are invited to submit questions, which will be referred to a consultant for an answer. The problems should not be highly specialized or unusual, nor should they be mundane. Questions are answered briefly, based largely on the judgment and personal experience of the consultant, although selected references may be cited to substantiate the consultant's advice.*

Use of H_2 histamine antagonists in allergic disorders

Question: When allergic disorders do not respond to chlorpheniramine or hydroxyzine, can an H_2 histamine antagonist be added to obtain a better response?

Answer: Histamine exerts its effects via stimulation of H_1 and H_2 histamine receptors. In some tissues, such as pulmonary vasculature and extravascular smooth muscle, stimulation of H_1 and H_2 receptors produces opposite effects.[1] However, in other tissues, stimulation of H_1 and H_2 receptors results in similar effects.[1] The role of H_1 antagonists in the management of allergic disorders is well known. A role for H_2 antagonists in the treatment of atopic conditions has been investigated over the past decade. Most studies conclude that H_2 antagonists used alone offer no clinical benefit in treating allergic diseases; however, the combination of H_1 and H_2 antagonists is beneficial in selected cases. Some of these studies are discussed below.

Smith et al.[2] measured the effects of cimetidine and chlorpheniramine on skin test reactivity. Each drug was administered alone or in combination at therapeutic doses for 24 hours before skin testing with histamine and an allergen to which the subject was sensitive. Chlorpheniramine decreased the skin test responses, whereas cimetidine had no effect. The combination of these two antihistamines significantly reduced the skin test reactions compared with chlorpheniramine alone.

In another study, hydroxyzine significantly reduced the skin test reaction to histamine.[3] Pretreatment with cimetidine had no effect on reactivity to histamine. The combination of these two agents significantly reduced the reaction compared with hydroxyzine alone. Each drug was given at usual therapeutic doses for 24 hours before skin testing. Doubling the dose of hydroxyzine hydrochloride to 50 mg every six hours was still less effective than the combination regimen.

The efficacy of combination therapy for chronic idiopathic urticaria has also been studied.[4] All study subjects had chronic urticaria that was refractory to conventional therapy. This was a double-blind randomized trial using hydroxyzine in combination with each of the following: placebo, terbutaline, cyproheptadine, chlorpheniramine, and cimetidine. Each combination was given for 7 to 10 days, and all subjects received the five combination treatments. Symptom scores were recorded twice daily by each subject as a measure of drug efficacy. Skin test reactivity to histamine was used as an objective measure of drug effectiveness. In 11 of 19 subjects, the combination of hydroxyzine plus cimetidine gave the greatest improvement in symptom scores and was significantly better than the other four combinations. Hydroxyzine plus cimetidine also significantly decreased skin test reactivity to histamine; the effect was better than that of all other combinations tested.

In summary, H_2 antagonists have no clinical benefit when used alone in the treatment of allergic diseases. However, these agents can act synergistically when administered with an H_1 antagonist. This combination has been studied primarily in various urticarial syndromes. Most studies agree that the combination is superior to use of an H_1 antagonist alone, although not all patients respond to combination therapy. Patients who fail to respond adequately to an H_1 antagonist may benefit from the addition of an H_2 antagonist. One caveat to bear in mind is that this combination may not be beneficial in treating allergic asthma. Stimulation of bronchial smooth muscle H_2 receptors causes bronchodilation, and receptor blockade may attenuate the beneficial effects of an H_1 antagonist in asthmatics.[5]

1. Douglas WW. Histamine and 5-hydroxytryptamine (serotonin) and their antagonists. In: Gilman AG, Goodman LS, Rall TW et al., eds. Goodman and Gilman's the pharmacologic basis of therapeutics. New York: Macmillan Publishing Co., Inc.; 1985:607–9.
2. Smith JA, Mansfield LE, deShazo RD. An evaluation of the pharmacologic inhibition of the immediate and late cutaneous reaction to allergen. *J Allergy Clin Immunol.* 1980; 65:118–21.
3. Harvey RP, Schocket AL. The effect of H_1 and H_2 blockade on cutaneous histamine response in man. *J Allergy Clin Immunol.* 1980; 65:136–9.
4. Harvey RP, Wegs J, Schocket AL. A controlled trial of therapy in chronic urticaria. *J Allergy Clin Immunol.* 1981; 68:262–6.
5. Nathan RA, Segall N, Schocket AL. A comparison of the actions of H_1 and H_2 antihistamines on histamine-induced bronchoconstriction and cutaneous wheal response in asthmatic patients. *J Allergy Clin Immunol.* 1981; 67:171–7.

JEFFREY C. DELAFUENTE, M.S., Associate Professor
Department of Pharmacy Practice, College of Pharmacy
Division of Clinical Immunology, Rheumatology and Allergy, College of Medicine
University of Florida
Gainesville, FL 32610

Letters

The Letters *column is a forum for rapid exchange of ideas among readers of* CP. *Liberal criteria are applied in the review of submissions to encourage contributions to this column.*

The Letters *column includes the following types of contributions: (1) comments, addenda, and minor updates on previously published work, (2) alerts on potential problems related to drug therapy or clinical research, (3) observations or comments on trends in drug therapy or clinical research, and (4) brief expressions of opinion about controversies in drug therapy or clinical research.*

Midazolam sedation and amnesia in elective cardioversion

Sodium thiopental was the intravenous anesthetic most commonly used for elective cardioversion until reports of the use of diazepam between 1965 and 1971 showed that adequate sedation and amnesia occurred with a benzodiazepine alone.[1,2] Diazepam has since been used most commonly; however, it has the disadvantages of a long half-life (20–50 hours) as well as active metabolites, pain on injection, thrombophlebitis, and occasionally increased ventricular irritability.[1,3] Midazolam is an injectable, water-soluble benzodiazepine with a rapid onset (1–2 minutes), short duration of action (half-life 1.2–6.0 hours), and potent anxiolytic, sedative, and amnesic effects. These properties make midazolam a very attractive agent for use in elective cardioversion. We evaluated prospectively the sedative and amnesic effects of midazolam given alone in four consecutive patients undergoing elective cardioversion. The results are shown in the table.

Effect of Midazolam Treatment during Elective Cardioversion

Parameter or Variable	Patient 1 (76 yr)[a]	Patient 2 (67 yr)	Patient 3 (75 yr)	Patient 4 (73 yr)
Heart rhythm[b]	Flutter	Fibr.[c]	Flutter	Flutter
Predose parameters				
Blood pressure				
Systolic	112	110	130	154
Diastolic	78	76	74	90
Heart rate	130	150	150	132
Respiratory rate	16	18	16	15
Midazolam dose (mg)	2	4	2	3
Postdose parameters				
Blood pressure				
Systolic	120	106	128	184
Diastolic	84	70	80	78
Heart rate	130	148	136	130
Respiratory rate	16	18	18	12
Onset of sedation (min)	1.5	9	6	6
Time to recovery (hr)	3.0	0.5	0.3	1.0
Amnesia present	Yes	Yes	No	Yes

[a] Patient's age in years.
[b] Refers to atrial rhythm.
[c] Fibr. = fibrillation.

To our knowledge this is the only report on the use of midazolam alone for sedation and amnesia in elective cardioversion. The onset of sedation adequate for performing the cardioversion (dysarthria, somnolence, loss of eyelid reflex) was quite variable and ranged from two to nine minutes. Midazolam has been reported to have minimal effects on the cardiovascular systems of patients with coronary artery disease.[4] We did not observe any changes in the vital signs of our patients that were clearly related to the administration of midazolam.

Amnesic effects with midazolam have been reported to occur in 70–90% of patients and are characterized by a short latency period of 2–3 minutes and a duration of 20–30 minutes.[5] Midazolam appears to induce anterograde amnesia more frequently than does diazepam.[6,7] We believed this property was particularly important for patients undergoing electrical cardioversion. Anterograde amnesia occurred in three of our four patients.

Proper dosing of midazolam requires slow titration to achieve the desired effect without inducing significant respiratory depression. We gave 1- to 2-mg doses at intervals of 2–3 minutes and did not observe any respiratory depression in these four elderly patients. Midazolam is three to four times as potent per milligram as diazepam and should not be given by rapid or single bolus intravenous injection.

Midazolam alone performed adequately as a sedative in four patients undergoing elective cardioversion. Direct comparisons with diazepam for this potential new indication may be warranted.

1. Ruskin J, Greenfield JC. Comparison of diazepam and sodium thiopental in cardioversion. *NC Med J*. 1970; 31(3):84–6.
2. Hendrix GH. Intravenous use of diazepam in cardioversion. *South Med J*. 1969; 62:483–4.
3. Barrett JS, Hey EB. Ventricular arrhythmias associated with the use of diazepam for cardioversion. *JAMA*. 1970; 214:1323–4.
4. Marty J, Nitenberg A, Blanchet F et al. Effects of midazolam on the coronary circulation in patients with coronary disease. *Anesthesiology*. 1986; 64:206–10.
5. Dundee JW, Wilson DB. Amnesic action of midazolam. *Anaesthesia*. 1980; 35:459–61.
6. Whitwam JG, al-Khudhairi D, McCloy RF. Comparison of midazolam and diazepam in doses of comparable potency during gastroscopy. *Br J Anaesth*. 1983; 55:773–77.
7. Cole SG, Brozinsky S, Isenberg KI. Midazolam, a new more potent benzodiazepine, compared with diazepam: a randomized, double blind study of preendoscopic sedatives. *Gastrointest Endosc*. 1983; 29:219–22.

Daniel W. Krichbaum, Pharm.D., Clinical Pharmacist Cardiology

Imtiaz Hamid, M.D., Invasive Cardiologist

Ingalls Memorial Hospital
Harvey, IL 60426

Drug Review

Clinical use of systemic antifungal agents

JOHN M. BENSON AND MILAP C. NAHATA

Abstract: The chemistry, pharmacology, pharmacokinetics, clinical uses, adverse effects, and drug interactions of amphotericin B, flucytosine, ketoconazole, and miconazole are reviewed.

Amphotericin B, a heptaene compound with poor water solubility, disrupts the fungal cell wall by binding to ergosterol. Ketoconazole and miconazole, imidazole derivatives, are poorly water soluble and inhibit the synthesis of ergosterol. Flucytosine is a readily water-soluble, fluorinated pyrimidine agent that may be metabolized to fluorouracil. The pharmacokinetics of amphotericin B is unique and has not yet been clearly defined. After oral administration, absorption of flucytosine from the gastrointestinal tract is rapid and nearly complete. In adults, oral administration of ketoconazole produces peak concentrations of drug one to two hours after the dose. Miconazole is administered only intravenously and distributes well into most tissues.

Amphotericin B remains the drug of choice for most systemic mycoses. Dosing of amphotericin B is often empiric and patient specific. Flucytosine is rarely used alone; the combination of flucytosine and amphotericin B exerts synergistic killing of many fungi. Ketoconazole is effective for treating many chronic fungal infections. Miconazole is seldom used because of the availability of agents that are equally effective, less toxic, or both. Nephrotoxicity can occur with amphotericin B therapy, while flucytosine is associated with gastrointestinal and hematologic toxicities. Ketoconazole is much less toxic than any of the other agents, while miconazole has a high incidence of adverse effects.

In addition to the need for more effective and less toxic agents, research is needed to clearly define the pharmacokinetics and pharmacodynamics of currently available antifungal drugs.

Index terms: Amphotericin B; Antifungals; Dosage; Drug interactions; Drugs; Flucytosine; Ketoconazole; Mechanism of action; Miconazole; Pharmacokinetics; Resistance; Toxicity
Clin Pharm. 1988; 7:424–38

Many serious and fatal fungal diseases became treatable after the introduction of amphotericin B in 1955.[1] This drug represented a major advance in the management of systemic fungal infections. Since that time, there have been few additions to the antifungal armamentarium, and none has replaced amphotericin B, despite its toxicity, as the drug of choice for most serious systemic fungal infections.[2] Only three other agents are available in the United States for the treatment of systemic fungal infections: flucytosine, ketoconazole, and miconazole.

The incidence of systemic fungal infections is increasing and may be attributed to recent increases in the use of intravascular catheters and other implanted devices, broad-spectrum antibiotics, and immunosuppressive agents, and in the prevalence of the acquired immunodeficiency syndrome (AIDS).[3] Although there are only a limited number of antifungal agents available, dosing recommendations for the treatment of systemic fungal infections vary from author to author and from clinician to clinician. Some reasons for this lack of uniformity include (1) limited pharmacokinetic data, especially in pediatric patients and (2) highly variable fungal minimum inhibitory concentration (MIC) results, which are greatly influenced by testing conditions and are poorly correlated with clini-

JOHN M. BENSON, PHARM.D., is Fellow in Infectious Disease Pharmacotherapy and MILAP C. NAHATA, PHARM.D., is Professor of Pharmacy and Pediatrics, Colleges of Pharmacy and Medicine, The Ohio State University and Childrens Hospital, Columbus.

Address reprint requests to Dr. Nahata at the College of Pharmacy, The Ohio State University, 500 West 12th Ave., Columbus, OH 43210.

This is **article 680-204-8809** in the **ASHP Continuing Education System;** it qualifies for 1.0 hour of continuing-education credit. See page 478 for learning objectives and test questions.

Copyright © 1988, American Society of Hospital Pharmacists, Inc. All rights reserved. 0278-2677/88/0601-0424$03.75.

cal outcome.[4,5]

The purpose of this article is to review each of the agents with respect to their individual features including mechanism of action, spectrum of activity, pharmacokinetics, clinical use, adverse effects, and drug interactions. The relative similarities, differences, advantages, and disadvantages of these agents will be emphasized.

Chemistry

Of the four commonly used antifungal agents, two (amphotericin B and flucytosine) are chemically distinct, and the other two (ketoconazole and miconazole) are similar to one another. Amphotericin B is a heptaene compound with very poor water solubility. It must be prepared as a colloidal suspension, using a desoxycholate bile salt surfactant. It cannot be mixed with any electrolyte solutions, such as sodium chloride, or aggregation will occur.[6] The colloid also aggregates if the final solution is too acidic (pH less than 5).[7] For systemic infections, amphotericin B is given only intravenously. Flucytosine is a fluorinated pyrimidine agent that, in contrast to the other agents, is readily water soluble. It is chemically similar to, and may be metabolized to, fluorouracil.

Miconazole and ketoconazole are both imidazole derivatives that are poorly water soluble. For systemic use, ketoconazole is available only as an oral tablet, while miconazole is available only as an intravenous colloidal dispersion, requiring the addition of polyethoxylated castor oil (Cremophor EL) for stabilization.

Mechanisms of Action

Amphotericin B acts by binding to ergosterol (the predominant sterol in the fungal cell wall), causing a mechanical disruption of the cell wall. The result is increased cell permeability or actual leakage of critical cytoplasmic contents.[8,9] Kotler-Brajtburg and colleagues[8] postulated that there are two types of amphotericin B binding. "Weak" binding, which is independent of energy and temperature, reversible, and nonlethal, may permit more amphotericin B to penetrate further into the cell membrane to facilitate "strong" binding, which is energy and temperature dependent, irreversible, and lethal. "Weak" binding also appears to enhance the diffusion of other molecules into the fungal cell, which may explain the synergism observed when amphotericin B is combined with certain other antimicrobials.[10] The "weak" binding of amphotericin B to the fungal cell membrane has been exploited by combining this agent with flucytosine in the treatment of certain fungal infections. In one study, two thirds of the strains of *Candida albicans* initially resistant to flucytosine were killed by the combination.[11] This effect of amphotericin B on the permeability of fungal cell walls has also been investigated with other agents.[12] Amphotericin B plus rifampin is synergistic against *C. albicans*, *Saccharomyces*, *Histoplasma capsulatum*, and *Blastomyces dermatitidis*, and amphotericin B plus tetracycline shows synergy against *Coccidioides immitis*.[10] This latter finding may be important since Hoeprich and Huston[13] reported primary resistance to amphotericin B in 20% of clinical isolates of *C. immitis*.

In addition to the direct action of amphotericin B on the fungal cell wall, there is evidence to suggest that amphotericin B also acts as an immunoadjuvant. Shirley and Little[14] showed that the administration of amphotericin B increased the cell-mediated response to dinitrobenzene sensitization in mice. They postulated that amphotericin B enhances antigen presentation to the body's immune system, probably by inhibition of a suppressive population of T-cells. Suppressor T-cells usually regulate the magnitude and duration of an immune response,[15] and inhibition of these suppressor T-cells results in an exaggerated host immune response to antigenic challenge. However, other studies have suggested that, depending on the timing of amphotericin B administration in relation to antigen exposure, the effect on the immune system can be either stimulation or depression. Amphotericin B can activate or depress macrophage and lymphocyte function, depending on the timing and amount of amphotericin B administered.[16] These effects may be responsible, at least in part, for the inconsistent correlation between in vitro susceptibility results and clinical response, since in vitro susceptibility testing does not account for immunologic effects.

Flucytosine, a pyrimidine analogue, acts by a mechanism different from that of amphotericin B. Flucytosine enters the fungal cell via the enzyme cytosine permease and is then converted either to fluorouracil, which is incorporated into RNA, or to 5-fluoro-2′-deoxyuridylate (floxuridine), which inhibits thymidylate synthetase, thereby interrupting DNA synthesis.[17] The latter pathway is now thought to be the primary mechanism of action of flucytosine, since the conversion of flucytosine to fluorouracil as a mechanism of action is not well supported by recent evidence.[18] Conversion to fluorouracil may, however, play a role in the toxicity of this agent.[19]

Ketoconazole and miconazole act by inhibiting the synthesis of ergosterol, via inhibition of the 14-demethylation step in the sterol synthesis pathway.[20] Direct binding to ergosterol, as seen with amphotericin B, does not appear to play an important role in the antifungal activity of the imidazoles. The inhibition of this step in sterol synthesis results in the accumulation of 14-methylsterols, which are incorporated into the cell membrane. Ketoconazole also increases the amount of saturated fatty acids in the fungal cell membrane. In the presence of ketoconazole, the structural integrity of the yeast membranes is completely disturbed, the uptake of certain molecules is hindered, there is leakage of cytoplasm, growth is inhibited, and the cell becomes increasingly susceptible to host defenses.[20,21] In dimorphous fungi, these effects occur in the mycelial and yeast phases.[21]

In recent years, ketoconazole and other imidazoles have been found to have potent inhibitory actions on steroidogenesis in humans.[22] This is not surprising since, in both organisms, the inhibited enzymes are in the cytochrome P-450 system. In humans, ketoconazole appears to inhibit 11β-hydroxylase and cholesterol side-chain cleavage in the hydrocortisone synthesis pathway, and 17,20-lyase in the testosterone synthesis pathway. In addition, ketoconazole is able to block corticosteroid action at the receptor level.[22] The importance of these actions is discussed under Adverse Effects and Drug Interactions.

Antifungal Spectrum

There are many similarities as well as important differences in the antifungal spectra of the antifungal agents. Amphotericin B is effective against most fungal isolates, including *Candida* species, *Cryptococcus neoformans, B. dermatitidis, H. capsulatum*, and *Torulopsis glabrata*, which generally have very low minimum inhibitory concentrations (MICs) (usually 0.05 to 1.6 μg/mL). It is also active against *Sporothrix schenckii*, and, although the drug is effective against *C. immitis, Aspergillus*, and *Mucor*, the MICs for these organisms are often much higher (usually 0.2 to greater than 20 μg/mL).[17,23-25] Amphotericin B is not active against *Pseudallescheria boydii.*

Flucytosine has a relatively narrow antifungal spectrum, with activity against *C. albicans, C. neoformans, Torulopsis glabrata*, and the dematiaceous fungi (imperfect fungi of the family Dematiaceae) that cause chromomycosis.[12,13,26,27] However, because of the high incidence of natural and acquired resistance that occurs with many of these organisms, flucytosine is seldom used alone, except in the treatment of chromomycosis and some fungal urinary-tract infections.[28,29] Depending on the organism, natural resistance to flucytosine occurs at different rates. For example, 7–8% of pretreatment isolates of *C. albicans* and *T. glabrata* are resistant to flucytosine. While only 1–2% of *C. neoformans* isolates show resistance to flucytosine initially, up to 22% of isolates of *Candida tropicalis* and *C. krusei* are initially resistant.[12] Fortunately, many initially resistant organisms are susceptible to the combination of flucytosine plus amphotericin B.

The spectrum of ketoconazole is relatively broad and includes dermatophytes, most isolates of *Candida* species (*C. tropicalis* is often resistant in vitro), *H. capsulatum, C. neoformans, B. dermatitidis, C. immitis, Paracoccidioides brasiliensis*, and *S. schenckii.*[28,30,31] Miconazole has a similar spectrum, but because of its greater toxicity and the necessity to administer it intravenously, it is seldom used. However, the recently identified *Malassezia furfur* has been consistently susceptible to miconazole while usually showing resistance to amphotericin B in vitro.[32] Further research is needed to demonstrate a correlation between these in vitro findings and clinical outcome.

Pharmacokinetics

The pharmacokinetic characteristics of the antifungal agents are quite diverse, and amphotericin B has the most unique pharmacokinetic characteristics. In adults receiving amphotericin B in doses of 5–50 mg, serum concentrations roughly correlate with the amount of drug given. However, at higher doses, tissue storage or inactivation mechanisms apparently disrupt this correlation with peak serum concentrations of the drug.[33] In adults, daily intravenous administration of amphotericin B 20–30 mg has resulted in serum concentrations of 0.3–6.24 μg/mL.[34,35] Doses of 0.9 to 1.1 mg/kg have produced peak serum concentrations of 1.5–2.1 μg/mL and trough concentrations of 0.1–0.15 μg/mL.[36] In a recent report, infants (less than three months of age) achieved peak serum concentrations of 0.31–2.08 μg/mL (mean, 0.96 μg/mL) at 30–45 minutes and trough concentrations of 0.08–0.55 μg/mL (mean, 0.28 μg/mL) after an infusion of 1 mg/kg of amphotericin B.[37] In this study, children 7.5 months to 15 years of age had peak and trough serum concentrations of 0.47–0.66 μg/mL (mean, 0.52 μg/mL) and 0.03–0.11 μg/mL (mean, 0.09 μg/mL), respectively, after a dose of 0.75 mg/kg.

During therapy, amphotericin B is detectable in various body fluids and tissues. The concentrations of amphotericin B in the cerebrospinal fluid (CSF) have been highly variable, and often undetectable. Perfect and Durack[38] have suggested, however, that the actual meningeal concentration of amphotericin B may be higher than that measured in the CSF. In adults, CSF concentrations after an intravenous dose of 20 mg/day ranged from 0.06 to 0.56 μg/mL.[34] In neonates, CSF concentrations were reported to be 40–90% of concomitant serum concentrations.[39] These values appear to be higher than those usually encountered in adults, but since the actual concentrations were not reported, an assessment of the clinical importance is not possible. Knee joint fluid has been reported to contain 0.08 μg of amphotericin B per milliliter with a concomitant serum concentration of 0.07 μg/mL.[37] Christiansen and colleagues[25] studied at autopsy various body tissues from eight patients who had received amphotericin B during their hospitalization and found the following mean tissue concentrations:

hepatic tissue, 70.2 μg/g; spleen, 44.5 μg/g; kidney, 14.3 μg/g; lung, 9.9 μg/g; esophagus, 3.1 μg/g; heart, 2.8 μg/g; fat, 1.0 μg/g; and muscle, 0.6 μg/g. Interpatient variability in tissue concentrations of amphotericin B was considerable. These findings demonstrate that amphotericin B is distributed into most tissues of the body, although penetration into closed cavities such as the central nervous system is considered poor.[12,17]

Amphotericin B appears to distribute largely into a slowly equilibrating peripheral compartment, which at steady state may account for two thirds of the total amount of drug in the body.[36] The apparent volume of distribution is approximately 4 L/kg. The primary tissue depots of amphotericin B in the body are the liver (14–41% of the total dose), the lungs (1.2–6%), and the kidney (0.3–2%). The liver and spleen acquire the highest concentrations of amphotericin B during therapy, possibly because of the micellar suspension of administered amphotericin B interacting with the reticuloendothelial system.[25] In the blood, amphotericin B is highly (>90%) bound to lipoproteins,[40] erythrocytes,[36] and cholesterol,[9] which may also account for the very large capacity of tissue storage for this agent. The finding that there is substantial accumulation of amphotericin B in tissues raises the question of whether a reduction in dosage after several days of therapy could reduce toxicity while still maintaining optimal efficacy. Clearly, this is an area that requires further research.

Amphotericin B is not appreciably metabolized. In adults, the elimination of amphotericin B is triexponential, with second- and third-phase elimination half-lives of 24 hours and 15 days, respectively. The terminal half-life is probably prolonged because of the extremely slow release of drug from peripheral tissue. Total body clearance averages 30 mL/min, with a mean renal clearance of 1 mL/min.[36] In dogs, the largest portion of the dose is eliminated in bile (19%) and urine (18%),[41] although in humans, only a small amount (2–5%) is recoverable in the urine.[17] Tissue accumulation appears to account for the majority of drug disposition, and amphotericin B can be detected in tissues such as liver and kidney for as long as 12 months after therapy has been terminated.[42] Because amphotericin B is not eliminated by the kidney, no dosage adjustment is necessary in patients with renal failure.

The pharmacokinetics of flucytosine is typical of a renally eliminated drug. After oral administration, absorption of flucytosine from the gastrointestinal tract is rapid and nearly complete.[43] Administration of 37.5 mg/kg every six hours (150 mg/kg/day) produces peak serum concentrations in the range of 50 to 100 μg/mL in adults with normal renal function. In neonates, oral doses of 25–100 mg/kg/day produced a mean peak serum concentration of 75 μg/mL.[39] Negligible protein binding and low molecular weight facilitate excellent penetration of flucytosine into nearly every tissue. Cerebrospinal fluid concentrations range from 53 to 80 μg/mL after doses of 150 mg/kg/day in patients with normal renal function.[34] The ability of flucytosine to penetrate into the CSF may be an additional reason for the improved results obtained when flucytosine and amphotericin B are combined in the treatment of cryptococcal meningitis. Flucytosine is not significantly metabolized, and approximately 90% of a dose is excreted unchanged in the urine.[26,44] In adults with normal renal function, the elimination half-life averaged approximately 3.2 hours,[43,44] while the mean elimination half-life in neonates was 12.8 hours, and highly variable.[39] Renal clearance of flucytosine is approximately equal to creatinine clearance,[45] and dosage adjustments are necessary in patients with renal failure. Schönebeck and colleagues[44] have recommended extending the dosing interval to 12 hours for patients with creatinine clearances of 20–40 mL/min, and to 24 hours when the creatinine clearance is 10–20 mL/min. Flucytosine is dialyzable; it has been recommended that patients on hemodialysis be given an additional dose of 25 to 50 mg/kg after dialysis.[45] These formulas, however, should not supplant serum drug concentration monitoring in patients at risk for drug accumulation. In all patients, the two-hour postinfusion serum concentration should be less than 100 μg/mL.

The imidazoles also have familiar pharmacokinetic characteristics. Ketoconazole is administered systemically as an oral tablet, and, in adults, it is well absorbed, producing peak serum concentrations of 1.5–3.1 μg/mL one to two hours after a 200-mg dose, and trough concentrations of 0.39–0.78 μg/mL 11 hours after a 200-mg dose.[46,47] Administration of 400 mg/day resulted in mean peak serum concentrations of 3.3–7.2 μg/mL, while 800 mg/day has produced mean peak concentrations of 6.2–27.5 μg/mL.[24,30,46,48,49] In two pediatric studies, ketoconazole doses of 4 to 6 mg/kg have produced peak serum concentrations of 0.8–4.4 μg/mL.[50,51] At equivalent doses, an investigational suspension of ketoconazole (Janssen Pharmaceutica, New Brunswick, NJ) produced peak serum concentrations that were nearly twice those achieved using crushed tablets,[51] possibly because of more rapid absorption. The absorption of ketoconazole is inversely related to the pH of the gastric contents, and administration with H_2-receptor antagonists, antacids, or meals may cause a clinically important decrease in the bioavailability.[17,46] The drug penetrates well into infected skin (10.7 μg/mL), joint spaces (0.2–0.9 μg/mL), tendon (2.0 μg/mL), and possibly saliva (although residue from oral administration of a suspension was not ruled out), but penetration into the CSF is usually poor (0.07–1.6 μg/mL).[46,52,53] Ketoconazole concentrations in bone have been reported to reach as high as 2.5 μg/

mL after doses of 400–800 mg/day but are often undetectable.[24,46,53] The elimination half-life of ketoconazole is approximately three hours, and may be concentration dependent.[46] It is metabolized primarily by the liver, with very little drug being excreted unchanged in the urine. Renal insufficiency and dialysis have minimal effects on serum concentrations of ketoconazole and therefore do not necessitate dosage adjustments.[46]

Miconazole is administered systemically only as an intravenous colloidal suspension. Peak serum concentrations have ranged from 5.0 to 13.4 μg/mL five minutes after one-hour infusions of 25 to 50 mg/kg/day in adult patients.[54] The drug distributes well into most tissues. A miconazole concentration of 1.2 μg/mL was detected in synovial fluid exudate from an infected knee (concomitant serum concentration, 4.0 μg/mL). A dose of 30 mg/kg/day resulted in only 0.26 μg/mL of miconazole in the CSF, indicating the need for intrathecal administration for CNS infections.[54] More than 90% of the drug in blood is bound to plasma proteins. Miconazole is predominantly metabolized in the liver, and less than 1% of a dose is excreted unchanged in the urine. The drug is eliminated in a triexponential fashion, with an initial half-life of 30 minutes, a second half-life of four hours, and a terminal half-life of approximately 20 hours.[17] No dosage adjustment is needed in patients with renal failure.

Clinical Uses

Amphotericin B. The drugs of choice for some common fungal pathogens are listed in Table 1. Dosage guidelines for antifungal agents, however, are often based on very limited data. Despite the fact that amphotericin B is the oldest agent in this group, dosing for this drug is often based on observed toxicity rather than on results from dose-finding studies that minimize toxicity while maximizing efficacy.[61] One reason for the lack of clinical studies defining optimal dosing guidelines for amphotericin B may be the hesitancy of investigators to alter recommended guidelines in patients with serious fungal disease because of the possibility of therapeutic failure, toxicity, or both. Fortunately, the current dosing guidelines are usually effective in eradicating fungal infections, and a majority of patients who develop toxicity do not have permanent sequelae.

Amphotericin B is indicated for the treatment of most serious systemic fungal infections and may also be used as a bladder irrigation for fungal cystitis. Amphotericin B therapy is usually started with a test dose of 0.1 mg/kg or 1 mg, diluted in 50–150 mL of 5% dextrose injection and given over 20–30 minutes.[28] The purpose of this test dose is to assess the degree of adverse effects that may be experienced by patients during drug administration. After the test dose, the daily dose is increased slowly to a total daily dose of 0.3–1.0 mg/kg/day, depending on clinical response, site of infection, pathogen, patient immune status, and severity of adverse effects. Several different regimens have been proposed to advance the dose to the desired therapeutic level.

Atkinson and Bennett[36] determined that giving a test dose of 1 mg followed by a conventional regimen of 5, 10, and 15 mg on each of the next three days did not achieve "therapeutic" serum concentrations until the fourth day of therapy. Even then, the serum concentration was considered therapeutic for only 10 hours. They recommended that patients with life-threatening infections be given a dose of 0.3 mg/kg on days 1 and 2. The dose should then be slowly increased over the next several days to 0.5–0.6 mg/kg/day. The authors predicted that, using these doses, "therapeutic" serum concentrations would be achieved on the first day and would be sustained throughout therapy. Weaknesses in these conclusions are that they were derived from pharmacokinetic data in one patient and that therapeutic outcomes are often poorly correlated with serum concentrations. In addition to dose, factors influencing steady-state concentrations include frequency of dosing (daily versus every other day), rate of dosage escalation, and rate of administration.

If the clinician desires to give a test dose of 0.1 mg/kg, this dose could be followed immediately by a second dose to give a total dose of 0.3 mg/kg on the first day. At our pediatric institution, for serious fungal infections requiring 1 mg/kg/day, we commonly administer a test dose of 0.1 mg/kg, followed by 0.4 mg/kg to provide a total of 0.5 mg/kg on the first day. This is followed by 0.5 mg/kg on day 2, 0.75 mg/kg on day 3, and 1 mg/kg/day thereafter. Test doses are often considered unnecessary in neonates,[37] although the reasons for this are not well documented. In our experience, newborn infants have a lower incidence of infusion-related adverse effects and are usually not given a test dose. The duration of treatment with amphotericin B is not well defined.

An effective dose of amphotericin B varies widely, depending on the type of infection, and is often empiric and patient specific. In general, though, doses of 0.4–0.6 mg/kg/day for 6 to 12 weeks achieve adequate clinical response. Doses of 1 mg/kg/day or more, and total doses of 2–4 g in adults, are usually required for serious infections (e.g., pneumonia or fungemia) caused by pathogens such as *Aspergillus* and *Coccidioides* or for infections in areas of poor antifungal penetration such as the central nervous system, joints, and heart valves. Conversely, Medoff and colleagues[62] achieved favorable results using lower-than-conventional doses of amphotericin B to treat patients with systemic *Candida* infections associated with intrave-

Table 1.
Drugs of Choice for Treating Infections with Major Fungal Pathogens

Pathogen or Condition	Adult Dosage[a]	Pediatric Dosage[a]	Alternative	Reference
Aspergillus species				
Amphotericin B	0.5–1.0 mg/kg/day for a total of 2–4 g	0.5–0.6 mg/kg/day	None reliable	55, 56
Blastomyces dermatitidis				
Amphotericin B or	0.3–1.0 mg/kg/day for a total of 1.5–2.5 g	1.0 mg/kg/day		55, 57
Ketoconazole	400–800 mg/day for 6–12 months			48
Candida species				
Life-threatening infection				
Amphotericin B with or without	0.5–1.0 mg/kg/day for a total of 2–4 g	0.5–1.0 mg/kg/day		57, 56
Flucytosine	37.5 mg/kg q6h	37.5 mg/kg q6h for four weeks		
Non-life-threatening infection[b]				
Amphotericin B or	100–200 mg over 7–10 days	0.5–1.0 mg/kg/day for two weeks		12, 57
Ketoconazole[c]	100–400 mg/day for six months	8–10 mg/kg/day for three to four months		50, 58
Chromomycosis				
Flucytosine	25–37.5 mg/kg q6h for four to eight weeks		Ketoconazole	55
Coccidioides immitis				
Life-threatening infection				
Amphotericin B	1.0–1.5 mg/kg/day for a total of 1.5–2 g	1.0 mg/kg/day for a total of 15–45 mg/kg		55, 57
Non-life-threatening infection				
Ketoconazole	200–800 mg/day for 6–12 months	5–22 mg/kg/day for several months after improvement	Amphotericin B	57, 59
Cryptococcus neoformans				
Meningitis				
Amphotericin B plus	0.3 mg/kg/day	Same as adult	Amphotericin B alone	57, 60
Flucytosine	37.5 mg/kg q6h for six weeks			
Nonmeningitis				
Amphotericin B with or without	0.3 to 0.6 mg/kg/day	Same as adult	Ketoconazole	55, 57
Flucytosine	37.5 mg/kg q6h			
Histoplasma capsulatum				
Disseminated				
Amphotericin B	0.6 mg/kg/day for a total of 2–3 g	1.0 mg/kg/day for a total of 35 mg/kg	Ketoconazole	55, 57
Chronic pulmonary				
Amphotericin B or	0.6 mg/kg/day for a total of 2–2.5 g			55
Ketoconazole	400 mg/day for 6–12 months			48
Malassezia furfur[b]				
Miconazole	400–1200 mg q6h			12
Mucor species				
Amphotericin B	1 mg/kg/day for two to three months or a total of 30–40 mg/kg		None reliable	55
Paracoccidioides brasiliensis				
Amphotericin B plus or followed by	0.3–1.0 mg/kg/day for a total of 1.2–3 g	0.3–1.0 mg/kg/day	Miconazole	55
Sulfadiazine or	4–6 g/day for three to five years	60–100 mg/kg/day for three to five years		55, 57
Ketoconazole	400 mg/day for six months			47
Pseudallescheria boydii				
Miconazole	400–1200 mg q8h	10 mg/kg q8h	Ketoconazole	12, 57
Sporothrix schenkii				
Lymphocutaneous				
Saturated solution of potassium iodide	3 mL daily, then increased to tolerance, or 24 mL daily		Amphotericin B	55
Pulmonary or disseminated				
Amphotericin B	0.5–1.0 mg/kg/day for a total of 2–3 g			57

[a] Usual dosage or until clinical and microbiologic cures are achieved.
[b] After conventional measures such as removal of catheters, discontinuation of antibiotics, or topical antifungal therapy have failed.
[c] Except in cases of infection with *C. tropicalis*.

nous catheters or previous antibiotic administration or mucocutaneous candidiasis unresponsive to topical antifungal therapy. Of 14 patients (3–82 years of age), 13 showed clinical improvement after total doses of 1–40 mg (median, 5 mg), and laboratory and clinical cure of infection was achieved in 13 patients after total doses of 10–355 mg (median, 77.5 mg) had been given over 4–18 days (median, 8.5 days). Most mucocutaneous infections responded within 48 hours, while three to four days of therapy was required for improvement in patients with candidal pneumonia or fungemia. The authors explained their results in part by the lower minimum inhibitory concentrations (MICs) of amphotericin B for *C. albicans* compared with other fungi (e.g., *C. immitis* or *Aspergillus* species). However, this is a report of published cases and does not represent an accurate estimate of the true response rate. This approach to therapy should be reserved for patients with superficial, catheter-associated, or other non-life-threatening mycoses for which more conservative measures, such as removal of catheters, discontinuation of antibiotics, or topical antifungal therapy, have failed.

Because of poor penetration into the CSF, amphotericin B occasionally must be given intrathecally in the treatment of fungal meningitis. Intrathecal administration of amphotericin B consists of 0.1 mg initially, increased gradually to a maximum of 0.5 mg every 48–72 hours.[28] The drug is usually dissolved in 10% dextrose injection, and the patient is placed in the Trendelenburg position after injection to facilitate cephalad flow. Alternate methods include cisternal or intraventricular injections via an indwelling reservoir. Intrathecal administration is usually required, in addition to intravenous injection, for coccidioidal meningitis, but is rarely needed for cryptococcal disease as discussed below (see Amphotericin B plus Flucytosine).

Flucytosine. Flucytosine is administered orally, and in contrast to amphotericin B, there are few variations in the recommended dosing of flucytosine. Currently, the dosage recommendation for flucytosine is 37.5 mg/kg given every six hours (150 mg/kg/day), except in neonates or patients with renal impairment.[28] Dosing in such patients should be determined by the degree of renal impairment and measured serum flucytosine concentrations. Because of the frequent resistance of many fungi to flucytosine,[12,28,56,63–65] it is useful as a single agent only in the treatment of chromomycosis and in some cases of uncomplicated candiduria. Flucytosine is commercially available in 250- and 500-mg capsules. Thus, for administration to pediatric patients, capsules must be opened and the drug must be mixed with a small amount of food (e.g., applesauce), or a suspension must be prepared extemporaneously. Currently, a 1% solution for intravenous administration is available from the manufacturer for compassionate use, but it is not marketed because of limited need.

Amphotericin B plus Flucytosine. The combination of amphotericin B and flucytosine was more rapidly curative than amphotericin B alone in the treatment of adults with cryptococcal meningitis.[60] In this study, Bennett and coworkers compared treatment with amphotericin B at 0.4 mg/kg/day for 10 weeks in 27 patients with treatment with amphotericin B at 0.3 mg/kg/day plus flucytosine at 37.5 mg/kg every six hours for six weeks in 24 patients. Eleven of 27 patients receiving amphotericin B alone and 16 of 24 patients receiving amphotericin B plus flucytosine were considered cured or improved. The authors concluded that the combination of amphotericin B plus flucytosine for six weeks is as effective as amphotericin B alone for 10 weeks. Weaknesses of this study include considerable variation in doses and treatment duration, and excessive doses of flucytosine may have been used (9 of 40 patients developed bone marrow toxicity). Despite these points, we believe that this combination is the treatment of choice for cryptococcal meningitis since it appears to be as effective as amphotericin B alone, sterilizes the cerebrospinal fluid more rapidly, and allows a shorter course of treatment. The combination of amphotericin B plus flucytosine has been shown in laboratory animals and in vitro to be synergistic against *C. neoformans*.[10,11]

There have also been reports of synergistic action of amphotericin B with flucytosine against chromomycosis and isolates of *Aspergillus, Candida*, and *Torulopsis*.[1,10,11,66–70] In a retrospective literature review, the use of 20–40 mg of amphotericin B per day plus flucytosine at 150–200 mg/kg/day for the treatment of *Candida* meningitis resulted in improvement or recovery in five of five adult patients. Amphotericin B (0.5–1 mg/kg/day) plus flucytosine (50–200 mg/kg/day) also was found to result in recovery in four of seven neonates (less than three months of age), and five of five infants and children (3.5 months to 12 years of age) with *Candida* meningitis.[63] However, these results must be interpreted with caution since case reports in the literature usually do not reflect a normal patient population and may overpredict efficacy. It must also be noted that not all fungi respond to antifungal combinations, and, in fact, in vitro antagonism between amphotericin B and both flucytosine and the imidazoles has been reported.[12,71,72] The clinical importance of these interactions remains undetermined.

Ketoconazole. Ketoconazole is the newest of the antifungal agents marketed in the United States. Its oral dosage form, low incidence of toxic effects, and favorable activity against many fungal pathogens make it one of the most important advances in antifungal chemotherapy in recent years. Dosage regimens for ketoconazole vary with the type of infection but generally require that the drug be given for 6–12 months. Because of relatively slow improvement during therapy, frequent treatment failures in immunocompromised hosts, and poor central nervous system (CNS) penetration, ketoconazole is generally not recommended for the treatment of severe systemic or CNS mycoses.[28]

Chronic mucocutaneous candidiasis in adults treated with 100–200 mg of ketoconazole per day showed improvement or resolution of all lesions after six months of therapy.[58] The use of higher doses (e.g., 400 mg/day), which may produce a more rapid response, was not studied. In children, treatment of candidiasis with ketoconazole resulted in clinical and mycologic cure in most of the patients treated.[50] Doses of ketoconazole 8–10 mg/kg/day were recommended to achieve adequate serum concentrations.

In the treatment of histoplasmosis (chronic cavitary [lung], localized, or disseminated) in adults, 400 mg of ketoconazole per day for six months was found to be as effective as 800 mg/day for the same duration.[48] Other studies using 400 mg of ketoconazole per day for periods of one month to a year reported similar benefit.[30,47,53,73]

In a controlled trial of ketoconazole comparing 400 mg/day with 800 mg/day for treatment of blastomycosis, adult patients were treated for six months or longer.[48] While 79% (27 of 33) of the patients treated with the low-dose regimen were considered cured, all (32 of 32) of the patients treated with the high-dose regimen were cured. Thus, the authors recommended that therapy with ketoconazole for blastomycosis be initiated at 400 mg/day and continued for at least six months; if necessary, the dose can then be increased to 600 or 800 mg/day. They suggested that therapy be continued until there is roentgenographic and microbiologic evidence of cure. Because of its lower toxicity relative to amphotericin B, ketoconazole is the drug of choice for the treatment of non-life-threatening blastomycosis requiring therapy.[49,74]

Successful treatment of coccidioidomycosis depends largely on host immune status; immunocompromised patients frequently experience relapses. In patients with no known immune deficiency, ketoconazole doses of 200 mg/day are usually curative in the treatment of soft-tissue coccidioidomycosis, while doses of 400–800 mg/day or more are often required for eradication of infection from pulmonary and skeletal sites.[24,30,59] Relapses are common among patients treated for less than six months, indicating the need for 6–12 months or longer of therapy. The optimal strategy may be for treatment to continue for six months after clinical improvement has been documented.[59] Ketoconazole has also been investigated in the treatment of infections caused by species of *Paracoccidioides* and *Cryptococcus*, with similarly favorable outcomes.[30,47]

Miconazole. Miconazole has been largely ignored in recent years because of the availability of other agents that have been more thoroughly studied and are either more effective, less toxic, or both.[75] Miconazole is the drug of choice only for the treatment of infections caused by *M. furfur* and possibly *P. boydii*.[28,32,54] Because of the possibility of serious adverse reactions, infusion of a 200-mg test dose under close supervision is recommended.[17,28] The recommended dose ranges from 400 to 1200 mg given every eight hours, depending on the susceptibility of the organism and clinical response.[12,17] The drug should be given in at least 200 mL of 5% dextrose or 0.9% sodium chloride injection and infused over one to two hours.[17,76] As with most antimycotic agents, the duration of treatment for miconazole is not well established, but 3–12 weeks has been suggested. Pediatric patients are treated with 20–40 mg/kg/day, although adequate studies of the efficacy and toxicity of miconazole in infants and children are lacking.[12,54]

Choosing an Agent. Although in vitro susceptibility can be demonstrated for these drugs against most fungi, the clinician must remember that the site of infection, host immune status, duration of therapy, underlying disease, and other factors will greatly influence the outcome of treatment. The poor correlation that often exists between in vitro susceptibility results and clinical response, even with demonstrably adequate serum concentrations, must be considered when choosing an antifungal regimen.

Investigational Agents

A number of investigational antimycotic agents are undergoing clinical trials in the United States and Europe (e.g., itraconazole, fluconazole, bifonazole, econazole, naftifine, terbinafine, amorolfine, fenpropimorph, and ambruticin), some of which may prove to be important additions to the antifungal armamentarium. Itraconazole, an oral agent that exhibits in vitro and in vivo activity against *S. schenkii* and *Aspergillus* species, appears to be promising.[3,77,78] Fluconazole is another oral agent that appears to be effective when used to treat cryptococcal meningitis and may be particularly useful for the treatment of this infection in patients with AIDS.[79]

Adverse Effects

Amphotericin B. The toxicity of antifungal agents, especially amphotericin B, has been a major area of research in recent years. The toxicity of amphotericin B can be divided into infusion-related adverse effects, which occur in nearly every patient and generally do not require alteration of therapy, and adverse effects that are not infusion-related, are often severe, and may necessitate a reduction or temporary cessation of therapy[80] (Table 2). Infusion-related reactions usually become less severe with continued therapy, although many patients may have severe reactions requiring treatment. Pretreatment with acetaminophen, aspirin, antihistamines, meperidine, or phenothiazine antiemetic agents is often effective in reducing these adverse effects.[17,80] In addition to these measures, 25–50 mg of hydrocortisone can be added directly to the infusion container.[81] Thrombophlebitis is also a common adverse effect associated with amphotericin B infusion. Slow infusion of the drug over four to six hours, rotation of the infusion site, application of hot packs, using inline filters (not less than 0.45 μm), and the addition of 500–1000 units of heparin to the infusion container may be useful measures in minimizing vein irritation.[80]

Table 2.
Adverse Effects of Systemic Antifungal Drugs

Drug	Adverse Effects
Amphotericin B, infusion-related	Fever
	Chills
	Nausea
	Vomiting
	Anorexia
	Headache
	Myalgias
	Arthralgias
	Phlebitis
	Ventricular fibrillation (anuric patients)
Amphotericin B, non-infusion-related	Renal dysfunction
	Hypokalemia
	Anemia
	Pulmonary dysfunction (with leukocyte infusions)
	Thrombocytopenia
	Leukopenia
	Grand mal seizures (rare)
	Cardiac arrest (rare)
	Anaphylaxis (rare)
Flucytosine	Anorexia
	Nausea
	Vomiting
	Abdominal pain
	Colitis
	Bone marrow suppression
	Rash
	Hepatic dysfunction (rare)
Ketoconazole	Nausea
	Vomiting
	Anorexia
	Rash
	Pruritus
	Endocrine suppression
	Menstrual irregularities
	Gynecomastia
	Hepatitis (rare)
Miconazole	Phlebitis
	Pruritus
	Rash
	Nausea
	Seizures
	Dyspnea
	Hypotension
	Hyponatremia
	Anemia
	Thrombocytopenia
	Cardiorespiratory arrest (rare)[a]
	Anaphylaxis (rare)[a]
	Hyperlipidemia (rare)[a]

[a] Probably attributable to the Cremophor EL stabilizer.

Renal function declines by 20–72% in nearly every patient treated with amphotericin B and is not infusion related.[12,17,82,83] Clinical manifestations of amphotericin B nephrotoxicity include renal tubular acidosis, loss of urine-acidifying capacity, presence of casts in the urine, azotemia, and oliguria.[80,83,84] In a study of eight patients treated with cumulative doses of 720–2000 mg of amphotericin B, Burgess and Birchall[83] found a decrease in the glomerular filtration rate of every patient. There was no correlation between the degree of renal impairment and the total administered dose of amphotericin B, although no patient received more than 2 g of drug. The authors speculated that severe permanent renal damage results from total doses in excess of 5 g, implying that serious nephrotoxicity may correlate with higher total doses of amphotericin B.

Several mechanisms for amphotericin B nephrotoxicity have been proposed. Heidemann et al.[82] have suggested that there is a tubuloglomerular feedback mechanism in the presence of sodium depletion, whereby a paradoxical increase in the delivery and reabsorption of monovalent ions in the distal tubule initiates a decrease in that nephron's glomerular filtration rate. In the presence of sodium loading, this feedback mechanism is minimized. They postulated that, in the sodium-depleted state, amphotericin B enhances the activity of this reflex arc by altering the permeability of the proximal tubule, thereby further increasing the delivery of monovalent ions to the distal tubule and further reducing the glomerular filtration rate. Burgess and Birchall[83] have suggested several other possibilities, including renal arteriolar spasm, calcium deposition during periods of ischemia, and direct tubular or renal cellular toxicity. The actual mechanism may be a combination of some or all of these.

Several modifications of the amphotericin B molecule have been made in an attempt to reduce adverse effects, particularly nephrotoxicity, while maintaining high antifungal activity. Amphotericin B methyl ester showed markedly reduced nephrotoxicity compared with amphotericin B but was subsequently found to be neurotoxic.[17] *N*-D-ornithyl amphotericin B methyl ester appears to have a similar spectrum and lower renal toxicity than amphotericin B. Studies in laboratory animals, however, have shown that doses much higher than those required with amphotericin B are necessary to achieve similar clinical results and that this ester is also neurotoxic.[38,85,86] Incorporating amphotericin B into phospholipid bilayer vesicles (liposomes) has been found to enhance the therapeutic index of amphotericin B by 20-fold.[87] Complete or partial remission of infection was achieved with liposomal amphotericin B in 8 of 12 immunocompromised cancer patients with fungal infections in whom conventional amphotericin B therapy had failed.[88]

Bullock and colleagues[84] investigated the effect of 1 g/kg of intravenous mannitol administered with amphotericin B. In this controlled study of 11 adult patients, mannitol did not prevent functional or histological nephrotoxicity from amphotericin B therapy. Sodium bicarbonate administration has also failed to prevent amphotericin B nephrotoxicity, although its use may be indicated in the presence of renal tubular acidosis.[80] In a study by Heidemann and colleagues[82] investigating their hypothesis of an enhanced tubuloglomerular feedback mechanism as a cause of nephrotoxicity, sodium depletion occurred in four of five patients receiving amphotericin B, and amphotericin B therapy was discontinued in four patients for one to four days. After the sodium in their diets was increased to 150–300 meq/day, all patients completed the amphotericin B course, with clinical resolution of their fungal infections and without further deterioration of kidney function. Whether hyponatremia is a risk factor for nephrotoxicity attributable to amphotericin B therapy, or whether sodium loading before therapy could protect against nephrotoxicity, as suggested in this study, requires further investigation. Currently, for adult patients, serum creatinine and BUN concentrations should be monitored regularly during treatment, and amphotericin B therapy should be discontinued for 24–48 hours if the serum creatinine concentration reaches 2.5–3.0 mg/dL, or if the BUN reaches 100 mg/dL.[80]

Hypokalemia occurs in nearly every patient treated with amphotericin B. The mechanism of this effect has yet to be determined but may be due to slight, infusion-related increases in serum potassium concentrations, documented in patients with renal failure,[89] which may result in transient increases in the excretion of potassium in patients with normal kidney function. Potassium loss may also be a result of direct damage to the distal tubule. This contrasts with the severe hyperkalemia seen in anuric patients, which will be discussed. Daily or every-other-day monitoring of serum potassium levels and aggressive potassium replacement are essential during treatment with amphotericin B. Serum magnesium levels may also decrease during therapy and should be monitored weekly.

Anemia is often associated with amphotericin B therapy. Maximal decreases in hemoglobin are observed after 3 to 10 weeks of therapy and are usually 18–35% below baseline. The anemia is usually normochromic and normocytic and is probably mediated by suppression of erythrocyte production, which may involve an inhibition of erythropoietin synthesis.[80] In most patients, the hemoglobin stabilizes and may even return to normal with no alteration in therapy. This differs substantially from the hematologic toxicities associated with flucytosine.

Other rare adverse reactions to amphotericin B therapy have been reported and deserve discussion. Ventricular fibrillation after rapid (less than one hour) infusions of amphotericin B has been reported in anuric adult patients. This complication is likely caused by the action of amphotericin B on cellular membranes, causing a release of intracellular potassium and resulting in a dramatic rise in serum potassium concentrations, up to 8.4 meq/L in one report.[89] The absence of this complication in patients with normal kidney function can be explained by their ability to excrete the released potassium renally, thereby maintaining the serum potassium concentration in the normal range. When amphotericin B is used in patients with renal failure, the drug should be administered during dialysis to remove the potassium (amphotericin B is poorly dialyzed); azotemic patients who are not on dialysis should receive slow infusions. Doses greater than 1 mg/kg, even in patients with normal renal function, should be given over four to six hours.[89] Close monitoring of the serum potassium level is indicated in all patients. Although it is rare, hepatotoxicity has been linked to amphotericin B therapy, possibly because of the desoxycholate bile salt used in the commercial preparation (Fungizone, E. R. Squibb & Sons, Inc.).[90] Thrombocytopenia,[91] leukopenia,[56] grand mal seizures, cardiac arrest,[83] and allergic reactions[80] have also been reported, but their relationship to amphotericin B therapy remains uncertain. Fatal pulmonary reactions after the administration of amphotericin B in conjunction with leukocyte transfusions have occurred[92] (see Drug Interactions, below).

Amphotericin B toxicity appears to be less common in infants and children than in adults and may be related to higher clearance seen in children. A recent study of 10 pediatric patients found only a modest rise in serum concentrations of creatinine and BUN, which resolved during therapy.[37] Other toxicities were uncommon. However, substantive data on amphotericin B in pediatric patients are limited.

Flucytosine. Flucytosine is associated with relatively few adverse effects, but some of these may be potentially lethal. In contrast to amphotericin B, many of the toxicities of flucytosine correlate with the serum concentration of the drug. The most common adverse reactions to flucytosine are gastrointestinal in origin (Table 2), occur in about 6% of patients, and usually are not severe.[17,26,27] Intestinal perforation has been attributed to flucytosine therapy but appears to be extremely rare, and the association is questionable.[93] Abnormal hepatic function occurs in approximately 5% of patients but is usually mild, transient, and does not require altering therapy.[26]

Perhaps the most alarming toxicity associated with flucytosine therapy is suppression of the bone marrow.[94] In a study of 15 adult patients receiving flucytosine, the four patients who developed bone marrow toxicity (neutropenia in three, pancytopenia in one) had serum concentrations of flucytosine in excess of 125 μg/mL for 2 to 14 days.[95] Three of four of these patients had renal impairment, and all had received previous or concurrent treatment with nephrotoxic drugs (amphotericin B or gentamicin). A reduction in serum concentrations of flucytosine resolved the neutropenia in three patients, but one patient died as a result of bone marrow aplasia.

Conversion of substantial amounts of flucytosine to the antimetabolite fluorouracil in the body has been demonstrated and may account for the severe gastrointestinal and hematologic toxicities seen in some patients.[19] In seven adults treated with flucytosine, all were found to have at least one serum sample with concentrations of fluorouracil in excess of 1 μg/mL, and five developed adverse effects to flucytosine therapy. Serum concentrations of fluorouracil at this level are commonly observed with antineoplastic doses of this drug and are known to be associated with gastrointestinal and hematologic toxicity. A good correlation between serum concentrations of flucytosine and fluorouracil was also found (correlation coefficient, 0.789). Although the mechanism for conversion of flucytosine to fluorouracil in humans is not yet understood, the intestinal flora may play a role.[95] Serious bone marrow suppression may be minimized by close monitoring of serum concentrations of flucytosine in patients (1) with renal compromise, (2) receiving nephrotoxic drugs concomitantly (especially amphotericin B), or (3) experiencing hematologic or gastrointestinal toxicity. Serum flucytosine concentrations should be maintained below 100 μg/mL, although periodic measurement of the white blood cell count is a more direct measure of toxicity and is often more accessible.[28,95] Adequate data on adverse effects of flucytosine in infants and children are lacking.

Ketoconazole. Ketoconazole is much less toxic and better tolerated than amphotericin B, and many patients experience no adverse effects from ketoconazole given orally. As with flucytosine, the most common adverse effects are gastrointestinal in origin (Table 2), occurring in 29% of patients.[48] These effects are dose related and are more common among patients receiving 600 to 800 mg or more of ketoconazole per day. Reactions involving the skin and the endocrine system occur in 5–16% of patients.[30,48,49,52,58,59,96–99] Suppression of endocrine hormone synthesis has been documented in several studies, although adverse effects associated with this suppression are unusual with lower or single daily doses, or both. This is probably because ketoconazole has a short half-life (three hours), which allows for a recovery of endocrine function between doses.[96,99] However, high or multiple daily doses of ketoconazole, or both, have been shown to cause substantial inhibition of steroidogenesis. These effects have been exploited in the use of ketoconazole for the treatment of Cushing's syndrome, prostate cancer, and precocious puberty.[22,100] The use of ketoconazole as an antifungal agent in children should be carefully considered in light of this potential adverse effect, and at least one group has advised against its use in pediatric patients.[74]

Hepatotoxicity has been reported with ketoconazole therapy in adult patients. Although this appears to occur only rarely, effects ranging from transient liver enzyme elevation to fulminant hepatitis resulting in death have been reported.[58,101–105] The incidence of hepatotoxicity has been estimated to be 1 in 10,000 treated patients, although the true incidence may be higher.[102] An apparent propensity for ketoconazole-induced hepatitis was found in elderly women with histories of adverse reactions to other antifungal agents.[98] However, these data were from a retrospective review of patient records and require further verification. It appears that ketoconazole hepatotoxicity is independent of dose and cannot be predicted from animal experiments.[105]

The few studies in pediatric patients indicate a lower incidence of adverse effects from ketoconazole therapy than is seen in adults.[50] Further research is needed to better define the toxicity of ketoconazole in children.

Miconazole. A relatively high incidence of adverse effects associated with miconazole and the availability of other agents with equal or superior antifungal activity are the probable reasons for the infrequent use of this drug in patients. However, miconazole is still used in certain situations, and clinicians should be aware of these adverse reactions, which may be serious. Infusion of miconazole is associated with phlebitis, pruritus, maculopapular rash, or nausea in 20–30% of treated adult patients.[54] Other adverse reactions (Table 2) occur with varying frequencies.[17,54] The occurrence of hyperlipidemia has been attributed to the Cremophor EL stabilizer in the intravenous formulation.[54] Cardiac and respiratory arrest and anaphylaxis associated with the first dose, which may also be due to the stabilizer rather than the drug, have been reported by Fainstein and Bodey.[76] In their study, the drug had been diluted in less than 200 mL of total volume in five of seven patients with toxicity. The manufacturer recommends dilution into at least 200 mL of diluent. When this guideline is followed and the drug is infused over at least two hours, cardiorespiratory arrest may be avoided.[76] As with ketoconazole, adverse effects in pediatric patients treated with miconazole are poorly understood, and further work is needed.

Drug Interactions

The effects of amphotericin B on host-cell membranes are similar to its effects on fungal cell walls, although much less pronounced. The result is an increase in the permeability of host cells to other agents, such as flucytosine, potentiating the toxicity of the second agent.[10,68] Amphotericin B may also enhance the toxicity of flucytosine by decreasing renal function, resulting in accumulation of flucytosine.[95] Additive toxicity of amphotericin B plus flucytosine has been well documented, but therapeutic benefits appear to outweigh the risks of this combination for most patients.[26,34,35,60]

Leukocyte transfusions given with amphotericin B infusions have been reported to result in serious and fatal pulmonary reactions. In rabbits, amphotericin B promoted aggregation of transfused leukocytes, which became entrapped in the microvasculature of the lung and resulted in pulmonary edema and hemorrhage.[106] In a review of patients treated over a period of six and one-half years, those who received amphotericin B with leukocyte transfusions were 10 times more likely to have respiratory deterioration than patients who received leukocytes alone.[92] The authors noted, however, that all patients developing respiratory distress also had gram-negative infections. The possibility of endotoxemia playing a role in the development of respiratory failure must be considered. In contrast, Dana and coworkers[107] found no difference in the incidence of respiratory deterioration in 23 patients receiving granulocytes with amphotericin B compared with 69 patients who received granulocyte transfusions without amphotericin B. However, this was a retrospective study, and there may be significant type II error in this analysis because of relatively small sample sizes. Thus, the combined use of amphotericin B and leukocytes should be avoided if possible. For patients who require both agents, (1) the two infusions should be given as far apart as possible; (2) the amphotericin B should be administered slowly; and (3) the patients should be monitored closely for respiratory deterioration.[92] If the infusions must be given close together, there is also a theoretical benefit of administering the amphotericin B first to allow for distribution of the amphotericin B (decreasing the serum concentration) before the leukocytes are administered.

The combination of amphotericin B and miconazole, for most fungi, is antagonistic.[12,71,72] This is probably due to a miconazole-induced reduction of ergosterol in the fungal cell wall, resulting in decreased binding sites for amphotericin B. This antagonism has been documented both in vitro and in vivo, and the combination should be avoided when possible. Ketoconazole appears to have a similar interaction with amphotericin B on some fungi, although there have been favorable reports of the use of this combination.[108,109]

Renal function should be assessed frequently in patients receiving flucytosine. However, measurement of serum creatinine using the Kodak Ektachem system has been reported to produce falsely elevated values in patients receiving flucytosine.[110] Flucytosine and creatinine are structurally similar molecules, and flucytosine apparently interferes with this assay. The authors suggested that the Jaffe method be used for the measurement of creatinine (which is not affected by flucytosine).

Ketoconazole undergoes hepatic metabolism and therefore interacts with several agents that undergo similar metabolic processes. In a patient with concomitant fungal and mycobacterial infections, treatment with a combination of ketoconazole, rifampin, and isoniazid failed to resolve either infection.[111] Serum concentrations of both rifampin and ketoconazole were markedly reduced. The proposed mechanisms are that rifampin and isoniazid induce the metabolism of ketoconazole, while ketoconazole inhibits the absorption of rifampin.[46,111] Ketoconazole has been reported to inhibit hepatic metabolism of cyclosporine, resulting in significantly increased serum cyclosporine concentrations and decreased renal function.[112] These data are supported by similar findings in laboratory animals.[113-115] Ketoconazole absorption may be inhibited by agents that increase gastric pH, such as antacids, H_2-receptor antagonists, and food,[46,47] while the corticosteroid-antagonist properties of ketoconazole may decrease the effects of exogenous steroid therapy.[22] The clinical importance of these interactions is not yet known, but they must be considered for any patient receiving any of these combinations, particularly if the therapeutic results are unexpected.

Ketoconazole and miconazole enhance the hypoprothrombinemic effect of oral anticoagulants, presumably by liver enzyme inhibition.[116] If imidazole therapy is started, stopped, or altered in patients receiving an oral anticoagulant, prothrombin time should be monitored closely and the anticoagulant dose should be adjusted as needed.

Selecting an Antifungal Agent

Many factors must be considered in selecting an appropriate agent to treat fungal infection. One of the most important considerations is early identification of the organism. As shown in Table 1, most organisms can be adequately treated with amphotericin B, so perhaps the next important question is: Can a less toxic agent be used? This is especially important to consider in patients who have received, or are receiving, other nephrotoxic agents. Many cancer patients are treated with myelosuppressive agents, and careful consideration needs to be given to the toxic effects of flucytosine on bone marrow before it is used in this population. In addition, the clinician must remember that renal function greatly influences the pharmacokinetics of flucytosine. Ketoconazole is usually given once daily, but with some infections requiring 800 mg/day or more, this is often not possible because of the high incidence of gastrointestinal discomfort associated with such doses. On the other hand, giving ketoconazole in divided daily doses may result in symptomatic suppression of the adrenal or other endocrine hormone systems. These effects must be weighed on an individual basis.

These are only a few examples of patient-specific conditions that must be considered in the decision-making process for selecting an antifungal regimen. Any antifungal regimen must be individualized with respect to organism, location of the infection, underlying disease and organ function (e.g., renal, hepatic, endocrine), concomitant medications, and adverse effects.

Conclusion

Amphotericin B, flucytosine, ketoconazole, and miconazole are antifungal agents currently available for the treatment of serious systemic fungal infections. Amphotericin B and miconazole are associated with a high incidence of adverse effects, and flucytosine results in frequent therapeutic failures when used alone. Several new agents are currently being evaluated; they represent urgently needed additions to the antifungal drug class. In addition to the need for more effective and less toxic agents, research is needed to (1) characterize the pharmacokinetics, pharmacodynamics, and adverse effects of currently available agents, particularly in pediatric patients; (2) define optimal dosing regimens for amphotericin B in treating various fungal infections at various sites; and (3) identify the predictors of amphotericin B nephrotoxicity.

References

1. Chesney PJ, Teets KC, Mulvihill JJ et al. Successful treatment of *Candida* meningitis with amphotericin B and 5-fluorocytosine in combination. *J Pediatr*. 1976; 89:1017–9.
2. Young LS. Current needs in chemotherapy for bacterial and fungal infections. *Rev Infect Dis*. 1985; 7(suppl 3):S380–S388.
3. Rippon JW. A new era in antimycotic agents. *Arch Dermatol*. 1986; 122:399–402.
4. Van Cutsem J. The antifungal activity of ketoconazole. *Am J Med*. 1983; 74(1B):9–15.
5. Odds FC. Problems in the laboratory assessment of antifungal activity. *Postgrad Med J*. 1979; 55:677–80.
6. Bennett JE. Antifungal agents. In: Principles and practice of infectious diseases. Mandell GL, Bennett JE, eds. New York: John Wiley & Sons, Inc.; 1985:264.
7. American hospital formulary service—drug information 87. McEvoy GK, ed. Bethesda, MD: American Society of Hospital Pharmacists, 1987:67.
8. Kotler-Brajtburg J, Medoff G, Schlessinger D et al. Characterization of the binding of amphotericin B to *Saccharomyces cerevisiae* and relationship to the antifungal effects. *Antimicrob Agents Chemother*. 1974; 6:770–6.
9. Kotler-Brajtburg J, Price HD, Medoff G et al. Molecular basis for the selective toxicity of amphotericin B for yeast and filipin for animal cells. *Antimicrob Agents Chemother*. 1974; 5:377–82.
10. Medoff G, Kobayashi GS. Amphotericin B: old drug, new therapy. *JAMA*. 1975; 232:619–20.
11. Medoff G, Comfort M, Kobayashi GS. Synergistic action of amphotericin B and 5-fluorocytosine against yeast-like organisms. *Proc Soc Exp Biol Med*. 1971; 138:571–4.
12. Medoff G, Kobayashi GS. Strategies in the treatment of systemic fungal infections. *N Engl J Med*. 1980; 302:145–55.
13. Hoeprich PD, Huston AC. Susceptibility of *Coccidioides immitis, Candida albicans,* and *Cryptococcus neoformans* to amphotericin B, flucytosine, and clotrimazole. *J Infect Dis*. 1975; 132:133–41.
14. Shirley SF, Little JR. Immunopotentiating effects of amphotericin B: I. Enhanced contact sensitivity in mice. *J Immunol*. 1979; 123:2878–82.
15. Shirley SF, Little JR. Immunopotentiating effects of amphotericin B: II. Enhanced in vitro proliferative responses of murine lymphocytes. *J Immunol*. 1979; 123:2883–9.
16. Thomas M, Medoff G, Kobayashi GF. Resistance to *Listeria monocytogenes* infections induced by amphotericin B. *J Infect Dis*. 1973; 127:373–7.
17. Koldin MH, Medoff G. Antifungal chemotherapy. *Pediatr Clin North Am*. 1983; 30:49–61.
18. Polack A. Effects of 5-fluorocytosine on protein synthesis and amino acid pool in *Candida albicans*. *Sabouraudia*. 1974; 12:309–19.
19. Diasio RB, Lakings DE, Bennett JE. Evidence for conversion of 5-fluorocytosine to 5-fluorouracil in humans: possible factor in 5-fluorocytosine clinical toxicity. *Antimicrob Agents Chemother*. 1978; 14:903–8.
20. Borgers M, Van den Bossche H, De Brabander M. The mechanism of action of the new antimycotic ketoconazole. *Am J Med*. 1983; 74(1B):2–8.
21. Van den Bossche H, Willemsens G, Cools W et al. In vitro and in vivo effects of the antimycotic drug ketoconazole on sterol synthesis. *Antimicrob Agents Chemother*. 1980; 17:922–8.
22. Feldman D. Ketoconazole and other imidazole derivatives as inhibitors of steroidogenesis. *Endocr Rev*. 1986; 7:409–20.
23. Fainstein V, Bodey GP, Elting L et al. Amphotericin B or ketoconazole therapy of fungal infections in neutropenic cancer patients. *Antimicrob Agents Chemother*. 1987; 31:11–5.
24. Graybill JR, Lundberg D, Donovan W et al. Treatment of coccidioidomycosis with ketoconazole: clinical and laboratory studies of 18 patients. *Rev Infect Dis*. 1980; 2:661–73.
25. Christiansen KJ, Bernard EM, Gold JWM et al. Distribution and activity of amphotericin B in humans. *J Infect Dis*. 1985; 152:1037–43.
26. Bennett JE. Flucytosine. *Ann Intern Med*. 1977; 86:319–22.
27. Harder EJ, Hermans PE. Treatment of fungal infections with flucytosine. *Arch Intern Med*. 1975; 135:231–7.
28. Anon. Drugs for treatment of systemic fungal infections. *Med Let Drugs Ther*. 1986; 28:41–4.
29. Fisher JF, Chew WH, Shadomy S et al. Urinary tract infections due to *Candida albicans*. *Rev Infect Dis*. 1982; 4:1107–18.
30. Dismukes WE, Stamm AM, Graybill JR et al. Treatment of systemic mycoses with ketoconazole: emphasis on toxicity and clinical response in 52 patients. *Ann Intern Med*. 1983;

98:13–20.
31. Shadomy S, White SC, Yu HP et al. Treatment of systemic mycoses with ketoconazole: in vitro susceptibilities of clinical isolates of systemic and pathogenic fungi to ketoconazole. *J Infect Dis.* 1985; 152:1249–56.
32. Powell DA, Aungst J, Snedden S et al. Broviac catheter-related *Malassezia furfur* sepsis in five infants receiving intravenous fat emulsions. *J Pediatr.* 1984; 105:987–90.
33. Polak A. Pharmacokinetics of amphotericin B and flucytosine. *Postgrad Med J.* 1979; 55:667–70.
34. Utz JP, Garriques IL, Sande MA et al. Therapy of cryptococcosis with a combination of flucytosine and amphotericin B. *J Infect Dis.* 1975; 132:368–73.
35. Bryan CS, McFarland JA. Cryptococcal meningitis: fatal marrow aplasia from combined therapy. *JAMA.* 1978; 239:1068–9.
36. Atkinson AJ, Bennett JE. Amphotericin B pharmacokinetics in humans. *Antimicrob Agents Chemother.* 1978; 13:271–6.
37. Starke JR, Mason EO, Kramer WG et al. Pharmacokinetics of amphotericin B in infants and children. *J Infect Dis.* 1987; 155:766–74.
38. Perfect JR, Durack DT. Comparison of amphotericin B and *N*-D-ornithyl amphotericin B methyl ester in experimental cryptococcal meningitis and *Candida albicans* endocarditis with pyelonephritis. *Antimicrob Agents Chemother.* 1985; 28:751–5.
39. Baley J, Meters C, Kliegman R et al. Pharmacokinetics of amphotericin B and 5-fluorocytosine in neonates. *Pediatr Res.* 1986; 20:201. Abstract.
40. Brajtburg J, Elberg S, Bolard J et al. Interaction of plasma proteins and lipoproteins with amphotericin B. *J Infect Dis.* 1984; 149:986–97.
41. Craven PC, Ludden TM, Drutz DJ et al. Excretion pathways of amphotericin B. *J Infect Dis.* 1979; 140:329–41.
42. Reynolds ES, Tomkiewicz ZM, Dammin GJ. The renal lesion related to amphotericin B treatment for coccidioidomycosis. *Med Clin North Am.* 1963; 47:1149–54.
43. Cutler RE, Blair AD, Kelly MR. Flucytosine kinetics in subjects with normal and impaired renal function. *Clin Pharmacol Ther.* 1978; 24:333–42.
44. Schönebeck J, Polak A, Fernex M et al. Pharmacokinetic studies on the oral antimycotic agent 5-fluorocytosine in individuals with normal and impaired kidney function. *Chemotherapy.* 1973; 18:321–36.
45. Block ER, Bennett JE, Livoti LG et al. Flucytosine and amphotericin B: hemodialysis effects on the plasma concentration and clearance. *Ann Intern Med.* 1974; 80:613–7.
46. Brass C, Galgiani JN, Blaschke TF et al. Disposition of ketoconazole, an oral antifungal, in humans. *Antimicrob Agents Chemother.* 1982; 21:151–8.
47. Negroni R, Robles AM, Arechavala A et al. Ketoconazole in the treatment of paracoccidioidomycosis and histoplasmosis. *Rev Infect Dis.* 1980; 2:643–9.
48. NIAID Mycoses Study Group. Treatment of blastomycosis and histoplasmosis with ketoconazole: results of a prospective randomized clinical trial. *Ann Intern Med.* 1985; 103(6, pt 1):861–72.
49. Bradsher RW, Rice DC, Abernathy RS. Ketoconazole therapy for endemic blastomycosis. *Ann Intern Med.* 1985; 103(6, pt 1):872–9.
50. Bardare M, Tortorano AM, Pietrogrande MC et al. Pharmacokinetics of ketoconazole and treatment evaluation in candidal infections. *Arch Dis Child.* 1984; 59:1068–71.
51. Ginsburg CM, McCracken GH, Olsen K. Pharmacology of ketoconazole suspension in infants and children. *Antimicrob Agents Chemother.* 1983; 23:787–9.
52. Goodpasture HC, Hershberger RE, Barnett AM et al. Treatment of central nervous system fungal infection with ketoconazole. *Arch Intern Med.* 1985; 145:879–80.
53. Drouhet E, Dupont B. Laboratory and clinical assessment of ketoconazole in deep-seated mycoses. *Am J Med.* 1983; 74(1B):30–47.
54. Hoeprich PD, Lawrence RM, Goldstein E. Treatment of coccidioidomycosis with miconazole. *JAMA.* 1980; 243:1923–6.
55. Mycoses. In: Mandell GL, Douglas RG, Jr, Bennett JE, eds. Principles and practice of infectious diseases, 2nd ed. New York: John Wiley & Sons, Inc.; 1985:1434–1504.
56. Hermans PE, Keys TF: Antifungal agents used for deep-seated mycotic infections. *Mayo Clin Proc.* 1983; 58:223–31.
57. Medoff G, Kobayashi GS. Fungal diseases. In: Feigin RD, Cherry JD, eds. Textbook of pediatric infectious diseases, 2nd ed. Philadelphia: W. B. Saunders Company; 1987:1925–2006.
58. Petersen EA, Alling DW, Kirkpatrick CH. Treatment of chronic mucocutaneous candidiasis with ketoconazole: a controlled clinical trial. *Ann Intern Med.* 1980; 93:791–5.
59. DeFelice R, Galgiani JN, Campbell SC et al. Ketoconazole treatment of nonprimary coccidioidomycosis: evaluation of 60 patients during three years of study. *Am J Med.* 1982; 72:681–7.
60. Bennett JE, Dismukes WE, Duma RJ et al. A comparison of amphotericin B alone and combined with flucytosine in the treatment of cryptococcal meningitis. *N Engl J Med.* 1979; 301:126–31.
61. Cherry JD, Lloyd CA, Quilty JF et al. Amphotericin B therapy in children: a review of the literature and a case report. *J Pediatr.* 1969; 75(6, pt. 1):1063–9.
62. Medoff G, Dismukes WE, Meade RH et al. A new therapeutic approach to candida infections. *Arch Intern Med.* 1972; 130:241–5.
63. Smego RA, Perfect JR, Durback DT. Combined therapy with amphotericin B and 5-fluorocytosine for candida meningitis. *Rev Infect Dis.* 1984; 6:791–801.
64. Block ER, Jennings AE, Bennett JE. 5-fluorocytosine resistance in *Cryptococcus neoformans. Antimicrob Agents Chemother.* 1973; 3:649–56.
65. Block ER, Jennings AE, Bennett JE. Variables influencing susceptibility testing of *Cryptococcus neoformans* to 5-fluorocytosine. *Antimicrob Agents Chemother.* 1973; 4:392–5.
66. Kitahara M, Seth VK, Medoff G et al. Activity of amphotericin B, 5-fluorocytosine, and rifampin against six clinical isolates of *Aspergillus. Antimicrob Agents Chemother.* 1976; 9:915–9.
67. Beggs WH, Sarosi GA, Walker MI. Synergistic action of amphotericin B and rifampin against *Candida* species. *J Infect Dis.* 1976; 133:206–9.
68. Montgomerie JZ, Edwards JE, Guze LB. Synergism of amphotericin B and 5-fluorocytosine for *Candida* species. *J Infect Dis.* 1975; 132:82–6.
69. Rabinovich S, Shaw BD, Bryant T et al. Effect of 5-fluorocytosine and amphotericin B on *Candida albicans* infection in mice. *J Infect Dis.* 1974; 130:28–31.
70. Ward RM, Sattler FR, Dalton AS. Assessment of antifungal therapy in an 800-gram infant with candidal arthritis and osteomyelitis. *Pediatrics.* 1983; 72:234–8.
71. Schacter LP, Owellen RJ, Rathbun HK et al. Antagonism between miconazole and amphotericin B. *Lancet.* 1976; 2:318.
72. Cosgrove RF, Beezer AE, Miles RJ. In vitro studies of amphotericin B in combination with the imidazole antifungal compounds clotrimazole and miconazole. *J Infect Dis.* 1978; 138:681–5.
73. Hawkins SS, Gregory DW, Alford RH. Progressive disseminated histoplasmosis: favorable response to ketoconazole. *Ann Int Med.* 1981; 95:446–9.
74. McManus EJ, Jones JM. The use of ketoconazole in the treatment of blastomycosis. *Am Rev Respir Dis.* 1986; 133:141–3.
75. Bennett JE, Remington JS. Miconazole in cryptococcosis and systemic candidiasis: a word of caution. *Ann Intern Med.* 1981; 94:708–9.
76. Fainstein V, Bodey GP. Cardiorespiratory toxicity due to miconazole. *Ann Intern Med.* 1980; 93:432–3.
77. Van Cutsem J, Van Gerven F, Van den Ven ME et al. Itraconazole, a new triazole that is orally active in aspergil-

losis. *Antimicrob Agents Chemother.* 1984; 26:527–34.

78. Restrepo A, Robledo J, Gómez I et al. Itraconazole therapy in lymphangitic and cutaneous sporotrichosis. *Arch Dermatol.* 1986; 122:413–7.
79. Dupont B, Drouhet E. Cryptoccal meningitis and fluconazole. *Ann Int Med.* 1987; 106:778. Letter.
80. Maddux MS, Barriere SL. A review of complications of amphotericin B therapy: recommendations for prevention and management. *Drug Intell Clin Pharm.* 1980; 14:177–81.
81. Trissel LA. Handbook on injectable drugs, 4th ed. Bethesda, MD: American Society of Hospital Pharmacists; 1986:44.
82. Heidemann HT, Gerkens JF, Spickard WA et al. Amphotericin B nephrotoxicity in humans decreased by salt repletion. *Am J Med.* 1983; 75:476–81.
83. Burgess JL, Birchall R. Nephrotoxicity of amphotericin B, with emphasis on changes in tubular function. *Am J Med.* 1972; 53:77–84.
84. Bullock WE, Luke RG, Nuttall CE et al. Can mannitol reduce amphotericin B nephrotoxicity? Double-blind study and description of a new vascular lesion in kidneys. *Antimicrob Agents Chemother.* 1976; 10:555–63.
85. Kobayashi GS, Little JR, Medoff G. In vitro and in vivo comparisons of amphotericin B and *N*-D-ornithyl amphotericin B methyl ester. *Antimicrob Agents Chemother.* 1985; 27:302–5.
86. Massa T, Sinha DP, Frantz JD et al. Subchronic toxicity studies of *N*-D-ornithyl amphotericin B methyl ester in dogs and rats. *Fundam Appl Toxicol.* 1985; 5:737–53.
87. Lopez-Berenstein G. Liposomal amphotericin B in the treatment of fungal infections. *Ann Int Med.* 1986; 105:130–1. Editorial.
88. Lopez-Berenstein G, Fainstein V, Hopfer R et al. Liposomal amphotericin B for the treatment of systemic fungal infections in patients with cancer: a preliminary study. *J Infect Dis.* 1985; 151:704–10.
89. Craven PC, Gremillion DH. Risk factors of ventricular fibrillation during rapid amphotericin B infusion. *Antimicrob Agents Chemother.* 1985; 27:868–71.
90. Miller MA. Reversible hepatotoxicity related to amphotericin B. *Can Med Assoc J.* 1984; 131:1245–7.
91. Chan CSP, Tuazon CU, Lessin LS. Amphotericin B-induced thrombocytopenia. *Ann Intern Med.* 1982; 96:332–3.
92. Wright DG, Robichaud KJ, Pizzo PA et al. Lethal pulmonary reactions associated with the combined use of amphotericin B and leukocyte transfusions. *N Engl J Med.* 1981; 304: 1185–9.
93. Harder EJ, Hermans PE. Treatment of fungal infections with flucytosine. *Arch Intern Med.* 1975; 135:231–7.
94. Meyer R, Axelrod JL. Fatal aplastic anemia resulting from flucytosine. *JAMA.* 1974; 228:1573.
95. Kauffman CA, Frame PT. Bone marrow toxicity associated with 5-fluorocytosine therapy. *Antimicrob Agents Chemother.* 1977; 11:244–7.
96. Tucker WS, Snell BB, Island DP et al. Reversible adrenal insufficiency induced by ketoconazole. *JAMA.* 1985; 253:2413–4.
97. DeFelice R, Johnson DG, Galgiani JN. Gynecomastia with ketoconazole. *Antimicrob Agents Chemother.* 1981; 19:1073–4.
98. Graybill JR. Summary: potential and problems with ketoconazole. *Am J Med.* 1983; 74(1B):86–90.
99. Pont A, Williams PL, Loose DS et al. Ketoconazole blocks adrenal steroid synthesis. *Ann Int Med.* 1982; 97:370–2.
100. Shepherd FA, Hoffert B, Evans WK et al. Ketoconazole: use in the treatment of ectopic adrenocorticotropic hormone production and Cushing's syndrome in small-cell lung cancer. *Arch Int Med.* 1985; 145:863–4.
101. Bercoff E, Bernau J, Degott C et al. Ketoconazole-induced fulminant hepatitis. *Gut.* 1985; 26:636–8.
102. Janssen PAJ, Symoens JE. Hepatic reaction during ketoconazole treatment. *Am J Med.* 1983; 74(1B):80–5.
103. Macnair AL, Gascoigne E, Heap J. Hepatitis and ketoconazole therapy. *Br Med J.* 1981; 283:1058. Letter.
104. Firebrace DAJ. Hepatitis and ketoconazole therapy. *Br Med J.* 1981; 283:1058–9. Letter.
105. Heiberg JK, Svejgaard E. Toxic hepatitis during ketoconazole treatment. *Br Med J.* 1981; 283:825–6.
106. Boxer LA, Ingraham LM, Allen J et al. Amphotericin-B promotes leukocyte aggregation of nylon-wool-fiber-treated polymorphonuclear leukocytes. *Blood.* 1981; 58:518–23.
107. Dana BW, Durie BGM, White RF et al. Concomitant administration of granulocyte transfusions and amphotericin B in neutropenic patients: absence of significant pulmonary toxicity. *Blood.* 1981; 57:90–4.
108. Fisher JF, Henson DM. Amphotericin B-resistance in *Candida. Ann Intern Med.* 1985; 102:563–4.
109. Goetz MB, Jones JM. Combined ketoconazole and amphotericin B treatment of acute disseminated histoplasmosis in a renal allograft recipient. *South Med J.* 1985; 78:1368–70.
110. Mitchell RT, Marshall LH, Lefkowitz LB et al. Falsely elevated serum creatinine levels secondary to the presence of 5-fluorocytosine. *Am J Clin Pathol.* 1985; 84:251–3.
111. Engelhard D, Stutman HR, Marks MI. Interaction of ketoconazole with rifampin and isoniazid. *N Engl J Med.* 1984; 311:1681–3.
112. Shepard JH, Simmons RL. Cyclosporine-ketoconazole: a potentially dangerous drug-drug interaction. *Clin Pharm.* 1986; 5:468.
113. Anderson JE, Blaschke TF. Ketoconazole inhibits cyclosporine metabolism in vivo in mice. *J Pharmacol Exp Ther.* 1986; 236:671–4.
114. White DJG, Blatchford NR, Cauwenbergh G. Cyclosporine and ketoconazole. *Transplantation.* 1984; 37:214–5.
115. Gumbleton M, Brown JE, Hawksworth G et al. The possible relationship between hepatic drug metabolism and ketoconazole enhancement of cyclosporine nephrotoxicity. *Transplantation.* 1985; 40:454–5.
116. Hansten PD. Drug interactions. 5th ed. Philadelphia: Lea & Febiger; 1985:88.

Stopping Antibiotic Therapy

“Unnecessary continuation of antibiotic therapy in neutropenic patients can result in increased toxicity as well as superinfection with resistant organisms. Antibiotic therapy can be stopped in certain situations despite the persistence of neutropenia. However, careful monitoring of these patients and a low threshold for restarting antibiotic therapy are mandatory. With this approach, patients will at worst end up where they started—stable on antibiotics—and many may be saved the hidden costs of prolonged antibiotic therapy.

—DiNubile MJ. Stopping antibiotic therapy in neutropenic patients. *Ann Intern Med.* 1988; 108:289–92.”

Research

Heparin sodium versus 0.9% sodium chloride injection for maintaining patency of indwelling intermittent infusion devices

ROBERT A. HAMILTON, JEANNINE M. PLIS, CAROL CLAY, AND LAWRENCE SYLVAN

Abstract: In a double-blind study, heparin sodium was compared with 0.9% sodium chloride injection for use in maintaining patency of indwelling devices for intermittent intravenous infusion.

Adult patients who required intermittent intravenous devices were randomly assigned to receive 1 mL of a heparin sodium 100 units/mL flush solution or a 0.9% sodium chloride flush solution. Observations were recorded for each catheter, rather than for each patient. Patients were evaluated daily for the development of phlebitis.

In the 160 patients for whom complete data on catheter patency were available, there were 307 observations (170 for the heparin group and 137 for the sodium chloride group). No significant difference in the duration of catheter patency or incidence of phlebitis was observed between the groups. A difference in the incidence of phlebitis could not be excluded with confidence, but inasmuch as there was no effect on duration of catheter patency, the clinical importance of this superficial venous phlebitis is questionable. The duration of patency was significantly greater in men than in women. The use of penicillins, cephalosporins, or clindamycin, alone or in combination, was significantly associated with the development of phlebitis for both treatment groups. No other factors were found to correlate with either the duration of catheter patency or incidence of phlebitis.

The results of this study indicate that heparin offers no advantage over 0.9% sodium chloride injection in maintaining the patency of intermittent intravenous devices.

Index terms: Antibiotics; Anticoagulants; Catheters; Cephalosporins; Clindamycin; Devices; Drug administration; Heparin sodium; Intravenous therapy; Penicillins; Phlebitis; Sex; Sodium chloride; Toxicity
Clin Pharm. 1988; 7:439–43

The use of dilute heparin solutions to maintain the patency of indwelling devices for intermittent intravenous infusion is accepted at a number of institutions. The large volume of use represents a considerable expense at many institutions. A literature review revealed one randomized, double-blind study, by Epperson,[1] that indicated that the use of heparin solutions did not significantly affect the duration of intravenous-device patency. Oral communication with several hospital pharmacy directors revealed that approximately equal numbers of hospitals use dilute heparin solutions or 0.9% sodium chloride injection.

We shared this limited information with the pharmacy and therapeutics committee and proposed to eliminate the use of heparin for maintaining the patency of intermittent intravenous devices. The initial proposal was not accepted for several reasons: the absence of information regarding the incidence of phlebitis with the use of 0.9% sodium chloride injection, the limited information provided by Epperson's study, the existence of only one study comparing the efficacy of the two solutions for maintaining the patency of these in-

ROBERT A. HAMILTON, PHARM.D., is Assistant Professor of Pharmacy, Department of Pharmacy Practice, Albany College of Pharmacy, Albany, NY. JEANNINE M. PLIS, M.S., is Nutritional Support Specialist; CAROL CLAY, M.S., is Director of Nursing Education; and LAWRENCE SYLVAN, M.S., is Director, Department of Pharmacy Services, Ellis Hospital, Schenectady, NY.
Address reprint requests to Dr. Hamilton at the Albany College of Pharmacy, 106 New Scotland Ave., Albany, NY 12208.

The contributions of Beverly Ciancetta, Phyllis VanWinkle, Mary Ann Schirmer, Minnie Fiorentino, and Aileen Teele in the collection of patient data are acknowledged.

Copyright © 1988, American Society of Hospital Pharmacists, Inc. All rights reserved. 0278-2677/88/0601-0439$01.25.

travenous devices, and the lack of acceptance of 0.9% sodium chloride injection for maintenance of patency by local hospitals. It was recommended that the pharmacy department conduct a study similar to that of Epperson, addressing issues not covered previously (e.g., phlebitis, the effect of heparin solutions on the incidence of phlebitis secondary to intravenous antibiotics, and potential confounding variables such as recent surgery or history of neoplastic disease).

The objective of this study was to compare heparin sodium 100 units/mL with 0.9% sodium chloride injection for use in the maintenance of intermittent intravenous devices. Study endpoints were (1) the duration of catheter patency, (2) the incidence of phlebitis, and (3) the determination of patient characteristics that correlated with the duration of catheter patency or the development of phlebitis.

Methods

All admitted adult patients who were to have an intermittent intravenous device inserted were considered eligible for this study. Patients admitted to the intensive-care units were excluded. Intermittent intravenous devices (either plastic catheters or steel needles [butterflies]) were inserted by the intravenous-therapy team, which was made up of registered nurses who received standardized training regarding the insertion of these devices. After the initial insertion, the device was flushed with dilute heparin sodium solution (100 units/mL). Patients were then randomly assigned, using a computer-generated assignment sheet, to receive heparin sodium flush solution or 0.9% sodium chloride flush solution. The study was conducted in a double-blind fashion. The assigned solutions were supplied in the standard manner used for all unit dose medications in the hospital.

The study solution (either heparin sodium or 0.9% sodium chloride injection) was used to flush the intermittent intravenous device every shift (every eight hours) if the patient received no intravenous medications. If the patient received intermittent intravenous medications, the device was flushed with a sodium chloride solution before and after the medication was administered. Then 1 mL of the study solution was used to flush the device. The patient continued to be assigned to the same study solution throughout the course of therapy with the intermittent intravenous device (i.e., a patient assigned to the sodium chloride group would continue to receive 0.9% sodium chloride injection if the intravenous device was replaced). For the purposes of the study, observations were recorded for each catheter, rather than each patient. This study was approved by the institutional review board.

The study solutions were prepared using empty 2-mL sterile cartridge–needle units (Carpuject, Winthrop Laboratories, lot MO63XE) and bacteriostatic 0.9% Sodium Chloride Injection, USP (benzyl alcohol preserved, Abbott Laboratories, lot 93-866-DK) or Heparin Lock Flush Solution, USP, 100 units/mL of heparin sodium (Hep-lock, Elkins-Sinn, Inc., lot 027006). The heparin lock flush solution was preserved with benzyl alcohol, as were the prefilled syringe cartridges that were used previously at the hospital. Each cartridge was filled with approximately 1.3 mL of either 0.9% sodium chloride injection or heparin lock flush solution. Each cartridge was labeled with a lot number and a solution letter. Four solution letters were used, two for heparin solutions and two for sodium chloride solutions. Two letters were used for each group to further protect the blinding of the study.

Table 1.
Phlebitis Grades

Grade 0	No pain, erythema, venous cord at site
Grade 1	Patient complains of pain but no obvious inflammation at the site
Grade 2	Visible evidence of phlebitis at the site (e.g., redness, palpable cord)

Patients were evaluated daily for the development of phlebitis by one of five registered nurses whose only contact with the patients resulted from their involvement in this study. These nurses were blinded to the group assignment. The daily evaluation included assessment of phlebitis using a modification of the method of Maddox et al.[2] (see Table 1). In addition to the grade of phlebitis, the following information was also recorded: the date and time the intravenous device was inserted; the type, manufacturer, and gauge of the device; patient diagnoses; type of nursing unit; history of recent surgery (i.e., during this hospitalization); and reason for discontinuation of the device. During the study period, the supplier of Teflon catheters to the hospital was changed, necessitating the recording of the manufacturer of each patient's catheter. Finally, concomitant drug therapy was recorded by pharmacy personnel.

Chi-square analysis or Student's t test for unpaired data was used to determine whether the use of heparin solution, 0.9% sodium chloride injection, or any of the variables recorded above were associated with duration of catheter patency or incidence of phlebitis. Student's t test was used for continuous variables, and chi-square analysis was used for dichotomous variables. The a priori level of significance was $p < 0.05$. The study hypothesis stated that no difference would be found between the two study groups. Preliminary sample size calculations indicated that the sample size should be 250 observations (125 per group) to achieve a beta error of 0.20 (alpha = 0.05, standard deviation = 18 hours, mean = 48 hours) by the method of Stolley and Strom.[3]

Results

A total of 241 patients were enrolled in the study. Incomplete data on the duration of catheter patency reduced that number to 160 patients. Reasons for not including observations or patients in the analysis are given in Table 2. In these 160 patients, there were a total of 307 observations, for an average of 1.92 catheters per patient. Table 3 shows the patient demographic data based on each observation or catheter (rather than individual patients). The study was designed to maintain patients in their assigned group as long as they continued to receive intermittent therapy through an intravenous catheter. This design stipulation resulted in an unequal distribution of the number of observations in the heparin group versus the sodium chloride group. This is reflected in the average number of catheters per patient in each group. The distribution of observations in men versus women between the two groups was significantly different. There were no other significant differences between the two groups.

Table 4 displays data on the duration of catheter patency in the heparin and sodium chloride groups. The mean duration of catheter patency in men was 47.8 hours, which was significantly different than that observed in women (42.5 hours). No significant differences were observed for any of the other variables examined. After adjustments were made for the difference in duration of catheter patency between men and women and the unequal distribution of the sexes between the heparin and sodium chloride groups, no significant difference in the duration of catheter patency between the heparin and sodium chloride groups was observed. The small number of patients who had steel needles (butterflies) as their intravenous device precludes any generalizations regarding patency and steel needles. Neither a history of cancer nor recent surgery significantly influenced the duration of catheter patency. Interestingly, there was no correlation between the duration of catheter patency and the grade of phlebitis.

Table 5 provides data on the incidence of phlebi-

Table 2.
Reasons for Not Including Observations in Analysis

Reason	No. Observations in Group	
	Sodium Chloride (*n* = 39)	Heparin (*n* = 58)
Device discontinued before observation[a]	16	19
Time of discontinuation not documented	10	20
Phlebitis grade 0	9	17
Phlebitis grade 1	0	1
Phlebitis grade 2	1	1
Grade not reported	0	1
I.V. therapy changed from intermittent to continuous infusion	12	17
Patient transferred to intensive-care unit	1	2

[a] Used less than 24 hours in all cases.

Table 3.
Patient Demographic Data

Characteristic	No. (%) Observations in Group[a]	
	Heparin (*n* = 170)	Sodium Chloride (*n* = 137)
Male	67 (39)	75 (55)
Female	103 (61)	62 (45)
Age of >60 years	132 (78)	104 (76)
Nursing unit		
Medical	86 (51)	81 (59)
Surgical	56 (33)	44 (32)
Orthopedic	21 (12)	11 (8)
Other	7(4)	1(1)
Drug use		
Penicillins	40 (24)	37 (27)
Cephalosporins	71 (42)	42 (31)
Clindamycin	9 (5)	8 (6)
Estrogens	5 (3)	1 (1)
Catheter or needle		
Plastic (Deseret, Hartford, CT)	89 (52)	70 (51)
Plastic (Terumo, Piscataway, NJ)	78 (46)	66 (48)
Butterfly	3 (2)	1 (1)
Mean ± S.D. no. catheters (range)	2.1 ± 1.3 (1–5)	1.7 ± 1.1 (1–7)
No. patients	80	80

[a] Percentages are based on the number of observations rather than the number of patients.

Table 4.
Duration of Catheter Patency

Characteristic	Mean (± S.D.) No. Hours of Patency	
	Heparin Group	Sodium Chloride Group
Overall	44.3 ± 18.6	45.4 ± 17.7
Drug use		
Penicillins	44.9 ± 23.7	42.9 ± 18.5
Cephalosporins	44.1 ± 17.7	43.4 ± 18.2
Clindamycin	39.9 ± 18.5	41.4 ± 17.2
Estrogens	40.2 ± 14.7	36
Gender		
Female	42.7 ± 17.8	41.5 ± 16.1
Male	46.9 ± 19.4	48.6 ± 18.2
Nursing unit		
Medical	43.8 ± 17.1	46.7 ± 18.7
Surgical	47.0 ± 19.7	45.0 ± 16.3
Orthopedic	45.1 ± 18.5	35.6 ± 10.4
Catheter or needle		
Plastic (Deseret)	43.6 ± 17.1	44.9 ± 17.5
Plastic (Terumo)	45.1 ± 20.1	45.9 ± 17.8
Butterfly	47.0 ± 18.0	68
Phlebitis grade		
0 (absent)	44.9 ± 18.8	45.1 ± 17.3
1 (pain only)	39.9 ± 16.4	48.8 ± 16.9
2 (visible)	44.6 ± 18.3	46.2 ± 17.8
Disease state		
Cancer	43.7 ± 11.2	47.0 ± 17.4
Recent surgery	48.6 ± 20.7	42.0 ± 14.6

tis. The incidence of grade 1 phlebitis was similar for the heparin (10%) and sodium chloride (9%) groups. A higher incidence of grade 2 phlebitis was observed in the sodium chloride group (18%) compared with the heparin group (11%), but this difference was not significant (chi square = 3.81, d.f. = 2, $p = 0.147$). However, a difference in the incidence of grade 2 phlebitis between the two groups cannot be excluded with confidence. The relative difference we could have detected was 106% (with alpha = 0.05 and beta = 0.2). Patient gender, device gauge, and history of cancer or recent surgery were not associated with phlebitis. The intravenous use of drugs commonly thought to induce phlebitis (i.e., penicillins, cephalosporins, or clindamycin) produced approximately twice as much phlebitis as that in patients not receiving these drugs. This increased incidence of phlebitis was statistically significant (chi square = 12.3, d.f. = 1, $p < 0.001$) and was not demonstrated to be affected by the concurrent use of 0.9% sodium chloride injection or heparin sodium flush.

The reason for discontinuing each intravenous device was also recorded (Table 6). No significant difference was observed between the two groups (chi square = 8.85, d.f. = 7, $p > 0.2$).

As noted previously, the supplier of plastic catheters to the hospital was changed during the study period. The data regarding duration of catheter patency and phlebitis grade are shown in Tables 4 and 5. Neither plastic catheter appeared to interact with the study flush solutions to affect duration of catheter patency or incidence of phlebitis.

Discussion

This investigation demonstrated that the use of 0.9% sodium chloride injection to maintain the patency of intermittent intravenous devices is as effective as heparin sodium 100 units/mL, when evaluated by the criterion of duration of catheter patency. The investigation did not demonstrate a significant difference in the incidence of phlebitis when intermittent intravenous devices were maintained with 0.9% sodium chloride injection versus heparin sodium. Patient gender was the only variable that correlated with the duration of catheter patency, with women having a slightly shorter (5.3 hours) duration of catheter patency. A trend toward an increased incidence of phlebitis was observed among patients who received penicillins, cephalosporins, or clindamycin, alone or in combination, through the intermittent intravenous device. This trend did not appear to be significantly influenced by the type of flush solution used.

The clinical importance of any undetected difference in the incidence of phlebitis between the heparin and sodium chloride groups is unknown. Even among patients who had grade 2 phlebitis, phlebitis was not cited frequently as the reason for discontinuation of the intravenous device. Likewise, the duration of catheter patency in the group of patients with grade 2 phlebitis was not significantly different from that in the group of patients with grade 0 phlebitis. Therefore, although we cannot exclude the possibility that the use of 0.9% sodium chloride injection is associated with a higher incidence of phlebitis, we also cannot ascribe any clinical importance to the development of phlebitis in these patients.

These data agree with those of Epperson,[1] who concluded that no benefit resulted from using heparin to maintain intermittent intravenous devices,

Table 5.
Factors Associated with Phlebitis

Factor	No. Observations of Phlebitis Grade 0 ($n = 234$)[a]	1 ($n = 30$)[a]	2 ($n = 43$)[a]
Treatment			
Heparin	135	17	18
Sodium chloride	99	13	25
Catheter			
Plastic (Deseret)	119	16	27
Plastic (Terumo)	115	14	16
Disease state			
Cancer	28	4	6
Surgery	50	8	9
Device gauge			
18	27	2	6
20	135	18	26
22	64	9	11
Other	8	1	0
Drug use			
Penicillins	56	8	13
Cephalosporins	88	7	19
Clindamycin	11	3	3
Other	86	14	9
Sex			
Male	112	13	18
Female	122	17	25
Age			
>60 Years	179	22	34
≤60 Years	55	8	9

[a] The n values refer to the number of observations rather than the number of patients.

Table 6.
Reasons for Discontinuation of Intermittent Intravenous Device

Reason	No. Observations in Group: Heparin ($n = 170$)	Sodium Chloride ($n = 137$)
Phlebitis	17	7
Loss of patency	10	11
Pulled by patient	2	2
Converted to continuous infusion	2	8
Standard 48-hour change	65	53
Medication discontinued	42	35
Patient discharged	18	12
Unknown	14	9

and also with the "common knowledge" that certain drugs cause a higher incidence of phlebitis than others. Dunn and Lenihan[4] recently published a study in which 112 catheters were maintained with one of two solutions (heparin sodium 100 units/mL or 0.9% sodium chloride injection) and one of two schedules (every 8 or every 24 hours). Their data indicated that no difference in duration of catheter use or incidence of phlebitis or infiltration existed between the two solutions regardless of the administration schedule. Information regarding intravenous medication administration was not provided, and the small sample size suggests the possibility of a large beta error. Despite this, their data are consistent with the results of this study.

The current practice standards of the Intravenous Nurses Society[5] (formerly the National Intravenous Therapy Association) recommend that if heparin is used to maintain the patency of intermittent intravenous devices it should be used only in amounts that do not affect systemic coagulation. This study provides further support for these guidelines.

The importance of these data is manifold. Incompatibilities between heparin and many drugs have been reported. If the use of heparin is eliminated, these incompatibilities became irrelevant. In the amounts conventionally used in intravenous catheters, heparin has little systemic pharmacologic effect. However, the possibility of hypersensitivity responses remains a potential complication of this use. Laster et al.[6] recently reported a fatality as the result of thrombocytopenia secondary to the use of heparin flush solutions. Although this is undoubtedly a severe and rare complication, our results indicate that it is a complication that is completely unnecessary.

Finally, the use of heparin may represent a large expense for an institution. More than 80% of our patients received intermittent intravenous injections through an indwelling device. According to our current policy, indwelling devices are flushed with sodium chloride solution and then with heparin sodium after each injection. We plan to eliminate use of heparin flush solution and increase the volume of 0.9% sodium chloride injection. This change will result in a substantial savings of time for nursing and pharmacy personnel and a reduction in the number of prefilled cartridges purchased by the pharmacy. Because the cost of prefilled cartridges is related to the cartridge, and not to the volume of its contents, we also anticipate a substantial reduction in drug expenditures. At our institution this will amount to approximately 2% of the pharmacy drug budget.

Conclusion

The results of this study indicate that heparin sodium offers no advantage over 0.9% sodium chloride injection in maintaining the patency of indwelling intermittent intravenous devices. A difference in the incidence of phlebitis could not be excluded with confidence, but inasmuch as there was no effect on duration of catheter patency, the clinical importance of this superficial (as opposed to deep) venous phlebitis is questionable.

References

1. Epperson EL. Efficacy of 0.9% sodium chloride injection with and without heparin for maintaining indwelling intermittent injection sites. *Clin Pharm*. 1984; 3:626–9.
2. Maddox RR, Rush DR, Rapp RP et al. Double-blind study to investigate methods to prevent cephalothin-induced phlebitis. *Am J Hosp Pharm*. 1977; 34:29–34.
3. Stolley PD, Strom BL. Sample size calculations for clinical pharmacology studies. *Clin Pharmacol Ther*. 1986; 39:489–90.
4. Dunn DL, Lenihan SF. The case for the saline flush. *Am J Nurs*. 1987; 87:798–9.
5. National Intravenous Therapy Association. Intravenous nursing standards of practice. Belmont, MA: National Intravenous Therapy Association; Nov 1981:12.
6. Laster J, Cikrit D, Walker N et al. The heparin-induced thrombocytopenia syndrome: an update. *Surgery*. 1987; 102:763–70.

Adjuvant Therapy for Breast Cancer

"The benefits of adjuvant chemotherapy for premenopausal women with histologically involved lymph nodes are unequivocal and substantial. Six months of combination therapy with cyclophosphamide, methotrexate, and fluorouracil can be accepted as a standard treatment for this group. Therapy with 20 mg of adjuvant tamoxifen daily for two to five years unequivocally prolongs the survival of postmenopausal women with positive nodes and should be standard for this group. Although the acceptable ratio of cost to benefit is likely to vary considerably among individual patients and their physicians, the data are insufficient to support the recommendation of other forms of therapy or the use of these therapies in other groups of patients except in an investigational setting.

—Henderson IC. Adjuvant therapy for breast cancer. *N Engl J Med*. 1988; 318:443–4. Editorial."

False-positive serum digoxin concentrations determined by three digoxin assays in patients with liver disease

JULIE FRISOLONE, LYNNE M. SYLVIA, JEFFREY GELWAN, SOMNATH PAL, AND CRESCENS PELLECHIA

Abstract: The incidence and magnitude of false-positive serum digoxin concentrations (SDCs) determined by three digoxin assays in patients with liver disease were studied.

Patients with biochemical evidence of liver disease were enrolled in the study if they had never received a cardiac glycoside, were not pregnant, were not receiving spironolactone, did not have moderate to severe renal impairment, and did not have transient elevations in liver function test results. Blood specimens from each patient were assayed for apparent SDCs in triplicate using a fluorescence polarization immunoassay (FPIA, TDx Digoxin II, Abbott) and a digoxin radioimmunoassay (RIA, GammaCoat I^{125}, Clinical Assays) and in duplicate using a fluorometric enzyme immunoassay (Dade Stratus, American Dade).

Forty-two patients met the study criteria. The percentage of patients exhibiting detectable apparent SDCs (≥0.2 ng/mL) was 57% with RIA, 55% with FPIA, and 28% with the fluorometric enzyme immunoassay. Apparent SDCs ranged from 0.2 to 0.6 ng/mL (RIA), 0.2 to 1.56 ng/mL (FPIA), and 0.2 to 0.38 ng/mL (fluorometric enzyme immunoassay). Values obtained using the fluorometric enzyme immunoassay were significantly different from the apparent SDCs determined using RIA and FPIA; however, no significant difference was found between the values obtained using RIA and FPIA. Significant correlations were found between the apparent SDCs determined using RIA and serum bilirubin values and between the apparent SDCs determined using the fluorometric enzyme immunoassay and alkaline phosphatase values.

Of the three assay methods tested, the fluorometric enzyme immunoassay showed the least cross-sensitivity to digoxin-like immunoreactive substance (DLIS). Clinicians should consider the possibility of DLIS interference when interpreting SDCs determined by RIA or fluorometric enzyme immunoassay in patients with liver disease exhibiting elevated total serum bilirubin (RIA) and alkaline phosphatase (fluorometric enzyme immunoassay) concentrations.

Index terms: Blood levels; Digoxin; Digoxin-like factor; Immunoassay; Liver diseases; Methodology; Radioimmunoassay; Tests, laboratory
Clin Pharm. 1988; 7:444–9

Previous investigations have shown that in patients with liver disease serum digoxin concentration (SDC) determinations can be inaccurate because of interference by an endogenous digoxin-like immunoreactive substance (DLIS); however, the incidence and magnitude of DLIS interference with digoxin assays in patients with liver disease have varied from study to study.[1-4] Rosenkranz and Frolich[1] found that 17 of 73 (23.3%) patients with liver disease had false-positive SDCs ranging from 0.3 to 3.6 ng/mL when the SDC was determined using radioimmunoassay (RIA). Gervais et al.[2] reported apparent SDCs of 0.2 to 1.4 ng/mL in 16 of 32 (50%) patients with liver disease when serum samples were analyzed using a digoxin RIA (NML Laboratories, Irving, TX 75015) known to exhibit a high degree of cross-sensitivity with DLIS. Other studies have demonstrated that cirrhotic patients receiving spironolactone,[3] patients with hyperbilirubinemia,[2] patients with hypoalbuminemia,[4] and patients with concomitant renal dysfunction[5] are most likely to exhibit false-positive SDCs that have been determined using various assay techniques.

According to a recent survey by the American Association of Clinical Chemistry,[6] approximately 45% of clinical laboratories use RIA when determining SDCs, whereas the TDx automated system for digoxin (Abbott Laboratories, North Chicago, IL 60064) is used by more than 40% of laboratories. DLIS interference with radioimmunoassay techniques has been shown to be substantial,[1,7] while minimal DLIS interference has been exhibited with the TDx Digoxin I method.[1,7,8] In late 1985, Abbott Laboratories introduced TDx Digoxin II, an immunoassay differing from TDx Digoxin I in its components used for protein precipitation and in its pretreatment solution.[5] TDx Digoxin I has been discontinued by the manufacturer. Preliminary data concerning the specificity of the TDx Digoxin

JULIE FRISOLONE, PHARM. D., is Resident in Clinical Pharmacy, Department of Pharmacy, Medical College of Virginia Hospitals, Richmond. At the time of this study, she was a Doctor of Pharmacy student, College of Pharmacy, St. John's University, Jamaica, NY. LYNNE M. SYLVIA, PHARM.D., is Assistant Clinical Professor, College of Pharmacy, St. John's University. JEFFREY GELWAN, M.D., is Fellow in Gastroenterology, Department of Medicine, Nassau County Medical Center, East Meadow, NY. SOMNATH PAL, PH.D., is Assistant Professor, Department of Pharmacy and Administrative Sciences, College of Pharmacy, St. John's University. CRESCENS PELLECHIA, M.D., is Chief, Division of Gastroenterology, Department of Medicine, Nassau County Medical Center, East Meadow, NY.

Address reprint requests to Dr. Sylvia at the College of Pharmacy, St. John's University, Grand Central and Utopia Parkways, Jamaica, NY 11439.

Presented at the Clinical Research Forum, 22nd Annual ASHP Midyear Clinical Meeting, Atlanta, GA, December 9, 1987.

Copyright © 1988, American Society of Hospital Pharmacists, Inc. All rights reserved. 0278-2677/88/0601-0444$01.50.

II method have revealed interference by DLIS, and false-positive SDCs determined using this system have been reported in three patients with combined hepatic and renal failure and in one patient with hepatic failure only, as well as in neonatal cord blood.[5] These apparent SDCs were higher than those reported when TDx Digoxin I and four different digoxin radioimmunoassays were used.[5] Because of the widespread use of the TDx automated system for digoxin and various RIA techniques, additional information concerning the incidence and magnitude of DLIS interference with these commonly employed methods in patients with liver disease is warranted. The degree of DLIS interference with other frequently used digoxin assays in patients with liver disease may also be clinically relevant.

We conducted this study to determine the incidence and magnitude of apparent SDCs using the TDx Digoxin II system, a digoxin RIA (GammaCoat I^{125} digoxin RIA, Clinical Assays, Baxter Travenol Diagnostics, Cambridge, MA 02139), and a fluorometric enzyme immunoassay (Dade Stratus, American Dade, Miami, FL 33152), with the intention of providing recommendations for the selection of digoxin assay methods and the interpretation of assay results in patients with liver disease. We also examined the relationships between apparent SDCs and specific biochemical indicators of liver function to identify patients most likely to exhibit apparent SDCs.

Methods

Patient Selection. Adult patients having clinical or biochemical evidence, or both, of chronic liver disease, who were admitted to a county medical center or seen at the liver disease clinic at the medical center between October 1, 1986, and December 31, 1986, were eligible for study entry. Clinical evidence of liver disease was determined by two gastroenterologists on the basis of biochemical indicators of liver function: alkaline phosphatase, aspartate aminotransferase (AST, also called SGOT), alanine aminotransferase (ALT, also called SGPT), gammaglutamyl transpeptidase (GGT), total bilirubin, serum albumin, total protein, prothrombin time (PT), and activated partial thromboplastin time (APTT). Patients were excluded from the study if they had ever received a cardiac glycoside, were pregnant, had transient elevations in liver function test results because of drugs, alcohol, or other nonhepatic diseases, were receiving spironolactone, or had moderate to severe renal impairment. Renal impairment was defined as a serum creatinine concentration greater than 2.0 mg/dL or an estimated creatinine clearance of 35 mL/min or less as determined using the method described by Cockcroft and Gault.[9] This cutoff value for serum creatinine was used in a previous investigation of DLIS interference.[10] The creatinine clearance value is the mean value representative of moderate renal impairment as defined by Wallach.[11]

For descriptive purposes only, patients were grouped according to the type of liver disease, as follows: (1) patients with alcoholic liver disease without complications, (2) patients with alcoholic liver disease and complications (presence of ascites, esophageal varices, coagulopathy, encephalopathy, or hypoalbuminemia), and (3) patients with nonalcoholic liver disease.

The study was approved by the institutional review board in September 1986.

Procedures. A 15-mL blood sample for determination of apparent SDC was collected from each patient after informed consent was obtained. Demographic data, including age, sex, type of liver disease, concurrent drug therapy, and concurrent disease states were obtained from the patients' medical records. The specific biochemical indicators of liver function, i.e., alkaline phosphatase, AST, ALT, GGT, total bilirubin, serum albumin, PT, and APTT, were also obtained from the medical records. The biochemical data were based on serum values determined using the Technicon SMAC system (Technicon Instruments Corporation, Tarrytown, NY 10591) on the day of study entry or within six days before the collection of the blood sample. When biochemical tests and apparent SDC determinations were performed on separate days, patients who received albumin during this interval or had fluctuations in biochemical test results during the previous six months were excluded.

Blood specimens were assayed in triplicate using a fluorescence polarization immunoassay (TDx Digoxin II, Abbott Laboratories, North Chicago, IL 60064, lot 91-675-AZ) and a digoxin RIA (GammaCoat I^{125} digoxin RIA, Clinical Assays, Baxter Travenol Diagnostics, Cambridge, MA 02139, lot H274) and in duplicate using a fluorometric enzyme immunoassay (Dade Stratus, American Dade, Miami, FL 33152, lots XDR-162 and XDK-175). Specimens were excluded from analysis if hemolyzed.

Once obtained, the samples were stored at 9 °C and batch analyzed within 24 hours using the fluorescence polarization immunoassay (FPIA) and the digoxin RIA. Specimens were then stored at −15 °C until thawed and batch analyzed within six days using the fluorometric enzyme immunoassay. The lower limits of detection of digoxin are 0.09 ng/mL (RIA), 0.2 ng/mL (FPIA), and 0.2 ng/mL (fluorometric enzyme immunoassay). The coefficients of variation for digoxin determination were 8.1% at 0.86 ng/mL and 8.3% at 2 ng/mL for RIA; 7.55% at 0.83 ng/mL, 5% at 1.35 ng/mL, and 3% at 2.76 ng/mL for FPIA; and 7.07% at 0.79 ng/mL for the fluorometric enzyme immunoassay. Detectable apparent SDCs using each assay were considered as those values greater than or equal to 0.2 ng/mL.

Statistical Analysis. Linear-regression analysis with determination of the correlation coefficient (Pearson's product–moment correlation coefficient) was used to evaluate whether the magnitude of apparent SDCs was related to the extent of liver disease as judged by biochemical indices (alkaline phosphatase, AST, ALT, GGT, total bilirubin, serum albumin, and total protein). Stepwise multiple linear-regression analysis was performed to identify those indices that best explained the observed variance in apparent SDC values. The covariance between the biochemical indices and the apparent SDC values was also examined. After log transformation of the apparent SDC values, observed differences among the assay results were analyzed using a one-way analysis of variance. If a difference was found, a two-tailed Student's t test was used to isolate the difference.

The a priori level of significance was set at $p < 0.05$. All data are reported as mean ± S.D.

Results

Forty-two patients met the study criteria. Demographic data are summarized in Table 1. The percentage of patients exhibiting detectable apparent SDCs (≥0.2 ng/mL) was 57% with RIA, 55% with FPIA, and 28% with the fluorometric enzyme immunoassay. Apparent SDCs ranged from 0.2 to 0.6 ng/mL using RIA, 0.2 to 1.56 ng/mL using FPIA, and 0.2 to 0.38 ng/mL using the fluorometric enzyme immunoassay, with 25%, 39%, and 0% of these values, respectively, being in the therapeutic range for digoxin (0.5 to 2 ng/mL). The mean detectable apparent SDCs obtained were 0.375 ± 0.13 ng/mL (RIA), 0.47 ± 0.35 ng/mL (FPIA), and 0.26 ± 0.06 ng/mL (fluorometric enzyme immunoassay). Considering the assay detection limit of RIA (0.09 ng/mL), 79% of the patients had apparent SDCs greater than the lower limit of detection at a mean of 0.307 ± 0.16 ng/mL. The biochemical indices and the apparent SDC values are presented according to patient group in Table 2.

Table 1.
Demographic Data for 42 Patients

Item	Value[a]
Clinical Variables	
Age (yr)	43 ± 14
Sex	31 men, 11 women
Diagnosis	
Alcoholic liver disease without complications	25
Alcoholic liver disease with complications	9
Nonalcoholic liver disease	8
Biochemical Indices	
Serum creatinine (mg/dL)	0.918 ± 0.19
Estimated creatinine clearance (mL/min/1.73 sq m)	85 ± 25.3
Alkaline phosphatase (U/L)	155.07 ± 76.65
Aspartate aminotransferase (IU/L)	141.12 ± 125.32
Alanine aminotransferase (IU/L)	90.26 ± 77.81
Gammaglutamyl transpeptidase (U/L)	230.67 ± 214.64
Total bilirubin (mg/dL)	2.66 ± 3.44
Serum albumin (g/dL)	2.89 ± 0.76
Total protein (g/dL)	6.96 ± 1.19
Detectable Apparent SDCs (ng/mL)[b]	
RIA (n = 24; 57%)	0.375 ± 0.13
FPIA (n = 23; 55%)	0.470 ± 0.35
FMEI (n = 12; 28.5%)	0.26 ± 0.06

[a] Expressed as mean ± S.D. or number of patients.
[b] SDCs = serum digoxin concentrations, RIA = radioimmunoassay, FPIA = fluorescence polarization immunoassay, FMEI = fluorometric enzyme immunoassay.

A significant difference ($F = 4.00$; d.f. = 2, 56; $p = 0.024$) was found between the apparent SDC values determined using the three assays. Values obtained using the fluorometric enzyme immunoassay were significantly different from the apparent SDCs determined using RIA ($p = 0.01$) and FPIA ($p = 0.016$); however, no significant difference was found between the values obtained using RIA and FPIA.

The correlations between the apparent SDCs as determined using each assay and the biochemical indices are presented in Table 3. Significant correlations were found between the apparent SDCs determined using RIA and serum bilirubin values ($r = 0.506$; $p = 0.01$) and between the apparent SDCs determined using the fluorometric enzyme immunoassay and alkaline phosphatase values ($r = 0.691$; $p = 0.02$); see Figures 1 and 2. No significant correlations were found between the FPIA-determined apparent SDCs and any of the biochemical indices. In the multiple regression models, alkaline phosphatase and serum albumin values collectively accounted for 55.8% of the variation observed in the RIA-determined apparent SDCs (y[ng/mL] = 0.018 [alkaline phosphatase, U/L] + 0.0235 [serum albumin, g/dL] + 2.495; $R^2 = 0.558$), whereas these values accounted for 99.9% of the variation in apparent SDCs as determined using the fluorometric enzyme immunoassay (y[ng/mL] = 0.0155 [alkaline phosphatase, U/L] + 0.0045 [serum albumin, g/dL] + 0.554; $R^2 = 0.999$).

Discussion

Limited data are available concerning the influence of liver disease on the incidence and magnitude of false-positive SDCs. Previous investigations have demonstrated that the incidence of apparent SDCs, as determined using RIA, may range from 0 to 75%[1,2,8]; however, interfering factors such as renal impairment and spironolactone administration may have contributed to the degree of DLIS interference. In a study by Gervais and associates,[2] 50% of patients with liver disease had apparent SDCs as determined using RIA. Although the difference between the serum creatinine values of the

Table 2.
Mean ± S.D. Biochemical Test Results and Apparent Serum Digoxin Concentrations in Patients with Liver Disease[a]

Variable	Group 1 (n = 25)	Group 2 (n = 9)	Group 3 (n = 8)
Biochemical Indices			
Alkaline phosphatase (U/L)	148.44 ± 79.5	138.66 ± 52.9	207.33 ± 83.82
Aspartate aminotransferase (IU/L)	207.04 ± 213.62	70.44 ± 39.77	112.12 ± 48.79
Alanine aminotransferase (IU/L)	105.58 ± 85.23	32.0 ± 17.66	109.88 ± 69.06
Gammaglutamyl transpeptidase (U/L)	249.0 ± 213.63	115.80 ± 69.56	379.0 ± 418.33
Total bilirubin (mg/dL)	1.61 ± 2.21	3.12 ± 1.63	2.33 ± 1.62
Serum albumin (g/dL)	7.24 ± 1.25	6.3 ± 1.23	7.3 ± 0.69
Total protein (g/dL)	3.2 ± 0.68	2.3 ± 0.68	3.1 ± 0.89
Apparent Serum Digoxin Concentration (ng/mL)[b]			
RIA	0.354 ± 0.132 (n = 13; 52%)	0.426 ± 0.09 (n = 6; 67%)	0.408 ± 0.15 (n = 4; 50%)
FPIA	0.49 ± 0.3 (n = 10; 40%)	0.58 ± 0.38 (n = 7; 77%)	0.45 ± 0.19 (n = 4; 50%)
FMEI	0.25 ± 0.04 (n = 9; 36%)	0.30 ± 0.14 (n = 3; 33%)	. . .[c]

[a] Group 1 = patients with alcoholic liver disease without complications, group 2 = patients with alcoholic liver disease with complications, group 3 = patients with nonalcoholic liver disease.
[b] RIA = radioimmunoassay, FPIA = fluorescence polarization immunoassay, FMEI = fluorometric enzyme immunoassay; values in parentheses are number and percentage of patients in groups 1, 2, and 3 in whom digoxin concentrations ≥ 0.2 ng/mL were detectable.
[c] Not detectable.

Table 3.
Correlations between Apparent Serum Digoxin Concentrations and Biochemical Indices

Biochemical Indices	Correlation Coefficients[a] RIA	FPIA	FMEI
Serum creatinine (mg/dL)	0.206	−0.024	−0.161
Alkaline phosphatase (U/L)	0.320	−0.316	0.691[b]
Aspartate aminotransferase (IU/L)	0.056	−0.112	−0.052
Alanine aminotransferase (IU/L)	0.016	0.017	−0.518
Gammaglutamyl transpeptidase (U/L)	−0.225	−0.264	−0.218
Total bilirubin (mg/dL)	0.506[b]	0.179	0.381
Serum albumin (g/dL)	0.357	−0.186	−0.635
Total protein (g/dL)	−0.284	−0.472	−0.589

[a] RIA = radioimmunoassay, FPIA = fluorescence polarization immunoassay, FMEI = fluorometric enzyme immunoassay.
[b] Significant at $p < 0.05$.

Figure 1. Total serum bilirubin concentration versus apparent serum digoxin concentration (SDC) determined using radioimmunoassay (RIA) (GammaCoat, Clinical Assays).

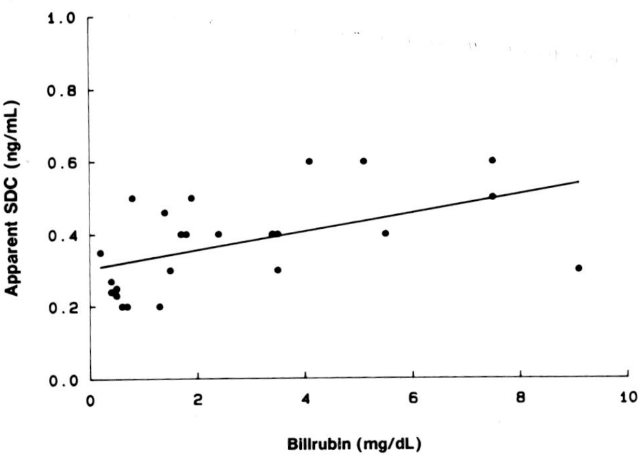

Figure 2. Alkaline phosphatase concentration versus apparent serum digoxin concentration (SDC) determined using fluorometric enzyme immunoassay (Dade Stratus, American Dade).

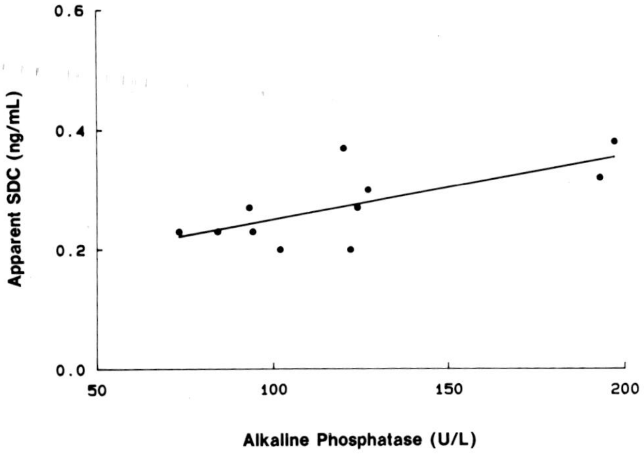

respondents (2.3 ± 2.1 mg/dL) and the nonrespondents (1.4 ± 0.9 mg/dL) was not significant, the possibility of DLIS interference from renal impairment cannot be overlooked. The magnitude of apparent SDC values may also be affected by the presence of renal impairment, as demonstrated by Rosenkranz and Frolich.[1] Higher assay results (mean SDC of 1.9 ng/mL) were noted in hepatically impaired patients with renal disease as compared with those patients having normal renal function (mean SDC of 0.6 ng/mL).

When patients with renal impairment (serum creatinine values ≥ 2 mg/dL) were excluded, Greenway and Nanji[8] reported a 75% incidence of false-positive SDCs as determined using RIA (Clinical Assays) in patients with liver disease. Apparent SDCs ranged from 0.3 to 1.2 nmol/L (0.23 to 0.92 ng/mL) with a mean SDC of 0.382 ± 0.157 ng/mL. Our results, revealing a 57% incidence of apparent SDCs (mean of 0.375 ± 0.13 ng/mL) determined using RIA (Clinical Assays), are consistent with these previous findings. In addition, our results confirm preliminary findings that the TDx Digoxin II system (Abbott Laboratories) exhibits a high degree of DLIS interference, with apparent SDCs determined using this system being comparable to those determined using RIA. However, the importance of this finding is questionable since Abbott Laboratories has subsequently changed the antibody pool of the TDx Digoxin II system. The formulation used in this study is no longer made available by Abbott Laboratories, and as of September 1987, distribution has been limited to the modified formulation.[a] Further study is necessary to determine whether a lesser degree of cross-sensitivity with DLIS will occur with the reformulated TDx system.

The type of liver disease may also influence the incidence and magnitude of apparent SDCs. When stratifying patients based on whether complications of liver disease were present, Nanji and Greenway[4] reported higher apparent SDCs (mean, 1.0 ± 0.6 nmol/L) in eight patients having ascites or edema as compared with nine patients with uncomplicated disease (mean, 0.3 ± 0.3 nmol/L); a significant difference ($p < 0.01$) between these SDC values was noted.[4] The majority of our patients had alcoholic liver disease without complications. Most patients had biochemical indicators consistent with mixed cholestatic–hepatocellular disease. Liver biopsy results were not available; thus, patients could not be stratified according to the type of liver disease. Because of the small size of our patient groups and the large disparity in the observed biochemical indices, a statistical analysis of the apparent SDCs by patient group was not performed.

Attempts have been made to determine whether any of the biochemical indicators of liver function influence the degree of DLIS interference, so that patients most likely to exhibit apparent SDCs may be identified. DiPiro et al.[3] found significant positive correlations between RIA-determined apparent SDCs and several indices of liver function, excluding total serum bilirubin and albumin. In contrast, Nanji and Greenway[4] reported a significant negative correlation ($r = -0.81$; $p < 0.001$) between apparent SDCs determined using RIA (NML Laboratories, Inc., Irving, TX 75015) and serum albumin, while a relationship between RIA-determined apparent SDCs (NML Laboratories) and serum total bilirubin ($r = 0.63$; $p < 0.05$) was recently reported by Gervais and associates.[2] Our results, which show that apparent SDCs determined using RIA (Clinical Assays) correlate positively with serum bilirubin concentrations, agree with those of Gervais and coworkers. The reported correlation coefficient, though significant, was not as strong as that reported by Gervais et al.,[2] which may be explained by our enrollment of patients with less severe liver disease. The mean total bilirubin concentration reported by these previous investigators was 4.2 ± 2.1 mg/dL, while that of our patients was 2.66 ± 3.44 mg/dL. However, in multiple regression models, more than 50% of the variability observed in the apparent SDCs determined using either RIA or the fluorometric enzyme immunoassay was explained by alkaline phosphatase and serum albumin values.

Both RIA and TDx are used frequently by clinical laboratories. RIA is considered a sensitive, precise, and inexpensive assay, whereas the TDx automated system is employed in more than 40% of laboratories because of its ease of use and sensitivity and the fact that it can be used to analyze icteric, lipemic, and hemolyzed specimens.[12] In terms of the potential for DLIS interference in patients with liver disease, both the RIA techniques, particularly the one marketed by NML Laboratories,[13] and the TDx automated Digoxin II system (Abbott Laboratories) exhibit a high degree of cross-sensitivity with DLIS. Based on this criterion alone, the fluorometric enzyme immunoassay appears to be preferable to these assay techniques; however, a substantial degree of lot-to-lot variation in SDCs determined using this assay has been reported in the literature.[6]

Conclusion

Of the three assay methods tested, the fluorometric enzyme immunoassay showed the least cross-sensitivity to DLIS; however, further evaluation of the fluorescence polarization immunoassay is needed because of assay modifications made since the study was conducted. When interpreting SDCs determined using RIA or the fluorometric enzyme immunoassay, clinicians should consider the possibility of DLIS interference in patients with liver disease exhibiting elevated total serum bilirubin (RIA) and alkaline phosphatase concentrations (fluorometric enzyme immunoassay).

---

[a] Stewart J, Abbott Laboratories, Inc. Personal communication. 1988 Apr 20.

References

1. Rosenkranz B, Frolich JC. Falsely elevated digoxin concentrations in patients with liver disease. *Ther Drug Monit.* 1985; 7:202–6.
2. Gervais A, Nanji AA, Greenway DC et al. Digoxin-like substance (DLIS) in liver disease: comparison of clinical and laboratory parameters in patients with and without DLIS. *Drug Intell Clin Pharm.* 1987; 21:450–2.
3. DiPiro JT, Cote JR, DiPiro CR et al. Spironolactone interference with digoxin radioimmunoassays in cirrhotic patients. *Am J Hosp Pharm.* 1980; 37:1518–21.
4. Nanji AA, Greenway DC. Correlation between serum albumin and digoxin-like immunoreactive substance in liver disease. *J Clin Pharmacol.* 1986; 26:152–3.
5. Gault MH, Vasdev S, Longerich L. Higher values for digitalis-like factors with TDx Digoxin II. *Clin Chem.* 1986; 32:2000–1. Letter.
6. Clark DR, Inloes RL, Kalman SM et al. Abbott TDx, Dade Stratus, and DuPont aca automated digoxin immunoassays compared with a reference radioimmunoassay method. *Clin Chem.* 1986; 32:381–5.
7. Nanji AA, Greenway DC. Falsely raised plasma digoxin concentrations in liver disease. *Br Med J.* 1985; 290:432–3.
8. Greenway DC, Nanji AA. Falsely increased results for digoxin in sera from patients with liver disease: ten immunoassay kits compared. *Clin Chem.* 1985; 31:1078–9.
9. Cockcroft DW, Gault MH. Prediction of creatinine clearance from serum creatinine. *Nephron.* 1976; 16:31–41.
10. Graves SW, Brown B, Valdes R. An endogenous digoxin-like substance in patients with renal impairment. *Ann Intern Med.* 1983; 99:604–8.
11. Wallach J. Specific laboratory examination. In: Wallach J, ed. Interpretation of diagnostic tests. A synopsis of laboratory medicine. Boston/Toronto: Little, Brown and Company; 1986:41–156.
12. Pleasants RA, Gadsen RH. A short course on drug assay methods. *US Pharm.* 1986; 11(5):1–16.
13. Seccombe DW, Pudek MR, Whitfield MF et al. Perinatal changes in digoxin-like immunoreactive substances. *Pediatr Res.* 1984; 18:1097–1099.

Endogenous digoxin-like immunoreactivity in elderly patients with normal serum creatinine concentrations

THOMAS E. LACKNER, BRAD W. C. LAU, CURTIS PARVIN, AND ROLAND VALDES, JR.

Abstract: The effect of digoxin-like immunoreactive substance (DLIS) on serum digoxin determinations in elderly patients with normal serum creatinine concentrations was studied.

Patients in the study group were over 70 years of age; the control population was under 55 years of age. All patients had serum creatinine concentrations of ≤1.5 mg/dL. Apparent digoxin content of serum samples from patients receiving digoxin and from patients in each age group who were not receiving digoxin was determined in duplicate by each of two radioimmunoassays: RIANEN (New England Nuclear), which detects DLIS, and Immophase (Corning Medical and Scientific), which is far less cross-reactive with DLIS. Results from the patients under 55 years of age were analyzed for inherent bias between the assay methods. In patients over 70 years of age, concentrations of DLIS (differences between serum digoxin concentrations measured by RIANEN and Immophase) were compared with creatinine clearance values.

No DLIS was detected in sera of patients who had not received digoxin. For patients who received digoxin, nearly all apparent digoxin concentrations were within the usual therapeutic range. For patients without liver or renal failure who received digoxin, no significant difference in digoxin concentrations was observed between the RIANEN and Immophase assays in either the young (n = 17) or elderly (n = 26) patients. There was no significant increase in the difference between the RIANEN and Immophase results with decreasing creatinine clearance.

In these elderly patients with normal serum creatinine concentrations, there was no evidence that measurement of serum digoxin concentration using the RIANEN and Immophase assays was compromised by DLIS.

Index terms: Age; Blood levels; Cardiac drugs; Digoxin; Digoxin-like factor; Geriatrics; Methodology; Radioimmunoassay; Tests, laboratory

Clin Pharm. 1988; 7:449–53

THOMAS E. LACKNER, PHARM.D., is Associate Professor of Clinical Pharmacy, St. Louis College of Pharmacy, and Clinical Pharmacist, Jewish Hospital of St. Louis, St. Louis, MO. BRAD W. C. LAU, PH.D., is Clinical Chemistry Research Fellow, Washington University School of Medicine, St. Louis, MO, and Jewish Hospital of St. Louis. CURTIS PARVIN, PH.D., is Assistant Professor of Pathology and Assistant Medical Director, Clinical Chemistry and Laboratory Computing, Washington University School of Medicine. ROLAND VALDES, JR., PH.D., is Assistant Professor of Pathology, Washington University School of Medicine, and Associate in Biochemistry, Jewish Hospital of St. Louis.

Address reprint requests to Dr. Lackner at the Jewish Hospital of St. Louis, 216 South Kingshighway Blvd., P.O. Box 14109, St. Louis, MO 63178.

Supported by the St. Louis College of Pharmacy Research Fund and in part by an NIH grant (#HL37074).

Presented at the Eighth Annual Meeting of the American College of Clinical Pharmacy, Austin, TX, July 21, 1987.

Copyright © 1988, American Society of Hospital Pharmacists, Inc. All rights reserved. 0278-2677/88/0601-0449$01.25.

Digoxin is the most commonly prescribed medication in the United States in people over 75 years of age.[1,2] More than 75% of all digitalis prescriptions are written for patients 65 years of age and older.[2]

Digoxin must be used judiciously because of its narrow therapeutic range (approximately 0.9 to 2.0 ng/mL) and potentially life-threatening toxicity.[3,4] The elderly patient is particularly at risk for toxicity from digoxin because of the high prevalence of predisposing conditions (i.e., hypokalemia, hypomagnesemia, hypercalcemia, metabolic acidosis or alkalosis, and hypoxia).[5–7] Furthermore, excessive serum digoxin concentrations are more likely to occur in the elderly because of unrecognized renal impairment.[8] For these reasons, the accurate measurement of serum digoxin concentrations is an integral component in the appraisal and modification of digoxin therapy.[9] However, serum digoxin concentrations may correlate poorly with clinical effect in the elderly.[10]

Research performed at our institution and elsewhere has identified one or more endogenous digoxin-like immunoreactive substances (DLISs) that cause erroneous digoxin measurement in patients with overt renal dysfunction.[11] Subclinical renal dysfunction (diminished renal function without an elevated serum creatinine concentration) is present in many elderly patients.[12] Therefore, DLIS might be present in the serum of elderly patients in the absence of recognized renal failure.

Discrepancies between calculated digoxin clearance and serum digoxin concentrations measured by radioimmunoassay have been reported for elderly patients with both normal and abnormal serum creatinine values.[13] Measured serum digoxin concentrations were significantly greater than the predicted value in 33% of elderly patients in the absence of conditions known to alter digoxin pharmacokinetics.[13] The presence of DLIS was suggested as a possible cause of this discrepancy.[14] The purpose of this study was to determine whether DLIS is present in serum of elderly patients without overt renal disease and to determine the effect of DLIS on digoxin quantitation in elderly patients.

Methods

Selection of Patients. Adult patients of either sex who had stable renal function within a normal reference range of 0.5 to 1.5 mg/dL for serum creatinine were studied; stable renal function was defined as a change in serum creatinine concentration of no more than 0.5 mg/dL within five days of sample collection for digoxin measurement. Patients older than 70 years of age were designated the "elderly" study population and patients younger than 55 years of age constituted the nonelderly control population. Serum samples from patients receiving digoxin and serum samples lacking digoxin (to serve as a control) were collected from routine laboratory specimens for analysis of digoxin content.

Patients receiving other digitalis products were excluded from the study. The use of other drugs that might interfere with digoxin measurement, such as spironolactone and corticosteroids, was noted, but therapy with these drugs was not a criterion for exclusion from the study. The medical records of all patients were reviewed to validate medication use. Women who were pregnant were ineligible for the study because of the high likelihood of DLIS in this population.[15] Patients with a clinical diagnosis of hepatic dysfunction were not excluded from enrollment in the study because liver disease was not fully recognized as a potential source of DLIS at the time the study was begun[16]; however, concentration data from these patients were excluded from statistical analysis. Similarly, patients with congestive heart failure and hypertension were not excluded from enrollment in the study.

Determination of Renal Function. Renal function was assessed by calculation of the creatinine clearance from serum creatinine by the method of Cockcroft and Gault and adjustment for body surface area.[17] This method has been documented to provide a reliable estimate of renal function in elderly patients.[18]

Serum Digoxin Assays. Digoxin was measured by two radioimmunoassays. Presence of DLIS was estimated by the difference in apparent digoxin concentrations obtained by RIANEN-Digoxin I 125 (New England Nuclear, North Billerica, CA), which exhibits high cross-reactivity with DLIS, and concentrations obtained by Immophase (Corning Medical and Scientific, Medfield, MA), which is much less cross-reactive with DLIS than is the RIANEN assay.[11] RIANEN measures digoxin by competitive displacement of digoxin I 125 from antidigoxin antibodies relative to digoxin. The displaced digoxin I 125 is separated from the antibody complex by a double antibody precipitation technique in which the rabbit antidigoxin antiserum is prereacted with goat antiserum to rabbit gammaglobulin. Immophase is a radioimmunoassay that is similar to RIANEN except that the antidigoxin antibodies are chemically immobilized on fine glass particles, allowing rapid and quantitative separation from the displaced digoxin I 125.

All serum samples were batch analyzed in duplicate by both immunoassays on the same day within six months of sample acquisition (samples were stored at −70 °C until analysis). Unpublished results from our laboratory indicate that DLIS in serum is stable under these storage conditions. Furthermore, DLIS is stable in urine for eight months at −20 °C.[19] Serum specimens that were lipemic, icteric, hemolyzed or obtained less than six hours after a digoxin dose was administered were excluded from the study. Serum digoxin concentrations are reported as the mean of duplicate analyses for each assay.

The lower limits of detection of digoxin in our laboratory with RIANEN and Immophase are 0.025 ng/mL and 0.02 ng/mL, respectively.[20,21] However, in this study, we designated 0.1 ng/mL as the lowest "detectable" concentration since false-positive serum digoxin concentrations lower than this are not clinically important.[22] All analyses for digoxin were performed within the same day. The within-assay coefficient of variation was less than 7% at concentrations between 0.5 and 3 ng/mL. The therapeutic range for serum digoxin concentrations at our institution is 0.5 to 2.0 ng/mL.

Statistical Analysis. The observed differences between serum digoxin concentrations measured by the RIANEN and the Immophase assays are assumed to have three possible components: (1) random error due to imprecision in the methods, (2) inherent bias between the analytical methods in the absence of DLIS, and (3) the presence of DLIS. The presence of DLIS in the elderly was estimated by calculating the difference in measured concentration between the RIANEN and the Immophase assays in patients older than 70 who were receiving digoxin, after adjusting for any expected difference due to inherent bias between the methods in the absence of DLIS.

To determine if there is any inherent bias between the analytical methods in the absence of DLIS, the paired data from patients 55 years of age or younger who were receiving digoxin were subjected to a method-comparison analysis.[23] This involved fitting a straight line by least-squares regression analysis to the paired data and examining the estimated slope and intercept. An intercept different from zero suggests a constant bias between the methods, and a slope different from one suggests a proportional bias between the methods. Student's *t* tests were used to determine the significance of the slope and intercept estimates. An a priori level of significance of $p < 0.05$ was assigned for all statistical tests.

The Student's *t* test was used to test the null hypothesis that the mean estimated DLIS concentration in patients over 70 years of age who were receiving digoxin was not significantly different from zero. Because the level of DLIS may be related to renal function, we examined the relationship between the concentration of DLIS (the difference between apparent serum digoxin concentrations measured by RIANEN and Immophase) in patients over 70 years of age who were receiving digoxin and their creatinine clearance value using linear regression analysis. A *t* test of the null hypothesis that the slope of the linear relationship between DLIS concentration and creatinine clearance was greater than or equal to zero (implying that the level of DLIS does not increase with a progressive decrease in creatinine clearance) was performed. Student's *t* test for unpaired data was used to compare calculated creatinine clearance between the two age groups.

Results

Eighty-seven patients were evaluated for the presence of DLIS. The statistical comparison of digoxin equivalents (digoxin plus DLIS) between assays excludes data from four patients with liver disease or cholecystitis who were enrolled in the study. Demographic characteristics of all 87 patients are presented in Table 1.

The mean serum creatinine concentration was similar between the young and the elderly patients. As expected based on the results of other studies, the calculated creatinine clearance of the older patients was significantly lower than that of the younger patients (48 versus 91 mL/min; $p < 0.0001$).

Nearly all serum digoxin concentrations in patients who had received digoxin were within the usual therapeutic range. DLIS was not detected (i.e., digoxin concentration <0.1 ng/mL) with the RIANEN or the Immophase assays in the serum of young or elderly patients who had not received digoxin.

Two patients received spironolactone (one young control and one elderly patient receiving digoxin) and another eight patients received corticosteroids (three young controls, two elderly controls, and three young patients receiving digoxin). None of the patients diagnosed with hepatic disease were receiving spironolactone or corticosteroids. There was no evidence of cross-reactivity of spironolactone or corticosteroids with either the Immophase or the RIANEN assays, since digoxin was not detectable in any of the control patients receiving these drugs. Also, digoxin concentrations measured by the two assays were similar in all patients who were receiving spironolactone or corticosteroids in addition to digoxin.

Table 1.
Description of Study Population[a]

Variable	Age > 70 Years		Age < 55 Years	
	Digoxin	No Digoxin	Digoxin	No Digoxin
No. patients	27	20	20	20
Sex (no. male/ no. female)	9/18	5/15	11/9	8/12
Age (yr)	78 ± 5	79 ± 8	45 ± 9	42 ± 10
SCr (mg/dL)	1.1 ± 0.2	1.1 ± 0.3	1.1 ± 0.3	1.0 ± 0.2
CL_{cr} (mL/min)	49 ± 14	47 ± 12	87 ± 25	94 ± 30

[a] Values for age, serum creatinine (SCr) and creatinine clearance (CL_{cr}) represent the mean ± standard deviation; values for four patients with liver disease or cholecystitis are included.

The method-comparison analysis between the RIANEN and the Immophase assays for the patients less than 55 years of age who were receiving digoxin is shown in Figure 1. The digoxin concentration was below the lower limit of Immophase sensitivity in a single patient. Excluding three patients with liver disease, serum digoxin concentrations (mean ± S.D., range in parentheses) were 0.82 ± 0.53 (0–2.3) ng/mL with Immophase and 0.85 ± 0.65 (0.04–2.9) ng/mL with RIANEN.

The regression equation for the data in Figure 1 is RIANEN = 0.001 + 0.99 Immophase, $r = 0.923$. The 95% confidence intervals for the y-intercept and slope are −0.187 to 0.190 and 0.77 to 1.22, respectively. The intercept and slope were not significantly different from zero and one, respectively, and no adjustment to the RIANEN values in the elderly group to account for the bias between methods was necessary; i.e., any observed difference in measured concentration between the RIANEN and the Immophase assays could be attributed to DLIS and random error.

The difference between the RIANEN and Immophase results for elderly patients who were receiving digoxin is plotted against creatinine clearance in Figure 2. The digoxin concentration was below the lower limit of RIANEN sensitivity in one patient over 70 years of age. Excluding one patient with liver disease, serum digoxin concentrations (mean ± S.D., range in parentheses), were 0.86 ± 0.56 (0.1–2.0) ng/mL with Immophase and 0.82 ± 0.49 (0.02–2.0) ng/mL with RIANEN. The slope of the regression line was 0.07 (95% confidence interval, 0.07 to 13.40), and the y-intercept was −3.93. The mean difference between assays (−0.064 ng/mL) was not significantly greater than zero (95% confidence interval = −0.165 to 0.037). Likewise, there was no significant increase in the difference between the RIANEN and the Immophase results with decreasing creatinine clearance. Surprisingly, a negative value for the difference in serum digoxin concentrations (RIANEN minus Immophase) was observed in several patients with a relatively low creatinine clearance. These differences appeared to be independent of the digoxin concentration.

A substantially higher mean (± S.D.) serum digoxin concentration was measured by the RIANEN assay (3.9 ± 1.5 ng/mL) than by the Immophase assay (2.4 ± 0.46 ng/mL) in four patients noted to have impaired liver function or cholecystitis.

Discussion

DLIS has been documented to interfere with the measurement of digoxin by numerous immunoassays. The magnitude of anomalous digoxin concentrations attributed to DLIS has ranged from negligible (0.1 ng/mL) to levels well above the usual upper limit of the therapeutic range of 2 ng/mL.[11] In addition, measurements of digoxin in serum between immunoassays have been reported to differ by as much as 3 ng/mL, indicating a risk for gross inaccuracy between results for any given patient.[11] Previous studies have demonstrated that erroneously elevated serum digoxin concentrations at-

Figure 1. Correlation of serum digoxin concentration (SDC) values determined by Immophase and RIANEN in patients less than 55 years of age and receiving digoxin ($n = 20$); 3/20 patients who had hepatic disease are denoted by open circles (O). The least-squares regression line is plotted.

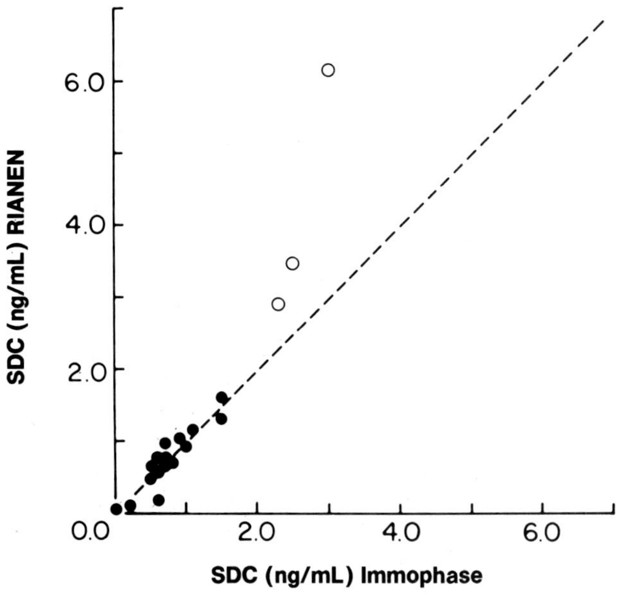

Figure 2. The mean difference between serum digoxin concentrations (SDCs) measured by Immophase and RIANEN assays is plotted as a function of normalized creatinine clearance for patients more than 70 years of age and receiving digoxin ($n = 27$); one patient who had hepatic disease is denoted by an open circle (O).

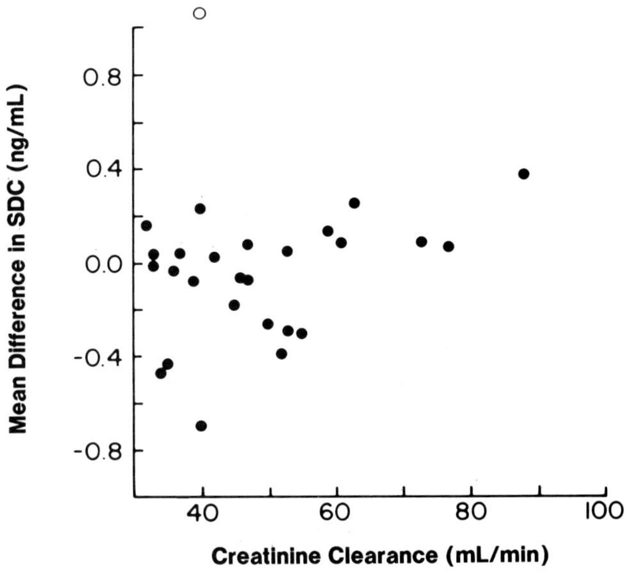

tributed to DLIS are not likely to be caused by cross-reacting digoxin metabolites or interfering drugs.[11]

DLIS is present in patients with overt renal disease and could jeopardize treatment with digoxin that is guided by serum-concentration monitoring. In fact, in a study of 54 patients with renal failure who did not receive digoxin, DLIS was detected in the serum of the majority of patients by several commonly used immunoassays for digoxin, including the RIANEN assay.[24] In the same study, DLIS was detected in only a single patient with the Immophase assay.[24]

Despite having serum creatinine values within the normal reference range, our elderly patients had lower creatinine clearance values than did the young control population. DLIS was not detected in elderly patients who were not receiving digoxin. Furthermore, the measurement of digoxin in serum of patients receiving digoxin was not compromised, as determined by comparison of digoxin equivalents measured by one assay that detects DLIS and another that is less sensitive to DLIS. The absence of DLIS in our elderly patients might be explained by their relatively mild renal impairment, compared with overt renal disease in which DLIS has been detected. The level of renal function in our patients is representative of renal function in hospitalized elderly patients without overt renal disease.[18]

We cannot explain the unexpected negative difference in serum digoxin measurement that we observed between the RIANEN and the Immophase assays in several patients with relatively low creatinine clearance values. This difference might represent differences in cross-reactivity between assays for one or more DLISs. Assay imprecision does not explain this observation, since this would be reflected by scatter of data points in both directions, in the demonstrated absence of bias between the two assays.

The concentration differences we found in four patients with cholecystitis or impaired liver function are consistent with previous findings.[25]

Conclusion

The diminished creatinine clearance associated with increased age does not appear to be independently associated with the presence of DLIS as determined by the difference in digoxin concentrations measured by the RIANEN and the Immophase assays. Our results suggest that use of these two assays to measure serum digoxin concentrations in elderly patients without overt renal disease is not compromised by DLIS.

References

1. Schocken DD, Robinson BE, Kruge-Fite J et al. Digitalis use in a retirement community. *J Am Geriatr Soc*. 1986; 34:504–6.
2. Baum C, Kennedy DL, Forbes MB et al. Drug utilization in the U.S. 1981: third annual review. Rockville, MD: Division of Drug Experience, National Center for Drugs and Biologics, Food and Drug Administration; 1982.
3. Smith TW, Digitalis toxicity: epidemiology and clinical use of serum concentration measurements. *Am J Med*. 1975; 58:470–6.
4. Smith TW, Haber E. Digoxin intoxication: the relationship of clinical presentation to serum digoxin concentration. *J Clin Invest*. 1970; 49:2377–86.
5. Smith TW, Haber E. Digitalis. *N Engl J Med*. 1973; 289:245–51, 1010–5, 1063–71, 1125–9.
6. Smith TW. Digitalis glycosides. *N Engl J Med*. 1973; 288:719–22, 942–6.
7. Rosen MR, Wit AL, Hoffman BF. Electrophysiology and pharmacology of cardiac arrhythmias, IV. Cardiac antiarrhythmic and toxic effects of digitalis. *Am Heart J*. 1975; 89:391–9.
8. Whiting B, Wandless I, Sumner DJ et al. Computer-assisted review of digoxin therapy in the elderly. *Br Heart J*. 1978; 40:8–13.
9. Duhme DW, Greenblatt DJ, Koch–Weser J. Reduction of digoxin toxicity associated with measurement of serum levels. *Ann Intern Med*. 1974; 80:516–9.
10. Sonnenblick M, Abraham AS. Digoxin treatment and control in the elderly. *Isr J Med Sci*. 1985; 21:276–8.
11. Valdes R. Endogenous digoxin-like immunoreactive factors: impact on digoxin measurements and potential physiological implications. *Clin Chem*. 1985; 31:1525–32.
12. Rowe JW, Andres R, Tobin JE et al. The effect of age on creatinine clearance in men: a cross-sectional and longitudinal study. *J Gerontol*. 1974; 31:155–63.
13. Mooradian AD, Wynn EM. Pharmacokinetic prediction of serum digoxin concentration in the elderly. *Arch Intern Med*. 1987; 147:650–3.
14. Reider C. Discrepancies between the calculated digoxin clearance and the serum digoxin level in elderly patients. *Arch Intern Med*. 1987; 147:1852–3.
15. Graves SW, Valdes R, Brown BA et al. Endogenous digoxin immunoreactive substance in human pregnancies. *J Clin Endocrinol Metab*. 1984; 58:748–51.
16. Nanji AA, Greenway DC. Falsely raised plasma digoxin concentrations in liver disease. *Br Med J*. 1985; 290:432–3.
17. Cockcroft DW, Gault MH. Prediction of creatinine clearance from serum creatinine. *Nephron*. 1976; 16:31–41.
18. Paladino JA, Kapfer JR, DiBona JR. Bedside estimation of creatinine clearance: which method is most accurate while least complex? *Hosp Formul*. 1986; 21:709–15.
19. Clerico A, Ghione S, Chicca MGD et al. Problems in standardization of digitalis-like substance assays by means of competitive immunological methods. *Clin Chem*. 1987; 33:340–1.
20. Valdes R Jr, Graves SW. Protein binding of endogenous digoxin-immunoreactive factors in human serum and its variation with clinical condition. *J Clin Endocrinol Metab*. 1985; 60:1135–43.
21. Skogen WF, Rea MR, Valdes R Jr. Endogenous digoxin-like immunoreactive factors eliminated from serum samples by hydrophobic silica-gel extraction and enzyme immunoassay. *Clin Chem*. 1987; 33:401–4.
22. Gault H, Vasdev S, Vlasses P et al. Interpretation of serum digoxin values in renal failure. *Clin Pharmacol Ther*. 1986; 39:530–6.
23. Westgard JO, Hunt MR. Use and interpretation of common statistical tests in method-comparison studies. *Clin Chem*. 1973; 19:49–57.
24. Graves SW, Brown B, Valdes R. An endogenous digoxin-like substance in patients with renal impairment. *Ann Intern Med*. 1983; 99:604–8.
25. Rosenkranz B, Frolich JC. Falsely elevated digoxin concentrations in patients with liver disease. *Ther Drug Monit*. 1985; 7:202–6.

Continuous i.v. infusion versus multiple bolus doses of metoclopramide for prevention of cisplatin-induced emesis

WILLIAM A. AGOSTINUCCI, RICHARD H. GANNON, GRANT R. GOLUB, ROBERT S. MARTIN, PETER K. SCHAUER, AND EMELIE B. DINONNO

Abstract: Continuous infusion of metoclopramide was compared with bolus dosing in a randomized, double-blind study in 27 patients receiving cisplatin therapy.

Hospitalized patients receiving their first course of cisplatin (120 mg/sq m administered i.v. over four hours) were randomized to receive either bolus doses or a continuous infusion of metoclopramide. In the infusion group (14 patients), a loading dose of metoclopramide 3 mg/kg (total body weight) as the hydrochloride salt was infused over one hour immediately before the administration of cisplatin, followed by a continuous infusion of metoclopramide 0.5 mg/kg/hr (as the hydrochloride salt) for 12 hours. Each patient received a total metoclopramide dose of 9 mg/kg over 13 hours. These patients also received five bolus doses of 5% dextrose injection (as placebo) over 15 minutes, with the first dose given one hour before the cisplatin and four more doses at two-hour intervals. In the bolus-dose group (13 patients), metoclopramide 2 mg/kg as the hydrochloride salt was added to each of the bolus doses, while the continuous infusion was a placebo of 5% dextrose injection. All patients also received dexamethasone 10 mg i.v. and diphenhydramine hydrochloride 50 mg i.v. Patients were monitored for 24 hours after initiation of metoclopramide administration for number of emesis episodes and for adverse effects.

In the infusion group, 11 of 14 (79%) patients had two or fewer episodes of emesis. In the bolus group, 10 of 13 (77%) had two or fewer vomiting episodes. Mild sedation occurred in both the infusion (79%) and bolus-dose (77%) groups. Despite the use of diphenhydramine, extrapyramidal reactions were seen in one bolus-dose patient and two infusion patients. Diarrhea was more common in the bolus group (38%) versus the infusion group (14%).

At the dosages used in this study, a continuous infusion of metoclopramide is as effective as the traditional bolus dosing for preventing cisplatin-induced emesis.

Index terms: Antiemetics; Antihistamines; Antineoplastic agents; Cisplatin; Dexamethasone; Diphenhydramine hydrochloride; Drug administration rate; Metoclopramide hydrochloride; Toxicity; Vomiting
Clin Pharm. 1988; 7:454–7

Metoclopramide is one of the most effective antiemetics available for preventing the nausea and vomiting induced by high-dose cisplatin.[1] Traditionally, metoclopramide has been given as an i.v. bolus varying from five doses of 2 mg/kg to two doses of 3 mg/kg.[2] High-dose oral metoclopramide has also been used successfully in patients receiving cisplatin.[3] We and others have successfully used continuous i.v. infusions of metoclopramide.[4–9] The bolus-dose method of administration for metoclopramide results in marked accumulation of metoclopramide and is labor intensive.[10] The oral route may also result in accumulation and is labor intensive. In addition, if the patient is experiencing nausea and vomiting, i.v. or i.m. antiemetics must be used. Based on a review of the literature and the use of pharmacokinetic modeling, we developed a loading-dose and continuous-infusion protocol that would theoretically maintain serum metoclopramide concentrations between 800 and 1200 ng/mL during a 12-hour continuous infusion.[4]

In this randomized, double-blind study, we compared five bolus doses of metoclopramide with a continuous infusion of metoclopramide to determine if a difference in efficacy or adverse effects existed.

Methods

Twenty-seven patients who were to receive their first course of cisplatin (120 mg/sq m) were randomized to receive either bolus doses or a continuous infusion of metoclopramide. Other concomi-

WILLIAM A. AGOSTINUCCI is Unit Pharmacist, Hartford Hospital, Hartford, CT. RICHARD H. GANNON, PHARM.D., is Assistant Director of Pharmacy, Hartford Hospital, and Assistant Clinical Professor, School of Pharmacy, University of Connecticut, Storrs. GRANT R. GOLUB, M.D., ROBERT S. MARTIN, M.D., and PETER K. SCHAUER, M.D., are Medical Oncologists, Department of Medicine, Hartford Hospital, and Clinical Associate Professors, School of Medicine, University of Connecticut, Farmington. EMELIE B. DINONNO is an oncology nurse, Hartford Hospital.

Address reprint requests to Mr. Agostinucci at the Department of Pharmacy Services, Hartford Hospital, 80 Seymour Street, Hartford, CT 06115.

The assistance of Ken Walters, the pharmacy staff, and the nurses on CCU-6 is acknowledged.

Supported by the Heublein Radiation Oncology Fund.

Copyright © 1988, American Society of Hospital Pharmacists, Inc. All rights reserved. 0278-2677/88/0601-0454$01.00.

tant antineoplastic therapy was considerably less emetogenic and consisted of vinblastine, etoposide, fluorouracil, and bleomycin. All patients were hospitalized during treatment, and administration of antineoplastic drugs was completed within 24 hours. Informed consent was obtained from all patients.

Cisplatin was administered as an intravenous infusion over four hours. All patients had a measured creatinine clearance greater than 60 mL/min and a total serum bilirubin concentration less than 2 mg/dL. Each patient required two infusion pumps and two i.v. sites, one for the delivery of metoclopramide and the other for the delivery of the antineoplastic agent and fluids for hydration.

In the infusion group, a loading dose of metoclopramide 3 mg/kg (total body weight) as the hydrochloride salt was infused over one hour immediately before the administration of the cisplatin. This was followed by a continuous infusion of metoclopramide 0.5 mg/kg/hr (total body weight) as the hydrochloride salt for 12 hours. Each patient received a total metoclopramide dose of 9 mg/kg over 13 hours. These same patients also received five bolus doses of 5% dextrose injection in an appropriate volume (as placebo) over 15 minutes, with the first dose given one hour before the cisplatin and four more doses at two-hour intervals. In the bolus-dose group, metoclopramide 2 mg/kg as the hydrochloride salt was added to each of the bolus doses, while the continuous infusion was a placebo of 5% dextrose injection. The study was blinded so that the physician, nurse, and patient did not know the method by which the metoclopramide was given.

The pharmacy department prepared all metoclopramide infusions in 5% dextrose injection at a concentration of 1 or 2 mg/mL. All infusions were protected from light during administration.

Before administration of the metoclopramide, dexamethasone 10 mg i.v. and diphenhydramine hydrochloride 50 mg i.v. were given to each patient to enhance the antiemetic efficacy of metoclopramide and to decrease the incidence of diarrhea and extrapyramidal reactions from metoclopramide. Dexamethasone doses were not repeated, and additional diphenhydramine was given only if an extrapyramidal reaction occurred. Administration of additional antiemetics was prohibited during the metoclopramide infusion.

Efficacy (measured by number of emesis episodes) and adverse effects (sedation, diarrhea, extrapyramidal reactions) were monitored for 24 hours after initiation of the metoclopramide. We defined a major response to antiemetic therapy as two or fewer emesis episodes, a partial response as three or four emesis episodes, and a treatment failure as more than four emesis episodes. Nausea was not included as a criterion for determining response because of the difficulty in grading the severity of nausea. Nausea was assessed as being present or absent.

Each patient's nurse recorded adverse effects, vital signs, and the time and number of emesis episodes every 4 hours for 24 hours after the cisplatin was given. One of the investigators interviewed each patient and reviewed his or her medical record before discharge. Data recorded by the nurses were confirmed in the interview. The investigator then recorded all clinical data pertinent to our study.

The number of episodes of vomiting in each group was compared using the Wilcoxon rank-sum test. The a priori level of significance was $p < 0.05$.

Results

A total of 27 patients were evaluated. Patient characteristics are described in Table 1. Men composed a majority of the study population, with lung cancer being the predominant cancer type. The average age for both groups was similar; however, the majority of patients treated in the infusion group (86%) were 51–70 years old, whereas 46% of the bolus-group patients were in that age range. Each patient was assigned a performance status, with 25 of 27 patients ranking between 80 and 100%.[11]

Antiemetic response and adverse effects for these patients are described in Table 2. Major responses to metoclopramide were observed in 10 of 13 (77%) bolus and 11 of 14 (79%) infusion regimens. The difference in the number of vomiting

Table 1.
Patient Characteristics

Characteristic	No. Patients (%) Receiving Bolus Dose (n = 13)	Receiving Infusion (n = 14)
Age (yr)		
20–30	1 (7.7)	1 (7.1)
31–40	3 (23.1)	0 (0.0)
41–50	2 (15.3)	1 (7.1)
51–60	3 (23.1)	6 (42.9)
61–70	3 (23.1)	6 (42.9)
71–80	1 (7.7)	0 (0.0)
Sex		
Male	11 (84.6)	10 (71.4)
Female	2 (15.4)	4 (28.6)
Performance status (%)[a]		
80–100	13 (100.0)	12 (85.8)
60–79	0 (0.0)	1 (7.1)
40–59	0 (0.0)	1 (7.1)
Cancer type		
Lung	8 (61.5)	9 (64.3)
Testicular	1 (7.7)	1 (7.1)
Head–neck	3 (23.1)	4 (28.6)
Rectal	1 (7.7)	0 (0.0)

[a] Based on criteria defined in reference 11.

Table 2.
Comparison of Antiemetic Response and Adverse Effects to Metoclopramide Given by Bolus Doses or Continuous Infusion

Item	No. Patients (%) Receiving Bolus Dose (n = 13)	Receiving Infusion (n = 14)
Response[a]		
Major (0, 1, or 2)		
0	6 (46.1)	6 (42.8)
1	2 (15.4)	3 (21.4)
2	2 (15.4)	2 (14.3)
Partial (3 or 4)		
3	1 (7.7)	0 (0.0)
4	1 (7.7)	0 (0.0)
Failure (5 or more)		
≥5	1 (7.7)	3 (21.4)
Adverse effect		
Sedation	10 (76.8)	11 (78.6)
Diarrhea	5 (38.5)	2 (14.3)
Extrapyramidal reactions	1 (7.7)	2 (14.3)

[a] Numbers in parentheses indicate the number of emesis episodes per response category.

episodes per patient between the two groups was not significant when compared by the Wilcoxon rank-sum test. In the bolus group, two patients had partial responses and treatment failed in one patient. In the infusion group, no patients had partial responses and treatment failed in three patients. Seven people in the bolus group (54%) versus eight people in the infusion group (58%) indicated nausea as being present.

The incidence of sedation was similar in both treatment groups. A single extrapyramidal reaction occurred in the bolus group, while two episodes occurred in the infusion group. Diarrhea was more predominant in the bolus group, with 5 of 13 (38%) patients having three or more diarrheal stools compared with 2 of 14 (14%) patients treated with metoclopramide administered via continuous infusion.

Discussion

The results of this study indicate that metoclopramide given by continuous infusion is an effective antiemetic at these dosages for cisplatin-induced vomiting. These results support a preliminary trial in which 12 patients were given metoclopramide via continuous infusion.[4] Furthermore, we have shown that the antiemetic effect of metoclopramide is equal using bolus or continuous-infusion techniques. With the number of patients in each treatment group, we could detect a 50% difference in response rates between bolus administration and continuous-infusion administration of metoclopramide, assuming a 75% major response rate in the bolus-dose group. This sample size ensures an 80% chance of detecting this difference if it exists, assuming an a priori level of significance of 0.05. We believed that to detect a 50% difference in response rate between groups would provide us with a clinically meaningful "difference."

Since we did not determine serum metoclopramide concentrations, we could not evaluate any potential concentration–response relationship. It would have been valuable to determine serum concentrations, especially in cases of treatment failure, to determine if response correlates with drug levels, as has been previously suggested.[7] In patients in whom metoclopramide therapy failed, inadequate serum metoclopramide concentrations may have accounted for the poor responses seen.[12] Metoclopramide clearance is highly variable, ranging from 0.2–1.3 L/kg/hr.[13] One of the infusion patients in whom treatment failed was a 21-year-old man with testicular cancer. We have treated subsequent young patients with testicular cancer with higher doses of metoclopramide and have observed major responses. There were no apparent reasons for the treatment failure with the bolus regimen.

Adverse effects were similar for both groups; however, there was a higher incidence of diarrhea in the bolus-treated group. This may be an additional advantage to the use of a continuous infusion. Sedation was common in both groups, but the use of intravenous diphenhydramine contributed to this effect. Patients did not complain of being oversedated. The number of extrapyramidal reactions was low and comparable to other published data. All extrapyramidal reactions responded well to additional doses of diphenhydramine.

Patients entered into the study were again randomized to the study upon readmission for further cisplatin therapy. Only 12 patients were evaluable during their second course of cisplatin. Results of these patients were analyzed separately to avoid any bias in results of the second course based on the first-course responses.[14] The number of major responders in each group was again similar: 100% (five of five) of the bolus group and 86% (six of seven) of the infusion group. Statistical analysis was not performed because of the small number of patients. Adverse-effect profiles were similar for both groups and both courses.

Of interest is that if patients vomited, they tended to do so at the end of the four-hour cisplatin infusion. Better responses may be achieved if an additional metoclopramide bolus dose is given before the end of the cisplatin infusion or if additional antiemetics are administered.

Pharmacy and nursing personnel favored the continuous metoclopramide infusion because it decreased pharmacy preparation and nursing administration time. No formal time studies were performed for either group.

Conclusion

The use of continuous-infusion metoclopramide is as effective in preventing cisplatin-induced vomiting as the bolus-dosing regimen. Ease of preparation and administration, as well as potentially fewer instances of diarrhea, favor the use of a continuous-infusion method at this dosage level. Because of the results of this study, our institution prevents cisplatin-induced emesis with a continuous infusion of metoclopramide.

References

1. Gralla RJ, Intri LM, Pisko SE et al. Antiemetic efficacy of high-dose metoclopramide in patients with chemotherapy induced nausea and vomiting. *N Engl J Med.* 1981; 305:905–9.
2. Kris MG, Gralla RJ, Tyson LB et al. Improved control of cisplatin-induced emesis with high-dose metoclopramide and with combinations of metoclopramide, dexamethasone, and diphenhydramine. *Cancer.* 1985; 55:527–34.
3. Anthony LB, Korzely MG, Woodward JG et al. Antiemetic effect of oral versus intravenous metoclopramide in patients receiving cisplatin: a randomized, double-blind trial. *J Clin Oncol.* 1986; 4:98–103.
4. Agostinucci WA, Gannon RG, Schauer PK et al. Continuous infusion of metoclopramide for prevention of chemotherapy-induced emesis. *Clin Pharm.* 1986; 5:150–3.
5. Joss RA, Galeazzi RL, Brunner KW. Continuous infusion of high-dose metoclopramide for the prevention of nausea and vomiting in patients receiving cancer chemotherapy. *Eur J Clin Pharmacol.* 1983; 25:35–9.
6. Taylor WB, Proctor SJ, Bateman DN. Pharmacokinetics and efficacy of high-dose metoclopramide given by continuous infusion for the control of cytotoxic drug-induced vomiting. *Br J Clin Pharmacol.* 1984; 18:679–84.
7. Saller R, Hellenbrecht D, Brieman L et al. Metoclopramide kinetics at high-dose infusion rates for prevention of cisplatinum induced emesis. *Clin Pharmacol Ther.* 1985; 37:43–7.
8. Cunningham D, Soukop M, Gilchrist NL et al. Randomized trial of intravenous high dose metoclopramide and intramuscular chlorpromazine in controlling nausea and vomiting induced by cytotoxic drugs. *Br Med J.* 1985; 290:604–5.
9. Dana BW, McDermott M, Everts E et al. A randomized trial of high-dose bolus metoclopramide versus low-dose continuous infusion metoclopramide in the prevention of cisplatin-induced emesis. *Am J Clin Oncol.* 1987; 10:253–6.
10. Taylor WB, Bateman DN. High dose metoclopramide—preliminary pharmacokinetic studies. *Br J Clin Pharmacol.* 1983; 16:341–2.
11. Karnofsky DA, Burchenal JH. In: MacLeod CM, ed. Evaluation of chemotherapeutic agents. New York: Columbia University Press; 1949:191.
12. Saller R, Hellenbrecht D, Hellstern A et al. Improved benefit/risk ratio of higher-dose metoclopramide therapy during cisplatin-induced emesis. *Eur J Clin Pharmacol.* 1985; 29:311–2.
13. McDermed JE, Cohen JL, Joseph C et al. Clinical pharmacokinetics of high-dose metoclopramide in cancer patients receiving cisplatin therapy. *J Clin Oncol.* 1985; 3:1400–8.
14. Oliver IN, Simon RM, Aisner J. Antiemetic studies: a methodological discussion. *Cancer Treat Rep.* 1986; 70:555–63.

Research Notes

Effect of pentoxifylline and its metabolites on three theophylline assays

IRA A. COHEN, CARY E. JOHNSON, LAURIE WESOLOWICZ, AND KATHLEEN CONVERSE-SWASTEK

Clin Pharm. 1988; 7:457–61

Pentoxifylline, 3,7-dimethyl-1-(5-oxohexyl)-xanthine, is approved for the treatment of intermittent claudication associated with chronic occlusive arterial disease. The recommended dose is one 400-mg controlled-release tablet three times a day with meals.[1]

Data regarding the pharmacokinetics of pentoxifylline are limited. After oral administration, the initial and major metabolite, metabolite I (3,7-dimethyl-1-(5-hydroxyhexyl)-xanthine) is formed by erythrocytes. However, hepatic metabolites are also produced, and at least six additional metabolites have been identified.[2] The plasma half-life of unchanged pentoxifylline in humans is 1.0 to 1.8 hours.[2] Approximately 95% of pentoxifylline and its metabolites are renally eliminated.[3] Only trace amounts of unchanged drug are found in the urine.[2] Metabolites I and V (3,7-dimethyl-1-(carboxybutyl)-xanthine) are found in the serum in concentrations exceeding that of the unchanged drug and appear to be equipotent to pentoxifylline.[1,3]

Hinze and coworkers[2] studied the pharmacokinetics of pentoxifylline in human subjects with normal renal and hepatic function. After administration of one 400-mg sustained-release pentoxifylline tablet three times a day for five days, the mean peak plasma concentration of pentoxifylline two to three hours after a dose was approximately 100 ng/mL. The mean peak concentration of metabolite I was reported to be 300 ng/mL.

In contrast to the work of Hinze, a study by Schaefer and coworkers[4] evaluated the elimination of only 98 mg of ^{14}C-labeled pentoxifylline administered as a single dose both to healthy adults and to subjects with chronic renal insufficiency (i.e., creatinine clearance of 3 to 38 mL/min). Serial determinations of radiolabeled pentoxifylline in plasma, presumably the total of unchanged drug and metabolites, were made over a 48-hour period. Serum concentrations four hours after dosing were 0.9 μg/mL in patients with normal renal function and 3.3 to 5.1 μg/mL in patients with renal insufficiency.

Some of the disparity in results obtained in the two studies may be attributed to the difference in dose and to the failure of Hinze et al. to quantitate additional metabolites, especially metabolite V. Also, the relatively high concentrations of pentoxifylline and metabolites identified by Schaefer and coworkers[4] may be explained, in part, by the relatively diminished renal function of their patients and by the researchers' possible failure to differentiate between unchanged drug and metabolites.

Pentoxifylline and its metabolites are structurally similar to other methyl-substituted xanthines (Figure 1). Of particular interest is their similarity to theophylline, since it possesses a low therapeutic index and is frequently monitored by serum assay. Methylxanthine compounds have been shown to variably cross-react both with a quantitative enzyme-multiplied immunoassay for theophylline[5] and with a fluorescence polarization immunoassay for the drug.[6] Interference with high-pressure liquid chromatography (HPLC) used for assaying theophylline content may also occur if other methylxanthine compounds have retention times similar to that of theophylline.

Cummings and coworkers[7] examined the potential influence of pentoxifylline and metabolite I on the results of three commercially available immunoassay systems for theophylline and on an HPLC assay. In their study, samples of pentoxifylline in concentrations of 50 and 100 ng/mL and metabolite I in concentrations of 200 and 400 ng/mL were prepared in serum and frozen until assayed. Although the authors concluded that there was a lack of interference under the conditions tested, they conceded that clinically important interference could occur if higher concentrations of pentoxifylline and its metabolites (consistent with an overdose) were used. In addition, their investigation did not evaluate the combined effect of (1) pentoxifylline plus metabolite I or (2) pentoxifylline or metabolite I, or both, plus theophylline on the theophylline assay results. Also, the potential effect of other pentoxifylline metabolites was not evaluated

Figure 1. Structural formulas of (top to bottom) pentoxifylline, metabolite I, metabolite V, and theophylline.

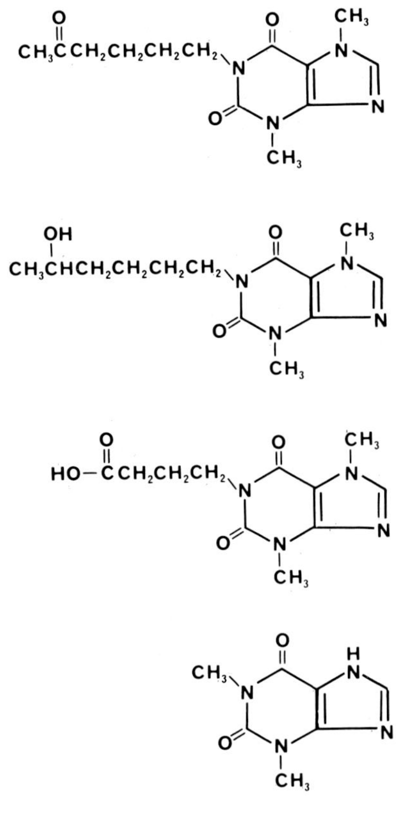

IRA A. COHEN, PHARM.D., is Clinical Research Scientist, Parke-Davis Pharmaceutical Research Division, Warner-Lambert Company, and Clinical Associate Professor of Pharmacy, College of Pharmacy, The University of Michigan, Ann Arbor; at the time of this study, he was Assistant Professor of Pharmacy, College of Pharmacy, The University of Michigan, and Clinical Pharmacist, Ann Arbor Veterans Administration Medical Center. CARY E. JOHNSON, PHARM.D., is Associate Professor of Pharmacy, College of Pharmacy, The University of Michigan, and Clinical Pharmacist–Pediatrics, The University of Michigan Medical Center, Ann Arbor. LAURIE WESOLOWICZ, PHARM.D., is Clinical Specialist–Drug Use Evaluation, Detroit Receiving Hospital and University Health Center, Detroit, MI, and KATHLEEN CONVERSE-SWASTEK, PHARM.D., is Drug Information Resident, Allegheny General Hospital, Pittsburgh, PA; at the time of this study, Wesolowicz and Converse-Swastek were Doctor of Pharmacy degree candidates, College of Pharmacy, the University of Michigan.

Address reprint requests to Dr. Cohen at Parke-Davis Pharmaceutical Research Division, Warner-Lambert Company, 2800 Plymouth Road, Ann Arbor, MI 48105-2430.

The assistance of Hoechst-Roussel Pharmaceuticals in supplying pentoxifylline and metabolite I; Abbott Laboratories, Diagnostics Division, in supplying TDx materials; and Syva Company in supplying EMIT materials used in this study is acknowledged.

Submitted in part to the College of Pharmacy, The University of Michigan, by Laurie (Hall) Wesolowicz and Kathy Converse-Swastek in partial fulfillment of the Doctor of Pharmacy degree requirements.

Copyright © 1988, American Society of Hospital Pharmacists, Inc. All rights reserved. 0278-2677/88/0601-0457$01.25.

in their in vitro study, which used spiked samples. The potential influence of freezing the samples before analysis on the assay results was also not reported.

Therefore, the purpose of this investigation was to evaluate the influence of a wide range of concentrations of pentoxifylline and metabolite I with and without the presence of other metabolites or theophylline, or both, on the results of three frequently used theophylline assay procedures.

Methods. *In Vitro Study of Theophylline Assay Cross-Reactivity.* This phase of the study involved an in vitro assessment of the cross-reactivity of pentoxifylline and metabolite I with theophylline as analyzed by a fluorescence polarization immunoassay (TDx, Abbott Laboratories, Diagnostics Division, Abbott Park, IL 60064), an enzyme-multiplied immunoassay system (EMIT, Syva Company, Palo Alto, CA 94303), and an HPLC method. Drug-free serum was obtained from a volunteer who gave his informed consent and abstained from substances known to contain substantial concentrations of methylxanthine (i.e., coffee, tea, other caffeinated beverages, and chocolate and other cocoa-containing foods and beverages[8]), as well as all medications, for seven days before the sample was obtained.

Stock solutions of pentoxifylline, metabolite I, and theophylline were prepared, and appropriate volumes of the stock solutions were added to the drug-free serum to yield the concentrations and combinations shown in Table 1. Samples containing 1.0×10^4 ng/mL or less of pentoxifylline or metabolite I, or both, reflect serum concentrations that might be achieved after long-term administration in patients, including those with renal insufficiency. The samples containing very high concentrations (i.e., greater than 1.0×10^4 ng/mL) are unlikely to occur clinically, except after overdoses of the drug. Each sample type was prepared in triplicate, with one sample set being used for each of the three assay systems. Before assay, samples were mixed in a Vortex mixer and incubated at 37.5 °C for 18 hours.

Serum theophylline assays were performed by the EMIT[5] and TDx[6] systems according to manufacturers' operating procedures. Intrarun theophylline controls of 15 μg/mL for the EMIT system (Sigma Chemical Company, St. Louis, MO 63178, lot 110f-0083) and both 7.0 and 26.0 μg/mL for the TDx system (TDx theophylline controls, Abbott Laboratories, Diagnostic Division, lot 74f-442AZ) were analyzed for each set of samples. Because of unexpected assay results when pentoxifylline and metabolite I concentrations exceeded 2.0×10^4 ng/mL, a second set of samples was prepared and analyzed by the EMIT system. Samples were analyzed using HPLC according to the method described by Orcutt et al.[9] Standard curves for all three assay systems were prepared just before sample analysis. Each sample was assayed in duplicate by each assay method.

The between-run coefficient of variation for the TDx theophylline assay was 3.0% at 7.0 μg/mL and 6.4% at 26.0 μg/mL. Evaluation of this system for the theophylline assay before the study revealed a within-run coefficient of variation of 4.1% at 5 μg/mL, 1.25% at 15 μg/mL, and 1.1% at 30 μg/mL. The within-run coefficients of variation for the EMIT and HPLC assays were 4.3% and 4.7%, respectively. The lower limits of detection for the EMIT, TDx, and HPLC assay methods used were 2.5, 0.3, and 0.1 μg/mL, respectively.

In Vivo Study of Theophylline Assay Cross-Reactivity. This phase of the study evaluated the potential theophylline cross-reactivity produced by concentrations of pentoxifylline and its metabolites, including metabolites II–V, found in the serum after oral administration of one 400-mg tablet of pentoxifylline (Trental, Hoechst-Roussel Pharmaceuticals Inc., Somerville, NJ 08876, lot RC1790) every eight hours for three days to a 34-year-old male volunteer who gave his informed consent. The volunteer adhered to the same dietary and drug restrictions described in the methods for the in vitro study. Serum was obtained 2.5 hours after the morning dose on the fourth day of pentoxifylline administration. Samples were assayed in duplicate by each of the aforementioned assay systems. In addition, theophylline was added to aliquots of the volunteer's serum to produce a final concentration of approximately 10 μg/mL, and these samples were also assayed as previously described.

Data Analysis. For samples containing pentoxifylline or metabolite I, or both, the mean concentration from the duplicate analysis by each assay method was compared with the concentration of samples of drug-free serum and with data for samples containing only theophylline (Table 1). When appropriate, the percentage increase of the assayed theophylline concentration over the expected (actual) theophylline concentration was calculated. For the purposes of this study, an increase of 30% or more was considered to be of potential clinical importance.

Results. The influence of pentoxifylline and its metabolites on theophylline assay results is presented in Table 1. The mean assayed concentration of theophylline by the TDx method for serum samples to which approximately 10 μg/mL of theophylline was added ranged from 9.29 to 10.42 μg/mL (range of 95.7 to 107.3% of expected concentration), despite the presence of pentoxifylline or metabolite I, or both, in concentrations ranging from 200 ng/mL to 1.0×10^6 ng/mL. Assayed theophylline concentrations were not quantifiable by the TDx system for samples containing only pentoxifylline or metabolite I, or both.

Similarly, assayed theophylline concentrations by the HPLC method did not exceed 104% of the

Table 1.
Effect of Pentoxifylline and Its Metabolites on Theophylline Assay Results

Theoretical Concentration			Measured Theophylline Concentration							
			EMIT Trial 1		EMIT Trial 2		TDx		HPLC	
Theophylline[a] (μg/mL)	Pentoxifylline[b] (ng/mL)	Metabolite I[c] (ng/mL)	Mean Assayed Concentration[d] (μg/mL), $n = 2$	% of Expected Concentration[e]	Mean Assayed Concentration[d] (μg/mL), $n = 2$	% of Expected Concentration[e]	Mean Assayed Concentration[d] (μg/mL), $n = 2$	% of Expected Concentration[e]	Mean Assayed Concentration[d] (μg/mL) $n = 2$	% of Expected Concentration[e]
0.0[f]	0.0	0.0	N.Q.[g]	N.A.[h]	N.Q.	N.A.	N.Q.	N.A.	N.Q.	N.A.
10.0	0.0	0.0	9.90 ± 0.14[i]	100.0	...	...	9.83 ± 0.14[i]	100.0	10.09 ± 0.10[i]	100.0
10.0	2.0×10^2	0.0	8.90 ± 0.42	89.9	...	...	9.89 ± 0.22	100.6	10.05 ± 0.08	99.6
10.0	1.0×10^3	0.0	9.20 ± 0.00	92.9	...	...	10.03 ± 0.28	102.0	10.13 ± 0.12	100.4
10.0	1.0×10^4	0.0	8.85 ± 0.35	89.4	...	...	10.10 ± 0.12	102.7	9.95 ± 0.07	98.6
10.0	0.0	2.0×10^2	9.00 ± 0.42	90.9	...	...	9.92 ± 0.08	100.9	10.07 ± 0.04	99.8
10.0	0.0	1.0×10^3	9.85 ± 0.35	99.5	...	...	9.98 ± 0.17	101.5	10.16 ± 0.11	100.7
10.0	0.0	1.0×10^4	9.55 ± 0.07	96.5	...	...	10.11 ± 0.32	102.8	10.04 ± 0.14	99.5
10.0	2.0×10^2	2.0×10^2	9.90 ± 0.14	100.0	...	...	10.07 ± 0.24	102.4	10.21 ± 0.08	101.2
10.0	1.0×10^3	1.0×10^3	9.85 ± 0.21	99.5	...	...	10.15 ± 0.16	103.3	10.17 ± 0.04	100.8
10.0	1.0×10^4	1.0×10^4	9.80 ± 0.14	99.0	...	...	9.96 ± 0.10	101.3	10.22 ± 0.02	102.3
0.0	2.0×10^2	0.0	N.Q.	N.A.	...	...	N.Q.	N.A.	N.Q.	N.A.
0.0	1.0×10^3	0.0	N.Q.	N.A.	...	...	N.Q.	N.A.	N.Q.	N.A.
0.0	1.0×10^4	0.0	N.Q.	N.A.	...	...	N.Q.	N.A.	N.Q.	N.A.
0.0	0.0	2.0×10^2	N.Q.	N.A.	...	...	N.Q.	N.A.	N.Q.	N.A.
0.0	0.0	1.0×10^3	N.Q.	N.A.	...	...	N.Q.	N.A.	N.Q.	N.A.
0.0	0.0	1.0×10^4	N.Q.	N.A.	...	...	N.Q.	N.A.	N.Q.	N.A.
0.0	2.0×10^2	2.0×10^2	N.Q.	N.A.	...	...	N.Q.	N.A.	N.Q.	N.A.
0.0	1.0×10^3	1.0 × 10.3	N.Q.	N.A.	...	...	N.Q.	N.A.	N.Q.	N.A.
0.0	1.0×10^4	1.0×10^4	N.Q.	N.A.	...	...	N.Q.	N.A.	N.Q.	N.A.
10.0	0.0	0.0	9.65 ± 0.07[i]	100.0	8.90 ± 0.28[i]	100.0	9.71 ± 0.08[i]	100.0	10.21 ± 0.11[i]	100.0
10.0	2.0×10^4	0.0	11.00 ± 0.14	114.0	11.00 ± 0.07	123.6	9.44 ± 0.36	97.2	10.37 ± 0.09	101.6
10.0	2.0×10^5	0.0	16.70 ± 0.14	173.1	17.30 ± 0.42	194.4	10.28 ± 0.24	105.9	10.58 ± 0.13	103.6
10.0	1.0×10^6	0.0	23.60 ± 0.14	244.6	23.70 ± 0.70	266.3	9.90 ± 0.24	102.0	10.55 ± 0.05	103.3
10.0	0.0	2.0×10^4	10.65 ± 0.07	110.4	10.20 ± 0.28	114.6	10.03 ± 0.48	103.3	10.20 ± 0.07	99.9
10.0	0.0	2.0×10^5	16.85 ± 0.06	174.6	14.55 ± 0.49	163.5	10.01 ± 0.23	103.1	10.62 ± 0.11	104.0
10.0	0.0	1.0×10^6	21.00 ± 0.70	217.6	20.65 ± 0.64	232.0	10.29 ± 0.10	106.0	10.36 ± 0.09	101.5
10.0	2.0×10^4	2.0×10^4	12.10 ± 0.07	125.4	11.65 ± 0.21	130.9	10.42 ± 0.48	107.3	10.28 ± 0.03	100.7
10.0	2.0×10^5	2.0×10^5	19.55 ± 0.07	202.6	18.55 ± 0.35	208.4	9.91 ± 0.05	102.1	10.26 ± 0.06	100.5
10.0	1.0×10^6	1.0×10^6	28.60 ± 0.61	296.4	25.95 ± 0.34	291.6	10.37 ± 0.27	106.8	10.44 ± 0.13	102.3
0.0	2.0×10^4	0.0	N.Q.	N.A.	N.Q.	N.A.	N.Q.	N.A.	N.Q.	N.A.
0.0	2.0×10^5	0.0	N.Q.	N.A.	N.Q.	N.A.	N.Q.	N.A.	N.Q.	N.A.
0.0	1.0×10^6	0.0	N.Q.	N.A.	N.Q.	N.A.	N.Q.	N.A.	N.Q.	N.A.
0.0	0.0	2.0×10^4	N.Q.	N.A.	N.Q.	N.A.	N.Q.	N.A.	N.Q.	N.A.
0.0	0.0	1.0×10^6	N.Q.	N.A.	N.Q.	N.A.	N.Q.	N.A.	N.Q.	N.A.
0.0	2.0×10^4	2.0×10^4	N.Q.	N.A.	N.Q.	N.A.	N.Q.	N.A.	N.Q.	N.A.
0.0	2.0×10^5	2.0×10^5	N.Q.	N.A.	N.Q.	N.A.	N.Q.	N.A.	N.Q.	N.A.
0.0	1.0×10^6	1.0×10^6	N.Q.	N.A.	N.Q.	N.A.	N.Q.	N.A.	N.Q.	N.A.
0.0[j]	0.0	0.0	N.Q.	N.A.	N.Q.	N.A.	N.Q.	N.A.	N.Q.	N.A.
10.0[k]	0.0	0.0	9.20 ± 0.71	95.3	8.45 ± 0.35	94.9	9.29 ± 0.15	95.7	10.39 ± 0.07	101.8

[a] Expected concentration after addition of theophylline to serum.
[b] Expected concentration after addition of pentoxifylline to serum.
[c] Expected concentration after addition of pentoxifylline's metabolite I to serum.
[d] Mean ± S.D.
[e] (Mean assayed theophylline concentration ÷ assayed concentration for theophylline control sample) × 100.
[f] Blank (drug-free) serum.
[g] Not quantifiable.
[h] Not applicable.
[i] Control sample; blank serum to which approximately 10 μg/mL of theophylline was added.
[j] Serum from volunteer taking pentoxifylline 400 mg orally every eight hours for three days; sample collected 2.5 hours after last dose.
[k] Serum from volunteer taking pentoxifylline to which approximately 10 μg/mL of theophylline was added.

expected concentration in the serum samples to which approximately 10 μg/mL of theophylline was added. As in the case of the TDx method, assayed theophylline concentrations were undetectable for serum samples containing only pentoxifylline or metabolite I, or both, in concentrations ranging from 200 ng/mL to 1.0×10^6 ng/mL.

Likewise, theophylline concentrations as assessed by the EMIT system were not quantifiable for serum samples containing only pentoxifylline or metabolite I, or both, and the mean assayed theophylline concentration for samples containing approximately 10 μg/mL of theophylline, but less than 1.0×10^4 ng/mL of pentoxifylline or metabolite I, or both, never exceeded 100% of the expected theophylline concentration. However, for samples containing approximately 10 μg/mL of theophylline in combination with high concentrations (i.e., 2.0×10^4 ng/mL or more) of pentoxifylline or metabolite I, or both, the EMIT method indicated theophylline concentrations ranging from 110.4 to 296.4% of the expected concentration. On the basis of these unusual results, a second set of samples was prepared and analyzed for theophylline concentration by the EMIT system. The original results were confirmed, and assayed theophylline concentrations for this second trial ranged from 114.6 to 291.6% of the expected concentration. Therefore, actual assayed concentrations exceeded expected theophylline concentrations by more than 30% for all samples containing 2.0×10^5 ng/mL or more of pentoxifylline or metabolite I, or both.

Theophylline concentrations by all three assay methods were undetectable when serum from the volunteer taking oral pentoxifylline 400 mg every eight hours for three days was analyzed. The assayed theophylline concentrations for the same samples to which approximately 10 μg/mL of theophylline was added were 9.20 and 8.45 μg/mL for EMIT trials 1 and 2, respectively. This was 95.3% (trial 1) and 94.9% (trial 2) of the expected theophylline concentration.

Discussion. Pentoxifylline or metabolite I, or both, in concentrations of up to 1.0×10^6 ng/mL of each does not interfere with the results of the TDx or HPLC assays for theophylline and does not interfere with the EMIT assay in concentrations of 1.0×10^4 ng/mL or less. These results substantiate those reported by Cummings and coworkers.[7] Although not previously evaluated, concentrations of pentoxifylline and its various metabolites achieved in the serum of a healthy volunteer taking the recommended dose of pentoxifylline also did not interfere with any of the three assay systems.

Interference with theophylline assay results occurred only with the EMIT system for samples containing very high concentrations of pentoxifylline or metabolite I, or both, and this interaction was evident only when theophylline was also present in the sample. The mechanism for this unexpected, but reproducible, finding is not apparent and deserves further investigation.

Conclusion. Theophylline assay results as determined by the TDx, EMIT, and HPLC methods are not influenced by the presence of usual clinically achievable concentrations of pentoxifylline and its metabolites. However, interference with EMIT theophylline assay results may occur if very high concentrations of pentoxifylline or metabolite I, or both, are achieved. Concern for potential pentoxifylline-associated theophylline assay interference appears to be limited to cases of pentoxifylline overdosage in theophylline-treated patients and only when the EMIT assay is employed.

References

1. Aviado DM, Dettelbach HR. Pharmacology of pentoxifylline, a hemorheologic agent for the treatment of intermittent claudication. *Angiology*. 1984; 35:407–17.
2. Hinze HJ, Grigoleit HG, Rethy B. Bioavailability and pharmacokinetics of pentoxifylline from 'Trental 400' in man. *Pharmatherapeutica*. 1976; 1:160–71.
3. Christ O, Gleixner K, Kellner HM et al. Pharmacokinetic investigations after oral administration of 3,7-dimethyl-1-(5'-oxohexyl)-xanthine-14C (BL 191)-14C) to rats, dogs and humans. *Arzneimittelforschung*. 1972; 22:1933–7.
4. Schaefer K, von Herrath D, Hensel A et al. Investigations on the pharmacokinetics of pentoxifylline in chronic renal failure. *Med Klin*. 1977; 72:204–6.
5. Syva Company. Emit-aad; for use in the quantitative enzyme immunoassay of theophylline in serum or plasma. Palo Alto, CA; 1979 May.
6. Abbott Laboratories, Diagnostics Division. Fluorescence polarization immunoassay for the determination of therapeutic drug levels in human plasma. Abbott Park, IL; 1982 Sep.
7. Cummings DM, Rocci ML, Green P et al. Interference potential of pentoxifylline and its major metabolite with theophylline assays. *Am J Hosp Pharm*. 1985; 42:2717–8.
8. Monks TJ, Caldwell J, Smith RL. Influence of methylxanthine containing foods on theophylline metabolism and kinetics. *Clin Pharmacol Ther*. 1979; 26:513–24.
9. Orcutt JJ, Kozak PP, Gillman SA et al. Micro-scale method for theophylline in body fluids by reversed-phase, high-pressure liquid chromatography. *Clin Chem*. 1977; 23:599–601.

Accuracy and time requirements for use of three rapid theophylline assay methods

G. DENNIS CLIFTON, MARK E. WEST, BERNARD A. HUNT, AND N. K. BURKI

Clin Pharm. 1988; 7:462-6

High-performance liquid chromatography (HPLC), enzyme-multiplied immunoassay (EMIT, Syva Corporation, Palo Alto, CA), and fluorescence polarization immunoassay (FPIA, TDx, Abbott Diagnostics, Irving, TX 75015) are the standard methods for determination of serum theophylline concentrations in most hospital and clinical laboratories. These methods are often too costly for practical use in small clinic or office practice settings. Furthermore, because of slow turnaround times by clinical laboratories that use these assays, results of serum theophylline determinations at a clinic visit are often not available until after the patient has departed. This necessitates time-consuming follow-up by telephone and may compromise patient care.

Three new devices, Acculevel (Syntex Medical Diagnostics, Palo Alto, CA 94304), Seralyzer (Ames Division, Miles Laboratories, Elkhart, IN 46515), and Vision (Abbott Diagnostics) are marketed specifically for use in these settings because of their ability to provide results within several minutes. All three devices use monoclonal antibody technology; however, Seralyzer and Vision are instrumented systems, whereas Acculevel is noninstrumented. All three devices have been compared with each of the standard methods (HPLC, EMIT, and FPIA).[1-4] The objective of this study was to compare these three commercially marketed devices with regard to performance, time requirements for use, and cost.

Methods. This was a nonblinded, nonrandomized evaluation of the three devices using TDx as the standard for comparison. The TDx analytical method for theophylline concentration determination has been demonstrated to be accurate, sensitive, specific, and precise, with within-run and between-run coefficients of variation (CVs) of 1.7–3.0%.[5,6] The study was approved by the University of Kentucky Medical Institutional Review Board.

Assay Systems. Vision (model 1436-01) is a fully automated system consisting of a centrifuge, spectrophotometer, microprocessor, and printer. A multichamber test pack (lot 01437A421) contains the reagent system: a theophylline conjugate complex, monoclonal antibody to theophylline, acetylcholinesterase, and substrate for acetylcholinesterase. Centrifugal force is used to separate the sample (if whole blood is used), measure the reagent and sample volumes, and complete all steps required for spectrophotometric analysis of the serum or plasma. Vision is capable of using whole blood, plasma, or serum for theophylline concentration determination. It is designed to measure theophylline concentrations above 0.2 μg/mL. Investigators using the Vision assay have reported within-run and between-run mean CVs of less than 8%.[7] Within-run and between-run CVs reported by Abbott are within the range of 4.4–6.2% (Data on file. Abbott Laboratories. 1988 Mar).

Acculevel is a noninstrumented system that uses whole blood for theophylline concentration determination. A chromatographic paper strip coated with monoclonal antibodies to theophylline (lot W02) is attached to the open center of a thermometer-like cassette. A sample of whole blood is added to an enzyme-labeled theophylline solution (lot W02), and the cassette is placed in the mixture. As fluid migrates up the strip, enzyme-labeled theophylline and theophylline from the sample bind to the immobilized antibody sites. Immersion of the cassette in the developing solution (lot W03) results in the formation of an insoluble blue product on the portion of the chromatographic paper to which enzyme-labeled theophylline is bound. The height of the color bar is measured and converted to a plasma theophylline concentration, using a result table. Although the assay uses whole blood, the result table uses a conversion factor (0.82) in order to give assay results in terms of serum or plasma concentration. Acculevel is designed to measure theophylline concentrations above 3.0 μg/mL. The within-run and between-run precision of the Acculevel assay has reported mean CVs of 6.9–8.1% and 5.0–7.9%, respectively.[8] Syntex reports within-run and between-run CVs of 4.7–7.8% and 2.9–6.7%, respectively.[9]

Seralyzer is a partially automated system designed for use with plasma or serum specimens. The assay uses a reagent strip (lots J134055 and M202066) impregnated with monoclonal antibodies to theophylline and a theophylline–enzyme conjugate complex. After centrifugation of a whole

G. DENNIS CLIFTON, PHARM.D., is Assistant Professor, Division of Clinical Practice, College of Pharmacy, University of Kentucky, Lexington. MARK E. WEST, PHARM.D., is Clinical Pharmacy Resident and BERNARD A. HUNT, PHARM.D., is Clinical Pharmacy Resident, University of Kentucky Medical Center, Lexington. N. K. BURKI, M.D., PH.D., is Professor and Chairman, Pulmonary Division, College of Medicine, University of Kentucky Medical Center, Lexington.

Address reprint requests to Dr. Clifton at University of Kentucky Medical Center Hospital, Room C-117, 800 Rose Street, Lexington, KY 40536-0084.

The technical assistance of Lena Richie in the preparation of this manuscript is acknowledged.

Presented at the 22nd Annual ASHP Midyear Clinical Meeting, Atlanta, GA, December 6, 1987.

Copyright © 1988, American Society of Hospital Pharmacists, Inc. All rights reserved. 0278-2677/88/0601-0462$01.25

blood sample, harvesting of the plasma or serum, and manual dilution, the sample is placed on the strip. Theophylline present in the sample displaces the conjugated theophylline, which reacts with the enzyme to form a colored compound. The color intensity of the strip is read by a reflectance photometer and converted to concentration by the instrument's microcomputer. Seralyzer is designed to measure theophylline concentrations above 3.0 μg/mL. Within-run CVs of 3.4–7.1% and between-run CVs of 4.6–11.5% have been reported by investigators using the Seralyzer assay.[4] Miles reports within-run CVs of 4.3–5.4% and between-run CVs of 3.5–4.4%.[10]

Procedure. Blood was collected from adult and pediatric outpatients at the Warren Wright Medical Plaza, University of Kentucky Medical Center. All patients were receiving maintenance dosages of theophylline products and were previously scheduled for theophylline concentration determination. Blood was collected by staff phlebotomists.

All blood was collected in heparin-containing tubes so that whole blood and plasma specimens could be obtained from a single sample. Plasma was used for the Seralyzer and whole blood for the Vision and Acculevel devices. Specimen type (whole blood or plasma) used for each of the three assays was chosen based on the type most likely to be used clinically. Heparin is reported to not interfere with any of the three test assays for theophylline.

Single analysis of all blood samples by the three test methods was performed by the investigators on the day of collection. Calibration and sample analysis were performed according to the methods recommended by each of the respective assay system manufacturers. Plasma theophylline concentration measurements by TDx were performed singly by the Medical Center's Therapeutic Drug Monitoring (TDM) laboratory. The TDM laboratory was blinded to which samples were being compared for assay results and time requirements. The mean interday CVs for control samples of theophylline analyzed by the laboratory during the months of the study were 2.88–5.76%.

Each assay was also compared with regard to time requirements. Time measurements for Vision, Acculevel, and Seralyzer began upon the initiation of sample preparation and ended when the result was reported (Vision, Seralyzer) or read (Acculevel). Because these assays are intended for use immediately after a specimen is collected, this time also represents turnaround time. Turnaround time for TDx was defined as the interval between the time that the blood sample was obtained and the time that the result was reported by the TDM laboratory.

Analysis of Data. Linear least-squares regression constants and the product-moment correlation coefficients (r) were determined from scatter plots of theophylline concentration measured by the test method versus that measured by TDx. The mean error (ME), a measure of bias, and root mean squared error (RMSE), a measure of precision, were calculated as follows[11]:

$$\mathrm{ME} = (1/n) \sum_{i=1}^{n} \mathrm{pe}$$

$$\mathrm{RMSE} = (1/n) \left(\sum_{i=1}^{n} (\mathrm{pe})^2 \right)^{1/2}$$

where pe is prediction error (test method concentration − TDx concentration) and n is the number of pairs of theophylline concentrations. Statistical inferences on continuous data were determined by one-way analysis of variance (ANOVA), while proportions were compared using chi-square analysis. The a priori level of significance was $p < 0.05$.

Results. A total of 44 blood samples were collected from 40 patients attending the medical center outpatient clinics. The patient population consisted of 15 males and 25 females ranging in age from 2 to 80 years (mean ± S.D., 36.4 ± 25.2 yr). All samples were assayed by the three rapid methods within six hours of blood collection (mean ± S.D., 2.6 ± 1.8 hr).

Theophylline concentrations according to TDx ranged from 0 to 26.0 μg/mL. Correlation coefficients for Vision, Acculevel, and Seralyzer versus TDx were 0.981, 0.982, and 0.974, respectively (all $p < 0.05$). Exclusion of values less than 3.0 μg/mL (according to TDx) resulted in very little change in the correlation coefficients (0.974, 0.980, 0.971 for Vision, Acculevel, and Seralyzer, respectively.)

The three assay methods varied in their bias (ME) and precision (RSME) (Table 1). When all data are included, Vision appears to produce the best balance of less bias and greater precision. By excluding the values less than 3.0 μg/mL (as measured by TDx), Acculevel and Seralyzer improve in both bias and precision.

Bias and precision data with respect to theophylline concentration ranges of 3.0 to 10.0 μg/mL, 10.1–20.0 μg/mL, and 20.1–26.0 μg/mL are also shown in Table 1. Overall, in terms of bias, Vision tended to underestimate, while both Acculevel and Seralyzer tended to overestimate plasma theophylline concentrations as compared with TDx. Seralyzer was both less biased and more precise than either of the other two methods for concentrations of 3.0 to 10.0 μg/mL. This difference, however, was not significant. In the 10.1 to 20.0 μg/mL concentration range (usual therapeutic range), Vision demonstrated the best balance between bias and precision. In this concentration range, Vision was more precise than Acculevel or Seralyzer ($p = 0.05$). The number of theophylline concentrations greater than 20 μg/mL was insufficient for statistical inference.

Table 1.
Predictive Performance[a] of Test Assay Method versus Reference in Various Theophylline Concentration Ranges

Assay	ME[b]	RMSE[b]
0.0–26 μg/mL (n = *44)*		
Vision	−0.40 (−0.83 to 0.31)	1.50 (0.77 to 2.23)
Acculevel	0.90 (0.47 to 1.33)	1.68 (1.13 to 2.23)
Seralyzer	0.90 (0.39 to 1.41)	1.93 (1.29 to 2.56)
3.0–26 μg/mL (n = *38)*		
Vision	−0.62 (−1.12 to 0.12)	1.63 (0.78 to 2.48)
Acculevel	0.61 (0.17 to 1.05)	1.47 (0.91 to 2.03)
Seralyzer	0.59 (0.03 to 1.15)	1.78 (1.08 to 2.48)
3.0–10 μg/mL (n = *18)*		
Vision	−0.71 (−1.69 to 0.27)	1.92 (0.30 to 3.54)
Acculevel	0.66 (0.06 to 1.26)	1.27 (0.49 to 2.05)
Seralyzer	0.23 (−0.33 to 0.79)	1.04 (0.35 to 1.73)
10.1–20 μg/mL (n = *13)*		
Vision	0.67 (−1.05 to 0.29)	0.90 (0.36 to 1.44)[c]
Acculevel	0.48 (−0.58 to 1.54)	1.77 (0.58 to 2.96)
Seralyzer	0.88 (−0.34 to 2.10)	2.14 (0.77 to 3.51)
20.1–26 μg/mL (n = *7[d])*		
Vision	−0.31 (−2.20 to 1.58)	1.93 (−0.33 to 4.19)
Acculevel	0.74 (−0.27 to 1.75)	1.25 (0.09 to 2.41)
Seralyzer	0.89 (−1.24 to 3.02)	2.32 (0.00 to 4.64)

[a] As indicated by mean error (ME), a measurement of bias, and root mean squared error (RMSE), a measurement of precision.

[b] Values in parentheses are 95% confidence interval.

[c] RMSE for Vision significantly different from Acculevel and Seralyzer (ANOVA).

[d] Insufficient sample size for statistical inference.

Frequency distributions of the prediction error of the three assay methods are shown in Figures 1, 2, and 3. Only concentrations greater than 3.0 μg/mL were included. Of the measurements by Vision (Figure 1), 76.3% were within 1.5 μg/mL of measurements by TDx. The corresponding values for Acculevel (Figure 2) and Seralyzer (Figure 3) were 68.4% and 60.5%, respectively. The differences between the three methods were not significant. Differences in measured theophylline concentrations of greater than 3.0 μg/mL occurred with all assays compared with TDx. This magnitude of difference occurred in 7.8, 2.6, and 7.8% of samples with Vision, Acculevel, and Seralyzer, respectively. No patients were using drugs known to cross-react with any of the assays. No other factors (e.g., hemolysis, anemia, uremia, age, or sex) could be identified to explain the outlying results.

Time requirements for the determination of theophylline concentration by each assay method are shown in Table 2. Of all samples, 48% (21) were run separately and 52% (23) were run as batches (two or more). The time for a single batch run of four samples could not be analyzed because of investigator error in timing. Vision was significantly more rapid than the other two systems in producing results. Acculevel was the least rapid, being significantly slower than Seralyzer as well.

Figure 1. Frequency distribution of the predicted error for Vision versus TDx (n = 38).

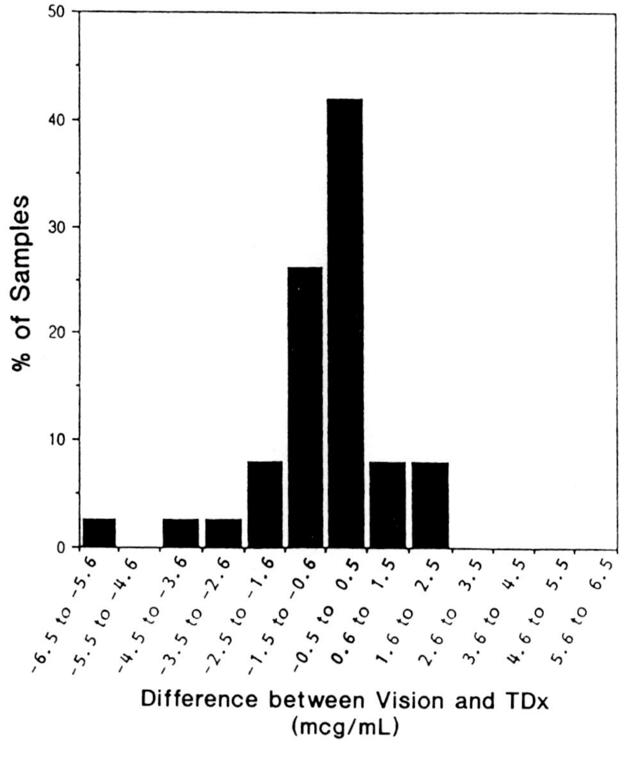

Figure 2. Frequency distribution of the predicted error for Acculevel versus TDx (n = 38).

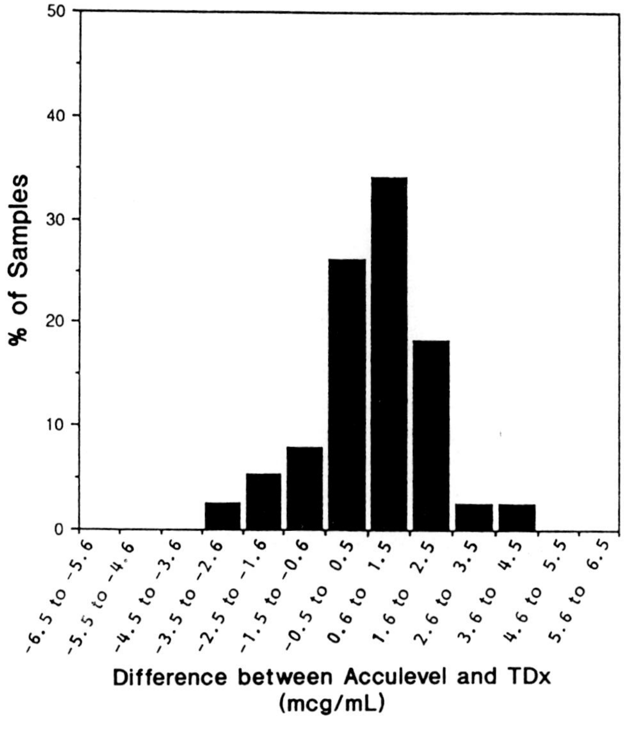

Figure 3. Frequency distribution of the predicted error for Seralyzer versus TDx (n = 38).

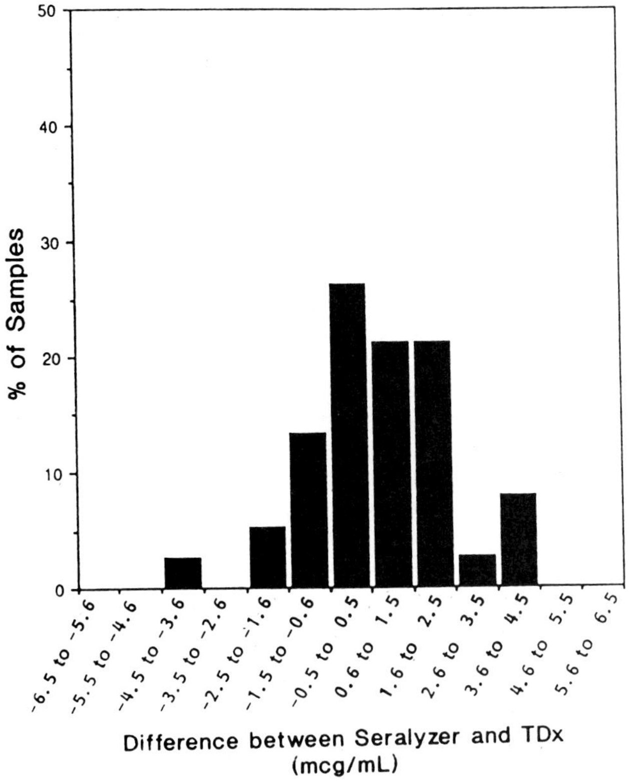

Table 2.
Time Requirements for Theophylline Concentration Determination

Assay[a]	Time (min) Single Samples (n = 21)	Time (min) Batched Samples[b] (n = 19)
Vision	17.8 ± 4.5[c]	18.7 ± 2.0[c]
Acculevel	28.7 ± 2.7	28.0 ± 3.2
Seralyzer	21.4 ± 4.9[d]	25.1 ± 4.2[d]

[a] Mean ± S.D. time required to perform TDx assay was 311.4 ± 286.2 minutes.
[b] Consisted of two or more samples. Time reported as minutes per batch.
[c] Significiantly different from values for Acculevel and Seralyzer (p < 0.05, ANOVA).
[d] Significantly different from value for Acculevel (p < 0.05, ANOVA).

Table 3 compares the total cost per theophylline sample for each of the three devices at selected usage levels over a one-month period. Assay costs refer to the cost of reagents or test packs necessary to analyze the desired number of samples. Vision and Seralyzer have fixed assay costs. Acculevel's assay costs were based on bulk purchasing of 48 test pack units at a time. Control and calibration costs were determined according to guidelines set by the manufacturers. All hardware costs were determined from price quotes by regional salespersons for each of the respective devices. Hardware (capital) expenditures for Vision and Seralyzer were amortized over a five-year period.

Total costs per sample for Vision and Seralyzer vary depending on the number of samples assayed per given time period. The difference in cost is directly related to the number of controls necessary per month. Both Vision and Seralyzer become less costly per sample when the average number per day increases. Acculevel requires only a single control per bulk package of assays. The control is provided at no cost by the manufacturer. Therefore, the cost per sample for Acculevel does not change with different volumes of use.

Discussion. All three methods—Vision, Acculevel, and Seralyzer—demonstrated very good to excellent performance for the measurement of plasma theophylline concentrations, as compared with TDx. Differences in measured theophylline concentrations of greater than 3.0 μg/mL occurred in less than 10% of specimens analyzed with each assay compared with TDx. Although it is unlikely in most patients, errors in measured theophylline concentrations of the magnitude seen in this study could be clinically important in some individuals. There was no significant difference among the three methods, except in the range of 10–20 μg/mL, where Vision was significantly more precise. The differences between assays, however, do not appear to be clinically important.

Our results are consistent with those of Chan et al.,[12] who showed excellent correlation of Vision to TDx. The only other published study comparing

Table 3.
Cost Analysis for Vision, Acculevel, and Seralyzer at Selected Usage Levels for One Month (20 Days)[a]

Cost Item	20 Samples/Month (Average 1/Day)			20 Samples/Month (Average 2/Day)			40 Samples/Month (Average 4/Day)		
	V	A	S	V	A	S	V	A	S
Assay[b]	120	300	60	120	300	60	240	600	120
Controls	120	...	60	60	...	30	60	...	30
Calibration	30	...	24	30	...	24	30	...	24
Hardware	208	...	36	208	...	36	208	...	36
Total cost	478	300	180	418	300	150	538	600	210
Average cost per sample	24	15	9	21	15	8	14	15	5

[a] All costs are in dollars; V = Vision, A = Acculevel, S = Seralyzer.
[b] Cost of reagents or test packs.

more than one of the test systems with TDx was by Fling et al.,[13] who compared Acculevel and Seralyzer with TDx. In their study, Acculevel proved accurate at all concentrations, while Seralyzer tended to underestimate serum theophylline concentrations (significant difference between Acculevel and Seralyzer). Busch and Virji[14] showed good correlation of the Seralyzer with TDx. Consistent with our findings, they noted the tendency for Seralyzer to overestimate (as compared with TDx). Busch and Virji attributed this overestimation to the effects of temperature on the reagents.

To our knowledge, this is the first published report evaluating and comparing all three systems. Unlike other investigators, we used bias and precision, as suggested by Sheiner and Beal.[11] Correlation coefficient, the sole measure used in many other reports, is not the best measure of predictive performance since it measures only the degree of association around the line of best fit. Precision and bias are better measures of predictive performance, as supported by numerous papers in the pharmacokinetics literature.[15-18]

The differences in the time to perform each assay were clinically important. However, it is important to realize that each device requires different levels of operator input and skill. Vision, the quickest system, requires little input from the operator and little technical knowledge. From start to finish, Acculevel is the most time consuming; however, little direct operator input is required. Seralyzer is more rapid overall than Acculevel but requires substantial manipulation by the operator. Seralyzer is the most difficult to use, requiring some basic laboratory skills on the part of the operator. An additional advantage for both the Vision and Acculevel systems is the ability to process whole blood obtained by either venipuncture or finger stick.

Cost is a highly variable factor in the choice between these systems. Based on low usage, Seralyzer is the least expensive. As usage increases, both the Vision and Seralyzer become less expensive, while Acculevel costs remain the same. The Vision and Seralyzer systems are capable of performing other drug and clinical chemistry assays in addition to theophylline assays. This may make these two systems more attractive for some practice sites.

Two aspects of our study design warrant discussion. Ideally, analyses by the reference method (TDx) should have been performed in duplicate to ensure that the results were correct. However, the relatively good precision characteristics of the TDx method when used by our laboratory personnel make inaccurate results less likely. The blinding procedure used to determine laboratory turnaround time precluded duplicate analyses. Evaluation of within-run and between-run variation of the three rapid theophylline assay methods was not performed as part of the study. Data from such an evaluation might have provided additional information for comparing the assay methods. These data would be valuable in further validating the findings of our clinical study.

Conclusion. Based on accuracy alone, all three devices are acceptable for measurement of theophylline concentrations in the clinical setting. Usage level of the assay and technical skill necessary for operation appear to be the most important criteria for device selection. Acculevel's fixed cost and technical simplicity may make it preferable at low usage levels. Vision and Seralyzer may be preferred at higher usage levels.

References

1. Rupchock P, Sommer R, Greenquist A et al. Dry reagent strips used for determination of theophylline in serum. *Clin Chem.* 1985; 31:737–40.
2. Amdall GG, Shapiro WW, Bierman CT et al. High pressure liquid chromatography vs Ames Seralyzer for serum theophylline determinations. *J Allergy Clin Immunol.* 1985; 128 (Suppl):74. Abstract.
3. Conboy C, Ellis E, Jenne J et al. Evaluation of a whole blood theophylline test requiring no instrument. *J Allergy Clin Immunol.* 1985; 128 (Suppl):75. Abstract.
4. Vaughan LM, Weinberger MW, Milavetz A. Evaluation of the Ames Seralyzer for therapeutic drug monitoring of theophylline. *Drug Intell Clin Pharm.* 1986; 20:118–21.
5. Oeltgen PR, Shank WA, Blouin RA et al. Clinical evaluation of the Abbott TDx fluorescence polarization immunoassay analyzer. *Ther Drug Monit.* 1984; 6:360–7.
6. Jolley ME, Stroupe SD, Schwenzer KS et al. Fluorescence polarization immunoassay. An automated system for therapeutic drug determination. *Clin Chem.* 1981; 27:1575–9.
7. Pesce MA, Giacomo DF, Fink D et al. Quantitation of theophylline with the Vision clinical analyzer. *Clin Chem.* 1986; 32:1071. Abstract.
8. Zuk RF, Ginsberg VK, Houts T et al. Enzyme immunochromatography—a quantitative immunoassay requiring no instrumentation. *Clin Chem.* 1985; 31:1144–50.
9. Syntex Medical Diagnostics. Acculevel product labeling. Palo Alto, CA; 1986.
10. Miles Laboratories. Seralyzer product labeling. Elkhart, IN; 1985 Jun.
11. Sheiner LB, Beal SL. Some suggestions for measuring predictive performance. *J Pharmacokinet Biopharm.* 1981; 9:503–12.
12. Chan KM, Walton KG, Koenig J et al. Evaluation of the theophylline procedure on the Abbott Vision analyzer. *Clin Chem.* 1986; 32:1051. Abstract.
13. Fling J, Olson P, Widish J et al. Two rapid methods for serum theophylline concentrations: a comparison. Paper presented to 43rd Annual Congress of the American Society of Allergists. Las Vegas, NV: 1987 Jan 17.
14. Busch RP, Virji MA. Serum theophylline assay by Ames Seralyzer compared with Abbott TDx in pediatric care. *Clin Chem.* 1985; 31:1247–8. Letter.
15. Burton ME, Chow MSS, Platt DR et al. Accuracy of Bayesian and Sawchuk–Zaske dosing methods for gentamicin. *Clin Pharm.* 1986; 5:143–9.
16. Bruno R, Iliadis A, Favre R et al. Dosage predictions in high dose methotrexate infusions. Part 2: Bayesian estimation of methotrexate clearance. *Cancer Drug Deliv.* 1985; 2:277–83.
17. Lalonde RL, Pao D. Correlation coefficient versus prediction error in assessing the accuracy of digoxin dosing methods. *Clin Pharm.* 1984; 3:178–83.
18. Rodvold KA, Paloucek FP, Zell M. Accuracy of 11 methods for predicting theophylline dose. *Clin Pharm.* 1986: 5:403–8.

Intraoperative serum, bile, and gallbladder-wall concentrations of cefmetazole in patients undergoing cholecystectomy

MATTHEW K. ITO, MARK A. GILL, FRANK C. CHENELLA, THOMAS V. BERNE, ALBERT E. YELLIN, PETER N. R. HESELTINE, AND MARIA D. APPLEMAN

Clin Pharm. 1988; 7:467–8

Antimicrobial prophylaxis is commonly used to prevent postoperative infections in cholecystectomy when risk factors such as jaundice, obesity, or recent episode of acute cholecystitis are present. Adequate tissue concentration of the antimicrobial agent during surgery is important for avoidance of postoperative infection.[1,2] First- and second-generation cephalosporins are the agents most commonly used for surgical prophylaxis. Cefmetazole is a new cephamycin-type injectable antimicrobial agent with activity against a wide variety of gram-positive and gram-negative organisms commonly found in the biliary tract. These bacteria include *Escherichia coli, Streptococcus faecalis,* and *Proteus* species. The objective of this study was to determine intraoperative concentrations of cefmetazole in serum, bile, and gallbladder wall to assess the agent's prophylactic utility in biliary surgery.

Methods. Tissue concentrations of cefmetazole were evaluated in 17 consecutive patients receiving cefmetazole as part of a comparative antibiotic trial. Informed consent was obtained from all patients. Patients 16 or more years of age who were undergoing elective cholecystectomy or cholecystectomy with common-duct exploration and who had one or more "high risk factors" were admitted to the study. High risk factors were defined as age ≥ 60 years, obesity (actual body weight ≥ 20% of ideal body weight), diabetes mellitus, recent acute cholecystitis (fever within two weeks), or presumed need for common-duct exploration (because of hyperbilirubinemia, hyperamylasemia, ultrasonic findings of common-duct stones or dilatation). Patients with one or more of the following conditions were excluded: type 1 hypersensitivity to penicillin or cephalosporins; therapy with any other antimicrobial agent within 72 hours before, during, or after surgery; white blood cell count less than 2000/cu mm; impaired renal function (serum creatinine greater than 2.0 mg/dL); hepatic dysfunction with alanine aminotransferase (ALT, also known as SGPT) and aspartate aminotransferase (AST, also known as SGOT) greater than 200 IU or bilirubin greater than 3 mg/dL; pregnancy; any concomitant known infections; history of severe hematological disease or host defense impairment; and temperature ≥ 38 °C during the 24 hours before surgery.

Cefmetazole 1 g (as cefmetazole sodium, The Upjohn Company) every eight hours for three doses administered by intermittent intravenous infusion was initiated approximately 30 minutes before surgery. During surgery no antibiotics were applied locally or added to any irrigating solutions and no drains through surgical wounds were allowed.

Intraoperative specimens of blood, gallbladder wall, and bile were obtained for analysis of cefmetazole. Serum was separated from the blood samples by centrifugation and was immediately frozen, along with the bile and gallbladder-wall specimens, at −70 °C. All specimens were assayed for determination of cefmetazole concentrations by microbioassay using Antibiotic Medium #1 (Difco) and *Clostridium perfringens* (UC 12074) as the test organism. Tissue samples (0.5 g) were ground with 2 mL of 0.1 M phosphate-buffered sodium chloride solution, pH 5.5, until a homogeneous suspension was obtained and then centrifuged to obtain the supernatant. Twenty-five μL of the supernatant, bile, or serum was dispensed onto Fisher's seeded agar disks and allowed to incubate at 35 °C for 18–24 hours under anaerobic conditions. The zones of inhibition were read on the Fisher-Lilly zone reader and converted to drug concentrations (in micrograms per milliliter or micrograms per gram) using a standard curve.

Results and Discussion. Seventeen patients (15 women, 2 men) were studied, with a mean ± S.D. age of 35.8 ± 14.0 years (age range of 21–63 years). Of these patients, 2 required common-bile-duct exploration, 10 were considered obese, 3 were elderly, 1 had diabetes mellitus, 1 had recent acute cholecystitis, and laboratory values revealed hyperbilirubinemia in 4 and hyperamylasemia in 7.

The mean ± S.D. cefmetazole dosage was 13.83 ± 1.86 mg/kg. A total of 42 specimens (17 serum, 10 bile, and 15 gallbladder wall) were obtained intraoperatively. The mean ± S.D. time between administration of the first dose given preoperatively and intraoperative specimen collection was 2.99 ± 1.14

MATTHEW K. ITO, PHARM.D., is Pharmacokinetics Fellow and Lecturer; MARK A. GILL, PHARM.D., is Associate Professor of Clinical Pharmacy; and FRANK C. CHENELLA, PHARM.D., is Assistant Clinical Professor, School of Pharmacy, University of Southern California, Los Angeles (USC–LA). THOMAS V. BERNE, M.D., and ALBERT E. YELLIN, M.D., are Professors of Surgery; PETER N. R. HESELTINE, M.D., is Associate Professor of Medicine, and MARIA D. APPLEMAN, PH.D., is Assistant Professor of Clinical Pathology, School of Medicine, USC–LA.

Address reprint requests to Dr. Gill at University of Southern California School of Pharmacy, 1985 Zonal Avenue, Los Angeles, CA 90033.

The technical assistance of Liliana Lucullo is acknowledged. Supported by a grant from The Upjohn Company.

Copyright © 1988, American Society of Hospital Pharmacists, Inc. All rights reserved. 0278-2677/88/0601-0467$00.50.

Table 1.
Concentrations of Cefmetazole in Serum, Bile and Gallbladder Wall

Patient No.	Time after First Dose[a]	Serum (μg/mL)	Bile (μg/mL)	Gallbladder Wall (μg/g)
1	4.5	30.9	. . .[b]	35.7
2	3.5	53.9	397.8	62.8
3	2.5	41.1	. . .	331.0
4	3.3	112.9	. . .	77.4
5	2.1	240.0	. . .	. . .
6	2.0	26.9	. . .	. . .
7	2.3	65.1	. . .	194.3
8	1.5	. . .	. . .	142.3
9	5.8	105.9	145.8	100.0
10	2.8	59.7	364.7	133.2
11	1.5	124.5	190.2	86.3
12	2.4	94.9	551.3	62.0
13	4.1	68.8	328.4	358.4
14	4.1	112.7	111.5	46.0
15	3.5	42.8	243.9	95.2
16	2.8	79.9	482.5	200.8
17	2.3	47.9	285.6	33.6

[a] In hours.
[b] Data not obtained.

hours. The mean ± S.D. concentrations of cefmetazole in serum, bile, and gallbladder wall were 76.94 ± 54.47 μg/mL, 310.10 ± 143.35 μg/mL, and 130.60 ± 101.08 μg/g, respectively (Table 1).

Preoperative antimicrobial prophylaxis is common practice in high-risk patients undergoing biliary-tract surgery. For effective prophylaxis, antimicrobial agents must be given within four hours of the first incision.[3,4] Agents such as cefoxitin that possess short elimination half-lives should be administered as close as possible to the time of incision.[5]

At the dosage studied, the overall cefmetazole concentrations in bile, serum, and gallbladder-wall tissue exceeded reported minimum inhibitory concentrations for the most commonly suspected organisms.[6,7] To ensure adequate concentrations of cefmetazole in bile, serum, and tissue at the time of incision and bacterial contamination, cefmetazole should be administered as close to the time of surgery as possible.

Conclusion. High bile and gallbladder-wall concentrations of cefmetazole are achieved after administration of cefmetazole 1 g to patients undergoing cholecystectomy.

References

1. Chisholm GD, Waterworth PM, Calnan JS et al. Concentration of antibacterial agents in interstitial tissue fluid. *Br Med J*. 1973; 1:569–73.
2. Demetrius HB, MacLowry J, Beazley RM et al. Antibiotic concentration in human wound fluid after intravenous administration. *Ann Surg*. 1978; 188:202–8.
3. Conte JE, Jacob LS, Polk HC. Surgery of the alimentary tract. In: Antibiotic prophylaxis. Philadelphia: J. B. Lippincott Company; 1984.
4. Burke JF. The effective period of preventing antibiotic action in experimental incisions and dermal lesions. *Surgery*. 1961; 50:161–8.
5. DiPiro JT, Vallner JJ, Bowden TA et al. Intraoperative serum concentrations of cefazolin and cefoxitin administered at different times. *Clin Pharm*. 1984; 3:64–7.
6. Jones RN, Barry AL, Fuchs PC et al. Antimicrobial activity of cefmetazole (Cs-1170) and recommendations for susceptibility testing by disk diffusion, dilution, and anaerobic methods. *J Clin Microbiol*. 1986; 24:1055–9.
7. Schell RF, Kurzynski TA, Le Frock JL et al. Antimicrobial activity of cefmetazole compared with those of other cephalosporins. *Chemotherapy*. Year; 32:431–8.

"

Treatment of Congestive Heart Failure

The hierarchy of therapeutic choices in the management of congestive heart failure and normal sinus rhythm has changed appreciably in recent years. The recognition that a sizable subset of patients have diastolic rather than systolic dysfunction has led to appropriate emphasis on treatment of the underlying causes of left ventricular hypertrophy or ischemia in this group, rather than on inotropic support with cardiac glycosides.

. . . . The current state of our knowledge allows few sweeping generalizations, apart from the importance of weighing each therapeutic decision in the balance of expected risk and benefit and of defining specific therapeutic objectives while maintaining close surveillance of each patient with heart failure.

—Smith TW. Digitalis: mechanisms of action and clinical use. *N Engl J Med*. 1988; 318:358–65.

"

Commentaries

Thrombolysis for acute myocardial infarction: Does a greater incidence of reperfusion justify preferential use of an agent?

PAUL E. NOLAN, JR.

Clin Pharm. 1988; 7:469–73

The Food and Drug Administration has recently approved alteplase (Activase, Genentech, Inc.), a recombinant tissue plasminogen activator, for lysis of coronary thrombi in the management of patients with clinical evidence of an evolving acute myocardial infarction (AMI). This approval resulted from a combination of clinical evidence that demonstrated (1) intravenously administered alteplase causes a relatively high incidence of clot lysis within the coronary circulation[1–3]; (2) thrombolytic therapy administered soon after the appearance of symptoms consistent with AMI can improve post-AMI survival at an acceptable level of risk[4–6]; and (3) the early intravenous administration of alteplase to patients having an AMI results in both improved left ventricular function and reduced incidence of post-AMI congestive heart failure.[7] It is hoped that the latter two observations will translate into improved long-term post-AMI survival.

The approval of alteplase has resulted in both scientific and economic questions about whether alteplase should become the fibrinolytic agent of choice in treating patients with an evolving AMI. Some of these questions include (1) Is alteplase more efficacious than other available thrombolytic agents (e.g., streptokinase) in lysing coronary thrombi and subsequently improving survival of patients? (2) Is alteplase a safer fibrinolytic agent than streptokinase? (3) If the responses to questions 1 and 2 are affirmative, does the use of alteplase in a patient with an evolving AMI represent a logical economic choice over streptokinase? Before these questions can be answered, a brief review outlining the rationale surrounding the use of thrombolytic agents in the management of an evolving AMI is warranted.

Rationale for Thrombolytic Therapy. The enthusiasm surrounding the use of thrombolytic agents in the management of an evolving AMI is predicated on several independent, but not unrelated, scientific observations. In 1980 DeWood and coworkers,[8] using coronary angiography, demonstrated that more than 87% of the patients evaluated within four hours of the onset of symptoms of a Q-wave AMI had complete thrombotic occlusion of the atherosclerotic, infarct-related artery. They also observed subtotal occlusion in an additional 10% of this subgroup of patients. Patients undergoing coronary angiography much later after the onset of symptoms had a significantly lower incidence of total occlusion. This finding suggested that spontaneous thrombolysis of the occluding coronary thrombus can occur in the setting of an evolving AMI. This investigation was instrumental in confirming the long-known, and almost equally long-debated, hypothesis that coronary thrombosis was the cause, rather than the result, of AMI.[9]

A few years before DeWood and coworkers' publication, Reimer et al.[10] had described a "wavefront" of irreversible ischemic myocardial cell death, which migrated from the subendocardium toward the subepicardium after acute coronary occlusion in dogs. The longer the duration of coronary occlusion, the greater was the extent of transmural necrosis. This finding demonstrated that abrupt coronary occlusion did not result in instantaneous, complete transmural necrosis. Rather, ischemic, but viable and potentially salvageable, myocardium remained for up to almost six hours after coronary occlusion. Thus, salvage of jeopardized myocardium was shown to depend on timely reperfusion of the ischemic area. Animal models and clinical studies have further demonstrated that recovery of biochemical, metabolic, and ultimately contractile properties are evident in the region of ischemic but salvaged (i.e., reperfused) myocardium when reperfusion is initiated within only a few hours of coronary occlusion.[11] These investigators have further suggested that the degree of function-

PAUL E. NOLAN, JR., PHARM.D., is Assistant Professor, Department of Pharmacy Practice, College of Pharmacy, University of Arizona, Tucson, AZ 85721.

Copyright © 1988, American Society of Hospital Pharmacists, Inc. All rights reserved. 0278-2677/88/0601-0469$01.25.

al recovery is also likely to depend on coronary collateral blood flow to the ischemic area, the size of the myocardial area at risk for necrosis after coronary thrombosis, and the extent of atherosclerotic disease in other, nonoccluded vessels.

The importance of limiting the size of the infarcted area was illustrated by Page and colleagues[12] in the early 1970s. Their postmortem findings indicated that patients who died from cardiogenic shock secondary to AMI had the greatest degree of necrosis of the left ventricle. Patients with AMI but without cardiogenic shock had less extensive loss of left ventricular myocardium. A clinical corollary to that study was evidenced in the post-AMI risk stratification and survival study by the Multicenter Postinfarction Research Group.[13] These investigators demonstrated that as the post-AMI global ejection fraction, a measure of overall cardiac mechanical function, fell below 0.40 (normal value, 0.67 ± 0.08, mean $\pm$ S.D.), the one-year cardiac mortality increased markedly. Thus, myocardial function, which partly depends on the degree of myocardial destruction, was shown to be a major determinant of post-AMI mortality. The use of combined global and regional (i.e., the contractile function of the area of infarct) left ventricular ejection fractions, as well as their relationship to long-term mortality, has been advocated as a means of evaluating thrombolytic therapy.[14]

It remained to be determined whether reperfusion of the thrombotic coronary artery could be accomplished by pharmacological (i.e., fibrinolytic) methods, since these certainly offered the most time-effective means for recanalization. Intracoronary thrombolysis with streptokinase was shown to be effective in restoring patency to the infarct vessel as well as in improving early and one-year post-AMI survival.[15,16] However, the time delays before coronary reperfusion inherent in this mode of fibrinolysis, coupled with the impracticality of this approach because of a relative lack of catheterization facilities, have been recognized.[17] Consequently, interest was diverted to the use of i.v. streptokinase. The early administration of i.v. streptokinase for an evolving AMI recently has been demonstrated to improve both short-term[4,5,18] and long-term[4-6] post-AMI survival, as well as global left ventricular function.[6,18]

Efficacy of Alteplase and Streptokinase. In spite of those and other, earlier clinical successes, streptokinase has little specific affinity for fibrin-bound plasminogen. Thus, streptokinase has a marked propensity to promote a systemic lytic state and possible severe, secondary hemorrhage. These pharmacological properties, along with streptokinase's potential to induce allergic and immunological reactions, have led to the development of thrombolytic agents such as alteplase, which has a relatively specific but dose-related affinity for fibrin-bound plasminogen as well as much less antigenic potential.[19] To validate some of its theoretical advantages, researchers have compared alteplase with streptokinase in two multicenter, prospective, randomized studies.[1-3]

Patency and Reperfusion. The European Cooperative Study Group[3] single-blind trial compared i.v. alteplase 0.75 mg/kg (old, double-strand alteplase formulation) administered over 90 minutes to 64 patients with i.v. streptokinase 1.5 million International Units (IU) given over one hour to 65 patients. Treatment with an i.v. bolus of heparin preceded the infusion of the thrombolytic agents. Therapy was initiated within six hours of symptoms in all patients, the majority of whom had treatment started within four hours of symptoms. The mean time from onset of symptoms to the initiation of thrombolytic therapy was three hours (range, 1.1 to 5.5 hours) for the alteplase-treated patients and 2.6 hours (range, 0.8 to 5.9 hours) for the streptokinase-treated group. Coronary angiography was performed within 75 to 90 minutes after the start of infusion of either alteplase or streptokinase. Seventy percent of the patients given alteplase and 55% of the patients given streptokinase were shown to have a patent infarct-related artery at angiography. The investigators did not provide information correlating patency to the time at which thrombolytic therapy was started. The rate of reocclusion for either therapy could not be determined because of the study design. Left ventricular function was not determined. However, the in-hospital mortality for each group was identical. Long-term follow-up data have not been published.

Streptokinase and alteplase were also compared in the double-blind Thrombolysis In Myocardial Infarction (TIMI) phase I trial in patients who sought treatment within seven hours of the onset of symptoms.[1,2] One hundred forty-three patients were given a fixed dose of double-strand alteplase 80 mg over three hours (40 mg over the first hour followed by 20 mg/hr for the subsequent two hours). Streptokinase 1.5 million IU over one hour was adminstered to 147 patients. The mean time from onset of symptoms to treatment was 4.75 hours for both the alteplase group (range, 1.3 to 8.3 hours) and the streptokinase group (range, 1.5 to 9.1 hours). Continuous infusion of heparin was started after treatment with the thrombolytic agents.

Pretreatment coronary angiography and sequential coronary angiography during infusion of the thrombolytic agents were performed in all patients. Among patients with baseline ineffective myocardial perfusion (grade 0, no perfusion; grade 1, some penetration of contrast material beyond the thrombotic obstruction but no distal perfusion), the 90-minute coronary angiogram revealed successful reperfusion in 62% (70/113) of those given alteplase versus 31% (37/119) of those given streptokinase. Seventy percent (100/143) of all patients treated with alteplase and 43% (63/147) of all patients treated with streptokinase showed successful reperfusion. When each hourly interval from the onset of symptoms to the initiation of therapy was analyzed for the percentage of recanalized infarct-related arteries, the patients receiving alteplase always had the greater percentage of successful reperfusions. This difference was most marked in patients treated more than four hours after onset of symptoms. Reocclusion of the reperfused artery at discharge occurred more frequently (24%) in those patients receiving alteplase who had successful reperfusion after ineffective baseline perfusion compared with a similar group of patients receiving streptokinase (14%). However, the estimated reocclusion rates for both agents would have been similar if all episodes of reinfarction or in-hospital death were assumed to be secondary to reocclusion. During the period of hospitalization, there were 7 deaths (5%) in the group receiving alteplase and 12 (8%) in the group receiving streptokinase. This difference was not statistically significant. To date, no long-term follow-up data have been published.

Left Ventricular Function. Sheehan and coworkers,[20] in a separate analysis of the TIMI phase I trial, reported the effects of alteplase and streptokinase on left ventricular function. Only 145 patients treated with thrombolytic agents (77 treated with alteplase and 68 with streptokinase) had both baseline and predischarge left ventricular function data. Of this group, the percentage of alteplase-treated patients showing successful reperfusion was twice that of the streptokinase-treated patients. However, there was no significant improvement in the global ejection fraction for either group, but the wall motion (i.e., contractile function) of the area of infarct improved in both groups. Greater recovery of left ventricular function was noted in those patients who had reperfusion within four hours of the onset of symptoms, however. Thus, there did not appear to be a correlation between reperfusion of the infarct-related artery and the extent of improvement in global or regional ventricular function. One possible explanation is the relatively long mean time (almost five hours) before the initiation of thrombolytic therapy in each treatment group. The mean time of actual reperfusion was approximately one hour later. Another important consideration is the group of 67 patients excluded from this analysis because paired ventricular function studies were not completed because of technical problems. Sixty-eight percent of these patients showed successful reperfusion. Although it was not reported, the majority of these 67 patients probably received alteplase because of the higher rate of successful reperfusion reported for those patients.[1,2]

Two recent investigations have shed some light on the efficacy of alteplase in preserving left ventricular function.[7,21] Investigators in both studies administered i.v. alteplase or placebo to patients within four hours of onset of symptoms. Guerci et al.[7] initially used the double-strand formulation of alteplase, 80 mg over three hours, and then switched to the newer single-strand formulation (the form that is currently marketed) of alteplase, 100 mg over three hours. These doses for the respective alteplase formulations have been thought to be clinically equivalent. The Australian Coronary Thrombolysis Group[21] used single-strand alteplase 100 mg given over three hours. All patients in both trials received continuous heparin infusions after administration of the study drug.[7,21]

The results from both trials were comparable. Coronary angiography performed one to six hours after drug infusion in the trial by Guerci et al.[7] revealed a patency rate of 66% for the patients given alteplase versus 24% for the group given placebo. Both alteplase- and placebo-treated patients were randomized to undergo elective angioplasty within 48 to 72 hours after AMI depending on the status of the initial angiograms. Ten days after the infarction, the resting ejection fraction improved significantly in the alteplase-treated group, independent of angioplasty, especially in those patients with an anterior AMI. The incidence of clinical congestive heart failure was also markedly reduced by alteplase. Ten-day mortality was lower in the alteplase-treated group. However, statistical inferences cannot be drawn because of the relatively small sample size. The incidence of presumed reocclusion before randomization for angioplasty, as evidenced by recurring chest pain or reinfarction, was similar in each group. These results appeared to relate reperfusion to both improved ventricular function and a better clinical outcome based on symptomatology.

An estimation of actual patency rates in the trial by the Australian Coronary Thrombolysis Group is difficult to provide because coronary angiography was not performed until one week after AMI.[21] However, global ejection fractions were greater in the alteplase-treated group, especially in the patients with anterior AMI and a patent infarct-related artery. The incidence of reocclusion was also difficult to assess because of the study design. Nonetheless, the one-week coronary angiogram revealed a patency rate of 70% in the group receiving alteplase and 41% in the group receiving placebo.

Safety of Alteplase and Streptokinase. Despite the potential or actual gains to be derived from thrombolytic therapy with either alteplase or streptokinase, the therapeutic risks associated with these agents must be acceptable before they can be considered standards of therapy. The predominant risk of thrombolytic therapy with either agent is hemorrhage.

The actual risk of bleeding associated with either alteplase or streptokinase therapy based on the two comparative trials is difficult to determine because of the invasive, interventional design of these investigations.[1-3] Both of these trials used the old, double-strand form of alteplase. In the European Cooperative Study, prolonged bleeding at puncture sites, hematoma, and hypotension were more common in the group receiving streptokinase.[3] However, there were no differences in the frequency of blood transfusions between treatment groups. One streptokinase-treated patient had an allergic reaction, and another was discharged with a neurological deficit. In the TIMI trial, bleeding complications, predominantly at the catheterization site, and transfusion requirements were virtually identical for both treatment groups.[1,2] The overall incidence of bleeding and the need for transfusion appeared greater in the TIMI investigation than in the European study, perhaps resulting from the use of a continuous infusion of heparin after thrombolytic therapy, as noted in the TIMI trial.[1-3] No intracranial hemorrhages were observed in the TIMI trial.[1,2]

The incidence of bleeding requiring transfusion in the study by Guerci et al.[7] was similar for both the alteplase (9.8%) and placebo (7.6%) group. This relatively high incidence may have occurred secondary to early catheterization after infusion of the study drug. This incidence was, however, lower than that observed in the TIMI trial, which may be related to differences in the formulation of alteplase.[1,2,22,23]

The Australian Coronary Thrombolysis Group[21] used single-strand alteplase followed by infusion of heparin for an unreported length of time but deferred coronary catheterization until five to seven days postinfarction. The bleeding complications, most of which were considered minor and located at arterial and venous puncture sites, occurred more frequently in the group receiving alteplase. No patients required transfusion therapy. However, there was one case of hemorrhagic stroke and two cases of retroperitoneal bleeding in the alteplase-treated group.

The hemorrhagic adverse-effect profiles from these placebo-controlled investigations of alteplase are not that different from those in trials that compared i.v. streptokinase therapy with either placebo[18] or matched controls.[4-6] However, the incidence of clinically important hypotension[4,5,18] and allergic reactions[4-6,18] is much greater in streptokinase-treated patients.

Economic and Therapeutic Implications. Depending on the institution, the cost of alteplase is currently 10 to 20 times greater than that of streptokinase. Because of this difference in price, justifiable economic concerns have been raised and a cost-effectiveness model for coronary thrombolysis/reperfusion has been developed to address the relative benefits and costs of alteplase, streptokinase, and related therapies.[24,25]

If alteplase is clearly more effective and safer than streptokinase, then the cost-related concerns can easily be dismissed. However, early (i.e., less than six hours from the onset of symptoms) administration of i.v. streptokinase reduces long-term mortality at an acceptable therapeutic level of risk, especially in patients with anterior AMI.[4-6] This reduction in mortality is most remarkable when streptokinase is administered within three hours of the onset of symptoms. Left ventricular function is also improved by the early administration of i.v. streptokinase.[6,18] The improvements in both survival and left ventricular function appear related to reperfusion of the infarct-related artery.[6,18] The additive effects of revascularization procedures after thrombolysis probably also play a role in improving clinical outcome.[6]

The higher reperfusion rates reported for alteplase and its relatively greater affinity for fibrin-bound plasminogen have not resulted in a superior clinical outcome for this agent.[1-3,20] Certainly study design and relatively small numbers of patients may partly explain this lack of enhanced benefit with alteplase. In addition, the dose and duration of the alteplase infusion may not have been optimal, based on more recent evidence.[22] Nonetheless, early (less than four hours from the onset of symptoms) administration of alteplase has been shown to improve left ventricular function and clinical outcome.[7,21] As with streptokinase, these two benefits were related to the restoration of patency to the infarct-related vessel.

At this time, the clinical evidence does not suggest that alteplase is the fibrinolytic agent of choice for treating most eligible patients with an evolving AMI because of the documented clinical efficacy and safety of streptokinase coupled with the relatively high cost of alteplase. Until more data become available that clearly demonstrate an advantage for alteplase over streptokinase, alteplase might be considered as the first-line thrombolytic agent for the following patient subgroups: (1) those for whom the time of onset of AMI symptoms cannot be clearly determined, since there is an increased likelihood of achieving reperfusion of the infarct-related vessel with alteplase; (2) patients who seek treatment relatively late (more than three to four hours) after the onset of symptoms and in whom thrombolytic therapy is thought to enhance clinical outcome because of the relatively greater recanalization rates seen with alteplase, especially late after the appearance of symptoms; (3) patients who have recently been given streptokinase, to avoid possible allergic reactions; (4) patients who are relatively hypotensive after the onset of AMI, to avoid the hypotensive effects of streptokinase; and (5) patients who have recently had a streptococcal infection.

Conclusion. The early administration of i.v. alteplase during an evolving AMI can frequently recanalize the infarct-related coronary artery, preserve left ventricular function, and decrease the incidence of post-AMI congestive heart failure. These therapeutic effects may result in improved long-term survival and decreased morbidity. However, it is difficult at this time to unequivocally recommend i.v. alteplase as the fibrinolytic agent of choice for all eligible AMI patients, because the early administration of i.v. streptokinase can also provide a similarly beneficial clinical outcome at a greater cost savings.

References

1. The TIMI Study Group. The Thrombolysis in Myocardial Infarction (TIMI) trial: phase I findings. *N Engl J Med*. 1985; 312:932–6.
2. Chesebro JH, Knatterud G, Roberts R et al. Thrombolysis in Myocardial Infarction (TIMI) trial, phase I: a comparison between intravenous tissue plasminogen activator and intravenous streptokinase. Clinical findings through hospital discharge. *Circulation*. 1987; 76:142–54.
3. Verstraete M, Bernard R, Borg M et al. Randomized trial of intravenous recombinant tissue-type plasminogen activator versus intravenous streptokinase in acute myocardial infarction. *Lancet*. 1985; 1:842–7.
4. Gruppo Italiano per lo Studio Della Streptochinasi Nell'Infarto Miocardico (GISSI). Effectiveness of intravenous thrombolytic treatment in acute myocardial infarction. *Lancet*. 1986; 1:397–402.
5. Gruppo Italiano per lo Studio Della Streptochinasi Nell'Infarto Miocardico (GISSI). Long-term effects of intravenous thrombolysis in acute myocardial infarction: final report of the GISSI study. *Lancet*. 1987; 2:871–4.
6. Kennedy JW, Martin GV, Davis KB et al. The Western Washington intravenous streptokinase in acute myocardial infarction randomized trial. *Circulation*. 1988; 77:345–52.
7. Guerci AD, Gerstenblith G, Brinker JA et al. A randomized trial of intravenous tissue plasminogen activator for acute myocardial infarction with subsequent randomization to elective coronary angioplasty. *N Engl J Med*. 1987; 317:1613–8.
8. DeWood MA, Spores J, Notske R et al. Prevalence of total coronary occlusion during the early hours of transmural myocardial infarction. *N Engl J Med*. 1980; 303:897–902.
9. Muller JE. Coronary artery thrombosis: historical aspects. *J Am Coll Cardiol*. 1983; 1:893–6.
10. Reimer KA, Lowe JE, Rasmussen MM et al. The wavefront phenomenon of ischemic cell death. 1. Myocardial infarct size vs duration of coronary occlusion in dogs. *Circulation*. 1977; 56:786–94.
11. Bergmann SR, Fox KAA, Ludbrook PA. Determinants of salvage of jeopardized myocardium after coronary thrombolysis. *Cardiology Clinics*. 1987; 5(Feb):67–77.
12. Page DL, Caulfield JB, Kastor JA et al. Myocardial changes associated with cardiogenic shock. *N Engl J Med*. 1971; 285:133–7.
13. The Multicenter Postinfarction Research Group. Risk stratification and survival after myocardial infarction. *N Engl J Med*. 1983; 309:331–6.
14. Verani MS, Roberts R. Preservation of cardiac function by coronary thrombolysis during acute myocardial infarction: fact or myth? *J Am Coll Cardiol*. 1987; 10:470–6.
15. Kennedy JW, Ritchie JL, Davis KB et al. The Western Washington randomized trial of intracoronary streptokinase in acute myocardial infarction: a 12-month follow-up report. *N Engl J Med*. 1985; 312:1073–8.
16. Simoons ML, Van Der Brand M, de Zwann C et al. Improved survival after early thrombolysis in acute myocardial infarction. *Lancet*. 1985; 2:578–81.
17. Ludbrook PA, Rentrop P. Coronary thrombolysis with intracoronary streptokinase. *Cardiology Clinics*. 1987; 5(Feb):79–90.
18. White HD, Norris RM, Brown MA et al. Effect of intravenous streptokinase on left ventricular function and early survival after acute myocardial infarction. *N Engl J Med*. 1987; 317:850–5.
19. Verstraete M. The search for the ideal thrombolytic agent. *J Am Coll Cardiol*. 1987; 10:4B–10B.
20. Sheehan FH, Braunwald E, Canner P et al. The effect of intravenous thrombolytic therapy on left ventricular function: a report on tissue-type plasminogen activator and streptokinase from the Thrombolysis in Myocardial Infarction (TIMI phase I) trial. *Circulation*. 1987; 75:817–29.
21. National Heart Foundation of Australia Coronary Thrombolysis Group. Coronary thrombolysis and myocardial salvage by tissue plasminogen activator given up to 4 hours after onset of myocardial infarction. *Lancet*. 1988; 1:203–8.
22. Mueller HS, Rao AK, Forman SA et al. Thrombolysis in Myocardial Infarction (TIMI): comparative studies of coronary reperfusion and systemic fibrinogenolysis with two forms of recombinant tissue-type plasminogen activator. *J Am Coll Cardiol*. 1987; 10:479–90.
23. Braunwald E, Knatterud GL, Passamani E et al. Update from the Thrombolysis in Myocardial Infarction trial. *J Am Coll Cardiol*. 1987; 10:970.
24. Rich MW. TPA: is it worth the price? *Am Heart J*. 1987; 114:1259–61.
25. Laffel GL, Fineberg HV, Braunwald E. A cost-effectiveness model for coronary thrombolysis/reperfusion therapy. *J Am Coll Cardiol*. 1987; 5:79B–90B.

Thrombolysis for acute myocardial infarction: Is proof of a reduction in mortality critical to drug selection?

JEFFREY A. GREEN

Clin Pharm. 1988; 7:473–7

Within the last decade, important advances have been made in the pharmacologic management of heart disease. This progress is exemplified by the development of thrombolytic agents for the treatment of acute myocardial infarction. Currently, this class of drugs includes streptokinase, tissue plasminogen activators (e.g., alteplase), and urokinase (listed alphabetically). Because myocardial infarction is a pressing and serious problem in our society, it is understandably surrounded by much

JEFFREY A. GREEN, PHARM.D., is Codirector, Cardiovascular Clinical Pharmacology Research Program, and Assistant Professor of Medicine, Case Western Reserve University School of Medicine, and Head, Pharmaceutical Product Development, Positron Emission Tomography Facility, University Hospitals of Cleveland, 2074 Abington Road, Cleveland, OH 44106.

Copyright © 1988, American Society of Hospital Pharmacists, Inc. All rights reserved. 0278-2677/88/0601-0473$01.25.

emotionalism and controversy. Moreover, the controversy is fueled by economic considerations, especially applicable to institutional pharmacy, because of the price differentials among these products. Thus, it is imperative that decisions regarding the selection of a thrombolytic agent are based on data obtained from controlled, scientific trials. The decision about which agent to use should not be made as the result of articles read in the *Wall Street Journal* or emphatic testimonials of influential health-care practitioners stating that one agent is twice as effective as another.

This commentary highlights some of the key facts regarding thrombolytic therapy that are scientifically based. The goal is to promote understanding of the decision-making process needed in the selection of a thrombolytic agent.

Rationale for Thrombolytic Therapy. Although it may seem surprising, the exact pathogenesis of acute myocardial infarction was unknown until 1980. Previously, there were various theories on how this disease state developed, including such hypotheses as vasospasm and acute increases in myocardial oxygen demand. Although such events cannot be ruled out as contributory factors, it is now known that acute coronary thrombosis is the precipitating event causing the vast majority of myocardial infarctions. In a classic study by DeWood and coworkers,[1] it was noted that an average of 86% of patients who underwent an angiogram within six hours of the onset of chest pain had an acute occlusion present in the coronary artery supplying the infarcting tissue. Also important is the fact that a lower percentage of patients demonstrated total occlusion when the interval from symptoms to angiogram extended beyond six hours. This demonstrates the efficiency of the endogenous fibrinolytic system and shows that "self-lysis," albeit delayed, does occur. This self-lysis justified the placebo-controlled design of early thrombolytic trials.

The second landmark investigation forming the foundation of rational thrombolytic intervention was that of Reimer et al.[2] Actually published three years before the occlusion mechanism was identified, this research concluded that myocardial cells undergoing ischemic death perish according to a "wavefront phenomenon." That is, subsequent to total occlusion, cells proximal to the interruption of blood flow die before those that are located distally. Additionally, there was a direct relationship between the duration of occlusion and the percentage of dead muscle quantitated via postmortem sections. A key finding of this study was the amount of viable muscle present in relation to the length of occlusion. Total coronary occlusion for six hours or longer usually resulted in a transmural (i.e., full-thickness) myocardial infarction and left as little as 20% of the involved muscle as potentially salvageable.

The following statements summarize why thrombolytic therapy came to be emphasized in the early 1980s.

1. The majority of acute myocardial infarctions are the result of acute occlusions in the coronary arteries. The majority of these occlusions are caused by thrombus formation.
2. Time is muscle. The longer the occlusion exists, the greater the chance myocardial cells will die.
3. The probability is low that a substantial amount of tissue can be saved if the occlusion exists for six hours or more (canine model).

Clinical Efficacy—Thrombolysis, Ventricular Function, and Mortality. Not long after publication of the developmental information presented in the preceding section, multiple trials were under way investigating all thrombolytic agents for the treatment of acute myocardial infarction. As was highlighted in the first commentary by Nolan,[3] alteplase and streptokinase are effective at causing lysis of coronary thrombi when administered intravenously. Streptokinase has been compared with both urokinase and alteplase. Streptokinase and urokinase have been found to be equally effective at initiating reperfusion,[4,5] with a success rate of approximately 60%. Alteplase has been compared with streptokinase only. Two comparative evaluations exist,[6,7] and each reports the consistent finding that alteplase caused reperfusion or patency in a greater proportion of patients than did streptokinase. The success rates of streptokinase and alteplase were 31% and 62%[6] and 55% and 70%,[7] respectively.

Several qualifications need to be made pertaining to these investigations. The first is a question of definition. The success rate in the Thrombolysis in Myocardial Infarction (TIMI) trial[6] for each drug was based on actual reperfusion. The success rate in the European Cooperative Study Group[7] trial was based on patency. To claim that reperfusion has taken place, the involved artery must undergo angiography both before and after treatment. Therefore, if an occlusive thrombus was present before thrombolytic therapy, and flow was restored after therapy, reperfusion occurred. Patency is defined differently. When only a posttreatment angiogram is performed to document the restoration of blood flow in the affected artery, it is not appropriate to use the term reperfusion, since one cannot prove the initial presence of a thrombus. In this instance, the term patency must be used.

It is important to understand these differences, because 14% of the patients in the study by DeWood et al.[1] who underwent angiography within six hours of classic signs and symptoms of an acute myocardial infarction, and who were ultimately diagnosed as such with enzyme changes, did not have a totally occlusive event. Although absence of an occlusion does not necessarily preclude use of a thrombolytic agent, it is interesting to speculate how this variable affected the patency statistics of the European Cooperative Study Group. Did a larger proportion of patients in either the streptokinase- or alteplase-treated groups belong to this 14% category, thereby falsely elevating the patency rate? Additionally, in the study by DeWood et al.[1] there was a 12% false-positive and a 25% false-negative rate for thrombus identification using angiography. Of the total of 322 patients, a thrombus was observed in 70%.[1] A total occlusion is not always the result of a thrombus; it could result from fragmented atherosclerotic plaques, platelet plugging, or sustained vasospasm—conditions that would not be amenable to thrombolytic therapy.

The second important point regarding these studies is the time delay from the onset of symptoms to treatment. In the TIMI trial this delay averaged 4.8 hours, whereas in the European Cooperative Study Group trial it was 3.0 hours for alteplase and 2.6 hours for streptokinase. In the case of the TIMI trial, this time delay resulted in a less-than-optimal comparison of the two agents because it is critically close to the "muscle salvage" window suggested by the canine model of Reimer et al.[2] Nonetheless, the success rate (pertaining only to reperfusion) of streptokinase declined precipitously in association with a longer treatment delay, and alteplase outperformed streptokinase at every separate treatment interval.[6]

The following are summary facts about reperfusion.

1. In the single trial designed to examine reperfusion, alteplase was a more effective thrombolytic agent than streptokinase.
2. This fact is supported by the superior patency rates for alteplase shown in the European Cooperative Study Group trial; however, the boundary conditions involved in defining reperfusion versus patency should always be kept in mind.

The variables surrounding reperfusion, patency, endogenous thrombolysis, and incidence of thrombus formation have led investigators and the FDA to search for other definitions of efficacy for the thrombolytic agents (i.e., changes in left ventricular function and mortality). The Western Washington trial demonstrated a significant reduction in 21-day mortality with streptokinase using the absolute qualifier of reperfusion versus no reperfusion.[8] However, using the same criterion, the mortality reduction at one year was not significant.[9] After statistical adjustment of other factors such as infarct location and ejection fraction, the results became statistically significant. Even though the number of patients in this study was relatively small ($n = 134$) the findings indicate that many factors contribute to infarct-related deaths and that perhaps an irrefutable endpoint (i.e., mortality) should be used for determining efficacy. Additionally, it was learned that stricter definitions of reperfusion should be used in future studies because in the 12-month follow-up evaluation[9] there was not even a suggestion that partial reperfusion was any more beneficial than no reperfusion ($p = 0.90$). This could very well indicate that reperfusion per se does not necessarily result in a lower mortality rate. Preliminary results from the TIMI trial may support this conclusion since the death rate at 21 days was 4% for the group receiving alteplase and 5% for the group receiving streptokinase.

The most impressive trial to date was the GISSI study.[10] This trial proved that thrombolytic therapy with streptokinase has a favorable effect on mortality at 21 days after an infarction. Treatment within three hours of the onset of symptoms had the greatest effect on mortality, whereas initiating treatment after six hours provided no benefit compared with controls. These results corroborated those of the canine model developed by Reimer et al.[2] almost a decade earlier. No significant difference in mortality was observed between streptokinase-treated and control patients exhibiting inferior-wall or lateral-wall myocardial infarctions. Likewise, no mortality reduction occurred in patients over 65 years of age. No studies currently exist that evaluate the beneficial effects on mortality of any other thrombolytic agent.

Improvement in left ventricular ejection fraction also has been examined as a measure of the efficacy of the thrombolytic agents. Although positive effects have been observed,[11] and although recognizing this improvement may aid in prolonging life through therapy with streptokinase (or other comparable agents), it is certainly a less sensitive and specific endpoint than death. Interestingly, in the TIMI trial analysis of left ventricular function, no significant difference was seen in pretreatment versus posttreatment ejection fractions for either streptokinase or alteplase.[12] Moreover, despite a doubling of successful reperfusions with alteplase, there was no difference in recoverable myocardial function between the two thrombolytic agents. This result substantiates the criticism that the treatment delay in this trial was an important limitation. Only time will tell whether the long-term mortality results in this trial will differ from those obtained in the GISSI study.

The following are summary facts about ventricular function and mortality.

1. Although therapy with thrombolytic agents has been shown to improve overall myocardial function, that improvement should be viewed as a secondary endpoint.
2. Streptokinase is the only thrombolytic agent proven to improve survival after an acute myocardial infarction.
3. No reduction in mortality has been shown for patients undergoing inferior-wall or lateral-wall myocardial infarctions.

4. It remains to be shown whether the relationship between reperfusion success and reduction in mortality is a continuous or an absolute association. In other words, is reduction in mortality proportional to the extent of reperfusion, or is total reperfusion required to achieve any reduction in mortality?
5. The ability of alteplase to reduce mortality from an acute myocardial infarction has not been demonstrated.

Adverse Effects. The major adverse effect of all thrombolytic agents is bleeding. However, there are important misconceptions about this event. Although alteplase is frequently described as a "clot-specific" agent, this characteristic does not portend a lower bleeding rate. In both comparative trials,[6,7] adverse events associated with bleeding were similar for streptokinase and alteplase irrespective of different declines in plasma fibrinogen levels. The GISSI study reported only a 3.5% incidence of major and minor episodes of bleeding.[10] This statistic is probably more indicative of future adverse-effect rates because, unlike the TIMI trial, the GISSI study involved no invasive procedures. Most patients who are candidates for thrombolytic therapy will no longer have immediate angiography or angioplasty. Urokinase was shown in one study to be associated with a significantly lower bleeding rate than streptokinase[4]; yet, when this presumably positive result was reported, many clinicians elected not to use urokinase because it was too expensive.

The following are summary facts about adverse effects.

1. With the exception of one study favoring urokinase, bleeding rates associated with the thrombolytic agents are not clinically different.
2. Anaphylaxis, a serious adverse effect, has been reported only for streptokinase.

Considerations in Selection of a Thrombolytic Agent. The pertinent clinical considerations regarding the thrombolytic agents can be summarized as follows: Alteplase causes reperfusion in a higher percentage of patients than streptokinase; only streptokinase has been shown to reduce mortality subsequent to a myocardial infarction; and bleeding rates are similar for streptokinase and alteplase.

The choice of a thrombolytic agent will depend on whether a clinician favors reperfusion or mortality as an endpoint. Clinicians who choose reperfusion must make a "leap of faith" in associating thrombolysis in general with lives and myocardium saved, regardless of the agent used. Some of the scientific evidence presented in this commentary questions whether a one-to-one relationship exists between reperfusion, salvage of myocardium, and improvement in mortality. The transitive law ($A = B$; $B = C$; therefore, $A = C$) is usually not thought to apply in clinical medicine, because all causes and effects are usually not known and few phenomena in physiological systems occur independently. For this reason, it has never been documented that antiarrhythmic agents save lives, even though they effectively reduce premature ventricular depolarizations, which have been shown to be harbingers of sudden death. The thrombolytic issue is analogous to this one.

However, death is an absolute endpoint. Although debate over the contribution of various pharmacologic effects to drug efficacy may continue, no extrapolation of results is necessary if mortality is used as the measure of efficacy, because the goal of therapy is prolongation of life.

A final point needs to be made about the dosage form of alteplase. The preparation used in the TIMI trial was a double-stranded molecule and the dosage was 80 mg.[13] The marketed preparation is a single-stranded molecule thought to be more clot specific.[13] Thus, the major trial providing the data for FDA approval used a different preparation than what is now available for patient therapy. The importance of this is unknown.

Conclusion. Given the available information, it is difficult to conclude that alteplase should be substituted for streptokinase in all cases. To favor alteplase, extrapolations must be made from two important investigations.[2,6] Data reported recently from the Second International Study of Infarct Survival (ISIS-II) bring into question one of these hypotheses; in this study, treatment of patients with streptokinase and aspirin provided a beneficial effect even when used 6 to 24 hours after the onset of an infarction. Thus, factors other than reperfusion per se apparently are operative in mortality reduction with thrombolytic agents and aspirin.[14] The volume of experience with and the subsequent effects on mortality of streptokinase cannot simply be dismissed. In general, "bandwagon-jumping" with regard to drug therapy is ill advised, and clinicians should be especially cautious of such a tendency with these thrombolytic agents. The ultimate mortality results from the TIMI trial will eventually indicate whether the superior reperfusion rates demonstrated for alteplase translate directly into a reduction in mortality compared with that associated with streptokinase therapy.

References

1. DeWood MA, Spores J, Notske R et al. Prevalence of total coronary occlusion during the early hours of transmural myocardial infarction. *N Engl J Med.* 1980; 303:897–902.
2. Reimer KA, Lowe JE, Rasmussen MM et al. The wavefront phenomenon of ischemic cell death. 1. Myocardial infarct size vs duration of coronary occlusion in dogs. *Circulation.* 1977; 56:786–94.
3. Nolan PE Jr. Thrombolysis for acute myocardial infarction: does a greater incidence of reperfusion justify preferential use of an agent? *Clin Pharm.* 1988; 7:469–73.
4. Tennant SN, Dixon J, Venable TC et al. Intracoronary thrombolysis in patients with acute myocardial infarction: comparison of the efficacy of urokinase with streptokinase. *Circulation.* 1984; 69:756–60.

5. Mathey DG, Schoffer J, Sheehan FH et al. Intravenous urokinase in acute myocardial infarction. *Am J Cardiol.* 1985; 55:878–82.
6. Chesebro JH, Knatterud G, Roberts R et al. Thrombolysis in Myocardial Infarction (TIMI) trial, phase I: a comparison between intravenous tissue plasminogen activator and intravenous streptokinase. Clinical findings through hospital discharge. *Circulation.* 1987; 76:142–54.
7. Verstraete M, Bory M, Collen D et al. Randomized trial of intravenous recombinant tissue-type plasminogen activator versus intravenous streptokinase in acute myocardial infarction. *Lancet.* 1985; 1:842–7.
8. Kennedy JW, Ritchie JL, Davis KB et al. Western Washington randomized trial of intracoronary streptokinase in acute myocardial infarction. *N Engl J Med.* 1983; 309:1477–82.
9. Kennedy JW, Ritchie JL, Davis KB et al. The Western Washington randomized trial of intracoronary streptokinase in acute myocardial infarction: a 12-month follow-up report. *N Engl J Med.* 1985; 312:1073–8.
10. Gruppo Italiano per lo Studio Della Streptochinasi Nell'Infarto Miocardico (GISSI). Effectiveness of intravenous thrombolytic treatment in acute myocardial infarction. *Lancet.* 1986; 1:397–402.
11. White HD, Norris RM, Brown MA et al. Effect of intravenous streptokinase on left ventricular function and early survival after acute myocardial infarction. *N Engl J Med.* 1987; 317:850–5.
12. Sheehan FH, Braunwald E, Canner P et al. The effect of intravenous thrombolytic therapy on left ventricular function: a report on tissue-type plasminogen activator and streptokinase from the Thrombolysis in Myocardial Infarction (TIMI phase I) trial. *Circulation.* 1987; 75:817–29.
13. Sherry S. Appraisal of various thrombolytic agents in the treatment of acute myocardial infarction. *Am J Med.* 1987; 83:31–46.
14. ISIS Collaborative Group. Results of a large randomized trial of intravenous streptokinase and oral aspirin in acute myocardial infarction. *J Am Coll Cardiol.* 1988; 11:232A. Abstract.

ARE YOU READY TO BE CHALLENGED?

The U.S. Public Health Service has just the pharmacy opportunities you're looking for...

☐ Prescriptive authority.
☐ Diversity of assignments.
☐ Patient counseling.
☐ Team partnership on clinical rounds.
☐ Advice on drug regimens.
☐ Opportunities for advancement.

If you're an entry-level pharmacist who wants to be on the leading edge, practicing high-tech pharmacy at its best, call us.

We need you in many areas: INDIAN HEALTH SERVICE, FOOD & DRUG ADMINISTRATION AND NATIONAL INSTITUTES OF HEALTH. And we have clinical, regulatory, administrative and research positions available nationwide.

Call or write Pharmacist Recruitment Officer
RM 7A-39 Parklawn Building
5600 Fishers Lane
Rockville, Maryland 20857
(301) 443-5740
U.S. Public Health Service

CP Continuing Education

The ASHP Continuing Education system gives readers a self-assessment mechanism for selected articles in Clinical Pharmacy *and the* American Journal of Hospital Pharmacy. *It also allows readers to obtain continuing-education credit for these articles.*

For the purpose of CE-credit enrollment a blank answer sheet is published at the end of each installment of the column for the CE articles in that issue. An enrollee accumulates these answer sheets until the enrollment is submitted, using the form that is published in the June and December issues of Clinical Pharmacy *and in the June and December issues of the* American Journal of Hospital Pharmacy. *Any combination of tests within a 18-month period, from both* Clinical Pharmacy *and* American Journal of Hospital Pharmacy, *may be included in an enrollment. More complete details about enrollment in the system will appear in the semiannual enrollment form.*

Article 680-204-8809 (see page 424)
Qualifies for 1.0 hour of CE credit

Clinical use of systemic antifungal agents

Learning Objectives

After studying this article, the reader should be able to

1. Explain the primary mechanism of action for each of the four antifungal drugs discussed.
2. Compare and contrast the pharmacokinetics of the four antifungal drugs.
3. Compare and contrast the adverse effects most frequently observed for each of the four antifungal drugs.
4. State two advantages of using ketoconazole instead of amphotericin B for a given susceptible fungal infection.
5. State two reasons for the infrequent use of miconazole for the treatment of fungal infections.

Self-assessment Questions

For each question there is one best answer only.

1. Synergism has been demonstrated in vivo and in vitro for which of the following antifungal drugs?
   a. Amphotericin B and miconazole.
   b. Amphotericin B and flucytosine.
   c. Ketoconazole and amphotericin B.
   d. Ketoconazole and flucytosine.

2. The imidazole antifungal drugs appear to inhibit the growth of fungi by
   a. Binding to ergosterol in the fungal cell wall.
   b. Inhibiting corticosteroid receptor sites on cell membranes.
   c. Inhibiting ergosterol synthesis in fungi.
   d. Binding to cholesterol in the fungal cell wall.

3. In patients with normal liver and kidney function, which of the following has the longest elimination half-life?
   a. Flucytosine.
   b. Ketoconazole.
   c. Miconazole.
   d. Amphotericin B.

4. Which of the following drug's serum concentrations would be most influenced by a change in kidney function?
   a. Flucytosine.
   b. Ketoconazole.
   c. Miconazole.
   d. Amphotericin B.

5. A decline in kidney function is observed in nearly every patient treated with which of the following?
   a. Flucytosine.
   b. Ketoconazole.
   c. Miconazole.
   d. Amphotericin B.

6. Gynecomastia is an adverse effect that occasionally results from treatment with
   a. Flucytosine.
   b. Ketoconazole.
   c. Miconazole.
   d. Amphotericin B.

7. One advantage of using ketoconazole instead of amphotericin B for susceptible infections is that
   a. Ketoconazole is marketed in oral as well as intravenous dosage forms.
   b. Ketoconazole can be given orally and is associated with less serious adverse effects than amphotericin B.

c. Ketoconazole causes less hepatotoxicity and has a shorter half-life than amphotericin B.
d. The duration of therapy with ketoconazole is usually shorter than that with amphotericin B and, therefore, results in fewer adverse effects.

8. To assess the potential for adverse effects in a given patient, a test dose is recommended for
   a. Miconazole and amphotericin B.
   b. Miconazole and flucytosine.
   c. Amphotericin B and flucytosine.
   d. Only for amphotericin B.

9. Why is intravenous miconazole used infrequently?
   a. Miconazole is available in an oral dosage form for systemic use, which has fewer adverse effects.
   b. Miconazole is poorly soluble in water and requires large volumes of fluid for administration.
   c. Miconazole has been poorly studied and is less effective or more toxic, or both, than other available agents.
   d. None of the above are correct.

10. The antifungal mechanism of action of flucytosine is probably due to
   a. Conversion to floxuridine.
   b. Inhibition of RNA synthesis.
   c. Conversion to fluorouracil.
   d. Inhibition of cholesterol side-chain cleavage.

Answer sheet

May 1988 *Clinical Pharmacy*

Note: An enrollment form for the ASHP Continuing-Education System appears in the June and December issues. Please accumulate all the answer sheets you wish to use in one enrollment and submit them at one time with a completed enrollment form.

Place an X in the box(es) at the top of the column(s) corresponding to the test(s) you are taking. Darken the boxes corresponding to the correct answers.

☐
680-204-8809
1.0 hour

	a	b	c	d
1.	☐	☐	☐	☐
2.	☐	☐	☐	☐
3.	☐	☐	☐	☐
4.	☐	☐	☐	☐
5.	☐	☐	☐	☐
6.	☐	☐	☐	☐
7.	☐	☐	☐	☐
8.	☐	☐	☐	☐
9.	☐	☐	☐	☐
10.	☐	☐	☐	☐

ASHP Use Only
(1.0)8809 ________ (3)

Critical Care Clinical Pharmacist

Miami Valley Hospital, located in Dayton, Ohio, is a 772-bed teaching facility. We are currently seeking a progressive, motivated professional to work primarily in ICU and NICU. In this position, you will provide drug related information to patients, physicians, nursing and pharmacy staff members. Responsibilities include pharmacokinetics, TPN monitoring, drug information, nursing, resident, and pharmacy inservices, and initiated and participating in pharmaceutical research. The clinical pharmacists work closely with staff pharmacists developing their clinical skills.

This very challenging position requires an advanced degree and Ohio licensure.

Miami Valley Hospital offers an excellent salary and benefits package to the qualified candidate. Please send your resume in confidence to Human Resources (SM). We are an Equal Opportunity Employer.

MVH MiamiValleyHospital
When you need us, we're there.

One Wyoming St. • Dayton, OH 45409

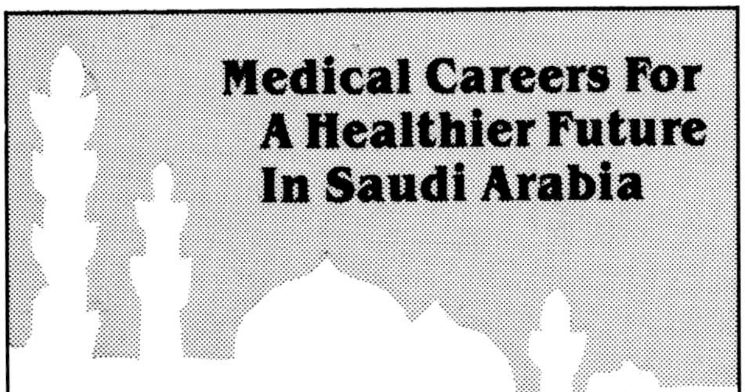

WITIKAR is Saudi Arabia's first and most prestigious hospital management firm. Vital openings are available for the following hospitals.

- National Guard Hospital—Riyadh
- Armed Forces Hospitals—Dhahran and Jeddah
- Ministry Of Health Hospitals—Southwest Region, (8 Locations)

Current Staff Needs Include:

Chief Pharmacists,
Pharmacy and Clinical Pharmacy Supervisors,
Clinical Pharmacists, and Pharmacists.
Hospital experience required.

An attractive TAX-FREE package is offered that includes rent-free accommodations, generous vacation and holiday leaves, exciting travel opportunities and professional growth in a multiculture environment.

For further information, please write enclosing CV to:

Witikar

Witikar Saudi Arabia Ltd.
2009 Massachusetts Ave. N.W.
Washington, DC 20036

ASHP CE instructions and enrollment form

Instructions

1. The system is flexible. You may select any combination of tests from the *American Journal of Hospital Pharmacy* and *Clinical Pharmacy* to give you the number of credits you need.
2. An Answer Sheet is published at the end of each installment of the CE column. An Enrollment Form is published in the June and December issues of *AJHP* and *CP*.
3. Complete only one Enrollment Form, but note on the form all the tests you are taking. Staple together all answer sheets for one enrollment.
4. Tests included in one enrollment must have been published within the past 18 months. Once a particular test is included in an enrollment, it may not be included in a subsequent enrollment.
5. The passing score on each test is 70%. Within four weeks of receiving your enrollment, ASHP will mail you a CE letter or notify you that certain tests were failed. Failed tests may be retaken only one time, without additional cost. There are no refunds for failed tests.
6. ASHP is approved by the American Council on Pharmaceutical Education as a provider of continuing pharmaceutical education (Provider Number 680-204). (The following states recognize ACPE-approved providers: AK, AR, AZ, CA, DE, FL, IA, ID, IL, IN, KS, KY, LA, MA, ME, MI, MN, MO, MS, MT, NE, NH, NM, NV, OH, OR, PA, RI, SD, TN, WA, and WY [also Puerto Rico].) Most states that recognize ACPE-approved providers will accept credit earned through journal CE programs; however, since some states have restrictions on the number of credit hours or CE units they will accept toward the total requirement, it is advised that readers check with their respective state board of pharmacy if they are uncertain about the board's regulations.
7. Send your Enrollment Form, Answer Sheet(s), and check (made payable to ASHP) to:

ASHP CE
American Society of Hospital Pharmacists
4630 Montgomery Avenue
Bethesda, MD 20814

Enrollment Form

Name____

Address______________________________________

City____________________State__________Zip________

Tests included in this enrollment must have been published within the past 18 months.

Test Number	*Hours of Credit*
________	______
________	______
________	______
________	______
________	______
________	______
________	______
________	______
________	______
________	______
________	______
________	______

(Write additional numbers and hours on a separate sheet and attach it to this form.)

Fee Schedule
$3.50/hour
$15.00 minimum/enrollment

Total hours ______

Total fee($) enclosed ______

Current Literature

Drug Reaction Alerts

Drug Reaction Alerts focuses primarily on serious, unlabeled reactions to new chemical entities. The citations are compiled monthly from International Pharmaceutical Abstracts, *which covers over 800 pharmacy and health-related journals worldwide. An address for reprints (when available) follows the name of the corresponding author in each citation.*

Anticoagulants

Pirson Y (Clinique Universitaires St Luc, Avenue Hippocrate 10, 1200 Brussels, Belgium), Honhon B, Cosyns JP et al. Cholesterol embolism in a renal graft after treatment with **streptokinase.** *Br Med J.* 1988; 296:394–5. Case. (56-year-old myocardial infarction patient; received streptokinase 1.5×10^6 IU over one hour by i.v. injection; concomitant azathioprine, prednisolone, β blocker, enalapril, and heparin; developed transient kidney failure attributed to cholesterol embolism of renal vessels induced by streptokinase; recovery without specific therapy)

Anticonvulsants

Gasperetti CM (Department of Medicine, Boston City Hospital, Boston, MA 02118). Conduction abnormalities complicating **carbamazepine** therapy. *Am J Med.* 1987; 82:381. Case. (87-year-old woman; received carbamazepine 100–200 mg twice daily; developed conduction abnormalities including atrioventricular block, hypotension, decreased mentation, congestive heart failure, and poor peripheral perfusion)

Antifungals

Best TR, Jenkins JK, Murphy FY et al. (Vesely DL, John L. McClellan Memorial VA Hospital 151, Little Rock, AK 72205). Persistent adrenal insufficiency secondary to low-dose **ketoconazole** therapy. *Am J Med.* 1987; 82:676–80. Case. (61-year-old woman with blastomycosis; received ketoconazole 400 mg/day orally; developed persistent adrenal insufficiency documented by endocrine testing; received oral hydrocortisone 20 mg in morning and 10 mg at night; adrenal insufficiency has not been reversible after two years of follow-up)

Antineoplastic Agents

Jacobs AD (Division of Hematology–Oncology, Department of Medicine, UCLA School of Medicine, Los Angeles, CA 90024), Levenson JE, Golde DW. Induction of acute corneal allograft rejection by **α_2-interferon.** *Am J Med.* 1987; 82:181–2. Case. (38-year-old male corneal allograft recipient with hairy cell leukemia; received subcutaneous α_2-interferon 4.6×10^6 units three times weekly for two weeks; developed allograft rejection; rejection episode resolved upon temporary discontinuation of α_2-interferon and administration of topical corticosteroid; negative rechallenge)

Cardiac Drugs

Gay RG (VA Medical Center, Tucson, AZ 85723), Fielder KL, Grogan TM. **Quinidine** induced reactive lymphadenopathy. *Am J Med.* 1987; 82:143–5. Case. (58-year-old man; received quinidine sulfate 200 mg four times daily for 2½ years; developed marked reactive lymphadenopathy; complete and rapid resolution of lymphadenopathy one month after drug withdrawal)

Cephalosporins

Csanyi P, Rado JP, Hormay M. Acute renal failure due to **cephamandole.** *Br Med J.* 1988; 296:433. Case. (76-year-old woman; received cefamandole 1 g four times daily for four days during cholelithiasis therapy; concomitant atropine, codeine, aminopyrine, and papaverine; developed acute renal failure; cefamandole therapy discontinued and furosemide and corticosteroid therapy unsuccessful; renal function returned without further drug therapy after 10 days of peritoneal dialysis)

Drug Interactions

Benetello P (Institute of Neurology, University of Padua, Via Giustiniani 5, 35128 Padua, Italy), Furlanut M. **Primidone-carbamazepine** interaction: clinical consequences. *Int J Clin Pharm Res.* 1987; 7:165–8. Case. (15-year-old boy with partial complex seizures; received oral primidone 12 mg/kg and carbamazepine 30 mg/kg without freedom from seizures; carbamazepine concentrations were low at 4.8 mg/mL; carbamazepine concentration increased and seizures controlled after gradual discontinuation of primidone)

Koren JF, Cochran DL (VA Medical Center, Salisbury, NC 28144), Janes RL. **Tolmetin-warfarin** interaction. *Am J Med.* 1987; 82:1278–9. Case. (64-year-old man; received three doses of tolmetin 400 mg; concomitant therapy with warfarin 2.5 mg/day; developed marked prolongation of prothrombin time to 70.2 seconds)

Zachariae H (Department of Dermatology, Marselisborg Hospital, University of Aarhus, 8000 Aarhus, Denmark). Dangers of **methotrexate/etretinate** combination therapy. *Lancet.* 1988; 1:422. Case. (47-year-old man with severe psoriasis; received etretinate 50 mg/day; concomitant oral methotrexate 15 mg/wk; developed severe drug-induced hepatitis; icterus slowly subsided and laboratory tests returned to normal two months after etretinate and methotrexate discontinued)

Gastrointestinal Drugs

Harvey RL (Division of Infectious Diseases, Hutzel Hospital, 4707 St. Antoine, Detroit, MI 48201), Luzar MJ. **Metoclopramide** induced agranulocytosis. *Ann Intern Med.* 1988; 108:214–5. Case. (61-year-old woman; received metoclopramide hydrochloride 10 mg four times daily for two weeks; concomitant antacids, ranitidine, and combination of oxycodone hydrochloride and aspirin; developed agranulocytosis; leukocyte count rose within six days of metoclopramide withdrawal; positive rechallenge)

Hypotensive Agents

Schubiger G (Kinderspital, CH-6000 Lucerne 16, Switzerland), Flury G, Nussberger J. **Enalapril** for pregnancy-induced hypertension: acute renal failure in a neonate. *Ann Intern Med.* 1988; 108:215–6. Case. (female neonate; developed acute renal failure after 34-year-old hypertensive mother received enalapril 10 mg twice daily for 17 days before delivery; anuria resolved after hemodialysis for 10 days)

Immunotherapy

Brox AG (Royal Victoria Hospital, 687 Pine Avenue West, Montreal, Quebec H3A 1A1, Canada), Cournoyer D, Sternbach M et al. Hemolytic anemia following intravenous **gamma globulin** administration. *Am J Med.* 1987; 82:633–5. Case. (30-year-old homosexual man with immune thrombocytopenia; received globulin immune intravenous 400 mg/kg/day for seven days; developed transient intravascular hemolysis mediated by anti-A antibody in the globulin immune; hemoglobin level normalized following discontinuation of immune globulin therapy, and Coomb's test result became negative)

Steroid, cortico-

Gutknecht DR (Department of General Internal Medicine, Geisinger Medical Center, Danville, PA 17822). Chemical meningitis following epidural injections of corticosteroids. *Am J Med.* 1987; 82:570. Case. (69-year-old woman; received one 80-mg and two 40-mg doses of **methylprednisolone** injection for lower back pain, sciatica, and inguinal pain; developed chemical meningitis)

Tranquilizers

Kanwar AJ (Division of Dermatology, Department of Medicine, Facility of Medicine, Al-Arab Medical University, Benghazi, Libya), Singh M, El-Sheriff AI et al. Fixed eruption due to **trifluoperazine** hydrochloride. *Br J Dermatol.* 1987; 117:798–9. Case. (30-year-old man with anxiety state; received trifluoperazine hydrochloride 5 mg twice daily for three days; developed fixed eruption)

The Merck Manual, Fifteenth Edition, edited by Robert Berkow and Andrew J. Fletcher. Published by Merck Sharp & Dohme Research Laboratories, Division of Merck & Co., Inc., Rahway, NJ 07065-0900, 1987. xxvii + 2696 p. Price $21.50, hardcover. Also available in a two-volume, softcover set: Volume I, $12.50; Volume II, $7.50.

Oral Sustained Release Formulations: Design and Evaluation, edited by Avraham Yacobi and Eva Halperin-Walega. Published by Pergamon Press, Maxwell House, Fairview Park, Elmsford, NY 10523, in cooperation with the American Pharmaceutical Association, 1988. xi + 252 p. Price $42.50.

Pharmaceutical Microbiology, Fourth Edition, edited by W. B. Hugo and A. D. Russell. Published by Blackwell Scientific Publications, P.O. Box 50009, Palo Alto, CA 94303, 1987. x + 511 p. Price $90, cloth; $48.50, paper.

Safer Prescribing: A Guide to Some Problems in the Use of Drugs, Fourth Edition, by Linda Beeley. Published by Blackwell Scientific Publications, 52 Beacon Street, Boston, MA 02108, 1987. Available from Year Book Medical Publishers, 35 East Wacker Drive, Chicago, IL 60601. vii + 99 p. Price $12.50 + $1.70 shipping and handling.

Self-assessment in Clinical Pharmacology, by Henry L. Elliott. Published by Blackwell Scientific Publications, 52 Beacon Street, Boston, MA 02108, 1987. Available from Year Book Medical Publishers, 35 East Wacker Drive, Chicago, IL 60601. viii + 154 p. Price $18.00 + $2.15 shipping and handling.

Topics in Pharmaceutical Sciences 1987: Proceedings of the 47th International Congress of Pharmaceutical Sciences of F.I.P., edited by D. D. Breimer and P. Speiser. Published by Elsevier Science Publications B. V., Amsterdam, the Netherlands, 1987. Distributed by Elsevier Science Publishing Company Inc., 52 Vanderbilt Ave., New York, NY 10017. x + 529 p. Price $158.

Books Received

Books are listed as soon as received; selected books may be reviewed in Book Reviews in subsequent issues.

Basic Clinical Pharmacokinetics, Second Edition, by Michael E. Winter, Mary Anne Koda-Kimble, and Lloyd Y. Young. Published by Applied Therapeutics, Inc., P.O. Box 1903, Spokane, WA 99210-1903, 1988. xviii + 416 p. Price $26.50, U.S. and Canada; $32.50, elsewhere; plus postage and handling.

Clinical Pharmacokinetics: The MCQ Approach, by Stephen H. Curry. Published by The Telford Press, Inc., 285 Bloomfield Ave., Caldwell, NJ 07006, 1987. iii + 185 p. Price $45; $27.50 paper.

Hospital Financial Reports: A Survey. Published by Healthcare Financial Management Association, 1900 Spring Rd., Suite 500, Oak Brook, IL 60521, 1987. vi + 94 p. Price $29.95 (HFMA members), $37.95 (nonmembers).

Manual of Antibiotics and Infectious Diseases, Sixth Edition, by John E. Conte, Jr., and Steven L. Barriere. Published by Lea & Febiger, 600 Washington Square, Philadelphia, PA 19106-4198, 1988. xvi + 392 p. Price $19.50.

Medical Decision Making, by Harold C. Sox, Jr., Marshal A. Blatt, Michael C. Higgins et al. Published by Butterworth Publishers, 80 Montvale Ave., Stoneham, MA 02180, 1988. x + 406 p. Price $24.95.

Advertising Index

American Society of Hospital Pharmacists
Database Services, 410
Handbook on Injectable Drugs, 420
Pharmacy Management Curriculum, 409
Beecham Laboratories
Timentin, 414–416
Eli Lilly and Company
Nebcin, 417–418
Tazidime, 411–412
Miami Valley Hospital
Position Available, 479
Roxane Laboratories, A Boehringer Ingelheim Company
Computer Program, 419
Intensols, 421
Stuart Pharmaceuticals, Division of ICI Americas, Inc.
Cefotan, inside back cover, outside back cover
U.S. Public Health Service
Positions Available, 477
Witikar Saudi Arabia Ltd.
Positions Available, 479
Wyeth Laboratories
Tubex, inside front cover

Our online databases

stand alone

in drug information.

ASHP® databases help you to locate a wide scope of drug information, including fultext drug monographs, patient counseling information and abstracts of articles.

rug Information Fulltext®

DIF

he DIF database contains detailed, mprehensive drug information presenting over 50,000 marketed ug products.

Consumer Drug Information™

CDIF

CDIF is a fulltext database with descriptions written for the patient's understanding. More than 3,000 brand name drug products are covered.

International Pharmaceutical Abstracts®

IPA

The IPA database is the practical, efficient way of locating information from over 800 pharmaceutical, medical, cosmetic and other health-related journals throughout the world. IPA's abstract/indexing system works to help you easily locate the information.

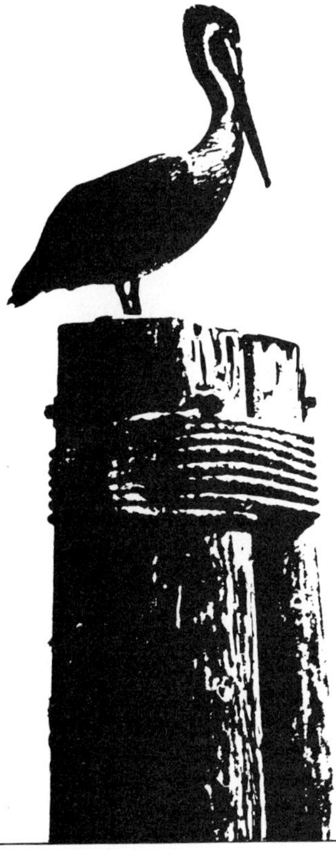

ASHP databases are available around the world through international online computer systems. For a brochure or more information, contact ASHP's Database Services at 301-657-3000, or write to:

Payments to ASHP are not deductible as charitable contributions for Federal Income Tax purposes. However, they may be deductible under other provisions of the Internal Revenue Code.

ASHP Database Services
4630 Montgomery Avenue
Bethesda, MD 20814

News

National committee recommends greater flexibility in stepped-care treatment of hypertension

Two additional classes of antihypertensive agents—the calcium antagonists and the angiotensin-converting enzyme inhibitors—should be considered as options in the initial drug therapy of high blood pressure, according to the 1988 Report of the Joint National Committee on Detection, Evaluation, and Treatment of High Blood Pressure. The committee also recommended use of smaller initial doses of most antihypertensive agents and more flexibility at each treatment step. Greater emphasis is placed on tailoring drug regimens to meet the needs of individual patients. The report is the fourth since 1976; major changes since the 1984 statement are summarized below. The committee was established under the auspices of the National Heart, Lung, and Blood Institute's National High Blood Pressure Education Program. The statement was published in the May 1988 issue of *Archives of Internal Medicine*.

Nonpharmacologic Therapy. The committee concluded that failure to control other risk factors for heart disease would reduce the health benefits of hypertension control. Thus, the revised document places greater emphasis on control of other cardiovascular risk factors. The nonpharmacologic therapies recommended for either hypertension control or risk-factor reduction include weight reduction, restriction of sodium intake, restriction of alcohol intake to no more than 30 mL of ethanol per day, cessation of smoking, and exercise. According to the report, data are insufficient to recommend modification of dietary fats for hypertension control, but such modifications "could be important for lowering blood cholesterol and reducing risk of developing coronary artery disease." The committee concluded that although fish consumption is recommended, the benefits of ω_3-fatty acid (fish-oil) capsules are unproven. The blood-pressure effects of cations other than sodium are also discussed. The data on calcium were deemed to be insufficient to merit specific recommendations.

Pharmacologic Therapy. The recommended stepped-care approach to drug therapy is outlined in the table. If mild hypertension has been controlled for at least one year, stepwise attempts to reduce drug dosages or the number of drugs are indicated, particularly if nonpharmacologic treatment recommendations are being followed. Also, when additional drugs are added to control blood pressure, later attempts at dosage reduction or elimination of the initial agent are appropriate. Other factors considered important in the selection of an antihypertensive agent for initial therapy are the patient's race, age, concomitant diseases and drug therapies, and lifestyle; the cost of therapy; and results of physiologic and biochemical tests. Guidelines for the management of isolated systolic hypertension, refractory hypertension, and hypertensive emergencies and urgencies are provided. Dosage ranges and precautions and special considerations in the use of individual antihypertensive agents are listed; for some agents recommended dosages have been lowered.

Individualized Stepped-Care Approach to Treatment of Hypertension

Step 1[a]
- Restrict sodium intake
- Restrict alcohol intake
- Control weight
- Control other cardiovascular risk factors

Step 2
- Begin drug therapy using a diuretic, β blocker, calcium antagonist, or angiotensin-converting enzyme inhibitor

Step 3
- Add a second drug from a different class, increase the dose of the first drug, or substitute another drug

Step 4
- Add a third drug of a different class or substitute a second drug

Step 5
- Evaluate possible reasons for lack of response, refer the patient for further evaluation, or add a third or fourth drug

[a] Some patients may require pharmacologic therapy initially. In these cases, nonpharmacologic approaches should be combined with drug therapy.

Other Considerations. Clinician–patient communication and patient involvement in treatment were stressed as important strategies for improving long-term compliance. The report lists many specific suggestions along these lines. Clinicians were urged to consider the effect of treatment on the patient's quality of life and to include all direct and indirect costs associated with therapy (not just the cost of the drug) in assessing the cost of care.

Special Populations. Discussion of hypertension in special populations is expanded in the 1988 report. These groups include patients who are black, elderly, young, or pregnant; patients who are surgical candidates; and those diagnosed as having cerebrovascular disease, coronary artery disease, congestive heart failure, left ventricular hypertrophy, peripheral vascular disease, diabetes mellitus, chronic obstructive pulmonary disease or asthma, hyperlipidemia, gout, or renal disease.

Community Programs. The committee concluded that mass screenings no longer need to be encouraged. According to the report, community efforts should be redirected to remove economic barriers to treatment and to provide follow-up services that complement medical management.

Procedures for reporting childhood-vaccine injuries announced

The Department of Health and Human Services has announced interim procedures for complying with the reporting requirements of the National Childhood Vaccine Injury Act. Health-care providers must maintain records on the administration of childhood vaccines, and health-care providers and manufacturers must report specified adverse events. The vaccines covered by this legislation and the adverse events that must be reported are listed in the table. Each health-care provider who administers one of these vaccines must ensure that the date of administration, the vaccine manufacturer and vaccine lot number, and the name and address and, if appropriate, the title of the health-care provider are recorded. Adverse events should be reported through local, county, or state health departments to the Centers for Disease Control if the vaccine was purchased using public funds; if the vaccine was purchased privately, adverse events should be reported to FDA using the agency's Adverse Reaction Report forms.

Reportable Adverse Events with Childhood Vaccines

Vaccine[a]	Event[b]
DTP, polio, DTP–polio combination, or other vaccine containing pertussis bacteria, extracted or partial cell bacteria, or specific pertussis antigens	Anaphylaxis or anaphylactic shock within 24 hours Encephalopathy or encephalitis within 7 days Shock collapse or hypotonic–hyporesponsive collapse Residual seizure disorder
Measles, mumps, or rubella, or a combination; DT; Td; or tetanus toxoid	Anaphylaxis or anaphylactic shock within 24 hours Encephalopathy or encephalitis within 15 days (mumps, measles, rubella) or 7 days (DT, Td, tetanus toxoid) Residual seizure disorder
Oral polio vaccine	Paralytic polio in a nonimmunodeficient recipient within 30 days, in an immunodeficient recipient within 6 months, or in a vaccine-associated community case (no time limit)
Inactivated polio vaccine	Anaphylaxis or anaphylactic shock within 24 hours

[a] DTP = diphtheria and tetanus toxoids and pertussis vaccine adsorbed, DT = diphtheria and tetanus toxoids adsorbed, and Td = tetanus and diphtheria tetanus toxoids adsorbed for adult use.

[b] For all vaccines listed, the following events are reportable: (1) any acute complication or sequela of the events listed above and (2) any contraindicating reaction to a vaccine that is specified in the product labeling.

Continued on page 490

NOW AVAILABLE

The Handbook on Injectable Drugs Fifth Edition

by Lawrence A. Trissel
Published by the American Society of Hospital Pharmacists

This popular reference covers a wide scope of injectable drugs used in admixtures. The fifth edition features completely revised monographs on 240 commercial drug products, plus information on investigational drugs. New dosage sections have been greatly expanded.

Monographs cover information on:

- products
- stability
- dosage
- compatibility

New drugs in this edition include:

- Aztreonam
- Imipenem-Cilastatin Sodium
- Ceftazidime
- Pentamidine Isethionate

Order your copy today.

ORDER FORM:

Handbook on Injectable Drugs, 5th Edition; 758 pp.

Please send me _____ copies of the *Handbook* (P276) @ $60.00.

☐ Enclosed is my check for $ _________ (Checks must be drawn on a U.S. bank.)

☐ Enclosed is our purchase order # _________ ; please issue an invoice and add postage and handling.

Charge $ _________ to my: ☐ MasterCard ☐ Visa

Acct. # _________________ Exp. _________ month/year

Signature _________________

Name _________________

Address _________________

City _____________ State _____ Zip _________

ASHP I.D.# _________________

Send to: **ASHP Publications Records Department**
4630 Montgomery Avenue
Bethesda, Maryland 20814

ASHP is a trademark of the American Society of Hospital Pharmacists, Inc.; Registered in the U.S. Patent and Trademark Office.

Payments to ASHP are not deductible as charitable contributions for Federal Income Tax purposes. However, they may be deductible under other provisions of the Internal Revenue Code.

Continued from page 489

FDA amends standards for nonsterile neomycin sulfate to specify oral use only

FDA has amended regulations establishing standards for nonsterile neomycin for prescription compounding. The product name has been changed to "neomycin sulfate for compounding oral products," and product labeling must state that the product is intended for oral use only. FDA's actions were prompted by recognition that the drug is being used for indications for which proof of efficacy is lacking (based on the Drug Efficacy Study Implementation [DESI] project findings) and for which there is a substantial risk of toxicity. These indications include the following uses: irrigation solutions for infected ulcers and wounds; prophylactic local use before, during, or after surgery; colonic or rectal irrigations or retention enemas; intrapleural instillation; use in wet dressings; aerosol inhalation; solutions for soaking grafts and silastic implants; and similar uses that may result in a substantial risk of toxicity. Certification of neomycin sulfate in sterile vials, a product labeled only for intramuscular administration in the treatment of certain urinary-tract infections, has been revoked.

FDA requires stronger warnings, imposes no limits on isotretinoin use

FDA will require Hoffmann-La Roche, Inc. to issue stronger warnings about the potential for isotretinoin (Accutane) to cause birth defects; the new warnings will be directed to both physicians and patients using the drug. Hoffmann-La Roche will be required to (1) double the type size of physician-directed warning statements, (2) include a picture of a deformed infant in the patient package insert, (3) use blister packs to ensure that patients receive warning materials with each prescription, (4) provide consent forms to be signed by patients and their physicians, (4) include a symbol of a pregnant woman crossed out on the blister packs and on materials sent to physicians and patients, and (5) warn physicians that they should provide patients with both oral and written warnings of the risk of birth defects. In addition, Hoffmann-La Roche will be required to conduct follow-up studies to assess the adequacy of these measures.

Continued reports of isotretinoin use by pregnant women prompted FDA to consider the need for new restrictions. A controversial report compiled by FDA scientists suggested to agency personnel that the number of birth defects and spontaneous abortions associated with isotretinoin are greatly underestimated by reports submitted to the agency. The teratogenic potential of isotretinoin also was the subject of a report in the March 25, 1988, issue of *Morbidity and Mortality Weekly Report*; the report described four cases of multiple, serious birth defects in infants born to women who had taken the drug during the first trimester of pregnancy.

On April 26, FDA's Dermatologic Drugs Advisory Committee voted by a margin of four to three to impose new restrictions but reaffirmed the importance of keeping the drug on the market. The panel recommended making product warning statements stronger and more prominent and requiring written informed consent from patients receiving the drug. A number of other mechanisms for limiting the use of isotretinoin were proposed. Challenges to FDA's legal authority to restrict use of isotretinoin were considered likely if FDA chose this course of action; such regulatory actions would have gone beyond the agency's usual regulation of the use of approved prescription drugs. Hoffmann-La Roche proposed a program that would strengthen product warnings, require written informed consent, and alter product packaging to limit the number of tablets and ensure that patients receive a warning with each prescription.

As of March 30, 1988, 62 cases of birth defects associated with isotretinoin use had been reported to FDA; however, the FDA report that focused attention on the use of isotretinoin by pregnant women estimated that the drug was responsible for severe birth defects in 900 to 1300 infants in the United States between September 1982 (when isotretinoin was first marketed) and the end of 1986. The number of spontaneous abortions that might have been caused by the drug were estimated at 700 to 1000. The report suggests that as many as 16,000 to 23,000 pregnant women might have been exposed to the drug. The reliability of these national estimates has been challenged because they were extrapolated from a review of the records of Michigan Medicaid patients. Of these patients, approximately 900 women of child-bearing age were exposed to the drug between 1982 and 1986 and approximately 50 took the drug during pregnancy.

Upcoming Specialty Meetings

Biology of Radionuclide Therapy . . . September 29–30 . . . Washington, DC . . . contact: American College of Nuclear Physicians, 1101 Connecticut Avenue, N.W., Suite 700, Washington, DC 20036; 202-857-1135.

American Venereal Disease Association . . . October 1–3 . . . Los Angeles, CA . . . contact: E. Hook III, Box 22349, San Diego, CA 92122; 619-233-2758.

American Academy of Family Physicians . . . October 3–6 . . . New Orleans, LA . . . contact: R. Graham, 1740 West 92nd Street, Kansas City, MO 64114; 816-333-9700.

National Perinatal Association . . . October 9–11 . . . San Diego, CA . . . contact: S. B. Whyte, National Perinatal Association, 101 South Union Street, Alexandria, VA 22314-3323; 703-549-5523.

American Society of Internal Medicine . . . October 13–16 . . . Atlanta, GA . . . contact: J. F. Boyle, 1101 Vermont Avenue, N.W., Suite 500, Washington, DC 20005; 202-289-1700.

American College of Gastroenterology . . . October 14–19 . . . New York, NY . . . contact: T. F. Fise, 13 Elm Street, Manchester, MA 01944; 617-927-8330.

American Epilepsy Society . . . October 15–19 . . . San Francisco, CA . . . contact: P. S. Bourgeois, 179 Allyn Street, Suite 304, Hartford, CT 06013; 203-246-6566.

Therapy Consultation

The Therapy Consultation *section provides brief advice, in question-and-answer format, on how to handle specific drug-therapy problems. Readers are invited to submit questions, which will be referred to a consultant for an answer. The problems should not be highly specialized or unusual, nor should they be mundane. Questions are answered briefly, based largely on the judgment and personal experience of the consultant, although selected references may be cited to substantiate the consultant's advice.*

Assistance in identifying Therapy Consultation *topics is provided by the drug information centers at the following institutions: Albert B. Chandler Medical Center and College of Pharmacy, University of Kentucky, Lexington; Arizona Health Sciences Center, Tucson; Medical College of Virginia Hospitals, Richmond; University of California Medical Center, San Diego; and University of Michigan Medical Center, Ann Arbor.*

Catecholamine selection for vasopressor-dependent patients

Question: Should current recommendations for the use of epinephrine in the treatment of cardiac arrest or anaphylaxis be modified for vasopressor-dependent patients who are receiving high doses of neuroleptic agents or α-adrenergic blockers?

Answer: Epinephrine, an endogenous catecholamine with both α- and β-adrenergic activity, is the catecholamine of choice for use during cardiopulmonary resuscitation (CPR) and during the treatment of anaphylactic shock, bronchospasm, and life-threatening angioedema. During CPR, epinephrine's potent α_1- and α_2-adrenergic effects improve cerebral blood flow by preventing arterial collapse and by increasing peripheral vasoconstriction.[1] The precise mechanisms by which epinephrine reverses rhinitis, urticaria, bronchoconstriction, and hypotension during anaphylaxis are not known.[2] These effects are attributed to concomitant β- and α-adrenergic agonist effects on the heart, lungs, and peripheral vasculature.[2,3] Preclinical studies and in vitro data have linked β-receptor activation by epinephrine to stimulation of adenylate cyclase, which results in an increased concentration of cyclic AMP and subsequent inhibition of histamine and other mediators.[3]

The end-organ effects of epinephrine depend on the dose and route of administration.[3] The optimal dose of epinephrine during CPR in humans is unknown. The current American Heart Association (AHA) recommendation of a 0.5- to 1.0-mg dose is based on studies in dogs weighing approximately 20 kg.[1] Preliminary data in humans suggest that epinephrine produces a dose-dependent vasopressor response; the data indicate that a 5-mg dose of epinephrine is needed to optimize blood pressure during CPR in humans.[4] Recommendations for dosage and rate of administration of epinephrine in anaphylactic reactions depend on the severity of the initial reaction.[3] In local anaphylactic reactions, subcutaneous injection of epinephrine 0.3 to 0.5 mg (0.01 mg/kg in children) as a 1:1000 solution is repeated every 15 to 20 minutes as needed. For patients in shock, intravenous epinephrine is advised. Although there is no consensus on the intravenous dose of epinephrine during anaphylactic shock, 0.1 mg of a 1:1000 solution can be mixed in 10 mL of 0.9% sodium chloride injection and administered over five to ten minutes.[3] Alternative recommendations are those given by the AHA.[1]

Drug interactions involving catecholamines have long been a topic of interest and controversy. Treatment decisions should be considered carefully when therapy for other medical problems could preclude or alter the anticipated responses to epinephrine and other adrenergic agonists.[2] Alpha-adrenergic blocking drugs would be expected to blunt the pressor response to catecholamines, whereas β-adrenergic blocking drugs would suppress the inotropic, dilatory, and metabolic effects of epinephrine. Phenothiazines block the reuptake of norepinephrine and serotonin and produce α-adrenergic blockade.[5] A common feature of phenothiazine toxicity, especially with chlorpromazine-like agents, is arterial hypotension.[6,7] Treatment with epinephrine results in profound hypotension because the α-adrenergic effects of epinephrine are blocked but the β-mediated vasodilatory effects remain unopposed.[6] Epinephrine should not be used in shock patients with recent exposure to phenothiazines.[7] Studies in animals show that small doses of epinephrine (0.33 μg/kg) do not interact with chlorpromazine but that larger doses (2.5 μg/kg) produce a

Continued on page 496

B fragilis group activity...

THE UNSURPASSED β-LACTAM CHOICE

TIMENTIN® *ticarcillin disodium/clavulanate potassium*

B fragilis group coverage superior to cephalosporins and penicillins

Susceptibility Pattern (%) of 531 *B fragilis* Group Isolates in a Nationwide *in vitro Study[1]**

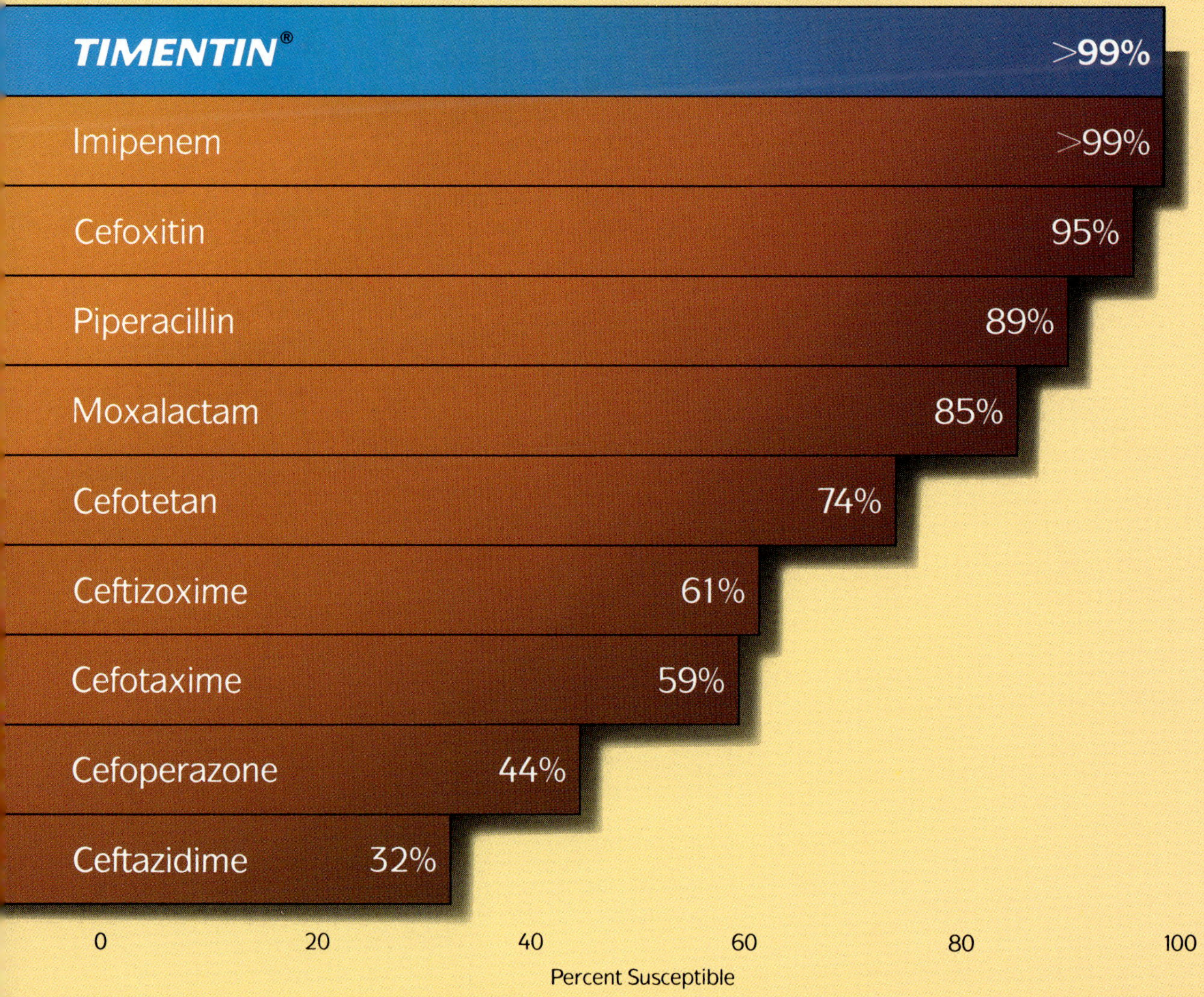

**In vitro* activity does not necessarily imply *in vivo* efficacy.

More active *in vitro** than traditional antianaerobic agents

Activity Against Clinical Isolates of *B fragilis* Group[2]		
Antibiotic	MIC_{50} (µg/mL)	MIC_{90} (µg/mL)
TIMENTIN†	≤1	4
Cefoxitin	8	32
Cefoperazone	32	128
Chloramphenicol	8	8
Clindamycin	0.5	8
Metronidazole	1	2

**In vitro* activity does not necessarily imply *in vivo* efficacy.
†Ticarcillin in the presence of a constant 2 µg/mL clavulanic acid.

More active *in vitro** than cefoxitin

Activity Against *B fragilis* Group[3]		
Organism (No. strains)	MIC_{90} (µg/mL)	
	TIMENTIN†	Cefoxitin
B fragilis (32)	0.5	16
B vulgatus (21)	1	16
B thetaiotaomicron (19)	2	32
B ovatus (16)	1	32
B distasonis (13)	8	64

**In vitro* activity does not necessarily imply *in vivo* efficacy.
†Ticarcillin in the presence of a constant 1 µg/mL clavulanic acid.

Destroys β-lactamases that limit the usefulness of other β-lactam choices

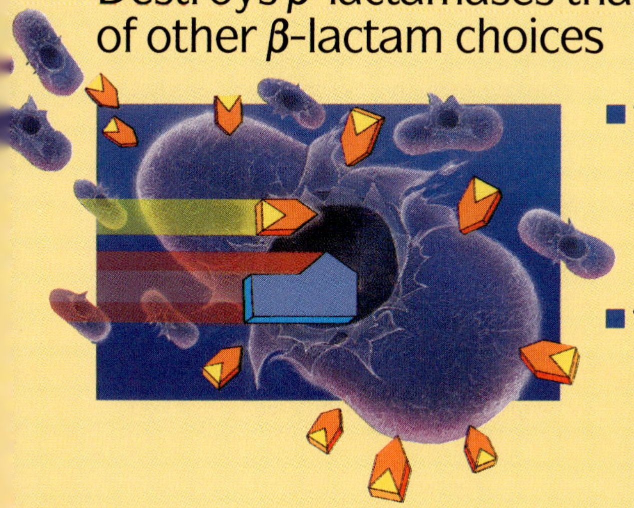

- "Most (90 percent) strains of B. fragilis produce constitutive beta-lactamases, which are primarily cephalosporinases. All other Bacteroides species probably produce beta-lactamases, but controversy exists concerning whether the enzymes are predominantly penicillinases or cephalosporinases."[4]
- "[Clavulanate potassium] inhibits the beta-lactamases of most Bacteroides species."[4]

△ Clavulanate potassium destroys most β-lactamases produced by Gram-positive and Gram-negative aerobes and anaerobes.
TIMENTIN destroys a broad range of aerobic and anaerobic bacteria regardless of β-lactamase production.

FOR ANAEROBIC CERTAINTY

TIMENTIN®

ticarcillin disodium/ clavulanate potassium

The unsurpassed β-lactam choice

Usual Dosage: 3.1 g every 4 to 6 hours.

Please see next page for brief summary of prescribing information.

THE CLAVULANATES Beecham laboratories BRISTOL, TENNESSEE 37620

© 1988, Beecham Laboratories.

BRIEF SUMMARY OF PRESCRIBING INFORMATION

TIMENTIN®

sterile ticarcillin disodium and clavulanate potassium
for Intravenous Administration

INDICATIONS AND USAGE: TIMENTIN® is indicated in the treatment of infections caused by susceptible strains of the designated organisms in the conditions listed below:

Bacterial Septicemia: including bacteremia, caused by β-lactamase producing strains of *Klebsiella* spp., *E. coli*, *Staphylococcus aureus* and *Pseudomonas aeruginosa* (and other *Pseudomonas* species).

Lower Respiratory Infections: caused by β-lactamase producing strains of *Staphylococcus aureus*, *Hemophilus influenzae* and *Klebsiella* spp.

Bone and Joint Infections: caused by β-lactamase producing strains of *Staphylococcus aureus*.

Skin and Skin Structure Infections: caused by β-lactamase producing strains of *Staphylococcus aureus*, *Klebsiella* spp., and *E. coli*.

Urinary Tract Infections (complicated and uncomplicated): caused by β-lactamase-producing strains of *E. coli*, *Klebsiella* spp., *Pseudomonas aeruginosa* (and other *Pseudomonas* species), *Citrobacter* spp., *Enterobacter cloacae*, *Serratia marcescens*, and *Staphylococcus aureus*. While TIMENTIN is indicated only for the conditions listed above, infections caused by ticarcillin susceptible organisms are also amenable to TIMENTIN treatment due to its ticarcillin content. Therefore, mixed infections caused by ticarcillin susceptible organisms and β-lactamase producing organisms susceptible to TIMENTIN should not require the addition of another antibiotic.

Appropriate culture and susceptibility tests should be performed before treatment in order to isolate and identify organisms causing infection and to determine their susceptibility to TIMENTIN. Because of its broad spectrum of bactericidal activity against Gram-positive and Gram-negative bacteria, TIMENTIN is particularly useful for the treatment of mixed infections and for presumptive therapy prior to the identification of the causative organisms. TIMENTIN has been shown to be effective as single drug therapy in the treatment of some serious infections where normally combination antibiotic therapy might be employed. Therapy with TIMENTIN may be initiated before results of such tests are known when there is reason to believe the infection may involve any of the β-lactamase producing organisms listed above; however, once these results become available, appropriate therapy should be continued.

Based on the *in vitro* synergism between TIMENTIN and aminoglycosides against certain strains of *Pseudomonas aeruginosa*, combined therapy has been successful, especially in patients with impaired host defenses. Both drugs should be used in full therapeutic doses. As soon as results of culture and susceptibility tests become available, antimicrobial therapy should be adjusted as indicated.

CONTRAINDICATIONS: TIMENTIN is contraindicated in patients with a history of hypersensitivity reactions to any of the penicillins.

WARNINGS: SERIOUS AND OCCASIONALLY FATAL HYPERSENSITIVITY (ANAPHYLACTOID) REACTIONS HAVE BEEN REPORTED IN PATIENTS ON PENICILLIN THERAPY. THESE REACTIONS ARE MORE LIKELY TO OCCUR IN INDIVIDUALS WITH A HISTORY OF PENICILLIN HYPERSENSITIVITY AND/OR A HISTORY OF SENSITIVITY TO MULTIPLE ALLERGENS. THERE HAVE BEEN REPORTS OF INDIVIDUALS WITH A HISTORY OF PENICILLIN HYPERSENSITIVITY WHO HAVE EXPERIENCED SEVERE REACTIONS WHEN TREATED WITH CEPHALOSPORINS. BEFORE INITIATING THERAPY WITH TIMENTIN, CAREFUL INQUIRY SHOULD BE MADE CONCERNING PREVIOUS HYPERSENSITIVITY REACTIONS TO PENICILLINS, CEPHALOSPORINS, OR OTHER DRUGS. IF AN ALLERGIC REACTION OCCURS, TIMENTIN SHOULD BE DISCONTINUED AND THE APPROPRIATE THERAPY INSTITUTED. **SERIOUS ANAPHYLACTOID REACTIONS REQUIRE IMMEDIATE EMERGENCY TREATMENT WITH EPINEPHRINE. OXYGEN, INTRAVENOUS STEROIDS, AND AIRWAY MANAGEMENT, INCLUDING INTUBATION, SHOULD ALSO BE PROVIDED AS INDICATED.**

PRECAUTIONS: While TIMENTIN possesses the characteristic low toxicity of the penicillin group of antibiotics, organ system functions should be assessed periodically during therapy.

Bleeding manifestations have occurred in some patients receiving β-lactam antibiotics. These reactions have been associated with abnormalities of coagulation tests such as clotting time, platelet aggregation and prothrombin time and are more likely to occur in patients with renal impairment. If bleeding manifestations appear, TIMENTIN treatment should be discontinued and appropriate therapy instituted.

TIMENTIN has only rarely been reported to cause hypokalemia. Periodic monitoring of serum potassium may be advisable in patients receiving prolonged therapy.

Pregnancy (Category B): Reproduction studies have been performed in rats given doses up to 1050 mg/kg/day and have revealed no evidence of impaired fertility or harm to the fetus due to TIMENTIN. There are, however, no adequate and well-controlled studies in pregnant women. Because animal reproduction studies are not always predictive of human response, this drug should be used during pregnancy only if clearly needed.

DOSAGE AND ADMINISTRATION: TIMENTIN should be administered by intravenous infusion (30 min.). Usual recommended dose for systemic and urinary tract infections for average (60 kg) adults is 3.1 Gm TIMENTIN (3.1 Gm vial containing 3 Gm ticarcillin and 100 mg clavulanic acid) given every 4 to 6 hours. In urinary tract infections, a dosage of 3.2 Gm TIMENTIN (3.2 Gm vial containing 3 Gm ticarcillin and 200 mg clavulanic acid) given every 8 hours is adequate. Please see official package insert for details on dosages for other patients, including those with renal insufficiency, and directions for use.

SUPPLIED: 3.1 Gm and 3.2 Gm Standard Vials; 3.1 Gm and 3.2 Gm Piggyback Bottles: 31 Gm Bulk Pharmacy Package: 3.1 Gm ADD-Vantage™ Antibiotic Vial.

7548/E-BS

References

1. Cuchural GJ, Tally FP, Jacobus NV, et al: Susceptibility of Bacteroides fragilis group clinical isolates to newer beta-lactam drugs, abstract No. 1B8. Presented to the 3rd Panamerican Congress of Infectious Diseases and Chemotherapy, San Juan, Puerto Rico, Dec 9-13, 1986.
2. Barry AL, Jones RN, Packer RR: *In vitro* susceptibility of the *Bacteroides fragilis* group to cefoperazone, ampicillin, ticarcillin, and amoxycillin combined with β-lactamase inhibitors. *J Antimicrob Chemother* 1986;17:125-127.
3. Bourgault AM, Lamothe F: In-vitro activity of amoxycillin and ticarcillin in combination with clavulanic acid compared with that of new β-lactam agents against species of the *Bacteroides fragilis* group. *J Antimicrob Chemother* 1986;17:593-603.
4. Neu HC: Contribution of beta-lactamases to bacterial resistance and mechanisms to inhibit beta-lactamases. *Am J Med* 1985;79(suppl 5B):2-12.

Beecham laboratories
BRISTOL, TENNESSEE 37620
© 1988, Beecham Laboratories.

Therapy Consultation *Continued from page 493*

significant reduction in mean arterial pressure.[6] Although chlorpromazine significantly reduced norepinephrine's pressor response, profound hypotension was not observed.[6] These findings underscore the need to use an α-adrenergic agonist in patients with phenothiazine-induced hypotension.

Lithium is an effective agent in the treatment of mania. Lithium increases the net uptake of amines and increases norepinephrine turnover and deamination.[8] Studies in lithium-treated patients show that lithium reduces norepinephrine's vasopressor response by 22%.[8] Two possible explanations for this effect are an increase in norepinephrine reuptake and a decreased sensitivity at the α receptor.

Unfortunately, no studies have examined the effect of α-blocking drugs or neuroleptics on epinephrine's vasopressor response during CPR. Yakaitis and coworkers[9] examined the effects of α blockade with phenoxybenzamine hydrochloride (2 mg/kg), β blockade with propranolol hydrochloride (0.5 mg/kg), and no adrenergic blockade on the success of CPR in dogs. Resuscitation efforts were 100% successful in restoring spontaneous circulation in dogs with blocked β receptors treated with phenylephrine and in dogs with unblocked receptors treated with epinephrine. Resuscitation with isoproterenol was successful in only 27% of dogs that had blocked α receptors. These data do not directly address the interaction between epinephrine and α-receptor blockade, but they highlight the importance of α-adrenergic stimulation during CPR.

Drug interactions are preventable adverse drug reactions. Protection of patients from harmful drug interactions begins with a careful drug history.[5] Unfortunately, there are no exact recommendations to follow in administering epinephrine to hypotensive patients receiving high doses of neuroleptic agents or α-adrenergic blockers. Because epinephrine may aggravate hypotension in these patients, I recommend the use of selective α-adrenergic agonists in patients who require vasopressor support and have been treated recently with α-adrenergic blockers or neuroleptic agents.

1. Anon. Pharmacology I. In: Jaffe AS, ed. Textbook of advanced cardiac life support. Dallas: American Heart Association; 1987; 97–114.
2. Morrow DH, Luther RR. Anaphylaxis: etiology and guidelines for management. *Anesth Analg.* 1976; 55:493–9.
3. Barach EM, Nowak RM, Lee TG et al. Epinephrine for treatment of anaphylactic shock. *JAMA.* 1984; 251:2118–22.
4. Gonzalez ER, Ornato JP, Garnett AR et al. Dose-dependent vasopressor response to epinephrine during CPR in humans. *J Am Coll Cardiol.* 1988; 11:42A. Abstract.
5. Cooke JE. Drug interactions in anesthesia. *Clin Plast Surg.* 1985; 12:83–9.
6. Yagiela JA, Duffin SR, Hunt LM. Drug interactions and vasoconstrictors used in local anesthetic solutions. *Oral Surg Oral Med Oral Pathol.* 1985; 59:565–71.
7. Inoue F. Adverse reactions of antipsychotic drugs. *Drug Intell Clin Pharm.* 1979; 13:198–208.
8. Fann WE, Davis JM, Janowsky DS et al. Effect of lithium on adrenergic function in man. *Clin Pharmacol Ther.* 1972; 13:71–7.
9. Yakaitis RW, Otto CW, Blitt CD. Relative importance of alpha and beta adrenergic receptors during resuscitation. *Crit Care Med.* 1979; 7:293–6.

EDGAR R. GONZALEZ, PHARM.D.
Assistant Professor of Pharmacy and Pharmaceutics, School of Pharmacy
Director, Critical Care Pharmacy Services, Medical College of Virginia Hospital
Virginia Commonwealth University
Richmond, VA 23298

Letters

The Letters *column is a forum for rapid exchange of ideas among readers of* CP. *Liberal criteria are applied in the review of submissions to encourage contributions to this column.*

The Letters *column includes the following types of contributions: (1) comments, addenda, and minor updates on previously published work, (2) alerts on potential problems related to drug therapy or clinical research, (3) observations or comments on trends in drug therapy or clinical research, and (4) brief expressions of opinion about controversies in drug therapy or clinical research.*

Letters need not be submitted with the journal's manuscript checklist. The following conditions, however, must be adhered to: (1) the body of the letter must be no longer than two typewritten pages, (2) the use of references, tables, and illustrations should be minimized, (3) the authors' names, affiliations, and mailing addresses must be typed at the end of the letter in the format used by CP, *and (4) the entire letter (including references, tables, and authors' names) must be typed double spaced on plain white paper (not letterhead). Following acceptance of a letter, the authors are required to sign an exclusive publication statement and a copyright-transferral form.*

Status of injectable calcium antagonists

The recent review of nicardipine, nitrendipine, and bepridil by Hasegawa[1] was well done and provided a balanced early evaluation of those agents. However, Hasegawa did not note that only nicardipine currently is undergoing Phase III investigation as an injectable dosage form. Injectable nicardipine has been used in the treatment of postoperative hypertension,[2] in the prevention of infarction following subarachnoid hemorrhage,[3] and in pharmacodynamic studies of experimental infarction and coronary hemodynamics.[4,5]

Clinical trials of injectable nitrendipine are not currently being conducted (Berkholder D, Miles Pharmaceutical. Personal communication. 1988 Mar). Injectable nifedipine is available in Europe, but neither Pfizer Laboratories nor Miles Pharmaceutical has any plans to market that dosage form in this country (Gerber F, Pfizer Laboratories, Personal communication, 1988 Mar, and Taylor R, Miles Pharmaceutical, Personal communication, 1988 Mar). Phase III trials of injectable nimodipine are scheduled to begin in three to four months (Kurtz N, Miles Pharmaceutical. Personal communication. 1988 Mar).

An injectable calcium antagonist without direct cardiovascular electrophysiological blocking properties could be useful.[6]

1. Hasegawa GR. Nicardipine, nitrendipine, and bepridil: new calcium antagonists for cardiovascular disorders. *Clin Pharm.* 1988; 7:97–108.
2. Casar G, Pool JL, Chelly JE et al. Intravenous nicardipine for treatment of postoperative hypertension. *Anesthesiology.* 1987; 67:A141. Abstract.
3. Adams H, Flamm E, Beck D et al. A study of nicardipine in prevention of infarction after subarachnoid hemorrhage. *Stroke.* 1987; 18:A281. Abstract.
4. Alps BJ, Calder C, Wilson A. Nicardipine in models of myocardial infarction. *Br J Clin Pharmacol.* 1985; 20(Suppl):29S–49S.
5. Lambert CR, Hill JA, Nichols WW et al. Coronary and systemic hemodynamic effects of nicardipine. *Am J Cardiol.* 1985; 55:652–6.
6. Matsui M, Nishiwaki H, Yoshino J et al. Effects of nicardipine hydrochloride on the conduction system of the heart in man. *Jpn Heart J.* 1982; 23:243–5.

DAVID M. ANGARAN, M.S., Director
Biomedical Research
United Hospital Heart Institute
201 Time Building
355 Sherman Street
St. Paul, MN 55102

Applicability of phenytoin predictive formulas to long-term-care facility residents

As three health professionals involved in the care of geriatric patients residing in a long-term-care facility, we were very interested in the recent work by Beck et al.[1] regarding the accuracy of three methods for predicting free (unbound) serum phenytoin concentrations. We often have questioned whether such predictive formulas would be applicable to our patients, since most of the formulas are generated by using data obtained from younger adult patients in acute-care settings.

We recently investigated the value of routine measurement of free phenytoin concentrations in 39 residents of the Wisconsin Veterans Home.[2] These patients generally were quite debilitated; 21 were not ambulatory. Like Beck et al., we measured unbound phenytoin concentrations using ultrafiltration and a fluorescence-polarization immunoassay (TDx Free Phenytoin, Abbott Laboratories, Irving, TX). We obtained the ultrafiltrate free fractions at 25 °C using a temperature-controlled centrifuge, and we obtained the ultrafiltrate for determination of free phenytoin concentration from each sample using an Amicon free-level filter (Amicon Corporation, Danvers, MA).

In an extension of our original analysis, we applied the predictive variables and equations reported by Beck et al. to our own data. Like Beck et al., we found good correlation between the percentage of free phenytoin and the albumin concentration, and the regression equations were surprisingly similar:

Beck et al.: Percent free phenytoin = 21.8 − (3.46 albumin)

Drinka et al.: Percent free phenytoin = 21.3 − (3.08 albumin)

The respective correlation coefficients were $r = -0.74$ (Beck et al.) and $r = -0.66$ (Drinka et al.). Our equation for the best model to predict the unbound phenytoin concentration (C_u) was also surprisingly similar to that of Beck et al.:

Beck et al.: $C_u = 1.53 + (0.09\ C_{PHT}) - (0.43 \text{ albumin})$

Drinka et al.: $C_u = 1.67 + (0.12\ C_{PHT}) - (0.51 \text{ albumin})$

where C_{PHT} = total phenytoin concentration. The respective coefficients of correlation were $R^2 = 0.77$ (Beck et al.) and $R^2 = 0.94$ (Drinka et al.).

We conclude that our results are in substantial agreement with those of Beck et al., despite the fact that we used data obtained from a chronic-care setting rather than an acute-care setting.

1. Beck DE, Farringer JA, Ravis WR et al. Accuracy of three methods for predicting concentrations of free phenytoin. *Clin Pharm*. 1987; 6:888–94.
2. Drinka PJ, Miller J, Voeks SK et al. Phenytoin binding in a nursing home. *J Geriatr Drug Ther*. 1988; in press.

Paul J. Drinka, M.D., Medical Director
Jan Miller, Medical Technologist
Susan K. Voeks, Ph.D., Research Analyst
Geriatric Evaluation Research and Education
Wisconsin Veterans Home
King, WI 54946

Pharmacy Practice in The PHS . . .
A Century of Service with Distinction

U.S. PUBLIC HEALTH SERVICE
1798

Call
1-301-443-5740
Or Write
Pharmacy Recruitment Officer
Room 7A-39
Parklawn Building
5600 Fishers Lane
Rockville, MD 20857

U.S. Public Health Service EOE/MF

Drug Review

Update on pentamidine for the treatment of *Pneumocystis carinii* pneumonia

FRANCINE R. SALAMONE AND BURKE A. CUNHA

Abstract: The chemistry, spectrum of activity, mechanism of action, pharmacokinetics, adverse effects, and dosage and administration of pentamidine are reviewed, and the role of the drug in treating *Pneumocystis carinii* infections in immunocompromised patients is discussed.

Pentamidine isethionate, an aromatic diamidine compound, is active against certain protozoan organisms. Used extensively in the tropics in the treatment of *Trypanosoma* and *Leishmania* infections, its value in the management of *Pneumocystis carinii* infections has been demonstrated in infected immunosuppressed children and adults. Recently, interest in pentamidine has increased with the rising number of patients with acquired immunodeficiency syndrome (AIDS) who have *P. carinii* pneumonia. Pentamidine's mechanism of action and pharmacokinetic profile are not completely understood. Pentamidine is distributed extensively after i.v. or i.m. administration, with a volume of distribution of 3 L/kg. Appreciable quantities of pentamidine concentrate in the urine, and drug levels are detectable for up to six to eight weeks after cessation of therapy. After aerosol administration, the drug is almost exclusively recovered from the lung, with little extrapulmonary distribution. Available data suggest that approximately 50% of patients who receive the drug by the i.v. or i.m. route will experience some drug toxicity (local pain, sterile abscesses at the intramuscular injection site, hypoglycemia, hypotension, or azotemia), while adverse effects after aerosol therapy include bronchial irritation but little systemic toxicity.

Regardless of the route of administration, pentamidine has emerged as a mainstay of therapy in the management of *P. carinii* pneumonitis in AIDS patients, especially in those who are allergic to the sulfa component of trimethoprim–sulfamethoxazole.

Index terms: Acquired immunodeficiency syndrome; Anti-infective agents; Dosage; Drug administration; Mechanism of action; Pentamidine isethionate; Pharmacokinetics; Pneumonia; Toxicity
Clin Pharm. 1988; 7:501–10

Pentamidine isethionate, synthesized in the 1930s, has substantially decreased the morbidity and mortality associated with a variety of protozoan infections. It first demonstrated its antiprotozoal efficacy when it was used successfully in the treatment of *Trypanosoma rhodesiense* and *Leishmania donovani* infections.[1-6] Subsequently, and before the introduction of trimethoprim–sulfamethoxazole (TMP–SMX), pentamidine was used extensively in Europe for an epidemic of infantile *Pneumocystis* pneumonia, where it reduced the mortality rate from 50% to 3.5%.[7,8] Pentamidine is especially efficacious in treating *Pneumocystis carinii* pneumonia (PCP), a common opportunistic infection in the immunocompromised host, which, if untreated, is associated with a mortality rate of 90–100%.[9-18] The use of pentamidine is associated with a reduction in mortality (25–50%) in patients with acquired immunodeficiency syndrome (AIDS) who are infected with the *P. carinii* organism.[19]

Infections caused by the protozoa *Leishmania*, particularly when unresponsive to therapy with pentavalent antimonial compounds and amphotericin B, are effectively treated with pentamidine. The World Health Organization (WHO) committee on leishmaniasis has recommended administration of an intramuscular dose of 4 mg/kg three times weekly for a period of up to 25 weeks as effective treatment for this disease.[20-22] Although ineffective against *Trypanosoma cruzi*, the causative organ-

FRANCINE R. SALAMONE, PHARM.D., is Clinical Pharmacist in Infectious Disease, Division of Pharmacy Services, Memorial Sloan Kettering Cancer Center, New York, NY. BURKE A. CUNHA, M.D., is Chief, Infectious Disease Division, and Vice Chairman, Department of Medicine, Winthrop University Hospital, Mineola, NY.

Address reprint requests to Francine R. Salamone, Pharm.D., Division of Pharmacy Services, Memorial Sloan Kettering Cancer Center, 1275 York Ave., New York, NY 10021.

Copyright © 1988, American Society of Hospital Pharmacists, Inc. All rights reserved. 0278-2677/88/0701-0501$02.50.

ism of Chagas's disease, pentamidine has demonstrated efficacy in the lymphatic stage of West African trypanosomiasis, producing a survival rate of 99% in more than 11,000 patients infected with *Trypanosoma gambiense*.[23,24] *Medical Letter* consultants consider pentamidine, in doses of 4–7 mg/kg/day for 7–10 days, an alternative to suramin in the treatment of infections that do not involve the nervous system.[22,24,25] Although routine prophylaxis in travelers from the United States is not recommended, administration of a single intramuscular injection (300–400 mg) every six months to individuals living in endemic areas affords protection against infection with certain *Trypanosoma* species.[23,26–28]

Most recently, the use of pentamidine has increased with the increasing number of AIDS patients who have pneumonia caused by the *P. carinii* organism.[29] More than 60% of patients with AIDS will develop PCP in their lifetime.[11] Approximately 100,000 cases of *P. carinii* pneumonitis are expected to occur in patients with AIDS in the United States by 1991.[30] Pentamidine is primarily used in the treatment of this infection as an alternative to trimethoprim–sulfamethoxazole (TMP–SMX).[31,32] Patients with AIDS and other opportunistic infections are often switched to pentamidine during a course of TMP–SMX treatment because of either lack of improvement or development of hypersensitivity reactions to the sulfa component.[33–35]

The purpose of this article is to update previously published reviews of pentamidine[28,36,37] and to discuss its role in the treatment of infections caused by the *P. carinii* organism in immunocompromised patients.

Chemical Properties

Pentamidine isethionate is chemically classified as an aromatic diamidine and is structurally related to synthalin.[38–41] Laboratory investigations in the late 1930s demonstrated that trypanosomes require glucose for metabolism, suggesting that a hypoglycemic agent such as synthalin might be trypanocidal.[1,41] Consequently, structural modifications of synthalin were evaluated, resulting in a variety of trypanocidal compounds, including pentamidine.[38,42]

Pentamidine is manufactured as either the isethionate salt or the methanesulfonate salt. However, the isethionate formulation is commercially available and used most frequently in the United States.[43,44] Major differences exist between the two formulations in terms of dosage, packaging, and perhaps toxicity. The dosages of the two salt forms are expressed differently based on differences in the amount of active drug. The isethionate form is labeled (and consequently dosed) to reflect both the amount of pentamidine base and salt, while the methanesulfonate form is expressed as the amount of pentamidine base only.[29,44] In addition, the risk of hypoglycemia may be greater in patients treated with the methanesulfonate salt form.[45]

Spectrum of Activity

The selective antiprotozoal effects of pentamidine are well documented.[1,23,38,41,46] *T. gambiense* and some strains of *T. rhodesiense* are highly susceptible.[23,38] Although the drug possesses activity against *L. donovani*, pentavalent antimony compounds remain the preferred drug for these infections.[20,47] *Babesia canis* and *Babesia microti* are susceptible to pentamidine in animals.[48] However, *B. microti* infections in humans do not respond to this drug.[49] Although in vitro studies suggest some antibacterial activity against *Staphylococcus aureus*, pentamidine is ineffective in vivo.[23,50] Additionally, pentamidine has no antifungal or antimalarial activity.[23] Its activity against the protozoan organism *P. carinii* has resulted in a dramatic increase in the drug's use since the 1950s.[29,51]

Mechanism of Action

The exact mechanism of the antiprotozoal effect of pentamidine has not been identified, although several theories have been proposed.[52–60] Pentamidine may inhibit protozoan dihydrofolate reductase and deplete folic acid.[52–54] Pentamidine may bind to extrachromosomal DNA and subsequently interfere with protozoan replication.[54] Other proposed mechanisms include the inhibition of the organisms' RNA polymerase,[55] ribosomal function,[56] and nucleic acid, protein, and phospholipid synthesis.[57,58] Pentamidine may interfere with aerobic glycolysis since the drug exerts its greatest activity against organisms that require glucose uptake and metabolism for respiratory processes.[60,61]

Pharmacokinetics

Data regarding the drug's pharmacokinetic disposition are variable.[61–66] Differences in techniques used for analysis of the compound in tissue and body fluids may account for some of the variability. Several investigators have developed methods for bioassay of the drug in both animals and humans.[61,62,67] The results of these pharmacokinetic studies in humans are presented in Table 1. As shown, Conte et al.[67] noted striking differences between intramuscularly and intravenously treated patients. After intramuscular and intravenous injections, peak plasma concentrations of 209 ng/mL and 612 ng/mL are obtained, respectively, within one hour after a 4-mg/kg dose of pentamidine isethionate. These concentrations are detected throughout a 24-hour dosing interval and decline biexponentially.[67] Plasma pentamidine concentrations do not appear to increase after multiple-dose administration.[61]

Table 1.
Summary of Pentamidine Pharmacokinetic Data in Human Subjects

Variable	Reference 62 (n = 3)	61 (n = 7)	67 (n = 6)	67 (n = 6)
Daily dosage of pentamidine isethionate (mg/kg)	4	4	4	4
Route of administration	I.V.	I.M.	I.M.	I.V.
Mean peak plasma concentration (μg/mL)	0.5–3.2	0.3–1.4	0.209 ± 0.048[a]	0.612 ± 0.371[a]
Mean ± S.D. distribution half-life (min)	17 ± 4	. . .[b]	54 ± 10.8[a]	18 ± 13.2[a]
Elimination half-life (hr)	. . .	. . .	9.36 ± 2.01[a]	6.4 ± 1.32[a]
Elimination rate–renal clearance (L/hr)	. . .	. . .	15.4 ± 14.9[a,c]	6.21 ± 3.63[a,d]
Estimated plasma clearance (L/hr)	. . .	. . .	305 ± 81[a]	248 ± 91[a]
Fraction of daily dose eliminated unchanged in the urine (%)	6	11–29	4.08[c]	2.46[d]
Assay procedure	Agar diffusion	Spectrophotofluorometry	HPLC[e]	HPLC[e]

[a] Mean (± S.D.) values for a two-compartment open model.
[b] Not determined.
[c] Value for five i.m.-treated patients.
[d] Value for four i.v.-treated patients.
[e] HPLC = high-performance liquid chromatography.

The volume of distribution of pentamidine is approximately 3 L/kg, suggesting that the drug is extensively taken up by most body tissues.[63] Studies in animals have demonstrated that after intramuscular administration, pentamidine concentrations found in the kidney are 5 to 10 times those found in the lung and approximately double the concentration found in hepatic tissue.[61,64] Conversely, aerosol administration of the drug in rats results in high intrabronchial levels and persistently low concentrations of pentamidine in the blood, kidney, and liver.[63] In another animal study, injection of liposome-encapsulated pentamidine resulted in higher and more persistent lung concentrations compared with levels achieved after injection of free drug.[65] Kidney levels of drug were significantly lower in the group treated with encapsulated pentamidine injection. Both free and encapsulated aerosolized pentamidine produced lung levels comparable to those obtained by intravenous injection, while markedly reduced extrapulmonary drug deposition occurred, with an up to 200-fold lower uptake in the kidney.[65]

Depending on the route of administration, approximately 2–29% of a daily dose may be excreted unchanged in the urine.[61,62,67] In one study, the total amount of pentamidine excreted was greatest within the first six hours after intramuscular administration of a dose, with urinary concentrations of drug averaging 20-25 μg of pentamidine base per milliliter. However, decreasing amounts of pentamidine were present in the urine for up to eight weeks after cessation of therapy.[61] This further supports the concept that the drug is extensively distributed in body tissues and slowly released from selected compartments.

Efficacy for *Pneumocystis carinii* Pneumonia

Congenital or Acquired Immune Deficiency. *Pneumocystis carinii* pneumonia (PCP) may occur in premature or debilitated infants (infantile *Pneumocystis* pneumonia) and older children and adults with congenital or acquired immunodeficiencies.[7,14,32,38,68] Infantile *Pneumocystis* pneumonia, when untreated, was associated with a mortality rate of approximately 50%.[7] Pentamidine was of unquestioned benefit in the European infantile *Pneumocystis* pneumonia epidemics of the 1940s and 1950s, since early intervention with pentamidine successfully reduced the fatality rate to 3.5% in infected infants.[7,68,69] Currently, use of pentamidine for this indication is rare since this entity is infrequently seen.[7]

The success of pentamidine in the treatment of PCP in patients with congenital or acquired immune deficiency (congenital hypogammaglobulinemia, lymphoproliferative malignancy, immunosuppressive therapy) is well documented.[70–87] In general, the survival rate is greatest when treatment with pentamidine is initiated early and continued for at least 10 days (Table 2).

There are a limited number of trials comparing the efficacy and toxicity of pentamidine with other treatment regimens in patients with PCP and underlying immune suppression other than AIDS.[32,35,80,87,88] In one prospective controlled study in 50 children with leukemia or other malignancies and *P. carinii* pneumonitis, patients were randomized to receive either intramuscular pentamidine isethionate therapy (4 mg/kg/day) or oral TMP-SMX (20 mg/kg/day of trimethoprim) for a total of 14 days.[80] Those patients found to be unresponsive to the first drug after three or more days

Table 2.
Summary of Treatment Results for Non-AIDS-Related *Pneumocystis carinii* Pneumonia in Immunocompromised Hosts[a]

Reference	No. of Patients Treated	Duration of Treatment (days)	No. of Recoveries (%)
14	14	10–14	10 (71%)
	8	<8	0 (0%)
78	43	≥9	33 (77%)
	32	1–8	3 (9%)
79	93	≥9	59 (63%)
	70	<9	10 (14%)
81	12	6–10	11 (92%)
	6	≤5	0 (0%)
82	17	14	7 (41%)
83	17	≥10	9 (53%)
84	31	10–14	25 (81%)
	25	<7	0 (0%)
85	8	10–14	5 (63%)
	4	≤6	0 (0%)

[a] Dosage of pentamidine isethionate was 4 mg/kg/day given intramuscularly or intravenously.

of therapy were changed to the alternate drug. Twenty (77%) of 26 patients initially treated with TMP–SMX therapy recovered, compared with 18 (75%) of 24 patients initially treated with pentamidine. Adverse effects (increase in blood urea nitrogen and creatinine values, hypoglycemia, and inflammation at the injection site) were observed in 14 of 15 patients treated with pentamidine alone, compared with only one case of an urticarial rash in a patient receiving TMP–SMX alone.[80]

In another prospective trial, Siegal and coworkers[32] compared the efficacy and toxicity of both drugs in 25 pediatric cancer patients with biopsy-confirmed *P. carinii* pneumonia. Patients were randomly assigned to receive either intramuscular pentamidine or oral TMP–SMX for 14 days. The authors noted no differences in the clinical or roentgenographic response between the two groups. The median number of days from the beginning of treatment to the presence of a normal chest roentgenogram was 13 for the pentamidine-treated group (n = 10), compared with 15 for those patients receiving TMP–SMX (n = 15). Additionally, a reduction in temperature (<38 °C) was observed between days 1 and 23 in the pentamidine-treated group and between days 0 and 22 in the alternate group. The number of patients experiencing toxicity was also similar for each drug. Rash (n = 5), mild elevations in liver enzymes (n = 2), and myelosuppression (n = 2) were observed in patients receiving TMP–SMX. Of the 10 patients receiving pentamidine, 3 had increases in their serum creatinine or urea nitrogen levels, or both; four experienced local reactions to the injections; and two experienced hypoglycemia.[32]

Based on the previous findings and those of other investigators, it appears that pentamidine and TMP–SMX are equally efficacious in treating *P. carinii* pneumonitis.[35,87,88] However, because of the lower frequency and severity of adverse effects, TMP–SMX is the preferred drug for the prophylaxis[89] and treatment of PCP in patients with underlying immunosuppressive disorders other than AIDS. Pentamidine is reserved for the treatment of those patients who are unresponsive or allergic to the sulfa component.

Acquired Immunodeficiency Syndrome. *Comparison with Trimethoprim–Sulfamethoxazole.* In an effort to determine the most appropriate place for pentamidine in the therapy of PCP in patients with AIDS, several investigators have compared it with TMP–SMX. In general, the drugs are of similar efficacy, as was previously observed in patients with malignancy and other forms of underlying immunosuppression.[90-99] However, patients with AIDS experience more adverse effects related to TMP–SMX.[31,34,88,91,92]

Leukopenia, fever, rash, eosinophilia, and hepatotoxicity are frequent and generally appear between days 7 and 14 of treatment.[31,34,88,91,92] Of 37 AIDS patients being treated with TMP–SMX in one retrospective review, only 5 patients completed their course of therapy and 2 patients died.[34] Severe toxicity occurred in 23 patients, and 19 required discontinuation of therapy. The incidence of skin rash (18 of 37) was almost 10 times greater than that reported for non-AIDS patients with PCP. Hepatic toxicity, generally rare with TMP–SMX, occurred in 20% of patients. Pentamidine toxicity occurred in 43% (12 of 30) of patients, which is similar to the 47% (189 of 404) reported by Walzer et al.[79] in their epidemiologic review of PCP in immunosuppressed patients who do not have AIDS.

In another retrospective review in a large series of patients, adverse reactions to TMP–SMX were significantly more common in AIDS patients compared with patients with other immunosuppressive disorders.[35] Of 34 AIDS patients, 22 (65%) developed some adverse reaction to therapy, the most frequent being rash (29%) and leukopenia (47%), compared with 12% of patients with other types of underlying immunosuppression (most frequently, leukopenia). The incidence of adverse reactions to pentamidine was similar for AIDS (47%) and non-AIDS patients (57%); the most frequent of these adverse effects was a rise in the serum creatinine concentration (more than 3.0 mg/dL).

Although a majority of AIDS patients with PCP initially receive treatment with a course of TMP–SMX, those given pentamidine experience similar rates of recovery. Indeed, AIDS patients who are switched from TMP–SMX therapy to pentamidine because of intolerable adverse effects to the former have a better chance of survival than those patients switched from TMP–SMX because of treatment failure.[33,88,93]

Small and coworkers[33] evaluated 44 episodes of PCP in 36 patients with AIDS. Initial therapy with TMP–SMX was successful in 18 of 40 episodes (45%), with adverse reactions occurring in 22 (65%) of the 34 patients treated. Fifteen patients (37.5%) failed to respond, with two deaths attributable to this lack of response. The remaining 13 patients, as well as seven patients who experienced adverse reactions to TMP–SMX therapy, were subsequently switched to pentamidine. Of the pentamidine-treated group (n = 24), the nine deaths that occurred were all patients who failed to respond to treatment with TMP–SMX. All seven patients who were switched to pentamidine because of an intolerable adverse reaction to TMP–SMX therapy improved, as did three patients who received pentamidine as initial therapy for an episode of PCP.

Similarly, Murray and coworkers[93] reported that 100% of patients (41 of 41) who were switched to pentamidine because of adverse reactions to TMP–SMX survived, compared with a survival rate of only 11% (4 of 37) in patients who were switched from TMP–SMX because of treatment failure.[93] In a large multicenter trial involving 27 medical centers, 71% (12 of 17) of AIDS patients who were switched to pentamidine because of adverse reactions to TMP–SMX survived for at least 90 days, compared with 37% (13 of 35) of patients who were switched to pentamidine as a result of treatment failure with TMP–SMX.[88]

There are few prospective studies comparing the efficacy and toxicity of both agents. In one randomized trial, 19 of 20 pentamidine-treated patients and 15 of 20 patients treated with TMP–SMX survived. Five patients treated initially with TMP–SMX died, compared with only one patient in the pentamidine-treated group. Adverse effects necessitating a change in therapy were observed in 10 patients treated with TMP–SMX and in 11 patients treated with pentamidine.[31] The authors concluded that the difference between these two drugs in terms of efficacy or adverse effects is not significant. However, the authors acknowledge the low power of their conclusions based on a small sample size. Correspondingly, the finding that more patients in the pentamidine group survived needs evaluation in a larger patient population.[94-99]

Although evaluated in only a small number of subjects, there appears to be no synergy or advantage in using both pentamidine and TMP–SMX in any type of patient. Combination therapy is no more effective than using either agent alone, or sequentially, and it increases the risk of adverse effects.[88,90,100] In one study of animals pretreated with steroids, 45% of rodents given the combination therapy died, compared with 48% and 21% for the pentamidine and TMP–SMX treatment groups, respectively. Although caution must be exercised in extrapolating animal data to human equivalents, the authors point out that a combination of TMP–SMX and pentamidine is probably no more effective than monotherapy with TMP–SMX and may, in fact, be harmful.[100]

Aerosolized Pentamidine. Most recently, a novel approach toward the treatment and prophylaxis of PCP in AIDS patients—using aerosolized pentamidine—has been evaluated. Since the *P. carinii* organism is highly concentrated in the alveoli of the lung, aerosolization would likely result in higher pentamidine concentrations at the infected site.[65,101,102] Indeed, animal and human studies suggest that aerosolized pentamidine may be an effective, site-specific, and less toxic mode of prevention and therapy of PCP.[65,101,102] Both ultrasonic and jet nebulizers have been used to deliver the drug in a particle size of 0.5 to 4 μm to ensure maximum pulmonary distribution.[103,104]

Several centers are currently evaluating the efficacy of such therapy as a form of treatment[103,105] and prophylaxis[104] of PCP in patients with AIDS. The results of one of the two published trials regarding the use of aerosolized pentamidine isethionate as treatment suggested benefit with such therapy. Of the 15 treated patients, 13 showed definite clinical improvement after inhalation of 300 mg daily for 21 days, and no patients experienced systemic adverse effects. Airway irritation resulting in cough was experienced by 12 subjects, with severe paroxysms reported by 3 patients, all of whom were smokers.[105] The lack of systemic toxicity is consistent with the significantly lower serum pentamidine concentrations (<10 ng/mL) attained after aerosolization, compared with the higher concentrations reached after i.m. or i.v. administration (>600 ng/mL).[67,105] Nevertheless, since this was an open study, further evaluation in a randomized controlled trial is warranted.

Conte and coworkers[103] compared the use of inhaled pentamidine and low-dose intravenous pentamidine in a small number of patients with mild PCP. Of 13 patients who received inhaled pentamidine isethionate (4 mg/kg/day in an ultrasonic nebulizer for two weeks), nine showed clinical and roentgenographic improvement; a serious adverse reaction (depressed white blood cell count) occurred in two patients. Eight of the nine patients given low-dose therapy administered intravenously or intramuscularly (3 mg/kg/day for two weeks) responded to therapy; serious toxicity (hepatotoxicity and neutropenia) occurred in two patients, and less serious adverse reactions occurred in four patients (elevated serum creatinine concentration in three patients, depressed white blood cell count in one, and rash in one). In general, pentamidine concentrations were lower in extrapulmonary sites and higher in bronchoalveolar fluid in patients who received aerosolized pentamidine compared with those who received systemic low-dose therapy.[103]

The results of the use of aerosolized pentamidine

in the prophylaxis of PCP appear promising. Of 120 patients evaluated in one ongoing large trial, a total of 1284 doses were administered using a hand-held nebulizer for 10–20 minutes. In the first trials, 30 mg of pentamidine isethionate was administered biweekly. In subsequent trials, patients were randomized to receive 30, 45, or 60 mg weekly for the first four weeks and then biweekly. All patients are currently receiving only the 60-mg dosage. All episodes of PCP were mild; these were most frequent with the 30-mg aerosolized dose (five episodes), compared with the 45-mg dose (two episodes) and the 60-mg dose (one episode). No adverse effects of aerosolized pentamidine were observed.[104]

Further evaluation is clearly essential to ascertain the most appropriate particle size, delivery method (nebulizer, baffling, gas pressure), total dose, and efficiency of nebulizer. However, from available data, it appears that aerosolized pentamidine may be of benefit in the prophylaxis of PCP in AIDS patients. It is now firmly established that prophylaxis is recommended in any patient at high risk for the development of PCP.[86,106] Although immunosuppressed patients without AIDS will benefit from prophylaxis with TMP–SMX administered either daily or three times weekly, the toxicity profile of pentamidine must be considered before it is used for prophylaxis in the AIDS population.[31,34,78,79,89] Similarly, pentamidine administered intravenously or intramuscularly is not without severe drug-related toxicity in any population.[78,79] Aerosolized pentamidine may have a role in the prevention of PCP and in the subsequent reduction in the duration and cost of hospitalization of AIDS patients. Further evaluation is clearly essential to determine the most appropriate dosage, dosage interval, and patients eligible for such prophylaxis.

Adverse Effects

The use of injectable pentamidine is associated with a variety of serious adverse effects in approximately 50% of treated patients (Table 3).[78] However, unlike therapy with TMP–SMX, these adverse effects do not appear to occur more frequently in AIDS patients compared with other immunosuppressed patients.[34,79] Local pain, swelling, and sterile abscess formation occur at the site of intramuscular injection in approximately 18% of patients.[78] Sterile abscess formation may be an immunologic and inflammatory response to the interaction between pentamidine and nucleic acids.[107] Several immediate reactions may occur in patients receiving intravenous pentamidine, the most frequent of which is hypotension.[67] Although originally associated with the intravenous route alone, severe hypotension may develop after either intramuscular or intravenous administration. It is now believed that the previously observed increased risk of hypotension with intravenous administration was associated with a rapid rate of infusion and that infusion of the drug over a minimum period of 60 minutes reduces the risk.[78,108,109] Less common immediate reactions include tachycardia, nausea and vomiting, facial flushing, hallucinations, unpleasant taste, and syncopal episodes.[19,78,79,110–112]

Hypoglycemia is a frequently reported dose-dependent adverse effect, with an incidence ranging from 6% to 40%.[35,78–80,113–116] Symptoms caused by inappropriately high insulin levels may be observed as early as two hours after an injection,[113] although the greatest depression of serum glucose is typically present after one week of therapy.[117] The severity and duration of hypoglycemia can extend beyond the initial occurrence and continue for several days after cessation of therapy.[117] It appears that the depression of blood glucose is due to a direct cytotoxic action of the drug on the β islet cells of the pancreas. Reports of the development of diabetes mellitus after pentamidine-induced hypoglycemia presumably resulting from a lack of insulin release after β-cell destruction by pentamidine further support this theory.[115,116,118–120] Additionally, several cases of pentamidine-associated pancreatitis have been observed.[121–123]

The most commonly reported systemic adverse effect of therapy is nephrotoxicity, which is observed in approximately 25% of treated patients.[79,80,124] This can occur in patients with no pre-existing renal disease or other possible causes of azotemia such as concurrent administration of nephrotoxic agents.[79] However, the results of one study suggest that volume depletion may have an

Table 3.
Toxicity Profile of Pentamidine

Adverse Effect	Incidence (%)	Reference[a]
Local pain or sterile-abscess formation at i.m. injection site	6–75	78–80, 107, 108
Skin rash or thrombophlebitis	1–2	79, 108
Nephrotoxicity	23–25	52, 79, 80, 107, 124–126
Hypoglycemia	6–40	35, 78–80, 99, 113–115, 117, 120
Hyperglycemia or diabetes mellitus	4–5	44, 115, 116, 118–119
Hypotension	9–10	35, 79, 108, 111
Neutropenia	14–15	74, 78, 79, 110, 111, 113
Thrombocytopenia	4	79, 112
Anemia	4	79
Abnormal liver enzymes	9–11	79
Hypocalcemia	1–2	79

[a] Adverse effects after i.v. or i.m. administration only.

important role in the incidence of nephrotoxicity occurring with pentamidine. Although it is usually mild and reversible, severe renal impairment leading to death has occurred.[23,125,126] The mechanism of renal toxicity is presumed to be related to the concentration of pentamidine in the kidneys, its binding with nucleic acids and depletion of the nucleotide pool essential for energy-dependent functions, and the subsequent production of insoluble precipitates.[107]

Hematologic adverse effects—especially leukopenia and neutropenia, anemia, and thrombocytopenia—have been noted.[74,78,98,111-113,125] The Centers for Disease Control (CDC) reported leukopenia in 14.5% of patients (26 of 179), with a 50% decrease in leukocyte counts from before therapy to during or after therapy. In 12 cases, pentamidine therapy had to be discontinued.[111]

Other less frequent adverse reactions include elevated serum aminotransferase levels, thrombophlebitis, skin rashes, hypocalcemia, decreased serum folic acid levels, and drug fever.[79,108] Case reports of rare adverse effects caused by pentamidine include a fatal Herxheimer-like reaction,[127] sciatic nerve damage,[128] toxic epidermal necrolysis leading to death,[129] and subcutaneous calcification seven years after intramuscular pentamidine therapy.[130]

Although only preliminary data exist, the previously described severe systemic adverse effects have not been observed after aerosol administration of the drug.[101-104] The major adverse effects experienced by most AIDS patients receiving aerosolized pentamidine have been bronchospasm, which can be alleviated by pretreatment with a bronchodilator, and a metallic bitter taste in the mouth caused by the drug, which can be reduced by keeping a peppermint or butterscotch candy in the mouth during treatment.[131]

Administration and Dosage

The suggested dosage regimen of pentamidine isethionate for adults and children with PCP (and underlying immunosuppression other than AIDS) is 4 mg/kg/day for 14 days.[132] Patients with AIDS and PCP often suffer from frequent relapses, and a treatment period of at least 21 days is generally recommended.[88] The preferred route of administration is intravenous, although intramuscular injection into the buttock is occasionally employed. The dose of pentamidine should be diluted in 50–250 mL of 5% dextrose injection and administered over a minimum of 60 minutes.[132] According to the manufacturer, prepared solutions for infusion are stable for 24 hours at room temperature, while the drug in unreconstituted form is stable for approximately six months if it is protected from light.[132]

Historically, the dosage of pentamidine has been adjusted in patients with renal failure, since the drug is excreted primarily by the kidneys. One possibility is to extend the dosing interval in patients with impaired renal function based on the glomerular filtration rate. A dose of 4 mg/kg has been recommended, with the dose being given every 48 hours if the creatinine clearance is less than 10 mL/min, every 36 hours if the clearance is 10–50 mL/min, and every 24 hours if the clearance is greater than 50 mL/min.[133] More recently, Conte and Lin[66] suggested that neither the elimination half-life nor the trough concentration of pentamidine is altered by renal failure and that in patients with creatinine clearances of ≥35 mL/min, dosage adjustments are unnecessary. Further evaluation is needed to more clearly define the pharmacokinetics of pentamidine, particularly in patients with renal disease.

Several indicators should be monitored during therapy to assess the development of toxicity. Laboratory studies indicated by the CDC, the manufacturer, and others include complete blood and platelet counts, blood urea nitrogen, serum creatinine, blood glucose, serum aminotransferase, and serum calcium and phosphorus levels.[132,134] In addition, blood pressure should be monitored closely, and patients should be placed in the supine position while receiving the drug.

Conclusion

There is little doubt that the use of pentamidine will substantially decrease the morbidity and mortality associated with certain protozoal infections, particularly *P. carinii* pneumonia in immunocompromised hosts. In immunosuppressed patients without AIDS, TMP-SMX is equally efficacious and less toxic than pentamidine in the treatment of PCP. However, since patients with AIDS frequently experience adverse reactions to sulfa drugs, the use of pentamidine for the treatment of PCP in this population will continue to increase. Clearly, the pharmacokinetics of both aerosolized and systemically administered pentamidine need further evaluation to promote the most appropriate use of this potent and useful agent.

References

1. Yorke W. Recent work on the chemotherapy of protozoal infections. *Trans R Soc Trop Med Hyg*. 1940; 33:463–82.
2. Lourie EM. Treatment of sleeping sickness in Sierra Leone. *Ann Trop Med Parasitol*. 1942; 36:113–131.
3. Saunders GFT. Preliminary report on the treatment of sleeping sickness by 4:4′-diamidinodiphenoxypentane. *Ann Trop Med Parasitol*. 1941; 35:169–74.
4. Saunders GFT, Holden JR, Hughes MH. Second report on the treatment of trypanosomiasis by pentamidine. *Ann Trop Med Parasitol*. 1944; 38:159–68.
5. Kirk R, Sati MH. The use of certain aromatic diamidines in the treatment of kala-azar. *Ann Trop Med Parasitol*. 1940; 34:181–97.
6. Adams ARD. Studies in chemotherapy. XXVI. A case of Indian kala-azar treated with 4:4′-diamidinodiphenoxypentane. *Ann Trop Med Parasitol*. 1941; 35:53–4.

7. Ivady G, Paldy L. Treatment of *Pneumocystis carinii* pneumonia in infancy. National Cancer Institute monograph. 1976; 201-5.
8. Hughes WT, McNabb PC, Makres TD et al. Efficacy of trimethoprim and sulfamethoxazole in the prevention and treatment of *Pneumocystis carinii* pneumonitis. *Antimicrob Agents Chemother.* 1974; 5:289-93.
9. Centers for Disease Control. Update: acquired immunodeficiency syndrome—United States. *MMWR.* 1985; 34:245-8.
10. Centers for Disease Control. Update on Kaposi's sarcoma and opportunistic infection in previously healthy persons—United States. *MMWR.* 1982; 31:294-301.
11. Centers for Disease Control. Acquired immunodeficiency syndrome (AIDS) update—United States. *MMWR.* 1983; 32:309-11.
12. Hughes WT, Price RA, Kim H et al. *Pneumocystis carinii* pneumonitis in children with malignancies. *J Pediatr.* 1973; 82:404-15.
13. Vogel CL, Cohen MH, Powell RD et al. *Pneumocystis carinii* pneumonia. *Ann Intern Med.* 1968; 68:97-108.
14. Burke BA, Good RA. *Pneumocystis carinii* infection. *Medicine.* 1973; 52:23-51.
15. Meuwissen JH, Tauber I, Leeuwenberg AD et al. Parasitologic and serologic observations of infection with *Pneumocystis* in humans. *J Infect Dis.* 1977; 136:43-9.
16. Kagan IG, Normal L. The laboratory diagnosis of *Pneumocystis carinii* pneumonia. *Health Lab Sci.* 1977; 14:155-63.
17. Hughes WT. *Pneumocystis carinii* pneumonia. *N Engl J Med.* 1977; 297:1381-3.
18. Hughes WT. Treatment of *Pneumocystis carinii* pneumonitis with trimethoprim-sulfamethoxazole. *CMS J.* 1975; 112:475.
19. Anon. Pentamidine for *Pneumocystis carinii* pneumonia. *Med Lett Drugs Ther.* 1985; 27(679):6-7.
20. Kager PA, Rees PH, Manguyo FM et al. Clinical, haematological and parasitological response to treatment of visceral leishmaniasis in Kenya; a study of 64 patients. *Trop Geogr Med.* 1984; 36:21-35.
21. WHO Expert Committee on Leishmaniasis. The leishmaniasis: technical report series 701. Geneva: World Health Organization; 1984.
22. Anon. Drugs for parasitic infections. *Med Lett Drugs Ther.* 1984; 26:27-34.
23. Pearson RD, Hewlett EL. Pentamidine for the treatment of *Pneumocystis carinii* pneumonia and other protozoal diseases. *Ann Intern Med.* 1985; 103:782-6.
24. Krogstad DJ, Walzer PD. Informational material for physicians, pentamidine isethionate (lomidine). Atlanta: Centers for Disease Control; 1971.
25. Eyckmans L. Trypanosoma species (African sleeping sickness). In: Mandell GL, Douglas RG Jr, Bennett JE, eds. Principles and practice of infectious diseases. New York: John Wiley & Sons; 1985:1537-40.
26. Sterner G, Nasander L. African trypanosomiasis: a danger for tourists visiting Gambia? *Scand J Infect Dis.* 1977; 9:154-6.
27. Willett KC. African human trypanosomiasis. In: Woodruff AW, ed. Medicine in the tropics. Edinburgh: Churchill-Livingstone, 1974:75-90.
28. Sands M, Keon MA, Brown RB. Pentamidine: a review. *Rev Infect Dis.* 1985; 7:625-34.
29. Centers for Disease Control. Pentamidine methanesulfonate to be distributed by CDC. *MMWR.* 1984; 33:225-6.
30. Public Health Service. Coolfont report: a PHS plan for prevention and control of AIDS and AIDS virus. *Public Health Rep.* 1986; 101:341-8.
31. Wharton JM, Coleman DL, Wofsy CB et al. Trimethoprim-sulfamethoxazole or pentamidine for *Pneumocystis carinii* pneumonia in the acquired immunodeficiency syndrome. *Ann Intern Med.* 1986; 105:37-44.
32. Siegel SE, Wolff LJ, Bachrer RL et al. Treatment of *Pneumocystis carinii* pneumonitis. A comparative trial of sulfamethoxazole-trimethoprim v. pentamidine in pediatric patients with cancer: report from the Children's Cancer Study Group. *Am J Dis Child.* 1984; 138:1051-4.
33. Small CB, Harris CA, Friedland GH et al. The treatment of *Pneumocystis carinii* pneumonia in the acquired immunodeficiency syndrome. *Arch Intern Med.* 1985; 145:837-40.
34. Gordin FM, Simon GL, Wofsy CB et al. Adverse reactions to trimethoprim-sulfamethoxazole in patients with the acquired immunodeficiency syndrome. *Ann Intern Med.* 1984; 100:495-9.
35. Kovacs JA, Heimerz JW, Macher AM et al. *Pneumocystis carinii* pneumonia: a comparison between patients with other immunodeficiencies. *Ann Intern Med.* 1984; 100:663-71.
36. Drake S, Lampasona V, Nicks HL et al. Pentamidine isethionate in the treatment of *Pneumocystis carinii* pneumonia. *Clin Pharm.* 1985; 4:507-16.
37. Goa KL, Campoli-Richards DM. Pentamidine isethionate. A review of its antiprotozoal activity, pharmacokinetic properties, and therapeutic use in *Pneumocystis carinii* pneumonia. *Drugs.* 1987; 33:242-58.
38. Briggaman RA. The aromatic diamidines. *Int J Dermatol.* 1977; 16:155-62.
39. Heathcote R. The diamidines, their pharmacologic actions and their therapeutic uses in some tropical diseases. *J Trop Med Hyg.* 1946; 44:1-8.
40. Schoenbach EB, Greenspan EM. The pharmacology, mode of action and therapeutic potentialities of stilbamadine, pentamidine, propamidine, and other aromatic diamidines—a review. *Medicine.* 1948; 27:327-77.
41. Lourie EM, Yorke W. Studies in chemotherapy: XXI. The trypanocidal action of certain aromatic diamidines. *Ann Trop Med Parasitol.* 1939; 33:289-304.
42. King H, Lourie EM, Yorke W. Studies in chemotherapy: XIX. Further report on new trypanocidal substances. *Ann Trop Med Parasitol.* 1938; 32:177-92.
43. Centers for Disease Control. U.S.-manufactured pentamidine isethionate cleared for investigational use. *MMWR.* 1984; 33:270.
44. Murdoch JK, Keystone JS. Two forms of pentamidine. *Can Med Assoc J.* 1983; 128:508.
45. Belehu A, Naafs B. Diabetes mellitus associated with pentamidine mesylate. *Lancet.* 1982; 1:1463-4. Letter.
46. Daubney R, Hudson JR. The action of two aromatic diamidines on *Trypanosoma congolense* infections in cattle. *Ann Trop Med Parasitol.* 1941; 35:175-86.
47. Jha TK. Evaluation of diamidine compound (pentamidine isethionate) in the treatment of resistant cases of kala-azar occurring in North Bihar, India. *Trans R Soc Trop Med Hyg.* 1983; 77:167-70.
48. Farwell GE, LeGrand EK, Cobb CC. Clinical observations on *Babesia gibsoni* and *Babesia canis* infections in dogs. *J Am Vet Med Assoc.* 1982; 180:507-11.
49. Francioli PB, Kiethly JS, Jones TC et al. Response of babesiosis to pentamidine therapy. *Ann Intern Med.* 1981; 94:326-30.
50. Gale EF, Folkes JP. Actions of pentamidine on the metabolism of *Staphylococcus aureus. Biochem Biophys Acta.* 1967; 144:467-70.
51. Hughes WT. *Pneumocystis carinii* pneumonitis. *Antibiot Chemother.* 1981; 30:257-71.
52. Waalkes TP, Makalu DR. Pharmacologic aspects of pentamidine. National Cancer Institute monograph. 1976:171-6.
53. Robbins JB. *Pneumocystis carinii* pneumonitis—a review. *Pediatr Res.* 1967; 1:131-8.
54. Williamson J. Effects of trypanocides on the fine structure of target organisms. *Pharmacol Ther.* 1979; 7:445-512.
55. Waring MJ. The effects of antimicrobial agents on ribonucleic acid polymerase. *Mol Pharmacol.* 1965; 1:1-13.
56. Wallis OC. The effect of pentamidine on ribosomes of the parasitic flagellate *Crithidia* (*Strigomonas*) *oncopelti. J Protozool.* 1966; 13:234-9.

57. Gutteridge WE. Some effects of pentamidine di-isethionate on *Crithidia fasiculata*. *J Protozool*. 1969; 16:306–11.
58. Bornstein RS, Yarbro JW. An evaluation of the mechanism of action of pentamidine isethionate. *J Surg Oncol*. 1970; 2:393–8.
59. Hill GC, Hutner SH. Effect of trypanocidal drugs on terminal respiration of *Crithidia fasiculata*. *Exp Parasitol*. 1968; 22:207–12.
60. Lourie EM, Yorke W. The action of certain aromatic diamidines on *Babesia canis* infections in puppies. *Ann Trop Med Parasitol*. 1939; 33:305–12.
61. Waalkes TP, Denham C, DeVita VT. Pentamidine: clinical pharmacologic correlations in man and mice. *Clin Pharmacol Ther*. 1970; 11:505–12.
62. Bernard EM, Maher M, Donnelly H. Use of a new bioassay to study pentamidine pharmacokinetics. *J Infect Dis*. 1985; 152:750–4.
63. Otterness IG, Torchia AJ, Doshan HD. Complement inhibition by amidines and guanidines—in vivo and in vitro results. *Biochem Pharmacol*. 1978; 27:1873–8.
64. Waldman RH, Pearce DE, Martin RA. Pentamidine isethionate in lung, liver and kidneys of rats after aerosol or intramuscular administration. *Am Rev Respir Dis*. 1973; 108:1004–6.
65. Debs RJ, Straubinger RM, Brunette EN et al. Selective enhancement of pentamidine uptake in the lung by aerosolization and delivery in liposomes. *Am Rev Respir Dis*. 1987; 135:731–7.
66. Conte JE, Lin ET. Pentamidine pharmacokinetics in AIDS patients with impaired renal function. Presented at the 27th Interscience Conference on Antimicrobial Agents and Chemotherapy. New York, NY: 1987 Oct 6.
67. Conte JE, Upton RA, Phelps RT et al. Use of a specific and sensitive assay to determine pentamidine pharmacokinetics in patients with AIDS. *J Infect Dis*. 1986; 154:923–9.
68. Redman JC. *Pneumocystis carinii* in an adopted Vietnamese infant. *JAMA*. 1974; 230:1561–3.
69. Dutz W, Post C, Jennings-Khodadad E et al. Therapy and prophylaxis of *Pneumocystis carinii* pneumonia. National Cancer Institute monograph. 1976:179–84.
70. Marshall WC, Weston HF, Bodian M. *Pneumocystis carinii* pneumonia and congenital hypogammaglobuminemia. *Arch Dis Child*. 1964; 39:18–25.
71. Robbins JB, Miller RH, Arean VM et al. Successful treatment of *Pneumocystis carinii* pneumonitis in a patient with congenital hypogammaglobulinemia. *N Engl J Med*. 1965; 272:708–13.
72. Rodgers TS, Haggie MHK. *Pneumocystis carinii* pneumonia associated with hypogammaglobulinemia responding to pentamidine. *Lancet*. 1964; 1:1042. Letter.
73. Patterson JH, Lindsey IL, Edwards ES et al. *Pneumocystis carinii* pneumonia and altered host resistance: treatment of one patient with pentamidine isethionate. *Pediatrics*. 1966; 38:388–97.
74. Smith E, Gasper IA. Pentamidine treatment of *Pneumocystis carinii* pneumonitis in an adult with lymphatic leukemia. *Am J Med*. 1968; 44:626–31.
75. Einzig S, Hong R, Sharp HL. Successful treatment of *Pneumocystis carinii* in an immunologically deficient acute lymphatic leukemia patient. *Cancer*. 1969; 23:658–62.
76. Cohen ML, Weiss EB, Monaco AP. Successful treatment of *Pneumocystis carinii* and *Nocardia asteroides* in a renal transplant patient. *Am J Med*. 1971; 50:269–76.
77. DeVita VT, Emmer M, Levine A et al. *Pneumocystis carinii* pneumonia. *N Engl J Med*. 1969; 280:287–91.
78. Western KA, Perera DR, Schultz MG. Pentamidine isethionate in the treatment of *Pneumocystis carinii* pneumonia. *Ann Intern Med*. 1970; 73:695–702.
79. Walzer PD, Perl DP, Krogstadt DJ et al. *Pneumocystis carinii* pneumonia in the United States. Epidemiologic, diagnostic and clinical features. *Ann Intern Med*. 1974; 80:83–93.
80. Hughes WT, Fedman S, Chaudhary SC et al. Comparison of pentamidine isethionate and trimethoprim–sulfamethoxazole in the treatment of *Pneumocystis carinii* pneumonia. *J Pediatr*. 1978; 92:285–291.
81. Goodell B, Jacobs B, Powell RD et al. *Pneumocystis carinii:* the spectrum of diffuse interstitial pneumonia in patients with neoplastic disease. *Ann Intern Med*. 1970; 72:337–40.
82. Rosen PP, Martin N, Armstrong D. *Pneumocystis carinii* pneumonia (PCP): diagnoses by lung biopsy. *Am J Med*. 1975; 58:794–802.
83. Johnson HD, Johnson WW. *Pneumocystis carinii* pneumonia in children with cancer. Diagnosis and treatment. *JAMA*. 1970; 214:1067–73.
84. Geelhoed GW, Hubbard SB, Powell RD et al. Clinical characteristics of *Pneumocystis carinii* pneumonia. *Am Surg*. 1979; 45:293–304.
85. Gentry LO, Ruskin J, Remington JS. *Pneumocystis carinii* pneumonia. Problems in diagnoses and therapy in 24 cases. *Calif Med*. 1972; 116:6–14.
86. Hughes WT, Kim HK, Price RA et al. Attempts of prophylaxis for murine *Pneumocystis carinii* pneumonitis. *Curr Ther Res*. 1973; 15:581–7.
87. Young LS. Trimethoprim-sulfamethoxazole in the treatment of adults with pneumonia due to *Pneumocystis carinii*. *Rev Infect Dis*. 1982; 4:608–13.
88. Haverkos HW. PCP Therapy Project Group: assessment of therapy for *Pneumocystis carinii* pneumonia. *Am J Med*. 1984; 76:501–8.
89. Hughes WT, Rivera GK, Schnell MJ et al. Successful intermittent chemoprophylaxis for *Pneumocystis carinii* pneumonia. *N Engl J Med*. 1987; 316:1627–32.
90. Engelberg LA, Lerner CW, Tapper ML. Clinical features of *Pneumocystis pneumonia* in the acquired immune deficiency syndrome. *Am Rev Respir Dis*. 1984; 130:689–94.
91. Jaffe HS, Abrams DI, Ammann AJ et al. Complications of co-trimoxazole in treatment of AIDS-associated *Pneumocystis carinii* pneumonia in homosexual men. *Lancet*. 1983; 2:1109–11.
92. Mitsuyasu R, Groopman J, Volberding P. Cutaneous reactions to trimethoprim-sulfamethoxazole in patients with AIDS and Kaposi's sarcoma. *N Engl J Med*. 1983; 308:1535.
93. Murray JF, Felton CP, Garay SM et al. Pulmonary complications of the acquired immunodeficiency syndrome. *N Engl J Med*. 1984; 310:1682–8.
94. Dennis T. Trimethoprim-sulfamethoxazole or pentamidine for *Pneumocystis pneumonia* in the acquired immunodeficiency syndrome. *Ann Intern Med*. 1986; 105:629–30. Letter.
95. Marantz PR. Trimethoprim-sulfamethoxazole or pentamidine for *Pneumocystis pneumonia* in the acquired immunodeficiency syndrome. *Ann Intern Med*. 1986; 105:630. Letter.
96. Begin P, Hanley J. Trimethoprim-sulfamethoxazole or pentamidine for *Pneumocystis carinii* pneumonia. *Ann Intern Med*. 1987; 106:474. Letter.
97. Polis MA, Blackwelder WC. Trimethoprim-sulfamethoxazole or pentamidine for *Pneumocystis carinii* pneumonia. *Ann Intern Med*. 1987; 106:475. Letter.
98. Ervan JK. Trimethoprim sulfamethoxazole or pentamidine for *Pneumocystis carinii* pneumonia. *Ann Intern Med*. 1987; 106:475. Letter.
99. Young RC, DeVita VT. Treatment of *Pneumocystis carinii* pneumonia: current status of the regimens of pentamidine isethionate and pyrimethamine-sulfadiazine. National Cancer Institute monograph. 1976: 193–8.
100. Kluge RM, Spaulding DM, Spain AJ. Combination of pentamidine and trimethoprim-sulfamethoxazole in the therapy of *Pneumocystis carinii* pneumonia in rats. *Antimicrob Agents Chemother*. 1978; 13:975–8.
101. Debs RJ, Blemenfeld W, Brunette EN et al. Successful treatment with aerosolized pentamidine for *Pneumocystis carinii* pneumonia in rats. *Antimicrob Agents Chemother*. 1987; 31:37–41.
102. Montgomery AB, Debs RC, Luce JM et al. Concentration of pentamidine in broncheoalveolar lavage fluid after aero-

sol and intravenous administration. *Am Rev Respir Dis.* 1987; 135:A167.
103. Conte JE, Hollander H, Golden JA. Inhaled or reduced-dose intravenous pentamidine for *Pneumocystis carinii* pneumonia: a pilot study. *Ann Intern Med.* 1987; 107:495–8.
104. Bernard E, Schmitt H, Pagel L et al. Safety and effectiveness of aerosol pentamidine for the prevention of PCP in patients with AIDS. Presented at the 27th Interscience Conference on Antimicrobial Agents and Chemotherapy. New York, NY: 1987 Oct 6.
105. Montgomery AB, Debs RJ, Luce JM et al. Aerosolized pentamidine as sole therapy for *Pneumocystis carinii* pneumonia in patients with the acquired immunodeficiency syndrome. *Lancet.* 1987; 2:480–3.
106. Hughes WT. *Pneumocystis carinii* pneumonitis. *N Engl J Med.* 1987; 317:1021–3.
107. Makalu DR, Walkes TP. Interaction between aromatic diamidines and nucleic acids: possible implications for chemotherapy. *J Natl Cancer Inst.* 1975; 54:305–9.
108. Navin TR, Fontaine RE. Intravenous versus intramuscular administration of pentamidine. *N Engl J Med.* 1984; 311:1701–2.
109. Helmick CG, Green JK. Pentamidine associated hypotension and route of administration. *Ann Intern Med.* 1985; 103:480.
110. Mallory DL, Parrillo JE, Bailey KR et al. Cardiovascular effects and safety of intravenous and intramuscular pentamidine isethionate. *Crit Care Med.* 1987; 15:503–5.
111. Centers for Disease Control. Severe neutropenia during pentamidine treatment of *Pneumocystis carinii* pneumonia in patients with acquired immunodeficiency syndrome—New York City. *MMWR.* 1984; 33:65–7.
112. Levy MA, Senior RM, Sneider RE. Severe thrombocytopenic purpura complicating pentamidine therapy for *Pneumocystis carinii* pneumonia. *Cancer.* 1974; 34:441–3.
113. Milder JE, Walzer PD, Powell RD Jr. Treatment of *Pneumocystis carinii* pneumonia with trimethoprim-sulfamethoxazole and pentamidine: efficacy and toxicity. *South Med J.* 1979; 72:1626–8.
114. Murdoch JK, Keystone JS. Pentamidine and hypoglycemia. *Ann Intern Med.* 1983; 99:879. Letter.
115. Bouchard PH, Sai P, Reach G et al. Diabetes mellitus following pentamidine-induced hypoglycemia in humans. *Diabetes.* 1982; 31:40–5.
116. Bryceson A. Pentamidine-induced diabetes mellitus. *East Afr Med J.* 1968; 45:110–7.
117. Stahl-Bayliss CM, Kalman CM, Laskin OL. Pentamidine-induced hypoglycemia in patients with the acquired immune deficiency syndrome. *Clin Pharmacol Ther.* 1986; 39:271–5.
118. Jha TK, Sharma VK. Pentamidine-induced diabetes mellitus. *Trans R Soc Trop Med Hyg.* 1984; 78:252–3.
119. Osei K, Falko JM, Nelson KP et al. Diabetogenic effects of pentamidine. In vitro and in vivo studies in a patient with malignant insulinoma. *Am J Med.* 1984; 77:41–6.
120. Yurdakok M. Diabetogenic effect of pentamidine. *JAMA.* 1987; 257:1177. Letter.
121. Murphey SA, Josephs AS. Acute pancreatitis associated with pentamidine therapy. *Arch Intern Med.* 1981; 141:56–8.
122. Zuger A, Wolf BZ, El-Sadr W et al. Pentamidine associated fatal acute pancreatitis. *JAMA.* 1986; 256:2383–5.
123. Salmeron S, Petitpretz P, Katlama C et al. Pentamidine and pancreatitis. *Ann Intern Med.* 1986; 105:140–1.
124. Stehr-Green JK, Helmick CG. Pentamidine and renal toxicity. *N Engl J Med.* 1985; 313:694–5.
125. Sensakovec JW, Suarez M, Perez G et al. Pentamidine treatment of *Pneumocystis carinii* pneumonia in the acquired immunodeficiency syndrome. Association with acute renal failure and myoglobinuria. *Arch Intern Med.* 1985; 145:2247.
126. Shuster M, Dunn M. Pentamidine and hematuria. *Ann Intern Med.* 1985; 105:146. Letter.
127. Stark FR, Crast F, Clemmer T et al. Fatal Herxheimer reaction after pentamidine in *Pneumocystis* pneumonia. *Lancet.* 1976; 1:1193. Letter.
128. Gutschi LM, Chandrasekar PH. Sciatic nerve damage associated with pentamidine. *Drug Intell Clin Pharm.* 1985; 19:762. Letter.
129. Want JJ, Freeman I, Gaeta JF et al. Unusual complications of pentamidine in the treatment of *Pneumocystis carinii* pneumonia. *J Pediatr.* 1970; 77:311–4.
130. Bellamy EA, Meller S, Westbury G et al. CT demonstration of calcified subcutaneous masses following parenteral pentamidine isethionate injection. *J Comp Assist Tomog.* 1985; 9:210–1.
131. Melamed AJ. The use of inhaled pentamidine for the prevention and treatment of *Pneumocystis carinii* pneumonia in AIDS patients. *Hosp Pharm.* 1988; 23:65–6.
132. LyphoMed Inc. Pentam 300 product literature. Melrose Park, IL:1984.
133. Bennett WM, Muther RS, Parker RA et al. Drug therapy in renal failure: dosing guidelines for adults. *Ann Intern Med.* 1980; 92:62–89.
134. Anderson RA, Boedicker M, Ma M et al. Adverse reactions associated with pentamidine isethionate in AIDS patients: recommendations for monitoring therapy. *Drug Intell Clin Pharm.* 1986; 20:862–8.

“

Reassessment of Interferon

Interferon has become the paradigm for the development of lymphokines and other protein products. Many of the molecular biologists who originally worked on interferon applied the technology used to develop that molecule to the development of others, such as interleukin-2, tumor necrosis factor, tissue plasminogen activator, growth hormone, and the colony-stimulating factors. In addition, clinical investigators can profit from insights gained with the use of interferon as an antitumor or antiviral agent. . . .

. . . [I]nterferon, both as a host-defense agent and a regulatory agent for normal cells, continues to intrigue basic-science and clinical investigators. Truly, it has given rise to as many new questions after its cloning as before.

—Merigan TC. Human interferon as a therapeutic agent. *N Engl J Med.* 1988; 318:1458–60.

”

Editorials

Infectious complications of AIDS

Infectious complications are the leading cause of death in AIDS patients.[1] Results from the first zidovudine trials revealed that recurrent opportunistic infections are not completely prevented by the best currently available treatment of human immunodeficiency virus (HIV) infection.[2] Therefore, until more effective therapies or a vaccine directed against HIV are developed, we will continue to be faced with AIDS patients who have a multiplicity of infectious diseases. It is not unusual to see patients in the terminal stages of their illness who are dying of disseminated infection caused by *Mycobacterium avium–intracellulare* as well as cryptococcal meningitis or encephalitis caused by *Toxoplasma gondii*. Such patients have chronically suffered from recurrent or persistent diarrhea caused by *Isospora belli* or *Cryptosporidium* and stomatitis caused by *Candida albicans*. Other opportunistic infections in these individuals include tuberculosis, histoplasmosis, cytomegalovirus retinitis or gastroenteritis, and severe localized outbreaks of herpes simplex or varicella zoster, to name just a few. All of these pathogens are usually controlled by an intact cellular immune system, which is deficient in patients with AIDS. This deficiency, which is almost complete, allows these individuals to be ravaged by infections seldom seen except in severely immunosuppressed individuals.

The papers in this issue of *Clinical Pharmacy* reflect the prevalence of the disease and its impact on health care in this country. They also reflect the futility experienced by health-care practitioners who try to manage the opportunistic infections of AIDS patients.

As we are developing vaccines and antiviral agents for the prevention and treatment of HIV infection, so are we exploring new ways to treat the infectious complications. Because cryptococcal meningitis is so prevalent and often inadequately treated with the conventional regimen of amphotericin B alone or combined with flucytosine, a great deal of effort is being directed to the development of more effective antifungal agents.[3] Fluconazole appears to be especially promising in this regard, principally because of excellent cerebrospinal-fluid penetration and good activity in experimental cryptococcal infection. Preliminary clinical trials are encouraging. A related triazole antifungal agent, itraconazole, is potentially valuable for other deep-seated mycoses such as histoplasmosis and coccidioidomycosis, both of which affect AIDS patients.[4]

One of the most frustrating diseases to manage is infection caused by *Mycobacterium avium* complex (MAC). Even in patients without AIDS, pulmonary or disseminated MAC infection is extraordinarily difficult to treat because of multidrug resistance and drug toxicity. Recommended therapy involves the concurrent use of four or five antimycobacterial agents and often includes several of the so-called second-line drugs that are inherently more toxic. In patients with AIDS, drug toxicity often limits antimycobacterial treatment and little benefit is demonstrable.[5] The recent availability of the antileprosy drug clofazimine appears to have contributed little, and rifabutin, a more potent analogue of rifampin, has not been found exceptionally effective either. Ciprofloxacin and newer fluoroquinolone analogues have activity against some MAC isolates.[5] Combinations such as a quinolone, rifabutin, clofazimine, and other active drugs such as imipenem and amikacin may offer some hope. Currently, the treatment of MAC infection remains inadequate.

One of the most prevalent infections in AIDS patients is *Pneumocystis carinii* pneumonia (PCP). Although the combination of trimethoprim–sulfamethoxazole (TMP–SMX) traditionally has been considered the therapy of choice, some authorities recommend the use of pentamidine as primary treatment. All of the available evidence from carefully performed, comparative trials in patients with and without AIDS suggests equivalence of these two forms of treatment.[6] Although adverse reactions are more common with TMP–SMX in patients with AIDS, toxic reactions to pentamidine often are more severe. For now, TMP–SMX should be used as initial therapy for first episodes of PCP.

Other agents that are either more effective or less toxic would be highly desirable. Eflornithine (DFMO) has undergone only limited testing, much of it uncontrolled, yet is recommended as an alternative by some authorities. Our local experience with the drug has not been as promising as originally described, and adverse effects

Copyright © 1988, American Society of Hospital Pharmacists, Inc. All rights reserved. 0278-2677/88/0701-0511$00.50.

have been frequent. Dapsone has been shown effective only in relatively healthy AIDS patients, and adverse effects have occurred in nearly all patients. Finally, trimetrexate and piritrexim have generated a great deal of interest, since the results from preliminary trials in humans and in animals have been promising. Trimetrexate, given with leucovorin "rescue," has produced cure rates comparable to those observed with TMP-SMX or pentamidine and has been well tolerated.

Prevention of PCP is also difficult because many patients cannot tolerate the sulfamethoxazole in TMP-SMX and sulfadoxine-pyrimethamine has been associated with a relatively high incidence of severe reactions such as Stevens-Johnson syndrome. The most interesting new method of managing and preventing PCP is the use of aerosolized pentamidine. As described by Salamone and Cunha,[7] this method of drug administration is theoretically optimal for delivering high concentrations of pentamidine to the alveoli. A key factor is the use of a device that can produce the correct particle size (0.5–2.0 μm). Notably, there is apparently only one commercially available "inline" nebulizer for treating patients who require mechanical ventilation. Despite only limited data demonstrating efficacy, the use of aerosolized pentamidine is widespread in many urban centers where AIDS is prevalent. This procedure is often performed in physicians' offices, and it is unclear whether all of the nebulizers being used are capable of producing the correct particle size, whether the dosage being given is too large or too small, and whether the frequency of dosing is appropriate. Controlled investigations to answer these questions are under way.

Infectious complications of AIDS continue to haunt us and daunt our efforts at controlling them.

1. Gold JWM, Armstrong D. Infectious complications of the acquired immunodeficiency syndrome. *Ann NY Acad Sci.* 1987; 437:383–93.
2. Hirsch M. Azidothymidine. *J Infect Dis.* 1988; 157:427–31.
3. Dismukes WE. Cryptococcal meningitis in patients with AIDS. *J Infect Dis.* 1988; 157:624–8.
4. Saag MS, Dismukes WE. Azole antifungal agents: emphasis on new triazoles. *Antimicrob Agents Chemother.* 1988; 32:1–8.
5. Young LS, Inderlied CB, Berlin OG et al. Mycobacterial infections in AIDS patients, with an emphasis on the *Mycobacterium avium* complex. *Rev Infect Dis.* 1986; 8:1024–33.
6. Wofsy CB. Use of trimethoprim-sulfamethoxazole in the treatment of *Pneumocystis carinii* pneumonia in patients with AIDS. *Rev Infect Dis.* 1987; 9(Suppl 2):S184–S193.
7. Salamone FR, Cunha BA. Update on pentamidine for the treatment of *Pneumocystis carinii* pneumonia. *Clin Pharm.* 1988; 7:501–10.

Steven L. Barriere, Pharm.D.
UCLA Medical Center
Los Angeles, CA 90024

What is the role of parenteral nutrition in AIDS?

The constellation of severe weight loss, diarrhea, and fever has been referred to as "Slim Disease" in Africa, and the World Health Organization considers these to be major clinical signs of acquired immunodeficiency syndrome (AIDS).[1] In developed countries as well, many patients with AIDS are underweight and have a decrease in body-cell mass and decreased serum concentrations of retinol-binding protein and albumin.[2] Zinc and selenium deficiencies have been found in AIDS patients, and deficiencies of other elements probably will be found.

The weight loss, diarrhea, lymphopenia, lack of response to common skin-test antigens, decreased levels of serum proteins, and subnormal anthropometric measurements in AIDS patients are likely to be picked up in routine nutritional screening. Clinicians' usual inclination would be toward the use of nutritional support to reverse these abnormalities. But can it? Although many of the objective signs of malnutrition seen in the AIDS patient are similar to those of protein-energy malnutrition (PEM), there are major differences in causation and response to feeding.

PEM is associated with a decrease in total lymphocytes, a lack of differentiation of pre-T lymphocytes, and a decrease in T4 cells. Refeeding patients who have PEM will reverse these lymphocyte abnormalities and the anergy to common skin-test antigens. However, in the AIDS patient these immunologic deficits are not reversed by nutritional intervention because the human immunodeficiency virus destroys the T4 lymphocytes and they are not repopulated. PEM is also associated with an increased incidence of infections, primarily bacterial bronchopneumonia and pulmonary tuberculosis, that are correctable by refeeding.[3] The opportunistic infections seen in AIDS are not seen even in the most severely malnourished patients unless the patients also have an underlying immunosuppressive disease such as cancer. There is no evidence that improving the nutritional status of the AIDS patient influences the occurence or severity of opportunistic infections. PEM is usually, although slowly, correctable by intensive feeding. Even during periods when AIDS patients are clinically stable, it is difficult to replete body cell mass and the malnourished state persists or progresses.[2]

Considering the lack of response to nutritional support in the AIDS patient and the complications and costs associated with total parenteral nutrition (TPN), is TPN ever indicated in patients with AIDS?

Key points to remember are that AIDS is always a rapidly fatal disease and that the only chance for cure hinges on effective antiretroviral drugs combined with reconstitution of the immune system. The available antiviral drugs are toxic and marginally effective, and all attempts at reconstituting the immune system have failed. The diagnosis of AIDS can also have devastating effects on patients' mental status; patients with AIDS were found to have a suicide risk 36 times that of men without this diagnosis.[4] Many patients also suffer neurological dysfunction (AIDS encephalopathy) that results

Copyright © 1988, American Society of Hospital Pharmacists, Inc. All rights reserved. 0278-2677/88/0701-0512$00.50.

in progressive cognitive, motor, and behavioral abnormalities, not unlike Alzheimer's disease.

In the face of an incurable disease, it is desirable to consider the costs to our health-care system of using TPN in large numbers of these patients. For both patients and third-party payers, AIDS is a very expensive disease to treat. Zidovudine is estimated to cost patients $8,000 to $10,000 per year, while treatments for each episode of an opportunistic infection cost at least that much. It is natural to want to do everything possible for young, terminally ill patients, but we need to sort out our feelings about the age of the patient and our psychological contiguity between feeding and love and concern. Patients should be fully informed regarding their disease and prognosis and the lack of proven benefit in giving them TPN; they should not be coerced into accepting TPN for purely cosmetic reasons. To maintain the idea that patients should be subjected to this futile sort of intervention because they have a negative nitrogen balance or decreased serum proteins is to lose sight of what medical care is all about.[5] Even if it were possible to improve the nutritional status of AIDS patients, it is unlikely that mortality would be affected. Fortunately, the courts are beginning to recognize the patient's right to refuse artificial feeding, and this is often the road taken by patients with AIDS.[6]

I propose that pharmacists working with AIDS patients adopt a sensible approach regarding TPN. The patient should be fully informed of the risks and costs of TPN and the probable futility of its use. However, when TPN is being used for a clearly defined purpose and for a specified period of time, its use should be encouraged. This would include perioperative TPN or TPN while a patient is undergoing radiation treatment that would make the gut unusable. After the gut again becomes usable, the urge to needlessly continue TPN because of a poor nutritional assessment or because the patient has diarrhea with enteral intake should be discouraged. TPN might also be used as part of a clearly defined study involving potentially curative therapy; however, this is unlikely in the near future. As the number of AIDS patients increases and the number of health-care dollars shrinks, both patients and providers will benefit from the judicious use of expensive and futile therapies.

1. Serwadda D, Mugerwa RD, Sewankambo NK et al. Slim disease: a new disease in Uganda and its association with HTLV-III infection. *Lancet*. 1985; 2:849–52.
2. Kotler DP, Wang J, Pierson RN. Body composition studies in patients with the acquired immunodeficiency syndrome. *Am J Clin Nutr*. 1985; 42:1255–65.
3. Helweg-Larsen P, Hoffmeyer H, Kieler J et al. Famine disease in German concentration camps: complications and sequels. *Acta Psychiatr Neurol Scand*. 1952; 27(Suppl 83):11–460.
4. Marzuk PM, Tierney H, Tardiff K et al. Increased risk of suicide in persons with AIDS. *JAMA*. 1988; 259:1333–7.
5. Lynn J, Childress JF. Must patients always be given food and water? *Hastings Cent Rep*. 1983; 13(5):17–21.
6. Steinbrook R, Lo B. Artificial feeding—solid ground, not a slippery slope. *N Engl J Med*. 1988; 318:286–90.

Alan W. Hopefl, Pharm.D.
St. Louis College of Pharmacy
St. Louis, MO 63110

“

Tumor Necrosis Factor

Is there a role for tumour necrosis factor in treating cancer? So far trials of recombinant tumour necrosis factor given systemically to patients with various types of cancer have yielded low response rates (less than 5%). Higher rates of remission (up to 40%) have, however, been reported after direct injection into the tumour. No deaths have occurred as a result of giving the factor, the most common side effects being fever, hypotension, headache, and occasional disturbances in the central nervous system. More effective regimens will probably exploit the known synergy between tumour necrosis factor and other cytokines such as interferon gamma and interleukin 2.

—Malik S, Balkwill FR. Tumour necrosis factor. *Br Med J*. 1988; 296:1214. Editorial.

”

Grand Rounds

Treatment of *Pneumocystis carinii* pneumonia in patients with AIDS

CINDY J. WORDELL AND STEPHEN P. HAUPTMAN

Abstract: A 44-year-old man with acquired immunodeficiency syndrome (AIDS) and *Pneumocystis carinii* pneumonia (PCP) who suffered adverse effects from treatment with trimethoprim–sulfamethoxazole (TMP–SMX) and was then treated with pentamidine isethionate is described, and approved and investigational drugs used in the management of PCP in the AIDS patient are discussed.

After taking TMP–SMX, 240 mg trimethoprim and 1200 mg sulfamethoxazole, four times a day orally for 10 days at home, the patient was hospitalized complaining of nausea, vomiting, diarrhea, and fever. Intravenous TMP–SMX was begun at a dosage of 18 mg/kg/day of trimethoprim. Four days later, his condition had deteriorated and he had elevations of liver enzymes and a decrease in white blood cell (WBC) count. TMP–SMX was discontinued and pentamidine isethionate was started at a dosage of 4 mg/kg/day i.v. His symptoms and fever subsided and his liver enzyme levels and WBC count improved. After nine days of pentamidine his WBC count decreased; pentamidine was suspected as the cause and discontinued; no further therapy was needed.

PCP was the initial infection that established this patient's diagnosis of AIDS. The patient did not have exertional dyspnea and nonproductive cough, which are usually seen in AIDS patients with PCP. TMP–SMX 20 mg/kg/day, based on the trimethoprim content, is the usual initial treatment for PCP. Adverse effects of TMP–SMX develop more frequently in AIDS patients than in non-AIDS patients with PCP. The recommended dose of pentamidine isethionate for the treatment of PCP is 4 mg/kg/day, im. or i.v. A few studies have shown good response to aerosolized pentamidine. Trials of investigational agents have excluded patients with severely compromised respiratory status; eflornithine, dapsone in combination with trimethoprim, and trimetrexate have been used. Corticosteroids should be considered a last effort until additional data are available. TMP–SMX may be used to prevent recurrence of PCP or to prevent the initial occurrence of PCP in AIDS patients. Intravenous or aerosol doses of pentamidine may be effective as prophylaxis. Sulfadoxine–pyrimethamine tried as prophylaxis produced adverse reactions.

Despite its higher incidence of serious adverse effects in the AIDS population, TMP–SMX is considered preferable to pentamidine for initial therapy. Pentamidine is preferred for patients with documented allergy to TMP–SMX or failure to respond to a five- to seven-day course of TMP–SMX.

Index terms: Acquired immunodeficiency syndrome; Anti-infective agents; Combined therapy; Dapsone; Eflornithine; Pentamidine isethionate; Pneumonia; Sulfamethoxazole; Sulfonamides; Sulfones; Toxicity; Trimethoprim
Clin Pharm. 1988; 7:514–27

The acquired immunodeficiency syndrome (AIDS) was first identified in 1981, and its incidence has increased since that time.[1–7] The surveillance definition established by the Centers for Disease Control (CDC) has been modified several times to reflect increasing knowledge about this disease.[4–7] Defects in both the T-cell (cellular) and B-cell (humoral) arms of the immune system have

CINDY J. WORDELL, PHARM.D., is Drug Information Supervisor, Drug Information and Research Division, Department of Pharmacy, and STEPHEN P. HAUPTMAN, D.O., is Professor of Medicine, Department of Medicine, and Director of the Tissue Typing and Clinical Immunology Laboratory, Thomas Jefferson University Hospital, Philadelphia, PA.

Address reprint requests to Dr. Wordell at the Department of Pharmacy, Thomas Jefferson University Hospital, 111 South 11th Street, Philadelphia, PA 19107.

Presented in part at the 22nd Annual ASHP Midyear Clinical Meeting, Atlanta, GA, December 9, 1987.

This is **article 680-204-8811** in the **ASHP Continuing Education System**; it qualifies for 1.0 hour of continuing education credit. See page 552 for learning objectives and test questions.

Copyright © 1988, American Society of Hospital Pharmacists, Inc. All rights reserved. 0278-2677/88/0701-0514$03.50.

been associated with AIDS.[8-9] Patients with AIDS, because of their immune deficiency, are susceptible to multiple opportunistic infections; these are associated with defects in both cellular and humoral immunity.[10-11]

Protozoal infections are frequently encountered in patients with AIDS. In particular, infection with *Pneumocystis carinii* occurs in approximately 80% of patients with AIDS at some time during their course of the disease; *Pneumocystis carinii* pneumonia (PCP) establishes the diagnosis of AIDS in approximately 60% of cases.[12-14]

In this paper, the clinical features, pathogenesis, diagnosis, and treatment of PCP in the AIDS patient are reviewed. Investigational agents that may serve as alternatives to the approved treatments for PCP are discussed in depth. A case report is presented to illustrate complications that may arise during treatment of PCP in an AIDS patient.

Papers in the Grand Rounds section are patient case reports and literature review combined in a way that gives them high educational value. The papers lead off with a well-documented case report of an unusual drug experience (e.g., adverse drug reaction or other unexpected drug response, experimental use of a drug). The case generally deals with a difficult therapeutic problem or dilemma that is commonly encountered but may be overlooked or misunderstood. (Esoteric or rare occurrences of minor importance do not make good Grand Rounds material.) A literature review puts the case in perspective with previously reported similar cases and alternative treatments. The review is integrated with related discussion of the case being reported.

CP readers are encouraged to use Grand Rounds for educational group discussions. For this purpose, discussion questions are printed at the end of Grand Rounds papers.

Case Report

A 44-year-old black man was admitted through a hospital emergency room with a history of AIDS, diagnosed one month before this admission. At the time AIDS was diagnosed, the patient's chief complaints were tiredness and recent weight loss. Outpatient workup included a chest roentgenogram that revealed bilateral infiltrates, a transbronchial biopsy with negative results, bronchoalveolar lavage that showed the presence of *P. carinii*, and a positive serum assay for antibodies to human immunodeficiency virus (HIV). The patient was started on a regimen of oral trimethoprim–sulfamethoxazole (TMP–SMX), 240 mg trimethoprim and 1200 mg sulfamethoxazole, four times a day. He was not admitted to the hospital at that time.

On the current admission he complained of nausea, vomiting, and diarrhea during the previous three days. He attributed these complaints to TMP–SMX, which he had taken for 10 days. He said his stools had become black during this time. He had stopped taking the TMP–SMX two days before admission. He also complained of temperatures at home as high as 104 °F. He denied cough, shortness of breath, sputum production, chest pain, hematemesis, hemoptysis, and hematochezia. He had noted a 20-pound weight loss during the last month.

Pertinent medical history included diagnosis of a hiatal hernia with gastroesophageal reflux one month before this admission; right-leg deep-vein thrombosis in 1980, which had been managed with warfarin; appendectomy in 1976; and a positive purified protein derivative of tuberculin (PPD) test in 1972, for which he had received prophylaxis with isoniazid for six months. His medical history did not include hepatitis or blood transfusions. His social history included homosexuality and a smoking habit of one pack per day for 32 years.

On admission his vital signs were as follows: temperature 37.4 °C orally; respirations 30/minute; blood pressure 90/50 mm Hg supine and 70/50 mm Hg sitting; pulse 104/minute supine and 132/minute sitting. He appeared cachectic and in mild distress. His admission weight was 52 kg (his usual weight was approximately 65 kg). His skin was warm and dry with no axillary sweat, poor turgor, and tenting. He had temporal wasting; mouth breathing; dry, cracked lips; dry oral mucosa; and noninjected pharynx. His lungs were clear on auscultation and percussion. Inguinal lymphadenopathy was present bilaterally. His stool was heme-negative. Nasogastric-tube aspirate had a coffee-grounds appearance; after lavage the gastric aspirate was clear fluid that initially contained flecks of blood.

Laboratory test findings on admission were within normal ranges with the following exceptions: arterial blood gas measurements (on room air) of pH 7.39, P_{O_2} 98 mm Hg, P_{CO_2} 25 mm Hg, and actual bicarbonate 15 meq/L; white blood cell (WBC) count 2200/cu mm with 66% segmented neutrophils, 15% bands, 10% lymphocytes, 4% atypical lymphocytes, 3% monocytes, and 2% eosinophils; platelet count 119,000/cu mm; serum creatinine concentration 1.7 mg/dL; urea nitrogen 29 mg/dL; prothrombin time ratio 1.21; lactate dehydrogenase (LDH) 957 IU/L; and aspartate aminotransferase (AST, also known as SGOT) 407 IU/L. Chest roentgenogram demonstrated bilateral upper-lobe infiltrates, with some improvement over the previous study.

The patient had been taking TMP–SMX (240 mg trimethoprim component) orally four times a day for 10 days. He was admitted with dehydration, probably secondary to vomiting and diarrhea induced by TMP–SMX, and worsening PCP. TMP–SMX was continued intravenously at a dose of 18 mg/kg/day (based on the trimethoprim component) in four divided doses. Other medications included ranitidine 150 mg (as the hydrochloride salt) orally twice a day, aluminum–magnesium hydroxide suspension 30 mL orally every four hours while awake, acetaminophen 650 mg as required for fever, and phytonadione 10 mg subcutaneously daily for three days. In addition, intravenous fluids were used for rehydration.

One day after admission, oral candidiasis was noted and therapy was begun with clotrimazole troches 10 mg orally five times a day. Five days into the hospitalization the patient experienced an episode of increased respiratory distress without the use of accessory muscles. On physical examination, rales at the bases of both lungs and small papules on the patient's back were noted. Arterial blood gas measurements on room air were pH 7.43, P_{O_2} 77 mm Hg, P_{CO_2} 22 mm Hg, and actual bicarbonate 14.4 meq/L. His hemoglobin had decreased with rehydration to 9.5 g/dL. A chest roentgenogram demon-

Table 1.
Liver Function Test Results[a] Correlated with Antipneumocystis Drug Therapy

Hospital Day	Drug Therapy[b]	ALP	GGTP	AST	ALT	LDH
1	TMP–SMX	59	. . .	407	. . .	957
2		125	. . .	39	. . .	852
5	TMP–SMX discontinued; pentamidine begun	. . .	. . .	. . .	. . .	. . .
6		170	. . .	410	. . .	1251
8		245	. . .	142	222	657
11		. . .	279	. . .	172	. . .
14		194	235	40	110	386
18		178	243	36	74	322
21	Pentamidine discontinued	143	214	43	69	271
3 Weeks after discharge		76	29	14	11	202

[a] ALP = Alkaline phosphatase (normal range, 25 to 95 IU/L), GGTP = γ-glutamyltransferase (normal range, 2 to 40 IU/L), AST = aspartate aminotransferase (normal range, 7 to 28 IU/L), ALT = alanine aminotransferase (normal range, 1 to 48 IU/L), LDH = lactate dehydrogenase (normal range, 70 to 186 IU/L).

[b] Throughout this admission the patient was receiving the following drugs: ranitidine 150 mg (as the hydrochloride salt) orally twice a day, aluminum–magnesium hydroxide suspension 30 mL orally every four hours while awake, acetaminophen 650 mg as needed for fever, phytonadione 10 mg subcutaneously daily for three days; clotrimazole troche 10 mg orally five times a day was begun on the second day of hospitalization.

Figure 1. White blood cell counts over 23 days. Trimethoprim–sulfamethoxazole was begun on day 1 and pentamidine on day 5.

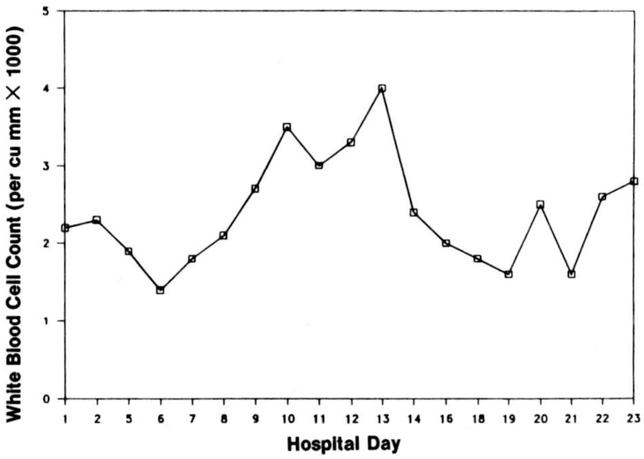

Figure 2. Patient's temperature curve over 23 days. Trimethoprim–sulfamethoxazole was begun on day 1 and pentamidine on day 5.

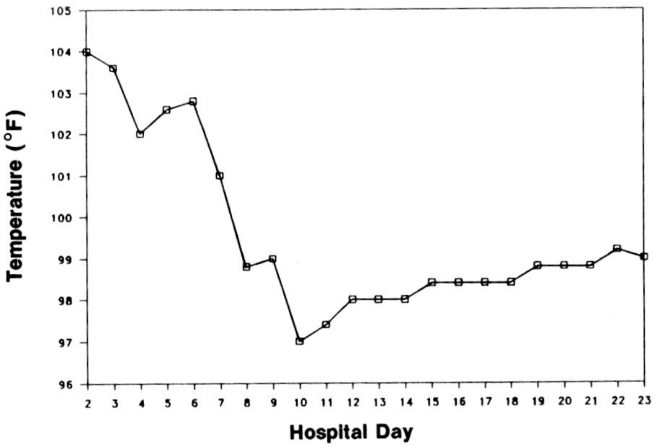

strated bilateral pulmonary interstitial infiltrates with Kerley-B lines at both bases; the infiltrates had increased since the admission study. During the initial five days of TMP-SMX therapy, the patient was noted to have elevations in LDH, AST, and alkaline phosphatase (ALP) (Table 1). In addition, the WBC count had decreased and the patient continued to be febrile (Figures 1 and 2). Trimethoprim-sulfamethoxazole was discontinued and pentamidine isethionate was begun at 4 mg/kg/day by intravenous infusion over one hour. Therapy was also begun with 30% oxygen by face mask. The patient improved, becoming afebrile after three days of pentamidine therapy (Figure 2). Over the next week, the WBC and platelet counts rose substantially (Figures 1 and 3). At this time the alanine aminotransferase (ALT, also known as SGPT), ALP, and γ-glutamyltransferase (GGTP) were noted to be elevated, at 170 IU/L, 222 IU/L, and 279 IU/L, respectively. A decline toward the normal

Figure 3. Platelet counts over 23 days. Trimethoprim–sulfamethoxazole was begun on day 1 and pentamidine on day 5.

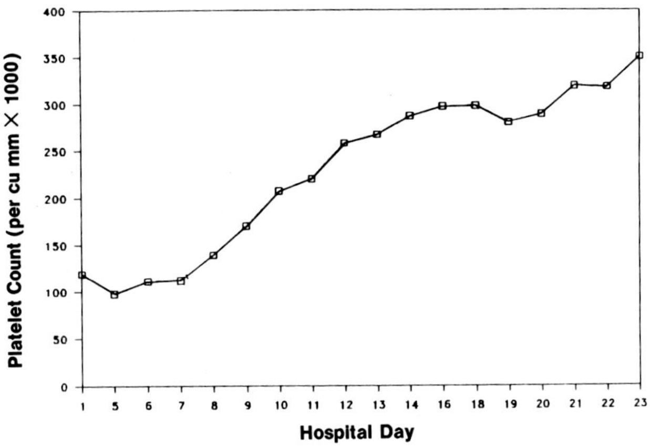

range was seen in the ALP, LDH, AST, ALT, and GGTP after TMP-SMX was discontinued and pentamidine isethionate was begun (Table 1).

After nine days of pentamidine therapy, a decrease was noted in the WBC count (Figure 1). This decrease continued and was attributed to pentamidine. After the patient had completed 21 days of antipneumocystis therapy, pentamidine was discontinued. The patient was discharged, and treatment with zidovudine was planned. A chest roentgenogram before discharge demonstrated residual infiltrates in the upper lobes of both lungs but improvement over previous studies.

Clinical Features

For this patient, like many patients with AIDS, *Pneumocystis carinii* pneumonia was the initial opportunistic infection that established the diagnosis of AIDS. PCP can be difficult to distinguish from other opportunistic pulmonary infections occurring in this patient group. Patients with PCP usually have fever, exertional dyspnea, and a nonproductive cough, although this patient did not. Because PCP is common in AIDS patients, it should be suspected in individuals with AIDS risk factors who have respiratory signs and symptoms. PCP may be identified later in the course of the infection in the AIDS patient than in the non-AIDS immunocompromised patient. Patients with AIDS often have a long history of a nonspecific illness with less acute signs and symptoms, as this patient did. In addition, a clinical response may take longer to occur in some patients with AIDS than in non-AIDS patients.[15]

Pathogenesis

Pneumocystis carinii can be classified as a protozoan, although its exact taxonomy has not yet been identified.[16] Unlike many of the other protozoan opportunistic infections (e.g., infections caused by *Cryptosporidium muris, Isospora belli, Toxoplasma gondii,* and *Giardia lamblia*) that occur in this population,[10,11] *P. carinii*, as well as the disease it causes, usually remains limited to the lung. Rarely, *P. carinii* has been reported to disseminate to areas outside the lung. Dissemination in AIDS patients has resulted in cotton wool spots on the retina, aural polyps, cutaneous lesions, thyroiditis, and splenic enlargement.[17-21]

Pneumocystis carinii is a prevalent organism in humans as well as in lower animals. Clinically, most *P. carinii* infections are not severe. Pneumonia due to *P. carinii* represents the reactivation of a latent infection because of the immunocompromised status of the host.[16] Therefore, PCP may be considered by some to be a reactivation disease as opposed to an opportunistic disease. Patients with AIDS are more likely to experience a relapse after treatment of PCP than are non-AIDS immunocompromised patients.

Diagnosis

Before the emergence of AIDS, the diagnosis of PCP was difficult, often requiring invasive procedures such as open-lung biopsy.[16,22] In the AIDS population, the diagnosis can frequently be made using less invasive procedures such as (1) sputum induction or (2) bronchoscopy to obtain specimens by transbronchial biopsy, bronchoalveolar lavage, or bronchial brushings.[23-27] Specimens are stained with Grocott–Gomori methenamine-silver or toluidine blue O stain to identify the cyst form (thick-walled structure to provide protection against the environment), or Giemsa or Weigert–Gram stain to identify the trophozoite form (actively feeding, growing, multiplying stage).[16] Even the gallium scan has been found to have diagnostic value in AIDS patients, although it will identify only an inflammatory process, not the pathogen. A gallium scan may demonstrate lung inflammation while the chest roentgenogram is still normal. The disadvantages of gallium scanning are cost and a two- to three-day lag time for study completion; this limits its usefulness as an initial study when fiberoptic bronchoscopy is available and the patient has typical clinical features. For the patient with a normal chest roentgenogram, gallium scanning may be a less invasive initial diagnostic study.[28] Open-lung biopsy should be reserved for patients who cannot be diagnosed with a less invasive procedure. The patient described in this report was diagnosed with an outpatient bronchoalveolar lavage.

Chest roentgenogram can be difficult to interpret, with PCP often appearing similar to other infectious processes in the lung. Typically, a chest roentgenogram would be similar to that seen in this patient, with diffuse bilateral alveolar and interstitial infiltrates. Commonly, these infiltrates begin in the perihilar areas and progress to the other areas of the lung.[15-16] Arterial blood gas (ABG) measurements may also be included in the evaluation of the patient, although the ABG of an AIDS patient, like the ABG for this patient, may not indicate the same degree of compromise as that observed in the non-AIDS immunocompromised patient with PCP.[15-16]

Treatment with Trimethoprim–Sulfamethoxazole

The initial outpatient therapy used in this patient was TMP–SMX 18 mg/kg/day of the TMP component. TMP–SMX is usually the initial agent used in the management of PCP in both AIDS and non-AIDS patients.[29]

TMP–SMX is a combination of a diaminopyrimidine (trimethoprim) and a sulfonamide (sulfamethoxazole). The antipneumocystis activity of TMP–SMX occurs by prevention of biosynthesis of tetrahydrofolic acid. This is accomplished by the trimethoprim reversibly inhibiting dihydrofolate reductase and the sulfamethoxazole competing with *para*-aminobenzoic acid in the production of dihydrofolate.[30]

The only prospective study comparing the use of TMP–SMX with pentamidine in the treatment of PCP in AIDS patients was reported by Wharton et al.[31] Forty patients were randomly assigned to receive either pentamidine isethionate or TMP–SMX for treatment of a first episode of PCP. The investigators noted no significant differences with regard to either the efficacy of the treatment regimen or the frequency of adverse effects. However, the size of this study population may have been insufficient to detect a difference in efficacy.[32–36] All patients in both groups experienced some toxicity. Major toxicity requiring discontinuation of initial drug therapy was noted in 10 of 20 patients treated with TMP–SMX and 11 of 20 patients in the pentamidine group. There is no definitive agent of choice in the treatment of PCP in patients with AIDS; current recommendations are to use TMP–SMX as initial therapy in patients with no history of intolerance or resistance to TMP–SMX.[29]

Therapy with TMP–SMX may be initiated by either the oral or the intravenous route. Although the intravenous route provides higher, more dependable serum concentrations, the oral route allows outpatient management of patients who would not otherwise require hospitalization,[16] such as the patient described in this case. The appropriate dosage for the treatment of PCP is 20 mg/kg/day (based on the trimethoprim component), divided into four equal doses.[16] Because of a slower response to therapy, the duration of treatment in the AIDS population may be longer than that used for management of the non-AIDS immunocompromised patient. An adequate trial may be defined as a five- to seven-day course, provided the patient's condition is not worsening and therapy is being tolerated. Because the AIDS population is often not as rapid to respond, this longer course is required to ensure that an adequate trial has been given. A complete course of therapy may be 14 to 21 days or may be extended to one month in some patients.[12]

Trimethoprim and sulfamethoxazole, as well as their metabolites, are primarily eliminated by the kidneys through glomerular filtration and tubular secretion. Patients with a creatinine clearance between 15 and 30 mL/min/1.73 sq m may receive one half of the usual dosage; use is not recommended in patients with a creatinine clearance less than 15 mL/min/1.73 sq m.[30] Serum drug concentration monitoring has been suggested to be of some benefit. Sulfamethoxazole and trimethoprim concentrations of 100–150 μg/mL and 3–5 μg/mL, respectively, two hours after administration have been considered therapeutic.[37]

When TMP–SMX is used for the routine management of bacterial infections, such as a urinary-tract infection, the most commonly encountered adverse reactions are gastrointestinal upset (3.0–3.5%) and allergic skin reactions (3–4%).[38,39] Serious reactions, such as increased serum creatinine (0.4%) and thrombocytopenia (<0.1%), occur less frequently.[38] Hepatotoxicity has been noted to occur rarely.[39] In 1121 patients who had received TMP–SMX for the treatment of common infections, the Boston Collaborative Drug Surveillance Program documented an adverse effect in only 91 (8%). When non-AIDS immunocompromised patients were treated with doses of TMP–SMX appropriate for the management of PCP, the same investigators observed an adverse reaction rate of 15%.[38] Unfortunately, the AIDS population has not experienced this same low incidence of adverse reactions.

Our patient experienced severe nausea, vomiting, and diarrhea as a result of oral TMP–SMX treatment. When therapy was changed to the intravenous route, he developed elevation in liver function enzymes, declines in the white blood cell and platelet counts, and a maculopapular rash. These effects are not unexpected in a patient with AIDS. Jaffe et al.[40] reported on a series of 18 homosexual men with AIDS and PCP treated with intravenous TMP–SMX. In this series, 8 of the 18 patients developed a symptom complex consisting of malaise and fever accompanied by nausea, headache, diffuse erythematous maculopapular rash, and, in some cases, hematologic reactions.

Later reports by several authors confirmed the findings of Jaffe et al. Gordin et al.[41] retrospectively reviewed the records of 38 patients with AIDS who were treated with TMP–SMX for an episode of PCP. Thirty-seven of the patients were initially treated with TMP–SMX; of these, only five were able to complete their course of therapy. Drug toxicity occurred in 29 patients and was serious enough in 19 patients to require a change in therapy. The most commonly seen toxic effects were rash, fever, leukopenia, thrombocytopenia, and hepatitis. Kovacs et al.,[15] in another retrospective review of patients treated for PCP, compared a group of 49 AIDS patients with 39 immunosuppressed non-AIDS patients. Adverse reactions occurred significantly more often (65%) in the patients with AIDS than in the non-AIDS population (12%). The most common adverse reactions were rash (29% of AIDS patients) and leukopenia (47% of AIDS patients versus 8% of non-AIDS patients). In addition, 21% of the AIDS patients had to have TMP–SMX discontinued because of adverse effects, compared with none of the non-AIDS patients. Finally, Small et al.[42] found a similar high incidence of adverse effects (65% incidence) secondary to TMP–SMX in AIDS patients being treated for PCP. This again was a retrospective review of patient records. The most common reactions were leukopenia (59%), hepatotoxicity (35%), fever (24%), and rash (18%). Treatment with TMP–SMX was successful in 18 of 40 episodes of PCP (45%) and was unsuccessful in 15 episodes (37.5%).

The mechanism by which TMP–SMX causes neutropenia has not been completely outlined. Antibodies directed against neutrophils have been identified in patients who developed neutropenia associated with TMP–SMX therapy. This potential mechanism is also supported by the lack of effect of folinic acid administration on the neutropenia, which would suggest that the neutropenia is not secondary to the effects of TMP–SMX on the folic acid pathways in the bone marrow.[12]

Rechallenge with TMP–SMX in a patient with documented hypersensitivity can be harmful and is not recommended.[12] Although successful treatment of PCP with TMP–SMX in combination with intravenous diphenhydramine and subcutaneous epinephrine has been reported, a severe anaphylactic reaction has also been documented secondary to rechallenge of a similar patient.[43,44]

Treatment with Pentamidine

This patient's therapy for PCP was changed to pentamidine because of both poor response and adverse effects from TMP–SMX. Pentamidine is the preferred alternative in this setting.[29]

Studies on the pharmacokinetics of pentamidine were summarized by Salamone and Cunha.[45] Additional comments on these studies are presented here. In the study reported by Conte et al.[46] comparing intramuscular and intravenous pentamidine (initial doses) in 12 patients with normal or near normal renal function, there was a significant difference between the two groups with regard to elimination half-life ($t_{1/2}$), volume of distribution in the central compartment (V_c) and the apparent volume of distribution at steady state (V_{ss}). However, the mean plasma clearance was not significantly different. The renal clearance was only 5% of the plasma clearance for intramuscular administration and 2.5% for the intravenous route. The study design of this investigation did not allow for randomization of patients to the intramuscular or intravenous route. Assignments were based on clinical features, which may have introduced selection bias. This may have played a role in the differences in pharmacokinetic values observed between the two routes of administration. Another factor that could play a role is delayed absorption from the intramuscular injection site, resulting in an overestimate of the $t_{1/2}$ and volume of distribution.

In another report, the pharmacokinetics of pentamidine was further characterized in 20 patients (5 with normal renal function, 13 with impaired function, and 2 children). Six of the patients were undergoing hemodialysis. All five with normal renal function received treatment by the intravenous route. Plasma pentamidine concentrations in those patients undergoing dialysis were not affected by dialysis. The data from this study indicate that dosage adjustments are not needed if the creatinine clearance is greater than 35 mL/min.[47]

After intravenous administration the mean $t_{1/2}$ for pentamidine is 6.22 to 6.40 hours (9.36 hours for the intramuscular route), V_c is 140 to 205 L (924 L for the intramuscular route), and V_{ss} is 821 to 1000 L (2724 L after intramuscular administration).[46,47]

Both of these studies used a high-performance liquid chromatographic (HPLC) assay that was more sensitive than previous assays. However, it may still not have been sensitive enough to accurately identify the terminal $t_{1/2}$. Metabolites that are not yet identified may account for a large portion of the dose administered and therefore may influence the pharmacokinetic profile. In addition, plasma samples were obtained for only 24 hours and may not characterize the entire elimination phase.

Determination of pentamidine concentrations in autopsy specimens from AIDS patients with PCP found that higher levels were achieved in liver, adrenal glands, kidney, and spleen than in the lung. Distribution of pentamidine to the lungs, the site of its activity against PCP, is poor. Pentamidine was detectable in the lung only after the fourth dose.[48] After aerosol administration to animals, pentamidine has been shown to provide sustained high levels in the lung.[49,50] Initial efficacy studies in rats have also demonstrated that aerosolized pentamidine not only resulted in sustained higher levels in the lung but was able to successfully treat PCP.[51,52]

Montgomery et al.[53] investigated the use of aerosolized pentamidine in the management of first episodes of PCP in 15 AIDS patients. This was an open trial in which all patients received daily treatments with approximately 300 mg of pentamidine isethionate for 21 days. (For each treatment, 600 mg of drug was dissolved in 6 mL of sterile water; approximately 300 mg was inhaled over 20 minutes.) Exclusion criteria limited the study population to those patients with an arterial P_{O_2} of 50 mm Hg or greater on room air. A lower arterial P_{O_2} has been associated with a greater risk of mortality from PCP in the AIDS patient.[54] Of the 15 patients in the study, 13 had some evidence of objective and subjective improvement as defined by the authors. One patient, also diagnosed as having tuberculosis, died because of worsening respiratory failure. Six days before death he had been switched to intravenous TMP–SMX. A second patient had to be switched to intravenous TMP–SMX because of deterioration after only one dose of pentamidine. No systemic adverse reactions were noted in any of the patients during treatment. Airway irritation occurred in most patients; 12 patients experienced cough, which was controlled in 9 by pretreatment with inhaled metaproterenol. All patients were able to receive at least part of their treatment as outpatients.

The only other published trial of aerosolized pentamidine was reported by Conte et al.[55] This was a prospective, nonrandomized, open trial comparing aerosolized pentamidine with reduced-dose intravenous pentamidine for the treatment of PCP in AIDS patients. Again, exclusion criteria limited the study population to patients with an arterial Po_2 of 55 mm Hg or greater on room air. Twenty-two patients were treated for a first episode (15 patients) or a repeat episode (7 patients) of PCP with either aerosolized (4 mg/kg) or intravenous (3 mg/kg) pentamidine isethionate for as long as the investigators thought the treatment was clinically indicated. Of the 13 patients in the inhalation group, nine had a good response, treatment failed in one, and three were unevaluable because of early discontinuation. Two patients in this group experienced a serious adverse effect, decreased leukocyte count, although they had low pretreatment counts and had been receiving zidovudine before entering the study. Three patients in this group suffered a recurrence that required readmission. Of the nine patients in the reduced-dose intravenous group, eight had a good response, as defined by the authors. Two patients in this group developed serious toxicity (hepatotoxicity and neutropenia); the neutropenic patient required a change in therapy. Minor toxicity, elevated serum creatinine (three patients) or decreased leukocyte count (one patient), occurred in four of the patients in the intravenous group; only one patient in the inhalation group had minor toxicity (rash). Bronchospasm occurred in five of the inhalation group. In addition, 8 of the 13 patients in this group had cough associated with drug administration.

Additional case reports of patients successfully treated with aerosolized pentamidine have also appeared in the literature.[53,56,57] Bronchospasm and cough, which have continued to be a problem during inhalation treatments, have been successfully managed in these cases by pretreatment with ipratropium or terbutaline.[56,57]

Pentamidine is available as the isethionate salt. The approved dose for the treatment of PCP is 4 mg/kg/day for 14 days, although it is recommended that AIDS patients receive a 14- to 21-day course.[29,58] Although some AIDS patients respond rapidly to treatment (in 10 to 14 days) some also have persistent symptoms after this treatment period. A portion of these patients eventually demonstrate improvement. In one retrospective study comparing survivors with PCP and AIDS with those with PCP without AIDS, the patients with AIDS were found to remain febrile longer (at least 10 days), although this difference was not significant.[15] The duration of therapy in the AIDS population requires further study.

Dosage guidelines for pentamidine in patients with renal dysfunction are lacking because of limited pharmacokinetic data in this population. Bennett et al.[59] have suggested that the dosage interval should be increased to 36 hours for a creatinine clearance of 10 to 50 mL/min and 48 hours in patients with a creatinine clearance less than 10 mL/min. However, the limited pharmacokinetic data available suggest that renal function plays a small part in the elimination of pentamidine.[46] Fitzsimmons and Luskin[60] have suggested that therapy in the patient with renal dysfunction be guided by the risk-to-benefit ratio of pentamidine treatment. If the risk of mortality due to PCP in a patient with renal failure outweighs the risk of pentamidine toxicity, the full-dose regimen is recommended. Patients who are clinically improved or have had their therapy changed to pentamidine because of toxicity of the initial agent used have a lowered risk of adverse effects if the pentamidine dosing interval is extended.

Administration may be either as an intramuscular injection or a one-hour intravenous infusion.[58] The intravenous route is preferred because of the potential for formation of a painful sterile abscess at the site of an intramuscular injection.[29] In a series of 165 AIDS patients treated with pentamidine, 32% developed renal toxicity after intramuscular administration, whereas only 14% who received therapy intravenously developed renal dysfunction. However, renal toxicity did occur more commonly in patients who also had diarrhea, suggesting that fluid imbalance may have been a contributing factor.[61]

Adverse reactions associated with pentamidine use in non-AIDS patients have included impaired renal function, elevated liver function test results, hyperglycemia, hypoglycemia, inflammation at the intramuscular injection site with sterile abscess formation, hematologic disturbances, hypotension, and pancreatitis.[62,63] Serious reactions to pentamidine have also been documented in the recent literature describing AIDS patients treated for PCP.[64–70] These have included pancreatitis, hypoglycemia, hyperglycemia, neutropenia, acute renal failure, arrhythmias, and increasing levels of liver function enzymes. Our patient experienced a decline in white blood cell count after nine days of pentamidine therapy.

Investigational Agents

Eflornithine. Eflornithine (α-difluoromethylornithine, DFMO) is a "suicide enzyme inhibitor."[71] It exerts its action by irreversibly binding and inactivating the enzyme ornithine decarboxylase. Ornithine decarboxylase is necessary for the production of polyamines required for the growth and reproduction of rapidly dividing mammalian and eukaryotic cells.[72]

Eflornithine has activity against protozoa (e.g., *Cryptosporidium muris*, trypanosomes, and *P. carinii*) and cytomegalovirus (in vitro); it has also shown activity against various cancers, although the results of initial trials have not been as good as originally expected.[72,73]

Clinical experience with eflornithine in the management of PCP has been documented in several reports. Four small studies are summarized in Table 2. McLees et al.[78] described a series of 345 AIDS patients with documented PCP treated in a compassionate-use protocol. As in the other studies, all patients had either failed to respond to or experienced intolerance to TMP–SMX or pentamidine, or both. The patients who were dependent on ventilators had a poorer chance of survival; only 10 of 101 (10%) patients treated for longer than four days survived, and 10 of 43 (23%) patients receiving more than 14 days of treatment survived. Those who were breathing spontaneously at study entry had a better outcome; 91 of 117 (78%) who received more than 14 days of treatment survived. For both groups, the clinical response was better than the survival rate. Of 74 patients examined for residual *P. carinii* after treatment, 30 (40%) had disappearance of cysts from the samples examined. This was significantly related to patient survival. The most frequent adverse effects were leukopenia, diarrhea, and neutropenia.

Therapy with eflornithine hydrochloride for the management of PCP is initiated with intravenous administration in a dose of 100 mg/kg infused over at least 20 minutes and administered every six hours. After the initial 10 days to two weeks of therapy, administration may be switched to the oral route. The usual dose is 75 mg/kg diluted in fruit juice or other beverage and administered every six hours. The maximum daily dose is 30 g. The dose may have to be decreased if adverse effects occur.[74-77]

Frequently encountered adverse reactions to eflornithine therapy include thrombocytopenia, neutropenia, gastrointestinal intolerance (particularly diarrhea), and ototoxicity. When hematologic toxicity occurs, eflornithine should be discontinued and the laboratory values should be allowed to return to baseline, after which eflornithine can be restarted at half the initial dose. Should gastrointestinal toxicity occur, the dose should be continued without change as long as normal intake can be maintained and symptoms can be controlled with antiemetics; otherwise, the dose should be decreased and then gradually increased back to the full dose as the patient can tolerate. If the patient has severe diarrhea, therapy should be continued with intravenous drug. If the patient is dehydrated because of the diarrhea, eflornithine should be stopped to allow recovery and then restarted at 50% of the original dose. Finally, all patients should undergo baseline audiometry, followed by monthly studies. Follow-up evaluations should occur if there is evidence that hearing impairment may be developing.[75-77] Data are not available for comparison of the clinical efficacy of eflornithine with that of other treatment regimens. There is a role for eflornithine as an alternative agent for patients in whom treatment with standard agents has failed or has not been tolerated.

Table 2.
Studies of Eflornithine

Study	No. of Patients[a]	No. of Responders (%)
Golden et al.[74]	6	6 (100)
Neibart et al.[75]	23	14 (61)[b]
Gilman et al.[76]	10	4 (40)
Paulson et al.[77]	18	7 (39)

[a] All patients had failed to respond to or had experienced an adverse reaction to pentamidine or trimethoprim–sulfamethoxazole, or both.

[b] Twelve patients had a definite response and two were classified as probable responders. One patient died from another opportunistic infection, and eight patients requiring mechanical ventilation did not respond to treatment.

Dapsone. A clinical trial evaluating the oral administration of dapsone in combination with trimethoprim in the treatment of PCP in AIDS patients has been reported by Leoung et al.[79] This series of 15 patients received dapsone 100 mg/day in combination with trimethoprim 20 mg/kg/day divided into four doses for a first episode of PCP. Exclusion criteria limited the patients to those who were not severely compromised. Thirteen of the 15 patients had arterial P_{O_2} evaluated before therapy was begun. All patients had a P_{O_2} of at least 55 mm Hg, except one with a value of 48 mm Hg. Drug therapy was administered for 21 days. Of the 15 patients, only two had to have therapy changed to pentamidine as the result of an adverse reaction. Six additional patients developed a rash that required a 50% decrease in the trimethoprim dose and a short course of diphenhydramine. Overall, 14 of 15 patients experienced some type of adverse effect, although these were often of minor severity. The adverse effects encountered included gastrointestinal effects such as nausea, vomiting, and elevated liver enzymes; hematologic effects including anemia, neutropenia, and thrombocytopenia; and skin rash.

A later study randomized a group of 58 AIDS patients with their first episode of PCP to receive either TMP–SMX (20 mg/kg/day TMP component) or dapsone 100 mg with TMP 20 mg/kg/day divided into four doses. Both regimens were administered for 21 days. The final week of treatment was administered as outpatient therapy. Again, patients were limited to those with a baseline P_{O_2} of at least 60 mm Hg on room air. If treatment failed or patients experienced severe toxicity, patients were switched to pentamidine, which was found to be equally effective. However, the sulfamethoxazole regimen had a higher incidence of decreased white blood cell count (5 of 29 versus 1 of 29 patients) and elevated liver function enzymes (6 of 20 versus 1 of 29 patients). All but three patients were followed for more than three months, with only seven relapses in the sulfamethoxazole group and four in the dapsone group.[80]

Clinical experience with dapsone in the management of PCP is limited. The experience of Leoung et al.[79] was in patients without serious compromise, early in their clinical course. Dapsone in combination with trimethoprim should be used cautiously as an alternative if treatment with TMP–SMX, pentamidine, or both, has failed. If dapsone is used, the patient must first be screened for glucose-6-phosphate dehydrogenase deficiency, which is a contraindication for dapsone use.[79] Dapsone has also been reported to cause methemoglobinemia in one AIDS patient with PCP.[81]

The potential for cross-sensitivity between dapsone and the sulfonamides has not yet been resolved.[12] Dapsone has been successfully administered to AIDS patients who experienced hypersensitivity to TMP–SMX.[82]

Trimetrexate. Trimethoprim and pyrimethamine are diaminopyrimidines, which, in combination with a sulfonamide, inhibit growth of *P. carinii*. As previously described, this provides a two-pronged approach. The diaminopyrimidines inhibit dihydrofolate reductase, while the sulfonamide blocks conversion of *p*-aminobenzoic acid to dihydrofolate by inhibiting dihydropteroate synthetase. This results in inhibition of de novo biosynthesis of folic acid, which is needed in the reproductive cycle of protozoa such as *P. carinii* and *Toxoplasma gondii*.[83]

Antineoplastic agents such as methotrexate also exert their effect through inhibition of dihydrofolate reductase. Methotrexate requires a folate-specific membrane carrier to enter cells. Although mammalian cells have this carrier, protozoal and bacterial cells do not; thus, the use of methotrexate as an antibacterial or antiprotozoal agent is limited. Trimetrexate is a highly lipophilic quinazoline analog of methotrexate that does not require this carrier. Trimetrexate can penetrate into mammalian, bacterial, and protozoal cells. Leucovorin (5-formyltetrahydrofolate), like methotrexate, requires a membrane carrier for transport into the cell, limiting its access to mammalian cells only. After trimetrexate administration, leucovorin can be given to "rescue" or protect the mammalian cells while not affecting activity against the protozoal cells.[83]

The potency of several inhibitors of *P. carinii* dihydrofolate reductase has been compared in vitro. The diaminopyrimidines trimethoprim and pyrimethamine, trimetrexate, and methotrexate were tested. Methotrexate and trimetrexate were more potent inhibitors of both *P. carinii* and mammalian dihydrofolate reductase than trimethoprim and pyrimethamine. Trimethoprim, although the most frequently used compound, was the weakest inhibitor. Trimetrexate was also more potent than the diaminopyrimidines in binding affinity for *P. carinii* dihydrofolate reductase.[83] In another in vitro study, trimetrexate was again found to be more potent than trimethoprim, pyrimethamine, or methotrexate in the ability to inhibit *P. carinii* dihydrofolate reductase.[84]

Few data are available regarding the pharmacokinetics of trimetrexate. Active metabolites of trimetrexate may interfere with the assay.[85,86] In a Phase I trial involving 11 patients treated with high doses of intravenous trimetrexate (60 to 210 mg/sq m) for management of metastatic cancer, trimetrexate was found to have a triphasic elimination curve with an alpha $t_{1/2}$ of 8±5 minutes, a beta $t_{1/2}$ of 102±48 minutes, and a terminal $t_{1/2}$ of 15.2±5.7 hours. The area under the serum concentration–time curve (AUC) was 373±336 μg·hr/mL, volume of distribution was 25.2±16.1 L/sq m, total clearance was 14±8 mL/min/sq m, and renal clearance was 8±6 mL/min/sq m. Patients with severe toxicity had a significant increase in terminal $t_{1/2}$ and AUC and a decrease in volume of distribution, total clearance, and renal clearance.[86] Allegra et al.[85] also evaluated the pharmacokinetics of trimetrexate during their trial in AIDS patients with PCP. Their data show a biphasic elimination curve with a terminal $t_{1/2}$ of 11 hours. Allegra et al. may have had insufficient data to accurately determine pharmacokinetic values; samples were obtained one hour after and one hour before administration, insufficient data points to characterize the distribution $t_{1/2}$. Ho et al.[86] had sufficient data-collection points, with data obtained soon enough after administration to identify a triexponential decay, and their assay methods differed from those of Allegra et al. Allegra et al. used both HPLC and competitive protein binding, while Ho et al. used only spectrophotometric inhibition of dihydrofolate reductase. Another difference between the two studies was the patient population. Ho et al. evaluated patients with metastatic cancer, while Allegra et al. studied AIDS patients.

Allegra et al.[85] reported the results of a pilot study to evaluate trimetrexate for the management of PCP in humans. Forty-nine patients with AIDS and PCP completed an open trial. The study population was divided into three groups: group I was patients in whom standard therapy either had failed or could not be tolerated (both pentamidine and TMP–SMX); group II had a history of past failure of or intolerance to sulfonamides, pentamidine, or both but were as yet untreated in this PCP episode; and group III included untreated patients who were eligible for standard therapy. All patients received trimetrexate 30 mg/sq m daily by intravenous infusion over 30 minutes for 21 days, in conjunction with leucovorin 20 mg/sq m every six hours by the intravenous or oral route for 23 days. Patients in group III also received sulfadiazine 1 g orally every six hours for 21 days.

Of the patients in group I, 69% (11 patients) were alive without support from a ventilator for a minimum of two weeks after completing therapy, 69% (11 patients) had positive responses, and none of the responders had a relapse during the three-month follow-up period. Eighty-eight percent (14 patients) of group II survived and 63% (10 patients) had a positive response; however, 60% of the responders suffered a relapse. Finally, group III had a 77% (13 patients) survival rate with a 71% (12 patients) response rate. One of the responders in group III suffered a relapse.[85]

Adverse effects were minimal. Twelve of the 49 patients had neutrophil counts less than 1,000/cu mm or platelet counts less than 100,000/cu mm. A reduction in trimetrexate dose to 15 mg/sq m allowed these counts to quickly rise. Although four patients had an increase in serum aspartate aminotransferase or alanine aminotransferase, these values returned to near normal with continued therapy. In addition, patients frequently had elevations in these enzymes at study entry. Rash occurred in one patient in group I, requiring discontinuation of trimetrexate. However, during a subsequent episode he was successfully treated with trimetrexate without recurrence. Rash was more common in group III (8 of 17 patients) but resolved when sulfadiazine was discontinued while trimetrexate was continued. Rare adverse effects were transient increase in serum creatinine (one patient), increased serum creatinine and bilirubin (one patient), and peripheral neuropathy (one patient) that resolved when therapy was discontinued.[85]

Although trimetrexate appears to be an efficacious agent, more clinical data are needed regarding its safety and efficacy. These trials are now under way in several centers.

Corticosteroids. Recently several reports have appeared in the literature describing a beneficial response to corticosteroid administration in patients with AIDS and PCP.[87–93] The largest series, reported by MacFadden et al.,[92] involved 18 AIDS patients with histologically proven PCP and lack of response to standard therapy. All patients continued to receive standard antipneumocystis therapy for PCP as well as standard supportive treatment, including ventilatory support if needed. Ten consecutive patients received corticosteroid therapy beginning with the onset of respiratory failure. One patient did not begin corticosteroid treatment until day 13 of ventilatory support. Methylprednisolone 40 mg intravenously every six hours for seven days was used in nine patients and prednisone 10 mg orally four times a day for seven days in one patient. Nine of the 10 patients survived respiratory failure, while only two of eight patients who were not treated with steroids survived. Although this was a prospective study, it was not conducted in a randomized, controlled design. Additional confirmation of this beneficial effect is needed from well-controlled, prospective, randomized trials.

Pneumocystis carinii pneumonia in AIDS patients has been reported to result in an inflammatory response, with destruction of lung tissue, including development of cavitary lesions and pneumothorax.[94] Examination of bronchoalveolar lavage fluid from two patients with AIDS and PCP showed that an active inflammatory response to the infection was occurring in the lung. Lavage fluid from the AIDS patients, when compared to lavage fluid from healthy controls, suggested that local antibody formation may occur in the lungs during episodes of PCP.[87] In contrast, a comparison of bronchoalveolar lavage fluid from a group of 36 AIDS patients and 11 non-AIDS, immune-suppressed patients with pneumonitis of various causes revealed that both groups had significant increases in lymphocytes, both as a percentage of total WBC count and in absolute number, compared with control subjects.[95] This occurred in the presence of peripheral lymphopenia. No difference was noted between various causes of pneumonitis. This has been supported by other reports with similar findings.[96,97]

The successful use of corticosteroids in the management of PCP in AIDS patients has been attributed to the inhibition of this inflammatory response to the infection and reduction of fibrosis and inflammation-associated destruction of lung tissue.[89,93] In addition, corticosteroids have been postulated to inhibit accumulation of mononuclear cells in the lung, which normally are present in response to infection.[90] Steroids reduce both chemotactic and phagocytic activity of polymorphonuclear neutrophils and reduce complement-mediated activation of these cells and production of leukocyte pyrogen, possibly resulting in a decreased inflammatory response in the lungs.[89,92]

Although there are data to support the use of corticosteroids in the management of PCP in AIDS patients, this should not be considered standard therapy. Controlled clinical trials are required before the risks and benefits of this therapeutic intervention can be evaluated. In case reports, patients with AIDS who received corticosteroids for management of another disease process rapidly developed PCP and deteriorated after discontinuation of the corticosteroid.[98] This therapy should be used with great caution, if at all, and should be considered a last effort until additional data are available.

Prophylaxis

When infection with *Pneumocystis carinii* is adequately treated and apparently resolved, the organism is not totally eliminated from the lungs of AIDS patients. *P. carinii* cysts and trophozoites have been recovered after treatment and clinical resolution have been documented.[99,100] The recurrent nature of this infectious process has led to the use of TMP–SMX as a prophylactic agent. Chemoprophylaxis with TMP–SMX has also been shown in a placebo-controlled trial to be effective in preventing the initial episode of PCP in recently diagnosed patients with biopsy-proven Kaposi's sarcoma and AIDS.[101] However, this may not be practical in many patients, such as our patient, because of the increased risk of adverse effects to this agent in this population. Our patient suffered adverse effects of both pentamidine and TMP–SMX. If tolerated, TMP–SMX may be used in a dose of one double-strength tablet twice a day.[12] Pentamidine isethionate has also been an effective prophylactic agent when administered at monthly intervals at a dose of 4 mg/kg/dose infused intravenously over one hour.[102] Administration of the same dose (4 mg/kg) at bimonthly intervals has also proven to be effective as prophylaxis against recurrence.[103] Aerosol administration of pentamidine isethionate has also been used for prophylaxis against recurrence. The data are limited; however, a dose of 60 mg by aerosol administration once weekly for four weeks, then every other week for an indefinite time, has initially proven to be effective as a prophylactic regimen.[104] However, the optimal dose and regimen have not yet been definitely established.

Finally, sulfadoxine–pyrimethamine (Fansidar, Hoffmann–La Roche Inc.) has been tried as prophylaxis in a once-weekly regimen. Gottlieb et al.[105] reported on a series of 12 patients with PCP and AIDS who were entered into a pilot study to evaluate sulfadoxine–pyrimethamine, one tablet (500 mg/25 mg) weekly, as prophylaxis against recurrence. All 12 patients had experienced adverse reactions to TMP–SMX. Nine patients tolerated the sulfadoxine–pyrimethamine treatment, while three patients had skin eruptions requiring discontinuation of therapy. None of the nine patients successfully treated had a recurrence during a 3- to 12-month follow-up period, while one of three who did not tolerate prophylaxis had a recurrence. Although initially promising, this regimen is not as effective as was originally thought.[106,107] In addition, the sulfonamide component of sulfadoxine–pyrimethamine has resulted in adverse reactions in AIDS patients, similar to reactions seen with TMP–SMX use. The rash may be particularly severe and has been reported to progress to Stevens–Johnson syndrome.[106]

Conclusion

Two drugs, pentamidine isethionate and TMP–SMX, have labeled indications for the treatment of PCP. Our case report illustrates the difficulty often encountered when treating PCP in the AIDS patient. Our patient's clinical features were not consistent with those usually seen in the AIDS population. During the course of TMP–SMX, he experienced serious adverse effects—gastrointestinal disturbances leading to dehydration, hematologic abnormalities, elevation in liver function test results, and the early stages of a maculopapular rash—while receiving no clinical benefit from therapy. When switched to pentamidine isethionate, he rapidly improved, although he began later to develop neutropenia from the pentamidine therapy.

Although there is a higher incidence of serious adverse effects from TMP–SMX therapy in the AIDS population than in the non-AIDS population, TMP–SMX is still considered the preferred agent for initial therapy.[29] Pentamidine isethionate is preferred for patients with documented allergy to TMP–SMX or failure to respond to a five- to seven-day course of TMP–SMX.[29] In the future, aerosolized pentamidine and trimetrexate may play an important role in the management of PCP. Although not warranted in every case, prophylaxis should be considered for patients with frequent recurrences.

Discussion Questions

1. Compare the clinical features of *Pneumocystis carinii* pneumonia (PCP) in this patient with those usually seen in an AIDS patient and a patient who does not have AIDS. What diagnostic tests may be used to identify *Pneumocystis carinii* as the causative organism?
2. Contrast the major advantages and disadvantages of using pentamidine and trimethoprim–sulfamethoxazole in the treatment of PCP. Which drug would you select as first-line therapy?
3. What is your recommendation for treatment of a refractory episode of PCP in an AIDS patient? Include investigational agents if appropriate.
4. Discuss the use of prophylactic therapy for prevention of recurrent PCP. What is your recommendation for therapy?

References

1. Centers for Disease Control. *Pneumocystis* pneumonia—Los Angeles. *MMWR*. 1981; 30:250–2.
2. Centers for Disease Control. Kaposi's sarcoma and *Pneumocystis* pneumonia among homosexual men—New York City and California. *MMWR*. 1981; 30:305–8.
3. Centers for Disease Control. Update: acquired immunodeficiency syndrome—United States. *MMWR*. 1986; 35:757–66.
4. Centers for Disease Control. Update on acquired immune deficiency syndrome (AIDS)—United States. *MMWR*. 1982;31:507–14.
5. Centers for Disease Control. Update: acquired immunodeficiency syndrome (AIDS)—United States. *MMWR*. 1984; 32:688–91.
6. Centers for Disease Control. Revision of the case definition of acquired immunodeficiency syndrome for national reporting—United States. *MMWR*. 1985; 34:373–5.
7. Centers for Disease Control. Revision of the CDC surveil-

lance case definition for acquired immunodeficiency syndrome. *MMWR*. 1987; 36(Suppl 1S):3s–15s.
8. Lane HC, Masur H, Edgar LC et al. Abnormalities of B-cell activation and immunoregulation in patients with the acquired immunodeficiency syndrome. *N Engl J Med*. 1983; 309:453–8.
9. Lane HC, Depper JM, Greene WC et al. Qualitative analysis of immune function in patients with the acquired immunodeficiency syndrome. *N Engl J Med*. 1985; 313:79–84.
10. Furio MF, Wordell CJ. Treatment of infectious complications of acquired immunodeficiency syndrome. *Clin Pharm*. 1985; 4:539–54.
11. Armstrong D, Gold JWM, Dryjanski J et al. Treatment of infections in patients with the acquired immunodeficiency syndrome. *Ann Intern Med*. 1985; 103:738–43.
12. Wofsy CB. Use of trimethoprim-sulfamethoxazole in the treatment of *Pneumocystis carinii* pneumonitis in patients with acquired immunodeficiency syndrome. *Rev Infect Dis*. 1987; 9(Suppl 2):S184–91.
13. Centers for Disease Control. Update: acquired immunodeficiency syndrome—United States. *MMWR*. 1985; 34:245–8.
14. Murray JF, Garay SM, Hopewell PC et al. Pulmonary complications of the acquired immunodeficiency syndrome: an update. Report of the second national Heart, Lung and Blood Institute workshop. *Am Rev Respir Dis*. 1987; 135:504–9.
15. Kovacs JA, Hiemenz JW, Macher AM et al. *Pneumocystis carinii* pneumonia: a comparison between patients with the acquired immunodeficiency syndrome and patients with other immunodeficiencies. *Ann Intern Med*. 1984; 100:663–71.
16. Hughes WT. *Pneumocystis carinii* pneumonitis. *Chest*. 1985; 6:810–3.
17. Kwok S, O'Donnell JJ, Wood IS. Retinal cotton-wool spots in a patient with *Pneumocystis carinii* infection. *N Engl J Med*. 1982; 307:184–5. Letter.
18. Schinella RA, Breda SD, Hammerschlag PE. Otic infection due to *Pneumocystis carinii* in an apparently healthy man with antibody to the human immunodeficiency virus. *Ann Intern Med*. 1987; 106:399–400.
19. Coulman CU, Greene I, Archibald RWR. Cutaneous pneumocystosis. *Ann Intern Med*. 1987; 106:396–8.
20. Pilon VA, Echols RM, Celo JS, et al. Disseminated *Pneumocystis carinii* infection in AIDS. *N Engl J Med*. 1987; 316:1410–1. Letter.
21. Gallant JE, Enriquez RE, Cohen KL et al. *Pneumocystis carinii* thyroiditis. *Am J Med*. 1988; 84:303–6.
22. Walzer PD, Perl DP, Krogstad DJ et al. *Pneumocystis carinii* pneumonia in the United States: epidemiologic, diagnostic, and clinical features. *Ann Intern Med*. 1974; 80:83–93.
23. Pitchenik AE, Ganjei P, Torres A et al. Sputum examination for the diagnosis of *Pneumocystis carinii* pneumonia in the acquired immunodeficiency syndrome. *Am Rev Respir Dis*. 1986; 133:226–9.
24. Bigby TD, Margolskee D, Curtis JL et al. The usefulness of induced sputum in the diagnosis of *Pneumocystis carinii* pneumonia in patients with the acquired immunodeficiency syndrome. *Am Rev Respir Dis*. 1986; 133:515–8.
25. Stover DE, Zaman MB, Hajdu ST et al. Bronchoalveolar lavage in the diagnosis of diffuse pulmonary infiltrates in the immunosuppressed host. *Ann Intern Med*. 1984; 101:1–7.
26. Broaddus C, Dake MD, Stulbarg MS et al. Bronchoalveolar lavage and transbronchial biopsy for the diagnosis of pulmonary infections in the acquired immunodeficiency syndrome. *Ann Intern Med*. 1985; 102:747–52.
27. Gal AA, Klatt EC, Koss MN et al. The effectiveness of bronchoscopy in the diagnosis of *Pneumocystis carinii* and cytomegalovirus pulmonary infections in acquired immunodeficiency syndrome. *Arch Pathol Lab Med*. 1987; 111:238–41.
28. Tuazon CU, Delaney MD, Simon GL et al. Utility of gallium[67] scintigraphy and bronchial washings in the diagnosis and treatment of *Pneumocystis carinii* pneumonia in patients with the acquired immune deficiency syndrome. *Am Rev Respir Dis*. 1985; 132:1087–92.
29. Anon. Treatment of *Pneumocystis carinii* pneumonia. *Med Lett Drugs Ther*. 1987; 29:103–4.
30. Roche Laboratories. Bactrim I.V. infusion package insert. Nutley, NJ: 1986 Sep.
31. Wharton JM, Coleman DL, Wofsy CB et al. Trimethoprim–sulfamethoxazole or pentamidine for *Pneumocystis carinii* pneumonia in the acquired immunodeficiency syndrome: a prospective randomized trial. *Ann Intern Med*. 1986; 105:37–44.
32. Dennis T. Trimethoprim–sulfamethoxazole or pentamidine for *Pneumocystis carinii* pneumonia in the acquired immunodeficiency syndrome. *Ann Intern Med*. 1986; 105:629–30. Letter.
33. Marantz PR. Trimethoprim–sulfamethoxazole or pentamidine for *Pneumocystis carinii* pneumonia in the acquired immunodeficiency syndrome. *Ann Intern Med*. 1986; 105:630. Letter.
34. Begin P, Hanley J. Trimethoprim–sulfamethoxazole or pentamidine for *Pneumocystis carinii* pneumonia. *Ann Intern Med*. 1987; 106:474–5. Letter.
35. Polis MA, Blackwelder WC. Trimethoprim–sulfamethoxazole or pentamidine for *Pneumocystis carinii* pneumonia. *Ann Intern Med*. 1987; 106:475. Letter.
36. Erban JK. Trimethoprim–sulfamethoxazole or pentamidine for *Pneumocystis carinii* pneumonia. *Ann Intern Med*. 1987; 106:475. Letter.
37. Hughes WT, Feldman S, Chaudhary SC et al. Comparison of pentamidine isethionate and trimethoprim–sulfamethoxazole in the treatment of *Pneumocystis carinii* pneumonia. *J Pediatr*. 1978; 92:285–91.
38. Jick H. Adverse reactions to trimethoprim–sulfamethoxazole in hospitalized patients. *Rev Infect Dis*. 1982; 4:426–8.
39. Lawson DH, Paice BJ. Adverse reactions to trimethoprim–sulfamethoxazole. *Rev Infect Dis*. 1982; 4:429–33.
40. Jaffe HS, Ammann AJ, Abrams DI et al. Complications of co-trimoxazole in treatment of AIDS-associated *Pneumocystis carinii* pneumonia in homosexual men. *Lancet*. 1983; 2:1109–11.
41. Gordin FM, Simon GL, Wofsy CB et al. Adverse reactions to trimethoprim–sulfamethoxazole in patients with the acquired immunodeficiency syndrome. *Ann Intern Med*. 1984; 100:495–9.
42. Small CB, Harris CA, Friedland GH et al. The treatment of *Pneumocystis carinii* pneumonia in the acquired immunodeficiency syndrome. *Arch Intern Med*. 1985; 145:837–40.
43. Gibbon R, Lindauer JA. Successful treatment of *Pneumocystis carinii* pneumonia with trimethoprim–sulfamethoxazole in hypersensitive AIDS patients. *JAMA*. 1985; 253:1259–60. Letter.
44. Arnold PA, Guglielmo BJ, Hollander H. Severe hypersensitivity reaction upon rechallenge with trimethoprim–sulfamethoxazole in a patient with AIDS. *Drug Intell Clin Pharm*. 1988; 22:43–5.
45. Salamone FR, Cunha BA. Update on pentamidine for the treatment of *Pneumocystis carinii* pneumonia. *Clin Pharm*. 1988; 7:501–10.
46. Conte JE, Upton RA, Phelps RT. Use of a specific and sensitive assay to determine pentamidine pharmacokinetics in patients with AIDS. *J Infect Dis*. 1986; 154:923–9.
47. Conte JE, Upton RA, Lin ET. Pentamidine pharmacokinetics in patients with AIDS with impaired renal function. *J Infect Dis*. 1987; 156:885–90.
48. Bernard EM, Rothkotter HE, Gold JWM et al. Distribution of pentamidine in humans. Twenty-Sixth Interscience Conference on Antimicrobial Agents and Chemotherapy. New Orleans, LA: American Society for Microbiology; 1986:696. Abstract.
49. Waldman RH, Pearce DE, Martin RA. Pentamidine isethionate in lungs, livers, and kidneys of rats after aerosol or

intramuscular administration. *Am Rev Respir Dis.* 1973; 108:1004–6.
50. Bernard EM, Donnelly HJ, Koo HP et al. Aerosol administration improves delivery of pentamidine to the lungs. Twenty-Fifth Interscience Conference on Antimicrobial Agents and Chemotherapy. Minneapolis, MN: American Society for Microbiology; 1985:552. Abstract.
51. Debs RJ, Blumenfeld W, Brunette EN et al. Successful treatment with aerosolized pentamidine of *Pneumocystis carinii* pneumonia in rats. *Antimicrob Agents Chemother.* 1987; 31:37–41.
52. Debs RJ, Straubinger RM, Brunette EN et al. Selective enhancement of pentamidine uptake in the lung by aerosolization and delivery in liposomes. *Am Rev Respir Dis.* 1987; 135:731–7.
53. Montgomery AB, Debs RJ, Luce JM et al. Aerosolised pentamidine as sole therapy for *Pneumocystis carinii* pneumonia in patients with acquired immunodeficiency syndrome. *Lancet.* 1987; 2:480–3.
54. Kales CP, Murren JR, Torres RA et al. Early predictors of in-hospital mortality for *Pneumocystis carinii* pneumonia in the acquired immunodeficiency syndrome. *Arch Intern Med.* 1987; 147:1413–7.
55. Conte JE, Hollander H, Golden JA. Inhaled or reduced-dose intravenous pentamidine for *Pneumocystis carinii* pneumonia: a pilot study. *Ann Intern Med.* 1987; 107:495–8.
56. Jesuthasan AJ, Datta AK, Hamilton R et al. Aerosolised pentamidine. *Lancet.* 1987; 2:971–2. Letter.
57. Heley A. Aerosolised pentamidine treatment at home. *Lancet.* 1987; 2:1092. Letter.
58. LyphoMed, Inc. Pentam 300 package insert. Melrose Park, IL: 1984 Sep.
59. Bennett WM, Aronoff GR, Golper TA et al. Drug prescribing in renal failure: dosing guidelines for adults. Philadelphia: American College of Physicians; 1987:26.
60. Fitzsimmons WE, Luskin SS. Pentamidine therapy in renal failure: case report and literature review. *Drug Intell Clin Pharm.* 1988; 22:25–8.
61. Stehr-Green JK, Helmick CG. Pentamidine and renal toxicity. *N Engl J Med.* 1985; 313:694–5.
62. Pearson RD, Hewlett EL. Pentamidine for the treatment of *Pneumocystis carinii* pneumonia and other protozoal diseases. *Ann Intern Med.* 1985; 103:782–6.
63. Murphey SA, Josephs AS. Acute pancreatitis associated with pentamidine therapy. *Arch Intern Med.* 1981; 141:56–8.
64. Salmeron S, Petitpretz P, Katlama C et al. Pentamidine and pancreatitis. *Ann Intern Med.* 1986; 105:140–1. Letter.
65. Zuger A, Wolf BZ, El-Sadr W et al. Pentamidine-associated fatal acute pancreatitis. *JAMA.* 1986; 256:2383–5.
66. Stahl-Bayliss CM, Kalman CM, Laskin OL. Pentamidine-induced hypoglycemia in patients with the acquired immune deficiency syndrome. *Clin Pharmacol Ther.* 1986; 39:271–5.
67. Centers for Disease Control. Severe neutropenia during pentamidine treatment of *Pneumocystis carinii* pneumonia in patients with acquired immunodeficiency syndrome—New York City. *MMWR.* 1984; 33:65–7.
68. Sensakovic JW, Suarez M, Perez G et al. Pentamidine treatment of *Pneumocystis carinii* pneumonia in the acquired immunodeficiency syndrome: association with acute renal failure and myoglobinuria. *Arch Intern Med.* 1985; 145:2247.
69. Wharton JM, Demopulos PA, Goldschlager N. Torsade de pointes during administration of pentamidine isethionate. *Am J Med.* 1987; 83:571–6.
70. Sattler FR, Waskin H. Pentamidine and fatal hypoglycemia. *Ann Intern Med.* 1987; 107:789–90. Letter.
71. Sjoerdsma A. Suicide enzyme inhibitors as potential drugs. *Clin Pharmacol Ther.* 1981; 30:3–22.
72. Sjoerdsma A, Schechter PJ. Chemotherapeutic implications of polyamine biosynthesis inhibition. *Clin Pharmacol Ther.* 1984; 35:287–300.
73. Gibson W, vanBreemen R, Fields A et al. D,L-alpha-difluoromethylornithine inhibits human cytomegalovirus replication. *J Virol.* 1984; 50:145–54.
74. Golden JA, Sjoerdsma A, Santi DV. *Pneumocystis carinii* pneumonia treated with alpha-difluoromethylornithine: a prospective study among patients with the acquired immunodeficiency syndrome. *West J Med.* 1984; 141:613–23.
75. Neibart E, Sacks HS, Hammer G et al. Difluoromethylornithine (DFMO) in the treatment of *Pneumocystis carinii* pneumonia (PCP). Twenty-Sixth Interscience Conference on Antimicrobial Agents and Chemotherapy. New Orleans, LA: American Society for Microbiology; 1986:693. Abstract.
76. Gilman TM, Paulson YJ, Boylen CT et al. Eflornithine treatment of *Pneumocystis carinii* pneumonia in AIDS. *JAMA.* 1986; 256:2197–8.
77. Paulson YJ, Gilman TM, Boylen CT et al. Eflornithine treatment of *Pneumocystis carinii* pneumonia in patients failing other therapy. Twenty-Sixth Interscience Conference on Antimicrobial Agents and Chemotherapy. New Orleans, LA: American Society for Microbiology; 1986:694. Abstract.
78. McLees BD, Barlow JLR, Kuzma RJ et al. Studies on successful eflornithine treatment of *Pneumocystis carinii* pneumonia (PCP) in AIDS patients failing conventional therapy. Third International Conference on AIDS. Washington, DC: U.S. Department of Health and Human Services and World Health Organization; 1987:TH.4.2. Abstract.
79. Leoung GS, Mills J, Hopewell PC et al. Dapsone–trimethoprim for *Pneumocystis carinii* pneumonia in the acquired immunodeficiency syndrome. *Ann Intern Med.* 1986; 105:45–8.
80. Medina I, Leoung G, Mills J et al. Oral therapy for *Pneumocystis carinii* pneumonia (PCP) in AIDS. A randomized double blind trial of trimethoprim sulfamethoxazole versus dapsone trimethoprim for first episode *Pneumocystis carinii* pneumonia in AIDS. Third International Conference on AIDS. Washington, DC: U.S. Department of Health and Human Services and World Health Organization; 1987:F.3.3. Abstract.
81. Reiter WM, Cimoch PJ. Dapsone-induced methemoglobinemia in a patient with *P. carinii* pneumonia and AIDS. *N Engl J Med.* 1987; 317:1740–1. Letter.
82. Edelson PJ, Metroka CE, Friedman-Kien A. Dapsone, trimethoprim–sulfamethoxazole, and the acquired immunodeficiency syndrome. *Ann Intern Med.* 1985; 103:963. Letter.
83. Allegra CJ, Kovacs JA, Drake JC et al. Activity of antifolates against *Pneumocystis carinii* dihydrofolate reductase and identification of a potent new agent. *J Exp Med.* 1987; 165:926–31.
84. Queener SF, Bartlett MS, Jay MA et al. Activity of lipid-soluble inhibitors of dihydrofolate reductase against *Pneumocystis carinii* in culture and in a rat model of infection. *Antimicrob Agent Chemother.* 1987; 31:1323–7.
85. Allegra CJ, Chabner BA, Tuazon CU et al. Trimetrexate for the treatment of *Pneumocystis carinii* pneumonia in patients with the acquired immunodeficiency syndrome. *N Engl J Med.* 1987; 317:978–85.
86. Ho DHW, Covington WP, Legha SS et al. Clinical pharmacology of trimetrexate. *Clin Pharmacol Ther.* 1987; 42:351–6.
87. Rankin JA, Walzer PD, Dwyer JM et al. Immunologic alterations in bronchoalveolar lavage fluid in the acquired immunodeficiency syndrome (AIDS). *Am Rev Respir Dis.* 1983; 128:189–94.
88. Foltzer MA, Hannan SE, Kozak AJ. *Pneumocystis carinii* pneumonia: response to corticosteroids. *JAMA.* 1985; 253:979. Letter.
89. MacFadden DK, Edelson JD, Rebuck AS. *Pneumocystis carinii* pneumonia in the acquired immunodeficiency syndrome: response to inadvertent steroid therapy. *Can Med Assoc J.* 1985; 132:1161–3.
90. El-Sadr W, Sidhu G, Diamond G et al. High-dose corticoste-

roids as adjunct therapy in severe *Pneumocystis carinii* pneumonia. *AIDS Res.* 1986; 2:349–55.
91. Rankin JA, Pella JA. Radiographic resolution of *Pneumocystis carinii* pneumonia in response to corticosteroid therapy. *Am Rev Respir Dis.* 1987; 136:182–3.
92. MacFadden DK, Edelson JD, Hyland RH et al. Corticosteroids as adjunctive therapy in treatment of *Pneumocystis carinii* pneumonia in patients with acquired immunodeficiency syndrome. *Lancet.* 1987; 1:1477–9.
93. Mottin D, Denis M, Dombret H et al. Role for steroids in treatment of *Pneumocystis carinii* pneumonia in AIDS. *Lancet.* 1987; 2:519. Letter.
94. Eng RHK, Bishburg E, Smith SM. Evidence for destruction of lung tissues during *Pneumocystis carinii* infection. *Arch Intern Med.* 1987; 147:746–9.
95. White DA, Gellene RA, Gupta S et al. Pulmonary cell populations in the immunosuppressed patient. Bronchoalveolar lavage findings during episodes of pneumonitis. *Chest.* 1985; 88:352–9.
96. Venet A, Dennewald G, Sandron D et al. Bronchoalveolar lavage in acquired immunodeficiency syndrome. *Lancet.* 1983; 2:53. Letter.
97. Wallace JM, Barbers RG, Oishi JS et al. Cellular and T-lymphocyte sub-population profiles in bronchoalveolar lavage fluid from patients with acquired immunodeficiency syndrome and pneumonitis. *Am Rev Respir Dis.* 1984; 130:786–90.
98. Shafer RW, Offit K, Macris NT et al. Possible risk of steroid administration in patients at risk for AIDS. *Lancet.* 1985; 1:934–5. Letter.
99. Shelhamer JH, Ognibene FP, Macher AM et al. Persistence of *Pneumocystis carinii* in lung tissue of acquired immunodeficiency syndrome patients treated for pneumocystis pneumonia. *Am Rev Respir Dis.* 1984; 130:1161–5.
100. El-Sadr W, Sidhu G. Persistence of trophozoites after successful treatment of *Pneumocystis carinii* pneumonia. *Ann Intern Med.* 1986; 105:889–90.
101. Fischl MA, Dickinson GM, La Voie L. Safety and efficacy of sulfamethaxazole and trimethoprim chemoprophylaxis for *Pneumocystis carinii* pneumonia in AIDS. *JAMA.* 1988; 259:1185–9.
102. Karaffa C, Rehm S, Calabrese L. Efficacy of monthly pentamidine infusions in preventing recurrent *Pneumocystis carinii* pneumonia (PCP) in the AIDS patient. Twenty-Sixth Interscience Conference on Antimicrobial Agents and Chemotherapy. New Orleans, LA: American Society for Microbiology; 1986:690. Abstract.
103. Johnson ES, Sulieman S, Perez G et al. Secondary prophylaxis of PCP in AIDS patients using bi-monthly parenteral pentamidine. Twenty-Seventh Interscience Conference on Antimicrobial Agents and Chemotherapy. New York, NY: American Society for Microbiology; 1987:943. Abstract.
104. Bernard E, Schmitt H, Pagel L et al. Safety and effectiveness of aerosol pentamidine for prevention of PCP in patients with AIDS. Twenty-Seventh Interscience Conference on Antimicrobial Agents and Chemotherapy. New York, NY: American Society for Microbiology; 1987:944. Abstract.
105. Gottlieb MS, Knight S, Mitsuyasu R et al. Prophylaxis of *Pneumocystis carinii* infection in AIDS with pyrimethamine-sulfadoxine. Lancet. 1984; 2:398–9. Letter.
106. Navin TR, Miller KD, Satriale RF et al. Adverse reactions associated with pyrimethamine-sulfadoxine prophylaxis for *Pneumocystis carinii* infections in AIDS. *Lancet.* 1985; 1:1332. Letter.
107. Fischl MA, Dickinson GM. Fansidar prophylaxis of pneumocystis pneumonia in the acquired immunodeficiency syndrome. *Ann Intern Med.* 1986; 105:629–30. Letter.

“

Treatment of Cytomegalovirus Disease in AIDS

. . . Cytomegalovirus retinitis, colitis, esophagitis, and gastritis are the commonest manifestations of severe cytomegalovirus end-organ disease. Extensive trials with intravenous ganciclovir, a nucleoside analogue with myelosuppressive toxicity, have shown that ganciclovir halts the progression of cytomegalovirus retinitis and gastrointestinal disease. Since relapse is common when therapy is discontinued, most patients with AIDS need life-long maintenance therapy. The clinical response to ganciclovir therapy is usually accompanied by diminished shedding of the virus. Based on limited data, foscarnet, a pyrophosphate analogue, also appears to have some efficacy in treating cytomegalovirus infection. Unlike ganciclovir, foscarnet does not cause myelosuppression. An important direction for future clinical research is the development of more effective and less toxic therapy, as well as orally bioavailable drugs for maintenance therapy.

—Jacobson MA, Mills J. Serious cytomegalovirus disease in the acquired immunodeficiency syndrome (AIDS). *Ann Intern Med.* 1988; 108:585–94.

”

Management of cryptococcal meningitis in patients with AIDS

JAN SAHAI

Abstract: A case of cryptococcal meningitis in a patient with the acquired immunodeficiency syndrome (AIDS) is described, as well as the epidemiology, pathogenesis, clinical manifestations, diagnosis, and therapeutic management of the disease.

In July 1987 a 38-year-old white man was admitted to the hospital because of confusion, disorientation, and headache. His medical history was notable for a positive human immunodeficiency virus test. Culture of the cerebrospinal fluid was positive for *Cryptococcus neoformans*. The patient was started on amphotericin B 16 mg/day (0.3 mg/kg/day) intravenously and flucytosine 2 g every six hours (150 mg/kg/day) orally. Despite premedication with diphenhydramine and acetaminophen, he experienced rigors that were treated with hydrocortisone and meperidine. Three weeks later he was discharged on flucytosine 2 g orally every six hours and amphotericin B 50 mg intravenously every other day. One week later the patient developed fever and chills; blood cultures were positive for methicillin-sensitive *Staphylococcus aureus*, and his peripheral leucocyte count was 1.8×10^3/cu mm. Flucytosine was discontinued, and he was treated with intravenous nafcillin while remaining on amphotericin B. In October the patient complained of nausea, vomiting, weakness, and agitation. A CSF latex agglutination titer for cryptococcal antigen was 1:32. He was treated with amphotericin B 50 mg daily until symptoms resolved and then continued on amphotericin B 50 mg twice weekly.

Cryptococcosis is the most common life-threatening fungal infection among AIDS patients. In contrast to immunocompetent hosts, this population invariably develops disseminated disease, with 85% having meningeal involvement. The most effective therapy for cryptococcal meningitis in patients with AIDS has not been established. Conventional therapy consists of amphotericin B and flucytosine. However, the bone-marrow-suppressive effects of flucytosine make administration of this drug difficult in AIDS patients. Because of the high relapse rates, maintenance therapy with amphotericin B is recommended. Relapse is associated with a mortality rate of 75–100%.

Therapeutic management of cryptococcal meningitis in patients with AIDS is problematic. Although many patients improve clinically during initial therapy with antifungal agents, cryptococcosis is difficult to eradicate.

Index terms: Acetaminophen; Acquired immunodeficiency syndrome; Amphotericin B; Antifungals; Combined therapy; Diphenhydramine; Dosage; Flucytosine; Hydrocortisone; Meningitis; Meperidine; Toxicity
Clin Pharm. 1988; 7:528–35

The acquired immunodeficiency syndrome (AIDS) results from infection with the human immunodeficiency virus (HIV),[1] originally designated as human T-cell lymphotropic virus type III (HTLV III)[2] and lymphadenopathy-associated virus (LAV).[3] The major defects associated with this syndrome are decreased numbers and abnormal function of CD4+ (T4+, or helper–inducer) T lymphocytes,[4] predisposing the patient to unusual neoplasms[5] and life-threatening opportunistic infections.[6,7] *Cryptococcus neoformans* is a virulent pathogen among patients with AIDS and is a common cause of meningitis in this population.[8-10] In this report I describe a patient with cryptococcal meningitis and discuss the epidemiology, pathogenesis, clinical manifestations, diagnosis, and therapy of the disease. The major focus is on the therapeutic management of cryptococcal meningitis; detailed reviews of agents used in the treatment of this disease have been published elsewhere.[11-15]

Case Report

On July 12, 1987, a 38-year-old white man was admitted to the Medical College of Virginia Hospitals because of confusion, disorientation, and headache. He had been well until one month earlier when he developed intermittent fever and a dull, constant headache that had progressively worsened during the two weeks before admission. Three days before admission the patient became anorexic, agitated, and confused. There were no reports of increased somnolence. The patient's medical history was notable for a positive HIV test (enzyme-linked immunosorbent assay) done two years before this admission. Social history was notable for homosexuality.

Physical examination revealed a thin, pale, white man who was alert but disoriented. Vital signs were as follows: blood pressure 130/76 mm Hg, pulse 80 per minute, respirations 20 per minute, and temperature 39.9 °C rectally. No cutaneous signs of rash or vasculitis were seen, and no lymphadenopathy was found. Examination of the head, ears, eyes, and nose was unremarkable. Scattered white plaques on the tongue and pharynx were

JAN SAHAI, PHARM.D., is ASHP Research and Education Foundation Fellow in Infectious Disease Pharmacotherapy, Antibiotic Research Unit, Department of Pharmacy and Pharmaceutics, Medical College of Virginia, Virginia Commonwealth University, P.O. Box 581, Richmond VA 23298-0581.

The assistance of Ronald Polk, Pharm.D., and Daniel Healy, Pharm.D., and the permission of Alison Berry, M.D., to report this case are acknowledged.

This is **article 680-204-8812** in the **ASHP Continuing Education System;** it qualifies for 1.0 hour of continuing-education credit. See page 553 for learning objectives and test questions.

Copyright © 1988, American Society of Hospital Pharmacists, Inc. All rights reserved. 0278-2677/88/0701-0528$02.00.

visible. The neck was supple. Lungs were clear on auscultation and percussion. Cardiac examination revealed a regular rate and rhythm with no murmurs, rubs, or gallops. The abdomen was relaxed and nontender, with normal bowel sounds; the liver and spleen were not felt. There was no peripheral edema, clubbing, or cyanosis, and articular examination was normal. Rectal examination was normal; a stool specimen gave a negative test for occult blood. Neurologic examination revealed fluctuating mental status. Cranial nerves II through XII, motor function, and sensation were intact. Tendon reflexes were ++ and equal; the plantar responses were flexor. Pulses were ++ throughout.

Chest roentgenogram revealed no apparent disease, and a computed axial tomography scan of the head showed no lesions or masses. Lumbar puncture showed an opening pressure of 20 cm of water with clear, colorless cerebrospinal fluid (CSF); 7 mL of CSF was obtained. CSF evaluation revealed a glucose of 63 mg/dL (serum glucose of 90 mg/dL), protein of 134 mg/dL, and a leukocyte count of 48/cu mm (40 lymphocytes, 8 polymorphonuclear leukocytes, and 2 monocytes). An India-ink test demonstrated many encapsulated budding yeast cells. A latex agglutination test for CSF cryptococcal antigen was positive (1:128). Culture of the CSF was positive for *C. neoformans*. Blood was not tested for antigen or cultured for the organism.

A Hickman catheter was inserted, and the patient was started on amphotericin B 16 mg/day (0.3 mg/kg/day) intravenously and flucytosine 2 g every six hours (150 mg/kg/day) orally. Despite premedication with diphenhydramine hydrochloride (50 mg orally) and acetaminophen (650 mg orally), he experienced rigors with amphotericin B infusion that subsequently resolved with administration of hydrocortisone (25 mg intravenously) and meperidine hydrochloride (50 mg intravenously). Three weeks later his mental status had returned to baseline, and a repeat lumbar puncture showed a decrease in cryptococcal antigen titer (1:16). The patient was discharged on daily oral flucytosine 2 g every six hours and amphotericin B 50 mg intravenously every other day.

One week after discharge, the patient came to the emergency room complaining of fever and chills. Blood cultures were positive for methicillin-sensitive *Staphylococcus aureus*. His peripheral leukocyte count had fallen to 1.8×10^3/cu mm (baseline 8.0×10^3/cu mm) and subsequently returned to normal 16 days after discontinuation of flucytosine. He was treated with intravenous nafcillin and remained on amphotericin B.

In October 1987, the patient returned to the emergency room complaining of nausea, vomiting, weakness, and agitation. A lumbar puncture was performed, which showed a CSF latex agglutination titer of 1:32 and a white blood cell count of 1/cu mm (one lymphocyte). The patient was treated with amphotericin B 50 mg daily with subsequent resolution of symptoms. After that he continued to receive amphotericin B 50 mg twice weekly.

Discussion

Etiology. The etiologic agent of cryptococcal meningitis, *Cryptococcus neoformans*, is an encapsulated yeast-like fungus.[16] The cell is spherical, usually 2–15 μm in diameter. The surrounding capsule may vary in size, depending on growth conditions.[17] Studies in mice indicate that size of the capsule is not related to virulence,[16] and there have been anecdotal reports of capsule-deficient *C. neoformans* causing infection in AIDS patients.[18]

Identification of the Organism. *C. neoformans* can be cultured in the clinical laboratory. The organism grows well on chocolate agar, Sabouraud's medium, and other fungal media, with smooth yellow or tan colonies appearing within four to seven days of inoculation.[17] Accuracy in identification is improved with greater volumes of CSF (10 to 40 mL)[19]; however, this is not usually practical in the clinical setting. The laboratory identification of *C. neoformans* is based on biochemical features of the organism. A rapid presumptive identification of the organism can be made within a few hours based on urease production[20] and the production of phenoloxidase.[19] The latter enzyme acts on certain substrates, such as caffeic acid and dihydroxyphenylalanine, to produce the brown pigment melanin.[21] There are four different serotypes of *C. neoformans:* A, B, C, and D.[22] Although these serotypes have different biochemical features and geographical distribution, it is unclear whether there is a difference in virulence.[16]

Epidemiology. *C. neoformans* is a ubiquitous organism and is frequently isolated from soil, pigeon feces, and other organic debris.[23,24] Animal-to-human and human-to-human transmission of the agent has not been described,[17,24] although there has been a case report of cryptococcal endophthalmitis resulting from a corneal transplant obtained from a donor who had active cryptococcosis.[25]

Accumulated epidemiologic data have placed cryptococcosis as the fourth most common opportunistic infection among patients with AIDS in the United States.[26,27] As in this patient, it may be the first clinical manifestation of the syndrome.[8–10,28,29] It is the most common life-threatening fungal infection, occurring in about 6–13% of patients with AIDS.[30–34] The mortality rate is 17–35% for the initial infection and increases to 75–100% in cases of relapse.[9,10]

Pathogenesis. *C. neoformans* is acquired by inhalation of the organism from environmental sources.[35,36] In most immunocompetent patients, the lesion is confined to the lung.[17,37] The organism produces no toxins and evokes only minimal tissue inflammatory response.[16,17,38] In cases of dissemination, large, focal collections of organisms may occur in the brain (cryptococcoma).[16] However, these are rare exceptions to the usual diffuse pattern of infection.[16]

Although human neutrophils and monocytes can ingest and kill cryptococci in vitro,[39] the polysaccharide capsule decreases the efficiency of phagocytosis by binding to the yeast surface and blocking recognition by phagocytes.[16] Efficient killing by macrophages requires an intact T-cell-mediated immune system.[39] Indeed, T lymphocytes as well as natural killer cells can directly inhibit growth of cryptococci in the absence of macrophages.[16] Several other studies[40–43] suggest that T-cell-dependent cellular immunity is an important defense mechanism against infection by *C. neoformans*. This hypothesis is supported by the predisposition to cryptococcal infection seen in patients with altered cell-mediated immunity, such as those with lymphoma[44–47] or sarcoidosis[48] or those receiving corticosteroids.[49–52] Patients with AIDS have a profound defect in cell-mediated immunity, and it is therefore not surprising that *C. neoformans* is an important pathogen in this population.

Although not tested in this patient, antibody to *C. neoformans* develops in approximately 50% of patients with cryptococcosis.[53] The exact role of antibody in containing the infection is not clear. In vitro studies have shown that anticryptococcal antibody does not appear to enhance phagocytosis of the organism.[39] However, antibody may enhance killing of large cryptococci by neutrophils and monocytes by a nonphagocytic mechanism.[40] The alternate complement pathway is thought to play a major role in opsonization of the organism, with the classical pathway allowing for optimal ingestion.[52,54]

The cryptococcal polysaccharide capsule may be immunosuppressive.[16] In humans, long after cure of cryptococcosis, patients often exhibit prolonged, specific immunologic (low titers of immunoglobulin G) unresponsiveness to cryptococcal polysaccharide.[16]

In contrast to immunocompetent hosts, patients with AIDS invariably develop disseminated disease, with 85% having meningeal involvement.[8–10] This was the case with the patient described here. Lung lesions in AIDS patients are often inapparent (as was true for this patient), suggesting that the current illness may be caused by reactivation of primary disseminated disease resulting from loss of T-cell-mediated immunity.[17] Several factors may account for persistence of *C. neoformans* in the central nervous system (CNS). The lack of complement on the surfaces of cryptococci recovered from infected CSF may contribute to the organisms' survival in the CNS.[52] Both serum and saliva have an anticryptococcal factor, whereas the CSF does not.[55] Furthermore, the growth of *C. neoformans* is supported in the rich nutritional medium of the CSF.[55]

Clinical Manifestations. Signs and symptoms of cryptococcal meningitis in patients with AIDS are presented in Table 1. These patients usually have typical signs and symptoms of meningitis (headache, nausea, vomiting, blurred vision, stiff neck), but the course is often more acute than that in non-AIDS patients.[56] However, some patients (as in this case report) have subtle, chronic symptoms (mild headache, personality changes, fever, confusion).[10] The duration of symptoms in the initial infection ranges from one day to four months, with a mean of 31 days; the duration of symptoms associated with relapse ranges from three days to three weeks, with a mean of 10 days.[9]

Headache (as seen in this patient) is often a prominent feature in AIDS and non-AIDS patients.[9,10] In patients with AIDS, it may begin several weeks before treatment is sought and increase in severity over time.[28] Fever is usually present[8–10,38]; however, it is infrequently one of the patient's major complaints.[28,57] Visual disturbances include blurred vision, diplopia, photophobia, and, rarely, blindness.[28] These complaints are often primary reasons for seeking treatment at a hospital.[28] Changes in mental status occur in about 20% of patients[8–10,28] but may also be due to CNS infection with HIV[58,59] or to adverse effects of drug therapy.[60] With respect to cranial nerve involvement, cranial nerve VI is most common.[28,57] Approximately 10–40% of AIDS patients with cryptococcal meningitis have no complaints referable to the CNS.[17,57] For this reason, the CSF should be examined whenever *C. neoformans* is isolated from any site.[17]

Diagnosis. The diagnosis of cryptococcosis can be made if characteristic yeast cells are found in body fluids.[19] The India-ink preparation is often used to identify the organism in the CSF.[19] However, because of the low sensitivity (60–72%), all negative India-ink tests should be confirmed by other tests such as latex agglutination and culture.[17,19] The India-ink test may remain positive for several months after successful treatment despite negative cultures.[57] In such cases, the latex agglutination test and culture of the organism should be used to confirm relapse of disease. Artifacts may be mistaken for cryptococci (false-positive result) when details of cell structure (doubly refractile cell wall, distinctly outlined capsule, and refractile inclusions in the cytoplasm) are ignored.[16]

When tissue specimens are obtained, *C. neofor-*

Table 1.
Frequency of Signs and Symptoms of Cryptococcal Meningitis in AIDS Patients[8–10,28]

Sign/Symptom	Incidence (%)
Fever	88
Headache	81–100
Nausea/vomiting	56
Malaise	38
Stiff neck	28–31
Photophobia	19–28
Mental status changes	19
Focal neurologic abnormalities	17
Seizures	8
Papilledema	5

mans may be seen in the histologic sections.[16] Methenamine silver or periodic acid–Schiff stains permit identification of the organism as a yeast that reproduces by formation of narrow-based buds.[16,17] *C. neoformans* may be distinguished from other fungi by Mayer's mucicarmine stain, which colors the cryptococcal capsule red but does not stain other fungi with similar morphologic characteristics.[16]

The serologic test of choice for the diagnosis of cryptococcosis is the latex agglutination test for antigen.[19] The test is sensitive (90%)[61] and highly specific (98.6%),[62] especially in cases of meningitis where the antigen is present in the CSF. However, low sensitivity of this test has been recently reported in a small number of non-AIDS patients.[63] False-positive results can occur in the presence of rheumatoid factor.[62] Use of reducing agents, such as mercaptoethanol, eliminates rheumatoid factor without affecting the ability to detect cryptococcal polysaccharide.[64] However, this test should always be verified by appropriate cultures for the fungus. The latex agglutination test is also helpful in the diagnosis of disseminated disease, in which case approximately 60% of patients have cryptococcal antigen in serum.[19] Patients with AIDS may have extraordinarily high serum titers, which may reflect a decreased ability of this population to eliminate the antigen.[8] At the present time, however, such a defect has not been identified.

It has been suggested that CSF titers of less than 1:8 are clinically unimportant[61]; however, many patients with documented cryptococcosis have titers of less than 1:8.[19] Thus, any titer should be considered important in predisposed patients having signs and symptoms consistent with cryptococcal disease.[19] Tests for anticryptococcal antibody are not recommended since this organism either fails to elicit an antibody response, or the response occurs too late during the course of illness to be of any value.[17]

The CSF findings in AIDS patients with cryptococcal meningitis are presented in Table 2. As seen in this patient, the CSF leukocyte count generally shows a predominance of lymphocytes.[8–10] However, many patients with AIDS have a leukocyte count of less than 20/cu mm.[9,10] About 60% of patients will have an increased opening pressure, elevated protein, and hypoglycorrhachia.[9,10] However, in up to 20% of patients with AIDS and cryptococcal meningitis CSF evaluation may be normal.[10,65] Therefore, it behooves the clinician to conduct tests specifically designed to detect *C. neoformans.*

Table 2.
Cerebrospinal Fluid (CSF) Findings in AIDS Patients with Cryptococcal Meningitis[8–10,28]

Finding	Incidence (%)
Positive CSF antigen	92
Positive CSF culture	92
Positive India-ink preparation	72
Leukocyte count of <20/cu mm	69
Glucose of <50 mg/dL	65
Opening pressure of >20 mm of water	62
Protein of >40 mg/dL	61

Cerebral computed axial tomography scans may show diffuse or local edema, cryptococcomas, or hydrocephalus.[57,66,67] However, as was the case with this patient, these conditions frequently are not found in patients with AIDS.[57]

Treatment. Patients with AIDS have an increased incidence of adverse reactions to many drugs,[68–70] and there is a danger of extrapolating data obtained from non-AIDS patients to this population. The most effective therapy for cryptococcal meningitis in patients with AIDS has not been established.

Amphotericin B Alone or with Flucytosine. Bennett et al.[71] conducted a prospective study in non-AIDS patients comparing six weeks of combination therapy consisting of amphotericin B (0.3 mg/kg/day) plus flucytosine (150 mg/kg/day) to eight weeks of amphotericin B alone (0.4 mg/kg/day for the first four weeks and 0.8 mg/kg/day for the second four weeks) for the treatment of cryptococcal meningitis. Of 24 patients, 16 (67%) were cured or improved clinically on combination therapy, compared with 11 of 27 (41%) treated with amphotericin B alone.

Although there was a trend favoring the combination, the difference was not statistically significant. The investigators concluded that combined flucytosine–amphotericin B therapy is the regimen of choice in cryptococcal meningitis.[71] Seven patients who experienced flucytosine toxicity subsequently improved or were cured with amphotericin B alone; these patients were excluded from the analysis.[17] In addition, the dose of amphotericin B may have been too low in the single-drug regimen to be curative. The question of whether combination therapy is equally efficacious as or less toxic than amphotericin B used in higher doses remains unanswered.

Although controlled trials have not been conducted in AIDS patients with cryptococcal meningitis, data generated from a small number of patients suggest that addition of flucytosine to a course of therapy with amphotericin B does not appreciably shorten the duration of therapy, does not alter the total amphotericin B dose administered, does not appear to have an important effect on patient relapse rate, and does not alter overall mortality.[9,10] In addition, flucytosine is difficult to administer to patients with AIDS because of its bone-marrow-suppressive[72] (as demonstrated in this patient) and gastrointestinal[73] adverse effects, which are often superimposed on symptoms caused by HIV.[74,75] However, Zuger et al.[9] were able to continue flucytosine until response or death in most of their patients.

Polsky et al.[76] conducted a retrospective study evaluating the use of intraventricular amphotericin B for the treatment of cryptococcal meningitis in non-AIDS patients. Death during therapy occurred in one of six patients who received intraventricular and systemic therapy and in six of seven patients who received systemic therapy alone. No major adverse effects were noted with intraventricular administration of amphotericin B. Although the data were retrospective, the authors suggested that early therapy that includes intraventricular amphotericin B may be beneficial and relatively safe in patients with cryptococcal meningitis and a poor prognosis. Preliminary data in patients with AIDS are not as encouraging. A limited number of AIDS patients have received intraventricular amphotericin B as part of the treatment regimen without therapeutic benefit.[9,10] The courses are often complicated by infection of the ventricular shunt and chemical arachnoiditis, consisting of fever, headache, and CSF pleocytosis. The adverse effects often necessitate premature discontinuation of intraventricular therapy.[9,10]

Therapy in full doses is typically continued for six weeks in patients who exhibit a prompt clinical response (decrease in cryptococcal antigen in the CSF, resolution of meningeal signs and symptoms).[9,10,56] In many cases, however, because of a lack of clinical improvement or persistently high levels of cryptococcal antigen in the CSF, therapy must be continued for longer periods of time.[9,10] Despite treatment the mortality rate resulting from cryptococcal meningitis in AIDS patients ranges from 17% to 35%,[9,10] and 25% of patients have persistently positive cultures.[10]

The types and incidence of adverse effects caused by amphotericin B in patients with AIDS have not been rigorously studied. Preliminary data suggest that adverse effects in this population are similar to those in non-AIDS patients.[9,10] These effects include infusion-related reactions (demonstrated in this patient), nephrotoxicity, and phlebitis. Although acetaminophen is widely used to premedicate non-AIDS patients receiving amphotericin B, many patients with AIDS and AIDS-related complex are being treated with zidovudine.[77] Since zidovudine and acetaminophen are both glucuronidated,[78] concomitant administration of both drugs may result in increased serum concentrations of zidovudine and increased hematologic toxicity.[79] Controlled studies are needed to evaluate other premedications that may be used to minimize infusion-related toxicities.

The rate of relapse of cryptococcal meningitis in AIDS patients ranges from 50% to 90%.[9,10] This is in contrast to non-AIDS patients, who have a relapse rate of 0% to 35%.[80-82] Zuger et al.[9] administered low weekly doses of amphotericin B (100 mg as a four-hour intravenous infusion) to seven AIDS patients who had responded initially to therapeutic doses of amphotericin B. This maintenance anticryptococcal therapy prevented relapse of infection in all seven patients, who were followed for nine months. This finding compared favorably with a historic control group of eight patients who received no maintenance treatment. Within six months, four patients from the latter group relapsed and died with active cryptococcal disease despite retreatment with amphotericin B. The type of study design used, the small number of patients, and brief period of follow-up do not allow firm conclusions to be made. However, it has become current practice to administer weekly maintenance doses of amphotericin B indefinitely to all AIDS patients with cryptococcal meningitis who have survived their first course of therapy.[56] The toxicity of such maintenance therapy has not been determined.

Imidazole Antifungal Agents. The efficacy of miconazole in treating cryptococcal meningitis has not been established. Because of miconazole's poor CSF penetration when given systemically, treatment of most fungal infections of the CNS require intrathecal administration.[83-86] In the murine model of cryptococcosis, miconazole was shown to have a delayed onset of antifungal activity compared with amphotericin B, and its antifungal activity was markedly inhibited by serum.[87] The clinical importance of these findings is currently unclear. Controlled, randomized trials are needed to define the role of miconazole in treating cryptococcal meningitis.

Limited data suggest that ketoconazole is not efficacious for the treatment of cryptococcal meningitis.[88] However, there is some evidence for synergy with amphotericin B in the animal model of disseminated cryptococcosis.[89] Further controlled, comparative studies are needed to define the role of ketoconazole in treating cryptococcal meningitis in patients with AIDS.

Oral Triazole Antifungal Agents. Fluconazole is an oral triazole antifungal agent that demonstrates good in vitro activity against *C. neoformans*.[90,91] In addition, this agent shows good penetration into the CSF in animals.[92] In an uncontrolled, open trial, Stern et al.[90] treated a small number of AIDS patients with fluconazole for cryptococcosis. The drug was effective in preventing relapses after the active disease was controlled with amphotericin B. However, the drug was not very effective in the doses used (50 to 100 mg per day) for the treatment of active cryptococcal disease. Adverse effects associated with fluconazole included an increase in hepatic function test values in one patient and seizures in another. These adverse effects necessitated discontinuation of the drug in both cases. A recent report described the successful use of fluconazole 150 mg/day in the treatment of cryptococcal meningitis in an AIDS patient who had not responded to initial therapy with amphotericin B.[93] Until more rigorous studies are conducted, the use of this drug cannot be recommended for the treatment of cryptococcosis in AIDS patients.

Itraconazole is another member of the triazole class of antifungal agents. Some benefit as maintenance therapy has been demonstrated.[94]

Studies investigating the efficacy of oral agents as maintenance therapy in patients who have initially responded to amphotericin B are under way.

Other Treatments. Transfer factor is a molecule contained in peripheral white blood cells that can transfer the immunologic competency of an individual to a nonimmunized person.[95] Administration of transfer factor has led to improvement in some non-AIDS patients with cryptococcal meningitis, but experience with this agent is limited.[95,96] In China, garlic has been used successfully for treatment of cryptococcal meningitis in non-AIDS patients.[97] I am unaware of widespread use of garlic for this indication in the United States.

Prognosis. In a study of 22 AIDS patients with cryptococcal meningitis, Zuger and associates[9] noted that the single factor most predictive of relapse was a CSF antigen titer of 1:8 or greater after treatment. However, since patients who relapsed were not maintained on amphotericin B, it is unclear whether this value is predictive of relapse in patients who continue to receive antifungal therapy. Several factors were found that predicted mortality.[9] A CSF cryptococcal antigen titer of 1:10,000 or greater was associated with a mortality rate of 100%, whereas titers less than 1:10,000 were associated with a mortality rate of 22%. However, Kovacs and associates[10] have reported the unreliability of the CSF cryptococcal antigen titer as a prognostic factor in patients with AIDS. Patients who had a relapse of cryptococcal meningitis similarly had a mortality rate of 100%.[9] In addition, patients who had a positive India-ink test at diagnosis had a significantly higher mortality rate than those with a negative test.[9]

Conclusion

The treatment of cryptococcal meningitis in patients with AIDS is problematic. Conventional therapy consisting of amphotericin B and flucytosine is complicated by the fact that AIDS patients cannot tolerate bone-marrow-suppressive drugs such as flucytosine. Furthermore, the available data suggest that the addition of flucytosine to amphotericin B therapy does not improve response. Although many patients improve clinically during initial therapy with antifungal agents, cryptococcosis is difficult to eradicate, resulting in high relapse rates. Accordingly, maintenance therapy with amphotericin B has been suggested to prevent relapse. New drugs have shown promising in vitro activity against *C. neoformans*, although it is clear that in vitro activity does not always predict in vivo efficacy. Widespread use of these agents must therefore be based on the results of well conducted clinical trials.

Discussion Questions

1. How do the signs and symptoms of cryptococcal meningitis differ between patients who have AIDS and those who do not?
2. Discuss the advantages and disadvantages of laboratory tests that are commonly used for identifying AIDS patients with cryptococcosis.
3. What are the advantages and disadvantages of adding flucytosine to amphotericin B in the initial management of an AIDS patient with cryptococcal meningitis?
4. Discuss the adverse effects of antifungal agents in patients with AIDS and cryptococcal meningitis. Which adverse effects are of particular concern in patients with AIDS?
5. What is the role of maintenance therapy in AIDS patients with cryptococcal meningitis who have initially responded to amphotericin B? What agents are being used or investigated for this indication?

References

1. Coffin J, Haase A, Levy JA et al. What to call the AIDS virus? *Nature.* 1986; 321:10.
2. Barre-Sinoussi F, Cherman JC, Rey F et al. Isolation of a T-lymphotropic retrovirus from a patient at risk for the acquired immune deficiency syndrome (AIDS). *Science.* 1983; 220:868–71.
3. Gallo RC, Salahuddin SZ, Popovich M et al. Frequent detection and isolation of cytopathic retroviruses (HTLV-III) from patients with AIDS and at risk for AIDS. *Science.* 1984; 224:500–3.
4. Fauci AS, Macher AM, Longo DL et al. Acquired immunodeficiency syndrome: epidemiologic, clinical, immunologic, and therapeutic considerations. *Ann Intern Med.* 1984; 100:92–106.
5. Groopman JE, Gottlieb MS. Kaposi's sarcoma: an oncologic looking glass. *Nature.* 1982; 299:103–4.
6. Gold JWM. Clinical spectrum of infections in patients with HTLV-III associated diseases. *Cancer Res.* 1985; 45:4652S–4654S.
7. Mildvan D, Mathur U, Enlow RW et al. Opportunistic infections and immunodeficiency in homosexual men. *Ann Intern Med.* 1982; 96 (Part 1):700–4.
8. Eng RHK, Bishburg E, Smith SM et al. Cryptococcal infections in patients with acquired immune deficiency syndrome. *Am J Med.* 1986; 81:19–23.
9. Zuger A, Louie E, Holzman RS et al. Cryptococcal disease in patients with the acquired immunodeficiency syndrome. *Ann Intern Med.* 1986; 104:234–40.
10. Kovacs JA, Kovacs AA, Polis M et al. Cryptococcosis in the acquired immunodeficiency syndrome. *Ann Intern Med.* 1985; 103:533–8.
11. Utz JP, Bennett JE, Brandriss MW et al. Amphotericin B toxicity. *Ann Intern Med.* 1964; 61:334–54.
12. Maddox MS, Barriere SL. A review of the complications of amphotericin B therapy: recommendations for prevention and management. *Drug Intell Clin Pharm.* 1980; 14:177–81.
13. Bennett JE. Flucytosine. *Ann Intern Med.* 1977; 86:319–22.
14. Graybill JR, Drutz DJ. Ketoconazole: a major innovation for treatment of fungal disease. *Ann Intern Med.* 1980; 93:921–3.

15. Sawyer PR, Brogden RN, Pinder RM et al. Miconazole: a review of its antifungal activity and therapeutic efficacy. *Drugs.* 1975; 9:406–23.
16. Diamond RD. *Cryptococcus neoformans.* In: Mandell GL, Douglas RG Jr, Bennett JE, eds. Principles and practice of infectious diseases. 2nd ed. New York: John Wiley & Sons; 1985:1460–8.
17. Sabetta JR, Andriole VT. Cryptococcal infection of the central nervous system. *Med Clin North Am.* 1985; 69:333–44.
18. Bottone EJ, Toma M, Johansson BE et al. Capsule-deficient *Cryptococcus neoformans* in AIDS patients. *Lancet.* 1985; 1:400.
19. Sarosi GA, Armstrong D, Davies SF et al. Laboratory diagnosis of mycotic and specific fungal infections. *Am Rev Respir Dis.* 1985; 132:1373–9.
20. Zimmer BL, Roberts GD. Rapid selection urease test for presumptive identification of *Cryptococcus neoformans. J. Clin Microbiol.* 1979; 10:380–1.
21. Rhodes JC, Polacheck I, Kwon-Chung KJ. Pheoloxidase activity and virulence in isogenic strains of *Cryptococcus neoformans. Infect Immun.* 1982; 36:1175–84.
22. Kaplan W, Bragg SL, Cune S et al. Serotyping *Cryptococcus neoformans* by immunofluorescence. *J Clin Microbiol.* 1981; 14:313–7.
23. Emmons CW. Saprophytic sources of *Cryptococcus neoformans* associated with the pigeon (*Columbia livia*). *Am J Hyg.* 1955; 62:227–32.
24. Litman ML, Walter JE. Cryptococcosis: current status. *Am J Med.* 1968; 45:922–32.
25. Beyt BE Jr, Waltman SR. Cryptococcal endopthalmitis after corneal transplantation. *N Engl J Med.* 1978; 298:825.
26. Fauci AS, Masur H, Gelmann EP et al. Acquired immunodeficiency syndrome: an update. *Ann Intern Med.* 1985; 102:800–13.
27. Masur H, Lane HC. The acquired immune deficiency syndrome. In: Remington JS, Swartz MN, eds. Current clinical topics in infectious disease. Vol. 6. New York: McGraw Hill; 1985:1–39.
28. Gibberson TP, Kalyan-Raman K. Cryptococcal meningitis: initial presentation of acquired immunodeficiency syndrome. *Ann Emerg Med.* 1987; 16:802–4.
29. Poon M, Cronin DC, Smith DA et al. Risk factors associated with primary cryptococcosis in AIDS patients residing in New York City. Paper presented to the 27th Interscience Conference on Antimicrobial Agents and Chemotherapy. Washington, DC:1987 Oct 6. Abstract 951.
30. Metroka CE, Cunningham-Rundles S, Pollack MS et al. Generalized lymphadenopathy in homosexual men. *Ann Intern Med.* 1983; 99:585–91.
31. Jaffe HW, Bregman DJ, Selik RK. Acquired immune deficiency syndrome in the United States. The first 1000 cases. *J Infect Dis.* 1983; 148:339–45.
32. Fauci AS, Macher AM, Longo DL et al. Acquired immune deficiency syndrome. *Ann Intern Med.* 1984; 100:92–106.
33. Reichert CM, O'Leary TJ, Levens DL et al. Autopsy pathology in the acquired immune deficiency syndrome. *Am J Pathol.* 1983; 112:357–82.
34. Welch K, Finkbeiner W, Alpers CE et al. Autopsy findings in the acquired immune deficiency syndrome. *JAMA.* 1984; 252:1152–9.
35. Neilson JB, Fromtling RA, Bulmer GS. *Cryptococcus neoformans:* size range of infectious particles from aerosolized soil. *Infect Immun.* 1977; 17:634–8.
36. Powell KE, Dahl BA, Weeks RJ et al. Airborne *Cryptococcus neoformans:* particles from pigeon excreta compatible with alveolar deposition. *J Infect Dis.* 1972; 125:412–5.
37. Duperval R, Hermans PE, Brewer NS et al. Cryptococcosis, with emphasis on the significance of isolation of *C. neoformans* from the respiratory tract. *Chest.* 1977; 72:13–19.
38. Anon. Case records of the Massachusetts General Hospital (case 41-1987). *N Engl J Med.* 1987; 317:946–53.
39. Diamond RD, Root RK, Bennett JE. Factors influencing killing of *Cryptococcus neoformans* by human leucocytes in vitro. *J Infect Dis.* 1972; 125:367–76.
40. Diamond RD, Allison AC. Nature of the effector cells responsible for antibody-dependent cell-mediated killing of *Cryptococcus neoformans. Infect Immun.* 1976; 14:716–20.
41. Schimpff SC, Bennett JE. Abnormalities in cell mediated immunity in patients with *Cryptococcus neoformans* infection. *J Allergy Clin Immunol.* 1975; 55:430–44.
42. Fung PYS, Murphy JW. In vitro interactions of immune lymphocytes and *Cryptococcus neoformans. Infect Immunol.* 1982; 36:1128–38.
43. Murphy JW, McDaniel DO. In vitro reactivity of natural killer (NK) cells against *Cryptococcus neoformans. J Immunol.* 1982; 128:1577–83.
44. Young RC, Bennett JE, Geelhoed GW et al. Fungemia with compromised host resistance—a study of 70 cases. *Ann Intern Med.* 1974; 80:605–12.
45. Hooper DC, Pruitt AA, Rubin RH. Central nervous system infection in the chronically immunosuppressed. *Medicine.* 1982; 61:166–88.
46. Kaplan MH, Rosen PP, Armstrong D. Cryptococcosis in a cancer hospital—clinical and pathologic correlates in forty-six patients. *Cancer.* 1977; 39:2265–74.
47. Lewis JL, Rabinovich S. The wide spectrum of cryptococcal infections. *Am J Med.* 1972; 53:315–22.
48. Schimpff SC, Bennett JE. Abnormalities in cell-mediated immunity in patients with *Cryptococcus neoformans* infection. *J Allergy Clin Immunol.* 1975; 55:430–41.
49. Wilson TS, Fleming WA, Robinson FLJ et al. Cryptococcal meningitis associated with steroid therapy. *J Clin Pathol.* 1970; 23:657–63.
50. Salaki JS, Louria DB, Chmel H. Fungal and yeast infections of the central nervous system. *Medicine.* 1984; 63:108–32.
51. Perfect JR, Durack DT, Gallis HA. Cryptococcemia. *Medicine.* 1983; 62:98–109.
52. Diamond RD, May JE, Kane MA et al. The role of the classical and alternate complement pathways in host defenses against *Cryptococcus neoformans* infection. *J Immunol.* 1974; 112:2260–70.
53. Diamond RD, Bennett JE. Prognostic factors in cryptococcal meningitis: a study in 111 cases. *Ann Intern Med.* 1974; 80:176–81.
54. Bobak DA, Washburn RG, Frank MM. Complement subcomponent C1q enhances the phagocytosis and killing of *Cryptococcus neoformans* blastospores by human monocytes. Paper presented to the 27th Interscience Conference on Antimicrobial Agents and Chemotherapy. Washington, DC: 1987 Oct 6. Abstract 586.
55. Ingel HJ, Bolande RP. Humoral defense mechanisms in cryptococcosis: substances in normal human serum, saliva, and cerebrospinal fluid affecting growth of *Cryptococcus neoformans. J Infect Dis.* 1966; 116:75–83.
56. Holmberg K, Meyer RD. Fungal infections in patients with AIDS and AIDS-related complex. *Scand J Infect Dis.* 1986; 18:179–92.
57. Tjia TL, Geow YK, Tan CB. Cryptococcal meningitis. *J Neurol Neurosurg Psychiatry.* 1985; 48:853–8.
58. Koenig S, Gendelman HE, Ornstein JM et al. Detection of AIDS virus in macrophages in brain tissue from AIDS patients with encephalopathy. *Science.* 1986; 233:1089–93.
59. Schrier RD, Nelson JA, Lampert PW et al. Cellular localization of human immunodeficiency virus within the brains of AIDS patients. *Proc Natl Acad Sci USA.* 1986; 83:7089–93.
60. Bach MC. Possible drug interaction during therapy with azidothymidine and acyclovir for AIDS. *N Engl J Med.* 1987; 316:547.
61. Snow RM, Dismukes WE. Cryptococcal meningitis—diagnostic value of cryptococcal antigen in cerebrospinal fluid. *Arch Intern Med.* 1975; 135:1155–7.
62. Stockman L, Roberts GD. Specificity of the latex test for cryptococcal antigen: a rapid, simple method for eliminating interfering factors. *J Clin Microbiol.* 1983; 17:945–7.
63. Cook P. Poor predictive value of the latex agglutination test for cryptococcal antigen in the management of renal transplant patients with cryptococcal infection. Paper presented

to the 27th Interscience Conference on Antimicrobial Agents and Chemotherapy. Washington, DC: 1987 Oct 6. Abstract 970.
64. Gordon MA, Lapa EW. Elimination of rheumatoid factor in the latex test from cryptococcosis. *Am J Clin Pathol.* 1974; 61:488–94.
65. Larsen RA, Leal ME, Evans S. *Cryptococcus neoformans* meningitis in patients with AIDS: lack of CSF abnormalities. Paper presented to the 27th Interscience Conference on Antimicrobial Agents and Chemotherapy. Washington, DC: 1987 Oct 6. Abstract 952.
66. DeWytt CN, Dickson PL, Holt GW. Cryptococcal meningitis: a review of 32 years experience. *J Neurol Sci.* 1982; 53:283–92.
67. Post MJD, Kursunoglu SJ, Hemsley GT et al. Cranial CT in acquired immunodeficiency syndrome—spectrum of diseases and optimal contrast enhancement technique. *Am J Roentgenol.* 1985; 145:929–40.
68. Greenberger PA, Patterson R. Management of drug allergy in patients with acquired immunodeficiency syndrome. *J Allergy Clin Immunol.* 1987; 79:484–8.
69. Gordin FM, Simon GL, Wofsky CB et al. Adverse reactions to trimethoprim-sulfamethoxazole in patients with acquired immunodeficiency syndrome. *Ann Intern Med.* 1984; 100:495–9.
70. Pearson RD, Hewlett EL. Pentamidine for the treatment of *Pneumocystis carinii* pneumonia and other protozoal diseases. *Ann Intern Med.* 1985; 103:782–6.
71. Bennett JE, Dismukes WE, Duma RJ et al. A comparison of amphotericin B alone and combined with flucytosine in the treatment of cryptococcal meningitis. *N Engl J Med.* 1979; 301:126–31.
72. Kauffman CA, Frame PT. Bone marrow toxicity associated with 5-flucytosine therapy. *Antimicrob Agents Chemother.* 1977; 11:244–7.
73. Dismukes WE, Cloud G, Gallis MA et al. Treatment of cryptococcal meningitis with combination amphotericin B and flucytosine for four as compared with six weeks. *N Engl J Med.* 1987; 317:334–41.
74. Donahue RE, Johnson MM, Zon LI et al. Suppression of in vitro haematopoiesis following human immunodeficiency virus infection. *Nature.* 1987; 326:200–3.
75. Kotler DP, Gaetz HP, Lange M et al. Enteropathy associated with the acquired immunodeficiency syndrome. *Ann Intern Med.* 1984; 101:421–8.
76. Polsky B, Depman MR, Gold JWM et al. Intraventricular therapy of cryptococcal meningitis via a subcutaneous reservoir. *Am J Med.* 1986; 81:24–8.
77. Fischl MA, Richman DD, Grieco MH et al. The efficacy of azidothymidine (AZT) in the treatment of patients with AIDS and AIDS-related complex. *N Engl J Med.* 1987; 371:185–91.
78. Anon. Azidothymidine (AZT) for AIDS. *Med Lett Drugs Ther.* 1986; 28:107–9.
79. Richman DD, Fischl MA, Grieco MH et al. The toxicity of azidothymidine (AZT) in the treatment of patients with AIDS and AIDS-related complex. *N Engl J Med.* 1987; 317:192–7.
80. Utz JP, Garriques IL, Sande ML et al. Therapy of cryptococcosis with a combination of flucytosine and amphotericin B. *J Infect Dis.* 1975; 132:368–73.
81. Diamond RD, Bennett JE. A subcutaneous reservoir for intrathecal therapy of fungal meningitis. *N Engl J Med.* 1973; 288:186–8.
82. Butler WT, Alling DW, Spickard A et al. Diagnostic and prognostic value of clinical and laboratory findings in cryptococcal meningitis. *N Engl J Med.* 1964; 270:59–67.
83. Bell WE. Treatment of fungal infections of the central nervous system. *Ann Neurol.* 1981; 9:417–22.
84. Sung JP, Campbell GD, Grendahl JC. Miconazole therapy for fungal meningitis. *Arch Neurol.* 1978; 35:443–7.
85. Deresinski SC, Lilly RB, Levine HB et al. Treatment of fungal meningitis with miconazole. *Arch Intern Med.* 1977; 137:1180–5.
86. Weinstein L, Jacoby I. Successful treatment of cerebral cryptococcoma and meningitis with miconazole. *Ann Intern Med.* 1980; 93:569–71.
87. Graybill JR, Mitchell L, Levine HB. Treatment of experimental murine cryptococcosis: a comparison of miconazole and amphotericin B. *Antimicrob Agents Chemother.* 1978; 13:277–83.
88. Perfect JR, Durack DT, Hamilton JD et al. Failure of ketoconazole in cryptococcal meningitis. *JAMA.* 1982; 247:3349–51.
89. Graybill JR, Williams DM, VanCutsan E et al. Combination therapy of experimental histoplasmosis and cryptococcosis with amphotericin B and ketoconazole. *Rev Infect Dis.* 1980; 2:551–8.
90. Stern J, Sharkey K, Hartman B et al. Fluconazole therapy in AIDS patients with cryptococcosis. Paper presented to the 27th Interscience Conference on Antimicrobial Agents and Chemotherapy. Washington, DC: 1987 Oct 6. Abstract 948.
91. Farrow PR, Brammer KW, Feczko JM. Fluconazole: a new treatment for oropharyngeal candidiasis in AIDS and malignancy. Paper presented to the 27th Interscience Conference on Antimicrobial Agents and Chemotherapy. Washington, DC: 1987 Oct 6. Abstract 949.
92. Perfect JR, Durack DT. Penetration of imidazoles and triazoles into the cerebrospinal fluid of rabbits. *J Antimicrob Chemother.* 1985; 16:81–6.
93. Byrne WR, Wajszczuk CP. Cryptococcal meningitis in the acquired immunodeficiency syndrome: successful treatment with fluconazole after failure of amphotericin B. *Ann Intern Med.* 1988; 108:384–5.
94. DeGans J, Schatternack JKM, VanKetel RJ. Itraconazole as maintenance treatment for cryptococcal meningitis in the acquired immunodeficiency syndrome. *Br Med J.* 1988; 296:339.
95. Conrad R, Lerner W. The use of transfer factor in a patient with chronic cryptococcal meningitis. *Clin Res.* 1973; 21:596.
96. Gross PA, Patel C, Spitler LE. Disseminated cryptococcosis treated with transfer factor. *JAMA.* 1978; 240:2460–2.
97. Anon. Garlic in cryptococcal meningitis: a preliminary report of 21 cases. *Chin Med J [Engl].* 1980; 93:123–6.

Parenteral nutrition in the management of gastrointestinal Kaposi's sarcoma in a patient with AIDS

DOUGLAS D. JANSON AND KATHLEEN M. TEASLEY

Abstract: A patient with acquired immunodeficiency syndrome (AIDS) who required aggressive nutritional intervention via home parenteral nutrition therapy is described, and nutritional status, etiology and therapeutic management of AIDS-associated malnutrition, role of nutrition support, and factors for consideration in using parenteral nutrition in AIDS patients are discussed.

Parenteral nutrition therapy was initiated in a 30-year-old AIDS patient with Kaposi's sarcoma lesions of the gastrointestinal tract because of rapid weight loss, low serum protein levels, and malnutrition. He had previously undergone a small-bowel resection and a jejunojejunostomy, and radiation and antineoplastic-drug therapy was planned. During parenteral nutrition therapy, the patient demonstrated increased physical strength and was able to care for himself during most of the time spent at home or in a long-term-care facility. Aggressive measures, including parenteral nutrition therapy, were discontinued 11 days before the patient's death. Complications of therapy included one episode of sepsis and a tear in the external catheter tubing.

Malabsorption and diarrhea mainly caused by gastrointestinal disease, reduced food intake because of oral and esophageal infections, adverse effects from medication, and depression are factors that can contribute to AIDS-associated malnutrition. Also, hypermetabolism resulting from infections and fevers may contribute to malnutrition in AIDS. The extent to which this malnutrition affects the underlying immune dysfunction occurring in the syndrome and the response to other more direct drug therapies in AIDS is not known. Available methods for nutritional intervention are based on clinical experience and anecdotal reports. Because of gastrointestinal disease, an oral diet, supplements, and enteral tube feedings may not meet nutritional goals for an AIDS patient.

In patients with AIDS who have protein–calorie malnutrition, parenteral nutrition support is an available treatment alternative. Continued research is needed to clarify the role of nutritional maintenance and restoration in AIDS.

Index terms: Acquired immunodeficiency syndrome; Health care; Nutrition; Sarcoma
Clin Pharm. 1988: 7:536–44

Severe weight loss and cachexia frequently develop during the course of acquired immunodeficiency syndrome (AIDS). Nutritional management of AIDS-associated malnutrition is a challenging problem. Home parenteral nutrition support has been recognized as a therapeutic modality in the management of malnutrition in AIDS patients with AIDS-associated enteropathy,[1] such as persistent gastrointestinal *Cryptosporidium* infection.[2,3]

Another potential candidate for parenteral nutrition support is the AIDS patient afflicted with complications from Kaposi's sarcoma (KS) of the gastrointestinal (GI) tract. KS, reported as the first sign of AIDS in approximately 30% of cases, is an aggressive multifocal neoplastic disease that involves the skin, mucosal surfaces, and lymph nodes. Systemic symptoms of the AIDS patient with KS include fever, weight loss, malaise, anorexia, and diarrhea.[4] Approximately 40% of AIDS patients with KS have been reported to have gastrointestinal lesions based on endoscopy of the upper GI tract and flexible fiber sigmoidoscopy.[5] Infrequent complications of gastrointestinal KS include obstruction and hemorrhage. In general, patients with AIDS who have KS have a better prognosis than those who have opportunistic infections, since KS can be easily treated and controlled with antineoplastic drugs and radiation therapy.[4]

In addition to a case report describing the use of parenteral nutrition support in an AIDS patient with gastrointestinal KS, this article reviews the medical literature that describes the nutritional status of AIDS patients and the etiology of AIDS-associated malnutrition. Also presented are factors that should be considered when parenteral nutrition is used as a therapeutic modality in AIDS-associated malnutrition.

Case Report

The Nutrition Support Service of the University of

DOUGLAS D. JANSON, PHARM.D., is Clinical Specialist in Nutrition Support, University of Minnesota Hospital and Clinic, and was a 1987–88 ASHP Research and Education Foundation Fellow in Nutrition Support, College of Pharmacy, University of Minnesota, Minneapolis. KATHLEEN M. TEASLEY, M.S., is Associate Professor, College of Pharmacy, University of Minnesota, and Director, Pharmacy Nutrition Support Service, University of Minnesota Hospital and Clinic.

Address reprint requests to Dr. Janson at Pharmaceutical Services, University of Minnesota Hospital and Clinic, Box 611, Harvard Street at East River Road, Minneapolis, MN 55455.

The contribution of Frank S. Rhame, M.D., as the patient's primary physician is acknowledged.

Presented at the 22nd Annual ASHP Midyear Clinical Meeting, Atlanta, GA, December 9, 1987.

Copyright © 1988, American Society of Hospital Pharmacists, Inc. All rights reserved. 0002-9289/88/0701-0536$02.25.

Minnesota Hospital and Clinic (UMHC) was consulted on April 9, 1987, to initiate home parenteral nutrition in a 30-year-old homosexual man who had positive results from a human immunodeficiency virus (HIV) test in October 1986. He also had KS lesions of the esophagus, jejunum, and rectum. Six days previously (April 3), he had undergone a 30-cm small-bowel resection, a jejuno-jejunostomy, and a biopsy of mesenteric lymph nodes at UMHC.

The patient initially came to UMHC in February 1985 because of viral dermatitis of the neck, trunk, and extremities. In June 1985, a lesion on the lower lip was diagnosed as *Verruca vulgaris*. The patient had furuncles on both thighs and the suprapubic and lower abdominal areas, as well as lymphadenopathy involving bilateral inguinal, bilateral axillary, and left cervical nodes in May 1986. AIDS was diagnosed in early November, when results of a bronchoscopy revealed *Pneumocystis carinii* and cytomegalovirus (CMV). The patient also was treated for oral candidiasis and perianal *Herpes simplex*. After the patient recovered from *Pneumocystis carinii* pneumonia (PCP), oral zidovudine therapy (200 mg every four hours) was initiated in early December 1986.

At this time, a lesion was found in the patient's right posterior nasopharynx that was believed to be KS. Because of intermittent nausea, decreased appetite, and stomach upset after eating, along with a hemoglobin concentration of 8.2 g/dL, the zidovudine dosage was decreased by one half. The patient reported less nausea and increased ability to eat. However, in early February 1987, he complained of upper midline chest pain, which increased in intensity with swallowing. During March, the month before admission, he experienced intermittent dysphagia with solids and liquids and occasionally vomited undigested food after swallowing. For two weeks before admission, he had been constipated. An esophagogastroduodenoscopy done on March 18, 1987, revealed a large vascular-appearing lesion involving 15 cm of mid-to-distal esophagus. Biopsy specimens of the esophageal lesion and the rectum showed a variant of KS. On April 1, 1987, a barium swallow test revealed a partial obstruction of the proximal jejunum. The patient was admitted to UMHC the next day, and surgery was performed on April 3.

Nutritional Assessment before Initiation of Therapy. During the course of this patient's HIV infection and other opportunistic infections (November 1987 to March 1988), he maintained a relatively constant weight at 89–94% reference weight for height based on Metropolitan Life Insurance Tables, 1959 (Table 1). For two to three months before surgery, the patient ingested an oral liquid dietary supplement (Ensure Plus, Ross Laboratories, Columbus, Ohio), which provided an estimated 1065–1420 calories and 39–52 g of protein per day. When his vomiting increased as a result of gastrointestinal KS, the patient had difficulty ingesting the supplement.

The result of a preoperative D-xylose test done on March 18, 1987, to determine whether malabsorption existed was 5.5 g per specimen (normal range, 5.0–8.5 g per specimen). Severe mixed protein–calorie malnutrition had developed by the time nutrition support was sought, six days postoperatively. The patient had lost 7.6 kg (11% of body weight) over the previous three weeks. Visceral proteins (albumin and transferrin) were substantially depleted over this period. Because of the patient's weight loss, low serum protein levels, and moderately malnourished state, as well as impending radiation and antineoplastic-drug therapy for esophageal KS, aggressive nutritional intervention was indicated. At this time, the patient still experienced occasional nausea and was able to ingest water, juices, and carbonated beverages; he was willing to ingest an oral supplement. Home parenteral nutrition was selected as a more desirable mode for nutrition support than enteral tube feeding (gastrostomy or jejunostomy) because of the presence of KS in the gastrointestinal tract. Also, because of the vascularity of KS lesions, enteral tube feeding could place the patient at risk for hemorrhage. Further, the establishment of central venous access for parenteral nutrition administration would facilitate antineoplastic-drug infusions and blood transfusions, if needed.

A double-lumen catheter was placed via a subcutaneous tunnel to obtain long-term central venous access for daily administration of parenteral nutrition therapy. A regimen formulated to meet both maintenance and restorative goals was initiated on April 11, 1987 (Table 2). Using the actual body weight of 60 kg, the estimated daily calories were approximately 2753–3146 based on

Table 1.
Nutritional Indicators before Initiation of Nutrition Therapy[a]

Date, Event	Weight (kg)	Albumin (g/dL)	Transferrin (mg/dL)	Total Protein (g/dL)
11/6/86: PCP[b] diagnosed	64.2	2.6	170	6.1
3/18/87: Endoscopy and biopsy; zidovudine stopped	67.7	2.5	203	4.8
4/8/87: Fourth postoperative day[c]	60.1	1.4	106	...

[a] The patient's height was 177.8 cm; his ideal body weight was 72 kg based on Metropolitan Life Insurance Table, 1959; and his usual body weight was 67 kg (i.e., when his health was good).
[b] *Pneumocystis carinii* pneumonia.
[c] The patient's preoperative weight (on 4/3/87) was 61.6 kg.

Table 2.
Parenteral Nutrition Regimen[a]

Component	Amount
Amino acids	126 g/day (2.1 g/kg/day)
Dextrose	360 g/day
Sodium chloride	63 meq/day
Potassium acetate	41 meq/day
Magnesium sulfate	29 meq/day
Potassium phosphate	27 mmol/day
Calcium gluconate	9 meq/day
Trace elements (Con Te Pak-4, SoloPak)	1 mL/day
Vitamins (M.V.C. 9+3 Injection, LyphoMed)	10 mL/day
Phytonadione	10 mg/wk
Zinc sulfate	15 mg/day
Lipid emulsion, 20%	500 mL/day

[a] Total calories per day were 2728 (175% of basal energy expenditure). The ratio of nonprotein calories to grams of nitrogen was 111:1. The percentage of total daily calories as fat was 37%. Dextrose–amino acid solution was administered as a cyclic infusion at a rate of 145 mL/hr for 12 hours and 60 mL/hr for 1 hour.

175–200% basal energy expenditure (BEE). Estimated protein need was 120 g of protein per day based on 2 g per kilogram of actual body weight per day. The majority of the patient's daily calorie and protein needs were met by the parenteral regimen, with the rest being met by ingested food and liquid dietary supplements as tolerated. Home parenteral nutrition training was initiated while the patient was hospitalized, and before discharge, the patient and his companion were observed for competency.

Clinical Course. Palliative radiation, 3000 rads in 15 fractions, as given from April 14 to May 6, and monthly antineoplastic therapy with etoposide, 150 mg/sq m for three consecutive days, was initiated on May 13. Radiation therapy was interrupted for several days when the patient was hospitalized on April 28 for sepsis caused by staphylococcal infection of the central venous catheter. The infection necessitated removal of the catheter and replacement with a single-lumen catheter. On May 25, 10 days after the initial course of etoposide therapy, the patient was hospitalized for fevers and hypotension. The next day, a bronchoscopy revealed PCP, which resolved with antimicrobial therapy.

The response of the esophageal tumor to radiation and antineoplastic-drug therapy was described as excellent based on the results of an upper GI endoscopy and a barium swallow test done in late June. However, by early July the patient began to sense increased fullness in his oropharynx, which caused choking and vomiting. Supraclavicular adenopathy and increasing back pain attributable to retroperitoneal lymph-node involvement was becoming more apparent, in addition to worsening KS lesions in the posterior oropharynx. Radiation therapy was reinitiated to the oropharyngeal area on July 30. By mid-August approximately one half of the total dose of radiation had been given; however, therapy was discontinued because of vocal cord irritation. Antineoplastic therapy was reinitiated on August 20 with vinblastine.

The patient was hospitalized from August 23 to 27 because of clumsiness and mental status changes, which were attributed to overmedication with morphine and diazepam by the patient at home. Also, *Clostridium difficile* toxin identified in the stool was treated. Three days after discharge, the external tubing of the patient's central venous catheter, which had been torn by needle puncture, was repaired in the emergency room. The patient was readmitted on September 7 because of increased diarrhea, weakness, and an inability to administer pain medication appropriately. The patient was discharged to a long-term-care facility on September 30 because of continued weakness and the amount of nursing care needed. However, with assistance from home health nursing, a Minnesota AIDS Project volunteer, and his companion, the patient was able to spend 29 days during November and December at his home. Parenteral nutrition continued as a part of this patient's regimen for a total of 250 days. During the course of parenteral nutrition, the patient spent 130 days at home, 73 days hospitalized, and 44 days in a long-term-care facility.

Disseminated KS continued to worsen. On December 15, the patient was admitted to UMHC for progressive confusion, pallor, and epistaxis. At this time, the patient and his companion desired only comfort measures, such as intravenous hydration and pain medication. Parenteral nutrition support was discontinued on December 17. The patient died on December 28, 1987.

Summary of Home Parenteral Nutrition Course

From the initiation of parenteral nutrition in April until September, nitrogen balances were zero or positive; visceral proteins were maintained in the lower range of normal limits; weight initially decreased, then gradually increased; and electrolyte and mineral status remained relatively sta-

Table 3.
Nutritional Data during Parenteral Nutrition (PN)[a]

Item	4/13	4/21	5/12	6/1	7/7	8/3	9/3	9/13	10/22	11/9	11/25
PN day no.	3	11	32	51	87	114	145	155	194	212	226
Wt (kg)	57.6	61.5	58.2	58.4	61.7	63.7	65.5	63.0	69.7	68.3	71.5
Albumin (g/dL)	1.9	2.9	3.1	1.8	3.3	3.4	2.8	2.6	2.0	2.2	2.2
Transferrin (mg/dL)	170	250	219	171	216	205	185	200	157	161	132
Magnesium (meq/L)	1.5	1.5	1.8	1.6	1.8	1.2	1.3	1.7	1.6	1.6	1.6
Phosphorus (mg/dL)	3.3	4.8	3.8	5.2	4.2	4.1	4.5	3.9	4.1	4.7	4.1
Calcium (mg/dL)	8.0	9.0	9.6	8.5	9.1	8.7	8.6	8.5	7.9	7.8	7.8
Zinc (μg/dL)	58		76			113	116		114		97
Nitrogen balance[b]		0	+2	+3	1	+4		0	−2[c]	−1	
UCr (mg/24 hours)[d]		1297	1200	1147	972	895		1168		1053	
% Expected UCr/24 hr[e]		81	75	72	61	56		73		66	
Triglyceride (mg/dL)		115	109	247[f]				119		175	300
Alkaline phosphatase (IU/L)	679	819	644	1960		841[g]	1057	791	937	874	888
AST[h] (IU/L)	33	25	32	91	25	29	41	42		43	
Total bilirubin (mg/dL)	0.3	0.5	0.3	0.7			0.6	0.5	0.8		

[a] All dates were in 1987.
[b] Based on urinary urea nitrogen.
[c] Nitrogen balance evaluated on 11/2/87.
[d] UCr = urinary creatinine.
[e] Based on Metropolitan Life Insurance Table, 1959.
[f] Serum drawn one hour after completion of lipid infusion.
[g] Serum drawn 7/28/87.
[h] AST = aspartate aminotransferase.

ble (Table 3). The patient demonstrated increased physical strength and was able to care for himself during the majority of this time spent at home on parenteral nutrition therapy. Use of total nutrient admixtures (three-in-one solutions) was initiated at home in early May to provide convenience for the patient. By early July, as the KS progressed to the oropharynx, all intake by mouth, including fluids, had severely diminished. At this time, an additional hydration infusion of 0.5–1 L was initiated as needed to prevent dehydration. Except for some fluid intake, the patient ingested essentially no liquid dietary supplement or food for the rest of his life. Selenium 100 μg/day was empirically added to the parenteral regimen in August because (1) the patient was not eating, (2) there was no selenium supplementation in the original parenteral formula, and (3) selenium deficiency has been reported in AIDS patients.[6] This selenium dosage has been used successfully to reverse deficiency symptoms in adult patients without AIDS who are being fed parenterally. Except for an occasional day of noncompliance, the patient received the regimen described in Table 2 through mid-October, therefore receiving 2728 calories (175% of BEE) and 126 g of protein daily (2.1 g/kg/day).

After September, nitrogen balances were negative, visceral proteins decreased, and the patient's weight dramatically increased (Table 3). The clinical instability exhibited after September may have contributed to the decrease in visceral proteins and negative nitrogen balances. Also, a dilutional effect resulting from edema may have lowered the level of visceral proteins. The increase in weight was primarily due to edema as a result of progressive KS involving the lymphatic system. An increase in body mass may have contributed to the weight gain. As a response, a mild diuresis and decrease in parenteral calories was initiated in mid-October. The daily parenteral calories were empirically decreased to 2238 calories per day (140% of BEE based on a weight of 63 kg) by decreasing the dextrose concentration to 12% (120 g/L) in the parenteral solution. No adjustment was made in the nitrogen content of the regimen. In early November, an indirect calorimetric assessment, measuring the resting energy expenditure (REE), was performed on the patient to more accurately determine the daily caloric requirement. The average steady-state REE was 2285 calories per day, or 140% of BEE compared with estimated requirements. No further caloric changes were made in the nutritional support regimen.

During the course of parenteral nutrition therapy, the patient exhibited changes in serum alkaline phosphatase (Table 3). In early June, during trimethoprim–sulfamethoxazole therapy for PCP, the alkaline phosphatase concentration increased to 2970 IU/L (normal range, 100–350 IU/L). This increase was attributed to the trimethoprim–sulfamethoxazole; therefore, pentamidine therapy was initiated as an alternative to PCP treatment. To what extent the nutritional support regimen caused an elevation in alkaline phosphatase is not known. A decrease in caloric support in mid-October did not cause any noticeable change in the serum alkaline phosphatase level.

As the patients's KS progressed, he became more anxious and depressed. A source of anxiety was his progressive inability to eat or drink and his dependency on intravenous therapy. However, maintenance of his nutritional status with home parenteral nutrition did alleviate his anxiety and concerns about progressive weight loss and cachexia. Catheter-related complications, sepsis, and a tear in the external tubing transiently added to his anxiety.

Nutritional Status in AIDS

"AIDS emaciation" describes the severe weight loss and cachexia, often unrelenting, that frequently accompany the clinical course of the syndrome. In some patients, weight loss may precede the development of opportunistic infections and cancers that point to a diagnosis of AIDS. No significant correlation between weight loss and disease duration has been observed.[6,7] An investigation of the long-term effect of AIDS on body composition revealed that a progressive depletion in body potassium and body cell mass is a common feature in AIDS patients.[8] Although weight maintenance has not been shown to increase survival time in AIDS patients, weight loss has been correlated with a poor prognosis in patients with KS.[7] Overall, there are limited data available that characterize the nutritional disorders of AIDS.

Estimates of the magnitude of weight loss in AIDS patients are variable. The percentage of ideal body weight of 13 AIDS patients was found to be significantly lower (80 ± 3%) compared with that of 11 homosexual controls (101 ± 5%).[9] Similarly, another group of AIDS patients was significantly underweight compared with the homosexual and laboratory control groups (82 ± 10, 101 ± 7, and 103 ± 6% of ideal body weight, respectively).[8] The mean (±S.D.) weight loss observed in 22 AIDS patients being evaluated for gastrointestinal manifestations of AIDS was 34 ± 10 pounds.[7] The weight loss in 20 AIDS patients with chronic diarrhea ranged from 5 to 32%, with a mean (±S.D.) of 14 ± 7.9%.[10] Body cell mass depletion, determined by measuring total body potassium/height and other indicators of body composition, was significantly lower in 15 AIDS patients with diarrhea than in 18 AIDS patients without diarrhea (62 ± 9 versus 74 ± 9% of normal total body potassium/height). Several AIDS patients with chronic diarrhea have been reported to have both marked malnutrition and a short survival in spite of aggressive management.[8]

Depletion of visceral protein has been reported

to occur in AIDS patients. Serum concentrations of albumin and retinol-binding protein and iron-binding capacities were significantly lower in AIDS patients than in controls.[8] Significantly lower serum albumin concentrations were reported in AIDS patients with diarrhea (2.2 ± 0.4 g/dL) than those without diarrhea (3.3 ± 0.2 g/dL).[9] However, in another study, in which diarrhea was significantly more prevalent in the group with documented infections (90%) than in the group without infection (25%), mean serum albumin concentrations were similar between both groups (3.3 ± 0.7 versus 3.4 ± 0.9 g/dL, respectively).[7] No significant correlation between serum albumin and disease duration has been observed.[6]

Decreased serum zinc concentrations and decreased concentrations of plasma and red blood cell selenium have been reported in AIDS patients. In one study, AIDS patients with chronic diarrhea had low or borderline zinc concentrations.[10] Mean (±S.D.) plasma selenium concentrations have also been shown to be significantly lower in AIDS patients (0.043 ± 0.01 μg/mL) than in controls (0.095 ± 0.016 μg/mL).[6] The exact cause of diminished blood selenium levels is not known, and its occurrence was independent of the presence or absence of malabsorption or disease duration.

Etiology of AIDS-Associated Malnutrition

Malabsorption and reduced food intake are two major factors that contribute to AIDS-associated malnutrition. Hypermetabolism, as a result of infection and fevers, may also contribute to malnutrition in AIDS.

Malabsorption. Malabsorption may occur because of mucosal abnormalities of the gastrointestinal tract and diarrhea caused by infectious agents, AIDS enteropathy in which no infectious agent is identified, and neoplasia.

The gastrointestinal tract is a major target organ in AIDS. Diarrhea and malabsorption frequently occur, both acutely and chronically, as a result of gastrointestinal opportunistic infections. Malabsorption based on clinical and quantitative laboratory evidence has been shown to accompany prominent gastrointestinal infections with parasites such as *Cryptosporidium, Isospora, Microsporidia,*[11,12] and *Mycobacterium avium–intracellulare*.[12,13] Malabsorption has been observed to be more prevalent in AIDS patients when gastrointestinal pathogens were identified.[7] *Cryptosporidium* can cause an intractable, profuse, secretory diarrhea that may last for months and often becomes a contributing factor in the death of AIDS patients. Diarrhea also manifests as a result of infection with cytomegalovirus, a common pathogen of the alimentary tract of AIDS patients; however, to what extent malabsorption occurs is not known.

Homosexuals with AIDS also may have diarrhea in association with the enteric bacterial pathogens *Shigella, Salmonella,* and *Campylobacter,* and occasionally *Entamoeba histolytica. Giardia lamblia* is frequently identified as a pathogen in homosexual men, causing diarrhea and malabsorption.[14] Drug therapy, often consisting of multiple drug regimens, used to treat the aforementioned pathogens is often unsuccessful in controlling or eradicating the infection. Furthermore, antibiotic therapy may also cause diarrhea, thereby increasing the difficulty of treating it.

In addition to infectious agents causing diarrhea and malabsorption in AIDS, many patients experience diarrhea and weight loss with no pathogens being identified.[7,9,10,14] The combination of malabsorption, steatorrhea, and nonspecific mucosal abnormalities based on the results of small-bowel biopsy, without identifiable infectious agent(s) or neoplasm, has been referred to as AIDS enteropathy.[9] Mucosal abnormalities and malabsorption (AIDS enteropathy) occurred more often in symptomatic AIDS patients—those with diarrhea and weight loss—than in asymptomatic patients.[9,10] Chronic diarrhea, malabsorption, and weight loss may be due to immunologic abnormalities predisposing the upper small intestine to colonization by bacteria that are not usually identified as pathogens.[15] Abnormal T-lymphocyte populations in the duodenal mucosa, which are similar to the abnormalities seen in the blood, have been reported in AIDS patients.[15,16] In AIDS patients who develop diarrhea for which no causative organism can be identified, Brinson[17] suggests that hypoalbuminemia should be considered as a possible etiology.

A theoretical cause of malabsorption in the AIDS patient is malnutrition itself. Malnutrition can lead to malabsorption. An unfed gastrointestinal tract can result in alterations in the gastrointestinal enzymes and in the structure of the villi, which may severely impede the absorption of nutrients. Malabsorption owing to malnutrition has been shown to be reversible by appropriate nutritional support in patients without AIDS.[18]

Gastrointestinal KS, reported to occur in 40% of AIDS patients who have KS, may also contribute to the malabsorption and diarrhea seen in the AIDS patient. Gastrointestinal KS in AIDS patients is reported to be rarely symptomatic; however, it remains to be determined whether more prominent manifestations of KS in the gastrointestinal tract might arise if improvements in therapy allow patients to survive longer.[5] Clinical and laboratory evidence of substantial malabsorption[19] and protein-losing enteropathy[20,21] accompanying KS has been reported in non-AIDS patients. Perhaps gastrointestinal complications as a result of KS, such as hemorrhage or obstruction requiring small-bowel resection, may contribute to malabsorption more frequently than protein-losing enteropathy.

Reduced Food Intake. Reduced food intake is

another major factor that leads to AIDS-associated malnutrition. Infection of several regions of the alimentary tract with herpes virus, cytomegalovirus, and *Candida albicans* may contribute to diminished oral intake. Oral and esophageal candidiasis is the most prevalent gastrointestinal infection in AIDS, causing dysphagia and odynophagia.[14] Herpetic esophagitis, cytomegalovirus esophagitis, and gastritis can also cause nausea and vomiting. Vomiting can occur as a result of KS lesions of the oropharyngeal and oral–esophageal region.

Diminished food intake can occur as an adverse effect of drug therapy. Both oral and intravenous drug therapy used to treat the numerous infections or neoplastic diseases in the AIDS patient can frequently produce gastrointestinal adverse effects such as nausea, vomiting, stomach pain, anorexia, and diarrhea. Fevers can also exacerbate anorexia.

Psychological (depression and anxiety) and neurological (encephalopathy and dementia) complications that can occur in AIDS patients[22] can threaten adequate nutritional intake.

Hypermetabolism. AIDS-associated malnutrition may be attributed to hypermetabolism as a result of infections and fevers. A pattern of wasting similar to that seen in stressed conditions such as sepsis, trauma, or surgery has been observed in AIDS patients.[8] The hypermetabolic state induced by sepsis is well documented and characterized.[23] In septic patients who do not have AIDS, muscle mass can rapidly disappear in a matter of days as a result of hypermetabolism, particularly if nutritional support is not a part of the clinical care regimen.[23] No information currently exists on the level of metabolic stress or energy requirement of the AIDS patient with or without sepsis.

Potential Role of Nutrition Support in AIDS

Similarities can be drawn between patients with recurrent, incurable cancers and patients with AIDS. For many cancer patients, loss of appetite, weight loss, and negative body image are primary means by which the disease threatens their sense of self and autonomy.[24] This also applies to the AIDS patient in whom each new symptom, infection, loss of weight, or fatigue is regarded as a sign of disease progression.[22] Parenteral or enteral nutrition support may affect morbidity and mortality attributable to malnutrition that develops as a result of the cancer or treatment and may substantially improve the quality of life in cancer patients.[25,26] An improvement in the quality of life demonstrated by increased physical strength, self-care status, decreased anxiety about disease cachexia, and a greater sense of psychosocial well-being may be realistic goals of aggressive nutrition support in some AIDS patients.

The extent of immune-system impairment and specific clinical problems varies among AIDS patients. These variations appear to affect the degree to which nutritional therapy can restore or even maintain nutritional integrity. In addition, the extent of protein–calorie malnutrition that exists before the initiation of aggressive nutrition support appears to affect the outcome of such therapy in an AIDS patient. It is not known whether aggressive nutritional intervention initiated before extensive weight loss and malnutrition occur can prevent or substantially retard the development of malnutrition and related physiologic impairment. At this time, we can only speculate on the cost-effectiveness of early intervention.

Other questions remain unanswered regarding the importance of nutritional status as it relates to AIDS. A major area of interest is the effect of AIDS-associated malnutrition on the underlying immunologic dysfunction occurring in the syndrome. HIV preferentially infects the T4 helper lymphocyte, causing both quantitative and qualitative abnormalities.[27] Malnutrition has been shown to alter both local factors that furnish barriers to invasion and mobile defenses of systemic resistance. Malnutrition impairs local resistance by disturbing epithelial structures, and thus abolishing the efficiency of cellular barriers, and by lowering secretory-immunoglobulin levels.[28] The effects of malnutrition on systemic resistance are most pronounced in the T-lymphocytes, with decreased numbers of T4 helper cells, poor primary and recall delayed cutaneous hypersensitivity responses, and depressed proliferation.[28,29] Several of the bacterial, viral, parasitic, and fungal infections identified by Chandra[30] as being influenced by nutritional status are commonly seen in AIDS. Obviously, the primary defect causing these opportunistic infections is the HIV infecting the T4 helper lymphocyte population; however, nutritional status may affect an AIDS patient's immune function. It is not known whether restoration of nutritional status can improve an AIDS patient's resistance to the environment nor what the importance of proper nutritional status is in achieving a favorable response to other more direct therapies in AIDS.[31]

It is possible that AIDS-associated malnutrition can alter the pharmacokinetic and pharmacodynamic responses to current drug therapies and future therapies used to halt viral replication, boost immune response, and treat opportunistic infections. For example, overhydration of the body by an increase in total body water and loss of body cell mass has been reported to occur because of AIDS-associated malnutrition.[8] Malnutrition, by altering the total body water, body composition, and drug binding, can lead to changes in the volume of distribution of a drug, depending on its physicochemical properties and its ability to bind to macromolecules. Also, the risk of susceptibility to drug toxicity may be increased because of malnutrition.[32] The effect of AIDS-associated malnutrition on the pharmacokinetic and pharmacodynamic responses to specific drug therapies are not known.

Therapeutic Management of AIDS-Associated Malnutrition

Limited information exists on how to effectively support the AIDS patient nutritionally. Hence, the available methods for nutritional intervention are based on clinical experience and anecdotal reports.[2,3,17,33]

Identifying the clinical status is an important factor in determining the nutritional status of any patient. Kotler[31] separates AIDS patients into two groups, clinically stable and clinically unstable. Clinically unstable patients often have active infectious complications. In such patients, poor intake, elevated metabolic rate, intestinal dysfunction with malabsorption, and protein exudation all may be present and contribute to progressive wasting. Clinically stable AIDS patients are relatively asymptomatic; their food intake appears normal, they have no signs of intestinal disease, and they may return to full employment.

Most AIDS patients will suffer from malnutrition and its associated morbidity and mortality. Therefore, evaluation of nutritional status and appropriate intervention should be addressed in the clinically stable patient and the unstable patient. Generally, weight loss is greater in the clinically unstable patient. The rate at which the loss occurs is also important, since rapid weight loss tends to be more detrimental than gradual changes in weight. A rapid weight loss often indicates a high degree of metabolic stress or a diet that is markedly deficient in calories, which is probably associated with inadequate intake of other essential nutrients.[34]

Caloric requirements can be estimated or measured directly. The estimated basal energy expenditure (BEE) can be determined by using the Harris–Benedict equation and multiplying by an appropriate factor based on repletion needs and metabolic stress. Indirect calorimetry, which measures the resting energy expenditure (REE), is another method of determining the caloric requirement. No data are currently available describing the energy requirements of AIDS patients as measured by indirect calorimetry.

In April 1987, we assessed the patient described in the case report as clinically unstable and estimated that an energy intake of at least 175% of BEE would be needed to meet repletion needs in the setting of an increased metabolic rate. The rapid rate at which weight was lost (11% lost in three weeks) led us to believe that in addition to a decreased oral intake, the patient's metabolic rate was increased because of the KS, febrile episodes, or both. Unfortunately, we were not able to obtain an indirect calorimetric measurement when home parenteral nutrition therapy was initiated. The indirect calorimetric measurement done in early November 1987 did reveal an elevation in metabolic rate, since the average steady-state REE was 140% of BEE and average steady-state oxygen consumption ($\dot{V}O_2$) was 170 mL/min/sq m (adult, normal range $\dot{V}O_2 = 90 \pm 10$ mL/min/sq m). When indirect calorimetry was performed, the patient had *Herpes simplex* proctitis, cellulitis of two digits on the right hand, and occasional fevers in addition to disseminated KS.

We estimated protein requirements based on the degree of metabolic stress and renal and hepatic function. Protein requirements may be higher in the clinically unstable patient to achieve a positive nitrogen balance. Nitrogen balances (Table 3), evaluated monthly, helped to validate the protein dosage (2.1 g/kg/day) given to our patient. Electrolyte, mineral, and trace element requirements are greatly increased in the AIDS patient with copious diarrhea.

Clinical experience suggests that an oral diet, even with high protein–calorie supplements, is rarely effective in meeting the nutritional needs of the AIDS patient with anorexia, nausea, dysphagia, malabsorption, and diarrhea. Before our patient developed gastrointestinal obstruction and the esophageal tumor, he received a liquid dietary supplement to help maintain a relatively constant weight and moderate protein stores (Table 1). Occasionally, an AIDS patient with low-volume diarrhea or documented steatorrhea may respond to dietary therapy; a low-fiber, lactose-free diet along with antidiarrheal agents or a low-fiber, low-fat, lactose-free diet has been used.[33] Selected AIDS patients may also respond to enteral feedings using a hydrolyzed, monomeric formula.[17] In general, because of gastrointestinal disease or intolerance, enteral feeding does not appear to be effective as a long-term method of nutritional support in AIDS.

In our opinion, parenteral nutrition is often the best method of support when intractable diarrhea, malabsorption, or gastrointestinal complications of Kaposi's sarcoma exists. As an AIDS patient continues to receive aggressive medical treatment for inhibiting viral replication, opportunistic infections, and neoplastic diseases, proper nutrition support should be incorporated in the treatment regimen. Peripheral parenteral nutrition can be used as a short-term supplement for orally or enterally fed patients during hospitalization. Central venous parenteral nutrition can generally supply the total nutrient and hydration needs of AIDS patients either in the hospital or at home. The potential risk of sepsis related to the central venous catheter in an immunocompromised AIDS patient is a valid concern. Data on the rate of catheter-related sepsis in AIDS are not available.

Home Parenteral Nutrition Support in AIDS

The decision to initiate home parenteral nutrition in a patient with AIDS requires the deliberation and consultation of all members of the health-care team and, most important, the participation of the patient. Careful attention must be given to patient-selection criteria for successful management of home parenteral nutrition in AIDS. Crucial issues to assess are the psychological status of the patient and the availability of a support system, the home environment, the ability of the patient to be trained and the patient's knowledge of the disease, and financial resources for such therapy. The potential risks and benefits need to be clearly presented and discussed with the patient and a designated caregiver, often a family member or companion. The patient must be motivated to go home with parenteral nutrition as a part of the daily routine. General guidelines for caring for AIDS patients at home have been identified to preserve a satisfactory quality of life for the patient and provide safety for the caregivers and family.[3] These guidelines can be incorporated into the home parenteral training program initiated in the hospital. Because of the often complex psychosocial and emotional issues surrounding this devastating illness, in which the patient progressively loses the ability to control his or her life, a multidisciplinary nutrition-support team can effectively provide a smooth transition from the hospital to the home. Generally, in patients with non-AIDS-related diseases who use home parenteral nutrition, the professional and technical support coordinated by a multidisciplinary clinical team is largely responsible for the success and low morbidity associated with this treatment modality.[35,36]

Home parenteral nutrition is usually not affordable without adequate insurance coverage or third-party reimbursement. In 1986, the estimated annual cost of such therapy to a patient was approximately $70,000.[37] Home parenteral nutrition may improve the quality of life in selected AIDS patients who cannot otherwise maintain a reasonably normal nutritional status. The effect of aggressive nutrition support on survival time is not known.

Conclusion

Persons with AIDS are at high risk for developing protein–calorie malnutrition caused by malabsorption and reduced food intake; hypermetabolism resulting from infections and fevers may be a contributory factor. The extent to which AIDS-associated malnutrition affects the underlying immune dysfunction occurring in the syndrome and the response of other more direct drug therapies in AIDS is not known. Continued research is needed to clarify the role of nutritional maintenance and restoration in AIDS.

Discussion Questions

1. What conditions can place AIDS patients at high risk for developing protein–calorie malnutrition?
2. Develop a treatment plan for managing progressive malnutrition in an AIDS patient. How would you assess the patient's nutritional status and estimate nutritional requirements? What factors would be important in determining nutrient composition and route of administration? How should therapy be monitored?
3. How might the nutritional status of an AIDS patient affect response to other forms of therapy?

References

1. American Society of Parenteral and Enteral Nutrition Board of Directors. Guidelines for use of total parenteral nutrition. *J Parenter Enter Nutr.* 1987; 11:342–4.
2. Domaldo TL, Natividad LS. Nutrition management of a patient with AIDS and cryptosporidium infection. *Nutr Support Serv.* 1986; 6(Apr):30–1.
3. Worthington P. Home TPN for the patient with AIDS. *Nutr Support Serv.* 1987; 7(Feb):37–8.
4. Safai B, Johnson KG, Myskowski PL et al. The natural history of Kaposi's sarcoma in the acquired immunodeficiency syndrome. *Ann Intern Med.* 1985; 103:742–50.
5. Friedman SL, Wright TL, Altman DF. Gastrointestinal Kaposi's sarcoma in patients with acquired immunodeficiency syndrome. *Gastroenterology.* 1985; 89:102–8.
6. Dworkin BM, Rosenthal WS, Wormser GP et al. Selenium deficiency in the acquired immunodeficiency syndrome. *J Parenter Enter Nutr.* 1986; 10:405–7.
7. Dworkin BM, Wormser GP, Rosenthal WS et al. Gastrointestinal manifestations of the acquired immunodeficiency syndrome: a review of 22 cases. *Am J Gastroenterol.* 1985; 80:774–8.
8. Kotler DP, Wang J, Pierson RN. Body composition studies in patients with the acquired immunodeficiency syndrome. *Am J Clin Nutr.* 1985; 42:1255–65.
9. Kotler DP, Gaetz HP, Lange M et al. Enteropathy associated with the acquired immunodeficiency syndrome. *Ann Intern Med.* 1985; 101:421–8.
10. Gillin JS, Shike M, Alcock N et al. Malabsorption and mucosal abnormalities of the small intestine in the acquired immune deficiency syndrome. *Ann Intern Med.* 1985; 102:619–22.
11. Modigliani R, Bories C, LeCharpentier Y et al. Diarrhea and malabsorption in acquired immune deficiency syndrome: a study of four cases with special emphasis on opportunistic protozoan infestations. *Gut.* 1985; 26:179–87.
12. Quinn TC. Clinical approach to intestinal infections in homosexual men. *Med Clin North Am.* 1986; 70:611–34.
13. Roth RI, Owen RL, Keren DF et al. Intestinal infection with *Myocobacterium avium* in acquired immune deficiency syndrome (AIDS)—histological and clinical comparison with Whipple's disease. *Dig Dis Sci.* 1985; 30:497–504.
14. Gelb A, Miller S. AIDS and gastroenterology. *Am J Gastroenterol.* 1986; 81:619–22.
15. Budhraja M, Levendoglu H, Kocka F et al. Abnormalities of duodenal mucosal T cells and bacterial cultures in acquired immune deficiency syndrome (AIDS). *Am J Gastroenterol.* 1986; 81:864.
16. Rodgers VD, Fassett R, Kagnoff MF. Abnormalities in intestinal mucosal T cells in homosexual populations including those with the lymphadenopathy syndrome and acquired immunodeficiency syndrome. *Gastroenterology.* 1986; 90:552–8.
17. Brinson BR. Hypoalbuminemia, diarrhea, and the acquired immunodeficiency syndrome. *Ann Intern Med.* 1985; 102:413.
18. Pimparker BD, Donde UM, Ambegaonkar SE et al. Malnutrition and malabsorption. *Am J Gastroenterol.* 1977; 67:580–8.
19. Bryk D, Farman J, Dalleman S et al. Kaposi's sarcoma of the

intestinal tract: roentgen manifestations. *Gastrointest Radiol.* 1978; 3:426–30.
20. Novis BH, King H, Bank S. Kaposi's sarcoma presenting with diarrhea and protein losing enteropathy. *Gastroenterology.* 1974; 67:996–1000.
21. Perrone V, Pergoal M, Abate G et al. Protein-losing enteropathy in a patient with generalized Kaposi's sarcoma. *Cancer.* 1981; 47:588–91.
22. Holland JC, Tross S. The psychosocial and neuropsychiatric sequelae of the acquired immunodeficiency syndrome and related disorders. *Ann Intern Med.* 1985; 103:760–4.
23. Cerra FB. Hypermetabolism, organ failure and metabolic support. *Surgery.* 1987; 101:1–13.
24. Peteet JR, Medeiros C, Slavin L et al. Psychological aspects of artificial feeding in cancer patients. *J Parenter Enter Nutr.* 1981; 5:138–40.
25. Weiss SM, Worthington PH, Prioleau M et al. Home parenteral nutrition in cancer patients. *Cancer.* 1982; 50:1210–3.
26. Teasley KT, Shronts EP, Lysne J et al. Nutritional/metabolic support: parenteral and enteral. In: Higby DJ, ed. Supportive care in cancer therapy. Boston: Martinus Nijhoff; 1983: 93–123.
27. Fauci AS, Masur H, Gelmann EP et al. The acquired immunodeficiency syndrome: an update. *Ann Intern Med.* 1985; 102:800–13.
28. Kahan BD. Nutrition and host defense mechanisms. *Surg Clin North Am.* 1981; 61:557–70.
29. Chandra RK, Gupta S, Singh H. Inducer and suppressor T cell subsets in protein-energy malnutrition: analysis by monoclonal antibodies. *Nutr Res.* 1982; 2:21–6.
30. Chandra RK. Nutrition, immunity and infection: present knowledge and future directions. *Lancet.* 1983; 1:688–91.
31. Kotler DP. Why study nutrition in AIDS? *Nutr Clin Pract.* 1987; 2:94–5.
32. Krishnawamy K. Drug metabolism and pharmacokinetics in malnutrition. *Clin Pharmacokinet.* 1978; 3:216–40.
33. Garcia ME, Collins CL, Mansell PWA. The acquired immune deficiency syndrome: nutritional complications and assessment of body weight status. *Nutr Clin Pract.* 1987; 2:108–11.
34. MacBurney M, Wilmore DW. Rational decision-making in nutritional care. *Surg Clin North Am.* 1981; 61:571–82.
35. Robinovitch AE. Home total parenteral nutrition: a psychosocial viewpoint. *J Parenter Enter Nutr.* 1981; 5:522–5.
36. Wesley JR. Home parenteral nutrition: indications, principles, and cost-effectiveness. *Compr Ther.* 1983; 9:29–36.
37. Rucker BB. The home drug delivery industry: an outlook. San Francisco, CA: Habrecht and Quist Incorporated; 1987.

"

Treatment of *Mycobacterium avium* Infection

The decision to treat *Mycobacterium avium* infection should be based on the physician's perception of whether it is a terminal complication of an inexorably progressive immunodeficiency state or whether the rapid and aggressive treatment of this opportunistic infection can provide the patient with an improved quality of life. . . .

. . . Inasmuch as AIDS is an immunodeficiency status that predisposes to this infection, one might postulate that ultimate control of *M. avium* infection will be related not only to the development and application of effective chemotherapeutic strategies but also to some efforts at restoring immune competence. Thus, attempts to deliver medications to the intracellular sites of infection, such as the use of liposome-encapsulated antibiotics, the use of antibiotics that penetrate phagocytic cells efficiently, and finally, the use of immunomodulators that can activate intracellular microbicidal mechanisms, represent combination approaches that appear to offer the best hope for the eventual control of this important systemic infection in patients with AIDS.

—Young LS. *Mycobacterium avium* complex infection. *J Infect Dis.* 1988; 157:863–7.

"

Treatment of nontuberculous mycobacterial infections in pediatric patients

ROBERT H. LEVIN AND ANN M. BOLINGER

Abstract: Two cases of *Mycobacterium avium-intracellulare* complex (MAC) infections are described, and the diagnosis, clinical features, and management of MAC infections are reviewed.

In case 1, a four-year-old boy was diagnosed as having both acquired immunodeficiency syndrome (AIDS) and disseminated MAC infection. He was treated with a combination of isoniazid, ethambutol hydrochloride, rifabutin, and clofazimine. Results of susceptibility testing showed that the MAC was susceptible to rifabutin and ethambutol with intermediate susceptibility to isoniazid. The child developed severe adverse effects that necessitated the discontinuation of rifabutin therapy. Despite therapy, blood cultures remained positive for MAC. The child died of disseminated human immunodeficiency virus and MAC infection. In case 2, a 20-month-old girl was found to have a prevertebral retropharyngeal mass caused by MAC. The child did not have evidence of immunologic deficiency. She was treated with streptomycin, ethambutol, clofazimine, and rifabutin. Streptomycin was discontinued after three months. After seven months the mass decreased in size, allowing for surgical resection. Intraoperative cultures were negative for mycobacteria. Ethambutol, rifabutin, and clofazimine were continued for a total of 12 months, at which time the child was determined to be clinically and radiologically cured.

Empiric multidrug antituberculous therapy should be initiated in patients with suspected disseminated nontuberculous mycobacterial infection because final isolation, identification, and susceptibility testing may take several weeks. Clofazimine and rifabutin, in combination with isoniazid and ethambutol, may be useful in the treatment of some MAC infections. At least four drugs are given, and regimens often consist of six drugs. However, long-term remission has not been reported for most patients with disseminated disease who have been treated with the currently recommended drugs. Since drug therapy is associated with many adverse effects, further studies are necessary to determine the most effective and least toxic regimen. Surgical resection of localized MAC infections often results in a good long-term prognosis.

These case studies illustrate the poor prognosis of a disseminated MAC infection in an AIDS patient and the relatively good prognosis of a localized infection in a patient not testing positive for the human immunodeficiency virus.

Index terms: Acquired immunodeficiency syndrome; Antituberculars; Clofazimine; Combined therapy; Ethambutol hydrochloride; Isoniazid; Mycobacterium infections; Pediatrics; Rifabutin; Streptomycin
Clin Pharm. 1988; 7:545–51

Mycobacterium avium–intracellulare complex (MAC; also abbreviated as MAI), which includes the atypical organisms *M. avium* and *M. intracellulare,* has been recognized as a cause of severe, disseminating disease in adult patients with acquired immunodeficiency syndrome (AIDS).[1] The atypical organisms are classified as a complex because they resemble each other closely. Although the organisms can be separated in the laboratory, serotyping is not generally available. Differentiation may be useful for epidemiologic review but is not usually helpful in the general management of infected patients. MAC is a common environmental contaminant, present in dust, dirt, fresh water, ocean water, and animal feed. It has also been identified in birds, eggs, dairy products, and meat.[2]

MAC infections appear to be more common in AIDS patients than in immunocompetent patients and in other immunocompromised patients.[3] Infections that occur in patients who do not have AIDS are usually uncomplicated, not disseminated, and often cured by surgical excision. However, in AIDS patients, MAC infections are typically disseminated and can occur in all organs including the bone marrow, lymph nodes, lungs, liver, spleen, bowel, skin, kidneys, and brain. In children, MAC infections most commonly affect the cervical lymph nodes.[4] The infections are often fatal, with evidence found only at postmortem examination.[5]

Before 1980, only 14 cases of disseminated MAC infections were reported, and these cases occurred primarily in men with chronic lung disease.[6] Many states do not require nontuberculous mycobacte-

ROBERT H. LEVIN, PHARM.D., is Clinical Professor, Division of Clinical Pharmacy, School of Pharmacy, University of California, San Francisco, and Coordinator of Clinical Pharmacy Services, San Francisco General Hospital. ANN M. BOLINGER, PHARM.D., is Assistant Clinical Professor, Division of Clinical Pharmacy, School of Pharmacy, University of California, San Francisco.

Address reprint requests to Dr. Levin at San Francisco General Hospital, Building 30, Room 3221, 1001 Potrero Avenue, San Francisco, CA 94110.

Peggy S. Weintraub, M.D., and Moses Grossman, M.D., were the principal physicians for case 1 and case 2, respectively. The editing and typing assistance of Lena Libatique and Lisa Crane also is acknowledged.

Presented in part at the 22nd Annual ASHP Midyear Clinical Meeting, Atlanta, GA, December 9, 1987.

Copyright © 1988, American Society of Hospital Pharmacists, Inc. All rights reserved. 0278-2677/88/0701-0545$01.75.

rial infections to be reported; therefore, it is difficult to determine the actual prevalence of MAC infections. However, nontuberculous mycobacterial infections have been diagnosed with increasing frequency over the last several years.[6] In 1985, the morbidity associated with tuberculosis did not continue to decline as it had over the last 32 years.[7] There was also an increase in the number of tuberculosis cases reported in the United States in 1986.[7] These changes have been attributed to the occurrence of tuberculosis among patients with AIDS. A total of 1214 pediatric patients were reported to have tuberculosis in 1986. It is not known how many of these children have AIDS or how many of the infections might have been caused by MAC.

Immunosuppression is a predisposing factor for developing opportunistic infections. Pulmonary involvement of opportunistic infections occurs frequently in pediatric AIDS patients. The two most common manifestations are pulmonary lymphoid hyperplasia secondary to previous infection with Epstein–Barr virus or infection with *Pneumocystis carinii*.[8] Cytomegalovirus and *Candida albicans* can also cause pulmonary infections in children who have AIDS, but these infections occur less often.[9,10] Pulmonary tuberculosis in patients infected with human immunodeficiency virus (HIV) is difficult to distinguish from other pulmonary infections on the basis of clinical and roentgenographic findings.[8] Although a tuberculin skin test should be administered, the immunosuppression associated with AIDS may cause the test to exhibit false-negative results.

The documentation of MAC infections in AIDS patients has brought more attention to the problem. Unfortunately, MAC infections respond poorly to therapy. The organism is resistant to many of the antimicrobial agents used in the treatment of *M. tuberculosis* infections. We report two cases of MAC infection in pediatric patients and review the information available regarding the treatment of MAC infection in AIDS patients.

Case Reports

Case 1. A four-year-old white boy, recently diagnosed as having AIDS, was admitted to the hospital for evaluation of night sweats, persistent fevers, cough, diarrhea, and weight loss. His medical history included intermediate-risk acute lymphocytic leukemia diagnosed at two years of age. His course of antineoplastic therapy was complicated by neutropenia, anemia, and thrombocytopenia requiring multiple blood and platelet transfusions. Additionally, his medical history included *Pneumocystis carinii* pneumonia and chronic mucocutaneous candidiasis. At age three, while in remission from leukemia, the child was found to have abnormal immune function with a decrease in the mixed lymphocyte count and T-cell rosettes. Initially he was diagnosed as having AIDS-related complex. However, several months later, HIV was cultured from his lymphocytes and the diagnosis was changed to AIDS, presumed to be secondary to multiple blood transfusions.

On physical examination the child appeared acutely ill. His vital signs were as follows: axillary temperature of 39 °C, pulse of 116 beats/min, respiratory rate of 24 breaths/min, and blood pressure of 85/35 mm Hg. The child was noted to have partial alopecia and cachexia (weight = 11.7 kg). The liver was mildly enlarged and nontender. Laboratory values included the following: hematocrit (Hct) 28%, hemoglobin (Hgb) 9.5 g/dL, and white blood cell (WBC) count 7300/cu mm with 35% segmented neutrophils, 33% bands, 7% lymphocytes, and 25% monocytes. His electrolytes, serum creatinine, and liver function tests were within normal limits. The chest roentgenogram did not show notable changes when compared with previous films. Cultures were obtained to rule out bacterial, viral, fungal, parasitic, and mycobacterial infections. Enteral tube feedings were started because the child was anorectic.

One month after admission, the blood culture results were reported as showing growth of *Mycobacterium avium–intracellulare*, and the child was given a presumptive diagnosis of infection with disseminated, nontuberculous mycobacteria. He was empirically given isoniazid 100 mg/day (9 mg/kg/day), ethambutol hydrochloride 100 mg/day (9 mg/kg/day), rifabutin 75 mg/day (6.5 mg/kg/day), and clofazimine 50 mg/day (4.3 mg/kg/day) pending results of susceptibility testing. Additionally, the child continued to receive trimethoprim–sulfamethoxazole for prophylaxis of *P. carinii* pneumonia and ketoconazole to control his chronic mucocutaneous candidiasis.

The patient was discharged from the hospital and returned to the clinic one month after starting therapy. His complaints included severe headaches, a productive cough, dry eyes, and continued diarrhea. On physical examination he was noted to have orange hair, orange urine, and a purple stain in the corner of his mouth. A lumbar puncture was performed to rule out meningitis as a cause for the headaches. Cerebrospinal fluid cultures were negative for bacteria, fungi, and acid-fast bacilli. Important laboratory values included the following: Hct 29%, Hgb 9.6 g/dL, WBC count 5600/cu mm (31% segmented neutrophils, 36% bands, 13.5% lymphocytes, 3.2% monocytes), aspartate aminotransferase (AST, also called SGOT) 89 IU/L, alanine aminotransferase (ALT, also called SGPT) 42 IU/L, lactate dehydrogenase 1388 IU/L, and alkaline phosphatase 259 IU/L. The Centers for Disease Control (CDC) reported that the organism was susceptible to rifabutin and ethambutol, with intermediate susceptibility to isoniazid. MAC susceptibility to clofazimine was not reported.

Two weeks later the patient developed a fever of 42 °C and a red, maculopapular rash over his buttocks and thighs. All medications were discontinued to rule out the possibility of a drug reaction. The patient defervesced to baseline fevers, and the rash disappeared within two days; he also stopped complaining of headaches. Drug therapy was restarted slowly, beginning with isoniazid and clofazimine. The child continued to have baseline fevers without signs of a rash. Two weeks later, trimethoprim–sulfamethoxazole therapy was restarted with no obvious sequelae. Rifabutin therapy was restarted one month later, and within two weeks the child developed a rash, high fevers, and vomiting. Rifabutin therapy was subsequently discontinued.

Six months after the initial diagnosis of MAC infection the child's condition appeared to be stable, without signs of a rash and with minimal complaints. Important laboratory values at this time included the following: Hct 28%, Hgb 8.4 g/dL, WBC count 4600/cu mm, AST 89 IU/L, and alkaline phosphatase 1069 IU/L. Blood cultures were repeated to determine whether MAC was present.

Four weeks later, the child's condition began to worsen. Despite appropriate therapy, blood cultures continued to be positive for MAC. A decision was made to provide only the medication necessary to keep the boy comfortable. He died within a few weeks. At autopsy, granulomatous inflammation was found in the lungs, bowel, bone marrow, and spleen, as well as the mediastinal and abdominal lymph nodes. The cause of death was listed as disseminating HIV and MAC infection.

Case 2. The patient was a previously well 16-month-old girl who developed low-grade fevers and enlarged, nontender, right anterior cervical lymph nodes near the angle of the mandible. These nodes continued to enlarge and included the ipsilateral nodes along the anterior and posterior aspects of the sternocleidomastoid muscle. The medical history showed that at one year of age the child developed adenitis. An old tuberculin (tine) test done at the time was negative, but a subsequent purified protein derivative of tuberculin (PPD) test (5 units) was positive, showing induration of 8 mm in diameter. The chest roentgenogram did not suggest pulmonary involvement. A presumptive diagnosis of nontuberculous mycobacterial infection was made and surgery was performed. Nodes in the superficial and deep jugular chain and at the angle of the jaw were excised. A large mass at the angle of the mandible was partially resected because it adhered to the carotid sheath. A culture of the neck mass grew *M. avium–intracellulare*, which was resistant to isoniazid, ethambutol, clofazimine, streptomycin, and rifampin. In spite of the culture results, the patient was started on isoniazid 10 mg/kg/day and rifampin 10 mg/kg/day.

Over the next six weeks, the patient had increased difficulty with swallowing. The mother decided to seek the help of a consultant and took her now 20-month-old child to San Francisco General Hospital for evaluation. A physical examination revealed a large mass in the right posterior oropharynx. A computed tomography (CT) scan showed a well delineated prevertebral retropharyngeal mass along the midline and the right side of the neck. This mass extended into the oropharynx and was 4 cm long and 3 cm wide. It was declared inoperable at this time because it extended around major vessels of the neck. Because of the extensive nature of this adenitis, the child was tested for an immunodeficiency syndrome. The mother had a history of i.v. drug abuse and the father was of Haitian origin; however, both the mother and the child had negative serologic tests for HIV. The child also had normal quantitative immunoglobulin levels and peripheral lymphocyte count and had a normal helper-to-suppressor lymphocyte ratio of 2.4.[11]

The isoniazid and rifampin were discontinued and treatment was changed to streptomycin 20 mg/kg/day (as the sulfate salt) three times weekly, ethambutol hydrochloride 8 mg/kg/day given in two doses, clofazimine 4 mg/kg/day (50 mg/day), and rifabutin 6 mg/kg/day (75 mg/day). Rifabutin was also the only antimicrobial agent to which the organism was susceptible in vitro.

Streptomycin was discontinued after three months of treatment. At seven months of therapy, the mass had decreased in size and was centrally liquefied. Additionally, a chin abscess and draining fistula developed at the previous surgical incision site. The patient had a second surgical procedure consisting of a modified radical neck dissection wherein the fistula, sternocleidomastoid muscle, internal jugular vein, and all involved lymph nodes were removed. Intraoperative cultures did not indicate the presence of mycobacteria.

Rifabutin, clofazimine, and ethambutol were discontinued after a total treatment period of one year. A repeat CT scan showed complete resolution of the mass, and clinically the child was cured. Six months later, the child developed acute meningitis that responded well to traditional treatment. Cultures for pyogenic bacteria and mycobacteria were negative. The child's immune status was tested and again proved to be normal. One year after cessation of treatment, there was no evidence of recurrence of disease.

Epidemiology and Clinical Features

M. avium–intracellulare was a pathogen in each of the patients. The organism is ubiquitous, with limited virulence in the immunocompetent host. Unlike *M. tuberculosis*, human-to-human transmission of nontuberculous mycobacteria has not been documented.

MAC infections in homosexuals and i.v. drug abusers were first documented in the literature in the early 1980s.[3,6,12,13] Over the last several years, MAC infections have been reported with increasing frequency, particularly in patients suffering from AIDS.[14] MAC infections have an insidious onset, and the actual incidence of disease is difficult to determine because many infections are not diagnosed until autopsy. This suggests that many infections may remain undiagnosed.

Typically, children with nontuberculous mycobacterial infections have lymphadenitis.[15] Pulmonary, skin, bone, joint, and disseminated infections are rare in children with normal immune systems.[15] Unfortunately, the AIDS epidemic has caused an increase in the incidence of life-threatening disseminated MAC disease in patients with HIV infection. Signs and symptoms of disseminated MAC infections are nonspecific. Chronic fevers, night sweats, weight loss, and cachexia are common complaints. Normocytic, normochromic anemia, abdominal pain, diarrhea, and malabsorption also may be present. Lymphadenopathy, hepatomegaly, and splenomegaly also have been reported in some patients.[16]

Diagnosis and Susceptibility Testing

In AIDS patients, MAC has been isolated from bone marrow, liver, spleen, lymph nodes, lung, gastrointestinal tract, urine, and blood. Sputum cultures must be carefully evaluated to rule out environmental contamination or colonization from disseminated disease.[14] Formation of granulomatous tissue requires a functioning immune system. Therefore, characteristic morphologic features of mycobacterial infection may not be present in tissue samples of immunocompromised patients. Even in the absence of granulomas, all tissue specimens obtained from patients with suspected infection should be tested for acid-fast bacilli.[14] Blood cultures have been useful in the detection of disseminated disease, and quantitative methods are available to measure the number of colony-forming units per milliliter of blood. These values may help to determine the response to therapy.[5] Stool cultures also are thought to correlate with dissemination of infection.[16]

Empiric multidrug antituberculous therapy should be initiated in patients with suspected disseminated nontuberculous mycobacterial infection because final isolation, identification, and susceptibility testing may take several weeks to complete. Tuberculin skin tests also take several weeks to complete; the tests should be done, but results may be of limited value in immunocompromised individuals.[1] Chest roentgenograms should be performed in patients with suspected pulmonary infections. However, MAC infections are difficult to differentiate from other mycobacterial infections and fungal infections by roentgenogram alone.[17] To date, the therapeutic response in cases of MAC infection has been poor, with a high failure rate caused by extensive drug resistance. Relapse has been reported in 25% of all adult patients who initially responded to therapy.[18]

In vitro susceptibility tests are indicated for nontuberculous mycobacterial infections, but the results should be used with caution since evidence supporting correlation of the tests with clinical response is not available.[12,13,19] Lack of standardization of MAC susceptibility testing may be one of the reasons in vitro drug susceptibility results do not reflect in vivo susceptibility of the organism. Although the organism is frequently resistant to high concentrations of individual drugs, multidrug combinations have demonstrated synergistic effects.[20] Therefore, modification of drug therapy based on in vitro susceptibility testing is controversial. Some clinicians prefer to modify therapy based on the clinical course of the infection.[19]

Treatment

Treatment of MAC infections frequently includes surgical resection in addition to drug therapy. Surgical resection of localized MAC infections often results in a good long-term prognosis.[7,14,15] Prolonged antitubercular therapy, however, is indicated when (1) surgery is not possible, (2) adenopathy or drainage persists after surgery, (3) the culture is positive for *M. tuberculosis*, (4) spontaneous or prominent drainage persists, or (5) the patient or a family member reacts to a PPD skin test for tuberculosis by developing induration of >15 mm in diameter or has equal reactions to PPD tests for tuberculosis and nontuberculous mycobacterial infections.[15]

Drug therapy for severe or disseminated MAC infections currently includes rifabutin, isoniazid, ethambutol, and clofazimine.[12,16] Rifampin, pyrazinamide, streptomycin, cycloserine, and amikacin have been used in various drug regimens.[14] Unfortunately, although some patients have had temporary clinical improvement, consistent, long-term remission has not been reported for most patients using the drugs that currently are recommended.[16]

The child in case 2 had adenitis that was surgically resected. She also received antituberculous drug therapy because initially the mass could not be resected and she had persistent drainage from the incision site. The combination of surgery and drug therapy led to an apparent cure. The child in case 1 was less fortunate. He had a diagnosis of both AIDS and disseminated MAC infection. Despite appropriate drug therapy, he continued to have positive blood cultures. Disseminated MAC infection also was found on autopsy.

Drug therapy in both cases involved a number of antimicrobial agents including isoniazid, rifampin, ethambutol, streptomycin, rifabutin, and clofazimine. The recommended pediatric dosages were used for isoniazid, ethambutol, rifampin, and streptomycin in both children. Pediatric dosages for rifabutin and clofazimine have not been established. Therefore, the dosages were estimated using Clarke's body area rule.[21] Generally, four to six agents are recommended for initial treatment of MAC infections.[13,15,22]

Isoniazid, Rifampin, Ethambutol, and Streptomycin

Isoniazid, rifampin, ethambutol, and streptomycin are standard therapy for *M. tuberculosis* infections. The usual dosage of isoniazid in children is 10–20 mg/kg/day but may go as high as 30 mg/kg/day.[23] In both cases, the children received approximately 10 mg/kg/day. The usual adult dosage is 300 mg/day. Adverse effects of isoniazid primarily involve the nervous system (peripheral neuritis, psychosis, confusion), liver (transient elevations in serum AST, ALT, and bilirubin), and hypersensitivity reactions.[24] The children did not appear to have any of the adverse effects associated with isoniazid therapy. In adults, the dosage of rifampin ranges from 300 to 600 mg/day, whereas the pediatric dosage ranges from 10 to 15 mg/kg/day.[23] Adverse effects attributed to rifampin include an orange coloration of all secretions. Rifampin also can cause dermatitis, flu-like symptoms, hepatitis, or nephritis.[24] The child in the second case received 10 mg/kg/day of rifampin for three months. Adverse effects of therapy were limited to an orange coloration of her secretions.

When indicated in pediatric patients, ethambutol hydrochloride is administered at a dosage of 10 to 25 mg/kg/day.[23] The adult dosage ranges from 600 to 1000 mg/day. Caution is recommended in treating children under 12 years of age because of the risk of optic neuritis and retrobulbar neuropathy.[15] Toxicity appears to be related to the dose and duration of therapy. Ethambutol should be used in children whose vision can be monitored closely. Children of all ages can be monitored for visual acuity and color vision, although it is more difficult to examine infants.[25] Vision testing should be done every month in patients receiving doses greater than 15 mg/kg/day. Because MAC infections are highly resistant to antitubercular drugs, both children received ethambutol. Neither child appeared to suffer from adverse effects.

Streptomycin is administered only by deep i.m. injection. The dose ranges from 10 to 25 mg/kg (as the sulfate salt) in both children and adults.[22] The drug is usually administered two to three times a week. Streptomycin is primarily added as adjunctive therapy in the treatment of miliary tuberculosis or infections of the central nervous system. In vitro studies have demonstrated synergistic effects when streptomycin is used in combination with isoniazid, rifampin, and ethambutol against MAC infections.[26] Adverse effects of streptomycin include pain on administration, ototoxicity (eighth cranial nerve damage), and nephrotoxicity.[24] Adverse effects on hearing and renal function are more likely to occur in patients who receive high doses or prolonged therapy, or who are receiving other drugs with similar adverse effects. The elderly are also at increased risk.[24] The child in the first case was at increased risk for toxicity based on his history of antineoplastic therapy and did not receive streptomycin. The culture susceptibility results were available later and indicated that the organism causing the child's infection was not susceptible to streptomycin. The second child received empiric therapy after diagnosis with streptomycin 10 mg/kg (as the sulfate salt) three times per week. Therapy was discontinued after three months when culture susceptibility results demonstrated resistance to streptomycin.

Rifabutin

Rifabutin (ansamycin, LM427) and clofazimine are two agents currently included in the treatment of resistant atypical, nontuberculous mycobacterial infections. When these children were first diagnosed, the drugs were not commercially available. Clofazimine (Lamprene, Ciba-Geigy Corporation) is now available in the United States. Rifabutin may be obtained on request by contacting the CDC drug service at 201-277-5787. Limited information is available regarding use of these drugs in the pediatric population. Therefore, until further information is available, dosing guidelines for these agents can be estimated from existing adult data.

Rifabutin is a semisynthetic rifamycin-S derivative. It is rapidly absorbed after oral administration, with peak blood levels occurring in 30 minutes. The drug is primarily excreted in the urine over an extended period of time.[27] The recommended adult dosage ranges from 150 to 300 mg/day. Dosage modifications are necessary in patients with renal impairment. In adults, the dosage should be decreased to 150 mg/day when the serum creatinine reaches 2 mg/dL, with further reduction to 75 mg every three days when the serum creatinine is >10 mg/dL. Extrapolation of this information to pediatric patients suggests that the dose should be decreased by 50% when the creatinine clearance falls to 50% of normal and should be decreased further when the creatinine clearance is less than 10% of normal.[27] Early pharmacokinetic studies in humans receiving oral doses of 75 mg and 150 mg demonstrated low peak plasma concentrations (0.15 μg/mL or less), with rifabutin detected in plasma up to 24 hours after a dose. The drug appears to concentrate in the lungs, although high levels also are found in the liver, spleen, eyes, and kidneys.[6] Therefore, it is postulated that tissue levels are higher than plasma levels and may reach concentrations 10 to 20 times the minimum inhibitory concentration (MIC) required for treating MAC infections. An MIC of 0.5 μg/mL is used to determine susceptibility of disseminated MAC infections, whereas concentrations of 2 μg/mL may be appropriate for lung isolates. Of 57 MAC isolates found in AIDS patients, only 28% were susceptible at an MIC of 0.5 μg/mL, whereas 92% of the isolates were found to be susceptible at an MIC of 2 μg/mL.[28] In vitro studies have shown susceptibility of MAC strains to rifabutin, with 81% of the organisms inhibited at a concentration of 1 μg/mL.[29] However, in vitro data also indicate that high plasma concentrations of rifabutin (2 to 32 μg/mL) are necessary to kill the MAC organism.[30] Rifabutin is very lipophilic, allowing for good penetration into bacteria. It inhibits all *M. tuberculosis* strains, including 30% of the strains that are resistant to rifampin (MIC for rifampin <10 μg/mL).[29]

The usual adult dosage of rifabutin is 150 to 300 mg/day administered as a single daily dose.[27] Currently, the drug is available only as 150-mg capsules. Each of the children in the case reports received 75 mg/day. Combination therapy with several antituberculous agents, including rifabutin and clofazimine, is currently recommended for optimal treatment of MAC infections.[26] The duration of therapy ranges from 6 to 24 months; ideally, therapy should be continued for 12 months after evidence of apparent remission.[15]

Rifabutin is associated with a number of adverse

effects. Like rifampin, it causes all secretions to turn orange.[27] Elevated liver enzymes have been reported in 30% of patients taking the drug.[27] Rifabutin should be discontinued if AST is greater than 500 IU/L or if total bilirubin is greater than 3 mg/dL. Liver function tests should be monitored weekly during the first two months of therapy and monthly thereafter.[27] Rifabutin also has been associated with a dose-dependent decrease in hematopoetic tissue, usually seen in patients receiving dosages of greater than 150 mg/day.[27] Thrombocytopenia and leukopenia may occur when the dosage exceeds 300 mg/day.[27] Rifabutin is contraindicated in patients with a WBC count of less than 1000/cu mm or a platelet count of less than 50,000/cu mm.[27] Complete blood counts (including WBC count with a differential, hematocrit, hemoglobin, and platelet count) should be monitored twice a week for the first month, weekly for the second month, and twice a month thereafter.[27] The boy in the first case had a number of adverse reactions that could be attributed to rifabutin. The reactions included orange discoloration of his secretions, skin, and hair; severe headaches; a maculopapular rash; high fevers; and vomiting. Additionally, his WBC count decreased from 7300/cu mm to 5600/cu mm within one month of therapy. Except for the orange discoloration, the adverse effects disappeared within 48 hours of discontinuing the drug. When the child was rechallenged, adverse reactions to rifabutin reappeared within two weeks and again forced discontinuation of the drug. Rifabutin was well tolerated by the second patient.

Clofazimine

Clofazimine is a phenazine aniline dye used in the treatment of *M. leprae*, the organism responsible for leprosy. Bioavailability is variable, with approximately 45–62% of the drug absorbed from a microcrystalline suspension and as much as 70% absorbed from an oil-wax base.[31] It is highly lipophilic, with minimal penetration into the central nervous system. Clofazimine is found in high concentrations in the liver, spleen, lung, adrenals, and adipose tissue.[32] The half-life of the drug is approximately 70 days; therefore, it may take several months to achieve the required inhibitory serum concentrations.[32] The MIC used in reporting MAC isolate susceptibility to clofazimine ranges from 0.3 to 5 μg/mL.[3] Serum concentrations of 1.8 to 3.5 μg/mL after two months of therapy have been reported.[33] A nonlinear correlation has been observed between the dose of clofazimine and serum concentrations. A small amount of the drug is eliminated in the urine (0.01–0.4%) within 24 hours; 5–11% is excreted in the feces within three days.[32]

The adult dosage of clofazimine used in the treatment of MAC infections ranges from 100 to 300 mg/day, administered in two to three doses. If the drug is tolerated, a dosage of 200–300 mg/day may be used; however, adverse effects may be less common if the dosage does not exceed 100 mg/day.[24,34] When these children were diagnosed as having MAC infections, clofazimine was available only as gelatin capsules containing 100 mg of the drug suspended in heavy oil. Clofazimine is currently available as both 50- and 100-mg capsules. Information on the stability of oral suspensions of clofazimine is not available. Both children were to receive a 50-mg dose and, as it was impossible to split the capsule, the contents were withdrawn, mixed with 5 mL of safflower oil, and administered as 2.5 mL each day. Clofazimine is a dye and causes permanent staining. Therefore, when preparing and administering a dose, special care is needed to avoid spilling the drug.

Clofazimine may cause gastrointestinal irritation producing nausea, vomiting, cramping, and diarrhea when large doses are used for a prolonged time. If severe gastrointestinal reactions develop, the dosage may be reduced or the drug may be administered three times a week.[24,34] Approximately 40–50% of patients receiving clofazimine have been reported to have gastrointestinal problems requiring discontinuation of therapy.[35] Additionally, the drug is a dye and within a few weeks of therapy, 75–100% of patients develop a red to black discoloration of the skin and conjunctiva. The lacrimal fluid, urine, sweat, and sputum also may be discolored. The skin discoloration reverses slowly after therapy is discontinued and may require years to become completely normal. Other adverse effects include dryness of the skin and eyes, pruritus, and photosensitivity. Dry skin may be alleviated with an oily liquid or petrolatum-based ointment. Topical steroids or oral antihistamines may help to control itching. Other adverse effects involve the central nervous system (dizziness, drowsiness, headache, neuralgia), the kidneys (discolored urine, cystitis), and the liver (increased AST, bilirubin); eosinophilia, hyperglycemia, and vascular pain also have been reported.[24] These adverse effects are dose dependent and transient in nature.[32] Adverse effects associated with clofazimine in these case reports were limited. The first child complained of dry eyes and had a purple stain in the corner of his mouth, caused by administration of the dye. The child in the second case developed skin discoloration during therapy.

Conclusion

The case studies reported outline typical management of MAC infections in the pediatric population. They illustrate the poor prognosis of a disseminated MAC infection in an AIDS patient and the relatively good prognosis of a localized infection in a patient who is HIV negative. Current therapy of MAC infections includes at least four and often six drugs. When infection is suspected, empiric therapy should be initiated pending culture susceptibility results. The initial assessment of various drug regimens has demonstrated that clofazimine and rifabutin, in combination with isoniazid and ethambutol, may be useful in the treatment of some MAC infections. Since drug therapy is associated with many adverse effects, further studies are necessary to determine the most effective and least toxic regimen.

Discussion Questions

1. Discuss the predisposing factors associated with MAC infection in both patients. What is the value of cultures in determining therapy?
2. What are the major complications associated with rifabutin and clofazimine therapy? How can these complications be minimized? Are the complications reversible?
3. Describe the importance of multidrug therapy. Should antimicrobial agents be added to therapy if the organism shows resistance?
4. Information available on the use of new and investigational agents in children is limited. How can dosing guidelines best be established?

References

1. Centers for Disease Control, U.S. Department of Health and Human Services. Diagnosis and management of mycobacteria infection and disease in persons with human immunodeficiency virus infection. *Ann Intern Med.* 1987; 106:254–6.
2. Chapman JS. The atypical mycobacteria and human mycobacteriosis. New York: Plenum Publishing Corp.; 1977:65.
3. Zakowski P, Fligiel F, Berlin OGW et al. Disseminated *Mycobacterium avium-intracellulare* infection in homosexual men dying of acquired immunodeficiency. *JAMA.* 1982; 248:2980–2.
4. Taka AM, Davidson PT, Bailey WC. Surgical treatment of atypical mycobacterial lymphadenitis in children. *Pediatr Infect Dis.* 1985; 4:664–7.
5. Macher AM, Kovacs JA, Gill V et al. Bacteremia due to *Mycobacterium avium-intracellulare* in the acquired immunodeficiency syndrome. *Ann Intern Med.* 1983; 99:782–5.
6. Greene JB, Sidhu GS, Lewin S et al. *Mycobacterium avium-intracellulare*: a cause of disseminated life-threatening infection in homosexuals and drug abusers. *Ann Intern Med.* 1982; 97:539–46.
7. Centers for Disease Control. Tuberculosis, final data—United States, 1986. *MMWR.* 1988; 36:817–20.
8. Rubinstein A, Morecki R, Silverman B et al. Pulmonary disease in children with acquired immune deficiency syndrome and AIDS-related complex. *J Pediatr.* 1986; 108:498–503.
9. Oleske J, Minneford A, Cooper R et al. Immune deficiency syndrome in children. *JAMA.* 1983; 249:2345–9.
10. Church JA, Allen JR, Stiehm ER. New scarlet letter(s), pediatric AIDS. *Pediatrics.* 1986; 77:423–7.
11. Center for Disease Control. Publication of revised case definition for AIDS surveillance. *MMWR.* 1987; 36(Suppl 1S):1–10.
12. Macher AM, Kovacs JA, Gill V et al. Bacteremia due to *Mycobacterium avium-intracellulare* in the acquired immunodeficiency syndrome. *Ann Intern Med.* 1983; 99:782–5.
13. Hawkins CC, Gold JWM, Whimbey E et al. *Mycobacterium avium* complex infections in patients with immunodeficiency syndrome. *Ann Intern Med.* 1986; 105:184–8.
14. Committee on *M. intracellulare* Disease. Disease due to *Mycobacterium avium-intracellulare. Chest.* 1985; 87(Suppl 2):139S–149S.
15. Margileth AM. Management of nontuberculosis (atypical) mycobacterial infections in children and adolescents. *Pediatr Infect Dis.* 1985; 4:119–21.
16. Snider DE, Hopewell PC, Mills J et al. Mycobacterioses and the acquired immunodeficiency syndrome. *Am Rev Respir Dis.* 1987; 136:492–6.
17. Sanders WE. Other mycobacterial species. In: Mandels GL, Douglas RG, Bennett SE, eds. Principles and practice of infectious diseases. 2nd ed. New York: John Wiley & Sons; 1985:1413–23.
18. Wolinsky E. Nontuberculosis mycobacteria and associated diseases. *Am Rev Respir Dis.* 1979; 119:107–43.
19. Lakshminarayan S, Sahn A. Disseminated infection caused by *Mycobacterium avium. Am Rev Respir Dis.* 1973; 108:123–6.
20. Zimmer BL, DeYoung DR, Roberts GD. In vitro synergistic activity of ethambutol, isoniazid, kanamycin, rifampin and streptomycin against *Mycobacterium avium-intracellulare* complex. *Antimicrob Agents Chemother.* 1982; 22:148–50.
21. Ansel HC. Calculation of doses for children. In: Stoklosa MJ, ed. Pharmaceutical calculations. Philadelphia: Lea & Febiger; 1980:98–103.
22. Davidson PT, Khanifo V, Goble M et al. Treatment of disease due to *Mycobacterium intracellulare. Rev Infect Dis.* 1981; 3:1064–7.
23. Levin RH, Zenk KE. Medication table. In: Rudolph AM, Hoffman JIE, eds. Pediatrics. 18th ed. East Norwalk, CT: Appleton and Lange; 1987: 1839.
24. Kastrup EK. Facts and comparisons. St. Louis: J. B. Lippincott; 1988.
25. Apt L, Gaffney WL. The eyes. In: Rudolph AM, Hoffman JIE, eds. Pediatrics. 18th ed. East Norwalk, CT: Appleton and Lange; 1987:1759.
26. Heifets LB. Synergistic effect of rifampin, streptomycin, ethionamide, and ethambutol on *Mycobacterium intracellulare. Am Rev Respir Dis.* 1982; 125:43–8.
27. Division of Tuberculosis Control of the Centers for Disease Control. Informational material for physicians–ansamycin LM-427. 1984:1–9.
28. Horsburgh CR Jr, Cohn DL, Roberts RB et al. *Mycobacterium avium–M. intracellulare* isolates from patients with or without acquired immunodeficiency syndrome. *Antimicrob Agents Chemother.* 1986; 30:955–7.
29. Woodley CL, Kilburn JD. In vitro susceptibility of *Mycobacterium avium* complex and mycobacterium tuberculosis strains to a spiro-piperidyl rifamycin. *Am Rev Respir Dis.* 1982; 126:586–7.
30. Yajko DM, Nassos PS, Hadley WK. Therapeutic implications of inhibition versus killing of *Mycobacterium avium* complex by antimicrobial agents. *Antimicrob Agents Chemother.* 1987; 31:117–20.
31. Levy L. Pharmacologic studies of clofazimine. *Am J Trop Hyg.* 1974; 23:1097–1109.
32. Weintraub M, Evan P. Clofazimine: an orphan drug approved for the treatment of leprosy that also has potential use in AIDS patients. *Hosp Formul.* 1987; 22:766–75.
33. Davidson PT, Goble M, Fernandez E et al. Clofazimine (B663) for the treatment of *M. intracellulare* infections in man. *Am Rev Respir Dis.* 1979; 119 (Suppl):398. Abstract.
34. U.S. Public Health Service hospital, Carville, LA. Fact sheet on clofazimine. 4th revision. 1979 Mar 21.
35. Moore VJ. A review of the side effects experienced by patients taking clofazimine. *Lepr Rev.* 1983; 54:327–35.

CP Continuing Education

The ASHP Continuing Education system gives readers a self-assessment mechanism for selected articles in Clinical Pharmacy *and the* American Journal of Hospital Pharmacy. *It also allows readers to obtain continuing-education credit for these articles.*

For the purpose of CE-credit enrollment a blank answer sheet is published at the end of each installment of the column for the CE articles in that issue. An enrollee accumulates these answer sheets until the enrollment is submitted, using the form that is published in the June and December issues of Clinical Pharmacy *and in the June and December issues of the* American Journal of Hospital Pharmacy. *Any combination of tests within a 18-month period, from both* Clinical Pharmacy *and* American Journal of Hospital Pharmacy, *may be included in an enrollment. More complete details about enrollment in the system will appear in the semiannual enrollment form.*

Article 680-204-8811 (see page 514)
Qualifies for 1.0 hour of CE credit

Treatment of *Pneumocystis carinii* pneumonia in patients with AIDS

Learning Objectives

After studying this article, the reader should be able to

1. Compare the clinical features of *Pneumocystis carinii* pneumonia in an AIDS patient with those in the immunocompromised patient without AIDS.
2. Identify the major adverse effects of pentamidine and trimethoprim–sulfamethoxazole in AIDS patients.
3. Outline a drug therapy plan, including the drug of choice and alternative agents for the management of *P. carinii* pneumonia in an AIDS patient.
4. Describe the pharmacologic mechanisms by which drugs that are active against *P. carinii* exert their effects.
5. Identify the role of investigational agents in the treatment of *P. carinii* pneumonia.

Self-assessment Questions

For each question there is one best answer only.

1. Which one of the following statements does not reflect current practices in the management of *P. carinii* pneumonia (PCP) in the AIDS population?
   a. Dapsone 100 mg/day has been used in combination with trimethoprim to treat PCP infections in AIDS patients.
   b. Eflornithine is effective in the management of PCP, but its use may be limited by hematopoietic and gastrointestinal toxicity.
   c. Pentamidine has been administered as an inhalation aerosol to enhance the concentration achieved in the lungs.
   d. Trimethoprim–sulfamethoxazole in a dose of 5 mg/kg/day (based on the trimethoprim component) is the preferred first-line therapy for management of PCP in AIDS patients.
2. Compared with patients who have PCP but do not have AIDS, patients with PCP and AIDS
   a. Seek health care earlier in the course of their illness.
   b. Have more acute initial signs and symptoms of a respiratory infection.
   c. Experience a high incidence of adverse reactions to trimethoprim–sulfamethoxazole.
   d. Have arterial blood gas values and chest roentgenograms that appear worse than their clinical condition.
3. Which of the following statements best describes the use of trimethoprim–sulfamethoxazole (TMP–SMX) in the treatment of PCP in AIDS patients?
   a. TMP–SMX exerts its antiprotozoal effects by inhibiting the breakdown of tetrahydrofolic acid.
   b. Because TMP–SMX is eliminated primarily by hepatic metabolism, dosage adjustment is not needed in patients who have renal failure.
   c. TMP–SMX is a safer drug than pentamidine because it has a lower incidence of adverse effects.
   d. TMP–SMX is effective when administered by either the oral or intravenous route.
4. One important advantage of administration of pentamidine by aerosol inhalation for treatment of PCP is
   a. A decreased incidence of serious systemic adverse reactions coupled with a good clinical response rate.
   b. Maintenance of therapeutic serum levels of pentamidine for a longer period of time.
   c. A decreased cost because doses are lower for inhalation therapy than for systemic administration.
   d. Improved distribution of pentamidine to the kidneys, spleen, and liver.
5. Inhibition of polyamine production is the mechanism for the antiprotozoal effect of
   a. Trimetrexate.
   b. Eflornithine.

c. Pentamidine.
d. Dapsone.

6. Eflornithine has activity, at least in vitro, against all of the following organisms except

a. *Cryptosporidium muris.*
b. *Pneumocystis carinii.*
c. *Mycobacterium avium–intracellulare.*
d. *Cytomegalovirus.*

7. When dapsone is considered for use as an alternative agent for treatment of PCP in an AIDS patient, the patient should first be screened to identify

a. Glucose-6-phosphate dehydrogenase deficiency.
b. Hypersensitivity to sulfonamides.
c. Pre-existing neutropenia.
d. Pre-existing abnormalities in the baseline audiogram.

8. Inhibition of dihydrofolate reductase is the mechanism for the antiprotozoal activity of

a. Trimetrexate, dapsone, and sulfamethoxazole.
b. Trimetrexate, pyrimethamine, and eflornithine.
c. Dapsone, eflornithine, and trimethoprim.
d. Trimethoprim, trimetrexate, and pyrimethamine.

9. Leucovorin is administered concurrently with trimetrexate to

a. Selectively rescue mammalian cells, while not affecting activity against protozoal cells.
b. Enhance penetration of trimetrexate into protozoal cells.
c. Protect the kidney from the nephrotoxic effects of trimetrexate.
d. Improve the affinity of trimetrexate for *P. carinii* dihydrofolate reductase.

10. Prophylaxis against recurrence of *P. carinii* pneumonia may be accomplished by administration of

a. Prednisone 10 mg orally once a day in the morning.
b. Eflornithine hydrochloride 75 mg orally twice a day.
c. Trimethoprim–sulfamethoxazole 160 mg/800 mg twice a day.
d. Pentamidine isethionate 600 mg in 6 mL of sterile water once a day by aerosol inhalation.

Article 680-204-8812 (see page 528)
Qualifies for 1.0 hr of CE credit

Management of cryptococcal meningitis in patients with AIDS

Learning Objectives

After studying this article, the reader should be able to

1. List the signs and symptoms of cryptococcal meningitis in AIDS patients.
2. Identify the advantages and disadvantages of the three laboratory tests that are commonly used to identify patients with cryptococcal meningitis.
3. Recommend an initial treatment regimen for an AIDS patient with cryptococcal meningitis.
4. Identify the agents that are used as maintenance therapy to prevent relapse of cryptococcal meningitis in patients with AIDS.
5. Describe the adverse effects of antifungal agents that are used for treating AIDS patients with cryptococcal meningitis.

Self-assessment Questions

For each question there is one best answer only.

1. The most frequent sign or symptom of cryptococcal meningitis in AIDS patients is

a. Stiff neck.
b. Photophobia.
c. A change in mental status.
d. Headache.

2. Which of the following diagnostic tests has the highest incidence of false-positive results?

a. Culture of the organism.
b. Latex agglutination test.
c. India-ink preparation.
d. Alternatives b and c are both correct.

3. The mortality rate for relapses of cryptococcal meningitis in AIDS patients is

a. 50–75%.
b. 75–100%.
c. 90–100%.
d. 25–50%.

4. Relapse rates of cryptococcal meningitis in AIDS patients range from

a. 10% to 25%.
b. 50% to 90%.
c. 30% to 50%.
d. 50% to 70%.

5. The initial treatment of choice for the management of an AIDS patient with cryptococcal meningitis is

a. Fluconazole alone.
b. Fluconazole plus amphotericin B.
c. Ketoconazole plus amphotericin B.
d. Amphotericin B alone.

6. Which one of the following drug regimens is currently recommended for maintenance therapy to prevent relapse of cryptococcal meningitis in patients with AIDS?

a. Amphotericin B 100 mg/day.
b. Amphotericin B 100 mg/week.
c. Amphotericin B 100 mg/week plus flucytosine 100 mg/day.
d. Fluconazole 150 mg/day.

7. Available data on the treatment of cryptococcal meningitis in AIDS patients suggest that the addition of flucytosine to amphotericin B therapy

a. Allows for a reduction in the total dosage of amphotericin B.
b. Reduces the relapse rate.
c. Does not alter overall mortality.

d. Is poorly tolerated because the drugs have similar toxicity profiles.

8. When patients have a prompt response to therapy for cryptococcal meningitis, treatment in full doses is typically continued for

a. 8 weeks.
b. 3 weeks.
c. 6 weeks.
d. 12 weeks.

9. Which of the following statements best describes amphotericin B toxicity in AIDS patients?

a. Amphotericin B causes a higher incidence of neutropenia in AIDS patients than in patients who do not have AIDS.
b. AIDS patients are more prone to renal toxicity than are patients who do not have AIDS.
c. The incidence of infusion-related toxicities is similar to that found in patients who do not have AIDS.
d. Life-threatening hypersensitivity reactions are more common in AIDS patients than in patients who do not have AIDS.

10. The most common toxicity of flucytosine in patients with AIDS is

a. Hepatotoxicity.
b. Nephrotoxicity.
c. Central nervous system toxicity.
d. Bone marrow suppression.

Answer sheet

July 1988 *Clinical Pharmacy*

Note: An enrollment form for the ASHP Continuing Education System appears in the June and December issues. Please accumulate all the answer sheets you wish to use in one enrollment and submit them at one time with a completed enrollment form.

Place an X in the box(es) at the top of the column(s) corresponding to the test(s) you are taking. Darken the boxes corresponding to the correct answers.

☐ 680-204-8811 1.0 hour	a b c d		a b c d	☐ 680-204-8812 1.0 hour	a b c d		a b c d
1.	☐☐☐☐	6.	☐☐☐☐	1.	☐☐☐☐	6.	☐☐☐☐
2.	☐☐☐☐	7.	☐☐☐☐	2.	☐☐☐☐	7.	☐☐☐☐
3.	☐☐☐☐	8.	☐☐☐☐	3.	☐☐☐☐	8.	☐☐☐☐
4.	☐☐☐☐	9.	☐☐☐☐	4.	☐☐☐☐	9.	☐☐☐☐
5.	☐☐☐☐	10.	☐☐☐☐	5.	☐☐☐☐	10.	☐☐☐☐

ASHP Use Only
(1.0)8811______(3)
(1.0)8812______(3)

PATIENT CARE • RESEARCH • CANCER PREVENTION • EDUCATION

It's Working At M.D. Anderson!

Patient Care, Research, Cancer Prevention and Education...words that are synonymous with M.D. Anderson Cancer Center in the renowned Texas Medical Center in Houston.

We're known worldwide for contributions in the battle against cancer, and comprehensive pharmaceutical services are a vital link in our commitment to provide the highest quality patient care. Our specialized focus allows us to offer you more sophisticated equipment, a wide range of experiences and more extensive training.

The Pharmacist is an important member of the highly specialized medical teams involved in the care of our patients. Pharmacists are deeply involved in patient care, patient education, drug information services, and drug-related research, both basic and clinical.

If you are a Pharmacist looking for a career opportunity that will have real impact on Patient Care, Research, Cancer Prevention and Education, consider M.D. Anderson. You'll find Houston a city of opportunity that offers diverse cultural and recreational activities as well as no state income tax.

M.D. Anderson offers a comprehensive benefits package and a competitive salary. We encourage you to call **(713)792-8001** for further information on our Pharmacy Opportunities, or send your resume to:
M.D. Anderson Cancer Center, 1515 Holcombe Blvd., HMB 205, Houston, Texas 77030.

THE UNIVERSITY OF TEXAS
MD ANDERSON
CANCER CENTER

We are an equal opportunity/affirmative action employer.
Targeting for a smoke-free workplace...non-smoking applicants encouraged to apply.

Current Literature

Drug Reaction Alerts

Drug Reaction Alerts focuses primarily on serious, unlabeled reactions to new chemical entities. The citations are compiled monthly from International Pharmaceutical Abstracts, *which covers over 700 journals. An address for reprints (when available) follows the name of the corresponding author in each citation.*

Antibiotics

Kline SS, Mauro VF (Department of Pharmacy, Medical College of Ohio, Toledo, OH 43699), Forney RB et al. **Cefotetan**-induced disulfiram-type reactions and hypoprothrombinemia. *Antimicrob Agents Chemother.* 1987; 31:1328–31. Study. (Double-blind, placebo-controlled; eight healthy men, aged 21–38 years; received three doses of cefotetan 2 g every 12 hours and ethanol 0.5/kg one hour after the third dose of cefotetan; five volunteers experienced flushing and increased heart rate; slight increase in prothrombin time with cefotetan)

Antineoplastic Agents

Goey SH (Free University Hospital, 1007 MB Amsterdam, Netherlands), Voerman HJ, Strack van Schijndel RJ et al. Swelling of metastatic tumors with high-dose **interleukin** therapy. *N Engl J Med.* 1988; 318:643–4. Case. (45-year-old woman with metastatic melanoma and 57-year-old man with bone metastasis from renal-cell carcinoma; first patient received interleukin-2 3×10^6 U/sq m on days 1 and 2 and 6×10^6 U/sq m on days 3 and 4 and second patient received interleukin-2 3×10^6 U/sq m for one day; both patients developed edema in metastatic tumors; symptoms resolved upon discontinuation of interleukin-2 and corticosteroid therapy)

Antivirals

Chuck AJ (Department of Rheumatology, Harlow Wood Hospital, Nottinghamshire, England), Lloyd Jones JK, Dunn NA. Is **inosine pranobex** contraindicated in autoimmune disease? *Br Med J.* 1988; 296:646. Case. (27-year-old woman with warts; received inosine pranobex 1 g four times daily for one week; exacerbation of polymyositis that had been controlled with prednisone 30 mg/day; substitution of azathioprine 150 mg/day for inosine pranobex controlled the symptoms of polymyositis and warts resolved after two months)

Cardiac Drugs

Falk RH (Boston City Hospital, Boston, MA 02118), Knowlton AA, Manaker S. **Verapamil**-induced atrial fibrillation. *N Engl J Med.* 1988; 318:640–1. Case. (26-year-old healthy man; received verapamil hydrochloride 10 mg i.v. over 10 minutes; developed atrial fibrillation three to five minutes after drug administration with ventricular response of 50 beats/min at rest; spontaneous return to sinus rhythm after 70 minutes)

Trohman RG (Cardiovascular Laboratory, VA Medical Center, University and Woodland Avenue, Philadelphia, PA 19104), Castellanos D, Castellanos A et al. **Amiodarone**-induced delirium. *Ann Intern Med.* 1988; 108:68–9. Case. (66-year-old man with ventricular tachycardia; received amiodarone 1 g/day orally for 17 days; developed delirium; mental status improved upon drug discontinuation; positive rechallenge)

Drug Interactions

D'Arcy PF (Department of Pharmacy, Queens University of Belfast, Medical Biology Centre, Lisburn Road, Belfast BT97BL, N. Ireland). Psychosis with combined **cimetidine** and **imipramine**. *Int Pharm J.* 1988; 2:44. Case. (38-year-old woman with major depression; received cimetidine 100 mg three times daily for one year and imipramine hydrochloride 10 mg on day 1 and 20 mg daily thereafter; became progressively more depressed and anxious and developed command and auditory hallucinations and paranoid delusions three days after start of imipramine therapy; depressive and psychotic symptoms resolved within 47–72 hours after discontinuation of cimetidine and imipramine; patient remained in remission after one year)

Huang SM (Research Laboratory, Ortho Pharmaceutical Corp., Raritan, NJ 08869), Weintraub HS, Marriott TB et al. **Etintidine–theophylline** interaction study in humans. *Biopharm Drug Dispos.* 1987; 8:561–9. Study. (Double-blind, two-way crossover; 10 healthy men, aged 21–41 years; received etintidine hydrochloride 400 mg twice daily and theophylline elixir 5 mg/kg; etintidine rapidly absorbed by placebo and etintidine-treated groups; C_{max} not altered significantly by etintidine; etintidine prolonged elimination half-life of theophylline)

Manolis AS (Cardiac Electrophysiology, Tufts/New England Medical Center, 750 Washington Street, Boston, MA 02111), Estes NA. Orthostatic hypotension due to **quinidine** and **atenolol**. *Am J Med.* 1987; 82:1083–4. Case. (56-year-old woman; received quinidine 300 mg four times daily and atenolol 50 mg once daily; developed orthostatic hypotension after previously tolerating each drug alone)

Smilkstein MJ (Rocky Mountain Poison and Drug Center, 645 Bannock Street, Denver, CO 80204), Smolinske S, Rumack BH. Case of MAO inhibitor/MDMA interaction: agony after ecstasy. *J Toxicol Clin Toxicol.* 1987; 25:149–59. Case. (50-year-old man; ingested one tablet of **3,4-methylene-dioxy-methamphetamine** and 15 mg of **phenelzine sulfate**; developed marked hypertension, diaphoresis, altered mental status, and hypertonicity lasting five to six hours)

Drugs, Adverse Reactions

Duhra P (Skin Hospital, Birmingham B15 1BR, England), Foulds IS. **Penicillin**-induced pemphigus vulgaris. *Br J Dermatol.* 1988; 118:307. Case. (71-year-old man with asymptomatic neurosyphilis; received procaine penicillin injection 2.4 g/day i.m. for 19 days; concomitant probenicid 2 g/day; devel-

Continued on page 556

Your Heritage

As a ***Pharmacist***
As a ***Professional***

IS PRESERVED, PROTECTED, AND EXPLORED BY

THE AMERICAN INSTITUTE OF THE HISTORY OF PHARMACY

JOIN by sending your name, address, and $25 tax-deductible dues to:
AIHP, Pharmacy Building, Madison, WI 53706-1508

PHARMACY PRACTICE / CLINICAL PHARMACOKINETICS POSITION COLLEGE OF PHARMACY WASHINGTON STATE UNIVERSITY

The Washington State University College of Pharmacy announces the availability of one or more annual, full time, tenured track positions in pharmacy practice/clinical pharmacokinetics. This position offers a special opportunity to an individual with an interest in teaching and research in clinical pharmacokinetics. The individual will be affiliated with a Spokane hospital, and will live and work in Spokane, Washington.

Varied responsibilities include teaching clinical pharmacokinetics to senior pharmacy students at WSU-Spokane, supervision of senior pharmacy students in clinical pharmacokinetics clerkships, participation in team-taught didactic pharmacy practice (clinical) courses in Spokane and Pullman, and research and contribution to the scientific and professional literature.

Qualifications required are a Pharm.D. or equivalent educational experience, training in clinical pharmacokinetics, and potential for research. A residency or fellowship in clinical pharmacokinetics is highly desirable.

Application deadline is July 1, 1988, or until the position is filled. The position is available September 1, 1988.

To apply, send letter of interest with a resume and three references to:

Danial E. Baker, Pharm.D.
Associate Professor of Pharmacy Practice
College of Pharmacy
Washington State University
Pullman, WA 99164-6510

Washington State University is an EO/AA educator and employer. Protected group members are encouraged to apply and to identify their status.

Current Literature *Continued from page 555*

oped pemphigus vulgaris; considerable improvement after treatment with potent corticosteroid ointment, but new lesions still erupting after one year)

Saven S (Albert Einstein Medical Center, York and Tabor Road, Philadelphia, PA 19141), Lippmann ML. **Aminophylline** allergy. *Am J Med.* 1987; 82:1092. Case. (83-year-old woman with emphysema; received aminophylline 300 mg i.v. as loading dose; developed diffuse urticaria with associated hypotension 10 minutes after receiving aminophylline)

Sympatholytic Agents

Larrey D (Iserm U 24, Hospital Beaujon, 92118 Clichy, France), Henrion J, Heller F et al. **Metoprolol**-induced hepatitis: rechallenge and drug oxidation phenotyping. *Ann Intern Med.* 1988; 108:67–8. Case. (56-year-old woman; received metoprolol tartrate 50 mg daily for two weeks for migraine; developed hepatitis; abdominal pains resolved within 48 hours and liver function tests returned to normal after drug discontinuation; positive rechallenge)

Books Received

Books are listed as soon as received; selected books may be reviewed in Book Reviews in subsequent issues.

Progress in Drug Metabolism, Volume 10, edited by J. W. Bridges, L. F. Chasseaud, and G. G. Gibson. Published by Taylor & Francis Inc., 242 Cherry St., Philadelphia, PA 19106-1906, 1987. x + 354 p. Price $88.

Therapeutic Pharmacology, by Glenn D. Appelt and Jennifer M. Appelt. Published by Lea & Febiger, 600 Washington Square, Philadelphia, PA 19106-4198, 1988. xiv + 503 p. Price $34.50.

Advertising Index

The American Institute of the History of Pharmacy
Institutional, 556
American Society of Hospital Pharmacists
Database Services, 487
Handbook on Injectable Drugs, 489
Pharmacy Management Curriculum, 499
Beecham Laboratories
Timentin, 494–496
Eli Lilly and Company
Nebcin, 491–492
M.D. Anderson Cancer Center
Positions Available, 554
Roxane Laboratories, A Boehringer Ingelheim Company
Intensols, 500
Marinol, inside back cover, outside back cover
U.S. Public Health Service
Positions Available, 498
The Upjohn Company
Cleocin Phosphate, 485–486
Washington State University
Positions Available, 556
Wyeth Laboratories
Tubex, inside front cover

CU trouble spot:
IG drug administration

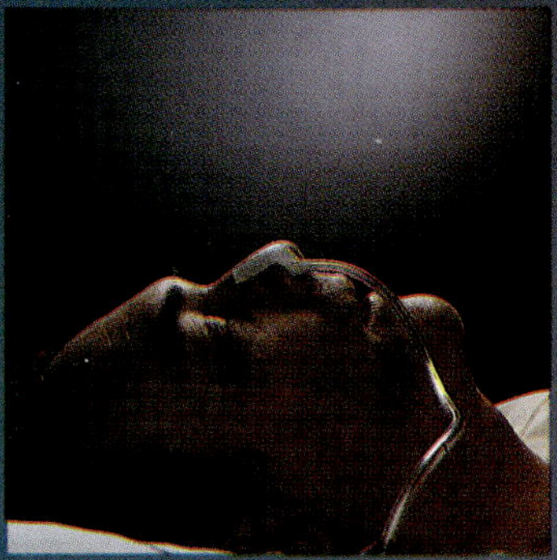

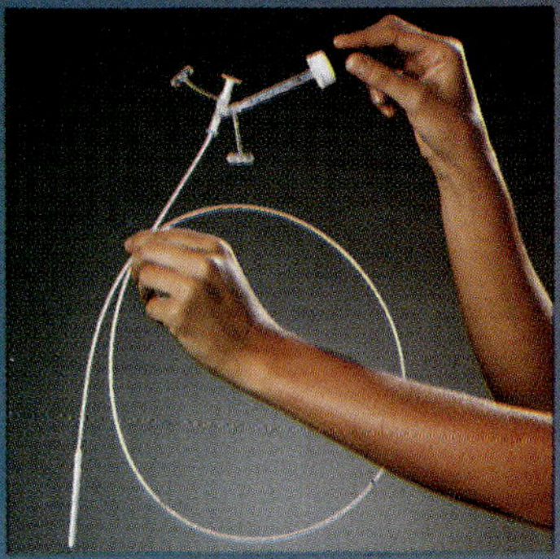

e solution is INTENSOLS™
oncentrated Oral Solutions

DEXAMETHASONE . . . . . . 1 mg/mL
PROPRANOLOL . . . . . . 80 mg/mL
PREDNISONE . . . . 5 mg/mL
DIAZEPAM . . . . 5 mg/mL

PALLIATIVE CARE AND CANCER PAIN PRODUCTS

Roxane
Laboratories, Inc.
Columbus, Ohio 43216

plifies drug ministration to sogastric patients

rsing benefits

- minates crushing tablets or dissolving psules
- ore accurate and consistent dose
- on't clog NG tubes
- ves nursing time for more productive tient care activities

rmacy benefits

- rrect dose is administered and sorbed by the patient
- ushing of sustained-release, sublingual, enteric-coated tablets is minimized
- ug/drug and acid/base interactions in ortar are avoided

y to dispense

ch bottle comes with a calibrated opper for accurate dosing and ation. Administering directly into NG e is possible.

Ideal for patients who have difficulty swallowing tablets

- Geriatric, pediatric, and cancer patients on high or variable doses
- Mixable with soft foods or liquids; most Intensols are tasteless so they won't alter the flavor
- Easy to swallow for improved compliance

Many Intensol-formulated drugs are available

- Prednisone, dexamethasone, diazepam, propranolol, and more
- Easy to switch from injectables to orals

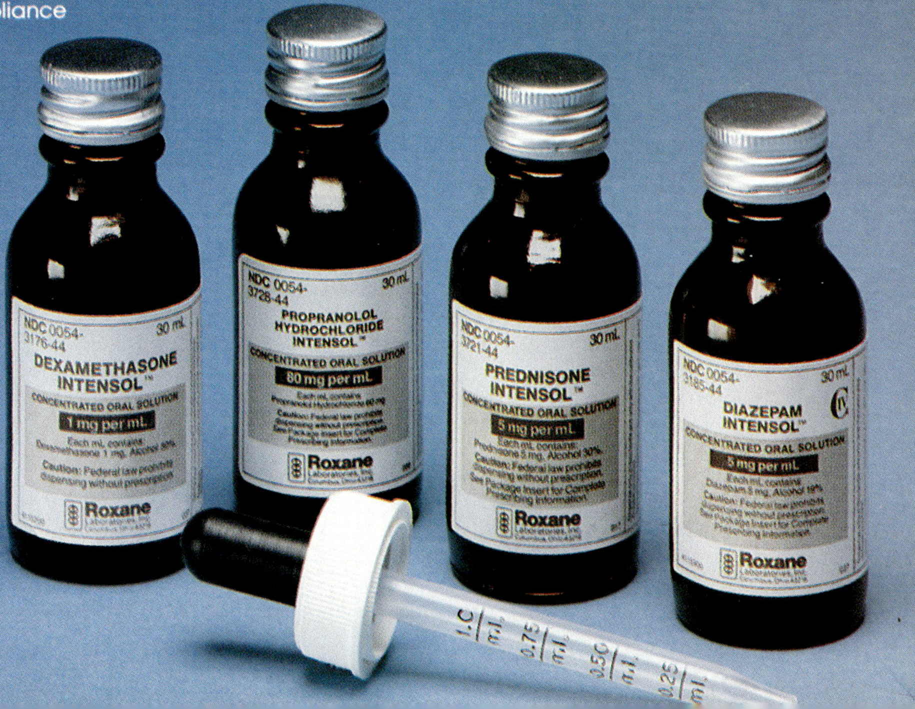

NTENSOLS™
olutions to tablet-taking problems

News

National Cancer Institute announces new study findings on breast-cancer treatment

Results of three unpublished studies on adjuvant therapy for node-negative breast cancer prompted the National Cancer Institute to inform practicing physicians of the findings and recommend that careful consideration be given to treating women with adjuvant hormonal or antineoplastic-drug therapy after surgery for breast cancer. Two of the studies were part of the National Surgical and Adjuvant Breast and Bowel Project; the third was a collaborative effort of the Eastern Cooperative Oncology Group and the Southwest Oncology Group. All three studies showed significant improvements in disease-free survival with adjuvant therapy after a median follow-up of three to four years. The studies used three different treatments—one hormonal regimen (tamoxifen) and two antineoplastic-drug regimens (one consisting of methotrexate, fluorouracil, and leucovorin and the other consisting of cyclophosphamide, methotrexate, fluorouracil, and prednisone). Disease-free survival rates were as follows: 82% with tamoxifen therapy versus 77% in the control group, 80% with the three-drug regimen versus 71% in the control group, and 84% with the four-drug regimen versus 67% in the control group. Both premenopausal and postmenopausal women benefited from adjuvant therapy in all three studies. Treatment was begun two to six weeks after primary therapy. The studies did not address the question of whether women who have had surgery for breast cancer in the past should now receive adjuvant therapy.

Fourth histamine antagonist, nizatidine, reaches U.S. market

FDA has approved nizatidine (Axid, Eli Lilly and Company) for the treatment of active duodenal ulcers and for use in the prevention of duodenal ulcer recurrence after ulcer healing. Nizatidine is the fourth histamine H_2 antagonist to be marketed in the United States.

Nizatidine is structurally related to ranitidine. It is rapidly absorbed after oral administration and is approximately 95% bioavailable. A volume of distribution of 1.5 L/kg and an elimination half-life of 1.6 hours have been reported. Nizatidine is metabolized to at least four compounds, one of which is about two thirds as active as nizatidine. About 95% of an oral dose is excreted in the urine as either the parent compound (60–65% of the dose) or metabolites (35%). Drug clearance is impaired by renal failure.

The drug is generally well tolerated. Preliminary data suggest that nizatidine does not inhibit the hepatic microsomal cytochrome P450 enzyme system. Antiandrogenic effects have not been reported.

The recommended dosage of nizatidine in the treatment of active duodenal ulcer disease is 300 mg at bedtime or 150 mg twice daily. A dosage of 150 mg at bedtime is recommended for maintenance therapy. Axid is available as 150- and 300-mg capsules. The suggested net trade price for bottles of 30 300-mg capsules is $54.77; the suggested price for bottles of 60 150-mg capsules is $56.62.

Preliminary study suggests role for clonidine in smoking cessation

Clonidine may have a role in smoking cessation, according to results of a preliminary double-blind, placebo-controlled randomized trial.[1]

Heavy smokers 18 to 55 years of age who wished to stop smoking and had failed in at least one previous attempt to stop were recruited to participate in the study. All participants received behavioral counseling based on the American Lung Association smoking cessation program. Clonidine hydrochloride was begun at least three days before the designated "quit day," and the dose was increased gradually to 200 μg/day by quit day. During the dosage titration period, participants were encouraged to taper their smoking. Only subjects who had reduced their smoking by at least 50% were entered in the study. During the four-week study period, the dosage of clonidine hydrochloride could be adjusted within the range of 150–300 μg/day. Clonidine therapy was withdrawn gradually after the four-week study period. Outcome was assessed by (1) self-report only, (2) self-report verified by serum cotinine concentration, and (3) a stricter standard of no relapses and verification by serum cotinine concentration.

Seventy-one subjects (33 in the clonidine group; 38 in the placebo group) were enrolled in the study. Average doses of clonidine during weeks 3 and 4, respectively, were 249 and 246 μg/day. During weeks 3 and 4, responders received an average daily dose of 244 μg, compared with 268 μg for nonresponders. Four of 33 subjects who began clonidine therapy withdrew from the study because of adverse effects.

Success rates were significantly higher (based on all three criteria) for the clonidine group. Based on the strictest outcome criterion, 52% of clonidine-treated patients and 21% of placebo recipients stopped smoking. Six months later, 27% of the clonidine group and 5% of the placebo group had not resumed smoking. Clonidine's effectiveness was limited to women.

Continued on page 562

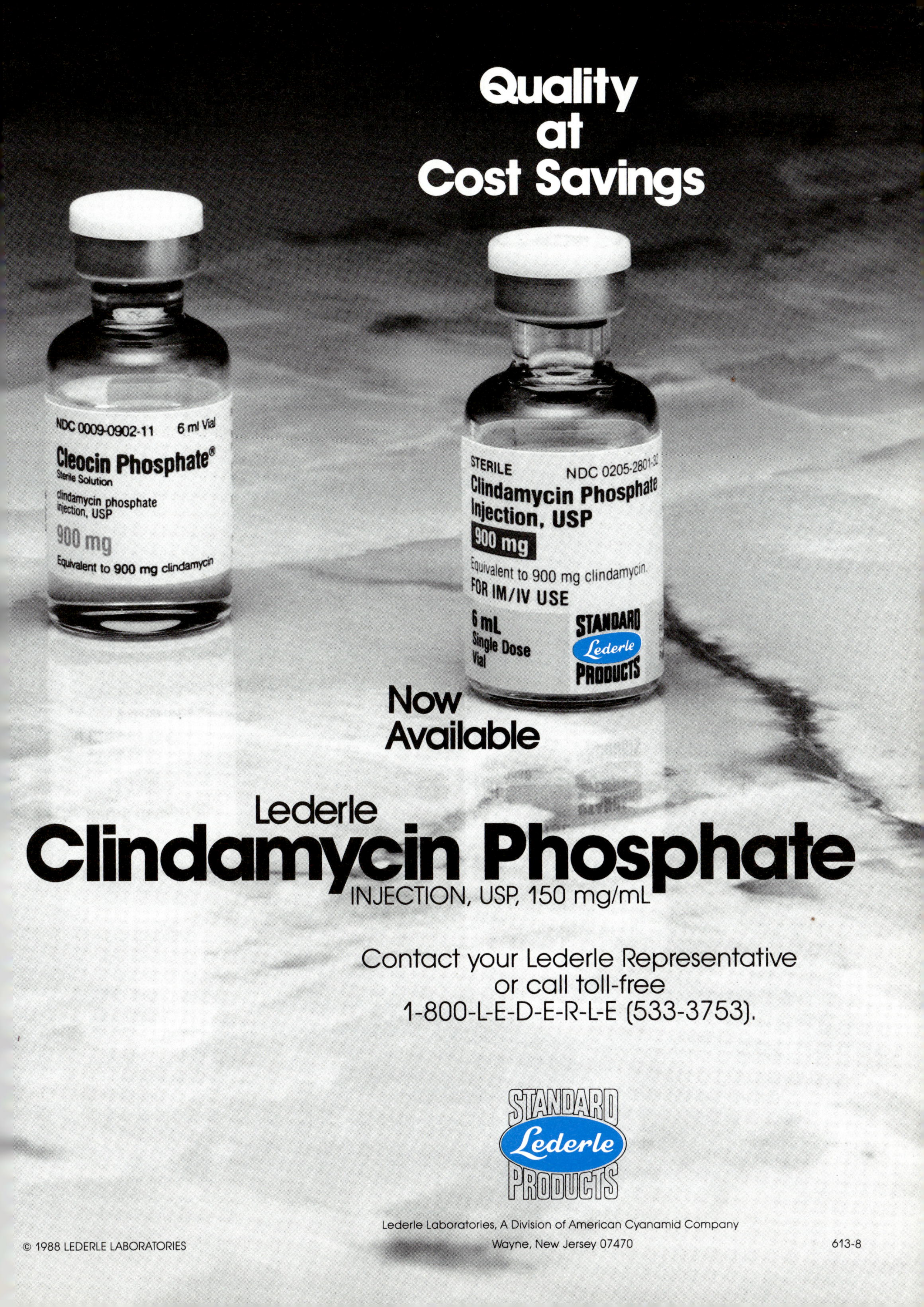

Quality
at
Cost Savings
NDC 0009-0902-11 6 ml Vial
Cleocin Phosphate®
Sterile Solution
clindamycin phosphate
injection, USP
900 mg
Equivalent to 900 mg clindamycin
STERILE NDC 0205-2801-32
Clindamycin Phosphate
Injection, USP
900 mg
Equivalent to 900 mg clindamycin.
FOR IM/IV USE
6 mL
Single Dose
Vial
STANDARD
Lederle
PRODUCTS
Now
Available
Lederle
Clindamycin Phosphate
INJECTION, USP, 150 mg/mL
Contact your Lederle Representative
or call toll-free
1-800-L-E-D-E-R-L-E (533-3753).
STANDARD
Lederle
PRODUCTS
Lederle Laboratories, A Division of American Cyanamid Company
Wayne, New Jersey 07470
© 1988 LEDERLE LABORATORIES
613-8

Continued from page 560

The study raises the issue of a possible association between smoking and major depression and highlights questions about how clonidine aids in nicotine withdrawal. The researchers noted an unexpectedly high prevalence (61%) of a history of major depression among study participants; in both the placebo and clonidine groups, success rates were significantly lower among individuals who had a history of depression.

1. Glassman AH, Stetner F, Walsh BT et al. Heavy smokers, smoking cessation, and clonidine: results of a double-blind, randomized trial. *JAMA*. 1988; 259:2863–6.

Overview of studies shows benefit of perioperative heparin use

Perioperative administration of heparin can reduce the risk of pulmonary emboli by about one half and prevent about two thirds of deep-vein thrombi, according to a systematic overview of more than 70 randomized trials of the efficacy of prophylactic use of subcutaneous heparin in general, urologic, or orthopedic surgery.[1] Most of the individual clinical trials have been too small to detect any effect of heparin prophylaxis on the incidence of pulmonary embolism.

General-surgery patients assigned to heparin therapy had a 67 ± 4% lower risk of deep-vein thrombosis than did control subjects. Risk reductions in orthopedic and urologic surgery were of similar magnitude. All trials used an every-8-hour or every-12-hour regimen and similar durations of therapy—5 to 7 days in the general-surgery trials and 7 to 10 days or until patients were ambulatory in the orthopedic surgery trials.

Findings of the overview confirmed the heparin-associated reduction in risk of fatal and nonfatal pulmonary emboli found in the International Multicentre Trial.[2-4] The overview showed a 40 ± 11% reduction in the risk of nonfatal pulmonary embolism and a 64 ± 15% reduction in the risk of fatal pulmonary embolism with heparin prophylaxis. There was no apparent increase in other causes of death.

Data on bleeding were incomplete in many trials, but there was evidence of an increased risk of bleeding among heparin recipients. The risk did not appear to be related to the frequency of heparin administration.

The authors concluded that routine perioperative administration of subcutaneous heparin should be considered, at least for patients who are at appreciable risk of thromboembolism.

1. Collins R, Scrimgeour A, Yusuf S et al. Reduction in fatal pulmonary embolism and venous thrombosis by perioperative administration of subcutaneous heparin: overview of results of randomized trials in general, orthopedic, and urologic surgery. *N Engl Med*. 1988; 318:1162–73.
2. Prevention of fatal postoperative pulmonary embolism by low doses of heparin: an international multicentre trial. *Lancet*. 1975; 2:45–51.
3. Gruber UF, Duckert F, Fridrich R et al. Prevention of postoperative thromboembolism by dextran 40, low doses of heparin, or xantinol nicotinate. *Lancet*. 1977; 1:207–10.
4. Prevention of fatal postoperative pulmonary embolism by low doses of heparin: reappraisal of results of International Multicentre Trial. *Lancet*. 1977; 1:567–9.

News Briefs

• **Interferon alfa-2b** (Intron A, Schering Corporation) has a new labeled indication for the treatment of selected cases of condyloma accuminata; intralesional administration of 1 million units three times a week for three weeks is recommended.

• Labeling indications for **captopril** (Capoten, E. R. Squibb & Sons, Inc.) have been expanded to include use in the treatment of mild to moderate congestive heart failure; the approved labeling previously specified use of captopril as an adjunct to digoxin and diuretic therapy.

• Based on antigenic analysis of recent influenza viruses, the World Health Organization and the U.S. Public Health Service have issued recommendations for updated type A(H3N2) and type B antigens for vaccines to be used during the 1988–1989 influenza season; **trivalent influenza vaccines** manufactured in the United States should contain A/Taiwan/1/86(H1N1), A/Sichuan/2/87(H3N2), and B/Victoria/2/87 antigens.

Upcoming Specialty Meetings

American College of Nutrition . . . September 14–16, . . . New Orleans, LA . . . contact: M. S. Seelig, M.D., 345 Central Avenue, Scarsdale, NY 10583; 914-723-4247.

Second Annual Aging Symposium: 1988 Drug Therapy and Nutrition in the Elderly . . . sponsored by Veterans Administration Medical Center, Martinez, CA, and Continuing Education in Pharmacy, University of California at San Francisco . . . September 17–18 . . . San Francisco, CA . . . contact: Continuing Education S/P, University of California, Box 0446, San Francisco, CA 94143; 415-476-4194.

American College of Chest Physicians . . . October 3–7 . . . Anaheim, CA . . . contact: A. Soffer, M.D., 911 Busse Highway, Park Ridge, IL; 312-698-2200.

Fiftieth Anniversary Symposium: Frontiers for Therapeutic Advance . . . coordinated by The Squibb Institute for Medical Research . . . October 31 . . . Princeton, NJ . . . contact: R. H. Jones; 609-921-4265.

American College of Clinical Pharmacology . . . October 31–November 2 . . . Orlando, FL . . . contact: W. F. Chaveas, 175 Strafford Avenue, Suite 1, Wayne, PA 19087; 215-687-7711.

American Association for the Study of Liver Disease . . . November 5–8 . . . Chicago, IL . . . contact: S. N. Crowley, Slack Inc., 6900 Grove Road, Thorofare, NJ 08086; 609-848-1000 ext. 210.

American Cancer Society . . . November 8–12 . . . New York, NY . . . contact: G. R. Gadberry, 90 Park Avenue, New York, NY 10016; 212-599-3600.

The First National Cholesterol Conference . . . November 9–11 . . . Arlington, VA . . . contact: The National Cholesterol Conference, 4733 Bethesda Avenue, Suite 530, Bethesda, MD 20814; 301-951-3275.

Therapy Consultation

The Therapy Consultation *section provides brief advice, in question-and-answer format, on how to handle specific drug-therapy problems. Readers are invited to submit questions, which will be referred to a consultant for an answer. The problems should not be highly specialized or unusual, nor should they be mundane. Questions are answered briefly, based largely on the judgment and personal experience of the consultant, although selected references may be cited to substantiate the consultant's advice.*

Assistance in identifying Therapy Consultation *topics is provided by the drug information centers at the following institutions: Albert B. Chandler Medical Center and College of Pharmacy, University of Kentucky, Lexington; Arizona Health Sciences Center, Tucson; Medical College of Virginia Hospitals, Richmond; University of California Medical Center, San Diego; and University of Michigan Medical Center, Ann Arbor.*

Treatment of acetaminophen overdose when oral acetylcysteine therapy is not tolerated

Question: A five-year-old girl who reportedly had ingested acetaminophen 200 mg/kg had a serum acetaminophen concentration of 240 μg/mL four hours after the ingestion. Oral acetylcysteine therapy was begun, but the patient vomited the first dose and complained of the unpleasant odor of the solution. What can be done when patients have difficulty tolerating oral acetylcysteine therapy and refuse subsequent doses? Is there an intravenous preparation available for use in the management of acetaminophen overdose?

Answer: Oral acetylcysteine is the approved antidote for the management of acetaminophen overdose in the United States. Because of the characteristic sulfurous odor and the large doses required for antidotal therapy, oral administration of acetylcysteine often results in nausea, vomiting, and other gastrointestinal adverse effects.

Complete gastric emptying, via emesis or lavage, and the administration of activated charcoal should be performed before oral acetylcysteine is given. (If activated charcoal is administered within one hour of acetylcysteine therapy, it should be removed before acetylcysteine is given to prevent binding of acetylcysteine in the gastrointestinal tract.) A loading dose of 140 mg/kg of acetylcysteine should be administered orally, followed by 17 maintenance doses of 70 mg/kg/dose given at four-hour intervals. Any dose that is vomited needs to be repeated.

Acetylcysteine is available as a 10% or a 20% solution. It should be diluted to at least 5%, which is approximately isotonic. Solutions should be administered within one hour after preparation. Water may be used as the diluent, but use of a flavored carbonated beverage, such as Fresca or a cola, or a citrus juice, such as orange or grapefruit juice, may increase the palatability. The use of iced or cold solutions may further improve the palatability. Having the patient pinch his or her nose and breathe through the mouth while drinking the solution may help. Use of a drinking straw may also minimize the unpleasant odor of acetylcysteine.

Alternatively, acetylcysteine may be administered, in the same dose and regimen, via a nasogastric tube. In this case, water should be used as the diluent, and the final concentration should be 5%. Vomiting that persists despite administration of the drug in this manner may be minimized if the nasogastric tube is advanced into the duodenum. Administration of acetylcysteine at a slow, continuous rate through the nasogastric tube may decrease the likelihood of emesis. If severe vomiting persists, metoclopramide hydrochloride 1 mg/kg (of metoclopramide) may be administered intravenously or intramuscularly.

Intravenous acetylcysteine is considered the drug of choice in the United Kingdom and Canada.[1,2] The 20-hour European protocol for intravenous acetylcysteine therapy consists of a 150-mg/kg dose (diluted in 200 mL of 5% dextrose injection) infused over 15 minutes, followed by acetylcysteine 50 mg/kg (in 200 mL of 5% dextrose injection) infused over the next 4 hours and 100 mg/kg (in 1000 mL of 5% dextrose injection) over the final 16 hours.

A sterile, pyrogen-free injectable formulation of acetylcysteine is not commercially available in the United States. Injectable acetylcysteine is available to eligible patients under two investigational protocols, one through the National Capital Poison Center and the other through the Rocky Mountain Poison Center. The regimen of acetylcysteine specified by the National Capital Poison Center protocol is identical to the 20-hour European regimen. The Rocky Mountain Poison Center protocol calls for administration of acetylcysteine over 48 hours. An initial dose of 140 mg/kg is given, followed by 12 doses of 70 mg/kg, administered as one-hour infusions every four hours. Acetylcysteine is supplied as a 0.2 g/mL solution in 30-mL vials; the solution should be diluted one-to-five with 5% dextrose injection.

Patients receiving intravenous acetylcysteine should be monitored carefully for adverse reactions. Flushing of the face or chest is relatively common.[3] Adverse reactions usually begin within 15 minutes after therapy is begun, but the onset may be delayed for up to one hour. Adverse reactions most commonly involve a generalized erythematous rash that may be accompanied by hypotension, tachycardia, nausea, vomiting, and dizziness. The incidence of anaphylaxis was 3% in one series of patients,[4] and one patient who received twice the recommended dose died.[5] Bronchospasm and precipitation of asthma have also been reported.[6] Adverse reactions usually resolve when therapy is discontinued, but patients may require supportive care.

Hepatotoxicity associated with acetaminophen overdose is usually transient in patients treated with acetylcysteine. It is characterized by marked increases in liver function test values and, in more serious cases, by a prolonged prothrombin time. With oral acetylcysteine therapy, the incidence of hepatotoxicity is 7% if therapy is begun within 10 hours after acetaminophen ingestion and 43% if treatment is begun within 10–24 hours.[7] With the 20-hour intravenous acetylcysteine protocol, incidence figures of 3% (treatment within 10 hours) and 67% (treatment within 10–24 hours) have been reported.[2] Fewer patients have received the 48-hour regimen. No cases of hepatotoxicity have been reported when this regimen was begun within 10 hours after acetaminophen ingestion; 15% of patients have developed hepatotoxicity when treatment was begun within 10–24 hours.[8]

Direct comparisons of intravenous and oral acetylcysteine therapy are lacking; thus, neither method has been proven to be superior.

1. Prescott LF. Treatment of severe acetaminophen poisoning with intravenous acetylcysteine. *Arch Intern Med.* 1981; 141:386–9.
2. Prescott LF, Illingworth RN, Critchley JAJH et al. Intravenous *N*-acetylcysteine: the treatment of choice for paracetamol poisoning. *Br Med J.* 1979; 2:1097–100.
3. Rumack BH, ed. Poisindex. 56th ed. Denver: Micromedix Inc.; 1988.
4. Mant TGK, Tempowski JH, Volans GN et al. Adverse reactions to acetylcysteine and effects of overdose. *Br Med J.* 1983; 287:876.
5. Anon. Death after *N*-acetylcysteine. *Lancet.* 1984; 1:1421.
6. Ho SWH, Beilin LJ. Asthma associated with *N*-acetylcysteine infusion and paracetamol poisoning: report of two cases. *Br Med J.* 1983; 287:876.
7. Rumack BH, Peterson RG, Koch GG et al. Acetaminophen overdose: 662 cases with evaluation of oral acetylcysteine treatment. *Arch Intern Med.* 1981; 141:880–5.
8. Bronstein AC, Linden GH, Hall AH et al. Intravenous *N*-acetylcysteine for acute acetaminophen poisoning. *Vet Hum Toxicol.* 1985; 28:316. Abstract.

KATHERINE V. MANN, PHARM.D.
Medical Information Resident
Philadelphia College of Pharmacy and Science
Philadelphia, PA 19104

Chair, Department of Pharmacy

The School of Pharmacy, State University of New York at Buffalo, is seeking a dynamic pharmaceutical scientist at the associate- or full-professor level to serve as Chair, Department of Pharmacy. Highly promising assistant professor candidates may also be considered. The department has 8 full-time and 18 part-time faculty and is responsible for both B.S. and Pharm. D. education. The successful candidate must have an active research program in an area of expertise, a solid publication record as documentation of accomplishment, and a record of commitment to excellence in teaching. The chair position presents an excellent opportunity for the continued conduct of scholarly activity as there is an established and smoothly functioning administrative support structure already in place.

Interested persons should send a curriculum vitae, a description of research and teaching activities and administrative experience, and the names of three references to Dr. Jerome J. Schentag, Professor of Pharmaceutics/Pharmacy, SUNY at Buffalo, and Director, The Clinical Pharmacokinetics Laboratory, 3 Gates Circle, Millard Fillmore Hospital, Buffalo, NY 14209. Inquiries 716-887-4917.

SUNY is an equal opportunity/affirmative action employer.

Consumer Drug Digest
Revised Edition

Consumer Drug Digest, Revised Edition, is a comprehensive, authoritative guide to common prescription and non-prescription drugs . . . helping patients to understand their medications and learn what they can do to be more aware of their drug therapy.

Written in layman's language, this drug information handbook contains over 250 of the most commonly prescribed drugs, which comprise over 95% of prescriptions written in the U.S. today. ***Consumer Drug Digest*** is easy to read and use. And, it's indexed by both brand names and generic names, so it's easy to locate information.

The ***Consumer Drug Digest*** is an excellent tool for patients and for pharmacy services areas.

Order your copy today.

☐ Please send me a brochure on **Consumer Drug Digest**

Name ______

Address ______

City ______ State ______ Zip ______

Send to: ASHP Publication Records Dept.,

4630 Montgomery Avenue, Bethesda, MD 20814

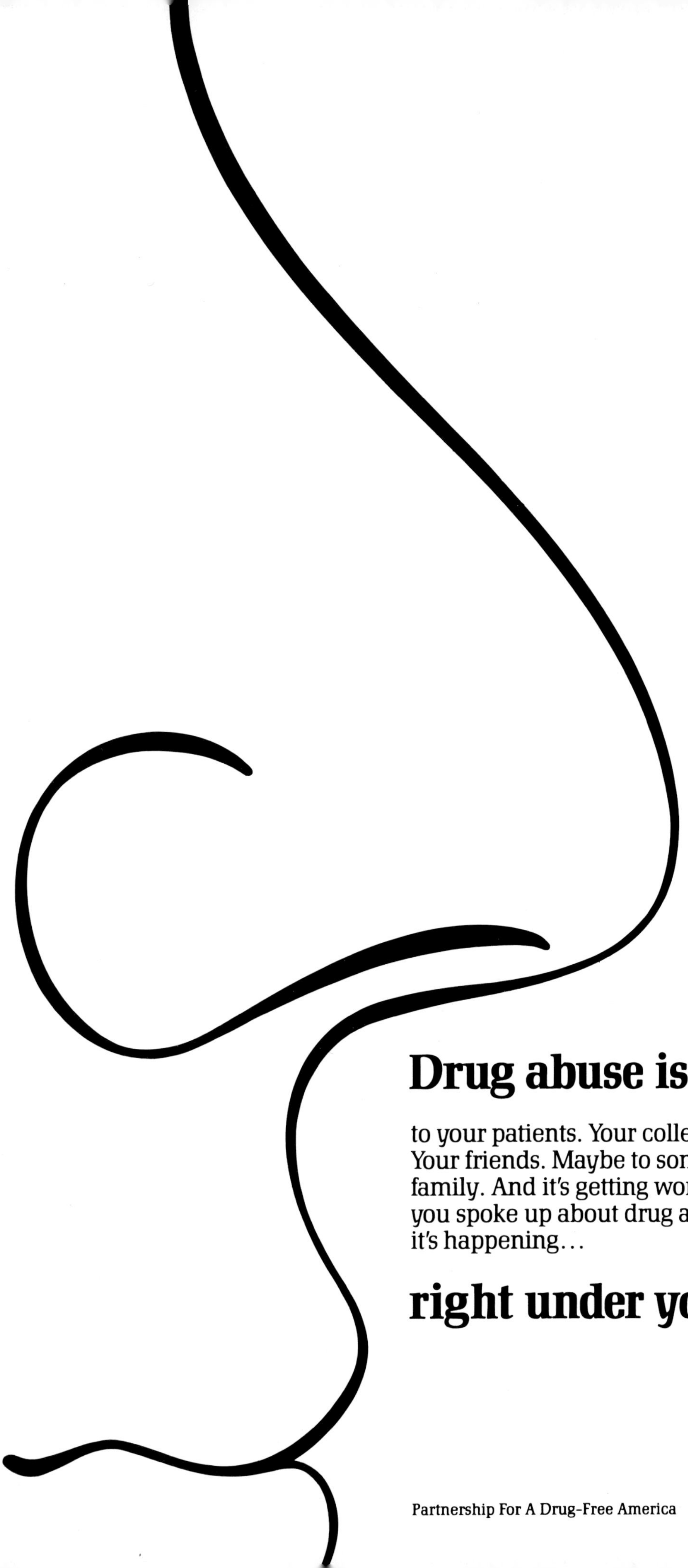

Drug abuse is happening...

to your patients. Your colleagues. Your friends. Maybe to someone in your family. And it's getting worse. Isn't it time you spoke up about drug abuse? Because it's happening...

right under your nose.

Partnership For A Drug-Free America

Letters

The Letters *column is a forum for rapid exchange of ideas among readers of* CP. *Liberal criteria are applied in the review of submissions to encourage contributions to this column.*

The Letters *column includes the following types of contributions: (1) comments, addenda, and minor updates on previously published work, (2) alerts on potential problems related to drug therapy or clinical research, (3) observations or comments on trends in drug therapy or clinical research, and (4) brief expressions of opinion about controversies in drug therapy or clinical research.*

Letters need not be submitted with the journal's manuscript checklist. The following conditions, however, must be adhered to: (1) the body of the letter must be no longer than two typewritten pages, (2) the use of references, tables, and illustrations should be minimized, (3) the authors' names, affiliations, and mailing addresses must be typed at the end of the letter in the format used by CP, *and (4) the entire letter (including references, tables, and authors' names) must be typed double spaced on plain white paper (not letterhead). Following acceptance of a letter, the authors are required to sign an exclusive publication statement and a copyright-transferral form.*

Sodium thiosulfate unproven as bromate antidote

In the recent Drug Experience report regarding bromate poisoning,[1] the patient was treated with sodium thiosulfate administered by intravenous drip. We encountered a similar case of sodium bromate poisoning in October 1984 that led us to question the use of sodium thiosulfate to prevent bromate-induced renal and aural toxicity.[2] We searched the literature at the time but failed to identify any controlled human or animal studies that have evaluated the use of sodium thiosulfate as an antidote for bromate poisoning. Only isolated anecdotal case reports exist.

The first documented use of sodium thiosulfate for the treatment of bromate poisoning was in 1949. Thompson and Westfall[3] contacted Toni (the manufacturer of the cold wave neutralizer involved in the case) and learned that "research is in progress to determine antidotes for this poison." Toni put Thompson and Westfall in contact with Michael G. Mulinos, M.D., Ph.D., the principal investigator in the aforementioned research. As Thompson and Westfall reported, Mulinos suggested that the stomach acidity be neutralized to prevent formation of the irritating hydrobromic acid and a sodium salt be used to either counteract "the toxic effects of potassium ion or substitute sodium bromate for potassium bromate." Mulinos also suggested that sodium thiosulfate be used to combat the oxidizing effect of the bromate ion. Thompson and Westfall did not cite any published literature to support this recommendation, just the personal communication with Mulinos.

The use of sodium thiosulfate was again recommended by a manufacturer in 1951.[4] The manufacturer also recommended emetics such as "a teaspoonful of mustard in a glassful of warm water or zinc sulfate, half teaspoonful in warm water" and demulcents such as "milk, flour and water, or cereal gruel." Although the latter recommendations are no longer considered to be acceptable therapy, sodium thiosulfate has been continually recommended in standard clinical toxicology texts,[5-10] and Poisindex, the standard reference used by most poison control centers, currently recommends its use.[11] None of these resources has cited original research on sodium thiosulfate. An author citation search that we conducted using *Science Citation Index* showed that Mulinos has published a great deal of original research, but none of the studies relates to bromate poisoning. Neither Redken, a recent manufacturer of bromate-containing hair products,[1] nor Gillette, parent company of Toni (the manufacturer originally contacted by Thompson and Westfall) has any unpublished data on file (King G, Redken, Personal communication, 1988 Mar 31, and Giovacchini RP, Gillette, Personal communication, 1988 Apr).

Although there is a theoretical basis for using a reducing agent such as sodium thiosulfate to treat the ingestion of a potent oxidizing agent such as bromate, current recommendations appear to be based purely on speculation. Empiric therapy is common in clinical toxicology because controlled clinical trials are rare[12]; however, treatment recommendations should be based on scientific facts. Bromate poisonings do not occur often, so it is unlikely in the near future that human studies will resolve the question of sodium thiosulfate efficacy. Animal studies probably should be conducted to initially determine sodium thiosulfate's potential as an antidote. Extrapolations from other areas of sodium thiosulfate use should be made cautiously; for example, although sodium thiosulfate has been used to prevent cisplatin-induced nephrotoxicity,[13] questions remain as to its mechanism of action and safety.[14] Until more data are available, we recommend that sodium thiosulfate not be used to treat human bromate poisoning.

1. Lue JN, Johnson ED, Edwards DL. Bromate poisoning from ingestion of professional hair-care neutralizer. *Clin Pharm.* 1988; 7:66–70.
2. Kearney TE, Redetzki HM, McElwee NE. Sodium bromate poisoning in an infant who ingested a home cold wave neutralizing solution. *Vet Hum Toxicol.* 1986; 28:482.
3. Thompson HC, Westfall SW. Potassium bromate poisoning: Report of a case due to ingestion of a "cold wave" neutralizer. *J Pediatr.* 1949; 34:362–4.
4. Parker WA, Barr JR. Potassium bromate poisoning. *Br Med J.* 1951; 1:1363.
5. Gleason MN, Gosselin RE, Hodge HC. Clinical toxicology of commercial products. Boston: Williams & Wilkins; 1957:123.

Continued on page 572

We Asked Pharmacists...

For several years, our researchers met with pharmacists in institutions both large and small, all across the country.

We asked about IV therapy in the ICU. And these were among the top priorities:

1. Simplified scheduling of multiple drugs

2. Simplified approach to drug compatibility

3. Reduced number of IV lines to the patient

4. Reduction in venipuncture sites needed

5. Reduced number of medications given at wrong times

6. Fewer IV pumps to manage

7. Reduced risk of sepsis/ infection due to touch contamination

8. Reduced time spent preparing IV medications

9. Reduced bedside clutter

10. Reduction in medications missed

Because a major breakthrough in IV management was on the horizon...

Baxter

Continued from page 570

6. Gleason MN, Gosselin RE, Hodge HC. Clinical toxicology of commercial products. 2nd ed. Boston: Williams & Wilkins; 1963:34.
7. Arena JM. Poisoning. 2nd ed. Springfield, IL: Charles C Thomas; 1970:163–4.
8. Arena JM. Poisoning. 3rd ed. Springfield IL: Charles C Thomas; 1974:163–4.
9. Driesbach RH. Handbook of poisoning: Diagnosis and treatment. 7th ed. Los Altos, CA: Lange; 1971:235–6.
10. Gosselin RE, Hodge HC, Smith RP et al. Clinical toxicology of commercial products. 4th ed. Boston: Williams & Wilkins; 1976:66.
11. Rumack BH, ed. Poisindex. 56th ed. Denver: Micromedex Inc.; 1988.
12. Mortensen ME. Clinical toxicology and epidemiology—A good match. *Pediatrics.* 1988; 81:163–4.
13. Markman M, Cleary S, Howells SB. Nephrotoxicity of high-dose intracavitary cisplatin with intravenous thiosulfate protection. *Eur J Cancer Clin Oncol.* 1985; 21:1015–18.
14. De Broe ME, Wedeen RP. Prevention of cisplatin-induced nephrotoxicity. *Eur J Cancer Clin Oncol.* 1986; 22:1029–31.

NEWELL E. MCELWEE, PHARM.D., Associate Director
Intermountain Regional Poison Center
College of Pharmacy
University of Utah
50 North Medical Drive, Building 428
Salt Lake City, UT 84132

THOMAS E. KEARNEY, PHARM.D., Executive Director
Delaware Valley Regional Poison Control Center
Children's Hospital of Philadelphia
One Children's Center
Philadelphia, PA 19104

FACULTY POSITION
DEPARTMENT OF PHARMACY PRACTICE
SCHOOL OF PHARMACY
UNIVERSITY OF WASHINGTON

The School of Pharmacy is seeking a full-time, tenure-tract, faculty member to participate in clinical research and education. Applicants should have a Pharm. D. degree and at least one year of postdoctoral or equivalent experience in a specialty area of adult internal medicine or surgery. A research fellowship or research experience is required.

The selected candidate will be expected to provide clinical and didactic instruction in baccalaureate and Doctor of Pharmacy programs, conduct clinical research, and actively participate in a progressive department of pharmacy practice. Salary and rank are commensurate with experience.

Interested applicants should submit a letter of application, curriculum vitae, and three letters of recommendation by November 1, 1988, to:

John R. Horn, Pharm.D.
Associate Professor
Department of Pharmacy Practice
Mail Stop SC-69
University of Washington
Seattle, WA 98195

The University of Washington is an
Affirmative Action/Equal Opportunity Employer.

I appreciate the comments and information provided by Drs. McElwee and Kearney concerning our case report. Retrospective review of case reports (descriptive epidemiology) is an accepted method of evaluating an empiric treatment approach that is not based on controlled clinical trials.[1] Unfortunately, the low incidence of pediatric bromate poisoning and the dearth of published reports of bromate poisoning managed with or without sodium thiosulfate essentially preclude this method of treatment evaluation. This leaves us with a very real and not uncommon therapeutic dilemma.

I compliment McElwee and Kearney for taking an absolute stand on the role of sodium thiosulfate in the management of bromate poisoning. However, I must question their final statement: "until more data are available . . . sodium thiosulfate [should] not be used for treatment of human bromate poisoning." They have not presented any clinical evidence to suggest that the drug is not effective. As practitioners, we must also consider the patient. When faced with the question of how to treat a child who has ingested a potentially lethal dose of sodium or potassium bromate, we must rapidly determine, on the basis of the available information, whether the potential benefits of sodium thiosulfate administration outweigh the potential risks. In addition to being used to prevent cisplatin-induced nephrotoxicity, injectable sodium thiosulfate has been used as an antidote for cyanide and iodine poisoning as well as to treat extravasation of antineoplastic agents such as dactinomycin and mechlorethamine.[2-4] Although extrapolations from this information must be made cautiously, the relative safety of sodium thiosulfate administration can be reasonably inferred.

Lack of harm may be an insufficient justification for adopting an unvalidated treatment,[1] and evaluative studies should be conducted. However, in the interim, I believe that the continued use of sodium thiosulfate in human bromate poisoning is rational, considering the morbidity and mortality associated with bromate poisoning and the high probability that sodium thiosulfate reduces bromate to bromide. Each practitioner faced with this clinical situation will have to use his or her own judgment to make the best decision possible.

1. Mortensen ME. Clinical toxicology and epidemiology—a good match. *Pediatrics.* 1988; 81:163–4.
2. Gosselin RE, Smith RP, Hodge HC et al. Clinical toxicology of commercial products. 5th ed. Baltimore: Williams and Wilkins; 1984:123–30.
3. Arena JM, Drew RH. Poisoning. 5th ed. Springfield, IL: Charles C Thomas; 1986:63.
4. Ignoffo RJ, Friedman MA. Therapy of local toxicities caused by extravasation of cancer chemotherapeutic drugs. *Cancer Treat Rev.* 1980; 7:17–27.

CARY E. JOHNSON, PHARM.D., Associate Professor and Clinical Pharmacist–Pediatrics
College of Pharmacy
The University of Michigan
428 Church Street
Ann Arbor, MI 48109-1065

Editor's note: According to McElwee and Kearney, Redken has discontinued the manufacture of bromate-containing neutralizers. The four Redken products listed in Table 1 of the Drug Experience report by Lue et al. have not been available commercially for several years. However, it is conceivable that these products may still be in the possession of consumers.

INTRODUCING

The MultiPlex™ Series 100 Fluid Management System

It gives you control over IV solutions

...and minimizes lost charges as well!

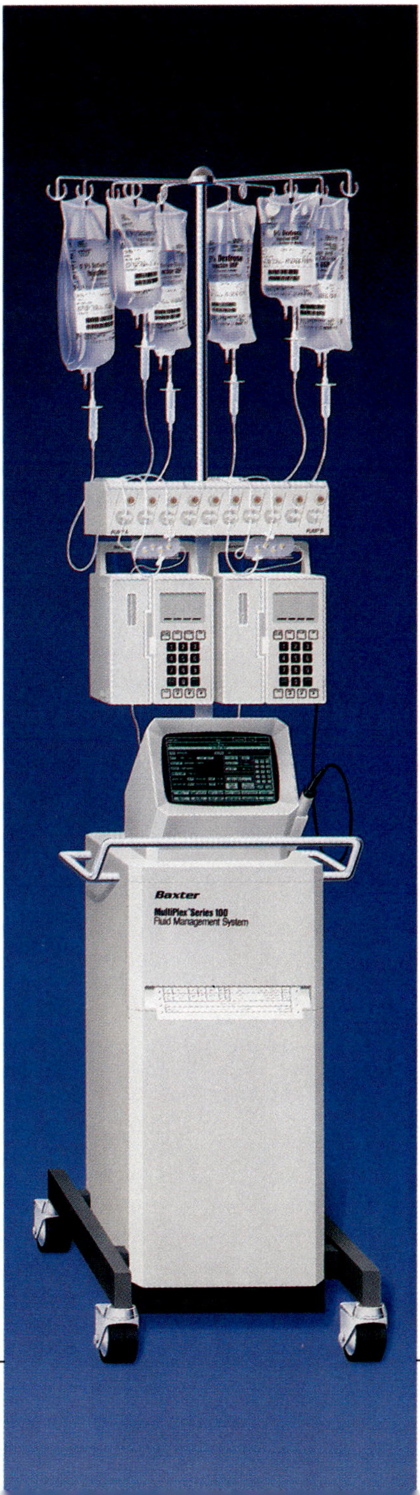

- Pharmacy generated bar codes — containing dose, rate and start times — enable entry of orders into the system and generate hard-copy documentation of solutions administered.
- Customized database at the patient's bedside contains your pharmacy's formulary — standard drugs, solutions, concentrations and dosages. Also, compatibility information.
- 24-hour programmability facilitates timely fluid delivery — supporting pharmacokinetics and providing multiple dose capabilities.

Want proof?
Call 1.800.527.2377
Right now!

Critical Care IV Therapy— An art becomes a science

Baxter Healthcare Corporation
MultiPlex Systems Division
Route 120 and Wilson Road
Round Lake, Illinois 60073
312.546.6311 ext. 5858

© Copyright 1988, Baxter Healthcare Corporation.
All rights reserved. Patent pending.

Baxter

Drug Review

Mitoxantrone: A novel anthracycline derivative

JIM KOELLER and MELODY EBLE

Abstract: The chemistry, pharmacology, pharmacokinetics, clinical efficacy, dosage and administration, and adverse effects of mitoxantrone are reviewed.

Mitoxantrone, an aminoanthraquinone that was synthesized in 1979, belongs to a new chemical class of agents known as the anthracenediones. It possesses antiviral, antibacterial, immunomodulatory, and antitumor activity. The drug's antitumor activity is attributed to its interaction with DNA topoisomerase II, and its interaction with human cells may also involve nonintercalary, electrostatic interactions. Mitoxantrone is poorly absorbed orally and is most commonly administered intravenously. The drug is rapidly distributed into the red blood cells, white blood cells, and platelets, followed by deep-tissue sequestration.

Mitoxantrone has demonstrated clinical efficacy in the treatment of leukemia, lymphoma, and breast cancer. As a single agent, mitoxantrone has a response rate of roughly 30% in acute nonlymphocytic leukemia or acute myeloid leukemia. In combination with other standard agents (cytarabine, vincristine, and prednisone), the response rate may reach 60%. In breast cancer, mitoxantrone's response rate as a single agent is 25–30%, while combination regimens produce response rates of 60% or more. The drug can cause cardiotoxicity with cumulative doses. Other adverse effects include myelosuppression, nausea and vomiting, stomatitis, mucositis, and alopecia. The cost of mitoxantrone is comparable to that of doxorubicin, but it is substantially more expensive than daunorubicin.

Mitoxantrone is an important new agent with antitumor activity in leukemia, lymphoma, and breast cancer. In most situations, mitoxantrone will be considered second-line treatment or a restricted-use item because of its high cost and because of the lack of FDA approval for indications other than acute nonlymphocytic leukemia.

Index terms: Antineoplastic agents; Breast neoplasms; Dosage; Drug administration; Leukemia; Lymphoma; Mitoxantrone; Pharmacokinetics; Toxicity

Clin Pharm. 1988; 7:574–81

For many years the anthracyclines have been the cornerstones of anticancer therapy. Doxorubicin and daunorubicin are the two anthracyclines that are commercially available in the United States. They are used in numerous protocols for both solid tumors and hematologic malignancies. This efficacy does not come without a cost. Although these agents are quite active against a variety of cancers, they also possess serious toxicity, which can even preclude subsequent treatment. At optimal doses, doxorubicin and daunorubicin can produce serious nausea and vomiting, myelosuppression, hair loss, and skin toxicity. Extravasation of these two drugs causes tissue necrosis. More important, these agents demonstrate cumulative cardiotoxicity, which is manifested by congestive heart failure, at total doses of more than 550 mg/sq m. This toxicity limits the duration of therapy for many patients and can necessitate a change to an agent that may be less active. Because of these difficulties, researchers have continued to look for newer, more active, less toxic derivatives, or new entities. Mi-

JIM KOELLER, M.S., is Associate Clinical Professor of Pharmacy, College of Pharmacy, The University of Texas at Austin; Associate Clinical Professor of Pharmacology and Medicine, The University of Texas Health Science Center, San Antonio; and Oncology Clinical Specialist, Audie L. Murphy Memorial Veterans' Hospital, San Antonio, TX. MELODY EBLE, PHARM.D., is Oncology Specialty Resident, Audie L. Murphy Memorial Veterans' Hospital, and Clinical Instructor, The University of Texas Health Science Center, San Antonio.

Address reprint requests to Mr. Koeller at Medical Oncology (111J), Audie L. Murphy Memorial Veterans' Hospital, 7400 Merton Minter Boulevard, San Antonio, TX 78284.

The assistance of Leslie Burk in preparing this manuscript is acknowledged.

Copyright © 1988, American Society of Hospital Pharmacists, Inc. All rights reserved. 0278-2677/88/0801-0574$02.00.

toxantrone is one such agent, which has recently been approved for use in acute nonlymphocytic leukemia.

Mitoxantrone (Novantrone, dihydroxyanthracenedione [DHAD], NSC-301739, Lederle Laboratories) is an intensely blue aminoanthraquinone, which was synthesized in 1979.[1,2] This drug belongs to a new chemical class of agents, known as the anthracenediones, that are structurally related to the anthracyclines but lack the sugar moiety and A ring of the tetracyclic structure of doxorubicin (Figure 1). Mitoxantrone was found to possess antiviral, antibacterial, immunomodulatory, and substantial antitumor activity.[3-5] The compound has since been proven efficacious in Phase II and Phase III trials. Mitoxantrone's activity has been previously reviewed.[6,7]

Figure 1. Chemical structures of doxorubicin, daunorubicin, and mitoxantrone.

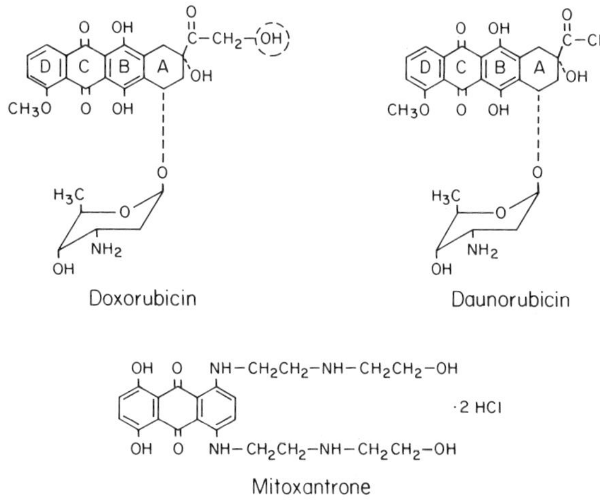

Mechanism of Action

It is now believed that the antitumor activity of mitoxantrone is due to its interaction with DNA topoisomerase II.[8] Topoisomerase II is an enzyme responsible for DNA helix supercoiling, which ultimately leads to cell death. The interaction of mitoxantrone with human cells may also involve nonintercalary, electrostatic interactions, such that protein and nonprotein DNA strand scission is induced.[9] The two alkyl residues present on the moiety (see Figure 1) preclude the molecule's smooth incorporation into DNA and may be largely responsible for mitoxantrone's activity and the lack of cross-resistance seen in doxorubicin-treated tumors.[10] It was once thought that mitoxantrone's mechanism of action was through intercalation of DNA.[11] Mitoxantrone is reportedly four to seven times more potent than doxorubicin at inhibiting the in vitro uptake of radiolabeled nucleosides.[12] In addition, mitoxantrone has been noted to lack cell-cycle phase specificity; thus, it kills both dividing and nondividing cells.[11] Of late, it has been noted that cell density may influence the ability of this agent to produce cell kill.[13] Additionally, the dose-intensity and dose-response relationship of the drug in relation to the tumor treated may be important.[14,15]

Additional mechanisms of antitumor activity may include immune modulation[16,17] and inhibition of prostaglandin synthesis and platelet aggregation.[18]

Preclinical Studies and Animal Toxicology

Mitoxantrone was shown to possess substantial antitumor activity against a broad spectrum of experimental mouse tumors in vitro.[19,20] Sensitive tumors included WiDr colon cancer, MCF7 breast cancer, IMR5 neuroblastoma, and MX breast cancer. In mice with P388 leukemia, L1210 leukemia, or solid-tumor colon cancer 26, mitoxantrone was more active than doxorubicin. Activity was also observed against B16 melanoma and M5076 ovarian cancer. Of note was the fact that tumors resistant to amsacrine were susceptible to mitoxantrone, which suggested incomplete cross-resistance of this drug with other DNA-binding agents.

In the human tumor clonogenic assay, mitoxantrone was found to be very effective against breast cancer, small-cell lung cancer, adenocarcinoma of the lung, lymphoma, and carcinoma of the biliary tract.[21] Moderate activity was also seen in head and neck carcinoma, pancreatic carcinoma, hepatoma, and ovarian carcinoma.

In animals receiving mitoxantrone, toxicity was seen in the lymph, bone marrow, and gastrointestinal tract (diarrhea, emesis).[22] Toxicology studies in beagles and rats focused on the potential cardiotoxicity of mitoxantrone. The beagle appeared to be the most sensitive animal model used in comparative cardiotoxicity studies.[23,24] In those animals treated with mitoxantrone alone, no electrocardiographic changes or congestive heart failure (CHF) was observed. Endomyocardial biopsy samples revealed none of the ultrastructural changes that are characteristic of the anthracyclines. The only major change seen was in the myocyte. The dilation of the sarcoplasmic reticulum observed was thought to be transient and independent of dose.

Pharmacokinetics

The published pharmacokinetic studies of mitoxantrone are summarized in Table 1.[25-32] Mitoxantrone is poorly absorbed after oral administration and is most commonly administered intravenously. The drug has been administered as a continuous infusion[33] and by the intra-arterial,[31,34] intrathecal,[35,36] and intraperitoneal[14] routes. The intrathecal route is not recommended by the manufacturer.

Animal studies first documented the extensive distribution of mitoxantrone into the bile, gallbladder, liver, spleen, and kidney but showed little penetration into the central nervous system.[37] Mitoxantrone disappears from the serum or plasma in a multiexponential fashion. Published studies have demonstrated both biphasic[25,26,32] and triphasic[27–31] elimination patterns. Those studies reporting biphasic pharmacokinetics were believed to lack sufficient early or late samples to adequately describe the kinetics. On the other hand, those studies that reported triphasic elimination have demonstrated that this model does not adequately characterize the pharmacokinetic variables in all patients. The large intersubject variability may be due in part to the clinical condition of the patient or, as demonstrated by Ehninger et al.,[30] concurrent drug therapy. Collectively, all studies indicate a rapid distribution of the drug into the red blood cells, white blood cells, and platelets. This initial distribution is then followed by a second distribution phase, which has been attributed to deep-tissue sequestration of mitoxantrone. The highest concentrations of mitoxantrone have been found in the thyroid, liver, heart, and red blood cells.[38] Estimates of the terminal half-life of mitoxantrone vary from 1 to 215 hours.[25–32] Using high-performance liquid chromatography (HPLC) and serum sampling for 28 days, a terminal elimination half-life of 215 hours was estimated.[30] This value is consistent with the prolonged urinary excretion and the persistence of mitoxantrone or its metabolites in tissue. In a patient who received 12 courses of mitoxantrone, pharmacokinetic values associated with the initial course remained the same throughout the treatment.[30] Mitoxantrone has been reported to bind to albumin (76%) and α_1-acid glycoprotein (66%) in in vitro studies.[37] This binding has thus far been independent of concentration and has not been found to be affected by methotrexate, doxorubicin, heparin, prednisone, or aspirin at the doses studied.[37]

Mitoxantrone is most likely metabolized in the liver to polar metabolites (the monocarboxylic and dicarboxylic acid derivatives). The glucuronide conjugates of mitoxantrone have been identified in the urine,[39] and the area under the curve is greater for the radiolabeled compound than for that measured by HPLC.[14] The bile may be the major route of elimination for mitoxantrone.[30] Liver dysfunction may lead to decreased rates of total body clearance of mitoxantrone.[26] Although this issue is still controversial, preliminary studies have shown that there may be a longer terminal half-life in patients with liver dysfunction than in healthy patients.[26] Attempts are being made to develop guidelines or methods to indicate that a dose of mitoxantrone should be reduced in patients with liver dysfunction.[40]

The primary route of mitoxantrone excretion in humans appears to be fecal. Elimination by the

Table 1.
Pharmacokinetics of Mitoxantrone

Study	No. of Patients	I.V. Dose (mg/sq m)	Mean Half-life (hours)			Mean Pharmacokinetic Values[a]
			α	β	γ	
Savaraj et al.[25]	6	1–3 (bolus)	0.228	37.4	. . .	V = 13.8 L/kg, CL = 230.7 mL/kg/hr
Saravaj et al.[26]	11 including 6 above, 5 with hepatic dysfunction	1–12 (bolus)	0.398	70.7	. . .	CL = 100.7 mL/kg/hr
Smyth et al.[27]	7	14	0.16	2.0	17.0	V = 24.5 L
Miser et al.[28]	17 children	12–20	0.057	0.378	3.87	V = 212.9 L/sq m
Alberts et al.[29]	5	12	0.1	1.0	42.6	V_c = 12.2 L/sq m, V = 1875 L/sq m, CL = 0.6 L/min/sq m, CL_r = 70 mL/min
Ehninger et al.[30]	7	14 (plus cyclophosphamide, no prior antineoplastic therapy)	0.14	3.12	214.8	V_{ss} = 2248 L/sq m; CL = 216.9 mL/min/sq m; CL_r = 15.4 mL/min/sq m
Van Belle et al.[31]	18	15	0.2	1.5	36.0	V_c = 26.2 L, V_{ss} = 1382 L, pleural fluid conc was six times the plasma conc[b]
Larson et al.[32]	22	10–12	0.16	29.3	. . .	V_c = 23.1 L/sq m, AUC = 484 ng · hr/mL, CL = 405 mL/min/sq m

[a] V = volume of distribution, CL = total body clearance, V_c = volume of central compartment, CL_r = renal clearance, V_{ss} = steady-state volume of distribution, AUC = area under the serum concentration–time curve.

[b] Hepatic infusion of mitoxantrone in one patient resulted in serum drug concentrations that were three times lower than those achieved after intravenous administration.

urinary route accounts for ≤10% of the total body clearance.[29]

Phase I Clinical Trials

Phase I studies of mitoxantrone were begun in 1979 in adults with solid tumors and in children with leukemia. These studies are summarized elsewhere.[6,7] The dose-limiting toxicity in those trials was myelosuppression (leukopenia), regardless of schedule. The most frequently studied schedule was a single dose given every 21 to 28 days. Continuous infusion, weekly doses for three weeks, or daily doses for five days were also studied. Mitoxantrone 12 to 14 mg/sq m every three weeks was the most commonly used dose and schedule for treating adults with solid tumors. In adult leukemia, higher doses given for five days were used, but the development of stomatitis and mucositis limited the dose that could be given. Pediatric patients tolerated higher doses of 18 to 24 mg/sq m every three to four weeks, or 5 to 8 mg/sq m on a weekly schedule.

Phase II and III Clinical Trials

Phase II trials conducted in adults and children with various types of tumors have also been previously reviewed.[6,7] Mitoxantrone is primarily active in the treatment of leukemia, lymphoma, and breast cancer but has also shown responses in other tumors (see Table 2).

Table 2.
Activity Profile of Mitoxantrone in Various Types of Cancer

Active	Ineffective
Leukemia	Renal cell
Lymphoma	Colorectal
Breast	Cervical
Modestly Active	Melanoma
Prostate	Small-cell lung
Hepatic	Pancreatic
Bladder	Gastric
Pediatric sarcoma	Esophageal
Myeloma	Germ cell
Head and neck	
Ovarian[a]	
Non-small-cell lung	

[a] Intraperitoneal administration.

Leukemia. Larson and associates[32] evaluated 22 patients with relapsed or refractory acute nonlymphocytic leukemia (ANLL) treated with mitoxantrone as a single agent for five days. Mitoxantrone 10 to 12 mg/sq m was given as a one-hour infusion. Of 13 patients who had a ≥95% reduction in their leukemic cell mass by day 6, 7 achieved a complete response. Of the 13 patients who had relapsed from previous therapy, 32% achieved a complete response. In contrast, only 8% of 9 patients who had refractory disease achieved a complete response. None of the 18 patients who did not have a ≥95% reduction in their tumor cell mass achieved a complete remission. In those 18 patients, 5-azacytidine was administered for five days with no apparent benefit. In this study, the major toxicity of mitoxantrone was bone marrow suppression.

In another study, Sanz and colleagues[41] used high-dose cytarabine and mitoxantrone in high-risk ANLL. Seventeen patients were treated with cytarabine 1000 mg/sq m for three days and mitoxantrone 12 mg/sq m for five days. Of the 16 patients evaluated, 8 had a complete response. None of 4 patients with refractory leukemia responded, whereas all of the patients with relapsed leukemia achieved a complete or partial response.

A large, drug-company-sponsored, multicenter trial involving 200 previously untreated patients with ANLL was performed. Mitoxantrone plus cytarabine, or daunorubicin plus cytarabine, was administered. These data are currently available only in the product brochure.[42] Cytarabine was given over seven days at a dose of 100 mg/sq m, while daunorubicin hydrochloride was given for three days at a dose of 45 mg/sq m (of daunorubicin) and mitoxantrone was given for three days at 12 mg/sq m. The complete response rate was 53% for the daunorubicin combination versus 63% for the mitoxantrone combination. These results were not significantly different. However, 89% of the patients treated with the mitoxantrone combination achieved their complete response after the first treatment course compared with 68% in the group treated with the daunorubicin combination. However, all other patients achieved their response by the end of the second course. Toxicity was not significantly different between the two study groups.

Hiddemann and coworkers[43] treated 40 patients with acute myeloid leukemia (AML) that was refractory to treatment with thioguanine, cytarabine, and daunorubicin (TAD-9) with a regimen containing high-dose cytarabine (3 g/sq m) and mitoxantrone (12 mg/sq m) on days 3 through 5. A total of 53% achieved a complete response, although 11 patients died from either aplasia, pericardial effusion, or cardiomyopathy. This study demonstrated that mitoxantrone had appreciable antileukemic effects. The investigators believed that this combination should be started earlier in the treatment of the disease. In another study by Paciucci and associates,[44] mitoxantrone was used as single-agent therapy or in combination in treating 47 patients with refractory acute leukemia. When mitoxantrone was used as a single agent (8–14 mg/sq m given every day for five days), there were responses in 5 of 12 patients with refractory acute lymphocytic leukemia (ALL). Of 12 patients with AML, one complete response and one partial response were observed. Two patients with chronic myelogenous leukemia in blast crisis also responded to mitoxantrone therapy. Dose-limiting mucositis was observed. Transient elevations of liver enzymes occurred in 50% of patients. When mitoxantrone was combined with vincristine and prednisone, five complete responses and three partial responses were observed in nine ALL and four AML patients. When combined with cytarabine, one partial and two complete responses in eight patients with AML were noted.

Because of the increased incidence of resistance to therapy and serious toxicity that can emerge with aggressive use of anthracyclines, the need for non-cross-resistant, effective, and less toxic agents for treatment of ANLL is evident. As a single agent, mitoxantrone has a response rate of roughly 30% (ranging from 9% to 64%) in ANLL or AML. In combination with other standard agents (cytarabine, vincristine, and prednisone), the response rate may be as high as 60%, which is comparable to rates associated with combinations containing anthracyclines. Results in patients with acute lymphocytic leukemia (ALL) are not as encouraging. The complete response rate is roughly 20% (ranging from 0% to 43%), although its efficacy in combination therapy continues to be evaluated. Trials have indicated that mitoxantrone will be a useful agent in the treatment of ANLL.

Lymphoma. Gams and colleagues,[45] in a Phase II Southeastern Cancer Study Group trial, studied mitoxantrone's effect in refractory lymphoma. A dose of 5 mg/sq m every week for six weeks was employed. Of the 51 patients entered in the trial, 28 patients were evaluated. In those patients, there were only three partial responses. This study was followed by the enrollment of 69 patients in a trial that employed a 14-mg/sq m dose every three weeks. Of the 30 patients evaluated, 4 achieved a complete response and 26 achieved a partial response.

Similar results were obtained in a Phase II Southwest Oncology Group study. Coltman and coworkers[46] reported the use of mitoxantrone at a dose of 12 mg/sq m every three weeks. Of 37 patients in this trial, 34 had previously received doxorubicin hydrochloride (mean dose, 240 mg/sq m). There were six partial responses and one complete response in 23 patients who had received up to three previous regimens. Four of 10 patients with small-cleaved-cell lymphoma and 1 of 9 patients with diffuse large-cell lymphoma responded to therapy. The investigators concluded that mitoxantrone was active against previously treated lymphomas and that this response was independent of previous doxorubicin administration.

The activity of mitoxantrone has been demonstrated in each histologic type of refractory lymphoma. Although the numbers are small, patients with low-grade lymphomas respond more consistently, and they respond to mitoxantrone despite previous exposure to doxorubicin. It appears that high-dose intermittent schedules of 12–14 mg/sq m every three weeks are appropriate. New uses for mitoxantrone may include salvage regimens for treating non-Hodgkins lymphoma.

Breast Cancer. Allegra and associates[47] studied the relative efficacy and toxicity of mitoxantrone and doxorubicin used as single agents in a randomized trial of 172 evaluable women with stage IV breast cancer who were not previously exposed to doxorubicin. Patients received either 14 mg/sq m of mitoxantrone or 75 mg/sq m of doxorubicin hydrochloride. The response rate for mitoxantrone was 25%, versus 35% for doxorubicin. For the two agents, the duration of remission was 5.1 months (mitoxantrone) versus 7.7 months (doxorubicin), and the time to treatment failure was 71 days (mitoxantrone) versus 106 days (doxorubicin). None of these differences were significant. Mucositis, stomatitis, nausea, vomiting, and alopecia were all less severe in the mitoxantrone treatment group. Cardiotoxicity was observed in four patients receiving doxorubicin but was not seen in those receiving mitoxantrone. In another trial, Neidhart and colleagues[48] randomized patients who had previously received a combination of cyclophosphamide, methotrexate, and fluorouracil (CMF) to be treated with either mitoxantrone or doxorubicin; response could be evaluated in 51 patients. The overall responses to mitoxantrone and doxorubicin were 27% and 40%, respectively. The incidence of myelosuppression was the same in both groups, while the incidence of nausea and vomiting, fatigue, and alopecia was lower in the mitoxantrone-treated group. The above studies have shown a lack of complete cross-resistance, with up to 15% of patients responding to mitoxantrone after being previously treated with doxorubicin.

Mitoxantrone's use in various combinations for advanced breast cancer has produced response rates ranging from 33% to 68%.[6] The most efficacious combination appears to be mitoxantrone combined with cyclophosphamide and fluorouracil (CNF). Holmes and coworkers[49] treated 55 newly diagnosed, estrogen-receptor-negative patients with metastatic breast cancer with mitoxantrone (10 mg/sq m), cyclophosphamide (500 mg/sq m), and fluorouracil (1000 mg/sq m) every three weeks. The response rate observed was 68%, with a seven-month duration of response. Myelosuppression was the major adverse effect. Four patients were withdrawn from the study, however, because of decreased ejection fractions and symptoms of CHF. Mild to moderate nausea and vomiting occurred in 76% of patients, and alopecia occurred in 88% of patients. Another multicenter trial reported by Bennett et al.[50] randomized patients to receive cyclophosphamide, mitoxantrone, and fluorouracil (CNF) or cyclophosphamide, doxorubicin, and fluorouracil (CAF). Of the 91 patients evaluated, 42% responded to CNF versus 45% for CAF. There was no significant difference between the two regimens for duration of response or time to treatment failure. There was less nausea and vomiting and alopecia reported with the mitoxantrone combination, and fewer dosage reductions were required. When patients were crossed over to receive the alternate therapy, 10% of those crossed over to doxorubicin treatment responded versus 21% of those who received mitoxantrone as second-line therapy.

Mitoxantrone's activity as a single agent in the treatment of breast cancer led to its use and the comparison of its activity in combination trials. The most common dose of mitoxantrone used in these trials was 10 to 12 mg/sq m every three weeks. The overall response to mitoxantrone appears to be less than that to doxorubicin in breast cancer, although the difference is not significant and the overall survival rate has not changed. However, mitoxantrone is associated with less toxicity.

Toxicity

Two excellent reviews of the toxicities of mitoxantrone have been previously published.[51,52]

Myelosuppression. Leukopenia is the dose-limiting adverse effect of mitoxantrone, although only 5% of patients had nadir leukocyte counts below 1000/cu mm.[51,52] The leukocyte nadir occurs by day 10 to 14, with recovery by day 21. Thrombocytopenia occurs less commonly, and only rarely do platelet counts fall below 100,000/cu mm. Red blood cells do not seem to be substantially affected.

Other Acute Toxicities. Nausea, vomiting, and stomatitis are the most frequent nonhematologic toxicities. Nausea and vomiting occur in roughly 40% of patients treated, but these symptoms are mostly mild to moderate.[51] Mucositis occurs in 10% of patients; severe cases are somewhat unusual, although in leukemic patients treated with a five-day course, mucositis is dose-limiting.[51] Alopecia occurs in less than 25% of patients.[52] Mitoxantrone has a lower incidence of these adverse effects than doxorubicin.

Extravasation of mitoxantrone has rarely been associated with tissue necrosis.[52] Phlebitis, allergic reactions, hypotension, urticaria, and rash have been reported but are also quite rare.[51] Patients should be informed of the skin, scleral, and urine discoloration that can occur with mitoxantrone administration. Elevated liver enzymes have been reported.[52] Since patients receiving mitoxantrone intrathecally have developed subsequent paralysis, this route is not recommended.[35]

Cardiotoxicity. Anthracycline-induced cardiotoxicity has been related to the ability of the quinone structure to form free-radical semiquinones, which can directly interact with oxygen, causing peroxidation of the lipid membranes of the heart. This type of reaction has not been demonstrated with mitoxantrone, although the potential for mitoxantrone-induced cardiotoxicity remains. Lederle has reported that in 6500 adult patients treated with mitoxantrone, 267 cardiac events have occurred.[37] Cardiac events that have been observed in patients treated with mitoxantrone include arrhythmias, decreased left ventricular function, CHF, tachycardia, ECG changes, and, rarely, myocardial infarction. A total of 59% of these patients had received doxorubicin previously, 36% had received radiation, and 50% had underlying cardiovascular disease. These factors and the age of the patients have been cited as predisposing factors in the development of mitoxantrone cardiotoxicity. In more than 300 pediatric patients, 21 cardiac events have been observed. All but one of these patients had received doxorubicin previously.[37]

The Southwest Oncology Group[53] reported data on 801 patients treated with mitoxantrone. Of those, 1.5% developed CHF, 1.5% had decreased left ventricular function, and 0.25% had a myocardial infarction. The data to date on mitoxantrone indicate an association between treatment with the drug and the development of decreased left ventricular function or CHF. Predisposing factors appear to be prior anthracycline therapy, prior cardiovascular disease, mediastinal irradiation, and age. The risk of developing CHF appears to be less than 3% if cumulative doses are less than 120 mg/sq m.[52] In patients with no prior treatment or risk factors, cumulative doses of up to 160 mg/sq m may be given.[52] Doses above these levels should be given cautiously, and cardiac ejection fractions should probably be monitored.

Cost

Mitoxantrone is marketed by Lederle under the trade name Novantrone. It is supplied as a sterile, dark-blue aqueous solution of mitoxantrone hydrochloride with a final concentration of 2 mg/mL of mitoxantrone. The drug is supplied in 20-mg vials ($363.42), 25-mg vials ($445.27), and 30-mg vials ($545.13) (direct prices from Lederle Laboratories). These vials do not contain a preservative and are stable for two years at room temperature.

Dosage and Administration

Mitoxantrone can be administered by a short intravenous infusion of 10 to 15 minutes. It also has been given by slow intravenous push.[46] Mitoxantrone has also been administered as a continuous infusion, intra-arterially, and intraperitoneally in various trials.[46] The most common dosage used in treating leukemia is 8 to 12 mg/sq m daily for five days, although the package insert recommends a starting dosage of 12 mg/sq m daily for three days. In solid tumors, the typical dosage is 12 to 14 mg/sq m every three to four weeks. The dose is generally reduced when the drug is used in combination or in patients who have received prior therapy.

FDA-Approved Labeling

Mitoxantrone is indicated for the initial treatment of adult acute nonlymphocytic leukemia (ANLL).

Formulary Considerations

Antineoplastic agents are specifically limited to the treatment of cancers; thus, the discussion of formulary or nonformulary status is not a major consideration. Consideration should be given to the criteria for use of such an agent. Mitoxantrone has demonstrated comparable efficacy to daunorubicin in combination with cytarabine for the treatment of ANLL. Acute toxicities are comparable. The differences between the cumulative cardiac toxicity of mitoxantrone and daunorubicin in this setting have not been established. A cost analysis is provided in Table 3. For the treatment of ANLL, mitoxantrone is almost four times more expensive than daunorubicin. Based on its comparable activity and toxicity but its much higher cost, mitoxantrone should be considered second-line treatment.

Mitoxantrone has also shown activity in lymphoma and breast cancer and has been used in the treatment of many other solid tumors. Based on comparable activity, an improved toxicity profile, and a potential for less cumulative cardiotoxicity, there will be a subset of patients who may benefit from the use of mitoxantrone (those in whom doxorubicin treatment has failed or those who cannot tolerate doxorubicin-associated toxicity). Since these indications are not FDA approved, doxorubicin would remain first-line treatment, with mitoxantrone being second line.

Table 3.
Cost Comparison between Mitoxantrone and Daunorubicin in the Treatment of Acute Nonlymphocytic Leukemia[a]

Drug	Dosage	Total Amount Used	Cost ($)
Mitoxantrone[b]	12 mg/sq m daily for three days	22 mg daily for three days, or 66 mg	17.80 per mg, or 1174.80
Daunorubicin[c]	45 mg/sq m daily for three days	81 mg daily for three days, or 243 mg	1.30 per mg, or 315.90

[a] Based on a patient with a body surface area of 1.8 sq m. Prices may vary depending on buying technique.
[b] Using 25-mg vials at $445 per vial.
[c] Using 20-mg vials at $26 per vial.

Conclusion

Mitoxantrone has demonstrated clinical efficacy in the treatment of leukemia, lymphoma, and breast cancer. In ANLL, mitoxantrone as a single agent produces response rates of 30% both in relapsed patients and in patients whose conditions are refractory to treatment. In combination, response rates have exceeded 60%, which is comparable to rates associated with current standard therapy. Mitoxantrone appeared most effective when given for five consecutive days. Responses have also been seen in patients who have relapsed after anthracycline therapy, indicating a lack of cross-resistance. Toxicities appear to be equivalent in this setting.

In lymphoma, mitoxantrone has shown good activity. Trials to determine its role in combination therapy are ongoing. The experience with mitoxantrone in acute lymphoblastic leukemia is less exciting, but some responses have been noted. Extensive testing in patients with breast cancer has also been done. Mitoxantrone's response rate as a single agent is 25–30%. Combination regimens produce response rates of 60% or more. Although mitoxantrone is slightly less active than doxorubicin-containing regimens, the incidence of acute toxicity is considerably less. There also is a lower risk of congestive heart failure.

Mitoxantrone is an important new agent with antitumor activity in leukemia, lymphoma, and breast cancer. Its place in cancer therapy will be based on this activity in light of minimal serious toxicity. The cost of mitoxantrone is comparable to that of doxorubicin, but it is substantially more expensive than daunorubicin. In most situations, mitoxantrone will be considered second-line treatment or a restricted-use item because of its high cost and because of the lack of FDA approval for indications other than ANLL.

References

1. Murdock KC, Child RG, Fabio PF et al. Antitumor agents: I. 1,4-bis[(aminoalkyl)amino]-9,10-anthracenediones. *J Med Chem.* 1979; 22:1024–30.
2. Johnson RK, Zee-Cheng RK-Y, Lee WW et al. Experimental antitumor activity of aminoanthraquinones. *Cancer Treat Rep.* 1979; 63:425–39.
3. White RJ, Durr FE. Development of mitoxantrone. *Invest New Drugs.* 1985; 3:85–93.
4. Sill AD, Andrews ER, Sweet FW et al. Bis-basic substituted polycyclic aromatic compounds, a new class of antiviral agents; 5 dibasic esters of anthraquinone dicarboxylic acids. *J Med Chem.* 1974; 17:965–8.
5. Cheng CC, Zee-Cheng RK. The design synthesis and development of a new class of potent antitumor quinone antineoplastics. *Prog Med Chem.* 1983; 20:83–118.
6. Shenkenberg TD, VonHoff DD. Mitoxantrone: a new antineoplastic agent with significant clinical activity. *Ann Intern Med.* 1986; 105:67–87.
7. Poirer TI. Mitoxantrone. *Drug Intell Clin Pharm.* 1986; 20:97–105.
8. Kapuscinski J, Darzynkiewicz Z, Traganos F et al. Interactions of a new antitumor agent, 1,4-dihydroxy-5,8-bis[(2-

{22-hydroxyethyl)amino]-9,10-anthracenedione, with nucleic acids. *Biochem Pharmacol*. 1981; 30:231–40.
9. Evenson DP, Darzynkiewicz Z, Stariano-Coico L et al. Effects of 9,10-anthracenedione, 1,4-bis[(2-{(2-hydroxyethyl)amino}-ethyl)amino]-diacetate on cell survival and cell cycle progression in cultured mammalian cells. *Cancer Res*. 1979; 39:2574–81.
10. Alberts DS, Peng YM, Bowden T et al. Mechanism of action and pharmacokinetics of Novantrone in intravenous and intraperitoneal therapy. In: The current status of Novantrone. Proceedings of a symposium. New York: John Wiley; 1985:15–21.
11. Durr FE, Wallace RE, Citapella RV et al. Molecular and biochemical pharmacology of mitoxantrone in cancer patients. *Cancer Treat Rep*. 1983; 10:3–11.
12. Traganos F, Evenson DP, Stariano-Coico L et al. Action of dihydroxyanthraquinone on cell cycle progression and survival of a variety of cultured mammalian cells. *Cancer Res*. 1980; 40:671–81.
13. Ohnuma T, Arkin H, Holland JF. Effects of cell density on drug induced cell kill kinetics in vitro (inoculum effect). *Br J Cancer*. 1986; 54:415–21.
14. Von Hoff DD, Clark GM, Weiss GR et al. Use of in vitro dose response effects to select antineoplastics for high dose or regional administration regimens. *J Clin Oncol*. 1986; 4:1827–34.
15. Hryniuk WM. Average relative dose intensity and the impact on design of clinical trials. *Semin Oncol*. 1987; 14:65–74.
16. Fidler JM, DeJoy SQ, Gibbons JJ. Selective immunomodulation by the antineoplastic agent mitoxantrone. I. Suppression of B lymphocyte function. *J Immunol*. 1986; 137:727–32.
17. Fidler TM, DeJoy SQ, Smith FR et al. Selective immunomodulation by the antineoplastic agent mitoxantrone. II. Nonspecific adherence suppressor cell derived from mitoxantrone treated mice. *J Immunol*. 1986; 136:2747–54.
18. Frank P, Novak RF. Effects of mitoxantrone and bisanthrene on platelet aggregation and prostaglandin, thromboxane biosynthesis in vitro. *Anticancer Res*. 1986; 6:941–8.
19. Wallace RE, Murdock KC, Angier RB et al. Activity of a novel anthracenedione against experimental tumors in mice. *Cancer Res*. 1979; 39:1570–41.
20. Fujimoto S, Ogawa M. Antitumor activity of mitoxantrone against murine experimental tumors: comparative analysis against various antitumor antibiotics. *Cancer Chemother Pharmacol*. 1982; 8:1570–82.
21. Cowan JD, Von Hoff DD, Clark GM et al. Comparative human tumor sensitivity to adriamycin, mitoxantrone, and bisantrene as measured by a human tumor cloning assay. *Proc Am Assoc Cancer Res*. 1982; 23:187.
22. Murray ED, Wallace RE. A novel antitumor agent. In: Crooke S, Reich SD, eds. Anthracyclines: current status and new developments. New York: Academic Press; 1980:397–402.
23. Henderson BM, Dougherty WJ, James VC et al. Safety assessment of a new anticancer compound. Mitoxantrone in beagle dogs: comparison with doxorubicin. *Cancer Treat Rep*. 1982; 66:1139–43.
24. Sparano BM, Gordon G, Hall C et al. Safety assessment of a new anticancer compound. Mitoxantrone in beagle dogs: comparison with doxorubicin. II. Histologic and ultrastructural pathology. *Cancer Treat Rep*. 1982; 66:1145–58.
25. Savaraj N, Lu K, Valdivieso M et al. Clinical kinetics of DHAD. *Clin Pharmacol Ther*. 1982; 31:3126.
26. Savaraj N, Lu K, Valdivieso M et al. Pharmacology of mitoxantrone in cancer patients. *Cancer Chemother Pharmacol*. 1982; 8:113–7.
27. Smyth JS, MacPherson JS, Ramsey M et al. Clinical and pharmacology studies of mitoxantrone. *Proc Am Assoc Cancer Res*. 1984; 25:162.
28. Miser JS, Malspeis L, Staubus AE et al. Plasma pharmacokinetics in pediatric patients. *Proc Am Assoc Cancer Res*. 1983; 24:132.
29. Alberts DS, Peng Y-M. Leigh S et al. Disposition of mitoxantrone in patients. *Cancer Treat Rep*. 1983; 10(Suppl B):23–7.
30. Ehninger G, Proksch B, Heinzel G et al. Clinical pharmacokinetics of mitoxantrone. *Cancer Treat Rep*. 1986; 70:1373–8.
31. Van Belle SJP, DePlanque MM, Smith IE et al. Pharmacokinetics of mitoxantrone in humans following single-agent infusion of intra-arterial injection therapy of combined-agent infusion therapy. *Cancer Chemother Pharmacol*. 1986; 18:27–32.
32. Larson RA, Daly KM, Choi KE. A clinical and pharmacokinetic study of mitoxantrone in acute nonlymphocytic leukemia. *J Clin Oncol*. 1987; 5(3):391–7.
33. Anderson KL, Garnick MB, Meshad MW et al. Phase I trial of mitoxantrone by 24 hour continuous infusions. *Cancer Treat Rep*. 1983; 67:435–8.
34. Shephard FA, Evans WK, Blackstein ME et al. Hepatic arterial infusion of mitoxantrone in the treatment of primary hepatocellular carcinoma. *J Clin Oncol*. 1987; 5:635–40.
35. LaPorte JP, Godefroy W, Verny A et al. Intrathecal mitoxantrone. *Lancet*. 1985; 2:160.
36. Lakhani AK, Zuiable AG, Pollard CM et al. Paraplegia after intrathecal mitoxantrone. *Lancet*. 1986; 2:1391.
37. Lederle Laboratories. Brochure for clinical investigators. Pearl River, NY; 1985 Oct.
38. Stewart DJ, Green RM, Mikhael NZ et al. Human autopsy tissue concentrations of mitoxantrone. *Cancer Treat Rep*. 1986; 70:1255–61.
39. Chiccarelli FS, Morrison JA, Cosulich DB et al. Identification of human urinary mitoxantrone metabolites. *Cancer Res*. 1986; 46:4858–61.
40. Chlebowski RT, Tong M, Woodward DL. Mitoxantrone administration in patients with hepatic dysfunction. In: The current status of Novantrone. Proceedings of a symposium. New York: John Wiley; 1985:23–8.
41. Sanz MA, Martinez J, Borreg D et al. High-dose cytosine arabinoside and mitoxantrone in high-risk acute non-lymphoblastic leukemia. *Semin Oncol*. 1987; 14:18–20.
42. Lederle Laboratories. Formulary brochure. Pearl River, NY; 1988 Feb.
43. Hiddemann W, Dreutzmann H, Straif K et al. High-dose cytosine arabinoside and mitoxantrone: a highly effective regimen in refractory acute myeloid leukemia. *Blood*. 1987; 69:744–9.
44. Paciucci PA, Cuttner J, Holland JF. Mitoxantrone as single agent and combination chemotherapy in patients with refractory acute leukemia. *Semin Oncol*. 1984; 11(3S1):36–40.
45. Gams RA, Steinberg J, Posner L. Mitoxantrone in malignant lymphoma. *Semin Oncol*. 1984; 11(3S1):47–9.
46. Coltman CA, Coltman TM, Balcerzak SP. Mitoxantrone in refractory non-Hodgkins lymphoma. A Southwest Oncology Group study. *Semin Oncol*. 1984; 11:50–3.
47. Allegra JC, Woodcock T, Woolf S et al. A randomized trial comparing mitoxantrone with doxorubicin in patients with stage IV breast cancer. *Invest New Drugs*. 1985; 3:153–61.
48. Neidhart JA, Gochnour D, Roach R et al. A comparison of mitoxantrone and doxorubicin in breast cancer. *J Clin Oncol*. 1986; 4:672–7.
49. Holmes FA, Yap H-Y, Espanza L et al. Mitoxantrone, cyclophosphamide, and 5-fluorouracil in the treatment of hormonally responsive metastatic breast cancer. *Semin Oncol*. 1984; 11:28–31.
50. Bennett JM, Byrne P, Desai A et al. A randomized multicenter trial of cyclophosphamide, Novantrone, and 5-fluorouracil (CNF) in patients with metastatic breast cancer. *Invest New Drugs*. 1985; 3:179–85.
51. Crossley RJ. Clinical safety and tolerance of mitoxantrone. *Semin Oncol*. 1984; 11(3S1):54–8.
52. Von Hoff DD, Turner JN, McConnell KI et al. The acute toxicities of Novantrone. In: The current status of Novantrone. Proceedings of a symposium. New York: John Wiley; 1985:29–34.
53. Mather FJ, Simon RM, Clark GM et al. Cardiotoxicity in patients treated with mitoxantrone: Southwest Oncology Group phase II studies. *Cancer Treat Rep*. 1987; 71(6):609–13.

Therapy Review

Drug therapy of hypertensive crises

Janice L. Stumpf

Abstract: The clinical features, pathogenesis, and pharmacologic management of hypertensive crises are reviewed, with emphasis on newer therapies.

Hypertensive crises may be divided into hypertensive emergencies and hypertensive urgencies. Hypertensive emergencies, in which acute organ damage exists, require blood pressure reduction within one hour. In hypertensive urgencies no acute end-organ damage has yet occurred; however, blood pressure should be controlled within 24 hours. Factors that may precipitate a hypertensive crisis include renovascular hypertension, acute glomerulonephritis, head injuries, renin- or catecholamine-secreting tumors, antihypertensive-therapy withdrawal syndromes, eclampsia, and ingestion of tyramine by patients receiving monoamine oxidase inhibitors.

The traditional drug of choice for therapy of hypertensive emergencies is sodium nitroprusside. Intravenous labetalol produces a prompt, controlled reduction in blood pressure and is a promising alternative. Other agents used are diazoxide, trimethaphan camsylate, hydralazine, nitroglycerin, and phentolamine. However, all these agents have disadvantages, including unpredictable antihypertensive effects, difficult blood pressure titration, and serious potential adverse effects such as profound hypotension, reduced renal blood flow, and increased myocardial workload. Most patients with hypertensive urgencies can be effectively treated with orally or sublingually administered agents. Older regimens of reserpine, methyldopa, or guanethidine, with their slow onsets and long durations of action, have been largely replaced by clonidine and nifedipine. Captopril and minoxidil have also been used with some success.

Despite the lack of comparative trials with traditional agents, demonstrated efficacy and desirable pharmacologic characteristics have made several new agents acceptable for therapy of hypertensive crises.

Index terms: Hypertension; Hypotensive agents; Sodium nitroprusside
Clin Pharm. 1988; 7:582–91

Hypertensive crisis describes a syndrome of greatly elevated blood pressure that, if untreated, results in irreversible organ damage or death within a short period of time. Hypertensive crises may be further delineated into hypertensive emergencies and hypertensive urgencies, classifications that determine the appropriate therapeutic intervention. Because of improved antihypertensive regimens, the incidence of hypertensive crises among patients with hypertension is less than 1%,[1] yet the associated morbidity and mortality make prompt recognition and treatment crucial. This article briefly reviews the clinical implications and management of hypertensive emergencies and urgencies, focusing on newer therapies.

In 1984, the Joint National Committee on the Detection, Evaluation, and Treatment of High Blood Pressure (JNC) differentiated between hypertensive emergencies and urgencies.[2] In hypertensive emergencies the elevated blood pressure should be reduced within one hour to diminish the risk of end-organ damage and death. Patients with a hypertensive emergency require hospitalization and closely monitored therapy with injectable agents. In contrast, the complications of hypertensive urgencies develop over days to weeks; there-

Janice L. Stumpf, Pharm.D., is Clinical Pharmacist, The University of Michigan Hospitals, and Clinical Assistant Professor, College of Pharmacy, The University of Michigan, Ann Arbor.

Address reprint requests to Dr. Stumpf at the Department of Pharmacy Services, The University of Michigan Hospitals, UH/B2D301/Box 0008, 1500 E. Medical Center Drive, Ann Arbor, MI 48109-0008.

Adapted from an article that appeared in the February 1988 issue of the *Michigan Drug Letter*, a publication of the Department of Pharmacy Services, University of Michigan Medical Center.

This is **article 680-204-8813** in the **ASHP Continuing Education System;** it qualifies for 1.0 hour of continuing education credit. See page 624 for learning objectives and test questions.

Copyright © 1988, American Society of Hospital Pharmacists, Inc. All rights reserved. 0278-2677/88/0801-0582$02.50.

fore, rapid blood pressure reduction is not as vital. The JNC recommends that blood pressure be controlled promptly, within an arbitrarily designated 24 hours.[3] In many cases, this may be achieved with oral therapy and without hospitalization.

Clinical Findings

Factors that may precipitate a hypertensive crisis include renovascular hypertension, acute glomerulonephritis, head injuries, renin- or catecholamine-secreting tumors, antihypertensive-therapy withdrawal syndromes, eclampsia, and ingestion of tyramine by patients receiving monoamine oxidase inhibitors.[4] Most often, the blood pressure of a patient with pre-existing hypertension suddenly rises because of noncompliance with drug therapy or other factors.[5] The rate at which the blood pressure rises, rather than an absolute blood pressure level, appears to be a critical factor in the development of hypertensive crises.[6,7] For example, patients with eclampsia may develop acute encephalopathic symptoms at relatively low blood pressure levels (<115 mm Hg).[8] In general, however, patients with hypertensive crises initially have a diastolic blood pressure of more than 120 to 130 mm Hg.

Hypertensive crises may be considered as a continuum from accelerated to malignant hypertension.[5,6,8,9] The accelerated phase consists of marked elevation of blood pressure over previously hypertensive levels, accompanied by retinal hemorrhages and exudates. This condition is usually managed as a hypertensive urgency, requiring prompt therapy to prevent potential progression to the malignant phase. Malignant hypertension is a medical emergency that is differentiated from accelerated hypertension by the presence of papilledema (grade 4 Keith–Wagener retinopathy). Papilledema, like the flame-shaped hemorrhages and cotton-wool exudates, usually resolves without sequelae several weeks after blood pressure is controlled. If the papilledema is protracted, however, optic atrophy and vision loss may result.

In addition to characteristic retinal findings, patients with untreated hypertensive crises may have damage to the renal, cardiovascular, and central nervous systems.[5-7,9] Rapid deterioration of renal function, as indicated by oliguria and progressive azotemia, may be the initial manifestation of a hypertensive crisis.[6,7,10] Urinalysis often reveals microscopic hematuria, proteinuria, and hyaline and granular casts. With appropriate antihypertensive therapy, renal damage is to some extent reversible; however, hemodialysis or peritoneal dialysis may be required for several months.

Cardiovascular complications originate from the increased afterload associated with the greatly elevated systemic blood pressure.[5,7,10] Left ventricular enlargement, noted by chest roentgenogram and electrocardiogram, may result in acute heart failure accompanied by an audible atrial gallop (S_4) and pulmonary edema. In addition, the increased cardiac workload may be particularly detrimental for patients with underlying coronary artery disease, potentially inducing angina or myocardial infarction.

The acute blood pressure rise of a hypertensive crisis may result in diffuse cerebral dysfunction ranging in severity from the generalized headache present in 85% of the patients to the somnolence and confusion of patients with hypertensive encephalopathy.[5-7,10] Focal neurologic deficits occur transiently and may consist of localized weakness, nystagmus, and visual blurring and blindness. Cerebral edema and elevated intracranial pressure are responsible for this central nervous system compromise that, if untreated, may progress to seizures, coma, and death within 48 hours.

Other manifestations of hypertensive crises include nausea, vomiting, microangiopathic hemolytic anemia, elevated plasma renin levels, and secondary hyperaldosteronism with hypokalemia.[7,10] Conditions classified as hypertensive emergencies and urgencies are presented in Table 1.[7,8,11]

Pathogenesis

The cause of the elevated blood pressure is most likely an increase in systemic vascular resistance resulting from the combination of chronic hyper-

Table 1.
Hypertensive Emergencies and Urgencies[7,8,11]

Hypertensive Emergencies (Severe Hypertension Accompanied by One of the Following)
Neurologic conditions
Hypertensive encephalopathy
Cerebrovascular accident
Intracranial or subarachnoid hemorrhage
Eclampsia
Cardiovascular conditions
Acute myocardial infarction
Unstable angina pectoris
Acute left ventricular failure
Dissecting aortic aneurysm
Renal conditions
Acute glomerulonephritis
Renovascular hypertension
Catecholamine-associated conditions
Pheochromocytoma
Antihypertensive-therapy withdrawal syndrome
Monoamine oxidase inhibitors + tyramine interaction
Miscellaneous conditions
Grade 3 or 4 Keith–Wagener funduscopic changes
Extensive burns
Disseminated vasculitis
Hypertensive Urgencies
Severe or accelerated hypertension with minimal or no end-organ damage and no impending complications
Perioperative hypertension
Severe hypertension in kidney transplant recipient

tensive changes and increased levels of vasoconstricting substances.[12] It has been suggested that chronic uncontrolled hypertension damages renal artery endothelia, thus increasing vascular reactivity.[7] Circulating vasoconstrictors (angiotensin II, norepinephrine, vasopressin) then induce constriction of the efferent renal arterioles, which raises glomerular capillary pressure and subsequently produces diuresis. The amounts of circulating vasoconstrictors are reflexly increased by the resultant hypovolemia and produce relative dilatation and constriction of the renal arteries, yielding a "sausage string" appearance. Excessive vasoconstriction induces additional endothelial damage with myointimal cell proliferation and narrowing of renal arteries. The cycle continues with further renin–angiotensin–aldosterone system activation, resulting in an overall increase in systemic vascular resistance and arterial blood pressure (Figure 1).

Autoregulation of Cerebral Blood Flow

The successful management of hypertensive crises depends on the rapid reduction of blood pressure to minimize organ damage. However, overzealous treatment may decrease perfusion to the cerebrovascular system, the heart, and the kidneys. Cerebral blood flow is autoregulated by arterial vasoconstriction and dilation to a constant level over a range of systemic blood pressures.[13] In the normotensive subject, stable cerebral perfusion is maintained as mean arterial blood pressure, varies from 60 to 160 mm Hg. As an adaptation to chronic uncontrolled hypertension, this range is elevated, with a mean lower limit of autoregulation of 120 mm Hg.[14] The development of arterial hypertrophy in the hypertensive patient accounts for the shift in the autoregulatory curve[14]; long-term antihypertensive therapy may reverse these structural changes and return the curve toward normal.[15]

Figure 1. Pathogenesis of a hypertensive crisis. (Reprinted with permission from reference 7.)

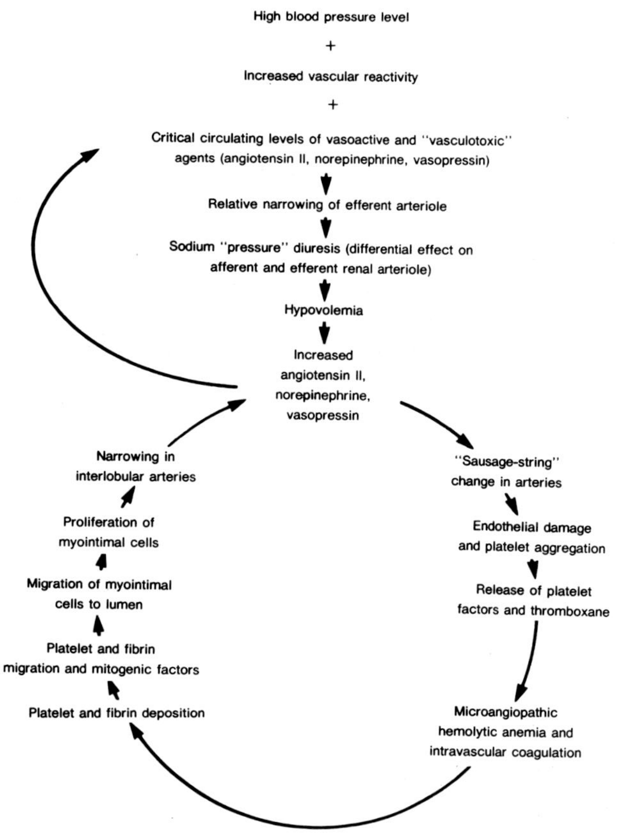

Because of the difference in cerebral blood flow set points, hypertensive encephalopathy may be induced in normotensive subjects at a lower absolute blood pressure level than in patients with hypertension.[14,16] Likewise, the rapid correction of blood pressure to normal levels in a hypertensive patient may produce cerebral hypoperfusion. Cerebral ischemia with resultant seizures and coma has been reported after aggressive antipressor therapy for hypertensive crises.[15–17]

With rapid blood pressure reduction, coronary perfusion may also be compromised, inducing myocardial ischemia, infarction, or arrhythmias.[16,18] Renal impairment may result when hypoperfusion is prolonged. Overall, the risks associated with rapid blood pressure reduction are generally less than those of continued end-organ damage in hypertensive emergencies.

Management of Hypertensive Emergencies

Because of the potential for cerebral, coronary, and renal hypoperfusion, the initial goal of therapy for hypertensive crises is a diastolic blood pressure of 100 to 110 mm Hg.[19,20] In cases of hypertensive emergencies, this blood pressure level should be maintained with injectable agents for one to two days. The injectable agent should then be tapered as the antihypertensive effects of newly initiated oral therapy are noted. Hypertensive crises are most often vasoconstrictive states with normal or low plasma volume; therefore, initiating therapy with a loop diuretic is not recommended. When used alone, diuretics are unlikely to be effective, but they are useful as adjuncts to potentiate other antihypertensive agents and to counter reflex sodium and fluid retention.[9,11,20] Since the primary hemodynamic defect is an increase in vascular resistance, therapy is often initiated with an injectable vasodilator. Dosage ranges, onsets and durations of action, and potential adverse effects of agents commonly used are listed in Table 2.

Sodium Nitroprusside. The traditional drug of choice for hypertensive emergencies is sodium ni-

Table 2.
Drugs for Treatment of Hypertensive Crises[2,9,11]

Drug	Adult Dosage	Onset of Action	Duration of Action	Adverse Effects
Sodium nitroprusside	0.5–8 μg/kg/min i.v. infusion (50–300 mg/L)	Seconds	3–5 min	Nausea, vomiting, muscle spasms, thiocyanate intoxication
Labetalol hydrochloride	20–80 mg i.v. bolus every 10–15 min 0.5–2 mg/min i.v. infusion (maximum cumulative dose of 300 mg)	5–10 min	3–6 hr	Nausea, vomiting, scalp tingling, orthostasis, dizziness
Diazoxide	50–150 mg i.v. bolus every 5–10 min 15–30 mg/min i.v. infusion	3–5 min	4–24 hr	Nausea, vomiting, hyperglycemia, flushing, hyperuricemia, hypotension, reflex tachycardia
Trimethaphan camsylate	0.5–5 mg/min i.v. infusion (500–1000 mg/L)	1–5 min	10 min	Bowel/bladder paresis, mydriasis, orthostasis, dry mouth
Hydralazine hydrochloride	10–50 mg i.m. 10–20 mg i.v. bolus	20–30 min 10–20 min	2–6 hr	Tachycardia, palpitations, flushing, headache, angina
Phentolamine mesylate	5–15 mg i.m. 5–15 mg i.v. bolus 0.2–5 mg/min i.v. infusion (200–400 mg/L)	Seconds	10 min	Tachycardia, flushing, nausea, vomiting
Nitroglycerin	0.5–10 μg/kg/min i.v. infusion	2–5 min	3–5 min	Bradycardia, tachycardia, flushing, headache
Clonidine hydrochloride[a]	0.2 mg orally initially, then 0.1 mg/hr up to 0.8 mg total	30–120 min	6–8 hr	Sedation, dry mouth
Nifedipine[a]	10–20 mg orally/sublingually/buccally	5–15 min	3–5 hr	Flushing, headache, orthostasis
Verapamil hydrochloride[a]	5–10 mg i.v. bolus	1–5 min	30–60 min	Hypotension, atrioventricular block
Captopril	6.5–50 mg orally	15 min	4–6 hr	Hypotension
Minoxidil	5–20 mg orally	30–60 min	12–16 hr	Tachycardia, fluid retention

[a] Not an FDA-labeled indication.

troprusside. This vasodilating agent acts on vascular smooth muscle to lower peripheral vascular resistance, but it is also a venodilator; its reduction of cardiac preload and afterload may benefit patients with concurrent heart failure.[6,21] Its effects on resistance vessels in the coronary circulation may be detrimental to patients with active coronary artery disease because of redistribution of blood flow away from areas of myocardial ischemia.[22]

Nitroprusside is the most rapid acting of the available vasodilators, producing an antihypertensive response within seconds.[21] As the duration of action is also short, continuous intravenous infusion and close monitoring are required for safe and effective titration. Sodium nitroprusside should be infused at an initial rate of 0.5 μg/kg/min, with the dosage increased as necessary at five-minute intervals until blood pressure is controlled.[9,11] Flushing, nausea, vomiting, muscle twitching, and profound hypotension may result when nitroprusside is administered too rapidly, but these effects are readily reversible after temporary discontinuation of the infusion. In general, patients receiving nitroprusside should be treated in an intensive-care setting because of the need for frequent blood pressure measurements.[8,11] Intra-arterial pressure monitoring is preferable, but not mandatory.

The principal metabolite of nitroprusside, cyanide, is hepatically converted to thiocyanate and may accumulate in patients with liver disease. Metabolic acidosis is the initial sign of cyanide toxicity, but this rarely occurs with short-term (<72 hours) infusions of less than 3 μg/kg/min. Toxic effects may be prevented or reversed by administration of sodium nitrite, sodium thiosulfate, or hydroxycobalamin.[21,23] Sodium nitrite induces the formation of methemoglobin, which then binds free cyanide ions. A potential disadvantage of this therapy is that the large amount of methemoglobin produced reduces oxygen delivery to the tissues. Sodium thiosulfate decreases circulating cyanide levels by acting as a sulfur donor, facilitating the enzymatic conversion of cyanide to thiocyanate. Continuous intravenous infusions of hydroxycobalamin may prevent the development of cyanide toxicity when administered concurrently with nitroprusside.[24] Hydroxycobalamin combines with cyanide to form the nontoxic, renally excreted compound cyanocobalamin (vitamin B_{12}). Although effective, these therapies are infrequently used since cyanide toxicity is relatively uncommon at usual nitroprusside dosages and discontinuation of the infusion is often adequate management.

If therapy is prolonged over 48 to 72 hours, thiocyanate may accumulate, especially in patients with renal impairment. Symptoms of thiocyanate toxicity—lethargy, convulsions, and psychosis—can be indistinguishable from those of hypertensive encephalopathy. Therefore, in patients who are receiving prolonged treatment with nitroprusside, thiocyanate concentrations should be monitored daily and the infusion should be discontinued if values exceed 10 mg/dL.[6,21] If clinically necessary, thiocyanate may be removed by hemodialysis.[23]

Sodium nitroprusside is available as a 50-mg vial of lyophilized powder that should be reconstituted with 5% dextrose injection to a final concentration of 50 to 300 mg/L.[11] The diluted solution is photosensitive and should be covered to avoid inactivation.[23] Discolored solutions should be discarded; however, when protected from light, solutions of nitroprusside are stable for up to 24 hours.

Diazoxide. The use of diazoxide for hypertensive emergencies is limited by unpredictable and long-lasting blood pressure reduction.[25] Severe hypotension inducing serious end-organ damage has been reported when this agent was administered as the previously recommended 300-mg intravenous bolus.[26] Smaller pulse boluses of 50 to 150 mg every 5 to 10 minutes or short continuous intravenous infusions of 15 to 30 mg/min allow a more controlled reduction in blood pressure that may require less frequent monitoring than that needed with sodium nitroprusside infusion.[25,27] The increase in cardiac output and reflex tachycardia caused by this arteriolar vasodilator may worsen myocardial infarction, dissecting aortic aneurysm, and angina; an agent other than diazoxide should be used for patients with these underlying conditions.[28]

Trimethaphan Camsylate. The ganglionic blocker trimethaphan camsylate, like sodium nitroprusside, has a rapid onset and short duration of antipressor action that necessitates continuous infusion and careful monitoring.[9,11] Elevating the patient's head by 8 to 10 inches enhances the predominantly postural antihypertensive effects of trimethaphan, presumably by reducing venous return.[29] Its principal indication is for hypertensive emergencies associated with dissecting aortic aneurysm because the agent reduces cardiac output and blood pressure without reflexly increasing ventricular rate. Trimethaphan is rarely used today because of the high incidence of such adverse effects as bowel and bladder atony (due to inhibition of the parasympathetic nervous system) and the rapid development of tachyphylaxis. In addition, the use of trimethaphan should be avoided in patients with renal insufficiency since it may reduce renal blood flow and, thereby, induce renal failure.[11]

Hydralazine, Nitroglycerin, and Phentolamine. Alternative injectable agents used for the management of hypertensive emergencies include hydralazine, nitroglycerin, and phentolamine. Hydralazine is the oldest of the available direct vasodilators.[19,30] With the advent of more predictable and rapid-acting antihypertensive agents, this drug is now primarily reserved for the treatment of pre-eclampsia and eclampsia. Hydralazine is unsuitable for patients who have coronary artery disease because it causes enhanced cardiac output and reflex tachycardia resulting in increased myocardial workload.[30] Beta-adrenergic blocking agents have been used as adjunct therapy to counter these hemodynamic effects, but combination therapy may induce excessive hypotension in some patients. Although hydralazine may be administered intramuscularly or intravenously, the latter route is preferred because intramuscular absorption may be erratic.[11]

Nitroglycerin, although not as potent an arterial dilator as sodium nitroprusside, has a comparable onset and duration of action, allowing controlled titration of blood pressure when administered as a 0.5- to 10-μg/kg/min continuous intravenous infusion.[19] This vasodilator is especially useful for conditions in which nitroprusside is relatively contraindicated, such as in hypertensive patients with advanced renal insufficiency or acute myocardial infarction.[22]

Phentolamine mesylate is an α-adrenergic blocker solely indicated for the management of hypertensive crises associated with increased levels of circulating catecholamines, e.g., pheochromocytoma, abrupt withdrawal of centrally acting α_2 agonists, and ingestion of tyramine by patients receiving monoamine oxidase inhibitors.[19] Intermittent intravenous doses of 5 to 15 mg or an intravenous infusion of 0.2 to 5 mg/min is commonly recommended. If tachycardia or arrhythmias accompany the elevated blood pressure, low doses of a β-adrenergic blocking agent may be used in conjunction with phentolamine.[31] Adequate α-adrenergic blockade must precede the addition of the β-receptor antagonist to prevent the potential aggravation of hypertension by exacerbating unopposed α-mediated vasoconstriction through inhibition of β_2 vasodilation. Sodium nitroprusside infusions also are effective for catecholamine-mediated hypertensive crises, and, in general, are preferable since blood pressure titration is often more manageable.[11]

Labetalol. A recent, potentially cost-effective alternative therapy for hypertensive emergencies is the adrenergic inhibitor labetalol. Labetalol competitively blocks both α- and β-adrenergic receptors, reducing peripheral vascular resistance and blood pressure with little change in heart rate or cardiac output.[32] Labetalol does not cause the reflex tachycardia and redistribution of coronary blood flow noted with nitroprusside. Therefore, it is especially useful for treating hypertensive emergencies in patients with underlying coronary artery disease or acute myocardial infarction. In addition, labetalol may be better tolerated than nitroprusside by patients with hepatic or renal insufficiency, in whom toxic metabolites could potentially accumulate. The drug has nonselective β-blocking activity and, therefore, is relatively contraindicated for patients with concurrent congestive heart failure, atrioventricular block, or asthma. To date, several studies have demonstrated that labetalol produces a prompt, controlled reduction in blood pressure.[33-39]

In the largest such trial, Wilson et al.[33] evaluated the antihypertensive effects of intermittent intravenous labetalol in 59 patients with hypertensive crises. Patients with a diastolic blood pressure (DBP) of 125 mm Hg or higher or a systolic blood pressure (SBP) of 200 mm Hg or higher were treated with an initial intravenous dose of labetalol hydrochloride 20 mg. Baseline mean blood pressure (MBP) decreased by 23.2 ± 2/14.2 ± 1 mm Hg 10 minutes after the injection. Further injections of 20 to 80 mg were administered at 10-minute intervals to attain one or more endpoints: a DBP reduction of at least 30 mm Hg, a supine DBP of 95 mm Hg, or a satisfactory response of SBP (as determined by the investigator). Labetalol therapy was effective in 53 patients (98%). Overall, the mean reduction in blood pressure was 55/33 mm Hg; the mean heart rate declined by three to four beats per minute ($p < 0.005$). The average dose needed was 186 mg; however, 24 patients (41%) required the maximum recommended dose of 300 mg. Adverse effects experienced by the subjects were mild and in no case necessitated withdrawal from the study. Reported adverse effects included nausea (14%), paresthesia (10%), vomiting (7%), and sweating (7%). Symptomatic hypotension occurred in two patients but resulted in no serious sequelae. The investigators concluded that intermittent intravenous labetalol is an effective, well-tolerated treatment for hypertensive emergencies.

In addition to intermittent injections, labetalol may be administered by continuous intravenous infusion.[32,40] A solution of 200 mg of labetalol hydrochloride diluted to a volume of 200 mL is infused at a rate of 0.5 to 2 mg/min. After adequate blood pressure response is obtained, the infusion is discontinued and may be repeated every six to eight hours as necessary to maintain blood pressure control. The maximum recommended dosage by either administration method is 300 mg.

A notable advantage of labetalol over other therapies for hypertensive crises is the availability of an oral formulation. Once blood pressure has been stabilized with intravenous therapy, therapy with oral labetalol hydrochloride 100 to 200 mg twice daily may be initiated. Because of large interpatient variability in first-pass hepatic metabolism, it is impossible to predict the precise dosage conversion between intravenous and oral therapies.[41]

Management of Hypertensive Urgencies

Distinguishing between hypertensive urgencies and emergencies may be difficult clinically because there are no differences in absolute blood pressure levels. Patients with hypertensive urgencies, however, do not have severe end-organ damage and impending complications of elevated blood pressure; therefore, most of these patients may be appropriately treated with oral agents. Over the last few years, several new approaches to the oral therapy of hypertensive urgencies have been introduced. Regimens of reserpine, methyldopa, or guanethidine were once widely used, but their slow onsets of antihypertensive effect and prolonged durations of action made them difficult to titrate in acute situations. In addition, the large doses necessary resulted in marked sedation and miosis, interfering with serial neurologic examinations. These agents have largely been replaced by clonidine and the calcium-channel blocker nifedipine. Minoxidil and the angiotensin-converting enzyme inhibitor captopril also have been used with some success. The choice of an agent for treatment of the acute hypertensive episode should be individualized, with consideration given to the possibility of continued therapy with the same agent.

Clonidine. Clonidine is a centrally acting, α_2-adrenergic agonist that diminishes sympathetic outflow and, after short-term administration, reduces cardiac output, heart rate, and blood pressure.[42] The agent's rapid absorption after oral administration and 30- to 60-minute onset of action permit its use for hypertensive urgencies as well as selected hypertensive emergencies. Oral loading-dose regimens facilitate dosage titration and are reported to be highly efficacious in achieving blood pressure control without causing serious adverse effects.[43-46]

The effectiveness and safety of oral clonidine for the treatment of hypertensive crises was first demonstrated in 1978 by Cohen and Katz.[43] Fifteen patients with blood pressures ranging from 170/105 to 195/128 mm Hg received an initial 0.1- or 0.2-mg dose of clonidine hydrochloride orally. Doses of 0.1 mg were then administered hourly until adequate blood pressure response had been achieved or a total of 0.5 mg of clonidine hydrochloride had been given. Mean baseline MBP fell from 141 ± 2 mm Hg to 108 ± 4 mm Hg ($p < 0.001$) after clonidine therapy in the 12 subjects (80%) who responded. Four patients complained of dry mouth, dizziness, and drowsiness; there were no cases of symptomatic orthostatic hypotension.

In a similar study Anderson et al.[44] established the efficacy of clonidine in 36 patients diagnosed as having hypertensive urgencies. All patients had a sustained DBP elevation above 120 mm Hg. Therapy was initiated with oral clonidine hydrochloride 0.2 mg followed by 0.1-mg hourly doses for a six-hour loading period (maximum dose of 0.7 mg) as needed to reduce DBP by at least 20 mm Hg or to a level below 110 mm Hg. A rapid, yet controlled, antihypertensive effect was noted in 34 (94%) of the 36 subjects. At six hours, mean baseline blood pressure was lowered from 212 ± 22/139 ± 11 mm Hg to 151 ± 21/103 ± 11 mm Hg ($p < 0.001$). Heart rate also fell by 10% to 20% in each patient. The total dose of clonidine hydrochloride required ranged from 0.2 to 0.7 mg with an average of 0.45 mg; mean response time was 2.8 hours. Sedation was the sole adverse effect described, yet it did not interfere with therapy. Clonidine therapy was subsequently continued in the 34 responders. However, maintenance doses based on the amount of drug required in the loading phase could not be retrospectively determined.

The average response rate for 139 patients with hypertensive crises treated with clonidine loading regimens is 92.6%.[46,47] Which patients will respond cannot be predicted based on clinical characteristics.[47] The consistently high response rates and lack of serious adverse effects make incremental clonidine regimens acceptable therapy for hypertensive urgencies.

Calcium-Channel Blockers. Therapy with calcium-channel blockers is one of the newest methods for treating acute hypertensive episodes. The antihypertensive effects of these agents result from inhibition of calcium influx in vascular smooth muscle, causing vasodilation and a reduction in total peripheral resistance. Nifedipine, the most potent vasodilator among the calcium-channel blockers currently available in the United States, consistently induces a mild compensatory increase in heart rate.[48] It also improves myocardial blood flow and cardiac output, which are favorable hemodynamic properties for some hypertensive patients with underlying ischemic heart disease or heart failure. Nifedipine is the best studied calcium-channel blocker for the treatment of hypertensive crises because of its relatively more potent and rapid-acting antihypertensive effects after oral dosing.[49–56]

In an early trial, Guazzi et al.[49] demonstrated the efficacy of orally and sublingually administered nifedipine in 26 patients with severe hypertension (DBP of >120 mm Hg). All patients responded to an initial 10-mg dose except for three subjects with hypertensive encephalopathy and left ventricular failure who required a total of 20 mg sublingually. In the 17 subjects receiving oral nifedipine, MBP fell a maximum of 36 mm Hg (24.3%) ($p < 0.05$), whereas heart rate increased 21.6%. Equivalent, yet more rapid, effects were produced after sublingual administration because of reduced absorption time. Oral nifedipine had an average onset of action of 20 minutes and maximal effect at 30 minutes compared with 5 and 15 minutes, respectively, for sublingual nifedipine. The incidence of adverse effects was similar with oral and sublingual therapy. Adverse reactions included headache (15%), palpitations (23%), premature ventricular contractions (19%), and facial and leg burning (27%), all of which resolved without treatment within 20 to 30 minutes.

The effects of nifedipine on blood pressure and cerebral blood flow in hypertensive emergencies were examined by Bertel et al.[50] in a single-blind, placebo-controlled trial. Nifedipine in 10- to 20-mg oral doses was effective in reducing mean blood pressure from 221 ± 22/126 ± 14 mm Hg to 152 ± 20/89 ± 12 mm Hg ($p < 0.001$) in all 25 study patients, whereas no changes were measured after placebo. As in other studies,[52–54,57] the absolute reduction in blood pressure was directly proportional to pretreatment blood pressure. Mean heart rate increased and was inversely related to patient age; younger patients had a greater compensatory increase in heart rate than older patients ($r = -0.65$, $p < 0.01$). Cerebral blood flow, as determined using xenon 133, was significantly increased after administration of nifedipine ($p < 0.01$) in four of five patients studied. The fifth patient showed a slight decrease. Alternatively, five patients randomized to receive 75-μg doses of intravenous clonidine had similar blood pressure responses, but up to 28% reductions in cerebral blood flow ($p < 0.01$). These results, although from a small patient population with normal baseline cerebral blood flow, imply that nifedipine, but not clonidine, may prevent cerebral ischemia in patients with hypertensive crises. Nifedipine has been previously demonstrated to cause a selective increase in cerebral circulation in animal models.[58] No serious adverse effects were observed; three patients treated with nifedipine reported flushing.

Nifedipine produces a consistent, predictable lowering of arterial blood pressure that is associated with few serious adverse reactions. Goal blood pressures were attained in 98% of 459 patients with severe hypertension or hypertensive emergencies reviewed by Houston.[59] MBP was reduced by 24.3%; pulse rate increased an average of 14.6%. The drug was equally effective by sublingual, oral, and buccal routes with maximal blood pressure lowering in 15, 30, and 40 minutes, respectively. Chewing or expelling the liquid contents from the punctured capsule sublingually results in more rapid absorption relative to oral administration and accounts for the faster onset of action. Although prompt blood pressure reduction is the goal, differences in times of onset and maximal effect between the sublingual, oral, and buccal routes are probably not of clinical importance in cases of hypertensive urgencies. Overall, the flexibility in administration and the rapid onset and relative safety are major advantages of nifedipine.

The use of intravenous verapamil hydrochloride

in doses of 5 to 10 mg has been evaluated in several hundred patients.[60] When the drug is given as an intravenous bolus injection over one to five minutes, maximal blood pressure response occurs two to five minutes later. Of the patients studied, only 0.2% did not respond to verapamil treatment. The major adverse effect reported in these trials was interference with atrioventricular conduction, manifested as heart block. Hypotension, gastrointestinal complaints, and drowsiness were also noted.

There is limited experience with diltiazem for hypertensive crises. In one study of five patients, a moderate response was seen after intravenous administration of escalating doses (5, 10, and 20 mg) of diltiazem hydrochloride.[60] An intravenous formulation of diltiazem is not yet commercially available in the United States.

Angiotensin-Converting Enzyme Inhibitors. As excessive activity of the renin–angiotensin–aldosterone system has frequently been implicated in causing severe hypertension,[61–63] the angiotensin-converting enzyme (ACE) inhibitors have been studied as potential therapy.[64–69] These agents, which include captopril, enalaprilat, teprotide, and lisinopril, block the conversion of angiotensin I to the aldosterone-stimulating vasoconstrictor angiotensin II.[70] The resulting reduction in peripheral vascular resistance is not accompanied by the reflex tachycardia seen with other vasodilators. Because of these hemodynamic effects, the ACE inhibitors are beneficial when coronary artery disease or congestive heart failure exists in the severely hypertensive patient. Therapy with the ACE inhibitors may produce severe hypotension and resultant organ damage in volume-depleted patients and in those receiving high doses of diuretics.

A study by Case and coworkers[64] of the acute effects of captopril in 10 patients with baseline DBP of >120 mm Hg and in 10 patients with malignant hypertension manifested by grade 3 or 4 neuroretinopathy is the most promising trial published to date. Blood pressure was reduced in all but 2 of the 20 subjects after a single 10- to 50-mg oral dose. Mean DBP fell from 132 ± 4 mm Hg to 107 ± 4 mm Hg ($p < 0.001$) 90 minutes after captopril administration, whereas heart rate remained unchanged. The onset of action of captopril was noted within minutes and reached a maximum within 30 to 90 minutes. The magnitude of blood pressure reduction correlated well with pretreatment plasma renin activity. Other investigators report a high incidence of nonresponse when captopril is used without diuretic therapy.[65]

Intravenous enalaprilat, the active moiety of the prodrug enalapril, has been evaluated for the treatment of hypertensive crises with disappointing results.[68,69] Enalapril itself is not useful for treatment of a hypertensive crisis because it has a delayed onset of action (two to four hours), the time required for conversion to enalaprilat.[71] One advantage of this regimen is that the same drug can be used for long-term oral therapy after blood pressure has been stabilized with the intravenous formulation. However, of the 19 patients studied,[68,69] blood pressure was controlled adequately in only 9 of them. Of these, five required intravenous furosemide to amplify the antihypertensive response. The antihypertensive effects of another oral ACE inhibitor, lisinopril, begin within two hours; therefore, this agent is not useful in treating hypertensive crises.[72] Because of the limited experience with and variable response to the ACE inhibitors, these agents currently are not recommended for the treatment of hypertensive urgencies.

Minoxidil. The effects of the potent direct-acting vasodilator minoxidil have been studied in patients with severe hypertension that is unresponsive to traditional agents.[73–75] Although minoxidil elicits a predictable and sustained blood pressure reduction, it, like the vasodilators hydralazine and diazoxide, may cause reflex tachycardia and fluid retention.[76] The efficacy of oral loading doses of minoxidil 20 mg in combination with propranolol and furosemide to counteract these compensatory mechanisms has been demonstrated.[73,74] Maximal blood pressure response occurs two to four hours after administration,[76] after which time subsequent "booster" 5- to 20-mg doses may be given. These regimens are successful in controlling blood pressure, and conversion to therapy with other agents that have fewer undesirable effects (e.g., hypertrichosis) is easily accomplished. Because of the relatively slow onset and necessity of a three-drug regimen for maximal effects, minoxidil should be reserved for hypertensive patients who do not respond to conventional therapies.

Conclusion

The selection of appropriate pharmacologic intervention for severe hypertension must be based on careful assessment of each patient's condition. Although it is not always possible to differentiate between hypertensive emergencies and urgencies, the outcome of therapy depends on a prompt and accurate diagnosis. The association of elevated blood pressure with new or progressive end-organ damage rather than absolute blood pressure readings should guide the clinician's choice of antihypertensive therapy.

Once the diagnosis is established, drug therapy should be individualized based on the patient's clinical symptoms as well as underlying disease states. An ideal agent for the management of hypertensive crises would have a rapid onset and short duration of action, facilitating blood pressure titration, a consistent and predictable effect, and flexibility in route of administration to permit ease in transition from short-term to long-term therapy, and would not cause hypotension and other serious adverse reactions. None of the antihypertensive agents discussed in this article possesses all of these characteristics. The drug of choice for true hypertensive emergencies remains sodium nitroprusside; however, labetalol is a promising alternative. New oral regimens of clonidine, nifedipine, and captopril have largely replaced older agents with their complicating adverse effects. Unfortunately, experience with many of these agents is still quite limited and there are few studies comparing them with traditionally used therapies.

References

1. Ledingham JGG. Management of hypertensive crisis. *Hypertension*. 1983; 5(Suppl 3):111–4.
2. Joint National Committee on Detection, Evaluation, and Treatment of High Blood Pressure. The 1984 report of the Joint National Committee. *Arch Intern Med*. 1984; 144:1045–57.
3. 1988 Joint National Committee. The 1988 report of the Joint National Committee on Detection, Evaluation, and Treatment of High Blood Pressure. *Arch Intern Med*. 1988; 148:1023–38.
4. Ram CVS. Hypertensive crisis: Part 2. Causes. *J Cardiovasc Med*. 1983; 8:781–9.
5. Alpert MA, Bauer JH. Hypertensive emergencies: recognition and pathogenesis. *Cardiovasc Rev Rep*. 1985; 6:407–13, 417–9, 423–5.
6. McRae RP, Liebson PR. Hypertensive crisis. *Med Clin North Am*. 1986; 70:749–67.
7. Houston M. Hypertensive emergencies and urgencies: pathophysiology and clinical aspects. *Am Heart J*. 1986; 111:205–10.
8. Ferguson RK, Vlasses PH. Hypertensive emergencies and urgencies. *JAMA*. 1986; 255:1607–13.
9. Meese RB, Ram CVS. Hypertensive cardiovascular emergencies. *Compr Ther*. 1985; 11:28–38.
10. Woods JW. Malignant hypertension: clinical recognition and management. *Cardiovasc Clin*. 1978; 9:311–21.
11. Burris JF, Freis ED. Hypertensive emergencies. *Cardiovasc Clin*. 1986; 16:163–79.
12. Kincaid-Smith P. Understanding malignant hypertension. *Aust NZ J Med*. 1981; 11(Suppl 1):64–8.
13. Olesen J. Quantitative evaluation of normal and pathologic cerebral blood flow regulation to perfusion pressure. *Arch Neurol*. 1973; 28:143–9.
14. Strandgaard S, Olesen J, Skinhoj E et al. Autoregulation of brain circulation in severe arterial hypertension. *Br Med J*. 1973; 1:507–10.
15. Strandgaard S. Autoregulation of cerebral blood flow in hypertensive patients. *Circulation*. 1976; 53:720–6.
16. Ledingham JGC, Rajagophalan B. Cerebral complications in the treatment of accelerated hypertension. *Q J Med*. 1979; 25:25–41.
17. Graham DI. Ischaemic brain damage of cerebral perfusion failure type after treatment of severe hypertension. *Br Med J*. 1975; 4:739.
18. Ross RS. Pathophysiology of coronary circulation. *Br Heart J*. 1971; 33:173–84.
19. Vidt DG. Current concepts in treatment of hypertensive emergencies. *Am Heart J*. 1986; 111:220–5.
20. Anderson RJ, Reed WG. Current concepts in treatment of hypertensive urgencies. *Am Heart J*. 1986; 111:210–9.
21. Cohn JN, Burke LP. Nitroprusside. *Ann Intern Med*. 1979; 91:752–7.
22. Mann T, Cohn PF, Holman L et al. Effect of nitroprusside on regional myocardial blood flow in coronary artery disease. *Circulation*. 1978; 57:732–40.
23. Schulz V. Clinical pharmacokinetics of nitroprusside, cyanide, thiosulphate and thiocyanate. *Clin Pharmacokinet*. 1984; 9:239–51.
24. Cotrell JE, Casthely P, Brodie JD et al. Prevention of nitroprusside-induced cyanide toxicity with hydroxycobalamin. *N Engl J Med*. 1978; 298:809–11.
25. Wilson DJ, Lewis RC, Vidt DG. Control of severe hypertension with pulse diazoxide. In: Vidt DG, ed. Cardiovascular therapy. Philadelphia: F. A. Davis; 1982:79–91.
26. Kumar GK, Dastoor FC, Robayo JR et al. Side effects of diazoxide. *JAMA*. 1976; 235:275–6.
27. Ram CVS, Kaplan NM. Individual titration of diazoxide dosage in the treatment of severe hypertension. *Am J Cardiol*. 1979; 43:627–30.
28. Koch-Weser J. Diazoxide. *N Engl J Med*. 1976; 294:1271–4.
29. Bhatia SK, Frohlich ED. Hemodynamic comparison of agents useful in hypertensive emergencies. *Am Heart J*. 1973; 85:367–73.
30. Koch-Weser J. Hydralazine. *N Engl J Med*. 1976; 295:320–3.
31. Bravo EL, Gifford RW. Pheochromocytoma: diagnosis, localization and management. *N Engl J Med*. 1984; 311:1298–1303.
32. MacCarthy EP, Bloomfield SS. Labetalol: a review of its pharmacology, pharmacokinetics, clinical uses and adverse effects. *Pharmacotherapy*. 1983; 3:193–219.
33. Wilson DJ, Wallin JD, Vlachakis ND et al. Intravenous labetalol in the treatment of severe hypertension and hypertensive emergencies. *Am J Med*. 1983; 75:95–102.
34. Cummings AMM, Brown JJ, Fraser R et al. Blood pressure reduction by incremental infusion of labetalol in patients with severe hypertension. *Br J Clin Pharmacol*. 1979; 8(Suppl 1):135S–140S.
35. Cressman MD, Vidt DG, Gifford RW et al. Intravenous labetalol in the management of severe hypertension and hypertensive emergencies. *Am Heart J*. 1984; 107:980–5.
36. Smith WB, Clifton GG, O'Neill WM et al. Antihypertensive effectiveness of intravenous labetalol in accelerated hypertension. *Hypertension*. 1983; 5:579–83.
37. Dal Palu C, Pessina AC, Semplicini A et al. Intravenous labetalol in severe hypertension. *Br J Clin Pharmacol*. 1982; 13(Suppl 1):97S–99S.
38. Cummings AMM, Brown JJ, Fraser R et al. Blood pressure reduction by incremental infusion of labetalol in patients with severe hypertension. *Br J Clin Pharmacol*. 1979; 8:359–64.
39. Lebel M, Langlois S, Belleau LJ et al. Labetalol infusion in hypertensive emergencies. *Clin Pharmacol Ther*. 1985; 37:615–8.
40. Vidt DG. Intravenous labetalol in the emergency treatment of hypertension. *J Clin Hypertens*. 1985; 2:179–86.
41. Vidt DG. Round table discussion. *Am Heart J*. 1986; 111:229–32.
42. Lowenstein J. Clonidine. *Ann Intern Med*. 1980; 92:74–7.
43. Cohen IM, Katz MA. Oral clonidine loading for rapid control of hypertension. *Clin Pharmacol Ther*. 1978; 24:11–5.
44. Anderson RJ, Hart GR, Crumpler CP et al. Oral clonidine loading in hypertensive urgencies. *JAMA*. 1981; 246:848–50.
45. Spitalewitz S, Porush JG, Oguagha C. Use of oral clonidine for rapid titration of blood pressure in severe hypertension. *Chest*. 1983; 83(Suppl):404–7.
46. Karachalios GN. Hypertensive emergencies treated with clonidine. *Eur J Clin Pharmacol*. 1986; 31:227–9.
47. Houston MC. Treatment of hypertensive emergencies and urgencies with oral clonidine loading and titration. *Arch Intern Med*. 1986; 146:586–9.
48. Sorkin EM, Clissold SP, Brogden RN. Nifedipine: a review of its pharmacodynamic and pharmacokinetic properties, and therapeutic efficacy, in ischemic heart disease, hypertension and related cardiovascular disorders. *Drugs*. 1985; 30:182–274.
49. Guazzi M, Olivari MT, Polese A et al. Nifedipine, a new antihypertensive with rapid action. *Clin Pharmacol Ther*.

1977; 5:528–32.
50. Bertel O, Conen D, Radu EW et al. Nifedipine in hypertensive emergencies. *Br Med J*. 1983; 286:19–21.
51. Huysmans FTM, Sluiter HE, Thien TA et al. Acute treatment of hypertensive crisis with nifedipine. *Br J Clin Pharmacol*. 1983; 16:725–7.
52. Ellrodt AG, Ault MJ, Riedinger MS et al. Efficacy and safety of sublingual nifedipine in hypertensive emergencies. *Am J Med*. 1985; 79(Suppl 4A):19–25.
53. Takekoshi N, Murakami E, Murakami H et al. Treatment of severe hypertension and hypertensive emergency with nifedipine, a calcium antagonistic agent. *Jpn Circ J*. 1981; 45:852–60.
54. Conen D, Bertel O, Dubach UC. An oral calcium antagonist for treatment of hypertensive emergencies. *J Cardiovasc Pharmacol*. 1982; 4(Suppl 3):S378–S382.
55. Cohan JA, Checcio LM. Nifedipine in the management of hypertensive emergencies. *Am J Emerg Med*. 1985; 3:524–30.
56. Haft JI, Litterer WE. Chewing nifedipine to rapidly treat hypertension. *Arch Intern Med*. 1984; 144:2357–9.
57. Kiowski W, Bertel O, Erne P et al. Hemodynamic and reflex responses to acute and chronic antihypertensive therapy with the calcium entry blocker nifedipine. *Hypertension*. 1983; 5:170–4.
58. Aboul-Khair M, Wicker P, Tarazi RC. Differences between the effects of hydralazine and a calcium antagonist (BAY e5009) on cerebral, renal and coronary blood flow. *Clin Res*. 1981; 29:704. Abstract.
59. Houston MC. Treatment of hypertensive urgencies and emergencies with nifedipine. *Am Heart J*. 1986; 111:963–9.
60. Frishman WH, Weinberg P, Peled H et al. Calcium entry blockers for the treatment of severe hypertension and hypertensive crisis. *Am J Med*. 1984; 77(Suppl 2B):35–45.
61. Case DB, Wallace JM, Keim JH et al. Possible role of renin in hypertension as suggested by renin-sodium profiling and inhibition of converting enzyme. *N Engl J Med*. 1977; 296:641–6.
62. Brunner HR, Gavras H, Laragh JH et al. Hypertension in man. Exposure of the renin and sodium components using angiotensin II blockade. *Circ Res*. 1974; 34(Suppl I):I35–I43.
63. Gavras H, Brunner HR, Laragh JH et al. An angiotensin converting enzyme inhibitor to identify and treat vasoconstrictor and volume factors in hypertensive patients. *N Engl J Med*. 1974; 291:817–21.
64. Case DB, Atlas SA, Sullivan PA et al. Acute and chronic treatment of severe and malignant hypertension with the oral angiotensin-converting enzyme inhibitor captopril. *Circulation*. 1981; 64:765–71.
65. Biollaz J, Waeber B, Brunner HR. Hypertensive crisis treated with orally administered captopril. *Eur J Clin Pharmacol*. 1983; 25:145–9.
66. Tifft CP, Gavras H, Kershaw GR et al. Converting enzyme inhibition in hypertensive emergencies. *Ann Intern Med*. 1979; 90:43–7.
67. Hauger-Klevene JH. Captopril in hypertensive crisis. *Lancet*. 1985; 2:732–3. Letter.
68. Strauss R, Gavras I, Vlahakos D et al. Enalaprilat in hypertensive emergencies. *J Clin Pharmacol*. 1986; 26:39–43.
69. DiPette DJ, Ferraro JC, Evans RR et al. Enalaprilat, an intravenous angiotensin-converting enzyme inhibitor, in hypertensive crises. *Clin Pharmacol Ther*. 1985; 38:199–204.
70. Edwards CRW, Padfield PL. Angiotensin-converting enzyme inhibitors: past, present, and bright future. *Lancet*. 1985; 1:30–4.
71. Sweet CS. Pharmacological properties of the converting enzyme inhibitor, enalapril maleate (MK-421). *Fed Proc*. 1983; 42:167–70.
72. Gomez HJ, Cirillo VJ, Moncloa F. The clinical pharmacology of lisinopril. *J Cardiovasc Pharmacol*. 1987; 9(Suppl 3):S27–S34.
73. Bauer JH, Alpert MA. Rapid reduction of severe hypertension with minoxidil. *J Cardiovasc Pharmacol*. 1980; 2(Suppl 2):S189–S199.
74. Alpert MA, Bauer JH. Rapid control of severe hypertension with minoxidil. *Arch Intern Med*. 1982; 142:2099–104.
75. Wood BC, Sharma JN, Crouch TT. Oral minoxidil in the treatment of hypertensive crisis. *JAMA*. 1979; 241:163.
76. Linas SL, Nies AS. Minoxidil. *Ann Intern Med*. 1981; 94:61–5.

“

Goals of Hypertension Therapy

. . . [I]t is not sufficient to reduce blood pressure in patients being treated for hypertension. It is also important to improve the status of the arterial wall. To achieve this goal, several possibilities have been proposed. The first is to treat hypertension with compounds that have no adverse effects on the arterial wall and even have ancillary properties, such as enhancement of arterial compliance, thus allowing improvement of the status of large arteries. The second is to propose treatments that, in combination with antihypertensive drugs, might have a specific beneficial effect on the arterial wall. To that end, intervention programs have recently established the value of controlling cholesterol, glucose, and even smoking, particularly in high-risk populations. Obviously, such approaches will be developed in the future but should be considered with caution for several reasons. The combination of several intervention programs is potentially susceptible to nonbeneficial interaction. . . . Another point to consider in clinical care is that the number of combined intervention programs in a large population of asymptomatic subjects favors noncompliance with treatment. . . .

—Safar M. Therapeutic trials and large arteries in hypertension. *Am Heart J*. 1988; 115:702–10.

”

Commentaries

Reassessment of the value of lowering serum cholesterol

Questioning the wisdom of widespread intervention

DUSTAN G. LABRECHE

Clin Pharm. 1988; 7:592–603

The National Cholesterol Education Program[1] was launched by the National Heart, Lung, and Blood Institute (NHLBI) in September 1987. NHLBI issued guidelines that establish diagnostic and treatment criteria for serum cholesterol concentrations greater than 200 mg/dL in persons 20 or more years of age. Initial treatment consists of dietary changes; pharmacologic intervention is recommended if dietary measures fail.[1,2] Lovastatin, the first of a new class of lipid-lowering agents, the 3-hydroxy-3-methylglutaryl-coenzyme A (HMG CoA) reductase inhibitors, reached the market at approximately the same time NHLBI issued its cholesterol recommendations. Lovastatin is markedly more effective than previously available agents in reducing serum cholesterol, particularly the low-density lipoprotein (LDL) fraction.

These two events, coupled with the results of the Lipid Research Clinics Coronary Primary Prevention Trial (LRC-CPPT)[3] and the Helsinki Heart Study,[4] seem certain to create a major effort by the public and the medical community to lower cholesterol. On the surface, there seems good reason for such steps. Ischemic heart disease is the leading cause of death in the United States today. Each year, 700,000 people are hospitalized with myocardial infarction,[5] and more than 550,000 per year die from coronary disease.[6] Elevated serum cholesterol has consistently and repeatedly been linked to increased morbidity and mortality from ischemic heart disease.[7] Logically, reductions in cholesterol by dietary or pharmacologic means, or both, should lead to reductions in the incidence of ischemic heart disease, but until recently there were no conclusive data supporting this hypothesis. The report of the LRC-CPPT was hailed as a source of authoritative answers. Its findings have been interpreted to mean that "the question is no longer whether to treat hypercholesterolemia but when and how to treat it."[8] With such overwhelming evidence, why would a distinguished panel of the National Academy of Sciences[9] recommend against such measures?

In this paper, numerous objections to a mass screening and intervention program are reviewed. It is hoped that this commentary, examined in the context of opposing viewpoints, will assist the reader in developing a balanced view of the expected benefits and risks of lowering plasma lipids. Objections to widespread intervention fall into several broad categories: (1) reservations about the results of past and recent lipid-lowering trials, (2) applicability of the LRC-CPPT results and other investigations to the population as a whole, (3) expected benefit from cholesterol reduction in a given individual, (4) cost-effectiveness of a national cholesterol reduction program relative to other risk-reduction strategies, (5) other potential risks of a lifelong program of cholesterol reduction using available agents, and (6) limitations on the interpretation of serum cholesterol measurements.

Diet and Drug Trials

Many epidemiologic investigations have associated progressive increments in serum cholesterol with increasing risk for development of ischemic heart disease. At least two dozen trials have been conducted over the past two decades to test the hypothesis that lowering serum cholesterol by dietary or pharmacologic means, or both, will reduce mortality from coronary disease. Of these investi-

DUSTAN G. LABRECHE, PHARM.D., is Assistant Professor of Pharmacy, School of Pharmacy, University of Connecticut, Storrs, and Assistant Professor of Medicine, University of Connecticut School of Medicine, Farmington.

Address reprint requests to Dr. Labreche at the University of Connecticut Health Center, Farmington, CT 06032.

Copyright © 1988, American Society of Hospital Pharmacists, Inc. All rights reserved. 0278-2677/88/0801-0592$03.00.

Table 1.
Prospective, Unifactorial Trials of Dietary Intervention To Lower Serum Cholesterol (SChol)

Ref No.	No. Subjects	Length of Follow-up (yr)	Type of Trial[a]	Baseline SChol (mg/dL)	% SChol Reduction[b]	Positive Effect in Females	CHD Mortality	Total Mortality
10	264	≤4	2	263	7.5	NS[c]	NC[d] in CHD deaths and nonfatal MI	NC
11	80	2	2	NR[e]	NQ[f]	NR	NC in CHD death and nonfatal MI[g]	Increased
12	393	2–6.75	2	272	6	NS	NC in CHD deaths and nonfatal MI	NR
13	846	≤8	3	233	12.7	NS	NC in SCD[h] or definite MI	NC
14	412	10	2	NR	NR	NS	Significant decrease in fatal MI	NC
15	I[i]	29,217[j]	3	266–278	12–18	No	Significant decrease in all CHD mortality	NC
16	458	2–7	2	281	3.9	NS	Significant increase in experimental group	NR

[a] 1 = Primary: no evidence of coronary heart disease (CHD); 2 = secondary: evidence of CHD, previous myocardial infarction (MI) or angina, or both; 3 = mixed: primary and secondary.
[b] Difference between control group and experimental group.
[c] Not studied.
[d] No change.
[e] Not reported.
[f] Cholesterol was reduced, but percentage was not quantified.
[g] Ischemic heart disease mortality increased in experimental group ($p > 0.05 < 0.1$).
[h] Sudden cardiac death.
[i] Indeterminate.
[j] Person years.

gations, 15 have been prospective, unifactorial trials testing cholesterol-lowering interventions and will be the focus of this commentary. Seven of the 15 tested dietary interventions[10–16] (Table 1), and eight were drug trials[3,4,17–22] (Table 2). The studies may be subdivided into primary trials, which studied subjects who exhibited no evidence of ischemic heart disease; secondary investigations, in which subjects who had angina or had suffered a myocardial infarction were studied; and mixed trials, which combined both types of subjects. Usually, reductions in morbidity and mortality from ischemic heart disease have been reported with both drug and dietary interventions. Most studies have been secondary investigations. All primary prevention trials have used drug therapy.

Because of various design flaws (e.g., inadequate controls or randomization, poor comparability of experimental and control groups, or small sample size), the early investigations were controversial and the value of lipid-lowering interventions remained in question. The recently completed LRC-CPPT was designed to provide the answer. A trial of diet alone for primary prevention was believed by some to be worthwhile because of the results of the pilot National Diet–Heart Study[23]; however, others believed such a trial would be too costly. Consequently, the LRC-CPPT compared diet alone with diet plus cholestyramine. It enrolled 3806 men who had serum cholesterol concentrations over 265 mg/dL and no evidence of ischemic heart disease. Approximately 38% of subjects in both groups were smokers at entry into the trial, and 25% had a known family history of ischemic heart disease. Subjects with diastolic blood pressures over 105 mm Hg or systolic blood pressures over 165 mm Hg on multiple visits were excluded.[24] The number of subjects who had mild hypertension was unreported. The primary endpoint was definite nonfatal myocardial infarction or death related to coronary heart disease (CHD).

After a mean of 7.4 years of follow-up, serum cholesterol concentration was reduced by 7.3% in the treatment group relative to the placebo group, from a value of 280.4 mg/dL after diet alone to 257.1 mg/dL after diet plus cholestyramine. Total serum cholesterol remained unchanged in the diet plus placebo group, at 279.2 mg/dL after diet and 277.3 mg/dL in the seventh year. The combined-event endpoint was significantly less frequent ($p < 0.05$ using a one-sided test) in the placebo group (8.6%) than in the cholestyramine group (7.0%), a relative difference of 19% but an absolute difference of only 1.6 percentage points. Definite

CHD death was 2.0% in the cholestyramine group and 1.6% in the placebo group. Neither the difference in nonfatal myocardial infarction nor the difference in CHD death was statistically significant, nor were differences in the development of angina or coronary artery bypass grafting.

At the beginning of the trial, it was considered unlikely that it could ever be repeated because of the time, magnitude, and costs involved; thus, it was essential "that any observed benefit of total cholesterol lowering was a real one."[25] Therefore, alpha was set at less than 0.01 using a one-sided test of significance.[25] By convention, two-sided tests of significance are used to evaluate a treatment. By looking for only the beneficial effects of a therapy, one-sided tests disregard the possible adverse effects of a therapy. As indicated by the World Health Organization trial of clofibrate,[19] lipid-lowering therapy can lead to an adverse outcome. Furthermore, smaller differences between groups will be found significant by one-sided tests of significance relative to two-sided tests of significance.

Kronmal[26] points out that after the data were analyzed, the LRC-CPPT investigators reneged and chose to accept an alpha less than 0.05 (one-sided test) as significant.[3] It is difficult to justify such a retrospective decision; using the original statistical criteria, the results were not significant. One could argue that this is statistical "hair-splitting." Indeed, many investigators and statisticians alike have criticized the arbitrarily accepted $p < 0.05$ as likely to obscure results of practical importance. Confidence intervals have been proposed as a means of overcoming such difficul-

Table 2.
Prospective, Unifactorial Trials of Pharmacologic Intervention To Lower Serum Cholesterol (SChol)

Ref. No.	No. Subjects	Length of Follow-up (yr)	Type of Trial[a]	Baseline SChol (mg/dL)	% SChol Reduction[b]	Positive Effect in Females	CHD Mortality	Total Mortality
Clofibrate								
17	497	5	2	242–268	11–16	No	Significant decrease in CHD deaths	NR[c]
18	717	6	2	259–272[d]	16	. . .	NC[e]	NR
19	15,745	5.3	1	248	9	NS[f]	Significant decrease in nonfatal MI	Significant increase
Niacin (N) or Clofibrate (C)								
20	2,222	≤5	2	NR	N 9.9 C 6.5	NS	Significant decrease in nonfatal MI with niacin	NC
Niacin and Clofibrate Combined								
21	555	≤5	2	NR	14	NR	Significant decrease in CHD deaths and nonfatal MI	Decreased
Colestipol								
22	2,278	1.9	3	301[g]	10.0	No	Significant decrease in all CHD deaths	NC
Cholestyramine								
3	3,806	7.4[h]	1	280	7.3	NS	Significant decrease in CHD deaths and nonfatal MI (when combined)	NC
Gemfibrozil								
4	4,081	5	1	270	9.4	NS	Significant decrease in nonfatal MI	NC

[a] 1 = Primary: no evidence of coronary heart disease (CHD); 2 = secondary: evidence of CHD, previous myocardial infarction (MI) or angina, or both; 3 = mixed: primary and secondary.
[b] Difference between control group and experimental group.
[c] Not reported.
[d] Cholesterol significantly greater in placebo group.
[e] No change.
[f] Not studied.
[g] Cholesterol in men significantly greater in colestipol group.
[h] Mean.

ties.[27,28] Yet when confidence intervals are applied to the LRC-CPPT data, the weakness of the findings remains apparent; the 95% confidence interval, −0.1% to +3.5%,[29] also showed a lack of significance.

Data from the LRC-CPPT were also analyzed retrospectively for a correlation between the percentage change in LDL or total cholesterol and the incidence of CHD events.[30] The percentage change in LDL or total cholesterol was taken as the difference between the baseline value and the average value over a two-year period. A significant positive correlation between the percentage reduction in total and LDL cholesterol and the primary endpoint was claimed. Kronmal[26] has pointed out that within the regression analysis model that was used, this ratio can lead to "spurious correlation." To illustrate, Kronmal said that if a group of individuals with a baseline LDL of 238 mg/dL has an average drop over two years of 30 mg/dL, this translates to a decrease of 12.6%. A group of similar individuals with a baseline LDL of only 190 mg/dL, having an identical 30-mg/dL drop over two years, would have a decrease of 15.8%. If a higher event rate was found in the group with a baseline LDL of 238 mg/dL, it would be due to the higher baseline LDL level rather than to the "spuriously" lower cholesterol reduction in this group compared with the group starting with a baseline LDL of only 190 mg/dL. Covariate analysis can solve such problems; however, this type of analysis may not be appropriate when the variables are interrelated, as are serum lipid levels. Because of this interrelationship, another problem, termed multicollinearity, may develop, in which the magnitude and direction of regression coefficients may become misleading. The implications are that without knowing the baseline levels of LDL and total cholesterol in relation to the absolute change in LDL and total cholesterol (information not provided by the LRC-CPPT), it is not possible to rule out a "spurious correlation," and a relationship may be assumed when there is none.[26]

In the Helsinki Heart Study[4] 4081 men met the entrance criteria of a non-high-density lipoprotein (non-HDL) cholesterol concentration of 200 mg/dL or greater and no evidence of heart disease. Total cholesterol was approximately 270 mg/dL in the study population, versus 245 mg/dL in the screened but excluded population. Approximately 36% of subjects were smokers, and 14% had hypertension. Subjects were randomized to receive gemfibrozil 600 mg twice daily or placebo. Fatal and nonfatal myocardial infarction and cardiac death combined was the principal endpoint. The trial was well designed, and the control and treatment groups were well matched for baseline risk characteristics. Total cholesterol was reduced by 8.5% and HDL was increased by 8.7% in those treated for at least 25 months. After five years of follow-up, the total number of cardiac endpoints was 4.14% in the placebo group and 2.73% in the gemfibrozil group, a 34% difference ($p < 0.02$ using a two-tailed test of significance) but an absolute difference of only 1.4%. The positive effect of gemfibrozil was limited to reduction in nonfatal myocardial infarction (2.19% versus 3.5%). There was no difference in fatal myocardial infarction and sudden cardiac death (5.4% in the gemfibrozil group versus 6.4% in the placebo group). Supporters of the LRC-CPPT already point to the Helsinki Heart Study as positive proof of the benefits of such lipid-lowering therapy.[31]

Total Mortality

A finding frequently dismissed in discussions of the LRC-CPPT was its failure to demonstrate a significant reduction in total mortality. Mortality from all causes was 3.6% in the cholestyramine group and 3.7% in the placebo group. An increase in suicide and violent deaths accounted for the difference. The investigators have rejected this finding as being due to chance, although Virkkunen[32] has cited data on a possible link between serum cholesterol and impulsive homicidal and suicidal behavior. If the failure to change total mortality was an isolated finding, most clinicians would be able to accept it as being a chance occurrence. However, as shown in Tables 1 and 2, of the 11 investigations reporting total mortality, only one,[21] a secondary trial, found a decrease. Indeed, two trials found an increase.[11,19] One could dismiss these findings on the basis of inadequate sample size that obscured the overall benefit of ischemic heart disease reductions. Yet, when the results were examined in the aggregate (more than 28,000 subjects), although significant reductions in ischemic heart disease mortality were noted, they were balanced by increases in noncardiac mortality.[33] Further evidence that this finding is not a chance occurrence comes from the Helsinki Heart Study.[4] As in previous trials, no change in total mortality was found in the gemfibrozil group (2.19% versus 2.07% in the placebo group). As in the LRC-CPPT, the Helsinki Heart Study found the excess of deaths in the gemfibrozil group to be due primarily to violence and accidents.

Some observers cite the long-term reduction in total mortality with niacin, reported by the Coronary Drug Projects,[20] as evidence of a beneficial effect of lipid-lowering agents. The Coronary Drug Project was designed to prospectively investigate the benefits of two levels of estrogen, dextrothyroxine, clofibrate, and niacin relative to placebo upon total mortality in men who had already suffered a myocardial infarction. The estrogen and dextrothyroxine trials were discontinued early because of excess mortality. The clofibrate and niacin groups showed no reduction in mortality after six years of treatment, although niacin was associated with significantly fewer nonfatal myocardial infarctions. Retrospectively, each of the six groups from the Coronary Drug Project was examined to determine postreatment mortality.[34] Information on cardiovascular surgery, nonfatal cardiovascular events, or other intercurrent treatments was not determined. The total mortality in the niacin group, to the exclusion of the other treatment groups, was found to be significantly reduced. The investigators believe this study proves that the beneficial effects of lipid lowering take years to become evident. It is difficult to evaluate this report because it is a retrospective review, the subjects had not taken niacin for almost nine years, and not all potentially influencing factors were accounted for in the analysis. The improved mortality could not be correlated with a reduction in nonfatal myocardial infarction that occurred years earlier while the subjects were receiving the drug. Decreases in the rate of nonfatal myocardial infarction could, at best, account for no more than 10 of the 69 fewer deaths found in the niacin group. The authors themselves suggest that, rather than providing evidence for taking a lipid-lowering drug, the findings could indicate a need for stopping niacin after a relatively brief exposure. If niacin had been continued, any adverse effect of the drug on mortality could also have persisted, leading to no reduction in total mortality.

At least some of the difference in total mortality noted by investigators has been attributed to an increase in cancer deaths. No one malignancy has emerged as predominant. Increased mortality at higher serum cholesterol levels is associated with increased coronary-related deaths, and increased mortality at the lower end of the cholesterol spectrum reportedly is associated with cancer[35] (Figure 1). The total mortality curve, as it relates to serum cholesterol, has been described as J-shaped.[36] Low serum cholesterol has been linked to occult malignancy.[37] When patients with low serum cholesterol at trial entry were eliminated, however, the association with malignancy persisted in some studies.[35,38] Other studies found a diminution of this relationship with time.[39,40] Whether there is a relationship between malignancy and cholesterol lowering or malignancy and baseline serum cholesterol awaits further investigation.

Figure 1. Age-adjusted nine-year death rates per 1000 by cause: (cancer, O; coronary heart disease, ●; and stroke, X) and serum cholesterol concentration in the Honolulu Heart Program. Reproduced, with permission, from reference 35.

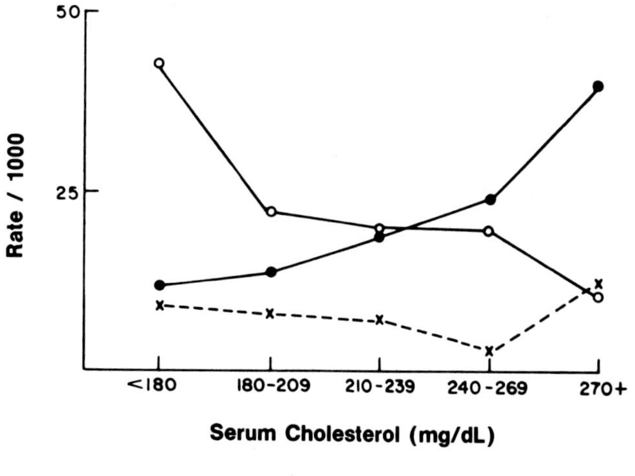

Applicability to the Population as a Whole

Based on the reportedly positive findings of the LRC-CPPT, the investigators recommended extension of drug treatment to men in other age groups, men with lower levels of cholesterol, and women. This recommendation has been attacked for a number of reasons. Typically, in preventive trials in which the number of events is low and these events develop over protracted periods of time, individuals at greatest risk are chosen as subjects. One is more likely to identify significant trends more quickly and with fewer numbers, reducing the cost of the study and the required duration of follow-up. The LRC-CPPT studied patients above the 95th percentile for serum cholesterol; 480,000 men had to be screened to identify 3,806 men who had no evidence of coronary disease but were considered to be at high risk on the basis of a serum cholesterol concentration above 265 mg/dL. The number studied represented only 0.8% of the nearly half-million men screened. The Helsinki Heart Study[4] had to screen 18,966 men to find 4,081 (21.5% of those screened) who were judged to be at greatest risk based on serum cholesterol.

The groups studied in both the LRC-CPPT and the Helsinki trial were men, predominantly white, between the ages of 35 and 59 years. Of the 15 unifactorial trials of cholesterol lowering summarized in Tables 1 and 2, only 5 included women. All three cholesterol-lowering investigations specifically reporting the effects in women found no benefit.[15,17,22] Like women, black men have not been systematically studied. Recent data from the Multiple Risk Factor Invervention Trial (MRFIT) screening program suggests that the risk of coronary disease in black men is less than that of the white population, unaccounted for by differences in risk factors.[41]

Expected Benefit to the Individual

One would expect that men at the greatest risk on the basis of their serum cholesterol concentrations would have a marked response to treatment. In both the LRC-CPPT and the Helsinki Heart Study, a substantial number of the subjects had multiple risk factors. One would expect that cholesterol-lowering interventions would have a proportionally greater benefit in this group than in the general population. Yet 250 men had to be treated with cholestyramine and diet for 7.4 years to prevent one coronary-related death and 300 men had to be treated to prevent one nonfatal myocardial infarction in the LRC-CPPT.[3] The Helsinki Heart Study[4] had comparable results; 300 men had to be treated for five years to prevent four nonfatal myocardial infarctions.

What would be the anticipated benefit in the population as a whole, the vast majority of whom would be at considerably less risk than those subjects studied thus far? The LRC-CPPT[3,30] suggested that for every 1% reduction in serum cholesterol, the risk of ischemic heart disease is reduced by 2%. Based on earlier comments, one could surely argue this point. Assuming, however, that a positive effect on ischemic heart disease mortality exists with cholestyramine, and disregarding increases in other causes of death, one would expect this estimation to hold only in that select group with the greatest levels of cholesterol. The most recent data, derived from the Multiple Risk Factor Intervention Trial, indicate that the relationship between serum cholesterol and coronary mortality is curvilinear[36] (Figure 2). Estimates of risk reduction provided by the LRC-CPPT are based on studies in subjects above the 95th percentile of serum cholesterol concentrations, the steepest part of the curve. As the serum cholesterol level declines, the benefit derived from any given reduction will also decline.

Figure 2. Age-adjusted six-year coronary heart disease (CHD) mortality and total mortality per 1000 men screened for the Multiple Risk Factor Intervention Trial according to serum cholesterol concentration. Reproduced, with permission, from reference 36. Entire cohort of 361,662 men was divided into approximate twentieths, and each point represents the mortality (either CHD or total) and the mean cholesterol concentration in one of those twentieths. Hand-fitted lines are drawn through the points.

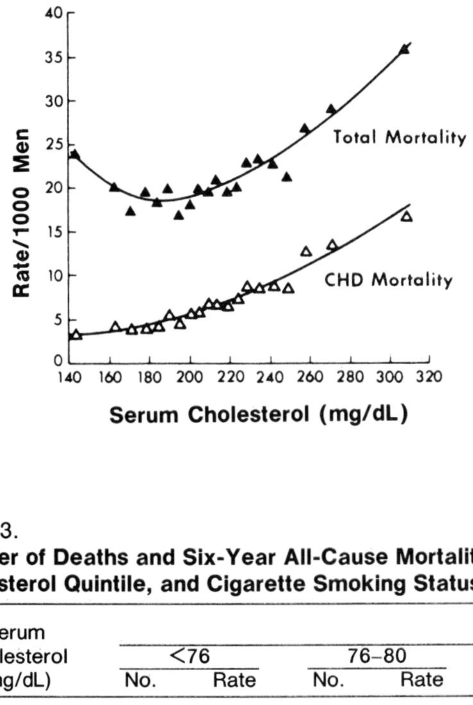

Data from MRFIT,[42] the Framingham study,[43] and the recent Nurses Health Study[44] indicate that reduction in serum cholesterol has comparatively little effect on coronary and total mortality except in the presence of other risk factors. As shown in Table 3,[42] when serum cholesterol is reduced from greater than 244 mg/dL to less than 182 mg/dL in a nonsmoker with a diastolic blood pressure of 76–80 mm Hg, six-year all-cause mortality is reduced from 22.2/1000 to 21.4/1000. Even if serum cholesterol remains greater than 244 mg/dL, by stopping smoking a patient in the same range of blood pressure reduces his risk from 46.3/1000 to 22.2/1000. Assuming that lowering blood pressure reduces the risk of CHD, lowering the blood pressure from greater than 91 mm Hg to 76–80 mm Hg in a nonsmoker with a serum cholesterol concentration greater than 244 mg/dL reduces a man's risk from 36.7/1000 to 22.2/1000. A hypertensive smoker would reduce his all-cause mortaility from 70.3/

Table 3.
Number of Deaths and Six-Year All-Cause Mortality Rates (per 1000) by Diastolic Blood Pressure Quintile, Serum Cholesterol Quintile, and Cigarette Smoking Status for MRFIT White Men Aged 46 to 57 Years[42,a]

Serum Cholesterol (mg/dL)	Diastolic Blood Pressure (mm Hg) <76		76–80		81–85		86–91		>91		Total	
	No.	Rate	No.	Rate	No.	Rate	No.	Rate	No.	Rate	No.	Rate
Nonsmokers												
<182	87	20.3	83	21.4	67	19.3	84	23.5	86	25.5	407	21.9
182–202	61	13.9	73	16.0	68	16.1	88	19.2	129	27.7	419	18.7
203–220	72	17.6	84	19.2	85	18.6	101	20.1	143	25.9	485	20.6
221–244	93	24.4	82	18.4	94	19.7	145	25.3	188	29.1	602	23.9
>244	62	19.9	93	22.2	127	26.5	178	29.2	296	36.7	756	28.8
Total	375	19.0	415	19.3	441	20.2	596	23.8	842	30.0	2669	23.0
Cigarette Smokers												
<182	119	46.1	79	40.7	62	39.0	76	48.6	74	51.3	410	45.0
182–202	87	33.3	86	37.8	76	39.0	77	38.3	119	59.4	445	41.0
203–220	81	32.6	77	32.4	80	38.1	110	48.8	143	63.6	491	42.8
221–244	94	38.4	95	38.4	83	34.8	130	50.5	172	61.3	574	45.3
>244	102	46.3	109	41.5	125	46.6	183	61.7	260	70.3	779	55.0
Total	483	39.2	446	38.1	426	39.8	576	50.7	768	63.0	2699	46.3

[a] Reprinted with permission from reference 42.

1000 to 51.3/1000 by reducing cholesterol from greater than 244 mg/dL to less than 182 mg/dL. If serum cholesterol concentration and blood pressure remained the same and the patient stopped smoking, his mortality would drop from 70.3/1000 to 36.7/1000.

Taylor et al.[45] have created a model using a multiple logistic equation to estimate the magnitude of the effect on life expectancy associated with reductions in serum cholesterol. The model takes into consideration the effects of age, sex, cigarette smoking, level of HDL, and blood pressure within a serum cholesterol range of 180 to 300 mg/dL. The authors assumed that reductions in ischemic heart disease mortality are not offset by proportional increases in other causes of death. For persons at low risk, depending upon age, sex, and initial cholesterol level, a lifelong dietary program to reduce serum cholesterol (assumed reduction in serum cholesterol of 6.7%) would increase life expectancy from three days to 3.1 months. A person at high risk, defined as systolic blood pressure, cigarette smoking habit, and total serum cholesterol each at the 90th percentile and HDL at the 10th percentile, would increase his life expectancy from 2 to 13 months. As shown in Table 4, reductions in serum cholesterol have less effect on life expectancy than do the elimination of cigarette smoking and the lowering of blood pressure, the effects of cholesterol reduction being most substantial in middle-aged to elderly hypertensive smoking women with cholesterol reductions of 20%. The conclusions of Taylor et al.[45] have been questioned by some investigators as erroneous and based on incorrect coefficients of risk.[46] Taylor et al. have made slight modifications in their originally published data; these are represented in Table 4. The adjustments did not substantively change their conclusions, which they have defended.[47,48]

Cost-effectiveness of a National Cholesterol Reduction Program

Spiraling health-care costs over recent years have led to increasing scrutiny of the cost-effectiveness of medical interventions. The financial burden of heart disease in the United States was estimated to top $87.5 billion in 1985,[49] representing 25% of all health-care expenditures. Should the National Cholesterol Education Program[1] lead to a reduction in health-care expenditures for CHD, one could make a strong argument for dietary or pharmacologic treatment, or both, of hypercholesterolemia.

Himmelstein and Woolhandler[50] contrasted the cost-effectiveness of cholestyramine treatment of hypercholesterolemia, based on the results of the LRC-CPPT, with that of the RAND experiment, which examined the benefit and cost of free health care. The RAND Health Experiment demonstrated a 21% reduction in mortality among the sickest 25% of the study population receiving free medical care when compared to the same group being required to share costs in some manner.[51,52] Greeted with as much enthusiasm as the LRC-CPPT, the RAND experiment was hailed as virtual proof that free care provided no additional health benefit over plans requiring patient contribution and was more expensive. Yet, in comparing the costs of "cradle-to-grave" free care with those of cholestyramine treatment, the authors found cholestyramine treatment to be 3 to 100 times more expensive per life saved

Table 4.
Months Added to Life Expectancy by Selected Changes in Risk Factors for Persons at High Risk[45,47,48,a,b]

Age (yr)	Cholesterol Reduction[c] 3%	Cholesterol Reduction[c] 6.7%	Cholesterol Reduction[c] 20%	Smoking Reduction[d] Program	Smoking Reduction[d] Quit	Blood Pressure Reduction[e]
Women						
20	2	4	13[f]	17	37	19
40	4	9	24	17	37	26
60	6[g]	13[h]	36[i]	11	23	22
Men						
20	2	4	11	32	70	24
40	3	7	18	29	63	34
60	1	2	5	15	32	24

[a] Adapted with permission from reference 45.
[b] High risk is defined as systolic blood pressure, cigarette smoking habit, and total serum cholesterol level each at the 90th percentile of the age- and sex-specific population distribution and high-density-lipoprotein cholesterol level at the 10th percentile of the age- and sex-specific population distribution.
[c] Reduction of total serum cholesterol level by 6.7% is the "base-case" assumption; reductions by 3% and 20% are the low and high amounts of cholesterol reduction considered in the sensitivity analyses (lag period for the achievement of full benefit = 3 years; discount rate = 0%).
[d] Program for smoking reduction is defined as a 46% reduction in cigarette smoking; quit is defined as a complete discontinuance of cigarette smoking (lag period for the achievement of full benefit = 3 years; discount rate = 0%).
[e] Reduction of systolic blood pressure by 14.3% (lag period for the achievement of full benefit = 3 years; discount rate = 0%).
[f] The figure reported in the original paper was 12 months.
[g] The figure reported in the original paper was 5 months.
[h] The figure reported in the original paper was 11 months.
[i] The figure reported in the original paper was 29 months.

than free health care. Cradle-to-grave health care ranged in cost from $420,000 to $726,000, while cholestyramine treatment of hypercholesterolemia, excluding the cost of physician visits and laboratory tests and the effects of inflation, ranged from $775,600 to $9,307,500 per life saved.

Himmelstein and Woolhandler's analysis has been criticized as using the packet price rather than the less expensive bulk powder price for cholestyramine resin and using the prescribed dose in the LRC-CPPT of 24 g rather than the dose most commonly taken, 15 g.[53] However, even when corrected for these failings, at the current retail price of $18.99 per 378-g bulk container of cholestyramine resin in the Hartford, Connecticut area, the cost is $1,374,275, still more than twice the greatest estimate for free health care.

Oster and Epstein[53] performed their own analysis and found that the cost-effectiveness of treatment ranged from $36,300 for a 35-year-old smoker with hypertension, diabetes, and a serum cholesterol concentration of 290 mg/dL to over $1,000,000 per year of life saved for a 70-year-old with a similar cholesterol concentration but no other risk factors. The authors based their estimation of benefit upon an 8.8% reduction in serum cholesterol, although the LRC-CPPT found an average decrease of only 6.8% with cholestyramine at seven years. Furthermore, Oster and Epstein based their cost estimates on epidemiologic data from the Framingham study, rather than on the actual observed benefit in recent trials. When the figures for the actual differences in mortality found in the LRC-CPPT are used, the cost per year of life saved more than doubles. The authors estimated that 30 to 35 years of cholestyramine therapy daily in a 35–39 year old with a serum cholesterol of 280 mg/dL would increase life expectancy by 7.2 months, similar to the increase estimated by Taylor et al.[45,47,48]

In an earlier analysis, Oster and Epstein concluded that lipid-lowering treatment was unlikely to produce substantial savings to the health-care system.[54] Similar analyses have resulted in comparable estimates and conclusions regarding cost-effectiveness.[55,56] Dietary treatment is also not cheap. As Fihn[57] points out, to achieve a 5.0% reduction in serum cholesterol at seven years, the LRC-CPPT investigators had to provide intensive dietary counseling every two months. Because the Helsinki Heart Study demonstrated a slight excess of deaths in the gemfibrozil group, there is no point in performing a cost analysis for this agent, nor when dietary or pharmacologic therapy is viewed in the aggregate is there any value to cost analysis. Since total mortality has not been shown to change, the tens of billions of dollars spent each year to lower serum cholesterol would be wasted.

How does the cost-effectiveness of cholesterol-lowering measures stack up to other risk-reduction measures? Treatment of mild to moderate hypertension has been estimated to cost $21,000 per year of life saved,[56] while nicotine gum as an aid to smoking cessation would cost between $4,113 and $13,112 per year of life saved.[58] This latter analysis is based upon a smoking cessation rate with nicotine gum alone of 1 in every 250 to 625 smokers. More recent data suggest that when counseling is combined with nicotine gum containing 4 mg of nicotine rather than the currently employed 2 mg, smoking cessation rates of 33% at two years may be achieved.[59] If this was confirmed, the cost-effectiveness of nicotine gum would be even more substantial.

Risks of Pharmacologic Reduction of Serum Cholesterol

The increase in mortality from causes other than CHD in the cholestyramine[3] and gemfibrozil[4] trials has already been discussed. Clofibrate use was associated with an actual increase in total mortality from a variety of causes in the World Health Organization (WHO) Cooperative Trial,[19] although this association was not found in other trials of clofibrate.[17,18] When examined individually, none of the causes emerged as predominantly responsible for the increase.

Lipid-lowering drugs have not proven innocuous. In the first year, 68% of patients receiving cholestyramine in the LRC-CPPT experienced at least one gastrointestinal adverse effect. A greater number of patients receiving cholestyramine required operations or procedures involving the nervous system (40 versus 23). There was a trend toward more gallstones and gallbladder operations in the cholestyramine group than in the placebo group, although it did not reach statistical significance. Similar findings were reported by the WHO investigators with clofibrate[19] and in the Coronary Drug Project.[20] Parallel to the LRC-CPPT, the Helsinki Heart Study of gemfibrozil[4] found an increased incidence of gallstone operations, and when hemorrhoidectomies were included, the number of gastrointestinal operations was significantly increased in the gemfibrozil group. Operations for cataracts were also somewhat more common in the gemfibrozil group.

Where does lovastatin fit in? As already mentioned, lovastatin is markedly more effective in lowering serum total and LDL cholesterol. Therefore, for any given dose, the cost-effectiveness with this medication should be greater. Oster and Epstein[54] have shown that although the cost-effectiveness of lipid-lowering therapy improves with greater percentage reductions in serum cholesterol, it does not keep pace with the rate of cholesterol reduction. Presumably, this is due to the curvilinear relationship between serum cholesterol and coronary mortality discussed earlier.

Relative to cholestyramine, clofibrate, or gemfibrozil, comparatively little experience has been gained with lovastatin. The maximum duration of lovastatin therapy reported to date has been only four years, and only 500 patients have taken the drug for more than one year.[60]

Because lovastatin is so well tolerated when compared with an agent such as cholestyramine, and markedly more effective, it is likely that it will enjoy widespread use despite the NHLBI's recommendation for cholestyramine as the agent of choice.[1,2] Nevertheless, certain adverse effects of lovastatin are worrisome, with so few patients studied to date. As pointed out by McKenney,[8] 5–7% of all patients have elevations in liver enzymes, and 1.9% of all patients require discontinuance of the drug because of elevations in aspartate aminotransferase (AST, formerly known as SGOT) to more than three times the upper limit of normal. Although no patient has developed signs or symptoms of serious hepatic dysfunction, when such small numbers of patients have been treated with lovastatin for so short a period, no firm conclusions can be drawn about the true risk of hepatitis. Merck Sharp & Dohme is recommending assay of liver enzymes every four to six weeks for 15 months and periodically thereafter.[61] Unfortunately, this will also escalate the cost of an already expensive drug.

Substantial attention has also been directed to a possible link between lovastatin and lens opacities. Current data are conflicting. Some studies have found the development of lens opacities in humans, while others have noted resolution of opacities found at baseline. The technique of slit-lamp examination may play a role in the discrepancies. Ongoing studies should resolve the dilemma. Nevertheless, the available data in dogs[60] suggest the need for caution. The possible increase in cataracts noted in the gemfibrozil group of the Helsinki Heart Study[4] suggests that ocular adverse effects may not be limited to HMG CoA reductase inhibitors. Until more is known, as suggested by the manufacturer, baseline and annual slit-lamp examination is necessary. Again, this reduces the cost-effectiveness of lovastatin therapy.

Myolysis has been reported in approximately 0.5% of patients treated with lovastatin.[8] In patients receiving cyclosporine concomitant with other immunosuppressive agents, the incidence may be as high as 30%.[62–64] When lovastatin is administered in combination with gemfibrozil, the incidence may increase to 5%.[63,64] In some cases, frank rhabdomyolysis has occurred. At least part of the cause may be due to inhibition of lovastatin elimination by cyclosporine.[63] The use of lovastatin under these conditions should be avoided if possible.

If the toxicities of lovastatin prove limited and additional studies conclusively demonstrate the value of cholesterol-lowering interventions upon total mortality, lovastatin will undoubtedly prove a remarkably valuable agent.

Interpretation of Serum Cholesterol Measurements

The lack of interlaboratory standards for serum cholesterol measurement presents an additional barrier to the NHLBI's recommendations. The most commonly employed methods have been found to consistently overestimate serum cholesterol by as much as 25 to 55 mg/dL.[65] When a serum sample was sent by the College of American Pathologists to 5000 laboratories in a 1985 survey, 47% of the determinations did not meet the desired goal of being within 5% of the "true" cholesterol value.[66]

Hegsted and Nicolosi[67] have found that intraindividual variations in serum cholesterol concentrations were substantial even in subjects and animals participating in diet-controlled metabolic studies. The standard deviation in serum cholesterol ranged from 7.0 to 17.8 mg/dL under metabolic ward conditions and from 10.1 to 48.0 mg/dL with no dietary control. Although the metabolic ward figures may seem small, the authors point out that, given a single sample from an individual with a serum cholesterol concentration of 220 mg/dL with a standard deviation of only 5% of the mean, the true value, assuming accurate methodology, can be expected to fall between 200 and 240 mg/dL. These are the very cutoff values defined by the NHLBI as being at low risk and at high risk, respectively. Multiple samples (as many as 5 to 10) would be necessary to be certain of the test's accuracy.[66]

More recently, the LRC investigators have reported cyclic alterations in plasma lipids, with the zenith occurring during the fall and winter months and the nadir in the spring and summer. As the investigators state, "The shift in this distribution resulting from a generalized 7.4 mg/dL seasonal shift in cholesterol levels could lead to a 30% increase in the frequency of referral in winter versus summer. Furthermore, one could not reliably assess the impact of intervention on cholesterol levels without a concurrent control group."[68] One can easily see how the difficulties with cholesterol measurement and interpretation will result in the institution of treatment in many individuals who do not meet the NHLBI guidelines and an inability to accurately assess treatment response in numerous others.

Establishing Priorities for Prevention of Ischemic Heart Disease

With ischemic heart disease the leading cause of suffering and death in this country today, efforts to reduce this burden are unassailable. Since the Surgeon General's report on smoking in 1964, emphasis has shifted from acute intervention to the reduction of mortality through prevention. In December 1984, an NIH Consensus Development conference concluded that the value of lowering serum cholesterol had been established beyond reasonable doubt and set forth treatment guidelines. Both the LRC-CPPT and the Helsinki Heart Study have been saluted in the medical literature and the popular press as providing the long-awaited answer linking cholesterol lowering and increased longevity. Although an association between ischemic heart disease and elevated serum cholesterol concentrations is undeniable, until a sufficient explanation for the paradoxical increase in noncardiac mortality is found or more protracted studies of lipid-lowering interventions demonstrate favorable effects on total mortality, support for cholesterol-lowering interventions is questionable.

As shown in this paper, such efforts probably will fail to influence total mortality. Becker[69] has suggested that cholesterol-lowering interventions are "analogous to stewards rearranging the deck chairs on the Titanic." There are currently no data other than epidemiologic observations to support extension of the most recent studies to blacks and women. For the general population with lower serum cholesterol levels, the benefit to be derived is considerably less than that in the high risk groups studied to date.[45,47,48] We should never be forced to place a dollar value on human life; the United States has steadfastly resisted all such efforts. Yet one cannot justify spending billions of dollars yearly pursuing a treatment with no proven benefit.

This view clearly goes against current "wisdom." The epidemiologic data linking cholesterol with heart disease are so convincing that it is unthinkable that lowering cholesterol could be anything but beneficial. One need only mention his or her concerns to a colleague to see the disbelief. It surfaces not only in personal communications but in the decision of the LRC-CPPT investigators to change study criteria after the fact[26] or in the refusal of the MRFIT investigators to accept the findings in their own study[70] of no benefit to a 6.7% cholesterol reduction.

NIH Consensus Development conferences wield enormous influence over the direction of health interventions in the United States and other countries. Some observers, however, have expressed concern that such conferences are called not to determine if there is consensus but to orchestrate consensus where there is none.[71,72] The "hear no evil, see no evil, speak no evil" attitude seems as likely to cut off further funding for investigation of the relationship between cholesterol and mortality as it is to promote lipid-lowering interventions. Despite the importance of the current issues, a firm policy of basing health recommendations to the public upon adequate sound scientific evidence may prove to be the greatest victim.[72] An uncritical approach has led to advocacy followed by immediate retreat by the medical profession from various health practices suggested to the general population.[69] With the increasing health-consciousness of the public, the media have been all too willing to trumpet every new study as "the answer" to long-sought-after questions. Without unbiased review and commentary by knowledgeable health professionals on what we know and don't know,[72] the health professions may soon be collectively perceived as a tower of Babel. This would further open the door to health care and health policy being dictated on the basis of economic or political considerations.

Preventive efforts to reduce ischemic heart disease need not falter. Cigarette smoking is widely recognized as the greatest single cause of premature preventable death.[73] Unlike cholesterol reduction measures, discontinuing smoking has been well documented to produce marked reductions in risk.[74-77] Although smoking is on the decline, nearly 30% of the population of the United States still smokes.[78] Measures to reduce smoking appear to be cost-effective. Rather than devoting precious resources to cholesterol-lowering measures, which are, at best, of borderline efficacy, efforts should be redoubled and extended to eliminate cigarette smoking. Despite the widely recognized risk associated with smoking, a recent study demonstrated that while 70% of smokers have contact with a physician, only 44% of smokers seeing a physician could recall their physician ever suggesting that they quit smoking,[79] regardless of the presence of other risk factors. Fielding[80] has suggested a number of steps for reducing cigarette use in the United States. Unfortunately, tobacco is a politically charged issue. Many government officials, not only in the United States, have found it politically inexpedient to support legislation controlling smoking and tobacco advertising. Perhaps the use of a method now employed in Australia—sending "smoking-death" cards to legislators informing them of constituents who have died as a result of smoking[81]—may apply some needed political pressure by the electorate upon legislators. Hypertension control clearly reduces causes of mortality other than coronary disease and may have merit in this disorder as well. Screening and treatment efforts should continue to be pursued.

Ischemic heart disease mortality is declining in this and other countries. The exact cause is unclear. Some, but not all, of the decline may be attributable to better cardiac care.[82] Although changes in diet leading to reductions in cholesterol have been cited as contributing to lowered mortality,[83] this is controversial.[84] A recent conference was unable to produce agreement on whether changes in serum cholesterol concentrations have actually occurred over the last two decades, despite data suggesting reductions in saturated fat intake.[85] A recent study in the black population hints that serum cholesterol has not changed meaningfully. The reductions in black mortality are ascribed primarily to decreases in cigarette smoking and hypertension.[86]

Conclusion

Is there a place for cholesterol-lowering therapy? Although no placebo-controlled data on outcome are available, drug treatment can be advocated in patients with heterozygous familial hypercholesterolemia and, when combined with liver transplantation, in patients with homozygous familial hypercholesterolemia because these groups are at such high risk. One would expect that in these groups the slowing or prevention of atherosclerosis would predominate over any paradoxic increase in other causes of death.

Future studies may prove these conclusions wrong. Perhaps studies of therapy employing longer periods of observation will demonstrate significant reductions in total mortality. Alternatively, trials employing more potent agents than heretofore investigated, such as lovastatin, may provide evidence of cost-effective reduction in total mortality. Until such time, committing millions of people to lifelong cholesterol-lowering interventions with unproven benefit and unknown risk is unwarranted.

References

1. National Heart Lung and Blood Institute. Draft report. National Cholesterol Education Program. Bethesda, MD: National Heart Lung and Blood Institute; 1987 Sep. 30.
2. The Expert Panel. Report of the National Cholesterol Education Program expert panel on detection, evaluation, and treatment of high blood cholesterol in adults. *Arch Intern Med*. 1988; 148:36-39.
3. Lipid Research Clinics Program. The Lipid Research Clinics Coronary Primary Prevention Trial results. I. Reduction in incidence of coronary heart disease. *JAMA* 1984; 251:351-64.
4. Frick MH, Elo O, Haapa K et al. Helsinki Heart Study: primary-prevention trial with gemfibrozil in middle-aged men with dyslipidemia. Safety of treatment, changes in risk factors, and incidence of coronary heart disease. *N Engl J Med*. 1987; 317:1237-45.
5. National Center for Health Statistics. Utilization of short-stay hospitals United States, 1984 annual summary. Hyattsville, MD: National Center for Health Statistics, 1986 Mar; DHHS publication no. (PHS) 86-1745. (Data from National Health Survey; series 13; no. 84).
6. National Center for Health Statistics. Vital statistics of the United States, 1982. Washington, DC: U.S. Government Printing Office; 1986 Dec. (DHHS publication no. (PHS) 87-1232).
7. Stamler J. Lifestyles, major risk factors, proof and public policy. *Circulation*. 1978; 58:3-19.
8. McKenney JM. Lovastatin: a new cholesterol-lowering agent. *Clin Pharm*. 1988; 7:21-36.
9. Kolata G. Heart panel's conclusions questioned. *Science*. 1985; 227:40-41.
10. Research Committee. Low-fat diet in myocardial infarction. A controlled trial. *Lancet*. 1965; 2:501-4.
11. Rose GA, Thomson WB, Williams RT. Corn oil in treatment of ischaemic heart disease. *Br Med J*. 1965; 1:1531-3.
12. Report of a Research Committee to the Medical Research Council. Controlled trial of soya-bean oil in myocardial infarction. *Lancet*. 1968; 2:693-700.
13. Dayton S, Pearce ML, Hashimoto S et al. A controlled clinical trial of a diet high in unsaturated fat in preventing complications of atherosclerosis. *Circulation*. 1969; 40:II-1-II-63.
14. Leren P. The Oslo diet-heart study. Eleven-year report. *Circulation*. 1970; 42:935-42.
15. Miettinen M, Turpeinen O, Karvonen MJ et al. Effect of cholesterol-lowering diet on mortality from coronary heart disease and other causes. A twelve-year clinical trial in men and women. *Lancet*. 1972; 2:835-8.
16. Woodhill JM, Palmer AJ, Leelarthaepin B. Low fat, low cholesterol diet in secondary prevention of coronary heart disease. *Adv Exp Med Biol*. 1978; 109:317-30.
17. Five-Year Study by a Group of Physicians of the Newcastle upon Tyne Region. Trial of clofibrate in the treatment of ischaemic heart disease. *Br Med J*. 1971; 4:767-75.
18. Report by a Research Committee of the Scottish Society of Physicians. Ischaemic heart disease: a secondary prevention trial using clofibrate. *Br Med J*. 1971; 4:775-84.
19. Report from the Committee of Principal Investigators. A co-operative trial in the primary prevention of ischaemic heart disease using clofibrate. *Br Heart J*. 1978; 40:1069-118.
20. The Coronary Drug Project Research Group. Clofibrate and niacin in coronary heart disease. *JAMA*. 1975; 231:360-81.
21. Rosenhamer G, Carlson LA. Effect of combined clofibrate-nicotinic acid treatment in ischaemic heart disease. *Atherosclerosis*. 1980; 37:129-38.
22. Dorr AE, Gundersen K, Schneider JC et al. Colestipol hydrochloride in hypercholesterolemic patients—effect on serum cholesterol and mortality. *J Chron Dis*. 1978; 31:5-14.
23. The National Diet-Heart Study. Final report. *Circulation*. 1968; 37(Suppl I):I-1-I-419.
24. The Lipid Research Clinics Program. Pre-entry characteristics of participants in the Lipid Research Clinics Coronary Primary Prevention Trial. *J Chron Dis*. 1983; 35:467-79.
25. Lipid Research Clinics Program. The Coronary Primary Prevention Trial. Design and implementation. *J Chron Dis*. 1979; 32:609-31.
26. Kronmal RA. Commentary on the published results of the Lipid Research Clinics Coronary Primary Prevention Trial. *JAMA*. 1985; 253:2091-3.
27. Gardner MJ, Altman DG. Confidence intervals rather than p values: estimation rather than hypothesis testing. *Br Med J*. 1986; 292:746-50.
28. Simon R. Confidence intervals for reporting results of clinical trials. *Ann Intern Med*. 1986; 105:429-35.
29. Pocock SJ. Current issues in the design and interpretation of clinical trials. *Br Med J*. 1985; 290:39-42.
30. Lipid Research Clinics Program. The Lipid Research Clinics Coronary Primary Prevention Trial Results. II. The relationship of reduction in incidence of coronary heart disease to cholesterol lowering. *JAMA*. 1984; 251:365-74.
31. Rifkind BM. Gemfibrozil, lipids, and coronary risk. *N Engl J Med*. 1987; 317:1279-81.
32. Virkkunen M. Lipid Research Clinics Coronary Primary Prevention Trial results. *JAMA*. 1985; 253:635-6.
33. Peto R, Yusuf S, Collins R. Cholesterol-lowering trial results in their epidemiologic context. *Circulation*. 1985; 72:III-451.
34. Canner PL, Berge KG, Wenger NK et al. Fifteen year mortality in Coronary Drug Project patients: long-term benefit with niacin. *J Am Coll Cardiol*. 1986; 8:1245-55.
35. Kagan A, McGee DL, Yano K et al. Serum cholesterol and mortality in a Japanese-American population. *Am J Epidemiol*. 1981; 114:11-20.
36. Martin MJ, Hulley SB, Browner WS et al. Serum cholesterol, blood pressure, and mortality: implications from a cohort of 361,662 men. *Lancet*. 1986; 2:933-6.
37. Rose G, Shipley MJ. Plasma lipids and mortality: a source of error. *Lancet*. 1980; 1:523-6.
38. Feinlieb M. On a possible inverse relationship between serum cholesterol and cancer mortality. *Am J Epidemiol*. 1981; 114:5-10.
39. International Collaborative Group. Circulating cholesterol level and risk of death from cancer in men aged 40 to 69 years. Experience of an International Collaborative Group. *JAMA*. 1982; 248:2853-9.
40. Sherwin RW, Wentworth DN, Cutler JA et al. Serum choles-

terol levels and cancer mortality in 361,662 men screened for the Multiple Risk Factor Intervention Trial. *JAMA*. 1987; 257:943–8.
41. Watkins LO, Neaton JD, Kuller LH (for the MRFIT Research Group). Racial differences in high-density lipoprotein cholesterol and coronary heart disease incidence in the usual-care group of the Multiple Risk Factor Intervention Trial. *Am J Cardiol*. 1986; 57:538–45.
42. Kannel WB, Neaton JD, Wentworth D et al. Overall and coronary heart disease mortality rates in relation to major risk factors in 325,348 men screened for the MRFIT. *Am Heart J*. 1986; 112:825–36.
43. Kannel WB, Castelli WP, Gordon T. Cholesterol in prediction of atherosclerotic disease. New perspectives based on the Framingham study. *Ann Intern Med*. 1979; 90:85–91.
44. Willett WC, Green A, Stampfer MJ et al. Relative and absolute excess risks of coronary heart disease among women who smoke cigarettes. *N Engl J Med*. 1987; 317:1303–9.
45. Taylor WC, Pass TM, Shepard DS et al. Cholesterol reduction and life expectancy. A model incorporating multiple risk factors. *Ann Intern Med*. 1987; 106:605–14.
46. Frommer PL, Verter J, Witters J et al. Cholesterol reduction and life expectancy. *Ann Intern Med*. 1988; 108:313. Letter.
47. Taylor WC, Pass TM, Shepard DS et al. Cholesterol reduction and life expectancy. *Ann Intern Med*. 1988; 108:313. Letter.
48. Taylor WC, Pass TM, Shepard DS et al. Correction: Appendix Table 1 in article on cholesterol reduction and life expectancy. *Ann Intern Med*. 1988; 108:314.
49. Harrison DC. Cost containment in medicine: why cardiology? *Am J Cardiol*. 1985; 56:10C–15C.
50. Himmelstein DU, Woolhandler S. Free care, cholestyramine, and health policy. *N Engl J Med*. 1984; 311:1511–4.
51. Brook RH, Ware JE Jr, Rogers WH et al. Does free care improve adults health? Results from a randomized controlled trial. *N Engl J Med*. 1983; 309:1426–34.
52. Newhouse JP, Manning WG, Morris CN et al. Some interim results from a controlled trial of cost sharing in health insurance. *N Engl J Med*. 1981; 305:1501–7.
53. Oster G, Epstein AM. Cost-effectiveness of antihyperlipemic therapy in the prevention of coronary heart disease. The case of cholestyramine. *JAMA*. 1987; 258:2381–7.
54. Oster G, Epstein AM. Primary prevention and coronary heart disease: the economic benefits of lowering serum cholesterol. *Am J Public Health*. 1986; 76:647–56.
55. Berwick DM, Cretin S, Keeler EB. Cholesterol, children, and heart disease. An analysis of alternatives. New York: Oxford University Press; 1980.
56. Weinstein MC, Stason WB. Cost-effectiveness of interventions to prevent or treat coronary heart disease. *Ann Rev Public Health*. 1985; 6:41–63.
57. Fihn SD. A prudent approach to control of cholesterol levels. *JAMA*. 1987; 258:2416–8.
58. Oster G, Huse DM, Delea TE et al. Cost-effectiveness of nicotine gum as an adjunct to physician's advice against cigarette smoking. *JAMA*. 1986; 256:1315–8.
59. Tonnesen P, Fryd V, Hansen M et al. Effect of nicotine chewing gum in combination with group counseling on the cessation of smoking. *N Engl J Med*. 1988; 318:15–8.
60. Tobert JA. New developments in lipid-lowering therapy: the role of inhibitors of hydroxymethylglutaryl-coenzyme A reductase. *Circulation*. 1987; 76:534–8.
61. Merck Sharpe & Dohme. Mevacor package insert. West Point, PA: 1987 Aug.
62. Norman DJ, Illingworth DR, Munson J et al. Myolysis and acute renal failure in a heart-transplant recipient receiving lovastatin. *N Engl J Med*. 1988; 318:46–7.
63. East C, Alivizatos PA, Grundy SM et al. Rhabdomyolysis in patients receiving lovastatin after cardiac transplantation. *N Engl J Med*. 1988; 318:47–8.
64. Tobert JA. Myolysis and rhabdomyolysis with lovastatin. *N Engl J Med*. 1988; 318:48. Letter.
65. Blank DW, Hoeg JM, Kroll MH et al. The method of determination must be considered in interpreting blood cholesterol levels. *JAMA*. 1986; 256:2767–70.
66. Roberts L. Measuring cholesterol is as tricky as lowering it. *Science*. 1987; 238:482–3.
67. Hegsted DM, Nicolosi RJ. Individual variation in serum cholesterol levels. *Proc Natl Acad Sci USA*. 1987; 84:6259–61.
68. Gordon DJ, Trost DC, Hyde J et al. Seasonal cholesterol cycles: the Lipid Research Clinics Coronary Primary Prevention Trial placebo group. *Circulation*. 1987; 76:1224–31.
69. Becker MH. The cholesterol saga: whither health promotion? *Ann Intern Med*. 1987; 106:623–6.
70. Stallones RA. Mortality and the Multiple Risk Factor Intervention Trial. *Am J Epidemiol*. 1983; 117:647–50.
71. Oliver MF. Consensus or nonsensus conferences on coronary heart disease. *Lancet*. 1985; 1:1087–9.
72. Ahrens EH. The diet–heart question in 1985: has it really been settled? *Lancet*. 1985; 1:1085–7.
73. Department of Health and Human Services, Public Health Service. The health consequences of smoking: chronic obstructive lung disease. A report of the Surgeon General, Washington, DC: Public Health Service; 1979. DHHS publication no. (PHS) 84-50205.
74. Gordon T, Kannel WB, McGee D et al. Death and coronary attacks in men after giving up cigarette smoking: a report from the Framingham study. *Lancet*. 1974; 2:1345–8.
75. Salonen JT. Stopping smoking and long-term mortality after acute myocardial infarction. *Br Heart J*. 1980; 43:463–9.
76. Friedman GD, Petitti DB, Bawol RD et al. Mortality in cigarette smokers and quitters: effect of base-line differences. *N Engl J Med*. 1981; 304:1407–10.
77. Rosenberg L, Kaufman DW, Helmrich SP et al. The risk of myocardial infarction after quitting smoking in men under 55 years of age. *N Engl J Med*. 1985; 313:1511–4.
78. Cigarette smoking in the United States, 1986. *MMWR*. 1987; 36:581–5.
79. Anda RF, Remington PL, Sienko DG et al. Are physicians advising smokers to quit? The patient's perspective. *JAMA*. 1987; 257:1916–9.
80. Fielding JE. Smoking and women. Tragedy of the majority. *N Engl J Med*. 1987; 317:1343–5.
81. Shean RE, Thompson PL, Armstrong BK. Smoking death-cards: making smoking a notifiable disease in Western Australia. *Med J Aust*. 1988; 148:58–9.
82. Pell S, Fayerweather WE. Trends in the incidence of myocardial infarction and in associated mortality and morbidity in a large employed population, 1957–83. *N Engl J Med*. 1985; 312:1005–11.
83. Goldman L, Cook EF. The decline in ischemic heart disease mortality rates. An analysis of the comparative effects of medical interventions and changes in lifestyle. *Ann Intern Med*. 1984; 101:825–36.
84. Gillum RF, Folsom AR, Blackburn H. Decline in coronary heart disease mortality. Old questions and new facts. *Am J Med*. 1984; 76:1055–65.
85. Havlik RJ, Feinleib M, eds. Public Health Service: proceedings of a conference on the decline in coronary heart disease mortality. Washington, DC: US Government Printing Office; 1979 May.
86. Rowlan ML, Fulwood R. Coronary heart disease risk factor trends in blacks between the first and second National Health and Nutrition Examination Surveys, United States, 1971–80. *Am Heart J*. 1984; 108:771–9.

Defending cholesterol-reduction efforts

ROBERT L. TALBERT

Clin Pharm. 1988; 7:604–5

Labreche's interesting and provocative review of cholesterol lowering and its relationship to coronary heart disease and total mortality[1] is an important reminder that data and conclusions from randomized clinical trials must be considered carefully and that interpretation of results from such studies is subject to individual or collective bias based on prior knowledge of the problem. Objections raised in Labreche's review concentrate on six general areas, with specific examples discussed to support each argument. Reservations concerning the acceptance of trial results are based on statistical endpoints. Although it is true that the absolute reduction in various endpoints was small in most studies—8.6% to 7.0% in combined-event endpoints in the Lipid Research Clinics Coronary Primary Prevention Trial (LRC-CPPT)[2] and 4.14% versus 2.73% in the Helsinki Heart Study,[3] the relative reduction in risk remains impressive and consistent between these studies. It should be noted that a similar trend and reporting of results exists for most major clinical trials (for example, with β blockers to reduce mortality or reinfarction after myocardial infarction[4]) and that this seeming disparity does not distract from the utility of the data derived from these studies. Use of a one-sided test of significance and alteration of the level of α from 0.01 to 0.05 are valid criticisms of the LRC-CPPT, and their occurrence is unfortunate.

Effect on Total Mortality

Lack of an effect on total mortality in most studies reflects an increase in exposure to other endpoints, in that reduction in cardiovascular risk may delay death but cannot prevent it. If an individual died of myocardial infarction at age 60, he is no longer at risk for cancer at age 65; conversely, if myocardial infarction is prevented at age 60, the risk of cancer or other endpoints continues to exist. If an intervention reduces cardiovascular mortality while noncardiovascular mortality is unaltered, a much larger sample size must be studied to demonstrate a reduction in total mortality that would be significant. Survival-curve analysis may demonstrate benefit at earlier points in the trial, but at some point the intervention group and control group curves will meet, emphasizing the importance of life-table analysis in the overall interpretation of outcome for a study. Of the two examples Labreche cited for increased mortality, the study of Rose et al.[5] included a very small number of patients and should not be considered in this discussion. The increased mortality observed with the WHO trial[6] is of concern and emphasizes that reductions in one endpoint, nonfatal myocardial infarction, may not outweigh the outcome of other endpoints.

Concern over the occurrence of cancer and accidental or suicidal death is important and warrants comment. Although population studies that have related low cholesterol to increased risk of cancer are interesting, it is not clear how these studies should be related to studies of cholesterol lowering because of the methodological differences in their conduct. Indeed, based on Figure 1[7] in Labreche's review, one could argue that no association exists if cholesterol is not lowered beyond the range recommended by the National Cholesterol Education Program (NCEP).[8] The review of Virkkunen[9] linking lower serum cholesterol to homicidal and suicidal behavior is based on studies that were performed in populations of alcoholics and prisoners, so an extrapolation to cholesterol-lowering studies is suspect.

Applicability to the Population as a Whole

As in any clinical trial, comments concerning the applicability of study results to the population as a whole are justified; these concerns form, in part, the basis for individualizing decisions to treat hypercholesterolemia and for tailoring therapy based on patient-specific risk factors and tolerability of drug therapy. The Helsinki Heart Study used population-based screening to identify study-eligible men; this strengthens the argument that the study results can be extrapolated to the general population (at least in Finland). Specific populations, women and blacks in particular, do deserve additional study to clarify who should be treated and how this can best be accomplished.

Expected Benefit to the Individual

Labreche's review appropriately points out that expected benefit to an individual is not based only on cholesterol but is also related to the presence and severity of other risk factors. Disregarding hypertension, family history of premature coronary heart disease, and smoking as concurrent risk factors is likely to lead to suboptimal results of treatment in an individual patient. Alteration in smoking and hypertension are more important than cholesterol lowering in terms of overall mortality, and modification of these risk factors should be part of a multifaceted approach to decreasing car-

ROBERT L. TALBERT, PHARM.D., is Professor of Pharmacy Practice, Department of Pharmacology, College of Pharmacy, The University of Texas Health Science Center at San Antonio, 7703 Floyd Curl Drive, San Antonio, TX, 78284-7765.

Copyright © 1988, American Society of Hospital Pharmacists, Inc. All rights reserved. 0278-2677/88/0801-0604$00.50.

diovascular risk. The prediction by Taylor et al.[10] of changes in life expectancy attributable to cholesterol reduction has created controversy but also provided information to aid in selection of patients who may benefit from treatment. Although one could use these data to suggest that treatment is not worthwhile or cost-effective, adding up to 29 months of life span (60-year-old man, 20% reduction in cholesterol) from an individual perspective would seem rational and justified.

Cost-effectiveness of Intervention

Inspection of the cost-effectiveness of any intervention—including cholesterol lowering—could lead one to the conclusion that few interventions are fiscally practical yet many are routinely undertaken. Undoubtedly, some of the variables used to estimate cost-effectiveness are in error, but the major implication remains valid: This intervention is expensive. Pharmacoeconomic studies are needed to determine the best approach to therapy; however, these studies would need to be very large to reach conclusions that would be reliable and could be generalized.

Conclusion

The approach of the NCEP—to lower cholesterol for the entire population and for individuals at highest risk—is a logical and pragmatic approach for long-term reduction in this risk factor for heart disease. Although the cut points chosen for decision-making could be argued and the specific approaches to therapy debated, decades of research and the weight of expert, considered opinion should lead one to the conclusion that cholesterol reduction is important and beneficial for cardiovascular risk reduction.

References

1. Labreche DL. Reassessment of the value of lowering serum cholesterol. *Clin Pharm.* 1988; 7:592–603.
2. Lipid Research Clinics Program. The Lipid Research Clinics Coronary Primary Prevention Trial results. I. Reduction in incidence of coronary heart disease. *JAMA.* 1984; 251:351–64.
3. Frick MH, Elo O, Haapa K et al. Helsinki Heart Study: primary-prevention trial with gemfibrozil in middle-aged men with dyslipidemia. Safety of treatment, changes in risk factors, and incidence of coronary heart disease. *N Engl J Med.* 1987; 317:1237–45.
4. The Norwegian Multicenter Study Group. Timolol-induced reduction in mortality and reinfarction in patients surviving acute myocardial infarction. *N Engl J Med.* 1981; 304:801–7.
5. Rose GA, Thomson WB, Williams RT. Corn oil in treatment of ischaemic heart disease. *Br Med J.* 1965; 1:1531–3.
6. Report from the Committee of Principal Investigators. A cooperative trial in the primary prevention of ischaemic heart disease using clofibrate. *Br Heart J.* 1978; 40:1069–118.
7. Peto R, Yusuf S, Collins R. Cholesterol-lowering trial results in their epidemiologic context. *Circulation.* 1985; 72:III-451. Abstract.
8. The Expert Panel. Report of the National Cholesterol Education Program expert panel on detection, evaluation, and treatment of high blood cholesterol in adults. *Arch Intern Med.* 1988; 148:36–69.
9. Virkkunen M. Lipid Research Clinics Coronary Primary Prevention Trial results. *JAMA.* 1985; 253:635–6.
10. Taylor WC, Pass TM, Shepard DS et al. Cholesterol reduction and life expectancy. A model incorporating multiple risk factors. *Ann Intern Med.* 1987; 106:605–14.

The questions are when and how to treat, not whether to treat, hypercholesterolemia

JAMES M. MCKENNEY

Clin Pharm. 1988; 7:605–7

Decisions in patient care are rarely black and white. More often they are made with incomplete knowledge and thus come down to the practitioner's judgment of what is best for the patient. This was the case with the recent recommendations for the detection and treatment of high blood cholesterol by the National Cholesterol Education Program.[1] These recommendations deserve careful consideration by every health professional, with especially critical appraisal of the scientific studies on which they are based. Labreche[2] has raised many of the key—and, frankly, quite thorny—issues relating to these recommendations. On the basis of his review of the literature, he advises treating only the severest forms of hypercholesterolemia (i.e., familial hypercholesterolemia). Based on my analysis of the same and related literature, I believe the question is no longer whether to treat hypercholesterolemia in the general population (i.e., both familial and nonfamilial forms) but when and how. I would like to briefly present my rebuttal to some of Labreche's positions.

Interpreting Clinical Trial Results in High-Risk Men

Labreche takes issue with the way that the results of treating high-risk men in the Lipid Research Clinics Coronary Primary Prevention Trial (LRC-CPPT)[3] were analyzed and extensively cites Kronmal's criticism[4] in his arguments. Labreche fails to cite the LRC-CPPT investigators' response[5] to Kronmal in which they point out that their reference to an alpha of 0.01 before the study was for the purpose of calculating the sample size. According to the LRC-CPPT investigators, use of a one-sided statistical test at the conclusion of the study

JAMES M. MCKENNEY, PHARM.D., FASHP, is Professor, Department of Pharmacy, School of Pharmacy, Virginia Commonwealth University, Box 581, MCV Station, Richmond, VA 23298.

Copyright © 1988, American Society of Hospital Pharmacists, Inc. All rights reserved. 0278-2677/88/0801-0605$00.75.

was determined by the one-sidedness of the hypothesis being tested and an alpha level of 0.05 was selected by convention. Further, they report that, in consultation with Kronmal, they reanalyzed the relationship between the change in measured low-density lipoprotein (LDL) cholesterol and coronary heart disease (CHD) incidence using proportional hazards coefficients and found a highly significant difference ($p < 0.001$), which gives even more credence to the benefit of treating high-risk men.

Labreche argues that since cholesterol-lowering therapy in the LRC-CPPT and Helsinki Heart Study[6] did not reduce total mortality in men with nonfamilial (polygenic) hypercholesterolemia, it cannot be recommended. Both of these trials showed a treatment-related reduction in the incidence of CHD but not in total mortality. This was primarily due to an increase in deaths from accidents and violence in the drug treatment group, which has led to speculation that cholesterol-lowering drugs may cause a central toxic effect that may have contributed to this outcome.[7] A recent examination of these data by one of the study groups reveals that most of these deaths were due to accidents and homicides unrelated to the study and that only two of the active-drug-treated patients committed suicide, compared with one placebo-treated patient.[8] This is hardly evidence of a drug-related event.

Neither the LRC-CPPT nor the Helsinki Heart Study was designed to determine whether cholesterol lowering would reduce total mortality or prolong life in men. This goal would have required a larger study population that was selected with different criteria and studied for a longer period. The studies were designed to determine whether cholesterol lowering reduced *premature* CHD in men with markedly elevated serum cholesterol levels. Both studies demonstrated a statistically significant and clinically important reduction in nonfatal myocardial infarctions, lending support to at least a narrow application of clinical trial results; that is treatment of men who are at high risk of CHD because they have serum cholesterol levels above 260 mg/dL (i.e., the approximate acceptance levels of the LRC-CPPT and Helsinki trials).

Applicability of Clinical Trial Results to Other Populations

Labreche takes the position that since the benefit of cholesterol-lowering treatment has been studied only in high-risk men, treatment recommendations should not be extended to men with lower cholesterol levels or to blacks, women, and the elderly. This obviously raises the question of how the results of the LRC-CPPT and the Helsinki Heart Study should be generalized to other populations. The basis of these trials was the strong epidemiologic evidence that CHD and cholesterol were positively linked in men.[9-13] The results of these clinical trials validated the cholesterol hypothesis; that is, not only does blood cholesterol define the level of risk, but it also defines the benefit of cholesterol-lowering therapy. The CHD reduction that occurred in these trials was predictable based on epidemiologic studies.[5,14] Furthermore, these studies showed that the greater the reduction in blood cholesterol, the greater the reduction in CHD incidence.[14,15] The consistency of the cholesterol–CHD relationship demonstrated in numerous epidemiologic studies, regardless of the methodologies employed or populations studied, and the close link between clinical trial data and predicted outcomes support the recommendation to treat all men at increased CHD risk because of elevated cholesterol levels.[1]

The same consistent epidemiologic relationship of blood cholesterol to CHD incidence is seen in women,[9] blacks,[16] and the elderly.[17] The relationship is continuous and graded, such that as serum cholesterol levels increase, CHD incidence increases. However, for any given cholesterol level, the CHD risk in these patient groups is less than that found in male populations.[9,16,17] This naturally leads to the assumption that effective treatment of elevated cholesterol levels in these patient populations would produce a proportionate (although somewhat smaller) reduction in CHD incidence. While the generalization to these populations is a matter of personal and professional judgment, I believe that recommending a low saturated fat diet for all patients at increased CHD risk because of cholesterol levels and offering drug therapy for those with levels in the top 10% who are not controlled with diet alone is prudent.

Association between Low Cholesterol Levels and Incidence of Cancer

The relationship of cholesterol and cancer is complex and poorly understood. Most observational studies have reported increased total mortality at low cholesterol levels, which is primarily due to an increased incidence of cancer.[18-23] No causal relationship has been demonstrated between lowering cholesterol and cancer, nor were there reports of increased cancer deaths in the two recent cholesterol-lowering trials.[3,6] When deaths caused by cancer two years after initiation of epidemiologic studies were dropped from analysis, the cholesterol–cancer relationship in most studies disappeared, suggesting that some of the patients may have had subclinical cancer at the time of entry into the study and that metabolic effects of undetected cancer may be responsible for the lower cholesterol level.[21-23] A precipitous drop in serum cholesterol has been identified as a poor prognostic sign,[24] possibly because tumor cells increase the clearance and degradation of the LDL cholesterol particle.[25] Until lowering cholesterol has been shown to cause cancer, there is no justification for withholding cholesterol therapy on this basis.

Selective Treatment of Smoking or High Blood Cholesterol Based on Cost-Effectiveness

Since the majority of patients with hypercholesterolemia can be treated with a low saturated fat diet alone, treatment of these patients should not be any more expensive than the time spent counseling and encouraging patients to cease smoking. Thus, the issue of cost that Labreche raises relates only to the use of drug treatment in the group of patients in the upper 10th percentile of cholesterol levels. These patients have a risk of CHD death equal to that caused by smoking one or more packs of cigarettes a day, and thus a theoretical equal benefit to treatment.[26] Could we then justify treating one patient group and not the other? I do not believe so. Patients with multiple risk factors have disproportionately higher risks of CHD and thus greater potential benefit from treatment. When high blood cholesterol and smoking coexist, it may be advisable to discuss the potential gain and costs of treating each risk factor with patients and to allow them to participate in the selection of treatment.

Conclusion

In making decisions about the application of knowledge to patient care, it is often advisable to view the evidence from a distance, rather than getting caught up in study details. With this broad perspective, one finds abundant evidence demonstrating a continuous and graded relationship between CHD and serum cholesterol, regardless of gender, race, or age. One also finds studies demonstrating that when cholesterol-lowering therapy is initiated in high-risk patients, premature CHD is reduced. Furthermore, the level of CHD risk for a given level of cholesterol predicts the benefit of cholesterol-lowering therapy. I believe these data support the treatment of hypercholesterolemia in the general population. For the majority of these individuals, a low saturated fat diet is sufficient. For those who are at highest risk because of very high cholesterol levels (upper 10% of the population), or who have other risk factors or CHD and are not adequately treated with diet (upper 25% of the population), drug therapy is recommended. In the final analysis, however, the decision to treat and how is a professional judgment based on assessment of the individual patient's needs.

References

1. The Expert Panel. Report of the National Cholesterol Education Program expert panel on detection, evaluation, and treatment of high blood cholesterol in adults. *Arch Intern Med*. 1988; 148:36–69.
2. Labreche DG. Reassessment of the value of lowering serum cholesterol: questioning the widsom of widespread intervention. *Clin Pharm*. 1988; 7:592–603.
3. Lipid Research Clinics Program. The Lipid Research Clinics Coronary Primary Prevention Trial results: I. Reduction in incidence of coronary heart disease. *JAMA*. 1984; 251:351–64.
4. Kronmal RA. Commentary on the published results of the Lipid Research Clinics Coronary Primary Prevention Trial. *JAMA*. 1985; 263:2091–3.
5. The Lipid Research Clinics Program Investigators. Reply to commentary by Richard Kronmal. *JAMA*. 1985; 254:263–4.
6. Frick MH, Elo O, Haapa K et al. Helsinki Heart Study: primary-prevention trial with gemfibrozil in middle-aged men with dyslipidemia. *N Engl J Med*. 1987; 317:1237–45.
7. Virkkunen M. Lipid Research Clinics Coronary Primary Prevention Trial results. *JAMA*. 1985; 253:635.
8. Frick MH, Heinonen OP, Huttunen JK et al. Gemfibrozil and coronary heart disease. *N Engl J Med*. 1988; 318:1275.
9. Lerner DJ, Kannel WB. Patterns of coronary heart disease morbidity and mortality in the sexes: a 26 year follow-up of the Framingham population. *Am Heart J*. 1986; 111:383–90.
10. Kannel WB, Castelli WP, Gordon T et al. Serum cholesterol, lipoproteins, and the risk of coronary heart disease. The Framingham Study. *Ann Intern Med*. 1971; 74:1–12.
11. Martin MJ, Hulley SB, Browner WS et al. Serum cholesterol, blood pressure, and mortality: implications from a cohort of 361,662 men. *Lancet*. 1986; 2:933–6.
12. Kannel WB, Neaton JD, Wentworth D et al. Overall and coronary heart disease mortality rates in relation to major risk factors in 325,348 men screened for the MRFIT. *Am Heart J*. 1986; 112:825–36.
13. Stamler J, Wentworth D, Neaton JD. Is relationship between serum cholesterol and risk of premature death from coronary heart disease continuous and graded? Findings in 356,222 primary screenees of the Multiple Risk Factor Intervention Trial (MRFIT). *JAMA*. 1986; 256:2823–8.
14. Lipid Research Clinics Program. The Lipid Research Clinics Coronary Primary Prevention Trial results II. The relationship of reduction in incidence of coronary heart disease to cholesterol lowering. *JAMA*. 1984; 251:365–74.
15. Tyroler HA. Review of lipid-lowering clinical trials in relation to observational epidemiologic studies. *Circulation*. 1987; 76:515–22.
16. Neaton JD, Juller LH, Wentworth D et al. Total and cardiovascular mortality in relation to cigarette smoking, serum cholesterol concentration, and diastolic blood pressure among black and white males followed up for five years. *Am Heart J*. 1984; 108:759–69.
17. Kannel WB, Vokonas PS. Primary risk factors for coronary heart disease in the elderly: the Framingham study. In: Wenger NK, Furbert CD, Pitt E, eds. Coronary heart disease in the elderly. New York: Elsevier; 1986; 60–95.
18. Williams RR, Sorlie PD, Feinleib M et al. Cancer incidence by levels of cholesterol. *JAMA*. 1981; 245:247–52.
19. Sorlie PD, Feinleib M. The serum cholesterol–cancer relationship: an analysis of time trends in the Framingham study. *J Natl Cancer Inst*. 1982; 69:989–96.
20. Miller SR, Tartter PI, Papatestas AE et al. Serum cholesterol and human colon cancer. *J Natl Cancer Inst*. 1081; 67:297–300.
21. Sherwin RW, Wentworth DN, Cutler JA et al. Serum cholesterol levels and cancer mortality in 361,662 men screened for the Multiple Risk Factor Intervention Trial. *JAMA*. 1987; 257:943–8.
22. Rose G, Shipley MJ. Plasma lipids and mortality: a source of error. *Lancet*. 1980; 523–6.
23. Mannes GA, Maier A, Thieme C et al. Relation between the frequency of colorectal adenoma and the serum cholesterol level. *N Engl J Med*. 1986; 315:1634–8.
24. Tornbert SA, Holm LE, Carstensen JM et al. Risks of cancer of the colon and rectum in relation to serum cholesterol and beta-lipoprotein. *N Engl J Med*. 1986; 315:1629–33.
25. Vitols S, Bjorkolm M, Gahrton G et al. Hypocholesterolemia in malignancy due to elevated low density-lipoprotein-receptor activity in tumor cells: evidence from studies in patients with leukemia. *Lancet*. 1985; 2:1150–4.
26. Goldman L, Cook EF. The decline in ischemic heart disease mortality rates. An analysis of the comparative effects of medical interventions and changes in lifestyle. *Ann Intern Med*. 1984; 101:825–36.

Aminoglycoside pharmacokinetic monitoring: An integral part of patient care?

KEITH A. RODVOLD, HUMPHREY ZOKUFA, AND JOHN C. ROTSCHAFER

Clin Pharm. 1988; 7:608–13

In the past decade, one of pharmacy's most notable achievements has been the development of clinical practice. Much of the success in creating a clinical role for pharmacists has involved the application of pharmacokinetic principles to drugs such as aminoglycosides. The introduction of several new β-lactam and quinolone antimicrobial agents has prompted a reassessment of the current and future role of aminoglycoside therapy. Because of the great variability in aminoglycoside pharmacokinetics and the narrow margin between effective and toxic concentrations, regular monitoring of serum aminoglycoside concentrations with appropriate adjustment of dose, dosage interval, or both is often recommended.[1-9]

Many facets of therapeutic monitoring of aminoglycosides remain controversial and unexplained. The purpose of this article is to summarize data evaluating the role and the impact of therapeutic monitoring of aminoglycosides.

Comparison of Aminoglycoside Dosing Methods

The goal of aminoglycoside pharmacokinetic monitoring is to maximize antimicrobial efficacy and minimize antimicrobial toxicity. To determine whether aminoglycoside pharmacokinetic monitoring is an integral part of patient care, several questions must be addressed. The first question is whether pharmacokinetic techniques outperform conventional methods of determining aminoglycoside dosages in the production of desired serum concentrations. If a particular aminoglycoside concentration range is desired, are pharmacokinetic techniques better than conventional methods for dosing aminoglycosides?

There is striking interpatient and intrapatient variation in the pharmacokinetics of the aminoglycosides for patients with normal and abnormal renal function.[1,10] This results in differences in peak concentration and drug clearance. The variation in serum aminoglycoside concentrations is dependent on renal function and on the volume of distribution, both of which are partially affected by patient factors including age,[11-13] weight,[14,15] gender,[1] fever,[16] and concurrent disease states.[17,18] If these factors are not considered or accounted for, the accuracy of any dosage calculation will be jeopardized.

There are many methods for determining aminoglycoside dosage. Some of the more common methods include empiric dosing ("rule of eights"),[19] dosage based on body weight (i.e., mg/kg/dose),[19] use of nomograms,[20-22] individualized pharmacokinetic models,[23,24] and Bayesian forecasting methods.[25,26] Empiric methods use a fixed dose and dosage interval but make no allowance for the patient's weight, age, or renal function. Dosing by body weight refines one aspect of empiric therapy but makes no allowance for age or renal function. Additionally, in obese patients, there is the dilemma of whether to use lean body weight or total body weight in calculating the aminoglycoside dose.

Nomograms use a statistical relationship between aminoglycoside elimination and measured creatinine clearance. The minimal information needed to use aminoglycoside dosing nomograms includes a patient's age, gender, weight, and serum creatinine concentration or creatinine clearance. Several investigators have found that aminoglycoside elimination half-life often correlates poorly with serum creatinine concentrations and estimates of creatinine clearance.[2,10] Although nomograms are based on measured creatinine clearance, most clinicians usually substitute a calculated creatinine clearance. In our experience, only 38% of the variance (r^2) in elimination rate is explained by differences in creatinine clearance.[27] Thus, other factors that are related to aminoglycoside disposition are not included in nomograms. This discrepancy reduces the usefulness of the statistical relationship between aminoglycoside elimination, creatinine clearance, and dosage calculation.

Individualized pharmacokinetic approaches attempt to measure the distribution volume and the elimination rate constant on a patient-by-patient basis. Using these pharmacokinetic values generat-

KEITH A. RODVOLD, PHARM.D., is Assistant Professor, Department of Pharmacy Practice and Clinical Pharmacokinetics Laboratory, College of Pharmacy, University of Illinois, Chicago. HUMPHREY ZOKUFA, PHARM.D., is Research Fellow and JOHN C. ROTSCHAFER, PHARM.D., is Associate Professor, Section of Clinical Pharmacology, St. Paul–Ramsey Medical Center, St. Paul, MN, and the College of Pharmacy, University of Minnesota, Minneapolis.

Address reprint requests to Dr. Rotschafer at the Section of Clinical Pharmacology, St. Paul–Ramsey Medical Center, 640 Jackson Street, St. Paul, MN 55101.

Presented at the 21st Annual ASHP Midyear Clinical Meeting, Las Vegas, NV, December 11, 1986.

Copyright © 1988, American Society of Hospital Pharmacists, Inc. All rights reserved. 0278-2677-88/0801-0608$01.50.

ed from measured serum concentration–time data, the clinician can determine the appropriate dose and dosage interval needed for an individual patient to achieve desired peak and trough concentrations. The method of Sawchuk and Zaske[23-28] has been used frequently for providing aminoglycoside pharmacokinetic dosing services.[29] This method permits rapid attainment of target steady-state serum aminoglycoside concentrations tailored to the patient's pharmacokinetic characteristics and clinical condition. This method has been tested widely in burn patients, geriatric patients, surgical patients, obstetric patients, gynecologic patients, obese patients, and patients with gram-negative infections.[1,13,14,17,30-32] The Sawchuk–Zaske method has been shown to be more accurate than empiric dosing or nomograms for predicting the aminoglycoside dose necessary to achieve specific serum concentrations.[27]

Recently, the design of individualized dosage regimens has focused on methods that incorporate Bayesian principles.[33] Before any measurements of drug concentrations for Bayesian forecasting, the patient is regarded as a typical member of a patient population in which all members have similar pharmacokinetic values. Once serum concentrations become available, the patient is regarded as a unique individual whose pharmacokinetic values are distinct from those of other patients. As additional serum concentrations accumulate, the base for patient assessment changes. Several investigators have demonstrated the effectiveness of this approach for predicting gentamicin, tobramycin, and amikacin doses to achieve therapeutic serum concentrations.[25,26,34-37] The Bayesian method can use one or more serum drug concentrations, whereas the Sawchuk–Zaske method requires two or more serum drug concentrations. Although these findings for the Bayesian method appear promising, prospective demonstration of cost-effectiveness and validation of performance are needed in large numbers of patients with a broad spectrum of clinical conditions.

Each of the methods described above has its own level of sophistication and advantages for aminoglycoside dosing. Empiric dosing, dosing by weight (i.e., mg/kg/dose), and nomograms have the obvious advantages of simplicity, lack of patient discomfort, and negligible cost associated with collecting blood samples and measuring aminoglycoside concentrations. Unfortunately, these predictive methods do not adequately account for individual patient characteristics such as variable distribution volumes and differences in aminoglycoside elimination. Most of these methods use a fixed dosage interval, which promotes drug accumulation in patients with age- or disease-related renal dysfunction. Additionally, all of these predictive methods result in a substantial number of aminoglycoside concentrations outside the therapeutic ranges because of the tendency to underdose patients. These methods may be useful for initiation of therapy; however, continued therapy must be followed with measurement of serum aminoglycoside concentrations and dosage adjustment to ensure therapeutic concentrations.

Because of the many variables that influence aminoglycoside disposition, the only way one can ensure adequate but nontoxic concentrations is to measure serum concentrations. Pharmacokinetic approaches, including those that incorporate Bayesian principles, account for individual patient variability in the design of aminoglycoside dosage regimens. The necessary components of these methods include supervised collection of serum concentration–time data, patient discomfort associated with phlebotomy, additional cost associated with the aminoglycoside concentration determinations, and sophisticated support and personnel to generate dosage recommendations. While these methods ensure that therapeutic and nontoxic concentrations are achieved, such highly individualized approaches to the monitoring of aminoglycoside therapy usually require establishment of a pharmacokinetic consultation service.[38-40] Although such a service potentially can improve quality control, it is not clear whether the added expense is justified.

Impact of Aminoglycoside Therapeutic Monitoring on Patient Outcome

The second question about therapeutic monitoring of aminoglycoside concentrations is whether an improvement in therapeutic response or reduction in toxicity can be demonstrated when desired aminoglycoside concentrations are achieved and maintained. Intuitively, it would seem logical that monitoring patients to maintain aminoglycoside levels within the desired peak and trough serum concentration range would be associated with a measurable improvement in efficacy and a minimization of drug toxicity. Ideally, a review of the literature should allow the reader to reach a conclusion as to whether aminoglycoside pharmacokinetic services are warranted. However, a review of the literature on cost-benefit analysis of serum aminoglycoside concentration monitoring is very difficult because there is very little to discuss.[41-44] Additionally, examination of these data (Table 1) identifies several uncontrolled variables that make conclusions difficult, if not impossible.

Vozeh[49] has recently reviewed the cost-effectiveness of therapeutic drug monitoring. His conclusions were as follows: (1) achievement of therapeutic concentrations is associated with increased efficacy, reduced frequency of adverse effects, or both; (2) without therapeutic drug monitoring, a large proportion of patients will have serum concentrations outside the therapeutic ranges; (3) per-

Table 1.
Studies Showing Uncontrolled Variables and Differences in Dosing Methods

	Study Design[a]	No. Patients	Infections Treated	TDM Point (hr)[b]	Days of Therapy[c]	Recommended Peak Conc. (mg/L)[d]	Definition of Peak (hr after dose)	Serum Sampling	Method of Dosing	Assay Method[e]	Stated Efficacy (%)
Arroyo et al.[45]	RCR	112	Mixed	≤72	NS	3.5–8 G&T; 15–30 A	NS	Trough/peak	House officer	EIA	42
Flint et al.[46]	P	68	Pneumonia	≤24	NS	6–10 G&T; 20–25 A	0.25 or 1	0.25, 1, 2, & 4 hr	LeFrock	FPI	78
Moore et al.[5]	RRPD	89	Bacteremia	≤48	8	5–10 G&T; 20–40 A	1	Trough/peak	Chan	REA	87
Noone et al.[4]	P	65	Mixed	≤72	NS	5–>8 G	1 i.m. 0.25 i.v.	Trough/peak	NS	Urease	84
Cipolle et al.[47]	P	26	Pneumonia	≤24	8	6–9 T	0	Series	Sawchuk-Zaske	RIA	88
Zaske et al.[48]	P	105	Burn	≤24	8	7–10 G	0	Series	Sawchuk-Zaske	RIA	86

[a] RCR = retrospective chart review; RRPD = retrospective review of prospective data; P = prospective.
[b] Time elapsed between initiation of therapy and therapeutic drug monitoring (TDM).
[c] Mean duration; NS = not stated.
[d] G = gentamicin; T = tobramycin; A = amikacin.
[e] EIA = Enzyme immunoassay (EMIT, Syva); FPI = fluorescence polarization immunoassay technique (Abbott); REA = radioenzymatic assay; RIA = radioimmunoassay technique (Monitor Science, Newport Beach, CA).

forming drug assays without therapeutic monitoring services does not improve the quality of treatment; and (4) dosage adjustment based on appropriate interpretation of drug concentrations reduces the proportion of patients with serum concentrations outside the therapeutic range. For the aminoglycosides, indirect evidence suggests that therapeutic monitoring may be cost-effective and improve the quality of care in the treatment of gram-negative infections.

As illustrated by the studies listed in Table 1, uncontrolled pharmacokinetic variables between investigators' protocols make comparisons of the impact of therapeutic drug monitoring difficult. The common practice of trough and peak determinations and application of a one-compartment pharmacokinetic model may skew the interpretation of serum concentration data. Theoretically, trough and peak concentrations must be determined when the patient has achieved steady-state concentrations. This may not be the case in a septic patient with progressive renal dysfunction or in an acute-care environment in which adherence to aminoglycoside dosage schedules may vary. Using trough and peak serum concentration–time data and a one-compartment pharmacokinetic model requires the trough be used twice, once to calculate distribution volume and again as the second postinfusion concentration to determine the elimination rate constant.

The aminoglycoside concentration measured before the administration of a dose may be affected by an increased or decreased ability on the part of the patient to eliminate the aminoglycoside or by early or late administration of the previous dose. Figure 1 illustrates the effects on serum concentrations when a patient receives an aminoglycoside dose one hour early, on time, and one hour late. A trough concentration blood sample obtained when the previous dose was given one hour late or one hour early will result in a trough concentration value that is twice or half the true value. If pharmacokinetic values are calculated from these serum concentration–time data, a 20–40% variation in half-life, a 6–7% variation in distribution volume, and a 6–11% variation in dosage recommendation are obtained. Investigators using trough and peak determinations in the evaluation of patients usually do not state whether they rigidly adhered to the conditions and circumstances of steady state under which trough and peak concentrations must be determined.

Another major difficulty in evaluating these data is the variability in serum-sampling strategies and reference points for peak serum aminoglycoside concentrations. While the true peak serum concentration occurs at the end of the intravenous infusion, several investigators report obtaining "peak" serum concentrations 15 to 60 minutes postinfusion[9,46] and attempting to adjust the serum concentrations obtained at these reference points to between 4 and 10 mg/L. They do not extrapolate the serum concentration–time data obtained 15 to 60 minutes postinfusion back to the time when the infusion stopped to determine the true peak concentration.

If a 60-minute-postinfusion serum concentration of 7 mg/L is desired, as illustrated in Figure 2, the true peak concentration is 14 mg/L. Thus, the true peak concentration is likely to be higher than the "peak" concentration that is reported in Table 1. The magnitude of this difference is a function of

Figure 1. Serum aminoglycoside concentrations when dose is given one hour early (light solid line), on time (dotted line), and one hour late (heavy solid line). Half-life = 1.0 hr; infusion time = 1.0 hr, dosage interval = 4.0 hr, dose = dose that will produce a 7-mg/L difference in peak and trough concentrations.

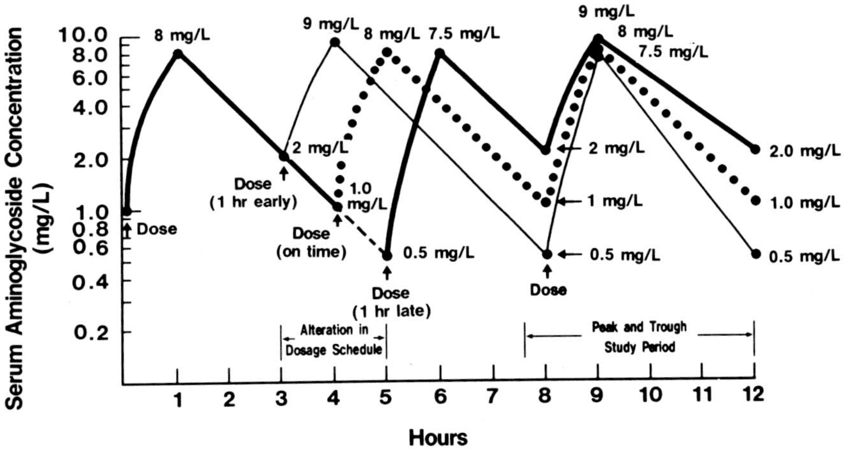

Figure 2. Plot of true peak versus one-hour-postinfusion serum concentration in a patient with a one-hour half-life. T = infusion time, τ = dosage interval.

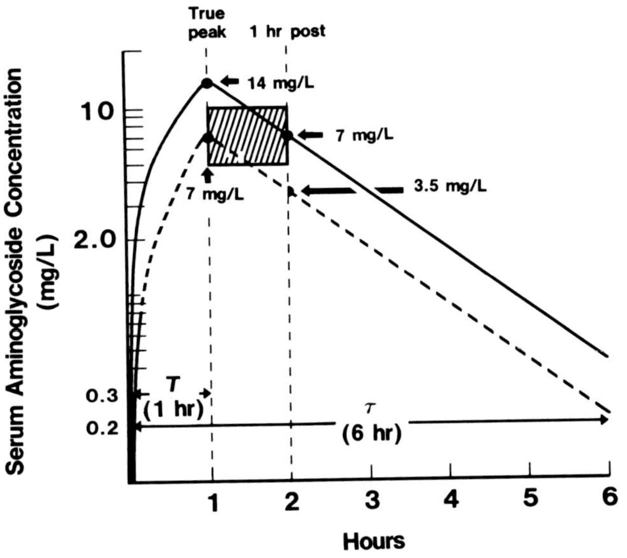

the patient's elimination rate constant, the time at which the blood sample for "peak" concentration is obtained relative to the true peak, the duration of the aminoglycoside infusion, and the magnitude of the desired concentration at that point.

A variable that often is not considered but may have a substantial impact on differences between studies is the use of different methods for quantitating serum aminoglycoside concentrations. In several investigations evaluating different aminoglycoside assay methods, a systematic bias for higher concentration values with one assay was observed.[50,51] The magnitude of assay bias increases with the serum concentration, resulting in different estimates for pharmacokinetic values and dosage recommendations. A 7–22% difference in distribution volume, a 6–10% difference in elimination rate constant, and a 9–20% difference in dosage recommendations have been observed.[50,51] The clinical practice of rounding dosages may further accentuate the differences in dosage recommendations.

The desired ranges for aminoglycoside concentrations proposed in the early 1970s were primarily derived using microbiologic assays, radioenzymatic assays, or radioimmunoassays. Desired serum aminoglycoside concentrations routinely used in clinical practice today have not changed since the early 1970s, despite substantial changes in assay technology. Institutions attempting to employ Bayesian pharmacokinetic principles must be assured that the a priori population value used in the forecasting technique was developed using an assay identical to that routinely used within their institution.

Many investigators measure trough and peak serum concentrations but do not employ a proven mathematical model or systematic method to adjust dose and dosage interval. In many studies, aminoglycoside dosage is not optimized for at least 48 hours, if at all (Table 1). Consequently, the time from the start of aminoglycoside therapy through obtaining serum concentration–time data, analysis of sera, and implementation of appropriate changes in dose and dosage interval could easily require three to four days, or 30–50% of the duration of aminoglycoside therapy.

There are very few reports of optimizing aminoglycoside therapy within 12 to 24 hours of the initial dose and systematically obtaining trough and peak serum concentrations throughout the course of aminoglycoside therapy. Uncontrolled variability in serum concentrations greatly reduces the ability of the investigators to make conclusive statements as to the effect of aminoglycoside serum concentrations on either efficacy or safety. How can legitimate claims be made about the relationship between serum aminoglycoside concentrations and efficacy or toxicity when aminoglycoside levels are essentially uncontrolled for up to half of the course of therapy?

Flint et al.,[46] attempting to measure the impact of aminoglycoside monitoring in a prospective study of 68 patients with bacterial pneumonia, concluded that monitoring may identify subtherapeutic concentrations but will not predict or avoid nephrotoxicity in critically ill patients. While these investigators obtained suitable serum aminoglycoside concentration–time data (trough, 0.25-, 1-, 2-, and 4-hour postinfusion serum samples) to individualize aminoglycoside therapy using a pharmacokinetic method, no such intervention was performed. The investigation by Flint et al. also contained a systematic problem in data collection. The authors commented that the peak concentration was defined as the higher of the 15-minute and one-hour postinfusion levels. The fact that the investigators' one-hour postinfusion sample was often larger than the 15-minute postinfusion sample indicates that sera collection and patient monitoring during intravenous administration were not rigidly supervised or controlled.

Arroyo et al.[45] attempted to measure the effect of serum assays on clinical decisions made by physicians and on renal toxicity. In this retrospective chart review there was no protocol for obtaining serum samples or for dosage adjustments. Patients received aminoglycosides for a variety of infections rather than for one specific type of infection. Patients in one group received aminoglycosides and were monitored for serum concentrations, while the other group received aminoglycosides but had no determinations of serum concentration. One potential problem of this retrospective study is that the physician may have requested determination of aminoglycoside levels only for patients considered to be at high risk or for those who had serious infections; the patients not having aminoglycoside determinations may have been considered low-risk patients with minor infections. These authors concluded that although serum concentration monitoring may have alerted physicians to subtherapeutic concentrations, it had no impact on predicting toxicity.

The studies of Flint et al. and Arroyo et al. lacked the necessary control and the prospective, systematic approach to collection of serum concentration data and adjustment of dosages to make valid conclusions. Specific pharmacokinetic guidelines to promote and ensure consistent collection of samples and interpretation of serum concentration–time data must be established before the impact of therapeutic drug monitoring can be assessed.

Conclusion

There are no reliable cost-effectiveness data from prospective, controlled studies in which pharmacokinetic dosing of the aminoglycosides was performed appropriately. Several problems still exist regarding the evaluation of the effect of therapeutic monitoring on aminoglycoside efficacy and toxicity.

Studies must be conducted that optimize aminoglycoside therapy at its onset and use a proven pharmacokinetic technique rather than trough and peak serum concentration monitoring with trial-and-error dosage adjustment. There must be consensus as to the accepted range of aminoglycoside concentrations and the point in the serum concentration–time curve at which these will be measured. Investigators trying to evaluate the efficacy or toxicity, or both, of aminoglycosides must operate with a protocol-based and systematic approach to data collection and evaluation.

References

1. Zaske DE, Cipolle RJ, Rotschafer JC. Gentamicin pharmacokinetics in 1640 patients: method for control of serum concentration. *Amtimicrob Agents Chemother.* 1982; 21:407–11.
2. Barza M, Brown RB, Shen D et al. Predictability of blood levels of gentamicin in man. *J Infect Dis.* 1975; 132:165–74.
3. Barza M, Lauermann M. Why monitor serum levels of gentamicin? *Clin Pharmacokinet.* 1978; 3:202–15.
4. Noone P, Parsons TMC, Pattison JR et al. Experience in monitoring gentamicin therapy during treatment of serious gram-negative sepsis. *Br Med J.* 1974; 1:477–81.
5. Moore RD, Smith CR, Lietman PS. The association of aminoglycoside plasma levels with mortality in patients with gram-negative bacteremia. *J Infect Dis.* 1984; 149:443–8.
6. Moore RD, Smith CR, Leitman PS. Association of aminoglycoside plasma levels with therapeutic outcome in gram-negative pneumonia. *Am J Med.* 1984; 77:657–62.
7. Dahlgren JG, Anderson ET, Hewitt WL. Gentamicin blood levels: a guide to nephrotoxicity. *Antimicrob Agents Chemother.* 1975; 8:58–62.
8. Moore RD, Smith RC, Lietman PS. Risk factors for the development of auditory toxicity in patients receiving aminoglycosides. *J Infect Dis.* 1984; 149:23–30.
9. Moore RD, Smith RC, Lipsky JJ et al. Risk factors for nephrotoxicity in patients treated with aminoglycosides. *Ann Intern Med.* 1984; 100:352–7.
10. Kaye D, Levison ME, Labovitz ED. The unpredictability of serum concentrations of gentamicin: pharmacokinetics of gentamicin in patients with normal and abnormal renal function. *J Infect Dis.* 1974; 130:150–4.
11. Bauer LA, Blouin RA. Influence of age on amikacin pharmacokinetics in patients without renal disease. Comparison with gentamicin and tobramycin. *Eur J Clin Pharmacol.* 1983; 24:639–42.
12. Matzke GR, Jameson JJ, Halstenson CE. Gentamicin disposition in young and elderly patients with various degrees of renal function. *J Clin Pharmacol.* 1987; 27:216–20.
13. Zaske DE, Irvine P, Strand LM et al. Wide interpatient variations in gentamicin dose requirements for geriatric patients. *JAMA.* 1982; 248:3122–6.
14. Sketris I, Lesar T, Zaske DE et al. Effect of obesity on gentamicin pharmacokinetics. *J Clin Pharmacol.* 1981; 21:288–93.
15. Bauer LA, Edwards WAD, Dellinger EP et al. Influence of weight on aminoglycoside pharmacokinetics in normal weight and morbidly obese patients. *Eur J Clin Pharmacol.* 1983; 24:643–7.

16. Pennington JE, Dale DC, Reynolds HY et al. Gentamicin sulfate pharmacokinetics: lower levels of gentamicin in blood during fever. *J Infect Dis.* 1975; 132:270–5.
17. Zaske DE, Sawchuk RJ, Gerding DN et al. Increased dosing requirements of gentamicin in burn patients. *J Trauma.* 1976; 16:824–8.
18. Gill MA, Kern JW. Altered gentamicin distribution in ascitic patients. *Am J Hosp Pharm.* 1979; 36:1704–6.
19. Physicians desk reference. Oradell, NJ: Medical Economics Co.; 1981:1607.
20. Chan RA, Benner EJ, Hoeprich RD. Gentamicin therapy in renal failure: nomogram for dosage. *Ann Intern Med.* 1978; 76:775–8.
21. Hull JH, Sarubbi FA. Gentamicin serum concentrations: pharmacokinetic prediction. *Ann Intern Med.* 1976; 85:183–9.
22. Sarubbi FA, Hull JH. Amikacin serum concentrations: prediction of levels and dosage guidelines. *Ann Intern Med.* 1978; 89:612–8.
23. Sawchuk RJ, Zaske DE. Pharmacokinetics of dosing regimens which utilize multiple intravenous infusions: gentamicin in burn patients. *J Pharmacokinet Biopharm.* 1976; 4:183–95.
24. Schentag JJ, Adelman MH. A microcomputer program for tobramycin consult services, based on the two-compartment pharmacokinetic model. *Drug Intell Clin Pharm.* 1983; 17:528–31.
25. Burton ME, Brater DG, Chen PS et al. A Bayesian feedback method of aminoglycoside dosing. *Clin Pharmacol Ther.* 1985; 37:349–57.
26. Murray KM, Bauer LA, Koup JR. Predictive performance of computer dosing methods for tobramycin using two pharmacokinetic models and two weighting algorithms. *Clin Pharm.* 1986; 5:411–4.
27. Lesar TS, Rotschafer JC, Strand LM et al. Gentamicin dosing errors with four commonly used nomograms. *JAMA.* 1982; 248:1190–3.
28. Sawchuk RJ, Zaske DE, Cipolle RJ et al. Kinetic model for gentamicin dosing with the use of individual patient parameters. *Clin Pharmacol Ther.* 1977; 21:362–9.
29. Matzke GR, Burkle WS, Lucarotti RL. Gentamicin and tobramycin dosing guidelines: an evaluation. *Drug Intell Clin Pharm.* 1983; 17:425–32.
30. Zaske DE, Cipolle RJ, Strate RG. Gentamicin dosage requirements: wide interpatient variations in 242 surgery patients with normal renal function. *Surgery.* 1980; 87:164–9.
31. Zaske DE, Cipolle RJ, Strate RG et al. Rapid gentamicin elimination in obstetric patients. *Obstet Gynecol.* 1980; 56:559–64.
32. Zaske DE, Cipolle RJ, Strate RG et al. Increased gentamicin dosage requirements: rapid elimination in 249 gynecology patients. *Am J Obstet Gynecol.* 1981; 139:896–900.
33. Sheiner LB, Beal SL, Rosenberg B et al. Forecasting individual pharmacokinetics. *Clin Pharmacol Ther.* 1979; 26:294–305.
34. Rodvold KA, Blum BA. Predictive performance of Sawchuk–Zaske and Bayesian dosing methods for tobramycin. *J Clin Pharmacol.* 1987; 27:419–27.
35. Burton ME, Chow MSS, Platt DR et al. Accuracy of Bayesian and Sawchuk–Zaske dosing methods of gentamicin. *Clin Pharm.* 1986; 5:143–9.
36. Hurst AK, Iseri KT, Gill MA et al. Comparison of four methods for predicting serum gentamicin concentrations in surgical patients with perforated or gangrenous appendicitis. *Clin Pharm.* 1987; 6:234–8.
37. Lacarelle B, Granthil C, Manelli JC et al. Evaluation of a Bayesian method of amikacin dosing in intensive care unit patients with normal or impaired renal function. *Ther Drug Monit.* 1987; 9:154–60.
38. Quebbeman EJ, Franson TR, Whipple JE et al. A quality control analysis of aminoglycoside management. *Arch Surg.* 1985; 120:1069–71.
39. Mason GE, Winter ME. Appropriateness of sampling times for therapeutic drug monitoring. *Am J Hosp Pharm.* 1984; 41:1796–801.
40. Whiting B, Kelman AW, Bryson SM et al. Clinical pharmacokinetics: a comprehensive system for therapeutic drug monitoring and prescribing. *Br Med J.* 1984; 288:541–5.
41. Bootman JL, Wertheimer AL, Zaske DE et al. Individualizing gentamicin dosage regimens in burn patients with gram-negative septicemia: a cost–benefit analysis. *J Pharm Sci.* 1979; 68:267–72.
42. Schloemer JH, Zagozen JJ. Cost analysis of an aminoglycoside pharmacokinetic dosing service. *Am J Hosp Pharm.* 1984; 41:2347–51.
43. Kimelblatt BJ, Bradbury K, Chodoff L et al. Cost–benefit analysis of an aminoglycoside monitoring service. *Am J Hosp Pharm.* 1986; 43:1205–9.
44. Sveska KJ, Roffe BD, Solomon DK et al. Outcome of patients treated by an aminoglycoside pharmacokinetic dosing service. *Am J Hosp Pharm.* 1985; 42:2472–8.
45. Arroyo JC, Milligan WL, Davis J et al. Impact of aminoglycoside serum assays of clinical decisions and renal toxicity. *South Med J.* 1986; 79:272–6.
46. Flint LM, Gott J, Short L et al. Serum level monitoring of aminoglycoside antibiotics. *Arch Surg.* 1985; 120:99–103.
47. Cipolle RJ, Seifert RD, Zaske DE et al. Hospital-acquired gram-negative pneumonias: response rate and dosage requirements with individualized tobramycin therapy. *Ther Drug Monit.* 1980; 2:359–63.
48. Zaske DE, Bootman JL, Solem LB et al. Increased burn patient survival with individualized dosages of gentamicin. *Surgery.* 1982; 91:142–9.
49. Vozeh S. Cost-effectiveness of therapeutic drug monitoring. *Clin Pharmacokinet.* 1987; 13:131–40.
50. Rotschafer JC, Morlock C, Strand L et al. Comparison of radioimmunoassay and enzyme immunoassay: methods in determining gentamicin pharmacokinetic parameters and dosages. *Antimicrob Agents Chemother.* 1982; 22:648–51.
51. Rotschafer JC, Berg HG, Nelson RB et al. Observed differences in gentamicin pharmacokinetic parameters and dosage recommendations determined by fluorescent polarization immunoassay and radioimmunoassay methods. *Ther Drug Monit.* 1983; 5:443–7.

Drug Experience

Straightforward reports of unusual drug experiences are included in this section. These may be confirmations of previously reported drug experiences or brief apparent first reports. While selected references may be cited, the purpose of a Drug Experience report is not to present an extensive review of the literature.

A related section, Grand Rounds, includes papers that are well-documented patient case reports with a thorough review of the important literature to help put the case in perspective.

Reversal of iatrogenic diazepam overdose with flumazenil

EMEKA O. C. UME AND ADRIAN W. GELB

Clin Pharm. 1988; 7:614–6

Benzodiazepine drugs are used clinically as anxiolytics, hypnotics, amnestics, sedatives, and anticonvulsants.[1] These features suit them for use in the intensive-care unit.[2] The unwanted adverse effects of these drugs are drowsiness, ataxia, dizziness, incoordination, and muscle weakness. Because of age-related reduction in clearance, diazepam tends to have a prolonged effect in the elderly (65 years of age and older).[3]

Several drugs including naloxone, physostigmine, and theophylline have been tried with only partial success in an attempt to reverse the central nervous system effects of benzodiazepines.[4] A newly synthesized imidazobenzodiazepine, flumazenil (Ro 15-1788, Hoffmann-La Roche Inc.; 8-fluoro-5,6-dihydro-5-methyl-6-oxo-4H-imidazo[1,5-a][1,4]-benzodiazepine-3-carboxylate), has been shown to specifically inhibit the central nervous system effects of benzodiazepines in humans by competitive inhibition at the benzodiazepine receptor site.[2,4–7] This is still an investigational drug in North America but has been released for clinical use in Europe. We present our experience using this compound in the diagnosis of the cause of coma in a patient in the intensive-care unit.

Case Report. A 74-year-old man with a two-year history of acute myelocytic leukemia was admitted to the hospital with a third relapse of the disease. Previous treatment with low-dose cytarabine and daunorubicin had resulted in two remissions. Other medical problems included a several-year history of parkinsonism and osteoarthritis involving his cervical and lumbar spine, knees, and shoulders. Medications at the time of admission included levodopa with carbidopa (Sinemet 10–100 every three hours while awake and Sinemet 25–250 at bedtime) and trihexyphenidyl hydrochloride 2 mg three times daily.

Physical examination revealed a 163-cm, 82-kg frail-appearing man in no apparent distress, with an oral temperature of 36.6 °C, pulse 84 beats per minute, respirations at a regular rate of 20 per minute, and blood pressure 100/60 mm Hg. On the second hospital day therapy was begun with cytarabine 20 mg subcutaneously every 12 hours for seven days and mitoxantrone hydrochloride 12 mg intravenously daily for three days. On the 11th hospital day his temperature rose to 39 °C, and cefazolin 1 g (as the sodium salt) intravenously every six hours, gentamicin 80 mg (as the sulfate salt) intravenously every eight hours, and ketoconazole 200 mg orally daily were added to the regimen.

On the 17th hospital day the patient developed a sore throat, inspiratory stridor, respiratory distress, right neck swelling, and a mass in his soft palate. In the operating room the patient was orally intubated, a submandibular abscess was incised, and he was then transferred to the intensive-care unit. Because blood cultures grew *Pseudomonas aeruginosa*, ceftazidime 1 g intravenously every six hours was given in addition to the other antimicrobial agents. The patient was returned to the operating room four days later for further debridement and incision of the abscess, which was now found to involve the right carotid artery.

Because of the discomfort associated with the dressing changes, the patient received diazepam

EMEKA O. C. UME, PHARM.D., is Clinical Pharmacist-Consultant, Jack Austin Drugs Limited, Downsview, Ontario; at the time of this report, he was Clinical Pharmacist, University Hospital, London, Ontario. ADRIAN W. GELB, M.B.CH.B., FRCP (C), is Associate Professor of Anaesthesia, University of Western Ontario, London, Ontario, and Deputy Coordinator, Intensive-Care Unit, University Hospital.

Address reprint requests to Dr. Gelb at the Department of Anaesthesia, University Hospital, P.O. Box 5339, Postal Station A, London, Ontario N6A 5A5, Canada.

The contribution of the patient's attending hematologist, R. M. Barr, M.D., is acknowledged.

Copyright © 1988, American Society of Hospital Pharmacists, Inc. All rights reserved. 0278-2677/88/0801-0614$00.75.

and morphine. During his first 11 days in the intensive-care unit he received 20 mg of diazepam and 34 mg of morphine sulfate intravenously. Although he was making continued but slow improvement, on the 29th hospital day he became agitated, combative, tachycardic, hypertensive, and tachypneic. Treatment with diazepam 2.5 mg intravenously every 15 minutes as needed was started; the patient received a total dose of 35 mg of diazepam on the 29th hospital day and an additional 17 mg over the next 24 hours. A total of 72 mg of diazepam and 54 mg of morphine sulfate was given intravenously during his stay in the intensive-care unit.

Before the 29th hospital day he had been drowsy but conscious. He became progressively more obtunded and eventually comatose. This condition was thought to be drug related, and the benzodiazepine therapy was stopped on hospital day 30. An additional 5 mg of morphine sulfate was given over the next two days. On day 34 he was still unconscious and had signs suggestive of a stroke involving the right cerebral hemisphere. Withdrawal in response to painful stimulation was much less vigorous on the left side, and the right pupil reacted slightly less than the left to light. We were concerned that he may have had septic emboli from the exposed right carotid artery. Two computed tomographic scans showed no evidence of a stroke. The neurologist recommended that magnetic resonance imaging be performed and that serious consideration be given to tying off the right carotid artery if the results suggested septic emboli. This would prevent further embolization but carried the risk of itself resulting in cerebral ischemia.

The intensive-care-unit staff was faced with two problems. First was the logistical problem of transporting a ventilated and very sick patient to the magnetic resonance imager and maintaining him in it, as well as the problems associated with trying to ventilate a patient in close proximity to such a powerful magnet. Second was the question of whether such high-risk surgery should be performed on a patient with an underlying malignancy, even if septic emboli were found.

As the patient's poor neurological status could have resulted from an iatrogenic drug overdose, naloxone 0.4 mg was given intravenously on hospital day 34 but did not change his neurological condition. Eighteen hours later an intravenous bolus of flumazenil 0.5 mg was administered. Within seconds, the patient opened his eyes, smiled, and stretched in bed. He regained full consciousness within two minutes, responded appropriately, and obeyed commands. Another 0.5-mg dose was administered 15 minutes later. Approximately half an hour after this last dose, the patient again became unconscious. The diagnosis of diazepam overdose was confirmed. The patient continued to make slow progress and was ultimately discharged home.

Discussion. Hepatic microsomal enzyme reactions are divided into phase I and phase II reactions. Phase I (preparative biotransformation reactions) includes oxidation (hydroxylation, *N*-dealkylation, and sulfoxidation), reduction, and hydrolysis.[3,8] These phase I reactions generally produce minor molecular modifications in compounds and make them more polar (water soluble).[3,8] The metabolites produced via this pathway often retain part or all of the pharmacological activity of the parent compound.[3] Phase II reactions involve conjugation or attachment of a drug molecule to a larger substituent, usually glucuronide, sulfate, or acetate.[3,8] The resulting conjugates usually have little or no pharmacological activity and are much more polar than the parent compound. They are generally excreted in the urine.[3]

During the aging process, the functional capacity as well as the size of the liver decreases.[8] There is little evidence to indicate a substantial age-dependent decline in efficiency of the hepatic phase II reactions or conjugation.[9] Conversely, efficiency of phase I reactions, most notably oxidation, decreases with age.[3,8,9] Diazepam is known to be metabolized through this latter pathway.[3] Therefore, the elimination half-life of the drug tends to be longer in the elderly. Failure to recognize this factor, coupled with the increased central nervous system sensitivity in the elderly, can result in intoxication or possibly coma in elderly patients receiving diazepam.

The benzodiazepines produce their pharmacological effects within the central nervous system by facilitating the inhibitory neurotransmitter γ-aminobutyric acid (GABA) in the opening of chloride channels on postsynaptic cells.[1,5,10] The most widely accepted hypothesis for the hypnotic effect of benzodiazepines is based on the existence of separate benzodiazepine and GABA receptors coupled to a common ionophore (chloride) channel. Occupation of both receptors facilitates opening of the channel and produces membrane hyperpolarization and neuronal inhibition.[10]

A new compound, flumazenil, has been shown to competitively antagonize benzodiazepines at the receptor level. The reversal of the central nervous system effects of diazepam in this patient took less than one minute. The short onset of action has been shown to result from the rapid distribution of flumazenil to the brain.[11] The half-life of the drug is 55 minutes,[11] which explains the drug's short duration of action of 2.5 hours. With long-acting benzodiazepines, e.g., diazepam and flunitrazepam, repeated boluses or continuous intravenous infusion of the antagonist is required to maintain consciousness and prevent respiratory depression.[2,12] On the other hand, when a short-acting benzodiazepine such as midazolam is used as an anaesthetic, an average dose of 0.4 mg of flumazenil is sufficient to reverse its effect and sedation does not recur.[5] The dose range that reverses the central nervous system effects of most benzodiazepine drugs is 0.2–0.8 mg.[5,12]

No adverse effects of the drug were observed in this patient, although nausea, vomiting, and sweating have been reported.[5] Two drug interactions may have contributed to this patient's coma. The oxidative hepatic metabolism of diazepam is decreased by ketoconazole, and the concurrent administration of narcotic analgesics with sedative properties may result in profound sedation or coma.[13]

In this patient, for whom the vital question of ischemic brain damage versus drug-induced coma had to be clarified, the antagonist proved to be extremely useful. Also, flumazenil's inhibition of the central nervous system effects of benzodiazepines has been shown to facilitate the weaning from mechanical ventilation of patients with acute respiratory failure and chronic obstructive pulmonary disease who had been on a ventilator for days or weeks.[2]

Conclusion. Preliminary experience suggests that flumazenil may be useful in the diagnosis and management of benzodiazepine overdoses.

References

1. Darragh A, Lambe R, Scully M et al. Investigation in man of efficacy of a benzodiazepine antagonist, Ro 15-1788. *Lancet.* 1984; 2:8–10.
2. Kleinberger G, Grimm G, Laggner A et al. Weaning patients from mechanical ventilation by benzodiazepine antagonist Ro 15-1788. *Lancet.* 1985; 2:268–9.
3. Greenblatt DJ, Sellers EM, Shader RI. Drug disposition in old age. *N Engl J Med.* 1982; 306:1081–8.
4. Geller E, Niv D, Rudick V et al. The use of Ro 15-1788: a benzodiazepine antagonist in the diagnosis and treatment of benzodiazepine overdose. *Anesthesiology.* 1984; 61:A135. Abstract.
5. Wolfe J, Carl P, Clansen TG et al. Ro 15-1788 for postoperative recovery: a randomized clinical trial in patients undergoing minor surgical procedure under midazolam anaesthesia. *Anaesthesia.* 1986; 41:1001–6.
6. Forster A, Rouiller M, Morel D et al. Double-blind randomized study evaluating a specific benzodiazepine antagonist. *Anesthesiology.* 1983; 59:A375. Abstract.
7. O'Boyle C, Lambe R, Darragh A et al. Ro 15-1788 antagonizes the effects of diazepam in man without affecting its bioavailability. *Br J Anaesth.* 1983; 55:349–55.
8. Henney HR III. Geriatric drug therapy. *US Pharm.* 1985; 10(Feb):41–50.
9. Schmucker DL. Drug disposition in the elderly: a review of the critical factors. *J Am Geriatric Soc.* 1984; 32:144–9.
10. Reves JG, Fragen RJ, Vinik R et al. Midazolam: pharmacology and uses. *Anesthesiology.* 1985; 62:310–24.
11. Roncan G, Ziegler WH, Guenter TW. Pharmacokinetics of the new benzodiazepine antagonist Ro 15-1788 in man following intravenous and oral administration. *Br J Clin Pharmacol.* 1986; 22:421–8.
12. Geller E, Niv D, Silbiger A et al. Ro 15-1788: a new benzodiazepine antagonist in the treatment of 34 intoxicated patients. *Anesthesiology.* 1985; 63:A157. Abstract.
13. Kastrup EK, Olin BR. Facts and comparisons. Loose-leaf drug information service. St. Louis: J. B. Lippincott Company; 1987.

Histamine-like reaction after a single intravenous dose of rifampin

PATTY FAN-HAVARD, MILAP C. NAHATA, WILLIAM J. BARSON, HENRY BARTKOWSKI, AND EDWARD KOSNIK

Clin Pharm. 1988; 7:616–20

Shunt infections remain a common postoperative complication of cerebrospinal fluid (CSF) shunt procedures, with a reported incidence of 6% to 27%.[1,2] *Staphylococcus epidermidis* is the most frequent causative pathogen and accounts for approximately 60% of all CSF shunt infections.[1] Furthermore, many strains of *S. epidermidis* have been isolated from patients with infected CSF shunts.[3] The use of antimicrobial prophylaxis for preventing CSF shunt infections remains unclear. Most of the clinical studies are retrospective, and many prospective studies contain methodologic flaws or improper selection of antimicrobial agents or lack sufficient sample size.[1,4–7] Therefore, conclusions cannot be drawn about the efficacy of antimicrobial prophylaxis in reducing CSF shunt infections.

Rifampin is one of the most active antimicrobials against staphylococci[8]; it may be a promising agent for prophylaxis in patients undergoing CSF shunt placement. Synergistic activity in vitro against methicillin-resistant staphylococci has been documented with rifampin and vancomycin and other antistaphylococcal agents.[8,9] Many clinical studies have demonstrated successful use of rifampin plus vancomycin or nafcillin to eradicate methicillin-resistant staphylococcal infections in patients with CSF shunts, prosthetic heart valves, orthopedic devices, or indwelling catheters.[10,11] However, there is only one published report on the prophylactic use of rifampin in CSF shunt procedures. Yogev et al.[12] reported a decrease in the incidence of ventriculoperitoneal (VP) shunt infections with oral rifampin in combination with intravenous nafcillin.

In the United States, the injectable form of rifampin is available only for compassionate use in criti-

PATTY FAN-HAVARD, PHARM.D., is Fellow in Infectious Disease Pharmacotherapy, College of Pharmacy; MILAP C. NAHATA, PHARM.D., is Professor of Pharmacy and Pediatrics, Colleges of Pharmacy and Medicine; WILLIAM J. BARSON, M.D., is Assistant Professor of Pediatrics, College of Medicine; HENRY BARTKOWSKI, M.D., is Associate Clinical Professor, Division of Neurologic Surgery, College of Medicine; and EDWARD KOSNIK, M.D., is Associate Professor, Division of Neurosurgery, College of Medicine, The Ohio State University and Children's Hospital, Columbus, OH.

Address reprint requests to Dr. Nahata at the College of Pharmacy, The Ohio State University, 500 West 12th Avenue, Columbus, OH, 43210.

Copyright © 1988, American Society of Hospital Pharmacists, Inc. All rights reserved. 0278-2677/88/0801-0616$01.25.

cally ill or comatose patients for whom oral administration is not feasible. Histamine-like reactions with cutaneous involvement after intravenous administration of rifampin have not been previously reported; however, cutaneous reactions associated with oral administration of rifampin have included the "red-man syndrome" after inadvertent overdosage and suicide attempts.[13-15] We describe an infant with no history of rifampin therapy who developed a histamine-like reaction similar to the red-man syndrome after a single intravenous dose of rifampin. This occurred during a double-blind, placebo-controlled study evaluating the efficacy and safety of intravenously administered rifampin for prevention of postsurgical CSF shunt infections.

Case Report. This nine-month-old, 11.5-kg, Caucasian boy was admitted to the hospital for evaluation of recurrent seizures and hydrocephalus. At four months of age, the infant had undergone a resection of a choroid plexus tumor. Postoperatively, seizures of a generalized tonic–clonic and petit mal nature developed, which were initially controlled with phenobarbital and phenytoin. The patient developed a rash that was attributed to phenytoin; phenytoin was discontinued and carbamazepine was added. Despite adequate concentrations of anticonvulsant agents, the infant continued to have seizures. One month before the present admission, a computed tomography (CT) scan revealed slight hydrocephalus. Therapy with acetazolamide (100 mg orally every eight hours) was instituted, and the anticonvulsant regimen was continued.

On this admission, the infant appeared well developed, well nourished, and in no acute distress. Findings of the neurological examination were normal except for mild papilledema and a mild right-sided hemiparesis. The serum concentrations of carbamazepine and phenobarbital on admission were 8.9 μg/mL (therapeutic range = 4–8 μg/mL) and 33.6 μg/mL (therapeutic range = 15–30 μg/mL), respectively. A CT scan of the infant's head demonstrated progressive hydrocephalus, which necessitated the placement of a right VP shunt.

The patient was enrolled in the study, which was approved by the Human Subjects Research Committee of Children's Hospital. The infant was randomized to receive a single dose of rifampin (Merrell Dow Pharmaceuticals, Inc., Cincinnati, OH) after informed consent was obtained from the parents. A total of 230 mg (20 mg/kg) of rifampin was infused over 60 minutes, via a syringe pump (Med-Fusion Systems Inc., Syringe Pump Model 1001), one hour before CSF shunt placement.

Five minutes after the end of drug infusion, the patient developed cutaneous eruptions and became irritable. His neck and head were intensely red and a faint red rash was present on his chest, abdomen, and back. Periorbital swelling was also noted. No respiratory distress was present and the vital signs had not changed from the preinfusion values (blood pressure 110/70 mm Hg, heart rate 140 beats per minute, respiratory rate 26 per minute). Diphenhydramine hydrochloride 15 mg was administered intravenously, which decreased the rash and swelling of the eyelids within five minutes. The rash was completely resolved within 30 minutes. Slight elevations of liver function test values were noted 24 hours after drug administration; these values returned to baseline by the time of discharge (Table 1). An orange-red discoloration of the urine was noted for 18 hours after the infusion. In a review of the pharmacist's records, no errors were found in the calculation or preparation of the rifampin for injection.

Discussion. Cutaneous reactions associated with intravenous rifampin are rare; however, thrombophlebitis has been associated with administration of rifampin by injection for longer than 30 days.[16] Pruritus involving the face and hands developed in three physicians and four nurses 30 to 60 min-

Table 1.
Changes in Liver Function Test Results after a Single Intravenous Dose of Rifampin

Test (Normal Range)[a]	Preoperative Value	24 Hours Postinfusion	7 Days Postinfusion[b]
Total bilirubin (0.2–1.3 mg/dL)	0.2	0.5	. . .
Alkaline phosphatase (90–350 U/L)	320	147	251
Lactate dehydrogenase (249–403 U/L)	255	138	. . .
Aspartate aminotransferase (13–65 U/L)	26	67	20
Alanine aminotransferase (0–45 U/L)	55	78	3
Gamma glutamyltransferase (0–18 U/L)	20	117	. . .

[a] Standard values reported by the clinical laboratory in pediatric patients ages 1 to 15 years.
[b] Day of discharge.

utes after they handled the rifampin powder.[17] One physician developed severe eczema 30 minutes after preparation of the rifampin solution; the eczema resolved after three days.[17] Three patients developed allergic rashes while receiving rifampin for treatment of nonmycobacterial infections; the onset and the characteristics of the cutaneous eruption and the dose of rifampin injected were not reported.[16] No mention was made of adverse effects in a group of 12 children treated with intravenous rifampin for staphylococcus-related shunt or catheter infections.[18]

Cutaneous reactions to oral rifampin occur frequently. The patients may have flushing, pruritus, erythema, urticaria, watering of the eyes, or redness involving the face, scalp, and shoulders. The incidence of cutaneous reactions has ranged from 0.5% to 28%[19,20]; the higher frequency is associated with larger doses of rifampin (900–1800 mg) given once or twice weekly for the treatment of tuberculosis.[19,21] The onset of cutaneous symptoms generally occurs during the first three months of therapy and around two to four hours after the administration of rifampin.[19]

Serious cutaneous complications after oral rifampin therapy are unusual. A case of recurrent Stevens–Johnson syndrome was reported in a 40-year-old African man diagnosed as having pulmonary tuberculosis. The antituberculous agents included daily oral rifampin 600 mg, ethambutol hydrochloride 800 mg, and intramuscular streptomycin 1 g (as the sulfate salt). All drugs were discontinued after the patient developed exfoliative dermatitis, buccal ulceration, fever, and anterior uveitis. These symptoms recurred when rifampin alone was reinstituted.[22] Chronic papular acneiform lesions on the face, neck, and shoulders were reported in 8 of 24 patients with urinary tuberculosis. The onset of lesions appeared around the fifth week after daily therapy with oral rifampin 100 mg, isoniazid 300 mg, and thioacetazone 150 mg was started. Complete resolution of lesions occurred within three weeks after discontinuation of rifampin in all patients.[23] A case of serious rifampin-induced purpura cutanea tarda was reported in a 55-year-old man with a tuberculous psoas abscess. The mechanism of this reaction was speculated to be an induction of hepatic delta-aminolevulinic acid synthetase by rifampin.[24]

Recently, the red-man syndrome has been described in 19 children after rifampin (100 mg/kg/day) overdose.[13] The syndrome was characterized by marked red discoloration of the skin, urine, feces, sweat, and tears. Other symptoms included periorbital and facial edema, pruritus of the head, vomiting, headache, diarrhea, fever, and transient elevation of total bilirubin. These symptoms were first noted one-half to four hours after the dose; they persisted from one to 78 hours.

The mechanisms for rifampin-induced cutaneous reactions remain unclear. Some possibilities may include amount of drug administered, infusion rate, excipients in the formulation, hypersensitivity or immunologic reactions, or histamine-like reaction. Two studies are available correlating the occurrence of cutaneous symptoms with serum concentrations of rifampin after oral administration.[21,25] Rifampin concentrations ranged from 9.8 to 48.4 μg/mL in patients with "flu-like" syndrome, pruritus, jaundice, rash, or dyspnea; concentrations were as high as 43.6 μg/mL in asymptomatic patients.[21] In a separate study, serum rifampin concentrations were compared in 29 asymptomatic patients and three symptomatic patients three, six, and eight hours after a single oral dose of rifampin 900 mg given six months after the initiation of therapy for tuberculosis. The adverse effects with rifampin included flu-like syndrome and gastrointestinal intolerance. The rifampin concentrations were five times higher after three hours, and five to 10 times higher after six to eight hours, in the symptomatic patients than in the asymptomatic patients.[25] The wide range in rifampin concentrations in these studies may be attributable to (1) intrapatient variability, (2) nonspecific microbiological assays, and (3) improper storage of rifampin samples. A recent study demonstrated that the degradation of rifampin is minimized by the addition of ascorbic acid to serum specimens immediately upon separation.[26] Based on these limited data and conflicting results, no conclusions can be drawn regarding the relationship between serum concentrations and the cutaneous adverse effects of rifampin.

Rifampin has been administered intravenously over various infusion periods. In one study, rifampin was administered as a bolus injection over five minutes, followed by an infusion over one hour, to 32 patients who had osteomyelitis or were undergoing an orthopedic surgical procedure.[27] In four separate studies, the duration of rifampin infusion has ranged from 0.5 to 3 hours.[18,28–30] Because no histamine-like reactions were reported in these studies, infusion rate may not be an important factor in causing such adverse effects.

According to the manufacturer of rifampin, the excipients in the solid dosage form for oral administration include magnesium stearate, sodium chloride, cornstarch, talc, gelatin, titanium dioxide, and dyes. For the injectable dosage form, the excipients include 0.2% polysorbate and sodium hydroxide, adjusted to a pH of 8.5.[a] Although the two preparations of rifampin have different excipients, no studies have compared the incidence of adverse effects caused by the oral versus the intravenous formulation.

Cutaneous symptoms can often be accompanied by other adverse effects such as flu-like symptoms, hematologic abnormalities, or gastrointestinal intolerance in patients receiving rifampin. These reactions have been speculated to be an immune response phenomenon. Rifampin antibodies have been detected in 31%, 21%, and 0.8% of patients receiving oral rifampin in once-weekly, twice-weekly, and daily regimens, respectively.[31] The onset of symptoms appears to occur at times when there are low levels of circulating antibodies, which may be attributable to the binding of antibodies to surface antigens.[25] In a review of the adverse effects of rifampin, Grosset and Leventis[32] suggested that the hemolytic anemia and thrombocytopenia may be associated with the capability of IgG and IgM to fix complement on erythrocytes or platelets in the presence of rifampin.

In our patient, the cutaneous symptoms were most likely a histamine-like reaction to rifampin. The symptoms appear to be similar to the red-man syndrome. Although blood samples were not drawn for determination of rifampin concentrations, it is unlikely that the administered dose resulted in toxic serum levels of rifampin, based on the results of pharmacokinetic studies in our previous patients.[33] A review of the pharmacy records documented no dosing errors. Eight additional patients received the same dose (20 mg/kg) and did not develop histamine-like reactions.

Conclusion. Based on this case presentation, a histamine-like reaction can occur with the first dose of injectable rifampin in patients with no history of rifampin therapy. Patients should be monitored closely during intravenous administration of rifampin. An antihistamine, such as diphenhydramine, appears to be effective in controlling the cutaneous symptoms. Further studies are needed to evaluate the mechanisms of rifampin-induced histamine-like reaction.

---

[a] Reavey-Cantwell N, Kenny MT, Hudak WJ, Merrell Dow Pharmaceuticals, Inc. Personal communication. 1988 May 26.

References

1. Schoenbaum SC, Gardner P, Shillito J. Infections of cerebrospinal fluid shunts: epidemiology, clinical manifestations and therapy. *J Infect Dis.* 1975; 131:543–52.
2. George R, Leibrock L, Epstein M. Long term analysis of cerebrospinal fluid shunt infections. A 25 year experience. *J Neurosurg.* 1979; 51:804–11.
3. Archer GL. Antimicrobial susceptibility and selection of resistance among *Staphylococcus epidermidis* isolates recovered from patients with infections with indwelling foreign devices. *Antimicrob Agents Chemother.* 1978; 14:353–9.
4. Odio C, McCracken GH, Nelson JD. CSF shunt infections in pediatrics: a seven year experience. *Am J Dis Child.* 1984; 138:1103–8.
5. Odio C, Mohs E, Sklar FH et al. Adverse reactions to vancomycin used as prophylaxis for CSF shunt procedures. *Am J Dis Child.* 1984; 138:17–9.
6. Haines SJ, Taylor F. Prophylactic methicillin for shunt operations: effects on incidence of shunt malfunction and infection. *Childs Brain.* 1982; 9:10–22.
7. Wang EL, Prober CG, Hendrick BE. Prophylactic sulfamethoxazole and trimethoprim in ventriculoperitoneal shunt surgery. A double blind, randomized placebo-controlled trial. *JAMA.* 1984; 251:1174–7.
8. Thornsberry C, Hill BC, Swenson JM et al. Rifampin: spectrum of antibacterial activity. *Rev Inf Dis.* 1983; 5(Suppl 3):S412–S417.
9. Ein ME, Smith NJ, Aruffo JF et al. Susceptibility and synergy studies of methicillin-resistant *Staphylococcus epidermidis. Antimicrob Agents Chemother.* 1979; 16:655–9.
10. Archer GL, Tenebaum MJ, Haywood HB. Rifampin therapy of *Staphylococcus epidermidis:* use in infections from indwelling artificial devices. *JAMA.* 1978; 240:751–3.
11. Faville RJ, Zaske DE, Kaplan EL et al. *Staphylococcus aureus* endocarditis: combined therapy with vancomycin and rifampin. *JAMA.* 1978; 240:1963–5.
12. Yogev R, Shinco F, McLone D. Prophylaxis for ventriculoperitoneal shunt surgery with nafcillin alone or in combination with rifampin. Paper presented to 23rd Interscience Conference on Antimicrobial Agents and Chemotherapy. Las Vegas, NV; 1983 Oct 25.
13. Bolan G, Laurie RE, Broome CV. Redman syndrome: inadvertent administration of an excessive dose of rifampin to children in a day care center. *Pediatrics.* 1986; 77:633–5.
14. Broadwell RO, Broadwell SD, Comer PB. Suicide by rifampin overdose. *JAMA.* 1978; 240:2283–4.
15. Wong P, Bottorff MB, Heritage RW et al. Acute rifampin overdose: a pharmacokinetic study and review of the literature. *J Pediatr.* 1984; 104:781–3.
16. Kissling M, Bergamini N, Xilinas M. Parenteral rifampicin in tuberculous and severe non-mycobacterial infections. *Chemotherapy.* 1982; 28:229–39.
17. Anker W, Bang FD. Long-term intravenous rifampin treatment: advantages and disadvantages. *Eur J Respir Dis.* 1981; 62:84–6.
18. Koup JR, Williams-Warren J, Weber A et al. Pharmacokinetics of rifampin in children. I. Multiple dose intravenous infusion. *Ther Drug Monit.* 1986; 8:11–6.
19. Aquinas M, Allan WGL, Horsfall PAL et al. Adverse reactions to daily and intermittent rifampicin regimens for pulmonary tuberculosis in Hong Kong. *Br Med J.* 1972; 1:765–71.
20. Dutt AK, Moers D, Stead WW. Undesirable side effects of isoniazid and rifampin in largely twice-weekly short course chemotherapy for tuberculosis. *Am Rev Respir Dis.* 1983; 128:419–24.
21. Pujet JC, Homberg JC, Decroix G. Sensitivity to rifampicin: Incidence, mechanism, and prevention. *Br Med J.* 1974; 2:415–8.
22. Nyirenda R, Gill GV. Stevens-Johnson syndrome due to rifampin. *Br Med J.* 1977; 2:1189.
23. Nwokolo U. Acneiform lesions in combined rifampicin treatment in Africans. *Br Med J.* 1974; 3:473.
24. Millar JW. Rifampin-induced porphyria cutanea tarda. *Br J Dis Chest.* 1980; 74:405–8.
25. O'Mahony MG, Kar CW. Relationships between rifampicin-dependent antibody scores, serum rifampin concentrations and symptoms in patients with adverse reactions to intermittent rifampin treatment. *Clin Allergy.* 1973; 3:353–62.
26. Weber A, Opheim KE, Smith AL et al. High pressure liquid chromatographic quantitation of rifampin and its two major metabolites in urine and serum. *Rev Inf Dis.* 1983; 5:S433–S439.
27. Roth B. Penetration of parenterally administered rifampicin into bone tissue. *Chemotherapy.* 1984; 30:358–65.
28. Koup JR, Williams-Warren J, Viswanathan CT et al. Pharmacokinetics of rifampin in children. II. Oral bioavailability. *Ther Drug Monit.* 1986; 8:17–22.
29. Houin G, Beucle A, Richelet S et al. Pharmacokinetics of rifampicin and desacetylrifampicin in tuberculous patients after different rates of infusion. *Ther Drug Monit.* 1983; 5:67–72.
30. Acocella G, Segre G, Conti R et al. Pharmacokinetic study on intravenous rifampicin in man. *Pharmacol Res Commun.* 1984; 16:723–36.
31. Wolledge S. Rifampin-induced antibodies. *Chemotherapy.* 1976; 4:273–8.

32. Grosset J, Leventis S. Adverse effects of rifampin. *Rev Inf Dis.* 1983; 5(Suppl 3):S440–S446.
33. Fan-Havard P, Nahata MC, Barson W et al. Serum and cerebrospinal fluid (CSF) concentrations after intravenous rifampin prophylaxis in pediatric patients undergoing CSF shunt surgery. *Clin Pharmacol Ther.* 1988; 43:154. Abstract PIIF-3.

Theophylline toxicity after iodine 131 treatment for hyperthyroidism

CARY E. JOHNSON AND IRA A. COHEN

Clin Pharm. 1988; 7:620–2

The rate of theophylline elimination has been reported to increase in patients with hyperthyroidism[1-3] and to decrease considerably in patients with hypothyroidism, which results in toxicity.[2,4,5] The pharmacokinetic characteristics of other drugs metabolized by hepatic microsomal enzymes also have been reported to be altered by thyroid dysfunction.[6,7] To our knowledge, theophylline toxicity after iodine 131 treatment for hyperthyroidism has not been reported.

Case Report. A 39-year-old white man came to the gastroenterology clinic with a two-month history of diarrhea. His medical history included asthma since the age of 22, which was well controlled by albuterol two inhalations four times a day and aminophylline 400 mg orally four times a day. He took no other medications and had never smoked.

The patient was thin, his blood pressure was 130/80 mm Hg, and his pulse rate was 110 beats/min. The results of a physical examination and laboratory studies, including a complete blood count, erythrocyte sedimentation rate, and urinalysis, were otherwise normal. Except for the presence of sinus tachycardia, an electrocardiogram and chest roentgenogram were normal. The patient's serum theophylline concentration was 16.8 μg/mL. Stool culture for pathogens and examination for ova and parasites were negative. Thyroid function test results, however, were markedly abnormal (Table 1). The patient was referred to the endocrinology and metabolism clinic for further evaluation and treatment.

On examination, the patient's thyroid was slightly enlarged and nontender. His hands were warm, moist, and tremulous, and reflexes were brisk. A test for thyroid microsomal antibodies was positive at a dilution of 1:6400 (normal, 0 to 1:400). A diagnosis of Graves' disease was made, and the patient was scheduled to receive ^{131}I treatment. Beta-blocker therapy was not initiated because of the patient's history of asthma.

The possibility that altered thyroid function would affect theophylline elimination was suggested.[1] The patient agreed to have blood samples taken for determination of his theophylline elimination rate before and after treatment of his hyperthyroidism.

The patient was instructed to continue taking aminophylline 400 mg orally every six hours to facilitate determination of the theophylline elimination rate. Two days before ^{131}I treatment, serial blood samples were obtained at 3, 6, 9, 12, 18, and 24 hours after the morning aminophylline dose, which was taken on an empty stomach (Table 2). Other scheduled aminophylline doses were withheld during this period. Serum theophylline concentrations were determined by high-performance liquid chromatography,[8] and the elimination rate constant was determined by log-linear regression (Figure 1).[9] The theophylline β-phase elimination half-life was subsequently calculated[9] (Table 1). The patient received sodium iodide I 131 solution on November 5, 1986, and was scheduled for a return visit to the clinic in three months. His aminophylline and albuterol therapy were continued and unchanged.

On return to the clinic on February 3, 1987, the patient complained of cold intolerance, muscle aches, and lethargy. His pulse rate was 60 beats/min and blood pressure was 120/80 mm Hg. His chest was clear, and the results of his cardiac evaluation were normal. The remainder of the physical examination revealed symptoms consistent with hypothyroidism. Thyroid function tests also indicated hypothyroidism (Table 1). The patient's diarrhea had initially improved but had returned with some cramping and nausea in the previous two weeks. His medications had remained unchanged and he had otherwise been well. Serial serum samples for reassessment of theophylline pharmacokinetic parameters were obtained as previously described (Table 2). Treatment with sodium levothyroxine 0.15 mg daily was initiated, and the patient was scheduled for a return visit in two months. Samples obtained during the February 3 clinic visit showed his estimated peak serum theophylline concentration to be in the toxic range (Table 2), and

CARY E. JOHNSON, PHARM.D., is Associate Professor of Pharmacy, The University of Michigan College of Pharmacy, and Clinical Pharmacist—Pediatrics, The University of Michigan Medical Center, Ann Arbor. IRA A. COHEN, PHARM.D., is Clinical Research Scientist, Parke-Davis Pharmaceutical Research Division, Warner-Lambert Company, Ann Arbor, and Clinical Associate Professor of Pharmacy, The University of Michigan College of Pharmacy; when this case report was prepared, he was Clinical Pharmacist in Oncology, St. Joseph Mercy Hospital, Catherine McAuley Health Center, Ann Arbor, and Clinical Associate Professor of Pharmacy, The University of Michigan College of Pharmacy.

Address reprint requests to Dr. Johnson at The University of Michigan College of Pharmacy, 428 Church Street, Ann Arbor, MI 48109-1065.

Copyright © 1988, American Society of Hospital Pharmacists, Inc. All rights reserved. 0278-2677/88/0801-0620$00.75.

Table 1.
Results of Thyroid and Theophylline Studies in a Patient with Hyperthyroidism before and after Treatment with Iodine 131[a]

Variable	Normal Range	Date of Study					
		10/15/86	11/3/86	2/3/87	2/10/87	4/7/87	4/10/87
Thyroid Studies							
Triiodothyronine uptake (%)	86–114	53				101	
Thyroxine (μg/dL)	4.4–11.6	13.9	17.4	<1.0		12.5	
Free thyroxine index	2.2–4.7	7.4					
^{131}I uptake (%/24 hr)	10–20		49.6				
Triiodothyronine (radioimmunoassay) (ng/dL)	90–190			39.0			
Thyroid-stimulating hormone (μU/mL)	<7.0		0.8	55.4		1.0	
Levothyroxine dosage (mg/24 hr)					0.15	0.15	0.15
Theophylline Studies							
Serum theophylline concentration (μg/mL)	8–20	16.8	15.2	30.9	16.1	6.4	13.9
Theophylline elimination rate constant (hr^{-1})			0.140	0.069	0.071	0.141	0.137
Theophylline terminal half-life (hr)			4.95	10.04	9.76	4.91	5.05
Aminophylline dosage (mg/24 hr)		1600	1600	1600	800	800	1600

[a] Sodium iodide I 131 solution administered on 11/5/86.

Figure 1. Semilogarithmic serum theophylline concentration versus time curve during β phase of elimination. (A) Hyperthyroid state: $y = 3.14 - 0.140x$; $R^2 = 0.9982$. (B) Hypothyroid state: $y = 3.61 - 0.069x$; $R^2 = 0.9955$. (C) Euthyroid state: $y = 2.28 - 0.141x$; $R^2 = 0.9995$.

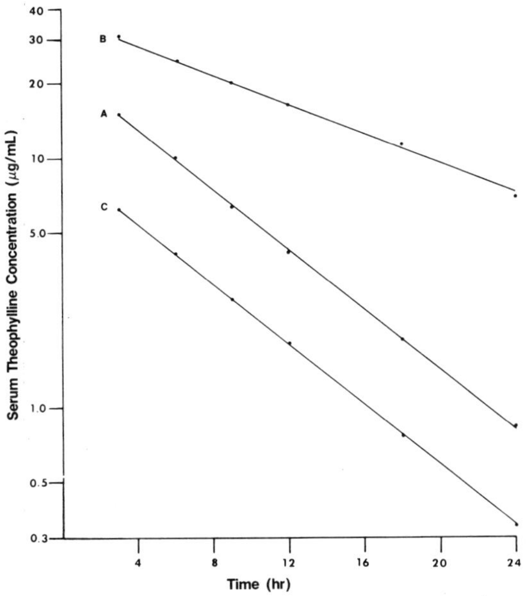

Table 2.
Patient's Serum Theophylline Concentrations (μg/mL) during Study Period

Time after Dose (hr)	Date				
	11/3/86	2/3/87	2/10/87	4/7/87	4/10/87
3	15.2	30.9	16.1	6.4	13.9
6	10.0	24.5	13.0	4.2	9.2
9	6.56	20.2	10.5	2.75	6.1
12	4.3	16.3	8.5	1.8	4.1
18	1.86	11.3	5.6	0.77	1.7
24	0.80	7.0	3.6	0.33	0.8

he was contacted and told not to take any aminophylline for 12 hours and to reduce his dosage to 200 mg orally every 6 hours. He returned to the clinic one week later, and his theophylline concentration and pharmacokinetic parameters were re-evaluated (Table 2). The nausea, cramping, and diarrhea had completely resolved, and the aminophylline dose was continued at 200 mg every six hours.

On a return visit April 7, the patient was clinically euthyroid; however, he complained of more frequent episodes of wheezing and shortness of breath. His estimated peak serum theophylline concentration was subtherapeutic, and the elimination rate constant had returned to the value determined before ^{131}I treatment (Tables 1 and 2). The previous aminophylline dosage of 400 mg orally every six hours was reinstituted, and the patient was asked to return to the clinic in three days for a final measurement of his theophylline elimination rate, which was determined to be unchanged (Tables 1 and 2). On return, the patient's medication was changed to sustained-release theophylline. Six months later, the patient remained clinically euthyroid with no gastrointestinal symptoms, and his asthma remained well controlled.

Discussion. Hyperthyroid patients who receive ^{131}I treatment frequently develop hypothyroidism. During the hypothyroid state these patients appear to be at risk for drug toxicity from theophylline and potentially from other drugs that are metabolized primarily by hepatic microsomal enzymes if the dosage received during the hyperthyroid state is not re-evaluated.[2,4–7] After replacement therapy with levothyroxine returns the patient to the euthyroid state, dosage adjustment may again be required. The magnitude of the theophylline half-life alterations caused by changing thyroid function did not appear to be dose dependent in this case (Table 1). It also appears that the linear relationship between percent change in serum thyroxine concentration and percent change in theophylline clearance reported by Vozeh et al.[1] plateaus as the thyroxine concentration increases beyond a certain value that may vary among individual patients; this requires further investigation.

Conclusion. Serum theophylline concentrations and potential symptoms of theophylline toxicity should be monitored closely during drug-induced alterations of thyroid function.

References

1. Vozeh S, Otten M, Staub JJ et al. Influence of thyroid function on theophylline kinetics. *Clin Pharmacol Ther.* 1984; 36:634–40.
2. Pokrajac M, Simic D, Varagic VM. Pharmacokinetics of theophylline in hyperthyroid and hypothyroid patients with chronic obstructive pulmonary disease. *Eur J Clin Pharmacol.* 1987; 33:483–6.
3. Bauman JH, Teichman S, Wible DA. Increased theophylline clearance in a patient with hyperthyroidism. *Ann Allergy.* 1984; 52:94–6.
4. Siefert CF, Covinsky JO, Hamburger S et al. Decreased theophylline clearance in a patient with severe hypothyroidism. *Drug Intell Clin Pharm.* 1987; 21:442–5.
5. Aderka D, Shavit G, Garfinkel D et al. Life-threatening theophylline intoxication in a hypothyroid patient. *Respiration.* 1983; 44:77–80.
6. Shenfield G. Influence of thyroid dysfunction on drug pharmacokinetics. *Clin Pharmacokinet.* 1981; 6:275–97.
7. Scott AK, Khir ASM, Bewsher PD et al. Oxazepam pharmacokinetics in thyroid disease. *Br J Clin Pharmacol.* 1984; 17:49–53.
8. Orcutt JJ, Kozak P, Gillman SA et al. Micro-scale method for theophylline in body fluids by reversed-phase, high-pressure liquid chromatography. *Clin Chem.* 1977; 23:599–601.
9. Winter ME, Katcher BS, Koda-Kimble MA. Basic clinical pharmacokinetics. San Francisco: Applied Therapeutics; 1980:36–8.

Use of fluconazole in a patient with documented malabsorption of ketoconazole

RICHARD H. DREW, JOHN R. PERFECT, AND HARRY A. GALLIS

Clin Pharm. 1988; 7:622–3

Ketoconazole is an orally administered imidazole agent with activity against a wide variety of fungal species. However, because of ketoconazole's dependency on an acidic environment for disintegration, dissolution, and absorption, serum concentrations may be reduced in some patients as a result of achlorhydria or concomitant administration of either antacids or histamine-H_2 antagonists (such as cimetidine or ranitidine).[1,2] This report describes a patient with documented impairment of ketoconazole absorption after oral administration who had favorable serum fluconazole concentrations after single-dose oral administration.

Case Report. A 39-year-old white woman with a clinical and microbiologic diagnosis of chronic mucocutaneous candidiasis of approximately 21 years' duration sought treatment for worsening mouth irritation, dysphagia, periodic vomiting, and vaginitis. Her medical history was otherwise notable only for pernicious anemia (with documented achlorhydria and gastrointestinal pH exceeding 8.0 on several occasions) and recurrent urinary-tract infections. Previous outpatient therapy for her fungal infection consisted mainly of nystatin-containing mouthwashes, nystatin vaginal suppositories, and oral oxycodone–acetaminophen for pain relief. However, the patient required hospitalization for intravenous amphotericin B therapy on several occasions because of severe oral, esophageal, and vaginal involvement. Although she had been receiving long-term suppressive therapy with ketoconazole for five to six years, her response was variable, with occasional exacerbations of disease. *Candida albicans* had been isolated while the patient was receiving ketoconazole doses of up to 600 mg. Coadministration of her dose with acidic beverages (e.g., carbonated cola beverages) failed to improve her clinical response.

Because of the patient's history of pernicious anemia and achlorhydria along with disease progression, her ability to absorb ketoconazole after oral administration was assessed. After one month of daily therapy with a single oral dose of ketoconazole 400 mg taken with approximately six ounces of a carbonated cola beverage, no ketoconazole could be detected in a serum sample obtained four hours after a dose (minimum detectable concentration 0.08 $\mu g/mL$ by the bioassay method described by Jorgensen et al.[3]). The test was repeated under similar conditions after a 600-mg dose was administered for one month and still failed to detect measurable ketoconazole levels. Ketoconazole therapy was discontinued, and the patient was placed on an investigational protocol to receive fluconazole 100 mg orally once daily.

Blood was obtained for measurement of the serum fluconazole concentration two hours after the seventh dose (approximately one week after ketoconazole therapy was discontinued). The concentration, determined by the bioassay technique,[3] was 3.1 $\mu g/mL$. The patient has been maintained on this dose. Although only moderate symptomatic improvement was demonstrated after one month of therapy, substantial reductions in dysphagia,

RICHARD H. DREW is Clinical Pharmacist; JOHN R. PERFECT, M.D., is Assistant Professor of Medicine; and HARRY A. GALLIS, M.D., is Associate Professor of Medicine, Division of Infectious Diseases, Department of Medicine, Duke University Medical Center, Durham, NC.

Address reprint requests to Mr. Drew at the Department of Medicine, Duke University Medical Center, Durham, NC 27710.

Copyright © 1988, American Society of Hospital Pharmacists, Inc. All rights reserved. 0278-2677/88/0801-0622$00.50.

oral mucosal lesions, and vaginitis occurred after two months.

Discussion. Absorption of ketoconazole after oral administration may be impaired in patients with elevated gastrointestinal pH values. Coadministration of dilute hydrochloric acid solutions has been proposed to enhance absorption of ketoconazole in such patients, but concomitant administration of 0.2 N hydrochloric acid solution to one patient via jejunostomy failed to achieve serum ketoconazole concentrations comparable to those of healthy volunteers.[4] Such data, however, must be interpreted in light of the known interpatient variability regarding absorption of ketoconazole.[5]

After oral administration of a single dose of fluconazole 100 mg to 10 healthy male volunteers, plasma concentrations reached a mean peak of 2.46 μg/mL (range 1.90–2.85 μg/mL) between 0.5 and 1.5 hours after administration (Pfizer, Inc., data on file; Peter Farrow, M.D., Pfizer, Inc., personal communication). Therefore, the serum fluconazole concentration obtained two hours after a dose in this patient (3.1 μg/mL) demonstrates that absorption was not impaired compared with that in healthy volunteers.

Fluconazole may provide effective oral antifungal therapy in patients whose absorption of ketoconazole is impaired. Based on initial evidence from this case and the different pKa values of fluconazole and ketoconazole (1.5 and 6.5, respectively), this would be especially true when such impairment is thought to be caused by an elevation in gastrointestinal pH. However, controlled clinical trials are needed that will define comparative absorptive profiles of these agents to account for potential influences such as rate of absorption, dosage formulation, concomitant medications, and disease states that may alter serum drug concentrations. Efficacy of fluconazole therapy in cases of chronic mucocutaneous candidiasis must be assessed over a longer period because of variability in this disease state over time.

Conclusion. Fluconazole appears to have provided effective oral antifungal therapy in a patient whose ability to absorb ketoconazole was impaired.

References

1. VanDerMeer JWM, Scheijground HW, Heykants J et al. The influence of gastric acidity on the bioavailability of ketoconazole. *J Antimicrob Chemother.* 1980; 6:552–4.
2. Carlson JA, Mann HJ, Canafax DM. Effect of pH on disintegration and dissolution of ketoconazole tablets. *Am J Hosp Pharm.* 1983; 40:1334–6.
3. Jorgensen JH, Alexander GA, Graybill JR et al. Sensitive bioassay for ketoconazole in serum and cerebrospinal fluid. *Antimicrob Agents Chemother.* 1981; 20:59–62.
4. Miyagawa CI. Hydrochloric acid given with ketoconazole through a jejunostomy tube. *Clin Pharm.* 1984; 3:205–7.
5. Brass C, Galgiani JN, Blaschke TF et al. Disposition of ketoconazole, an oral antifungal, in humans. *Antimicrob Agents Chemother.* 1982; 21:151–8.

“

Metabolic Effectiveness of Insulin

There is increasing evidence that the metabolic effectiveness of insulin may be a function not only of its absolute level but also of the rate of change in the level. Studies in patients with insulin-dependent diabetes have suggested that hepatic sensitivity to insulin may play a pivotal part in glucose metabolism, and that the liver is possibly more responsive to insulin pulses than to the steady-state level of insulin. Part of the difficulty of mimicking the normal process with standard insulin therapy may result from the inability to provide portal-vein levels of insulin and pulsatile patterns by means of peripheral administration of the agent. These ideas need further investigation and certainly have therapeutic implications.

—Cahill GF Jr. Beta-cell deficiency, insulin resistance, or both? *N Engl J Med.* 1988; 318:1268–9. Editorial.

”

CP Continuing Education

The ASHP Continuing Education system gives readers a self-assessment mechanism for selected articles in Clinical Pharmacy *and the* American Journal of Hospital Pharmacy. *It also allows readers to obtain continuing-education credit for these articles.*

For the purpose of CE-credit enrollment a blank answer sheet is published at the end of each installment of the column for the CE articles in that issue. An enrollee accumulates these answer sheets until the enrollment is submitted, using the form that is published in the June and December issues of Clinical Pharmacy *and in the June and December issues of the* American Journal of Hospital Pharmacy. *Any combination of tests within a 18-month period, from both* Clinical Pharmacy *and* American Journal of Hospital Pharmacy, *may be included in an enrollment. More complete details about enrollment in the system will appear in the semiannual enrollment form.*

Article 680-204-8813 (see page 582)
Qualifies for 1.0 hour of CE credit

Drug therapy of hypertensive crises

Learning Objectives

After studying this article, the reader should be able to

1. Differentiate between hypertensive emergencies and urgencies on the basis of clinical features and principles of management.
2. Describe the proposed pathogenesis and potential end-organ complications of hypertensive crises.
3. List the advantages and disadvantages of intravenous labetalol compared with the injectable antihypertensive agents traditionally used to treat hypertensive emergencies.
4. List the advantages and disadvantages of clonidine, calcium-channel blockers, angiotensin-converting enzyme inhibitors, and minoxidil in the therapy of hypertensive urgencies.

Self-assessment Questions

For each question there is one best answer only.

1. Hypertensive urgencies are characterized by
   a. Severe, acute end-organ damage.
   b. A blood pressure level that is lower than that seen in hypertensive emergencies.
   c. Papilledema and retinal hemorrhages.
   d. A high likelihood of renal, cardiovascular, and central nervous system complications if the blood pressure is not controlled.

2. The elevation of blood pressure in hypertensive crises is most likely the result of
   a. An increase in systemic vascular resistance resulting from the combined effects of chronic hypertension and increased levels of circulating catecholamines.
   b. Hypervolemia.
   c. Acute damage of the renal artery endothelium.
   d. The combined effects of hypervolemia and chronic hypertension.

3. In the treatment of hypertensive emergencies, the initial goal of therapy is
   a. A diastolic blood pressure of 90–100 mm Hg.
   b. A diastolic blood pressure of 100–110 mm Hg.
   c. A systolic blood pressure of 110–120 mm Hg.
   d. A systolic blood pressure of 120–130 mm Hg.

4. The treatment of choice for hypertensive emergencies is
   a. Intravenous bolus doses of furosemide.
   b. Intravenous infusion of sodium nitroprusside.
   c. Diazoxide given by a series of short continuous intravenous infusions.
   d. Reinstitution of the patient's usual antihypertensive regimen.

5. The primary indication for use of trimethaphan camsylate in the treatment of hypertensive emergencies is in patients who have
   a. Renal insufficiency.
   b. Dissecting aortic aneurysm.
   c. Angina.
   d. Acute myocardial infarction.

6. Compared with sodium nitroprusside, labetalol
   a. Is more likely to cause reflex tachycardia and redistribution of coronary blood flow in patients with coronary-artery disease.
   b. May be better tolerated by patients with hepatic insufficiency.
   c. Has the advantage of precise, predictable conversion from the intravenous to the oral dosage form.
   d. May be better tolerated by patients who have congestive heart failure.

7. Which one of the following properties of antihypertensive agents is not desirable in a drug used in the treatment of hypertensive urgencies?
   a. Rapid onset of action.
   b. Lack of central nervous system adverse effects.
   c. Available as an oral formulation.
   d. Consistent hypotensive effects.
   e. Prolonged duration of action.

8. Oral antihypertensive agents that can be used alone in treating hypertensive urgencies include
   a. Clonidine, lisinopril, and captopril.
   b. Nifedipine, clonidine, and enalapril.
   c. Nifedipine, enalapril, and minoxidil.
   d. Nifedipine, clonidine, and captopril.

9. In the treatment of hypertensive urgencies, nifedipine
   a. Has a more rapid onset of action if it is administered orally than if it is given sublingually.
   b. Is effective in approximately 50% of cases.
   c. Consistently lowers arterial blood pressure and may increase cerebral blood flow.
   d. Produces maximal antihypertensive effects more rapidly after buccal administration than after oral administration.

10. The oral loading-dose regimens of clonidine that are used to treat hypertensive urgencies
   a. Facilitate dosage titration.
   b. Allow for accurate prediction of a maintenance dose of clonidine.
   c. Are effective in 75–80% of patients.
   d. Typically have an onset of action of 15 to 30 minutes.

Answer sheet

August 1988 ***Clinical Pharmacy***

Note: An enrollment form for the ASHP Continuing-Education System appears in the June and December issues. Please accumulate all the answer sheets you wish to use in one enrollment and submit them at one time with a completed enrollment form.

Place an X in the box(es) at the top of the column(s) corresponding to the test(s) you are taking. Darken the boxes corresponding to the correct answers.

☐
680-204-8813
1.0 hour

	a b c d		a b c d e
1.	☐☐☐☐	6.	☐☐☐☐
2.	☐☐☐☐	7.	☐☐☐☐☐
3.	☐☐☐☐	8.	☐☐☐☐
4.	☐☐☐☐	9.	☐☐☐☐
5.	☐☐☐☐	10.	☐☐☐☐

ASHP Use Only
(1.0)8813_______(3)

Enhance your clinical practice skills and earn CE credit with a new self-study course from ASHP

Concepts in Clinical Pharmacokinetics

A Self-Instructional Course

Written by a trio of pharmacy professors, this book provides an orientation to pharmacokinetic concepts and procedures. It can help prepare you for pharmacokinetics courses of instruction, or serve as a handy reference and refresher course. With it you can earn up to 20 hours of ACPE-approved continuing education credit.

Input topics include:
- therapeutic drug monitoring
- compartmental models
- clearance
- volume of distribution
- loading dose
- elimination rate constant

Order your copy today!

The American Society of Hospital Pharmacists is approved by the American Council on Pharmaceutical Education as a provider of continuing pharmaceutical education.

Order Form

Concepts in Clinical Pharmacokinetics: A Self-Instructional Course (P275); 1988; approx. 150 pp; $50.00

☐ Please send me _____ copies of **Concepts in Clinical Pharmacokinetics: A Self-Instructional Course** (P275) at $50.00 each; 1988; 140 pp.

☐ Enclosed is my check for $__________. (Checks must be drawn on a U.S. bank and made payable to ASHP.)

☐ Enclosed is our purchase order #__________; please issue an invoice and add postage and handling.

Charge $__________ to my ☐ VISA ☐ MasterCard

Account #____________________

Exp. ________ *month/year* Signature ________________

Name ____________________

Institution ____________________

Address ____________________

City ____________ State ____ Zip ________

ASHP ID #____________________

Send to: ASHP Publications Records Dept.
4630 Montgomery Avenue
Bethesda, MD 20814

Payments to ASHP are not deductible as charitable contributions for Federal Income Tax purposes. However, they may be deductible under other provisions of the Internal Revenue Code.

© 1988 American Society of Hospital Pharmacists

For accurate and up-to-date information on injectable drug products, health professionals reach for . . .

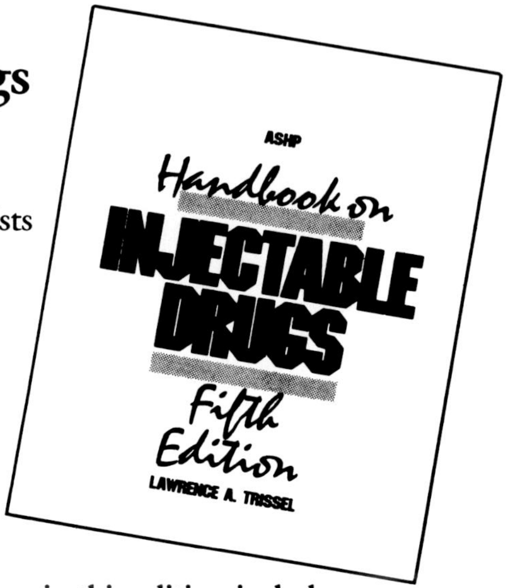

The Handbook on Injectable Drugs Fifth Edition

by Lawrence A. Trissel
Published by the American Society of Hospital Pharmacists

The most respected reference on stability and compatibility of injectable drug products, the *Handbook on Injectable Drugs* features 240 commercial drugs used in admixtures, plus information on investigational drugs.

Monographs in this volume are:

- completely revised to cover product, stability and compatibility information, as well as greatly expanded sections on dosage and administration
- presented in a standardized format, with easy-to-use compatibility tables
- extensively referenced to the primary literature, with cross-indexing among monographs.

New drugs in this edition include:

- Aztreonam
- Ceftazidime
- Imipenem-Cilastatin Sodium
- Pentamidine Isethionate

Order your copy today.

Order Form

Please send me: ________ copies of the *Handbook on Injectable Drugs* (P276) at $60.00 each.

☐ Enclosed is my check for $ ________ . (Checks must be drawn on a U.S. bank and made payable to ASHP.)

☐ Enclosed is our purchase order # ________ ; please issue an invoice and add postage and handling.

OR: Charge to ☐ Visa ☐ MasterCard

Account # ________________ Exp. ____________

Signature ______________________________

Send to: **ASHP Publications Records Dept.**
4630 Montgomery Avenue
Bethesda, MD 20814

The *Handbook on Injectable Drugs*, Fifth Edition; hardbound; 758 pages; $60.00

Name ______________________________

Institution ______________________________

Address ______________________________

City ______________________________

State ____________________ Zip ____________

ASHP I.D. # ______________________________

ASHP is a trademark of the American Society of Hospital Pharmacists, Inc.; Registered in the U.S. Patent and Trademark Office.

Payments to ASHP are not deductible as charitable contributions for Federal Income Tax purposes. However, they may be deductible under other provisions of the Internal Revenue Code.

Current Literature

Drug Reaction Alerts

Drug Reaction Alerts focuses primarily on serious, unlabeled reactions to new chemical entities. The citations are compiled monthly from International Pharmaceutical Abstracts, *which covers over 700 journals. An address for reprints (when available) follows the name of the corresponding author in each citation.*

Antilipemic Agents

Arellano F (Department of Clinical Pharmacology, Hospital Marques de Valdecilla, 39008 Santander, Spain), DeCos MA, Valiente R et al. **Gemfibrozil** induced headache. *Lancet.* 1988; 1:705. Case. (46-year-old woman with hypercholesterolemia; received gemfibrozil 600 mg twice daily; developed frontotemporal headache accompanied by dry mouth 30–90 minutes after ingestion of gemfibrozil; headache easily relieved by analgesics until gemfibrozil discontinued)

Antineoplastic Agents

Ascher DP (Department of Pharmacy, Regional Medical Center, Clark Air Force Base, Philippines), Delaney RA. Acute dystonia from **etoposide.** *Drug Intell Clin Pharm.* 1988; 22:41–2. Case. (11-year-old boy with acute lymphoblastic leukemia relapse; received etoposide 250 mg/sq m alternated weekly with cytarabine as maintenance therapy; developed dystonic facial reactions during etoposide infusion on 54th week of therapy; dystonic reactions resolved promptly with administration of diphenhydramine 25 mg i.v.; positive rechallenge on week 56; premedication with diphenhydramine during subsequent courses of etoposide resulted in cessation of reaction)

Antivirals

Harris PJ (1759 Que Street, N.W., Washington, DC 20009), Caceres CA. **Azidothymidine** in the treatment of AIDS. *N Engl J Med.* 1988; 318:250. Case. (43-year-old man with antibodies to human immunodeficiency virus; received zidovudine 200 mg every four hours; developed grand mal epileptic seizures; patient also experienced nausea, diarrhea, diffuse headache, myalgia, and insomnia; positive rechallenge with decrease in zidovudine dosage to 100 mg every four hours while receiving nearly therapeutic concentrations of phenytoin sodium; seizures, nausea, diarrhea, and headaches resolved upon discontinuation of zidovudine)

Anti-inflammatory Agents

Turner M, Laitt R. (Department of Surgery, Hope Hospital, Salford M6 8HD, England). **Benzydamine** oral rinse and rash. *Br Med J.* 1988; 296:1071. Case. (21-year-old man with mouth ulcer; received benzydamine hydrochloride 10 mL four times daily for three days; concomitant ranitidine; developed generalized dermatitis attributed to either benzydamine or one of the dyes in solution; resolution of rash 48 hours after withdrawal of benzydamine)

Benzodiazepine Antagonists

Short TG, Maling T, Galletly DC (Department of Anesthesia, Wellington School of Medicine, Wellington, New Zealand). Ventricular arrhythmia precipitated by **flumazenil.** *Br Med J.* 1988; 296:1070–1. Case. (30-year-old woman; received flumazenil 0.5 mg by i.v. injection to antagonize oxazepam overdose; concomitant chloral hydrate; developed ventricular tachycardia; no response after two i.v. bolus doses of lidocaine 50 mg; arrhythmia settled slowly after 20 minutes)

Central Nervous System Stimulants

Trugman JM (Department of Neurology, University of Virginia Medical Center, Charlottesville, VA 22908). Cerebral arteritis and oral **methylphenidate.** *Lancet.* 1988; 1:584–5. Case. (12-year-old boy with attention deficit disorder and hyperactivity; received methylphenidate 10 mg orally for seven years; developed cerebral arteritis and infarction; recovery upon drug withdrawal with some residual paralysis)

Drug Interactions

Tilkemeier P, Thompson PD (Miriam Hospital, Providence, RI 02906). Acute pancreatitis possibly related to **enalapril.** *N Engl J Med.* 1988; 318:1275–6. Case. (69-year-old man; received two doses of enalapril 5 mg; developed pancreatitis; symptoms occurred shortly after ingestion of second dose along with **ethanol** contained in one bottle of beer; resolution of symptoms upon withdrawal of enalapril)

Drugs, Adverse Reactions

Black RJ, Dawson TA (Department of Dermatology, Craigavon, Craigavon Area Hospital, Craigavon BT63 5QQ, Northern Ireland). **Erythromycin** and nightmares. *Br Med J.* 1988; 296:1070. Case. (21-year-old woman with acne; received erythromycin 250 mg once daily for one month; developed nightmares; nightmares stopped after drug withdrawal)

Marini JC (Human Genetics Branch/NICHD, Building 10, Room 8C-429, 9000 Rockville Pike, Bethesda, MD 20892), Hill S, Zasloff MA. Dense metaphyseal bands and growth arrest associated with **isotretinoin** therapy. *Am J Dis Child.* 1988; 142:316–8. Case. (9-year-old boy with fibrodysplasia ossificans progressiva; received isotretinoin 5 mg/kg/day for five months; developed dense metaphyseal bands and growth arrest; metaphyseal bands decreased gradually and clinical growth resumed after isotretinoin discontinuation)

Vexiau P (Hospital Saint Louis, 75475 Paris, France), Gourmel B, Julien R et al. Severe acne-like lesions caused by **amineptine** overdose. *Lancet.* 1988; 1:585. Cases. (five women, aged 27–62 years; received self-administered overdoses of amineptine aminoheptanoic acid 200–1000 mg/day for up to 36 months; developed severe acne-like lesions; no improvement after therapy with isotretinon 0.5 mg/kg/day for 6–18 weeks while amineptine therapy continued; withdrawal of amineptine led to slight improvement in some patients and complete recovery in one patient)

Gastrointestinal Drugs

Haboubi N (Alastair Fraser and John Squire, Clinical Investigation Unit, E. Birmingham Hospital, Birmingham B9 5ST, England), Asquith P. Rash mediated by immune complexes associated with **ranitidine.** *Br Med J.* 1988; 296:896. Case. (three men with duodenal ulcers, aged 60–79 years; received ranitidine 150 mg twice daily for two to four weeks; developed vasculitic skin diseases; resolution upon drug withdrawal)

Sulfonamides

Hoo JJ (University of Illinois, Chicago, IL 60612), Hadro TA, Von Behren P. Possible teratogenicity of **sulfasalazine.** *N Engl J Med.* 1988; 318:1128. Case. (male infant born with ventricular septal defect and coarctation of the aorta; mother received sulfasalazine 500 mg three times daily throughout pregnancy; defects gradually resolved and did not require surgical intervention)

Book Reviews

Psychotropic Drug Handbook, 5th Edition

By Paul J. Perry, Bruce Alexander, and Barry I. Liskow. Published by Harvey Whitney Books, 4906 Cooper Rd., P.O. Box 42696, Cincinnati, OH 45242, 1988. vi + 346 p. Price $15.00.

I approached my review of this book in two ways: first as a specialist in psychiatric pharmacy to assess the accuracy of the information, and, second from the perspective of a general pharmacy practitioner to assess the handbook's usefulness. For the latter purpose, I placed the book on my desk for one month and used it for every question that was referred to me at my hospital.

The handbook is pocket-sized and spiral bound. The book is divided into 14 chapters and concludes with patient-information sheets for each drug category covered in the book. As would be expected, there are chapters on antipsychotics, antidepressants, anxiolytics, hypnotics, and the drugs used in treating extrapyramidal adverse effects. Additional chapters cover disulfiram, drug interactions, management and treatment of drug overdose, management of drug withdrawal, the amobarbital interview, and electroconvulsive therapy. The chapters on drug categories are divided into the following sections: indications, efficacy, mechanism of action, dosage, pharmacokinetics, adverse effects, principles of rational prescribing, product listings (drug, dosage form, dosage range, and cost), and references.

The use of bold-face headings and key words has made this edition more useful as a quick reference than as a textbook. The advantages of this edition over previous editions are updated information, a darker and more readable type style, and more referencing. The indexing, however, is not as handy as the authors describe, because drugs alone are indexed. For instance, lithium augmentation of antidepressant therapy is found in the antidepressant chapter, is not discussed at all in the antimanic drug chapter, and is not found in the index. The use of triiodothyronine as an adjunct antidepressant agent is also not found in the index.

The authors continue to rely on review articles and textbooks as references, instead of using original research reports. The pharmacokinetics of antipsychotics, antidepressants, and lithium are covered extensively, and some of the sections are designed to be helpful in the choice of dosing regimens. "Newer" drugs, such as carbamazepine, L-tryptophan, and buspirone, are included.

The chapter on antipsychotics attempts to rationally discuss the empiric nature of drug dosing of antipsychotics. The authors ignore the standard dosage conversions from oral to depot fluphenazine. The discussion of antipsychotic adverse effects, especially in management, is excellent. There is no discussion of clozapine (Clozaril), an antipsychotic that reportedly does not cause tardive dyskinesia and may be approved and marketed during the lifetime of this edition. The section on neuroleptic malignant syndrome needs greater depth, specifically in regard to which symptoms may benefit from drug therapy. The section on neurological adverse effects of antipsychotics is very good; however, it lacks any discussion of drug therapy proposed for tardive dyskinesia.

The chapter on antidepressants does not contain any information on fluoxetine (Prozac), an antidepressant that has been marketed since early this year. This is an unfortunate and ironic exclusion, because the fourth edition contained information on bupropion, an antidepressant that was close to being approved but subsequently was not approved.

The drug interaction chapter uses the categories established in the standard textbooks on the subject and is very complete. It lacks any mention of the carbamazepine–antipsychotic interaction, first described in 1980. The treatment of drug overdose is covered in a separate chapter to facilitate inclusion of basic overdose management principles. Overdose with the standard psychotropics and with some common drugs of abuse is adequately discussed.

The disadvantages of this handbook are many. The authors focus on approved indications for drugs instead of the more commonly used target-symptom approach. There are no sections on child, adolescent, or geriatric psychopharmacology, including the treatment of dementia. There is no information on the use of stimulants. Very few alternative indications for psychotropic drugs, which are not specifically on the FDA-approved labeling, are discussed. Other notable omissions are the treatment of aggression (with carbamazepine or propranolol) and the use of verapamil in bipolar disorder. There is little mention of possible combination regimens for unresponsive schizophrenics or unipolar or bipolar disorder patients. There is not much discussion of controversies, such as the never ending debate on anticholingeric prophylaxis of acute extrapyramidal side effects. Broader discussions of teratogenicity with psychiatric drugs should be essential, but what is discussed is brief and cursory.

The authors do not use diagnostic criteria from *Diagnostic and Statistical Manual of Mental Disorders, 3rd Edition-Revised* (*DSM-III-R*) in their discussions. *DSM-III-R* is considered the "bible" of psychiatric diagnosis and has been used since mid-1987. However, it was probably not included because of the delay between the time the handbook was written and the time it was published.

I can remember when I, as a recently trained pharmacist, needed quick answers to questions about psychiatric pharmacotherapy. For the most part, with some familiarization with the layout, this book can be used to answer the majority of questions about psychiatry.

Very few references adequately summarize rational psychiatric pharmacotherapy. Other references of this nature have typically been plagued with authors' opinions and have lacked referencing. The handbook is recommended as a good general reference for psychiatric pharmacotherapy. It should appeal most to pharmacy practitioners who serve psychiatric patients. Unfortunately, it covers only the standard uses of psychotropic drugs. Because psychiatry is often subjective, a handbook with a conservative stance is helpful to those without much background in the field. General principles of psychiatric pharmacotherapy are emphasized and rational prescribing is summarized at the end of each chapter. I would recommend that the *Psychotropic Drug Handbook* be included in drug information libraries.

For those who may be searching for a general psychiatric pharmacotherapy reference, I hope that this review does not discourage you from purchasing the book. The handbook is very inexpensive, and I have yet to see another that fulfills this book's purpose.

Reviewed by Peter G. Dorson, Pharm.D., Clinical Pharmacology Service, Austin State Hospital and College of Pharmacy, The University of Texas, Austin, TX 78712.

Manual of Antibiotics and Infectious Diseases, Sixth Edition

Edited by John E. Conte, Jr., and Steven L. Barriere.

Published by Lea & Febiger, 600 Washington Square, Philadelphia, PA 19106-4198, 1988. xvi + 392 p. Price $19.50 U.S., $26.00 Canada.

Manual of Antibiotics and Infectious Diseases was designed and published for students, house staff, practicing physicians, and other health-care professionals involved in the day-to-day care of patients with infectious diseases.

Contrary to what the authors state, this edition has been divided into seven sections, not eight: (1) antibiotics, (2) empiric antibiotic therapy, (3) therapy of established infection, (4) antibiotic susceptibilities, (5) prophylactic antibiotics, (6) availability and clinical use of immunobiologic agents and antiparasitic drugs, and (7) treatment guidelines for sexually transmitted diseases. A well-organized index is included.

On the technical side, the book contains only a few spelling errors, as would be expected of a book that has been through several editions. The book reads quite well and is easy to comprehend. In the section on empiric antibiotic therapy, the authors list the antibiotics of choice for various infections in penicillin-allergic patients but do not state the type of penicillin allergy in question and substitute vancomycin for the penicillin in each case. It should be noted that only Type I (immediate-type) allergic reactions are contraindications for cephalosporins, while in other types of reactions cephalosporins can be used with caution. There is an error on page 97, which is repeated on page 111, regarding the treatment of prosthetic valve endocarditis; the drugs of choice for empiric treatment of prosthetic valve endocarditis are vancomycin with an aminoglycoside, not peni-

Continued on page 630

When you're trying to document the cost-effectiveness of pharmaceutical services, it helps to know what others have done. Now you can, with the

Resource Book on Progressive Pharmaceutical Services

Published by ASHP

Whether your pharmacy is introducing new clinical services or expanding existing ones, the *Resource Book* directs you to the literature describing what's been accomplished, in terms of implementing and evaluating progressive pharmaceutical services.

The book's first section lists and organizes articles according to pharmacy practice area. The second section features abstracts on all of the literature listed.

The ***Resource Book*** can help you make more efficient use of your pharmacy department's resources. **Order today!**

Order Form

Please send me ____ copies of the *Resource Book* at $15.00 each. 110 pp: softbound

☐ Enclosed is my check for $ ________.

☐ Enclosed is our purchase order # ________; please issue an invoice and add postage and handling.

Charge $ ________ to my
☐ MasterCard ☐ VISA
(minimum charge of $25 required)

Account # ____________________

Exp. ________ Signature ____________________
(month/year)

Name ____________________

Institution ____________________

Address ____________________

City ____________ State ____ Zip ________

ASHP ID# ____________________

Send to: ASHP Publications Records Dept.
4630 Montgomery Avenue
Bethesda, MD 20814

Payments to ASHP are not deductible as charitable contributions for Federal Income Tax purposes. However, they may be deductible under other provisions of the Internal Revenue Code.

Continued from page 629

cillin G with nafcillin and gentamicin. In addition, the treatment of choice for documented methicillin-resistant *Staph. epidermidis* prosthetic-valve infection is vancomycin with an aminoglycoside and rifampin, not vancomycin and rifampin alone. In several sections of the book the authors suggest rather low dosing of pencillin G for serious infections. For example, on page 110, the antibiotics of choice for documented acute bacterial endocarditis caused by *Strep. faecalis* are stated to be penicillin G and gentamicin, and the recommended daily dosage of penicillin G is only 12 million units. Finally, throughout the book (e.g., pages 110, 120, 121, 156) gentamicin and tobramycin are used interchangeably as aminoglycosides of choice, without regard as to which one should be given preference in various conditions.

In comparison with the fifth edition, the style of the book has changed. The authors have attempted, and succeeded, in making the book easier to read (especially sections six and seven). The organization of the book has changed slightly, with the incorporation of the fifth edition's section on viral hepatitis into the sixth edition's section on availability and clinical use of immunobiologic agents and antiparasitic drugs. The section on antibiotics has been updated with the additions of cefotetan, clavulanic acid, imipenem–cilastatin, and the quinolones and the deletion of cefmenoxime. The sections on empiric antibiotic therapy and therapy of established infection have been updated, with second- and third-generation cephalosporins replacing (for certain infections) previously recommended combination therapy or more toxic aminoglycoside therapy. The section on antibiotic susceptibilities has been updated with more extensive and detailed susceptibility criteria for various antibiotics and a table displaying the antimicrobial activity of several quinolones. The section on prophylactic antibiotics remains essentially unchanged, except that malaria chemoprophylaxis has been updated and moved to the section on availability and clinical use of immunobiologic agents and antiparasitic drugs, which has been changed considerably. The sections on pneumococcal vaccine and varicella-zoster immune globulin have been completely revised; that on zoster immune plasma has been deleted. The section on viral hepatitis has been revised and information on delta hepatitis and non-A, non-B hepatitis has been included. The treatment guidelines for sexually transmitted diseases have been greatly expanded and acquired immunodeficiency syndrome (AIDS) has been added.

The strength of the book is that it is easy to read and understand. Information on various aspects of antibiotics and infectious diseases can be located quickly. The section on antibiotic susceptibilities is put together well, displaying several tables with minimum inhibitory concentrations for various bacteria when tested against most of the commonly used antimicrobials. The section entitled "Immunobiologic Agents and Antiparasitic Drugs," which deals mainly with vaccines, is excellent and well referenced.

The book does have several weaknesses. There is no section that discusses the treatment of tuberculosis, and several of the new antitubercular agents are not mentioned (e.g., clofazimine, ansamycin). The section on fungal infections and antifungal agents needs to be expanded. The AIDS section needs to be completely revised to include information on zidovudine and treatment of the various opportunistic infections. Finally, with the exception of the section on vaccines, several sections are poorly referenced, and some of the references are out of date.

I believe that this book is a valuable reference for drug information centers that answer a variety of questions on the subjects of antibiotics and treatment of infectious diseases. It is also a valuable reference for students who possess a limited knowledge of these subjects. As far as house staff, practicing physicians, and clinical pharmacists involved in patient care are concerned, I believe that the book offers little extra when compared with Sanford's *Guide to Antimicrobial Therapy*—except for added bulk.

Reviewed by George G. Zhanel, Pharm.D., Faculty of Pharmacy, University of Manitoba, Winnipeg, Manitoba, Canada R3T 2N2.

Books Received

Books are listed as soon as received; selected books may be reviewed in Book Reviews in subsequent issues.

Annual Reports in Medicinal Chemistry, Volume 22, Denis M. Bailey, Editor-in-Chief. Published by Academic Press, Inc., Orlando, FL 32887, 1987. xiii + 384 p. Price $55.

Drugs for Children. Published by the World Health Organization Regional Office for Europe, Copenhagen, Denmark, 1987. Available from WHO Publications Center USA, 49 Sheridan Ave., Albany, NY 12210. xi + 185 p. Price Sw.fr.30.

A Primer of Drug Action, Fifth Edition, by Robert M. Julien. Published by W. H. Freeman and Company, 41 Madison Ave., New York, NY 10010, 1988. xiv + 364 p. Price $24.95 (cloth), $14.95 (paper).

Advertising Index

American Society of Hospital Pharmacists
Concepts in Clinical Pharmacokinetics, 625
Consumer Drug Digest, 564
Handbook on Injectable Drugs, Fifth Edition, 626
Resource Book on Progressive Pharmaceutical Services, 629
Baxter Healthcare Corporation, MultiPlex Systems Division
MultiPlex Fluid Management System, 571, 573
Lederle Laboratories, A Division of American Cyanamid Company
Clindamycin Phosphate, 561
Eli Lilly and Company
Tazidime, 565–566
Partnership for a Drug-Free America
Institutional, 569
Roxane Laboratories, A Boehringer Ingelheim Company
Intensols, 559
State University of New York at Buffalo
Position Available, 564
Stuart Pharmaceuticals, Division of ICI Americas, Inc.
Cefotan, inside back cover, outside back cover
University of Washington
Position Available, 572
The Upjohn Company
Cleocin Phosphate, 567–568
Wyeth Laboratories
Tubex, inside front cover

Reduce the multiple problems of skin antigen testing...

to one simple, standardized test.

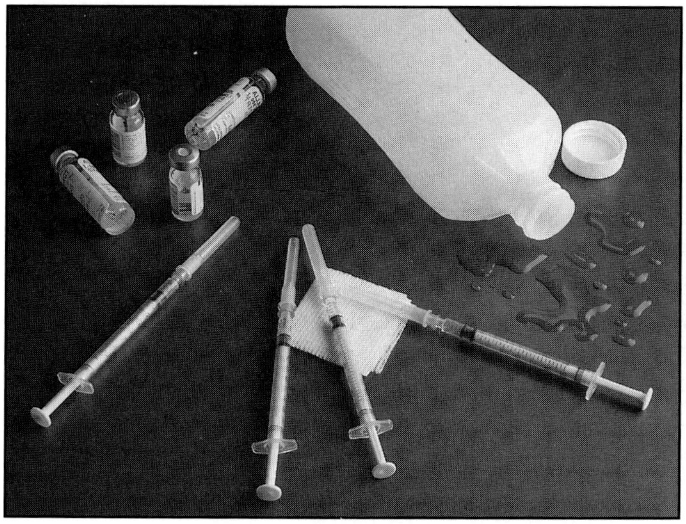

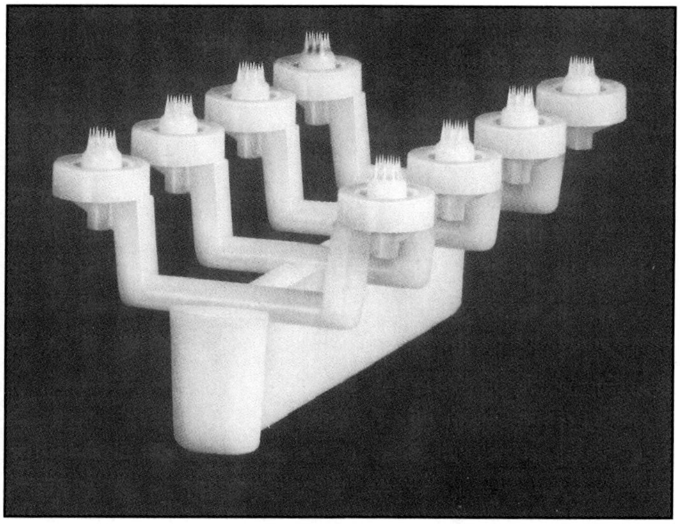

Multitest® CMI™

(skin test antigens for cellular hypersensitivity)

For improved accuracy...

Sensitive, standardized, reproducible.

For greater convenience, comfort and economy.

Seven antigens and one control on one easy-to-apply multipuncture test.

Distributed by
MERIEUX INSTITUTE, INC.
P.O. Box 52-3980
Miami, Florida 33152-3980

Manufactured by
INSTITUT MERIEUX
Lyon—France
U.S. Lic. No. 384

For more information, write or call:
Toll-free: **800-327-2842** In Florida, Alaska or Hawaii, call collect: **305-593-9577**

© 1987, Merieux Institute, Inc.

BRIEF SUMMARY

DESCRIPTION
Skin Test Antigens for Cellular Hypersensitivity, MULTITEST® CMI™ is a disposable plastic applicator consisting of eight sterile test heads preloaded with the following seven delayed hypersensitivity skin test antigens and glycerin negative control for percutaneous administration: Tetanus Toxoid Antigen, Diphtheria Toxoid Antigen, Streptococcus Antigen, Old Tuberculin, Candida Antigen, Trichophyton Antigen, and Proteus Antigen.

INDICATIONS
For detection of anergy (nonresponsiveness to antigens) by means of delayed hypersensitivity skin testing.

CONTRAINDICATIONS
Do not apply at sites involving acneiform, infected or inflamed skin. Although severe systemic reactions to diphtheria and tetanus antigens are rare, persons known to have a history of systemic reactions should be tested with MULTITEST® CMI™ only after the test heads containing these antigens have been removed.

PRECAUTIONS

General:
Discard the MULTITEST® CMI™ applicator after use. DO NOT REUSE. The sterility of MULTITEST® CMI™ is guaranteed only when the seals on the individual test heads are intact. Do not attempt to resterilize the applicator as this may result in transmission of hepatitis and/or other infections.
If periodic testing is done more frequently than every two months, then the test sites should be rotated so that retesting is not conducted at the same site sooner than two months.

Reactivity to delayed hypersensitivity skin test antigens may decrease or disappear temporarily as a result of: febrile illness; measles and other viral infections; live virus vaccination including measles, mumps, rubella, and poliomyelitis vaccines.
Individuals may acquire skin testing sensitivity resulting from either immunization or infection.
Epinephrine should be available in case of severe reactions.

Information for patients:
Patients should be informed of the types of test site reactions that may be expected.

Drug/Drug Interactions:
It is possible to observe loss of reactivity in patients undergoing treatment with drugs or procedures that suppress immunity such as: corticosteroids, chemotherapeutic agents, antilymphocyte globulin, and irradiation.

Drug/Laboratory Test Interactions:
The effect of repeated skin testing on specific antibody levels is not yet known, consequently those doing *in vitro* testing must be cognizant of the fact that repeated skin testing may alter antibody levels.

Pregnancy Category C:
Animal reproduction studies have not been conducted with MULTITEST® CMI™ It is also not known whether MULTITEST® CMI™ can cause fetal harm when administered to a pregnant woman or can affect reproduction capacity. MULTITEST® CMI™ should be given to a pregnant woman only if clearly needed.

ADVERSE REACTIONS
Vesiculation, ulceration, or necrosis may occur in highly sensitive subjects at the test site. Pain or pruritus at the test site may be relieved by topical glucocorticoids or ice pack.

News

Pediatrics academy issues recommendations on use of *Haemophilus influenzae* type b conjugate vaccine

Recommendations for the use of *Haemophilus influenzae* type b conjugate vaccine have been issued by the Committee on Infectious Diseases of the American Academy of Pediatrics.[1] The vaccine, a conjugate of the capsular polysaccharide of *H. influenzae* type b and diphtheria toxoid, is the result of efforts to develop a vaccine that would be more immunogenic than the polysaccharide vaccines. A conjugate vaccine (ProHIBiT, Connaught Laboratories, Inc.) was licensed by FDA in December 1987.

The committee's recommendations are as follows:

- All children should receive a single dose of the conjugate vaccine at 18 months of age; special efforts to immunize children, such as those in day care, who are at high risk of acquiring invasive *H. influenzae* type b disease are warranted.
- Children who received a dose of polysaccharide vaccine at 18–23 months of age should receive a single dose of the conjugate vaccine; the two vaccine doses should be separated by at least two months.
- Children 19–23 months of age who have not been immunized against *H. influenzae* type b disease should receive one dose of the conjugate vaccine.
- Immunization against *H. influenzae* type b disease is recommended for children up to 60 months of age. Children between 24 and 60 months of age who have not been immunized should receive one of the vaccines; the conjugate vaccine is preferred, but either vaccine is acceptable.
- Children who were at least 24 months old when they received a dose of polysaccharide vaccine do not need to be immunized with the conjugate vaccine.
- Children who had invasive *H. influenzae* type b disease before they were 24 months old should receive a dose of the conjugate vaccine because the disease may not have left them immune. If the child was older when the disease occurred, a disease-induced immune response is more likely, and vaccine administration is not necessary.
- The conjugate vaccine may be administered simultaneously (at separate sites) with either diphtheria and tetanus toxoids and pertussis vaccine adsorbed (DTP) or polio vaccine inactivated (IPV).
- A booster dose of the conjugate vaccine is not currently recommended.
- The conjugate vaccine is not a substitute for diphtheria immunization.
- Rifampin prophylaxis is recommended for all appropriate contacts of individuals with invasive *H. influenzae* type b disease regardless of immunization status. Appropriate contacts include household contacts and others who spent at least four hours with the index patient for at least five of the seven days before the patient's hospitalization.
- The conjugate vaccine is also indicated for children five years of age or older who have chronic diseases that place them at increased risk for *H. influenzae* type b disease. Included are children with sickle-cell disease and anatomic or functional asplenia and those who have undergone splenectomy. Patients with Hodgkin's disease should be immunized in the manner recommended for the polysaccharide vaccine—at least 10–14 days before initiation of antineoplastic-drug therapy or, if this is not possible, at least three months after therapy.
- Protection cannot be expected for the first one to two weeks after administration of the conjugate vaccine. Serious adverse reactions and cases of invasive disease occurring at any time after vaccine administration should be reported to state and local health departments, the vaccine manufacturer, FDA, or the Centers for Disease Control.
- Although preliminary data suggest that conjugate vaccines may be effective in children younger than 18 months of age, use of the vaccine in children less than 18 months old is not currently recommended.

1. Committee on Infectious Diseases. *Haemophilus influenzae* type b conjugate vaccine. *Pediatrics.* 1988; 81:908–11.

Study finds similar reperfusion rates with intravenous APSAC and intracoronary streptokinase in acute myocardial infarction

Early intravenous administration of anisoylated plasminogen–streptokinase activator complex (APSAC, Beecham Pharmaceuticals) may be as effective as intracoronary infusion of streptokinase in achieving reperfusion after acute myocardial infarction, according to results of a randomized multicenter trial.[1]

A total of 240 patients met all clinical, angiographic, and electrocardiographic criteria and were randomized to treatment with APSAC (123 patients) or streptokinase (117 patients). All patients had grade 0 or 1 coronary occlusion (based on the criteria used in the Thrombolysis in Myocardial Infarction trial). APSAC 30 units was administered intravenously over two to four minutes. Streptokinase was administered by the intracoronary route. An initial bolus dose of 20,000 units was followed by a continuous infusion of 2000 units/minute for 60 minutes; a reloading bolus dose of 10,000 units was administered after each arteriogram. The mean total dose of streptokinase was 156,000 units. Reperfusion was assessed angiographically at 15-minute intervals for 90 minutes. Reperfusion was defined as advancement from flow grade 0 or 1 to grade 2 or 3. The mean time from onset of symptoms to treatment was 204 ± 60 minutes (range, 23–359 minutes).

Continued on page 638

Does so much for so much less than cefoxitin

A retrospective chart review of four antibiotic regimens was conducted in an 800-bed hospital on a total of 141 patients. CEFOTAN was compared with cefoxitin as well as combination antibiotic therapy. The clinical success rate and incidence of adverse reactions were similar with CEFOTAN and cefoxitin.

Equally as effective as combination antibiotic therapy with a cost advantage

When CEFOTAN was compared with the ampicillin/aminoglycoside/clindamycin combination and the ampicillin/aminoglycoside/metronidazole combination, results were comparable.

40%

savings over cefoxitin

Clinical efficacy

Infection	CEFOTAN Success/Total	(%)	Cefoxitin Success/Total	(%)
OB/GYN	10/11	(91)	24/26	(92)
Abdominal	10/11	(91)	3/4	(75)
Miscellaneous	6/8	(75)	4/5	(80)
Prophylaxis	2/2	(100)	3/3	(100)
Total	28/32	(88)	34/38	(89)

—adapted from Sochalski et al, p 98

However, using CEFOTAN costs approximately 40% less than cefoxitin.

Clinical efficacy

Infections	CEFOTAN Success/Total	(%)	Amp/Ag/Clin Success/Total	(%)	Amp/Ag/Met Success/Total	(%)
OB/GYN, abdominal, miscellaneous, and prophylaxis	19/21	(90)	27/29	(93)	17/21	(81)

—adapted from Sochalski et al, p 98

Cost comparisons showed that CEFOTAN was more cost-effective than the clindamycin- or metronidazole-containing regimens.

In intra-abdominal and gynecologic infection due to indicated organisms

CEFOTAN® IM/IV
(cefotetan disodium)

Does so much for so much less than cefoxitin.

REFERENCE: Sochalski A, Sullman S, Andriole VT: Cost-effectiveness study of cefotetan versus cefoxitin and cefotetan versus combination antibiotic regimens. *Am J Surg* 1988;155(5A):96-101.

© 1988 ICI Americas Inc.

Continued from page 634

Reperfusion was achieved at any time within the 90-minute evaluation period in 67 (55%) of 122 APSAC-treated patients and in 73 (64%) of 114 streptokinase-treated patients. Reperfusion rates were 51% at 90 minutes after APSAC administration and 60% at the end of the 60-minute streptokinase infusion. The mean time to initial reperfusion was significantly different (43 ± 23 minutes, APSAC; 31 ± 17 minutes, streptokinase). A plateau in the rate of coronary reperfusion was reached after 45–60 minutes with streptokinase therapy but not until after 90 minutes with APSAC.

Reperfusion success rates with both treatments were related to the initial coronary flow grade. Reperfusion occurred in 78% of patients with grade 1 flow and in 48% of those with grade 0 flow. Success rates with intravenous APSAC, but not intracoronary streptokinase, were dependent on the delay between onset of symptoms and initiation of therapy. APSAC was successful in 60% of patients treated within four hours but in only 33% of patients treated after four hours. Streptokinase success rates were 60% for treatment within four hours and 61% when treatment was begun later. Reocclusion occurred during the 90-minute evaluation period in 6 (9%) of 67 APSAC-treated patients and 11 (15%) of 73 streptokinase-treated patients. Additional intervention was required by 39% of the APSAC group and 58% of the streptokinase group. In-hospital mortality rates were low in both treatment groups (five deaths, APSAC group; nine deaths, streptokinase group).

Blood pressure was decreased initially after administration of either agent; the reduction was generally mild to moderate but was greater with APSAC than with streptokinase. In the dosages given, APSAC had a greater effect on fibrinogen and plasminogen levels than did streptokinase. Bleeding was reported in 29% of the APSAC group and in 14% of the streptokinase group. Other adverse reactions occurred at a similar frequency in both treatment groups.

1. Anderson JL, Rothbard RL, Hackworthy RA et al. Multicenter reperfusion trial of intravenous anisoylated plasminogen streptokinase activator complex (APSAC) in acute myocardial infarction: controlled comparison with intracoronary streptokinase. *J Am Coll Cardiol.* 1988; 11:1153–63.

Guidelines issued on treatment of pediatric bacterial meningitis

Cephalosporins may be used as first-line drugs for the treatment of meningitis, and, in some cases, shorter courses of therapy may be appropriate, according to a report issued by the Committee on Infectious Diseases of the American Academy of Pediatrics.[1]

Initial Empiric Therapy. The committee concluded that ampicillin plus an aminoglycoside or a cephalosporin (cefotaxime or ceftazidime) can be used for initial empiric therapy of meningitis in neonates. Ceftazidime would be preferred over cefotaxime in hospitalized low-birth-weight premature infants in whom *Pseudomonas* is a possible pathogen. For older infants and children, either ampicillin and chloramphenicol or one of the newer cephalosporins—cefuroxime, cefotaxime, moxalactam, or ceftriaxone—would be equally acceptable. However, single-drug therapy with moxalactam was not recommended because moxalactam has limited activity against group B streptococci and *Streptococcus pneumoniae.* In addition, during the first six to eight weeks of life, ampicillin should be given in addition to a cephalosporin because of the possibility that meningitis could be caused by *Listeria* or enterococcus.

Subsequent Therapy. According to the committee's report, penicillin G or ampicillin is preferred for the treatment of meningitis caused by group B streptococcus, *Neisseria meningitidis,* and susceptible strains of *Strep. pneumoniae.* Penicillin-resistant strains of *Strep. pneumoniae* should be treated with chloramphenicol or vancomycin until susceptibility testing is completed. Meningitis caused by *Listeria monocytogenes* or β-lactamase-negative strains of *Haemophilus influenzae* is best treated with ampicillin. Chloramphenicol or one of the new cephalosporins is preferred for treating β-lactamase-producing strains of *H. influenzae.* In cases of neonatal meningitis caused by gram-negative enteric bacilli, antimicrobial selection should be based on the results of susceptibility testing.

Duration of Therapy. A 14-day course of therapy is usually satisfactory for cases of neonatal meningitis caused by group B streptococci or *L. monocytogenes.* In contrast, infants with meningitis caused by gram-negative enteric bacilli should receive at least three weeks of antimicrobial therapy; four to six weeks of therapy may be indicated if sterilization of cerebrospinal-fluid cultures is delayed. Uncomplicated *H. influenzae* meningitis in infants and children generally responds to 7–10 days of therapy. Seven days of antimicrobial therapy is adequate for meningococcal meningitis. A 10-day course of therapy is preferred for pneumococcal meningitis.

Home Therapy. Although some physicians may choose to complete the treatment course by home administration of oral chloramphenicol or intramuscular ceftriaxone, the committee declined to endorse this practice. If the decision is made to complete the treatment course using oral chloramphenicol, the adequacy of drug absorption should be documented before the patient is discharged. The committee concluded that experience with intramuscular ceftriaxone is insufficient to support this route of administration.

1. Committee on Infectious Diseases. Treatment of bacterial meningitis. *Pediatrics.* 1988; 81:904–7.

Wider use of clomipramine approved by FDA

A treatment IND protocol for use of the experimental drug clomipramine (Anafranil, Ciba-Geigy Pharmaceuticals) in the treatment of severe cases of obsessive–compulsive disorder has been approved by FDA. Recent clinical studies have indicated that the drug is effective in controlling symptoms in some patients with severe disease. Clomipramine may increase the risk of seizures; a seizure rate of 0.7% has been reported. Submission of a new drug application is not expected before next year. Clomipramine will be distributed by Ciba-Geigy to physicians of eligible patients. Patients must be 18 to 70 years of age and must have had symptoms that interfere with day-to-day functioning for at least one year. Information about the program can be obtained by calling 1-800-842-2422 (201-277-5000 in New Jersey).

FDA requires new, permanent Reye's syndrome warning on aspirin products

All aspirin-containing products marketed after December 9, 1988, must contain the statement, "WARNING: Children and teenagers should not use this medicine for chicken pox or flu symptoms before a doctor is consulted about Reye syndrome, a rare but serious illness reported to be associated with aspirin." Based on results of a Public Health Service study showing an association between Reye's syndrome and aspirin ingestion during chicken pox and influenza, the previously required warning was modified to contain the phrase "reported to be associated with aspirin." The current warning statement continues in effect until December 1988. In addition, for one year all nonprescription aspirin products must contain a prominent statement that includes the words "new" and "warning" to draw attention to the revised, permanent warning.

News Briefs

• A new synthetic allylamine topical antifungal agent, **naftifine hydrochloride 1% cream** (Naftine, Herbert Laboratories), has been approved by FDA and is available in 15- and 30-g sizes.

• **Pancrelipase capsules** containing small (2-mm diameter) enteric-coated microtablets of enzyme concentrate (Pancrease MT, McNeil Pharmaceutical) are now available. In vitro tests conducted under simulated physiologic conditions indicate that more than 90% of the enzyme activity of Pancrease MT is released within 15 minutes, with peak enzyme activity (97% of Pancrease MT activity) occurring at 30 minutes. The capsules contain amylase and protease, each in a three-to-one ratio to lipase. Three capsule strengths (expressed according to lipase content) are available: Pancrease MT 4 (4,000 U.S.P. units), Pancrease MT 10 (10,000 U.S.P. units), and Pancrease MT 16 (16,000 U.S.P. units).

• Audiotapes of a symposium entitled, **"Hospice: An In-depth Perspective on Pain,"** are available for purchase separately or as a complete set of four tapes. The conference, which was held January 27, 1988, under the sponsorship of Long Island Jewish Medical Center, The Jewish Institute for Geriatric Care, and Islip Friends to Promote Hospice, Inc., examined the psychosocial, physical, and spiritual aspects of pain. For further information, contact the Office of Continuing Education, Long Island Jewish Medical Center, New Hyde Park, NY 11042.

• **"Inspiration," a resource booklet intended for use by asthmatic patients and their parents,** is available at no charge from Fisons Corporation; the booklet lists information sources—books, newsletters, organizations and support groups, hospitals, asthma and allergy disease centers, equipment, and a videotape—and briefly describes each source. For a free copy, send name and address to Inspiration, FISONS, 307 Silver Street, Coventry, CT 06238.

• Single copies of the consensus statement from the **National Institutes of Health Consensus Development Conference on Magnetic Resonance Imaging** may be obtained by writing to Michael J. Bernstein, Office of Medical Applications of Research, National Institutes of Health, Building 1, Room 216, Bethesda, MD 20892.

• Revised guidelines for clinical investigations of nonsteroidal anti-inflammatory drugs and disease-modifying antirheumatic drugs have been issued by FDA. Copies of the document, entitled **"Guidelines for the Clinical Evaluation of Anti-inflammatory and Antirheumatic Drugs (Adults and Children),"** (GPO stock no. 017-012-00333-8), can be purchased from the Superintendent of Documents, U.S. Government Printing Office, Washington, DC 20402.

Upcoming Specialty Meetings

National Conference on Chronic Disease Prevention and Control (3rd) . . . October 19–21 . . . Denver, CO . . . contact: M. S. Brocato, Division of Chronic Disease Control, Center for Environmental Health and Injury Control, Centers for Disease Control (F10), Atlanta, GA 30333; 404-488-4251.

Applied Research Ethics National Association . . . October 26 . . . Boston, MA . . . contact: Public Responsibility in Medicine and Research, 132 Boylston Street, 4th Floor, Boston, MA 02116; 617-423-4112 or 1099.

American Academy of Child and Adolescent Psychiatry . . . October 26–30 . . . Seattle, WA . . . contact: V. Anthony, AACP, 3615 Wisconsin Aveune, N.W., Washington, DC 20016; 202-966-7300.

IRBs at the Crossroads: Expanding Roles and Expanded Problems . . . October 27–28 . . . Boston, MA . . . contact: Public Responsibility in Medicine and Research, 132 Boylston Street, 4th Floor, Boston, MA 02116; 617-423-4112 or 1099.

Association of Clinical Scientists . . . November 10–13 . . . Newport Beach, CA . . . contact: F. William-Sunderman, Jr., M.D., Department of Laboratory Medicine, University of Connecticut Health Center, Farmington, CT 06032; 203-679-2328.

American College of Allergy and Immunology . . . November 12–16 . . . Los Angeles, CA . . . contact: J. R. Slawny, 800 East Northwest Highway, #1080, Palatine, IL 60067; 312-359-2800.

American Heart Association . . . November 14–17 . . . Washington, DC . . . contact: D. H. Hafner, 7320 Greenville Avenue, Dallas, TX 75231; 214-373-6300.

Gerontological Society of America . . . November 18–22 . . . San Francisco, CA . . . contact: J. M. Cornman, 1411 K Street N.W., Suite 300, Washington, DC 20005; 202-393-1411.

American Society for Cancer Education . . . November 29–December 2 . . . San Diego, CA . . . contact: S. Brown, Jr., Ed.D., Office of Educational Research and Development, 401 Community Health Services Building, University of Alabama at Birmingham, Birmingham, AL 35294; 205-934-7442.

American Society of Hematology . . . December 3–6 . . . San Antonio, TX . . . contact: I. J. Weiss, 6900 Grove Road, Thorofare, NJ 08086; 609-845-0003.

Therapy Consultation

The Therapy Consultation *section provides brief advice, in question-and-answer format, on how to handle specific drug-therapy problems. Readers are invited to submit questions, which will be referred to a consultant for an answer. The problems should not be highly specialized or unusual, nor should they be mundane. Questions are answered briefly, based largely on the judgment and personal experience of the consultant, although selected references may be cited to substantiate the consultant's advice.*

Use of tamoxifen in stage I breast cancer

Question: A 54-year-old woman was recently diagnosed as having stage I breast cancer. After resection and biopsy, the tumor was found to be estrogen-receptor positive, poorly differentiated, and of high nuclear grade and growth fraction. It was localized to the breast with no lymph node involvement. The tumor was identified as infiltrating ductal carcinoma. Use of adjuvant therapy was considered, but the patient was deemed a poor candidate for therapy with antineoplastic agents. Is tamoxifen useful as adjuvant therapy in patients with stage I disease?

Answer: The term adjuvant therapy refers to any form of treatment that is used to prolong disease-free or overall survival after primary treatment with surgery or radiation therapy, or both. Until recently, adjuvant therapy was reserved almost exclusively for patients with node-positive (stage II) disease. Patients with node-negative (stage I) breast cancer were usually followed without further treatment. However, 25–35% of patients with stage I disease die within 10 years after mastectomy, usually as a direct result of cancer recurrence at distant sites.[1] This raises the question of adjuvant therapy for this group of patients.

Factors associated with a high risk of recurrence include large tumor size, negative estrogen- and progesterone-receptor status, poor differentiation of the tumor, high nuclear grade, high thymidine labeling index or high growth fraction, and aneuploid tumors. The patient described in the question may be at high risk of recurrence because several of these factors are present. Generally, adjuvant combination antineoplastic-drug therapy is considered for those patients with node-negative (stage I) disease who are at high risk of recurrence; however, this patient was deemed to be a poor candidate for antineoplastic-drug therapy.

In 1985, the National Institutes of Health convened a Consensus Development Conference to develop guidelines for the use of adjuvant therapy. The panel advocated use of tamoxifen as the treatment of choice for postmenopausal women with positive lymph nodes and positive hormone-receptor levels. The panel's recommendation led to the recent FDA approval of tamoxifen for this indication. The panel made no recommendations regarding the use of tamoxifen for stage I breast cancer. However, two studies suggest a potential benefit from tamoxifen, given as a single adjuvant agent, in patients who have stage I disease with either estrogen-receptor positive or negative tumors.

The six-year results of a controlled trial of tamoxifen as a single adjuvant agent in the management of early breast cancer were reported in 1985 by the Nolvadex Adjuvant Trial Organization (NATO).[2] After primary treatment with total mastectomy and either axillary node removal or nodal sampling, 1285 patients were randomized to receive tamoxifen 10 mg (as the citrate salt) twice daily or no further treatment. Treatment was initiated eight weeks after mastectomy and was continued for two years or until relapse.

At a maximum follow-up of six years (median = 45 months), a significant benefit was seen in tamoxifen-treated patients regardless of menopausal, estrogen-receptor, or nodal status. There were 152 events (first recurrence or death) in the tamoxifen group compared with 220 events in the control group; the treatment failure rate was 41% lower for tamoxifen-treated patients than for control patients (95% confidence interval = 27–53%; log-rank analysis, $p < 0.0001$). The survival rate was also significantly greater in the tamoxifen group; 34% fewer deaths occurred in the tamoxifen group than in the control group (95% confidence interval = 16–49%; chi-square analysis, $p = 0.0019$).

Recently, the Breast Cancer Trials Committee of the Scottish Cancer Trials Office reported the results of a study of 1312 patients with early breast cancer.[3] In contrast to the NATO study, premenopausal as well as postmenopausal women with node-negative tumors were included in the trial. The duration of adjuvant tamoxifen therapy was five years, and follow-up was from 2.5 to 8 years.

At the time of the report, recurrent disease had developed in 61 (16%) of 377 node-negative and 84 (39%) of

Continued on page 643

Continued from page 640

213 node-positive patients who received adjuvant tamoxifen therapy compared with 104 (28%) of 374 node-negative and 129 (60%) of 215 node-positive patients who received no adjuvant treatment. Overall, recurrent disease developed in 157 (24%) of 661 patients randomized to the adjuvant tamoxifen group compared with 250 (38%) of 651 patients in the control group. These percentages include some patients in whom nodal status was not identified. The authors concluded that tamoxifen delayed recurrence in node-negative as well as node-positive patients. Death with or from recurrent disease occurred in 117 (18%) of 661 treated patients and in 151 (23%) of 651 control patients. Significant increases in overall survival (p = 0.002), disease-free survival (p = 0.0001), and distant-disease-free survival ($p < 0.0001$) were also observed for the treatment group. Similar to the NATO study, the improvement in disease-free survival did not differ significantly with respect to nodal, menopausal, or estrogen-receptor status. In both studies, adjuvant tamoxifen therapy was generally well tolerated, with 4% of patients discontinuing treatment because of adverse effects.

Although limited data suggest a potential benefit (delayed disease recurrence and improved survival with minimal toxicity) from adjuvant tamoxifen therapy in patients with stage I disease, recommendations pertaining to tamoxifen use in this population have not been established, and this indication has not received FDA approval. Furthermore, the optimum duration of treatment with tamoxifen has not yet been determined. Additional studies with longer follow-up periods are needed to determine the optimum duration of therapy and to assess the full long-term effects of tamoxifen therapy in patients with stage I disease. However, use of tamoxifen may currently be warranted in certain cases: Patients, such as the one described in this question, who are at increased risk of recurrence and are poor candidates for antineoplastic-drug therapy may benefit from tamoxifen therapy.

1. Henderson IC, Canellos GP. Cancer of the breast (part one). *N Engl J Med*. 1980; 302:17–30.
2. Baum M, Brinkley DM, Dossett JA et al. Controlled trial of tamoxifen as a single adjuvant agent in management of early breast cancer. *Lancet*. 1985; 1:836–40.
3. Report from the Breast Cancer Trials Committee, Scottish Cancer Trials Office. Adjuvant tamoxifen in the management of operable breast cancer: the Scottish Trial. *Lancet*. 1987; 1:171–5.

MYRNA Y. MUNAR, PHARM.D.
Fellow in Pharmacokinetics/Oncology
Philadelphia College of Pharmacy and Science (PCPS)

JEAN M. SCHOLTZ, PHARM.D.
Clinical Pharmacist in Oncologic Chemotherapy, Hospital of the University of Pennsylvania
Clinical Assistant Professor of Pharmacy, PCPS

Woodland Avenue at 43rd Street
Philadelphia, PA 19104

DRUG INFORMATION SCIENTIST

Lorex Pharmaceuticals represents an on-going partnership committed to the development and commercialization of the highest quality ethical pharmaceuticals. To realize this commitment, we depend on the skills, expertise and professional attitude of individuals who take pride in their achievements and who function best as a member of a team that is dedicated to our common goals and objectives.

An outstanding career opportunity currently exists at Lorex for a Drug Information Scientist. Responsibilities of this position include determining the types of technical literature searches and sources of information required to satisfy the scientific information needs of our researchers and staff. The selected candidate will conduct searches of technical literature, analyze and evaluate data and extract and prepare all pertinent information; will keep abreast of all new developments in areas of interest to our company, periodically consulting with researchers and other information users to ensure maximum usefulness and service. The qualified candidate shall be able to write reviews, monographs and pertinent publications in the area of cardiovascular and central nervous system therapeutics. These activities will be key to our on-going research effort.

Qualified candidates will possess a Master's or Pharm.D in Drug Information Sciences, along with experience in using Med-Line, SCI, Drug Dex, etc.

This position offers excellent compensation and benefits. For confidential consideration, send your resume to:

Janet M. Pavlich
Director, Personnel Operations

LOREX
PHARMACEUTICALS
4930 W. Oakton Street
Skokie, IL 60077

Equal Opportunity Employer M/F/H/V

University of Alberta
Edmonton

Dean
Faculty of Pharmacy and Pharmaceutical Sciences

The University of Alberta invites applications and nominations for the position of Dean of the Faculty of Pharmacy and Pharmaceutical Sciences. Located in Edmonton, Alberta, the University of Alberta is a comprehensive public university with an enrolment of approximately 30,000 full-time and part-time students. The appointment will take effect July 1, 1989 or as soon as possible thereafter. The present Dean has advised that he will not be a candidate for the position.

The Faculty of Pharmacy and Pharmaceutical Sciences offers a four-year undergraduate program leading to the Bachelor of Science in Pharmacy Degree. Programs leading to the M.Pharm., M.Sc., and Ph.D. degrees in various disciplines in Pharmacy are also available. Current enrolment is approximately 420 undergraduate students and 45 graduate students. There are 20 full-time academic staff and 12 support staff. The Faculty also maintains a strong research program including cooperative projects with the Faculty of Medicine, University of Alberta Hospitals and the Cross Cancer Institute, in addition to an international collaborative research program.

The Dean is responsible to the Vice-President (Academic) for the supervision and administration of the academic program, budget, and all activities of the Faculty. Candidates should have a demonstrated capacity for collegial leadership, strong academic qualifications, and proven administrative ability. Knowledge of pharmacy in Canada is desirable.

Written nominations or applications for the position, accompanied in the latter case by a resume of qualifications and experience, and the names of three referees, should be submitted by December 1, 1988 to:

Dr. J. Peter Meekison
Vice-President (Academic)
Third Floor University Hall
University of Alberta
Edmonton, Alberta
Canada
T6G 2J9

The University of Alberta is committed to the principle of equity in employment.

Clinical Pharmacist Faculty Position University of North Carolina at Chapel Hill and the Area L Area Health Education Center

The School of Pharmacy, University of North Carolina at Chapel Hill, and the Area L Area Health Education Center (AHEC), Rocky Mount, NC, are recruiting a clinical pharmacist faculty member.

Based at the Area L AHEC, this individual will coordinate the experiential education of baccalaureate and doctor of pharmacy students and the continuing-education and inservice programs for pharmacists throughout the five-county AHEC region. Responsibilities also include implementing a clinical pharmacy practice at an affiliated hospital for the purpose of precepting students in clinical clerkship rotations. Development of personal scholarship is expected.

The applicant should possess a Pharm.D. or M.S. degree, a residency or equivalent experience, teaching skills, and scholarship ability. Salary and rank are commensurate with training and experience.

Letters of application accompanied by a curriculum vitae and three letters of recommendation should be sent by October 15, 1988, to:

David M. Webb, Ed.D.
Director, Area L AHEC
P.O. Drawer 7368
Rocky Mount, NC 27804-0368
Phone: 919-972-6958

The Area L AHEC and the University of North Carolina at Chapel Hill are Equal Opportunity/Affirmative Action Employers

The VA Medical Center, Syracuse, New York, has an immediate opening for a clinical pharmacist interested in adult ambulatory-care medicine. Responsibilities include evaluating drug regimens, making dosage recommendations, providing drug information to professional staff, instructing resident staff concerning the concepts of effective prescribing, and drug-use evaluation. The Syracuse VA Medical Center is a 329-bed acute-care facility that is affiliated with the SUNY College of Medicine and operates many ambulatory-care clinics representing all major surgical and medical subspecialities.

A Pharm.D. or equivalent professional degree is required; residency experience is preferred. Two or more years of work experience in a clinical capacity is desirable, but the major requirement is a motivated individual with strong professional and interpersonal skills. Salary is commensurate with qualifications and experience. Salary range is $33,218 to $43,181 per year.

If you are interested in a challenging practice within a dynamic outpatient setting, we want to know more about you. Qualified candidates should send resumes to:

VA Medical Center
Personnel Service (05)
800 Irving Avenue
Syracuse, NY 13210
315-476-7461, ext. 2311

Equal Opportunity Employer

Drug Reviews

Teicoplanin: An investigational glycopeptide antibiotic

RANDY D. PRYKA, KEITH A. RODVOLD, AND JOHN C. ROTSCHAFER

Abstract: The chemistry, mechanism of action, antimicrobial spectrum, pharmacokinetics, adverse effects, and clinical uses of teicoplanin are reviewed.

Teicoplanin, a novel glycopeptide that is similar to vancomycin, was isolated in the mid-1970s. A fermentation product of *Actinoplanes teicomyceticus*, teicoplanin is a structurally complex compound made up of six fatty-acid components attached to a common aglycone. Teicoplanin's mechanism of action, like that of vancomycin, is inhibition of cell-wall biosynthesis. In vitro activity is comparable to that of vancomycin and includes staphylococci, streptococci, corynebacterium, listeria, and anaerobic cocci. Resistance to teicoplanin has been reported with coagulase-negative staphylococci. Teicoplanin is 50 to 100 times more lipophilic than vancomycin. Teicoplanin is poorly absorbed after oral administration but is 90% bioavailable when administered intramuscularly. The drug distributes widely into body tissue and is eliminated primarily renally. Optimal dosing regimens and therapeutic serum drug concentrations have not been well established. Reported adverse effects have included irreversible ototoxicity, allergic reactions with maculopapular rash and eosinophilia, pain at intramuscular injection site, and elevation of aminotransferases. Initial clinical trials have yielded conflicting results in gram-positive bacteremia, endocarditis, osteomyelitis, and soft-tissue infections. Teicoplanin has shown promise in surgical and dental prophylaxis.

Comparative trials with vancomycin and other antimicrobial agents must be completed before teicoplanin's role as a therapeutic agent in the treatment of systemic gram-positive infections is defined.

Index terms: Antibiotics; Dosage; Drug administration; Mechanism of action; Pharmacokinetics; Teicoplanin; Toxicity
Clin Pharm. 1988; 7:647–58

Vancomycin is the only glycopeptide antibiotic currently marketed in the United States. The increased incidence of methicillin-resistant isolates of *Staphylococcus aureus* and *Staphylococcus epidermidis*[1,2] has prompted the development of alternative antimicrobials from the glycopeptide class. Teicoplanin is currently under clinical investigation by Merrell Dow Pharmaceuticals for the treatment of various gram-positive infections. Teicoplanin has a novel structure and unique pharmacokinetic properties. A preliminary review of the current literature is provided; and the structure, mechanism of action, antimicrobial spectrum, pharmacokinetics, toxicity, and clinical use of teicoplanin as an addition to the glycopeptide class of antibiotics will be discussed.

Chemistry

Since the late 1950s antibiotics of the glycopeptide class have been available for use, the major representative being vancomycin. Numerous other glycopeptides are in various stages of research and development. These antibiotics typically have the same basic structural characteristics, consisting of one or more amino sugars plus one or more basic

RANDY D. PRYKA, PHARM.D., is Clinical Research Fellow, Department of Pharmacy Practice and Clinical Pharmacokinetics Laboratory, and KEITH A. RODVOLD, PHARM.D., is Assistant Professor, Departments of Pharmacy Practice and Pharmacodynamics, Clinical Pharmacokinetics Laboratory, College of Pharmacy, University of Illinois at Chicago. JOHN C. ROTSCHAFER, PHARM.D., is Associate Professor, College of Pharmacy, University of Minnesota, Minneapolis, and Department of Clinical Pharmacology, St. Paul-Ramsey Medical Center, St. Paul, MN.

Address reprint requests to Dr. Rodvold at the College of Pharmacy, Room 244, University of Illinois m/c 886, 833 South Wood Street, Chicago, IL 60612.

The assistance of Marion Sitt in preparing the illustration is acknowledged.

This is **article 680-204-8814** in the **ASHP Continuing Education System.** See page 702 for learning objectives and test questions.

Copyright © 1988, American Society of Hospital Pharmacists, Inc. All rights reserved. 0278-2677/88/0901-0647$03.00.

sugars arranged around a central complex amino acid moiety.[3]

In the mid-1970s, Parenti and colleagues[4] isolated two potential antimicrobials—teichomycin $A_1(TA_1)$ and teichomycin A_2 (TA_2)—during a screening process for antimicrobial-producing strains of Actinoplanaceae. Both teichomycin compounds are fermentation products of *Actinoplanes teicomyceticus*. Teichomycin A_1 was eventually determined to be a phosphoglycopeptide antibiotic, structurally unrelated to TA_2. Teichomycin A_1, while demonstrating some activity against gram-negative organisms, was shown to be considerably less active than TA_2 against gram-positive species, and further development of TA_1 was abandoned.[5] Teichomycin A_2, now commonly known as teicoplanin, is a glycopeptide antibiotic complex consisting of five major components—$TA_{2\text{-}1}$ through $TA_{2\text{-}5}$—plus a more polar sixth component designated TA_3, arranged around a common aglycone.[6-8] The $TA_{2\text{-}1}$ through $TA_{2\text{-}5}$ components account for 89% to 95% of the teicoplanin complex; these components have different lipid side chains at the R position (Figure 1).[6-8] The TA_3 component is more polar because hydrogen, rather than a fatty acid chain, occupies the R position. Teicoplanin has several unique structural differences from vancomycin. The presence of an acyl chain allows for the variance of the five members of the teicoplanin complex. Also, the presence of D-glucosamine and D-mannose differentiates teicoplanin from other members of the glycopeptide antibiotics including vancomycin (Figure 1).

Physicochemically, teicoplanin is an ivory-colored, amorphous powder that melts and decomposes at 260 °C. The $TA_{2\text{-}1}$ through $TA_{2\text{-}5}$ components range in molecular weight from 1875 to 1891, while the molecular weight of the TA_3 component is 1562. The teicoplanin complex is soluble in water and water–methanol mixtures at pH >7 but is insoluble in nonpolar organic solvents. The complex has four phenolic groups and six ionizable groups, yielding an isoelectric point of 5.1. Vancomycin, a basic molecule, has an isoelectric point of 8.0.[9] Parenti[9] found that in similar chemical environments, teicoplanin was 50 to 100 times more lipophilic than vancomycin. This difference in lipophilicity results from the fatty acid moieties on teicoplanin.

Mechanism of Action

Structural similarities between teicoplanin and vancomycin and preliminary evidence of comparable antimicrobial spectra suggested that teicoplanin inhibits cell-wall synthesis, as does vancomycin. Somma and colleagues[10] proved this assumption valid by demonstrating that teicoplanin inhibited the polymerization of peptidoglycan by binding to the D-alanyl-D-alanine terminal end of the peptidoglycan molecule or a precursor. The exact step inhibited has not yet been clearly described. Unlike vancomycin, teicoplanin was shown not to interfere with the synthesis of microbial DNA or RNA.[11] Spontaneous variants of some bacteria can produce L-forms, which are small cells with deficient or totally absent cell-wall processes. In contrast to vancomycin, L-form bacteria are not affected by teicoplanin's cell-wall-specific mechanism of action.[4] L-forms, including L-forms of *Staph. aureus*, are primarily limited to laboratory findings and are not usually clinically important.

Figure 1. Structures of teicoplanin (left) and vancomycin.

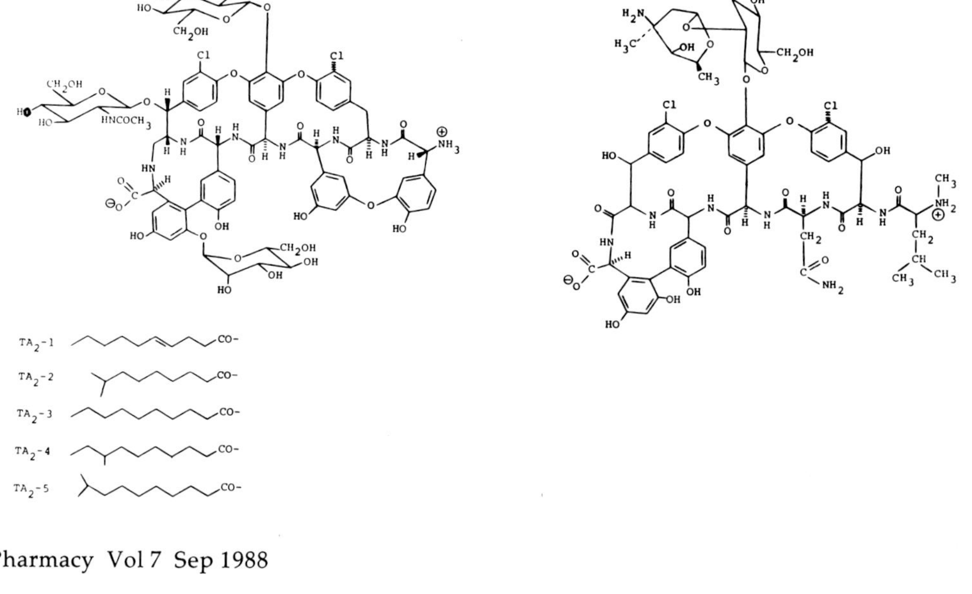

Antimicrobial Spectrum

Teicoplanin's antimicrobial activity has been evaluated in more than 3000 isolates of various aerobic and anaerobic organisms. Early studies demonstrated that the spectrum of teicoplanin is restricted to gram-positive organisms, with most common gram-negative species having minimum inhibitory concentration (MIC) values of 100 mg/L or greater.[4,10] Common pathogenic gram-positive organisms and respective MIC data are presented in Table 1.

Effects of pH, Inoculum Size, and Methods of MIC Evalution. Most in vitro studies evaluated antimicrobial activity of teicoplanin using inoculum sizes of 10^4 to 10^5 colony-forming units (CFU)/mL at physiologic pH. Teicoplanin is only slightly affected by changes in pH, with modest changes in MICs over a pH range of 6.4 to 8.4.[21] Data regarding inoculum effects are conflicting. Increasing inoculum sizes from 10^3 to 10^7 CFU/mL only slightly affected MIC values for most clinical isolates, increasing MICs by fourfold or less. Notable exceptions were isolates of *Staph. epidermidis* and enterococcus, which demonstrated 8- to 16-fold increases in MICs.[21,22] Greenwood and colleagues[23] recently demonstrated the presence of inoculum effect for some staphylococcus and streptococcus isolates when inocula were increased from 10^3 to 10^7 CFU/mL.

Increasing bovine serum concentration from 5% to 70% had no effect on MIC values.[21] Differences in culture media have only occasionally been reported to affect MIC determinations, with agar dilution techniques yielding slightly higher MICs than microtiter techniques.[21,22] Quality control limits for teicoplanin susceptibility testing correlating zone size with MICs based on a disk diffusion method have recently been established.[24] Disk susceptibility zone sizes of less than 10 mm and greater than 14 mm, using a 0.03-mg teicoplanin disk, correspond to resistance and susceptibility, respectively. The interpretive MIC breakpoints used for susceptibility and resistance were less than 4 mg/L and greater than 8 mg/L, respectively.[24,25]

Staphylococci. The minimum inhibitory concentration of teicoplanin for 50% and 90% of isolates (MIC_{50} and MIC_{90}) of *Staph. aureus* ranged from 0.2 to 0.8 mg/L and 0.2 to 1.6 mg/L, respectively.[12-16,21,22] Methicillin-susceptible and methicillin-resistant isolates, including strains resistant to multiple antibiotics had similar MIC_{50} and MIC_{90} values.[13,17-20,22,26] All MIC values for teicoplanin were found to be similar, with most reports suggesting two- to fourfold lower MICs as compared with those associated with vancomycin.[11-16,21,22] Specific phage typing or geographical location of clinical isolates did not affect susceptibility to teicoplanin.[27]

Table 1.
Mean In Vitro Susceptibility of Various Gram-Positive Organisms to Teicoplanin and Vancomycin[a]

Organism	Antibiotic	MIC_{50}[b]	MIC_{90}[c]	MIC (Range)	MBC[d] (Range)
Methicillin-susceptible *Staphylococcus aureus*	Teicoplanin	0.5	1.0	0.25–1.6	0.16–3.1
	Vancomycin	1.0	1.0	0.03–3.2	0.25–5.0
Methicillin-resistant *Staphylococcus aureus*	Teicoplanin	0.5	1.0	0.6–6.3	0.6–6.25
	Vancomycin	1.0	1.0	0.2–6.3	0.78–6.4
Methicillin-susceptible *Staphylococcus epidermidis*	Teicoplanin	1.0	2.0	0.5–1.6	0.25–4.0
	Vancomycin	1.0	2.0	0.5–3.1	0.125–4.0
Methicillin-resistant *Staphylococcus epidermidis*	Teicoplanin	1.0	2.0	0.5–12.5	0.2–16.0
	Vancomycin	1.0	2.0	0.25–10.0	0.25–25.0
Streptococcus faecalis	Teicoplanin	0.5	1.0	0.4–2.0	0.12– >128
	Vancomycin	2.0	4.0	0.125–4.0	0.2– >128
Clostridium difficile	Teicoplanin	0.12	0.12	0.12–1.56	...
	Vancomycin	0.25	0.5	0.12–3.2	...
Listeria monocytogenes	Teicoplanin	0.05	0.8	0.05–0.8	6.2–12.5
	Vancomycin	0.4	1.6	0.25–1.6	12.5–25.0
JK diphtheroids	Teicoplanin	1.6	1.6	0.1– <25.0	...
	Vancomycin	0.8	0.8	0.1–6.25	...

[a] Adapted from references 10–20. All values are expressed in milligrams per liter.
[b] Minimum inhibitory concentration in 50% of isolates.
[c] Minimum inhibitory concentration in 90% of isolates.
[d] Minimum bactericidal concentration.

Coagulase-negative staphylococci are routinely less sensitive to teicoplanin than are *Staph. aureus* isolates. *Staph. epidermidis* MIC_{50} values range from 0.5 to 1.6 mg/L, and MIC_{90} values range from 1.6 to 12.5 mg/L,[12-16,21,22] with methicillin-resistant species accounting for the higher MIC_{90} values. In comparison, vancomycin MIC values are one- to twofold lower and are unaffected by methicillin resistance. MICs for *Staphylococcus haemolyticus* ranged from 0.25 to 32 mg/L, with a minimum bactericidal concentration (MBC) up to 32 mg/L.[28,29] Twelve isolates of unspeciated coagulase-negative staphylococci have also been found to have MICs of 12.5 mg/L.[30]

Streptococci. Streptococcal species are very susceptible to teicoplanin, with MICs two- to eightfold lower than those for vancomycin.[12-16,21,22] The MIC values of teicoplanin against *Streptococcus pneumoniae* commonly ranged from 0.05 mg/L to 0.78 mg/L.[12-16,21,22] The MICs of teicoplanin against enterococci ranged from 0.04 to 2.0 mg/L.[12-14,22,31] Teicoplanin demonstrated MICs that were fourfold lower than those associated with ampicillin.[32] Pallanza et al.[16] compared eight commonly used antibiotics for *Streptococcus faecalis* and found teicoplanin to have the lowest MICs (0.05 to 0.8 mg/L). The evaluation of the bactericidal effects of teicoplanin against enterococci produced conflicting results. MBC-to-MIC ratios for teicoplanin against enterococci ranged widely, from 1 to 64, reflecting tolerance or a relative bacteriostatic activity.[18,31-33]

Miscellaneous. *Corynebacterium* species, including group JK diphtheroids, are routinely resistant to many antimicrobials. Teicoplanin showed excellent activity against 98 strains of JK diphtheroids, with MIC_{50} and MIC_{90} values of 0.78 mg/L and 1.56 mg/L, respectively.[34] The MICs for vancomycin were one- to twofold lower than teicoplanin MICs.

Clostridium difficile isolates were uniformly inhibited by <0.1 mg/L of teicoplanin, and *Clostridium perfringens* isolates were routinely inhibited at <0.2 mg/L.[14,16,35-37] No clostridium species demonstrated an MIC value of >1.56 mg/L, representing a 2- to 16-fold decrease in MIC compared with that of vancomycin. Like vancomycin, teicoplanin does not appear to be sporicidal.[36]

Propionibacterium were inhibited by less than 0.2 mg/L of teicoplanin. MIC_{50} and MIC_{90} values for *Listeria monocytogenes* were identical at 0.8 mg/L of teicoplanin.[15]

Synergy and Antagonism. Numerous in vitro synergy studies have been completed.[15,33,38-46] In most studies, MICs and minimum bactericidal concentrations (MBCs) for the combination of rifampin or rifapentine with teicoplanin were not sufficiently different from those for teicoplanin alone to result in synergy or antagonism. Less than 1% of staphylococcal or streptococcal strains demonstrated synergy.[33,39,42] However, Watanakunakorn et al.[46] did report a synergistic effect on 29 of 50 isolates using this combination. Despite the lack of documented synergy, teicoplanin and rifampin combinations have been shown to prevent emergence of rifampin-resistant isolates.[16] In vitro antagonism has only rarely been reported with the addition of rifampin or ampicillin to teicoplanin.[41,43]

Gentamicin in combination with teicoplanin resulted in 42% of *Staph. aureus* and 33% of *Staph. epidermidis* isolates showing synergy.[15] Enterococcal isolates predominantly showed no synergy or antagonism to this antibiotic combination.[15] The lack of synergy against enterococcal isolates is in contrast to the results of other investigators who reported high rates of synergy.[33,41] Amikacin and netilmicin appear synergistic against enterococci when used in combination with teicoplanin.[45] Using the combination of imipenem and teicoplanin, Debbia et al.[44] found that 23 of 76 and 11 of 42 isolates of enterococci demonstrated synergistic effects, depending on the methods used. In a second paper by the same author, 70% of enterococcal isolates showed synergy.[45]

Results of in vitro tests of antibiotic combinations have provided variable results that are greatly dependent on the method used to test synergy. Clinical trials will be required to resolve these in vitro discrepancies.

Resistance. Teicoplanin exhibits a very low spontaneous mutation rate of 10^{-10} per cell per generation[16] and does not increase the frequency of plasmid transfer.[47] Despite limited clinical use, several incidents of teicoplanin resistance have been reported in isolates of coagulase-negative staphylococci.[16,28-30,48] Arioli and Pallanza[29] compared teicoplanin and vancomycin in vitro against several species of coagulase-negative staphylococci isolated from hospitalized patients. The activities of both agents were similar for all species except *Staph. haemolyticus*, which demonstrated increased resistance to teicoplanin. The MIC_{90} for 29 strains of *Staph. haemolyticus* was 32 mg/L for teicoplanin and 4 mg/L for vancomycin. Also, a recent report of a vancomycin-resistant isolate of *Staph. haemolyticus* was also shown to be intrinsically resistant to teicoplanin, suggesting a possible common mechanism of resistance to glycopeptides.[48] Clinically, these reports are of questionable importance, since *Staph. haemolyticus* is rarely pathogenic in humans.

Of greater concern is the paucity of information on resistance patterns of *Staph. epidermidis* because of the failure of some reports to identify the staphylococcal species. Grant and colleagues[30] isolated 25 strains of unspeciated coagulase-negative staphylococci with MICs of >6.4 mg/L from hospitalized patients who were being treated with vancomycin or gentamicin. Minimum inhibitory concentrations for 12 of the 25 isolates ranged from 12.5 to 25 mg/L for teicoplanin and from 0.8 to 3.2

mg/L for vancomycin. Brumfitt and Hamilton-Miller[49] isolated 8 methicillin-resistant and 11 methicillin-susceptible strains of coagulase-negative staphylococci from patients undergoing continuous ambulatory peritoneal dialysis. The methicillin-resistant organisms were less susceptible to teicoplanin than were the methicillin-susceptible strains, with geometric mean MICs of 5.2 mg/L and 2.0 mg/L, respectively. Isolates also demonstrated decreased susceptibility to vancomycin, with geometric mean MICs of 4.4 mg/L and 2.4 mg/L for methicillin-resistant and methicillin-susceptible strains, respectively. Again, no speciation of isolates was performed. Further information is needed to evaluate the teicoplanin-resistance patterns of *Staph. epidermidis*.

Pharmacokinetics

The pharmacokinetic profile of teicoplanin has been evaluated extensively in both animals[50,51] and humans. Human data were primarily generated in healthy volunteers.[52-56] Four investigators have studied the effects of various degrees of renal impairment in noninfected patients.[57-60] Teicoplanin has been shown to demonstrate first-order pharmacokinetics.[52] Traina and Bonati,[52] using traditional pharmacokinetic modeling, found intravenous teicoplanin disposition to be best described using a three-compartment open pharmacokinetic model. Data from intramuscular administration have been fitted to a two-compartment pharmacokinetic model.[53] Pharmacokinetic variables for teicoplanin and vancomycin[61] are shown in Table 2.

Assay Methods. The majority of pharmacokinetic studies and early chemical and analytical work quantified teicoplanin concentrations using a *Bacillus subtilis* agar diffusion method. This assay, while quite sensitive (0.1-0.2 mg/L), lacked specificity, determining only the concentration of the parent compound.[52,53] High-performance liquid chromatography (HPLC) can determine the concentrations of each component of the six-part teicoplanin complex (TA_{2-1} through TA_{2-5} and TA_3), with the lower limit of detection of the major component being 0.05 mg/L.[62,63] However, none of the HPLC studies have used pure standards of each component to quantitate actual concentration or have correlated HPLC activity with microbiological activity. No studies have determined whether possible metabolites of teicoplanin were present. Two newly developed competitive binding assays, a solid-phase enzyme receptor assay (SPERA) and a receptor-antibody sandwich assay (RASA) have been shown to correlate well with the original agar assay.[64-66] The 0.03-mg/L detection limit of the RASA assay is 16-fold lower than that of the SPERA assay.[64,66] Both new methods offer the advantage of a less labor-intensive assay, increasing clinical usefulness.

Table 2.
Pharmacokinetic Variables for Teicoplanin and Vancomycin[a]

Variable[b]	Teicoplanin[c]	Vancomycin[d]
Bioavailability (%)		
after i.m. administration	90	...
V_c (L/kg)	0.08–0.11	0.10–0.55
V_{ss} (L/kg)	0.68–1.17	0.24–1.25
k_{12} (hr^{-1})	0.69–2.19	0.21–2.05
k_{21} (hr^{-1})	0.60–2.01	0.11–1.18
k_{13} (hr^{-1})	0.31–0.85	...
k_{31} (hr^{-1})	0.05–0.10	...
k_{10} (hr^{-1})	0.05–0.27	0.03–0.72
$t_{1/2_\alpha}$ (hr)	0.17–0.51	0.11–1.52
$t_{1/2_\beta}$ (hr)	1.62–4.40	2.82–39.7
$t_{1/2_\gamma}$ (hr)	31.9–157	...
CL (mL/min/kg)	0.27–0.35	0.19–1.71
CL_R (mL/min/kg)	0.12–0.21	0.11–2.37

[a] Adapted from references 52, 53, 60, 61.
[b] V_c = apparent volume of the central compartment; V_{ss} = apparent volume of distribution at steady state; k_{12} = the rate constant for drug movement from compartment 1 to 2; k_{21} = the rate constant for drug movement from compartment 2 to 1; k_{13} = the rate constant for drug movement from compartment 1 to 3; k_{31} = the rate constant for drug movement from compartment 3 to 1; k_{10} = the rate constant for elimination of drug from compartment 1; CL = total body clearance; CL_R = renal clearance.
[c] Values for teicoplanin, except for bioavailability, reflect ranges of mean values.
[d] Values for vancomycin reflect ranges of values.

Absorption. Like vancomycin, teicoplanin shows negligible absorption after oral administration. The possibility of accumulation after oral dosing in patients with renal insufficiency remains to be examined. In sharp contrast to vancomycin, teicoplanin's highly lipophilic nature and acidic charge at physiologic pH promote i.m. absorption. After single i.m. and i.v. doses of teicoplanin of 3 mg/kg in healthy adult male volunteers, i.m. bioavailability was found to be 90%.[53]

Traina and Bonati[52] obtained peak concentrations immediately after a 30-minute i.v. infusion of 12.7 to 19.5 mg/L and 20.3 to 23.5 mg/L from doses of 2 mg/kg and 3 mg/kg of teicoplanin, respectively. Verbist and colleagues[53] found mean peak concentrations of 53.5 mg/L and 111.8 mg/L immediately after i.v. bolus administration of 3 mg/kg and 6 mg/kg, respectively.

Distribution. Bernareggi et al.[50] found an apparent steady-state volume of distribution of 0.28 L/kg in male rats. Tissue concentrations correlated with blood flow; lung, kidney, heart, and adrenal gland tissue had the highest concentrations of teicoplanin. The deep-tissue compartment consisted of liver, kidney, fat, and skin tissue.[50]

Human data demonstrated that teicoplanin distributes widely into body fluids and tissues. Three-compartment pharmacokinetic analysis yielded apparent steady-state volumes of distribution (V_{ss}) ranging from 0.68 to 1.17 L/kg, with volumes of the central compartment (V_c) ranging from 0.08 to 0.11 L/kg.[52,53,60] The major components of teicoplanin (TA_{2-1} through TA_{2-5}) are 90% to 95% bound to serum albumin.[67]

Simulating penetration of the drug into inflammatory exudates, McNulty et al.[54] found that 77% of teicoplanin available systemically penetrated into blister fluid, with the maximal concentration being present within two to three hours after a dose. Seven of eight meningitis patients receiving a one-time i.v. dose of 400 mg had cerebrospinal fluid (CSF) concentrations of less than 0.3 mg/L. The highest CSF teicoplanin concentration obtained in the eight patients was 1.3 mg/L.[68] Published data evaluating diffusion into human erythrocytes are not available. Teicoplanin does penetrate into both macrophages and polymorphonuclear leukocytes; however, this has not correlated with intracellular killing of microorganisms.[69]

Elimination. Preliminary data suggested the possibility of both renal and nonrenal routes of elimination, with total body clearance and renal clearance of teicoplanin found to be substantially lower than endogenous creatinine clearance (CL_{cr}).[52-54] In addition, urinary recovery from a 96-hour collection interval ranged from 48% to 52% of the total teicoplanin dose.[52,53] No data are available that document possible nonrenal routes of elimination or the presence of metabolites of teicoplanin. Assandri and Bernareggi[67] have demonstrated that the difference in teicoplanin clearance and CL_{cr} could be accounted for by passive glomerular filtration alone, caused by the high degree of protein binding.

Elimination half-life has ranged from 32 hours to more than 150 hours, depending on the length of sample collection.[52-54,70] Two authors using three-compartment open pharmacokinetic models found mean terminal half-lives of 40 to 47 hours.[52,53] These data were the result of a 96-hour serum and urine collection. However, when serum and urine collection times were extended to 600 hours, terminal half-life increased to greater than 180 hours in patients who had normal renal function.[70] The authors did not report extent of drug recovery from this extended urinary recovery time.

Falcoz and colleagues[60] evaluated teicoplanin pharmacokinetics in three groups of volunteers with six to seven subjects in each group. The apparent volume of distribution appeared unaffected by changes in renal function. Teicoplanin's renal clearance and total body clearance were greatly reduced with diminishing renal function. Mean terminal half-life in patients with moderate (mean CL_{cr}, 57 mL/min) and severe (mean CL_{cr}, 9.9 mL/min) renal insufficiency increased to 96 hours and 111 hours, respectively. Bonati and colleagues[58] further evaluated the effects of renal dysfunction by subdividing patients into five groups based on CL_{cr}, including patients on hemodialysis and peritoneal dialysis. The concentration data for all patients were fitted to a three-compartment model. The mean terminal half-life increased from 41 hours in the group of healthy volunteers to 163 hours in anuric patients on hemodialysis. Both total and renal clearance decreased in a linear fashion with creatinine clearance. Hemodialysis or peritoneal dialysis had little effect on drug elimination, since relatively little drug was recovered in the dialysis fluids.[57,58] In a study of critically ill patients with various degrees of renal function, pharmacokinetic data obtained after several days of therapy showed wide interpatient variability, but the results agreed with previously reported data.[59] To date, there are no published data evaluating the effects of hepatic dysfunction.

Several important points must be mentioned in considering the pharmacokinetic data. Most of the information has been gained from single-dose studies, mainly in volunteers. In addition, discrepancies in elimination half-life data may be due in part to the available assay methods that measure parent drug but do not account for any possible metabolites.[58] Improved assay methods and multiple-dose pharmacokinetic studies in patient populations are needed.

Clinical Trials

Treatment of endocarditis, osteomyelitis, and septicemia has been evaluated in animal models.[16,71-77] There is a lack of human data evaluating teicoplanin for the treatment of documented infection.[78-86] Data on the use of teicoplanin in prophylaxis are based on healthy volunteers and one large trial of preoperative cardiac surgery patients.[87-89] Results of open clinical trials are summarized in Table 3.

Animal Trials. The first published animal data evaluated teicoplanin against six other antibiotics including vancomycin in the treatment of experimentally induced septicemia.[16] Three groups of 10 mice were inoculated with *Staph. aureus*, *Streptococcus pyogenes*, and *Strep. pneumoniae*, respectively. Teicoplanin was found to have the lowest effective dose for 50% of isolates (ED_{50}) of *Staph. aureus* and *Strep. pneumoniae*, and only ampicillin and cephaloridine showed lower ED_{50} values against *Strep. pyogenes*. Carper et al.[71] evaluated teicoplanin 33 mg/kg, vancomycin 33 mg/kg (as the hydrochloride salt), or rifampin 13 mg/kg for *Staph. aureus* bacteremia and deep-seated visceral infections in mice. Vancomycin was found to be least effective, with survival rates not significantly different from those associated with placebo (72% versus 50%). Teicoplanin's survival rate (82%) was significantly better than that of placebo, while rifampin demonstrated a 96% survival rate.

The most extensive animal data are in the area of endocarditis. Chambers and Sande[72] evaluated rab-

Table 3.
Clinical Trials of Teicoplanin as a Single Agent

Reference	No. of Patients	Dosing Regimen[a]	% Demonstrating Clinical Response[b]			
			Cure	Improvement	Relapse	Failure
78	47	400 mg LD 200 mg MD	47 (50)	17	4 (4)	32 (46)
79	6	400 mg LD 200 mg MD	0	0	50	50
80	69	400 mg LD 200–400 mg MD	61 (73)	25	0	14 (27)
81	85	400 mg LD 200 mg MD	90 (79)	0	0	10 (21)
82	19	400–600 mg LD 200–600 mg MD	61 (46)	15	5 (5)	15 (30)
83[c]	12	400 mg LD 200 mg MD	58	0	34	8

[a] LD = loading dose; MD = maintenance dose given every 24 hours; ranges represent variable maintenance doses.
[b] The percentage of patients demonstrating microbiological response is shown in parentheses in cases in which microbiological response was tested.
[c] Several patients in this study also received concomitant antibiotics.

bits with experimentally induced aortic valve endocarditis. Teicoplanin, nafcillin, or placebo for methicillin-susceptible organisms and teicoplanin, vancomycin, or placebo for methicillin-resistant infections were compared. Serum concentrations of all antibiotics were above the MIC for the entire dosing interval. Teicoplanin was as effective as nafcillin in eliminating organisms from valve sites, and survival rates were comparable (89% versus 80%). Bacteriologic cure rates for methicillin-resistant organisms for vancomycin and teicoplanin were 40% and 16%, respectively. These data are in contrast to those of Arioli et al.,[73] who found teicoplanin superior to vancomycin in reducing vegetation counts. Ten-day survival showed no difference between teicoplanin (80%) and vancomycin (100%).

A 14-day treatment regimen of placebo, teicoplanin alone, rifampin alone, or teicoplanin plus rifampin for methicillin-susceptible *Staph. epidermidis* endocarditis was evaluated in rabbits.[74] Animals were killed three days after the end of therapy. Rifampin plus teicoplanin was significantly superior to teicoplanin alone in producing sterile vegetation (67% versus 7%). Survival rates using teicoplanin plus rifampin (83%) and rifampin alone (82%) were equivalent, and both were significantly better than rates associated with teicoplanin alone (64%) or placebo (27%). Galetto et al.[75] examined the efficacy of several regimens against methicillin-resistant *Staph. epidermidis* endocarditis in a rabbit model. Animals were treated for three days and killed 12 hours or 7 days after the last dose. Gentamicin, rifampin, or gentamicin and rifampin were added to teicoplanin or vancomycin. Combination therapy was significantly superior in reducing vegetation titers over single-agent therapy with teicoplanin or vancomycin. When the regimens were evaluated at seven days after the last dose, teicoplanin and vancomycin were not significantly different in producing sterile vegetations (77% versus 54%).

Sixty-eight rabbits with *Strep. faecalis* endocarditis were treated for four days with either teicoplanin or ampicillin in combination with gentamicin.[76] The combination of gentamicin and teicoplanin was as effective as gentamicin plus ampicillin in reducing vegetation titers.

Teicoplanin was evaluated for treatment of experimentally induced *Staph. aureus* osteomyelitis in rabbits.[77] The 28-day treatment course was initiated 14 days after infection. Despite adequate bone concentrations, the results of bone cultures in 100% of rabbits in both the control and the teicoplanin groups were positive on day 70. MICs and MBCs were 16- to 32-fold higher under anaerobic conditions, offering a possible explanation for the lack of teicoplanin efficacy in the anaerobic environment of bone infections.

Human Trials. Glupczynski and colleagues[78] evaluated 47 patients with gram-positive infections including endocarditis, pneumonia, septicemia, and bone and soft-tissue infections. Patients were given a 400-mg loading dose of teicoplanin, followed by 200 mg every 24 hours via i.v. or i.m. routes. Mean peak concentrations of teicoplanin were 10.4 mg/L, and mean trough concentrations were 2.7 mg/L. Peak concentrations were obtained one hour after the end of a one-hour infusion. The predominant pathogen isolated was *Staph. aureus* (including methicillin-resistant strains). A total of 47% of patients were considered cured, and 17% of patients improved, providing an overall favorable outcome of 64%. Relapse occurred in two patients (4%), one patient with methicillin-susceptible *Staph. aureus* osteomyelitis and one with endocarditis caused by a strain of *Strep. faecalis*. Bacteremic patients had a 50% favorable outcome rate, compared with 83% in the nonbacteremic patients. Gram-negative superinfections were reported in six patients.

A prospective randomized trial of teicoplanin compared with flucloxacillin in the treatment of severe gram-positive infections was terminated prematurely because the first six patients randomized to treatment with teicoplanin had unfavorable outcomes.[79] The two treatment groups were comparable at the initiation of therapy. Wide variation in serum teicoplanin concentrations were reported. Peak concentrations one hour after the second dose ranged from 2.2 to 23.0 mg/L, and trough concentrations ranged from 1.0 to 12.0 mg/L 24 hours after the first dose. Dose and dosing interval in this study were the same as those in the study by Glupczynski et al.[78] Treatment failures may have been caused by inadequate loading doses of teicoplanin, low peak and trough concentrations early in therapy, and the high degree of teicoplanin protein binding.

Pauluzzi and associates[80] evaluated 69 patients with 71 episodes of gram-positive infections. The dose of teicoplanin used in this trial (200 mg to 400 mg i.v. every 24 hours) was higher than that in previous reports. Peak (one hour after administration) and trough concentrations were similar to those reported in the previous studies. The microorganisms isolated, as well as the type and severity of infections, were similar to those in the previous studies. The overall clinical cure rate was 61%, and the improvement rate was 25%, producing a favorable outcome rate of 86%.

Using the same protocol as that used by Glupczynski et al.[78] and Calain et al.,[79] Williams et al.[81] found clinical cure rates of 90% in 85 evaluable patients treated for gram-positive infections. All patients treated for soft-tissue infections, septicemia, urinary-tract infections, chest infections, and osteomyelitis demonstrated 100% clinical cure rates. Patients with infections associated with Hickman catheters and patients with endocarditis demonstrated clinical cure rates of 70%. The overall bacteriologic cure rate was 79%. Bibler and colleagues[82] evaluated 19 patients with serious gram-positive infections, with an overall favorable outcome rate of 76%. Bacteriologic cure rates in this study were less favorable than those in the previous study, with only 46% of treated patients having bacteriologic cures, regardless of the site of infection.

Only one clinical trial to date has focused on endocarditis.[83] Twelve patients with either prosthetic-valve or native-valve endocarditis resulting from infection with *Staph. aureus*, *Staph. epidermidis*, *Strep. faecalis*, or *Strep. viridans* were treated with teicoplanin alone or in combination with aminoglycosides, rifampin, or flucloxacillin. All cases of endocarditis caused by either penicillin-susceptible staphylococci or enterococcal isolates were cured. Both patients treated for enterococcal infections received concurrent gentamicin therapy, while two of the five patients with staphylococcal infections received concurrent gentamicin therapy. None of the three patients with *Staph. epidermidis* endocarditis were cured; one patient succumbed to the infection. These data suggest that teicoplanin may be effective in the treatment of gram-positive endocarditis, but concomitant therapy with aminoglycosides or rifampin may be required.

Teicoplanin has been evaluated in immunocompromised hosts in a prospective randomized trial for acute febrile episodes in leukemic patients.[84] Twenty-two patients were randomized to receive teicoplanin in combination with amikacin and ceftazidime, and 25 patients were treated with amikacin and ceftazidime only. Overall improvement rates were not significantly different; however, the sample size was small, and a trend favoring the teicoplanin group did exist (82% versus 56%). Analysis of patients by degree of neutropenia showed no significant difference between the two treatment regimens, but the most severely neutropenic patients showed an 83% rate of improvement with teicoplanin compared with 30% with standard therapy. Bacteremic patients receiving teicoplanin demonstrated an 89% improvement rate compared with 57% for conventional therapy; however, this difference was not significant. Webster et al.[85] also evaluated teicoplanin therapy in the immunocompromised host. Teicoplanin was found to be effective in the treatment of Hickman-catheter-related infections, with all 16 patients being able to retain the catheter after treatment.

Use of teicoplanin for the treatment of ventriculoperitoneal and external ventricular shunt infections caused by methicillin-susceptible *Staph. aureus* and methicillin-resistant *Staph. epidermidis* has produced promising results in three patients.[86] Teicoplanin was given by either the intravenous or intraventricular route. Intraventricular administration of 20 mg/day was well tolerated and produced mean CSF concentrations of 26.4 mg/L. All patients were cured with teicoplanin therapy either alone or in combination with antibiotics.

The prophylactic utility of teicoplanin has been evaluated in a small number of trials for prevention of bacteremia after dental procedures and prevention of sternal and leg wound infections after cardiac surgery.[87-89] The two evaluations of effectiveness in decreasing the number of bacteremic episodes after dental procedures produced different results.[87,88]

In patients undergoing cardiac surgery, teicoplanin was evaluated against a combination of flucloxacillin and tobramycin for prevention of infections in sternal and leg wounds.[89] The trial was ongoing at the time of this report, with 195 patients evaluated thus far. The dose of teicoplanin used was 400 mg intravenously at the induction of anesthesia and 200 mg 24 hours later. Flucloxacillin 500 mg (as the sodium salt) and tobramycin 1.5 mg/kg (as the sulfate salt) were given at the induction of anesthesia and every eight hours for five days. No significant differences between the two treatment regimens exist at this time. Superinfections, appearing as gram-negative urinary-tract infections, were more common in the teicoplanin treatment group.

No published trials have evaluated the use of teicoplanin for the treatment of infections caused by anaerobic gram-positive cocci, including pseudomembranous colitis caused by *Clostridium difficile*.

Adverse Reactions

Animal and In Vitro Data. Evaluations of vestibular and cochlear ototoxicity using a guinea pig model have yielded conflicting results.[90,91] Cazals et al.[90] found teicoplanin to be a vestibular and cochlear toxin at doses of 90 mg/kg/day, while Brummett et al.[91] found no evidence of ototoxicity using a dose of 75 mg/kg/day. Teicoplanin showed evidence of nephrotoxicity when given to rats in doses of 40 mg/kg/day for one month.[92] No published information is available on the type of nephrotoxicity or methodologies used in these reports. Teicoplanin was shown to inhibit in vitro platelet function only at very high serum concentrations (5,000–10,000 mg/L).[93,94]

Clinical Trials. Teicoplanin has been administered to a total of 294 patients in clinical trials.[78–86] Development of a maculopapular rash, which occurred in six patients, was the most common adverse reaction. No infusion-related reactions resembling the vancomycin "red-neck" or "red-man" syndrome have been reported.[80,82]

Eosinophilia in association with formation of a maculopapular rash has been noted in five patients.[78,82] Pauluzzi et al.[80] noted bronchospasm in two patients experiencing anaphylaxis-like reactions. Evidence of cross-sensitivity between teicoplanin and vancomycin is controversial. One patient has been reported to demonstrate cross-sensitivity between vancomycin and teicoplanin, with rash and other symptoms of an allergic reaction to vancomycin occurring when the patient subsequently received teicoplanin.[95] However, other recent reports suggest that patients may be successfully treated with teicoplanin despite vancomycin allergy.[a,96]

Pain at the site of intramuscular injection (four patients), mild thrombophlebitis (two patients), and pruritus (one patient) have been reported.[78,80,82] Teicoplanin has been reported to cause reversible neutropenia in two patients.[79,80] One report of the production of circulating inhibitor to factor VIII is noted in the literature, but the patient also had other possible causes, including staphylococcal septicemia.[97] Elevation of aminotransferase values to three to five times baseline has been noted in five patients receiving teicoplanin; values returned to normal upon cessation of therapy.[82,85]

There are three reports in the current literature of possible teicoplanin-associated ototoxicity.[82,83,98] A 39-year-old patient with Down's syndrome developed asymptomatic high-frequency hearing loss that did not improve with the discontinuation of teicoplanin. This patient may have been more susceptible to the ototoxic effects of teicoplanin because premature neuronal aging is common in adults with Down's syndrome.[98] The second report involved a patient who showed evidence of nonreversible vestibular toxicity after 59 days of intravenous teicoplanin therapy. This patient also received gentamicin concomitantly. The third patient with potential ototoxicity had received 3 g of teicoplanin over a seven-day period.

Nephrotoxicity has been reported to occur in 5% of patients treated with vancomycin alone and in up to 35% of patients receiving vancomycin plus an aminoglycoside.[99] Nephrotoxicity has not been reported to date in any clinical trial with teicoplanin. The number of patients treated is too small to allow comparison of the incidence of adverse reactions to teicoplanin or vancomycin.

Because of limited patient exposure and the fact that many patients treated with teicoplanin were not receiving concomitant medications, little information is currently available regarding drug-drug interactions with teicoplanin. An in vitro evaluation of the effect of cholestyramine on the antimicrobial activity of vancomycin and teicoplanin found that almost 100% of teicoplanin was bound to cholestyramine.[36]

Dosage and Administration

Teicoplanin is still an investigational drug and is available only in experimental protocols or on a compassionate-use basis. The manufacturing, testing, and marketing of this product in the United States is done by Merrell Dow Pharmaceuticals. Expected date of release is not known at this time. Teicoplanin has been used in many varied dosing regimens; however, the most effective regimen has not been determined. Early reports of possibly inadequate or variable serum concentrations provided by a dosage regimen including a 400-mg loading dose, followed by 200 mg every 24 hours, prompted a change in dosage regimens used in experimental protocols.[60,79] The dosage regimen currently used in investigations for patients with systemic infections and normal renal function is 6 mg/kg every 12 hours for three doses, then 6 mg/kg every 24 hours. The investigational dose for patients with endocarditis has been increased to 15 mg/kg twice daily.[a]

The drug can be administered safely by either intramuscular or intravenous routes. Teicoplanin has been infused intravenously over five minutes without adverse reactions; however, most trials used 30-minute infusions. Therapeutic serum drug concentrations and adequate dosing regimens for patients with renal disease are not clearly established. One investigator recommended the usual loading doses, followed by 6 mg/kg every 48 hours for moderate renal impairment and 6 mg/kg every 72 hours for patients with severe renal impairment.[58]

Conclusion

Teicoplanin is a new glycopeptide antibiotic, similar to vancomycin, with a spectrum of activity encompassing a wide variety of gram-positive microorganisms. Teicoplanin's unique structure allows for approximately 90% absorption after intramuscular administration; the drug can also be given safely via intravenous bolus administration. Teicoplanin is thus easy to administer in patients with limited venous access or in outpatients and can be prepared and administered inexpensively.

The toxicity profile of teicoplanin is similar to that of vancomycin; however, relative incidence rates cannot be compared at this time. While the extended half-life of teicoplanin may offer advantages in administration, the management of adverse effects may be complicated by this factor.

Teicoplanin is a potent antibiotic; however, an adequate dosing regimen and therapeutic serum concentrations need to be more clearly identified. Although most open clinical trials have found overall favorable outcome rates, which are similar to those reported for vancomycin, conflicting results have also been reported, with one trial requiring early termination because of unfavorable outcomes. An erratic serum concentration profile coupled with a high degree of protein binding may account for these findings. Another discouraging finding is the reports of resistant coagulase-negative staphylococci, namely *Staph. haemolyticus*, despite rather limited clinical use of this agent.

Possible uses of teicoplanin in the future are still unclear. Teicoplanin's efficacy in the treatment of pseudomembranous colitis caused by *Clostridium difficile* remains to be explored, but in vitro data are promising, as evidenced by relatively lower MICs and higher stool concentrations than are found with vancomycin. Teicoplanin may provide an easily administered alternative in surgical and dental prophylaxis, offering the advantage of sustained serum concentrations after a one-time dose. The place of teicoplanin in the treatment of systemic gram-positive infections with respect to other antibiotics, including vancomycin, awaits the results of comparative clinical trials.

[a] Rios I, Merrell Dow Research Institute. Written communication. 1988 May 11.

References

1. Sheagren JN. *Staphylococcus aureus:* the persistent pathogen. *N Engl J Med.* 1984; 310:1368–73, 1437–42.
2. Blum RA, Rodvold KA. Recognition and importance of *Staphylococcus epidermidis. Clin Pharm.* 1987; 6:464–75.
3. Hunt AH, Molloy RM, Occolowitz JL et al. Structure of the major glycopeptide of the teicoplanin complex. *J Am Chem Soc.* 1984; 106:4891–95.
4. Parenti FG, Beretta G, Berti M et al. Teichomycins, new antibiotics from *Actinoplanes teichomyceticus* nov. sp. I. Description of the producer strain, fermentation studies and biological properties. *J Antibiot.* 1978; 31:276–83.
5. Bardone MR, Paternoster M, Coronelli C. Teichomycins, new antibiotics from *Actinoplanes teichomyceticus* nov. sp. II. Extraction and chemical characterization. *J Antibiot.* 1978; 31:170–7.
6. Borghi A, Coronelli C, Faniuolo L et al. Teichomycins, new antibiotics from *Actinoplanes teichomyceticus* nov. sp. IV. Separation and characterization of the components of teichomycin (teicoplanin). *J Antibiot.* 1984; 37:615–20.
7. Barna JC, Williams DH, Stone DJ et al. Structure elucidation of the teicoplanin antibiotics. *J Am Chem Soc.* 1984; 106:4895–902.
8. Barna JC, Williams DH, Strazzolini P et al. Structure and conformation of epimers derived from the antibiotic teicoplanin. *J Antibiot.* 1984; 37:1204–8.
9. Parenti F. Structure and mechanism of action of teicoplanin. *J Hosp Infect.* 1986; 7(Suppl A):79–83.
10. Somma S, Gastaldo L, Corti A. Teicoplanin, a new antibiotic from *Actinoplanes teichomyceticus* nov. sp. *Antimicrob Agents Chemother.* 1984; 26:917–23.
11. Peters G, Pulverer G. Antibacterial activity of teichomycin, a new glycopeptide antibiotic, in comparison to vancomycin. *J Antimicrob Chemother.* 1983; 11:94–5.
12. Cynamon MH, Granato PA. Comparison of the in vitro activities of teichomycin A_2 and vancomycin against staphylococci and enterococci. *Antimicrob Agents Chemother.* 1982; 21:504–5.
13. Fainstein V, LeBlanc B, Bodey GP. Comparative in vivo study of teichomycin A_2. *Antimicrob Agents Chemother.* 1983; 23:497–9.
14. Gruneberg RN, Ridgway GL, Cremer AWF et al. The sensitivity of gram-positive pathogens to teichomycin and vancomycin. *Drugs Exp Clin Res.* 1983; 9:139–41.
15. Neu HC, Labthavikul P. In vitro activity of teichomycin compared with those of other antibiotics. *Antimicrob Agents Chemother.* 1983; 24:425–8.
16. Pallanza R, Berti M, Goldstein BP et al. Teichomycin in-vitro and in-vivo evaluation in comparison with other antibiotics. *J Antimicrob Chemother.* 1983; 11:419–25.
17. Guenthner SH, Wenzel RP. In vitro activities of teichomycin, fusidic acid, flucloxacillin, fosfomycin, and vancomycin against methicillin-resistant *Staphylococcus aureus. Antimicrob Agents Chemother.* 1984; 26:268-9.
18. Dixson S, Brumfitt W, Hamilton-Miller JMT. In vitro activity of six antibiotics against multiresistant staphylococci and other gram-positive cocci. *Eur J Clin Microbiol.* 1985; 4:19–23.
19. Dixson S, Brumfitt W, Hamilton-Miller JMT. In vitro activity of combinations of antibiotics against *Staphylococcus aureus* resistant to gentamicin and methicillin. *Infection.* 1985; 13:35–46.
20. Moorhouse EC, Mulvihill TE, Jones L et al. The in-vitro activity of some antimicrobial agents against methicillin-resistant *Staphylococcus aureus. J Antimicrob Chemother.* 1985; 15:291–5.
21. Bauernfeind A, Petermuller C. In vitro activity of teicomy-

cin A_2 in comparison with penicillin and vancomycin against gram-positive cocci. *Eur J Clin Microbiol.* 1982; 1:278–81.
22. Fietta A, Bersani C, Mangiarotti P et al. In vitro activity of teichomycin against isolates of gram-positive bacteria. *Chemotherapy.* 1983; 29:275–82.
23. Greenwood D, Bidgood K, Turner M. A comparison of the responses of staphylococci and streptococci to teicoplanin and vancomycin. *J Antimicrob Chemother.* 1987; 20:155–64.
24. Barry AL, Jones RN, Gavan TL et al. Quality control limits for teicoplanin susceptibility tests and confirmation of disk diffusion interpretive criteria. *J Clin Microbiol.* 1987; 25:1812–14.
25. Barry AL, Thornsberry C, Jones RN. Evaluation of teicoplanin and vancomycin disk susceptibility tests. *J Clin Microbiol.* 1986; 23:100–3.
26. Berti M, Pallanza R, Arioli V. In vitro and in vivo activity of teicoplanin against multiply-resistant staphylococci. In: Mitsuhashi S, Krcmery V, eds. Transferable antibiotic resistance plasmid and gene, gene manipulation. New York: Springer-Verlag; 1984:69–73.
27. Aldridge KE, Janney A, Sanders CV. Comparison of the activities of coumermycin, ciprofloxacin, teicoplanin and other non-B-lactam antibiotics against clinical isolates of methicillin-resistant *Staphylococcus aureus* from various geographical locations. *Antimicrob Agents Chemother.* 1985; 28:634–8.
28. Wilson APR, O'Hare MD, Felmingham D et al. Teicoplanin-resistant coagulase-negative staphylococcus. *Lancet.* 1986; 2:973. Letter.
29. Arioli V, Pallanza R. Teicoplanin-resistant coagulase-negative staphylococci. *Lancet.* 1987; 1:39. Letter.
30. Grant AC, Lacey RW, Brownjohn AM et al. Teicoplanin-resistant coagulase-negative staphylococcus. *Lancet.* 1986; 2:1166–7. Letter.
31. Varaldo PE, Schito GC. Teichomycin A_2, in vitro antibacterial activity against streptococci and staphylococci and comparison with vancomycin. *Drugs Exp Clin Res.* 1983; 9:437–40.
32. Chandrasekar PH, Price S, Levine DP. In-vitro evaluation of cifpirome (HR 810), teicoplanin and four other antimicrobials against enterococci. *J Antimicrob Chemother.* 1985; 16:179–82.
33. Tuazon CU, Miller H. Comparative in vitro activities of teichomycin and vancomycin alone and in combination with rifampin and aminoglycosides against staphylococci and enterococci. *Antimicrob Agents Chemother.* 1984; 25:411–2.
34. Jadeja L, Fainstein V, LeBlanc B et al. Comparative in vivo activities of teichomycin and other antibiotics against JK diphtheroids. *Antimicrob Agents Chemother.* 1983; 24:145–6.
35. Glupczynski Y, Labbe M, Crokaert F et al. In vitro activity of teicoplanin and vancomycin against anaerobes. *Eur J Clin Microbiol.* 1984; 3:50–1.
36. Pantosti A, Luzzi I, Cardines R et al. Comparison of the in vitro activities of teicoplanin and vancomycin against *Clostridium difficile* and their interactions with cholestyramine. *Antimicrob Agents Chemother.* 1985; 28:847–8.
37. Traub WH, Karthein J, Spohr M. Susceptibility of *Clostridium perfringens* type A to 23 antimicrobial drugs. *Chemotherapy.* 1986; 32:439–45.
38. Klastersky J, Van der Auwera P. Cephalosporins, vancomycin, aminoglycosides and other drugs especially in combination, for the treatment of methicillin-resistant staphylococcal infections. *J Antimicrob Chemother.* 1986; 17(Suppl A):19–24.
39. Varaldo PE, Debbia E, Schito GC. In vitro activity of teichomycin and vancomycin alone and in combination with rifampin. *Antimicrob Agents Chemother.* 1983; 23:402–6.
40. Dixon S, Brumfitt W, Hamilton-Miller JMT. Activity of rifampicin against staphylococci, with special reference to multiresistant strains. *J Antimicrob Chemother.* 1984; 13(Suppl C):7–16.
41. Chen HY, Williams JD. The activity of vancomycin and teicoplanin alone and in combination with gentamicin or ampicillin against *Streptococcus faecalis. Eur J Clin Microbiol.* 1984; 3:436–8.
42. Varaldo PE, Debbia E, Schito GC. In vitro activities of rifapentine and rifampin, alone and in combination with six other antibiotics, against methicillin-susceptible and methicillin-resistant staphylococci of different species. *Antimicrob Agents Chemother.* 1985; 27:615–8.
43. Hackbarth CJ, Chambers HF, Sande MA. Serum bactericidal activity of rifampin in combination with other antimicrobial agents against *Staphylococcus aureus. Antimicrob Agents Chemother.* 1986; 29:611–3.
44. Debbia E, Varaldo P, Schito GC. In vitro activity of imipenem against enterococci and staphylococci and evidence for high rates of synergism with teicoplanin, fosfomycin, and rifampin. *Antimicrob Agents Chemother.* 1986; 30:813–5.
45. Debbia E, Pesce A, Schito GC. In vitro interactions between teicoplanin and other antibiotics against enterococci and staphylococci. *J Hosp Infect.* 1986; 7(Suppl A):73–7.
46. Watanakunakorn C. In-vitro activity of teicoplanin alone and in combination with rifampicin, gentamicin or tobramycin against coagulase-negative staphylococci. *J Antimicrob Chemother.* 1987; 19:439–43.
47. Barr V, Barr K, Millar MR et al. Beta-lactam antibiotics increase the frequency of plasmid transfer in *Staphylococcus aureus. J Antimicrob Chemother.* 1986; 17:409–13.
48. Schwalbe RS, Stapleton JT, Gilligan PH. Emergence of vancomycin resistance in coagulase-negative staphylococci. *N Engl J Med.* 1987; 316:927–31.
49. Brumfitt W, Hamilton-Miller JMT. Activity of teicoplanin against coagulase-negative staphylococci isolated from patients undergoing continuous peritoneal dialysis. *Eur J Clin Microbiol.* 1986; 5:48–9.
50. Bernareggi A. Cavenaghi L, Assandri A. Pharmacokinetics of ^{14}C-teicoplanin in male rats after single intravenous dose. *Antimicrob Agents Chemother.* 1986; 30:733–8.
51. Marre R. Teicoplanin renal toxicity and pharmacokinetics in a rat model. *J Antimicrob Chemother.* 1987; 20:697–701.
52. Traina GL, Bonati M. Pharmacokinetics of teichoplanin in man after intravenous administration. *J Pharmacokinet Biopharm.* 1984; 12:119–128.
53. Verbist L, Tjandramaga B, Hendrickx B et al. In vitro activity and human pharmacokinetics of teicoplanin. *Antimicrob Agents Chemother.* 1984; 26:881–6.
54. McNulty CM, Garden GM, Wise R et al. The pharmacokinetics and tissue penetration of teicoplanin. *J Antimicrob Chemother.* 1985; 16:743–9.
55. Lagast H, Dodion P, Klastersky J. Comparison of pharmacokinetics and bactericidal activity of teicoplanin and vancomycin. *J Antimicrob Chemother.* 1986; 18:513–20.
56. Wise R, Donovan IA, McNulty AM et al. Teicoplanin, its pharmacokinetics, blister and peritoneal fluid penetration. *J Hosp Infect.* 1986; 7(Suppl A):47–55.
57. Traina GL, Gentile MG, Fellin G et al. Pharmacokinetics of teicoplanin in patients on continuous ambulatory peritoneal dialysis. *Eur J Clin Pharmacol.* 1986; 31:501–4.
58. Bonati M, Traina GL, Villa G et al. Teicoplanin pharmacokinetics in patients with chronic renal failure. *Clin Pharmacokinet.* 1987; 12:292–301.
59. Domart Y, Pierre C, Clair B et al. Pharmacokinetics of teicoplanin in critically ill patients with various degrees of renal impairment. *Antimicrob Agents Chemother.* 1987; 31:1600–4.
60. Falcoz C, Ferry N, Pozet N et al. Pharmacokinetics of teicoplanin in renal failure. *Antimicrob Agents Chemother.* 1987; 31:1255–62.
61. Rodvold KA, Blum RA, Fischer JH et al. Vancomycin pharmacokinetics in patients with various degrees of renal function. *Antimicrob Agents Chemother.* 1988; 32:848–52.
62. Joos B, Luthy R. Determination of teicoplanin concentrations in serum by high-pressure liquid chromatography. *Antimicrob Agents Chemother.* 1987; 31:1222–24.
63. Levy J, Truong BL, Goignau H et al. High pressure liquid

chromatographic quantitation of teicoplanin in human serum. *J Antimicrob Chemother.* 1987; 19:533–9.
64. Corti A, Rurali C, Borghi A et al. Solid-phase enzyme-receptor assay (SPERA): a competitive-binding assay for glycopeptide antibiotics of the vancomycin class. *Clin Chem.* 1985; 31:1606–10.
65. Cavenaghi L, Corti A, Cassani G. Comparison of the solid phase enzyme receptor assay (SPERA) and the microbiological assay for teicoplanin. *J Hosp Infect.* 1986; 7(Suppl A):85–9.
66. Corti A, Cavenaghi L, Giani E, et al. A receptor-antibody sandwich assay for teicoplanin. *Clin Chem.* 1987; 33:1615–8.
67. Assandri A, Bernareggi A. Binding of teicoplanin to human serum albumin. *Eur J Clin Pharmacol.* 1987; 33:191–5.
68. Stahl JP, Croize J, Wolff M et al. Poor penetration of teicoplanin into cerebrospinal fluid in patients with bacterial meningitis. *J Antimicrob Chemother.* 1987; 20:141–2. Letter.
69. Pascual A, Tsukayama D, Kovarik J et al. Uptake and activity of rifapentine in human peritoneal macrophages and polymorphonuclear leukocytes. *Eur J Clin Microbiol.* 1987; 6:152–7.
70. Carver P, Nightingale CH, Quintiliani R. Single and multiple dose pharmacokinetics. Abstract presented to 26th Interscience Conference on Antimicrobial Agents and Chemotherapy. New Orleans, LA: 1986 Oct 1.
71. Carper HT, Sullivan GW, Mandell GL. Teicoplanin, vancomycin, rifampicin: in-vivo and in-vitro studies with *Staphylococcus aureus. J Antimicrob Chemother.* 1987; 19:659–62.
72. Chambers HF, Sande MA. Teicoplanin versus nafcillin and vancomycin in the treatment of experimental endocarditis caused by methicillin-susceptible or resistant *Staphylococcus aureus. Antimicrob Agents Chemother.* 1984; 26:61–4.
73. Arioli V, Berti M, Candiani G. Activity of teicoplanin in localized experimental infections in rats. *J Hosp Infect.* 1986; 7(Suppl A):91–9.
74. Tuazon CU, Washburn D. Teicoplanin and rifampicin singly and in combination in the treatment of experimental *Staphylococcus epidermidis* endocarditis in the rabbit model. *J Antimicrob Chemother.* 1987; 20:233–7.
75. Galetto DW, Boscia JA, Kobasa WD et al. Teicoplanin compared with vancomycin for treatment of experimental endocarditis due to methicillin-resistant *Staphylococcus epidermidis. J Infect Dis.* 1986; 154:69–75.
76. Sullam PM, Tauber MG, Hackbarth CJ et al. Therapeutic efficacy of teicoplanin in experimental enterococcal endocarditis. *Antimicrob Agents Chemother.* 1985; 27:135–6.
77. Norden CW, Niederreiter K, Shinners EM. Treatment of experimental chronic osteomyelitis due to *Staphylococcus aureus* with teicoplanin. *Infection.* 1986; 14:136–8.
78. Glupczynski Y, Lagast H, Van Der Auwera P et al. Clinical evaluation of teicoplanin for therapy of severe infections caused by gram-positive bacteria. *Antimicrob Agents Chemother.* 1986; 29:52–7.
79. Calain P, Krause KH, Vaudaux P et al. Early termination of a prospective, randomized trial comparing teicoplanin and flucloxacillin for treating severe staphylococcal infections. *J Infect Dis.* 1987; 155:187–91.
80. Pauluzzi S, Del Favero A, Menichetti F et al. Treatment of infections by staphylococci and other gram-positive bacteria with teicoplanin: an open study. *J Antimicrob Chemother.* 1987; 20:431–8.
81. Williams AH, Gruneberg RN, Webster A et al. Teicoplanin in the treatment of infections caused by gram-positive organisms. *J Hosp Infect.* 1986; 7(Suppl A):101–4.
82. Bibler MR, Frame PT, Hagler DN et al. Clinical evaluation of efficacy, pharmacokinetics, and safety of teicoplanin for serious gram-positive infections. *Antimicrob Agents Chemother.* 1987; 31:207–12.
83. Webster A, Wilson AR, Williams AH et al. The use of a new glycopeptide antibiotic, teicoplanin, in the treatment of bacterial endocarditis. *Postgrad Med J.* 1987; 63:621–4.
84. Del Favero A, Menichetti F, Guerciolini R et al. Prospective randomized clinical trial of teicoplanin for empiric combined antibiotic therapy in febrile, granulocytopenic acute leukemia patients. *Antimicrob Agents Chemother.* 1987; 31:1126–9.
85. Webster A, Russell SJ, Souhami RL et al. Use of teicoplanin for Hickman catheter associated staphylococcal infection in immunosuppressed patients. *J Hosp Infect.* 1987; 10:77–82.
86. Masserati R, Cruciani M, Azzini M et al. Teicoplanin in the therapy of staphylococcal neuroshunt infections. *Int J Clin Pharm Res.* 1987; 7:207–13.
87. Maskell JP, Carter JLB, Boyd RB et al. Teicoplanin as a prophylactic antibiotic for dental bacteraemia. *J Antimicrob Chemother.* 1986; 17:651–9.
88. Shanson DC, Shehata A, Tadayon M et al. Comparison of intravenous teicoplanin with intramuscular amoxycillin for the prophylaxis of streptococcal bacteraemia in dental patients. *J Antimicrob Chemother.* 1987; 20:85–93.
89. Wilson AR, Gruneberg RN, Treasure T et al. A clinical trial of teicoplanin compared with a combination of flucloxacillin and tobramycin as antibiotic prophylaxis for cardiac surgery: the use of a scoring method to assess the incidence of wound infection. *J Hosp Infect.* 1986; 7(Suppl A):105–12.
90. Cazals Y, Erre JP, Aurousseau C et al. Ototoxicity of teicoplanin in the guinea pig. *Br J Audiol.* 1987; 21:27–30.
91. Brummett RE, Fox KE, Warchol M et al. Absence of ototoxicity of teichomycin A_2 in guinea pigs. *Antimicrob Agents Chemother.* 1987; 31:612–3.
92. Williams AH, Gruneberg RN. Teicoplanin. *J Antimicrob Chemother.* 1984; 14:441–8.
93. Porta M, Ricchetti I. A study of the possible interactions between human platelets and the antibiotic MDL-507 (teicoplanin). *Int J Clin Pharmacol Ther Toxicol.* 1986; 24:661–4.
94. Agnelli G, Longetti M, Guerciolini R et al. Effects of the new glycopeptide antibiotic teicoplanin on platelet function and blood coagulation. *Antimicrob Agents Chemother.* 1987; 31:1609–12.
95. McElrath MJ, Goldberg D, Neu HC. Allergic cross-reactivity of teicoplanin and vancomycin. *Lancet.* 1986; 1:47. Letter.
96. Schlemmer B, Falkman H, Boudjadja A et al. Teicoplanin for patients allergic to vancomycin. *N Engl J Med.* 1988; 318:1127–28. Letter.
97. Legrand JC, Van Der Auwera P, Bailly A et al. Circulating inhibitor of factor VIII during treatment with teicoplanin and rifampicin. *J Antimicrob Chemother.* 1987; 19:850–2. Letter.
98. Maher ER, Hollman A, Gruneberg RN. Teicoplanin-induced ototoxicity in Down's syndrome. *Lancet.* 1986; 1:613. Letter.
99. Farber BF, Moellering RC. Retrospective study of the toxicity of preparations of vancomycin from 1974 to 1981. *Antimicrob Agents Chemother.* 1983; 23:138–41.

Lisinopril: A nonsulfhydryl angiotensin-converting enzyme inhibitor

TERESA A. NOBLE AND KIM M. MURRAY

Abstract: The chemistry, pharmacology, pharmacokinetics, clinical use, adverse effects, and dosage of lisinopril are reviewed.

Lisinopril, a new nonsulfhydryl angiotensin-converting-enzyme (ACE) inhibitor, is absorbed in its active form. Like the other ACE inhibitors, it lowers peripheral vascular resistance, with a resultant decrease in blood pressure. Approximately 29% of lisinopril is absorbed after oral administration. No measurable metabolism occurs, and excretion is primarily renal. Accumulation of lisinopril occurs in patients with renal dysfunction; however, dosage adjustment is necessary only when the creatinine clearance is less than 30 mL/min. Lisinopril has been shown to be an effective antihypertensive agent at doses of 10 to 80 mg given once daily in patients with essential and secondary hypertension caused by renal artery stenosis. The effectiveness of lisinopril is comparable to that with diuretics, β blockers, and calcium-channel antagonists. In patients who are unresponsive to maximal doses of lisinopril alone, addition of another antihypertensive agent may be beneficial. Limited information suggests that lisinopril may be comparable to captopril for the treatment of congestive heart failure. Adverse effects associated with lisinopril are relatively minor and are comparable to those associated with enalapril. Hematological abnormalities have not been reported with lisinopril. Class-related adverse effects include cough, azotemia, angioedema, hypotension, and hyperkalemia.

Lisinopril appears to be comparable to other ACE inhibitors for the treatment of hypertension and may be as effective as its predecessors for the treatment of congestive heart failure. Further study is needed to better define a therapeutic niche for lisinopril.

Index terms: Dosage; Hypotensive agents; Lisinopril; Pharmacokinetics; Toxicity
Clin Pharm. 1988; 7:659–69

Lisinopril (MK-521) received approval from the Food and Drug Administration for the treatment of hypertension in December 1987 and was marketed in January 1988 under a joint marketing agreement with Merck Sharp & Dohme (Prinivil) and Stuart Pharmaceuticals (Zestril). Lisinopril is the latest of the oral angiotensin-converting-enzyme (ACE) inhibitors approved in the United States. Captopril (Capoten, E.R. Squibb & Sons), marketed in 1980, was the first ACE inhibitor for the treatment of hypertension. It was labeled in 1981 for the treatment of congestive heart failure. Enalapril maleate (Vasotec, Merck Sharp & Dohme), marketed in 1985, was the next ACE inhibitor for the treatment of hypertension. It was labeled for the treatment of congestive heart failure in June 1988. The purpose of this paper is to review current available literature regarding the pharmacology and proposed therapeutic uses of lisinopril and to compare lisinopril with the other available oral ACE inhibitors to assist practitioners in rational drug selection.

Chemistry

The chemical name for lisinopril is N^2-(1-carboxy-3-phenylpropyl)-L-lysyl-L-proline.[1] The structures of lisinopril, enalaprilic acid, enalaprilat, and captopril are shown in Figure 1.[1,2] Lisinopril and enalapril were developed without the sulfhydryl moiety in an attempt to eliminate certain adverse reactions—disturbance of taste perception, rash, oral mucosal ulcers, and proteinuria caused by immune-complex membranous glomerulopathy—associated with captopril.[3] These adverse reactions were thought to be related to the sulfhydryl moiety of captopril but more recently have been associated with nonsulfhydryl ACE inhibitors. Enalapril is a prodrug that is converted by ester hydrolysis to enalaprilat, a potent ACE inhibitor. Lisinopril is a lysine analog of enalaprilat. It is absorbed in the active form and does not require metabolic activation for activity.[2]

Pharmacology

ACE Inhibition. The activity of angiotensin-converting enzyme is markedly reduced during therapy with lisinopril, resulting in decreased formation of angiotensin II from angiotensin I.[4] In 12 healthy adult male volunteers, the plasma convert-

TERESA A. NOBLE, PHARM.D., is Assistant Professor and Director of the Drug Information Service, College of Pharmacy, University of South Carolina (USC), Columbia. KIM M. MURRAY, PHARM.D., is Assistant Professor, College of Pharmacy, and Adjunct Assistant Professor, School of Medicine, USC, and Clinical Faculty in Internal Medicine, Richland Memorial Hospital, Columbia, SC.

Address reprint requests to Dr. Noble at the College of Pharmacy, University of South Carolina, Columbia, SC 29208.

Copyright © 1988, American Society of Hospital Pharmacists, Inc. All rights reserved. 0278-2677/88/0901-0659$02.50.

ing-enzyme activity was decreased 4–10 hours after the oral administration of 10 mg of enalapril and 10 mg of lisinopril. Similarly, in patients with hypertension and congestive heart failure, plasma converting-enzyme activity and angiotensin II decreased,[5,6] and plasma renin activity and angiotensin I increased.[6,7] Accumulated angiotensin I has been attributed to the rise in renin activity rather than to decreased conversion of angiotensin I to angiotensin II[8] (Figure 2).

Cardiovascular Effects. ACE inhibitors are used in the treatment of hypertension and congestive heart failure because they inhibit the renin–angiotensin system. Short-term administration of lisinopril to normotensive volunteers,[9] hypertensive patients,[5] and patients with congestive heart failure[6] resulted in a maximal decrease in diastolic blood pressure of 10% (lisinopril 10 mg), 13% (lisinopril 5–20 mg), and 17.5% (lisinopril 1.25–10 mg), respectively. During short-term therapy (four to eight days), doses beyond 5 mg were not associated with an increased hypotensive effect but were associated with an increased duration of antihypertensive activity.[6] Heart rate was not affected with short-term administration of lisinopril.[5,6,9] Limited information regarding the long-term use of lisinopril suggests that the blood-pressure-lowering effects were maintained in patients who received lisinopril alone (14% reduction) and in combination with hydrochlorothiazide (17% reduction) over a 28-week open-label continuation of an evaluative antihypertension study.[10] However, during long-term therapy, a 9.3% reduction in heart rate was observed in patients who were treated with lisinopril alone. No change in heart rate was observed in the patients treated with combination therapy. In normotensive patients with congestive heart failure, lisinopril has been shown to decrease pulmonary capillary wedge pressure and systemic vascular resistance and increase cardiac output.[6]

Other Effects. Inhibition of angiotensin-converting enzyme, also known as kininase II, prevents the inactivation of bradykinin, a vasodilator.[11] The role of this inhibition by ACE inhibitors and the subsequent degree of the hypotensive effects attributable to bradykinins and prostaglandins is yet to be determined. It is known that indomethacin decreases the hypotensive effects of ACE inhibitors.[12,13] However, the exact mechanism of bradykinin and prostaglandin involvement with the pharmacological effects of ACE inhibition has not been fully elucidated (Figure 2).

The effects of ACE inhibitors on intrarenal hemodynamics have also been an area of investigation, specifically in progressive diabetic glomerular hyperfiltration.[14] Taguma et al.[15] studied the effects of ACE inhibition in azotemic diabetics and observed decreased proteinuria without appreciable changes in blood pressure or glucose. Although not substantiated by this study, the decreased proteinuria may be associated with an altered permeability of the glomerular capillary wall and changed intrarenal hemodynamics. Further inves-

Figure 1. Chemical structures of lisinopril, enalaprilic acid, enalaprilat, and captopril.

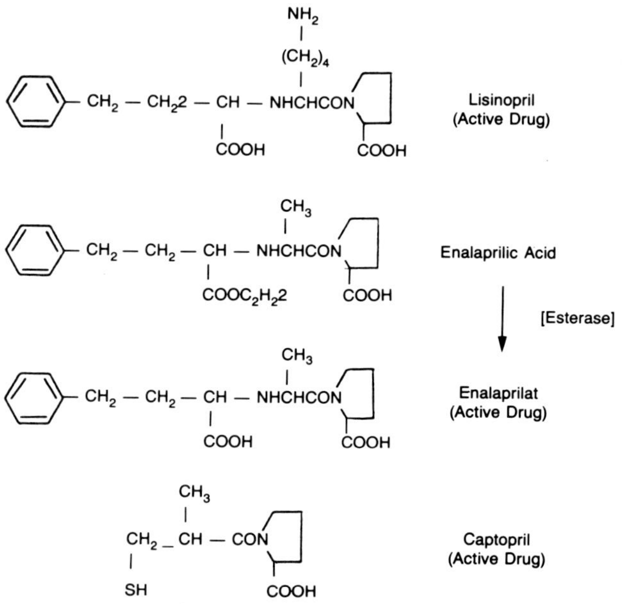

Figure 2. Representation of the renin–angiotensin–aldosterone and kallikrein–kinin–prostaglandin systems. Angiotensin, increased blood pressure, and increased intravascular volume exert negative effects on renin. The degree to which bradykinin affects prostaglandins has not been established.

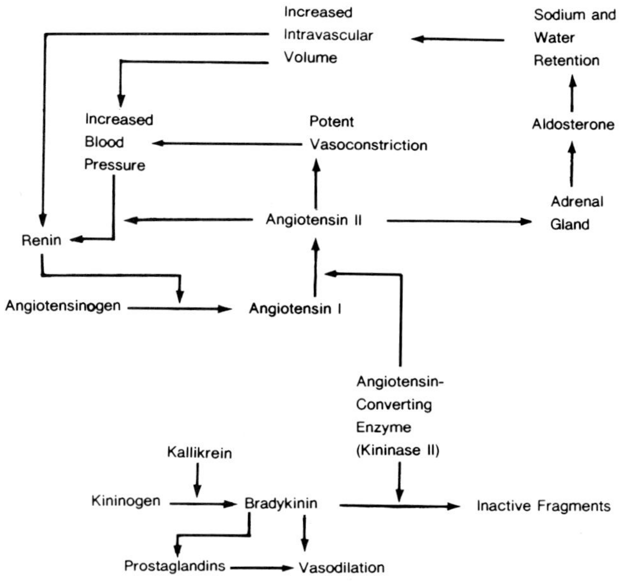

tigation is warranted to determine the clinical application of ACE inhibitors in diabetic patients with azotemia.

Pharmacokinetics

Assay Methods. Lisinopril concentrations have been measured in the serum, urine, and feces by a competitive inhibitor-binding assay (CIBA) estimation method,[16-18] a radioimmunoassay (RIA) method using antibodies to lisinopril harvested from rabbits,[16,19] and the fluorescent enzymatic method of Tocco et al.[20] The CIBA method is used to determine the relationship between serum ACE activity and serum lisinopril concentration. During long-term ACE inhibitor therapy, the production of ACE is induced, resulting in increased radioinhibitor binding and an altered activity–concentration relationship. Therefore, CIBA is limited to use in short-term experimental dosing situations; RIA may be preferred in evaluating long-term ACE inhibitor therapy.[16]

Lisinopril exhibits a concentration-dependent relationship between the ACE inhibitor concentrations and the serum ACE activity.[16,21] Maximum blockade is achieved at serum concentrations of 10 ng/mL. Apparently, no significant increase in ACE inhibition can be achieved at higher serum concentrations.[21] Serum samples may be frozen before the determination of the ACE inhibitor concentration.[18]

Absorption. Twelve healthy male volunteers received 10 mg (25 μmol) of lisinopril orally. Serum, urine, and fecal samples were collected at timed intervals after the dose.[22] The absorption of lisinopril was slow and incomplete in the subjects studied. The mean peak serum concentration was reported as 95 nM at six to eight hours after the dose. Approximately 98% of the dose administered was recovered.[22] Between 6% and 60% (mean 29%) was recovered as unchanged drug in the urine, and a mean of 69% was recovered as unchanged drug in the feces. In older patients the area under the concentration–time curve and serum concentrations are doubled; thus, the dosage may need to be adjusted.[23]

The influence of food on the extent and rate of absorption was studied in 18 healthy, normotensive subjects.[24] The subjects received a single 20-mg oral dose of lisinopril either in a fasting state or immediately after a standardized breakfast and were crossed over after a 14-day washout period. Timed blood and urine samples were collected after each dose was administered. No significant differences were found between the fasting and fed states. The area under the curve from time zero to 120 hours (AUC_{0-120}) was 1231 ± 620 ng · hr/mL in the fasting state and 1029 ± 254 ng · hr/mL in the fed state. The peak serum concentrations were 86 ± 48 ng/mL and 69 ± 19 ng/mL at 6.2 ± 1.1 hours and 6.8 ± 1.0 hours, respectively, for the fasting and fed states. The mean urinary recovery was 27.2 ± 15% for the fasting state and 25.7 ± 10% after the standardized breakfast. Therefore, lisinopril may be administered regardless of meals.

Distribution. Ajayi et al.[25] studied the pharmacokinetics of oral lisinopril using the nonlinear mixed effects model (NONMEM) computer program of Beal and Sheiner.[26] This program provided mean population parameter estimates using a one-compartment open model. The apparent volume of distribution (V) was derived using the relative bioavailability (F) since data on intravenous administration were not obtained. The mean V/F was 124 ± 16 L. Lisinopril does not appear to bind to plasma proteins other than ACE.[11] The clinical importance of the lack of protein binding is yet to be determined.

Metabolism and Excretion. Lisinopril undergoes no measurable metabolism.[22] In contrast, enalapril, a prodrug, is metabolized by esterolysis to enalaprilat, a potent ACE inhibitor,[27] and captopril is metabolized to form disulfide bonds with the sulfhydryl groups of endogenous compounds, including proteins.[28] Approximately 98% of unchanged lisinopril is recovered (29% in urine and 69% in feces) and 94% of enalapril and enalaprilat are recovered (61% in urine and 33% in feces).[22]

Lisinopril has a polyphasic elimination curve with a prolonged terminal phase and a terminal elimination half-life of approximately 30 hours.[22] During multiple dosing, lisinopril has an accumulation half-life of approximately 12 hours. After a 10-mg dose of either lisinopril or enalapril maleate in healthy volunteers, mean renal clearances were 106 ± 13 mL/min (lisinopril) and 158 ± 46 mL/min (clearance of enalaprilat after enalapril administration).[22]

Influence of Renal Disease. Lisinopril accumulation depends on the degree of renal insufficiency present.[29,30] In six patients with CL_{cr} < 30 mL/min, serum blood concentrations were significantly ($p <$ 0.01) higher at 24 and 96 hours than in nonrenally impaired patients after a single 5-mg oral dose of lisinopril.[29] The single-dose evaluation was followed by a seven-day study of lisinopril 5 mg administered daily. Lisinopril accumulated to a serum concentration 12-fold that of patients without renal dysfunction and sixfold that of patients with mild renal dysfunction (CL_{cr}, 30–60 mL/min). At 168 hours, ACE activity was inhibited by 60% in patients with severe renal impairment, 25% in patients with mild impairment, and only 5% in healthy subjects. Similar antihypertensive responses were observed regardless of renal function in this small open trial.[29] Donohoe et al.[30] studied the antihypertensive effects of lisinopril in 23 renally impaired patients (mean glomerular filtration rate = 38 ± 16.4 mL/min at baseline, 41 ± 21 mL/min at 12 weeks). Patients maintained a significant ($p < 0.001$) reduction in blood pressure (standing diastolic blood pressure, 106 ± 10.5 mm Hg at baseline, 89 ± 10.9 mm Hg at 12 weeks) on a mean daily dose of 10 mg of lisinopril (range, 2.5–40 mg). The manufacturer recommends that patients with moderate and severe renal impairment should initially receive 5 mg; patients on dialysis should receive 2.5 mg.[23]

Comparative Pharmacokinetics of Lisinopril, Enalapril, and Captopril. The pharmacokinetics of lisinopril, enalapril, and captopril are compared in Table 1. Captopril is the least potent ACE inhibitor and has less affinity for ACE.[31] Lisinopril and enalapril have similar potency and equal affinity for ACE[22] but have different bioavailabilities, approximately 29%[22] and 65%,[38] respectively. The equivalent dose of lisinopril is approximately twice that of enalapril. This should be considered when comparing the two agents. Lisinopril is given once daily and can be administered with food.[23] Enalapril can also be given with food[32,33] and is usually administered once or twice per day. Captopril is given two or three times per day on an empty stomach.[24,32] Lisinopril is eliminated unchanged in the urine (29%) and the feces (69%).[22] Enalapril and enalaprilat are eliminated in the urine (18% and 43%) and in the feces (6% and 27%), respectively.[22] Captopril and its metabolites are recovered to a larger degree in the urine (67.5%) and to a lesser degree in the feces (18.3%).[28]

Table 1.
Pharmacokinetics of Lisinopril, Enalapril, and Captopril

Variable	Lisinopril	Enalapril	Captopril
Absorption	Slow[22]	Rapid[22]	Rapid[31]
Time of peak serum conc (hr)	6–8[22]	0.5–1.5[22]	0.5–1.5[28,31,37]
Bioavailability (%) (F)	6–60[22]	53–74[32]	68–75[28,33]
Effect of food on F	None[23]	None[32,33]	Absorption decreased 30–40%[23,32]
Peak effect (hr)	6–8[22]	3–4[24,32]	1–1.5[32]
Active metabolite	None[24]	Enalaprilat[22]	None[32]
Time of peak serum conc of active metabolite (hr)	. . .	2.5–5.5[22]	. . .
Volume of distribution (V)	124 ± 16 L[25,a]	93 ± 12 L[25,a] (37.2, enalaprilat)[25]	0.7 L/kg[23,b]
Urinary excretion (% of dose)	29[22]	18, as enalapril[22] (43, as enalaprilat)[22]	67.5[28]
Renal clearance	6.36 L/hr[22]	9.48 L/hr[22] (enalaprilat)	0.72 L/kg · hr[34]
Serum half-life (hr)			
Healthy	12[23,c]	11[35]	2–3[35]
Renal dysfunction	. . .	. . .	3.5–32[36]

[a] Reported as V/F.
[b] Steady-state volume of distribution.
[c] A terminal half-life of 30 hours has been reported.[22]

Hypertension

Currently, the only FDA-labeled indication for lisinopril is hypertension. Clinical trials are summarized in Tables 2 and 3. The tables include studies of lisinopril alone and lisinopril in combination or in comparison with diuretics, β-adrenergic inhibitors, calcium-channel antagonists, and other ACE inhibitors. Few long-term evaluative studies are published, although results of long-term studies are expected. Limited information exists on the comparative effects of lisinopril and calcium-channel antagonists in animals[43] and humans.[27] Selected studies of lisinopril for the treatment of hypertension will be discussed.

Mild to Moderate Hypertension. The short-term effects of lisinopril have been studied in hypertensive patients in open trials over a period of one to eight weeks.[5,7] In an initial evaluation of lisinopril in hypertension, oral doses of 2.5–20 mg were studied.[5] All doses reduced standing diastolic blood pressure (SDBP) from baseline. The mean reduction was from 101 ± 7 mm Hg to 94 ± 7 mm Hg after 2.5 mg of lisinopril and from 101 ± 7 mm Hg to 88 ± 8 mm Hg after doses of 5 mg and greater. In a subsequent two-week open trial, SDBP was reduced at one hour to a maximal decrease at six hours after a 20-mg daily dose of lisinopril. On day 14 of therapy, the lisinopril group had a mean SDBP of 95 ± 10 mm Hg, which was significantly different from that associated with placebo at 106 ± 8 mm Hg ($p < 0.05$). The hypotensive effect was maintained over 24 hours.[7]

Lisinopril has also been compared with other antihypertensive therapies used alone and in combination. When lisinopril is administered as a single agent, blood pressure control is similar to that associated with hydrochlorothiazide[7,10,38] and nifedipine.[40] There has been some variability among studies with regard to the relative effects of various monotherapy regimens on systolic blood pressure (SBP). In preliminary results from a multicenter study ($n = 175$),[41] lisinopril caused a significantly ($p < 0.01$) larger decrease in SBP (−20 mm Hg) than metoprolol (−13 mm Hg). The authors did not indicate whether the systolic blood pressure measurements were taken with the patient standing or sitting. In a smaller ($n = 35$), poorly designed study with only black and Indian patients, both lisinopril and atenolol were found to reduce blood pressure. The report did not include a statistical analysis of the differences between lisinopril and atenolol with regard to systolic or diastolic blood pressure.[39] As expected, the overall antihypertensive effect of

Table 2.
Clinical Studies of Lisinopril in Patients with Mild to Moderate Essential Hypertension

Study	Study Design[a]	Daily Drug Dose[b]	Duration of Therapy (wk)	Mean BP Reduction (mm Hg)[c] SBP	DBP	% Patients Achieving DBP ≤ 90 mm Hg
Rotmensch et al.[5]	Open	L 2.5–20 mg ($n = 9$)	1	. . .	13	. . .
Rotmensch et al.[7]	Open	L 20 mg ($n = 10$)[d]	8	. . .	11[e,f]	. . .
		HCTZ 50 mg ($n = 10$)		. . .	11[e,f]	. . .
		L 20 mg plus HCTZ 50 mg ($n = 10$)		. . .	18[e]	. . .
Kochar et al.[10]	R, DB, parallel	L 20–80 mg ($n = 10$)	28	21[g]	15[g]	. . .
		HCTZ 12.5–50 mg ($n = 10$)		9[g]	13[g]	. . .
		L 20–80 mg plus HCTZ 12.5–50 mg ($n = 4$)		3[g]	14[g]	. . .
Pool[38]	R, DB, parallel	L 20–80 mg ($n = 162$)	24	16.6[h,i]	12.5[h,i]	82[j]
		HCTZ 12.5–50 mg ($n = 155$)		10.4[h,i]	6.8[h,i]	67[j]
		L 20–80 mg plus HCTZ 12.5–50 mg ($n = 74$)		23.9[h,i]	18.2[h,i]	84[j]
Seedat and Parag[39]	R, DB, parallel	L 20–80 mg ($n = 24$)	24	31[e]	18[e]	61
		A 50–200 mg ($n = 12$)		18[e]	11[e]	33

[a] R = randomized, DB = double blind.
[b] L = lisinopril, HCTZ = hydrochlorothiazide, A = atenolol.
[c] BP = blood pressure, SBP = systolic blood pressure, DBP = diastolic blood pressure.
[d] A total of 10 subjects were studied. Each patient received all three treatment regimens in a crossover manner.
[e] Represents a significant change ($p \leq 0.05$).
[f] Blood pressure reductions with lisinopril or hydrochlorothiazide were not significantly different.
[g] Blood pressure reductions for responders only at week 28.
[h] Represents a significant change ($p \leq 0.01$).
[i] Blood pressure reductions at week 12. An optional open continuation was available up to 100 weeks.
[j] Standing diastolic blood pressure ≤85 mm Hg.

Table 3.
Clinical Studies of Lisinopril in Patients with Severe and Renovascular Hypertension

Study	Study Design[a]	Daily Drug Dose[b]	Duration of Therapy (wk)	Mean BP Reduction (mm Hg)[c] SBP	DBP	% Patients Achieving DBP ≤90 mm Hg
Mild to Severe Essential Hypertension						
Morlin et al.[40]	R, DB, parallel	L 20–80 mg ($n = 88$)	14	25[d,e]	19[d,e]	82[f]
		N 20–80 mg ($n = 47$)		25[d,e]	15[d,e]	79[f]
Moderate to Severe Essential Hypertension						
Zachariah et al.[41,g]	R, DB, parallel	L 40–80 mg ($n = 115$)	8	18[d,h]	14[d,h]	38
		M 100–200 mg ($n = 60$)		12[d,h]	11[d,h]	27
Renovascular Hypertension						
Karlberg et al.[42]	Open	L 1.25–80 mg ($n = 10$)	12	33[i]	22[i]	. . .
		E 1.25–80 mg ($n = 12$)		42[i]	17[i]	. . .

[a] R = randomized, DB = double blind.
[b] L = lisinopril, N = nifedipine, M = metoprolol tartrate, E = enalapril maleate.
[c] BP = blood pressure, SBP = systolic blood pressure, DBP = diastolic blood pressure.
[d] Represents a significant change ($p \leq 0.01$).
[e] Blood pressure reductions with lisinopril and nifedipine were not significantly different.
[f] DBP decreased to ≤90 mm Hg or by ≥10 mm Hg.
[g] Preliminary report of first eight weeks of single-drug therapy. Study also evaluated hydrochlorothiazide plus lisinopril or metoprolol and the combination of hydrochlorothiazide, hydralazine, and either lisinopril or metoprolol.
[h] Blood pressure reduction after four weeks of therapy.
[i] Represents a significant change ($p \leq 0.05$).

lisinopril was enhanced with increased doses of the drug, with a maximal effect at 80 mg daily. Further decreases in blood pressure were observed when a second antihypertensive agent was added to lisinopril.[7,10,38] Studies are summarized in Table 2.

In comparison with hydrochlorothiazide, SDBP reductions with lisinopril alone and in combination were significantly less in blacks than in nonblacks.[38] However, similar antihypertensive effects of lisinopril given with hydrochlorothiazide compared with atenolol given with hydrochlorothiazide have been reported regardless of race.[39] Further, nonblacks responded significantly better ($p < 0.01$) to lisinopril alone (−17 mm Hg) than to metoprolol alone (−11 mm Hg).[41] Similar blood pressure reductions have been reported in all adult age groups studied.[38,41]

Moderate to Severe Essential Hypertension. Zachariah and coworkers[41] are currently investigating the effects of lisinopril alone and in combination with hydrochlorothiazide and hydralazine in patients with moderate to severe essential hypertension. Preliminary results of the first eight weeks of lisinopril monotherapy in comparison with metoprolol have been reported[41] (Table 3). Comparable antihypertensive effects were observed with lisinopril and nifedipine in patients with SDBPs ranging from 95 to 135 mm Hg at baseline; study participants were classified as having mild to severe hypertension.[40] Further investigation of the effectiveness of lisinopril alone and in combination regimens for the treatment of severe hypertension is warranted.

Secondary Forms of Hypertension. Lisinopril was compared with enalapril in 22 patients with renovascular hypertension (unilateral and bilateral renal artery stenosis).[42] Both ACE inhibitors equally reduced blood pressure and angiotensin II and aldosterone levels over 24 hours. No change in heart rate or renal function was observed.

Congestive Heart Failure

FDA labeling for lisinopril currently does not include congestive heart failure (CHF). There are relatively few studies with a limited number of patients that address the therapeutic use of lisinopril for this indication. Table 4 summarizes selected studies and abstracts of lisinopril in CHF.

Dickstein et al.[6] studied 12 patients, with a New York Heart Association (NYHA) rating of III and IV, who had no previous history of myocardial infarction and who had been stabilized on digitalis and diuretic therapy for at least three months. On days 1 and 3 at 0800, a single dose of lisinopril was administered orally. The dose administered on day 3 was determined by the response to the first dose. Hemodynamic effects monitored over the four-day study period are shown in Table 4. Mean arterial pressure, mean pulmonary capillary wedge pressure, and systemic vascular resistance were reduced, and the cardiac index was increased. Heart rate did not change. Effects of therapy on NYHA class, exercise tolerance times, and other noninvasive measurements were not addressed.

Two studies evaluated the efficacy and safety of lisinopril in patients with symptomatic congestive heart failure. A double-blind, randomized, placebo-controlled multicenter study was performed in CHF patients (NYHA class III or IV).[45] After 12 weeks of therapy, the increase in exercise time was significantly greater ($p < 0.01$) for lisinopril than placebo. Significant improvement ($p < 0.01$) was seen in 59% of lisinopril-treated patients, while only 22% of placebo-treated patients showed improvement. Lisinopril in doses of 2.5–20 mg/day orally may be effective for the treatment of CHF.

Only one study comparing lisinopril with another ACE inhibitor in CHF patients has been published. In a multicenter, randomized, double-blind study of patients with CHF (NYHA classes II–IV), 64 patients received lisinopril 5–20 mg/day orally once daily and 65 received captopril 35–150 mg/day orally divided into three daily doses.[46] Preliminary data demonstrated a significantly ($p < 0.05$) greater improvement in exercise time after 12 weeks of therapy with lisinopril than with captopril. Sixteen patients in each group showed improvements in NYHA class rating, two patients in the captopril group worsened, and the remainder demonstrated no change. The preliminary data in this study showed that, using these dosage regimens in patients with symptomatic CHF, lisinopril exhibits superior improvements in exercise tolerance times compared with captopril.

Currently, labeling for captopril and enalapril includes use in the treatment of CHF; these agents are being used extensively to achieve afterload reduction and relief of symptoms. An early study by Davis and associates[47] in 10 patients with stable but poorly controlled CHF (NYHA classes III and IV)

Table 4.
Clinical Studies of Lisinopril in Patients with Congestive Heart Failure

Study	Study Design	Patient Population[b]	Dose	Mean Change in Hemodynamic Parameters[a]: HR	MAP (%)	Mean PCWP (%)	CI (%)	SVR (%)
Dickstein et al.[6]	Open	NYHA III ($n = 8$) NYHA IV ($n = 4$)	1.23–10 mg	NS	17.2[c]	27.9[c]	10.2	25 (4 hr)[d]; 4 (48 hr)[d]
Uretsky et al.[44]	Open	NYHA III–IV ($n = 8$)	NR	. . . . . .	12.8[d,e] −1.2[f]	. . . . . .	11.1[e] 4.8[f]	17.4[e] 10[f]

[a] HR = heart rate, MAP = mean arterial pressure, mean PCWP = pulmonary capillary wedge pressure, CI = cardiac index, SVR = systemic vascular resistance, NR = not reported, NS = not significant.
[b] NYHA = New York Heart Association classification.
[c] $p < 0.05$.
[d] $p < 0.01$.
[e] After 24 hours.
[f] After 12 weeks.

showed favorable hemodynamic effects, including improved cardiac index and decreased pulmonary capillary wedge pressure and mean arterial pressure, with captopril therapy. Follow-up studies included a placebo-controlled trial in 92 CHF patients over 12 weeks.[48] Of the patients treated with captopril, an increase in exercise performance and an improvement in NYHA functional class and alleviation of symptoms of dyspnea, fatigue, orthopnea, and edema were observed.

Further investigation ensued after the release of enalapril to establish its effectiveness in the treatment of CHF. Packer et al.[49] reported that enalapril and captopril produced similar hemodynamic effects in patients with severe congestive heart failure. In this study, enalapril was associated with a higher frequency of hypotension, syncope, decreased creatinine clearance, and increased serum potassium concentration. These effects are probably attributable to the relatively large initial doses of enalapril maleate (10 mg orally) administered and its longer half-life compared with that of captopril.

A recent evaluation of enalapril for the treatment of severe CHF was the first study to demonstrate a decrease in the mortality of patients treated with ACE inhibitors[50] and led to its recent FDA labeling for the treatment of CHF. After patients received treatment with enalapril, mortality was reduced by 31% at one year, and a significant improvement in NYHA class was observed (p = 0.001). Patients initially received enalapril maleate 5 mg twice daily, with a withdrawal rate associated with hypotension of 11.8%. A subsequent decrease in the initial dose of enalapril to 2.5 mg daily resulted in a reduction of the withdrawal rate to 3.3%. These and other studies have left little doubt of the usefulness and safety of ACE inhibitors for the treatment of CHF when low initial doses are used.

Lisinopril may also be a treatment option for CHF patients; its long duration of action allows for once-daily dosing, and hepatic bioconversion is not required for activation.[22] Hepatic congestion in many CHF patients could theoretically alter the metabolism of enalapril and other drugs that are dependent on hepatic function for activation, metabolism, or elimination.[51] Schwartz et al.[52] compared the peak effect and clearance of enalapril and its metabolite enalaprilat in hypertensive patients and patients with CHF. Results indicate that a longer duration of action, with a slower onset of action, is expected with enalapril or enalaprilat in CHF patients. Further investigation is needed to establish the role of lisinopril in the treatment of CHF.

Use in Pregnancy and Lactation

In animal studies, no associated teratogenicity or toxic effects on the fetus were observed when saline supplementation was administered with lisinopril.[23] However, in sheep, rabbits, and dogs, an increased occurrence of stillbirths has been reported when lisinopril is administered without saline supplementation. The increased death rate in these animals has been attributed to the hemodynamic effects of the ACE inhibitors.[23,53] Cases of captopril-associated intrauterine effects have been reported in humans. A woman who received captopril throughout pregnancy delivered a male infant by cesarean section who was small for gestational age.[54] The infant required endotracheal intubation and treatment for symptomatic hypotension and persistent patent ductus arteriosus.[54] Although no information is available on lisinopril use during human pregnancy, the manufacturer recommends that lisinopril be reserved for use in pregnant women when the benefits clearly outweigh the risks.

There is no information available regarding the secretion of lisinopril into human breast milk. Therefore, it is recommended that lisinopril be administered with caution in breast-feeding mothers. Captopril is excreted in low concentrations in human breast milk. However, no effects have been reported in breast-feeding infants, and captopril is considered compatible with breast-feeding by the American Academy of Pediatrics.[55,56]

Adverse Effects

Lisinopril has been used in more than 2000 patients during clinical trials, and, in general, adverse effects were mild and transient.[5,7,9,10,30,42] Of these 2000 patients, 420 were also being treated with digitalis or diuretic therapy, or both, for congestive heart failure. Discontinuation of therapy was required in only 6% of the patients studied. Safety and effectiveness in children have not been established. Lisinopril appears to be well tolerated in the elderly, and adverse effects appear to be mild.[41]

Adverse effects have been evaluated in hypertensive patients receiving lisinopril alone and in combination with other antihypertensive agents.[41,46,57] Rush and Merrill[57] reported adverse experiences from clinical trials (n = 1165) for this patient population. The most commonly reported adverse effects with lisinopril alone are dizziness (5.6%), headache (6.2%), cough (3.4%), and diarrhea (3.1%).[57] The incidence of dizziness was twice as frequent in the patients receiving lisinopril and hydrochlorothiazide compared with the lisinopril-only groups; the lisinopril-only groups had a greater frequency of adverse effects than the control group.[57] Incidences of headache and diarrhea appeared similar in these groups and in the placebo group. Cardiovascular adverse effects include orthostatic changes and hypotension, usually in patients who were severely volume depleted or salt depleted, or both. The incidence of hypotension and orthostatic effects during lisinopril therapy is low (0.3%).[57] Adverse effects that occur with greater frequency in CHF patients than in patients with hypertension include dizziness (9.6%), diarrhea (6.1%), and hypotension (4.8%).[57]

Patients receiving enalapril, a structurally similar compound, have displayed adverse effects such as proteinuria and hematological abnormalities including neutropenia, agranulocytosis, eosinophilia, and thrombocytopenia. To date, these abnormalities have not been associated with lisinopril therapy, but patient experience is much less than that with enalapril. Likewise, proteinuria or other symptoms of nephrotoxicity have not been described.

Coughing has been associated with lisinopril[58] and other ACE inhibitors. The cough is described as an annoying, ticklish, dry cough—irritating but not disabling. The four patients who had this symptom, as described in the report by Nash,[58] were all women, but a higher incidence of this adverse effect in women has not been established. No permanent pulmonary dysfunction or alteration in pulmonary function tests was observed. This should be considered when evaluating pulmonary congestion and cough in a patient with congestive heart failure. Other pulmonary findings include upper respiratory symptoms (3.0%) and dyspnea (1.1%).

Other adverse effects that have been reported with relatively low incidences include gastrointestinal complaints of nausea (2.3%) and vomiting (1.3%), as well as rash (1.5%), asthenia (1.3%), and chest pain (1.3%).

Adverse Effects of Lisinopril, Enalapril, and Captopril. One of the primary features used to compare the current ACE inhibitors is their adverse-effect profiles. Differences in study groups must be considered when these agents are compared. Populations in the studies of lisinopril and enalapril included more healthy control subjects, whereas the population in the captopril studies had more patients with abnormal renal function. Abnormal renal function may increase serum concentrations, which may be associated with a higher frequency of adverse effects. Also important, the higher doses of captopril originally studied were associated with higher incidences of the following adverse effects: taste alterations, membranous glomerulopathy, mucocutaneous lesions, pemphigus, and hematologic reactions.[3] After dose reductions, the more serious adverse reactions were no longer found.[3]

ACE inhibitors tend to be devoid of adverse effects commonly associated with other antihypertensive agents, such as hypokalemia, hyperuricemia, glucose intolerance, bronchospasm, sexual dysfunction, and depression.[32] Cough, azotemia, angioedema, hypotension, and hyperkalemia appear to be class-related adverse reactions, appearing with equal frequency among the three agents.[11,57] In Table 5, the relative incidences of the most common adverse reactions to the three ACE inhibitors are compared.

Table 5.
Incidence of Adverse Effects of Lisinopril, Enalapril, and Captopril[a]

Adverse Effect	Lisinopril[23]	Enalapril	Captopril
Dizziness	6.3	4.6[35]	6.0[49]
Headache	5.3	4.8[35]	2.9[60]
Fatigue	3.3	2.8[35]	2.7[59,60]
Diarrhea	3.2	1.6[35]	0.5–2.0[61]
Cough	2.9	1.3[60]	0.5–2.0[61,62]
Rash	1.5	1.5[35]	10.0[61]
Taste disturbance	NR[b]	0.5[35,61]	7.0[61]
Neutropenia	NR	0.06[35]	0.3[61]
Proteinuria	NR	0.6[59]	1.2[61]
Hypotension	1.8	2.4[59]	2.5[32]

[a]Values represent the percentage of patients who had the indicated adverse effect.
[b] NR = not reported.

Drug Interactions

Lisinopril alone and in combination with hydrochlorothiazide has been studied.[7,10,38] No severe hypotensive effects attributable to the combination have been described. However, patients being treated with combination therapy including lisinopril and hydrochlorothiazide should be monitored carefully because of the possible additive hypotensive effect. Additionally, lisinopril has been reported to decrease the degree of potassium lost in patients who were initially treated with hydrochlorothiazide alone.[7] Potassium-sparing diuretics and potassium supplements should be administered cautiously in patients treated with ACE inhibitors because of the probable development of hyperkalemia.[63,64]

The antihypertensive effect of ACE inhibitors has been shown to be decreased with concomitant use of nonsteroidal anti-inflammatory agents (NSAIAs), including indomethacin and aspirin.[12,65] An interaction with sulindac is likely, regardless of the selective inhibition of systemic prostaglandin synthesis.[66] The contribution of prostaglandin production to the therapeutic effects of ACE inhibitors and their interaction with NSAIAs warrant further investigation.

Lisinopril has been studied in patients with congestive heart failure who were treated with multiple drug therapies including digoxin.[6] No clinically important increases in digoxin levels have been reported in patients treated with lisinopril and digoxin. Cleland et al.[67] reported increased digoxin concentrations (1.4 mmol/L, placebo; 1.7 mmol/L, digoxin; $p < 0.05$) in patients with severe CHF

(NYHA classes III and IV) treated with captopril and digoxin. No patient studied developed signs of toxicity. Digoxin concentrations and signs of toxicity should be monitored when ACE inhibitors are used concomitantly with digoxin in patients with severe CHF and decreased renal function.

Dosage

In clinical trials, lisinopril has been initiated for the treatment of hypertension at a dose from 1.25 mg to 20 mg orally.[5,7,10,41] In the initial evaluation of lisinopril in hypertensive humans, further decrease in blood pressure was not observed when the dose was increased beyond 5 mg daily. However, the duration of clinical effect increased proportionately.[5] In contrast, more recent studies with larger patient populations showed an effective decrease in blood pressure at dosages beyond 5 mg up to 80 mg daily. Enhanced antihypertensive effect was also observed with combination therapy.[7,10] In practice, the initial lisinopril dose for hypertension is 10 mg, compared with a 5-mg dose of enalapril maleate.[23] Although the products are equipotent, the difference in the initial dose is due to enalapril's increased absorption and bioactivation relative to lisinopril.[22] Dosages should be increased based on clinical response and duration of antihypertensive effect.

A lower initial dose of lisinopril has been used in studies involving patients with CHF. Initial doses have ranged from 1.25 to 5 mg (mean, 3.4 mg) on day 1, and doses were increased to a range of 1.25 to 10 mg on day 3 based on the initial response.[6] Further study is necessary for dosage recommendations in patients with congestive heart failure, although a lower initial recommended dose is expected.

Lisinopril accumulates in cases of severe renal impairment ($CL_{cr} < 30$ mL/min).[29] Lisinopril is an effective antihypertensive agent in renally impaired patients, but therapy should be initiated at lower doses.[30] The manufacturer recommends an initial dosage of 5 mg per day in patients with $CL_{cr} < 30$ mL/min and 2.5 mg for dialysis patients.[23] Doses should be titrated, and the patients should be monitored for excessive hypotensive responses, hyperkalemia, and changing renal function during lisinopril therapy.

Cost and Availability

Lisinopril is available as Prinivil by Merck Sharp & Dohme as 5-mg (white, scored, MSD 19), 10-mg (light yellow, MSD 106), and 20-mg (peach, MSD 207) tablets and as Zestril by Stuart Pharmaceuticals as 5-mg (pink, scored, Zestril 5, 130), 10-mg (pink, Zestril 10, 131), and 20-mg (red, Zestril 20, 132) tablets. At the time this review was written, the institutional cost and suggested direct price of the 5-, 10-, and 20-mg tablets were equivalent between manufacturers for each strength.[68] The costs of lisinopril, enalapril, and captopril are compared in Table 6.

Table 6.
Cost of Lisinopril, Enalapril, and Captopril

Drug Regimen	Cost ($) per 30 Days[a]
Lisinopril	
5 mg q.d.	11.94
10 mg q.d.	13.26
20 mg q.d.	13.92
Enalapril maleate	
5 mg q.d.	15.28
10 mg q.d.	16.05
20 mg q.d.	22.83
5 mg b.i.d.	30.56
10 mg b.i.d.	32.10
20 mg b.i.d.	45.66
Captopril	
12.5 mg b.i.d	17.44
25 mg b.i.d.	19.20
50 mg b.i.d.	32.01
12.5 mg t.i.d.	26.16
25 mg t.i.d.	28.80
50 mg t.i.d.	48.01

[a] Suggested direct price (reference 68).

Formulary Considerations

Lisinopril is comparable to enalapril as an antihypertensive agent and is less expensive than enalapril and captopril. Additionally, lisinopril may be preferable to enalapril in patients with altered hepatic metabolic activity. However, further research is needed to document the efficacy of lisinopril in CHF and clinical usefulness in patients with hepatic dysfunction. Enalapril has reduced the mortality rate and improved the New York Heart Association classification in patients with CHF. Therefore, for an institution with only captopril on its formulary, it is recommended that enalapril be added if a once-daily ACE inhibitor is desired. Lisinopril should not be added to the formulary until its beneficial effects and therapeutic usefulness in comparison with the other ACE inhibitors can be assessed.

Conclusion

Lisinopril is the third oral ACE inhibitor available for use in the United States. This agent is a nonsulfhydryl lysine analog of enalaprilat. The therapeutic advantage of lisinopril compared with the other ACE inhibitors is yet to be determined. Lisinopril has been shown to be comparable to the other ACE inhibitors and other antihypertensive agents for the treatment of essential and renovascular hypertension. When dosed appropriately, captopril and enalapril have proven efficacy for the treatment of CHF, regardless of the duration of action. Lisinopril may be as effective as its predecessors for the beneficial hemodynamic effects exhibited in patients with heart failure, but further investigation and documentation are required. At this time, there is no clear reason to choose lisinopril over the other ACE inhibitors. The only distinction between lisinopril and enalapril is the need for enalapril to be hepatically activated. A clinically important therapeutic niche for lisinopril may be identified with further study.

References

1. Wu MT, Douglas AW, Ondeyka DL et al. Synthesis of N^2-[(S)-1-Carboxy-3-phenylpropyl-]-L-lysl-L-proline (lisinopril). *J Pharm Sci.* 1985; 74:352–4.
2. Fyhrquist F. Clinical pharmacology of the angiotensin converting enzyme inhibitors. *Drugs.* 1986; 32:33–9.
3. Jaffe IA. Adverse effects profile of sulfhydryl compounds in man. *Am J Med.* 1986; 80:471–6.
4. Brunner DB, Desponds G, Biollaz J et al. Effect of a new angiotensin converting enzyme inhibitor MK 421 and its lysine analogue on the components of the renin system in healthy subjects. *Br J Clin Pharmacol.* 1981; 11:461–7.
5. Rotmensch HH, Vincent M, Vlasses PH et al. Initial evaluation of the nonsulfhydryl containing converting enzyme inhibitor MK-521 in hypertensive humans. *Fed Proc.* 1984; 43:1333–5.
6. Dickstein K, Aarsland T, Woie L et al. Acute hemodynamic and hormonal effects of lisinopril (MK-521) in congestive heart failure. *Am Heart J.* 1986; 112:121–9.
7. Rotmensch HH, Vlasses PH, Swanson BW et al. Antihypertensive efficacy of once daily MK-521, a new nonsulfhydryl angiotensin-converting enzyme inhibitor. *Am J Cardiol.* 1984; 53:116–9.
8. Nussberger J, Brunner WB, Biollaz J et al. Lack of angiotensin I accumulation after converting enzyme blockade by enalapril or lisinopril in man. *Clin Sci.* 1987; 72:387–9.
9. Hodsman GP, Zabludowski JR, Zoccali C et al. Enalapril (MK-421) and its lysine analogue (MK-521): a comparison of acute and chronic effects on blood pressure, renin angiotensin system and sodium excretion in normal subjects. *Br J Clin Pharmacol.* 1984; 17:233–41.
10. Kochar MS, Bolek G, Kalbfleisch JH et al. A fifty-two week comparison of lisinopril, hydrochlorothiazide and their combination in hypertension. *J Clin Pharmacol.* 1987; 27:373–7.
11. Gomez HJ, Girillo VJ, Mondoa F. The clinical pharmacology of lisinopril. *J Cardiovasc Pharmacol.* 1987; 9(Suppl 3):S27–S34.
12. Abe K, Ito J, Sato M et al. Role of prostaglandins in the antihypertensive mechanism of captopril in low renin hypertension. *Clin Sci.* 1980; 59:141s–144s.
13. Moore TS, Crantz FR, Hollenberg NK et al. Contribution of prostaglandins to the antihypertensive action of captopril in essential hypertension. *Hypertension.* 1981; 3:168–73.
14. Dunn BR, Anderson S, Brenner BM. The hemodynamic basis of progressive renal disease. *Semin Nephrol.* 1986; 6:122–38.
15. Taguma Y, Kitamoto Y, Futaki G et al. Effect of captopril on heavy proteinuria in azotemic diabetics. *N Engl J Med.* 1985; 313:1617–20.
16. Jackson B, Cubela R, Johnston CI. Measurement of angiotensin converting enzyme inhibitors in serum by radioinhibitor binding displacement assay. *Biochem Pharmacol.* 1987; 36(8):1357–60.
17. Johnston DI, Cubela R, Sakaguchi K et al. Angiotensin converting enzyme inhibition in plasma and tissues. *Clin Exp Hypertens.* 1987; 9(2–3):307–21.
18. Gronhogen-Riska C, Tikkanen I, Fyhrquist F. Competitive inhibitor binding assay (CIBA) of ACE inhibitors. *Acta Med Scand.* 1986; 714(Suppl):43–7.
19. Hichens M, Hand EL, Mulcamy WS. Radioimmunoassay for angiotensin converting enzyme inhibitors. *Ligand Q.* 1981; 4:43.
20. Tocco DJ, de Luna FA, Duncan AEW et al. The physiological disposition and metabolism of enalapril maleate (MK-421) in laboratory animals. *Drug Metab Dispos.* 1982; 10:15–9.
21. Biollaz J, Schelling JL, Jacot Des Combes B et al. Enalapril maleate and lysine analogue (MK-521) in normal volunteers; relationship between plasma drug levels and the renin angiotensin system. *Br J Pharmacol.* 1982; 14:363–8.
22. Ulm EH, Hichens M, Gomez HJ et al. Enalapril maleate and a lysine analogue (MK-521): disposition in man. *Br J Clin Pharmacol.* 1982; 14:357–62.
23. Merck Sharp & Dohme, Division of Merck & Co., Inc., Prinivil package insert. West Point, PA: 1987 Dec.
24. Mojaverian P, Rocci ML Jr, Vlasses PH et al. Effect of food on the bioavailability of lisinopril, a non-sulfhydryl angiotensin-converting enzyme inhibitor. *J Pharm Sci.* 1986; 75:395–7.
25. Ajayi AA, Campbell BC, Kelman AW et al. Pharmacodynamics and population pharmacokinetics of enalapril and lisinopril. *Int J Clin Pharm Res.* 1985; 6:419–27.
26. Beal SL, Sheiner LB. NONMM users guide, part 1. Los Angeles: University of California; 1979.
27. Patchett AA, Harris E, Tristan EW. A new class of angiotensin converting enzyme inhibitors. *Nature.* 1980; 288:280–3.
28. Kripalani KJ, McKinstry DN, Singhvi SM. Disposition of captopril in normal subjects. *Clin Pharmacol Ther.* 1980; 27:636–41.
29. Van Schaik BAM, Geipkes GG, Boer P. Lisinopril in hypertensive patients with and without renal failure. *Eur J Clin Pharmacol.* 1987; 32:11–6.
30. Donohoe JF, Laher M, Doyle GD et al. Lisinopril in hypertension associated with renal impairment. *J Cardiovasc Pharmacol.* 1987; 9(Suppl 3):S66–S68.
31. Jarrott B, Drummer O, Hooper R et al. Pharmacokinetic properties of captopril after acute and chronic administration to hypertensive subjects. *Am J Cardiol.* 1982; 49:1547–9.
32. Materson BJ. Advances in the management of hypertension: ACE inhibitor therapy. *Intern Med.* 1986; 7(9):175–92.
33. Swanson BN, Vlasses PH, Ferguson RK et al. Influence of food on the bioavailability of enalapril. *J Pharm Sci.* 1984; 73:1655–7.
34. Duchin KL, Pierides AM, Heald A et al. Elimination kinetics of captopril in patients with renal failure. *Kidney Int.* 1984; 25:942–7.
35. Borek M, Charlap S, Frishman W. Enalapril: a long acting angiotensin converting enzyme inhibitor. *Pharmacotherapy.* 1987; 7:133–48.
36. Duchin KL, Singhvi SM, Willard DA et al. Captopril kinetics. *Clin Pharmacol Ther.* 1982; 31:452–8.
37. Cody RJ, Covit A, Schaer G et al. Captopril pharmacokinetics and the acute hemodynamic and hormonal response in patients with severe chronic congestive heart failure. *Am Heart J.* 1982; 104:1103–8.
38. Pool JL, Gennari J, Goldstein R et al. Controlled multicenter study of the antihypertensive effects of lisinopril, hydrochlorothiazide and lisinopril plus hydrochlorothiazide in the treatment of 394 patients with mild to moderate essential hypertension. *J Cardiovasc Pharmacol.* 1987; 9(Suppl 3):S36–S42.
39. Seedat YK, Parag KB. A comparison of lisinopril and atenolol in black and Indian patients with mild to moderate essential hypertension. *S Afr Med J.* 1987; 71:149–53.
40. Morlin C, Baglivo H, Boeijnga JK et al. Comparative trial of lisinopril and nifedipine in mild to severe essential hypertension. *J Cardiovasc Pharmacol.* 1987; 9(Suppl 3):S48–S52.
41. Zachariah PK, Bonnet G, Chrysant G et al. Evaluation of antihypertensive efficacy of lisinopril compared to metoprolol in moderate to severe hypertension. *J Cardiovasc Pharmacol.* 1987; 9(Suppl 3):S53–S58.
42. Karlberg BE, Fyhrquist F, Gronhagen-Riska C et al. Enala-

pril and lisinopril in renovascular hypertension—antihypertensive and hormonal effects of two new angiotensin converting enzyme (ACE) inhibitors. *Scand J Urol Nephrol.* 1984; (Suppl)79:103–6.
43. Sweet CS, Ludden CT, Adkins E et al. Enalapril in experimental hypertension and acute heart failure: comparison with calcium channel blockers. *J Cardiovasc Pharmacol.* 1986; 9(Suppl 3):S15–S19.
44. Uretsky BF, Lawless CE, Rahko PS et al. Treatment of severe heart failure with lisinopril: acute and chronic hemodynamic echocardiographic and clinical responses. *Circulation.* 1985; 72(4 Pt 2):III–406. Abstract.
45. Chalmers JP, West MJ, Cyran J et al. Placebo-controlled study of lisinopril in congestive heart failure: a multicentre study. *J Cardiovasc Pharmacol.* 1987; 9(Suppl 3):S89–S97.
46. Powers ER, Chiaramida A, DeMaria N et al. A double-blind comparison of lisinopril with captopril in patients with symptomatic congestive heart failure. *J Cardiovasc Pharmacol.* 1987; 9(Suppl 3):S82–S88.
47. Davis R, Ribner HS, Klung E et al. Treatment of chronic congestive heart failure with captopril, an oral inhibitor of angiotension converting enzyme. *N Engl J Med.* 1979; 301:117–21.
48. The Captopril Multicenter Research Group. A placebo-controlled trial of captopril in refractory chronic congestive heart failure. *J Am Coll Cardiol.* 1983:755–63.
49. Packer M, Lee HL, Yushak M et al. Comparison of captopril and enalapril in patients with severe chronic heart failure. *N Engl J Med.* 1986; 315:847–53.
50. The CONSENSUS Trial Study Group. Effects of enalapril on mortality in severe congestive heart failure. *N Engl J Med.* 1987; 316:1429–35.
51. Johnston CI, Jackson BJ, Larmour I et al. Plasma enalapril levels and hormonal effects after short and long-term administration in essential hypertension. *Br J Clin Pharmacol.* 1984; 18:233S–239S.
52. Schwartz JB, Taylor A, Abernethy D et al. Pharmacokinetics and pharmacodynamics of enalapril in patients with congestive heart failure and patients with hypertension. *J Cardiovasc Pharmacol.* 1985; 7:767–76.
53. Pipkin FB, Turner SR, Sigmond EM. Possible risk with captopril in pregnancy: some animal data. *Lancet.* 1980; 2:1256.
54. Boutroy MJ, Verb P, de Ligny BH. Captopril administration in pregnancy impairs fetal angiotensin converting enzyme activity and neonatal adaptation. *Lancet.* 1984; 2:935–6.
55. Devlin FL, Huss PM. Captopril in human blood and breast milk. *J Clin Pharmacol.* 1981; 21:110–3.
56. American Academy of Pediatrics Committee on Drugs. The transfer of drugs and other chemicals into human breast milk. *Pediatrics.* 1983; 72:375–83.
57. Rush JE, Merrill DB. The safety and tolerability of lisinopril in clinical trials. *J Cardiovasc Pharmacol.* 1987; 9(Suppl 3):S99–S107.
58. Nash DT. Lisinopril cough. *Postgrad Med J.* 1986; 80(1):40. Letter.
59. Davis RO, Irvin JD, Kramsch DK et al. Enalapril worldwide experience. *Am J Med.* 1984; 77(Suppl 2A):25–35.
60. Merck Sharp & Dohme, Division of Merck & Co., Inc., Vasotec package insert. West Point, PA: 1986 Oct.
61. E. R. Squibb and Sons, Inc. Captopril package insert. Princeton, NJ: 1985 Sep.
62. Inman WHW. Enalapril induced cough. *Lancet.* 1986; 2:1218.
63. Warren SE, O'Conner DT. Hyperkalemia resulting from captopril administration. *JAMA.* 1980; 244:2551–2.
64. Burnakis TG, Mioduch HJ. Combined therapy with captopril and potassium supplementation, a potential for hyperkalemia. *Arch Intern Med.* 1984; 144:2371–2.
65. Moore TJ, Crantz FR, Hollenberg NK et al. Contribution of prostaglandins to the antihypertensive action of captopril in essential hypertension. *Hypertension.* 1981; 3:168–73.
66. Salvetti A, Pedrinelli R, Magagna A et al. Differential effects of selective and non-selective prostaglandin synthesis inhibition on the pharmacological responses to captopril in patients with essential hypertension. *Clin Sci.* 1982; 63:261S–263S.
67. Cleland JGF, Dargie HJ, Pettigrew A. The effects of captopril on serum digoxin and urinary urea and digoxin clearances in patients with congestive heart failure. *Am Heart J.* 1986; 112:130–5.
68. Cardinale VA, Thurlow RM, eds. Drug Topics redbook annual pharmacists' reference. Oradell, NJ: Medical Economics Company, Inc.; 1988:579.

"

Obstacles to an AIDS Vaccine

The development of a safe and effective vaccine for AIDS is proving to be a formidable task. . . .

A persistent dilemma confounds the research. People infected with the live AIDS virus develop antibodies that inactivate it in laboratory tests, yet they become sick and die anyway. This leaves researchers in the position of trying to design a vaccine without knowing what kinds of immune responses will protect a person from infection with the AIDS virus. . . .

[A] unifying strategy has been to make a vaccine that stimulates the production of antibodies against the envelope protein that surrounds HIV. Theoretically, these antibodies should prevent virus particles from infecting cells if a person is exposed to HIV. The approach worked with the polio, measles, and hepatitis B vaccines, but it is not working for AIDS, at least so far. HIV is elusive because it can be transmitted in infected cells as well as by free particles. Thus, researchers must design a vaccine that also triggers the immune system to destroy HIV-infected cells.

—Barnes DM. Obstacles to an AIDS vaccine. *Science.* 1988; 240:719–21.

"

Use of ipratropium bromide in obstructive lung disease

KATHERINE V. MANN, ANN L. LEON, AND KAREN J. TIETZE

Abstract: The chemistry, pharmacology, pharmacokinetics, clinical efficacy, adverse effects, and dosage of ipratropium bromide are reviewed.

Ipratropium bromide, a synthetic quaternary isopropyl derivative of atropine, interrupts vagally mediated bronchoconstriction by inhibiting the cyclic guanosine 3′,5′-monophosphate system at parasympathetic nerve endings. Ipratropium bromide is poorly absorbed after oral and inhaled administration but diffuses rapidly into tissue after i.v. or i.m. administration. The elimination half-life is 3.2–3.8 hours. After inhalation, the drug is eliminated in the urine and feces. The bronchodilatory effect of ipratropium bromide in stable chronic obstructive pulmonary disease appears to be comparable, and may be superior, to that of the β-sympathomimetic agents. In acute exacerbations, ipratropium bromide is useful but may not be the preferred agent because of a delayed onset of action (within 15 minutes; mean dose-dependent duration of effect, three to five hours). Combination therapy with other bronchodilating drugs has proved useful. Ipratropium bromide may be a useful adjunctive agent in the treatment of asthma. Since the onset of action is delayed, ipratropium bromide should not be used as single-drug therapy in an acute asthmatic exacerbation. Reported adverse effects, including cough, nausea, palpitations, dry mouth, nervousness, gastrointestinal distress, and dizziness, have been mild. The usual dosage is two inhalations (36 μg) four times daily, and the maximum number of doses per day should not exceed 12.

Although ipratropium bromide is currently indicated only for maintenance therapy in stable chronic bronchitis and emphysema, it may be useful as adjunctive therapy in asthma and in the management of acute exacerbations of chronic bronchitis and asthma. Additional experience in a variety of chronic obstructive pulmonary disorders will help to clarify the role of ipratropium bromide in the treatment of obstructive pulmonary disease.

Index terms: Bronchodilators; Dosage; Ipratropium bromide; Lung diseases; Pharmacokinetics; Toxicity
Clin Pharm. 1988; 7:670–80

Ipratropium bromide (Atrovent, Boehringer Ingelheim Pharmaceuticals, Inc.), a synthetic anticholinergic (parasympatholytic) drug available in Europe for several years, was released for marketing in the United States in April 1987. Although anticholinergic agents have been used to treat obstructive pulmonary disease for more than 4000 years,[1] these drugs were associated with serious anticholinergic adverse effects, which limited their clinical utility. The availability of the synthetic quaternary derivative, ipratropium bromide, has renewed interest in this class of drugs and has stimulated extensive evaluation of the clinical usefulness of ipratropium bromide in the treatment of obstructive pulmonary disease.

Chemistry and Stability

Ipratropium bromide, *N*-isopropylnortropine tropic acid ester methylbromide, a tropane alkaloid, is the synthetic quaternary isopropyl derivative of atropine. It is a white, crystalline substance with a bitter taste that is freely soluble in water and lower alcohols but insoluble in lipophilic solvents such as ether, chloroform, or fluorohydrocarbons.[2,3] Ipratropium bromide is fairly stable in neutral and acid solutions but is rapidly hydrolyzed in alkaline solutions.[2,3]

Pharmacology

The major neural control of the airways is through the parasympathetic system, with efferent and afferent impulses carried through the vagal nerves.[4–6] Parasympathetic nerve endings release acetylcholine, which binds to cholinergic receptors and stimulates the enzyme guanyl cyclase to produce cyclic guanosine 3′,5′-monophosphate (cGMP). Increased concentrations of cGMP appear to favor bronchoconstriction.

In a recent review of the cholinergic and neurogenic mechanisms in obstructive pulmonary disease, Bleecker[5] described the primary parasympathetic pulmonary reflexes. These reflexes, which consist of the rapidly adapting, the slowly adapting, and the type "J" or "C" fiber receptors, are

KATHERINE V. MANN, PHARM.D., is Resident in Pharmacy Practice, Philadelphia College of Pharmacy and Science (PCPS), Philadelphia, PA. ANN L. LEON, PHARM.D., is Copywriter, Integrated Communications Corp., Morris Plains, NJ. When this review was prepared, Drs. Mann and Leon were Doctor of Pharmacy candidates at PCPS. KAREN J. TIETZE, PHARM.D., is Assistant Professor of Clinical Pharmacy, PCPS.

Address reprint requests to Dr. Tietze at the Department of Pharmacy Practice/Pharmacy Administration, Philadelphia College of Pharmacy and Science, 43rd and Kingsessing Mall, Philadelphia, PA 19104.

Copyright © 1988, American Society of Hospital Pharmacists, Inc. All rights reserved. 0278-2677/88/0901-0670$02.75.

activated by mechanical stimulation, chemical irritants, increases in lung volume or transpulmonary pressure, and by histamine and other mediators, resulting in smooth-muscle contraction, cough, hyperventilation, inhibition of inspiration, lengthening of the expiratory pause, hyperpnea, and smooth-muscle constriction.[5]

Anticholinergic drugs interrupt vagally mediated bronchoconstriction by inhibiting the cGMP system at parasympathetic nerve endings.[7,8] In addition to the interruption of vagally mediated bronchoconstriction, the anticholinergic drugs may inhibit the release of mast-cell-derived mediators by competitive antagonism of acetylcholine at the postganglionic neuromuscular junction.[7]

Although there is general agreement that β-sympathomimetic drugs act directly on smooth muscles distributed throughout the large and small airways regardless of the route of administration,[9-11] there is disagreement on the exact site of action of the anticholinergic drugs. Vagal control appears to be important in the large airways (trachea down to bronchioles of 0.55 mm in diameter).[12] Most investigators consider the site of action of the anticholinergic drugs to be the large central airways.[9,10,13-16] Some investigators[17-22] found that the site of action was both the large and small airways. Differences in dose, degree of bronchoconstriction, and route of administration may account for the discrepancies reported in the literature.[23-25] Additional well-designed studies in patients with a variety of obstructive pulmonary diseases are needed to determine the exact site of action of the anticholinergic drugs.

The acute oral toxic dose of ipratropium bromide in all animal species is greater than 1 g/kg.[7,26] The dose of intravenous ipratropium bromide that is lethal to 50% of animals (LD_{50}) is between 10 and 20 mg/kg.[7,26] The lethal dose of ipratropium bromide administered as a metered aerosol in rats could not be determined because it was not possible to administer a high enough dose.[26] No teratogenic effects have been demonstrated in animals.

Pharmacokinetics

Ipratropium bromide has poor systemic absorption after oral and inhaled administration. The absolute amount of ipratropium bromide in the blood after oral administration is approximately 0.5% of the administered dose[2]; blood concentrations after inhalation of the drug are about 1000 times lower than concentrations achieved after oral administration of equipotent bronchodilatory doses.[27] Although specific data regarding the distribution of inhaled ipratropium bromide are not available, the drug diffuses rapidly into tissues after i.v. or i.m. administration.[28] Ipratropium bromide is partially metabolized to eight metabolites (six in very small quantities) that have little if any anticholinergic effect.[2,27] The main metabolite is the quaternary tropinium salt formed by enzymatic hydrolysis of the ester. The elimination half-life for all routes of administration is 3.2–3.8 hours.[27] After inhalation, the parent drug and metabolites are eliminated in the urine and feces, with approximately 3.2% recovered in the urine and 69% recovered in the feces after six days.[28]

Evaluation of Clinical Trials

Numerous clinical trials evaluating the efficacy and safety of ipratropium bromide in the treatment of chronic obstructive pulmonary disease (COPD) and asthma have appeared in the medical literature. Comparative evaluation of published studies is difficult because of small and variable patient populations, differences in baseline disease severity, and diverse study methodology. Major inconsistencies include the variable patient populations; the methodologies for assessment of pulmonary function; and the dose, route, time, and sequence of drug administration. Despite these problems, some trends are apparent.

Treatment of Chronic Bronchitis

The bronchodilatory effects of ipratropium bromide in COPD appear to be comparable, and may be superior, to those of the β-sympathomimetic agents.[18,29-34] The onset of action is within 15 minutes, with a mean dose-dependent duration of effect of three to five hours.[29,35] The peak bronchodilatory effect occurs between one and two hours after inhalation of the drug, with 50% of the eventual maximum bronchodilation occurring by three minutes and 80% occurring within thirty minutes after doses of 40–160 μg.[36,37] Maximal changes in objective measures of pulmonary function are evident within one to two hours and persist for at least four hours.[36,37] Although increasing the dose of ipratropium bromide from 40 to 160 μg does not substantially increase the degree of bronchodilation, a dose-duration relationship exists.[34,37] Nebulized doses of 80 to 500 μg have been reported to have a duration of action up to six hours.[31,34,37,38]

The efficacy of ipratropium bromide as single-agent therapy in the treatment of stable chronic obstructive pulmonary disease is comparable or superior to that of conventional sympathomimetic agents (Table 1). Ipratropium bromide 40–120 μg produces comparable[32,39-41] or superior[18,34,42] bronchodilation compared with albuterol 200–600 μg. The degree of bronchodilation and duration of effect of ipratropium bromide 80 μg were superior to those associated with isoproterenol hydrochloride 75–150 μg[30] and fenoterol 400 μg.[33] This relationship may not be true in unstable disease. Lees et al.[49] found that ipratropium bromide 80 μg was only comparable to albuterol 400 μg in hospitalized

Table 1.
Studies of Ipratropium Bromide (IPBR) in the Treatment of Chronic Obstructive Pulmonary Disease

Reference	Year	No. Patients	Drug and Dose[a]	Results[b]
32	1975	8	IPBR 40 μg Albuterol 200 μg	No difference in mean change in FEV_1 or SG_{aw} over 240 min with single or combination therapy
30	1977	7	IPBR 10, 20, 40, 80 μg Isoproterenol hydrochloride 75, 150 μg	FEV_1 and FVC increased within 5 min after all doses of both drugs; values remained significantly higher for 1 hr after isoproterenol hydrochloride 75 or 150 μg, for 3–4 hr after IPBR 10, 20, and 40 μg, and for 5 hr after IPBR 80 μg
39	1978	24	IPBR 40 μg Albuterol 200 μg	Combination therapy produced largest increase in 12MD, FEV_1, and FVC, but values were not significantly different from those for either drug alone
40	1978	10	IPBR 40 μg q.i.d. for 3 days Albuterol 200 μg q.i.d. for 3 days Prednisolone 10 mg t.i.d.	Comparable improvement in FEV_1 with single-drug therapy; increase in FEV_1 more than doubled with combination therapy; no additional improvement with addition of prednisolone
18	1979	21	IPBR 80 μg Albuterol 200 μg	IPBR increased FEV_1 from 0.58 to 0.73 L and FVC from 1.45 to 1.83 L; albuterol increased FEV_1 from 0.58 to 0.69 L and FVC from 1.5 to 1.84 L; FEV_1 significantly greater with IPBR than with albuterol; increase in FEV_1 greater with combination therapy (IPBR plus albuterol 3 hr later) than with monotherapy
52	1979	32	IPBR 40 μg q.i.d. for 5 mo	Oral steroid dose reduced by 50% in 11 patients and 30% in 6 patients
49	1980	63	IPBR 80 μg Albuterol 400 μg	FEV_1 increased 18.5% with IPBR and 13.5% with albuterol (significantly different); no difference in percentage of patients with >20% increase in PEFR and FEV_1
42	1982	20	IPBR 40 μg q.i.d. for 1 yr	Significant increases in FEV_1 at 6 and 9 mo and in FVC at 12 mo
33	1982	12	IPBR 40μg Fenoterol 400 μg	VC significantly greater at 15 min with fenoterol than with IPBR and at 60 min with fenoterol plus IPBR than with IPBR; FEV_1 significantly greater at 60 and 90 min with IPBR and IPBR plus fenoterol than with fenoterol; VC significantly greater at 90 min than at 15 min with IPBR and IPBR plus fenoterol; VC plateau reached at 15 min with fenoterol
51	1982	15	IPBR 40 μg Fenoterol 5 mg p.o. Oxtriphylline 400 mg p.o.	Three-drug combination produced larger increase in FEV_1 and FVC than fenoterol plus oxtriphylline but not larger than with IPBR alone
29	1986	261	IPBR 40 μg q.i.d. for 3 mo Metaproterenol sulfate 1500 μg	Mean peak FEV_1 was higher with IPBR than with metaproterenol on days 1 (1.45 versus 1.38 L), 45 (1.47 versus 1.32 L), and 90 (1.39 versus 1.30 L); mean duration of ≥15% increase in FEV_1 was longer with IPBR than with metaproterenol on days 1 (5 versus 4 hr), 45 (3 versus 1 hr), and 90 (3 versus 1 hr)
41	1986	11	IPBR 80 and 40 μg plus albuterol 200 μg at 2 hr Albuterol 400 and 200 and 200 μg plus IPBR 80 μg at 90 min	No significant difference in percentage change in FEV_1, SG_{aw}, FVC, and FRV with combination maximum dose therapy
50	1987	10	IPBR 80 μg Fenoterol 200 μg Albuterol 200 μg	Mean percentage improvement in FEV_1, FVC, and PEFR 2–5 hr after dose was significantly greater with IPBR plus fenoterol than with albuterol
43	1987	51	IPBR 0.5 mg Fenoterol 1.25 mg	FEV_1, FVC, MMEFR, and PEFR improved significantly with IPBR, fenoterol, and IPBR plus fenoterol (no significant difference between treatments); maximum improvement noted at 90 min (mean change from baseline: 26.5%, FEV_1; 25%, FVC; 32.6%, MMEFR; and 38.5%, PEFR)

[a] All studies were single-dose studies unless otherwise indicated. Doses were administered via inhalation unless an alternate route is specified.
[b] SG_{aw} = specific airways conductance, FEV_1 = one-second forced expiratory volume, FVC = forced vital capacity, 12MD = 12-minute walking distance, PEFR = peak expiratory flow rate, VC = vital capacity, FRV = functional residual volume, MMEFR = maximal midexpiratory flow rate.

patients who had recently recovered from acute exacerbations of chronic bronchitis. Rebuck et al.[43] found that ipratropium bromide 500 μg was comparable to but not better than fenoterol 1.25 mg in patients with acute exacerbations of COPD who were treated in the emergency room.[43]

Numerous studies document the short- and long-term efficacy of ipratropium bromide in COPD. Tashkin et al.[29] compared the efficacy of ipratropium bromide 40 μg and metaproterenol sulfate 1500 μg in a 90-day multicenter study of 261 patients with chronic bronchitis.[29] Ipratropium bromide had the greater short- and long-term efficacy. Peak and overall time-averaged bronchodilatory response was significantly greater, and the duration of action was longer, with ipratropium bromide than with metaproterenol. Tolerance to the bronchodilatory effect of ipratropium bromide did not develop over the three-month observation period, whereas tachyphylaxis with metaproterenol was evident. Other reports support the long-term (five weeks to more than four years) efficacy of ipratropium bromide.[42,44–48]

In summary, currently available literature supports the use of ipratropium bromide as a first-line therapeutic agent in stable COPD. In acute exacerbations, ipratropium bromide is useful but may not be the preferred agent because of a delayed onset of action compared with inhaled sympathomimetic agents.

Combination Treatment in COPD. Additional clinical benefit is gained when ipratropium bromide is combined with other bronchodilating drugs (Table 1). Douglas et al.[18] found that the sequential administration of albuterol 200 μg three hours after ipratropium bromide 80 μg to patients with stable COPD resulted in a significant increase in mean forced expiratory volume in one second (FEV_1) compared with either drug given as a single agent.[18] The bronchodilatory effect from simultaneous[49] or sequential[39] administration of single doses of ipratropium bromide and albuterol or successive administration of fenoterol and albuterol[33] was comparable to that of either agent alone, although Lightbody et al.[40] did demonstrate a significant increase in pulmonary function with the concomitant administration of ipratropium bromide and albuterol in a multiple-dose study.[40] Easton et al.[41] evaluated the effect of single and sequential maximal doses of aerosolized ipratropium bromide (120 μg) and albuterol (400 μg).[41] Easton et al.[41] concluded that the two drugs were usually equipotent in maximal doses and that the addition of the second drug was of no value. Other studies support an increase in duration but not degree of bronchodilatory effect when ipratropium bromide is given concomitantly with β sympathomimetics.[32,38,50]

Few studies have evaluated the combination of methylxanthines and ipratropium bromide in COPD. Lefcoe et al.[51] found that the addition of ipratropium bromide 40 μg to the combination of oral fenoterol 5 mg and oxtriphylline 400 mg (equivalent to approximately 254 mg of anhydrous theophylline) was superior to the combination of fenoterol and oxtriphylline. A similar but nonsignificant improvement in FEV_1 was noted for the three-drug combination when compared with the effect of ipratropium bromide alone.

The effects of ipratropium bromide used in conjunction with corticosteroids have been assessed to a limited degree. Lightbody et al.[40] found that the addition of prednisolone did not add to the effect of ipratropium bromide in patients with COPD. However, there is evidence that administration of ipratropium bromide allows some patients to substantially decrease their daily doses of corticosteroids[52] and therefore may be a useful adjunct in steroid-dependent patients.

In summary, the evidence suggests that combination of ipratropium bromide with β sympathomimetics produces greater bronchodilatory effects when ipratropium bromide is administered at least two hours before the β-sympathomimetic agent. This may relate to time of peak efficacy of ipratropium bromide coinciding with time of maximal β-sympathomimetic activity or may relate to the enhanced deposition of β sympathomimetics as a result of ipratropium-induced bronchodilation.

Treatment of Asthma

Numerous studies evaluating the efficacy of ipratropium bromide in asthma have appeared in the literature (Table 2). Unfortunately, there are few well-designed, long-term, large-scale efficacy studies involving specific types of asthma (i.e., intrinsic, extrinsic, and exercise-induced). Since the efficacy of ipratropium bromide may depend on the specific type of asthma, these study design issues are important. Despite major limitations, certain trends for the use of ipratropium bromide in the management of asthma are apparent.

A review of the studies of ipratropium bromide in asthma reveals that 40 μg of ipratropium bromide by metered-dose inhaler may be as effective as standard doses of metaproterenol or albuterol.[14,30,53–55] Ipratropium bromide has a slower onset of effect (mean 10 minutes) and a longer duration of action (up to four hours) than the β_2-sympathomimetic agents.[30,53,56–58]

Emirgil et al.[59] compared 40 μg of ipratropium bromide and isoproterenol hydrochloride 150 μg (aerosol). Bronchodilation, as measured by flow rate, improved in one to three minutes with ipratropium bromide and in one minute with isoproterenol. Bronchodilation with ipratropium bromide was still increasing at the end of one hour, when the study was terminated, while the effects of isoproterenol peaked at six minutes and fell

Table 2.
Studies of Ipratropium Bromide (IPBR) in the Treatment of Asthma

Reference	Year	No. Patients	Drug and Dose[a]	Results[b]
56	1975	10	IPBR 40, 80 μg Isoproterenol hydrochloride 150 μg	IPBR 40 and 80 μg produced significant changes in FEV_1 at 5 min (duration = 4 hr); onset of isoproterenol action was within 5 min (duration = 2 hr); both drugs had similar effects on MMEFR; both had significant effects on $\dot{V}max_{50}$ within 30 min (IPBR duration = 2 hr, isoproterenol duration = 1 hr); neither drug had a significant effect on $\dot{V}max_{75}$
58	1975	11	IPBR 20 μg and 40 μg 1 hr later	VC, FEV_1, and $\dot{V}max_{50}$ progressively increased after IPBR 20 μg, with further increase after 40-μg dose; maximum values reported 2 hr after 40-μg dose
		13	IPBR 40, 80, 160 μg at 30-min intervals	PEFR increased significantly with each dose from control PEFR of 173 L/min to 244 L/min 0.5 hr after last dose
35	1975	10	IPBR 10, 20, 40, 80 μg Isoproferenol hydrochloride 75, 150 μg	Onset of 715% increase in FEV_1 and MMEFR for IPBR was between 15 and 30 min vs. 5 min for isoproterenol; duration was 4 hr for IPBR and 1 hr for isoproterenol; maximum bronchodilation was comparable with either drug
59	1975	10	IPBR 40 μg Isoproterenol hydrochloride 150 μg	Time to ≥15% increase in FEV_1 was 1 min with isoproterenol (+436.3 mL) and 3 min with IPBR (+230.1 mL); similar time course for MEFR; MEFR increased from 40% at 3 min to 88% at 60 min after IPBR dose
60	1976	10	IPBR 40, 80 μg Isoproterenol hydrochloride 150 μg	Comparable bronchodilation with both drugs, but duration was longer with IPBR; FEV_1 was maximal at 15 min with isoproterenol and at 120 min with IPBR; FEV_1 was >15% of baseline value at 15–60 min with isoproterenol, at 30–180 min with IPBR 40 μg, and at 15–180 min with IPBR 80 μg
30	1977	10	IPBR 10, 20, 40, 80 μg Isoproterenol hydrochloride 75, 150 μg	Duration of significant improvement in FEV_1 was <15 min with IPBR 10 μg, 30 min with IPBR 20 μg and isoproterenol hydrochloride 75 μg, 1 hr with isoproterenol hydrochloride 150 μg, and up to 4 hr with IPBR 40 and 80 μg
54	1977	25	IPBR 40 μg Albuterol 200 μg	FEV_1 significantly increased over baseline value 30–90 min after albuterol and 90–180 min after IPBR; increase in FEV_1 with albuterol exceeded that with IPBR for first 3 hr, but effects were not different 4–8 hr after dose; FEV_1 was significantly increased for up to 3 hr after albuterol dose in atopic patients (*n* = 12) and for 1 hr in nonatopic patients (*n* = 13)
53	1978	23[c]	IPBR 40 μg Metaproterenol sulfate 10 mg p.o.	No significant difference in PEFR, $\dot{V}max_{50}$, or FEV_1 between single-drug and combination therapy
69	1978	9[c]	IPBR 80 μg	IPBR prevented methacholine-induced bronchoconstriction but had no effect on histamine-induced bronchoconstriction
64	1979	8	IPBR 40 μg Fenoterol 400 μg	Mean percentage change in FEV_1 was significantly greater with IPBR plus fenoterol (59.5 ± 10.5%) than with IPBR (32.6 ± 5%) or fenoterol (51.1 ± 9.8%); AUC for FEV_1 versus time was significantly greater with IPBR plus fenoterol than with IPBR or fenoterol
65	1981	12	IPBR 40 μg q.i.d. for 2 weeks Oxtriphylline	Greater mean increase in FEV_1 at 1 hr with oxtriphylline plus IPBR (0.4 L) than with IPBR (0.27 L) or oxtriphylline (0.07 L); greater mean increase in MMEFR at 1 hr with combination therapy (0.45 L/sec) than with IPBR (0.24 L/sec) or oxtriphylline (0.12 L/sec)
70	1982	12[c]	IPBR 40 μg	IPBR prevented bronchoconstriction induced by hyperventilation, methacholine, histamine, or allergen
61	1983	22	IPBR 40 μg q.i.d. for 1 mo Fenoterol 200, 400 μg Oxtriphylline 200 mg p.o.	30-day PEFR was similar for fenoterol plus oxtriphylline and three-drug regimen; values for both regimens were significantly better than those for IPBR plus oxtriphylline; AUCs for FEV_1, VC, and $\dot{V}max_{50}$ versus time were greater for three-drug regimen
67	1983	16[c]	IPBR 40, 80 μg Metaproterenol sulfate 1.25, 2.5 mg	FEV_1, FEF_{25-75}, and SG_{aw} were significantly better with IPBR 40 μg plus metaproterenol sulfate 1.25 mg than with IPBR, metoproterenol, or IPBR 40 μg plus metaproterenol sulfate 1.25 mg; combination therapy produced 48% peak increase in FEV_1 1 hr after metaproterenol dose, and FEV_1 was still increased by 25% at 5 hr

(Continued on next page)

Table 2 (*continued*).

Reference	Year	No. Patients	Drug and Dose[a]	Results[b]
57	1984	17	IPBR 7.5, 25, 75, 250 μg	All doses resulted in significant increases in FEV_1 (0.15–0.4 L, 11–31% increase) as early as 15 min after dose, with plateau extending to 120 min; dose-dependent bronchodilation was evident at 75-μg dose
62	1985	28	IPBR 0.5 mg q6h for 2 days Fenoterol 1 mg q6h for 2 days	Mean change in FEV_1 at 15, 30, 45, 60, and 75 min was significantly greater with fenoterol than with IPBR; addition of fenoterol 90 min after first dose of fenoterol or after IPBR resulted in significantly greater mean change in FEV from 120 to 180 min (15.9 ± 5.5% versus 20.8 ± 7.1%)
66	1985	8[c]	IPBR 1 mg Albuterol 200 μg Cromolyn sodium 20 mg	Bronchodilation was comparable with IPBR and albuterol (FEV_1 increased 4.4% with albuterol and 3.2% with IPBR; SG_{aw} increased 49.2% with albuterol and 45.7% with IPBR); IPBR had no effect on airway or mediator response to allergen challenge
63	1985	28	Albuterol 150 μg/kg, then 50 μg/kg every 20 min for six doses plus IPBR 250 μg at 1 hr	Addition of IPBR at 1 hr resulted in further gradual improvement; FEV_1 was improved 40 min after IPBR dose, with peak effect noted at 1 hr (20.6% increase in FEV_1); effect was maintained to end of study (90 min)
55	1986	164	IPBR 40 μg q.i.d. for 3 mo Metaproterenol sulfate 1500 μg	≥15% increase in FEV_1 occurred in ≤15 min on days 1, 45, and 90 with IPBR and in <5 min on days 1, 45, and 90 with metaproterenol; on day 90, FEV_1 remained ≥15% above baseline for 5 hr with IPBR and 2 hr with metaproterenol (significantly different)
68	1987	48[c]	IPBR 0.025%; 1 mL, 2 mL Albuterol 0.5%; 0.01 mL/kg, 0.02 mL/kg	Increase in FEV_1 and FEF_{25-75} with albuterol or albuterol plus IPBR was almost twice that with IPBR (difference not always significant); duration of significant improvement in bronchodilation was 6 hr with albuterol; duration of IPBR effect was variable

[a] Studies were single-dose studies unless otherwise indicated. All doses were administered via inhalation unless an alternate route is specified.

[b] FEV_1 = one-second forced expiratory volume, MMEFR = maximum midexpiratory flow rate, $\dot{V}max_{50}$ = maximum expiratory flow at 50% vital capacity, $\dot{V}max_{75}$ = maximum expiratory flow rate at 75% vital capacity, VC = vital capacity, PEFR = peak expiratory flow rate, AUC = area under the curve, FEF_{25-75} = forced expiratory flow over 25–75% vital capacity, SG_{aw} = specific airways conductance.

[c] Patients had atopic (extrinsic) asthma.

thereafter. Another study, with a longer evaluation period, showed that ipratropium bromide significantly increased airway conductance for up to 240 minutes, whereas the effect of isoproterenol lasted for only 60 minutes.[60]

Studies evaluating ipratropium bromide in combination with β-sympathomimetic drugs in asthma are limited.[54,61–63] In a well-designed, randomized, double-blind parallel study of 148 asthmatics, Rebuck et al.[61] compared the efficacy of single or combination therapy using 500 μg of nebulized ipratropium bromide and 1.25 mg of nebulized fenoterol. The combination of ipratropium bromide and fenoterol resulted in the greatest improvement; moreover, the improvement was significantly greater than that associated with either treatment alone. Improvement was greatest in patients with the greatest degree of pretreatment airway obstruction. Bryant[62] found that bronchodilation from the combination of fenoterol 1000 μg and ipratropium bromide 500 μg administered by nebulizer was significantly better than that achieved with fenoterol alone. Ruffin et al.[54] found that the combination of ipratropium bromide 40 μg and albuterol 200 μg showed a greater duration of bronchodilation than either drug alone; similar results were observed in children when ipratropium bromide was given one hour after albuterol.[63] Marlin et al.[64] found similar additive effects when fenoterol 400 μg was administered two hours after ipratropium bromide 40 μg. In addition, the duration of action (three and six hours) from the sequential doses was prolonged when compared with that of either drug alone.[64]

There is limited information on long-term combination therapy with ipratropium bromide and oral methylxanthines. Oral oxtriphylline (mean serum concentration 13.8 mg/L) in combination with ipratropium bromide 40 μg administered by metered-dose inhaler, resulted in significantly greater bronchodilation, which was sustained over a two-week period, than that achieved with either drug alone.[65] The long-term (four-week) administration of inhaled ipratropium bromide, inhaled fenoterol, and oral oxtriphylline showed greater bronchodilation than the combination of ipratropium bromide and oxtriphylline or fenoterol and oxtriphylline alone.[61]

Ipratropium Bromide Therapy of Extrinsic Asthma. Few studies evaluating single and combination therapy with ipratropium bromide in extrinsic asthmatics have been published. Ipratropium bromide, as single-drug therapy in the treatment of extrinsic asthma, appears to be comparable, but not superior, to β-sympathomimetic agents. Maximum bronchodilation with ipratropium bromide (10–1000 μg) was significantly greater than that associated with placebo,[35,36] was comparable to that associated with albuterol (200 μg),[66] and was comparable to, but did not reach, that associated with isoproterenol hydrochloride (75–150 μg).[66] Lin et al.[53] suggested that ipratropium bromide may have the greatest bronchodilatory effects in patients with the most severe baseline bronchospasm.

Lin et al.[53] compared ipratropium bromide 40 μg by aerosol alone and in combination with a single 10-mg oral dose of metaproterenol sulfate and found a greater, though not significantly different, bronchodilatory effect with the combined drug therapy. A double-blind randomized study evaluated the bronchodilatory effect of the sequential combination of inhaled ipratropium bromide 40 μg and metaproterenol sulfate 1.25 mg in 10 patients with extrinsic asthma.[67] The second of each combination was given one hour after the first drug. The additive bronchodilatory effect achieved with ipratropium bromide followed by metaproterenol was significantly greater than that associated with ipratropium bromide or metaproterenol alone, two consecutive metaproterenol inhalations, or metaproterenol followed by ipratropium bromide. The bronchodilatory effect was maintained for five hours. The greater bronchodilatory effect of ipratropium bromide on large airways may enhance metaproterenol deposition when metaproterenol is given as the second drug. Alternatively, this may be the result of the peak effect of each drug coinciding when ipratropium bromide is given one hour before metaproterenol.

The combination of ipratropium bromide and β sympathomimetics may allow for lower anticholinergic and β-sympathomimetic doses in patients who are intolerant of the dose-related adverse effects of β-sympathomimetic drugs. The effect of albuterol and ipratropium bromide administered alone or in combination at different doses in a randomized double-blind study of 48 children with extrinsic asthma was evaluated by Boner et al.[68] The concurrent administration of smaller aerosolized doses of albuterol (0.01 mL/kg of a 5% solution) and ipratropium bromide (1 mL of a 0.025% solution) achieved bronchodilation comparable to that produced by large doses of albuterol (0.02 mL/kg of a 5% solution) or ipratropium bromide (2 mL of a 0.025% solution) as single-drug therapy.[68] Additional long-term studies are needed to verify the effectiveness and clinical usefulness of low-dose combination therapy.

The protective effects of ipratropium bromide against allergen-induced bronchospasm are variable. Ipratropium bromide, in doses up to 1000 μg, appears to have little effect against mast-cell-mediator release.[66] Ipratropium bromide did protect against methacholine-induced bronchospasm[69,70] but did not protect against bronchoconstriction with histamine challenge.[69] Histamine response is therefore unlikely to be vagally mediated. Although ipratropium bromide appears to have some bronchodilatory effect in extrinsic asthma, the effect is not specific against allergen-induced bronchospasm.

Ipratropium Bromide Therapy of Exercise-Induced Asthma. Ipratropium bromide appears to have variable efficacy in exercise-induced bronchospasm (Table 3). Several investigators[71–74] have reported that ipratropium bromide protected against exercise-induced bronchospasm; however, exercise was performed 15–20 minutes after drug administration, which was near the time of expected maximal bronchodilation. Thus, the study design makes it difficult to distinguish the prophylactic effect from the bronchodilatory effect. Wolkove et al.[75] and Larsson[76] found that ipratropium bromide failed to prevent exercise-induced bronchospasm, although pulmonary function immediately after exercise was superior to that achieved with placebo. Although ipratropium bromide does not protect against exercise-induced bronchospasm, it does appear to have a bronchodilatory effect both before and after exercise-induced spasm[77] and therefore may be a useful adjunctive agent.

High-Dose Ipratropium Bromide. Studies of the effect of higher than recommended doses of ipratropium bromide in asthma have shown a dose-response relationship for doses of 80 μg,[30] 120 μg,[58,78] and 500 μg.[79] Studies by Wegener and Hendenstrom[80] and Davis et al.[57] suggest that ipratropium bromide may affect small airways in a dose-dependent manner. High-dose ipratropium bromide may be beneficial for patients who are unresponsive to conventional doses.

Summary. Ipratropium bromide may be a useful adjunctive agent in the management of asthma. Since the onset of action is delayed, ipratropium bromide should not be used as single-drug therapy of an acute exacerbation of asthma. Ipratropium bromide may be a useful alternative drug for patients who are intolerant of β sympathomimetics or who are at risk for adverse cardiovascular effects from standard therapy. The combination of ipratropium bromide and lower doses of β-sympathomimetic agents or methylxanthines may be better tolerated without compromising therapeutic benefit.

Table 3.
Studies of Ipratropium Bromide (IPBR) for Prevention of Exercise-Induced Asthma

Reference	Year	No. Patients	Drug and Dose[a]	Results[b]
72	1973	24	IPBR 40 μg Albuterol 200 μg	No difference between drugs in postexercise reduction in PEFR
71	1977	9	IPBR 80 μg Cromolyn sodium 20 mg	IPBR and cromolyn prevented EIA (measured as maximum percentage change in FEV_1) in the majority of patients
75	1981	8	IPBR 40 μg	FEV_1 and MMEFR were significantly better pre-exercise (1 hr postdose) with IPBR; FEV_1 and MMEFR were significantly better in early postexercise period (0, 5, and 10 min) with IPBR
76	1982	8	IPBR 40 μg Oxitropium bromide 100 μg Fenoterol 400 μg	Fenoterol completely prevented postexercise bronchoconstriction (FEV_1 >85% of baseline); IPBR and oxitropium did not prevent bronchoconstriction
77	1985	6	IPBR 250 μg	IPBR significantly increased FEV_1 (+12 ± 4%) and $\dot{V}max_{50}$ (+36 ± 12%) but did not prevent EIA
74	1987	15	IPBR 500 μg Cromolyn sodium 20 mg Verapamil 5 mg	D FEV_1 was significantly less with cromolyn (15.3 ± 11.7%) and IPBR (21.7 ± 17.7%); verapamil had no significant effect on D FEV_1

[a] Single doses were given, and drugs were administered via inhalation.
[b] PEFR = peak expiratory flow rate, EIA = exercise-induced asthma, FEV_1 = one-second forced expiratory volume, MMEFR = maximum midexpiratory flow rate, $\dot{V}max_{50}$ = maximal expiratory flow at 50% vital capacity, D FEV_1 = maximum percentage decrease in FEV.

Adverse Effects

In contrast to atropine, which is well absorbed from mucosal surfaces, crosses the blood–brain barrier, and is associated with substantial systemic effects, inhaled ipratropium bromide is highly specific and virtually free of severe adverse effects.[81–83] Inhaled ipratropium bromide has no marked deleterious effect on mucociliary clearance rate or sputum viscosity or volume.[6,65,84,85] It has no effect on micturition[86] or cardiovascular function.[87,88] Although there is one case report of elevated intraocular pressure after a regimen of inhaled ipratropium bromide at a dose of 40 μg four times daily for one week,[89] studies of doses of up to 0.8 mg in volunteers and patients with glaucoma documented no effect on intraocular pressure.[90–92]

Adverse effects reported by study volunteers and patients throughout the literature are relatively mild and infrequent. Adverse effects reported by Tashkin et al.[29] in a 90-center, controlled clinical trial included cough (4.6%), nausea (3.8%), palpitations (3%), dry mouth (2.3%), nervousness (1.5%), gastrointestinal distress (1.52%), and dizziness (0.8%). Adverse effects reported by the manufacturer include cough (5.9%), nervousness (3.1%), nausea (2.8%), dizziness (2.4%), headache (2.4%), gastrointestinal distress (2.4%), dry mouth (2.4%), exacerbation of symptoms (2.4%), palpitations (1.8%), irritation from aerosol (1.6%), rash (1.2%), and blurred vision (1.2%).[93] Accommodation disturbances may occur if the aerosol is inadvertently sprayed in the eyes.

There are no reported adverse drug interactions.

Dosage and Cost

The usual dosage is two inhalations (36 μg) four times daily. Patients may take additional inhalations as needed, but the maximum number of inhalations per 24 hours should not exceed 12.[93]

The 14-g canister (200 inhalations) costs $14.38 (average wholesale price).[94] Total cost of therapy may increase if ipratropium bromide is simply added to a pre-existing drug regimen; total cost of therapy will decrease if ipratropium bromide replaces or decreases the use of other therapeutic agents.

Patient Instructions

Patients should be told that ipratropium bromide will not work as quickly as the sympathomimetic amines and that it is not indicated for the initial treatment of an acute asthma attack. Patients should be counseled on proper techniques for using metered-dose inhalers and should be advised to use the closed-mouth technique (i.e., to seal their lips around the mouthpiece when inhaling the drug) to avoid spraying the drug in the eyes.

FDA-Labeled Indications

Ipratropium bromide is indicated for maintenance treatment of bronchospasm associated with chronic obstructive pulmonary disease, including chronic bronchitis and emphysema. Safety and efficacy in children less than 12 years of age have not been established.

Formulary Recommendation

Ipratropium bromide, as a bronchodilator with few adverse effects and a unique mechanism of action, is indicated for maintenance therapy in stable chronic bronchitis and emphysema and may be useful as adjunctive therapy in allergen- and exercise-induced asthma and intrinsic asthma and in the management of acute severe exacerbations of chronic bronchitis and asthma. Therefore, we recommend that ipratropium bromide be added to hospital formularies but that it not replace other bronchodilator drugs.

Conclusion

Ipratropium bromide is an exciting new therapeutic agent. Although the current indications are somewhat limited, additional experience in a wide variety of acute and chronic obstructive pulmonary disorders will help clarify the role of ipratropium bromide in the treatment of obstructive pulmonary disease.

References

1. Gandevia B. Historical review of the use of parasympatholytic agents in the treatment of respiratory disorders. *Postgrad Med J*. 1975; 51(Suppl 7):13–20.
2. Deckers W. The chemistry of new derivatives of tropane alkaloids and the pharmacokinetics of a new quaternary compound. *Postgrad Med J*. 1975; 51(Suppl 7):76–81.
3. Rominger KL. Chemistry and pharmacokinetics of ipratropium bromide. *Scand J Respir Dis*. 1979; 103(Suppl):116–29.
4. Gross NJ, Skorodin MS. Anticholinergic, antimuscarinic bronchodilators. *Am Rev Respir Dis*. 1984; 129:856–70.
5. Bleecker ER. Cholinergic and neurogenic mechanisms in obstructive airways disease. *Am J Med*. 1986; 81(Suppl 5A):93–102.
6. Wanner A. Effect of ipratropium bromide on airway mucociliary function. *Am J Med*. 1986; 81(Suppl 5A):23–7.
7. Engelhardt A. Pharmacology and toxicology of Atrovent. *Scand J Respir Dis*. 1979; 103(Suppl):110–5.
8. Nadel JA. Parasympathetic regulation of lungs and airways. *Postgrad Med J*. 1975; 51(Suppl 7):86–90.
9. Hensley MJ, O'Cain CF, McFadden ER Jr et al. Distribution of bronchodilation in normal subjects: beta agonist versus atropine. *J Appl Physiol*. 1978; 45:778–82.
10. Ingram RH, Wellman JJ, McFadden ER Jr et al. Relative contributions of large and small airways to flow limitation in normal subjects before and after atropine and isoproterenol. *J Clin Invest*. 1977; 59:696–703.
11. Vanden Brink FG. The pharmacology of bronchodilator muscle relaxation. *Bull Physiol Pathol Respir*. 1972; 8:475–6.
12. Widdicombe JG. Studies on afferent airways innervation. *Am Rev Respir Dis*. 1977; 115(Suppl):99–105.
13. Storms WW, DoPico GA, Reed CE. Aerosol Sch 1000. *Am Rev Respir Dis*. 1975; 111:419–22.
14. Firstater E, Mizrachi E, Topilsky M. The effect of vagolytic drugs on airway obstruction in patients with bronchial asthma. *Ann Allergy*. 1981; 46:332–5.
15. Ashutosh K, Mead G, Dickey JC Jr et al. Density dependence of expiratory flow and bronchodilator response in asthma. *Chest*. 1980; 77:68–75.
16. McFadden ER Jr, Ingram RH Jr, Haynes RL et al. Predominant site of flow limitation and mechanisms of postexertional asthma. *J Appl Physiol*. 1977; 42:746–52.
17. Partridge MR, Saunders KB. Site of action of ipratropium bromide and clinical and physiological determinants of response in patients with asthma. *Thorax*. 1981; 36:530–3.
18. Douglas NJ, Davidson I, Sudlow MF et al. Bronchodilatation and the site of airway resistance in severe chronic bronchitis. *Thorax*. 1979; 34:51–6.
19. Diamond L, O'Donnell M. A comparative study of two parasympatholytic bronchodilator agents: ipratropium bromide and diphemanil methylsulfate. *J Pharmacol Exp Ther*. 1981; 216:1–5.
20. Douglas NJ, Sudlow MF, Flenley DC. Effect of an inhaled atropinelike agent on normal airway function. *J Appl Physiol*. 1979; 46:256–62.
21. Frith PA, Thomas PD, McEvoy RD et al. Factors contributing to bronchodilatation induced by ipratropium bromide in asthmatics. *Aust NZ J Med*. 1982; 12:686. Abstract.
22. Molho M, Benzaray S, Lidji M et al. Salbutamol versus atropine. Site of bronchodilation in asthmatic patients. *Respiration*. 1987; 51:26–34.
23. Holtzman MJ, McNamara MP, Sheppard D et al. Intravenous versus inhaled atropine for inhibiting bronchoconstrictor responses in dogs. *J Appl Physiol*. 1983; 54:134–9.
24. Shepard D, Epstein J, Holtzman MJ et al. Effect of route of atropine delivery on bronchospasm from cold air and methacholine. *J Appl Physiol*. 1983; 54:130–3.
25. Weiss JW, McFadden ER Jr, Ingram RH Jr. Parenteral vs. inhaled atropine: density of maximal expiratory flow. *J Appl Physiol*. 1982; 392–6.
26. Engelhardt A, Klupp H. The pharmacology and toxicology of a new tropane alkaloid derivative. *Postgrad Med J*. 1975; 51(Suppl 7):82–4.
27. Adlung Von J, Hohle KD, Zeren S et al. Untersuchungen zur Pharmakokinetik und Biotransformation von Ipratropiumbromid am Menschen. *Arzneimittelforschung*. 1976; 26:1005–10.
28. Wahl D. Pharmacokinetics (absorption-distribution-metabolism-excretion) of ^{14}C-labeled Sch 1000 administered by inhalation, orally and intravenously. *Postgrad Med J*. 1975; 51(Suppl 7):93–6. Abstract.
29. Tashkin DP, Ashutosh K, Bleecker ER et al. Comparison of the anticholinergic bronchodilator ipratropium bromide with metaproterenol in chronic obstructive pulmonary disease. *Am J Med*. 1986; 81(Suppl 5A):81–90.
30. Baigelman W, Chodash S. Bronchodilator action of the anticholinergic drug, ipratropium bromide (Sch 1000), as an aerosol in chronic bronchitis and asthma. *Chest*. 1977; 71:324–8.
31. Jenkins CR, Chow CM, Fisher BL et al. Comparison of ipratropium bromide and salbutamol by aerosolized solution. *Aust NZ J Med*. 1981; 11:513–6.
32. Petrie GR, Palmer KNV. Comparison of aerosol ipratropium bromide and salbutamol in chronic bronchitis and asthma. *Br Med J*. 1975; 1:430–2.
33. Hughes JA, Tobin MJ, Bellamy D et al. Effects of ipratropium bromide and fenoterol aerosols in pulmonary emphysema. *Thorax*. 1982; 37:667–70.
34. Poppius H, Salorinne Y. Comparative trial of a new anticholinergic bronchodilator Sch 1000 and salbutamol in chronic bronchitis. *Br Med J*. 1973; 24:134–6.
35. Gross NJ. Sch 1000: a new anticholinergic bronchodilator. *Am Rev Respir Dis*. 1975; 112:823–7.
36. Loddenkemper R. Dose and time-response of Sch 1000 on total (R_T) and expiratory (R_E) airways resistance in patients with chronic bronchitis and emphysema. *Postgrad Med J*. 1975; 51(Suppl 7):97. Abstract.

37. Allen JC, Campbell AH. Dose response of ipratropium bromide assessed by two methods. *Thorax*. 1979; 35:137–9.
38. Howarth PH, Stainforth JN, Holgate ST. Bronchodilator efficacy of nebulised salbutamol and ipratropium bromide in chronic airflow obstruction. *Thorax*. 1982; 37:789.
39. Leitch AG, Hopkin JM, Ellis DA et al. The effect of aerosol ipratropium bromide and salbutamol on exercise tolerance in chronic bronchitis. *Thorax*. 1978; 33:711–13.
40. Lightbody IM, Ingram LG, Legge JS et al. Ipratropium bromide, salbutamol and prednisolone in bronchial asthma and chronic bronchitis. *Br J Dis Chest*. 1978; 72:181–6.
41. Easton PA, Jadue C, Dhingra S et al. A comparison of the bronchodilating effects of a beta-2 adrenergic agent (albuterol) and an anticholinergic agent (ipratropium bromide), given by aerosol alone or in sequence. *N Engl J Med*. 1986; 315:735–9.
42. Cockcroft DW, Cotton DJ, Berscheid BA. Long-term efficacy and safety of inhaled Sch 1000, an anticholinergic bronchodilator. *Curr Ther Res*. 1982; 31:138–47.
43. Rebuck AS, Chapman KR, Abboud R et al. Nebulized anticholinergic and sympathomimetic treatment of asthma and chronic obstructive airways disease in the emergency room. *Am J Med*. 1987; 82:59–64.
44. Ulmer WT. Repeated measurements of total airways resistance (R_t), intrathoracic gas volume (TGV), PaO_2, $PaCO_2$ and clinical features in patients with chronic obstructive lung disease during long-term treatment with Sch 1000 inhalation. *Postgrad Med J*. 1975; 51(Suppl 7):133. Abstract.
45. Brinkman O. The results of long-term treatment with Sch 1000 MDI on repeated measurements of FEV_1, total airways resistance (R_t), haematological and biochemical tests in patients with chronic bronchitis and emphysema. *Postgrad Med J*. 1975; 51(Suppl 7):130. Abstract.
46. Haslreiter E. Haematological and biochemical monitoring during long-term treatment with Sch 1000 MDI in patients with chronic bronchitis and emphysema. *Postgrad Med J*. 1975; 51(Suppl 7):130–1. Abstract.
47. Jilg J. Long-term treatment with Sch 1000 MDI in outpatients with chronic bronchitis. *Postgrad Med J*. 1975; 51(Suppl 7):131. Abstract.
48. Cummiskey J, Keelan P. Study of Sch 1000 MDI used in therapeutic doses in patients with chronic bronchitis. *Postgrad Med J*. 1975; 51(Suppl 7):130. Abstract.
49. Lees AW, Allan GW, Smith J. Nebulized ipratropium bromide and salbutamol in chronic bronchitis. *Br J Clin Pract*. 1980; 34:340–2.
50. Crane J, Gamble S, Purdie G. Comparison of a fenoterol/ipratropium combination with salbutamol from MDI in subjects with chronic partially reversible airways obstruction. *Aust NZ Med J*. 1987; 100:385–7.
51. Lefcoe HM, Toogood JH, Blennerhassett G et al. The addition of an aerosol anticholinergic to an oral beta agonist plus theophylline in asthma and bronchitis. *Chest*. 1982; 82:300–5.
52. Ajewski Z, Popiak B. The relation between permanent administration of Atrovent and the dose of steroids in chronic bronchitis. *Scand J Respir Dis*. 1979; 103(Suppl):205.
53. Lin MT, Lee-Hong E, Collins-Williams C. A controlled trial of the bronchodilator effect of Sch 1000 aerosol in asthmatic children. *Ann Allergy*. 1978; 40:326–32.
54. Ruffin RE, Fitzgerald JD, Rebuck AS. A comparison of the bronchodilator activity of Sch 1000 and salbutamol. *J Allergy Clin Immunol*. 1977; 59:136–41.
55. Storms WW, Bodman SF, Nathan RA et al. Use of ipratropium bromide in asthma: results of a multi-clinic study. *Am J Med*. 1986; 81(Suppl 5A):61–6.
56. Storms WW, DoPico GA, Reed CE. Aerosol Sch 1000: an anticholinergic bronchodilator. *Am Rev Respir Dis*. 1975; 111:419–22.
57. Davis A, Vickerson F, Worsley G et al. Determination of dose-response relationship for nebulized ipratropium in asthmatic children. *J Pediatr*. 1984; 105:1002–5.
58. Simonsson BG, Jonson B, Strom B. Bronchodilatory and circulatory effects of inhaling increasing doses of an anticholinergic drug, ipratropium bromide (Sch 1000). *Scand J Respir Dis*. 1975; 56:138–49.
59. Emirgil C, Dwyer K, Baskette P et al. A new parasympatholytic bronchodilator: a study of its onset of effect after inhalation. *Curr Ther Res*. 1975; 17:215–24.
60. Yeager H, Weinberg RM, Kaufman LV et al. Asthma: comparative bronchodilator effects of ipratropium bromide and isoproterenol. *J Clin Pharmacol*. 1976; 16:198–204.
61. Rebuck AS, Gent M, Chapman KR. Anticholinergic and sympathomimetic combination therapy of asthma. *J Allergy Clin Immunol*. 1983; 71:317–23.
62. Bryant DH. Nebulized ipratropium bromide in the treatment of acute asthma. *Chest*. 1985; 88:24–9.
63. Beck R, Robertson C, Galdes-Sebaldt M et al. Combined salbutamol and ipratropium bromide by inhalation in the treatment of severe acute asthma. *J Pediatr*. 1985; 107:605–8.
64. Marlin GE, Berend N, Harrison AC. Combined cholinergic antagonist and β_2-adrenoreceptor agonist bronchodilator therapy by inhalation. *Aust NZ J Med*. 1979; 9:511–4.
65. Kreisman H, Frank H, Wolkove N et al. Synergism between ipratropium and theophylline in asthma. *Thorax*. 1981; 36:387–91.
66. Howarth PH, Durham SR, Tak HL et al. Influence of albuterol, cromolyn sodium, and ipratropium bromide on the airway and circulating mediator responses to allergen bronchial provocation in asthma. *Am Rev Respir Dis*. 1985; 132:986–92.
67. Bruderman I, Cohen-Aronovski R, Smorzik J. A comparative study of various combinations of ipratropium bromide and metaproterenol in allergic asthmatic patients. *Chest*. 1983; 83:208–10.
68. Boner AL, DeStefano G, Niero E et al. Salbutamol and ipratropium bromide solution in the treatment of bronchospasm in asthmatic children. *Ann Allergy*. 1987; 58:54–8.
69. Woenne R, Katan M, Orange RP et al. Bronchial hyperreactivity to histamine and methacholine in asthmatic children after inhalation of Sch 1000 and chlorpheniramine maleate. *J Allergy Clin Immunol*. 1978; 62:119–24.
70. Clarke PS, Jarrett RG, Hall GJL. The protective effect of ipratropium bromide aerosol against bronchospasm induced by hyperventilation and the inhalation of allergen, methacholine and histamine. *Ann Allergy*. 1982; 48:180–3.
71. Chan-Yeung M. The effect of Sch 1000 and disodium cromoglycate on exercise-induced asthma. *Chest*. 1977; 71:320–3.
72. Poppius H, Salorinne Y. Comparative trial of salbutamol and an anticholinergic drug, Sch 1000, in prevention of exercise-induced asthma. *Scand J Respir Dis*. 1973; 54:142–7.
73. Thomson NC, Patel KR, Kerr JW. Sodium cromoglycate and ipratropium bromide in exercise-induced asthma. *Thorax*. 1978; 33:694–9.
74. Boner AL, Antolini I, Andreoli A et al. Comparison of the effects of inhaled calcium antagonist verapamil, sodium cromoglycate and ipratropium bromide on exercise-induced bronchoconstriction in children with asthma. *Eur J Pediatr*. 1987; 146:408–11.
75. Wolkove N, Kreisman H, Frank H et al. The effect of ipratropium bromide on exercise-induced bronchoconstriction. *Ann Allergy*. 1981; 47:311–5.
76. Larsson K. Oxitropium bromide, ipratropium bromide and fenoterol in exercise-induced asthma. *Respiration*. 1982; 43:57–63.
77. Pasterkamp H, Tal A, Leahy F et al. The effect of anticholinergic treatment on postexertional wheezing in asthma studies by phonopneumography and spirometry. *Am Rev Respir Dis*. 1985; 132:16–21.
78. Burge PS, Haries MG, I'Anson E. Comparison of atropine with ipratropium bromide in patients with reversible airways obstruction unresponsive to salbutamol. *Br J Dis Chest*. 1980; 74:259–62.
79. Ward MJ, Fentem PH, Smith WHR et al. Ipratropium bromide in acute asthma. *Br Med J*. 1981; 282:598–600.

80. Wegener T, Hendenstrom J. Effect of nebulized ipratropium bromide on lung function in nonallergenic bronchial asthma. *Respiration*. 1987; 52:1–6.
81. Cugell DW. Clinical pharmacology and toxicology of ipratropium bromide. *Am J Med*. 1986; 81(Suppl 5A):18–22.
82. Pakes GE, Brogden RN, Heel RC et al. Ipratropium bromide: a review of its pharmacological properties and therapeutic efficacy in asthma and chronic bronchitis. *Drugs*. 1980; 20:237–66.
83. Gross NJ, Skorodin MS. Anticholinergic, antimuscarinic bronchodilators. *Am Rev Respir Dis*. 1984; 129:856–70.
84. Bell JA, Bluestein DM, Danta I et al. Effect of inhaled ipratropium bromide on tracheal mucociliary transport in bronchial asthma. *Mt Sinai J Med*. 1984; 51:215–7.
85. Ghafouri MA, Patil KD, Kass I. Sputum changes associated with the use of ipratropium bromide. *Chest*. 1984; 86:387–93.
86. Molkenboer JFW, Lardenoye JG. The effect of Atrovent in micturition function, double blind cross-over study. *Scand J Respir Dis*. 1979; 103(Suppl):154–8.
87. Sackner MA, Friedman M, Silva G et al. The pulmonary hemodynamic effects of aerosols of isoproterenol and ipratropium in normal subjects and patients with reversible airway obstruction. *Am Rev Respir Dis*. 1977; 116:1013–22.
88. Chervinsky P. Double-blind study of ipratropium bromide, a new anticholinergic bronchodilator. *J Allergy Clin Immunol*. 1977; 59:22–30.
89. Holst PE, Gebbie T, Martin PD et al. A long-term trial of ipratropium in asthmatic patients. *Aust NZ J Med*. 1976; 6:367–8.
90. Thumm HW. Ophthalmic effects of high doses of Sch 1000 MDI in healthy volunteers and patients with glaucoma. *Postgrad Med J*. 1975; 51(Suppl 7):132–3. Abstract.
91. Lichterfeld A. Safety of Atrovent. *Scand J Respir Dis*. 1979; 103(Suppl):143–7.
92. Scheufler G. Ophthalmotonometry, pupil diameter and visual accommodation following repeated administration of Sch 1000 MDI in patients with glaucoma. *Postgrad Med J*. 1975; 51(Suppl 7):134. Abstract.
93. Boehringer Ingelheim Pharmaceuticals, Inc. Atrovent package insert. Ridgefield, CT; 1986 Dec.
94. Cardinale VA, Thurlow RM, eds. Drug Topics redbook annual pharmacists' reference. Oradell, NJ: Medical Economics Co., Inc.; 1988:175.

“

The Future of Fish Oil Supplements

Clinical trials of fish oil in the prevention of coronary thrombosis have yet to be published. With appropriate clinical endpoints such as death or myocardial infarction, they will necessarily be large and time consuming. Nevertheless, they will be of great interest both because of the favourable effect of fish oil on the prostacyclin-thromboxane axis and because of the effects on blood lipids, whole-blood viscosity, fibrinolytic activity, and vascular reactivity. Several clinical trials of fish oils in diseases with an inflammatory component—eg, rheumatoid arthritis, asthma, and most recently, psoriasis—have been reported.

. . . What of the future? Studies with fish oil have already imparted important information about lipid-derived mediators and seem likely to yield further insights into the role of these local hormones in a wide array of common and severe human diseases. Therapeutically, despite the encouraging findings in psoriasis, it seems unlikely that fish oil will make a dramatic impact in inflammatory disease unless long-term studies show that it influences disease progression. However, it may well prove to be a useful adjunct to more conventional therapy, particularly in patients who cannot tolerate large doses of nonsteroidal drugs. On the vascular front, it is just possible that a modest intake of, say, mackerel pâté will prove to be a safer and more efficacious alternative to mass prophylaxis with aspirin—only appropriately constructed and executed clinical trials will tell.

—Anon. Fish oil. *Lancet*. 1988; 1:1081–3. Editorial.

”

Research

Predicting need for pharmacokinetic consultation follow-up using discriminant analysis

DIANE E. BECK, EDWIN L. BRADLEY, AND JOHN A. FARRINGER

Abstract: A discriminant function that predicts whether a patient will require more than one intervention by the pharmacokinetic consultation service (PCS) was derived and evaluated prospectively.

In phase 1, peak and trough serum aminoglycoside concentrations were evaluated for each of the 150 patients. The patients were then classified into either group 1 or group 2. Group 1 patients required a change in regimen after the initial recommended regimen was begun, while patients in group 2 did not require a change in regimen. Forty-seven variables of group 1 and group 2 were compared by univariate analysis. Stepwise discriminant analysis was then used to develop a model for classifying patients into either group 1 or group 2. In phase 2, the discriminant function derived in phase 1 was applied to a new group of 47 patients.

In phase 1, significant variables of the derived discriminant function, in decreasing order of significance, were leukemia, serum creatinine concentration, location in an intensive-care unit (ICU), male sex, actual volume of distribution, therapeutic trough concentration, and number of days in the ICU before consultation. In phase 2, 6 (23%) of the 26 patients who actually required a change were classified into group 2, and 8 (38%) of the 21 patients who were assigned to group 1 for continuous monitoring did not actually require a regimen change.

Although the results of the derived discriminant function were significant, the function's clinical utility in predicting the need for a second dosing intervention was poor.

Index terms: Aminoglycosides; Blood levels; Dosage schedules; Hospitals; Methodology; Models; Pharmacokinetics
Clin Pharm. 1988; 7:681–8

With the increasing emphasis on cost containment in health care, pharmacists are finding it necessary to demonstrate that their services are beneficial to the patient and are being provided in the most economical manner. Studies have shown that pharmacokinetic monitoring improves patient care.[1,2] However, there are few data assessing the efficient use of a pharmacokinetic consultation service (PCS).

The major costs of providing pharmacokinetic monitoring include laboratory charges and personnel time.[3,4] PCSs usually include providing an initial patient assessment and then calculating a dosage regimen. In addition, the PCS team usually continues to monitor the patient daily and provide new dosing recommendations when indicated. The provision of this continuous monitoring can be quite time consuming and therefore increase personnel costs.

Some patients who are monitored daily by our team do not require a change in their aminoglycoside regimen after the initial recommendation is made. If such patients could be identified upon initial consultation, the pharmacist could selectively monitor only those who would benefit from continuous monitoring. The goals of this study

DIANE E. BECK, PHARM.D., is Associate Professor, School of Pharmacy, Auburn University, Auburn University, AL, and Clinical Pharmacist–Pharmacokinetics Consult Service, Department of Pharmacy, University of Alabama Hospital, Birmingham. EDWIN L. BRADLEY, PH.D., is Professor, Department of Biostatistics and Biomathematics, University of Alabama at Birmingham. JOHN A. FARRINGER, PHARM.D., is Assistant Director, Department of Pharmacy, University of Alabama Hospital, Birmingham, and Assistant Professor, School of Pharmacy, Auburn University.

Address reprint requests to Dr. Beck at the University of Alabama Hospital, Department of Pharmacy, 619 South 19th Street, Birmingham, AL 35233.

Presented at the 23rd Annual ASHP Midyear Clinical Meeting, Atlanta, GA, December 9, 1987.

Copyright © 1988, American Society of Hospital Pharmacists, Inc. All rights reserved. 0278-2677/88/0901-0681$02.00.

were to (1) derive a discriminant function for predicting which patients will require more than one adjustment to their aminoglycoside dose during treatment and (2) prospectively validate this discriminant function and assess its clinical utility.

Methods

Phase 1. A total of 150 patients who received either gentamicin, tobramycin, or amikacin and were monitored by the PCS team were retrospectively selected for study. These patients had been monitored during the months of October and November 1984 and February, March, October, and December 1986. Upon initial consultation, aminoglycoside concentrations were obtained. A trough serum concentration was determined within five minutes before the dose. The dose was then infused over one-half hour. The peak serum concentration was drawn one-half hour after the end of the infusion. A third sample, obtained at least one half-life after the peak concentration, was drawn if concentrations had not reached steady state. All samples were assayed by fluorescence polarization immunoassay (TDx, Abbott Laboratories, Irving, TX 75015). This assay method exhibited a coefficient of variation of less than 5%.

Before serum concentrations were obtained, pharmacokinetic values were calculated. Creatinine clearance was estimated using the Hull equation.[5] The Dettli equation was used to calculate the population rate of elimination (k).[6] The population volume of distribution (V) was determined by the following equation: $V(\text{L}) = 0.25$ L/kg [IBW + 0.5(ABW − IBW)], where IBW = ideal body weight and ABW = actual body weight.[7,8] For each patient, disease states or other factors affecting these values were considered in the evaluation of serum concentrations and calculation of dosages but not in the discriminant analysis.[7]

Using the Sawchuk–Zaske equation, pharmacokinetic values were derived from the measured concentrations.[9,10] These data had to agree with population data or have been verified by another set of serum concentrations. Twelve patients were excluded from the study because this criterion was not met. Based on patient-specific data, a dosage regimen was determined using the Sawchuk–Zaske equation. The patient's physician must have accepted and ordered the regimen recommended by the team.

Each patient was monitored from the time of initial consultation until the drug was discontinued, the patient was discharged, or the patient died. Patients were then classified into two groups. Patients in group 1 were those who had required a change in their aminoglycoside regimen. These patients required a second intervention because of either a change in pharmacokinetic values, type of aminoglycoside, or desired peak and trough concentrations. Patients in group 2 did not require a change in regimen after the initial regimen was implemented.

The values of 47 variables, known at the time of consultation, were recorded. These variables were tested for individual predictive power using methods of univariate analysis.[11] Specifically, categorical data were evaluated using chi-square analysis and Fisher's exact test. Continuous data were analyzed by the two-tailed Student's t test. In each case, the null hypothesis was that the variable tested did not affect assignment of a patient to the appropriate group.

Definitions

For each patient, the prediction error for the elimination rate constant was determined by subtracting the patient's actual elimination rate constant from the population elimination rate constant. The prediction error for volume of distribution was calculated in a similar manner. Acute renal failure was defined as a rise in serum creatinine concentration greater than 0.5 mg/dL in less than 24 hours. If the patient's serum creatinine concentration increased or decreased by 0.3 mg/dL or more within three days before the initial consultation, the patient was considered to have a fluctuating serum creatinine concentration. A patient was determined to have a hypotensive episode if, at the time of consultation, a sympathomimetic agent was required to maintain the blood pressure. Liver disease was present if at least three of the following criteria were met: an aspartate aminotransferase concentration >40 IU/L, an alanine aminotransferase concentration >40 IU/L, a total bilirubin concentration >2.5 mg/dL, diagnosis of liver disease, and presence of ascites. Cachexia was defined as a total body weight less than 80% of ideal body weight. The variable "other medications" was the total number of other scheduled medications the patient was receiving.

A model for classifying patients into either group 1 or group 2 was then derived by stepwise discriminant analysis.[12,13] This analysis selects the best subset of variables for classifying patients into one of two groups. For each patient, this discriminant model assumes that all variables are known simultaneously. This model (see appendix) is described by a mathematical equation called the discriminant function. The discriminant function can be used to calculate a discriminant score for a patient as follows:

$$Di = d_{i1}Z + d_{i2}Z_2 + \ldots d_{in}Z_n$$

where Di is the discriminant score for a given patient, d_{in} are the discriminant weights or coefficients, and Z_n are the discriminating variables.[12] The discriminant score categorizes a patient into one of two groups and may be used to determine the probability that the patient has been assigned to the correct group. For all statistical analyses, the a priori level of significance was $p < 0.05$. Statistical analyses were performed using SAS software (SAS System, SAS Institute, Inc., Cary, NC 27512).

Phase 2. The discriminant function derived in the phase 1 study was then prospectively evaluated in 47 new patients. Phase 2 was conducted during April and May 1987. These patients were required to meet the criteria described in the phase 1 study. At the time of consultation, the following variables were documented for each patient: sex, serum creatinine concentration, actual volume of distribution, diagnosis of leukemia, whether the trough concentration was in the therapeutic range (0.5–2.0 mg/L), whether the patient was in an intensive-care unit (ICU) at the time of consultation and, if so, the number of days the patient had been in the ICU before entry into the study. These variables were recorded because they were significant in the discriminant function derived during the phase 1 study.

A discriminant score was calculated for each patient by using the discriminant function derived in phase 1. The probability of a patient's requiring a regimen change was then determined by the following equation[12,13]:

$$P = 1/1 + e^{-Di}$$

where P is the probability of requiring a regimen change and Di is the patient's discriminant score. A probability score of 0.5 or greater was considered to predict that a change in regimen would be necessary.

Sensitivity was calculated by dividing the number of patients for whom a change in dosage regimen was correctly predicted by the total number of patients who actually required a regimen change. Specificity was calculated by dividing the number of patients for whom it was correctly predicted that a regimen change was not required by the total number of patients who actually did not require a regimen change. For both phases, approval for study was granted by the hospital's investigational review board.

Results

Phase 1. Forty-five percent (67 of 150) of patients required a second intervention by the PCS team for aminoglycoside dosing and therefore were classified into group 1. The remaining 83 patients were classified into group 2. Results of a comparison of these two groups by univariate analysis are shown in Tables 1 and 2. The demographic variables age, sex, and race, when tested for individual power, were not significantly different between the two groups. Patients in groups 1 and 2 received an aminoglycoside for a mean (±S.D.) of 1.9 ± 3.5 days and 1.5 ± 3.1 days, respectively, before consultation ($p > 0.05$).

Table 1.
Variables Evaluated by Chi-Square Test (Categorical Data)

Variable	*n* Group 1	*n* Group 2	*p* Value
Sex			0.28
Male	32	47	
Female	35	36	
Race			0.16
Black	20	34	
White	47	49	
Number of ICU patients	34	12	<0.0001
Presence of			
Fluctuation in serum creatinine concentration	25	13	0.009
Acute renal failure	18	7	0.01
Hypotensive episode	9	5	0.13
Hemodialysis	9	0	0.001
Peritoneal dialysis	1	0	0.28
Condition			
Chronic renal failure	16	6	0.01
Urinary-tract infection	12	24	0.14
Soft-tissue infection	17	22	0.77
Sepsis	32	27	0.03
Pneumonia	29	26	0.24
Other types of infection	1	3	0.47
Congestive heart failure	4	3	0.22
Leukemia	7	4	0.19
Other types of cancer	8	23	0.007
Liver disease	3	6	0.42
Ascites	0	1	0.37
Postpartum	1	4	0.26
Thermal injury	2	3	0.83
Chronic bedridden state	14	14	0.11
Paralysis	3	10	0.16
Cachexia	5	5	0.93
History of aminoglycoside toxicity	2	0	0.27
Therapeutic peak concentration	44	57	0.39
Therapeutic trough concentration	49	68	0.34
Number of patients receiving another nephrotoxic drug	9	6	0.11
Temperature[a]			0.57
Increased	1	0	
Decreased	11	17	
No change	17	17	
White blood cell count[a]			0.21
Increased	2	2	
Decreased	9	6	
No change	11	7	
Culture results[a]			0.18
Positive	12	9	
Negative	2	5	
Pending	9	5	

[a] Determined if patient was receiving aminoglycosides before the consultation.

The team spent a greater amount of time monitoring and calculating new dosages for the group 1 patients. Of these patients, 67% (45 of 67) required a dosage decrease, and 20.9% (14 of 67) required a dosage increase; 8 (11.9%) were changed to another aminoglycoside. Patients in group 1 were followed by the PCS team for 15.7 ± 11.9 days, and patients

Table 2.
Variables Evaluated by the Two-tailed Student's *t* Test

Variable[a]	*p* Value	Group 1 $n = 67$		Group 2 $n = 83$	
		Mean ± S.D.	Range	Mean ± S.D.	Range
Age (yr)	0.15	56.64 ± 17.23	26.00–84.00	52.10 ± 20.76	18.00–90.00
Serum creatinine concentration (mg/dL)	0.0027	2.4 ± 2.5	0.4–13.0	1.4 ± 1.1	0.3–9.0
Calculated creatinine clearance (mL/min)	0.051	66.62 ± 54.24	3.07–254.60	83.76 ± 51.86	4.82–357.00
Height (in)	0.57	67.3 ± 3.5	60.0–75.0	66.9 ± 4.1	54.0–76.0
Ideal body weight (kg)	0.74	64.5 ± 9.7	45.5–84.5	63.9 ± 11.0	31.7–86.8
Total body weight (kg)	0.63	71.3 ± 16.1	39.0–110.7	69.9 ± 17.4	33.0–132.7
k Population (hr^{-1})	0.051	0.17 ± 0.13	0.02–0.62	0.21 ± 0.12	0.02–0.87
k Actual (hr^{-1})	0.012	0.14 ± 0.11	0.01–0.53	0.18 ± 0.09	0.03–0.41
k Prediction error (hr^{-1})	0.91	0.03 ± 0.08	−0.18–0.30	0.03 ± 0.08	−0.11–0.55
V population (L)	0.53	17.06 ± 2.97	11.40–27.70	16.75 ± 3.05	8.25–24.85
V actual (L)	0.59	20.98 ± 6.24	10.30–37.00	20.38 ± 6.71	11.00–46.00
V prediction error (L)	0.30	−4.33 ± 5.74	−9.30–3.53	−3.30 ± 5.71	−20.90–7.00
Albumin concentration (g/dL)	0.14	2.7 ± 0.7	1.4–4.9	2.9 ± 0.6	1.3–4.5
Other medications (no.)	<0.0001	6.4 ± 3.5	0.0–14.0	4.2 ± 2.5	1.0–14.0
Days of therapy before consultation	0.4	1.9 ± 3.5	0.0–20.0	1.5 ± 3.2	0.0–25.0
No. of days in ICU	0.0001	9.3 ± 15.3	0.0–69.0	1.3 ± 4.2	0.0–29.0

[a] *k* = elimination rate constant, *V* = volume of distribution, ICU = intensive-care unit.

in group 2 were followed for 8.4 ± 4.8 days ($p < 0.0001$). Additional serum concentrations interpreted during the study interval for groups 1 and 2 were 7.7 ± 5.3 and 3.4 ± 2.3, respectively ($p < 0.0001$).

The majority of variables that were significantly different between the two groups were related to either renal function or critical-care status. By univariate analysis, the following variables were significant and occurred more frequently in the group that required a change in regimen: fluctuating serum creatinine concentrations, acute renal failure, hemodialysis, sepsis, chronic renal failure, location in an ICU, and trough aminoglycoside concentration that was outside the therapeutic range. In addition, these patients had significantly higher serum creatinine concentrations and lower rates of elimination and received a larger number of scheduled medications. The incidence of cancer, other than leukemia, was higher in the group that did not require a change in regimen ($p < 0.007$).

By univariate analysis, there was no significant difference in the actual volume of distribution, population volume of distribution, or volume of distribution prediction error between the two groups. Both groups demonstrated an actual volume of distribution that was greater than predicted. The mean volume of distribution in groups 1 and 2 was 0.32 ± 0.10 L/kg IBW and 0.31 ± 0.09 L/kg IBW, respectively ($p > 0.05$). The following variables were not significantly different between the two groups: height, ideal body weight, total body weight, cachexia, albumin concentration, presence of ascites, and diagnosis of thermal injury.

For those patients receiving aminoglycosides before consultation, treatment duration, temperature, white blood cell count, and culture results were not significantly different between the two groups.

Sepsis was diagnosed more frequently in group 1 according to univariate analysis ($p < 0.03$). However, there was no significant difference in the incidence of urinary-tract infections, soft-tissue infections, pneumonia, and other types of infection between groups 1 and 2. Also, there were no significant differences between the two groups in the number of patients who had had a hypotensive episode at the time of consultation, or who had congestive heart failure, liver disease, or paralysis, or who were bedridden or postpartum. Other variables that were not significantly different included prior history of aminoglycoside toxicity, peak aminoglycoside concentration, and administration of other nephrotoxic drugs.

The results of stepwise discriminant analysis from the phase 1 study are shown in Table 3. Significant variables of the derived discriminant model, in decreasing order of significance, were leukemia, serum creatinine concentration, location in ICU, sex, actual volume of distribution, trough aminoglycoside concentration, and number of days in the ICU before consultation. Patients with diagnoses of leukemia, increased serum creatinine concentration, increased volume of distribution, or critical-care status were more likely to require a second intervention. Men and patients with therapeutic trough concentrations were less likely to require a second intervention. When the discriminant function (see Table 3) was retrospectively applied to the phase 1 patients, 79% of patients were correctly assigned to the appropriate group.

Phase 2. A change in aminoglycoside regimen was necessary in 55.3% (26 of 47) of patients in phase 2. The discriminant function derived in the phase 1 study correctly predicted assignment to group 1 or group 2 in 70.2% (33 of 47) of the patients. Figure 1 is a histogram of the probability values calculated for the phase 2 patients.

In phase 2, the sensitivity of the discriminant function was 76.9%, which indicates that for 20 of the 26 patients who required a change in aminoglycoside dosage, such a change was predicted correctly. Twenty-one phase 2 patients did not require a change in their aminoglycoside regimen, and 13 of these patients were correctly assigned to group 2. Therefore, the discriminant function demonstrated a specificity of 61.9% (13 of 21).

Table 3.
Stepwise Discriminant Analysis[a]

Variable	Coefficient	p Value
Leukemia	3.1789	0.0002
Intensive-care unit patient	1.8276	0.0044
Serum creatinine concentration (mg/dL)	0.3921	0.0009
Actual V^b (L)	0.0844	0.0159
Number of days in intensive-care unit	0.0537	0.03
Therapeutic trough concentration	−1.2085	0.0198
Male sex	−1.2651	0.006
Constant	−2.0935	

[a] The following equation, called the discriminant function, is used to calculate a discriminant score for the patient: $Di = 3.1789(X1) + 1.8276(X2) + 0.3921(X3) + 0.0844(X4) + 0.0537(X5) - 1.2085(X6) - 1.2651(X7) - 2.0935$, where Di = discriminant score, X1 = diagnosis of leukemia (no = 0; yes = 1), X2 = location in an intensive-care unit (no = 0; yes = 1), X3 = serum creatinine concentration (mg/dL), X4 = volume of distribution (L), X5 = number of days in an intensive-care unit before the consultation, X6 = therapeutic trough concentration (no = 0; yes = 1), X7 = sex (females = 0; males = 1).

[b] V = volume of distribution.

Discussion

The univariate analysis identified individual variables that were significantly different between the two groups. However, the greatest discrimination between groups 1 and 2 was provided by the combination of variables included in the discriminant model. A major advantage of discriminant analysis is its ability to determine those variables that contribute additional information beyond that of other variables.[12,13] For example, of the six renal-related variables identified as significant by individual evaluation, the serum creatinine concentration contributed the most information according to discriminant analysis. Stepwise discriminant analysis also identified two variables related to patient location in an ICU. Each of these variables was contributing different information in the model.

Most variables involved in the discriminant function have been previously reported to cause interpatient or intrapatient variability in aminoglycoside pharmacokinetic values. Diagnosis of leukemia was the variable that contributed most to the discrimination of groups 1 and 2. Other investigators have demonstrated that cancer patients have an altered volume of distribution for aminoglycosides and altered clearance.[14,15] However, intrapatient variability involving leukemia patients has not been elucidated.

The derived discriminant function indicated that patients in an ICU were more likely to require a second intervention by the PCS team. In addition, those who had been there longer were more likely to require a change in regimen. The effect of

Figure 1. For each patient in phase 2 (n = 47), the probability of requiring a second dosing intervention by the pharmacokinetic consultation services team was calculated as described in the Methods section. A probability score of 0.5 or greater indicated that the patient would require a change in aminoglycoside regimen. ■ = patients who did not actually require a change in regimen; □ = patients who actually required a change in regimen. An ideal model would have classified all patients who did not require a change in regimen to the left of 0.5 and all patients who did require a change in regimen to the right of 0.5 on the x-axis.

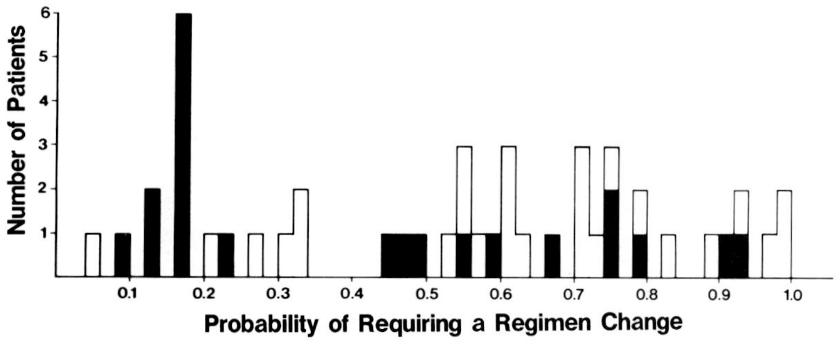

critical-care status on aminoglycoside pharmacokinetics is well documented in the literature.[16-20] Fuhs et al.[16] demonstrated significant intrapatient variability in aminoglycoside pharmacokinetic values in critically ill surgery patients with sepsis. This variability did not correlate with physiologic variables such as central venous pressure or creatinine clearance. Of their patients, 90% required at least one change in dosage regimen during the course of treatment. These investigators concluded that such patients should be closely monitored with serum aminoglycoside concentration analysis every three to four days. Niemiec et al.[17] reported an increased volume of distribution of aminoglycosides in surgical intensive-care patients. These investigators also found that changes in renal function and volume of distribution significantly altered dosage requirements during the course of treatment. In our study, actual volume of distribution and serum creatinine concentration significantly contributed to the discrimination of groups 1 and 2. In the discriminant model, these two variables were contributing information beyond that accounted for by the two variables related to critical-care status (i.e., presence in an ICU and length of time in an ICU before pharmacokinetic consultation).

The discriminant function also indicates that males and patients with therapeutic serum aminoglycoside concentrations were less likely to require a change in dosage regimen during the course of treatment. Interestingly, Moore et al.[21] found that males were less likely to develop nephrotoxicity. Elevated trough concentrations have been associated with a higher risk of nephrotoxicity by some studies.[22] However, it must be emphasized that the goal of our study was not to identify risk factors for nephrotoxicity but to identify a subset of variables that predict whether a patient will require a change from the initial recommended regimen. Our patients could have also required a second dosing intervention because of a change in desired concentrations or type of aminoglycoside.

Lampasona and Crass[23] suggested criteria for selecting patients who would most benefit from serum gentamicin concentration determinations. Serum creatinine concentration, leukemia, and volume of distribution were significant variables in our discriminant model and were also components of criteria described by these investigators. Our study documents that not only would these patients benefit from serum concentration analysis but that they are likely to require more than one dosing intervention.

Young et al.[24,25] performed a similar study to derive a discriminant function for identifying patients who would benefit most from pharmacist monitoring. In their study, a model was developed to predict patients for whom pharmacist intervention would result in a written communication about the patient's drug therapy. When this discriminant function was prospectively evaluated, 66% of patients were correctly classified. In these patients, the model demonstrated a sensitivity of 68.5% and a specificity of 54.0%. These investigators suggested use of the model for selectively monitoring patients and determining pharmacy staffing for a hospital.

Prospectively, the sensitivity and specificity of our model were better than those of the model derived by Young et al. However, our model's clinical utility in predicting the need for dosing intervention was poor. Twenty-three percent of the phase 2 patients who actually required a regimen change were incorrectly classified into group 2. In addition, eight patients were assigned to group 1 for continuous monitoring but never actually required a regimen change.

When the discriminant function was retrospectively applied to the phase 1 patients, 79% of patients were correctly classified. In the phase 2 study, 70% of patients were correctly assigned when this function was prospectively applied. This demonstrates that the discriminant function was consistent between the two phases.

Reasons for the model's poor clinical utility are unclear. This study demonstrated that critically ill patients were more likely to require a second intervention. Critically ill patients are also more likely to die. A regimen change was predicted for one study patient who was critically ill but who died shortly after the initial consultation. Actually, he did not require a change in regimen. However, had he lived, he might have required a second intervention. If a patient at the time of the initial consultation was not critically ill, he was more likely to be classified as not requiring a regimen change (group 2). However, if the patient developed complications after the initial workup, his clinical status might have become critical. This could have altered the patient's dosing requirements, resulting in an incorrect assignment to group 2.

During phase 1, both groups exhibited a volume of distribution of 0.31–0.32 L/kg IBW. A mean volume of distribution of 0.25 L/kg has been demonstrated in average patients.[7,22] However, values of 0.3–0.4 L/kg have been reported in surgical patients and in patients who are below ideal body weight, obese, critically ill, burned, postpartum, paraplegic, and quadriplegic.[22,26-29] A slightly larger than average volume of distribution would be expected in the study patients, since most of them exhibited at least one of these conditions.

Several investigators have studied pediatric patients to assess the need for routine pharmacokinetic monitoring.[30,31] Massey et al.[30] found that patients who were three months to 18 years of age did not have a rise in aminoglycoside trough concentration unless the duration of therapy was greater than 10 days. However, none of their patients were receiving other nephrotoxic drugs or had impaired renal function. In addition, none of their patients had a change in desired serum concentrations or type of aminoglycoside.

Our study evaluated adult patients and derived a model for predicting patients who would require a second dosing intervention. Before our study, we proposed that only patients for whom a second dosing intervention was predicted would need routine monitoring by the PCS team. Statistically, this could be concluded from our study. However, routine monitoring was not predicted for 23% of patients in phase 2, but these patients actually benefited from such monitoring.

Our data document that a large subgroup of our patients require daily monitoring for almost twice as long as other patients. For these patients, the pharmacist must interpret a greater number of serum aminoglycoside concentrations and make new dosing recommendations based on these data. This finding should be considered in determining reimbursement for pharmacokinetic monitoring.

This study was conducted in the practice setting. For most patients, a two-point sampling method (peak and trough serum concentrations) was used to calculate patient pharmacokinetic values, which could have biased the study results. However, a recent study at our institution found no significant difference in aminoglycoside pharmacokinetic values calculated by either the two-point or four-point method.[32] In addition, Torres et al.[9] compared the maintenance dosages calculated using two-point, three-point, and four-point methods and found no significant difference. Therefore, we believe it is unlikely that use of a two-point method biased the calculation of dosages in this study. Improper timing of blood sampling or improper sampling technique could have caused bias with the two-point method. However, the times of all blood sampling and drug administration were carefully recorded. In addition, when the derived pharmacokinetic data did not agree with population data, repeat peak and trough serum aminoglycoside concentrations were obtained to verify the initial data. Twelve patients were excluded from study because their initial data could not be verified.

Conclusion

This study demonstrates that some variables are significantly different between patients who require more than one dosing intervention by the PCS and those who do not. Although the derived discriminant model was significant, clinically it exhibited poor sensitivity and specificity. Because of this, clinical use of a discriminant function to predict whether an adult patient will require more than one aminoglycoside dosing intervention is not suggested.

References

1. Zaske DE, Cipolle RJ, Rotschafer JC et al. Gentamicin pharmacokinetics in 1,640 patients: method for control of serum concentrations. *Antimicrob Agents Chemother*. 1982; 21:407–11.
2. Sveska KJ, Roffe BD, Solomon DK et al. Outcome of patients treated by an aminoglycoside pharmacokinetic dosing service. *Am J Hosp Pharm*. 1985; 42:2472–8.
3. Schloemer JH, Zagozen JJ. Cost analysis of an aminoglycoside pharmacokinetic dosing program. *Am J Hosp Pharm*. 1984; 41:2347–51.
4. Rich DS, Pelter MA, Jeffrey LP. Pharmacokinetic consultation services: 1979 versus 1983. *Am J Hosp Pharm*. 1984; 41:56.
5. Hull JH, Hak LJ, Kock CG. Influence of range of renal function and liver disease on predictability of creatinine clearance. *Clin Pharmacol Ther*. 1981; 29:516–21.
6. Dettli LC. Drug dosage in patients with renal disease. *Clin Pharmacol Ther*. 1974; 16:274–80.
7. Zaske DE, Shikuma LR, Tholl DA. Aminoglycosides. In: Taylor WJ, Diers Caviness MH, eds. A textbook for the clinical application of therapeutic drug monitoring. Irving, TX: Abbott Laboratories; 1986:285–320.
8. Sketris I, Lesar T, Zaske DE et al. Effect of obesity on gentamicin pharmacokinetics. *J Clin Pharmacol*. 1981; 21:288–93.
9. Torres MJ, Kern JW, Gill MA et al. Comparison of serum sampling methods for estimating gentamicin pharmacokinetic variables. *Clin Pharm*. 1983; 2:353–5.
10. Sawchuk RJ, Zaske DE. Pharmacokinetics of dosing regimens which utilize multiple intravenous infusions: gentamicin in burn patients. *J Pharmacokinet Biopharm*. 1976; 4:183–95.
11. Marks, RG. Analyzing research data—the basics of biomedical research methodology. Belmont, CA: Lifetime Learning Publications; 1982.
12. Zelnio RN, Simmons SA. Interpretation of research data: other multivariate methods. *Am J Hosp Pharm*. 1981; 38:369–76.
13. Kleinbaum DG, Kupper LL, Muller KE. Applied regression analysis and other multivariable methods. Boston, MA: PWS-Kent Publishing Co.; 1988.
14. Higa GM, Murray WE. Alterations in aminoglycoside pharmacokinetics in patients with cancer. *Clin Pharm*. 1987; 6:963–6.
15. Kramer WG, Cleary T, Frankel LS et al. Multiple-dose amikacin kinetics in pediatric oncology patients. *Clin Pharmacol Ther*. 1979; 26:635–40.
16. Fuhs DW, Mann HJ, Kubajak CA et al. Intrapatient variation of aminoglycoside pharmacokinetics in critically ill surgery patients. *Clin Pharm*. 1988; 7:207–13.
17. Niemiec PW, Allo MD, Miller CF. Effect of altered volume of distribution on aminoglycoside levels in patients in surgical intensive care. *Arch Surg*. 1987; 122:207–12.
18. Lacarelle B, Granthil C, Manelli JC et al. Evaluation of a Bayesian method of amikacin dosing in intensive care unit patients with normal or impaired renal function. *Ther Drug Monit*. 1987; 9:154–60.
19. Flint LM, Gott J, Short L et al. Serum level monitoring of aminoglycoside antibiotics. Limitations in intensive care unit-related bacterial pneumonia. *Arch Surg*. 1985; 120:99–103.
20. Mann HJ, Fuhs DW, Awang R et al. Altered aminoglycoside pharmacokinetics in critically ill patients with sepsis. *Clin Pharm*. 1987; 6:148–53.
21. Moore RD, Smith CR, Lipsky JJ et al. Risk factors for nephrotoxicity in patients treated with aminoglycosides. *Ann Intern Med*. 1984; 100:352–7.
22. Zaske DE. Aminoglycosides. In: Evans WE, Schentag JJ, Jusko WJ, eds. Applied pharmacokinetics—principles of therapeutic drug monitoring. Seattle: Applied Therapeutics; 1986:331–81.
23. Lampasona V, Crass RE. Patient selection for serum genta-

micin levels. *Ther Drug Monit*. 1983; 5:255–62.
24. Young WW, Bell JE, Bouchard VE et al. Clinical pharmacy services: prognostic criteria for selective patient monitoring, part I. *Am J Hosp Pharm*. 1974; 31:562–8.
25. Young WW, Bell JE, Bouchard VE et al. Clinical pharmacy services: prognostic criteria for selective patient monitoring, part II. *Am J Hosp Pharm*. 1974; 31:667–76.
26. Kloth DD. Altered gentamicin pharmacokinetics during the perioperative period. *Clin Pharm*. 1985; 4:182–5.
27. Segal JL, Gray DR, Gordon SK et al. Pharmacokinetics of gentamicin in patients with spinal cord injury. *Clin Pharm*. 1984; 3:418–20.
28. Gardner DK, Schneider PJ. Gentamicin dosage requirements in postpartum patients. *Clin Pharm*. 1984; 3:416–8.
29. Tointon MM, Job ML, Peltier TT et al. Alterations in aminoglycoside volume of distribution in patients below ideal body weight. *Clin Pharm*. 1987; 6:160–2.
30. Massey KL, Hendeles L, Neims A. Identification of children for whom routine monitoring of aminoglycoside serum concentrations is not cost effective. *J Pediatr*. 1986; 109:897–901.
31. Green TP, Mirkin BL, Peterson PK et al. Tobramycin serum level monitoring in young patients with normal renal function. *Clin Pharmacokinet*. 1984; 9:457–68.
32. McClellan S, Farringer J. Evaluation of the Sawchuk-Zaske method using two serum levels. Paper presented to 45th ASHP Annual Meeting. San Francisco, CA: 1988 Jun 6.

Appendix—Instructions for Using the Discriminant Model

1. Using the discriminant function, calculate a discriminant score for the patient.
   Discriminant function:
   $$Di = 3.1789(X1) + 1.8276(X2) + 0.3921(X3) + 0.0844(X4) + 0.0537(X5) - 1.2085(X6) - 1.2651(X7) - 2.0935$$
   where Di = discriminant score for the patient, X1 = diagnosis of leukemia (no = 0; yes = 1), X2 = location in an ICU (no = 0; yes = 1), X3 = serum creatinine concentration (mg/dL), X4 = volume of distribution (L), X5 = number of days in an ICU before the consultation, X6 = therapeutic trough concentration (no = 0; yes = 1), X7 = Sex (female = 0; male = 1).
2. Calculate the probability that the patient will require a regimen change using the equation below:
   $$P = 1/(1 + e^{-Di})$$
   where P = the probability score for the patient, and Di = the discriminant score for the patient.
3. A probability score of 0.5 or greater indicates that a change in regimen will be needed.

Research Note

Predictability of unbound antiepileptic drug concentrations in children treated with valproic acid and phenytoin

Michael V. Miles, O. Carter Snead III, and Michael D. Thorn

Clin Pharm. 1988, 7:688–93

Monitoring unbound (free) antiepileptic drug concentrations has been recommended for drugs that are highly protein bound, that have a poor dose–effect relationship, and for which unbound and total concentrations are weakly correlated.[1] Differences in plasma protein binding of valproic acid and phenytoin have been reported between neonates and adults.[2,3] The need for monitoring unbound concentrations of highly bound drugs such as valproic acid and phenytoin may be more important in children than in adults because of the changes in tissue binding, distribution, and elimination characteristics of drugs that occur during childhood.[4]

Baird-Lambert et al.[5] evaluated the influence of several factors that could affect the variability of phenytoin binding, including hypoalbuminemia, other concurrent medications, age over 65 years, liver or renal disease, and pregnancy. Although their results included data from seven children less than 12 years of age, only age over 65 years was considered as a possible age-related factor in their data analysis. Advanced age was not shown to significantly affect phenytoin binding in this study. Other studies of phenytoin and valproic acid binding in children have not characterized the interindividual variability and possible age-related effects of the interaction between these antiepileptic agents.[6–11]

We studied the plasma protein-binding characteristics of phenytoin and valproic acid in epileptic children to determine whether age affects the predictability of unbound concentrations and whether unbound concentrations are more reliable than total concentrations for monitoring phenytoin and valproic acid therapy in pediatric patients.

Methods. This study was approved by the institutional review board. Thirty-five consecutive pa-

Michael V. Miles, Pharm.D., is Assistant Professor, School of Pharmacy, and Clinical Assistant Professor, School of Medicine, The University of North Carolina, Chapel Hill. O. Carter Snead III, M.D., is Professor, School of Medicine, The University of Alabama at Birmingham, AL. Michael D. Thorn, M.S., is a statistician for the Burroughs Wellcome Company, Research Triangle Park, NC.

Address reprint requests to Dr. Miles at the School of Pharmacy, CB # 7360, Beard Hall, University of North Carolina, Chapel Hill, NC 27599.

Copyright © 1988, American Society of Hospital Pharmacists, Inc. All rights reserved. 0278-2677/88/0901-0688$01.50.

tients who had been taking both phenytoin and valproic acid for more than two months and were being seen in the pediatric neurology clinic were selected for the study. None was taking the enteric-coated form of valproic acid. After informed consent was obtained, parents were asked to bring their children to the hospital laboratory at approximately 0800 to have a 3-mL blood sample drawn. Immediately after blood samples were obtained, patients were given their usual medication doses. Most took their medications after an overnight fast, but some were fed to minimize the upsetting gastrointestinal effects of valproic acid. Another blood sample was drawn three to four hours after the first, to allow for most of the valproic acid to be absorbed and to approximate peak effects. Patients were taking no drugs that might affect the plasma protein binding of phenytoin or valproic acid. None had evidence of renal or hepatic dysfunction, although several had mildly elevated serum aspartate aminotransferase concentrations.

Protein-free serum samples were obtained by ultrafiltration of 0.5–1.0 mL of serum using methods described earlier.[12,13] Unbound and total phenytoin and valproic acid serum concentrations were measured in duplicate the same day by fluorescence polarization immunoassay (TDx, Abbott Laboratories, Chicago, IL). The sensitivity ranges for free phenytoin and valproic acid were 0.5–4.0 mg/L and 2.0–25.0 mg/L, respectively. For total concentrations the ranges were 2.5–40.0 mg/L for phenytoin and 12.5–150 mg/L for valproic acid. The within-run and day-to-day precision determinations for unbound and total concentrations for both agents were <6.0%. The fraction of unbound drug, expressed as a percentage, was calculated by dividing unbound drug concentration by total drug concentration.

Student's t tests for paired data and unpaired data were used for group comparisons (within group and between group comparisons, respectively). Data were fitted to multiple linear regression models,[14] and 90% prediction limits were calculated[14,15] to evaluate the effects of various factors on unbound concentrations and free fractions of phenytoin and valproic acid. Specifically, four statistical models (using unbound concentrations and free fractions of each antiepileptic agent separately) were tested as linear functions of age, weight, sex, the presence or absence of encephalopathy, and total concentrations of antiepileptic drug. Unbound concentrations and free fractions of valproic acid also were tested against unbound and total phenytoin concentrations to assess what effect the saturable binding properties of valproic acid might have on phenytoin binding. All statistical analyses were performed using the Statistical Analysis System.[16,17] To assess age-related maturational effects, patients were divided into two groups: children <10 years old (group 1) and adolescents ≥10 years old (group 2).

Results. Twenty-six patients were included in the data analyses. Five patients were excluded because their total phenytoin concentrations were <2.5 mg/L, two because their total valproic acid concentrations were <12.5 mg/L, one because the morning dose was not administered properly, and one because no postdose blood sample was taken. Clinical information for groups 1 and 2 is summarized in Table 1.

The dosages of both agents, corrected for weight, were significantly higher in group 1 (Table 1). This was expected because of the higher dosage requirement, based on weight, for children. No significant differences in predose concentrations, postdose concentrations, or free fractions of phenytoin and valproic acid were found between groups (Table 2).

Within-group comparisons, however, showed statistically significant increases in unbound phenytoin and valproic acid concentrations (Table 2). The increase in the mean free fraction of phenytoin was from 11.94% to 14.76% for group 1 ($p <$ 0.001), and from 12.16% to 14.28% for group 2 ($p <$ 0.001). The mean free fraction of valproic acid increased from 7.56% to 9.76% for group 1 ($p = 0.002$), and from 6.98 to 8.59% ($p = 0.003$) for group 2. Similar changes in concentrations and free fractions have been reported previously, although the patient population was smaller ($n = 7$) and included both children and adults.[18] Our results confirm these earlier findings.

Age, sex, weight, the presence of encephalopathy, and total concentrations were identified as possible modifiers of unbound drug concentrations. Total predose and postdose serum phenytoin and valproic acid concentrations were the only factors related to the respective predose and postdose concentrations of unbound drug in both groups. The correlations of predose unbound drug concentrations with total drug concentrations were significant for phenytoin ($r = 0.94$; $p < 0.0001$; $y = 0.110x + 0.086$) and valproic acid ($r = 0.89$; $p < 0.0001$; $y = 0.082x - 0.308$). The postdose correlations between unbound and total drug concentrations were $r = 0.91$; $p < 0.0001$; $y = 0.134x + 0.086$ for phenytoin and $r = 0.90$; $p < 0.0001$; $y = 0.125x - 1.874$ for valproic acid. In these equations, x equals total drug concentration and y equals the predicted unbound drug concentration.

Age, weight, sex, and presence of encephalopathy were used in a multiple linear regression model to test dependency with unbound and total drug concentrations and free fractions of each antiepileptic agent. No models could be fitted, which suggests that none of these factors is related to the concentrations or free fractions of either agent.

Predose and postdose free fractions of phenytoin and valproic acid were widely variable. Free phenytoin fractions for most patients remained within the range of 8% to 18%; however, one (patient 24)

Table 1.
Patient Characteristics and Medication Use

Patient No.	Age (yr)	Weight (kg)	Sex	Seizure Classification	Medications[a] Valproic Acid (mg/kg/day)	Phenytoin (mg/kg/day)	Other
Group 1							
1	4.2	16.2	M	Tonic–clonic	29.6	7.7	PB
2	5.5	12.5	M	Tonic–clonic	36.0	8.0	PB
3	4.6	16.1	F	Tonic–clonic	65.2	4.6	CBZ
4	8.0	30.9	F	Myoclonic	24.3	8.1	PB, CLP
5	8.0	27.5	F	Tonic–clonic	27.3	8.2	PB, CLP
6	6.9	25.9	M	Complex partial	50.2	6.8	PB
7	1.6	9.0	M	Tonic–clonic	27.8	11.1	PB
8	6.8	21.1	M	Myoclonic	47.4	5.9	None
9	0.6	10.2	M	Tonic–clonic	23.5	4.9	PB
10	7.4	22.6	M	Myoclonic	60.1	6.6	None
11	8.0	22.7	M	Tonic–clonic	49.6	6.6	PB
12	9.3	20.0	F	Tonic–clonic	50.0	8.8	PB
13	5.0	18.6	F	Mixed	64.5	7.4	None
Mean ± S.D.	5.8 ± 2.6	19.5 ± 6.6			42.7 ± 15.4	7.3 ± 1.7	
Group 2							
14	15.0	60.9	M	Complex partial	36.9	3.3	PB, CBZ
15	12.5	39.5	M	Tonic–clonic	15.8	4.3	PB
16	11.5	60.9	F	Tonic–clonic	16.4	4.5	PB
17	16.0	66.4	F	Tonic–clonic	22.6	4.5	PB, CBZ, CLP
18	14.0	54.8	M	Mixed	27.4	3.6	CBZ
19	19.0	46.4	M	Complex partial	16.2	4.3	CBZ
20	19.0	62.7	M	Tonic–clonic	12.0	4.8	PB
21	10.1	31.2	M	Tonic–clonic	46.5	7.2	PB, ACZ
22	13.0	40.2	F	Tonic–clonic	37.3	7.5	CBZ, MB
23	14.3	45.5	F	Tonic–clonic	49.5	8.8	PB
24	14.0	52.7	M	Tonic–clonic	32.7	4.7	CBZ, PMD
25	15.7	54.0	M	Complex partial	13.9	3.7	CBZ
26	15.9	57.3	F	Tonic–clonic	17.5	5.2	None
Mean ± S.D.	14.6 ± 2.6	51.7 ± 10.5			26.5 ± 12.8[b]	5.1 ± 1.7[c]	

[a] PB = phenobarbital; CBZ = carbamazepine; CLP = clonazepam; ACZ = acetazolamide; MB = mephobarbital; PMD = primidone.
[b] $p = 0.008$.
[c] $p = 0.003$.

Table 2.
Predose and Postdose Unbound and Total Concentrations and Free Fractions of Phenytoin and Valproic Acid[a]

Drug	Group 1[b] Predose	Group 1[b] Postdose	Group 2[c] Predose	Group 2[c] Postdose
Unbound serum phenytoin concentration (mg/L)	1.25 ± 0.57	1.42 ± 0.68	1.27 ± 0.54	1.43 ± 0.59
Total serum phenytoin concentration (mg/L)	10.50 ± 4.58	9.62 ± 4.08	10.91 ± 4.92	10.34 ± 4.52
% Unbound phenytoin	11.94 ± 1.33	14.76 ± 2.47	12.16 ± 3.15	14.28 ± 4.01
Unbound serum valproic acid concentration (mg/L)	2.79 ± 1.46	6.57 ± 3.41	2.75 ± 0.92	5.73 ± 2.81
Total serum valproic acid concentration (mg/L)	35.59 ± 16.59	64.18 ± 22.91	39.14 ± 8.45	64.56 ± 22.60
% Unbound valproic acid	7.56 ± 1.28	9.76 ± 2.79	6.98 ± 1.53	8.59 ± 1.62

[a] All values are reported as mean ± S.D.
[b] Age <10 years.
[c] Age ≥10 years.

had values of 20.8% to 26.8% (Figure 1). Unbound valproic acid concentrations fluctuated consistently between 5% and 15% (Figure 2).

To evaluate the predictability of unbound drug concentrations, the difference between the unbound concentration predicted from the regression model and the observed unbound concentration was plotted against the observed unbound concentration (Figures 3 and 4). This method is more appropriate for comparison of clinical data than the correlation coefficient and techniques such as regression analysis, which may be misleading.[19] The 90% prediction limits were ±0.32 mg/L and ±0.44 mg/L for predose and postdose unbound phenytoin concentrations, respectively. Predose unbound phenytoin concentration predictions fell outside the 90% prediction limits for five individuals; postdose unbound concentration val-

Figure 1. Predose and three-hour postdose free fractions of phenytoin for each patient (n = 26).

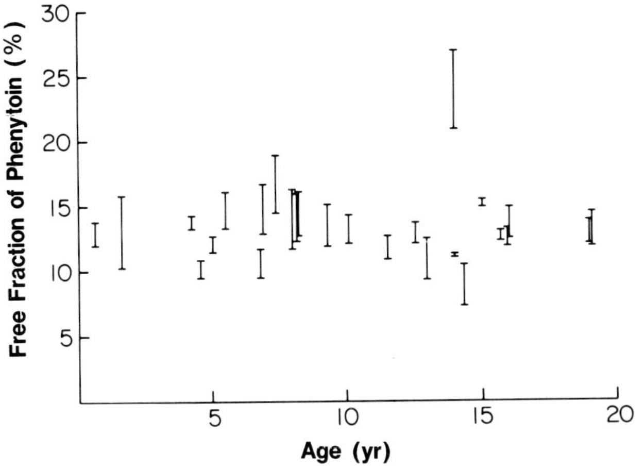

Figure 2. Predose and three-hour postdose free fractions of valproic acid for each patient (n = 26).

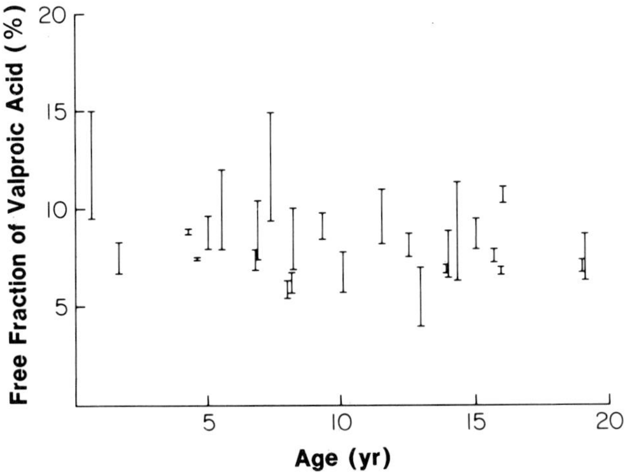

ues were outside the prediction limits for two individuals (Figure 3). The 90% prediction limits were ±0.89 mg/L and ±2.28 mg/L for predose and postdose unbound valproic acid concentrations, respectively. Predose unbound valproic acid concentration predictions fell outside the 90% prediction limits for only two individuals, and postdose values for three individuals were outside the prediction limits (Figure 4). Although relatively few in number, the outliers for both antiepileptic agents were approximately evenly split between groups 1 and 2.

Discussion. It is a fundamental principle that only unbound drug is pharmacologically active. The free fraction, or ratio of unbound to total concentration, depends on the association constant of the drug–binding site interaction and the availability or concentration of binding sites. The unbound drug concentration, however, is directly related to dosage and inversely related to intrinsic clearance.[20]

Valproic acid and phenytoin are highly bound to plasma proteins and compete for closely related binding sites. The time course of this interaction, studied in eight patients ranging in age from 5 to 51 years, showed a 12% to 36% increase in unbound phenytoin concentration, whereas total phenytoin concentrations decreased slightly.[18] This study was weakened because the control and study groups were poorly matched, and two patients were included in both treatment and control groups. We attempted to characterize the interaction of valproic acid and phenytoin by determining simultaneous unbound and total concentrations before the first morning dose and then again approximately

Figure 3. Differences between observed and model-predicted predose (A) and postdose (B) unbound phenytoin concentrations plotted against observed concentrations. Dashed lines indicate 90% prediction limits. ▲ = group 1; ● = group 2.

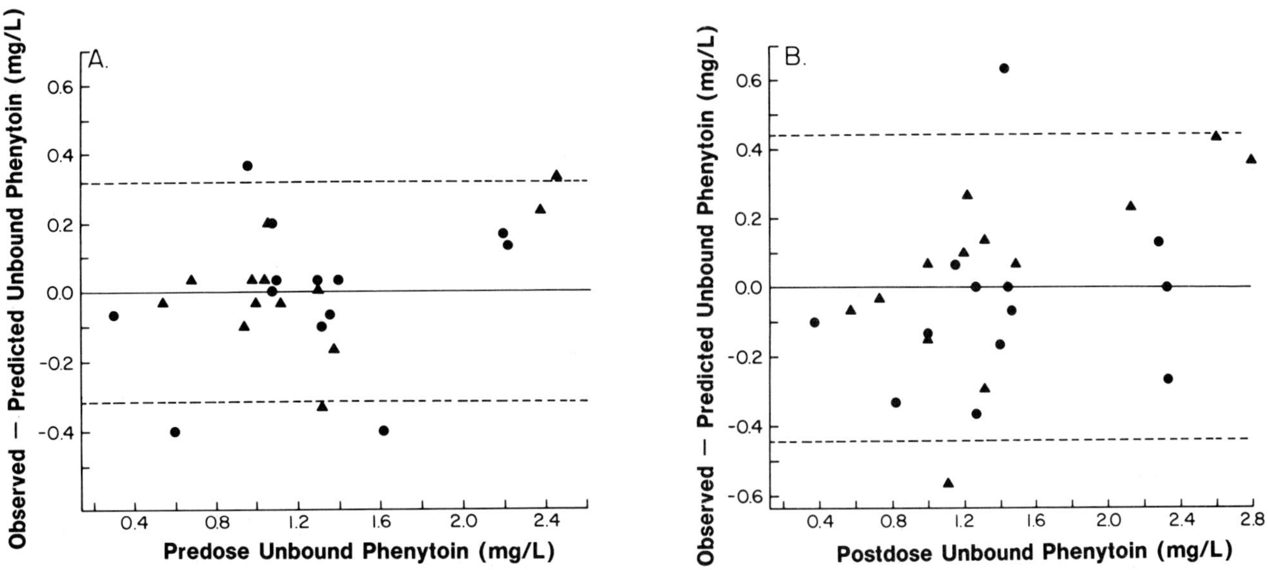

Figure 4. Differences between observed and model-predicted predose (A) and postdose (B) unbound valproic acid concentrations plotted against observed concentrations. Dashed lines indicate 90% prediction limits. ▲ = group 1; ● = group 2.

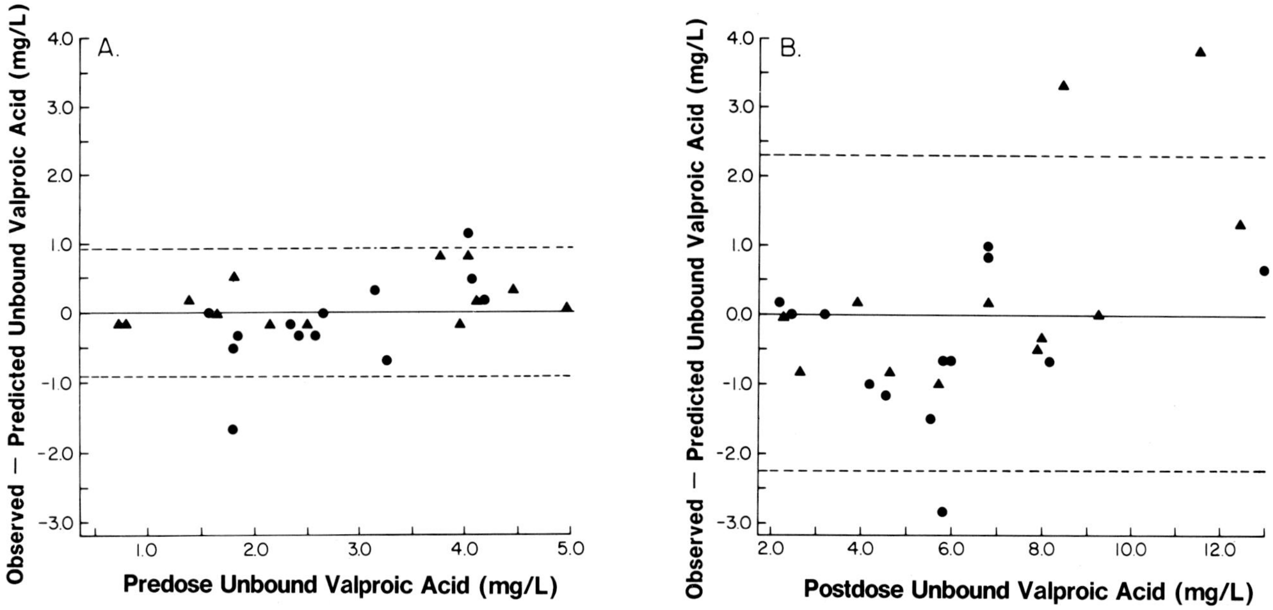

three hours later, when valproic acid concentrations and phenytoin displacement from binding sites would be near maximum. During the three-hour postdose period, mean unbound phenytoin concentrations increased 13.6% and 12.6% in groups 1 and 2, respectively (Table 2). Mean total phenytoin concentrations decreased 8.6% and 4.4% in groups 1 and 2, respectively. Mean free fractions of phenytoin increased 24.4% in group 1 and 17.2% in group 2 after the morning dose. Changes between groups were comparable for valproic acid (Table 2), since mean predose unbound concentrations increased 235.5% and 208.4% in groups 1 and 2, respectively. Mean total valproic acid concentrations increased 180.3% in group 1 and 167.5% in group 2. Mean free fractions of valproic acid increased 29.1% and 23.1% in groups 1 and 2, respectively. The interindividual variability in the free fractions of both phenytoin and valproic acid binding is particularly notable (Figures 1 and 2). None of the factors that have been cited[20] as interfering with phenytoin and valproic acid protein binding was present in any of our patients.

Although many studies have reported good correlations between unbound and total concentrations of phenytoin and valproic acid, few have involved children. Using stepwise regression analysis, Baird-Lambert et al.[5] found no relationship between patient age (≤65 years and >65 years) and unbound phenytoin concentration in 314 serum samples. We did not find a significant difference in the plasma protein-binding characteristics for either phenytoin or valproic acid between two younger age groups, children <10 and ≥10 years. These data are consistent with other evidence that the protein-binding characteristics of phenytoin and valproic acid are constant throughout life after infancy.[4]

Poor predictability of unbound and total drug concentrations has been suggested as justification for monitoring unbound drug concentrations. Using the method of Armitage[15] for the calculation of 90% prediction limits, predose unbound phenytoin concentrations can be expected to be within ±0.32 mg/L of the value calculated using the equation $y = 0.110x + 0.086$ 90% of the time, and postdose unbound phenytoin concentrations should be within ±0.44 mg/L of the value calculated using the equation $y = 0.134x + 0.086$ 90% of the time. Predose unbound valproic acid concentrations can be expected to be within ±0.89 mg/L of the value calculated using the equation $y = 0.082x + 0.308$ 90% of the time, and postdose unbound valproic acid concentrations should be within ±2.28 mg/L of the equation $y = 0.125x - 1.874$ 90% of the time.

Realization that 10% of the time unbound phenytoin concentrations will vary by more than 0.3–0.4 mg/L from the best possible statistical prediction of unbound concentration provides evidence that unbound phenytoin concentrations should be monitored in certain patients. Although the pharmacodynamics of unbound valproic acid is not as well defined as that for unbound phenytoin, it should be noted that the 90% prediction limits for unbound valproic acid, calculated using predose (trough) concentrations, are less than 50% of those occurring three to four hours after a dose. Predose unbound and total valproic acid concentrations, therefore, should be considerably more reliable for patient monitoring.

Conclusion. We studied the effects of dosing, age, sex, weight, and the presence of encephalopathy on unbound concentrations and free fractions of phenytoin and valproic acid in a pediatric population. None of these factors was found to affect the unbound concentrations or free fractions of either drug. Wide interpatient variability in free fractions and poor predictability of the unbound concentrations of both phenytoin and valproic acid indicate that unbound concentrations should be monitored. We found no evidence to suggest that unbound phenytoin and valproic acid concentrations are less predictable in younger children than they are in older children; therefore, age beyond the infancy period is not a factor for the clinician to consider when deciding whether to monitor unbound concentrations of these antiepileptic agents.

References

1. Levy RH, Moreland TA. Rationale for monitoring free drug levels. *Clin Pharmacokinet*. 1984; 9(Suppl 1):1–9.
2. Gal P, Oles KS, Gilman JT et al. Valproic acid efficacy, toxicity, and pharmacokinetics in neonates with intractable seizures. *Neurology*. 1988; 38:467–71.
3. Besunder JB, Reed MD, Blumer JL. Principles of drug biodisposition in the neonate. *Clin Pharmacokinet*. 1988; 14:189–216.
4. Stewart CF, Hampton EM. Effect of maturation on drug disposition in pediatric patients. *Clin Pharm*. 1987; 6:548–64.
5. Baird-Lambert J, Manglick MP, Buchanan N. Identifying patients who might benefit from free phenytoin monitoring. *Ther Drug Monit*. 1987; 9:134–8.
6. Bruni J, Gallo JM, Lee CS, et al. Interactions of valproic acid with phenytoin. *Neurology*. 1980; 30:1233–6.
7. Farrell K, Orr JM, Abbott FS et al. The effect of acetylsalicylic acid on serum free valproate concentrations and valproate clearance in children. *J Pediatr*. 1982; 101:142–4.
8. DeMonaco HJ, Lawless LM. Variability of phenytoin protein binding in epileptic patients. *Arch Neurol*. 1983; 40:481–3.
9. Riva R, Albani F, Franzoni E et al. Valproic acid free fraction in epileptic children under chronic monotherapy. *Ther Drug Monit*. 1983; 5:197–200.
10. Otten N, Hall K, Irvine-Meek J et al. Free valproic acid: steady-state pharmacokinetics in patients with intractable epilepsy. *Can J Neurol Sci*. 1984; 11:457–60.
11. Yu H. Clinical implications of serum protein binding in epileptic children during sodium valproate maintenance therapy. *Ther Drug Monit*. 1984; 6:414–23.
12. Argyle JC, Kinniburgh DW, Costa R et al. Evaluation of an ultrafiltration–fluorescence polarization immunoassay for monitoring unbound phenytoin. *Ther Drug Monit*. 1984; 6:117–20.
13. March C, Blanke RV. Determination of free valproic acid concentrations using the Amicon Micropartition MPS-1 ultrafiltration system. *Ther Drug Monit*. 1985; 7:115–20.
14. Draper NR, Smith H. Applied regression analysis. 2nd ed. New York: John Wiley & Sons; 1981:141–280.
15. Armitage P. Statistical methods in medical research. Oxford: Blackwell Scientific Publications; 1971:147–66.
16. SAS Institute. SAS user's guide: statistics, version 5. Cary, NC: SAS Institute, 1985:655–710.
17. SAS Institute. SUGI: supplemental library user's guide, version 5. Cary, NC: SAS Institute; 1986:269–94.
18. Riva R, Albani F, Contin M. Time-dependent interaction between phenytoin and valproic acid. *Neurology*. 1985; 35:510–5.
19. Bland JM, Altman DG. Statistical methods for assessing agreement between two methods of clinical measurement. *Lancet*. 1986; 1:307–10.
20. Levy RH, Schmidt D. Utility of free level monitoring of antiepileptic drugs. *Epilepsia*. 1985; 26:199–205.

“

Vasodilator Therapy for Heart Failure

. . . The evidence suggests that at least some vasodilator regimens—particularly the angiotensin converting-enzyme inhibitors, which have been most thoroughly studied—can accomplish symptom relief in a large percentage of patients. Thus, the physician has strong inducements and few risks in instituting vasodilator therapy in all of his/her patients with heart failure. Only ongoing large-scale trials and new ones yet to be initiated can satisfactorily answer the question of *which* vasodilator regimen should be initiated in *which* patient. In the meantime, however, the patient with heart failure should be the beneficiary of the extensive research effort to date.

—Cohn JN. Vasodilator therapy for heart failure: what have we learned from controlled clinical trials? *JAMA*. 1988; 259:3456–7. Editorial.

”

Commentary

How many subjects are required for a study?

Jerry W. McLarty

Clin Pharm. 1988; 7:694–6

The number of subjects required for a study (henceforth called sample size) is easily and often overlooked by Institutional Review Boards (IRBs) as an ethical issue. After all, sample size is a scientific question usually reviewed by others before the IRB gets involved. Moreover, it is a statistical, almost mystical, concept that most members do not understand. However, as I will try to demonstrate, estimation of sample size is an important ethical issue. Although highly mathematical in practice, sample size determination is based on commonsense principles that are within the grasp of the least mathematically trained IRB member.

Why is sample size so important? For several reasons. Using too many subjects can result in unnecessary exposure of humans to risk; valuable resources, both human and monetary, can be wasted. If too few subjects are used, totally wrong inferences can be drawn from the experiment. One of the most common mistakes in human studies is to underestimate the number of participants needed to answer the scientific questions that are the purpose of the study. As a result, there are no clear-cut answers at the conclusion of the study. In effect, nothing has been learned. For example, if a new drug has been tested and no response was observed, either the drug didn't work or too few persons were tested to prove it works. After all, humans are complicated, highly variable organisms, some of whom may respond where others won't. The consequence is that a good drug could have been prematurely discarded. This is termed a false negative conclusion. How many "penicillins" of the future are missed like this?

Jerry W. McLarty is Chairman and Professor of Epidemiology/Biomathematics, University of Texas Health Center, Tyler, TX.

Copyright © 1987, The Hastings Center. Reprinted with permission from *IRB: A Review of Human Subjects Research.* 1987; 9(Sep–Oct):1–3.

Because of inconclusive results, the study may be repeated, exposing more humans to needless potential risk.[1] A fair question to ask is the following: If too few persons were tested to prove that the drug works, why not just recruit more patients until statistical significance is attained? The statistical objections to this procedure are complicated[2] but the basic objections are that the significance levels (p values, discussed later) must be adjusted for multiple testing and, perhaps more important, that investigators would be tempted to continue the study until they obtained any answer they wanted. Sequential trials with multiple analysis of the data can be legitimately performed, but usually entail a much more sophisticated study design and analysis.[3]

Another possibility, perhaps worse than a false negative conclusion, is a false positive one; that is, a worthless (or even harmful) drug may be declared effective. Many exciting new discoveries that are later found not to work are the result of studies performed with too few subjects. The costs in dollars, human hopes, and lives are incalculable.

Using too many subjects minimizes the chance of false negative or positive conclusions, but leads to the more obvious ethical violations, unnecessarily exposing humans to potential risk and wasting resources. Human studies are inherently expensive and time-consuming. One of the major obstacles to many important human studies is the availability of eligible subjects; unnecessarily large sample sizes deplete this pool of subjects for other important studies, wasting financial resources and time for all involved.

Estimation of Sample Size

The calculation of the required number of subjects is a complicated procedure involving mathematical and statistical concepts that are under continual discussion and development by professional statisticians. However, most such calculations have a common basis of several easily understood principles. Furthermore, published charts and tables[4,5] make calculations easily accessible to researchers who are not familiar with the underlying mathematical formulas. Sample size is directly determined by four factors: variability of the outcome measurement (end-point) of the study; magnitude of the expected outcome; power of the study to reach a true positive conclusion; and the willingness of the investigator to accept the risk of a false positive conclusion.

Variability of Endpoint. Every study has a measurable endpoint, such as change in some physiologic variable (e.g., blood pressure, survival time, percent response). The more precisely an endpoint can be measured, the fewer the required number of subjects. On the other hand, measurements that show extreme variability between subjects (or even from time to time in the same subject) require more subjects for study. Such imprecise measurements are invariably encountered in human studies; some endpoints are either impossible to measure accurately (I.Q., for example) or they vary considerably (pulse rate, for example, which is quite different in different individuals and changes constantly depending upon what we are doing, what we are thinking, or what is being done to us). The loss of information to such variability can be overcome only by making more measurements or adding more individuals to the study.

Magnitude of Response. The second factor that dramatically affects sample size is the magnitude of the response under investigation. As an extreme example, if a cure is sought for a previously untreatable, fatal disease, only a single successfully treated patient is required to demonstrate the value of the new treatment. However, in most human research we are not so fortunate. Cancer chemotherapy, for example, has often advanced by finding therapeutic regimens with only small (say, 5% or 10%) improvements over previous regimens; such studies often require hundreds of patients, recruited from many different institutions. The investigator is expected to know, in advance, what magnitude of response to expect or at least what would be considered of scientific (clinical) merit.

Power To Reach True Positive Results. Power, in the narrowly defined statistical sense, is the probability of getting the right answer, e.g., finding a positive result if one really exists. A study with a statistical power of 50% is just as likely (and no more) to obtain a correct answer as could be obtained by simply tossing a coin. It is incredible but true that many studies are conducted (with full IRB approval)[6] that could be better answered by tossing a coin (just as effective, much cheaper, and without putting humans at risk)! Of course, absolute certainty (power of 100%) is unattainable, since all subjects in the population would have to be used in the study, i.e., a virtually infinite sample size. Setting power requirements for a study (80–90% are common) requires an explicit value judgment for the investigator: How important is it that an important positive effect not be missed, i.e., what are the consequences of a false negative conclusion?

Statistical Significance. The final consideration in sample size calculation is statistical significance. Significance, as quantified by the commonly used p value, is simply the probability of coming to a false positive conclusion, e.g., saying a procedure is effective or better than the comparison procedure when it is not. A significance (p value) of .05, which is commonly used, means that 5% of the time, 1 out of 20 experiments, an experiment can be expected to give erroneous results, just by chance. The smaller the desired p value, i.e., the more certainty, the more subjects required. Again, virtual certainty ($p = 0$) is unattainable, but reasonable judgments can be made. For example, an investigator may be willing to take a 1 in 10 chance ($p = .10$) of being in error by declaring that a headache remedy, with minor side effects, is effective. On the other hand, for an anticancer drug with potentially fatal side effects, he or she would want to be sure, say, a 1 in 100 chance of error ($p = .01$) in concluding the drug was effective.

Once decisions about power, significance, and expected magnitude of response have been made and variability of the measurements ascertained, the required number of subjects can be calculated. The details of the calculations are intimidating, but fortunately, published charts and tables[4,5,7] and, more recently, user-friendly computer programs[8,9] make such calculations relatively easy. Blindly using such aids is justifiable in many circumstances but where the costs are high in terms of dollars, time, resources, or human risk, professional help should be sought. It is a false economy to sacrifice ethical considerations, and to risk wasting resources to avoid a short consultation with a statistician.

Common Excuses

If sample size determination is so important, both scientifically and ethically, then why is it so often not properly done? Reasons (or excuses) frequently given include: not understanding the statistics of the process and not knowing how to do the calculations; not enough information available to make the calculations; the study is of such low risk no harm will be done even if the sample size is improperly small or large; and, many other studies have been published with the same sample size or smaller.

"I don't know how to do it." This first excuse is especially weak. As already discussed, published tables and graphs and software packages are readily available to make the calculations and most research centers employ statisticians to help as requested. There are now many books with excellent expositions of the subject.[10]

"Not enough information available to make the calculation." The second excuse often comes under the guise of a "pilot" study. Only rarely is the information needed to make the calculations (e.g., variabil-

ity, magnitude of the response) not available. The scientific literature often contains similar experiments with the needed information. Sometimes data must be extrapolated from animal experiments or clinical experience. Investigators should be sufficiently knowledgeable in their field of research to make educated guesses if hard data are not available.

Asking "what if" type questions is common in the early exploratory phases of study design. Numbers can be generated and judgments made on reasonable assumptions. For example, an investigator may not know what magnitude of response to expect from a new drug to lower blood pressure; but he or she can compute sample sizes for a range of responses, e.g., 10%, 20% reduction, etc. Or he or she can ask the question, "If the drug significantly lowered the pressure in half the patients, how many subjects would it take to detect this change?" and calculate sample size appropriately. In short, the data for sample size estimation are usually available; if not, it is better to make reasonable assumptions about the data and calculate sample size from these assumptions than to just pick an arbitrary sample size (10 patients is common) based on wishful thinking.

"The study is of such low risk no harm will be done." As discussed previously, a study with too few patients may lead to erroneous conclusions with potentially disastrous results; good drugs or procedures may be discarded or bad ones accepted into common practice. Too large a sample size wastes resources that could be better used. So, even low-risk studies should be carefully planned and executed.

"Many published studies used the same number of subjects, or less." This is an especially insidious reason. There is an unfortunate trend in almost all areas of applied research that only "significant" results get published.[11,12] However, as we have seen, small numbers of subjects lead to the danger of falsely significant results. With the conventional p value of .05, at least five out of a hundred studies will be declared significant, when in fact they are not! With a selective publishing policy, these five may be published and the other 95 rejected or not even submitted for publication. The result is that wrong results often do get published; if the sample size was inadequate, other investigators are led into following a bad example.

The IRB's Role

Imprecision in measurement, small effects, and high likelihood of drawing correct conclusions all demand a penalty—more subjects. It is the investigator's job to balance this penalty against the risk to subjects, the cost of the research, and the anticipated benefits. It is the IRB's job to verify that he or she has documented these decisions properly and that the benefits do exceed the risks.

IRBs are rightfully concerned about the informed consent process. Perhaps truly informed consent would require investigators to explain statistical power considerations to patients as well. Should we require statements like the following? "It has been explained to me that the study in which I am being asked to participate has only a 50–50 chance of reaching a correct conclusion, or perhaps any conclusion at all." Sample size considerations are vital to good research and human subjects have an expectation and a right to participate in only well-designed studies. If it is not good science, it is not ethical.

References

1. Frieman JA, Chalmers TC, Smith H Jr et al. The importance of beta, the type II error and sample size in the design and interpretation of the randomized control trial. *N Engl J Med.* 1978; 299:690–4.
2. McPherson K. Statistics: the problems of examining accumulating data more than once. *N Engl J Med.* 1974; 290:501–2.
3. Whitehead J. The design and analysis of sequential clinical trials. Chichester: Ellis Horwood Limited; 1983.
4. Cohen J. Statistical power analysis for the behavioral sciences, 2nd ed. Orlando: Academic Press; 1977.
5. Fleiss JL. Statistical methods for rates and proportions, 2nd ed. New York: Wiley and Sons; 1981.
6. Giammona M, Glantz SA. Poor statistical design in research on humans: the role of committees on human research. *Clin Res.* 1983; 31:572–8.
7. Young MJ, Bresnitz EA, Strom BL. Sample size nomogram for interpreting negative clinical studies. *Ann Intern Med.* 1983; 99:248–51.
8. Brown B, Herson J. STPLAN, a computer system for performing statistical calculations needed to plan a study. *Am Statistician.* 1981; 35:164.
9. Rothman KJ, Boice JD. Epidemiological analysis with a programmable calculator, 2nd ed. Boston: Epidemiology Resources, Inc.; 1982.
10. Friedman LM, Furberg CD, Demets DL. Fundamentals of Clinical Trials. Boston: John Wright–PSG Inc.; 1983.
11. Simes RJ. Confronting publication bias: a cohort design for meta-analysis. *Stat Med.* 1987; 6:11–29.
12. Zelen M. Guidelines for publishing papers on cancer clinical trials: responsibilities of editors and authors. *J Clin Oncol.* 1983; 1:164–9.

Diagnosis and treatment of neuroleptic malignant syndrome

RAWLEY M. GUERRERO AND KENNETH A. SHIFRAR

Abstract: A patient who developed neuroleptic malignant syndrome (NMS) from the use of several neuroleptic agents and the therapeutic interventions used to reverse the syndrome are described, and the clinical presentation and treatment of NMS are reviewed.

Fever, leukocytosis, seizures, delirium, and elevated serum creatine phosphokinase levels developed in a 17-year-old girl who was receiving perphenazine and haloperidol. The patient was admitted to a hospital for treatment of atypical psychosis and received haloperidol and, later, thioridazine. Autonomic disturbances, altered consciousness, and muscular rigidity developed. Thioridazine was discontinued in favor of perphenazine because of anticholinergic adverse effects. Symptoms persisted despite treatment with benztropine and diphenhydramine. After the diagnosis of NMS was made, all neuroleptics were discontinued, and the patient began therapy with dantrolene sodium and bromocriptine. Dramatic improvement in the patient's condition followed.

NMS has four characteristic signs: hyperthermia, muscular rigidity, altered consciousness, and autonomic dysfunction. Mechanisms believed to cause NMS include alteration of central neuroregulatory mechanisms and neuroleptic-induced imbalance between central dopaminergic and γ-aminobutyric acid neurotransmitter systems. Bromocriptine, amantadine, dantrolene sodium, and electroconvulsive therapy have been used effectively in the treatment of NMS.

NMS is a rare but potentially fatal adverse drug reaction that occurs in situations that make diagnosis difficult. Dramatic, favorable responses can be achieved with early diagnosis and appropriate treatment.

Index terms: Antihistamines; Benztropine; Bromocriptine; Combined therapy; Dantrolene sodium; Diphenhydramine; Haloperidol; Neuroleptic malignant syndrome; Perphenazine; Prolactin inhibitors; Skeletal muscle relaxants; Smooth-muscle relaxants; Thioridazine; Toxicity; Tranquilizers
Clin Pharm. 1988; 7:697–701

Neuroleptic malignant syndrome (NMS) is a rare but potentially fatal adverse drug reaction associated with the use of dopamine antagonists and, in particular, neuroleptic drugs. If the reported incidence of NMS in patients treated with neuroleptic drugs (0.5–1.4%)[1,2] is accurate, the syndrome often is unrecognized or misdiagnosed.[3–5] Mortality has been estimated at 20–30%.[3,6–9] Treatment has consisted of supportive measures and attempts to affect the postulated central and peripheral pharmacological mechanisms. Early diagnosis is essential, and recognition of this syndrome and intervention by the pharmacist providing service to the patient may expedite therapy and avoid potentially fatal complications. We report a case in which the patient was successfully treated with bromocriptine and dantrolene sodium.

Case Report

A 17-year-old white girl was admitted to the medical intensive care unit on October 12, 1987, from a community psychiatric institute (CPI) with a postpartum diagnosis of atypical psychosis, acute upper respiratory tract infection, and possible CNS infection. During her three-day CPI stay she received neuroleptic therapy and had increasing delirium, fever, an elevated white blood cell

RAWLEY M. GUERRERO, PHARM.D., is Associate Director, Department of Pharmacy Services, University Hospital, University of Utah Health Sciences Center, and Adjunct Assistant Professor of Clinical Pharmacy, College of Pharmacy, University of Utah, Salt Lake City. KENNETH A. SHIFRAR is Staff Pharmacist, Department of Pharmacy Services, University Hospital.

Address reprint requests to Dr. Guerrero at the Department of Pharmacy Services (A-050), University Hospital, University of Utah Health Sciences Center, 50 North Medical Drive, Salt Lake City, UT 84132.

Presented at the 45th ASHP Annual Meeting, San Francisco, CA, June 8, 1988.

Copyright © 1988, American Society of Hospital Pharmacists, Inc. All rights reserved. 0278/2677/88/0901-0697$1.25.

Papers in the Grand Rounds section are patient case reports and literature review combined in a way that gives them high educational value. The papers lead off with a well-documented case report of an unusual drug experience (e.g., adverse drug reaction or other unexpected drug response, experimental use of a drug). The case generally deals with a difficult therapeutic problem or dilemma that is commonly encountered but may be overlooked or misunderstood. (Esoteric or rare occurrences of minor importance do not make good Grand Rounds material.) A literature review puts the case in perspective with previously reported similar cases and alternative treatments. The review is integrated with related discussion of the case being reported.

CP *readers are encouraged to use Grand Rounds for educational group discussions. For this purpose, discussion questions are printed at the end of Grand Rounds papers.*

count, seizures, and increasing serum creatine phosphokinase (CPK) levels. Medications at the time of admission included phenytoin sodium 100 mg p.o. b.i.d., lorazepam 1 mg p.o. or i.m. every six hours as needed, acetaminophen 650 mg p.o. every four hours as needed, haloperidol 2 mg p.o. t.i.d., benztropine mesylate 1 mg p.o. t.i.d., and perphenazine 4 mg p.o. t.i.d.

Admission laboratory data included a white blood cell count of 14,000 cells/cu mm and a serum CPK concentration of 1829 IU/L. Vital signs were temperature, 38 °C; pulse, 100 per minute; respirations, 22 per minute; and blood pressure, 160/90 mm Hg. Treatment was started with phenytoin sodium 300 mg i.v. at bedtime, diphenhydramine hydrochloride 25–50 mg i.v. every two to four hours as needed for hypertonus, midazolam 1–2 mg (as the hydrochloride salt) i.v. every two to four hours as needed for agitation, and penicillin G potassium 4 million units i.v. every four hours. Within six hours, midazolam was discontinued, and diazepam 2–6 mg i.v. every one to four hours was ordered for agitation. On day 2, diazepam was discontinued in favor of haloperidol 2 mg i.m. (as the lactate salt) every four to six hours for severe agitation and combativeness. The patient responded well to haloperidol and was transferred to a neurology unit. Bacterial cultures of blood, urine, sputum, and cerebrospinal fluid were negative and a test for human immunodeficiency virus was negative, but the patient demonstrated positive herpes simplex virus type 1 titers, at 0.30 outer diameter (low positive) by the enzyme-linked immunosorbent assay method. The patient was hyperreflexic and had episodes of tachycardia and elevated blood pressure. Medications included phenytoin sodium 300 mg p.o. at bedtime, haloperidol 1–2 mg (as the lactate salt) i.m. or i.v. every six hours as needed for agitation.

On day 6, because of dystonic reactions, haloperidol was discontinued and replaced with thioridazine hydrochloride 100 mg p.o. every eight hours and 25–50 mg p.o. every eight hours as needed for agitation and benzotropine mesylate 1–2 mg p.o. every eight hours as needed. On day 7, the routine dose of thioridazine hydrochloride was increased to 100 mg p.o. every six hours. Pulse was 132 per minute, and respirations were 20 per minute. The patient was hyperreflexic (5+), with bilateral sustained clonus. After being transferred to a psychiatric unit, the patient had to be restrained because of continued agitation and combativeness. The mental status of the patient fluctuated from lucidity to delirium. She was disoriented most of the time and responded only intermittently to simple commands.

On day 11, the patient became drowsy and had a short attention span. Because of suspected anticholinergic effects, thioridazine was replaced by perphenazine 12 mg p.o. b.i.d. Dystonia was observed two days later, with rigidity and posturing, and was treated with diphenhydramine hydrochloride 25 mg i.m. Dystonia persisted and was unresponsive to repeated doses of diphenhydramine and to benztropine. The patient was transferred to the neurological critical care unit (NCCU), and all neuroleptics were discontinued.

On day 14, the patient demonstrated widely fluctuating respiration rate, temperature, and blood pressure. The diagnosis of NMS was made, and dystonia was treated with lorazepam 1 mg i.v. every four hours as needed. Dantrolene sodium therapy was initiated at 70 mg i.v. every four hours, and improvement was noted within the first 11 hours. Over the next 96 hours, the patient received 2380 mg of dantrolene sodium in both oral and injectable form.

On day 15, bromocriptine 5 mg (as the mesylate salt) p.o. every eight hours was initiated and given concurrently with dantrolene sodium therapy. The dosage of bromocriptine was increased to 10 mg p.o. every eight hours on day 16. Laboratory findings included a serum CPK concentration of 701 IU/L on day 15, which increased to 742 IU/L on day 16. Within the first 96 hours of dantrolene therapy and the first 72 hours of bromocriptine therapy, blood pressure, pulse, respiration, and temperature were normal, rigidity was resolved, and the patient was oriented to time and place. The patient remained in the NCCU for 40 days for the resolution of other problems and was eventually transferred to a separate rehabilitation unit.

Discussion

NMS has four characteristic signs: hyperthermia, muscular rigidity, altered consciousness, and autonomic dysfunction, but characteristic symptoms are not always present in all cases.[1,6,10] Hyperthermia, with a temperature as high as 42 °C, results in profuse diaphoresis, dehydration, and often acute renal failure.[6] Muscular rigidity has been described as "lead-pipe" or "plastic" rigidity. Additionally, muscular dystonia has been reported as pseudoparkinsonism, opisthotonos, dysphagia, sialorrhea, chorea, trismus, akathisia, and rhabdomyolysis. Altered consciousness has appeared as stupor, akinesia, mutism, coma, seizure activity, and aspiration. The level of consciousness often fluctuates from an alert to a delirious state.[11] Autonomic dysfunction has included tachycardia, pallor, labile blood pressure, incontinence, dyspnea, and pulmonary congestion with respiratory stridor. Tachypneic hypoventilation and respiratory distress may occur as a result of neuromuscularly induced decreased chest-wall compliance, necessitating mechanical ventilation.[9,12] Our patient demonstrated persistent and, at times, sustained dystonic episodes with posturing and hyperreflexia. Also present were minor episodes of tachycardia, increased respiration rate, blood pressure changes, and hyperthermia, as well as varying levels of consciousness and awareness. In this case, profound hyperthermia and profuse diaphoresis were not observed.

NMS usually begins soon after the initiation of neuroleptic therapy or after an elevation in dosage. In this case, several neuroleptics were used: haloperidol, perphenazine, and thioridazine, with multiple dosage adjustments and changes in agents used.

Once it has begun, NMS progresses rapidly over 24 to 72 hours.[1] Manifestations of rigidity and hyperthermia typically are the first symptoms to appear. Duration of symptoms may be from several days to weeks after discontinuation of the neuroleptic agent, with duration being substantially increased in patients treated with long-acting injectable neuroleptic agents. The most frequently encountered complications are those due to respiratory, renal, or cardiac failure.[12] Death has occurred up to 30 days after initial onset of symptoms, resulting from respiratory failure, aspiration pneumonia, thromboembolism, renal failure, or cardiovascular complications.[10]

Laboratory abnormalities, including leukocytosis and elevated aspartate aminotransferase, alanine aminotransferase, lactate dehydrogenase, and alkaline phosphatase levels, have been reported, but they are mostly nonspecific. Serum CPK levels are often dramatically increased and may exceed 16,000 IU/L.[1,14,15] Laboratory findings may be useful to help rule out infections or neoplastic, traumatic, vascular, or toxic–metabolic conditions that may appear to be NMS[6,12]; however, postmortem histopathologic studies of the brain have not demonstrated specific structural changes.[3,6,13] Our patient demonstrated substantially elevated white blood cell counts and CPK levels, and CPK levels remained persistently elevated during hospitalization.

The occurrence of NMS has been strongly associated with the use of phenothiazines, butyrophenones, thioxanthenes, and dibenzoxazepines, in therapeutic doses rather than toxic doses.[1,4,6,13,16–20] Additionally, abrupt discontinuation of antiparkinsonian agents and dopamine-depleting agents has been reported to result in NMS.[10,21] A drug's potential to induce NMS may parallel its antidopaminergic potency.[1] Rechallenge with the neuroleptic agent has not frequently resulted in NMS, suggesting that the neuroleptic alone may not be sufficient to cause the syndrome.[1,6] Other contributing factors in the development of NMS may include physical exhaustion, dehydration, organic brain syndrome, initiation of neuroleptic treatment at high dosage levels, rapid increases in dosage, and the use of long-acting depot agents.[1,10] In our patient, NMS developed after treatment with haloperidol and perphenazine and persisted and progressed after thioridazine was replaced with perphenazine on day 11.

An alteration of central neuroregulatory mechanisms involving the hypothalamus and the basal ganglia, and complicated by the induction of hypertonia, has been postulated as the most plausible explanation for the emergence of NMS.[1,6,12,13,22] Dopamine receptor sites in the hypothalamus and limbic structures are involved in the regulation of muscle tone and body temperature, with central regulation of temperature involving thermodetection by the preoptic hypothalamus and the generation of effector signals by the posterior hypothalamus. Hyperpyrexia can result from elevation of the hypothalamic set point, impaired heat dissipation, or excessive heat production.[13]

Neuroleptics have been demonstrated to antagonize the ability of intracerebrally injected dopamine to induce hypothermia in animals.[23] The presentation of profuse diaphoresis with vasoconstriction implies that peripheral temperature regulatory mechanisms remain intact.[9,24] While muscle contraction can raise body temperature, the muscular rigidity associated with parkinsonism does not typically cause hyperthermia. Hyperthermia and rigidity have been observed after abrupt discontinuation of antiparkinsonian drugs[13,21,25–27] and after the use of dopamine-depleting drugs in Huntington's chorea.[28] Additionally, neuromuscular blockade producing flaccid paralysis has not been successful in reducing fever[3,6]; however, sodium nitroprusside was successful in a case of NMS characterized by pronounced vasoconstriction and without substantial rigidity that was previously unresponsive to therapy with dantrolene sodium.[29] These observations strongly suggest the involvement of contributory mechanisms.[6,13]

Neuroleptic-induced imbalance between central dopaminergic and γ-aminobutyric acid (GABA) neurotransmitter systems has been postulated as another possible primary or contributory pharmacological mechanism for NMS.[14] Dopamine-receptor blockade with haloperidol has been demonstrated to decrease GABA levels in the nigrostriatal neurons of rats, thereby possibly activating the increased turnover of dopamine in the striatum.[30] NMS was successfully reversed by diazepam administration in two reported cases of neuroleptic-induced NMS, presumably by a GABA-mediated effect on dopamine turnover.[14] Sangal and Dimitrijevic[31] reported a case of NMS in which the combination of pancuronium bromide and diazepam was used successfully. Diazepam 4 mg every four to six hours as needed was administered for the intended purpose of sedation while the patient was mechanically ventilated. The patient received a total of 64 mg of diazepam during the 48-hour period of mechanical ventilation. The apparent efficacy of benzodiazepines in some cases and failure in others, as well as the lack of evidence to support a more substantial role for benzodiazepines, suggests a probable secondary role for GABA in the development of NMS.

Treatment

Dopamine-receptor agonists have demonstrated success in the treatment of NMS, including three cases of NMS successfully treated with bromocriptine.[32–34] The patients had hyperthermia, muscular rigidity, autonomic dysfunction, and various manifestations of altered CNS function. Initial bromocriptine dosages ranged from 2.5 mg t.i.d. to 5 mg every four hours. In all cases, dosages were adjusted during the course of therapy to a range of 5–10 mg t.i.d. In two cases, rigidity and blood pressure improved within hours of bromocriptine administration. In all cases, substantial or complete response was noted within two to three days of initiation of therapy, including reduction in serum CPK levels, blood pressure, and temperature. A single case involving the prior administration of a long-acting neuroleptic agent by depot injection necessitated a second period of increased dosage of bromocriptine, with a subsequent improvement.[34] The rapid and substantial response of NMS to bromocriptine administration supports the hypothesis that the pathogenesis of NMS involves central dopaminergic blockade or hypoactivity.[32,33]

Additionally, amantadine has also been reported to be effective in the treatment of NMS.[16,35] McCarron et al.[35] reported a case of a patient with fluphenazine-induced NMS who was treated with amantadine hydrochloride 100 mg b.i.d.[35] Marked improvement, consisting of reduction in rigidity and intermittent tremor, reduction of fever to 37 °C, no diaphoresis, and an oriented and cooperative demeanor, was noted after two doses of amantadine. Discontinuation of the drug after 72 hours of treatment resulted in a return of symptoms, necessitating reinstitution of the previous regimen and continuation for a total of 21 days of therapy. Amdurski et al.[16] reported a case of haloperidol-induced NMS successfully treated with amantadine hydrochloride 200 mg/day and diazepam 15 mg/day, with the patient improving gradually over a period of days.[16] Amantadine causes the release of dopamine from central neurons in the nigrostriatum and has also been shown to delay the reuptake of dopamine from neural cells.[36]

Because NMS resembles the syndrome of malignant hyperthermia associated with the use of anesthetic agents, dantrolene sodium has been used in some cases. Goulon et al.[37] observed a relationship between temperature decrease and muscle relaxation and suggested that fever in NMS may have a muscular origin. The recurrence of muscle rigidity and fever after the discontinuation of neuroleptic therapy and after a single dose of i.v. dantrolene sodium suggests that muscle contraction can be triggered by remaining amounts of the neuroleptic agent.[38] Oral regimens have ranged from 100 to 300 mg daily in divided doses for two to three days, and intravenous doses in the range of 1.25 to 1.5 mg/kg as single doses have been reported.[39]

Electroconvulsive therapy (ECT) is an alternative treatment modality that has been used in situations in which there has been difficulty in differentiating between NMS and an evolving catatonic state.[7,37,40] Jessee and Anderson[39] described two cases, and Lazarus[38] described one case, in which ECT resulted in general clinical improvement when it was used to treat patients with hyperthermia, rigidity, and a history of neuroleptic use. Clinical response generally consisted of rapid reduction of fever and gradual improvement in the manifestations of muscular rigidity. Patients demonstrated rapid and dramatic reduction of symptoms after initial treatments with ECT. Subjects eventually received between two and five total ECT treatments during their hospital stay. Treatment with ECT has not been without attributed complications. In 2 of 14 cases reviewed by Addonizio and Susman,[7] brief atrial arrhythmias, which resolved spontaneously, were associated with ECT; however, single cases of ventricular fibrillation and cardiac arrest have also been reported. The mechanism by which ECT reverses the effects of NMS is unclear but may involve enhanced nigrostriatal dopaminergic function.[7]

Conclusion

NMS is a rare but potentially fatal adverse drug reaction that occurs in situations that make diagnosis difficult. The incidence is not well documented, but data suggest that the syndrome may be frequently misdiagnosed. NMS has a high mortality rate, but dramatic, favorable responses can be achieved with early diagnosis and appropriate treatment.

Discussion Questions

1. What is the presumed mechanism by which NMS evolves?
2. What are some physiological conditions that may contribute to the evolution of NMS?
3. What are the four characteristic signs of NMS?
4. What therapeutic measures have been used successfully in the treatment of NMS?
5. What are the consequences of unrecognized and untreated NMS?

References

1. Caroff S. The neuroleptic malignant syndrome. *J Clin Psychiatry*. 1980; 41:79–83.
2. Cohen BM, Baldessarini RJ, Pope HG Jr et al. Neuroleptic malignant syndrome. *N Engl J Med*. 1985; 313:1293. Letter.
3. Morris H, McCormick W, Reinarz J. Neuroleptic malignant syndrome. *Arch Neurol*. 1980; 37:462–3.

4. Delay J, Deniker P. Drug induced extrapyramidal syndromes. In: Vinken PJ, Bruyn GW, eds. Handbook of clinical neurology. Vol 6. Diseases of the basal ganglia. Amsterdam: North Holland Publishing. 1968:248–66.
5. Diamond JM, Santos AB. Unusual complications of antipsychotic drugs. *Am Fam Phys*. 1982; 26:153–7.
6. Smego R Jr, Durack D. The neuroleptic malignant syndrome. *Arch Intern Med*. 1982; 142:1183–5.
7. Addonizio G, Susman V. ECT as a treatment alternative for patients with symptoms of neuroleptic malignant syndrome. *J Clin Psychiatry*. 1987; 48:102–5.
8. Greenberg L, Gujavarty K. The neuroleptic malignant syndrome: review and report of three cases. *Compr Psychiatry*. 1985; 26(1):63–70.
9. Szabaldi E. Neuroleptic malignant syndrome. *Br Med J*. 1984; 288:1399–1400.
10. Guze B, Baxter L. Neuroleptic malignant syndrome. *N Engl J Med*. 1985; 313:163–6.
11. Vincent F, Zimmerman J, Van Haren J. Neuroleptic malignant syndrome complicating closed head injury. *Neurosurgery*. 1986; 18:190–3.
12. Lazarus A. The neuroleptic malignant syndrome: a review. *Can J Psychiatry*. 1986; 31:132–7.
13. Henderson V, Wooten G. Neuroleptic malignant syndrome: a pathogenic role for dopamine receptor blockade? *Neurology*. 1981; 31:132–7.
14. Lew T-Y, Tollefson G. Chlorpromazine-induced neuroleptic malignant syndrome and its response to diazepam. *Biol Psychiatry*. 1983; 18: 1441–8.
15. Anon. Neuroleptic malignant syndrome. *Lancet*. 1984; 1:545–6.
16. Amdurski S, Radwan M, Levi A et al. A therapeutic trial of amantadine in haloperidol induced neuroleptic syndrome. *Curr Ther Res*. 1983; 33:225–9.
17. Dosani R. Haloperidol-induced neuroleptic malignant syndrome. *South Med J*. 1983; 76:546. Letter.
18. Cruz F, Thiagarajan D, Harney J. Neuroleptic malignant syndrome after haloperidol therapy. *South Med J*. 1983; 76:684–6.
19. McAllister RG Jr. Fever, tachycardia, and hypertension with acute catatonic schizophrenia. *Arch Intern Med*. 1978; 138:1154–6.
20. Ewert AL, Kloek J, Wells B et al. Neuroleptic malignant syndrome associated with loxapine. *J Clin Psychiatry*. 1983; 44:37–8.
21. Friedman J, Feinberg S, Feldman R. A neuroleptic malignant-like syndrome due to levodopa therapy withdrawal. *JAMA*. 1985; 254:2792–5.
22. Pearlman C. Neuroleptic malignant syndrome: a review of the literature. *J Clin Psychopharmacol*. 1986; 6:257–73.
23. Weinberg S, Twersky RS. Neuroleptic malignant syndrome. *Anesth Analg*. 1977; 165:263–8.
24. Martin ML, Lucid EJ, Walker RW. Neuroleptic malignant syndrome. *Ann Emerg Med*. 1985; 14:354–8.
25. Simpson DM, Davis SC. Case report of neuroleptic malignant syndrome associated with withdrawal from amantadine. *Am J Psychiatry*. 1984; 141:796–7.
26. Sechi GP, Tanda F, Mutani R. Fatal hyperpyrexia after withdrawal of levodopa. *Neurology*. 1984; 34:249–51.
27. Toru M, Matsuda O, Makiguchi K et al. Neuroleptic malignant syndrome-like state following a withdrawal of antiparkinsonian drugs. *J Nerv Ment Dis*. 1981; 169:324–7.
28. Burke RE, Fahy S, Mayeux R et al. Neuroleptic malignant syndrome caused by dopamine-depleting drugs in a patient with Huntington disease. *Neurology*. 1981; 31:1022–6.
29. Blue M, Schneider S, Noro S et al. Successful treatment of neuroleptic malignant syndrome with sodium nitroprusside. *Ann Intern Med*. 1986; 104:56–7.
30. Kim J-S, Hassler R. Effects of acute haloperidol on the gamma-aminobutyric acid system in rat striatum and substantia nigra. *Biol Res*. 1975; 88:150–3.
31. Sangal R, Dimitrijevic R. Neuroleptic malignant syndrome: successful treatment with pancuronium. *JAMA*. 1985; 254:2795–6.
32. Mueller P, Vester J, Fermaglich J. Neuroleptic malignant syndrome: successful treatment with bromocriptine. *JAMA*. 1983; 249:386–8.
33. Dhib-Jalbut S, Hesselbrock R, Brott T et al. Treatment of the neuroleptic malignant syndrome with bromocriptine. *JAMA*. 1983; 250:484–5.
34. Zubenko G, Pope H. Management of a case of neuroleptic malignant syndrome with bromocriptine. *Am J Psychiatry*. 1983; 140:1619–20.
35. McCarron MM, Boettger ML, Peck JJ. A case of neuroleptic malignant syndrome successfully treated with amantadine. *J Clin Psychiatry*. 1982; 43:381–2.
36. Bianchine JR. Drugs for Parkinson's disease, spasticity, and acute muscle spasms. In: Goodman and Gilman, eds. The pharmacological basis of therapeutics. 7th ed. New York: Macmillan Publishing Co.; 1985: 473–90.
37. Goulon M, Rohan-Chabot P, Elkharrat D et al. Beneficial effects of dantrolene in the treatment of neuroleptic malignant syndrome: a report of two cases. *Neurology*. 1983; 33:516–8.
38. Lazarus A. Treatment of neuroleptic malignant syndrome with electroconvulsive therapy. *J Nerv Ment Dis*. 1986; 174:47–9.
39. Jessee S, Anderson F. ECT in the neuroleptic malignant syndrome: case report. *J Clin Psychiatry*. 1983; 44:186–8.
40. Birkhimer L, DeVane C. The neuroleptic malignant syndrome: presentation and treatment. *Drug Intell Clin Pharm*. 1984; 18:462–5.

“

Use of Thiazide Diuretics as Initial Therapy for Hypertension

The role of thiazide diuretics in initial antihypertensive therapy has been recently challenged, and their range of application has been somewhat narrowed. Today, several possible first-choice agents are available, and treatment can be tailored to specific patient needs. The selection of a first drug depends on a consideration of demographic factors as well as on associated illnesses and potential side effects. As therapeutic approaches to the management of mild hypertension are broadened, the need for a rational application of nonpharmacologic and pharmacologic methods is clearly evident. With care, the risks of antihypertensive drug therapy are less than the benefits.

—Khair GZ, Kochar MS. Mild hypertension, diuretics, and cardiac arrhythmias: consensus amid controversy? *Am Heart J*. 1988; 116:216–21. Editorial.

”

CP Continuing Education

The ASHP Continuing Education system gives readers a self-assessment mechanism for selected articles in Clinical Pharmacy *and the* American Journal of Hospital Pharmacy. *It also allows readers to obtain continuing-education credit for these articles.*

For the purpose of CE-credit enrollment a blank answer sheet is published at the end of each installment of the column for the CE articles in that issue. An enrollee accumulates these answer sheets until the enrollment is submitted, using the form that is published in the June and December issues of Clinical Pharmacy *and in the June and December issues of the* American Journal of Hospital Pharmacy. *Any combination of tests within a 18-month period, from both* Clinical Pharmacy *and* American Journal of Hospital Pharmacy, *may be included in an enrollment. More complete details about enrollment in the system will appear in the semiannual enrollment form.*

Article 680-204-8814 (see page 647)
Qualifies for 1.0 hour of CE credit

Teicoplanin: An investigational glycopeptide antibiotic

Learning Objectives

After studying this article, the reader should be able to

1. State the mechanism of action of teicoplanin.
2. Describe the antimicrobial spectrum of teicoplanin, including resistance patterns and synergy information.
3. Compare the pharmacokinetic properties of teicoplanin with those of vancomycin, with specific emphasis on absorption, distribution, and elimination.
4. List the most likely types of infection teicoplanin will be used to treat given its antibiotic class and antimicrobial spectrum.
5. List the current dosing guidelines based on site of infection.
6. Describe the current adverse-effect profile of teicoplanin.

Self-assessment Questions

For each question there is only one best answer.

1. The structure of teicoplanin can be best described as a
   a. Phosphoglycopeptide structurally related to vancomycin.
   b. Glycopeptide complex consisting of five major components plus a sixth more polar component.
   c. Lipopeptide antibiotic complex closely related to vancomycin.
   d. Alternatives b and c are both correct.
2. The mechanism of action of teicoplanin against gram-positive microorganisms is
   a. Inhibition of DNA-dependent RNA synthesis.
   b. Binding to penicillin-binding protein (PBP) 3.
   c. Inhibition of peptidoglycan and cell-wall synthesis.
   d. Inhibition of amino acid uptake by bacterial cells.
   e. Alternatives a and b are both correct.
3. Which of the following statements regarding the pharmacokinetics and administration of teicoplanin is not correct?
   a. Teicoplanin has negligible absorption after oral administration.
   b. Like vancomycin, teicoplanin cannot be given intramuscularly.
   c. The elimination half-life of teicoplanin has varied from 33 to more than 100 hours.
   d. Teicoplanin is approximately 90% bound to serum albumin.
4. The most common adverse effect reported with teicoplanin is
   a. Nephrotoxicity, especially when administered with other nephrotoxic medications.
   b. Dose-related ototoxicity.
   c. Infusion reactions resembling the vancomycin "red-neck" syndrome.
   d. Development of a maculopapular rash.
5. The dosage of teicoplanin currently used in investigational trials for patients with normal renal function is
   a. A 400-mg loading dose followed by 200 mg every 24 hours.
   b. 6 mg/kg every 12 hours for three doses, then 6 mg/kg every 24 hours.
   c. 15 mg/kg twice daily for patients with endocarditis.
   d. Alternatives b and c are both correct.

6. Teicoplanin is active in vitro against all of the following organisms except
   a. *Streptococcus pneumoniae.*
   b. *Pseudomonas aeruginosa.*
   c. *Clostridium difficile.*
   d. *Staphylococcus aureus.*
   e. Alternatives b and c are both correct.
7. Possible areas of clinical use for teicoplanin include all of the following except
   a. Surgical and dental procedure prophylaxis for patients with prosthetic heart valves.
   b. Acute or chronic osteomyelitis caused by *Staphylococcus aureus.*
   c. Chronic urinary-tract infections caused by *Escherichia coli.*
   d. Prosthetic-valve endocarditis caused by *Staphylococcus epidermidis.*
   e. Alternatives a and c are both correct.
8. Resistance to teicoplanin
   a. Occurs at a spontaneous mutation rate of 10^{-4} per cell per generation.
   b. Has been reported for strains of *Staphylococcus haemolyticus.*
   c. Has been commonly reported with methicillin-susceptible and methicillin-resistant *Staphylococcus aureus.*
   d. Is uniformly noted in β-lactamase-producing strains of *Streptococcus faecalis.*
9. Which of the following statements comparing vancomycin to teicoplanin is correct?
   a. Teicoplanin has a considerably shorter elimination half-life than vancomycin, requiring multiple daily dosing.
   b. Both teicoplanin and vancomycin have been shown to be effective in vitro against methicillin-resistant *Staphylococcus aureus.*
   c. Teicoplanin can be used orally for systemic infections, while vancomycin must be given intravenously.
   d. Teicoplanin offers the advantage of greatly increased gram-negative coverage compared with vancomycin.
   e. None of the above alternatives is correct.
10. Teicoplanin and other glycopeptides are being tested because
   a. Of the increasing prevalence of methicillin-resistant staphylococci.
   b. Vancomycin is the only glycopeptide currently marketed in the United States.
   c. Of increasing reports of toxicity to vancomycin.
   d. Alternatives a and b are both correct.

Answer sheet

September 1988 *Clinical Pharmacy*

Note: An enrollment form for the ASHP Continuing-Education System appears in the June and December issues. Please accumulate all the answer sheets you wish to use in one enrollment and submit them at one time with a completed enrollment form.

Place an X in the box(es) at the top of the column(s) corresponding to the test(s) you are taking. Darken the boxes corresponding to the correct answers.

☐
680-204-8814
1.0 hour

	a	b	c	d	e
1.	☐	☐	☐	☐	
2.	☐	☐	☐	☐	☐
3.	☐	☐	☐	☐	
4.	☐	☐	☐	☐	
5.	☐	☐	☐	☐	
6.	☐	☐	☐	☐	☐
7.	☐	☐	☐	☐	☐
8.	☐	☐	☐	☐	
9.	☐	☐	☐	☐	☐
10.	☐	☐	☐	☐	

ASHP Use Only
(1.0)8814______(3)

Consumer Drug Digest
Revised Edition

Consumer Drug Digest, Revised Edition, is a comprehensive, authoritative guide to common prescription and non-prescription drugs . . . helping patients to understand their medications and learn what they can do to be more aware of their drug therapy.

Written in layman's language, this drug information handbook contains over 250 of the most commonly prescribed drugs, which comprise over 95% of prescriptions written in the U.S. today. ***Consumer Drug Digest*** is easy to read and use. And, it's indexed by both brand names and generic names, so it's easy to locate information.

The ***Consumer Drug Digest*** is an excellent tool for patients and for pharmacy services areas.

Order your copy today.

☐ Please send me a brochure on **Consumer Drug Digest**

Name ________________

Address ________________

City ________ State ______ Zip ______

Send to: ASHP Publication Records Dept.,
4630 Montgomery Avenue, Bethesda, MD 20814

Current Literature

Drug Reaction Alerts

Drug Reaction Alerts focuses primarily on serious, unlabeled reactions to new chemical entities. The citations are compiled monthly from International Pharmaceutical Abstracts, *which covers over 800 pharmacy and health-related journals worldwide. An address for reprints (when available) follows the name of the corresponding author in each citation.*

Antidepressants

Banerjee AK (St. Thomas's Hospital, London SE1 7EH, England). Recovery from prolonged cerebral depression after **fluvoxamine** overdose. *Br J Med.* 1988; 296:1774. Case. (74-year-old woman with depression; became comatose after overdose of fluvoxamine maleate 3 g and temazepam 250 mg; regained consciousness after fluvoxamine blood concentration fell below 0.7 g/L)

Anti-infective Agents

Karboski JA, Godley PJ (University of Texas, Austin, TX 78712). Inhaled **pentamidine** and hypoglycemia. *Ann Intern Med.* 1988; 108:490. Case. (45-year-old man with acquired immunodeficiency syndrome; received pentamidine 300 mg once daily as solution by oral inhalation via nebulizer over 30 minutes for *Pneumocystis carinii* pneumonia; developed hypoglycemia; hypoglycemia resolved despite pentamidine continuation)

Kristenson M, Fryden A (University Hospital, Kinkoping, Sweden). Pneumonitis caused by **metronidazole.** *JAMA.* 1988; 260:184. Case. (42-year-old woman with vaginitis; received metronidazole for two days; developed pneumonitis; recovery upon drug withdrawal; positive rechallenge five months later)

Anti-inflammatory Agents

Kollef MH, Irvine T, Cragun WH (Madigan Army Medical Center, Tacoma, WA 98431-5088). Nonbacterial thrombotic endocarditis associated with gold induced pulmonary disease. *Ann Intern Med.* 1988; 108:903–4. Case. (63-year-old woman with rheumatoid arthritis; received four i.m. injections of **gold sodium thiomalate** over two months; developed nonbacterial thrombotic endocarditis; therapy with methylprednisolone, prednisone, dopamine, dobutamine, mezlocillin, and gentamicin unsuccessful and patient died after seven days)

Presley AP. **Penicillamine** induced rhinitis. *Br Med J.* 1988; 296:1332. Case. (78-year-old man with rheumatoid arthritis; received penicillamine 125 mg three times daily for two years; developed nasal pemphigus foliaceus; therapy with intranasal beclomethasone, flunisolide, and xylometazoline and oral ephedrine unsuccessful; symptoms resolved upon withdrawal of penicillamine

Antineoplastic Agents

Hardy R (Department of Internal Medicine, Meharry Medical College, 1005 D. B. Todd Boulevard, Nashville, TN 37208) et al. *Pneumocystis carinii* pneumonia following **5-fluorouracil** administration. *J Natl Med Assoc.* 1987; 79:1205–9. Case. (54-year-old black man with gastrointestinal neoplasm; received five-day courses of fluorouracil every 28 days for one year; pneumonia successfully treated with sulfamethoxazole 100 mg/kg–trimethoprim 20 mg/kg)

Hitchins RN, Hocker GA, Thomson DB (Princess Alexandra Hospital, Ipswich Road, Woolloongabba, Queensland 4102, Australia). **Chlorambucil** allergy—series of three cases. *Aust N Z J Med.* 1987; 17:600–2. Cases. (Three patients with non-Hodgkin's lymphoma, aged 58–72 years; received chlorambucil 4–8 mg/day for three to six weeks; concomitant furosemide, allopurinol, metoprolol, diazepam, and ibuprofen; after chlorambucil withdrawal, rash resolved in one patient; second patient responded to oral and topical corticosteroid therapy; third patient died of erythema multiforme despite therapy with prednisone 100 mg/day)

Antivirals

Sirota P (Yehuda Abarbanel Mental Health Center, Bat-Yam, Israel), Stoler M, Meshulam B. Major depression with psychotic features associated with **acyclovir** therapy. *Drug Intell Clin Pharm.* 1988; 22:306–8. Case. (63-year-old man with herpes simplex dermatitis; received acyclovir 500 mg three times daily for six days by i.v. injection; developed major depression and delusions; psychiatric symptoms resolved after acyclovir withdrawal and therapy with haloperidol 7.5 mg/day for two days and maprotiline up to 125 mg/day)

Anxiolytics, Sedatives and Hypnotics

El Sayed S, Symonds RP (Beatson Oncology Center, Belvidere Hospital, Glasgow G31 4PG, Scotland). **Lorazepam** induced pancytopenia. *B Med J.* 1988; 296:1332. Case. (47-year-old woman with insomnia; received lorazepam 1 mg/day for three weeks; developed pancytopenia; concomitant thyroxine, diphenoxylate hydrochloride, and radiation therapy; blood cell count resolved after lorazepam withdrawal)

Cardiac Drugs

Moots RJ, Banerjee A (Northwick Park Hospital, Harrow, Middlesex, England). Exfoliative dermatitis after **amiodarone** treatment. *Br Med J.* 1988; 296:1332–3. Cases. (two men with arrhythmias, aged 68 and 78 years; received amiodarone 200 mg/day for five weeks and amiodarone 200 mg/day three times daily for six weeks, respectively; developed dermatitis exfoliativa; rash resolved upon withdrawal of amiodarone and therapy with topical corticosteroids in one patient and with i.v. fluids, corticosteroids, and antihistamines in the other)

Drug Interactions

Achumba JI (Department of Clinical Pharmacy and Biopharmacy, College of Medicine, University of Lagos, Idi-Araba, Lagos, Nigeria), Ette EI, Thomas WO et al. **Chloroquine** induced acute dystonic reactions in the presence of **metronidazole.** *Drug Intell Clin Pharm.* 1988; 22:308–10. Case. (30-year-old woman with malaria; received single i.m. injection of chloroquine phosphate 5 mL [equivalent to 200 mg chloroquine base] for malaria and metronidazole 400 mg three times daily for five days for postsurgical prophylaxis; developed acute dystonia; concomitant ampicillin; acetaminophen, and diphenhydramine hydrochloride; symptoms subsided after withdrawal of chloroquine and administration of diazepam 5 mg i.v.)

Corpier CL, Jones PH, Suki WN (Renal Section, Methodist Hospital, 6565 Fannin, MS F505, Houston, TX 77030) et al. Rhabdomyolysis and renal injury with **lovastatin** use: report of two cases in cardiac transplant recipients. *JAMA*. 1988; 260:239–41. Cases. (two cardiac transplant patients, aged 36 and 46 years; received lovastatin 40 mg twice daily and **cyclosporine** 120 or 150 mg twice daily; developed acute kidney failure and rhabdomyolysis; withdrawal of lovastatin and reduction in cyclosporine dosage led to resolution of symptoms in both patients; negative rechallenge in one patient)

Drugs, Adverse Reactions

Krohn KD, Slowman-Kovacs S, Leapman SB (Indiana University Medical Center, Indianapolis, IN 46223). **Cocaine** and rhabdomyolysis. *Ann Intern Med*. 1988; 108: 639–40. Case. (34-year-old man; self-administered cocaine by i.v. injection; developed rhabdomyolysis; received therapy with sodium chloride solution only; recovery after several days)

Zamora-Quazeda JC, Dinerman H (New England Medical Center, Rheumatology Division, Box 406, 750 Washington Street, Boston, MA 02111), Stadecker MJ et al. Muscle and skin infarction after free-basing **cocaine** (crack). *Ann Intern Med*. 1988; 108:564–6. Case. (20-year-old woman; developed necrosis of peripheral skin and muscle after smoking cocaine [crack]; received prednisone 80 mg/day initially and tapered over nine months; recovery with residual hyperpigmentation and scarring of skin)

Steroids, Cortico-

Al Mahdy H, Hall M (Caerphilly District Miners Hospital, Caerphilly, Mid Glamorgan CFB 2WW, Wales). Anaphylaxis and **hydrocortisone.** *Ann Intern Med*. 1988; 108:487–8. Case. (23-year-old patient with acute asthma; received hydrocortisone sodium phosphate 300 mg i.v.; concomitant albuterol; developed anaphylaxis and died)

Vaccines

Patel U, Bradley JR, Hamilton DV (Department of Renal Medicine, W. Norwich Hospital, Norwich NR2 3TU, England). Henoch-Schoenlein purpura after influenza vaccination. *Br Med J*. 1988; 296:1800. Case. (77-year-old man; received **influenza vaccine** 0.5 mL; developed Schoenlein-Henoch purpura; recovery after four weeks and therapy with prednisolone 60 mg/day)

Book Reviews

Immunology, Immunopathology, and Immunity

By Stewart Sell.

Published by Elsevier Science Publishing Company, Inc., 52 Vanderbilt Ave., New York, NY 10017, 1987. xvii + 852 p. Price $55.

The discipline of immunology is a vast and rapidly expanding field. It is often difficult for pharmacists to keep abreast of even the basic concepts involved with immunology because research continues to expand the breadth and depth of knowledge. The fourth edition of *Immunology, Immunopathology and Immunity*, by Stewart Sell, provides the reader with a good basic understanding of concepts involved with immunology.

The book itself is easy to read, and it has numerous tables and illustrations that enhance the reader's understanding of the topic. As the author states in the preface, the book was not written with the detail needed by a scientist working in the field of molecular biology or immunobiology. Dr. Sell emphasizes the relationship between the immune system and disease processes. The author has divided the book into three sections—immunology, immunopathology, and immunity.

The first section of the book, "Immunology," covers basic concepts in this area. Terms pertaining to immunology are discussed in detail, providing the reader with a good background for future chapters. This section also discusses the various components of the immune system, and chapters pertaining to antibodies and cells of the immune system are included.

"Immunopathology," the second section of the book, discusses diseases involving the immune system. Chapters in this section emphasize the mechanism by which the immune system causes disease. The author does touch on symptoms, diagnosis, and treatment of these diseases; however, these discussions are superficial. Topics in this section that would be of particular interest to pharmacists include serum sickness, glomerulonephritis, atopic or anaphylactic reactions, and autoallergic diseases.

In the final section, "Immunity," mechanisms of host resistance and diseases that can result when these mechanisms are destroyed or fail are explained. Included in this section is a well-written chapter on tumor immunity. One chapter in this section also contains a short but interesting discussion on acquired immunodeficiency syndrome.

Immunology, Immunopathology, and Immunity contains several chapters that are particularly relevant to the practice of pharmacy. These chapters include drug allergy, immunizations, and immune deficiency disease. In the chapter on immunodeficiency, the author discusses medications that are prescribed to suppress the immune system. However, the emphasis is on the mechanisms involved in producing suppression; very little information is included on the application to the clinical setting. An extensive glossary has also been provided for the reader, which should be extremely helpful to students reading the book.

In summary, *Immunology, Immunopathology, and Immunity* is a well-written book that provides the reader with a background in immunology. This book would be an excellent textbook for students taking immunology or as initial reading for the pharmacist who would like to develop a better understanding of the immune system.

Reviewed by Michael D. Parr, Pharm.D., Assistant Professor, College of Pharmacy, University of Kentucky, Lexington, KY 40536-0082.

Therapeutic Pharmacology

By Glenn D. Appelt and Jennifer M. Appelt.

Published by Lea & Febiger, 600 Washington Square, Philadelphia, PA 19106-4198, 1988. xiv + 503 p. Price $34.50.

Therapeutic Pharmacology is a small book that attempts to "provide health professionals with a clear understanding of the use of drugs from a clinical standpoint." In comparison with other books of this type, and by virtue of its size, the application of drugs in disease management is limited and often superficial.

The book, which is divided into 10 chapters, is arranged by organ system. These are the central nervous, autonomic nervous, cardiovascular, circulatory and reticuloendothelial, renal, endocrine, respiratory, digestive and gastrointestinal, reproductive and genitourinary, and integumentary and connective tissue systems. The book concludes with appendices containing six tables of drug classes, each listing available products within the drug class, corresponding trade names, and supplementary information about each drug.

The introduction to each chapter is prefaced by objectives, ranging in number from 10 to 50, which serve to outline the chapter contents. After the introduction, the anatomy and physiology of the organ is examined, followed by a consideration of disorders commonly affecting the organ. Then, the pharmacology of the drugs used in the treatment of these disorders is discussed. Each chapter concludes with a section on drug interactions, a summary, suggested readings (the book contains no references), and a chapter examination. The chapter examination consists of multiple-choice questions that are based on briefly presented clinical practice situations. The pharmacology discussion is arranged similarly in that the mechanism of drug action is examined followed by the clinical indications for the drug and its major adverse effects or precautions.

A useful feature of this book is the anatomy and physiology sections, which give pharmacists quick reviews of perhaps forgotten areas. The brief sketches of pathophysiological conditions are also worthwhile and serve to orient pharmacists to patient problems and system dysfunctions. Many clearly drawn diagrams help to reinforce the conceptual points covered in the well-written text. Suitable tables, which often contain lists of available drug products, trade names, and daily dosage ranges, are presented. The typeface is easily read on the high quality bond paper.

A book of this size (503 pages) is bound to suffer by comparison with similar but larger and more all-encompassing texts. Information in this text is either omitted or mentioned with or without detailed explanation. For example, condylomata acuminata (venereal warts) is a major public health problem. However, neither the disease nor its traditional treatment method (podophyllin) is mentioned. The fact that prazosin "does not routinely produce reflex tachycardia . . ." is mentioned, but no explanation for this fact is forthcoming. As to why the clinical effects of tricyclic antidepressants are not seen for two to three weeks after treatment administration, the authors simply state that "adaptive alterations in monoamine receptor function or topography possibly also contribute to the antidepressant activity."

New chemical entities approved through 1986 are contained in the book. Pharmacological sketches of drugs released in that year include buspirone hydrochloride, encainide, etretinate, famotidine, guanfacine hydrochloride, ipratropium bromide, and norfloxacin. There is no information about drugs approved after 1986.

Therapeutic Pharmacology is not a resource book. Little pharmacological profiling exists to assist in choosing a drug product. However, hospital pharmacies may wish to purchase this book to have on hand as a ready reference for quick reviews of anatomy and physiology of organ systems, pathophysiology, and synopses about the clinical use of drugs.

Reviewed by Norman L. Katz, Department of Pharmacodynamics, College of Pharmacy, University of Illinois at Chicago, Chicago, IL 60612.

Books Received

Books are listed as soon as received; selected books may be reviewed in Book Reviews in subsequent issues.

Clinical Progress in Nutrition Research, edited by A. Sitges-Serra, A. Sitges-Creus, S. Schwartz-Riera. Published by S. Karger AG, P.O. Box, CH-4009 Basel, Switzerland, 1988. viii + 281 p. Price $78.

Enteral Feeding: Scientific Basis and Clinical Applications. Report of the 94th Ross Conference on Pediatric Research. Published by Ross Laboratories, 625 Cleveland Ave., Columbus, OH 43215, 1988. viii + 161 p.

The Pharmacologic Approach to the Critically Ill Patient, Second Edition, Bart Chernow, editor. Published by Williams & Wilkins, 428 East Preston St., Baltimore, MD 21202, 1988. xx + 975 p. Price $116.50.

Practical Clinical Psychopharmacology, Third Edition, by William S. Appleton. Published by Williams & Wilkins, 428 East Preston St., Baltimore, MD 21202, 1988. xiii + 199 p. Price $26.95.

Advertising Index

American Society of Hospital Pharmacists
Consumer Drug Digest, 703
Eli Lilly and Company
Nebcin, 641–642
Lorex Pharmaceuticals
Position Available, 643
Merieux Institute, Inc.
Multitest CMI, 633
Roxane Laboratories Inc., A Boehringer Ingelheim Company
Intensols, inside front cover
Marinol, inside back cover, outside back cover
Stuart Pharmaceuticals, Division of ICI Americas, Inc.
Cefotan, 635–637
University of Alberta (Edmonton)
Position Available, 644
University of North Carolina at Chapel Hill
Position Available, 644
The Upjohn Company
Cleocin Phosphate, 645–646
Veterans Administration Medical Center (Syracuse)
Position Available, 644

CU trouble spot: IG drug administration

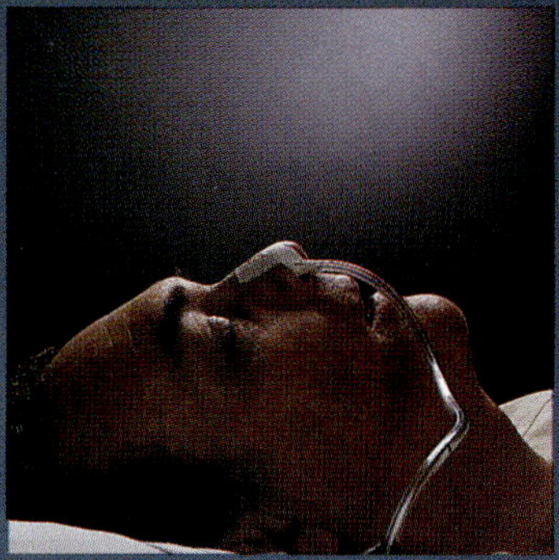

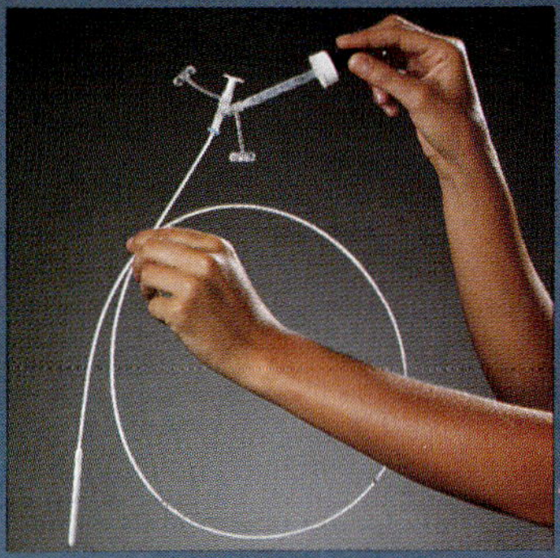

ie solution is INTENSOLS™ oncentrated Oral Solutions

DEXAMETHASONE . . . . . . 1 mg/mL
PROPRANOLOL . . . . . . 80 mg/mL
PREDNISONE . . . . 5 mg/mL
DIAZEPAM . . . . 5 mg/mL

PALLIATIVE CARE AND CANCER PAIN PRODUCTS

Roxane Laboratories, Inc. Columbus, Ohio 43216

ıplifies drug ministration to sogastric patients

ırsing benefits

- minates crushing tablets or dissolving ıpsules
- ore accurate and consistent dose
- on't clog NG tubes
- ıves nursing time for more productive ıtient care activities

ırmacy benefits

- orrect dose is administered and osorbed by the patient
- ushing of sustained-release, sublingual, enteric-coated tablets is minimized
- ug/drug and acid/base interactions in ortar are avoided

y to dispense

ch bottle comes with a calibrated opper for accurate dosing and ation. Administering directly into NG be is possible.

Ideal for patients who have difficulty swallowing tablets

- Geriatric, pediatric, and cancer patients on high or variable doses
- Mixable with soft foods or liquids; most Intensols are tasteless so they won't alter the flavor
- Easy to swallow for improved compliance

Many Intensol-formulated drugs are available

- Prednisone, dexamethasone, diazepam, propranolol, and more
- Easy to switch from injectables to orals

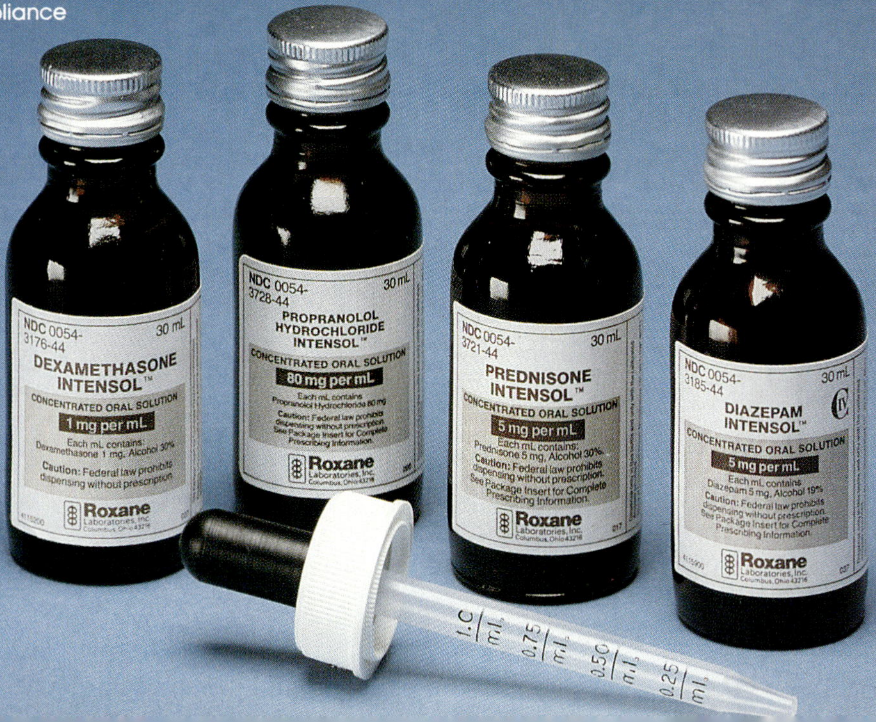

ITENSOLS™

olutions to tablet-taking problems

News

Future applications of biotechnology explored by ACCP speakers

Several educational sessions at the Ninth Annual Meeting of the American College of Clinical Pharmacy (ACCP) in Philadelphia, Pennsylvania, July 24–27, 1988, focused on potential applications of biotechnology-derived products in the areas of oncology, diabetes mellitus, and infectious disease.

Cancer Treatment and Imaging. In the Therapeutic Frontiers Award Lecture, Paul A. Bunn, M.D., University of Colorado Health Sciences Center, Denver, discussed potential diagnostic and therapeutic applications of monoclonal antibodies in cancer therapy. In contrast to conventional cytotoxic therapy, monoclonal antibodies offer the possibility of treatment that is specific for tumor cells.

In assessing the current status of work in this area, Bunn identified a number of obstacles that must be overcome. Among these are questions of where the antibody goes after it is injected into the body and how it is cleared. If antigen is shed from the cancer cell into the blood stream, the monoclonal antibody binds first to free antigen in the serum. Therefore, the amount of antibody administered must be enough to ensure that it reaches the targeted cancer cells. Even if antibody reaches the cancer cell, the antigen–antibody complex may be internalized, or the complex may be shed into the circulation. In either case, antigen or antibody is no longer on the cell surface, and the immune system does not recognize the cell as being a different type of cell. This process is called antigen modulation.

If modulation occurs because of internalization of the antigen–antibody complex, imaging is still possible using a radiolabeled antibody. However, nonspecific uptake by the liver and spleen occurs and is an important problem to be overcome. Bunn presented data on the KC4 antibody, an antibody directed against a high-molecular-weight mucin antigen produced by many solid tumors, as an example of the problems of circulating antigen–antibody binding and nonspecific uptake of radiolabeled antibody. The sensitivity and specificity of antibody products are not yet adequate for more imaging agents to be available. With the KC4 antibody, only large lesions can be visualized.

Bunn noted that the use of murine antibodies is also a problem. An "antimouse" response can develop, especially with repeated exposure to the antibody. This response will change the kinetics of the antibody and may inhibit the antibody's effect.

According to Bunn, use of unlabeled antibodies alone is insufficient for cancer treatment. Cells must be killed quickly; otherwise, the tumor may mutate or the patient may develop an immune reaction to the administered antibody, limiting the number of doses that can be given.

Bunn also pointed out that tumor cells can secrete peptide hormone growth factors. Antibodies that are specific for the hormone can bind to the hormone and inhibit tumor cell growth during monoclonal antibody therapy. This approach is analogous to hormonal therapy. The treatment is cytostatic, not cytotoxic. The possibility of making antibodies to growth-factor receptors also holds promise. Other approaches that are being studied include augmentation of the immune system response and use of antibodies that bind to tumor cells and improve cell killing.

Diabetes Mellitus. An overview of the applications of biotechnology to diabetes research was presented by Ronald Chance, Ph.D., Lilly Research Laboratories, Indianapolis, Indiana. Chance noted that the new gene technologies have provided scientists with opportunities to perform structure–activity relationship studies of insulin and to modify the insulin molecule. Through such modifications it may be possible to alter the duration or onset of action of insulin. Chance predicted that insulin analogues that have different properties may be available in the near future. Studies at the molecular level of the interactions between insulin and its receptor may lead to work on lower-molecular-weight agents that can interact with the insulin receptor.

The newer technologies have also improved understanding of islet cell physiology. These advances could have important implications in transplantation. In the future it may be possible to transfer islet cells and grow them in cultures to provide material for transplantation. Chance also noted that identification of patients who are likely to develop type I or type II diabetes mellitus may be possible.

Infectious Disease. Endotoxin monoclonal antibodies appear to be the most promising of the current biotech-

Continued on page 713

Continued from page 710

nology strategies in the area of infectious disease, according to Jerome J. Schentag, Pharm.D., Millard Filmore Hospital, Buffalo, New York. Monoclonal antibodies are directed against the endotoxin lipid A fragment that is common to gram-negative bacteria. Three of these products are currently under investigation.

Researchers have also used enhanced endogenous products—purified or enhanced intravenous immune globulin and pseudomonas immune globulin—to confer passive immunity. However, these products may cause allergic reactions and pose a risk of transmitting infectious agents.

According to Schentag, the timing of the intervention may be critical. Few of these agents work after tissue damage has occurred. To be cost-effective, an agent would need to act before the onset of shock. Schentag reviewed the difficulties faced by investigators working with these monoclonal agents. Currently, clinical trials are examining short-term use of monoclonal antibodies, although production of secondary mediators of sepsis (interleukins, tumor necrosis factor, and prostaglandin E) is continuous. The challenge will be to prove that the monoclonal antibody products provide greater benefit than antimicrobial therapy alone.

JANE L. MILLER

Biotechnology-based drug products grow in importance

Biotechnology product development has become an important part of pharmaceutical research and development, according to survey results released in July 1988 by the Pharmaceutical Manufacturers Association (PMA). According to PMA, 81 biotechnology-based drugs and vaccines are under development in the United States; 67 of these are undergoing clinical trials and 14 are awaiting approval by FDA. The data are based on a study commissioned by PMA to analyze the trends in biotechnology research in the United States.

According to PMA, 206 of the 1476 biotechnology patents issued by the United States Office of Patents and Trademarks in 1987 involved genetic engineering; the remainder involved techniques such as fermentation with microorganisms. Of the 206 patents, 96% were in the pharmaceutical or health-care industry, and 80% originated in the United States.

The genetic engineering patents primarily involved three techniques: recombinant DNA technology (104 patents), monoclonal-hybridoma technology (81 patents), and DNA probe technology (14 patents). Recombinant DNA techniques were among the earliest genetic engineering methods used; according to PMA, these methods now have an established role in protein production. According to the survey results, monoclonal-hybridoma technology is the principal technique used in developing diagnostic products. This technique also is being used increasingly in drug development to isolate and purify proteins (e.g., human growth hormone, interferon, tissue plasminogen activator). Use of monoclonal-hybridoma technology in vaccine development also is increasing. DNA probe technology is being used to make diagnostic agents that are specific to certain segments of DNA or RNA. Products that will detect infectious agents, genetic mutations, or cancer are being developed. Other products are intended for use in transplantation and forensic medicine.

PMA noted that 40 of the 81 drugs and vaccines under development are in the area of cancer treatment. Numerous approaches are being studied, including colony-stimulating factors, interferons, interleukins, monoclonal antibodies, and tumor necrosis factors. Vaccines against hepatitis B, *Haemophilus influenzae*, respiratory viruses, and cancer are being tested.

PMA classified the patents into the following categories: diagnostic agents, 52; therapeutic agents, 37; vaccines, 20; diagnostic or therapeutic agents (both uses possible), 15; techniques that advance the technology of genetic engineering, 68; and other uses, 7.

According to PMA, 50 companies have biotechnology-based pharmaceutical products in clinical research, and nearly every major pharmaceutical company in the United States is involved in biotechnology research. Many companies are developing similar products, although questions of how patent law applies to genetically engineered products persist.

CDC updates influenza recommendations for 1988–1989 season

Recommendations for prevention and control of influenza have been updated by the Centers for Disease Control (CDC).[1] Virus strains in the trivalent vaccine have been modified, and greater emphasis is placed on vaccination of health-care workers and prevention of influenza in patients with AIDS.

Vaccination. Vaccination of persons infected with the human immunodeficiency virus (HIV) is described in the CDC guidelines as being prudent, because infection could result in serious illness in some HIV-infected patients. In addition, the guidelines stress the need for vaccination of persons who have extensive contact with high-risk persons. The statement notes that efforts to protect high-risk individuals who might have low antibody responses to influenza vaccine (e.g., elderly persons, transplant recipients, AIDS patients) may be enhanced if the chance of exposure to influenza through their care providers is reduced. Thus, the CDC recommends vaccination of the following groups: health-care personnel who have extensive contact with high-risk patients; providers of home care to high-risk persons; and all household members, including children.

The CDC statement encourages health-care facilities to establish procedures for making vaccine readily available to staff members at their worksites to improve staff vaccination rates.

Use of Amantadine. Amantadine prophylaxis is recommended as a supplement to vaccination for high-risk patients who may have a poor antibody response to the vaccine. CDC noted that although adults with AIDS would be expected to have some residual immunity to influenza from previous infections, children who have AIDS may have little or no immunity. Thus, the guidelines recommend that amantadine prophylaxis be considered during epidemics, especially for children with AIDS. However, the CDC cautioned that decisions should be made on a case-by-case basis and should take into account amantadine's adverse-effect profile, particularly in patients who have central nervous system involvement.

1. Centers for Disease Control. Prevention and control of influenza. *MMWR.* 1988; 37:361-4.

Study supports previous findings of colchicine activity in primary biliary cirrhosis

Results of a recent double-blind, randomized, placebo-controlled study on colchicine use in primary biliary cirrhosis lend support to other clinical trials suggesting that colchicine has a beneficial effect.[1]

Fifty-seven patients with a history of chronic cholestatic liver disease and liver biopsy results compatible with primary biliary cirrhosis were randomized to receive either colchicine 0.6 mg twice daily or placebo. Other supportive medications were continued. The study duration was five years; the mean follow-up for all patients was 30 months. Ten patients (five in the colchicine group) were noncompliant and withdrew from the trial; four patients (three in the colchicine group) withdrew because of diarrhea.

Mean alkaline phosphatase values in colchicine-treated patients decreased from 281 IU/L to 112 IU/L, whereas the values for placebo recipients fluctuated within the range of 215–273 IU/L (initial mean value, 273 IU/L). Mean alanine aminotransferase values decreased significantly in the colchicine group from 129 IU/L to 86 IU/L; values in the placebo group rose from 129 IU/L to 160 IU/L. Mean bilirubin and IgM values tended to be lower in the colchicine group but did not differ significantly between treatment groups. Five patients in the placebo group and one patient in the colchicine group had rapid increases in bilirubin concentration. This pattern is usually seen in the later stages of the disease and is a prognostic indicator of survival. Additional information on the outcome of these patients was not available. Despite stabilization or improvement of biochemical test values with colchicine therapy, no difference in clinical signs or symptoms or histological progression of the disease was noted.

As noted by Boyer in an accompanying editorial, the lack of symptomatic improvement and the inconsistency between biochemical and histological effects are of concern.[2] For these reasons and because there is uncertainty as to colchicine's effects on long-term survival, additional controlled studies are needed. Demonstration of a beneficial effect of therapy is complicated by the variable prognosis of primary biliary cirrhosis, the need for long-term follow-up in assessing drug effects, the increasing number of patients who have undergone liver transplantation, the small number of patients with primary biliary cirrhosis treated at any one medical center, and the fact that clinical trials conducted thus far have included asymptomatic patients as well as patients with progressive disease.

1. Bodenheimer H Jr, Schaffner F, Pezzulio J. Evaluation of colchicine therapy in primary biliary cirrhosis. *Gastroenterology.* 1988; 95:124–9.
2. Boyer JL. Definitive therapy for primary biliary cirrhosis—fact or fiction? *Gastroenterology.* 1988; 95:242–5. Editorial.

New AIDS reference service available through National Library of Medicine

The National Library of Medicine (NLM) and the National Institutes of Health Office of AIDS Research have announced the availability of AIDSLINE, a new database containing about 13,000 references to scientific articles on AIDS. The database will be available through NLM's online network. Articles published since 1980 on the clinical and research aspects and epidemiology of AIDS and health policy issues will be covered. The database is updated twice monthly. References are currently being drawn from NLM's MEDLINE database. Beginning in early 1989 AIDSLINE will be expanded to include references from NLM's CANCERLIT and the Health Planning and Administration database. Inquiries about AIDSLINE may be directed to NLM's MEDLARS Management Section, 301-496-6193 (toll free: 800-638-8480).

FDA issues consumer warning, announces crackdown on bogus Retin A products

FDA has warned consumers about indiscriminate use of tretinoin (Retin A, Ortho Pharmaceutical Corporation) to reduce or prevent wrinkles and has announced plans to work with other government agencies to curb illegal imitation products. The agency is investigating a number of firms that are advertising and selling products based on antiwrinkle claims.

In his caution to consumers, FDA Commissioner Frank E. Young cited the lack of long-term studies of the antiwrinkling effects of Retin A and the known adverse effects of the formulation. Consumers were advised of several problems with imitation products. First, products that differ from Retin A in the amount of tretinoin are being compounded, promoted, or sold by some dermatologists, pharmacists, and unlicensed manufacturers. Second, some products (often sold as cosmetics) have names similar to Retin A or retinoic acid but do not contain retinoic acid as the active ingredient.

Papers sought for National Conference on High Blood Pressure Control

Papers are being solicited for the National Conference on High Blood Pressure Control, scheduled for May 6–9, 1989, in Lake Buena Vista, Florida. The conference organizers seek papers on new approaches to the detection, treatment, and long-term management of hypertensive patients, particularly special populations such as blacks, Hispanics, the elderly, children, pregnant women, or patients with hypertension-related diseases. Further information about the conference, guidelines regarding specific areas for papers, and rules for submitting abstracts can be obtained from the National Conference on

Continued on page 717

News *Continued from page 714*

High Blood Pressure Control, 4733 Bethesda Avenue, Suite 530. Bethesda, MD 20814; 301-951-3275.

News Briefs

• Clinicard (Chem-Elec, Inc., North Webster, IN), a **device designed to rapidly estimate serum cholesterol concentrations**, has been approved by FDA. The device is intended for use as a preliminary screening technique. Results are not accurate enough to be used for diagnosis or for monitoring cholesterol-lowering therapy; the device indicates a range of values (<200 mg/dL, 200–300 mg/dL, or >300 mg/dL) in which the test sample concentration falls.

• Labeling indications for **enalapril maleate** (Vasotec, Merck Sharp & Dohme) have been expanded to include use with digoxin and diuretics in the treatment of congestive heart failure.

• **Clindamycin hydrochloride** (Cleocin HCl, The Upjohn Company) is now available as a 300-mg capsule for use in the treatment of serious infections caused by susceptible anaerobic bacteria and susceptible strains of streptococci, pneumococci, and staphylococci.

Upcoming Specialty Meetings

Regulation of the Acute Phase and Immune Responses: A New Cytokine . . . New York, NY . . . December 12–14 . . . contact: Conference Department, New York Academy of Science, 2 East 63rd Street, New York, NY 10021; 212-838-0230.

Southern Society for Pediatric Research . . . New Orleans, LA . . . February 1–3 . . . contact: R. F. Jacobs, M.D., Arkansas Children's Hospital, 800 Marshall Street, Little Rock, AR 72202; 501-370-1416.

Advances in Gene Technology: Molecular Neurobiology and Neuropharmacology, Miami Bio/Technology Winter Symposium . . . Miami, FL . . . February 6–10 . . . contact: S. Black, Miami Bio/Technology Winter Symposium, P.O. Box 016129, Miami, FL 33101-6129.

American Academy of Allergy and Immunology . . . San Antonio, TX . . . February 24–March 1 . . . contact: M. Fogarty, Director of Medical Education, 611 East Wells Street, Milwaukee, WI 53202; 414-272-6071.

The International Symposium on Drugs Affecting Lipid Metabolism . . . Houston, TX . . . November 8–11, 1989 . . . contact: L. C. Smith, International Meetings Managers, Inc., 4550 Post Oak Place, Suite 248, Houston, TX 77027; 713-965-0566.

The University of Illinois at Chicago General and Specialized Residencies and Fellowships

General clinical pharmacy and specialized residencies and fellowships are being offered by the College of Pharmacy, University of Illinois at Chicago. The general clinical residency is a 12-month ASHP-accredited program designed to develop well-rounded clinical practitioners. This program emphasizes innovative comprehensive pharmacy practice through participation in clinical rotations and ongoing administrative research projects. All rotation sites will be at the University of Illinois Hospital and Clinics and the Veterans Administration West Side Medical Center.

The specialized residency/fellowship is a two-year program designed to develop the individual as a clinical scientist. The first year of the specialized residency/fellowship emphasizes clinical practice and advanced specialization through clinical rotations and participation in a 24-hour, inhouse, on-call program. The second year's emphasis is on clinical research, with the fellow serving as an investigator on at least one research project. Areas of specialization include administration, adult internal medicine, cardiology, clinical research, clinical pharmacokinetics, dermatology, drug information, emergency medicine, nephrology–transplantation, neurology–neurosurgery, oncology, pediatrics, psychiatry, and surgery. The administration, adult internal medicine, drug information, pediatrics, and oncology specialized residencies are ASHP-accedited.

Residents will receive formal and informal instruction in clinical research and pharmacotherapeutics. Each resident will have a teaching appointment in the College of Pharmacy and have the opportunity to develop didactic and clerkship teaching skills. All applicants must possess a Pharm.D. degree or be enrolled in a program leading to the Pharm.D. degree. For more information, please contact Donald L. Kendzierski, Pharm.D., The University of Illinois at Chicago, College of Pharmacy, 833 S. Wood Street, m/c 886, Chicago, IL 60612; 312-996-4033.

The University of Illinois is an Equal Opportunity/Affirmative Action Employer.

CLINICAL PHARMACISTS OWEN HEALTHCARE - YOUR CONNECTION TO A QUALITY CAREER

Owen Healthcare, Inc., a national hospital pharmacy management company, is looking for **Clinical Pharmacy Managers** for the following hospitals:

Maryland General Hospital - Baltimore, Maryland
Good Shepherd Medical Center - Longview, Texas
Sam Houston Memorial Hospital - Houston, Texas
Rosewood Medical Center - Houston, Texas

Qualified candidates must have an advanced degree with previous hospital clinical pharmacy experience. Because Owen serves more than 150 hospitals in 30+ states, we offer well-defined, upward mobility and opportunities uncommon to those traditionally offered to pharmacists. Owen offers competitive salaries and excellent benefits including: an employee stock ownership plan; semi-annual evaluations; and medical, dental, and life insurance. Owen offers attractive honorariums and encourages its employees to participate in clinical pharmacy seminars and hospital pharmacy society meetings. For more information, please contact **Robert Jordin, R. Ph., at 800-231-9807 or (713) 777-8173** inside Texas. Equal opportunity employer.

Therapy Consultation

The Therapy Consultation *section provides brief advice, in question-and-answer format, on how to handle specific drug-therapy problems. Readers are invited to submit questions, which will be referred to a consultant for an answer. The problems should not be highly specialized or unusual, nor should they be mundane. Questions are answered briefly, based largely on the judgment and personal experience of the consultant, although selected references may be cited to substantiate the consultant's advice.*

Assistance in identifying Therapy Consultation *topics is provided by the drug information centers at the following institutions: Albert B. Chandler Medical Center and College of Pharmacy, University of Kentucky, Lexington; Arizona Health Sciences Center, Tucson; Medical College of Virginia Hospitals, Richmond; University of California Medical Center, San Diego; and University of Michigan Medical Center, Ann Arbor.*

Treatment of metronidazole-resistant cases of vaginal trichomoniasis

Question: A woman who has received a seven-day course of metronidazole for vaginal trichomoniasis complains that despite compliance with therapy her infection has not been eradicated. Have cases of trichomoniasis resistant to metronidazole been reported? How should refractory cases be treated?

Answer: Recommended therapy for vaginal trichomoniasis consists of either a single 2-g oral dose of metronidazole or metronidazole 250 mg orally three times daily for seven days. These regimens have proven remarkably efficacious (92–96%) in numerous clinical trials. The efficacy of metronidazole given in lower single doses (1.5 or 1.75 g) or in short courses (250 mg three times daily for five days) has been studied in small numbers of patients with conflicting results. These regimens are not currently recommended.[1]

Reports of *Trichomonas vaginalis* infections refractory to metronidazole appeared as early as 1961, but these reports were initially discounted because anaerobic testing indicated that the organisms were susceptible to metronidazole.[2] The reasons most commonly offered to explain treatment failures with metronidazole include noncompliance, lack of drug absorption, inactivation of the drug by intestinal or vaginal bacteria,[3,4] increased hepatic inactivation of the drug,[5] reinfection, and lack of assay sensitivity.[1]

In 1979, Meingassner and Thurner[6] reported that resistant strains of *T. vaginalis* could be detected by testing under aerobic conditions, rather than the usual anaerobic conditions. Since that time, several other reports have confirmed these findings.[7–10] The mechanism and frequency of resistance to metronidazole are unclear at this time, but resistance may be caused by deficiencies in the anaerobic metabolic pathway that provides electrons for activation of metronidazole within the protozoan.[1]

There are no firm guidelines for the management of refractory trichomoniasis. In the largest series of refractory cases reported to date, Lossick et al.[10] described the aerobic and anaerobic susceptibility data for 53 resistant isolates of *T. vaginalis* and the clinical responses of patients to treatment. Clinical and microbiologic resistance varied from mild to severe. Anaerobic minimum inhibitory concentrations (MICs) provided the best indicator of clinical resistance. Although higher anaerobic MICs generally correlated with more severe clinical resistance, other factors such as drug concentration at the site of infection, intravaginal redox potential, and vaginal microflora were also thought to influence the rate of cure. Most patients were cured with daily dosages of 2 to 4 g of metronidazole, and a faster clinical response was usually observed with concomitant intravaginal administration of metronidazole tablets.[10]

Although the small number of metronidazole-resistant cases reported to date precludes the recommendation of predictably effective treatment regimens, Lossick[1] has suggested the following guidelines. Because clinical resistance is usually mild, the patient may be retreated with metronidazole at the same dosage that was given initially. If the patient's infection does not respond to retreatment, a higher dose regimen may be used. Most resistant infections appear to respond to daily administration of metronidazole 2 or 3 g orally plus 500 mg intravaginally for 7 to 14 days. Although high-dose therapy with intravenous metronidazole has been used in some cases, it should be reserved for patients who do not tolerate oral therapy, since this treatment requires hospitalization and is associated with a higher incidence of adverse reactions. The duration of treatment should be determined by the time required for complete resolution of symptoms and conversion to a negative culture.

The use of alternative agents such as nimorazole, tinidazole, or ornidazole (none of which is currently available in the United States) cannot be recommended at this time. Although clinical trials have demonstrated efficacy in the treatment of vaginal trichomoniasis equivalent to that of metronidazole, these agents have not been evaluated in cases of refractory vaginitis. Like metronidazole, these agents are nitroimidazole derivatives; it is unclear whether cross-resistance will be observed.[1]

1. Lossick JG. Treatment of *Trichomonas vaginalis* infections. *Rev Infect Dis.* 1982; 4(Suppl):S801–S818.
2. Kane PO, McFadzean JA, Squires S. Absorption and excretion of metronidazole. Part II. Studies on primary failures. *Br J Vener Dis.* 1961; 37:276–7.

3. Larsen B, Wilson AH, Glover DD et al. Implications of metronidazole pharmacodynamics for therapy of trichomoniasis. *Gynecol Obstet Invest*. 1986; 21:12–8.
4. Nicol CS, Evans AJ, McFadzean JA et al. Inactivation of metronidazole. *Lancet*. 1966; 1:441. Letter.
5. Mead PB, Gibson M, Schentag JJ et al. Possible alteration of metronidazole metabolism by phenobarbital. *N Engl J Med*. 1982; 306:1490. Letter.
6. Meingassner JG, Thurner J. Strain of *Trichomonas vaginalis* resistant to metronidazole and other 5-nitroimidazoles. *Antimicrob Agents Chemother*. 1979; 15:254–7.
7. Muller M, Meingassner JG, Miller WA et al. Three metronidazole-resistant strains of *Trichomonas vaginalis* from the United States. *Am J Obstet Gynecol*. 1980; 138:808–12.
8. Kulda J, Vojtechovska M, Tachezy J et al. Metronidazole resistance of *Trichomonas vaginalis* as a cause of treatment failure in trichomoniasis. *Br J Vener Dis*. 1982; 58:394–9.
9. Krajden S, Lossick JG, Wilk E et al. Persistent *Trichomonas vaginalis* infection due to a metronidazole-resistant strain. *Can Med Assoc J*. 1986; 134:1373–4.
10. Lossick JG, Muller M, Gorrell TE. In vitro drug susceptibility and doses of metronidazole required for cure in cases of refractory vaginal trichomoniasis. *J Infect Dis*. 1986; 153:948–55.

PEGGY L. CARVER, PHARM.D.
Assistant Professor of Pharmacy, College of Pharmacy
The University of Michigan

PAMALA COLBURN, PHARM.D.
Advanced Resident in Infectious Diseases
The University of Michigan Hospitals

Ann Arbor, MI 48109

Staff Pharmacist

The Bristol Bay Area Health Corporation, Kanakanak Hospital, in Dillingham, Alaska, is seeking a staff pharmacist. Hospital pharmacy experience is required, knowledge of unit dose desired. Excellent opportunity to experience Alaska wilderness while providing inpatient and outpatient services as well as clinic services and traveling to 28 villages of the Bristol Bay Area. National Park, National Monument, National Wildlife Refuge, and largest state park in the United States located within our service unit. World class fishing location. Close working relationship with physicians and village health aides.

Candidate must be a graduate of an accredited school of pharmacy with Alaska state license or eligibility to become state licensed. Excellent benefits. Will assist with relocation expenses. Interested?

Contact:

Bristol Bay Area Health Corporation

Personnel Dept.
Bristol Bay Area Health Corp.
Kanakanak Hospital
P.O. Box 130
Dillingham, AK 99576
907-842-5201, ext. 324
EOE

Your Heritage

As a ***Pharmacist***
As a ***Professional***

IS PRESERVED, PROTECTED, AND EXPLORED BY

THE AMERICAN INSTITUTE OF THE HISTORY OF PHARMACY

JOIN by sending your name, address, and $25 tax-deductible dues to:
AIHP, Pharmacy Building, Madison, WI 53706-1508

PHARMACIST

The University of Alabama Hospital, UAB, Department of Pharmacy, is seeking decentralized pharmacists for its Clinical Division. Support services include centralized cartfill, i.v. admixture, and drug information services. Areas of opportunity are pharmacokinetics, rounding, ASHP residency, and Pharm.D instruction.

University Hospital, located in Birmingham, is an 800-bed medical center and teaching institution offering opportunities for professional development as well as competitive salaries and an excellent benefits program. Interested candidates should contact Scott Brown at 205-934-6321, or forward résumé to:

Personnel Administration
University of Alabama Hospital
619 South 19th Street
Birmingham, AL 35233

University of Alabama Hospital

Affirmative Action/Equal Opportunity Employer UAB

Letters

The Letters *column is a forum for rapid exchange of ideas among readers of* CP. *Liberal criteria are applied in the review of submissions to encourage contributions to this column.*

The Letters *column includes the following types of contributions: (1) comments, addenda, and minor updates on previously published work, (2) alerts on potential problems related to drug therapy or clinical research, (3) observations or comments on trends in drug therapy or clinical research, and (4) brief expressions of opinion about controversies in drug therapy or clinical research.*

Letters need not be submitted with the journal's manuscript checklist. The following conditions, however, must be adhered to: (1) the body of the letter must be no longer than two typewritten pages, (2) the use of references, tables, and illustrations should be minimized, (3) the authors' names, affiliations, and mailing addresses must be typed at the end of the letter in the format used by CP, *and (4) the entire letter (including references, tables, and authors' names) must be typed double spaced on plain white paper (not letterhead). Following acceptance of a letter, the authors are required to sign an exclusive publication statement and a copyright-transferral form.*

Phlebitis associated with vancomycin therapy

Postinfusion phlebitis was commonly recognized as a problem with the early preparations of vancomycin.[1-3] More recently, Farber and Moellering[4] noted an incidence of only 13% in a retrospective study. Vancomycin preparations have undergone additional purification since the time of Farber and Moellering's study, and many expert sources now state that phlebitis occurs infrequently when currently available preparations are diluted adequately.[5-8]

While conducting a prospective, randomized, double-blind study of intermittent i.v. lock flush solutions, we noticed a much higher incidence of vancomycin-induced phlebitis than has been reported recently. The study took place from March to June 1987, and the most recently purified preparation of Vancocin HCl (vancomycin hydrochloride, Eli Lilly and Company) was administered to six patients. The pharmacy department prepared all doses in a laminar-airflow hood using aseptic technique; 500-mg doses were diluted in 100 mL of 5% dextrose injection (5 mg/mL), and 1-g doses were diluted in 250 mL of 5% dextrose injection (4 mg/mL). The admixtures were infused at rates that did not exceed 1 g per 60 minutes. The i.v. lock sites were evaluated by an experienced nurse at least every 24 hours. Phlebitis was defined as one or more of the following: erythema with a radius of 2 cm or more from the i.v. lock site, induration, or a palpable cord.

A total of 35 i.v. locks were used to administer vancomycin to the six patients. A 20-gauge Teflon catheter was inserted in 33 of the sites by an experienced i.v. team. A 1-g dose of vancomycin was administered through 32 of the sites, and 500-mg doses were administered through the remaining three. Phlebitis occurred at 32 (91.4%) of the 35 sites. Infiltration was noted at four sites; two of these developed phlebitis concurrently. Loss of patency occurred at the final site, thus resulting in 100% site loss for the 35 sites. Pain and erythema each were noted in 30 (85.7%) of the sites, induration was noted in 21 (60%) of the sites, and a palpable cord was found at 5 (14.3%) of the sites. The typical i.v. lock site remained usable for a mean (± S.D.) of 25.3 ± 16.3 hours in the six patients.

Sorrell and Collignon[9] also reported a high incidence of phlebitis when vancomycin was infused through peripheral catheters. Eight of the patients in their study required placement of a central venous catheter so that therapy could be completed after severe phlebitis developed. Although phlebitis is rarely dangerous, it does cause substantial patient discomfort; also, once phlebitis develops, hospital personnel must devote time to frequently changing the peripheral i.v. locks. Clinicians should keep the possibility of phlebitis in mind when prescribing or recommending vancomycin. In addition, researchers should seek methods for reducing vancomycin-induced phlebitis.

1. Geraci JE, Heilman FR, Nichols DR et al. Some laboratory and clinical experiences with a new antibiotic, vancomycin. *Proc Staff Meet Mayo Clin (Antibiot Ann)*. 1956; 31:90–106.
2. Geraci JE, Heilman FR, Nichols DR et al. Antibiotic therapy of bacterial endocarditis VII. Vancomycin for acute micrococcal endocarditis. *Proc Staff Meet Mayo Clin (Antibiot Ann)*. 1958; 33:172–81.
3. Woodley DW, Hall WH. The treatment of severe staphylococcal infections with vancomycin. *Ann Intern Med*. 1961; 55:235–49.
4. Farber BF, Moellering RC. Retrospective study of the toxicity of preparations of vancomycin from 1974 to 1981. *Antimicrob Agents Chemother*. 1983; 23:138–41.
5. Anon. New Preparations of Vancomycin. *Med Lett Drugs Ther*. 1986; 28(729):121–22.
6. Cook FV, Farrar WE. Vancomycin revisited. *Ann Intern Med*. 1978; 88:813–8.

7. Cheung RPF, DiPiro JT. Vancomycin: an update. *Pharmacotherapy*. 1986; 6(4):153–69.
8. Cunha BA, Ristuccia AM. Clinical usefulness of vancomycin. *Clin Pharm*. 1983; 2:417–24.
9. Sorrell TC, Collignon PJ. A prospective study of adverse reactions associated with vancomycin therapy. *J Antimicrob Chemother*. 1985; 16:235–41.

JAMES C. GARRELTS, PHARM.D., Coordinator of Clinical Pharmacy Services
DALE F. SMITH, JR., M.S., Director of Pharmacy
DAN AST, Assistant Director for I.V. Therapy
JOANNE LAROCCA, M.N., Clinical Nurse Specialist

St. Francis Regional Medical Center
929 North St. Francis
Wichita, KS 67214

JERRY D. PETERIE, M.D., FACP, Clinical Assistant Professor
University of Kansas School of Medicine-Wichita
1010 North Kansas
Wichita, KS 67214

Aseptic meningitis associated with muromonab-CD3 therapy

Patients who receive solid organ transplants also must receive multiple immunosuppressive agents to prevent and treat allograft rejection. These agents include cyclosporine, azathioprine, antilymphoblast globulin, and prednisone. When acute rejection of a transplanted organ occurs, treatment includes high doses of corticosteroids, antilymphocyte globulin (ALG), or muromonab-CD3 (Orthoclone OKT3, Ortho Pharmaceutical Corporation). Muromonab-CD3, commonly referred to as OKT3, is effective in the treatment of acute renal allograft rejection and is being studied for use in the treatment of acute rejection of liver, heart, and pancreas transplants.[1-3] The usual adult dose of OKT3 is 5 mg/day for 10 to 14 days. Administration of OKT3 often is followed by flu-like symptoms including fever, chills, dyspnea, chest pain, vomiting, wheezing, nausea, diarrhea, and tremor.[1] Although these symptoms may be common during the first two days of treatment, they diminish as therapy continues.[1]

Relatively few patients had received muromonab-CD3 when the drug received FDA approval, and greater clinical experience with this drug has revealed a previously unanticipated adverse effect. At least 143 cases of aseptic meningitis syndrome or cerebrospinal fluid inflammation have been reported in patients who have received muromonab-CD3 for the treatment of acute allograft rejection.[4-7] Most of these cases have been associated with symptoms of fever (reported in 87% of cases), headache (42%), stiff neck (13%), photophobia (10%), and confusion. In cases where the patient's cerebrospinal fluid was analyzed, the findings included leukocytosis with predominant neutrophils, elevated protein, and negative bacterial, fungal, and viral cultures.

We observed a recent case of what we believe was aseptic meningitis induced by muromonab-CD3 therapy. The patient was a 24-year-old woman with an 18-year history of insulin-dependent diabetes complicated by severe nephropathy and severe proliferative retinopathy. She had undergone regular hemodialysis since 1986 and had received cadaveric renal and pancreas allografts in July 1987. The patient was admitted to our hospital for evaluation of abdominal pain, nausea, and hematuria. The patient received muromonab-CD3 5 mg for the treatment of apparent acute pancreas allograft rejection. After the first dose was administered, the patient's temperature increased to 102.5°F and she became disoriented; evidence of meningeal irritation was found. A neurologist recommended that we perform a lumbar puncture. The results showed a total white blood cell count of 838 cells/cu mm with 99% neutrophils, protein 65 mg/dL, and glucose 72 mg/dL, with a corresponding serum glucose concentration of 153 mg/dL. Cerebrospinal fluid cultures for virus, bacteria, and fungi were negative. Muromonab-CD3 therapy was discontinued after the first dose because of suspected aseptic meningitis, and the patient's neurological and meningeal symptoms resolved rapidly following discontinuation of therapy.

Patients who are treated with muromonab-CD3 should be monitored closely for symptoms suggestive of meningeal irritation. Muromonab-CD3 therapy should be discontinued if such symptoms develop. The symptoms usually will resolve within one to two days after therapy is discontinued. In some patients who received muromonab-CD3 to treat acute rejection of liver transplants, the symptoms of cerebrospinal fluid inflammation resolved despite continued therapy; however, the patients experienced symptoms for as long as five days.[4] A prospective postmarketing surveillance program currently is underway to determine the incidence of OKT3-associated aseptic meningitis syndrome.

1. Canafax DM, Draxler CA. Monoclonal antilymphocyte antibody (OKT3) treatment of acute renal allograft rejection. *Pharmacotherapy*. 1987; 7:121–4.
2. Burke GW, Simmons RL, Canafax DM et al. Initial experiences with OKT3 for prophylaxis and treatment of rejection in kidney, liver and pancreas allografts. *Transplant Proc*. 1988; 20(Suppl):252–3.
3. Ortho Multicenter Transplant Study Group. A clinical trial of OKT3 monoclonal antibody for acute rejection of cadaveric renal transplants. *N Engl J Med*. 1985; 313:337–42.
4. Roden J, Klintman GB, Husberg BS et al. Cerebrospinal fluid inflammation during OKT3 therapy. *Lancet*. 1987; 2:272.
5. Emmons C, Smith J, Flanigan M. Cerebrospinal fluid inflammation during OKT3 therapy. *Lancet*. 1986; 2:510–1.
6. Ortho Pharmaceutical Corporation. Orthoclone OKT3 package insert. Raritan, NJ; 1986 Jun.
7. Thistlethwaite JR, Gaber AO, Haag BW et al. OKT3 treatment of steroid-resistant renal allograft rejection. *Transplantation*. 1987; 43:176–84.

MARTHA E. JOY, PHARM.D., Director of Drug Information and Assistant Professor
MARCIA L. MICHALS, PHARM.D.
DANIEL M. CANAFAX, PHARM.D., Associate Professor

Department of Pharmacy Practice
College of Pharmacy
University of Minnesota
5-130 Health Sciences Unit F
308 Harvard Street, S.E.
Minneapolis, MN 55455

Diminishing bioavailability of oral leucovorin calcium

I read with great interest the article by McGuire et al.[1] about the pharmacokinetics of leucovorin calcium. It is unfortunate, however, that the reader is left with the impression that the bioavailability of oral leucovorin calcium is always "comparable" to that of injectable formulations. I do not dispute the authors' conclusion that the bioavailability of 25-mg doses is comparable, but I believe that McGuire et al. should have emphasized that larger, single oral doses demonstrate diminishing bioavailability when compared with i.v. doses.

In another recent study, McGuire and colleagues[2] reported that the bioavailability percentages of 20-, 40-, 60-, 80-, 100-, and 200-mg single oral doses of leucovorin calcium when compared with a 200-mg i.v. dose in the same subjects were 98%, 76%, 61%, 48%, 41%, and 31%, respectively. Based on these data, the bioavailabilities of oral and parenteral doses of leucovorin calcium greater than 20 mg do not appear to be "comparable." It does appear that patients who need single doses of more than 20–25 mg should receive the drug by injection to ensure systemic availability of the full dose.

I have already been frightened by the impact of advertisements and sales representatives who emphasize to prescribers the "complete bioavailability" of oral tablet formulations. Although this may be true for a single tablet because of the low tablet strengths commercially available, it is not made clear that single oral doses of more than 20–25 mg are *not* completely bioavailable. Therefore, for many patients it may not be advisable to administer several tablets as a single dose.

When leucovorin calcium is administered as a potential rescue or antidote, there should be no doubt in the clinician's mind for the need to administer leucovorin calcium only by injection until the patient is stabilized.

1. McGuire BW, Sia LL, Leese PT et al. Pharmacokinetics of leucovorin after intravenous, intramuscular, and oral administration. *Clin Pharm.* 1988; 7:52–8.
2. McGuire BW, Sia LL, Haynes JD et al. Bioavailability of oral leucovorin calcium. Wayne, NJ: Lederle Laboratories; 1987.

JOSEPH G. ROSSI, PHARM.D., Clinical Pharmacy Specialist
Overlook Hospital
99 Beauvoir Avenue at Sylvan Road
Summit, NJ 07901

We agree with Dr. Rossi's comment about the bioavailability of large oral doses of leucovorin. However, we do not agree with his conclusion that doses of 20–25 mg fall within the range of doses that must be administered intravenously. The labeling of Lederle's leucovorin calcium tablets (the preparation that was used in the second study cited by Dr. Rossi) states that "doses greater than 25 mg should be given parenterally."[1] Straw et al.[2] reported the absolute bioavailability of a 25-mg leucovorin dose to be 97%. We obtained very similar results in our study; we found the absolute bioavailability of a 25-mg dose to be 92%. A concurrent dose-proportionality study demonstrated that the intestinal absorption of leucovorin is a saturable process.[3] It was an oversight on our part that no reference was made to this phenomenon. Our study of the comparative pharmacokinetics of leucovorin after intravenous, intramuscular, and oral administration necessitated the choice of a dose known to be completely absorbed.

The leucovorin rescue regimen given in the Lederle methotrexate product labeling is standard: 15 mg every six hours for 10 doses when methotrexate elimination is normal.[4] This empiric dose is a safe and effective rescue for methotrexate doses as high as 12 g/sq m and is well within the range in which leucovorin is well absorbed.[5] The Lederle labeling for both methotrexate and leucovorin states that when higher doses of leucovorin are needed, leucovorin must be given intravenously.[1,4] The Lederle product advertising is consistent with this labeling and does not suggest that oral leucovorin has "complete bioavailability" at higher doses.

We very much appreciate Dr. Rossi's close review and comment on both of our leucovorin pharmacokinetics studies. Each study had different objectives and consequently different emphases; however, both were designed to provide clinicians with information about rational leucovorin dosing regimens.

1. Lederle Laboratories. Leucovorin calcium tablets package insert. Pearl River, NY: 1987 Feb.
2. Straw JA, Szapary D, Wynn WT. Pharmacokinetics of the diastereoisomers of leucovorin after intravenous and oral administration to normal subjects. *Cancer Res.* 1984; 44:3114–9.
3. McGuire BW, Sia LL, Haynes JD et al. Absorption kinetics of orally administered leucovorin calcium. *Natl Cancer Inst Monogr.* 1987; 7:47–56.
4. Lederle Laboratories. Methotrexate package insert. Pearl River, NY: 1988 May.
5. Link MP, Goorin AM, Miser AW et al. The effect of adjuvant chemotherapy on relapse-free survival in patients with osteosarcoma of the extremity. *N Engl J Med.* 1986; 314:1600–2.

RICHARD STEFFAN, M.D.
Professional Medical Services

JOSEPH DE VITO, PHARM.D.
Professional Pharmaceutical Services

Lederle Laboratories
North Middletown Road
Pearl River, NY 10965

BRIAN W. MCGUIRE, PH.D., Clinical Project Manager
Clinical Research Department
Alpha Therapeutic Corporation
5555 Valley Boulevard
Los Angeles, CA 90032

Consumer Drug Digest
Revised Edition

Consumer Drug Digest, Revised Edition, is a comprehensive, authoritative guide to common prescription and non-prescription drugs . . . helping patients to understand their medications and learn what they can do to be more aware of their drug therapy.

Written in layman's language, this drug information handbook contains over 250 of the most commonly prescribed drugs, which comprise over 95% of prescriptions written in the U.S. today. ***Consumer Drug Digest*** is easy to read and use. And, it's indexed by both brand names and generic names, so it's easy to locate information.

The ***Consumer Drug Digest*** is an excellent tool for patients and for pharmacy services areas.

Order your copy today.

☐ Please send me a brochure on **Consumer Drug Digest**

Name ____________________

Address ____________________

City ____________ State ________ Zip ________

Send to: ASHP Publication Records Dept.,
4630 Montgomery Avenue, Bethesda, MD 20814

Drug Review

Therapeutic evaluation of omeprazole

MARIJKE H. ADAMS, JOHN D. OSTROSKY, AND CRAIG F. KIRKWOOD

Abstract: The pharmacology, pharmacokinetics, clinical efficacy, adverse effects, and dosage and administration of omeprazole are reviewed.

Omeprazole, a substituted benzimidazole, has a unique site and mechanism of action because it inhibits the proton pump—i.e., hydrogen, potassium adenosine triphosphatase (H^+,K^+-ATPase)—and consequently blocks the final common step in the gastric acid secretory pathway. Omeprazole inhibits basal and histamine-, gastrin- and pentagastrin-stimulated gastric hydrochloric acid secretion. It produces a dose-dependent reduction in gastric acidity, gastric acid output, and gastric juice volume and has variable effects on pepsin secretion. Omeprazole has no documented effect on esophageal motility or lower esophageal sphincter pressure. Omeprazole is variably absorbed from the gastrointestinal tract, and food appears to decrease the rate, but not the extent, of drug absorption. The drug is approximately 95% bound to plasma proteins and is metabolized to inactive components that are enterohepatically or renally eliminated. Omeprazole is more effective (in most studies) than H_2-receptor antagonists in treating duodenal ulcer, at least as effective in treating benign gastric ulcer, and more effective in treating reflux esophagitis. Omeprazole has been used successfully in patients with Zollinger–Ellison syndrome refractory to treatment with H_2-receptor antagonists. Gastrointestinal complaints (nausea and diarrhea) are the most commonly reported adverse effects associated with omeprazole therapy. The most frequently reported laboratory abnormality occurring with omeprazole use is elevation of serum aspartate aminotransferase and alanine aminotransferase concentrations.

Omeprazole will serve a valuable role in the management of gastrointestinal tract ulcers and hypersecretory conditions.

Index terms: Dosage; Esophagitis; Gastrointestinal drugs; Omeprazole; Pharmacokinetics; Toxicity; Ulcers; Zollinger–Ellison syndrome
Clin Pharm. 1988; 7:725–45

Omeprazole represents a new class of drugs for use in the treatment of peptic ulcer disease and hypersecretory conditions. Current medical management of these disorders includes the histamine H_2-receptor antagonists, which substantially reduce acid secretion but do not abolish it. Omeprazole blocks the proton pump of the parietal cell, believed to be the final common step in the acid secretory pathway,[1] and therefore abolishes acid secretion in response to any type of stimulation. Omeprazole was developed by AB Astra of Sweden and is under investigation in the United States and in other countries. It is distributed for compassionate use in the United States by Merck Sharp & Dohme under the brand name Losec.

Description and Chemistry

Omeprazole is the generic name for 5-methoxy-2-[[(4-methoxy-3,5-dimethyl-2-pyridinyl)methyl]

MARIJKE H. ADAMS is a Doctor of Pharmacy candidate and Doctor of Philosophy student in the Department of Pharmacy and Pharmaceutics, Medical College of Virginia–Virginia Commonwealth University (MCV–VCU), Richmond. JOHN D. OSTROSKY, PHARM.D., is Drug Information Specialist, Department of Pharmacy Services, Medical College of Virginia Hospitals, and Assistant Clinical Professor, Department of Pharmacy and Pharmaceutics, MCV–VCU. CRAIG F. KIRKWOOD, PHARM.D., is Director, Drug Information Service, Department of Pharmacy Services, Medical College of Virginia Hospitals, and Assistant Professor, Department of Pharmacy and Pharmaceutics, MCV–VCU.

Address reprint requests to Dr. Ostrosky at Medical College of Virginia Hospitals, Box 42 MCV Station, Richmond, VA 23298-0042.

This is article **680-204-8815** in the **ASHP Continuing Education System.** See page 775 for learning objectives and test questions.

Copyright © 1988, American Society of Hospital Pharmacists, Inc. All rights reserved. 0278-2677/88/1001-0725$05.25.

sulfinyl]-1H-benzimidazole (Figure 1), a substituted benzimidazole with a molecular weight of 345. While substituted benzimidazoles resemble the H_2-receptor antagonists in structure, their sites and mechanisms of action are quite different.

Omeprazole is an ampholyte with pK_a values of approximately 4 and 8.8.[2] Although only very slightly soluble in water, omeprazole is very soluble in alkaline solutions as the negatively charged ion. It degrades rapidly at low pH in aqueous solutions. Below pH 4, the degradation half-life is less than 10 minutes; at pH 6.5, the half-life of degradation is 18 hours.[2]

Site and Mechanism of Action

Secretion of hydrochloric acid from the parietal cell is stimulated by activation of membrane receptors for histamine, gastrin (a peptide), or acetylcholine (Figure 2). Stimulation of the histamine receptor activates adenylate cyclase, resulting in an increased intracellular concentration of cyclic adenosine 3′,5′ monophosphate (cAMP), which in turn stimulates hydrochloric acid secretion.[1,3] Peptide hormone and cholinergic agonists stimulate gastric secretion of hydrochloric acid by increasing the intracellular concentration of free calcium. The final, common step in the acid secretory pathway is believed to be the enzyme hydrogen, potassium adenosine triphosphatase (H^+,K^+-ATPase), also called a proton pump, which transports hydrogen ions into the secretory canaliculus of the parietal cell in exchange for potassium ions. If H^+,K^+-ATPase is indeed the final step, then its blockade would prevent acid secretion stimulated either by receptor agonists (e.g., histamine) or by postreceptor secretagogues (i.e., cAMP). Histamine phosphate, pentagastrin (a synthetic analog of gastrin), and derivatives of cAMP have been used clinically or experimentally to stimulate gastric hydrochloric acid secretion.

Figure 1. Structural formula of omeprazole.

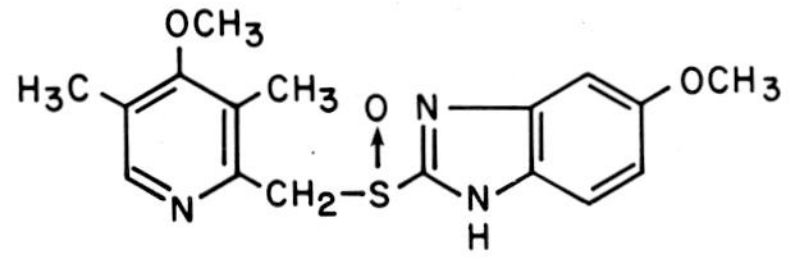

Parietal cells are located deep within the mucosa of the body of the stomach and are the source of both hydrochloric acid and intrinsic factor, a cobalamin-binding protein. The resting parietal cell contains many smooth-walled vesicular membranes (tubulovesicles) and an intracellular membrane structure with few microvilli along the extracellular face (the secretory canaliculus). When the cell is stimulated and actively secreting, the tubulovesicles disappear and the secretory surface becomes deeply invaginated to form channels that are covered with numerous long microvilli.[3,4] H^+,K^+-ATPase, unique to the parietal cell, is located at the canalicular microvilli (Figure 2) and is the site of omeprazole's action.[1,3,4] Each canaliculus can be viewed as an invaginated extracellular compartment of approximately pH 1. This is an environment that should readily accumulate weak bases, such as omeprazole, with a pK_a higher than the pH of the gastric compartment. Limited permeability of omeprazole in an acid environment should make its actions relatively specific to the parietal cell, although one in vitro study has shown that, at low pH, omeprazole also inhibits adenylate cyclase in guinea pigs and sodium, potassium adenosine triphosphatase in dog kidneys.[5]

Omeprazole is activated by protonation at a low pH.[6] The proton-activated derivative then reacts with and binds to sulfhydryl groups associated with gastric H^+,K^+-ATPase, resulting in inhibition of the pump. An alternative mechanism proposes

Figure 2. A model of the actively secreting parietal cell and mechanisms controlling gastric acid secretion.

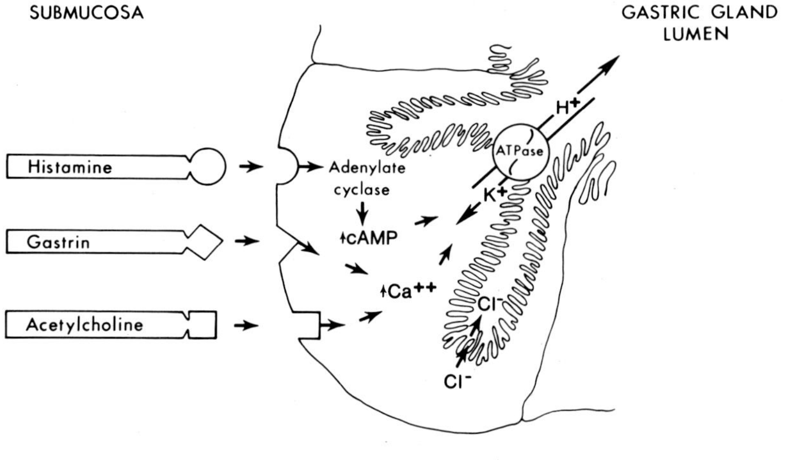

that essential sulfhydryl groups of gastric H^+,K^+-ATPase may react with activated omeprazole to form an *N*-sulfenylated complex, rather than a disulfide complex.[7] Regardless of mechanism, activated omeprazole binds tightly with the enzyme, which may explain the prolonged acid inhibition in the absence of detectable plasma concentrations. Whether restoration of acid secretion requires reactivation of H^+,K^+-ATPase by endogenous sulfhydryl compounds or synthesis of new enzyme is unknown.[6] Guinea pig parietal cells exposed to omeprazole in vitro or in vivo have shown that inhibition of acid secretion is reversible,[8] but in vitro studies of gastric glands from rabbits and dogs exposed to omeprazole in vivo demonstrated irreversible inhibition.[9]

The degree of gastric acid inhibition observed may be related to the activity of the parietal cells at the time of omeprazole administration. In rats and dogs, the inhibitory effect of omeprazole was diminished when the drug was administered after a resting state for acid production was induced by cimetidine or somatostatin.[7,10] When omeprazole was administered to animals in an acid-stimulated state, its inhibitory effects were increased.

Omeprazole may possess other pharmacologic activity of interest. Gastric cytoprotective effects have been observed after oral administration of proton pump inhibitors,[11,12] although the mechanism is unknown. Studies with rats have reported increases in gastric mucosal blood flow after omeprazole treatment[11,13] and an increase in mucosal prostaglandin E_2 concentration after administration of a proton pump inhibitor.[12] Omeprazole in vitro inhibits human polymorphonuclear neutrophilic granulocyte chemotaxis, superoxide anion generation, and degranulation but not cytochrome b translocation, which suggests potential anti-inflammatory activity.[14] These reported effects will not be reviewed.

Pharmacologic Effects

Omeprazole has produced significant inhibition of gastric acid secretion in animal studies. In vitro experiments using isolated gastric glands from rabbits demonstrated omeprazole 10^{-5} M reduced acid secretion in unstimulated glands by 64% to 77%, as measured by ^{14}C-aminopyrine accumulation.[1] In glands stimulated by histamine or a cAMP mimetic, acid secretion was reduced by a mean of 59% to 75% and 59% to 64%, respectively, compared with acid secretion in unstimulated glands. These decreases persisted for the 60-minute study period. In vivo studies in dogs with gastric fistulas reported that omeprazole (1 mg/kg) given by i.v. bolus injection before histamine i.v. infusion (40 μg/kg/hr) almost completely inhibited subsequent acid secretion.[15] Omeprazole injected during histamine infusion produced a mean 65% reduction in gastric acid secretion (approximately 11 mmol/30 minutes, histamine alone; approximately 4 mmol/30 minutes, omeprazole plus histamine). Duration of acid inhibition was not measured.

Several physiologic changes are observed in humans after omeprazole administration, apparently because of its effect on gastric acid secretion. Omeprazole produces a substantial dose-dependent inhibition of gastric acid secretion after either single or multiple dosing, and it decreases the volume of gastric juice. Changes in gastric pepsin concentration are variable; increases, decreases, and no significant change have been reported. Increases in serum pepsinogen concentration have been observed. Intrinsic factor secretion and cobalamin absorption are unchanged by omeprazole, while intragastric bile acid concentration is substantially increased. Short-term studies with omeprazole demonstrate an increase in serum gastrin concentration that returned to baseline when omeprazole was discontinued. Variable changes in serum gastrin concentration have been reported after longer treatment with omeprazole.

Gastric Acid. Omeprazole produces a long-lasting, dose-dependent inhibition of gastric acid secretion after both single and multiple doses in patients with peptic ulcer disease and in healthy volunteers. Single doses of omeprazole 20 to 60 mg p.o. reduce acid secretion by 36% to 90%, with effects persisting for 24 to 72 hours. Multiple doses of omeprazole 10 to 40 mg p.o. daily for 5 to 28 days reduce acid secretion by 32% to 100%.[16–22]

In vitro studies have examined the response of human gastric glands and purified H^+,K^+-ATPase, obtained from either healthy subjects or gastric ulcer patients, to omeprazole.[23] Omeprazole 10^{-5} M almost totally inhibited basal acid production in glands from both sources, as measured by aminopyrine accumulation. In glands from healthy subjects, omeprazole produced a 91% inhibition in maximal response to dibutyryl cAMP 1 mM. In glands from gastric ulcer patients, omeprazole produced a 90% inhibition in maximal response to either dibutyryl cAMP 1 mM or to histamine 50 μmol. H^+,K^+-ATPase activity was inhibited by 75% in the presence of omeprazole 10^{-5} M.[23]

Healthy Subjects. Duration of acid inhibition has been studied in healthy volunteers after single doses of omeprazole 20 or 40 mg or placebo oral suspension.[16] Mean acid response to pentagastrin stimulation (91 μg i.v. over one hour) at 2, 24, 48, and 72 hours after dosing was 7.4, 9.0, 9.6, and 9.5 mmol/15 min after placebo; 3.6, 6.4, 7.9, and 8.7 mmol/15 min after omeprazole 20 mg; and 0.9, 4.3, 6.3, and 7.9 mmol/15 min after omeprazole 40 mg. When it was measured 14 days after dosing, acid response was not significantly different from that associated with placebo for either dose.

Numerous studies have reported the extent of acid inhibition with omeprazole use. Comparison of these studies is difficult because of variations in study design and measurement method. Gastric acidity was measured under basal conditions at 0.9, 1.5, and 2 hours after a single i.v. dose of either omeprazole 80 mg or placebo in healthy volunteers.[17] When subjects received omeprazole, acid concentration was decreased (median: 22–32 mmol/L after placebo, 0 mmol/L after omeprazole; $p < 0.001$), and gastric aspirate pH was increased (median: pH 2 after placebo, approximately pH 7 after omeprazole; $p < 0.001$), at each measurement. In 14 of 17 subjects, aspirate pH was greater than 6.0 at 1.5 and 2 hours after administration of omeprazole.

Ten healthy subjects who received single intravenous doses of omeprazole and oral omeprazole at 0800 for seven days experienced a significant decrease in acid concentration.[18] During the daytime (0800 to 2200), mean hourly acid concentration after no drug; i.v. omeprazole 10, 20, 40, and 80 mg; and oral omeprazole 20 mg/day was 21.26, 9.04, 6.62, 1.01, 0.28, and 2.79 mmol/L, respectively. Nighttime (2300 to 0700) acidity was 46.94, 27.36, 20.54, 11.77, 9.91, and 13.18 mmol/L, respectively. No significant differences were observed between i.v. omeprazole 40 or 80 mg and oral omeprazole 20 mg for seven days.

Single doses of omeprazole oral suspension 20, 40, 60, and 80 mg in healthy volunteers produced 36%, 65%, 90%, and 99% mean reductions (Table 1) in gastric acid secretion, respectively, during pentagastrin i.v. infusion.[16] The degree of inhibition remained constant for the three study hours. Howden et al.[19] studied healthy subjects receiving oral omeprazole 10 mg or placebo daily for seven days. These subjects experienced no significant change in either basal or pentagastrin-stimulated acid output as compared with placebo after the first dose of omeprazole (Table 1). After the seventh dose of omeprazole, however, basal acid output was decreased by a mean of 93% ($p < 0.02$), and pentagastrin-stimulated acid output was decreased by a mean of 67% ($p < 0.01$).

Duodenal Ulcer Patients. Substantial decreases in intragastric acidity have also been observed after omeprazole administration in patients with duodenal ulcers (DUs). Omeprazole administered intravenously produces a rapid inhibition of acid secretion: Within one hour of an 80-mg dose, the lowest gastric pH recorded has been 4.0.[20] Omeprazole 160 mg i.v. daily, given in two or three divided doses, was required to produce acid inhibition similar to that reported after omeprazole 30 mg p.o. daily. Mean hourly acid concentrations (measured over 22 hours) after the two i.v. omeprazole dosage regimens were 1.1 and 0.5 mmol/L, respectively. The authors speculate that this anomaly may be the result of comparing single-day i.v. treatment with repeated-dose oral treatment or that a local effect in the stomach before absorption or an active metabolite in the gastrointestinal tract might exist.

Intragastric acidity was measured over a 24-hour period after eight days of treatment with either oral omeprazole 20 mg or placebo in ten DU pa-

Table 1.
Inhibition of Acid Secretion after Oral Placebo and Omeprazole Administration in Healthy Subjects

			Mean Acid Output (mmol/15 min)		
			Basal	Pentagastrin Stimulation	
Reference	No. of Subjects	Drug and Dose (mg)	After Treatment	Before Treatment	After Treatment
16	6[a]	Placebo	. . .	7.1	6.4
		Omeprazole[b] 20	. . .	7.6	4.3
		Omeprazole 40	. . .	6.6	2.1
		Omeprazole 60	. . .	7.4	0.57
		Omeprazole 80	. . .	6.8	0.06
19	6[c]	Placebo	0.63[e]	. . .	5.83[e]
		Omeprazole[d] 10			
		Day 1	0.35[e]	. . .	5.78[e]
		Day 7	0.05[e]	. . .	1.95[e]
16	6[f]	Placebo			
		Day 1	. . .	9.3	8.3
		Day 3	. . .	8.9	7.6
		Day 5	. . .	8.5	7.3
		Omeprazole[b] 15			
		Day 1	. . .	9.3	4.3
		Day 3	. . .	5.9	1.8
		Day 5	. . .	5.1	1.4

[a] Subjects received pentagastrin 30 μg/hr as i.v. infusion.
[b] As suspension.
[c] Subjects received pentagastrin 1.2 μg/kg i.v.
[d] As capsule.
[e] Derived from reference; originally reported as millimoles per hour.
[f] Subjects received pentagastrin 91 μg/hr as i.v. infusion.

tients.[21] For each observation, the median pH value was higher after omeprazole than after placebo treatment (overall, median pH 4.8 versus 1.6, respectively). The mean 24-hour intragastric acid concentration decreased from 34 mmol/L with placebo to 9.2 mmol/L with omeprazole (73% decrease). In six patients, acid concentration was decreased from 5.2–38.1 mmol/L with placebo to 0.0–0.3 mmol/L with omeprazole and from 35.1–54.4 mmol/L after placebo to 18.3–27.7 mmol/L after omeprazole in the remaining four patients.

Gastric acid output was measured before and after four weeks of treatment with oral omeprazole in DU patients.[22] Under basal, sham feed (in which food is chewed and then spit out, rather than swallowed), and pentagastrin-stimulated conditions, acid output was increased by 1% and decreased by 63% and 47%, respectively, after omeprazole 20 mg. Omeprazole 40 mg resulted in decreases of 100%, 98%, and 84%, respectively ($p < 0.01$). Median values were not reported.

"Weekend therapy" has been evaluated in DU patients as a potential maintenance regimen.[24] Eight weeks of omeprazole 20 mg/day for three days each week resulted in a basal acid output of 7.6, 1.4, 3.6, and 2.1 mmol/L when measured before and 24 hours after weekend 1 and 8, respectively.

Gastric Juice Volume. Omeprazole decreases the volume of gastric juice secreted, although not to the same extent as it inhibits acid secretion. After single doses of omeprazole 20, 40, and 60 mg, the volume of gastric output after pentagastrin stimulation was reduced by a mean of 19%, 37%, and 70%, respectively, compared with gastric output associated with placebo.[16] Oral omeprazole 10 mg daily for seven days produced a mean 27% reduction ($p < 0.02$, compared with placebo) in volume of basal secretions but no significant change in the volume of pentagastrin-stimulated secretions.[19] The volume of basal gastric secretion in six subjects with advanced chronic renal failure was unchanged by single-dose omeprazole 30 mg either with or without hemodialysis on the same day.[25] During pentagastrin stimulation, gastric secretion volume in these subjects was reduced by a mean of 51% without dialysis and 64% with dialysis. In DU patients receiving omeprazole daily for four weeks, the volume of gastric secretions under basal, sham feed, and pentagastrin-stimulated conditions was altered by a mean of +6%, −6%, and −20%, respectively, after 20 mg; corresponding values after the 40-mg dose were −32%, −22%, and −48%, respectively.[22]

Pepsin and Pepsinogen. Changes in pepsin secretion after omeprazole administration are less consistent than effects on gastric acid output. Healthy subjects receiving oral omeprazole 10 mg daily for seven days experienced no significant change in pepsin output under basal conditions or during pentagastrin stimulation.[19] In nine DU patients who received omeprazole daily for four weeks, pepsin concentration with omeprazole 20 mg ($n = 4$) was reduced by approximately 45% (difference was not significant) under either basal or sham feed conditions.[22] Pepsin concentration in the five patients who received omeprazole 40 mg was reduced by 62% ($p < 0.05$) under basal conditions and by 46% (difference was not significant) under sham feed conditions. Pepsin output (units/hr) was not significantly decreased after omeprazole 20 mg daily, but significant decreases were observed after 40 mg (71%, $p < 0.01$, basal conditions; 58%, $p < 0.05$, sham feed). Pepsin concentration and pepsin output increased under pentagastrin treatment after omeprazole 20 and 40 mg daily, but the increases were not significant. Results for this study were presented graphically for individual subjects; median data were not provided.

Elevation of fasting serum pepsinogen I concentration has been reported in one study after a regimen of omeprazole 30 mg daily for 14 days in healthy volunteers.[26] A maximal increase of 126% of baseline concentration was observed after 14 days, and fasting concentrations of pepsinogen I were still elevated two and four days after omeprazole was discontinued. In contrast, no significant increase in serum pepsinogen I concentration was observed after a test meal in these subjects. Pepsinogen I represents a group of pepsinogens found in chief and mucous cells in the body and fundus of the stomach.[27] In an acid environment, inactive pepsinogens are cleaved to active pepsin. Pepsinogen I is normally found in plasma, and there is a high correlation between serum concentrations of pepsinogen I and maximal gastric acid secretion. Generally, agents that stimulate acid secretion also stimulate pepsinogen secretion. The clinical importance of these observations with omeprazole is unknown.

Intrinsic Factor. No significant changes have been observed in intrinsic factor concentration, intrinsic factor output, or cobalamin absorption after omeprazole use. Intrinsic factor secretion has been studied in 17 healthy volunteers after a single i.v. infusion of omeprazole 80 mg.[17] The median unbound intrinsic factor concentration in gastric juice was slightly but not significantly increased after omeprazole compared with that associated with placebo. Effects on cobalamin absorption in the study were variable, with both increased and decreased absorption observed after omeprazole administration; however, median cobalamin absorption after omeprazole was not significantly reduced ($p = 0.52$) compared with that associated with placebo.

After seven and nine days of oral omeprazole 60 mg daily, basal and pentagastrin-stimulated (1.5 μg/kg/hr) peak intrinsic factor output were unchanged from baseline in eight healthy volunteers.[28] To differentiate direct effects of omeprazole on intrinsic factor from hypochlorhydria, subjects received 0.9 N sodium chloride or 0.1 M hydrochloric acid perfusion during testing. Steady-state stimulated intrinsic factor secretion was not significantly different from baseline during sodium chloride perfusion (mean 10.8 μg/hr baseline, 10.7 μg/hr sodium chloride perfusion) but was significantly decreased during hydrochloric acid perfusion (mean 10.5 μg/hr baseline, 4.1 μg/hr hydrochloric acid perfusion; $p < 0.001$). The authors concluded that omeprazole did not affect intrinsic factor secretion, but they were unable to explain the observed decrease in intrinsic factor secretion during hydrochloric acid perfusion.

Cobalamin absorption has been studied in eight volunteers with a history of acid-peptic disease who received 10 days of treatment with omeprazole 20 or 40 mg.[29] Based on excretion data, absorption of protein-bound cobalamin was decreased after omeprazole, but absorption of unbound cobalamin was not significantly different from baseline.

Bile Acids. Intragastric bile acid concentrations were determined in DU patients after placebo or omeprazole 20 mg daily for eight days.[21] The median 24-hour bile acid concentration increased from 221 μmol/L after placebo to 290 μmol/L after omeprazole ($p < 0.05$). This increase was a result of reduced acidity and reduced volume of gastric secretions.

Gastrin. Although single-dose studies in humans have shown no significant effect on serum gastrin concentrations, short-term clinical trials have demonstrated an increase in mean fasting and postprandial serum gastrin levels. In healthy volunteers, mean fasting serum gastrin concentration was essentially unchanged after a single 30-mg dose of omeprazole, but increased from 27 pg/mL to 44 and 42 pg/mL after 7 and 14 days of treatment with omeprazole 30 mg daily, respectively.[26] Two days after omeprazole was discontinued, mean fasting serum gastrin concentration was not significantly different from baseline. Serum gastrin concentrations were measured in 10 DU patients receiving placebo or omeprazole 20 mg daily for eight days.[21] After omeprazole, both fasting and postprandial mean serum gastrin concentrations were increased when compared with placebo treatment, but the differences were not significant. In 3 of the 10 patients, no increase in the postprandial serum gastrin concentration was observed after omeprazole. Fasting serum gastrin concentrations were elevated after omeprazole treatment (study duration unspecified) in 102 DU patients receiving omeprazole 20 mg p.o. daily.[30] Fasting serum gastrin concentrations increased from a mean of 39.9 to 73.5 pg/mL and increased to more than 150 pg/mL in 12.5% of patients. Two weeks after discontinuation of omeprazole, fasting serum gastrin concentration had decreased to 49.7 pg/mL.

Serum gastrin concentrations have been reported for patients receiving more than two weeks of omeprazole treatment. In patients with chronic gastric or esophageal peptic ulcers, mean fasting serum gastrin concentrations increased significantly (from 103 to 205 pg/mL) during the first 12 weeks of treatment with omeprazole 20 to 60 mg daily for 13 to 21 months.[31] No subsequent increases were observed. Seventy-three patients with severe reflux esophagitis received omeprazole 40 mg daily for 4 to 12 weeks, then omeprazole 20 mg daily as maintenance.[32] Median serum gastrin concentrations demonstrated considerable variability at each measurement time. Fasting plasma gastrin concentration has also been measured after "weekend therapy" with omeprazole.[24] In DU patients who received eight weeks of omeprazole 20 mg/day for three days each week, median fasting plasma gastrin concentrations were 17, 25, 22, and 31 pmol/L when measured before and 24 hours after weekend 1 and 8, respectively (reference range <50 pmol/L). Two weeks after omeprazole was discontinued, the median fasting plasma gastrin concentration was 20 pmol/L.

Increases in fasting serum gastrin concentration also occur with other antisecretory agents. In 309 DU patients who received omeprazole 20 mg p.o. daily or ranitidine hydrochloride 150 mg (of ranitidine) p.o. twice daily for four weeks,[33] mean fasting serum gastrin concentrations before treatment, after two and four weeks of treatment, and two weeks after treatment was discontinued were 34.4, 66.7, 72.7, and 52.3 pg/mL, respectively, for omeprazole and 47.6, 57.1, 56.1, and 48.1 pg/mL, respectively, for ranitidine. Gastrin concentrations after both treatments were significantly different from baseline values at two and four weeks; increases with omeprazole treatment were also significantly greater than increases with ranitidine.

Hypergastrinemia is most likely triggered by a pronounced decrease in intragastric acidity. In addition to stimulating gastric acid secretion, gastrin promotes the growth and proliferation of endocrine or enterochromaffin-like (ECL) cells in the gastric fundus or oxyntic gland area, although most evidence of this trophic action in humans is indirect.[34] Clinical conditions involving elevated serum gastrin concentrations, such as atrophic gastritis and Zollinger–Ellison syndrome (ZES), are associated with ECL cell hyperplasia.[34–36] ECL cell neoplasia has been associated with hypergastrinemia,[35] although gastric carcinoids are uncommon.[37] (See also Contraindications and Precautions.) For a discussion of the relationships between gastric acid, gastrinemia, and gastric carcinoids, see references 34–36.

Miscellaneous. Omeprazole has no direct effect on the lower esophageal sphincter (LES) pressure or the frequency of hourly LES relaxations.[38] Additionally, omeprazole has no effect on gastrointestinal motility.[39]

Pharmacokinetics

Absorption. Several oral formulations of omeprazole have been used in clinical trials, since the drug degrades rapidly in acidic solutions. Early studies used aqueous suspensions of omeprazole with methylcellulose and sodium bicarbonate, or with polyethylene glycol.[2,16,40] Sodium bicarbonate solutions were usually administered with and after the suspension for several doses to reduce acid degradation.

In one randomized, crossover trial, an oral omeprazole suspension in doses of 10 and 40 mg (given with multiple doses of sodium bicarbonate) demonstrated a mean systemic availability of 40% and 58%, respectively.[40] Mean area under the plasma concentration versus time curve (AUC) and peak plasma concentration were increased disproportionally to the omeprazole dose. Considerable variability was observed in the data, but the results suggest a saturation of the first-pass effect, since the plasma clearance of omeprazole given i.v. was unaffected by dose.

A more recent formulation, enteric-coated granules of drug in a hard gelatin capsule, has overcome many of the problems of oral administration, but absorption from this formulation is unpredictable and variable. One report estimates the systemic availability of the encapsulated enteric-coated granules, compared with the solution, as 70%.[41] After initial and multiple dosing of oral omeprazole, the time to peak plasma concentration has been variable, with a range of 0.5 to 7 hours.[42,43] Absorption was delayed when the capsules were given with a meal[2]; however, insufficient data have been collected to evaluate the extent of absorption. A comparison of omeprazole administered 2 minutes versus 15 minutes before breakfast demonstrated no difference in the total amount absorbed, as measured by the AUC.[2] With a buffered suspension used as a reference, the AUC for 2-minute and 15-minute prebreakfast dosing was 66.6% and 65.5%, respectively.

Omeprazole appears to enhance its own bioavailability, since peak plasma concentration and AUC are increased with repeated doses. In subjects receiving oral omeprazole daily for seven days,[42] mean peak plasma concentration after an initial dose of 30 and 60 mg was 558 μg/L (range, 223 to 1160 μg/L) and 1670 μg/L (range, 860 to 3830 μg/L), respectively. After the seventh dose, peak plasma omeprazole concentrations had increased to a mean of 712 μg/L (range, 239 to 1260 μg/L) with 30 mg and 2070 μg/L (range, 1310 to 3180 μg/L) with 60 mg. Plasma omeprazole concentrations were undetectable 24 hours after a dose (limit of detection, 10 μg/mL), and omeprazole AUC was consistently increased after repeated dosing ($p < 0.01$). Elimination half-life did not change significantly, but the absorption rate constant substantially increased with repeated dosing (for 60 mg, the absorption rate constant = 0.36 hr^{-1} after first dose, 7.06 hr^{-1} after seventh dose). Other studies have also reported an increase in peak concentration and AUC after multiple dosing.[19,43] Since omeprazole is acid labile, this enhanced bioavailability may be due to less inactivation of the drug as gastric pH increases. This effect stabilizes in three to five days, based on gastric acid secretion.

In healthy subjects receiving omeprazole 15 mg or placebo daily for five days, maximal acid response to i.v. pentagastrin when measured two hours postdose on days 1, 3, and 5 was inhibited by 47%, 75%, and 80%, respectively, relative to placebo (Table 1).[16] Plasma omeprazole concentrations were undetectable before drug administration on study days 3 and 5 (lower limit of detection estimated at 0.3 μmol/L).

Distribution. Plasma omeprazole concentration data after both i.v. and p.o. administration have been fitted to a two-compartment model, using nonlinear analysis.[40,44] After i.v. administration, omeprazole's mean distribution half-life is approximately three to seven minutes.[40,44]

The initial volume of distribution for omeprazole after an i.v. dose has been described as 0.05–0.24 L/kg.[40,44] At distribution equilibrium, the volume of distribution increases to 0.19–0.48 L/kg and is comparable to the extracellular fluid volume.[40,44]

In vitro ultrafiltration studies have shown that omeprazole is approximately 95% bound in human plasma at 20 °C.[40] The extent of omeprazole binding in plasma was virtually unchanged by a 100-fold variation in the drug concentration. When added to a physiologic solution of purified human serum albumin and α_1-acid glycoprotein, therapeutic concentrations of omeprazole were approximately 95% bound and 94% bound at 20 °C and 37 °C, respectively, suggesting that omeprazole is bound primarily to these plasma proteins. In patients with chronic renal insufficiency, mean plasma protein binding was 95% (range, 94% to 96%), which was not significantly different from that in healthy subjects.[44]

In vitro and in vivo, the ratio between whole blood and plasma omeprazole concentration is approximately 0.6 in humans, indicating that omeprazole has limited distribution into red blood cells.[40] No information is available regarding excretion of omeprazole into breast milk.

The results of one study in eight elderly subjects, age 75–80 years, suggest that changes may occur in omeprazole's distribution with age.[41] Further study is needed to verify this observation and to determine the clinical importance of observed changes.

Metabolism. At least three metabolites have been identified in human plasma,[40–41] but none is believed to contribute to acid inhibition. Hydroxyomeprazole and omeprazole sulfone are the major plasma metabolites, and omeprazole sulfide appears in low concentration. Plasma omeprazole sulfone concentration is greater than plasma omeprazole concentration four hours after omeprazole administration and is still measurable after nine hours.[45] Peak plasma concentration and AUC for omeprazole sulfone increase after repeated dosing.[43] At least six different metabolites have been identified in human urine[41]; hydroxy-omeprazole and its corresponding carboxylic acid are the most abundant urinary metabolites. At least 10 urinary metabolites of omeprazole have been isolated in rats and dogs.[46] Structures have been determined for 7 of the 10 metabolites.[47]

Elimination. Omeprazole has a plasma half-life of approximately 60 minutes after i.v. administration and two to three hours after oral administration.[40,42] Plasma omeprazole concentrations are undetectable at six hours after i.v. administration and at eight hours after oral administration (lower limit of detection, 50 nmol/L).[44]

Omeprazole's rapid elimination is primarily due to metabolic processes, since insignificant amounts of unchanged drug are excreted in the urine and stool.[40] Approximately 80% of an i.v. or p.o. (as suspension) dose is excreted as urinary metabolites over a four-day period, and approximately 60% of a radiolabeled dose appears in the urine within the first six to eight hours after administration.[41] A minor fraction (<1%) of the omeprazole dose is excreted via the kidneys as the sulfone metabolite, although it is present in plasma in a relatively high concentration.[40] This may be due to further metabolism before renal excretion or to nonrenal elimination, such as biliary excretion. Fecal excretion accounts for 19% (i.v.) and 18% (p.o.) of an administered dose. Studies conducted in rats have demonstrated that a considerable amount of the drug appears in the feces after absorption from the gastrointestinal tract, which strongly suggests biliary excretion.[46] Biliary recovery over a six-hour period (approximately 62% of the dose) was higher compared with fecal excretion over 72 hours (approximately 49% of the dose), possibly indicating enterohepatic recycling of omeprazole metabolites in rats.

No significant difference was noted in AUC or extent of acid inhibition when omeprazole was administered to patients with chronic renal failure on regular hemodialysis.[25] Patients were hemodialyzed for four hours, starting 1.5 hours after omeprazole administration. Dialysate samples were taken at one-hour intervals; omeprazole was not detected in the dialysis fluid. Urinary excretion of metabolites was significantly altered in patients with impaired renal function (defined as creatinine clearance between 10 and 62 mL/min/1.73 sq m), although the disposition characteristics of omeprazole were within the range reported for young, healthy subjects.[44] Mean total urinary recovery over four days was approximately 50% in these subjects compared with approximately 80% in healthy individuals.

Therapeutic Plasma Concentration. A therapeutic range for omeprazole concentration in plasma has not been established and may not be important, since degree of acid inhibition is not directly related to plasma concentration. Extent of acid inhibition does correlate with total omeprazole plasma AUC.[16,21,48]

Clinical Trials

Because of its dose-dependent inhibition of gastric acid secretion, omeprazole has been studied in the short-term treatment of active peptic (duodenal and gastric) ulcer, reflux esophagitis, and hypersecretory conditions, such as ZES. With the exception of ZES, omeprazole has been compared with H_2-receptor antagonists in each disorder. Other potential uses of omeprazole include the prophylaxis of aspirin-induced ulcer, prophylaxis of stress ulcer, and treatment of acute upper gastrointestinal bleeding.

Duodenal Ulcer

Studies in DU patients conducted to date have produced fairly consistent results. Omeprazole in doses of 20 to 60 mg daily results in healing rates of 60% to 100% after two weeks and 90% to 100% after four weeks. Omeprazole is effective in the treatment of patients with ulcers refractory to treatment with H_2-receptor antagonists.[49-51] Tables 2 and 3 summarize the methodology and results of variable-dose studies[52-55] and of comparative clinical trials[33,56-60] with omeprazole, respectively, in the treatment of duodenal ulcer. No studies conducted to date have compared omeprazole with antacids or misoprostol in the treatment of duodenal ulcer disease.

A cooperative study compared different doses of omeprazole for DU treatment in a multicenter, four-week, open trial.[53] Forty-four outpatients with symptomatic ulcers verified by endoscopy were enrolled in the study. Each study center compared either omeprazole 20 mg with 40 mg, or omeprazole 30 mg with 60 mg, and patients were randomly assigned to a treatment group. Duodenal ulceration healed in 41 of 43 patients (95%) who completed the study. The proportion of patients healed in each treatment group was similar (Table 2). All patients had pain before starting treatment: 42 with daytime pain and 31 with pain at night. After seven days of omeprazole therapy, seven patients reported daytime pain, and five patients reported pain at night. Pain relief was not evaluated by treatment group. Of the patients whose ulcers had healed after four weeks of treatment, 29%, 27%, 43%, and 27% of those subjects in the omeprazole

Table 2.
Variable-Dose Omeprazole Trials in Patients with Endoscopically Proven Duodenal Ulcer

Reference	Study Design	Daily Dose of Omeprazole (mg)[a]	No. of Evaluable Patients	% Healed at Indicated Time[b] 2 Weeks	4 Weeks
52	Randomized, double-blind	20	15	63	93
		60	16	100[c]	100
53	Randomized, open, multicenter	20	10	...	90
		30	12	...	100
		40	10	...	90
		60	11	...	100
54	Randomized, double-blind	10	30	50	83
		30	36	78[d]	94[e]
55	Randomized, double-blind, multicenter	20	57	79.0	96.5
		30	55	72.7	92.7

[a] Omeprazole therapy was continued for four weeks in all studies.
[b] Evaluated by endoscopy.
[c] $p < 0.02$.
[d] $p < 0.03$.
[e] Not significant.

Table 3.
Comparative Trials of Omeprazole and H_2-Receptor Antagonists in Patients with Endoscopically Proven Duodenal Ulcer[a]

Reference	Duration of Therapy (wk)	Drug and Dose (mg)	% Healed at Indicated Time[b] 2 Weeks	4 Weeks	6 Weeks	8 Weeks
56	4	Omeprazole 30 daily	73 (49/67)	92 (55/60)	...	...
		Cimetidine 200 t.i.d. and 400 at bedtime	46 (30/65)[d]	74 (43/58)[e]	...	...
57	6	Omeprazole 20 daily	60 (49/81)[g]	87 (71/82)[g]	93 (75/81)[g]	...
		Cimetidine 600 b.i.d.	46 (39/84)[h]	84 (67/80)[g]	95 (75/79)[g]	...
58	8	Omeprazole 20 daily	83 (24/29)	97 (32/33)	...	100 (33/33)
		Omeprazole 40 daily	83 (30/36)	100 (36/36)	...	100 (36/36)
		Ranitidine 150 b.i.d.[j]	53 (17/32)[f]	82 (27/33)[f]	...	94 (31/33)
59	6	Omeprazole 20 daily	66 (40/61)	97 (59/61)	100 (61/61)	...
		Ranitidine 150 b.i.d.[j]	53 (32/60)[e]	85 (51/60)[c]	92 (55/60)[c]	...
60	4	Omeprazole 20 daily	72 (105/146)	96 (139/145)	...	...
		Ranitidine 150 b.i.d.[j]	59 (94/160)[c]	92 (143/156)	...	...
33	4	Omeprazole 20 daily	42 (N.R.)[i]	82 (N.R.)	...	...
		Ranitidine 150 daily[j]	34 (N.R.)	63 (N.R.)[d]	...	...

[a] All trials were randomized, double-blind, multicenter.
[b] Evaluated by endoscopy. Reported as percentage of evaluable subjects.
[c] $p < 0.012$.
[d] $p < 0.01$.
[e] $p < 0.05$.
[f] $p < 0.007$.
[g] Nonevaluable patients were not included in results reported.
[h] $p = 0.056$.
[i] Number of patients per group was not reported.
[j] Given as ranitidine hydrochloride.

20, 30, 40, and 60 mg daily treatment groups, respectively, had a symptomatic and endoscopically diagnosed relapse within six months after treatment was discontinued.

Comparison with Cimetidine. Lauritsen and colleagues[56] compared the efficacy of omeprazole and cimetidine in a four-center, double-blind, randomized trial. Because of reports of carcinoid tumors in rats upon long-term administration of omeprazole, the trial was discontinued prematurely, with 118 patients completing four weeks of treatment (10 others completed two weeks, and 4 subjects withdrew). Inclusion criteria were the presence of an ulcer upon endoscopy within four days before the start of treatment, age between 18 and 80 years, and pain for at least three days during the preceding two weeks. Exclusion criteria included treatment with an H_2-receptor antagonist during the preceding two weeks; presence of pyloric stenosis, gastric ulcer, or prepyloric ulcer; history of gastric surgery; concurrent therapy or disease complicating the evaluation (not defined); and inadequate contraception or pregnancy or lactation in women. Patients were instructed to record pain in a diary, and noncompliant subjects, defined as those who had not taken the study drug for more than three days per two-week period, were excluded from analysis. Study findings are summarized in Table 3. Ulcer healing rates at two and four weeks were significantly higher in the omeprazole group than in the cimetidine group. The differences in duration of ulcer pain (days until pain ceased) and average hours of pain (cumulative) between the groups were not significant. The absence of ulcer pain did not correlate with healing at two weeks.

Upon complete healing, patients were followed for up to six months for asymptomatic and symptomatic recurrence. If a patient experienced ulcer pain on four days during a one-week period, endoscopy was performed. Patients were withdrawn from the follow-up study if an ulcer was found. All remaining patients, regardless of symptoms, were evaluated by endoscopy at six months. By six months after completion of therapy, 45% of the omeprazole-treated patients and 59% of the cimetidine-treated patients had recurrence of an endoscopically proven, symptomatic ulcer; this difference was not significant. Upon endoscopy at this time, six asymptomatic patients in each group demonstrated an ulcer.

In general, the study was well conducted; however, a few minor flaws are worthy of comment. In following through on the phases of the study, particularly from the efficacy to recurrence sections, it is impossible to account for all subjects. As with any multicenter study, consistency in evaluations among centers could not be substantiated. In reporting the findings, the authors were consistent in noting results that favored omeprazole compared with cimetidine, even though these differences were not significant. Regardless of this bias, the authors' results and conclusions appear valid.

Comparison with Ranitidine. Bardhan et al.[58] compared omeprazole with ranitidine in 105 patients with DU (≥5 mm in diameter) proven by endoscopy. Exclusion criteria included treatment with antiulcer drugs for more than three days during the previous two weeks, continuous treatment with nonsteroidal anti-inflammatory drugs, pregnancy, breast-feeding, clinically important laboratory abnormalities in the pretreatment screening, and any concurrent disease or treatment likely to make drug evaluation difficult. Treatment was started within four days of diagnosis. Patients with unhealed ulcers at four weeks were treated for an additional four weeks; treatment was considered to have failed in patients who were unhealed at the end of eight weeks of therapy.

There were no significant differences in patient characteristics between the groups. At two weeks, ulcers were healed in significantly more patients receiving either dose of omeprazole compared with those who received ranitidine (Table 3).

Patients receiving omeprazole had significantly fewer days with pain (median values: two days for omeprazole 20 mg, one day for omeprazole 40 mg, seven days for ranitidine), and they used significantly fewer antacid tablets. There was no significant difference in the relapse patterns of the three groups. Median time to relapse for all patients was similar in two of the three groups, with a higher proportion of patients relapsing after healing on omeprazole 40 mg (82.6%, median 84 days) than on omeprazole 20 mg (58.3%, median 154 days) or ranitidine (60%, median 84 days).

More recently, Barbara et al.[59] compared the efficacy of omeprazole 20 mg with ranitidine hydrochloride 150 mg (of ranitidine) twice daily. Inclusion and exclusion criteria were similar to those described in the previous studies. Seven of 128 subjects withdrew before the two-week assessment because of persistent pain while receiving omeprazole (three), rash attributed to ranitidine (one), and failure to report for evaluation (three subjects randomized to receive ranitidine). Healing rates after two, four, and six weeks of treatment were significantly higher for the omeprazole group compared with rates for the placebo group (Table 3). No significant differences in pain relief or antacid use were noted between groups.

The major problems with this study concern methodology and statistical analysis. Since the number of omeprazole and ranitidine subjects was the same at the start of this multicenter study, block randomization was probably used; therefore, a perfect randomization was not conducted. The authors did not state whether the statistical tests employed were one-tailed or two-tailed, and two-tailed analyses should have been conducted. The pain scores were averaged, which is incorrect for rank data, and the presentation of the antacid usage is difficult to evaluate.

In summary, the efficacy of omeprazole 20 mg daily may be comparable to that associated with ranitidine hydrochloride 150 mg (of ranitidine) twice daily in the treatment of duodenal ulcer.

Recurrence after Omeprazole Therapy. Duodenal ulcer recurrence was studied in 55 patients who were successfully treated with omeprazole 10 or 30 mg daily for four weeks.[61] Of the 45 patients who completed the 12-month study, 18 had received omeprazole 10 mg and 27 had received omeprazole 30 mg. Twenty patients remained symptom free; however, ulcers were detected upon endoscopy in five (four who received omeprazole 10 mg and one who received 30 mg) of 11 patients who consented to the examination. The remaining 25 patients experienced symptomatic recurrence, which was confirmed by endoscopy. For the 10- and 30-mg treatment groups, the median time to relapse was 39 and 50 weeks, respectively. The differences between the treatment groups were not significant, and the results generally agree with previous findings after treatment with H_2-receptor antagonists. Although a study of the benefits of a maintenance regimen in duodenal ulcer has not been reported to date, such an evaluation is warranted.

Benign Gastric Ulcer

Omeprazole doses of 20 to 40 mg/day have been studied in the management of benign gastric ulcer.[60,62–64]

Comparison with Ranitidine. In a randomized, double-blind multicenter trial, omeprazole 20 mg p.o. before breakfast was compared with ranitidine hydrochloride 150 mg (of ranitidine) p.o. twice daily for eight weeks in 184 adult outpatients having endoscopically confirmed gastric ulcers.[60] Concomitant use of antacids or other antiulcer agents was not permitted. Patients were appropriately matched for age, gender, smoking status, current dyspepsia, recurrent ulcerations, duration of ulcer disease, number and location of ulcers, maximal ulcer diameter, and epigastric pain. Thirty patients were unevaluable because of study withdrawal before the two-week ($n = 6$) or eight-week ($n = 4$) follow-up period or because of an incomplete follow-up examination ($n = 20$). On follow-up endoscopic examination, there was no significant difference in the ulcer healing rate between the omeprazole- and ranitidine-treated patients at two weeks (36 of 83, or 43%, versus 33 of 74, or 45%, respectively), four weeks (67 of 83, or 81%, versus 59 of 74, or 80%, respectively), or eight weeks (77 of 81, or 95%, versus 66 of 73, or 90%, respectively). Although symptomatic relief was "equally good" with either drug, no comparison was made of the mean time to obtain symptomatic relief.

In a randomized, multicenter trial, omeprazole 20 mg daily was compared with ranitidine hydrochloride 150 mg (of ranitidine) twice daily for eight weeks in 167 patients with gastric ulcers.[62] Regardless of ulcer size, the ulcer healing rate was significantly greater at two, four, and eight weeks in the omeprazole-treated group compared with the ranitidine-treated group. Symptomatic relief was reportedly faster and more extensive in the omeprazole group than in the ranitidine group.

Omeprazole 20 and 40 mg daily was compared with ranitidine hydrochloride 150 mg (of ranitidine) twice daily for eight weeks in 602 patients with benign gastric or prepyloric ulcers.[63] Both omeprazole groups exhibited significantly faster symptomatic relief (actual data not reported) and higher healing rates at four weeks than the ranitidine group. At eight weeks, the healing rate was significantly greater with omeprazole 40 mg than with either omeprazole 20 mg or ranitidine. Six months after discontinuation of therapy, significantly more patients in the omeprazole 40 mg group remained in symptomatic and endoscopic remission than in the ranitidine group. No data were reported on the difference in remission rates between the two omeprazole regimens.

These studies suggest that omeprazole 20 mg daily is at least as effective as ranitidine hydrochloride 150 mg (of ranitidine) twice daily in the treatment of benign gastric ulcer. Higher doses of omeprazole may provide faster relief of ulcer pain and may reduce ulcer recurrence.

Comparison with Cimetidine. In a randomized, double-blind multicenter trial, Lauritsen et al.[64] compared the efficacy of omeprazole 30 mg daily with cimetidine 1000 mg/day (as 200 mg p.o. t.i.d. and 400 mg at bedtime) for six weeks in 176 patients with prepyloric gastric ulcers. Patients were permitted concomitant antacid use (actual consumption not reported). On follow-up endoscopic examination, there was no significant difference in ulcer healing between the evaluable omeprazole- and cimetidine-treated patients at two weeks (45 of 82, or 55%, versus 33 of 78, or 42%, respectively), four weeks (66 of 78, or 85%, versus 56 of 73, or 77%, respectively), or eight weeks (62 of 70, or 89%, versus 59 of 69, or 86%, respectively).

Although no significant difference in healing rate between or within groups occurred when data were analyzed by gender, smoking status, or length of ulcer history, patients with ulcers less than 9 mm in diameter had a significantly higher healing rate with omeprazole therapy than patients with larger ulcers. During the first week of therapy, 13 (19%) of 68 initially symptomatic patients receiving omeprazole were pain free, compared with 4 (5%) of 73 symptomatic patients receiving cimetidine ($p < 0.05$); however, at the end of the study no difference in symptomatic relief between groups existed. Additionally, the mean number of hours that patients were in pain between treatment groups was similar throughout the entire study period.

Esophagitis

Omeprazole has been evaluated in the treatment of erosive (grade 2) and ulcerative (grade 3) esophagitis,[38,65–71] hemorrhagic esophagitis,[72] and Barrett's esophagitis,[73] a complication of chronic reflux esophagitis. Short-term, open, uncontrolled trials[38,74] with omeprazole have yielded favorable results. To date, seven comparative trials[65–71] address the symptomatic, endoscopic, or histologic response to omeprazole given in daily doses of 20 to 60 mg in the treatment of esophagitis. Omeprazole has been compared with H_2-receptor antagonists but has not been compared with metoclopramide or other gastrointestinal motility stimulants (cisapride or bethanecol) in the treatment of reflux esophagitis.

In a randomized, double-blind, placebo-controlled trial, Dent et al.[65] studied the efficacy of omeprazole 20 or 40 mg daily in 63 adults with erosive or ulcerative esophagitis. At four weeks, 25 (81%) of the 31 omeprazole-treated patients had endoscopically documented esophageal healing, compared with 2 (6%) of the 32 placebo-treated patients ($p < 0.001$). The comparative efficacy of the two omeprazole dosing regimens was not reported. Heartburn resolved in 64% of the omeprazole group versus 14% of the placebo group ($p < 0.001$). Of 24 healed patients, 50% developed recurrence (endoscopic and symptomatic) of esophagitis at one month and 67% developed recurrence at three months after cessation of omeprazole therapy. No significant adverse effects could be attributed to omeprazole therapy.

A randomized, double-blind comparison of two dosage regimens of omeprazole—20 and 40 mg daily—in 164 patients with erosive or ulcerative esophagitis showed no significant difference in healing rate between the two regimens at eight weeks.[66] The investigators suggested that the 40-mg dose produced endoscopic healing more quickly at four weeks ($p = 0.05$, one-tailed test); however, when the data are reanalyzed via a two-tailed analysis, the difference is not significant.

Comparison with Ranitidine. Omeprazole 60 mg daily and ranitidine hydrochloride 150 mg (of ranitidine) twice daily were compared in a randomized, double-blind study of 51 outpatients with endoscopically confirmed esophageal erosions or ulcerations.[67] Exclusion criteria included pregnancy, lactation, concomitant peptic ulcer, Barrett's ulcer and esophageal stricture, previous esophageal and gastric surgery, severe systemic disease, and clinically important abnormal laboratory findings. Patients had received no other medications for relief of esophagitis for at least two weeks before the study period. The healing rate (evaluated by endoscopy) with omeprazole was significantly greater than that with ranitidine. At four weeks, 19 of 25 (76%) patients receiving omeprazole were healed, compared with 7 of 26 (27%) patients receiving ranitidine ($p = 0.002$). At eight weeks, 22 of 25 (88%) in the omeprazole group were healed, compared with 10 of 26 (38%) in the ranitidine group ($p = 0.001$). Omeprazole was notably more effective than ranitidine in the treatment of ulcerative (grade 3) esophagitis. Heartburn was the most frequent symptom in patients before study. Based on self-assessment results, omeprazole-treated patients showed a more rapid and profound relief of heartburn at four weeks than those who received ranitidine ($p = 0.0001$). No significant difference was found between the groups for regurgitation or dysphagia. Although the authors stated that antacid tablet use was similar in both groups, the actual amounts of antacid used were not reported. After two weeks of treatment, 92% (23 of 25) of the omeprazole-treated patients reported their reflux symptoms had resolved or had improved, compared with 65% (17 of 26) in the ranitidine group ($p = 0.01$). Of 15 ranitidine nonresponders, 13 attained esophageal healing after receiving an eight-week course of omeprazole. Healing was achieved in one of three omeprazole nonresponders who were switched to ranitidine therapy. No clinically important laboratory changes were observed, and no difference in adverse-effect frequency was noted between groups.

In a randomized, stratified double-blind controlled trial, 162 outpatients with confirmed reflux esophagitis (grades 1–3) received either omeprazole 40 mg daily with evening placebo ($n = 80$) or ranitidine hydrochloride 150 mg (of ranitidine) twice daily ($n = 82$) for a maximum of 12 weeks.[68] The groups were comparable in age, gender, and disease extent and duration; however, there were more smokers in the omeprazole-treated group (35 versus 25). At the four-week follow-up period, patients treated with omeprazole had significantly fewer symptoms, a shorter duration of treatment, less mucosal inflammation on repeat biopsy, a higher rate of healing (documented by endoscopy), and less frequent use of antacid. Regardless of the severity of esophagitis and the handling of study dropouts, cumulative healing rates were at all times higher in the omeprazole-treated group ($p < 0.0001$).

Similar results were obtained in a study comparing omeprazole 40 mg daily with ranitidine hydrochloride 150 mg (of ranitidine) twice daily for four weeks in 61 patients with ulcerative reflux esophagitis.[69] Cumulative healing rates at four and eight weeks were 74% and 81% in the omeprazole group, respectively, and 43% and 50% in the ranitidine group, respectively ($p < 0.01$). A significantly greater number of omeprazole-treated patients obtained symptomatic relief of heartburn during therapy.

On the other hand, Blum et al.[70] found no difference in lesion healing rate in 164 reflux esophagitis patients who received either omeprazole 40 mg daily or ranitidine hydrochloride 150 mg (of ranitidine) twice daily for three weeks. After data were regrouped, a significantly lower failure rate was associated with omeprazole therapy (13%) versus ranitidine therapy (33%; $p < 0.025$).

In a double-blind multicenter trial comparing omeprazole 20 mg daily ($n = 76$) with ranitidine hydrochloride 300 mg (of ranitidine) daily ($n = 80$) for up to nine weeks in patients (mean age, 56 years) with endoscopically proven erosive or ulcerative esophagitis, 50 of the 62 evaluable omeprazole-treated patients (81%) had healed lesions at four weeks. At eight weeks, the cumulative healing rate in the omeprazole group was 95% (58 of 61). In contrast, the ranitidine group achieved lesion healing rates of 45% (31 of 69; $p < 0.001$) and 65% (40 of 61; $p < 0.001$) at four and eight weeks, respectively.

These studies demonstrate that omeprazole affords superior efficacy over H_2-receptor antagonists in the management of reflux esophagitis. The effect of omeprazole on the rate of esophageal lesion recurrence relative to H_2-receptor antagonists remains unknown.

Cases Refractory to Treatment with H_2-Receptor Antagonists. Several case reports describe the efficacy of omeprazole in esophagitis refractory to treatment with H_2-receptor antagonists. A 61-year-old man with protracted hemorrhagic esophagitis refractory to treatment with high-dose H_2-receptor antagonists (ranitidine 300 mg twice daily) and antacids obtained ulcer healing after an eight-week regimen of omeprazole 40 mg daily.[72] By the third treatment month, the patient's hemoglobin level returned to within normal limits (>14 g/dL) for the first time in more than a year. With continued omeprazole therapy (20 mg daily), the patient remained healed (as confirmed by endoscopy) at the 18-month follow-up examination.

Hameeteman and Tytgat[73] described three patients each with Barrett's ulcer who were unresponsive to treatment with H_2-receptor antagonists; one patient was also unresponsive to treatment with antacids. After a nine-week course of omeprazole 40 mg daily, all three patients had documented endoscopic healing of the ulcer. Thereafter, each patient resumed a maintenance regimen with an H_2-receptor antagonist; however, within two to six months all three patients had ulcer recurrence. This report suggests the potential utility of omeprazole in the short-term management of Barrett's ulcers and the need for long-term gastric acid suppression in such patients to minimize or prevent ulcer recurrence.

Suppressive Therapy with Omeprazole. The optimal dose of omeprazole to provide suppressive prophylaxis in patients who experience recurrent episodes of reflux esophagitis has not yet been established. Preliminary work has been done in 73 patients with refractory reflux esophagitis who had ulcer healing while receiving omeprazole 40 mg daily and who then received maintenance therapy with omeprazole 20 mg daily.[32] Fifty-nine (81%) remained ulcer free for at least six months during suppressive therapy (mean, 13 months; range, 6–23 months). Fourteen patients had endoscopic recurrences after a mean six months of therapy (range, 1–15 months). These patients required an increase in omeprazole dosage (40 mg, $n = 12$; 60 mg, $n = 2$) to obtain ulcer healing.

Zollinger–Ellison Syndrome

Zollinger–Ellison syndrome (ZES) is a severe form of peptic ulcer disease that is characterized by hypersecretion of gastric acid and the presence of gastrinomas. The condition may be present in up to 0.1% of all DU patients in the United States.[75] Several open studies with relatively small numbers of subjects have been conducted in patients with ZES, particularly in patients whose conditions are resistant to treatment with H_2-receptor antagonists.[48,76–86]

Lamers et al.[48] conducted both a single-dose and a long-term study in one of the first trials of omeprazole in symptomatic ZES. Inclusion and exclusion criteria were not described, and some patients participated in both studies. For the single-dose study, therapy with H_2-receptor antagonists was discontinued for at least 36 hours before evaluation. Oral administration of omeprazole 80 mg, as four 20-mg capsules of enteric-coated granules, produced inhibition of gastric acid secretion in all five patients studied. Three patients with omeprazole AUC >2 μmol·hr/L were achlorhydric at the six-hour evaluation. The remaining two patients had 26% and 30% acid inhibition, with omeprazole AUC <1 μmol·hr/L. At 24 hours after drug ingestion, gastric acid secretion in all patients was inhibited by 76% to 100%. The plasma omeprazole concentration at that time was below the detection limit of the assay (50 nmol/L). No adverse effects or laboratory abnormalities were observed.

The long-term study described seven patients treated for 8 to 19 months (mean, 14 months) with omeprazole. The dosage was adjusted to maintain a basal acid output (BAO) of less than 10 mmol/hr. At the end of the study period, five patients received 30 to 80 mg daily, while two patients received 100 or 120 mg daily in twice-daily schedules. Omeprazole was found to be a potent and long-acting antisecretory drug in these patients. Inhibition of acid secretion was pronounced on the first day, and the degree of inhibition did not change during the first month of treatment. Symptoms improved within one to two weeks, and peptic ulcers or esophagitis were healed, as determined by endoscopy, in all patients after one month of treatment. Omeprazole did not affect serum gastrin concentrations, and laboratory abnormalities or adverse effects were not reported. In one patient, an elevated serum creatinine concentration attributed to previous cimetidine treatment returned to normal during omeprazole treatment.

In a subsequent symposium, Lamers[76] reviewed the effect of omeprazole in patients with ZES and included an update on the seven patients in the long-term study. Data presented included duration of treatment (range, 18 to 27 months; mean, 24 months), daily dose (range, 20 to 100 mg), and BAO. During this extended period with regular measurements of BAO, the daily omeprazole dose remained the same for four patients, was decreased for two patients, and was increased for one patient. No adverse effects were related to treatment.

McArthur and colleagues[77] evaluated the short-term and long-term (up to nine months) efficacy of omeprazole in patients with ZES. Eleven patients participated in the studies, which evaluated the acute effect on BAO, the maintenance-dose requirement, the duration of drug action, and the long-term-dose requirements. In all patients, previous therapy with H_2-receptor antagonists was titrated to reduce predose gastric acid secretion to less than 10 mmol/hr; additional treatment with an anticholinergic agent was necessary in three patients. After the discontinuation of previous therapy (i.v. cimetidine for 12 hours, oral cimetidine and ranitidine p.o. for 24 hours, and anticholinergic agents for 72 hours) and the baseline measurement of BAO, gastric acid secretion was measured from two to eight hours and once at 24 hours after the administration of omeprazole 60 mg in nine patients. To determine a maintenance dose, all 11 patients received omeprazole daily in the morning, and the dosage was adjusted as necessary to achieve a predose gastric secretion of less than 10 mmol/hr. The initial dose was 60 mg daily, and, if a patient required a dose of omeprazole greater than 200 mg, the daily dose was divided and given every 12 hours. The duration of action of omeprazole was determined in five patients, who each had received a minimum of two months of treatment, by measuring gastric acid secretion at eight-hour intervals for 48 hours (or until an acid output of greater than 30 mmol/hr was achieved) after discontinuing therapy. The long-term-dose requirements were evaluated in all patients at one week, three weeks, and two, four, six, and nine months by measuring the acid secretion for one hour before the next dose. If necessary, the dose was adjusted to achieve a gastric acid secretion of less than 10 mmol/hr.

For the patients in the acute efficacy evaluation, BAO was inhibited by a mean of 50%, 78%, and 86% at three, four, and eight hours, respectively, after the 60-mg dose (actual values not reported). In two of the nine patients, the acid secretion was more than 20 mmol/hr after eight hours and a second dose was required, according to the study protocol. For the remaining seven patients, the mean inhibition of gastric acid secretion was 80% at 24 hours. For all 11 patients, the mean maintenance dose was 70 mg (range, 20–160 mg). The authors reported significant positive correlations between the omeprazole maintenance dose and the previous maintenance dose of cimetidine or ranitidine (r = 0.936 and 0.913, respectively), the BAO (r = 0.713), and maximal acid output (r = 0.611); however, these data and the statistical tests used were not provided. For the five patients in whom the duration of action was being evaluated, the mean dose was 56 mg (range, 20–100 mg). The BAO was inhibited by greater than 80% and 50% (mean values; actual values not reported) at 24 and 48 hours, respectively, after discontinuation of omeprazole, and only one subject achieved his pretreatment BAO by 48 hours. In the evaluation of long-term-dose requirements, the mean duration of therapy at the end of the study was five months. The conditions of nine of the patients were controlled by the initial maintenance dose, while one subject each required an increase or decrease in the daily dose. Clinical and laboratory assessment during treatment showed no adverse effects attributable to omeprazole therapy.

These investigators subsequently reported on the long-term use of omeprazole in 27 patients with ZES, with at least one patient being treated for 30 months.[78] The mean maintenance dose, determined by the method previously described, was 75 mg daily (range, 20 mg daily to 60 mg every 12 hours). Gastric acid secretion was controlled in all patients, and only two patients required an increase in dose during the study (individual treatment duration not reported). Unlike the results in the initial study, the dose of omeprazole did not correlate with the BAO or maximal acid output but did correlate significantly with the dose of the previous H_2-receptor antagonist ($r = 0.70$, $p < 0.001$). Hematological and biochemical testing, conducted before and after 6, 12, 18, and 24 months of treatment, demonstrated no evidence of adverse effect, and plasma gastrin concentrations did not change significantly during treatment. Endoscopy demonstrated no mucosal abnormalities, and biopsy of gastric tissue revealed no evidence of carcinoid tumors.

Patients noted in a recently published review of ZES[79] coauthored by members of this research group were probably the subjects from the latter two studies.[77,78]

After their initial report of efficacy of intravenous omeprazole in acute ZES,[80] Delchier et al.[81] studied omeprazole in seven patients who had ZES that was resistant to treatment with H_2-receptor antagonists, with or without anticholinergic therapy. Despite treatment with high doses of cimetidine (167 to 200 mg/hr by i.v. infusion) or ranitidine (19 mg/hr i.v.; 600 to 1200 mg/day p.o.) either alone or combined with pirenzepine (20 to 50 mg/8 hr), symptoms related to overproduction of gastric acid persisted and BAO was more than 10 mmol/hr. The five patients who were free of complications received omeprazole 60 mg p.o. at 2000, two hours after the evening meal, with current medication unchanged. BAO was measured the next morning at 0800 before a second dose of omeprazole. Previous therapy was discontinued when BAO was less than that measured on day 1. BAO was measured at 0800 on day 3; if it was lower than 10 mmol/hr, control of acid secretion was considered adequate, and the dose was continued at 60 mg once daily. If BAO was zero, the daily dose was decreased to 40 mg, and if BAO was greater than 10 mmol/hr, the dosage was increased to 80 mg once daily. The two patients with ZES complications received higher doses to achieve rapid control of gastric acid secretion. One patient, perhaps the individual from the original case report, received 60 mg i.v. every eight hours, while the other received 60 mg p.o. b.i.d. Endoscopy was performed before omeprazole treatment and on day 22 for all patients.

Three of the five patients without ZES complications had a BAO of <2 mmol/hr on day 2, which remained unchanged on days 3, 8, and 22, although previous therapy had been discontinued. BAO increased in one patient after previous therapy was discontinued and was not under control until day 8. The fifth patient's BAO was controlled by day 22 with omeprazole 80 mg twice daily. The four patients with duodenal or duodenojejunal lesions at pretreatment endoscopy attained ulcer healing on day 22. Seven patients were followed for 4 to 24 months (mean, 15 months). Some dosage adjustments were required to maintain adequate control of acid secretion for four of the seven patients. One patient tolerated a decrease in dosage (from 180 to 60 mg/day), while three patients required increases (two from 60 to 80 mg/day; one from 80 to 120 mg/day). Symptoms or endoscopic lesions recurred in no patients during follow-up. No adverse effects were observed, and serum gastrin levels did not change. This study demonstrated effective control of gastric acid output by omeprazole in ZES patients.

Bardram and Stadil[82] evaluated the short-term efficacy of omeprazole in nine ZES patients whose conditions were inadequately controlled by H_2-receptor antagonists. The methods employed and results achieved were similar to those in the aforementioned studies; however, a twice-daily dosing regimen was employed more frequently. According to the study protocol, the divided regimen was used when the daily omeprazole dose exceeded 80 mg, and four patients reached this dose during the first two months. Upon completion of the study (treatment duration range, 2–27 months), two of these four subjects had daily doses of 60 mg or less but remained on twice-daily (every 12 hours) regimens. The authors concluded that the total daily doses required, which were lower than those reported by others, were due to the use of the twice-daily schedule. Further study is necessary to determine the merits of a twice-daily (every 12 hours) regimen when a single daily dose is sufficient to maintain the predose acid secretion at less than 10 mmol/hr.

The long-term efficacy and safety of omeprazole in 80 ZES patients for up to four years (mean, 19 months) has been reported in a multicenter summary.[83] The decline in symptoms, including resolution of diarrhea, and healing of ulcers followed the maintenance of acid secretion at less than 10 mmol/hr. The median daily dose of omeprazole was 60–70 mg. A daily dose of omeprazole of 120 mg or less controlled the conditions of 90% of the patients, and tachyphylaxis was not observed. One third of the patients required a divided dosage regimen, with omeprazole 120 mg t.i.d. being the highest dosage. The treatment was reportedly well tolerated. Thirteen patients died during therapy, but none of these deaths were drug related.

Other Indications

Although omeprazole 5 to 10 mg daily does not appear to be effective in preventing aspirin-induced gastric lesions in healthy subjects,[87] higher daily doses of omeprazole may prove beneficial. Bigard[88] compared the mucosal protective effects of a four-day pretreatment regimen of omeprazole 60 mg daily with placebo in healthy volunteers who received a single dose of aspirin 1000 mg. No omeprazole-treated subject had more than 10 hemorrhages (defined as the upper limit of clinically important mucosal protection) on endoscopic examination compared with 14 of 15 placebo-treated subjects ($p < 0.0001$). Additional studies are needed to confirm the utility and optimal dosing of omeprazole in the prevention of aspirin-induced gastric lesions.

Contraindications and Precautions

Omeprazole is contraindicated in patients who are hypersensitive to the compound. No information is available regarding its use in pediatric patients, and information about its use in geriatric patients is limited. It should, therefore, be used with caution in these groups.

Gastric Hypertrophy and Carcinoid Tumors. General hypertrophy of the oxyntic mucosa was observed in chronic-toxicity studies conducted in rats receiving omeprazole 400 μmol/kg/day (138 mg/kg/day) for 14 days to six months.[89] The hypertrophy was reversed one month after omeprazole withdrawal, and mucosal thickness was not different from that of the control group six months after discontinuation of treatment. In the 24-month carcinogenicity study, rats developed generalized gastric mucosal hypertrophy, as well as spontaneous hyperplasia of enterochromaffin-like (ECL) cells in the basal region of the gastric glands. In the control group (treated with vehicle), hyperplasia was observed more often in females (18%) than in males (8%); hyperplasia was reportedly increased by omeprazole treatment.

Changes in gastric endocrine cells were studied in rats receiving omeprazole 40 mg/kg, famotidine 3 mg/kg, or a control solution daily for 60 days.[90] Significant increases in mean argyrophilic cell volume density (control, 1.42%; famotidine, 2.18%; omeprazole, 3.92%) and mean argyrophilic cell count (control, 410 cells/sq mm; famotidine, 554 cells/sq mm; omeprazole, 1059 cells/sq mm) were observed after treatment with the drugs compared with control values. Most argyrophilic cells are considered to be ECL cells.[34]

Increases in ECL density have also been observed in rats after ranitidine treatment. Daily treatment for 10 weeks with omeprazole 10 or 400 μmol/kg (3.45 or 138 mg/kg), ranitidine 700 μmol/kg (220 mg/kg), or vehicle resulted in approximately 210, 560, 340, and approximately 190 ECL cells per visual field, respectively.[91] Increases in ECL cell density after both omeprazole (high dose) and ranitidine were significant compared with values for the vehicle alone.

Carcinogenicity studies in rats involving large doses of omeprazole—40 to 400 μmol/kg/day (equivalent to 13.8 to 138 mg/kg/day)—for 24 months have shown that a significant percentage of animals developed gastric carcinoid tumors (with 400 μmol/kg/day, 10% of males and 40% of females versus no tumors in control groups).[89] Carcinoid tissue did not develop in mice receiving the same dose (40 to 400 μmol/kg/day) for 18 months.

Current evidence suggests that the tumors were not directly induced by omeprazole but were a physiologic response to hypergastrinemia caused by a profound, long-term inhibition of gastric acid secretion.[92] Modest, reversible elevations in serum gastrin concentration have been noted in humans during short-term omeprazole treatment of duodenal and gastric ulcers, but these elevations were small compared with those reported in the animal toxicology studies. The dosage in these animal studies was at least three times that used to date for humans with ZES and 10 to 100 times greater than human doses for treatment of duodenal ulcer. No increase in ECL cell volume density was observed in patients with reflux esophagitis; esophageal, gastric, or duodenal ulcer; or ZES who received omeprazole 20 to 120 mg/day for four weeks to four years.[31-32,93-95] Gastric carcinoid tumors have not been reported to date in humans receiving omeprazole[93-96]; however, it is not likely that a tumor would be detected in the limited number of subjects that have been studied thus far. The issue of carcinoid tumor formation is a controversial aspect of omeprazole use.[92,97-100] The data suggest that omeprazole does not represent a carcinogenic risk for short-term use. The long-term risk of gastric carcinoid tumors occurring with long-term omeprazole use is not certain.

Bacterial Overgrowth. Bacterial overgrowth in the gastrointestinal tract with long-term use of omeprazole has raised concern.[97] Overgrowth of various microorganisms introduced into the stomach by ingested foods or fluids may occur with reduced hydrochloric acid secretion.[3] Intragastric bacteria may reduce nitrate to nitrite and facilitate formation of nitrosamine compounds, which are carcinogenic in a variety of organs and in many animal species.[35,101]

One investigator studied intragastric bacterial activity before, during, and after treatment with omeprazole 30 mg daily for two weeks in 10 healthy volunteers.[101] During the night after the 14th dose, the mean nocturnal intragastric acidity was decreased from 44.1 to 11.0 meq/L ($p < 0.001$). In gastric juice, significant increases in bacterial count and in nitrite and nitrosamine concentrations were noted 22 hours after the last omeprazole dose. A decrease in nitrate concentration was observed, although this difference was not significant. The changes were completely resolved three days after omeprazole was discontinued. Results of this study are difficult to extrapolate, since the specific gravity of gastric secretions was not measured and the variables measured were all reported in terms of concentration (nanomoles per gram of gastric juice) rather than amount. The observed changes may be more closely associated with a reduction in secretion volume, although this would not explain the decrease in nitrate concentration. The clinical importance of these changes with omeprazole is unknown.

An additional potential risk of bacterial overgrowth in the gastrointestinal tract is the development of nosocomial pneumonia, as a result of aspiration of gastric contents. Antacids and H_2-receptor antagonists have been implicated in increasing the frequency of nosocomial pneumonia, although studies to date have not consistently demonstrated that a correlation exists.[102-104] No infection related to bacterial overgrowth in patients treated with omeprazole has been reported, yet no studies have been performed that specifically address this issue with omeprazole use.

Mutagenicity. Omeprazole has shown no mutagenic potential in microbial studies or in in vitro and in vivo studies in mice. Reproduction studies performed in rats and rabbits have shown no embryotoxic, teratogenic, or direct fetotoxic effects related to omeprazole treatment.[89] A slight increase in fetal loss was seen in rabbit studies at higher doses (200 and 400 μmol/kg/day); however, this loss was considered to be due to maternal toxicity manifested as anorexia and reduced water intake. The anorexia was most likely related to severe constipation seen in rabbits receiving high doses of omeprazole.

Drug Interactions

Cytochrome P-450 System. Numerous reports have shown imidazole and benzimidazole derivatives to be inhibitors of oxidative metabolism by the cytochrome P-450 system.[105-107] It is not surprising, then, that omeprazole inhibits oxidative drug metabolism.[45,108] The effects of omeprazole on the metabolism of 7-ethoxycoumarin were examined in vitro using human liver tissue.[45] Addition of either omeprazole 0.5 mM or cimetidine 0.5 mM inhibited 7-ethoxycoumarin de-ethylase activity, with a 24% greater inhibition with omeprazole than with cimetidine (based on high-affinity V_{max} estimates). Omeprazole and cimetidine inhibited both high- and low-affinity components of the enzyme.

In a study of eight healthy volunteers who received diazepam 0.1 mg/kg i.v. two weeks before and on day 7 of treatment with omeprazole 40 mg p.o. daily for nine days, total plasma clearance of diazepam decreased (mean 54%, $p < 0.01$) and plasma elimination half-life of diazepam increased in every person (mean elimination half-life: 37 hours before omeprazole treatment, 85 hours with omeprazole treatment; $p < 0.01$).[45] Diazepam plasma protein binding and volume of distribution were unchanged by omeprazole administration. Plasma concentrations of diazepam were increased, and concentrations of desmethyldiazepam, a diazepam metabolite, were reduced after omeprazole use for the 72 hours studied.

Gugler and Jensen[45] also examined changes in phenytoin pharmacokinetics with omeprazole treatment. Eight subjects received a single i.v. infusion of phenytoin 250 mg two weeks before and on day 7 of treatment with omeprazole 40 mg p.o. daily for eight days. A small but consistent increase in phenytoin concentration was observed with omeprazole treatment during the 48 hours studied, and phenytoin clearance was reduced in all subjects (mean clearance: 25.1 mL/kg/hr before omeprazole treatment, 21.4 mL/kg/hr with omeprazole treatment; $p < 0.05$). The mean plasma elimination half-life was prolonged from 20.7 hours before omeprazole treatment to 26.3 hours with omeprazole treatment ($p < 0.05$). No change in phenytoin volume of distribution, protein binding, or urinary excretion of the major metabolite, 5-(*p*-hydroxyphenyl)-5-phenylhydantoin, was observed.

Prichard et al.[109] performed a similar study with single-dose oral phenytoin. Ten subjects received omeprazole 40 mg or placebo each morning for nine days and took phenytoin sodium 300 mg with the seventh dose. The peak plasma phenytoin concentration was greater with omeprazole than with placebo, although the difference was not significant. Mean phenytoin AUC (from 0 to 72 hours) increased by 19% ($p < 0.01$), although the AUC decreased in one subject and was minimally changed in another. The apparent elimination half-life of phenytoin was prolonged, primarily because of one subject who had a phenytoin half-life of 42.7 hours with placebo and 98.4 hours with omeprazole. When this subject was excluded, mean elimination half-life was not significantly different (mean, 15.2 hours with placebo, 17.9 hours with omeprazole treatment; $p < 0.1$).

A limitation of the two phenytoin interaction studies is that only single-dose phenytoin was investigated. Since phenytoin exhibits dose-dependent pharmacokinetics, studies involving steady-state phenytoin, with single or short-term dosing with omeprazole, are needed to better define the clinical importance of the interaction between the two agents.

Henry et al.[108] tested omeprazole at 30- and 60-mg oral doses for interactions with antipyrine and aminopyrine. Omeprazole 60 mg daily for 14 days prolonged the half-lives of antipyrine and aminopyrine by 10% and 21%, respectively. Omeprazole 30 mg daily for 14 days resulted in no significant change in aminopyrine half-life and no alteration in antipyrine metabolism.

These reports suggest that drug interactions are less likely when omeprazole is used at lower doses, but interactions between omeprazole and therapeutically important compounds that undergo hepatic metabolism (e.g., warfarin, theophylline, phenobarbital) should be investigated. Omeprazole sulfone, the major plasma metabolite, may be a more important inhibitor of drug-metabolizing enzymes than omeprazole itself.[45] Patients receiving omeprazole for treatment of hypersecretory states should be monitored for potential interactions.

Gastrointestinal Tract. Interaction between omeprazole enteric-coated granules in capsules and an antacid combination product (aluminum hydroxide, magnesium hydroxide, and magnesium carbonate) has been studied, and no significant influence on omeprazole AUC has been demonstrated.[2] No difference in omeprazole peak plasma concentration or AUC occurred when omeprazole encapsulated enteric-coated granules were given with magnesium hydroxide antacid, as compared with omeprazole alone.[110]

Concomitant omeprazole therapy may diminish the gastrointestinal inactivation of exogenously administered pancreatic enzymes. Two patients with pancreatic insufficiency demonstrated a reduction of steatorrhea when treated with omeprazole (40 and 80 mg daily, respectively), despite no alteration in their pancreatic enzyme dosage regimen.[111] Hence, when omeprazole is used in combination with an effective pancreatic enzyme replacement regimen, a dosage reduction of pancreatic enzyme may be necessary.

Omeprazole may decrease the gastrointestinal absorption of drugs such as ketoconazole and tetracycline, which require an acidic environment for gastrointestinal absorption. As a result, a decrease in the efficacy of ketoconazole or tetracycline may occur when used in combination with omeprazole. This drug–drug interaction is theoretical and requires additional investigation.

Adverse Reactions and Toxicity

Therapeutic trials conducted to date have shown omeprazole to be well tolerated. No individual adverse effect appears to be related to omeprazole dose, ulcer type, or hypersecretory condition. Volunteers and patients (n = 2480) who participated in phase I to phase III studies reported 28 serious adverse effects, nine of which were possibly due to omeprazole administration.[112] These latter effects included four reports of skin rashes and one report of each of the following: increased serum alanine aminotransferase (ALT) concentration; deep-vein thrombosis; sweating attacks, vertigo, and menopausal symptoms; diarrhea; and leukopenia. Seventy-two ZES patients were included in the previous group, and of the 17 adverse reactions reported among them, none was attributed solely to omeprazole therapy.

Collectively, gastrointestinal effects have occurred in approximately 4% of the patients with DU (n = 256) who received omeprazole in variable-dose studies[52–55] and in 1.8% of DU patients (n = 277) enrolled in comparative trials.[56,59,60] Gastrointestinal effects have included diarrhea or loose stools, constipation, nausea, and abdominal colic. Central nervous system effects of headache, dizziness or vertigo, tiredness, and somnolence have been reported.[49–56,59–61,83] However, insufficient data are available to estimate the frequency of these effects. Omeprazole use has been infrequently associated with other adverse effects, such as dry mouth, stuffy nose, skin rash, eczema, feeling of coldness, a "swollen" feeling, numbness of fingertips, and palpitations.

Transient, reversible elevations in serum ALT and aspartate aminotransferase (AST) concentrations during omeprazole use have been noted.[49–56,59–60,81,112–113] Leukopenia,[112] eosinopenia, and elevated alkaline phosphatase concentrations[56] have been reported rarely with omeprazole use.

In comparative trials, the frequency of reported adverse effects and laboratory abnormalities associated with the use of omeprazole has not been significantly different from that occurring with the H_2-receptor antagonists; the adverse-effect profile of omeprazole has not included thrombocytopenia, endocrine effects (e.g., gynecomastia or impotence), or renal effects (e.g., increased serum creatinine concentration) to date.

Omeprazole has been used for up to 48 months and in doses up to 360 mg/day to treat patients with ZES.[83,93] No serious adverse effects or irreversible variations in laboratory values have been reported with such doses to date.

Toxicology studies with omeprazole have suggested a wide margin of safety between the therapeutic dose for humans (0.6–3 μmol/kg/day) and the toxic dose in animals (>12 mmol/kg/day).[89] Patients in clinical trials have received up to 360 mg/day with no observed signs of acute toxicity. Intentional overdosage has not been reported, and no information is available regarding treatment of overdosage.

Dosage and Administration

The usual oral adult dosage of omeprazole for treatment of peptic ulcers (gastric and duodenal) is 20 mg once daily before breakfast. Patients with reflux esophagitis should receive 40 mg once daily. Morning administration is preferred over evening administration based on gastric acid inhibition.[43] Treatment should be continued until ulcers are healed, which is usually two to four weeks for duodenal ulcers and four to eight weeks for gastric ulcers and reflux esophagitis. Data demonstrating a need for longer treatment duration in patients who smoke or who have large ulcers, as shown with H_2-receptor antagonists, are equivocal with omeprazole.[54–56,60]

Patients having recurrent episodes of peptic ulcer disease or esophagitis may conceivably benefit from maintenance omeprazole therapy. Omeprazole 10 mg daily may be suitable for management of peptic ulcer, based on extent of acid inhibition and duodenal ulcer healing rate.[19,54] "Weekend therapy" in which patients receive omeprazole for three days per week has also been proposed.[24] Patients with recurrent reflux esophagitis may require suppressive therapy with omeprazole 20 mg daily. The most appropriate dosage regimen to employ in such situations requires further study.

In the management of ZES with omeprazole, total daily doses of up to 360 mg have produced substantial symptomatic improvement and marked inhibition of gastric acid secretion. Omeprazole is often given as a single daily dose, but a divided regimen (b.i.d. or t.i.d.) may be employed, especially when the daily dose exceeds 120 mg. Dosage should be individualized to maintain a predose acid secretion of <10 mmol/hr.

Insufficient information is available to recommend dosages in pediatric patients at this time. Most studies have involved young adults, and no studies involving subjects less than 18 years old have been reported. There is no information at present that indicates dosage adjustment is required in patients with chronic renal failure. Although no information is available yet regarding dosage in the presence of impaired hepatic function, omeprazole's extensive metabolism suggests an empiric dosage reduction may be appropriate.

Formulary Considerations

In evaluating omeprazole for addition to a hospital formulary, efficacy, safety, and cost-effectiveness must be examined with the characteristics of each institution's patient mix in mind. The efficacy of omeprazole has been shown to be comparable or superior to conventional treatments for several conditions. Considering the efficacy and safety of H_2-receptor antagonists, the potential for omeprazole to cause gastric carcinoid tumors in humans should be further resolved before a role is established. For ZES, in which hypergastrinemia is present and gastrinomas may be metastatic, the relative risk-to-benefit ratio favors omeprazole as first-line therapy. Although the development of carcinoid tumors has not been demonstrated in patients who received omeprazole, the designs of the trials and number of patient-month exposures are inadequate to appropriately study this adverse effect. The cost of omeprazole has not been established to date, therefore the cost-efficacy of therapy cannot be determined. The standard for prospective and historical comparisons with omeprazole in most conditions was (and should be) H_2-receptor antagonists; therefore, the cost of this drug will likely be similar to that of the H_2-receptor antagonists. If the cost of treatment is in this range and if safety in humans is further substantiated, omeprazole will be used commonly in the treatment of various peptic ulcer diseases.

Conclusion

Omeprazole will serve a valuable role in the treatment of gastrointestinal tract ulcers and hypersecretory conditions. It represents a new class of therapeutic agents that produce potent and sustained inhibition of gastric acid secretion with once- or twice-daily oral doses. In most studies omeprazole is superior to cimetidine or ranitidine for treating duodenal ulcers in terms of decreased time to onset of healing and pain relief. Omeprazole is at least as effective as H_2-receptor antagonists in treating gastric ulcers but is more effective in the treatment of esophagitis; in esophagitis, omeprazole demonstrates a significantly faster healing rate than that associated with ranitidine. Omeprazole offers an effective treatment for patients with ZES refractory to treatment with H_2-receptor antagonists; further studies are needed to compare omeprazole with H_2-receptor antagonists as initial treatment for ZES.

Adverse effects from omeprazole treatment appear to be infrequent and mild. The risk for gastric carcinoid tumors and bacterial overgrowth exists; however, current evidence suggests that these effects may not be of clinical concern with short-term use. Drug interactions with omeprazole have been noted, and patients receiving other drugs concurrently should be monitored for potential interactions.

References

1. Zdon MJ, Ballantyne GH, Schafer DE et al. Proton pump inhibition—the ultimate control of acid secretion? *J Surg Res*. 1986; 40:353–61.
2. Pilbrant A, Cederberg C. Development of an oral formulation of omeprazole. *Scand J Gastroenterol*. 1985; 108(Suppl): 113–20.
3. Granger DN, Barrowman JA, Kvietys PR. Clinical gastrointestinal physiology. Philadelphia: W.B. Saunders Company; 1985:66–95.
4. Rabon E, Cuppoletti J, Malinowska D et al. Proton secretion by the gastric parietal cell. *J Exp Biol*. 1983; 106:119–33.
5. Beil W, Sewing KF. Acid activation makes omeprazole a specific K^+/H^+-ATPase inhibitor. *Gastroenterology*. 1985; 88:1320. Abstract.
6. Lorentzon P, Eklundh B, Brandstrom A et al. The mechanism for inhibition of gastric (H^+-K^+)-ATPase by omeprazole. *Biochim Biophys Acta*. 1985; 817:25–32.
7. Im WB, Sih JC, Blakeman DP et al. Omeprazole, a specific inhibitor of gastric (H^+-K^+)-ATPase, is a H^+-activated oxidizing agent of sulfhydryl groups. *J Biol Chem*. 1985; 260:4591–7.
8. Sewing KF, Beil W, Hannemann H. The in vitro inhibitory effect of omeprazole on parietal cell H^+-transport is reversible. *Gastroenterology*. 1985; 88:1581. Abstract.
9. Berglindh T, Hansen D, Bergqvist E. Irreversible inhibition by omeprazole. The in vivo–in vitro connection. *Gastroenterology*. 1985; 88:1322. Abstract.
10. De Graef J, Woussen-Colle M-C. Influence of the stimulation state of the parietal cells on the inhibitory effect of omeprazole on gastric acid secretion in dogs. *Gastroenterology*. 1986; 91:333–7.
11. Tanimura H, Sato N, Kawano S et al. The effect of proton pump inhibitor on gastric mucosal hemodynamics. *Gastroenterology*. 1988; 94:A455. Abstract.
12. Satch H, Arakawa T, Sakuma H et al. Cytoprotection by proton-pump inhibitors in rat gastric mucosa. A possible role of endogenous prostaglandins (PG). *Gastroenterology*. 1988; 94:A400. Abstract.
13. Chan BW, Hui WM, Lam SK et al. Effect of misoprostol and omeprazole on gastric mucosal blood flow in rats—a comparative study by laser-doppler flowmetry. *Gastroenterology*. 1988; 94:A64. Abstract.
14. Wandall JH. Effect of omeprazole on polymorphonuclear leucocyte chemotaxis, superoxide anion (O_2) generation and degranulation. *Gastroenterology*. 1988; 94:A486. Abstract.
15. Stachura J, Konturek SJ, Cieszkowsky M et al. Comparison of the effect of omeprazole—a substituted benzimidazole—and ranitidine—a potent H_2-receptor antagonist—on histamine-induced gastric acid secretion and the ultrastructure of canine parietal cells. *Hepatogastroenterology*. 1983; 30:205–10.
16. Lind T, Cederberg C, Ekenved G et al. Effect of omeprazole—a gastric proton pump inhibitor—on pentagastrin stimulated acid secretion in man. *Gut*. 1983; 24:270–6.
17. Kittang E, Aadland E, Schjonsby H et al. The effect of omeprazole on gastric acidity and the absorption of liver cobalamins. *Scand J Gastroenterol*. 1987; 22:156–60.
18. Dammann HG, Kangah R, Dreyer M et al. Substantial decrease of 24 hours intragastric acidity by a single intravenous omeprazole application in man. *Gastroenterology*. 1988; 94:A85. Abstract.
19. Howden CW, Forrest JAH, Meredith PA et al. Antisecretory effect and oral pharmacokinetics following low dose omeprazole in man. *Br J Clin Pharmacol*. 1985; 20:137–9.
20 Walt RP, Reynolds JR, Langman MJS et al. Intravenous omeprazole rapidly raises intragastric pH. *Gut*. 1985; 26:902–6.
21. Naesdal J, Bankel M, Bodemar G et al. The effect of 20 mg omeprazole daily on serum gastrin, 24-h intragastric acidity, and bile acid concentration in duodenal ulcer patients. *Scand J Gastroenterol*. 1987; 22:5–12.
22. Thompson JN, Barr JA, Collier N et al. Basal, sham feed and pentagastrin stimulated gastric acid, pepsin and electrolytes after omeprazole 20 mg and 40 mg daily. *Gut*. 1985; 26:1018–24.
23. Elander B, Fellenius E, Leth R et al. Inhibitory action of omeprazole on acid formation in gastric glands and on H^+,K^+-ATPase isolated from human gastric mucosa. *Scand J Gastroenterol*. 1986; 21:268–72.

24. Hewson EG, Angus PW, Yeomans ND et al. Effect of "weekend therapy" with omeprazole on acid secretion and fasting plasma gastrin in duodenal ulcer patients. *Gastroenterology*. 1987; 92:1434. Abstract.
25. Howden CW, Payton CD, Meredith PA et al. Antisecretory effect and oral pharmacokinetics of omeprazole in patients with chronic renal failure. *Eur J Clin Pharmacol*. 1985; 28:637–40.
26. Festen HPM, Thijs JC, Lamers CBHW et al. Effect of oral omeprazole on serum gastrin and serum pepsinogen I levels. *Gastroenterology*. 1984; 87:1030–4.
27. McGuigan JE. Peptic ulcer. In: Braunwald E, Isselbacher KJ, Petersdorf RG et al., eds. Harrison's principles of internal medicine. 11th ed. New York: McGraw-Hill; 1987: 1239–53.
28. Tuynman H, Festen H, Hollander W et al. Repeated high oral doses of omeprazole do not affect intrinsic factor secretion: proof of a selective mode of action. *Gastroenterology*. 1988; 94:A469. Abstract.
29. Festen H, Tertoolen J. Malabsorption of protein-bound but not unbound cobalamin during treatment with omeprazole. *Gastroenterology*. 1988; 94:A125. Abstract.
30. Graham DY, McCullough A, Sklar M et al. Omeprazole in duodenal ulcer: the U.S. experience. *Gastroenterology*. 1988; 94:A152. Abstract.
31. Creutzfeldt W, Lamberts R, Brunner G. Serum gastrin concentrations and gastric endocrine cell population during longterm treatment with omeprazole in man. *Gut*. 1987; 28:A1341. Abstract.
32. Klinkenberg-Knol EC, Jansen JBMJ, de Bruyne JW et al. Longterm efficacy and safety of omeprazole (OME) on healing and prevention of resistant reflux esophagitis. *Gastroenterology*. 1988; 94:A230. Abstract.
33. Van Deventer GM, Cagliola A, Whipple J et al. Duodenal ulcer healing with omeprazole: a multicenter, double-blind, ranitidine controlled study. *Gastroenterology*. 1988; 94:A476. Abstract.
34. Johnson LR. Regulation of gastrointestinal mucosal growth. *Physiol Rev*. 1988; 68:456–502.
35. Penston J, Wormsley KG. Achlorhydria: hypergastrinemia: carcinoids—a flawed hypothesis? *Gut*. 1987; 28:488–505.
36. Bordi C, Creutzfeldt W, Hakanson R et al. Achlorhydria: carcinoids—a flawed hypothesis. *Gut*. 1987; 28:1189–91. Letter.
37. MacDonald WC, Rubin CE. Gastric tumors, gastritis, and other gastric diseases. In: Braunwald E, Isselbacher KJ, Petersdorf RG, et al., eds. Harrison's principles of internal medicine. 11th ed. New York: McGraw-Hill; 1987:1256.
38. Dent J, Downton J, Buckle P et al. Omeprazole heals peptic esophagitis by elevation of intragastric pH. *Gastroenterology*. 1985; 88:1363. Abstract.
39. Horowitz M, Hetzel DJ, Buckle PJ et al. The effect of omeprazole on gastric emptying in patients with duodenal ulcer disease. *Br J Clin Pharmacol*. 1984; 18:791–4.
40. Regardh C-G, Gabrielsson M, Hoffman K-J et al. Pharmacokinetics and metabolism of omeprazole in animals and man—an overview. *Scand J Gastroenterol*. 1985; 108(Suppl): 79–94.
41. Regardh C-G. Pharmacokinetics and metabolism of omeprazole in man. *Scand J Gastroenterol*. 1986; 118(Suppl):99–104.
42. Howden CW, Meredith PA, Forrest JAH et al. Oral pharmacokinetics of omeprazole. *Eur J Clin Pharmacol*. 1984; 26:641–3.
43. Prichard PJ, Yeomans ND, Mihaly GW et al. Omeprazole: a study of its inhibition of gastric pH and oral pharmacokinetics after morning or evening dosage. *Gastroenterology*. 1985; 88:64–9.
44. Naesdal J, Andersson T, Bodemar G et al. Pharmacokinetics of [^{14}C] omeprazole in patients with impaired renal function. *Clin Pharmacol Ther*. 1986; 40:344–51.
45. Gugler R, Jensen JC. Omeprazole inhibits oxidative drug metabolism. *Gastroenterology*. 1985; 89:1235–41.
46. Hoffmann K-J, Renberg L, Olovson S-G. Comparative metabolic disposition of oral doses of omeprazole in the dog, rat, and mouse. *Drug Metab Dispos*. 1986; 14:336–40.
47. Hoffmann K-J. Identification of the main urinary metabolites of omeprazole after an oral dose to rats and dogs. *Drug Metab Dispos*. 1986; 14:341–8.
48. Lamers CBHW, Lind T, Moberg S et al. Omeprazole in Zollinger-Ellison syndrome: effects of a single dose and of long-term treatment in patients resistant to histamine H-2 receptor antagonists. *N Engl J Med*. 1984; 310:758–61.
49. Bardhan KD, Dhande D, Hinchliffe RFC et al. Omeprazole in the treatment of ultra refractory duodenal ulcer. *Gastroenterology*. 1988; 94:A22. Abstract.
50. Pen JH, Michelsen PP, Pelckmans PA et al. Omeprazole in the treatment of H2-resistant gastroduodenal ulcers. *Gastroenterology*. 1988; 94:A348. Abstract.
51. French Cooperative Study. Omeprazole versus ranitidine in duodenal ulcer patients unhealed after six weeks treatment with H2-receptor antagonists. *Gut*. 1987; 28:A1341. Abstract.
52. Gustavsson S, Adami HO, Loof L et al. Rapid healing of duodenal ulcers with omeprazole: double-blind dose-comparative trial. *Lancet*. 1983; 2:124–5.
53. Omeprazole in duodenal ulceration: acid inhibition, symptom relief, endoscopic healing, and recurrence. Cooperative study. *Br Med J*. 1984; 289:525–8.
54. Prichard PJ, Rubinstein D, Jones DB et al. Double blind comparative study of omeprazole 10 mg and 30 mg daily for healing duodenal ulcers. *Br Med J*. 1985; 290:601–3.
55. Huttemann W, Rohner HG, DuBosque G et al. 20 versus 30 mg omeprazole once daily: effect on healing rates in 115 duodenal ulcer patients. *Digestion*. 1986; 33:117–20.
56. Lauritsen K, Rune SJ, Bytzer P et al. Effect of omeprazole and cimetidine on duodenal ulcer: a double-blind comparative trial. *N Engl J Med*. 1985; 312:958–61.
57. Archambault AP, Pare P, Bailey RJ et al. Omeprazole (20 mg daily) versus cimetidine (1200 mg daily) in duodenal ulcer healing and pain relief. *Gastroenterology*. 1988; 94:1130–4.
58. Bardhan KD, Porro GB, Bose K et al. A comparison of two different doses of omeprazole versus ranitidine in treatment of duodenal ulcers. *J Clin Gastroenterol*. 1986; 8:408–13.
59. Barbara L, Blasi A, Cheli R et al. Omeprazole vs. ranitidine in the short-term treatment of duodenal ulcer: an Italian multicenter study. *Hepatogastroenterology*. 1987; 34:229–32.
60. Classen M, Dammann HG, Domschke W et al. Omeprazole heals duodenal, but not gastric ulcers more rapidly than ranitidine. Results of two German multicentre trials. *Hepatogastroenterology*. 1985; 32:243–5.
61. Brook CW, Yeomans ND, McCarthy PG et al. Relapse of duodenal ulceration after healing with omeprazole. *Med J Aust*. 1987; 147:595–7.
62. Barbara L, Saggioro A, Olsson J et al. Omeprazole 20 mg om and ranitidine 150 mg bd in the healing of benign gastric ulcers—an Italian multicenter study. *Gut*. 1987; 28:A1341. Abstract.
63. Walan A, Bader JP, Classen M et al. Effect of omeprazole and ranitidine on ulcer healing and relapse rates in gastric ulcer patients. An international multicenter study. *Gastroenterology*. 1988; 94:A484. Abstract.
64. Lauritsen K, Rune SJ, Wulff HR et al. Effect of omeprazole and cimetidine on prepyloric gastric ulcer: double blind comparative trial. *Gut*. 1988; 29:249–53.
65. Dent J, Hetzel DJ, Reed WD et al. Healing of peptic esophagitis with omeprazole. *Gastroenterology*. 1986; 90:1392. Abstract.
66. Hetzel DJ, Dent J, Reed W et al. Healing of peptic esophagitis with omeprazole. *Gastroenterology*. 1987; 92:1434. Abstract.
67. Klinkenberg-Knol EC, Jansen JMBJ, Festen HPM et al. Double-blind multicentre comparison of omeprazole and

ranitidine in the treatment of reflux oesophagitis. *Lancet*. 1987; 1:349–51.
68. Havelund T, Laursen LS, Skoubo-Kristensen E et al. Omeprazole and ranitidine in treatment of reflux oesophagitis: double blind comparative trial. *Br Med J*. 1988; 296:89–92.
69. Vantrappen G, Coenegrachts JL, Rutgeerts L et al. Omeprazole (40 mg) is superior to ranitidine in the short term treatment of ulcerative reflux esophagitis. *Gastroenterology*. 1987; 92:1681. Abstract.
70. Blum AL, Riecken EO, Dammann HG et al. Comparison of omeprazole and ranitidine in the treatment of reflux esophagitis. *N Engl J Med*. 1986; 314:716. Letter.
71. Zeitoun P, Desjars De Keranroue N, Isal JP. Omeprazole versus ranitidine in erosive oesophagitis. *Lancet*. 1987; 2:621–2. Letter.
72. Hetzel DJ, Bonnin M. Long term management of hemorrhagic esophagitis with cimetidine and omeprazole. *Aust NZ J Med*. 1986; 16:226–8.
73. Hameeteman W, Tytgat GN. Healing of chronic Barrett ulcers with omeprazole. *Am J Gastroenterol*. 1986; 81:764–6.
74. Dent J, Heddle R, Downton J et al. Omeprazole heals ulcerative peptic esophagitis. *Gastroenterology*. 1984; 86:1062. Abstract.
75. Wolfe MW, Jensen RT. Zollinger–Ellison syndrome. Current concepts in diagnosis and management. *N Engl J Med*. 1987; 317:1200–9.
76. Lamers CBHW. Present experiences with omeprazole in the Zollinger–Ellison syndrome. *Scand J Gastroenterol*. 1986; 118(Suppl):123–7.
77. McArthur KE, Collem MJ, Maton PA et al. Omeprazole: effective, convenient therapy for Zollinger–Ellison syndrome. *Gastroenterology*. 1985; 88:939–44.
78. Maton P, McArthur K, Wank S et al. Long-term efficacy and safety of omeprazole in patients with Zollinger–Ellison syndrome (ZES). *Gastroenterology*. 1986; 90:1537. Abstract.
79. Maton PN, Frucht H, Vinayek R et al. Medical management of patients with Zollinger–Ellison syndrome who had previous gastric surgery: a prospective study. *Gastroenterology*. 1988; 94:294–9.
80. Blanchi A, Delchier JC, Soule JC et al. Control of acute Zollinger–Ellison syndrome with intravenous omeprazole. *Lancet*. 1982; 2:1223–4.
81. Delchier JC, Soule JC, Mignon M et al. Effectiveness of omeprazole in seven patients with Zollinger–Ellison syndrome resistant to histamine H-2 receptor antagonists. *Dig Dis Sci*. 1986; 31:693–9.
82. Bardram L, Stadil F. Omeprazole in the Zollinger–Ellison syndrome. *Scand J Gastroenterol*. 1986; 21:374–8.
83. Lloyd-Davies KA, Rutgerson K, Sovell L. Omeprazole in Zollinger–Ellison syndrome: four-year international study. *Gastroenterology*. 1986; 90:1523. Abstract.
84. Corlato V, Puoti M, Annibalo M et al. Loss of efficacy of famotidine (FMT) in the control of gastric acid secretion in patients with Zollinger–Ellison syndrome (ZES), reversed by omeprazole (OMP). *Gastroenterology*. 1988; 94:A79. Abstract.
85. Hirschowitz BI, Deren J, Raufman JP et al. A multicenter U.S. study of omeprazole treatment of Zollinger–Ellison syndrome (ZES). *Gastroenterology*. 1988; 94:A188. Abstract.
86. Griffith J, Hirschowitz BI. Omeprazole treatment in Zollinger–Ellison syndrome (ZES): relative effects on acid, pepsin, chloride, and volume secretion. *Gastroenterology*. 1988; 94:A157. Abstract.
87. Simon B, Dammann HG, Muller P. Gastroduodenal tolerability of nonsteroidal antiinflammatory agents (NOSAC) in man: endoscopic comparative studies with antiulcer drugs. *Gastroenterology*. 1986; 90:1635. Abstract.
88. Bigard MA. Complete prevention by omeprazole of aspirin induced gastric lesions in healthy subjects. *Gastroenterology*. 1988; 94:A34. Abstract.
89. Ekman L, Hansson E, Havu N et al. Toxicological studies on omeprazole. *Scand J Gastroenterol*. 1985; 108(Suppl):53–69.
90. Stockmann F, Bernhard F, Mostar F et al. Morphological changes of gastric endocrine cells during treatment with omeprazole and famotidine. *Gastroenterology*. 1988; 94:A445. Abstract.
91. Larsson H, Carlsson E, Mattsson H et al. Plasma gastrin and gastric enterochromaffinlike cell activation and proliferation. *Gastroenterology*. 1986; 90:391–9.
92. Clissold SP, Campoli-Richards DM. Omeprazole: a preliminary review of its pharmacodynamic and pharmacokinetic properties, and therapeutic potential in peptic ulcer disease and Zollinger–Ellison syndrome. *Drugs*. 1986; 32:15–47.
93. Maton PN, Lack E, McArthur KE et al. Effects of long term omeprazole on gastric acid secretion and mucosal histology in patients with Zollinger–Ellison syndrome (ZES). *Gastroenterology*. 1988; 94:A288. Abstract.
94. Karvonen A-L, Keyrilainen O, Uusitalo A et al. Effects of omeprazole in duodenal ulcer patients. *Scand J Gastroenterol*. 1986; 21:449–54.
95. Helander HF. Stereological data on parietal and endocrine cells of the gastric corpus in patients treated with omeprazole. *Gastroenterology*. 1985; 88:1416. Abstract.
96. Pen JH, Michielsen PP, Pelckmans PA et al. Omeprazole in the treatment of H_2-resistant gastro-duodenal ulcers. *Gastroenterology*. 1988; 94:A348. Abstract.
97. Friedman G. Omeprazole. *Am J Gastroenterol*. 1987; 82:188–91.
98. Anon. Omeprazole. *Lancet*. 1987; 2:1187–8. Editorial.
99. Wormsley KG. Omeprazole. *Lancet*. 1987; 2:1467. Letter.
100. Colin-Jones DG. Omeprazole. *Lancet*. 1987; 2:1467. Letter.
101. Sharma BK, Santana IA, Wood EC et al. Intragastric bacterial activity and nitrosation before, during, and after treatment with omeprazole. *Br Med J*. 1984; 289:717–9.
102. Driks MR, Craven DE, Celli BR et al. Nosocomial pneumonia in intubated patients given sucralfate as compared with antacids or histamine type 2 blockers. The role of gastric colonization. *N Engl J Med*. 1987; 317:1376–82.
103. Tryba M. Risk of acute stress bleeding and nosocomial pneumonia in ventilated intensive care unit patients: sucralfate versus antacids. *Am J Med*. 1987; 83(Suppl 3B):117–24.
104. Crabbe S, Ostrosky JD, Hopkins LE. Development of nosocomial pneumonia with antiulcer agents. *Drug Intell Clin Pharm*. 1986; 20:951–2.
105. Holder GM, Little PJ, Ryan AJ et al. Inhibitors of hepatic mixed function oxidases. II. Some benzimidazole, benzoxazole and benzothiazole derivatives. *Biochem Pharmacol*. 1976; 25:2747–50.
106. Little PJ, Ryan AJ. Inhibitors of hepatic mixed-function oxidases. 4. Effects of benzimidazole and related compounds on aryl hydrocarbon hydroxylase activity from phenobarbitone and 3-methylcholanthrene induced rats. *J Med Chem*. 1982; 25:622–6.
107. Murray M, Ryan AJ, Little PJ. Inhibition of rat hepatic microsomal aminopyrine *N*-demethylase activity by benzimidazole derivatives. Quantitative structure–activity relationships. *J Med Chem*. 1982; 25:887–92.
108. Henry DA, Somerville KW, Kitchingman G et al. Omeprazole: effects on oxidative drug metabolism. *Br J Clin Pharmacol*. 1984; 18:195–200.
109. Prichard PJ, Walt RP, Kitchingman GK et al. Oral phenytoin pharmacokinetics during omeprazole therapy. *Br J Clin Pharmacol*. 1987; 24:543–5.
110. Tuynman HARE, Festen HPM, Rohss K et al. Lack of effect of antacids on plasma concentrations of omeprazole given as enteric-coated granules. *Br J Clin Pharmacol*. 1987; 24:833–5.
111. Lamers CBHW, Jansen JBMJ. Omeprazole as adjunct to enzyme replacement treatment in severe pancreatic insufficiency. *Br Med J*. 1986; 293:994.
112. Solvell L. Safety aspects of omeprazole. *Scand J Gastroenterol*. 1986; 118(Suppl):129–35.
113. Lewis JH. Hepatic effects of drugs used in the treatment of peptic ulcer disease. *Am J Gastroenterol*. 1987; 82:987–1003.

Therapy Review

Management and prevention of bacterial diarrhea

JEANETTE SUAREZ AND FRANCINE R. SALAMONE

Abstract: The etiology, pathogenesis, transmission and communicability, diagnosis, and management of infectious diarrhea are reviewed.

Infectious diarrhea is common in both industrialized and unindustrialized areas of the world. Better understanding of the etiology and pathogenesis and identification of "new" enteric pathogens has resulted in the use of a variety of drugs to relieve symptoms or to effect a clinical cure. Both host and microbial virulence factors are key in the acquisition of diarrheal illness. Host factors such as extreme age, a dysfunctional gastrointestinal tract, or underlying immunodeficiency enhance the risk of illness after ingestion of a pathogen or its toxins. Microbial virulence factors (the pathogen's ability to invade or produce enterotoxins, neurotoxins, or cytotoxins) characterize the type of illness manifested and the symptom complex (e.g., acute watery diarrhea versus chronic dysentery). Supportive care is indicated in the majority of cases of infectious enteritis, and rehydration is considered the mainstay of therapy in any diarrheal illness accompanied by dehydration. Antimicrobial therapy is beneficial in the treatment of severe diarrhea caused by *Shigella*, *Campylobacter* spp., *Vibrio cholerae*, *Escherichia coli*, and *Clostridium difficile*.

Infectious diarrhea is common but is often self-limited and of short duration. Therapy frequently consists of symptomatic relief and fluid replacement.

Index terms: Adsorbents; Antibiotics; Antidiarrheal agents; Diarrhea; Oral rehydration compound; Replacement solutions
Clin Pharm. 1988; 7:746–59

Infectious diarrhea, one of the most common debilitating diseases worldwide, remains the third most frequent syndrome seen in the United States in the outpatient setting.[1,2] In the tropical developing world, diarrheal illness constitutes the greatest single cause of morbidity and mortality in children.[3-5] Correspondingly, traveler's diarrhea is the most frequent and dreaded health problem of international tourists, with an incidence of greater than 50%.[6] Most recently, the incidence of colonization and disease with newly recognized pathogens such as *Cryptosporidium, Isospora belli,* and *Giardia lamblia* has increased coincident with the increasing number of cases of the acquired immunodeficiency syndrome (AIDS).[7,8]

The purpose of this review is to familiarize the clinician with the epidemiology and pathogenesis of infectious diarrhea, with special emphasis on prevention, supportive care, and the most appropriate role of anti-infective therapy.

Pathogenesis

Host Factors. After exposure to a pathogen, the manifestation and severity of diarrheal disease are determined in part by specific host factors, such as age, personal hygiene, and barriers of the gastrointestinal tract (gastric acid, intestinal motility, normal bowel microflora, and immunoglobulin secretion).[9-12] Age plays a role in the susceptibility to enteric infection, since adults and children often acquire different forms of disease or manifest the same syndrome differently.[12] Rotavirus and enteropathogenic *Escherichia coli*, for example, are frequent causes of infectious diarrhea in children but are relatively uncommon in older individuals.[13,14]

JEANETTE SUAREZ is Clinical Pharmacist and FRANCINE SALAMONE, PHARM.D., is Pharmacy Specialist in Infectious Disease, Division of Pharmacy Services, Memorial Sloan-Kettering Cancer Center, New York, NY.

Address reprint requests to Dr. Salamone at the Division of Pharmacy Services, Memorial Sloan-Kettering Cancer Center, 1275 York Avenue, New York, NY 10021.

This is **article 680-204-8816** in the **ASHP Continuing Education System.** See page 776 for learning objectives and test questions.

Copyright © 1988, American Society of Hospital Pharmacists, Inc. All rights reserved. 0278-2677/88/1001-0746$03.50.

Similarly, children less than one year of age develop *Salmonella* bacteremia after *Salmonella* gastroenteritis more frequently than adults, in whom positive blood cultures are rarely observed after intestinal illness.[15] In addition, children often have prolonged intestinal carriage of this organism after gastrointestinal symptoms have ceased.[15]

Since acquisition of nearly all forms of diarrheal disease depends on the ingestion of specific organisms, and most intestinal pathogens originate in other mammalian (human and animal) intestinal tracts, poor personal hygiene and improper sanitation are important contributing factors in the fecal-oral route of disease transmission.[12,16] Bacterial enteric infections occurring in the immunocompetent patient usually require the ingestion of large quantities (large infectious doses) of the organism to overcome the host's natural protective barriers. Large concentrations of certain pathogens (e.g., *Salmonella, Vibrio* spp., *E. coli*) are generally found in improperly prepared or refrigerated food.[12] Conversely, infections with *Shigella* and *Campylobacter* develop after ingestion of lower infectious doses and are frequently transmitted through person-to-person contact. Such infections are commonly observed in young children in day-care centers and in hospitalized patients (e.g., immunosuppressed hosts).[12]

The gastrointestinal tract of a healthy host is capable of reducing the virulence of a majority of ingested pathogens. Virtually all ingested bacteria are destroyed within 30 minutes at normal gastric pH, whereas more than one hour is required for pathogen destruction in achlorhydric patients or in patients who habitually ingest neutralizing agents (e.g., sodium bicarbonate, antacids) or H_2-receptor antagonists.[9,17] The natural motility of the gastrointestinal tract promotes the proper distribution and flow of indigenous bowel flora, facilitates the rapid passage of pathogens through the gastrointestinal tract, and aids in the fluid reabsorptive process.[12,18,19] Drugs that slow peristalsis, such as opiates and anticholinergic agents, cause a delay in the transit and excretion of pathogens and are generally not recommended for use in the symptomatic relief of diarrhea.[10,19] Indigenous microbes resist the colonization of potential pathogens by virtue of their occupation of mucosal receptor sites.[11,20-22] Patients with defects in the normal bowel microflora are at high risk for a variety of serious enteric infections, as are patients receiving prolonged antimicrobial therapy.[11,20] The immune system of the host plays an important role in disease prevention.[23-28] Intestinal secretion of antigen-specific immunoglobulins has a bactericidal, neutralizing, or opsonic effect on gut pathogens.[12,23] Hereditary or acquired alterations in intestinal secretion of immunoglobulins (e.g., hereditary telangiectasia, hypogammaglobulinemia) appear to be directly related to the increased prevalence of diarrheal disease and malabsorption observed in these patients.[24-28] Further, there is an increased risk of gram-negative and viral intestinal infections in recipients of bone marrow transplants and patients with malignancy.[28]

Microbial Virulence Factors. In addition to host factors, microbial virulence factors (Table 1) are important determinants of the physical manifestations of specific diarrheal syndromes.[12,23,29] After resisting destruction by the gastrointestinal tract, a pathogen will adhere to and colonize the mucosal lining of the intestine.[30] After adhesion and colonization, pathogens invade the bowel wall, destroying mucosal epithelial cells (ulceration and sloughing), or produce toxins (enterotoxins, cytotoxins, neurotoxins), or both. Enterotoxins are noninflammatory microbial products that exert a direct functional effect on the intestinal mucosa, resulting in a net increase in fluid secretion.[31,32] This is the characteristic mechanism of most forms of traveler's diarrhea (e.g., *E. coli*) and food poisoning caused by *Clostridium perfringens* and "long-incubation" *Bacillus cereus*. Cytotoxigenicity refers to the ability of an organism to elaborate an inflammatory toxin that causes structural damage to the mucosal surface, resulting in colitis and dysentery (watery stool containing blood, pus, and mucus).[12,23,33] Several pathogens have the ability to produce toxins outside of the intestinal tract, and disease development depends on ingestion of these performed toxins rather than ingestion of the organism itself. Neurotoxins, the preformed toxins associated with certain types of food poisoning, have a direct effect on the central nervous system rather than the gastrointestinal tract. The abrupt onset of upper gastrointestinal symptoms within six hours after ingestion of neurotoxin is most commonly observed with *Staphylococcus aureus* or "short-incubation" *Bacillus cereus* food poisoning.[12,23]

Diagnosis

The diagnosis of infectious diarrhea is primarily dependent upon a careful history, physical assessment, and microbiologic examination of the stool specimen (Table 2).[34-36] Information regarding geographic location of the host at the time of infection (e.g., recent travel outside the United States, to the seacoast, or to mountainous areas) must be obtained.[12,23] Additionally, the possibility of an apparent epidemic illness among family or friends or in a particular neighborhood should be considered.[12,23] Predominant physical symptoms are especially important in pathogen identification. An enteroinvasive organism that causes structural damage (e.g., certain serotypes of *E. coli*) is suspected as the etiologic pathogen when a patient has dysentery and fever. Conversely, chronic watery diarrhea often indicates infection with a protozoan

Table 1.
Determinants of the Development of Enteric Infection: Microbial Virulence Factors[12,23,29]

Pathogen	Enterotoxigenic	Cytotoxigenic	Enteroinvasive
Bacteria			
Vibrio cholerae	x		
Vibrio parahemolyticus	x	x	x
Escherichia coli (ETEC, EPEC)[a]	x		x
E. coli serotype 0157.H7		x	
Salmonella spp.	x	x	x
Shigella spp.			x
Clostridium perfringens	x	x	
Clostridium difficile		x	x
Clostridium botulinum[b]	x		
Bacillus cereus[b]	x		
Staphylococcus aureus[b] (preformed toxin)	x		
Staph. aureus (enterocolitis)			x
Yersinia enterocolitica		x	x
Aeromonas hydrophilia		x	x
Campylobacter jejuni		x	x
Protozoa			
Giardia lamblia	x		
Cryptosporidia	x		
Entamoeba histolytica		x	x
Isospora belli			x
Viruses			
Cytomegalovirus		x	x
Rotavirus	x		
Norwalk-like virus	x		

[a] ETEC = enterotoxigenic, EPEC = enteropathogenic.
[b] Neurotoxigenic.

organism such as *Giardia* or *Cryptosporidium* (Table 2).

When history or physical findings suggest the presence of serious illness, laboratory examination of a fresh stool is clearly indicated.[34,37,38] Since special enriching techniques and optimal conditions of temperature and atmosphere are required for identification of a variety of pathogens and their toxins, the clinician must be specific in requests to the microbiology laboratory. Correspondingly, microbiology personnel must be alerted to the patient's recent use of drugs or other chemicals, since many compounds (e.g., antiamebic drugs, antibiotics, antimalarial drugs, barium, bismuth, castor oil, iodine preparation, iron, mineral oil, and psyllium[29]) will interfere with pathogen identification for up to one month after ingestion.[29] Gram's stain of the stool is of benefit in the diagnosis of infectious gastroenteritis, particularly when *Staph. aureus* enterocolitis is suspected in a patient recently treated with broad-spectrum antibiotics.[29] Perhaps one of the most valuable diagnostic aids in the examination of the fresh stool of a patient who has a diarrheal illness is the presence of fecal leukocytes.[39] Since damage to the mucosal lining results in an outpouring of white blood cells, the presence of fecal leukocytes is most commonly associated with the presence of enteroinvasive disease or certain enterotoxigenic pathogens (Table 3).

Role of Supportive Care in the Treatment of Infectious Diarrhea

Rehydration. Since infectious diarrhea is often self-limited and of short duration, therapy frequently consists of symptomatic relief and fluid replacement. Although intravenous fluid replacement is essential in the management of the dehydrated patient with prolonged symptoms and in extremely old or young patients, oral fluid replacement is satisfactory in mild to moderate dehydration. Oral rehydration has gained importance in developing countries, since it is a simpler, less expensive, and more available means of replacement therapy than intravenous fluid.[40–44]

Regardless of the degree of intestinal hypersecretion associated with a particular diarrheal illness, the proper concentrations of glucose and sodium in an oral rehydration solution will result in maximum fluid reabsorption by the patient. A key ingredient in oral rehydration therapy is glucose, which facilitates the absorption of sodium and water across mucosal cells of the small bowel.[42] In the absence of glucose, the simple solution of salts and water may aggravate severe gastroenteritis.[44] Optimum sodium and water reabsorption occurs with oral rehydration solutions containing 1–2% glucose.[42,44] Solutions consisting of greater than 3% glucose have little caloric benefit and appear to

Table 2.
Differential Diagnosis of Infectious Causes of Diarrhea[12,23,34–36]

Organism	History/Epidemiology	Symptom Complex	Incubation Period
Salmonella (not *Salmonella typhi*)	Ingestion of improperly prepared or unrefrigerated poultry, dairy products or meat; homosexual males	Acute dysentery	>8 hr
Shigella	Human fecal contamination; homosexual males	Acute dysentery	>8 hr
Escherichia coli[a]	Recent travel to an underdeveloped area; infantile diarrhea in the tropics	Acute watery diarrhea	>12 hr
E. coli (0157:H7)	Ingestion of fast-food hamburgers	Hemorrhagic colitis	>8 hr
E. coli (invasive)	Ingestion of imported cheese	Dysentery, acute fever	>12 hr
Yersinia enterocolitica	Ingestion of water, milk, or food contaminated with animal feces	Acute dysentery, fever	>8 hr
Campylobacter jejuni	Ingestion of water, milk, or food contaminated with animal feces; homosexual males	Acute dysentery	>8 hr
Vibrio cholerae	Ingestion of water and raw mollusks contaminated with human feces	Acute watery diarrhea	>8 hr
Vibrio parahemolyticus	Ingestion of contaminated raw mollusks and crustaceans	Acute dysentery	>8 hr
Clostridium difficile	Prolonged antibiotic use	Acute dysentery	>8 hr
Bacillus cereus or *Clostridium perfringens*	Ingestion of rice, cereal, or foods containing cornstarch that were heated and kept warm for hours	Acute vomiting, watery diarrhea	>12 hr
Staphylococcus aureus (preformed toxin)	Ingestion of unrefrigerated (>4 hr) pastries, dairy products, meats	Acute vomiting, acute watery diarrhea	>12 hr
Entamoeba histolytica	Human fecal cyst contamination; homosexual males	Chronic dysentery and fever	>12 hr
Giardia lamblia	Ingestion of water contaminated with human or animal (beaver) feces; travelers; day-care centers; homosexual males; AIDS[b]	Chronic watery diarrhea	>7 days
Cryptosporidium	Tropical areas; homosexual males; AIDS	Chronic watery diarrhea	>7 days
Isospora belli	Ingestion of water contaminated with human feces	Chronic watery diarrhea, malabsorption	>7 days
Enteric viruses	Infant winter diarrhea; ingestion of water contaminated with feces	Acute watery diarrhea, fever, vomiting	>12 hr

[a] Enterotoxigenic or enteropathogenic.
[b] Acquired immunodeficiency syndrome.

reverse the osmotic gradient with a subsequent increase in the symptoms of the diarrheal illness.[45]

The oral rehydration solution recommended by the World Health Organization (WHO) was originally formulated for the treatment of enteritis caused by *Vibrio cholerae* in underdeveloped areas and is now commonly used for all types of diarrheal disease.[46,47] This solution is also the base formula for several commercially available oral rehydration solutions.[43] The preparation and electrolyte composition of the WHO oral rehydration solution are detailed in Table 4.[12,23,46–48] For rehydration therapy, the WHO solution is administered in a volume to replace the estimated deficit (e.g., weight loss); this generally results in reversal of dehydration within eight hours.[43,49]

Homemade electrolyte solutions are useful as rehydration therapy in patients who develop diarrheal disease during travel to unindustrialized areas (Table 5).[50] In industrialized areas, commercial beverages (juices, colas, ginger ale) can be administered to a mildly dehydrated patient in the approximate equivalent (Table 4).[48]

Antimotility and Antisecretory Agents. The role of antimotility agents (e.g., opiates, anticholinergic agents) in the symptomatic relief of diarrhea is controversial.[10,29,51,52] Although frequently used, anticholinergic agents do not appear to be of benefit in the treatment of infectious diarrheal disease. Although these agents relieve abdominal cramping and decrease the number of diarrheal episodes, they may delay the clearance of infecting organisms, resulting in an increase in the duration and severity of illness.[10,29,37,51–54] In general, most authorities advise against the use of antimotility preparations in patients with fever or dysentery, or both, or in those patients whose condition worsens with therapy.[37,53] Conversely, since most cases of infectious diarrhea, regardless of etiology, involve increased small-bowel secretion, antisecretory drugs such as loperamide and bismuth subsalicylate are recommended to block the diarrheagenic

Table 3.
Pathogens Associated with the Presence of Fecal Leukocytes[29,39]

Bacteria (Invasive)
- *Escherichia coli*
- *Campylobacter fetus* subsp. *jejuni*
- *Aeromonas hydrophilia*
- *Salmonella* spp.
- *Shigella* spp.
- *Yersinia enterocolitica*
- *Vibrio parahemolyticus*
- *Clostridium difficile*

Bacteria (Enterotoxigenic)
- *Escherichia coli*
- *Bacillus cereus*
- *Clostridium perfringens*
- *Vibrio cholerae*
- *Staphylococcus aureus* (enterocolitis)

Viruses
- Rotavirus
- Parvovirus

Parasites
- *Giardia lamblia*
- *Entamoeba histolytica*
- *Cryptosporidium*

Table 4.
Electrolyte Composition and Oral Rehydration Therapy of Infectious Diarrhea[12,23,46-48]

	Solution Composition (meq/L)		
Liquid	Sodium	Potassium	Chloride
World Health Organization Solution[a]	90.0	20.0	80.0
Coca-Cola	1.0	<1.0	600.0
Ginger ale	>3.0	<1.0	553.0
Jello	30.0	<1.0	1000.0
Pepsi-Cola	2.0	<1.0	672.0
7-UP	>3.0	<1.0	532.0
Orange juice	<1.0	190.0	644.0
Gatorade	23.0	>2.0	318.0
Apple juice	2.0	100.0	N.A.[b]

[a] Content of solution: sodium chloride, 3.5 g; sodium bicarbonate, 2.5 g; potassium chloride, 1.5 g; glucose, 20 g; distilled water in a sufficient quantity to make 1000 mL of solution.
[b] Not available.

Table 5.
Formula for Treatment of Diarrheal Disease (Homemade Rehydration Solutions)[50]

Ingredient	Amount
Glass 1[a]	
Orange, apple, other fruit juice	8 oz.
Honey or corn syrup	½ tsp.
Table salt	1 pinch
Glass 2	
Water (carbonated or boiled)	8 oz.
Baking soda	¼ tsp.

[a] Patient is to drink alternately from each glass until thirst is quenched.

effects of bacterial pathogens.[55-58] Loperamide is occasionally recommended, since it is effective in delaying intestinal stool passage and is not associated with anticholinergic adverse effects.[37] Bismuth subsalicylate, another antisecretory compound, is suggested in the treatment of diarrhea in mild to moderately ill adults and in children more than three years of age.[55,56,59] Further, it is advocated in the short-term prophylaxis of traveler's diarrhea so long as the period of therapy does not exceed two weeks.[59] Although the mechanism of action is still debated, most authorities agree that the bismuth salts appear to be antibacterial,[60] while the salicylate is systemically absorbed.[58] Despite the widespread use of bismuth subsalicylate, no clinically important adverse effects have been associated with its use in the United States.[59]

Adsorbent Drugs. Adsorbent drugs used in the management of infectious diarrhea probably have little effect on the natural course of the disease. However, adsorbent drugs, such as kaolin–pectin and aluminum hydroxide, improve the patient's formation of stool and consequently allow for better control and timing of evacuation.[37,61] Thus, adsorbent drugs may help to relieve the symptoms of infectious enteritis.

Anti-infective Therapy of Common Bacterial Infections

Therapy with appropriate anti-infective agents has been shown to reduce the severity and duration of diarrheal illnesses caused by a variety of enteric bacterial pathogens (Table 6).[37,53,62-66] Conversely, specific antiviral agents are not deemed effective in the management of viral forms of gastroenteritis. The following discussion summarizes anti-infective therapy of bacterial enteritis and empiric treatment of diseases presumably caused by bacterial pathogens (e.g., traveler's diarrhea).

Salmonellosis

Salmonella typhi, Salmonella choleraesuis, and *Salmonella enteritidis* are frequently implicated strains of salmonellae responsible for gastroenteric infection.[67] Symptoms of vomiting, headache, myalgia, abdominal cramps, fever, and chills usually appear within 48 hours after ingestion of contaminated food or water.[29] Salmonella enterocolitis is almost always mild and self-limited and spontaneously resolves within three to five days without therapy, whereas in the presence of a febrile illness the course of treatment may be prolonged.[29] In addition, it has been shown that the use of antimicrobial agents prolongs the excretion of salmonella organisms in the stool (e.g., development of the carrier state) and promotes the emergence of resis-

Table 6.
Oral Antimicrobial Therapy of Common Bacterial Enteric Infections[37,53,62–66]

Organism	Recommended Treatment
Shigella	Trimethoprim–sulfamethoxazole 160 mg[a] every 12 hours for 5 days
Campylobacter jejuni	Erythromycin 50 mg/kg/day every 6 hours in divided doses for 7 days
Vibrio cholerae	Tetracycline hydrochloride 500 mg every 6 hours for 5 days
Escherichia coli	
Enterotoxigenic or traveler's diarrhea	Trimethoprim–sulfamethoxazole 160 mg[a] b.i.d. for 5 days and/or bismuth subsalicylate 60 mL q.i.d. for 5 days
Enteropathogenic or neonatal	Colistin 10 mg/kg/day (as the sulfate salt) for 5 days
Enteroinvasive	Ampicillin 500 mg orally q.i.d. for 5 days
Clostridium difficile (antibiotic-associated colitis)	Vancomycin 125 mg (as the hydrochloride salt) four times daily for 10 days

[a] Dose based on trimethoprim component.

tance.[68,69] Since no clinically important reduction in the duration of fever or severity of disease has been demonstrated after the use of antimicrobial agents, most authorities consider anti-infective therapy ineffective in salmonella gastroenteritis.[37]

Conversely, since salmonella bacteremia with its long febrile course can lead to serious metabolic and vascular complications, patients with signs of enteric or metastatic infection should be treated with anti-infective therapy.[37,70–72] Therapy with oral chloramphenicol (50 mg/kg/day) usually results in a reduction of temperature within three days[29] if the organism is susceptible. More frequently, chloramphenicol-resistant strains are observed, and ampicillin (150 mg/kg/day) is the preferred drug administered either orally, intravenously, or intramuscularly.[29,73] As an alternative to chloramphenicol and ampicillin therapy, a 14-day course of trimethoprim–sulfamethoxazole (TMP–SMX) in daily dosages of 320–640 mg of the trimethoprim component is efficacious.[29,74]

The chronic carrier state (positive stool cultures for more than six months) that develops in 1–3% of adults with typhoid fever also requires antimicrobial therapy. The persistence of the organism results from biliary-tract carriage, which, when associated with biliary calculi, requires cholecystectomy. Milder cases respond to treatment with oral ampicillin (4–6 g daily) or amoxicillin (6 g daily) for four to six weeks.[29,75] The new quinolone antimicrobial agents appear promising in the treatment of the asymptomatic salmonella carrier state, and isolated cases in which ciprofloxacin[76] and norfloxacin[77] were beneficial have been reported.

Shigellosis

Shigellae, the nonmotile gram-negative bacteria of the family Enterobacteriaceae, are frequent causes of bacillary dysentery in the United States.[29] Symptoms of bloody mucoid diarrhea, abdominal pain, and high fever generally begin one to two days after ingestion of contaminated food or water and may persist for seven days if left untreated.[12,23,29] Although several authorities consider this syndrome to be self-limited, requiring only supportive care, antibiotic therapy is indicated in the majority of cases.[78,79] It is well documented that antibiotic treatment reduces the duration of this disease, shortens the period of pathogen excretion (and communicability), and decreases the rate of relapse.[30,80,81] Unfortunately, a large number of antimicrobial agents possessing in vitro activity against shigellae (neomycin, amoxicillin, tetracycline, polymyxin B sulfate, furazolidone, cephalosporins) have only minimal effectiveness in vivo.[80,82–84] Further contributing to the dilemma is the constant emergence of resistant strains. In the 1970s, the preferred treatment of shigellosis was ampicillin (2 g daily for five days) with TMP–SMX (10 mg/kg of the trimethoprim component for five days) reserved for patients with ampicillin-resistant disease.[80,84] Currently, greater than 50% of shigella strains demonstrate resistance to ampicillin.[53] Changes in susceptibility patterns have resulted in the more frequent use of TMP–SMX and the search for other useful antimicrobial agents. The nonabsorbable investigational agent bicozamycin was as effective as TMP–SMX in shortening the clinical course of shigellosis in several patients.[66,79,85] Preliminary data also exist supporting the use of norfloxacin in shigellosis.[86,87] However, until available evidence suggests that such expensive drugs are unequivocally superior, TMP–SMX remains the drug of choice in the treatment of shigellosis.[37,53]

Escherichia coli Infections

Several *Escherichia coli* serotypes, collectively referred to as diarrheagenic *E. coli*, are recognized as major causes of diarrheal disease.[88] Enteropathogenic *E. coli* (EPEC), formerly responsible for the severe infantile diarrhea epidemics in the United States and abroad (1940–1950), remains an important cause of infantile diarrhea in underdeveloped countries.[14] In the early 1970s, strains of *E. coli* were identified as causes of diarrhea in military personnel stationed in the Middle East and Southeast Asia. These new strains were shown to produce cholera-like toxins or heat-stable toxins and therefore termed enterotoxigenic *E. coli* (ETEC). Like EPEC, enterotoxigenic *E. coli* is an important cause of diarrhea in infants in tropical developing areas. In addition, it is considered one of the most frequently isolated strains of diarrheagenic *E. coli* in persons traveling from industrialized to unindustrialized areas of the world.[88] When a large series of diarrhea outbreaks occurred in the United States after the ingestion of Camembert and Brie cheese, it was learned that the particular strain of *E. coli* responsible for disease possessed a shigella-like invasiveness (enteroinvasive *E. coli*). Aside from these outbreaks, invasive *E. coli* has not been shown to be an important cause of diarrhea in the United States, although it is a common pathogen in South America.[88] The most recently identified strain of diarrheagenic *E. coli*, 0157:H7 serotype, was responsible for the hemorrhagic colitis observed after ingestion of contaminated hamburger meat at a popular fast-food chain in 1982.[79,85,88] Approximately 40 people were affected with this syndrome, characterized by grossly bloody diarrhea. As with invasive *E. coli*, however, diarrhea caused by the 0157:H7 strain does not appear to constitute a major cause of enteritis to date.[88]

Treatment regimens for the various strains of diarrheagenic *E. coli* have been evaluated. Enteropathogenic *E. coli* (EPEC) infections in young children can be severe, and most authorities recommend the use of antimicrobial therapy. However, there are few data to substantiate the usefulness of any one agent. Neomycin, colistin, and gentamicin have each been used with some success; however, the development of resistance to these agents has occurred.[65,89-92] Oral, rather than intravenous or intramuscular, antimicrobial therapy appears to be of greater benefit, although in one double-blind study, neither oral nor intravenous nor intramuscular ampicillin significantly improved the cure rate of children with diarrhea caused by EPEC.[92] If systemic infection occurs, intravenous or intramuscular therapy should be initiated and tailored to the susceptibility pattern of the infecting pathogen.[23,93]

The role of antimicrobial therapy in the treatment of traveler's diarrhea (ETEC) is controversial. Several investigators suggest a favorable outcome of ETEC enteric infection after the use of TMP–SMX, tetracycline, bicozamycin, or the new quinolones, although the emergence of resistance has substantially complicated therapy.[37,53,62,66,94-99] Similarly, both TMP–SMX and ampicillin are considered efficacious in hemorrhagic colitis caused by the 0157:H7 serotype and enteroinvasive *E. coli*, although no placebo-controlled studies have been reported thus far.[65]

Campylobacteriosis

Campylobacter jejuni is one of the newly recognized yet most common causes of bacterial diarrhea throughout the world.[37,100] Recent laboratory studies indicate that *C. jejuni* is more frequently isolated from the stool culture of a patient with diarrhea than either *Salmonella* or *Shigella*.[100] The organism is a known commensal in the gastrointestinal tract of many animals (fowl, chickens) and is commonly spread to humans through contact with contaminated animal feces. Diagnosis requires a special selective medium, and routine cultures only occasionally reveal the presence of the organism in the stools of bacteremic patients.[29] Common symptoms of *C. jejuni* enteritis include diarrhea, fever, malaise, and abdominal pain; these symptoms rarely persist beyond one week.[100]

Although campylobacteriosis is a self-limited syndrome, patients who are ill enough to seek medical attention generally benefit from a course of antimicrobial therapy. In vitro susceptibility testing suggests sensitivity to a number of antimicrobial agents including erythromycin, tetracycline, chloramphenicol, clindamycin, and the newer quinolones, although few clinical trials have been published to date.[62,101] Of special note, campylobacteriosis does not respond to TMP–SMX. This may complicate empiric therapy of a patient who has diarrhea, since campylobacteriosis is clinically indistinguishable from shigellosis, which, as previously described, responds to TMP–SMX.[37,53]

Because of its apparent usefulness and lack of toxicity, erythromycin is recommended as the antibiotic of choice in *C. jejuni* enteritis.[102-105] One group of investigators evaluated the efficacy of erythromycin (50 mg/kg/day) in a placebo-controlled double-blind study of children with *C. jejuni* enteritis.[102] The mean number of days of diarrhea after initiation of therapy was 2.5, compared with 4.2 for patients receiving placebo. Similarly, patients continued to excrete the organism for an average of 0.5 and 2.2 days when given erythromycin and placebo, respectively. These results were superior to those achieved by other investigators who used erythromycin 40 mg/kg/day.[104,105] The investigators concluded that early high-dose therapy with erythromycin is of benefit in treating *C. jejuni* enteritis.[102]

Yersinia enterocolitica Enteritis

Yersinia enterocolitica, a gram-negative coccobacillus, is indigenous to a variety of animals including sheep, cattle, horses, and domestic animals.[106] Foodborne transmission has been suggested, since the organism has been isolated from a number of foods including meats, mussels, oysters, ice cream, bean curd, and milk.[107] The incidence of this disease appears to have increased dramatically in recent years, probably owing to the development of specialized culture techniques and improved detection.[106,108]

Y. enterocolitica enterocolitis causes symptomatology that varies with age and the physical state of the host.[106] Overall, the symptoms of fever, abdominal pain, and diarrhea lasting one to three weeks are commonly present in more than half of the diagnosed cases.[29,106,107,109] The value of anti-infective agents in this disease is unclear, since symptoms spontaneously remit in most cases. In vitro susceptibility tests demonstrate the organism's susceptibility to a variety of antimicrobial agents, including the aminoglycosides, chloramphenicol, tetracycline, TMP-SMX, and the third-generation cephalosporins.[110] The results of one placebo-controlled trial using TMP-SMX have been reported. Although TMP-SMX did not shorten the duration of illness, the period of pathogen excretion in the stool was significantly reduced. Of notable importance, the duration of illness before antimicrobial therapy was more than five days. The investigators concluded that further studies using TMP-SMX early in the course of illness are necessary to ascertain the merit of such therapeutic intervention in *Yersinia enterocolitica* infection.[105]

Infections Caused by *Vibrio* spp.

Vibrio parahemolyticus and *Vibrio cholerae* are the two major vibrio pathogens associated with human disease.[111] *Vibrio* spp. are ubiquitous in coastal waters throughout the world and most often transmitted through the ingestion of contaminated seafood.[111] *Vibrio parahemolyticus* has been implicated in major outbreaks along the Atlantic and Gulf coasts of the United States, on Caribbean cruise ships, and, most recently, in underdeveloped countries.[111] *V. parahemolyticus*, by virtue of its ability to invade the colon, can produce symptoms varying from mild gastroenteritis to a full dysenteric syndrome. Since *V. parahemolyticus* infection is often self-limited, supportive therapy is generally the only type of treatment necessary.[111] Antimicrobial therapy is not indicated, since it has not been shown to shorten the duration of illness or the period of pathogen excretion.[111,112]

Vibrio cholerae, one of the most potent causes of infectious diarrhea, was responsible for the high incidence of mortality and morbidity in Europe, Asia, and America in the nineteenth century and remains a major health problem in several areas today.[111] Compared with *Vibrio parahemolyticus*, *Vibrio cholerae* is a noninvasive pathogen with enterotoxigenic properties affecting the small intestine.[111] Cholera may appear asymptomatically or as the typical "full-blown" syndrome, which, when severe, rapidly leads to dehydration and death.[113] Interestingly, there is little clinical difference in the presentation of the patient with cholera compared with a patient infected with enterotoxigenic *E. coli* or noncholera vibrio organisms.[113] Initially, the patient experiences an increase in peristalsis, followed by several watery bowel movements often described as having a fishy odor.[113] In advanced disease, hypotension, shock, renal failure, hypokalemia, and other electrolyte imbalances may occur because of the extreme volume depletion. In severe disease it is not infrequent for greater than 70% of total body weight to be purged within seven days.[113,114]

Clearly, rehydration therapy is indicated in cholera for volume replacement and correction of hypoglycemia, electrolyte imbalances, and hypotension. In addition, antimicrobial therapy has been shown to significantly decrease diarrhea and stool volume and duration of vibrio excretion.[115-119] The preferred drug for the management of this disease is tetracycline hydrochloride (1-2 g daily for two to five days) or its congener (doxycycline).[65,113] In rare cases of tetracycline resistance, furazolidone may be used.[118] Effective alternative antimicrobial agents include chloramphenicol, erythromycin, TMP-SMX, kanamycin, and streptomycin.[65,113] In pregnant patients, cholera generally leads to spontaneous abortion, and, although not proven to decrease this risk, ampicillin (1 g daily for five days) may be the preferred drug.[113] Interestingly, because of the superiority of tetracycline in *Vibrio cholerae* infection, several experts consider it the treatment of choice in infected children and adults. Such a short course of therapy does not seem to be associated with the drug's known effects on the tooth and bone development of children.[65]

Although of little concern historically, it is now accepted that non-O1 serogroup *Vibrio cholerae* are also capable of producing diarrheal illness, which may range from mild traveler's diarrhea to a severe syndrome indistinguishable from that produced by *V. cholerae*. Non-O1 *Vibrio cholerae* result in enteric infection after ingestion of large quantities of contaminated food or drink. Antimicrobial therapy is not indicated in the majority of infected patients, since it has not been shown to reduce the duration of illness.[111] Electrolyte replacement therapy is recommended, however, in those patients who are severely fluid depleted.[111]

Food Poisoning

The diagnosis of food poisoning is considered when an enteric or neurologic illness develops in more than two patients who have consumed the same meal in the past 72 hours.[93] Since food poisoning can result from the ingestion of any one of a variety of virulent microbes, as well as from ingestion of certain chemicals (e.g., heavy metals), the reader is referred to an in-depth review of this topic elsewhere.[93,120] This discussion will be limited to three major bacterial pathogens commonly implicated in the development of food poisoning.

Ingestion of food containing a preformed toxin is responsible for the development of *Staphylococcus aureus* food poisoning.[93] This heat-stable toxin is most commonly elaborated by the organism in improperly stored dairy products or meats and is unaffected by common cooking and reheating temperatures.[29] Clinical onset of symptoms, including severe nausea, vomiting, and diarrhea, follows a relatively short incubation period of approximately two to six hours after ingestion of the preformed toxin.[29]

Bacillus cereus food poisoning can be either of two varieties.[93] Disease may result from ingestion of food containing a preformed toxin similar to that previously described with *Staph. aureus* (short-incubation "emetic" syndrome) or ingestion of the pathogen in food may result in enterotoxin production in the intestine.[121,122] The latter syndrome is associated with a longer incubation period (long-incubation "diarrhea" syndrome) and is not considered an intoxication.[93]

Similar to the "long-incubation" *B. cereus* food poisoning, *Clostridium perfringens* food poisoning also results from ingestion of the organism, which elaborates its toxin in vivo.[93] Once in the bowel, *C. perfringens* organisms multiply and produce a diarrhea-forming enterotoxin.[93] Although nausea may occur, the most common symptoms of *C. perfringens* food poisoning are diarrhea and abdominal cramps.[93]

Since all three diarrheal illnesses spontaneously remit within one day, most experts recommend supportive care (oral rehydration) as the mainstay of therapy in most cases of food poisoning.[29,93] In addition, since *Staph. aureus* and short-incubation *B. cereus* food poisoning are considered intoxications rather than infections, antimicrobial therapy is of little value.[29,93]

Clostridium difficile Enteritis

Antibiotic-associated diarrhea is an intestinal syndrome that may occur as an adverse effect of therapy with almost any antimicrobial agent, regardless of the route of administration.[29,123] This disease ranges from a benign self-limiting entity associated with an alteration in normal bowel flora that readily reverses upon discontinuation of the offending agent, to a more serious and potentially fatal form known as pseudomembranous colitis (PMC).[123] Although severe cases were originally attributed to *Staph. aureus* infection, *Clostridium difficile* is now the most frequently recognized cause of PMC in high-risk groups (e.g., the elderly, women, and immunocompromised hosts).[124-126] *Clostridium difficile* elaborates toxins (A or B) and other antigenic substances within the intestinal lumen that are responsible for the typical pseudomembranous inflammatory lesions of PMC.[29,126]

The range of symptoms of *C. difficile* colitis (PMC) vary widely.[126] Profuse watery or mucoid-green foul-smelling diarrhea may develop during the course of antibiotic therapy, although in more than 30% of cases, symptoms do not begin until after treatment has been discontinued.[123,126] Diagnosis of *C. difficile* diarrhea is confirmed by laboratory tests assaying for the presence of toxins in the stool.[29,123] Isolation of the organism itself from the stool is of little value, since a majority of healthy newborns and adults may be asymptomatic carriers.[123,124]

While treatment of antibiotic-associated (benign) diarrhea simply involves removal of the offending agent(s), management of PMC requires eradication of the causative organism, *C. difficile*.[127] In vitro susceptibility testing has demonstrated reliable inhibition of *C. difficile* by bacitracin, erythromycin, tetracycline, ampicillin, and several cephalosporins, although the agent considered most effective is oral vancomycin.

Clinical studies suggest that a 10-day course of oral vancomycin (125–250 mg as the hydrochloride salt every six hours) suppresses *C. difficile* and shortens the course of illness, since improvement of symptoms is usually observed within 24 hours.[29,123,128-130] Relapses, which occur in up to 25% of treated patients, are managed effectively with a repeat course of oral vancomycin.[29,131] Intravenous vancomycin is of little value because of its minimal distribution to the bowel after this route of administration.[128-130]

Metronidazole, in doses of 1 g daily for 10 days, is a less expensive alternative treatment.[132,133] However, unlike oral vancomycin, oral metronidazole is systemically absorbed, thereby decreasing the concentration of drug at the site of action and increasing the risk of the development of adverse effects. Further, metronidazole has been implicated as a cause of antibiotic-associated colitis and should therefore be reserved as a second-line agent in mildly to moderately ill patients who cannot receive vancomycin.[134]

Cholestyramine resin, an anion exchange resin originally used as the primary agent in managing antibiotic-associated colitis, binds and inactivates *C. difficile* toxin in the bowel.[29,135] It is also suggested that cholestyramine resin firms the stool through its natural moisture-absorbing ability.[29,135] However, since this form of treatment does not eliminate the pathogen itself, it is reserved as a third-line drug for mild forms of disease.[29,123] Additionally, since cholestyramine resin may bind concurrently administered antimicrobial agents, combination therapy with a drug such as vancomycin should be avoided.[136]

Several patients with *C. difficile* colitis have responded to treatment with oral bacitracin (100,000 units daily in four equally divided doses) administered for 7 to 19 days. Although it is less expensive than the other agents, bacitracin must be specially prepared in capsule form for oral consumption. From a clinical perspective, there have been suggestions that strains resistant to bacitracin may exist.[123] In addition, the safety and degree of absorption in patients with inflamed intestinal mucosa are not well documented; therefore, other forms of therapy are more frequently prescribed.[123]

Prophylaxis of Traveler's Diarrhea

It is well documented that enteric infection of travelers at high risk can be minimized.[43,84,96,137–139] Available data suggest that definite protection is afforded the person previously treated with nonantimicrobial therapy such as bismuth subsalicylate,[138] or antimicrobial therapy such as doxycycline,[43] TMP-SMX,[139] norfloxacin,[79,85] and bicozamycin.[79,85] The advantage of using doxycycline is its long half-life, which permits daily dosing. Bicozamycin has limited absorption and may not cause serious systemic adverse effects. A benefit in using either bicozamycin or the quinolones is that both are active against *Campylobacter* species, a frequent pathogen.[62,79,85] Table 7 outlines the dosing schedules for prophylaxis with these agents. Protection lasts for only as long as the drugs are being taken, however.[140] Regardless of the apparent merit associated with prophylaxis of the traveler, a National Institutes of Health consensus development panel suggested that travelers should not be encouraged to use chemoprophylaxis in preventing diarrhea.[141] Such recommendations were developed based on the known incidence of adverse effects associated with the various agents employed and the potential for the development of resistant strains after their use.[37] The data, however, are continuously being re-evaluated and are admittedly anecdotal.[140,142] In general, chemoprophylaxis is recommended for a traveler at high risk (e.g., achlorhydric patients and those using antacids or H_2-receptor antagonists) when the period of risk will not exceed two weeks.[37] Beyond two weeks, such prophylaxis may be associated with an increased risk of adverse effects or elimination of normal intestinal flora. Further, the patient should be informed of the potential for adverse effects associated with the agent employed (Table 7).

Table 7.
Chemoprophylaxis of Traveler's Diarrhea[44,85,86,97,138–140]

Agent	Oral Dosage[a]	Major Adverse Effects
Doxycycline	100 mg (daily)	Nausea, vomiting, abdominal cramping, increased skin sensitivity to sunlight
Trimethoprim–sulfamethoxazole	160 mg (daily)[b]	Diarrhea, skin rash
Trimethoprim	200 mg (daily)	Skin rash, headache
Bismuth subsalicylate	60 mL (4 times daily) or 1.05 g (3 tablets daily)	Dizziness, nausea, constipation, tinnitus

[a] Treatment should continue for duration of trip and at least two days after returning home; period of prophylaxis should not exceed two weeks.
[b] Dose based on trimethoprim component.

Protection from enteric infection while traveling also involves behavioral modification. Travelers are advised to assume that tap water and ice are not safe for consumption unless specifically deemed otherwise by the proper health authorities.[143] Water for drinking can be disinfected by boiling (three to five minutes) or by adding either 5% chlorine bleach (two drops or 1 mL) or 2% tincture of iodine (0.25 mL).[143] Wine, beer, other nonmixed alcoholic beverages, and carbonated bottled beverages are generally considered safe. Similarly, coffee and tea are safe if consumed while very hot.[143] The traveler should also be informed that contaminated water can be ingested while swimming.[143]

Food should be well cooked and hot when served. Boiling and baking eliminate several well-known intrinsic food pathogens, although preformed toxins (*Staph. aureus*) resist common cooking temperatures, as previously described.[143] Vegetables and fruits are considered safe for consumption if they are peeled before ingestion. Travelers should be warned against consuming dairy products unless assured by the proper authorities that the products have been properly pasteurized and refrigerated.[143]

Future Modalities

Novel strategies are being employed in the prevention and treatment of enteric infections. Bacteriophages have been effective in preventing experimentally induced EPEC infections in animals,[144] although their value in the treatment of human infections requires additional study.[145] Several authorities hypothesize that expansion of the antimicrobial spectrum of activity of the bacteriophage will enhance its future usefulness in the management of enteric infection.[146]

The antidiarrheal properties of a number of compounds have been evaluated and include nicotinic acid,[147] indomethacin,[148] phenothiazines and thioxanthines,[149,150] berberine,[151] glucocorticoids,[152] amphotericin B,[153] somatostatin,[154] and α agonists.[155,156] Of these preparations, berberine, α-adrenergic agonists, and enkephalins appear promising. Berberine, a plant alkaloid, was an ancient remedy that recently regained attention when its use resulted in improvement in infections caused by ETEC and *V. cholerae*.[151,157] The newly developed α-adrenergic agonist lidamidine appears to reduce stool volume and frequency in infectious diarrhea of various etiology. Moreover, lidamidine rarely produces cardiovascular adverse effects typically observed with other compounds of its class.[155,156,158] An enkephalin anologue (BW-942C) may have a physiologic role in the control of intestinal ion transport with its ability to reduce stool frequency and abdominal cramping. Further, it appears to be well tolerated in the high doses required for treatment.[159]

Finally, the new era of genetic engineering has resulted in the unfolding of a number of promising new vaccines against enteric infection. Recent work has resulted in the development of new vaccines or improvement of currently available vaccines against cholera,[14,160,161] typhoid fever,[162] shigellosis,[163] rotavirus,[164] and infections caused by various strains of *E. coli*.[165,166] Future research will determine the most appropriate role, if any, of these newly developed vaccines.

Conclusion

Infectious diarrhea is common in both industrialized and nonindustrialized areas of the world. Host factors such as extreme age, gastrointestinal-tract dysfunction, and immunodeficiency states increase the risk of illness after ingestion of a pathogen or its toxin. Microbial virulence factors—the pathogen's ability to invade the bowel wall or produce enterotoxins, neurotoxins, or cytotoxins—are important determinants of the clinical manifestations of diarrheal syndromes. Infectious diarrhea is often self-limited and of short duration. Thus, therapy frequently consists of symptomatic relief and fluid replacement. Rehydration is the mainstay of therapy. Antimicrobial therapy is beneficial in the treatment of severe diarrhea caused by *Shigella*, *Campylobacter* spp., *Vibrio cholerae*, *Escherichia coli*, and *Clostridium difficile*.

References

1. Walsh JA, Warren KW. Selective primary health care: an interim strategy for disease control in developing countries. *N Engl J Med*. 1979; 301:967–74.
2. Hodgkin K. Towards earlier diagnosis. A family doctor's approach. Baltimore: Williams & Wilkins; 1963.
3. Anon. The ten leading causes of death for selected countries in Africa, South and Central America and Asia. *World Health Stat Rep*. 1974; 27:150–2.
4. Black RE, Merson MH, Huq I et al. Incidence and severity of rotavirus and *E. coli* diarrhea in rural Bangladesh. Implications for vaccine development. *Lancet*. 1981; 1:141–3.
5. Guerrant RL, Kirchhoff LV, Sheilds DS et al. Prospective study of diarrheal illness in northeastern Brazil: patterns of disease, nutritional impact, etiologies and risk factors. *J Infect Dis*. 1983; 148:986–97.
6. Steffen R, Van der Linde F, Gyr K et al. Epidemiology of diarrhea in travelers. *JAMA*. 1983; 249:1176–80.
7. Gottlieb MS, Groopman JE, Weinstein WM et al. The acquired immunodeficiency syndrome. *Ann Intern Med*. 1983; 99:208–20.
8. Soave R, Danner RL, Honig CI et al. Cryptosporidiosis in homosexual men. *Ann Intern Med*. 1984; 100:504–11.
9. Giannella RA, Broitman SA, Zamcheck N. Gastric acid barrier to ingested microorganisms. Studies in vivo and in vitro. *Gut*. 1972; 13:251–6.
10. DuPont HL, Homick RB. Adverse effect of Lomotil therapy in shigellosis. *JAMA*. 1973; 226:1525–8.
11. Price DJE, Sleigh JD. Control of infection due to *Klebsiella aerogenes* in a neurosurgical unit by withdrawal of all antibiotics. *Lancet*. 1970; 2:1213–5.
12. Guerrant RL. Principles and definition of syndromes. In: Mandell GL, Douglas RG Jr, Bennett JE, eds. Principles and practice of infectious disease. New York: John Wiley & Sons; 1985: 635–46.
13. Gurwith J, Wenamm W, Hinde D et al. A prospective study of rotavirus infection in infants and children. *J Infect Dis*. 1981; 144:218–24.
14. Levine MM, Edelman R. Enteropathogenic *Escherichia coli* of classic serotypes associated with infant diarrhea: epidemiology and pathogenesis. *Epidemiol Rev*. 1984; 6:31–51.
15. Anon. Salmonella surveillance summary for 1980. Atlanta: Centers for Disease Control; 1982.
16. Gordon AG. Breast feeding. *JAMA*. 1986; 256:3215.
17. Hornick RB, Musik SI, Wenzel R et al. The Broad Street pump revisited: response of volunteers to ingested cholera vibrios. *Bull NY Acad Med*. 1971; 47:1181–91.
18. Higgins JA, Code CF, Orvis AL. The influence of motility on the rate of absorption of sodium and water from the small intestine of healthy persons. *Gastroenterology*. 1956; 31:708–16.
19. Formal SB, Abrams GD, Schneider H et al. Experimental *Shigella* infections. VI. Role of the small intestine in an experimental infection in guinea pigs. *J Bacteriol*. 1963; 85:119–25.
20. Mentzing LO, Ringertz O. Salmonella infection in tourists. 2. Prophylaxis against salmonellosis. *Acta Pathol Microbiol Scand*. 1968; 74:405–13.
21. Bohnhoff M, Miller CP, Martin WR. Resistance of the mouse's intestinal tract to experimental salmonella infections. *J Exp Med*. 1964; 120:805–16.
22. Schrank GD, Verwey WF. Distribution of cholera organisms in experimental *Vibrio cholerae* infections: proposed mechanisms of pathogenesis and antibacterial immunity. *Infect Immun*. 1976; 13:195–203.
23. Guerrant RL, Hughes JM. Nausea, vomiting, and non-inflammatory diarrhea. In: Mandell GL, Douglas RG Jr, Bennett JE, eds. Principles and practice of infectious disease. New York: John Wiley & Sons; 1985:646–55.
24. Jones EG, Brown WR. Serum and intestinal fluid immunoglobulins in patients with giardiasis. *Am J Dig Dis*. 1974; 19:791–6.
25. Zinneman HH, Kaplan AP. The association of giardiasis with reduced intestinal secretory immunoglobulin A. *Am J Dig Dis*. 1972; 17:793–7.
26. Ament ME, Ochs HD, Davis SD. Structure and function of the gastrointestinal tract in primary immunodeficiency syndromes. A study of 9 patients. *Medicine*. 1973; 52:227–48.
27. Hermans PE, Huizenga KA, Hoffman HN et al. Dysgammaglobulinemia associated with nodular lymphoid hyperplasia of the small intestine. *Am J Med*. 1966; 40:78–89.
28. Yolken RH, Bishop CA, Townsend TR et al. Infectious gastroenteritis in bone-marrow-transplant recipients. *N Engl J Med*. 1982; 306:1009–12.
29. Hruska JF. Gastrointestinal and intraabdominal infections. In: Reese RE, Douglas RG Jr, eds. A practical approach to infectious diseases. Boston: Little, Brown and Company; 1986:284–326.
30. Salit IE, Gostchlich EC. Type 1 *Escherichia coli* pili: characterization of binding to monkey kidney cells. *J Exp Med*. 1977; 146:1182–94.
31. Chen LC, Rohde JE, Sharp GWG. Intestinal adenyl-cyclase activity in human cholera. *Lancet*. 1971; 1:939–41.
32. Guerrant RL, Chen LC, Sharp GWG. Intestinal adenyl-cyclase in canine cholera: correlation with fluid accumulation. *J Infect Dis*. 1972; 125:377–81.
33. Johnson WM, Lior H, Bezanson GS. Cytotoxic *Escherichia coli* 0157:H7 associated with hemorrhagic colitis in Canada. *Lancet*. 1983; 1: 76. Letter.
34. Guerrant RL, Shields DS, Thorson SM et al. Evaluation and diagnosis of acute infectious diarrhea. *Am J Med*. 1985; 78:91–8.
35. Cantey JR. Infectious diarrhea. Pathogenesis and risk factors. *Am J Med*. 1985; 78:65–75.
36. Nelson JD. Etiology and epidemiology of diarrheal disease in the United States. *Am J Med*. 1985; 78:76–80.

37. DuPont HL. Nonfluid therapy and selected chemoprophylaxis of acute diarrhea. *Am J Med*. 1985; 78(Suppl 6B):81–90.
38. Guerrant R. Diagnosis and fluid therapy of acute diarrhea. *Am J Med*. 1985; 78(Suppl 6B):91–8.
39. Harris JC, Dupont HL, Hornick RB. Fecal leukocytes in diarrheal illness. *Ann Intern Med*. 1972; 76:697–703.
40. Sack RB, Pierce NF, Sirschorn N. The current status of oral therapy in the treatment of acute diarrheal illness. *Am J Clin Nutr*. 1978; 31:2251–7.
41. Santosham M, Daum RS, Dillman L et al. Oral rehydration therapy of infantile diarrhea. *N Engl J Med*. 1982; 306:1070–6.
42. Hirschhorn N. The treatment of acute diarrhea in children. A historical and physiological perspective. *Am J Clin Nutr*. 1980; 33:637–9.
43. Sack RB. Antimicrobial prophylaxis of traveller's diarrhea: a summary of studies using doxycycline or trimethoprim and sulfamethoxazole. *Scand J Gastroenterol*. 1982; 18:111–7.
44. Nalin DR, Cash RA. Oral therapy for diarrhea. *Lancet*. 1977; 1:1059–60.
45. Kjelmann B, Ronge E. Oral solutions for gastroenteritis—optimal glucose concentration. *Arch Dis Child*. 1982; 57:313–5.
46. Nalin DR, Levine MM, Mata L et al. Oral rehydration and maintenance of children with rotavirus and bacterial diarrhoeas. *Bull WHO*. 1979; 57:453–9.
47. Anon. Treatment of cryptosporidiosis in patients with acquired immunodeficiency syndrome (AIDS). *MMWR*. 1984; 33:117–9.
48. Vanderhoof JA, Hovancsak CF, Baldwin JN. Acute vomiting and diarrhea in infancy. *US Pharmacist*. 1981; 6:33–40.
49. Finberg L. The role of oral electrolyte-glucose solutions in hydration for children—international and domestic aspects. *J Pediatr*. 1980; 96:51–4.
50. U.S. Department of Health and Human Services. Health information for the international traveler. Washington, DC: U.S. Government Printing Office, 1987; HHS publication no. (CDC) 85-8280.
51. Johnson PC, Ericsson CD, DuPont HL et al. Comparison of loperamide with bismuth subsalicylate for the treatment of acute traveler's diarrhea. *JAMA*. 1986; 255:757–60.
52. Kachel G, Ruppin H, Hagel H et al. Human intestinal motor activity and transport: effects of a synthetic opiate. *Gastroenterology*. 1986; 90:85–93.
53. DuPont HL. Shigella species (bacillary dysentery). In: Mandell GL, Douglas RG Jr, Bennett JE, eds. Principles and practice of infectious disease. New York: John Wiley & Sons, 1985:1269–74.
54. Reves R, Bass P, DuPont HL et al. Failure to demonstrate effectiveness of an anticholinergic drug in the symptomatic treatment of acute traveler's diarrhea. *J Clin Gastroenterol*. 1983; 5:223–7.
55. DuPont HL, Sullivan P, Pickering LK et al. Symptomatic treatment of diarrhea with bismuth subsalicylate among students attending a Mexican university. *Gastroenterology*. 1977; 73:715–8.
56. Merson M, Morris GK, Sack DA et al. Travelers' diarrhea in Mexico: a prospective study of physicians and family members attending a congress. *N Engl J Med*. 1976; 294:1299–305.
57. Ericsson CD, Evans DG, DuPont HL et al. Bismuth subsalicylate inhibits activity of crude toxins of *Escherichia coli* and *Vibrio cholerae*. *J Infect Dis*. 1977; 136:693–6.
58. Pickering LK, Feldman S, Ericsson CD et al. Absorption of salicylate and bismuth from a bismuth subsalicylate-containing compound (Pepto-Bismol). *J Pediatr*. 1981; 99:654–6.
59. DuPont HL. Bismuth subsalicylate in the treatment and prevention of diarrheal disease. *Drug Intell Clin Pharm*. 1987; 21:687–93.
60. Graham DY, Estes MK, Gentry LO. Double-blind comparison of bismuth subsalicylate and placebo in the prevention and treatment of enterotoxigenic *Escherichia coli*-induced diarrhea in volunteers. *Gastroenterology*. 1983; 85:1017–22.
61. Portnoy D, Whiteside ME, Buckley E III et al. Treatment of intestinal cryptosporidiosis with spiramycin. *Ann Intern Med*. 1984; 101:202–4.
62. Carlson JR, Thornton SA, DuPont HL et al. Comparative in vitro activity of ten antimicrobial agents against bacterial enteropathogens. *Antimicrob Agents Chemother*. 1983; 24:509–13.
63. Anders B, Lauer BA, Paisley JW et al. Double-blind placebo controlled trial of erythromycin for treatment of campylobacter enteritis. *Lancet*. 1982; 1:131–2.
64. Merson MH, Sack RB, Islam S et al. Disease due to enterotoxigenic *E. coli* in Bangladeshi adults: clinical aspects and a controlled trial of tetracycline. *J Infect Dis*. 1980; 141:702–11.
65. Levine MM. Antimicrobial therapy for infectious diarrhea. *Rev Infect Dis*. 1986; 8(Suppl 2):S207–16.
66. DuPont HL, Reves RR, Galindo E et al. Treatment of traveler's diarrhea with trimethoprim/sulfamethoxazole and with trimethoprim alone. *N Engl J Med*. 1982; 307:841–4.
67. Schulman JA, Schlossberg D. Differential diagnosis of infectious causes of diarrhea. In: Handbook for differential diagnosis of infectious diseases. New York: Appleton-Century-Crofts; 1980:57–67.
68. Rosenthal SJ. Exacerbation of salmonella enteritis due to ampicillin. *N Engl J Med*. 1969; 280:147–8.
69. Aserkoff B, Bennett JV. Effect of antibiotic therapy in acute salmonellosis on the fecal excretion of salmonellae. *N Engl J Med*. 1969; 281:636–40.
70. Glaser JB, Morgon-Kute L, Berger SR et al. Recurrent *Salmonella typhimurium* bacteremia associated with the acquired immunodeficiency syndrome. *Ann Intern Med*. 1985; 102:189–93.
71. Hook EW. Salmonellosis: certain factors influencing the interaction of salmonella and the human host. *Bull NY Acad Med*. 1961; 37:499–512.
72. Cherubin CE, Neu HC, Imperato PJ et al. Septicemia with non-typhoid salmonella. *Medicine*. 1974; 53:365–76.
73. Pillay N, Adams EB, Coombes DN. Comparative trial of amoxycillin and chloramphenicol in treatment of typhoid fever in adults. *Lancet*. 1975; 2:333–5.
74. Snyder MJ, Perroni J, Gonzalez O et al. Trimethoprim-sulfamethoxazole in the treatment of typhoid and paratyphoid fevers. *J Infect Dis*. 1973; 128(Suppl):S734–7.
75. Nolan CM, White PC Jr. Treatment of typhoid carriers with amoxicillin. Correlates of successful therapy. *JAMA*. 1978; 239:2352–4.
76. Hudson SJ, Ingham HR, Snow MH. Treatment of *Salmonella typhi* carrier state with ciprofloxacin. *Lancet*. 1985; 1:1047. Letter.
77. Bryan JP, Rocha H, Scheld WM. Problems in salmonellosis: rationale for clinical trials with newer beta lactam agents and quinolones. *Rev Infect Dis*. 1986; 8:189–207.
78. Weissman JB, Gangaroasa EJ, DuPont HL et al. Shigellosis: to treat or not to treat. *JAMA*. 1974; 229:1215–6.
79. DuPont HL, Ericsson CD, Reves RR et al. Antimicrobial therapy for traveler's diarrhea. *Rev Infect Dis*. 1986; 8(Suppl 2):S217–22.
80. Haltalin KC, Nelson JD, Hinton LV et al. Comparison of orally absorbable and nonabsorbable antibiotics in shigellosis: a double-blind study with ampicillin and neomycin. *J Pediatr*. 1968; 72:708–20.
81. Cheever FS. The treatment of shigellosis with antibiotics. *Ann NY Acad Sci*. 1952; 55:1063–9.
82. Haltalin KC, Nelson JD. Failure of furazolidine therapy in shigellosis. *Am J Dis Child*. 1972; 123:40–4.
83. Nelson JD, Haltalin KC. Comparative efficacy of cephalexin and ampicillin for shigellosis and other types of acute diarrhea in infants and children. *Antimicrob Agents Chemother*. 1975; 7:415–20.
84. Barada FA Jr, Guerrant RL. Sulfamethoxazole/trimethoprim versus ampicillin in the treatment of acute invasive diarrhea in adults. *Antimicrob Agents Chemother*. 1980; 17:961–4.

85. DuPont HL, Ericsson CD, Johnson PC et al. Antimicrobial agents in the prevention of traveler's diarrhea. *Rev Infect Dis.* 1986; 8:S167–71.
86. Rogerie F, Ott D, Vandepitte J et al. Comparison of norfloxacin and nalidixic acid for treatment of dysentery caused by *Shigella dysenteriae* type 1 in adults. *Antimicrob Agents Chemother.* 1986; 29:883–6.
87. Feldman A. Southwestern Internal Medicine Conference: traveler's diarrhea. *Am J Med Sci.* 1984; 288:136–48.
88. DuPont HL. Gastrointestinal infections. In: Stein JH, eds. Internal medicine. Boston/Toronto: Little, Brown, and Company, 1987:1511–20.
89. Nelson JD. Duration of neomycin therapy for enteropathogenic *Escherichia coli* diarrheal disease: a comparative study of 113 cases. *Pediatrics.* 1971; 48:248–58.
90. South MA. Enteropathogenic *Escherichia coli* disease: new developments and perspectives. *J Pediatr.* 1971; 79:1–11.
91. Thoren A, Wolde-Mariam T, Stintzing G et al. Antibiotics in the treatment of gastroenteritis caused by enteropathogenic *E. coli. J Infect Dis.* 1980; 141:27–31.
92. De Olarte GD, Trujillo H, Agudelo N et al. Treatment of diarrhea in malnourished infants and children. A double-blind study comparing ampicillin and placebo. *Am J Dis Child.* 1974; 127:379–88.
93. Hughes JM. Food poisoning. In: Mandell GL, Douglas RG Jr, Bennett JE, eds. Principles and practice of infectious disease. New York: John Wiley & Sons; 1985:680–91.
94. Black R, Levine MM, Clements ML et al. Treatment of experimentally induced enterotoxigenic *Escherichia coli* diarrhea with trimethoprim, trimethoprim/sulfamethoxazole, or placebo. *Rev Infect Dis.* 1982; 2:540–5.
95. DuPont HL, West AH, Evans DG et al. Antimicrobial susceptibility of enterotoxigenic *Escherichia coli. J Antimicrob Chemother.* 1978; 4:100–2.
96. Ericsson CD, DuPont HL, Sullivan P et al. Bicozamycin, a poorly absorbable antibiotic, effectively treats traveler's diarrhea. *Ann Intern Med.* 1983; 98:20–5.
97. Echeverria P, Verhaert L, Ulyangco CV et al. Antimicrobial resistance and enterotoxin production among isolates of *Escherichia coli* in the Far East. *Lancet.* 1978; 2:589–92.
98. Echeverria P, Murphy JR. Enterotoxigenic *Escherichia coli* carrying plasmids coding for antibiotic resistance and enterotoxin production. *J Infect Dis.* 1980; 142:273–8.
99. Sack RB, Santosham M, Froehlich JL et al. Doxycycline prophylaxis of traveler's diarrhea in Honduras, an area where resistance to doxycycline is common among enterotoxigenic *Escherichia coli. Am J Trop Med Hyg.* 1984; 33:460–6.
100. Blaser MJ, Reller B. Campylobacter enteritis. *N Engl J Med.* 1981; 305:1444–52.
101. Pichler HET, Diridl G, Stickler K et al. Clinical efficacy of ciprofloxacin compared with placebo in bacterial diarrhea. *Am J Med.* 1987; 82:S329–32.
102. Salazar-Lindo E, Sack RB, Chea-Woo E et al. Early treatment with erythromycin of *Campylobacter jejuni*-associated dysentery in children. In: Proceedings of the 21st Joint Conference (U.S.-Japan). Bethesda, MD: Cooperative Medical Science Program on Cholera; 1985.
103. Schwartz RH, Bryan RC, Rodriguez WJ et al. Experience with the microbiological diagnosis of campylobacter enteritis in an office laboratory. *Pediatr Infect Dis.* 1983; 2:298–301.
104. Robins-Browne RM, Mackenjee MKR, Bodasing MN et al. Treatment of campylobacter-associated enteritis with erythromycin. *Am J Dis Child.* 1983; 137:282–5.
105. Pai CH, Gillis F, Tuomanen E et al. Erythromycin in the treatment of campylobacter enteritis in children. *Am J Dis Child.* 1983; 137:286–8.
106. Boyce JM. *Yersinia* species. In: Mandell GL, Douglas RG Jr, Bennett JE, eds. Principles and practice of infectious disease. New York: John Wiley & Sons; 1985:1296–1301.
107. Black RE, Jackson RJ, Tsai T et al. Epidemic *Yersinia enterocolitica* infection due to contaminated chocolate milk. *N Engl J Med.* 1978; 298:76–9.
108. Kohl S. *Yersinia enterocolitica.* A significant "new" pathogen. *Hosp Pract.* 1978; 13:81–5.
109. Marks MI, Pai CH, LaFleur L et al. *Yersinia enterocolitica* gastroenteritis. A prospective study of clinical, bacteriologic, and epidemiologic features. *J Pediatr.* 1980; 96:26–31.
110. Scribner RK, Marks MI, Weber et al. *Yersinia enterocolitica:* comparative in vitro activities of seven new beta lactam antibiotics. *Antimicrob Agents Chemother.* 1982; 22: 140–1.
111. Carpenter CCJ. Other pathogenic vibrios. In: Mandell GL, Douglas RG Jr, Bennett JE, eds. Principles and practice of infectious disease. New York: John Wiley & Sons, 1985:1218–21.
112. Bolen JL, Zamiska SA, Greenough WB. Clinical features in enteritis due to *Vibrio parahemolyticus. Am J Med.* 1974; 57: 638–41.
113. Greenough WB III. *Vibrio cholerae.* In: Mandell GL, Douglas RG Jr, Bennett JE, eds. Principles and practice of infectious disease. New York: John Wiley & Sons, 1985:1209–18.
114. Hirschorn N, Kinzie JL, Sachar DB et al. Decrease in net stool output during intestinal perfusion with glucose-containing solutions. *N Engl J Med.* 1968;279:176–81.
115. Carpenter CCJ, Barua D, Wallace CK et al. Clinical studies in Asiatic cholera. IV. Antibiotic therapy in cholera. *Bull Johns Hopkins Hosp.* 1966; 118:216–29.
116. Glass RI, Huq I, Alim ARM et al. Emergence of multiply antibiotic-resistant *Vibrio cholerae* in Bangladesh. *J Infect Dis.* 1980; 142:939–42.
117. Pierce NF, Banwell JG, Mitra RC et al. Controlled comparison of tetracycline and furazolidine in cholera. *Br Med J.* 1968; 3:277–80.
118. Mhalu FS, Mmari PW, Ijumba J. Rapid emergence of El Tor *Vibrio cholerae* resistant to antimicrobial agents during the first six months of fourth cholera epidemic in Tasmania. *Lancet.* 1979; 1:345–7.
119. Wallace CK, Anderson PN, Brown TC et al. Optimal antibiotic therapy in cholera. *Bull WHO.* 1968; 39:239–45.
120. Sours HE, Smith DG. Outbreak of foodborne disease in the United States, 1972-1978. *J Infect Dis.* 1980; 142:122–5.
121. Mortimer PR, McCann G. Food poisoning episodes associated with *Bacillus cereus* in fried rice. *Lancet.* 1974; 1:1043–5.
122. Terranova W, Blake PA. *Bacillus cereus* food poisoning. *N Engl J Med.* 1978; 298:143–4.
123. Fekety R. Antibiotic-associated colitis. In: Mandell GL, Douglas RG Jr, Bennett JE, eds. Principles and practice of infectious disease. New York: John Wiley & Sons, 1985:655–60.
124. Fekety R, Kim KH, Brown D et al. Epidemiology of antibiotic associated colitis. Isolation of *Clostridium difficile* from the hospital environment. *Am J Med.* 1981; 70:906–8.
125. Larson HE, Price AB, Honour P et al. *Clostridium difficile* and the aetiology of pseudomembranous colitis. *Lancet.* 1978; 1:1063–6.
126. Bartlett JG. Antibiotic-associated pseudomembranous colitis. *Rev Infect Dis.* 1979; 1:530–9.
127. Keighley MRB, Burdon DW, Arabi Y et al. Randomised controlled trial of vancomycin for pseudomembranous colitis and postoperative diarrhea. *Br Med J.* 1978; 2:1667–9.
128. Fekety R, Silva J, Toshniwal R et al. Antibiotic-associated colitis. Effects of antibiotics upon *Clostridium difficile* and the disease in hamsters. *Rev Infect Dis.* 1979; 1:386–97.
129. Silva J, Batts DH, Fekety R. Treatment of *Clostridium difficile* colitis and diarrhea with oral vancomycin. *Am J Med.* 1981; 71:815–22.
130. Tedesco F, Markham R, Gurwith M et al. Oral vancomycin for antibiotic associated pseudomembranous colitis. *Lancet.* 1978; 2:226–8.
131. Bartlett JS. Treatment of antibiotic-associated pseudomembranous colitis. *Rev Infect Dis.* 1984; 6:S235–41.
132. Cherry RD, Portnoy D, Jabbari M et al. Metronidazole: an alternate therapy for antibiotic-associated colitis. *Gastroenterology.* 1982; 82:849–51.
133. Teasley DG, Gerding DN, Olsen MM et al. Prospective

randomized trial of metronidazole versus vancomycin for *Clostridium difficile*-associated diarrhea and colitis. *Lancet*. 1983; 2:1043–6.
134. Saginur R, Hawler CR, Bartlett JG. Colitis associated with metronidazole therapy. *J Infect Dis*. 1980; 141:772–4.
135. Kreutzer EW, Milligan FD. Treatment of antibiotic-associated pseudomembranous colitis with cholestyramine resin. *Johns Hopkins Med J*. 1978; 143:67–72.
136. King CY, Barriere SL. Analysis of the in vitro interaction between vancomycin and cholestyramine. *Antimicrob Agents Chemother*. 1981; 19:326–7.
137. Kean BH. The diarrhea of travelers to Mexico: summary of five year study. *Ann Intern Med* 1963; 59:605–14.
138. DuPont HL, Sullivan P, Evans DG et al. Prevention of traveller's diarrhea (emporiatric enteritis): prophylactic administration of subsalicylate bismuth. *JAMA*. 1980; 243:237–41.
139. DuPont HL, Galindo E, Evans DG et al. Prevention of traveler's diarrhea with trimethoprim-sulfamethoxazole and trimethoprim alone. *Gastroenterology*. 1983; 84:75–80.
140. Sack RB. Antimicrobial prophylaxis of traveler's diarrhea: a selected summary. *Rev Infect Dis*. 1986; 8:S160–6.
141. Anon. Consensus conference: traveler's diarrhea. *JAMA*. 1985; 253:2700–4.
142. Forestier C, Darfeuille-Michaud A, Jolly B. Effects of antibiotics on adhesion of enterotoxigenic *Escherichia coli* strains. *Eur J Clin Microbiol*. 1984; 3: 427–32.
143. Blaser MJ. Environmental interventions for the prevention of traveler's diarrhea. *Rev Infect Dis*. 1986; 8:S142–9.
144. Smith HW, Huggins MB. Effectiveness of phages in treating experimental *Escherichia coli* diarrhoea in calves, piglets and lambs. *J Gen Microbiol*. 1983; 129:2659–75.
145. Marcuk LM, Nikiforov VN, Scerbak JAF et al. Clinical studies of the use of bacteriophage in the treatment of cholera. *Bull WHO*. 1971; 45:77–83.
146. Edelman R. Prevention and treatment of infectious diarrhea. *Am J Med*. 1985; 78(Suppl):99–106.
147. Rabbani GH, Butler T, Bardhan PK et al. Reduction of fluid loss in cholera by nicotinic acid: a randomized controlled trial. *Lancet*. 1983; 2:1439–42.
148. Giannella RA, Gots RE, Charney AN et al. Pathogenesis of salmonella-mediated intestinal fluid secretion: activation of adenylate cyclase and inhibition by indomethacin. *Gastroenterology*. 1975; 69:1238–45.
149. Rabbani GH, Greenough WB III, Holmgren J et al. Controlled trial of chlorpromazine as antisecretory agent in patients with cholera hydrated intravenously. *Br Med J*. 1982; 284:1361–4.
150. Donowitz M, Elta G, Bloom SR et al. Trifluoperazine reversal of secretory diarrhea in pancreatic cholera. *Ann Intern Med*. 1980; 93:284–5.
151. Lahiri SC, Dutta NK. Berberine and chloramphenicol in the treatment of cholera and severe diarrhea. *J Indian Med Assoc*. 1967; 48:1–11.
152. Charney AN, Donowitz M. Prevention and reversal of cholera enterotoxin-induced intestinal secretion by methylprednisolone induction of Na+-K+-ATP-ase. *J Clin Invest*. 1976; 57:1590–9.
153. Chen LC, Guerrant RL, Rhode JE et al. Effect of amphotericin B on sodium and water movement across normal and cholera toxin-challenged canine jejunum. *Gastroenterology*. 1973; 65:252–8.
154. Dharmsathaporn K, Binder HJ, Dobbins JW. Somatostatin stimulates sodium and chloride absorption in the rabbit ileum. *Gastroenterology*. 1980; 78:1559–65.
155. Field M, McCall I. Ion transport in rabbit ileal mucosa. III. Effects of catecholamines. *Am J Physiol*. 1973; 225:852–7.
156. McArthur KE, Anderson DS, Durkin TE et al. Clonidine and lidamidine to inhibit watery diarrhea in a patient with lung cancer. *Ann Intern Med*. 1982; 96:323–5.
157. Amin AH, Subbaiah TV, Abbasi KM. Berberine sulfate: antimicrobial activity, bioassay, and mode of action. *Can J Microbiol*. 1969; 15:1067–76.
158. Martin L, Guadron O, Ortiz M del C et al. Experimental diarrhea: evaluation and safety of WHR-1142A in healthy volunteers. *IRCS Med Sci*. 1981; 9:1052–3.
159. Dobbins J, Racusen L, Binder HJ. Effect of d-alanine methionine enkephalin amide on ion transport in rabbit ileum. *J Clin Invest*. 1980; 66:19–28.
160. Levine MM, Black RE, Clements ML et al. Duration of infection-derived immunity to cholera. *J Infect Dis*. 1981; 143:818–20.
161. Mekalanos JJ, Swartz DJ, Pearson GDN et al. Cholera toxin genes: nucleotide sequence, deletion analysis, and vaccine development. *Nature*. 1983; 306:551–7.
162. Levine MM, Kaper JB, Black RE et al. New knowledge on pathogenesis of bacterial enteric infections as applied to vaccine development. *Microbiol Rev*. 1983; 47:510–50.
163. Formal SB, Baron LS, Kapecko DJ et al. Construction of a potential bivalent vaccine strain: introduction of *Shigella sonnei* from I antigen genes into the gas E *Salmonella typhi* Ty21a typhoid vaccine strain. *Infect Immun*. 1981; 34:746–50.
164. Wyatt RG, James WD, Bohl EH et al. Human rotavirus type 2: cultivation in vitro. *Science*. 1980; 207:189–91.
165. Baldini MM, Kaper JB, Levine MM et al. Plasmid-mediated adhesion in enteropathogenic *Escherichia coli*. *J Pediatr Gastroenterol Nutr*. 1983; 2:534–8.
166. O'Brien AD, LaVeck GD, Thompson MR et al. Production of *Shigella dysenteriae* type 1-like cytotoxin by *Escherichia coli*. *J Infect Dis*. 1982; 146:763–9.

“

Evaluation of Thrombolytic Agents

Current data do not support the concepts that fibrin selectivity endows thrombolytic agents with a major advance over nonfibrin-selective agents or that fibrin selectivity serves as a decisive factor determining clinical benefit. Each of the agents within these two classes of activators differs in many respects and will require evaluation on an individual basis. However, in view of the public health importance of thrombolytic therapy in the treatment of an acutely evolving myocardial infarction, and the necessity to avoid conflicting claims based on marketing strategy and public relations programs in contrast to science, it would be desirable to evaluate all of the five current agents against each other in a trial designed to compare their effects on mortality and safety. Also, in view of current information, it no longer makes sense to spend public money primarily on the development of a single agent that may or may not be in the best interest of the patient at risk.

—Sherry S. Unresolved clinical pharmacologic questions in thrombolytic therapy for acute myocardial infarction. *J Am Coll Cardiol*. 1988; 12:519–25.

”

Research

Postinfusion phlebitis after intravenous push versus intravenous piggyback administration of antimicrobial agents

JAMES C. GARRELTS, DAN AST, JOANNE LAROCCA, DALE F. SMITH, JR., AND JERRY D. PETERIE

Abstract: The incidence and severity of phlebitis associated with the i.v. push method versus the i.v. piggyback method of administration of antimicrobial agents were evaluated.

All patients admitted to two nursing units of an 886-bed, tertiary-care hospital from March through June 1987 who received intravenous cephalosporins or extended-spectrum penicillins were considered for inclusion in the study. The method of administration, either i.v. push or i.v. piggyback, was randomly assigned. Each patient's catheter site was evaluated every 24 hours according to standardized definitions of phlebitis and patency. Information on each patient and venipuncture site also was collected.

A total of 319 catheter sites were studied in 155 patients. There was no significant difference in the incidence or severity of postinfusion phlebitis between the i.v. push and the i.v. piggyback groups (41% versus 47%). When studying only those catheter sites discontinued because of phlebitis, the time until development of phlebitis averaged 45 ± 20.5 hours in the i.v. push group, compared with only 36.2 ± 17.6 hours in the i.v. piggyback group; this difference was significant. The fact that the catheter sites lasted significantly longer in the i.v. push group, combined with elimination of the cost of syringe infusion pumps or i.v. tubing and minibags, suggests that use of the i.v. push method may result in substantial cost savings. Other advantages associated with the i.v. push method include time savings for nursing personnel and patients and greater ease in scheduling doses of multiple antimicrobial agents.

Administration of cephalosporins and extended-spectrum penicillins by i.v. push does not appear to produce phlebitis at a rate any greater than that observed with the traditional piggyback method of administration.

Index terms: Catheters; Cephalosporins; Drug administration; Drug administration sites; Injections; Intravenous therapy; Penicillins; Phlebitis; Toxicity
Clin Pharm. 1988; 7:760–5

The most popular method of administering injectable antimicrobial agents since the 1970s has been by i.v. piggyback, in which 50–150 mL of 5% dextrose or 0.9% sodium chloride injection is used as the diluent and doses are infused over 30–60 minutes.[1] Syringe infusion pumps have been shown to be considerably less expensive than the traditional piggyback method of antimicrobial administration.[2–4] They also have been evaluated for their ability to cause postinfusion phlebitis.[5–9] Most studies have found no difference in the incidence of postinfusion phlebitis, although some have found a small increase with the syringe infusion pump.

JAMES C. GARRELTS, PHARM.D., is Coordinator, Clinical Pharmacy Services, St. Francis Regional Medical Center, Wichita, KS, and Adjunct Assistant Professor of Medicine, The University of Kansas School of Medicine–Wichita. DAN AST is Assistant Director for I.V. Therapy; JOANNE LAROCCA, M.N., is Clinical Nurse Specialist; and DALE F. SMITH, JR., M.S., is Director of Pharmacy Services, St. Francis Regional Medical Center. JERRY D. PETERIE, M.D., F.A.C.P., is Clinical Assistant Professor, The University of Kansas School of Medicine–Wichita.

Address reprint requests to Dr. Garrelts at the Department of Pharmacy, St. Francis Regional Medical Center, 929 North St. Francis, Wichita, KS 67214.

The technical assistance of Vanessa Petersen and the assistance of the pharmacy staff, the nursing staffs on the study units, and the i.v. therapy team are acknowledged.

This study was supported by a grant from the Midwest Heart and Vascular Institute, Inc.

Copyright © 1988, American Society of Hospital Pharmacists, Inc. All rights reserved. 0278-2677/88/1001-0760$01.50.

An alternative method of antimicrobial administration is manual i.v. push using a syringe. This method avoids the cost of syringe infusion pumps, i.v. tubing, and minibags. However, before it can be widely adopted, it must be shown to be as safe as standard methods of administration. Therefore, we undertook this prospective, randomized study to evaluate the incidence and severity of postinfusion phlebitis occurring with the i.v. push method versus the i.v. piggyback method of administration.

Methods

The study was conducted in an 886-bed, tertiary-care hospital over a four-month period, from March 1987 through June 1987. Two 35-bed general medical and surgical nursing units were used to obtain a broad-based patient sample while still allowing tight control over study procedures. All patients receiving one of the study antimicrobial agents (Table 1) were considered for inclusion in the study. Written informed consent was obtained from all patients or their legal guardians. Only patients who were 18 years of age or older were eligible to participate. Excluded from the study were patients concurrently receiving the following i.v. drugs, which are known or thought to produce a substantial degree of phlebitis: antineoplastic agents, potassium chloride administered intravenously at a rate of ≥8 meq/hour, phenytoin, vancomycin, amphotericin B, tetracycline, doxycycline, erythromycin, sulfamethoxazole–trimethoprim, penicillins other than piperacillin or mezlocillin, or any investigational drug.

All antimicrobial doses were prepared in the pharmacy, using a laminar-airflow hood and aseptic technique. During preparation, a 5-μm filter was used in both the syringe and piggyback groups to standardize the amount of particulate matter present. Antimicrobial agents in the piggyback group were administered with i.v. tubing that did not contain an inline filter. Sterile water for injection was used as the diluent for all antimicrobial agents in syringes. The antimicrobials administered by small-volume injection were diluted with sterile water and then injected into Viaflex minibags containing either 5% dextrose injection or 0.9% sodium chloride injection, as shown in Table 1. The concentrations and administration rates for different doses were simply direct increments of those shown in Table 1 (e.g., cefazolin 2 g/20 mL administered over two to four minutes). Osmolality was determined in duplicate for each sample using an automated freezing-point method (Advanced Micro-Osmometer, Advanced Instruments Inc., Needham Heights, MA 02194).

The method of administration, either i.v. push or piggyback, was randomly assigned. Before initiation of the study, eight sealed envelopes were prepared, four containing the words "i.v. push" and four with "i.v. piggyback." A person not associated with the study opened the envelopes and matched the method of antimicrobial administration to a particular nursing unit for a given month.

Most of the i.v. catheters in the study were inserted by an experienced i.v. therapy team (91% in the i.v. push group and 90.4% in the piggyback group). The use of an i.v. therapy team has been shown to significantly reduce the incidence of phlebitis compared with that occurring after insertion by other medical personnel.[10] Since the type of i.v. catheter used may itself affect the incidence of phlebitis,[11] all patients had a Teflon Cathlon-IV catheter (Critikon Division, Johnson and Johnson, Tampa, FL) inserted (Table 2). A Click-Lock extension set (ICU Medical Inc., Huntington Beach, CA) was then inserted into the metal hub of the Cathlon-IV to serve as an injection site or as a receptacle for i.v. tubing hooked to a continuous large-volume injection. The setup was securely taped in place on the patient's arm to minimize mechanical phlebitis resulting from catheter movement.

Each patient's catheter site was evaluated at least once every 24 hours by one of three experienced

Table 1.
Concentrations, Administration Rates, and Osmolalities of Antimicrobial Agents Included in the Study

Antimicrobial Agent	I.V. Push Group: Concentration	I.V. Push Group: Administration Rate	I.V. Push Group: Osmolality (mOsm)	I.V. Piggyback Group[a]: Concentration	I.V. Piggyback Group[a]: Administration Time (min)	I.V. Piggyback Group[a]: Osmolality (mOsm)
Cefazolin	1 g/10 mL	1–2 min/g	340	1 g/50 mL D5W[b]	30	298
Cefuroxime	750 mg/10 mL	1–2 min/g	447	750 mg/50 mL D5W	30	301
Cefoxitin	1 g/10 mL	1–2 min/g	525	1 g/50 mL D5W	30	320
Cefamandole	1 g/10 mL	1–2 min/g	604	1 g/50 mL D5W	30	336
Cefotaxime	1 g/10 mL	1–2 min/g	440	1 g/50 mL D5W	30	300
Ceftriaxone	1 g/10 mL	1–2 min/g	423	1 g/50 mL D5W	30	306
Ceftazidime	1 g/10 mL	1–2 min/g	435	1 g/50 mL NS[b]	30	304
Cefoperazone	1 g/10 mL	1–2 min/g	235	1 g/50 mL D5W	30	284
Piperacillin	1 g/5 mL	3–5 min/dose	587	2 g/50 mL D5W	30	286
Mezlocillin	1 g/10 mL	3–5 min/dose	230	2 g/50 mL D5W	30	335

[a] All drugs were administered over a 30-minute period.
[b] D5W = 5% dextrose injection, NS = 0.9% sodium chloride injection.

Table 2.
Demographic Characteristics and Factors That Might Affect Phlebitis Rates

Variable	I.V. Push Group	I.V. Piggyback Group	Statistical Analysis
Inserted by i.v. team	91%	90.4%	NS[a]
Catheter gauge			
20	76.3%	58.2%	$p < 0.001$
22	12.7%	30.1%	$p < 0.001$
18	9.8%	11.0%	NS
16	0.6%	0.7%	NS
24	0.6%	0.0%	NS
Age (yr)	56.8 ± 20.2	58.9 ± 16.6	NS
Weight (kg)	66.1 ± 20	75.8 ± 24.4	$p < 0.02$
Sex	57% Male	39% Male	$p < 0.025$
Race	76% White, 17% black	76% White, 13% black	NS
Number of doses given/site	7.2 ± 5.3	6.7 ± 4.7	NS
Large-volume injection (LVI) infused through site[b]	60%	51%	NS
Potassium chloride in LVI	57%	66%	NS
Dextrose in LVI	94%	92%	NS

[a] NS = Not significant.
[b] LVI (≥250 mL) infused through the catheter during part or all of the time that it lasted.

nurses employed for the duration of the study. Regardless of the reason for discontinuing use of the site, each site was evaluated by one of the study nurses before discontinuation. The nurses used carefully standardized definitions of phlebitis and patency when assessing i.v. catheter sites (appendix). Before initiation of the study, interrater reliability was established and defined as 100% agreement between evaluators on at least 15 patient observations of phlebitis and loss of patency.

All nursing and ancillary personnel on the two study units received inservice education before initiation of the project. The inservice education session included the rationale for the study as well as specific steps to be taken during its progress. Only registered nurses administered medications and solutions through the i.v. catheters. For patients who had an indwelling intermittent injection site (i.v. lock), the device was routinely flushed with 2 mL of 0.9% sodium chloride injection before and after antimicrobial administration to avoid incompatibilities. In patients receiving a continuous large-volume injection, antimicrobials were administered through an injection port in the unfiltered i.v. tubing. Unless the patient refused or initial needle placement was extremely difficult, i.v. catheters were changed every 72 hours, even if phlebitis was not present. In determining the incidence of phlebitis, the status of the catheter at 72 hours was used. The percentages of catheters not changed at 72 hours for the i.v. push and piggyback groups were 13.9% and 9.6%, respectively, a difference that was not significant.

In addition to evaluating the i.v. catheter site, the study nurses collected the following information on each patient and site, using a standardized data collection form: demographic characteristics, disease states, surgical procedures, medications and i.v. solutions administered to the patient, information concerning the cause of site loss, and the time that each site lasted.

Nominal data were evaluated statistically using chi-square analysis with Yates correction, or Fisher's exact test when expected frequencies were less than five. Interval data were evaluated using the unpaired *t* test. Time to development of phlebitis also was evaluated with a Kaplan–Meier curve and the Mantel–Haenszel test. Comparisons were considered to be significant if p was <0.05. All results were reported as a percentage or as mean ± S.D.

Results

A total of 319 i.v. catheter sites and 155 patients were included in the study. There were 173 sites studied in 88 patients in the i.v. push group and 146 sites in 67 patients in the piggyback group. The difference in the number of sites per patient (1.97 versus 2.18) was not significant. The groups were similar in terms of demographic characteristics and the distribution of factors that might affect the phlebitis rate (Table 2). A larger catheter gauge was used more frequently in the i.v. push group; this should have favored the development of phlebitis in these patients. Although there were significant differences in weight and sex between the groups, these variables have not been identified as risk factors for phlebitis. The distribution of medications administered through the catheters was similar in the two groups (Table 3).

There was no significant difference between the two groups in terms of site loss caused by postinfusion phlebitis (Table 4). The overall incidence of phlebitis was 41% in the i.v. push group and 47% in the group receiving antimicrobials via small-volume injection. The large sample size in this study provided excellent power; the ability to correctly identify a 10% difference in incidence of phlebitis between groups was 75%, and it was 99% for a 20% difference. When examining the subgroup of patients whose catheter was used for infusion of i.v. fluids, there still was no significant difference in phlebitis rates. In catheters that were used only as indwelling intermittent i.v. locks, the incidence of phlebitis was 36% in the i.v. push group, compared with 44% in the i.v. piggyback group. No significant difference was noted between the groups in terms of other causes of site loss (Table 4). There also were no differences between the i.v. push and piggyback groups in individual measures of the severity of phlebitis (pain, erythema, cord, and induration) (Table 4).

Catheter sites in the i.v. push group tended to last longer (48 ± 27.7 hours versus 42.4 ± 31.7 hours, $p < 0.10$), but the difference was not significant. Because phlebitis was our primary outcome variable, and since miscellaneous causes of site loss (e.g., pulled out by patient, physician discontinued antimicrobial drug therapy) could have affected the time that sites lasted differently in each group, we decided to evaluate this variable only for sites discontinued because of phlebitis. In addition, because the policy of changing sites at least every 72 hours was not followed in every patient, we substituted a value of 72 hours in our calculations for sites lasting longer than that. We believed that these changes would provide the most accurate indicator of how the method of antimicrobial administration affected the time that the site lasted. Under these conditions, there was a significant difference between groups in the time that sites lasted. The time until development of phlebitis averaged 45 ± 20.5 hours in the i.v. push group, compared with only 36.2 ± 17.6 hours in the i.v. piggyback group ($p < 0.01$). The probability of survival of the site is shown in the Kaplan–Meier plot in Figure 1. Again there was a significant difference in favor of the i.v. push group ($p < 0.001$).

Table 3.
Percentage of Catheters through Which the Listed Drugs Were Administered

Drug	No. (%) of Catheters: I.V. Push Group	I.V. Piggyback Group
Cefazolin	61 (35.3)	69 (47.3)
Cefamandole	4 (2.3)	8 (5.5)
Cefoxitin	30 (17.3)	31 (21.2)
Cefuroxime	17 (9.8)	13 (8.9)
Cefotaxime	20 (11.6)	14 (9.6)
Ceftazidime	27 (15.6)	1 (0.7)
Cefoperazone	7 (4.0)	2 (1.4)
Ceftriaxone	9 (5.2)	7 (4.8)
Mezlocillin	0 (0.0)	4 (2.7)
Piperacillin	2 (1.2)	0 (0.0)

Discussion

Numerous risk factors for the development of postinfusion phlebitis have been identified and reviewed.[11–13] Briefly, these risk factors include the type of cannula used, skill of the personnel inserting and maintaining the catheter, duration of cannula placement, medications or solutions administered through the catheter (osmolality, pH, particulate matter, inherent irritant properties), and infection. The i.v. push and piggyback groups in this study were well matched with respect to these risk factors.

The i.v. push method of administering antimicrobial agents has been avoided in the past because of concern about giving a hypertonic solution over

Table 4.
Incidence and Causes of Site Loss, Individual Measures of Phlebitis, and Time That Sites Lasted

Characteristic	No. (%) of Catheters: I.V. Push Group	I.V. Piggyback Group	Statistical Analysis
Phlebitis (all sites)	71 (41)	69 (47)	NS[a]
Phlebitis (large-volume injection sites)	46 (44)	37 (50)	NS
Phlebitis (i.v. lock sites)	25 (36)	32 (44)	NS
Loss of patency	10 (5.8)	14 (9.6)	NS
Infiltration	26 (15)	19 (13)	NS
Miscellaneous causes	57 (33)	40 (27.4)	NS
Time that the site lasted (all sites)	48 ± 27.7 hr[b]	42.4 ± 31.7 hr[b]	NS
Time that the site lasted in those patients developing phlebitis, substituting 72 hr for those sites lasting longer	45 ± 20.5 hr[b]	36.2 ± 17.6 hr[b]	$p < 0.01$
Indicators of phlebitis			
Pain	61 (35.3)	54 (37)	NS
Erythema	74 (42.8)	67 (45.9)	NS
Cord	10 (5.8)	8 (5.5)	NS
Induration	32 (18.5)	35 (24)	NS

[a] NS = Not significant.
[b] Mean ± S.D.

Figure 1. Kaplan–Meier plots showing the probability of survival of the i.v. lock site over time for the i.v. push (□) and i.v. piggyback (+) groups.

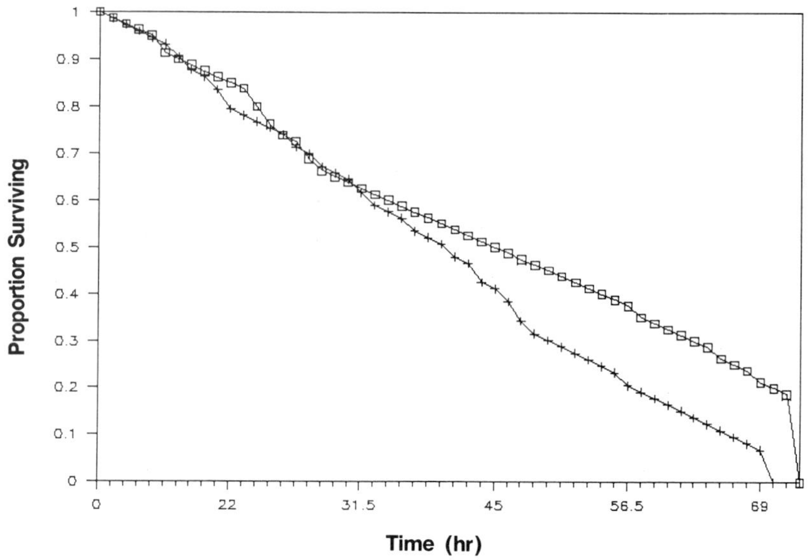

a short period of time and the effect this might have on postinfusion phlebitis. However, recent evaluations indicate that increasing osmolality does not increase the incidence of phlebitis, at least not until very high values are reached.[14,15] Massar and coworkers[14] found equal phlebitis rates with 5% dextrose (369 mOsm/L), crystalline amino acids (450–500 mOsm/L), and 5% dextrose with crystalline amino acids (713–763 mOsm/L). On the other hand, Gazitua and associates[15] found similar phlebitis rates for solutions with an osmolality of <600 mOsm/L, but a 100% incidence when a value of >600 mOsm/L was reached. In addition, Daly and coworkers[16] noted equivalent phlebitis rates for solutions with an osmolality of either 600 or 900 mOsm/L. The results of the current study support these observations, since osmolality for the 10 antimicrobial agents averaged 439 mOsm/L in the i.v. push group, compared with only 309 mOsm/L in the i.v. piggyback group; however, the incidence of phlebitis was not significantly different between the two groups.

Rate of administration also has been a concern that has precluded i.v. push administration of antimicrobial agents. For some antimicrobials, such as vancomycin, rapid administration has been reported to result in severe systemic adverse reactions.[17] However, systemic adverse reactions have not been noted after rapid administration of cephalosporins and extended-spectrum penicillins. In three years of administering antimicrobial agents by i.v. push at our institution, not one complaint or report of an adverse reaction related to the method of administration has been received. This leaves only the concern over increased local vein irritation that might occur because of rapid administration. However, other investigators have noted more vein irritation with slow i.v. infusion of fluids than when the same volume was infused over a short period of time.[18] Our work supports this finding, although we administered a smaller volume in the i.v. push group than in the i.v. piggyback group.

Our finding that incidence of site loss from phlebitis or other causes was similar for the i.v. push and i.v. piggyback methods of administration of antimicrobial agents is important in the current era of limited health-care resources. Although we do not have a good explanation for the finding, the fact that i.v. sites lasted significantly longer in the i.v. push group increases the potential economy of this method of antimicrobial administration. An additional advantage to i.v. push administration has been noted by the nursing staff. They have found that the one to two minutes required to administer a cephalosporin antimicrobial agent by i.v. push can be spent talking to the patient. Setting up and regulating the drip rate for piggyback administration does not allow such use of time and may be more time consuming. Nurses must "check" the piggyback solution once or twice during infusion, which requires additional trips to the patient's room. If the solution is not flowing at the desired or expected rate, additional time must be spent solving the problem. Our nursing staff immediately believed that i.v. push administration was less time consuming than the i.v. piggyback method. Furthermore, with piggyback or syringe infusion pump administration, the patient must stay in bed or near an i.v. pole for at least 30 minutes every time a dose is administered. This may be especially important in cases of outpatient antimicrobial administration, where i.v. push administration may result in substantial time savings for the patient.

Despite the advantages of i.v. push administration, it is not appropriate for all antimicrobial agents. Many antimicrobials are associated with undue toxicity when administered too rapidly. However, cephalosporins and extended-spectrum penicillins currently constitute approximately 60% to 65% of all antimicrobial use at many large hospitals, meaning that other methods of antimicrobial administration will have to be used in one-third of the cases. When a nurse must schedule administration of doses of two or three different antimicrobial agents, being able to give several of those doses by i.v. push over 1 to 4 minutes each, instead of 30 minutes, is advantageous. Although these data are not included in the study, we currently administer aztreonam by i.v. push as well. Its osmolality is 487 when diluted 1 g/10 mL in a syringe.

Conclusion

Administration of cephalosporins and extended-spectrum penicillins by i.v. push does not appear to produce postinfusion phlebitis at a rate greater than that seen with the traditional piggyback method.

References

1. Turco SJ. Intravenous piggyback—a new dimension in unit dose. *J Parenter Drug Assoc.* 1978; 32(Jan–Feb):50–3.
2. Colangelo A, Clark ST, Janousek JP. Implementation and cost analysis of a syringe pump system for intermittent i.v. drug delivery. *Am J Hosp Pharm.* 1985; 42:581–4.
3. Goudreau JB, Morrisey JM. Pharmacy-initiated implementation of a syringe pump infusion system. *Am J Hosp Pharm.* 1985; 42:584–7.
4. Fiorenzo VJ, Kelly WN. A financial evaluation of the Becton-Dickinson 360 Infuser System. *Hosp Pharm.* 1987; 22:563–6.
5. Baptista RJ, Gallagher JA, Sesin GP et al. Infusion system tested for phlebitis potential. *IV Ther News.* 1984; 11:14–6.
6. Rapp RP, Powers P, Tolbert V et al. Postinfusion phlebitis associated with a syringe system versus minibags. *Clin Pharm.* 1986; 5:408–11.
7. DeMonaco HJ, Cronin CM, Dempsey MJ et al. Comparison of phlebitis rates with Buretrol and Harvard Mini-Infuser for administration of i.v. piggyback medications. *NITA.* 1986; 9:475–7.
8. Jarrard C, Goodner W, Piazza JA et al. The syringe infusion pump system. Its effect on phlebitis rates. *NITA.* 1987; 10:29–33.
9. Baptista RJ, Driscoll DF, Gallagher JA et al. Infusion phlebitis associated with a programmable syringe-pump system versus gravity-feed minibottles. *Clin Pharm.* 1987; 6:314–8.
10. Tonford JW, Hershey CO, McLaren CE et al. Intravenous therapy team and peripheral venous catheter-associated complications. A prospective controlled study. *Arch Intern Med.* 1984; 144:1191–4.
11. Turnidge J. Hazards of peripheral intravenous lines. *Med J Aust.* 1984; 14:37–40.
12. Turco SJ. Infusion phlebitis: a review of the literature. *Parenterals.* 1987; 14:37–40.
13. Fricker MP. Infusion phlebitis. *Infusion.* 1981; 4:33–4.
14. Massar EL, Daly JM, Copeland EM et al. Peripheral vein complications in patients receiving amino acid/dextrose solutions. *J Parenter Enter Nutr.* 1983; 7:159–62.
15. Gazitua R, Wilson K, Bistrian BR et al. Factors determining peripheral vein tolerance to amino acid infusions. *Arch Surg.* 1979; 114:897–900.
16. Daly JM, Massar E, Hansen L et al. Peripheral vein infusion of dextrose/amino acid solutions ± 20% fat emulsion. *J Parenter Enter Nutr.* 1985; 9:296–9.
17. Garrelts JC, Peterie JD. Vancomycin and the "Red Man's Syndrome." *N Engl J Med.* 1985; 312:245. Letter.
18. Hessov I, Bojsen-Moller M. Experimental infusion thrombophlebitis: importance of infusion rate. *Eur J Intensive Care Med.* 1976; 2:103–5.

Appendix—Definition of Phlebitis and Loss of Patency

A. **Definition of Phlebitis**

1. Erythema in a 2-cm or greater radius present around the i.v. lock site, or
2. Presence of induration around the i.v. lock site, or
3. A palpable cord present around the i.v. lock site.

B. **Assessment and Definition of Loss of Patency**

1. Apply tourniquet to obstruct venous flow. Aspirate the i.v. lock for a blood return using a 3-mL syringe and 23-gauge, 1-inch needle.
2. If no blood return is obtained, attempt to flush the i.v. lock with 1 mL of 0.9% sodium chloride injection.
3. If significant resistance to flushing is encountered, remove the i.v. catheter and flush with 1 mL of 0.9% sodium chloride injection onto white blotting paper and examine for the presence of a clot or fibrin strand.

Inability to complete any portion of the sequence will be considered to be loss of patency.

Grand Rounds

Sulindac-induced toxic epidermal necrolysis

RALPH E. SMALL AND WILLIAM R. GARNETT

Abstract: A case of sulindac-induced toxic epidermal necrolysis (TEN) is described; the etiology, symptoms, and treatment of TEN are reviewed; and sulindac's pharmacokinetic characteristics and other adverse effects are discussed.

A 62-year-old black woman was given a prescription for sulindac 150 mg twice daily to relieve pain associated with degenerative joint disease. She also had a nine-year history of type II diabetes mellitus that was being managed with tolbutamide 500 mg once daily. After two weeks of sulindac therapy she developed a rash that spread over her entire body. Sulindac therapy was discontinued, and one day later the patient was admitted to the hospital with a temperature of 104.6 °F, conjunctivitis, and an erythematous macular rash over 60% of her body. Initially, therapy included prednisone 160 mg orally every day, applications of silver sulfadiazine cream four times daily for two days, and methylcellulose 0.5% ophthalmic solution (two drops four times daily) for the conjunctivitis. She also received intravenous hydration. By the fifth hospital day the patient's skin lesions and conjunctivitis had improved to the point that the prednisone dosage was tapered to 120 mg, then to 80 mg, and then to nothing over the following three days. Her diabetes was managed by short-term treatment with NPH insulin; however, before discharge, tolbutamide therapy was reinstituted, and insulin was discontinued. At follow-up four weeks after discharge, the patient's skin was largely clear.

TEN has multiple etiologies, but the basic mechanism of injury is believed to be an immunological reaction directed at the basal cell layer. Drug-induced TEN causes more serious skin damage than staphylococcal TEN, with a mortality rate of about 25% to 50%. Because both types of TEN resemble a severe partial-thickness burn, fluid and electrolyte replacement is critical. Use of high-dose corticosteroids remains controversial because controlled studies are not available. The most frequent adverse reactions to sulindac therapy are gastrointestinal; severe dermatological reactions are rare. Five other cases of TEN attributable to sulindac have been reported in the literature. Other reported adverse reactions include pancreatitis, hepatotoxicity, and meningitis.

Clinicians should be aware of the risk of TEN with sulindac and should monitor patients appropriately for dermatological reactions.

Index terms: Anti-inflammatory agents; Drugs, adverse reactions; Epidermal necrolysis; Methylcellulose; Prednisone; Silver sulfadiazine; Skin and mucous membrane preparations; Solutions, ophthalmic; Sulindac
Clin Pharm. 1988; 7:766–71

Sulindac (Clinoril, Merck Sharp & Dohme) is a nonsteroidal anti-inflammatory drug (NSAID) that may offer the advantage of less renal toxicity in some patients.[1] It is a widely prescribed drug, ranking 44th in the number of new and refill prescriptions filled in 1987.[2] The large number of patients exposed to the drug means that we can expect to see more adverse drug reactions. This case report illustrates a relatively infrequent, but serious, adverse reaction to sulindac.

Case Report

A 62-year-old black woman had a five-year history of degenerative joint disease that had been treated with aspirin. She also had a nine-year history of type II diabetes mellitus that was being managed with tolbutamide 500 mg once daily. One month before admission, she noted increasingly severe knee and ankle pain that interfered with her ability to work and caused her to visit the company physician. She was given a prescription for sulindac 150 mg twice daily and received good relief of

RALPH E. SMALL, PHARM.D., is Associate Professor of Pharmacy and Pharmaceutics and Associate Professor of Medicine (Rheumatology, Allergy, and Immunology), Medical College of Virginia, Virginia Commonwealth University (MCV/VCU), Richmond. WILLIAM R. GARNETT, PHARM.D., is Professor of Pharmacy and Pharmaceutics, MCV/VCU.

Address reprint requests to Dr. Small at Box 581, MCV Station, Medical College of Virginia/VCU, Richmond, VA 23298-0581.

Copyright © 1988, American Society of Hospital Pharmacists, Inc. All rights reserved. 0278-2677/88/1001-0766$01.50.

pain for two weeks.

Three days before admission, the patient noted an erythematous rash over her neck and forearms. Within one day, the rash had spread over her entire body. Her temperature spiked to 102 °F, she felt weak and confused, and she was unable to go to work. Administration of diphenhydramine produced no change in her condition. Sulindac therapy was discontinued because of a suspected adverse reaction. When there was no improvement after 24 hours, she was admitted to the hospital for evaluation.

On examination, the patient was a well developed, well nourished black woman who was in obvious acute distress. Her temperature was 104.6 °F, pulse 76 (regular), respirations 18/min, and blood pressure 120/78. Important findings noted during the examination were crusting of the eyes, presumed to be conjunctivitis, and a diffusely distributed erythematous macular rash over 60% of her body, with confluence in areas over the arms, legs, back, and face (Figure 1). Several of these areas had bullae formation and serous discharge. The patient's throat was erythematous, with white papules over the mucous membrane and soft and hard palate. During the examination she mentioned that her mouth was tender. The remainder of the physical examination was within normal limits.

Notable laboratory findings were serum creatinine concentration 1.9 mg/dL, blood urea nitrogen (BUN) 35 mg/dL, uric acid 6.7 mg/dL, total protein 7.1 g/dL, albumin 2.7 g/dL, hemoglobin 10.2 g/dL, hematocrit 32.9%, and blood sugar 198 mg/dL. All other hematology and chemistry tests were within normal limits. The histological view of the biopsy specimen, which showed subepidermal and dermal cleavage, is shown in Figure 2. The provisional diagnosis was toxic epidermal necrolysis (TEN) secondary to sulindac therapy.

Figure 1. Denuded skin of patient with sulindac-induced toxic epidermal necrolysis.

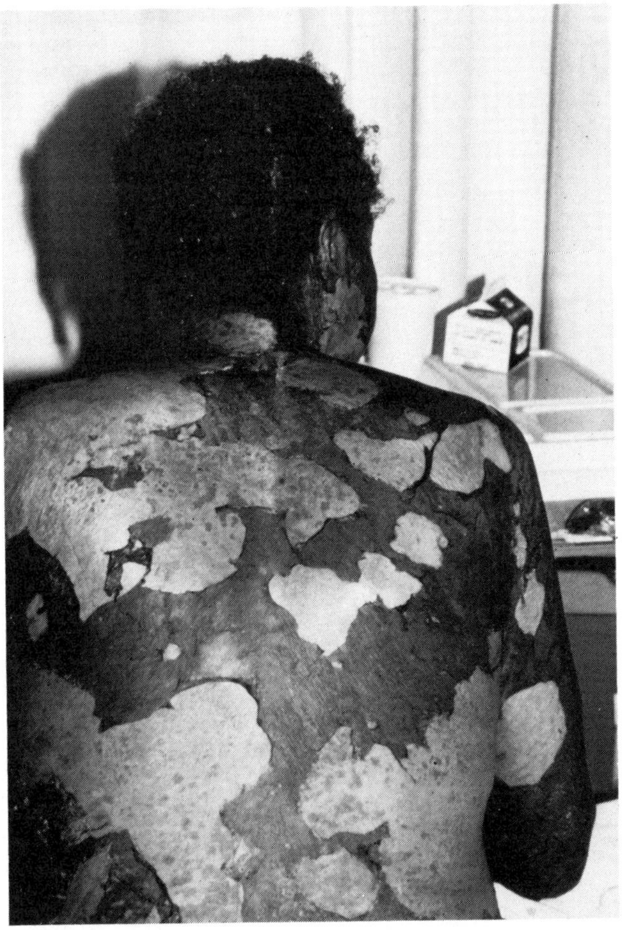

Papers in the Grand Rounds section are patient case reports and literature review combined in a way that gives them high educational value. The papers lead off with a well-documented case report of an unusual drug experience (e.g., adverse drug reaction or other unexpected drug response, experimental use of a drug). The case generally deals with a difficult therapeutic problem or dilemma that is commonly encountered but may be overlooked or misunderstood. (Esoteric or rare occurrences of minor importance do not make good Grand Rounds material.) A literature review puts the case in perspective with previously reported similar cases and alternative treatments. The review is integrated with related discussion of the case being reported.

CP *readers are encouraged to use Grand Rounds for educational group discussions. For this purpose, discussion questions are printed at the end of Grand Rounds papers.*

The initial treatment plan for the skin lesions was prednisone 160 mg orally every day, with rapid tapering of the dosage once the lesions started to heal; applications of silver sulfadiazine cream four times daily to the broken skin areas for two days; and good hygiene. Methylcellulose 0.5% ophthalmic solution (two drops four times daily) was used to treat the patient's conjunctivitis. Medications taken before admission were discontinued.

On the first day after admission no new maculopapular lesions were found. The bullous lesions on the back, buttocks, and arms began sloughing. Her oral mucosa was dry and forming a yellow crust. The patient was afebrile and lethargic but less confused, and she was not in pain. Her fasting blood sugar had increased to 454 mg/dL, and urine tests detected 4+ sugar and negative acetone. No treatment was instituted, since it was believed that these conditions were caused by steroid administration and lack of diabetic medications.

During the next three days the patient continued to receive 160 mg of prednisone daily and wound care. Hubbard tank treatments twice daily were also initiated.

Figure 2. Subepidermal bulla covered by necrotic epidermis.

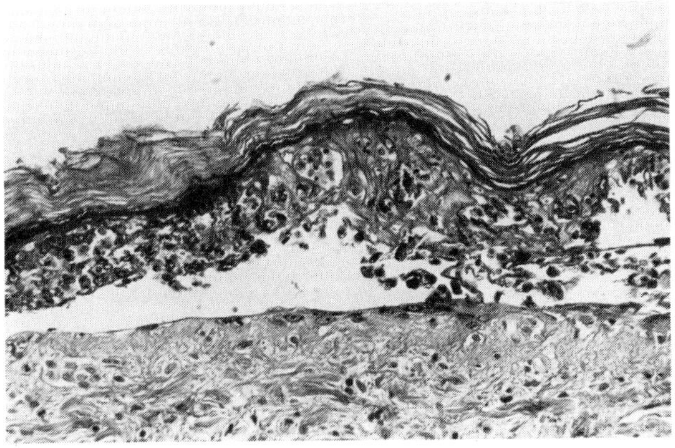

Her skin continued to slough at pressure points, with the formation of necrotic, dry, clean skin on the back. No new bullous lesions were found. Her conjunctivitis improved. With intravenous hydration the BUN returned to normal. She remained afebrile; however, her albumin concentrations decreased to 2.1 g/dL because of lack of nutrition and tissue sloughing. She was given albumin 25 g intravenously once, and the American Diabetes Association (ADA) diet was increased from 2000 to 4000 calories. Her albumin concentration was corrected to 3.0 g/dL over four days. On the fifth day the tank treatments and intravenous fluids were discontinued. The prednisone dosage was tapered to 120 mg, then to 80 mg, and then to nothing over the following three days. She continued to progress, with most areas becoming re-epithelialized. Her remaining problem was diabetes, with fasting blood sugars of about 335 mg/dL caused by steroid administration. Once the prednisone was stopped and the ADA diet was reduced in calories, short-term treatment with NPH insulin was begun. Tolbutamide therapy was reinstituted, and insulin was discontinued before discharge. She was discharged on the 15th day after admission on only the methylcellulose 0.5% ophthalmic solution. Follow-up four weeks later in the dermatology clinic revealed that her skin was virtually clear except for some residual desquamation on her feet.

Discussion

Etiologic Factors and Symptoms Associated with TEN. Toxic epidermal necrolysis was first described in 1956 and has been associated with many different etiologic factors (Table 1).[3] TEN also is known as Lyell's disease, scalded skin syndrome, acute epidermal necrolysis, Ritter's disease, dermatitis exfoliativa neonatorum, and staphylococcal scarlatiniform eruption. Drug-induced TEN is a serious condition, with a mortality rate of about 25% to 50% despite treatment.[4] The actual mechanism of the injury is still open to speculation, but it is believed to be an immunologic reaction directed at the basal cell layer.

In TEN (staphylococcal and drug induced) the patient may have a prodromal period of malaise, fever, arthralgias, and irritability, with exquisite tenderness of the skin or the onset of a generalized erythema. Patients with TEN (both types) usually have an acute onset of a morbilliform rash on the head and neck between a few hours and two days later and may have extensive involvement of the skin surface, with detachment of the epidermis resembling that occurring after scalding. Moist, glistening, denuded areas will remain. Loss of fingernails, hair, eyebrows, or toenails is also seen. In some cases of drug-induced TEN, there is extensive involvement of the mucous membranes, including those of the eyes, nose, oropharynx, trachea, bronchial tree, urethra, gastrointestinal tract, and vagina. This involvement may result in conjunctivitis, pharyngitis, and erosions of the oral mucous membranes.[5]

Table 1.
Etiological Factors Implicated in Toxic Epidermal Necrolysis

Drug allergy—see Table 3 for list of implicated drugs
Viral infection—measles, varicella, zoster, herpes simplex
Bacterial infection—*Escherichia coli* septicemia
Fungal infection—pulmonary aspergillosis
Vaccination—smallpox, measles, tetanus, poliomyelitis, diphtheria
Neoplastic diseases—lymphomas, leukemias
Graft versus host reaction—renal, liver, skin, heart
Beverages—tonic water
Airborne toxins—carbon monoxide, fumigants

Because of the extensive denuded skin areas, the patient is susceptible to massive fluid losses, electrolyte imbalances, shock, and infection.[5] Liver involvement (with or without jaundice), pneumonitis, and bronchiolitis have been reported.[5] Bone marrow depression, especially thrombocytopenia and granulocytopenia, and CNS and renal effects also have been described.[5] Elevated blood urea nitrogen, leukopenia (granulocytopenia), and neutropenia are associated with a poorer prognosis, which may assist the clinician in deciding the course or aggressiveness of therapy.[6] Recovery of the granulocyte count seems to herald a more favorable course of the disease.

With the idea that an immunologically mediated reaction may be occurring, human lymphocyte antigen (HLA) phenotypes have been quantified to assess possible links between their presence and an increased risk of severe skin reactions to medications.[7] A significant increase of HLA B-12 has been found in those patients with drug-induced TEN. Furthermore, results within subgroups suggest that the susceptibility to drug-induced TEN may be related to different HLAs. HLA associations within the sulfonamide subgroup are significant for A29 plus B12 and for B12 plus DR7, whereas cases of TEN related to the oxicam NSAIDs are linked to A2 and B12. To date, these findings have only theoretical implications, but they suggest that drug-induced TEN is immunologically mediated.

In the drug-induced type of TEN, widespread macular erythema and stomatitis may be prominent features, with epidermolysis occurring only in limited areas. The differences between drug-induced TEN and idiopathic TEN are shown in Table 2. Since drug-induced TEN causes cleavage and exfoliation at a deeper level of the epidermis or at the subepidermal level, the consequences of skin loss are more serious. Basal cell degeneration and spongiosis (intercellular edema of the spongy layer of the skin) may be marked. The dermal inflammatory infiltrate is sparse, and vasculitis is absent. A positive Nikolsky's sign or ease in rubbing off the epidermis with light pressure is found. As many as 40% of patients may follow a progressive course with deepening lethargy, fever, necrolysis, and death during the first two to five days of illness.[5] If re-epithelization occurs, it is slow and tends to

Table 2.
Differentiation between Staphylococcal and Drug-Induced Disease[3,4]

Variable	Staphylococcal Scalded Skin Syndrome Toxic Epidermal Necrolysis (TEN)	Nonstaphylococcal (Drug-Induced) TEN
Histology	Cleavage is high in epidermis	Subepidermal blister
	Basal layer intact	Necrosis of basal layers (immunoglobulin G deposited)
	Minimal dermal inflammation	Lack of inflammatory reaction in dermis
Predominance	Children, infants (female:male = 1:1)	Adult (female:male = 3:2)
Prognosis	10% Mortality	25%–50% Mortality
Clinical manifestations	Acute onset	Acute onset
	Scarlatiniform eruption to epidermal wrinkling to bullae formation	Prodrome—fever, erythema
		Morbilliform rash
	Denuded areas	Denuded areas of >10% of body surface area
	Face, neck, groin first	Moderate tenderness
	Marked tenderness	Mucous membrane involvement
	Superficial desquamation and healing in five to seven days	Two- to three-week course
Treatment	Antibiotics (sepsis)	Stop offending agent
	Electrolytes, albumin	Electrolytes, albumin
	Fluids, plasma	Fluids, plasma
	Topical antiseptics	Topical antiseptics
	Oral hygiene	Oral hygiene
	Postural drainage	Postural drainage
	Avoid steroids	Corticosteroids (?)
	Grafting	Grafting
	Low-dose heparin	Low-dose heparin
	Analgesics, tranquilizers	Analgesics, tranquilizers
	Plasmapheresis	Plasmapheresis

produce scarring. Sequelae of scarring include symblepharon, entropion and ectropion, trichiasis, corneal opacities, scarring alopecia, and anonychia.

The group 2, phage type 71 staphylococcal type of TEN predominates in infants and children under the age of 10.[7] When it occurs in the neonate, it is usually not present at birth. This type of TEN is rare in the adult and, when observed, may reflect defective host defense mechanisms. Drug-induced TEN is somewhat more common in women than in men (3:2); it has been noted at all ages but is seen more frequently in adults.[5] Examples of medications causing TEN are listed in Table 3. There is no racial preponderance.

Table 3.
Drugs Causing Toxic Epidermal Necrolysis (TEN)[12,18]

Causal Relationship to TEN	Drugs
Frequently implicated	Butazones, sulfonamides, chlorpropamide, barbiturates, phenytoin, phenolphthalein, tolbutamide
Infrequently implicated	Acetazolamide, allopurinol, neomycin, salicylates, penicillin, tetracycline, brompheniramine, gold salts, nitrofurantoin, pentazocine, quinine, chlorpromazine, plicamycin, dapsone, triamterene, hydrochlorothiazide, reserpine, hydralazine, carbenicillin, piroxicam, chloramphenicol, carbamazepine

Treatment. In many respects, TEN (staphylococcal or drug-induced) resembles a severe partial-thickness burn, and treatment is the same for both conditions. Fluid and electrolyte replacement for the massive transudate and insensible losses is critical. Body temperature, serum electrolytes, and hematology laboratory tests should be carefully monitored. Topical antiseptics help prevent infection, but sulfa-based antiseptics are obviously contraindicated in patients whose TEN may have been induced by a sulfa drug. The skin should be treated gently and kept moist with saline or 0.25% silver nitrate compresses. Silver sulfadiazine should be avoided, since sulfonamides are frequently indicated in TEN and silver sulfadiazine has been thought to cause neutropenia in some patients with TEN.[6] Vaporizers or tents with cold steam may be helpful.

In the desquamative phase the skin should be kept lubricated with bland ointments. The use of high-dose corticosteroids (prednisone 60 mg/sq m/day) remains somewhat controversial, since controlled studies are not available. In those patients with tracheobronchial involvement, physiotherapy and postural drainage are useful. In cases of severe shock with acute renal failure, dialysis may be necessary.[8] The pain associated with the denuded areas and use of dressings is treated with mild to moderate analgesics.

Characteristics and Adverse Effects of Sulindac. Sulindac was first marketed in the United States in 1978. It is an indoleacetic acid nonsteroidal drug related to indomethacin. Sulindac is usually taken in doses of 150–200 mg twice daily for the treatment of rheumatoid arthritis, osteoarthritis, acute gouty arthritis, ankylosing spondylitis, and acute bursitis. Sulindac is considered a prodrug, since most of its efficacy can be attributed to its reduction to the sulfide metabolite. After oral administration, sulindac is rapidly absorbed from the gastrointestinal tract. Approximately 90% of an oral dose is absorbed in fasting subjects. The parent compound has a mean half-life of about 7 to 8 hours, whereas the mean half-life of the active sulfide metabolite is about 16.4 hours. Sulindac and its metabolites undergo extensive enterohepatic recirculation and are more than 90% bound to plasma proteins. Sulindac is eliminated via the urine primarily as the inactive oxidized metabolite sulfone and the parent sulfoxide. The active sulfide metabolite of sulindac is not present in the urine; this has been postulated to be why sulindac appears to have fewer renal adverse effects than other NSAIDs.[9,10]

The most frequent adverse reactions occurring with sulindac are gastrointestinal. These include abdominal pain (10%), dyspepsia, nausea, diarrhea, and constipation (3–9%).[11] Other reactions occurring in 3–9% of patients are dizziness, headache, and rash. Reactions seen in 1–3% of patients include anorexia, vomiting, flatulence, gastrointestinal cramps, pruritus, nervousness, tinnitus, vertigo, and edema.[9,11] Listed under incidence less than 1% are the following dermatological reactions: erythema multiforme, stomatitis, toxic epidermal necrolysis, sore or dry mucous membranes, Stevens–Johnson syndrome, and exfoliative dermatitis.[11,12]

Cutaneous reactions to sulindac are infrequent. However, the most common reaction is morbilliform drug eruptions, which often occur in patients with toxic hepatitis or other systemic hypersensitivity reactions. Pruritus is also common and may occur without a rash or as a clinical symptom of erythema multiforme, TEN, anaphylaxis, or a morbilliform drug eruption. Other cutaneous reactions that have been reported with sulindac use are petechiae, exfoliative erythroderma, photosensitivity, serum sickness, facial and oral erythema, urticaria, and stomatitis.[13]

NSAIDs in the same chemical class often produce similar adverse cutaneous reactions. Those drugs, of the heterocyclic acetic acid class, similar to sulindac are indomethacin and tolmetin.

Incidence of Sulindac-Induced TEN. A review of the literature revealed four reports (five cases) of TEN attributed to sulindac.[14–17] As in the case reported here, sulindac therapy was instituted 14–16 days before onset of symptoms in all five cases. Four of the five previous cases had fatal outcomes, but these were complicated by toxic hepatitis in one patient and bone marrow suppression in another. Descriptions of all cases are provided in Table 4. All patients were women who took normal doses of sulindac and had similar clinical manifestations.

One additional article was published describing serious adverse reactions associated with sulindac.[11] The four patients described in this article had fever and involvement of one or more organs after therapy with sulindac. These patients had pancreatitis, hepatotoxicity, and meningitis, which are other potentially fatal adverse effects. None of these patients were diagnosed as having sulindac-induced TEN.

Conclusion

A patient taking sulindac developed an erythematous maculopapular pruritic rash that later became a blistering, erosive cutaneous reaction diagnosed as TEN. The case had the typical histological features of drug-induced disease. Drug-induced TEN is not a single disease but involves clinical manifestations of several unrelated disease processes.[18] Clinicians should be aware of the risk of TEN with sulindac and should monitor patients appropriately for dermatological reactions.

Discussion Questions

1. What are the major differences between staphylococcal scalded skin syndrome and drug-induced toxic epidermal necrolysis?
2. Describe the pathophysiology, clinical presentation, complications, prognosis, and treatment of drug-induced TEN.
3. List some of the drugs that are known to cause TEN.
4. What criteria should be used by clinicians for assessing and monitoring patients who receive drugs that are known to cause TEN?

References

1. Roberts DG, Gerber JG, Barnes JS et al. Sulindac is not renal sparing in man. *Clin Pharmacol Ther.* 1985; 38:258–65.
2. Anon. The top 200 prescription drugs of 1987. *Am Drug.* 1988; 197(Feb):40–52.
3. Lyell A. Toxic epidermal necrolysis (the scalded skin syndrome): a reappraisal. *Br J Dermatol.* 1979; 100:69–86.
4. Elias PM, Fritsch PO. Toxic epidermal necrolysis. *Arch Dermatol.* 1977; 113:207–10.
5. Anon RB, Dimond RL. Toxic epidermal necrolysis: rapid differentiation between staphylococcal and drug-induced disease. *Arch Dermatol.* 1975; 111:1433–7.
6. Westly ED, Wechsler HL. Toxic epidermal necrolysis: granulocytic leukopenia as a prognosis indicator. *Arch Dermatol.* 1984; 120:721–6.
7. Roujeau JC, Huynh TN, Bracq C et al. Genetic susceptibility to toxic epidermal necrolysis. *Arch Dermatol.* 1987; 123:1171–3.
8. Pearson RW. Advances in the diagnosis and treatment of blistering diseases: a selective review. In: Malkinson FD, Pearson RW, eds. *1977 Year Book of Dermatology.* Chicago: Year Book Medical Publishers, Inc.; 1977: 7.
9. Brogden RN, Heel RC, Speight TM et al. Sulindac: review of its pharmacological properties and therapeutic efficacy in rheumatic diseases. *Drugs.* 1978; 16:97–114.
10. Duggan DE, Hare IE, Ditzler CA et al. The disposition of sulindac. *Clin Pharmacol Ther.* 1977; 21:326.

Table 4.
Case Reports of Sulindac-Induced Toxic Epidermal Necrolysis

Reference	Patient Age (yr)	Sex	Race	Dose/Day (mg)	Clinical Manifestations	Onset (Days after Start of Sulindac Therapy)	Treatment	Outcome	Associated Diseases
This study	62	F	B	300	Fever, erythematous rash on neck, mucous lesions, conjunctivitis, bullae, pruritus	14	Antihistamines, fluids, electrolytes, steroids	Recovered	Adult-onset diabetes
Levitt and Pearson[14]	39	F	W	400	Fever, erythematous maculopapular rash on chest, sloughing, pruritus, mucous lesions	15	Antihistamines, antibiotics, fluids, steroids	Recovered	None
Klein and Khan[15]	52	F	W	400	Fever, malaise, mouth ulcers, erythema	16	Antihistamines, antibiotics, fluids, steroids	Fatal[a]	Adult-onset diabetes, hypertension, toxic hepatitis
Breton et al.[16]	80	F	W	200	Flu-like syndrome, rash (erythema, vesicobullous)	14	Fluids, antibiotics, analgesics	Fatal[b]	Senile dementia, bone marrow suppression (neutropenia, leukopenia, thrombocytopenia)
Stern and Bigby[17]	81	F	W	400	Fever, rash	14	Bed rest, fluids antibiotics	Fatal[a]	None
	82	F	W	400	Fever, rash, sloughing	14	Bed rest, fluids antibiotics	Fatal[b]	None

[a] Death occurred 22 days after start of sulindac therapy.
[b] Death occurred 20 days after start of sulindac therapy.

11. Park GD, Spector R, Headstream T et al. Serious adverse reactons associated with sulindac. *Arch Intern Med.* 1982; 142:1292–4.
12. Husain Z, Runge LA, Jabbs JM et al. Sulindac-induced Stevens-Johnson syndrome. Report of 3 cases. *J Rheumatol.* 1981; 8:176–9.
13. Bigby M, Stern R. Cutaneous reactions to non-steroidal anti-inflammatory drugs. *J Am Acad Dermatol.* 1985; 12:866–76.
14. Levitt L, Pearson RW. Sulindac-induced Stevens-Johnson toxic epidermal necrolysis syndrome. *JAMA.* 1980; 243:1262–3.
15. Klein SM, Khan MA. Hepatitis, toxic epidermal necrolysis and pancreatitis in association with sulindac therapy. *J Rheumatol.* 1983; 10:512–3.
16. Breton JC, Pibouin M, Allain H et al. Sulindac: toxic epidermal necrolysis. *Therapie.* 1985; 40 (Jan–Feb):67–8.
17. Stern RS, Bigby M. An expanded profile of cutaneous reactions to nonsteroidal anti-inflammatory drugs. *JAMA.* 1984; 252:1433–7.
18. Guillaume JC, Roujeau JC, Revuz J et al. The culprit drugs in 87 cases of toxic epidermal necrolysis (Lyell's syndrome). *Arch Dermatol.* 1987; 123:1166–70.

"

Ethical Basis of Treatment Decisions

. . .The quality of medical care already has improved dramatically through two scientific advances: the development of exciting new possibilities for effective intervention in many diseases and the documentation through rigorous clinical trials that these interventions do in fact lead to demonstrable benefits. Clinical decisions about whether to apply these interventions, however, inevitably involve questions of values—whether the benefits of intervention are judged to outweigh any associated burdens. According to the doctrine of informed consent, this determination must be made from the perspective of the patient.

Improvements in the care of patients thus depend not only on advances in science but also on attention to contemporary medical ethics, in which engaging the patient as an active participant in medical decision making is seen as particularly important.

—Forrow L, Wartman SA, Brock DW. Science, ethics, and the making of clinical decisions. *JAMA.* 1988; 259:3161–7.

"

Drug Experience

Straightforward reports of unusual drug experiences are included in this section. These may be confirmations of previously reported drug experiences or brief apparent first reports. While selected references may be cited, the purpose of a Drug Experience report is not to present an extensive review of the literature.

A related section, Grand Rounds, includes papers that are well-documented patient case reports with a thorough review of the important literature to help put the case in perspective.

Rebound hypertension after discontinuation of transdermal clonidine

GARY R. SCHMIDT AND ARTHUR A. SCHUNA

Clin Pharm. 1988; 7:772–4

An uncommon but serious consequence of discontinuing oral clonidine therapy is a rebound syndrome characterized by a rapid rise in blood pressure to levels greater than pretreatment values.[1,2] Upon discontinuation of central α_2 stimulation (which inhibits release of norepinephrine), high levels of plasma catecholamines and increased sensitivity of peripheral adrenergic receptors result in a hyperadrenergic state. This condition is characterized by headache, diaphoresis, tachycardia, insomnia, and tremor. The syndrome appears to be more common in patients with relatively severe hypertension who receive high doses of clonidine for a long time. Clonidine is now available in a dosage form that delivers a more constant blood level of clonidine via percutaneous drug delivery. These patches (Catapres-TTS, Boehringer Ingelheim Pharmaceuticals) are designed to provide a constant amount of drug via transdermal absorption when applied weekly. The transdermal system may decrease the incidence and severity of adverse effects commonly associated with oral clonidine. It was proposed that a rebound syndrome would not occur after Catapres-TTS dosing because the low doses of clonidine used are less likely to induce withdrawal reactions, and serum clonidine levels decrease more slowly after patches are removed from the skin (half-life of drug elimination = 20 hours).[3,4] After a study designed to evaluate the safety and efficacy of transdermal clonidine in elderly male patients with mild hypertension, we noted one instance of rebound hypertension accompanied by hyperadrenergic symptoms.

Case Report. A 64-year-old white man entered the active phase of a transdermal clonidine study after a four-week placebo phase. While he used placebo patches his blood pressure averaged 167/91 mm Hg when it was measured at the clinic. His highest blood pressure reading at home during the placebo phase was 180/100 mm Hg, and the highest blood pressure reading at the clinic was 172/92 mm Hg. He attained good control of his blood pressure with Catapres-TTS-2 (0.2 mg/24 hours), which kept his systolic blood pressure under 150 mm Hg for eight weeks (average clinic blood pressure, 148/91 mm Hg). Ten weeks into the study, his transdermal clonidine dose was further titrated to control his blood pressure. A Catapres-TTS-3 patch (programmed to deliver 0.3 mg of clonidine per day) was applied, and he wore a patch of this strength for the remaining four weeks of the study. The patient complained of a dry mouth, which started three days after application of the Catapres-TTS-3 patch. After two weeks of Catapres-TTS-3 therapy, he also complained of pruritus under and around the patch. When the patch was replaced in the clinic, the patch site was erythematous. These symptoms persisted throughout the last four weeks of the study. The patient achieved good control of his blood pressure during Catapres-TTS-3 therapy, with an average clinic blood pressure of 141/86

GARY R. SCHMIDT is Hypertension Research Pharmacist and Clinical Instructor and ARTHUR A. SCHUNA, M.S., is Clinical Pharmacy Coordinator, William S. Middleton Memorial Veterans' Hospital, and Clinical Associate Professor, School of Pharmacy, The University of Wisconsin, Madison.

Address reprint requests to Mr. Schmidt at the Pharmacy Service, William S. Middleton Memorial Veterans' Hospital, 2500 Overlook Terrace, Madison, WI 53705.

The contribution of the patient's physician, Theodore L. Goodfriend, M.D., is acknowledged.

Supported in part by a grant from Boehringer Ingelheim Pharmaceuticals, Inc., Ridgefield, CT 06877.

Presented at the 22nd Annual ASHP Midyear Clinical Meeting, Atlanta, GA, December 7, 1987.

Copyright © 1988, American Society of Hospital Pharmacists, Inc. All rights reserved 0278-2677/88/1001-0772$00.75.

mm Hg and an average radial pulse of 66. The patient continued to take sulindac 200 mg once a day throughout the study. He completed the protocol after 14 weeks of transdermal therapy: two weeks on Catapres-TTS-1, eight weeks on Catapres-TTS-2, and four weeks on Catapres-TTS-3.

Immediately after discontinuation of Catapres-TTS, the patient entered the placebo lead-in phase of a second study. On May 31, two days after discontinuing patch therapy and starting placebo antihypertensive tablets, the patient was examined by an emergency room physician (not the investigator), complaining of headache, increased perspiration, and increased blood pressure (measured at home). The patient noted a peak home blood pressure of 210/113 mm Hg. The emergency room physician recorded a blood pressure of 170/110 mm Hg and a radial pulse of 100 (Figure 1). The patient was described as anxious and distraught. The emergency room physician treated the patient with sublingual nifedipine, since he did not know the patient had previously been receiving transdermal clonidine. The patient's blood pressure responded to nifedipine. On June 1, the third day after Catapres-TTS-3 therapy was discontinued, the patient was examined in our clinic. His blood pressure was 154/102 mm Hg, with a radial pulse of 112, and he was complaining of headache and increased perspiration. He reported that symptoms started about 36 hours after discontinuation of transdermal clonidine therapy. A clonidine hydrochloride 0.2-mg tablet was administered by mouth to the patient in the clinic. After one and one-half hours, the patient's headache and diaphoretic symptoms were markedly improved; his blood pressure was 132/88 mm Hg, with a radial pulse of 102. He was given a prescription for clonidine hydrochloride 0.1 mg #15, with instructions to take one tablet twice a day for five days, followed by one tablet daily for five days. He was also instructed to take hydrochlorothiazide 50 mg daily for 10 days. The patient had previously been treated successfully with a diuretic. On June 12, he returned to the clinic with a blood pressure of 152/92 mm Hg and a radial pulse of 76. He had no complaints at this visit. The patient was examined again 14 days later. At this time he had no complaints; his blood pressure was 164/92 mm Hg, with a radial pulse of 80. During these last two weeks he had taken only placebo medication for his hypertension, which he began taking as part of another study.

Discussion. We observed a rapid rise in blood pressure after discontinuation of transdermal clonidine monotherapy, which the patient had been receiving for 14 weeks. Blood pressure values recorded at home and by the emergency room physician were greater than those recorded before therapy. This appears to be a true "overshoot" and not a reversal of therapeutic effect. Rebound hypertension was accompanied by symptoms of a hyperadrenergic state, including diaphoresis, headache, and tachycardia. Symptoms were intense two to three days after discontinuation of transdermal clonidine therapy. Metz et al.[5] observed a rapid rise in blood pressure to levels above control readings in three elderly hypertensive patients who were followed sequentially after discontinuation of transdermal clonidine monotherapy. These investigators did not observe an overshoot of plasma norepinephrine levels or symptoms of β-adrenergic overactivity. All three of their patients had blood pressure levels exceeding pretreatment val-

Figure 1. Mean blood pressure (taken at a clinic) of one patient in a pilot study to evaluate the safety and efficacy of transdermal clonidine (Catapres-TTS). The arrow indicates the initiation of oral clonidine therapy administered in the clinic. HCTZ = hydrochlorothiazide; Catapres-TTS-1 = 0.1 mg/24 hr, Catapres-TTS-2 = 0.2 mg/24 hr, Catapres-TTS-3 = 0.3 mg/24 hr.

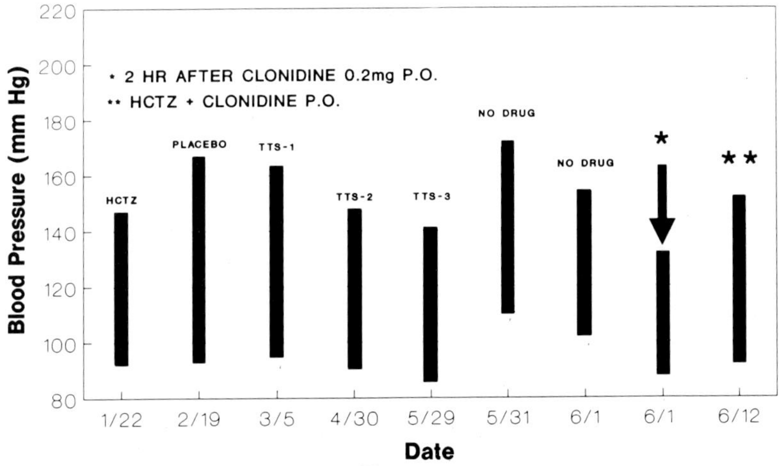

ues by the third to seventh day after the last patch was removed. White and Guidry[6] reported that a 67-year-old woman experienced rebound hypertension while taking furosemide 20 mg daily and atenolol 100 mg daily while a Catapres-TTS-2 patch remained in place. They noted the presence of contact dermatitis with edema, erythema, and vesicle formation beneath the patch. It was postulated that the clonidine was not absorbed because of inflammation associated with a type IV allergic reaction, and the rebound hypertension was exacerbated by the coadministration of a β blocker. Therapy with β blockers results in unopposed α receptors throughout the sympathetic nervous system. Increased serum catecholamines will stimulate these α receptors to cause vasoconstriction, resulting in an acute increase in total peripheral resistance and blood pressure. In the three patients in the study by Metz et al.,[5] White and Guidry's patient, and our patient, a state of α-adrenergic hyperresponsiveness was probably induced by the suppression of norepinephrine release during therapy. Metz et al. treated one 65-year-old patient for 15 months and two 70-year-old patients for 12 months. Weber et al.[7] reported that after discontinuation of transdermal clonidine, blood pressure returned smoothly to pretreatment levels in 12 patients. The patients in the study by Weber and associates were younger and were treated for only three months. Serial blood pressure measurements were obtained only in the 3 of his 12 patients who stopped patch therapy.

Conclusion. This is the first report of rebound hypertension and symptoms of a hyperadrenergic state (diaphoresis, headache, and tachycardia) in a patient taking transdermal clonidine for only 14 weeks. In discontinuing transdermal clonidine therapy, it may be prudent to use a gradual tapering regimen with oral clonidine or to slowly reduce the patch strength, rather than abruptly stopping therapy. Additionally, other oral adrenergic inhibitors such as methyldopa or guanabenz could be used to reduce the likelihood of rebound hypertension.

References

1. Hunyor SN, Hansson L, Harrison TS et al. Effects of clonidine withdrawal: possible mechanisms and suggestions for management. *Br Med J*. 1973; 2:209–11.
2. Hamilton BP, Mersey JH, Hamilton J et al. Withdrawal phenomena in subjects with essential hypertension on clonidine or tiamenidine. *Clin Pharmacol Ther*. 1984; 36:628–33.
3. Lowenthal DT, Saris S, Paran E et al. Efficacy of clonidine as transdermal therapeutic system: the international clinical trial experience. *Am Heart J*. 1986; 112:893–900.
4. Arndts D, Arndts K. Pharmacokinetics and pharmacodynamics of transdermally administered clonidine. *Eur J Clin Pharmacol*. 1984; 26:79–85.
5. Metz S, Klein C, Morton N. Rebound hypertension after discontinuation of transdermal clonidine therapy. *Am J Med*. 1987; 82:17–9.
6. White TM, Guidry JR. Rebound hypertension associated with transdermal clonidine and contact dermatitis. *West J Med*. 1986; 145(1):104.
7. Weber MA, Brewer DD, Drayer JM et al. Transdermal continuous antihypertensive therapy. *Lancet*. 1984; 1:9–11.

“

Replication of Scientific Findings

Given the wide variety of reasons two studies of the same therapeutic agent may differ in their conclusions, how should the clinician view the first report of a favorable result with a new drug? The approach taken by the FDA (when it assesses the benefits and risks of a new drug) is to review data derived from the individual case report forms submitted on each patient enrolled in all studies of a new drug; the FDA does not rely on the published data of a single trial. Because the results of various studies are frequently conflicting or raise additional questions, the FDA generally requires the submission of two well-controlled trials that support the efficacy of a new drug before it will consider the agent to have potential therapeutic value. Replication is an essential element in advancing scientific knowledge—a principle physicians may wish to keep firmly in mind before accepting recommendations from a single published report.

—Packer M. Clinical trials in congestive heart failure: why do studies report conflicting results? *Ann Intern Med*. 1988; 109:3–5. Editorial.

”

CP Continuing Education

The ASHP Continuing Education system gives readers a self-assessment mechanism for selected articles in Clinical Pharmacy *and the* American Journal of Hospital Pharmacy. *It also allows readers to obtain continuing-education credit for these articles.*

For the purpose of CE-credit enrollment a blank answer sheet is published at the end of each installment of the column for the CE articles in that issue. An enrollee accumulates these answer sheets until the enrollment is submitted, using the form that is published in the June and December issues of Clinical Pharmacy *and in the June and December issues of the* American Journal of Hospital Pharmacy. *Any combination of tests within a 18-month period, from both* Clinical Pharmacy *and* American Journal of Hospital Pharmacy, *may be included in an enrollment. More complete details about enrollment in the system will appear in the semiannual enrollment form.*

Article 680-204-8815 (see page 725)
Qualifies for 1.0 hour of CE credit

Therapeutic evaluation of omeprazole

Learning Objectives

After studying this article, the reader should be able to

1. Contrast the chemistry and mechanism of action of omeprazole with H_2-receptor antagonists.
2. List the principal pharmacologic effect of omeprazole on gastric acid secretion, gastric juice volume, pepsin and pepsinogen concentrations, and gastrin secretion.
3. Describe the pharmacokinetics and dosing recommendations of omeprazole.
4. Describe the role of omeprazole, based on clinical trials, in the treatment of the following conditions: duodenal ulcer, benign gastric ulcer, esophagitis, and Zollinger–Ellison syndrome.
5. List five common adverse drug reactions of omeprazole.

Self-assessment Questions

For each question there is one best answer only.

1. Which of the following statements best describes the proposed mechanism of action of omeprazole?
   a. Inhibition of cyclic adenosine 3′,5′-monophosphate (cAMP) production in the parietal cell.
   b. Inhibition of the H^+,K^+-ATPase proton pump.
   c. Competitive binding for the acetylcholine receptor.
   d. Inactivation of gastrin in the canaliculi.

2. Which of the following is not a pharmacologic effect of omeprazole?
   a. Gastric acid secretion is significantly inhibited.
   b. Serum gastrin concentrations increase after repeated dosing.
   c. The volume of gastric juice secretions is reduced.
   d. Secretion of intrinsic factor is inhibited.

3. Which of the following statements regarding the pharmacokinetics of omeprazole is incorrect?
   a. Omeprazole has a plasma half-life of two to three hours after oral administration.
   b. Omeprazole is approximately 95% bound to plasma proteins; protein binding is not altered by chronic renal insufficiency.
   c. The degree of gastric acid inhibition is directly related to plasma omeprazole concentration.
   d. The rate of omeprazole absorption increases after repeated oral doses.

4. Which of the following statements regarding the efficacy of omeprazole in the treatment of duodenal ulcer has been demonstrated in comparative clinical trials?
   a. Omeprazole is more efficacious than antacids in terms of pain relief.
   b. Omeprazole is more efficacious than H_2-receptor antagonists in terms of onset of healing.
   c. Omeprazole is less efficacious than H_2-receptor antagonists in terms of onset of healing.
   d. Omeprazole is more efficacious than antacids in terms of healing rates.

5. Which of the following statements regarding the efficacy of omeprazole in the treatment of benign gastric ulcer has been demonstrated in comparative clinical trials?
   a. Omeprazole is more efficacious than antacids in terms of pain relief.
   b. Omeprazole is as efficacious as H_2-receptor antagonists in terms of onset of healing.
   c. Omeprazole is less efficacious than H_2-receptor antagonists in terms of onset of healing.
   d. Omeprazole is more efficacious than antacids in terms of healing rates.

6. Which of the following statements regarding the efficacy of omeprazole in the treatment of esophagitis has been demonstrated in comparative clinical trials?
   a. Omeprazole is more efficacious than antacids in terms of pain relief.
   b. Omeprazole is more efficacious than H_2-receptor antagonists in terms of onset of healing.
   c. Omeprazole is less efficacious than H_2-receptor antagonists in terms of onset of healing.

d. Omeprazole is more efficacious than antacids in terms of healing rates.

7. Which of the following statements regarding the efficacy of omeprazole in the treatment of Zollinger–Ellison syndrome has been demonstrated in clinical trials?

a. Omeprazole is more efficacious than ranitidine as initial therapy.
b. Omeprazole is efficacious for patients who become refractory to therapy with an H_2-receptor antagonist.
c. Omeprazole is less efficacious than H_2-receptor antagonists in terms of resolution of symptoms.
d. Omeprazole and H_2-receptor antagonist dosages must be increased during long-term therapy at comparable rates.

8. The recommended initial dosage of omeprazole for the treatment of duodenal or gastric ulcer is

a. Omeprazole 40 mg once daily before breakfast.
b. Omeprazole 20 mg twice daily with food.
c. Omeprazole 40 mg once daily with food at bedtime.
d. Omeprazole 20 mg once daily before breakfast.

9. Studies in humans have demonstrated drug–drug interactions between omeprazole and

a. Ketoconazole.
b. Diazepam.
c. Theophylline.
d. Antacids.

10. The most common adverse effects of omeprazole include all of the following except

a. Diarrhea.
b. Headache.
c. Rash.
d. Anterograde amnesia.

Article 680-204-8816 (see page 746)
Qualifies for 1.0 hour of CE credit

Management and prevention of bacterial diarrhea

Learning Objectives

After studying this article, the reader should be able to

1. List host and microbial characteristics that are important determinants of the severity of diarrheal disease.
2. Describe the appropriateness of oral or intravenous fluid replacement in the treatment of diarrheal illnesses and list the essential components of rehydration solutions.
3. Identify advantages and disadvantages of using antimotility agents, antisecretory drugs, and adsorbent drugs in the treatment of infectious diarrhea.
4. List bacterial diarrheal diseases for which antimicrobial therapy is indicated and recommend an antimicrobial regimen for each.
5. List nondrug measures and drug therapies that can be used to protect travelers against acquiring enteric infections.

Self-assessment Questions

For each question there is one best answer only.

1. The severity of diarrheal disease after ingestion of a pathogen is influenced by

a. The patient's age.
b. The quantity of organisms ingested.
c. Alterations in intestinal secretion of immunoglobulins.
d. Abnormalities in the microflora of the bowel.
e. All of the above alternatives are correct.

2. An inflammatory toxin that causes structural damage to the intestinal mucosal surface, resulting in colitis and dysentery, is a

a. Cytotoxin.
b. Enterotoxin.
c. Neurotoxin.
d. Endotoxin.

3. A diagnosis of infectious diarrhea is based on

a. The patient's history.
b. The symptoms present.
c. Microbiologic examination of a stool specimen.
d. The presence of fecal leukocytes.
e. All of the above alternatives are correct.

4. To promote maximal reabsorption from the gastrointestinal tract, oral rehydration solutions should contain

a. Sodium in a concentration of 20 meq/L.
b. Glucose 3–4%.
c. Glucose 1–2%.
d. Sodium in a concentration of 50 meq/L.

5. A chronic carrier state requiring antimicrobial therapy can develop in patients who have bacterial diarrhea caused by

a. *Salmonella typhi*.
b. Enterotoxigenic *Escherichia coli*.
c. *Vibrio cholerae*.
d. *Yersinia enterocolitica*.

6. Patients who have dysentery or diarrhea accompanied by fever should not take

a. Bismuth subsalicylate.
b. Loperamide.
c. Diphenoxylate plus atropine.
d. Kaolin–pectin.

7. Which one of the following antimicrobial agents has not been shown to protect against traveler's diarrhea?

a. Doxycycline.
b. Ampicillin.
c. Trimethoprim–sulfamethoxazole.
d. Norfloxacin.

8. Infectious diarrhea occurring during prolonged antimicrobial therapy can be caused by

a. *Isospora belli.*
b. Cryptosporidium.
c. *Clostridium difficile.*
d. *Giardia lamblia.*

9. Acute dysentery is caused by all of the following organisms except

a. *Clostridium difficile.*
b. *Campylobacter jejuni.*
c. *Shigella* spp.
d. *Isospora belli.*
e. *Yersinia enterocolitica.*

10. Trimethoprim–sulfamethoxazole is recommended for the treatment of enteric infections caused by

a. Enteropathogenic *Escherichia coli.*
b. *Campylobacter jejuni.*
c. *Vibrio cholerae.*
d. *Shigella* spp.

Answer sheet

October 1988 *Clinical Pharmacy*

Note: An enrollment form for the ASHP Continuing-Education System appears in the June and December issues. Please accumulate all the answer sheets you wish to use in one enrollment and submit them at one time with a completed enrollment form.

Place an X in the box(es) at the top of the column(s) corresponding to the test(s) you are taking. Darken the boxes corresponding to the correct answers.

	☐ 680-204-8815 1.0 hour		☐ 680-204-8816 1.0 hour
	a b c d		a b c d e
1.	☐☐☐☐	1.	☐☐☐☐☐
2.	☐☐☐☐	2.	☐☐☐☐
3.	☐☐☐☐	3.	☐☐☐☐☐
4.	☐☐☐☐	4.	☐☐☐☐
5.	☐☐☐☐	5.	☐☐☐☐
6.	☐☐☐☐	6.	☐☐☐☐
7.	☐☐☐☐	7.	☐☐☐☐
8.	☐☐☐☐	8.	☐☐☐☐
9.	☐☐☐☐	9.	☐☐☐☐☐
10.	☐☐☐☐	10.	☐☐☐☐

ASHP Use Only
(1.0)8815________(3)
(1.0)8816________(3)

When you're trying to document the cost-effectiveness of pharmaceutical services, it helps to know what others have done. Now you can, with the

Resource Book on Progressive Pharmaceutical Services

Published by ASHP

Whether your pharmacy is introducing new clinical services or expanding existing ones, the *Resource Book* directs you to the literature describing what's been accomplished, in terms of implementing and evaluating progressive pharmaceutical services.

The book's first section lists and organizes articles according to pharmacy practice area. The second section features abstracts on all of the literature listed.

The ***Resource Book*** can help you make more efficient use of your pharmacy department's resources. **Order today!**

Order Form

Please send me ____ copies of the *Resource Book* at $15.00 each. 110 pp: softbound

☐ Enclosed is my check for $ ________.

☐ Enclosed is our purchase order # ________; please issue an invoice and add postage and handling.

Charge $ ________ to my
☐ MasterCard ☐ VISA
(minimum charge of $25 required)

Account # ________________

Exp. ________ *(month/year)* Signature ________________

Name ________________

Institution ________________

Address ________________

City ________ State ____ Zip ________

ASHP ID# ________________

Send to: ASHP Publications Records Dept.
4630 Montgomery Avenue
Bethesda, MD 20814

Payments to ASHP are not deductible as charitable contributions for Federal Income Tax purposes. However, they may be deductible under other provisions of the Internal Revenue Code.

Current Literature

Drug Reaction Alerts

Drug Reaction Alerts focuses primarily on serious, unlabeled reactions to new chemical entities. The citations are compiled monthly from International Pharmaceutical Abstracts, *which covers over 800 journals. An address for reprints (when available) follows the name of the corresponding author in each citation.*

Anthelmintics

Homeida MM, Bagi IA, Ghalib HW et al. (Sheikh HE, Department of Medicine, Dermatology, Pharmacology, Pathology, and Surgery, Facility of Medicine, University of Khartoum, P.O. Box 102, Khartoum, Sudan.) Prolongation of prothrombin time with **ivermectin**. *Lancet*. 1988; 1:1346–7. Cases. (two men, aged 40 and 16 years; received oral ivermectin 150 μg/kg for onchocerciasis; developed hematomatous swellings on thigh and right side of chest 27 and 30 days after treatment, respectively; swelling started spontaneously and enlarged over three to four days and prothrombin time prolonged in both patients; first patient recovered in one week without treatment and second patient received transfusion of freshly prepared blood and recovered within same period of time)

Anti-inflammatory Agents

Novis BH (Meir General Hospital, 44281 Kfar-Saba, Israel) Korzets Z, Chen P. Nephrotic syndrome after treatment with **5-aminosalicylic acid.** *Br Med J*. 1988; 96:1442. Case. (61-year-old woman with colitis; received mesalamine [5-aminosalacylic acid] 800 mg three times daily for five months; developed nephrotic syndrome; withdrawal of mesalamine and therapy with prednisone 1 mg/kg/day initially and tapered over four months led to resolution of syndrome within six weeks; no rechallenge)

Antineoplastic Agents

Ford MR, Turner MJ, Wood C et al. (Soutter WP, Institute of Obstetrics and Gynecology, Royal Postgraduate Medical School, Hammersmith Hospital, Du Cane Road, London W12 OHS, England.) Endometriosis developing during **tamoxifen** therapy. *Am J Obstet Gynecol*. 1988; 158:1119. Case. (54-year-old woman with benign breast disease; received tamoxifen 20 mg twice daily for five months; developed endometriosis; recovery after drug withdrawal and total hysterectomy)

Cardiac Drugs

Owen J (Department of Obstetrics and Gynecology, University Station, Birmingham, AL 35294), Colvin EV, Davis RO. Fetal death after successful conversion of fetal supraventricular tachycardia with **digoxin** and **verapamil**. *Am J Obstet Gynecol*. 1988; 158:1169–70. Case. (28-year-old pregnant woman with supraventricular tachycardia; received digoxin 2.5 mg/day depending on fetal response and verapamil 80 mg three times daily initially then 120 mg three times daily for four weeks; fetus died)

Drug Interactions

Erice A, Rhame FS, Chinnock B et al. (Balfour HH, University of Minnesota AIDS Clinical Trials Unit, Minneapolis, MN). Neutropenia in an HIV-1 infected renal transplant recipient treated with **zidovudine**. *JAMA*. 1988; 259:3407–8. Case. (28-year-old renal transplant patient with human immunodeficiency virus type 1; received zidovudine 200 mg every four hours for one week; concomitant azathioprine and **sulfamethoxazole–trimethoprim**; developed neutropenia; white blood cell count improved after zidovudine withdrawal; neutropenia recurred when zidovudine reinstituted at 100 mg every eight hours initially and increased to 100 mg every six hours over two weeks; white blood cell count recovered upon withdrawal of sulfamethoxazole–trimethoprim and no further episodes of neutropenia occurred)

Falkenberg HM. Possible interaction report. *Can Pharm J*. 1988; 121:294. Cases. (two women, aged 43 and 70 years; first patient received **nifedipine** 10 mg three times daily for angina pectoris and one 60-mg **terfenadine** tablet for seasonal rhinitis and second patient received verapamil 80 mg three times daily and identical dosage of terfenadine; first patient suffered acute angina attack and second patient developed lethargy, headache, and confusion; recovery upon withdrawal of terfenadine in both patients; no rechallenge)

Ragni MV, Tama G, Lewis JH et al. (Ho M, Department of Microbiology and Infectious Disease, Graduate School of Public Health, Pittsburgh, PA 15219). Increased frequency of hemarthroses in hemophilic patient treated with **zidovudine**. *Lancet*. 1988; 1:1454–5. Case. (48-year-old man with AIDS and hemophilia A; received zidovudine 200 mg five times daily for four weeks then 100 mg four times daily; concomitant ibuprofen for painful joint bleeding; fourfold increase in spontaneous hemorrhages, primarily of knees and elbows)

Kolski GB (Department of Pediatrics, Mary Imogene Bassett Hospital, Cooperstown, NY 13326), Cunningham AS, Niemiec PW et al. Hypokalemia and respiratory arrest in an infant with status asthmaticus. *J Pediatr*. 1988; 112:304–7. Case. (11-month-old girl with asthma; received **theophylline** sustained release 50 mg twice daily and **albuterol** 1 mg three to four times daily orally; developed life-threatening respiratory arrest, marked hyponatremia, and profound hypokalemia; positive rechallenge)

Kunzendorf U, Brockmoller J, Jochimsen F et al. (Offermann G, Klinikum Steglitz, Free University of Berlin, 1000, Berlin 45, FRG). **Cyclosporin** metabolites and central nervous system toxicity. *Lancet*. 1988; 1:1223. Case. (53-year-old kidney transplant recipient with tuberculosis; received cyclosporine 120–180 mg/day; concomitant isoniazid; developed mental disturbance; mental state improved after trough concentration of metabolite 17 fell)

Immunoglobulins

Kato E, Shindo S, Eto Y et al. (Hiyoshi Y, St. Mary's Hospital, Kurume, Japan). Administration of **immune globulin** associated with aseptic meningitis. *JAMA*. 1988; 259:3269–70. Case. (two-year-old girl with idiopathic thrombocytopenic purpura; received immune globulin intravenous 0.4 mg/kg/day; concomitant hydrocortisone; developed aseptic meningitis attributed to polyethylene glycol in immune globulin injection; positive reaction 20 days later after receiving sulfonated immune globulin injection)

Potter M, Stockley R, Storry J et al. (Slade R, Department of Hematology, Southmead Hospital, Bristol BS10 5NB, England). ABO alloimmunization after intravenous **immunoglobulin** infusion. *Lancet*. 1988; 1:932–3. Case. (29-year-old pregnant woman with thrombocytopenic purpura; received immune globulin 0.4 g/kg for three days when platelet count dropped to 32 x 10^9/L; patient went into spontaneous labor when platelet count rose to 80 x 10^9/L; delivered live infant vaginally with minimum blood loss; newborn diagnosed with ABO hemolytic disease, received exchange transfusion, and made good recovery)

Topical Preparations

Pazmino P (Texas Technical University, Health Science Center, El Paso, TX). Topical **tretinoin** for photoaged skin. *JAMA*. 1988; 259:3271. Case. (63-year-old man; received tretinoin topically on alternate days for two months; developed dermatitis and kidney function abnormalities; resolution of symptoms when drug withdrawn)

Vaccines

Osanto S, Cluitmans FH, Franks CR et al. (Bosker H, Department of Clinical Oncology and Cardiology, University Hospital, 2300RC Leiden, Netherlands). Myocardial injury after **interleukin 2** therapy. *Lancet*. 1988; 2:48–9. Case. (29-year-old woman with metastatic melanoma; received two cycles of interleukin-2 at daily dosage of 3 x 10^6 U/sq m for five days; infusion interrupted on day 3 because of slight fall in blood pressure and patient received higher dosage of interleukin-2 on day 4 to compensate for interruption; after completion of interleukin-2 therapy on day 6, ECG showed ST-segment elevations in leads V2–V4 and ventricular extrasystoles; elevated serum creatine kinase and other cardiac enzymes consistent with acute myocardial injury)

Cox NH, Moss C, Forsyth A (Contact Dermatitis Investigation Unit, Belvidere Hospital, Glasgow, Scotland). Cutaneous reactions to **aluminium in vaccines**: avoidable problem. *Lancet*. 1988; 2:43. Case. (3.5-year-old boy; developed three itchy lesions on right buttock at sites of previous DPT triple vaccine injections; positive reaction at 48 hours to patch testing, which resolved after seven days)

Vasodilating Agents

Shaw DR (Department of Medicine, Royal Adelaide Hospital, Adelaide, SA 5000, Australia) Misan GM, Johnson RD. **Nifedipine** hepatitis. *Aust N Z J Med*. 1987; 17:447–8.Case. (80-year-old woman; received nifedipine 10 mg three times daily for one day, then 20 mg three times daily for one day; developed acute hepatitis characterized by fever, chills, anorexia, nausea, liver tenderness, hepatitic liver function tests, and peripheral blood eosinophilia; no rechallenge)

Book Reviews

Basic Clinical Pharmacokinetics, Second Edition

By Michael E. Winter, Mary Anne Koda-Kimble, and Lloyd Y. Young.

Published by Applied Therapeutics, Inc., P.O. Box 1903, Spokane, WA 99210-1903, 1988. xviii + 416 p. Price $26.50, U.S. and Canada; $32.50 elsewhere; plus postage and handling.

It was with considerable interest that we reviewed the second edition of *Basic Clinical Pharmacokinetics*. The first edition has either been required or recommended as a text for our introductory pharmacokinetics course since its publication in 1980. When the first edition was initially published, the availability of pharmacokinetics texts was somewhat limited. Numerous books on the general subject now exist, enhancing the need to be selective and to choose cost-effective references and learning guides. The first edition of *Basic Clinical Pharmacokinetics* was reviewed in *AJHP* in 1981.[1] For a comprehensive and historical approach, we will occasionally refer to that review.

The second edition, again in paperback form, has grown to 416 pages, almost double the original 231. It is still divided into two sections, the first dealing with basic principles of pharmacokinetics (pages 7–99) and the second dealing with individual drugs (by chapter). The format for the drug section remains about the same as that in the first edition, with a summary of key variables and a discussion of population values, including a discussion of the time to sample. This is followed by case examples that are in a format similar to the cases in *Applied Therapeutics*.[2] The number of cases varies depending on the extent to which the individual drug's clinical pharmacokinetic characteristics are known.

In the basic principles section, the authors have expanded the portion on creatinine clearance estimation (considered a deficient area by the reviewer of the first edition). Several methods of predicting clearance have been added, along with sections on creatinine values at non-steady state and time to reach steady-state creatinine concentration. A new section on dialysis and estimating dialyzability potential also has been added.

In addition to the original eight drugs—gentamicin, digoxin, lidocaine, procainamide, quinidine, theophylline, phenobarbital, and phenytoin—the following drugs were added: carbamazepine, ethosuximide, lithium, methotrexate, primidone, salicylates, valproic acid, and vancomycin. Additionally, the gentamicin chapter was changed to "aminoglycosides" and covers gentamicin, tobramycin, and amikacin. Three appendices contain nomograms for body surface area, a list of equations used, and a glossary of terms and abbreviations.

We consider this book to be a very useful tool for teaching or for learning basic pharmacokinetic principles, and it is a useful basic reference and learning text for the therapeutic monitoring of drugs. The authors are particularly adept at clearly and concisely explaining important concepts (e.g., half-life, volume of distribution, and clearance) that can be difficult for those unfamiliar with pharmacokinetics to grasp. We believe that this book is one of the better texts in terms of providing a combination of basic pharmacokinetics and information on therapeutic monitoring. A description on the book cover states, "This book is an essential addition to the library of anyone involved in the interpretation of drug levels in the patient-care setting." At its relatively inexpensive price, we tend to agree, because very few practitioners will routinely monitor all of the drugs covered in the text. However, pharmacists with considerable experience in pharmacokinetic monitoring would derive limited benefits from the chapters on nonfamiliar drugs, because the text does not provide in-depth analysis of the variability in therapeutic drug monitoring. With the availability of computer software covering some of the drugs, the utility of the drug section may also decrease. However, few software packages cover all the drugs discussed in the text, and the basic section would remain beneficial to the novice.

For the next edition we would suggest that the authors give more attention to pediatric and neonatal considerations and the underlying premises associated with Bayesian forecasting. This text remains a valuable addition to the literature for the teacher and the new learner of pharmacokinetics and therapeutic drug monitoring. There are many useful suggestions gleaned from Dr. Winter's years as a practicing pharmacokineticist. The text is a basic reference for drugs not routinely monitored and for teaching purposes. We will continue to require or suggest this text to our students.

1. Rich DS. Basic clinical pharmacokinetics. 1st Ed. *Am J Hosp Pharm*. 1981; 38:1241–2. Book Review.
2. Katcher BS, Young LY, Koda-Kimble MA, eds. Applied therapeutics: the clinical use of drugs, 3rd Ed. Spokane, WA: Applied Therapeutics, Inc.; 1983.

Reviewed by John E. Murphy, Pharm.D., and David R. Collette, Pharm.D., Mercer University Southern School of Pharmacy and Georgia Baptist Medical Center, Atlanta, GA 30312.

Clinical Pharmacokinetics: The MCQ Approach

By Stephen H. Curry
Published by the Telford Press, Inc. 285 Bloomfield Ave., Caldwell, NJ 07006, 1987. iii + 185 p. Price $45; $27.50 paper.

This book is a well-organized collection of examination questions that students typically encounter in their initial pharmacokinetics courses. The reader's first challenge is to discover what the MCQ approach is. The author presents all of the problems as multiple-choice questions—hence the MCQ. It is necessary that the reader be familiar with basic pharmacokinetics concepts before using this text.

The introduction is a summary of useful pharmacokinetic equations, too brief to be of instructional value but useful for answering the questions in the following five chapters. The first chapter consists of problems requiring the drawing of graphs, and many examples of rectilinear and logarithmic graphs are provided. Familiarity with the basic pharmacokinetic equations presented in the introduction is required to answer the computational problems in chapter two. Many questions would require extensive reading of other texts and related primary literature before the average pharmacist could answer the questions. The third and fourth chapters are a collection of true-and-false statements covering various pharmacokinetic issues such as protein binding, absorption, and induction. Again, additional reading is required to answer these questions. The final chapter asks questions about specific references that can be answered only after reading the referenced scientific papers. While the appendix lists 28 well-selected references that contain enough information to answer any of the questions in the book, the references and questions are not specifically linked, which makes it difficult for the reader to know which references to consult for an in-depth answer to a particular question.

This book is best used as an instructional tool. The questions are provocative enough to encourage further reading and study and comprehensive enough to be used as a gauge of one's understanding of basic pharmacokinetics. However, it lacks the detailed information necessary in a reference or textbook. As such, it would be the last book bought by students or pharmacists to test their mastery of elementary pharmacokinetics, or the first book bought by instructors as an aid in designing examination questions.

Reviewed by Donald P. Hill, Jr., Pharm.D., and Michael E. Burton, Pharm.D., Veterans Administration Medical Center (11E), Dallas, TX 75216 and The University of Texas at Austin, College of Pharmacy.

Books Received

Books are listed as soon as received; selected books may be reviewed in Book Reviews in subsequent issues.

Atherosclerosis Reviews, Volume 18. Hypercholesterolemia: Clinical and Therapeutic Implications, edited by Joseph Stokes III and Mario Mancini. Published by Raven Press, Ltd., 1185 Avenue of the Americas, New York, NY 10036, 1988. xv + 202 p. Price $65.

Boyd's Introduction to the Study of Disease, Tenth Edition, by Huntington Sheldon. Published by Lea & Febiger, 600 Washington Square, Philadelphia, PA 19106-4198, 1988. vii + 702 p. Price $32.50.

Handbook of Clinical Drug Data, Sixth Edition. James E. Knoben and Philip O. Anderson, editors. Published by Drug Intelligence Publications, Inc., 1241 Broadway, Hamilton, IL 62341, 1988. xvi + 790 p. Price $39.50.

Medicinal Chemistry: A Biochemical Approach, Second Edition, by Thomas Nogrady. Published by Oxford University Press, 200 Madison Ave., New York, NY 10016, 1988. x + 514 p. Price $49.95, cloth; $32.50, paper.

Advertising Index

The American Institute of the History of Pharmacy
Institutional, 719
American Society of Hospital Pharmacists
ASHP Membership, 723
Consumer Drug Digest, 722
Resource Book on Progressive Pharmaceutical Services, 777
Baxter Healthcare Corporation, MultiPlex Systems Division
MultiPlex Fluid Management System, inside front cover
Bristol Bay Area Health Corporation, Kanakanak Hospital
Position Available, 719
Lemmon Company
Clindamycin, 724
Eli Lilly and Company
Tazidime, 715–716
Owen Healthcare, Inc.
Positions Available, 717
Roxane Laboratories Inc., A Boehringer Ingelheim Company
Intensols, 709
Stuart Pharmaceuticals, Division of ICI Americas, Inc.
Cefotan, inside back cover, outside back cover
The University of Alabama Hospital
Positions Available, 719
University of Illinois at Chicago
Positions Available, 717
The Upjohn Company
Cleocin Phosphate, 711–712

News

FDA approves marketing of diclofenac

FDA recently approved marketing of the nonsteroidal anti-inflammatory agent diclofenac (Voltaren, Ciba-Geigy Corporation) for use in the treatment of rheumatoid arthritis, osteoarthritis, and ankylosing spondylitis.

Diclofenac, a phenylacetic acid derivative, is completely absorbed from the gastrointestinal tract after oral administration. Peak plasma concentrations occur two to three hours after a dose. Administration with food delays the rate but not the extent of absorption. First-pass metabolism reduces systemic availability to about 50%. Diclofenac is more than 99% bound to plasma albumin. The terminal elimination half-life is approximately two hours. Diclofenac is eliminated via metabolism and subsequent renal and biliary elimination of sulfate and glucuronide conjugates of the metabolites.

Gastrointestinal complaints were reported by 20% of patients who participated in controlled clinical trials; symptoms led to discontinuation of therapy in 3% of patients. Serum aminotransferase concentrations increased to greater than three times the upper limit of normal in 2% of patients during the first two months of treatment; marked elevations occurred in about 1% of patients treated for two to six months. Aminotransferase abnormalities were more common among patients who had osteoarthritis. Postmarketing drug surveillance in other countries indicates that serious or fatal hepatic reactions are rare. Headache and dizziness occur at rates of 7% and 3%, respectively.

As with other nonsteroidal anti-inflammatory agents, labeled precautions include renal toxicity and fluid retention. Use of diclofenac in patients with hepatic porphyria is not recommended.

The recommended dosage for patients with osteoarthritis is 100–150 mg/day, given in divided doses two or three times daily. In rheumatoid arthritis, the recommended dosage is 150–200 mg/day, given as 50 mg three or four times daily or 75 mg twice daily. Dosages of 100–125 mg/day (25 mg four times daily and an additional 25 mg at bedtime, if needed) are recommended in the treatment of ankylosing spondylitis.

Voltaren is available as enteric-coated tablets containing 25, 50, or 75 mg of diclofenac. The drug is supplied in bottles of 60 and 100 tablets and unit dose boxes of 100 tablets. The 50- and 75-mg tablets are also available in bottles of 1000. The average retail cost for one month of therapy is $45 to $60.

Study suggests added benefit from combined aspirin–streptokinase therapy after myocardial infarction

Combined use of aspirin and streptokinase may result in a greater reduction in mortality after myocardial infarction than use of either agent alone, according to results of the Second International Study of Infarct Survival (ISIS-2).[1]

A total of 17,187 patients with suspected acute myocardial infarction were enrolled in the randomized, placebo-controlled multicenter study comparing the separate and combined effects of streptokinase 1.5 million units infused intravenously over one hour and aspirin 160 mg/day orally for one month. Patients were enrolled within 24 hours of the onset of symptoms; ECG changes were not required for study entry. Effects on mortality were analyzed according to intention-to-treat.

Both streptokinase alone and aspirin alone produced significant five-week reductions in mortality from vascular causes (mortality rates: streptokinase, 9.2%, or 791 of 8592 patients, and placebo injection, 12.0%, or 1029 of 8595 patients; aspirin, 9.4%, or 804 of 8587 patients, and placebo tablets, 11.8%, or 1016 of 8600 patients). The mortality rate with combination therapy (8.0%, or 343 of 4292 patients) was significantly lower than that with either agent alone. Reductions in mortality with aspirin therapy were similar with either early or late onset of therapy, whereas the benefits of streptokinase were greatest when therapy was begun within four hours.

Streptokinase therapy was associated with more episodes of minor bleeding, hemorrhage requiring transfusion, and cerebral hemorrhage than was placebo; other types of strokes were less common and nonfatal reinfarction was reported slightly more often with streptokinase therapy. Compared with the placebo group, patients receiving aspirin alone had fewer nonfatal reinfarctions and strokes and more minor bleeding episodes but no increase in major hemorrhage or cerebral hemorrhage. An excess of major bleeds and cerebral hemorrhage and a lower incidence of other types of strokes and reinfarction were reported with combination therapy.

Median follow-up at the time of the report was 15 months; longer follow-up will be required to determine how long the early benefits of treatment persist.

An international study involving as many as 40,000 patients is currently being planned. This study will compare alteplase with streptokinase; both drugs will be given in combination with aspirin. Completion of this trial is likely to take three years.

1. ISIS-2 Collaborative Group. Randomised trial of intravenous streptokinase, oral aspirin, both, or neither among 17187 cases of suspected acute myocardial infarction: ISIS-2. *Lancet*. 1988; 2:349–60.

FDA approves treatment IND protocols for selegiline and pentostatin

Two treatment IND protocols recently approved by FDA will permit broader use of pentostatin, an anticancer agent, and selegiline. Selegiline will be used as an adjunct to levodopa in the treatment of severe Parkinson's disease; studies have suggested that concomitant use of selegiline may permit a reduction in the dosage of levodopa. Information on the protocol for selegiline use can be obtained from Somerset Pharmaceuticals, Inc., Denville, New Jersey; 201-586-2310. Pentostatin will be made available for the treatment of cases of hairy cell leukemia unresponsive to interferon alfa. Information on the pentostatin protocol can be obtained from the National Cancer Institute, Bethesda, Maryland; 800-422-6237.

Design of future thrombolytic studies explored by speaker

Changes in the design of future trials evaluating the efficacy and safety of thrombolytic agents in acute myocardial infarction can be expected, according to Craig Pratt, M.D., chairman of the FDA Cardiovascular Advisory Committee. Speaking at the Ninth Annual Meeting of the American College of Clinical Pharmacy in Philadelphia, Pennsylvania, August 24–27, Pratt outlined important considerations in the design and interpretation of clinical trials of this class of agents.

Study Design Issues. According to Pratt, placebo control groups may not be used much longer because of the benefits that have been achieved with thrombolytic therapy. In their place will be active-treatment control groups with prospectively designated subsets of patients. Pratt estimated that trials comparing thrombolytic agents probably need to include at least 15,000–20,000 subjects to detect any differences between treatments. Pratt stated that recent studies have demonstrated the importance of control groups: Mortality rates of control groups in various parts of the world have differed substantially. In many of these trials, concomitant therapy has differed.

Pretreatment catheterization studies may also become less common because extensive baseline evaluations delay treatment. In studies comparing alteplase with streptokinase, such delays may favor alteplase.

Endpoint of Therapy. Use of either patency or left-ventricular function as a surrogate for mortality requires a "leap of faith." If left-ventricular function is used as the endpoint, timing (early or late after treatment) is an important factor, as is evaluation of global versus segmental left ventricular function. Recent studies have brought into question the adequacy of left-ventricular function as a surrogate for mortality. The magnitude of the difference in ejection fractions has not always correlated with differences in mortality. Thus, many other factors must be important. According to Pratt, one of these factors is probably concomitant therapy. Analysis of subsets of data is extremely important for identifying subsets of patients who may experience dramatic improvements that may be obscured in the overall analysis.

As noted by Pratt, use of patency as the therapeutic endpoint requires the greatest leap of faith. Some spontaneous effect will become apparent if the evaluator simply waits long enough. Thus, timing of therapy, angiographic evaluation, and concomitant therapy are critical to interpretation of study results.

Reimbursement for contraception counseling, initial pregnancy test included in isotretinoin program

Hoffmann–La Roche has announced that, as part of a program aimed at preventing use of isotretinoin (Accutane) by pregnant women, the company will reimburse physicians and clinical laboratories for contraception counseling and initial pregnancy tests. The program will allow for referral of patients to consulting physicians for counseling. Kits to be supplied to all dermatologists and other prescribers of isotretinoin will describe the program; outline new prescribing guidelines; and provide patient consent forms, self-evaluation forms for assessing patients' understanding of the risks associated with therapy, and patient information brochures on isotretinoin and birth control.

News Briefs

- Single copies of **"The 1988 Report of the Joint National Committee on Detection, Evaluation, and Treatment of High Blood Pressure"** may be obtained free of charge from The National High Blood Pressure Education Program, Information Center, 4733 Bethesda Avenue, Suite 530, Bethesda, MD 20814; 301-951-3260.

- **"CPR for Everyone,"** a 90-minute instructional videotape on cardiopulmonary resuscitation and emergency choking procedures for the infant, child, and adult, is available at a cost of $29.95 plus postage and handling; for further information, contact CPR for Everyone, 7 Evergreen Way, Stratham, NH 03885; 603-778-3010.

- FDA has withdrawn approval for the combination of **sulfanilamide, aminacrine hydrochloride, and allantoin** (AVC Cream, Merrell Dow Pharmaceuticals, Inc.) because evidence of efficacy for the labeled indication is lacking; reformulation of the product as sulfanilamide alone was approved.

- Labeling indications for **ticarcillin–clavulanate potassium** (Timentin, Beecham Laboratories) have been expanded to include use in the treatment of endometritis.

Continued on page 788

CU trouble spot:
IG drug administration

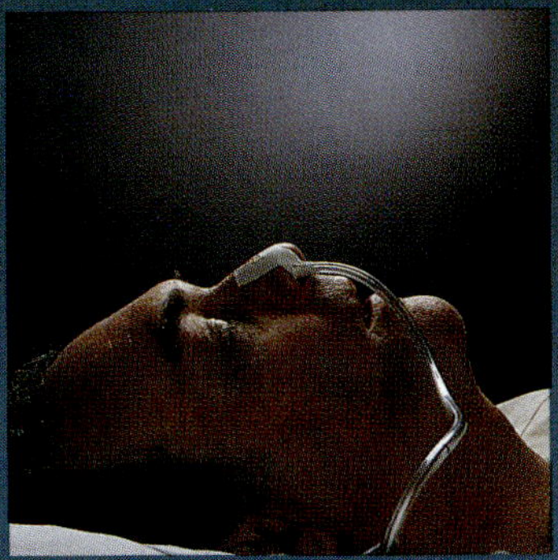

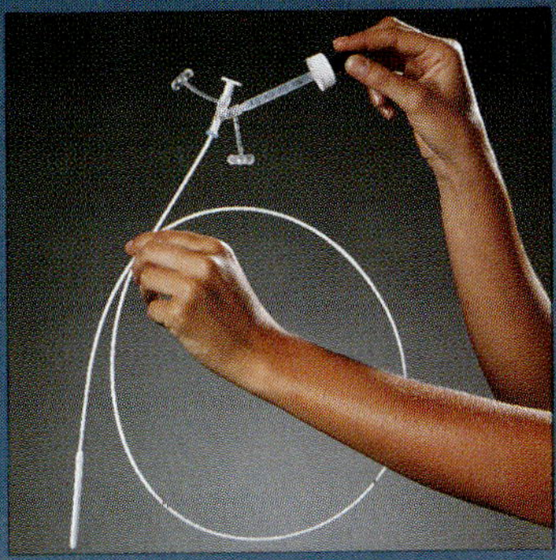

e solution is INTENSOLS™
oncentrated Oral Solutions

DEXAMETHASONE . . . . . . 1 mg/mL
PROPRANOLOL . . . . . . 80 mg/mL
PREDNISONE . . . . 5 mg/mL
DIAZEPAM . . . . 5 mg/mL

PALLIATIVE CARE AND CANCER PAIN PRODUCTS

Roxane Laboratories, Inc. Columbus, Ohio 43216

nplifies drug ministration to sogastric patients

rsing benefits

iminates crushing tablets or dissolving apsules
lore accurate and consistent dose
/on't clog NG tubes
aves nursing time for more productive atient care activities

armacy benefits

orrect dose is administered and bsorbed by the patient
rushing of sustained-release, sublingual, r enteric-coated tablets is minimized
rug/drug and acid/base interactions in ortar are avoided

sy to dispense

ach bottle comes with a calibrated ropper for accurate dosing and ration. Administering directly into NG be is possible.

Ideal for patients who have difficulty swallowing tablets

- Geriatric, pediatric, and cancer patients on high or variable doses
- Mixable with soft foods or liquids; most Intensols are tasteless so they won't alter the flavor
- Easy to swallow for improved compliance

Many Intensol-formulated drugs are available

- Prednisone, dexamethasone, diazepam propranolol, and more
- Easy to switch from injectables to orals

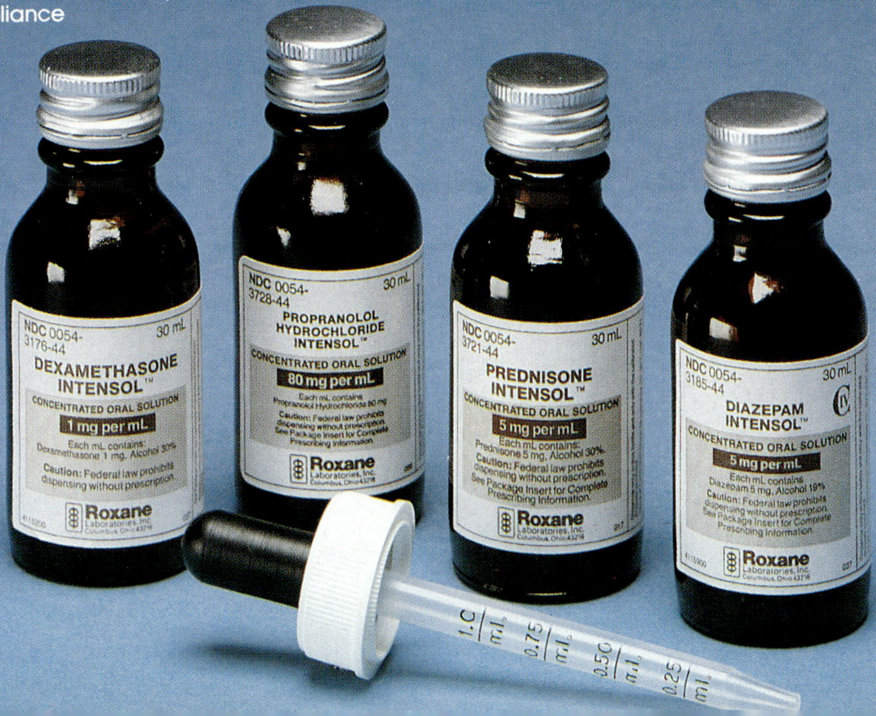

NTENSOLS™
solutions to tablet-taking problems

The University of Illinois at Chicago General and Specialized Residencies and Fellowships

General clinical pharmacy and specialized residencies and fellowships are being offered by the College of Pharmacy, University of Illinois at Chicago. The general clinical residency is a 12-month ASHP-accredited program designed to develop well-rounded clinical practitioners. This program emphasizes innovative comprehensive pharmacy practice through participation in clinical rotations and ongoing administrative research projects. All rotation sites will be at the University of Illinois Hospital and Clinics and the Veterans Administration West Side Medical Center.

The specialized residency/fellowship is a two-year program designed to develop the individual as a clinical scientist. The first year of the specialized residency/fellowship emphasizes clinical practice and advanced specialization through clinical rotations and participation in a 24-hour, inhouse, on-call program. The second year's emphasis is on clinical research, with the fellow serving as an investigator on at least one research project. Areas of specialization include administration, adult internal medicine, cardiology, clinical research, clinical pharmacokinetics, dermatology, drug information, emergency medicine, nephrology–transplantation, neurology–neurosurgery, oncology, pediatrics, psychiatry, and surgery. The administration, adult internal medicine, drug information, pediatrics, and oncology specialized residencies are ASHP-accedited.

Residents will receive formal and informal instruction in clinical research and pharmacotherapeutics. Each resident will have a teaching appointment in the College of Pharmacy and have the opportunity to develop didactic and clerkship teaching skills. All applicants must possess a Pharm.D. degree or be enrolled in a program leading to the Pharm.D. degree. For more information, please contact Donald L. Kendzierski, Pharm.D., The University of Illinois at Chicago, College of Pharmacy, 833 S. Wood Street, m/c 886, Chicago, IL 60612; 312-996-4033.

The University of Illinois is an Equal Opportunity/Affirmative Action Employer.

CALL FOR ABSTRACTS
1989 Annual Meeting
AMERICAN COLLEGE OF CLINICAL PHARMACY
August 6–9, 1989

All investigators in the field of clinical pharmacy and therapeutics are invited to submit abstracts of papers to be considered for Original or Encore presentation at the 10th Annual Meeting of the American College of Clinical Pharmacy, August 6–9, 1989, at the Westin Crown Center Hotel, Kansas City, Missouri. This will be an especially exciting meeting to commemorate ACCP's tenth anniversary.

Papers must describe original research in therapeutics, clinical pharmacokinetics, pharmacodynamics, innovations in clinical pharmacy practice, or cost analyses of clinical pharmacy services or drug therapy. In vitro and animal studies will be considered only if they represent innovative pharmacologic or pharmacokinetic principles that cannot be demonstrated in humans for ethical reasons.

ORIGINAL Presentations must neither have been published in abstract or complete form nor presented elsewhere prior to presentation at the 10th Annual Meeting.

ENCORE Presentations may have been presented elsewhere or published in abstract form only prior to presentation at the 10th Annual Meeting. Encore papers must not have been published in complete form.

All abstracts must be submitted on an official abstracts form and must be postmarked no later than January 15, 1989. Contact:

American College of Clinical Pharmacy
3101 Broadway, Suite 350
Kansas City, Missouri 64111
816-531-2177

accp
American College of Clinical Pharmacy

News *Continued from page 786*

Upcoming Specialty Meetings

Cardiology for the Clinician: Practical Guidelines for Merging Advances in Cardiology with Bedside Medicine . . . Snowmass, CO . . . March 5–10 . . . contact: Jane Whitener, University of Illinois at Chicago, Conferences and Institutes (M/C 607), Box 6998, Chicago, IL 60680; 312-996-5751.

American Society for Clinical Pharmacology and Therapeutics . . . Nashville, TN . . . March 8–10 . . . contact: E. Galasso, 1718 Gallagher Road, Norristown, PA 19401; 215-825-3838.

Pan American Allergy Society . . . San Antonio, TX . . . March 8–12 . . . contact: B. Kahler, 229 Parking Way, Lake Jackson, TX 77566; 405-297-5636.

American College of Cardiology . . . Anaheim, CA . . . March 19–23 . . . contact: W. D. Nelligan, CAE, 9111 Old Georgetown Road, Bethesda, MD 20814; 1-800-253-4636.

American Society for Clinical Nutrition . . . New Orleans, LA . . . March 19–24 . . . contact: S. Schiaffino, ASCN, 9650 Rockville Pike, Bethesda, MD 20814; 301-530-7110.

International Workshop on Clinical Pharmacy Epidemiology of Antibiotic Drug Use, in conjunction with the 16th International Congress of Chemotherapy . . . Herzlia on Sea, Israel . . . June 18–20 contact: Avraham Kreiser, P.O.B. 983, Jerusalem 91009 Israel.

C O N S I D E R
NEW BEDFORD
C O N S I D E R
ST. LUKE'S

Consider a beautiful seacoast city, home to one of New England's great harbors and graced with fine Victorian architecture. Consider a vibrant, multicultural city that's close to Boston, Providence, and Cape Cod, yet with its own distinct identity. Consider New Bedford.

New Bedford is where you'll find St. Luke's Hospital, a 433-bed community hospital that's provided quality healthcare to the Greater New Bedford Community for over a century. Join us, and you'll find that we provide our staff with an environment that encourages collaboration, supports professional development, and recognizes achievement. If you're looking for a better career in a better place, consider this currently available position:

Staff Pharmacist

In this outstanding position, you'll be part of a dynamic professional pharmacy staff caring for patients in our 433-bed acute care hospital. You'll provide a full range of services, including unit dose and IV Admixtures, and you'll participate in satellite operations involving med/surg, oncology, and mental health. Qualified applicants will be Massachusetts registered pharmacists interested in expanding their clinical roles.

St. Luke's offers highly competitive salaries and extensive benefits, including health and dental insurance; generous tuition assistance; pension plan; and credit union. Please send resume or direct inquiries to: **Personnel Department, St. Luke's Hospital, 101 Page Street, New Bedford, MA 02741-3003, (508) 997-1515, ext. 2125.**

St. Luke's Hospital of New Bedford
An Equal Opportunity Employer

Therapy Consultation

The Therapy Consultation *section provides brief advice, in question-and-answer format, on how to handle specific drug-therapy problems. Readers are invited to submit questions, which will be referred to a consultant for an answer. The problems should not be highly specialized or unusual, nor should they be mundane. Questions are answered briefly, based largely on the judgment and personal experience of the consultant, although selected references may be cited to substantiate the consultant's advice.*

Conversion from oral to intravenous verapamil therapy

Question: A hospitalized patient with supraventricular tachyarrhythmias controlled by oral verapamil can no longer take oral medication. How would you determine the dosage of intravenous verapamil that should be given?

Response: The approach to take when converting a patient from oral to intravenous verapamil therapy depends on the type and severity of the supraventricular arrhythmia.

Patients who have chronic atrial fibrillation or flutter may be treated with intermittent intravenous bolus doses of verapamil. However, despite rapid control of the ventricular rate, the duration of effect can be relatively short and sometimes highly variable (30–60 minutes to several hours). Some patients may require numerous and frequent doses. Therefore, in some cases continuous infusion of verapamil hydrochloride may be the best method for maintaining adequate control of the ventricular rate. Verapamil infusion therapy is generally safe and effective.[1,2] In our experience, an infusion rate of 5 to 10 mg/hr is sufficient to control the ventricular rate in most patients. The infusion should be titrated to achieve the desired response in each patient and minimize adverse effects. Generally, for patients with atrial fibrillation or flutter, the dose should be titrated to maintain a ventricular rate of less than 100 beats/minute. The infusion should be continued until appropriate oral therapy can be resumed, at which time the infusion can be tapered. Although relatively expensive, verapamil infusions have been continued for as long as 33 days.[3]

The approach to treating patients with re-entrant paroxysmal supraventricular tachycardia (PSVT) depends not only on the severity, but also on the frequency, of the arrhythmia. Patients who suffer from infrequent and well-tolerated episodes may best be treated with intermittent intravenous bolus doses given on an as-needed basis. Scheduled maintenance therapy is probably not warranted. A bolus dose of 5 to 10 mg of verapamil hydrochloride administered intravenously over two to five minutes provides rapid control of atrial tachyarrhythmias. About 80% of PSVT episodes will revert to sinus rhythm within five minutes of i.v. verapamil therapy. If the patient does not adequately respond to the initial dose, a second dose can be administered 15 minutes after the first. This method of control may not be suitable for patients suffering from frequent or clinically severe episodes of PSVT. These latter patients require preventive therapy; their arrhythmias may best be controlled with an i.v. bolus dose followed by a continuous infusion of verapamil. An initial bolus dose may not be necessary if oral therapy has been discontinued very recently. The bolus dose and infusion rate are the same as previously discussed.

Some may question whether plasma verapamil concentrations can be used to guide the conversion from oral to intravenous therapy. However, the pharmacokinetic and pharmacodynamic differences between the oral and intravenous dosage forms preclude equating plasma concentrations after oral and intravenous therapy. Verapamil undergoes extensive first-pass metabolism after oral administration; this process appears to be stereoselective in that clearance of the L-isomer is significantly greater than that of the D-isomer. This results in a relatively low ratio of L-isomer to D-isomer in the plasma after oral administration. This stereoselective first-pass phenomenon is further complicated by the fact that the L-isomer is 6 to 10 times more potent in depressing AV nodal conduction than the D-isomer. Intravenous administration avoids this extensive first-pass metabolism, resulting in a greater ratio of L-isomer to D-isomer. Because of the difference in potency of the two isomers, the total plasma concentration of verapamil may be an unreliable indicator of drug response.

1. Barbarash RA, Bauman JL, Lukazewski AA et al. Verapamil infusions in the treatment of atrial tachyarrhythmias. *Crit Care Med.* 1986; 14:886–8.
2. Iberti TS, Benjamin E, Paluch TA et al. Use of constant-infusion verapamil in the treatment of postoperative supraventricular tachycardia: a prospective study. *Crit Care Med.* 1986; 14:283–4.
3. Weber RJ, Dasta JF, Traetow WD. Long-term verapamil infusion in paroxysmal supraventricular tachycardia. *Crit Care Med.* 1984; 12:465–6.
4. Hoon TJ, Bauman JL, Rodvold KA et al. The pharmacodynamic and pharmacokinetic differences of the D- and L-isomers of verapamil: implications in the treatment of paroxysmal supraventricular tachycardia. *Am Heart J.* 1986; 112:396–403.

Marieke Dekker Schoen, Pharm.D.
Fellow, Cardiovascular Pharmacotherapy

Jerry L. Bauman, Pharm.D.
Associate Professor

Departments of Pharmacy Practice and Medicine, Section of Cardiology
University of Illinois at Chicago
Chicago, IL 60680

Letters

The Letters *column is a forum for rapid exchange of ideas among readers of* CP. *Liberal criteria are applied in the review of submissions to encourage contributions to this column.*

The Letters *column includes the following types of contributions: (1) comments, addenda, and minor updates on previously published work, (2) alerts on potential problems related to drug therapy or clinical research, (3) observations or comments on trends in drug therapy or clinical research, and (4) brief expressions of opinion about controversies in drug therapy or clinical research.*

Letters need not be submitted with the journal's manuscript checklist. The following conditions, however, must be adhered to: (1) the body of the letter must be no longer than two typewritten pages, (2) the use of references, tables, and illustrations should be minimized, (3) the authors' names, affiliations, and mailing addresses must be typed at the end of the letter in the format used by CP, *and (4) the entire letter (including references, tables, and authors' names) must be typed double spaced on plain white paper (not letterhead). Following acceptance of a letter, the authors are required to sign an exclusive publication statement and a copyright-transferral form.*

Storing extra calibration curves in the TDx assay system

The Abbott TDx drug assay system provides memory space for one calibration curve for each specific drug assay. If the concentration of a specific drug is to be determined in samples from more than one biological medium (e.g., serum and urine), separate calibration curves should be used; polarization readings vary depending on the medium, and inaccurate concentrations can be obtained if separate calibration curves are not used. Unfortunately, there is no simple way to access unused memory space within the TDx computer system to enter the second calibration curve under an alias.

We used a nonlinear curve-fitting program (PCNONLIN) to expand the capability of the TDx system without substantially increasing assay costs or limiting access to the calibration curve for serum samples. Serum samples from patients receiving tobramycin as part of a clinical trial were analyzed using TDx in the usual fashion. To determine the concentration of tobramycin in urine samples from these patients, standard solutions with tobramycin concentrations of 0.5 mg/L to 10 mg/L were prepared from fresh urine on the day of analysis and assayed in duplicate with the patient samples. The serum standard solutions were also assayed with the urine samples to ensure that the TDx system was functioning properly. The net polarization values for the urine standard solutions and samples were recorded. The net polarization values for the standard solutions of known tobramycin concentration were fitted using PCNONLIN to a four-parameter equation similar to that used internally by the TDx system.[1] This model (Figure 1) must be stored under a library name (e.g., TDXMOD>LIB), and the library name must be referenced in the data set to be analyzed by PCNONLIN. We then wrote a BASIC program that would calculate the concentration of tobramycin in the urine samples based on the standard curve concentration values and the net polarization values of the urine samples (Figure 2). The values obtained using PCNONLIN are substituted for x in lines 50 to 80. The values should not be rounded off, and the symbol # should be typed after each number.

Although this method is time consuming, it eliminates the need to re-enter the calibration curve for serum samples after every urine assay procedure.

1. Statistical Consultants, Inc. PCNONLIN and NONLIN84:

Figure 1. PCNONLIN program.

```
METHOD 3
MODEL 1
COMM
NPARM 4
PNAMES 'A', 'B', 'C', 'D'
WT -2
END
TEMP
A=P(1)
B=P(2)
C=P(3)
D=P(4)
END
FUNC1
IF X>0 THEN
F=A+B/(C+X**D)
ELSE
F=A+B/C
END IF
END
EOM
```

Figure 2. Program for determining drug concentrations from TDx polarization values.

```
10 REM PROGRAM FOR DRUG CONCENTRATION BASED UPON TDx
   POLARIZATION VALUES
20 REM A, B, C, D, are parameter values determined by PCNONLIN
30 REM Y = polarization value from TDx assay, X = drug concentration
40 CLS
50 LET A =    xx.xxxxxx#
60 LET B = xxxx.xxxxxx#
70 LET C =     x.xxxxxx#
80 LET D =     x.xxxxxx#
90 PRINT TAB(10); "Enter polarization value: ":INPUT" ",Y
100 X = EXP(LOG(B/(Y-A)-C)/D)
110 PRINT TAB(10); "The concentration is: ";X
120 PRINT TAB(30); "Continue? (Y/N)"; TAB(50);:INPUT" ",R$
130 PRINT:PRINT
140 IF R$="Y" THEN 80
150 IF R$="y" THEN 80
160 IF R$="N" THEN 180
170 IF R$="n" THEN 180
180 END
```

software for the statistical analysis of nonlinear models. *Am Stat*. 1986; 40:52.

DAVID E. NIX, PHARM.D.
CHARLES A. PELOQUIN, PHARM.D.

Clinical Pharmacokinetics Laboratory
Millard Fillmore Hospital
3 Gates Circle
Buffalo, NY 14209

Clinical Pharmacist / Pharmacologist

Texas Department of Mental Health and Mental Retardation

San Antonio State School

The 360-bed developmental disability facility is seeking a clinical pharmacist/pharmacologist. Pharm.D. required and completion of an accredited residency in clinical psychiatric pharmacy, or previous experience. Requires Texas license in pharmacy. Facility appointment and excellent fringe benefits that include no state income tax, state-paid partial social security payment, and tax deferred retirement contributions.

Interested persons should send résumé or call **Personnel Office, P.O. Box 14700, Harlandale Station, San Antonio, TX 78214; 512-532-9610.** An Equal Opportunity/Affirmative Action Employer.

When you're trying to document the cost-effectiveness of pharmaceutical services, it helps to know what others have done. Now you can, with the

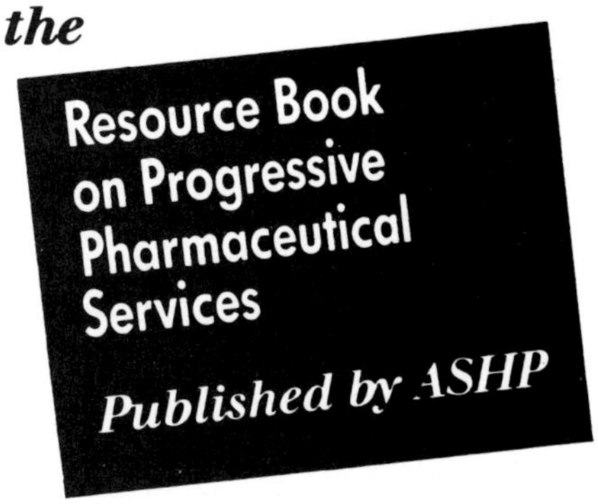

Whether your pharmacy is introducing new clinical services or expanding existing ones, the *Resource Book* directs you to the literature describing what's been accomplished, in terms of implementing and evaluating progressive pharmaceutical services.

The book's first section lists and organizes articles according to pharmacy practice area. The second section features abstracts on all of the literature listed.

The ***Resource Book*** can help you make more efficient use of your pharmacy department's resources. **Order today!**

Order Form

Please send me _____ copies of the *Resource Book* at $15.00 each. 110 pp: softbound

☐ Enclosed is my check for $ __________.

☐ Enclosed is our purchase order # __________; please issue an invoice and add postage and handling.

Charge $ __________ to my
☐ MasterCard ☐ VISA
(minimum charge of $25 required)

Account # ____________________

Exp. __________ Signature ____________________
(month/year)

Name ____________________

Institution ____________________

Address ____________________

City __________ State ____ Zip __________

ASHP ID# ____________________

Send to: ASHP Publications Records Dept.
4630 Montgomery Avenue
Bethesda, MD 20814

Payments to ASHP are not deductible as charitable contributions for Federal Income Tax purposes. However, they may be deductible under other provisions of the Internal Revenue Code.

THERE IS ONLY ONE REASON YOU NEED TO JOIN ASHP

YOUR COMMITMENT TO QUALITY IN PATIENT-ORIENTED PHARMACEUTICAL SERVICES

ASHP is the national professional association dedicated to advancing rational drug therapy in organized health-care settings. ASHP members have come to expect quality products and services including • timely journals, videotapes, software programs and special publications • top-flight continuing education programs • special member registration fees and prices • and multiple opportunities for networking with colleagues.

There is a membership category to suit just about every need. There are, however, two major categories. *Active Membership* is for any pharmacist licensed to practice in the United States, who supports the goals of ASHP. *Student Membership* is for students enrolled full-time in undergraduate or graduate pharmacy programs in accredited U.S. colleges of pharmacy. There's also an ASHP Pledge Program (for new graduates), plus Associate, International, Joint (husband/wife), Retired and Technician member categories.

ASHP membership offers an easy way to gain the knowledge you need to keep professionally current, improve your pharmacy services and multiply your opportunities for professional success — join ASHP today!

Become a part of ASHP today!
Here's how:

Name ______________________________
First M.I. Last

Address ______________________________
(include name of institution if this is a business address)

____

____

____
City State Zip

Is this your ☐ home or ☐ business/school address?

Date of Birth ______________ ☐ Male ☐ Female
month/day/year

Students: School of Pharmacy ______________

Anticipated Graduation Date: ______________
month/year

$30 of dues are for a subscription to *AJHP* and $3 for a subscription to the *ASHP Newsletter*

Please check the category for which you are applying:

☐ **Active** (H) $85

☐ **Student** (S) $20

☐ Send me a membership brochure with information on all categories.

☐ My check for $ __________ is enclosed (payable to ASHP)

Or, charge $ __________ to ☐ VISA ☐ MasterCard

Account # ______________ Exp. Date ________
month/year

Signature ______________________________

Mail to:
ASHP • Membership Records • 4630 Montgomery Avenue • Bethesda, Maryland 20814

Payments to ASHP are not deductible as charitable contributions for Federal Income Tax purposes. However, they may be deductible under other provisions of the Internal Revenue Code.

©1988 American Society of Hospital Pharmacists

Drug Review

Biological mechanisms and cardiovascular effects of omega-3 fatty acids

BRUCE A. MUELLER AND ROBERT L. TALBERT

Abstract: The mechanisms and cardiovascular effects of omega-3 fatty acids are reviewed.

Omega-3 polyunsaturated fatty acids are the major ingredient found in commercially available fish oil products. The incidence of many diseases, including coronary heart disease, diabetes mellitus, and psoriasis, is lower in Eskimos, who ingest diets rich in omega-3 fatty acids, compared with European controls. Potential mechanisms by which these fatty acids cause their many physiologic effects include competing with omega-6 fatty acids for prostaglandin and leukotriene pathways and enhancing cell membrane fluidity by virtue of the high degree of unsaturation. Numerous studies have documented longer bleeding times and decreased platelet aggregation in subjects ingesting omega-3 fatty acids. Omega-3 fatty acids may reduce serum cholesterol concentrations by decreasing the synthesis of very low density lipoprotein and, therefore, low-density lipoprotein. Blood viscosity is significantly and uniformly lower in subjects receiving omega-3 fatty acids compared with controls. Potential risks of supplementation with fish oils include hypervitaminosis A and D, vitamin E deficiency, increased bleeding times, decreased platelets, and ingestion of contaminated fish. Supplementation with moderate amounts of omega-3 fatty acids appears to be relatively safe. Possible adverse effects include nausea, diarrhea, and a "fishy" taste.

Properly controlled, long-term clinical trials are needed to determine whether supplementation with omega-3 fatty acids would be therapeutically beneficial in various patient populations and disease states.

Index terms: Acids, fatty; Antilipemic agents; Fish oil; Hypercholesterolemia; Mechanism of action; Toxicity
Clin Pharm. 1988; 7:795–807

Although present in the diet of certain cultures for eons, fish oils have been recently popularized by lay and medical media, and health professionals now frequently receive questions about this dietary supplement. Although these substances have been ingested by humans for thousands of years, only recently have the biological mechanisms and effects been identified. Fish oils, as they are known to the public, or omega-3 fatty acids, as they are referred to in the scientific literature, do have a wide spectrum of potential therapeutic uses. The intent of this article is to explain the mechanisms by which the omega-3 fatty acids exert their effects and to describe the cardiovascular responses observed with omega-3 fatty acid dietary supplementation.

It has been estimated that more than 1000 articles were published about omega-3 fatty acids and fish oils between 1975 and 1985.[1] Interest in this topic blossomed after Bang, Dyerberg, and Nielsen published their classic study in 1971 of Greenlandic Eskimos. These authors found profound differences in lipoprotein profiles between the Eskimos and age-matched and sex-matched Danish con-

BRUCE A. MUELLER, PHARM.D., is Assistant Professor of Clinical Pharmacy, Department of Pharmacy Practice, School of Pharmacy and Pharmacal Sciences, Purdue University, West Lafayette, IN. ROBERT L. TALBERT, PHARM.D., is Professor of Pharmacy, College of Pharmacy, University of Texas at Austin, and Departments of Pharmacology and Medicine, University of Texas Health Science Center at San Antonio.

Address reprint requests to Dr. Mueller at the Pharmacy Department, N-109-A, Indiana University Hospital, 926 West Michigan, Indianapolis, IN 46223.

This is **article 680-204-8817** in the **ASHP Continuing Education System.** See page 851 for learning objectives and test questions.

Copyright © 1988, American Society of Hospital Pharmacists, Inc. All rights reserved. 0278-2677/88/1101-0795$03.75.

trols.[2] Very low density lipoprotein (VLDL) and low-density lipoprotein (LDL) levels were strikingly lower in the Eskimos than in the Danes. High-density lipoprotein (HDL) levels were significantly higher in Eskimo men than in Danish men. Serum triglyceride and cholesterol levels were also found to be lower in the Eskimos than in the Danes. These lipoprotein differences were surprising, because the average daily Eskimo cholesterol intake was found to be twice that of the Danes.

In an epidemiologic study, Kromann and Green[3] found markedly different incidences of disease in Eskimos compared with European controls. As shown in Table 1, Eskimos had a higher frequency of stroke and epilepsy but a lower frequency of acute myocardial infarction, diabetes mellitus, asthma, multiple sclerosis, and psoriasis than the European population. A health report of this district of Greenland noted that only three cases of "atherosclerotic heart disease including coronary arterial disease" were found in a population of 1350 inhabitants between the years 1963 and 1967.[4] Only one confirmed case of diabetes mellitus was discovered in an epidemiological survey of 4249 Eskimos living in Greenland.[5] These profound differences between Eskimos and Europeans were likely due to either genetics or the Eskimo lifestyle and diet. Expatriated Eskimos living in Denmark and leading a European lifestyle were found to have the same frequency of disease as Europeans[2]; therefore, the theory of a disease-resistant Eskimo genetic profile was less likely. The Eskimo diet was then examined to determine whether it was the reason for the differences in disease state noted. Greenlandic Eskimos are primarily carnivorous, eating an average of 400 g of whale and seal meat per day per person.[6] Sea birds and fish, primarily halibut, capelin, and salmon, are also commonly eaten.[2] This diet was found to be rich in polyunsaturated fatty acids of the omega-3 class, compared with the Danish diet, which is rich in polyunsaturated fatty acids of the omega-6 class.[6]

Table 1.
Relative Disease Incidence in Eskimos versus Europeans[3]

Disease	Observed No. of Cases (1950–1974)	Expected No. of Cases Based on European Controls
Acute myocardial infarction	3	40
Asthma	1	25
Cancer (all forms)	46	53
Diabetes mellitus	1	9
Epilepsy (grand mal)	16	8
Multiple sclerosis	0	2
Peptic ulcer disease	19	29
Psoriasis	2	40
Stroke	25	15
Thyrotoxicosis	0	7

Disease prevalence has been investigated in other societies that have diets rich in omega-3 fatty acids, but the results are not as striking as are the Eskimo data. Turks who eat fish and marine animals were found to have a lower incidence of coronary artery disease than their "well-fed" controls.[7] Unlike the Greenlandic Eskimo findings, a study of Vancouver Island Indians found an increased prevalence of connective tissue and rheumatoid diseases.[8] Despite this lack of conclusive corroborating evidence, polyunsaturated fatty acids, especially of the omega-3 class, have spurred intensive research over the last decade.

Classification of Polyunsaturated Fatty Acids

The polyunsaturated fatty acids can be categorized into three major classes: oleic acid (omega-9 fatty acids), linoleic acid (omega-6), and linolenic acid (omega-3). None of these classes of polyunsaturated fatty acids can be metabolically converted to another in vivo. The omega (ω) number indicates the location of the first double bond counting from the methyl end of the fatty acid. These fatty acids differ in their sources, major metabolites, biological effects, and degree of saturation. The chemical structures of arachidonic acid, an important omega-6 fatty acid, and eicosapentaenoic acid (EPA) and docosahexaenoic acid (DHA) are shown in Figure 1.

Members of the omega-3 and omega-6 fatty acid classes are considered to be essential fatty acids, because they cannot be synthesized by humans and must be ingested via the diet. A knowledge of the differences between these two classes is fundamental to understanding the biological changes that occur when omega-3 fatty acids are administered in the form of marine fish oils in attempts to treat a variety of disease states.

Omega-6 fatty acids originate from oils derived from seeds and nuts, as well as from animal fats, all of which come from land. By definition, omega-6 fatty acids have their first double bond six carbon atoms from the methyl end. In omega-3 fatty acids, the first double bond is located three carbon atoms from the methyl end; therefore, omega-6 fatty acids are a more saturated species than their omega-3 counterparts. This distinction is noteworthy, because the sources of omega-3 fatty acids are quite different from the sources of omega-6 fatty acids. Omega-3 fatty acids are derived from marine phytoplankton. Teleologically, the phytoplankton require a more polyunsaturated fatty acid to keep their membranes fluid in the cold environment in which they live. The colder the environment of the phytoplankton, the more likely that their membranes will contain omega-3 fatty acids. Because these phytoplankton are at the bottom of the food chain, they are the prime source of polyunsaturat-

Figure 1. Classes of polyunsaturated fatty acids.

Fatty Acid Class	Parent Fatty Acid	Major Metabolite	Chemical Structure
Omega-9	oleic acid C18:1 ω-9	eicosatrienoic acid C20:3 ω-9	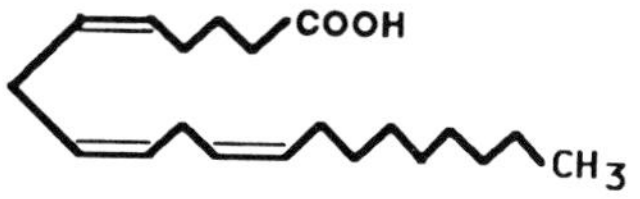
Omega-6	linoleic acid C18:2 ω-6	arachidonic acid C20:4 ω-6	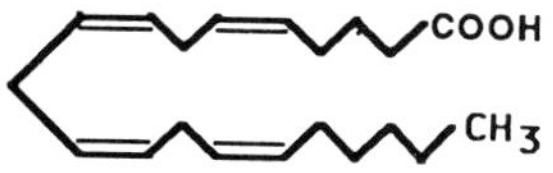
Omega-3	linolenic acid C18:3 ω-3	eicosapentaenoic acid [EPA] C20:5 ω-3	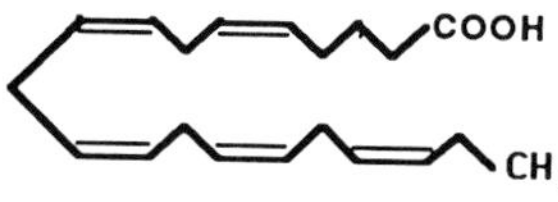
		docosahexaenoic acid [DHA] C22:6 ω-3	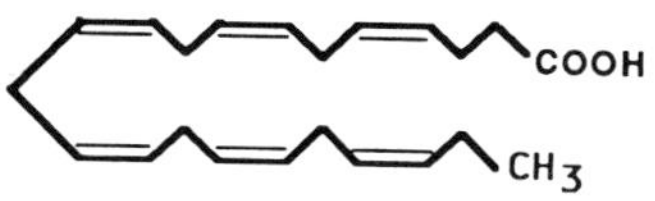

ed fatty acids for higher organisms in the food chain, such as fish and sea mammals.

Specialized human tissues such as the nervous system contain omega-3 fatty acids, even in people who are not actively supplementing their diet with omega-3 fatty acids. Omega-3 fatty acids are also found in human colostrum and mature breast milk.[9] EPA and DHA are the primary omega-3 fatty acids found in oils derived from fish, although other omega-3 fatty acids can be found in these oils in lesser amounts. EPA and, to a lesser extent, DHA are the two most studied omega-3 fatty acids. Constituents of marine fish oils other than omega-3 fatty acids are not well studied but may have important physiologic roles.

Proposed Mechanisms for the Effect of Omega-3 Fatty Acids on Omega-6 Prostaglandin and Leukotriene Pathways

Linoleic acid is the precursor for arachidonic acid, which in turn is the major substrate for human prostaglandin and leukotriene synthesis. The typical Western diet primarily consists of polyunsaturated fatty acids from the omega-6 class, with only small amounts of omega-3 fatty acids ingested. Marine omega-3 fatty acids are derived from linolenic acid instead of linoleic acid. Although linolenic acid can serve as the substrate for prostaglandin and leukotriene synthesis, this does not usually occur because so little omega-3 fatty acid is ingested in the Western diet. As a result, the Western human prostaglandin and leukotriene pathways are based on omega-6 fatty acids, with omega-3 fatty acids contributing only negligibly to production. Prostaglandin and leukotriene pathways that are dependent on omega-3 fatty acids develop with a diet high in omega-3 fatty acids and low in omega-6 fatty acids, as in the diet of Greenlandic Eskimos. Different types of prostaglandins and leukotrienes are formed when EPA is used as a precursor instead of arachidonic acid.

Ingestion of omega-3 fatty acids leads to an incorporation of EPA and DHA into tissue phospholipids, including platelet and erythrocyte membranes, plasma, and adipose tissue.[10-22] Galloway et al.[11] found that the EPA concentration in the platelet phospholipids, phosphatidylcholine and phosphatidylethanolamine, increased significantly on a diet supplemented with 1.8 g of EPA per day for four weeks. As EPA content increased in these phospholipids, arachidonic acid content decreased concurrently. Knapp et al.[12] found similar EPA incorporation into platelet phospholipids but also found a significant change in erythrocyte membrane fatty acid configuration when 10 g of EPA per day were added to the diet. By the end of four weeks of EPA supplementation, the ratio of EPA to arachidonic acid had risen from a baseline value of 0.08 to 1.24 in erythrocyte phosphatidylcholine in the six adult male patients with atherosclerosis who were studied.

Arachidonic acid stored in tissue phospholipids is the substrate for prostaglandin and leukotriene biosynthesis in the typical Western diet. Replacing arachidonic acid with EPA in these phospholipids results in the formation of EPA-derived prostaglandins and leukotrienes, rather than the typical arachidonic acid pathway. DHA does not appear to alter prostaglandin (PG) synthesis by changing the type of prostaglandin formed; however, DHA is a powerful competitive inhibitor of arachidonic acid conversion to PGG_2, PGH_2, and thromboxane A_2, all of which are potent platelet-aggregating agents.[23] Effects of omega-3 fatty acids on the typical Western omega-6-dependent prostaglandin and leukotriene pathways are seen in Figure 2. The administration of omega-3 fatty acids leads to a less thrombogenic state overall, because of the formation of the less reactive prostaglandins and leukotrienes based on omega-3 fatty acids. Additionally, unlike arachidonic acid, a potent platelet-aggregating factor, EPA does not induce platelet aggregation in vitro.[24]

In vitro studies have shown EPA to compete with arachidonic acid for platelet cyclooxygenase.[25] Inhibition by EPA of arachidonic-acid-derived prostaglandins via cyclooxygenase occurs through both reversible and irreversible actions on cyclooxygenase.[26] Human umbilical arteries were observed to convert EPA to the EPA-derived PGI_3 rather than the typical arachidonic-acid-derived prostaglandin PGI_2 (prostacyclin) that is associated with the Western diet.[27] In vivo evidence for the formation of prostaglandins not derived from omega-6 fatty acids during omega-3 fatty acid supplementation was reported by Fischer and Weber.[28] They found urinary metabolites of PGI_3 in the urine of subjects receiving omega-3 fatty acid supplementation in the form of cod liver oil or a diet rich in mackerel. PGI_3-M, the major urinary metabolite of PGI_3, was detected in subjects receiving single doses of purified EPA or DHA, suggesting that DHA can be converted to EPA in vivo and then incorporated into prostaglandins.[29] In another study, PGI_3 metabolites increased fourfold after four weeks in subjects taking 10 g of EPA per day.[12] Additionally, excretion of thromboxane B_3, the dinor metabolite of thromboxane A_3, was detected after four weeks, while none was found at baseline. Thromboxane A_3 is an omega-3-based compound and is less vasoactive than thromboxane A_2, an omega-6-derived, potent vasoconstrictive agent. Concurrently, the excretion of thromboxane B_2, a metabolite of the active compound thromboxane A_2, was significantly lowered. This decline of thromboxane A_2 formation was not seen when the EPA dose was reduced to 1 g per day. Available evidence indicates that omega-3 fatty acid supplements may influence qualitatively prostaglandin production when ingested in sufficient quantities.

In a similar vein, omega-3 fatty acid ingestion influences leukotriene biosynthesis. Leukotriene formation during the typical Western omega-6-fortified diet uses arachidonic acid that is stored in tissue phospholipids as the substrate for 5-lipoxygenase to form leukotriene B_4. Leukotriene B_4 is a potent chemotactic and platelet-aggregating substance. Although DHA does not seem to affect leukotriene B_4 production in vitro,[23] EPA supplementation has been shown to alter the human leukotriene profile, also shown in Figure 2. Leukotriene B_5, an EPA-derived leukotriene, has been found in neutrophils from volunteers who had been supplementing their diet with omega-3 fatty acids.[30-32] Leukotriene B_5 is much less potent than leukotriene B_4 as a chemotactic factor or aggregating agent. Leukotriene B_5 seems to be produced at the

Figure 2. Effects of omega-3 fatty acids on the typical Western omega-6-dependent prostaglandin and leukotriene pathways. EPA = eicosapentaenoic acid, AA = arachidonic acid, LTB = leukotriene B, PG = prostaglandin, TXA = thromboxane A.

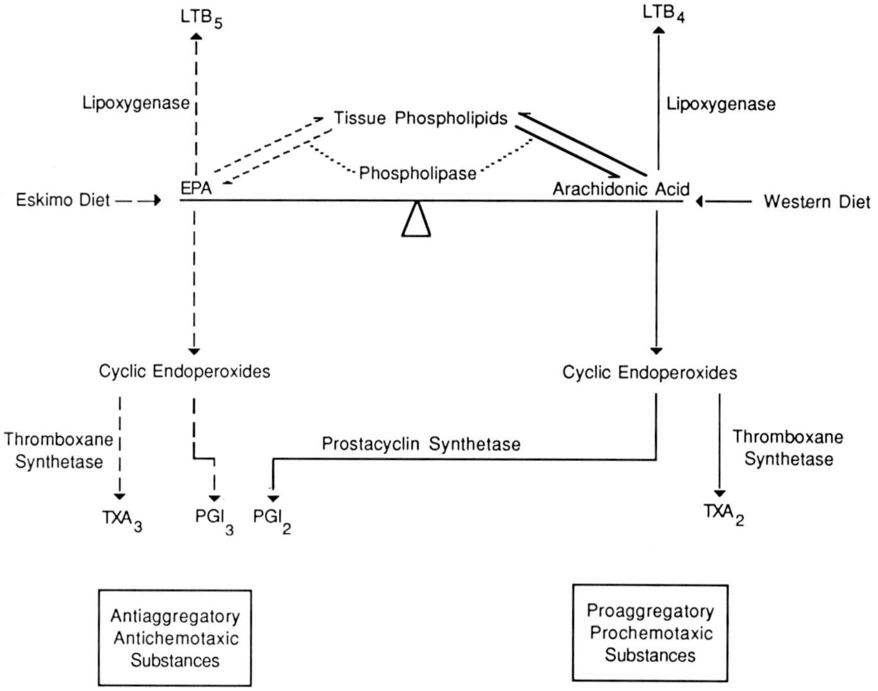

expense of leukotriene B_4, possibly because an oxygenated EPA metabolite inhibits leukotriene B_4 production by inhibiting leukotriene A hydrolase, the enzyme responsible for leukotriene B production.[32]

Consequences of the Effects of Omega-3 Fatty Acids on Prostaglandin and Leukotriene Pathways

Because omega-3 fatty acids alter both the prostaglandin and leukotriene pathways in humans, changes in neutrophil and platelet function might be expected. These changes are observed and form the basis for some proposed uses for omega-3 fatty acids in the treatment of various disease states. The decreased incidence of myocardial infarction, psoriasis, and other diseases observed in Eskimos may be explained now that some of the mechanisms by which omega-3 fatty acids interfere with prostaglandin and leukotriene formation have been delineated. Diminished platelet aggregation would be expected in a high omega-3 fatty acid state, because of the decreased amount of potent platelet-aggregating agents, thromboxane A_2 and leukotriene B_4, and the increased amount of thromboxane A_3 and leukotriene B_5, weak aggregating agents, that are formed. In fact, Eskimos have drastically lengthened bleeding times, a measure of platelet function, compared with those of Danish controls.[33] Numerous studies have documented longer bleeding times[12,13,20,34,35] and decreased platelet aggregation[13,18,19,20,22,36,37] as measured by in vitro testing in subjects supplementing their diet with omega-3 fatty acids. Concurrent aspirin administration can lengthen bleeding time even further.[18]

Macrophages play an important role in the pathogenesis of atherosclerotic heart disease.[38,39] Monocytes attach to vessel endothelium and secrete substances, including leukotriene B_4, which promotes atherogenesis. In vitro neutrophil adherence to bovine endothelial cell monolayers and leukotriene B_4 release from monocytes are reduced in subjects consuming a diet fortified by omega-3 fatty acids.[31] This may partially explain the decreased incidence of myocardial infarction observed in Eskimos. Because omega-3-derived leukotriene B_5 is a less potent chemotactic factor than omega-6-derived leukotriene B_4, numerous clinical trials have been designed to capitalize on this effect through dietary supplementation of patients suffering from a variety of disease states, including rheumatoid arthritis[40,41] and psoriasis.[42,43]

Not all of the touted biological effects of omega-3 fatty acids are necessarily due to changes in prostaglandin and leukotriene production. Barcelli and colleagues[44] reported a significant increase in concentrations of vascular plasminogen activator and decreases in plasmin inhibitor and inhibitor of plasminogen activation in healthy volunteers ingesting a diet supplemented with omega-3 fatty acids. The authors offer no explanation of the mechanism of this phenomenon, but this also may be an important factor in the development of coronary heart disease. Another example of a biological effect of the omega-3 fatty acids that may not be due to an alteration in prostaglandin and leukotriene production and function are the frequently observed hypolipidemic effects.

Proposed Mechanisms for the Effects of Omega-3 Fatty Acids on Lipids

Serum triglyceride concentrations of the Greenlandic Eskimos have been found to be significantly lower than those of Danish controls for every age range studied regardless of gender, despite the high-fat diet of the Greenlandic Eskimo people.[2] A hypotriglyceridemic effect of omega-3 fatty acids has been found in numerous clinical trials. Many mechanisms have been proposed to explain this triglyceride-lowering effect of omega-3 fatty acids.

The best-substantiated mechanism for the hypotriglyceridemic effects of the omega-3 fatty acids is a reduction of VLDL synthesis in the liver (Figure 3). Evidence for this mechanism comes from a study by Nestel and associates,[45] who compared the daily production of VLDL apoprotein B using ^{125}I-labeled lipoprotein in six subjects during three weeks of dietary supplementation with safflower oil, an oil rich in omega-6 fatty acids, or a diet similarly enriched with fish oils.[45] Each diet contained 30% of daily calories as one of the two oils. Production of VLDL apoprotein B was significantly lower in subjects consuming fish oil compared with those consuming safflower oil. The irreversible fractional removal rate of VLDL apoprotein B was increased negligibly in healthy subjects and decreased in hyperlipidemic subjects, suggesting that the fish oil affected VLDL production more than VLDL removal. Sanders et al.[46] reported similar results: no increase in VLDL catabolism rate but a decrease in serum triglyceride concentrations. A diet supplemented with omega-3 fatty acids prevented the normally increased production of VLDL triglyceride after a high-carbohydrate meal.[47] Presumably, this effect was due to an inhibition of hepatic VLDL synthesis by the fish oil diet. Saynor et al.[34] also have reported results consistent with a decrease in VLDL synthesis caused by omega-3 fatty acids.

Because both exogenous intake of triglycerides in the diet and endogenous secretion of VLDL contribute to circulating triglyceride levels, it follows that factors that alter adipose tissue lipolysis will affect serum triglyceride levels. Prostaglandin E_2 has been shown to inhibit lipolysis of rat adipocytes in vitro,[48] but altering the dietary ratio of polyunsaturated to saturated fatty acids in rats has not been shown to influence lipolysis.[49] Prosta-

Figure 3. Hypotriglyceridemic effects of omega-3 fatty acids. The ingestion of omega-3 fatty acids results in a decreased production of VLDL and consequently LDL under certain conditions. VLDL that is synthesized during ingestion of diets supplemented with omega-3 fatty acids contains less triglyceride and may be a better substrate for enzyme activity. VLDL = very low density lipoprotein, LDL = low density lipoprotein, FA = fatty acid.

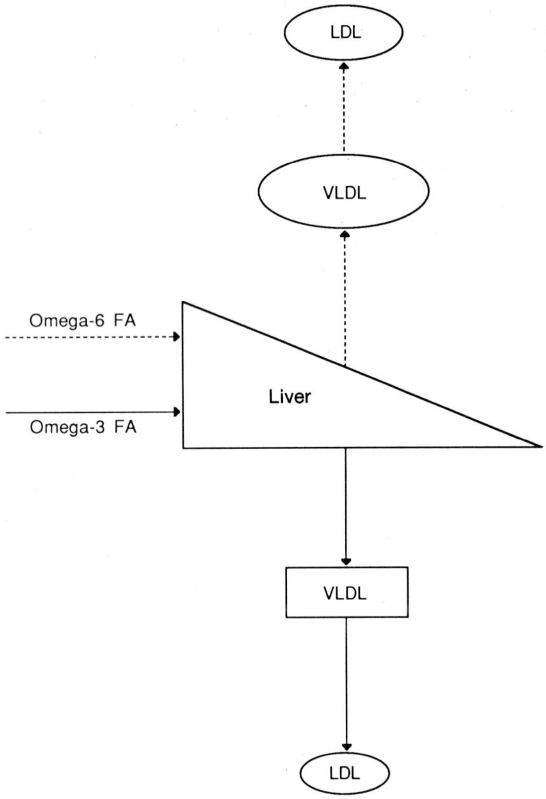

glandins derived from omega-3 fatty acids may have a role in lipolysis inhibition that has not yet been described.[50]

VLDL particles that contain omega-3 fatty acids may be of a different conformation than VLDL particles that contain omega-6 fatty acids. VLDL from subjects ingesting a diet supplemented by omega-3 fatty acids contains less triglyceride and cholesterol than VLDL from these same subjects before dietary supplementation.[45] Omega-3 fatty acids are incorporated into the VLDL of hypertriglyceridemic subjects ingesting 15 g of fish oil daily.[46] Omega-3 fatty acids are less saturated than omega-6 fatty acids and therefore could change the shape of the lipoprotein. This could potentially make omega-3-derived VLDL a better substrate for lipolytic enzymes, although evidence for this is lacking. Phillipson and colleagues[51] reported that lipoprotein lipase activity did not increase after a heparin infusion during a fish oil diet. This evidence suggests that the hypotriglyceridemic effects of omega-3 fatty acids are not due to an increase in lipolytic enzyme activity or an increase in the fractional catabolic rate of VLDL; rather, these effects are more likely due to a better substrate–enzyme interaction or, more likely, a decrease in VLDL synthesis.[52]

The hypocholesterolemic mechanisms of omega-3 fatty acids are less well described than the hypotriglyceridemic effects. Many of the hypocholesterolemic hypotheses are the same as the ones used to explain the triglyceride changes seen. The relatively more unsaturated omega-3 fatty acids may change the conformation of lipoproteins, thus changing the lipoprotein's affinity for lipolytic enzymes. As mentioned earlier, VLDL synthesis is decreased by omega-3 fatty acids. VLDL serves as the biological precursor for LDL. One mechanism by which omega-3 fatty acids may reduce serum cholesterol concentrations is by decreasing VLDL synthesis and, therefore, LDL synthesis. Illingworth and associates[53] found a lowering of LDL and a decrease in LDL synthesis in healthy volunteers fed omega-3 fatty acids. Serum LDL concentrations, however, do not decline in all clinical trials. Sullivan and colleagues[54] reported an increase in LDL apoprotein B levels in hypertriglyceridemics and healthy subjects ingesting a diet enriched by omega-3 fatty acids. This was presumably due to a change in the triglyceride content of VLDL. VLDL formed in the course of a diet enriched by omega-3 fatty acids contains relatively fewer triglycerides than VLDL formed in the course of a diet enriched by omega-6 fatty acids. These smaller and denser triglyceride-poor VLDL particles are more easily converted to LDL. Further study needs to be done to determine the effects of omega-3 fatty acids on serum LDL concentrations, because of the potential for an increased risk of coronary artery disease caused by an increase in serum LDL concentrations.[55]

Experimental studies in rats indicate that biliary secretion of cholesterol is increased when a diet rich in fish oil is instituted.[56] Biliary secretion of cholesterol was higher in rats fed fish oil than in rats fed equivalent amounts of safflower oil (rich in omega-6 fatty acids) or coconut oil. In humans, a diet supplemented with omega-3 fatty acids has been shown to increase fecal sterol excretion, compared with a control saturated-fat diet or a diet supplemented with omega-6 fatty acids.[52]

Hypotriglyceridemic and hypocholesterolemic effects are associated with ingestion of omega-3 fatty acids and omega-6 fatty acids; however, differences exist between them for these effects. Omega-3 fatty acids decrease triglyceride concentrations in a dose-related fashion[45] and with no relationship to the number of bonds in their structures. Double bonds, or "unsaturatedness," are more common in omega-3 fatty acids, approximately 2.7 times so, than in omega-6 fatty acids. The amount of unsaturation is related to cholesterol-lowering potency, and when equivalent amounts of omega-6 fatty acids are given to compensate for the number of double bonds found in omega-3 fatty acids, comparable hypocholesterolemic effects are noted.[57]

An explicit explanation of the effects of omega-3 fatty acids on serum cholesterol levels is not available yet, but it appears that the mechanisms include a change in cholesterol excretion from the body and diminished synthesis of LDL derived from VLDL.

Consequences of the Effects of Omega-3 Fatty Acids on Lipids

Numerous clinical trials have been conducted to examine the effect of various omega-3 fatty acid dosing regimens on serum lipids. Although the intent of this paper is not to review all of these trials, a summary of the results of these experiments follows. Serum triglyceride levels, almost universally, decrease substantially. Total cholesterol levels generally decline in most, but not all, studies. Levels of VLDL, primarily composed of triglycerides, also universally and significantly decline. Studies involving supplementation with omega-3 fatty acids have reported no change,[22,58] a significant increase,[36,51,59] and a significant decrease[34,57] in LDL cholesterol concentrations. Like the LDL results, HDL concentrations have been reported to remain the same,[22,51,58] significantly increase,[60,61] and significantly decrease[47,62] compared with controls. Firm conclusions on the effects of omega-3 fatty acids on LDL cholesterol and HDL cholesterol cannot be reached at this time. Subpopulations of patients reacting differently to these agents or dosing differences between the studies may account for these discordant results, although there is no conclusive evidence.

Many of the early studies examining the hypocholesterolemic effects of fish oils did not show the striking effects on serum cholesterol that are seen in some of the more recent studies. Investigators often did not control for the cholesterol that was contained in the fish oil itself.[63,64] The hypocholesterolemic effects of the fish oils were blunted because of the large cholesterol load administered by the researchers in the form of fish oil. More recent studies have described some profound changes in serum cholesterol as a result of dietary supplementation with omega-3 fatty acids.

Other than observations made in the Eskimos, no long-term trials examining the effects of omega-3 fatty acids on morbidity and mortality have been conducted in humans. Without carefully controlled longitudinal clinical studies, the explanations of the different disease profile observed in the Eskimos cannot be confirmed. To determine whether lifelong supplementation with omega-3 fatty acids would be antiatherogenic, Weiner et al.[65] fed two groups of swine a diet high in saturated fat and cholesterol for eight months. One of the groups also received 30 mL of cod liver oil daily. Three weeks into the diet, all animals underwent cardiac catheterization, at which time their proximal left anterior descending coronary artery was abraded to accelerate coronary atherosclerosis. At the end of the eight-month feeding period, the animals were killed, and the coronary arteries of the two groups were compared. Swine fed cod liver oil had significantly less luminal encroachment and smaller atherosclerotic lesions in all vessels, including those not surgically abraded, than the control animals. Microscopic calcification of vessels occurred significantly more often in control swine. These findings indicate that omega-3 fatty acids may slow or inhibit the formation of atherosclerotic plaque. Whether this antiatherogenesis is due to the effects of omega-3 fatty acids on lipids or a change in neutrophil and platelet function is not described. These antiatherogenic effects may be species specific. Thiery and Seidel[66] reported that a high-cholesterol diet supplemented with fish oil increased aortic atherosclerosis in rabbits, compared with a high cholesterol diet alone, although the methodology for this study has been criticized recently.[67] Extrapolation of the results from these animal trials to humans may not be possible.

Although evidence for a hypolipidemic and antithrombogenic effect in humans of a diet supplemented with fish oil is mounting, surprisingly few studies have examined the usefulness of fish oil in carefully controlled clinical trials in patients with coronary heart disease. In an unblinded study, Saynor et al.[34] published one of the earliest attempts to assess the effects of supplementation with omega-3 fatty acids for up to two years in 92 patients with coronary heart disease. In addition to observing the expected effects of omega-3 fatty acids on serum lipids, bleeding time, and platelet count, these authors noted a dramatic decline in weekly nitroglycerin tablet consumption by the participants of the study. No objective measures of myocardial ischemia were reported. In contrast to the previous study, Kristensen et al.[68] reported no difference in angina attacks or nitroglycerin use in 36 subjects receiving fish oil for 12 weeks. In addition to nitroglycerin use, Mehta et al.[58] objectively monitored myocardial ischemia in eight men with stable coronary heart disease in a double-blind, placebo-controlled trial. Systolic blood pressure and double product were lower during the fish-oil-supplementation phase than during the placebo phase. After both three and six minutes of exercise, heart rate, double product, and systolic pressure were lower in those receiving fish oil than in those receiving placebo. However, no significant difference was noted in angina frequency, nitroglycerin use, or exercise time.

Incorporating Omega-3 Fatty Acids into Erythrocyte Membranes

Because the highly unsaturated omega-3 fatty acids are incorporated into erythrocyte membranes, these membranes become more fluidic, much like the omega-3-rich membranes of the cold-water marine phytoplankton. This increase in membrane fluidity allows the red blood cell to become more deformable and able to flow better through vessels. A positive correlation exists between red blood cell membrane incorporation of omega-3 fatty acids and red blood cell deformability.[37] The study of this phenomenon is called blood rheology; one method by which the rheology of blood can be quantified is by measuring blood viscosity. Blood viscosity is significantly and uniformly lower in subjects receiving omega-3 fatty acids compared with controls.[21,37,69,70] This observation explains why some investigators have examined the effects of omega-3 fatty acids in subjects with peripheral vascular diseases such as intermittent claudication.[70] In this trial, a two-week diet enriched with 1.8 g of omega-3 fatty acids per day was compared with a diet supplemented with corn oil or olive oil in patients with intermittent claudication. Whole-blood viscosity significantly declined in the omega-3 fatty acid group, but no statistical analysis on measures of claudication was performed. The efficacy of these fatty acids in treating vascular diseases has not been confirmed.

Interpreting the Literature on Omega-3 Fatty Acids

Most studies examining the biological effects of omega-3 fatty acids use fish or refined marine fish oil as the source of omega-3 fatty acids. Often the authors of these studies emphasize only the EPA content of the fish product and disregard other omega-3 fatty acids and other components found in fish and fish oil. Because fish oils contain many other fatty acids, as well as other non-fatty-acid constituents, studies need to be conducted to determine which of the ingredients are beneficial and which are potentially harmful. The effects of pure EPA have been investigated by using a concentrated EPA ethylester product that eliminates most of the other components found in fish oil. Changes in platelet aggregation in human dietary supplementation trials[22,37] with purified EPA ethylester are similar to the changes seen when fish oil is the source of omega-3 fatty acids, suggesting that EPA is responsible for at least some of the biological effects attributed to fish oil. Clinical trials with other purified omega-3 fatty acids, including DHA, are lacking.

Omega-3 fatty acids may occur in the *cis* and the *trans* form. Omega-3 fatty acids ingested in the typical Western diet are typically *trans* and unnatural *cis* isomers, whereas Eskimos ingest primarily naturally occurring *cis* forms. The *trans* and *cis* isomers that do not occur in nature may well have different biological properties than the naturally occuring *cis* isomers.[71] Few authors report the concentrations of *cis* and *trans* forms used in their trials. Discrepancies in the results of trials using omega-3 fatty acids may be attributable in part to the isomers used.[72] It has been proposed that other constituents of fish oil may have some important biological effects of their own.[59,73] The trace element selenium may be one of the components in fish that have important biological activity.[74]

An important consideration when placebo-controlled trials of the effects of omega-3 fatty acids are critically examined is the ingredients of the placebo.[75] Frequently, the identical-looking, oil-filled placebos used in these trials contain olive oil. Olive oil, rich in monounsaturated fatty acids, has long been thought to be without hypolipidemic properties. However, Mattson and Grundy[76] reported that a diet high in monounsaturated fatty acids significantly reduced serum cholesterol and LDL cholesterol concentrations, compared with a diet high in saturated fats. At least one author has suggested that placebos be made from a blend of oils that more closely approximates the fatty acid composition of the typical Western diet so that the placebo has no intrinsic effect on lipids.[75]

The quantities of fish and fish oils used in most clinical trials examining the effects of omega-3 fatty acids are quite high and have been designed to mimic the Eskimo diet. Examinations of the potential effects of the fish diet ingested by other populations have been performed. Many longitudinal dietary studies have been published examining the relationship between fish consumption and morbidity and mortality in European and North American populations. Kromhout et al.[77] examined the relationship between fish consumption of 852 middle-aged men from Zutphen, the Netherlands, and 20-year mortality from coronary heart disease. A significant inverse relationship was noted between these two factors. Coronary heart disease mortality was more than 50% lower among those who consumed 30 g of fish per day than among those who did not eat fish at all. These authors concluded that as little as one to two fish meals per week could protect against coronary heart disease.[77] Results of the Western Electric Study in the United States also showed that fish consumption was significantly inversely related to a 25-year risk of coronary death and total mortality in 1931 middle-aged men.[78] No significant relationship between deaths from coronary heart disease and fish consumption was noted in a Norwegian study of 11,000 men[79] or in a cohort of 7,615 men from the Honolulu Heart Program.[80] Differences in data collection may account for the discrepancy of results among these trials. It is important to point out that the subjects in all of these studies were men. Little information exists relating fish consumption and long-term mortality data in women.

Potential Hazards of Fish Oil Use

Dietary supplementation with fish oils can carry potential risks if the source of the product is not carefully examined. Cod liver oil has long been touted as a health food and, in fact, is a rich source of omega-3 fatty acids. However, cod liver oil also contains high concentrations of vitamins A and D. One teaspoonful contains 100% of the recommended dietary allowance (RDA) of each vitamin. The potential for hypervitaminosis A and D has been recognized by most investigators[50,81]; therefore, other products rich in omega-3 fatty acids without the high vitamin A and D content have been developed. A second potential toxicity concerning vitamins involves the potential for vitamin E deficiency induced by the ingestion of large amounts of fish oils. This concern has been raised because EPA and DHA are prone to peroxidation and therefore may increase the biological requirements for antioxidants.[72] This problem appears to have been solved, because vitamin E is added to most commercial fish oil products as an antioxidant to stop the oil from becoming rancid. Most of the information on vitamin E deficiency comes from animal data, because diseases caused by vitamin E deficiency in humans are rare.[82] Vitamin E deficiency as a result of fish oil consumption in humans has never been reported.[83] Another toxicity of high-dose fish oil that has been reported in animals, but never in humans, is myocardial lipidosis as a result of ingestion of the gadoleic and cetoleic acids contained in the oil.[84]

Other adverse effects include the previously mentioned increase in bleeding time caused by omega-3 fatty acids and the relatively consistent decrease in platelet count observed in clinical trials. The platelet count of subjects supplementing their diets with omega-3 fatty acids often declines. The magnitude of this fall can be as great as 35%.[20] Usually the platelet count does not fall below the lower limit of normal, but occasionally a greater decline is noted.[20] Subjects continuing supplementation with omega-3 fatty acids often normalize their platelet count over many months.[34] It may take four to six weeks after dietary supplementation is discontinued for the platelet count to return to normal; thus, this may be an important consideration in crossover studies. Despite a decreased platelet count, Hay et al.[85] reported an increased platelet survival time. These authors theorized that, in light of this evidence, observed thrombocytopenia induced by omega-3 fatty acids is due to decreased thrombopoiesis rather than increased platelet destruction.

An exacerbation of the diabetic state in six untreated adult male patients with non-insulin-dependent diabetes mellitus after receiving 5.5 g of omega-3 fatty acids daily for four weeks was reported by Glauber et al.[86] During treatment, a significant worsening of fasting blood glucose levels, basal hepatic glucose output, results of glucose tolerance tests, and glycosylated hemoglobin levels was observed compared with baseline values. Fasting and postprandial insulin levels during fish oil administration were also lower than they were at baseline. In contrast to this study, Popp-Snijders et al.[87] reported a decrease in fasting blood glucose levels and increased metabolic clearance of glucose at the steady state of an insulin sensitivity test in six subjects with non-insulin-dependent diabetes mellitus who received 3 g of omega-3 fatty acids daily for eight weeks. This suggests that omega-3 fatty acids improve insulin sensitivity in this population; however, plasma insulin levels during this test were significantly lower than baseline levels. Whether omega-3 fatty acids are harmful or beneficial in non-insulin-dependent diabetes mellitus is not resolved, but it appears that close monitoring is imperative if supplementation with omega-3 fatty acids is to be instituted in this population.

Even omega-3 fatty acids ingested in the form of fish can carry a potential for toxicity if pesticides or other pollutants are endemic to where the fish live. Yet, despite the potential toxicities listed here, dietary supplementation with moderate amounts of omega-3 fatty acids appears to be relatively safe. The Conference on the Health Effects of Polyunsaturated Fatty Acids in Seafoods stated that there is no appreciable evidence of toxicity in patients or healthy subjects with doses of 20 g daily of EPA-enriched preparations.[88]

Sources of Omega-3 Fatty Acids

Although omega-3 fatty acids are found in trace amounts in wild game, such as deer or buffalo,[89] the most obvious source for dietary supplementation with omega-3 fatty acids is increased fish consumption. Unfortunately, not all fish contain omega-3 fatty acids in equal amounts. Recall that omega-3 fatty acids are derived from phytoplankton found in very cold environments. Because these phytoplankton are the primary source, it follows that only those animals at the top of the food chain in cold climates will contain appreciable amounts of omega-3 fatty acids. Indeed, higher concentrations of EPA and DHA are found in fish caught in colder environments than in warm-water species. Whether the fish are from salt water or fresh water does not seem to matter as much as the temperature of their environment.[90] Lastly, "oily or fatty" fish such as salmon, herring, and mackerel have more available omega-3 fatty acids for human ingestion than lean fish such as cod, because they store their fat in muscle rather than in viscera.[81] The EPA and DHA content in various seafoods are listed in Table 2. The amount of omega-3 fatty acids in other foods is listed in Table 3.[91-93]

For various reasons, many do not eat enough fish to experience the physiologic changes that occur when omega-3 fatty acids are ingested in relatively high amounts. Numerous products to supplement the diet with omega-3 fatty acids have become

Table 2.
Eicosapentaenoic Acid (EPA) and Docosahexaenoic Acid (DHA) Content in Seafood [a, 91–93]

Food	EPA	DHA
Fish		
Channel catfish	0.1	0.2
Cod, Atlantic	0.1	0.2
Haddock	0.1	0.1
Herring, Atlantic	0.7	0.9
Mackerel, Atlantic	0.9	1.6
Salmon, Atlantic	0.3	0.9
Salmon, Coho (Pacific)	0.82	0.94
Snapper, Red	Trace	0.2
Trout, Rainbow	0.1	0.4
Tuna, Albacore (canned)	0.63	1.7
Shellfish		
Crab, Alaskan King (legs and claws)	0.33	0.15
Lobster	0.2	0.1
Oyster, Eastern (flesh)	0.17	0.17
Scallop (flesh)	0.12	0.14
Shrimp, Atlantic	0.2	0.2

[a] Expressed as grams per 100-gram edible raw portion.

Table 3.
Omega-3 Fatty Acid Content in Various Food Products[a, 92]

Food	Omega-3 Fatty Acid (g)	Cholesterol (mg)
Cured bacon	0.8	67
Beans, common, dry	0.6	0
Ground beef	0.2	85
Butter	1.2	219
Cheddar cheese	0.4	105
Chicken, light meat, without skin	Trace	58
Lard	1.0	95
Whole milk	0.1	14
Italian salad dressing (regular)	3.3	0
Soybeans, green, raw	3.2	0
Seaweed, spirulina, dried	0.8	0
Black walnuts	3.3	0
Wheat germ	0.7	0
Egg yolk, chicken, raw	0.1	1602

[a] Expressed as grams or milligrams per 100-gram edible portion.

Table 4.
Selected Commercial Products and Their Contents[94]

Trade Name	Manufacturer	Contents (mg)[a]	Cost/100 ($)
Cardi-Omega-3	SevenSeas Health Care	EPA, 180; DHA, 120	10.71
Promega	Parke-Davis	EPA, 350; DHA, 150	21.23
Promega Pearls	Parke-Davis	Omega-3 fatty acids, 300	10.62
Proto-chol	Squibb	EPA, 180; DHA, 120	11.17

[a] EPA = eicosapentaenoic acid, DHA = docosahexaenoic acid.

commercially available for those who would like to increase their intake of these fatty acids without ingesting large amounts of fish in their diet. These products are derived from oil from commercially caught fish. Unlike earlier products, most now have eliminated any cholesterol in the oil-filled capsules. Because of the tendency for fish oil to go rancid, vitamin E is added to most of the products as an antioxidant. This is beneficial to those who ingest high-dose fish oil because of the theoretical concern that omega-3 fatty acids may induce a vitamin E deficiency. A list of selected commercially available products and their average wholesale prices is found in Table 4.[94]

Patient Counseling

Frequently, patients and other health-care providers ask pharmacists about the merits of omega-3 fatty acid supplementation. As these products become more widely used for a variety of disease states, pharmacists should be able to describe the rationale and potential adverse effects that might be experienced. Nausea, diarrhea, and a "fishy" taste are often encountered. Potential complications including thrombocytopenia, lengthened bleeding time, and alterations in lipoprotein profile make it imprudent for a pharmacist to recommend the supplementation with high-dose omega-3 fatty acids to a patient without physician approval and appropriate laboratory monitoring. Additionally, patients should be cautioned about the concomitant use of nonsteroidal anti-inflammatory agents because of the potential for further prolonging bleeding time. Questions are frequently asked about the caloric content of the available commerical products. Like other fats, the omega-3 fatty acids contain 9 kilocalories per gram of fatty acid. This may be an important consideration in those ingesting high daily doses of these products and in patients with diabetes mellitus.

The public's recent concern about the link between hyperlipidemia and coronary heart disease is due in large part to the National Cholesterol Education Program. The Expert Panel's recommendations for a national cholesterol screening program for all adults and earlier treatment of hypercholesterolemia will result in a heightened public awareness of the problem and in the treatment of more hyperlipidemic Americans than ever before.[95] Many of them will hear of the supposed benefits of dietary supplementation with omega-3 fatty acids despite the fact that the National Cholesterol Education Program Expert Panel specifically does not recommend their use in the treatment of high-risk cholesterol levels. The Expert Panel's rationale for not endorsing their use has to do with a lack of extended trials investigating efficacy and toxicity of these fatty acids.

Conclusion

Although the use of omega-3 fatty acids is considered by many to be a fad, the physiological alterations observed in those who ingest large amounts of omega-3 fatty acids are real. It appears that many of the changes may be beneficial in humans; however, no well-controlled long-term studies measuring objective outcomes with respect to morbidity and mortality have been performed. For example, it is possible that omega-3 fatty acid supplementation would benefit hypertriglyceridemic patients, but because of the unpredictable changes in HDL and LDL concentrations seen with omega-3 fatty acid supplementation, cardiovascular risk may be higher in these patients, despite the lowering of serum triglyceride concentrations. Additionally, the potentially beneficial antiaggregating effects on neutrophils and platelets may be outweighed by risks caused by a possible increase in bleeding. The therapeutic index of the omega-3 fatty acids is high, although a decline in platelet count and lengthened bleeding time are observed in most people. Properly controlled, long-term clinical trials are needed to determine whether supplementation with omega-3 fatty acids would be therapeutically beneficial in various patient populations and disease states.

Addendum

Since this manuscript was submitted for publication, a report describing what may represent an important use of the omega-3 fatty acids was published. In a randomized unblinded trial, Dehmer et al.[96] added 3.2 g of EPA, in the form of fish oil, daily to a standard regimen of aspirin and dipyridamole in one group of adult male patients who had received percutaneous transluminal coronary angioplasty (PTCA). A control group of adult male patients received the same regimen without fish oil. Coronary angiography was performed three to four months after PTCA, and the degree of restenosis in each group was compared. The patients receiving supplementation with omega-3 fatty acids had a significantly lower rate of restenosis than did the control group, on both a per-patient and a per-vessel basis. No major adverse effects were reported. These authors concluded that omega-3 fatty acids may have an important role in the prevention of early restenosis after PTCA.

References

1. Swanson DR. Fish oil, Raynaud's syndrome, and undiscovered public knowledge. *Perspect Biol Med*. 1986; 30:7–17.
2. Bang HO, Dyerberg J, Nielsen AB. Plasma lipid and lipoprotein pattern in Greenlandic West-Coast Eskimos. *Lancet*. 1971; 1:1143–6.
3. Kromann N, Green A. Epidemiological studies in the Upernavik District, Greenland. *Acta Med Scand*. 1980; 208:401–6.
4. State Board of Health in Greenland. Annual report from the chief medical officer, 1963–67.
5. Sagild U, Littauer J, Jespersen CS et al. Epidemiological studies in Greenland 1962–1964. I. Diabetes mellitus in Eskimos. *Acta Med Scand*. 1966; 179:29–39.
6. Bang HO, Dyerberg J, Sinclair HM. The composition of the Eskimo food in northwestern Greenland. *Am J Clin Nutr*. 1980; 33:2657–61.
7. Yotakis LDO. The preventative effect of the polyunsaturated fats on thrombosis. *Thromb Haemostas*. 1981; 46:65. Abstract.
8. Atkins CJ, Caira L, Ward RH et al. Unusual rheumatic diseases in the Nootka Indians of British Columbia. *BC Med J*. 1982; 24:20–3.
9. Gibson RA, Kneebone GM. Fatty acid composition of human colostrum and mature human milk. *Am J Clin Nutr*. 1981; 34:252–7.
10. Siess W, Roth P, Scherer B et al. Platelet-membrane fatty acids, platelet aggregation, and thromboxane formation during a mackerel diet. *Lancet*. 1980; 1:441–4.
11. Galloway JH, Cartwright IJ, Woodcock BE et al. Effects of dietary fish oil supplementation on the fatty acid composition of the human platelet membrane: demonstration of selectivity in the incorporation of eicosopentaenoic acid into membrane phospholipid pools. *Clin Sci*. 1985; 68:449–54.
12. Knapp HW, Reilly MB, Alessandrini P et al. In vivo indexes of platelet and vascular function during fish-oil administration in patients with atherosclerosis. *N Engl J Med*. 1986; 314:937–42.
13. Lorenz R, Spengler U, Fischer S et al. Platelet function, thromboxane formation and blood pressure control during supplementation of the Western diet with cod liver oil. *Circulation*. 1983; 67:504–11.
14. Wood DA, Butler S, Riemersma RA et al. Adipose tissue and platelet fatty acid and coronary heart disease in Scottish men. *Lancet*. 1984; 2:117–21.
15. Sinclair H, Gale M. Eicosapentenoic acid in fat. *Lancet*. 1987; 1:1202. Letter.
16. Katan MB, van de Bovenkamp P. Eicosapentaenoic acid in fat. *Lancet*. 1987; 1:862–3. Letter.
17. Hirai A, Hamazaki T, Terano T. Eicosapentaenoic acid and platelet function in the Japanese. *Lancet*. 1980; 2:1132–3.
18. Thorngren M, Gustafson A. Effects of 11-week increase in dietary eicosapentaenoic acid on bleeding time, lipids, and platelet aggregation. *Lancet*. 1981; 2:1190–3.
19. von Schacky C, Fischer S, Weber PC. Long-term effects of dietary marine ω-3 fatty acids upon plasma and cellular lipids, platelet function, and eicosanoid formation in humans. *J Clin Invest*. 1985; 76:1626–31.
20. Goodnight SH, Harris WS, Connor WE. The effects of dietary omega-3 fatty acids on platelet composition and function in man: a prospective, controlled study. *Blood*. 1981; 58:880–5.
21. Cartwright J, Pockley AG, Galloway JH et al. The effects of dietary ω-3 polyunsaturated fatty acids on erythrocyte membrane phospholipids, erythrocyte deformability and

blood viscosity in healthy volunteers. *Atherosclerosis.* 1985; 55:267–81.
22. Nagakawa Y, Orimo H, Harasawa M et al. Effect of eicosapentaenoic acid on the platelet aggregation and composition of fatty acid in man. *Atherosclerosis.* 1983; 47:71–5.
23. Corey EJ, Shih C, Cashman JR. Docosahexaenoic acid is a strong inhibitor of prostaglandin but not leukotriene biosynthesis. *Proc Natl Acad Sci USA.* 1983; 76:3581–4.
24. Dyerberg J, Bang HO, Stoffersen E. Eicosapentaenoic acid and prevention of thrombosis and atherosclerosis? *Lancet.* 1978; 2:117–9.
25. Needleman P, Raz A, Minkes MS et al. Triene prostaglandins: prostacyclin and thromboxane biosynthesis and unique biological properties. *Proc Natl Acad Sci.* 1979; 76:944–8.
26. Culp BR, Titus BG, Lands WEM. Inhibition of prostaglandin biosynthesis by eiscosapentaenoic acid. *Prostaglandins Med.* 1979; 3:269–78.
27. Dyerberg J, Jorgensen KA, Arnfred T. Human umbilical blood vessel converts all *cis*-5,8,11,14,17 eicosapentaenoic acid to prostaglandin I_3. *Prostaglandins.* 1981; 22:857–62.
28. Fischer S, Weber PC. Prostaglandin I_3 is formed in vivo in man after dietary eicosapentaenoic acid. *Nature.* 1984; 307:165–8.
29. Fischer S, Vischer A, Preac-Mursic V et al. Dietary docosahexaenoic acid is retroconverted in man to eicosapentaenoic acid, which can be quickly transformed to prostaglandin I_3. *Prostaglandins.* 1987; 34:367–75.
30. Strasser T, Fischer S, Weber PC. Leukotriene B_5 is formed in human neutrophils after dietary supplementation with icosapentaenoic acid. *Proc Natl Acad Sci USA.* 1982; 82:1540–3.
31. Lee TH, Hoover RL, Williams JD et al. Effect of dietary enrichment with eicosapentaenoic and docosahexaenoic acids on in vitro neutrophil and monocyte leukotriene generation and neutrophil function. *N Engl J Med.* 1985; 312:1217–24.
32. Prescott SM, Zimmerman GA, Morrison AR. The effects of a diet rich in fish oil on human neutrophils: identification of leukotriene B_5 as a metabolite. *Prostaglandins.* 1985; 30:209–27.
33. Dyerberg J, Bang HO. Haemostatic function and platelet polyunsaturated fatty acids in Eskimos. *Lancet.* 1979; 2:433–5.
34. Saynor R, Verel D, Gillott T. The long-term effect of dietary supplementation with fish lipid concentrate on serum lipids, bleeding time, platelets and angina. *Atherosclerosis.* 1984; 50:3–10.
35. Dyerberg J, Mortensen JZ, Nielsen AH et al. n-3 polyunsaturated fatty acids and ischaemic heart disease. *Lancet.* 1982; 2:614.
36. Haines AP, Sanders TAB, Imeson JD et al. Effects of a fish oil supplement on platelet function, haemostatic variables and albuminuria in insulin-dependent diabetics. *Thrombosis Res.* 1986; 43:643–55.
37. Terano T, Hirai A, Hamazaki T et al. Effect of oral administration of highly purified eicosapentaenoic acid on platelet function, blood viscosity and red cell deformability in healthy human subjects. *Atherosclerosis.* 1983; 46:321–31.
38. Ross R. The pathogenesis of atherosclerosis—an update. *N Engl J Med.* 1986; 314:488–500.
39. Schwartz CJ, Valente AJ, Sprague EA et al. Monocyte-macrophage participation in atherogenesis: inflammatory components of pathogenesis. *Semin Thromb Hemost.* 1986; 12:79–86.
40. Kremer JM, Jubiz W, Michalek A et al. Fish-oil fatty acid supplementation in active rheumatoid arthritis. *Ann Intern Med.* 1987; 106:497–503.
41. Kremer JM, Bigauoette J, Michalek AV et al. Effects of manipulation of dietary fatty acids on clinical manifestations of rheumatoid arthritis. *Lancet.* 1985; 1:184–7.
42. Ziboh VA, Cohen KA, Ellis CN et al. Effects of dietary supplementation of fish oil on neutrophil and epidermal fatty acids. *Arch Dermatol.* 1986; 122:1277–82.
43. Bittiner SB, Tucker WFG, Cartwright I et al. A double-blind, randomised, placebo-controlled trial of fish oil in psoriasis. *Lancet.* 1988; 1:378–80.
44. Barcelli U, Glas-Greenwalt P, Pollak VE. Enhancing effect of dietary supplementation with ω-3 fatty acids on plasma fibrinolysis in normal subjects. *Thrombosis Res.* 1985; 39:307–12.
45. Nestel PJ, Connor WE, Reardon MF et al. Suppression by diets rich in fish oil of very low density lipoprotein production in man. *J Clin Invest.* 1984; 74:82–9.
46. Sanders TAB, Sullivan DR, Reeve J et al. Triglyceride-lowering effect of marine polyunsaturates in patients with hypertriglyceridemia. *Arteriosclerosis.* 1985; 5:459–65.
47. Harris WS, Connor WE, Inkeles SB et al. Dietary omega-3 fatty acids prevent carbohydrate-induced hypertriglyceridemia. *Metabolism.* 1984; 33:1016–9.
48. Dalton C, Hope H, Martikes L. Prostaglandin inhibition of cyclic-AMP accumulation and rate of lipolysis in fat cells. *Prostaglandins.* 1974; 7:319–26.
49. Lipinski BA, Mathias MM. Prostaglandin production and lipolysis in isolated rat adipocytes as effected by dietary fat. *Prostaglandins.* 1978; 16:957–63.
50. Goodnight SH, Harris WS, Connor WE et al. Polyunsaturated fatty acids, hyperlipidemia, and thrombosis. *Arteriosclerosis.* 1982; 2:87–113.
51. Phillipson BE, Rothrock DW, Connor WE et al. Reduction of plasma lipids, lipoproteins, and apoproteins by dietary fish oils in patients with hypertriglyceridemia. *N Engl J Med.* 1985; 312:1210–6.
52. Connor WE, Lin DS, Harris WS. A comparison of dietary polyunsaturated ω-6 and ω-3 fatty acids in humans: effects upon plasma lipids, lipoproteins and sterol balance. *Arteriosclerosis.* 1981; 1:363a. Abstract.
53. Illingworth DR, Harris WH, Connor WE. Inhibition of low density lipoprotein synthesis by dietary omega-3 fatty acids in humans. *Arteriosclerosis.* 1984; 4:270–5.
54. Sullivan DR, Sanders TAB, Trayner IM et al. Paradoxical elevation of LDL apoprotein B levels in hypertriglyceridaemic patients and normal subjects ingesting fish oil. *Atherosclerosis.* 1986; 61:129–34.
55. Lipid Research Clinics Program. The Lipid Research Clinics Primary Prevention Trial Results. II. The relationship of reduction in incidence of coronary heart disease to cholesterol lowering. *JAMA.* 1984; 251:365–74.
56. Balasubramaniam S, Simons LA, Chang S et al. Reduction in plasma cholesterol and increase in biliary cholesterol by a diet rich in N-3 fatty acids in the rat. *J Lipid Res.* 1985; 26:684–9.
57. Harris WS, Connor WE, McMurry MP. The comparative reductions of the plasma lipids and lipoproteins by dietary polyunsaturated fats: salmon oil versus vegetable oils. *Metabolism.* 1983; 32:179–84.
58. Mehta JL, Lopez LM, Lawson D et al. Dietary supplementation with omega-3 polyunsaturated fatty acids in patients with stable coronary disease. *Am J Med.* 1988; 84:45–52.
59. Atkinson PM, Wheeler MC, Mendelsohn D et al. Effects of a 4-week freshwater (trout) diet on platelet aggregation, platelet fatty acids, serum lipids, and coagulation factors. *Am J Hematol.* 1987; 24:143–9.
60. Saynor R, Verel D. Effect of a fish oil diet on blood lipids and coagulation. *Thromb Haemostas.* 1981; 46:65. Abstract.
61. Tamura Y, Hirai A, Terano T et al. Effects of eicosapentaenoic acid on hemostatic function and serum lipids in humans. *Adv Prostaglandin Thromboxane Leukotriene Res.* 1985; 15:265–7.
62. Nestel PJ. Fish oil attenuates the cholesterol-induced rise in lipoprotein cholesterol. *Am J Clin Nutr.* 1986; 43:752–7.
63. Bronte-Stewart B, Antonis A, Eales L et al. Effects of feeding different fats on serum cholesterol levels. *Lancet.* 1956; 1:521–6.
64. Keys A, Anderson JT, Grande F. "Essential" fatty acids, degree of unsaturation and effect of corn (maize) oil on the serum-cholesterol level in man. *Lancet.* 1957; 1:66–8.

65. Weiner BH, Ockene IS, Levine PH. Inhibition of atherosclerosis by cod liver oil in a hyperlipidemic swine model. *N Engl J Med*. 1986; 315:843–6.
66. Thiery J, Seidel D. Fish oil feeding results in an enhancement of cholesterol-induced atherosclerosis in rabbits. *Atherosclerosis*. 1987; 63:53–6.
67. Sanders TAB. *Atherosclerosis*. 1987; 67:91–3. Letter.
68. Kristensen SD, Schmidt EB, Andersen HR et al. Fish oil in angina pectoris. *Atherosclerosis*. 1987; 64:13–9.
69. Kobayashi S, Hirai A, Terano T et al. Reduction in blood viscosity by eicosapentaenoic acid. *Lancet*. 1981; 2:197.
70. Woodcock BE, Smith E, Lambert WH et al. Beneficial effect of fish oil on blood viscosity in peripheral vascular disease. *Br Med J*. 1984; 288:592–4.
71. Booyens J, Louwrens CC. The Eskimo diet. Prophylactic effects ascribed to the balanced presence of natural *cis* unsaturated fatty acids and to the absence of unnatural *trans* and *cis* isomers of unsaturated fatty acids. *Med Hypothesis*. 1986; 21:387–408.
72. Meydani SN, Siguel E, Shapiro AC et al. Fish consumption and mortality from coronary heart disease. *N Engl J Med*. 1985; 313:822. Letter.
73. Kromhout D. *N Engl J Med*. 1985; 313:824. Letter.
74. Salonen JT, Alfthan G, Huttunen JK et al. Association between cardiovascular death and myocardial infarction and serum selenium in a matched-pair longitudinal study. *Lancet*. 1982; 2:175–9.
75. von Schacky C. Prophylaxis of atherosclerosis with marine omega-3 fatty acids. *Ann Intern Med*. 1987; 107:890–9.
76. Mattson FH, SM Grundy. Comparison of effects of dietary saturated, monounsaturated, and polyunsaturated fatty acids on plasma lipids and lipoproteins in man. *J Lipid Res*. 1985; 26:194–202.
77. Kromhout D, Bosschieter EB, Coulander CL. The inverse relation between fish consumption and 20-year mortality from coronary heart disease. *N Engl J Med*. 1985; 312:1205–9.
78. Shekelle RB, Missill L, Paul O et al. Fish consumption and mortality from coronary heart disease. *N Engl J Med*. 1985; 313:820. Letter.
79. Vollset SE, Heuch I, Bjelke E. Fish consumption and mortality from coronary heart disease. *N Engl J Med*. 1985; 313:820–82. Letter.
80. Curb JD, Reed DM. Fish consumption and mortality from coronary heart disease. *N Engl J Med*. 1985; 313:821–2. Letter.
81. Dyerberg J. Linolenate-derived polyunsaturated fatty acids and prevention of atherosclerosis. *Nutr Rev*. 1986; 44:125–34.
82. Dormandy TL. Free radical oxidation and antioxidants. *Lancet*. 1978; 1:647–50.
83. Phillipson BE, Rothrock DW, Connor WE et al. Fish consumption and mortality from coronary heart disease. *N Engl J Med*. 1985; 313:824. Letter.
84. Ackman RG, Eaton CA, Dyerberg J. Marine docosenoic acid isomer distribution in the plasma of Greenland Eskimos. *Am J Clin Nutr*. 1980; 33:1814–7.
85. Hay CRM, Durber AP, Saynor R. Effect of fish oil on platelet kinetics in patients with ischaemic heart disease. *Lancet*. 1982; 1:1269–72.
86. Glauber H, Wallace P, Griver K et al. Adverse metabolic effect of omega-3 fatty acids in non-insulin-dependent diabetes mellitus. *Ann Intern Med*. 1988; 108:663–8.
87. Popp-Snijders C, Shouten JA, Heine RJ et al. Dietary supplementation of omega-3 polyunsaturated fatty acids improves insulin sensitivity in non-insulin-dependent diabetes. *Diabetes Res*. 1987; 4:141–7.
88. Simopoulos AP. Summary of the Conference on the Health Effects of Polyunsaturated Fatty Acids in Seafoods. *J Nutr*. 1986; 116:2350–4.
89. French JK, McColl SR, Cleland LG. Fish oils and coronary heart disease. *NZ Med J*. 1986; 99:962. Letter.
90. Skorepa J, Todorovicova H, Mares P. Carp as a source of eicosapentaenoic acid. *Lancet*. 1983; 1:717. Letter.
91. Exler J, Weihrauch JL. Comprehensive evaluation of fatty acids in foods. *J Am Diet Assoc*. 1976; 69:243–7.
92. Hepburn FN, Exler J, Weihrauch JL. Provisional tables on the content of omega-3 fatty acids and other fat components of selected foods. *J Am Diet Assoc*. 1986; 86:788–93.
93. Exler J, Weihrauch JL. Comprehensive evaluation of fatty acids in foods. *J Am Diet Assoc*. 1977; 71:518–21.
94. Drug Topics redbook annual pharmacists' reference. Cardinale VA, ed. Oradell, NJ: Medical Economics Company, Inc., 1988.
95. The Expert Panel. Report of the National Cholesterol Education Program Expert Panel on detection, evaluation, and treatment of high blood cholesterol in adults. *Arch Intern Med*. 1988; 148:36–69.
96. Dehmer GJ, Popma JJ, van den Berg EK et al. Reduction in the rate of early restenosis after coronary angioplasty by a diet supplemented with ω-3 fatty acids. *N Engl J Med*. 1988; 319:733–40.

"

Understanding the Mechanisms of Proarrhythmic Effects

Little definitive information is available regarding the cellular mechanisms of proarrhythmia. It is thought that the mechanisms underlying the induction of clinical arrhythmias—namely, conduction block, reentry, and abnormal impulse initiation—also produce proarrhythmia. These mechanisms may be induced by toxic effects of the antiarrhythmic agents. The toxicity may well represent an extension of the therapeutic effects of these drugs, as well as an interaction with an arrhythmogenic substrate present in diseased hearts. Exciting but inconclusive studies have suggested that one particular type of electrophysiologic abnormality—early afterdepolarizations and triggered activity—may be the cause of torsades de pointes. In general, however, our understanding of the cellular mechanisms of proarrhythmia is rudimentary.

In the past several years, progress has been made in the study of proarrhythmia. Much of this work has been descriptive, but such a foundation is necessary for more definitive studies in the future. For now, however, the dark side of antiarrhythmic therapy must be accepted along with its benefits.

—Horowitz LN. Proarrhythmia—taking the bad with the good. *N Engl J Med*. 1988; 319:304–5.

"

Therapy Review

Combination drug therapy for ventricular arrhythmias

Daniel W. Krichbaum

Abstract. The role of drug combinations for the treatment of patients with ventricular arrhythmias is reviewed.

The use of single drugs to suppress ventricular arrhythmias is often unsatisfactory; a drug may be ineffective or cause intolerable adverse effects. Simultaneous use of antiarrhythmic agents with different but compatible electrophysiologic effects may control arrhythmias refractory to single-drug therapy. Patients may tolerate combination therapy fairly well because dosages in combination therapy are often lower than those employed when either drug is used alone.

Although comparison of drug trials is hampered by nonuniformity among study protocols, the data suggest that drug combinations can be effective in treating some patients. Pairs of drugs showing the most promise have been a class IA drug (procainamide, quinidine, or disopyramide) with a class IB drug (usually mexiletine), and a class IA drug with a β blocker. Amiodarone should be combined with a class I drug only as a last resort. There is little evidence to support the simultaneous use of two class IA drugs. Selection of a drug combination should be guided by consideration of the patient's medical history, concurrent disease states, and risk of sudden cardiac death. The efficacy of combination therapy should be evaluated by electrophysiologic testing or ambulatory electrocardiography.

Combination antiarrhythmic therapy should be reserved for patients in whom single-drug therapy has been ineffective or poorly tolerated. More studies are needed to further define the efficacy, safety, and role of drug combinations in the treatment of ventricular arrhythmias.

Index terms: Amiodarone; Arrhythmia; Cardiac drugs; Combined therapy; Disopyramide; Dosage; Mexiletine; Procainamide; Protocols; Quinidine; Sympatholytic agents; Toxicity
Clin Pharm. 1988; 7:808–19

There are currently 10 oral antiarrhythmic drugs approved for the treatment of ventricular arrhythmias in the United States. The recent expansion in the number of available antiarrhythmic drugs has created the need for a more sophisticated approach to the selection of these agents. Patients are typically given a single drug and then undergo some form of objective testing of drug efficacy, such as 24-hour ambulatory electrocardiography, electrophysiologic (EP) testing, or exercise electrocardiography. Frequently, however, single agents induce intolerable toxicity or fail to control the arrhythmias. A number of studies have been performed to assess combination antiarrhythmic therapy in the treatment of ventricular tachyarrhythmias. The use of antiarrhythmic combinations at relatively low drug dosages may circumvent problems of toxicity and result in increased efficacy. In this paper the literature on oral combination regimens for ventricular arrhythmias is reviewed and a role for their place in therapy is proposed.

Ventricular Arrhythmias

The identification of patients with ventricular arrhythmias who require drug therapy is an important and controversial topic. Ventricular arrhythmias are generally of four types: premature ventricular contractions (PVCs), nonsustained ventricular tachycardia (ns-VT), sustained ventricular

Daniel W. Krichbaum, Pharm.D., is Clinical Pharmacist in Cardiology, Ingalls Memorial Hospital, Harvey, IL, Clinical Assistant Professor of Pharmacy Practice, University of Illinois at Chicago, and Affiliate Assistant Professor of Pharmacy Practice, Purdue University, West Lafayette, IN.

Address reprint requests to Dr. Krichbaum at Ingalls Memorial Hospital, 1 Ingalls Drive, Department of Pharmacy Services, Harvey, IL 60426.

The assistance of Tamara Small, Pharm.D., with the initial stages of manuscript preparation is acknowledged.

Copyright © 1988, American Society of Hospital Pharmacists, Inc. All rights reserved. 0278-2677/88/1101-0808$03.00.

tachycardia (s-VT), and ventricular fibrillation (VF). Bigger[1] has devised a classification for ventricular arrhythmias, along with objectives for treatment of each type (Table 1). The decision to treat a patient with complex PVCs or ns-VT should include an assessment of the symptoms resulting from the arrhythmia, an evaluation of underlying heart disease, including left ventricular function, and the status of any electrolyte abnormalities. Asymptomatic patients who have complex ventricular ectopy (multiformed complexes, repetitive or alternating patterns, or the R on T phenomenon) but are otherwise healthy may not require antiarrhythmic therapy.[2] In fact, no studies have proved that antiarrhythmic agents given to asymptomatic patients with complex ventricular ectopy alone prevent sudden death. However, complex ventricular ectopy is thought to be an independent risk factor for sudden cardiac death in patients with chronic ischemic heart disease,[3,4] recent myocardial infarction,[5-8] hypertensive left ventricular hypertrophy,[9] cardiomyopathy,[10,11] or poor left ventricular function.[4,12] In these patients, antiarrhythmic therapy seems warranted, particularly when the arrhythmia causes symptoms. Cardiac arrest that occurs outside of the hospital and is not associated with an acute myocardial infarction (AMI) carries the poorest prognosis and requires aggressive evaluation and treatment.[13,14]

Approximately one million people suffer AMI annually in the United States. The management of ventricular arrhythmias that develop after hospital discharge is a challenging problem. Patients with ventricular arrhythmias recorded 7 to 21 days after AMI have a higher mortality risk over the subsequent two years than similar patients without ventricular arrhythmias.[5-8] However, no study to date has included enough patients to test the hypothesis that reducing or eliminating ventricular arrhythmias with antiarrhythmic drugs after AMI reduces mortality. Results of the ongoing Cardiac Arrhythmia Suppression Trial (CAST) may help clarify this issue. This placebo-controlled study will assess patients with AMI who have asymptomatic ventricular arrhythmias and reduced myocardial function.

Table 1.
Bigger Classification of Ventricular Arrhythmias[a,b]

Definition	Treatment Objectives
Benign	
Infrequent PVCs; no repetitive PVCs; good LV function	Relieve symptoms; allay anxiety; avoid adverse effects
Potentially Malignant	
Frequent PVCs; repetitive PVCs; poor LV function	Reduce PVC frequency; abolish PVC runs; prevent VT or VF
Malignant	
Sustained VT or VF; poor LV function	Abolish malignant rhythm; prevent recurrences

[a] Reprinted from reference 1, with permission.
[b] PVC = premature ventricular complex, LV = left ventricle, VT = ventricular tachycardia, VF = ventricular fibrillation.

Evaluating Antiarrhythmic Efficacy

How to best predict drug efficacy has been a controversial subject over the past few decades. Much has been said of 24-hour ambulatory electrocardiography versus electrophysiologic testing.[15,16] In the only randomized, prospectively conducted study comparing EP testing with 24-hour ambulatory electrocardiography, programmed electrical stimulation, a form of EP testing, was more often effective in identifying a therapy that prevented recurrence of ventricular tachyarrhythmias.[17] The EP approach, however, required more drug trials and longer hospitalization. In addition, not all patients have an inducible ventricular arrhythmia during EP testing. It is now clear that each technique has a place in the management of ventricular arrhythmias.[18]

Electrophysiologic Testing. Programmed electrical stimulation has evolved substantially as a diagnostic and therapeutic tool since it was first described in 1968. EP studies are performed invasively by cardiologists who position electrode catheters within the heart to record electrical activity. Programmed stimulation is performed by electronically pacing the atrium or ventricle and then introducing critically timed extra beats in an attempt to induce the clinically documented arrhythmia. If the clinical arrhythmia can be reproduced in the laboratory, the patient undergoes serial drug testing using programmed electrical stimulation. Drug efficacy is suggested if the clinical arrhythmia can no longer be induced with the patient receiving a specific antiarrhythmic drug regimen. A lack of efficacy is suggested when the regimen does not prevent induction of the arrhythmia.

Interpretation of studies in which EP testing has been used is limited by the heterogeneity of patient populations, the differences in the stimulation protocols used, and the variable drug-administration techniques employed. The best candidates for EP testing have life-threatening or infrequent symptomatic arrhythmias, such as sustained monomorphic ventricular tachycardia, ventricular fibrillation, or out-of-hospital cardiac arrest.

Ambulatory Electrocardiography. Ambulatory 24-hour electrocardiography has been used to assess drug efficacy for more than 30 years. The usefulness of this technique, in which recordings made before and during drug therapy are compared, is limited by the spontaneous variability in the occurrence of arrhythmia during the assessment periods. The end point of therapy based on

24-hour monitoring periods should be a greater than 75% to 83% reduction in the number of PVCs, a greater than 90% reduction in ventricular couplets, and complete elimination of VT.[19,20] Monitoring the ECG during exercise may help identify effective drug therapy in patients whose ventricular arrhythmias can be exercise-induced. The best candidates for ambulatory electrocardiography have frequent complex PVCs, ns-VT, or both.

Pharmacology

The modified Vaughan Williams[21] classification of antiarrhythmic agents is shown in Table 2. The electrophysiologic properties of antiarrhythmic agents are listed in Table 3. The class IA drugs are considered "first generation" agents, whereas tocainide, mexiletine, flecainide, encainide, and amiodarone have been labeled "second generation" agents.[23] The difference in designation stems from the more rigorous preapproval evaluation process that was required by the FDA for the latter group of drugs and from the different electrophysiologic properties of those agents. The mechanisms by which antiarrhythmic agents act are not entirely known. Proposed explanations include suppression of automaticity, reduction of conduction velocity, prolongation of action potential duration, and lengthening of refractoriness. These actions may interfere with one of the mechanisms of arrhythmogenesis—re-entry, enhanced automaticity, and triggered automaticity. The electrophysiologic rationale for combination therapy will be presented in each category below.

Class IA with Class IA Combinations

The electrophysiologic properties of the class IA agents quinidine, procainamide, and disopyramide are similar (Table 3). Prior to the recent approval of numerous new antiarrhythmic agents, clinicians were limited to selecting the class IA agents alone or in combination. In two studies, investigators have used different methods to evaluate the combination of two class IA agents. Kim et al.[24] used ambulatory electrocardiography to evaluate the combination of quinidine and procainamide in 19 patients with recurrent s-VT or symptomatic ventricular arrhythmias; the patients served as their own controls. High doses of the single agents frequently caused intolerable gastrointestinal effects, but the combination of quinidine and procainamide, given in lower doses, was well tolerated. An effective drug regimen was defined as one causing >83% reduction in PVC occurrence and complete abolition of VT during a 24-hour period. At maximum dosages, quinidine alone was effective in five patients (26%) and procainamide alone was effective in four patients (21%); the combination of quinidine and procainamide in reduced dosages of each was effective in 14 (74%) patients ($p <$ 0.01).

Table 2.
Modified Vaughan Williams[21] Classification of Oral Antiarrhythmic Agents

Class I.	Sodium-channel blocking agents	
	A.	Quinidine[a]
		Procainamide[a]
		Disopyramide[a]
	B.	Mexiletine[a]
		Tocainide[a]
		Phenytoin
		Aprindine[b]
	C.	Encainide[a]
		Flecainide[a]
		Propafenone[b]
		Lorcainide[b]
Class II.	Beta-adrenergic blocking agents	
		Acebutolol[a]
		Atenolol
		Labetolol
		Metoprolol
		Nadolol
		Pindolol
		Propranolol[a]
		Sotalol[b]
		Timolol
Class III.	Inhibitors of repolarization	
		Amiodarone[a]
		Sotalol[b]
Class IV.	Calcium-channel modulating agents	
		Verapamil
		Diltiazem

[a] FDA-approved labeling includes an indication for treatment of ventricular arrhythmias.
[b] Currently investigational in the United States.

Duffy and associates[25] used EP testing to assess the efficacy of combinations of quinidine, procainamide, and disopyramide in nine patients; these agents, used singly, had previously failed to prevent the induction of s-VT in these patients. The addition of intravenous procainamide to high dosages of either quinidine or disopyramide failed to prevent the induction of s-VT in all nine patients. Although the tachycardia cycle length was increased with the combination regimen, the induction of VT during EP testing was easier. None of the patients in this study received long-term combination therapy.

The simultaneous use of two class IA agents is based on the premise that smaller than usual dosages of each drug can be effective and that dosage-related toxicity of individual agents can be reduced. However, not all adverse effects are dosage-related, and proarrhythmia may occur more often during combination than single-drug therapy. Until more data are available, there is little rationale for using two class IA drugs, especially because many new agents are now available. Recently, the addition of quinidine to procainamide therapy has been reported to cause steady-state procainamide concentrations to rise 70% above the concentrations measured when procainamide was used alone at the same dosage.[26]

Table 3.
Electrophysiologic Properties of Antiarrhythmic Agents[a,b]

Drug	Conduction Velocity	Refractory Period	Automaticity	AV Nodal Conduction	Surface ECG PR	Surface ECG QRS	Surface ECG QT_c
Class IA[c]					0/↑	↑	↑↑
Disopyramide	↓↓	↑↑	↓↓	↑			
Procainamide	↓↓	↑↑	↓↓	↑/↓			
Quinidine	↓↓	↑↑	↓↓	↑/↓			
Class IB[c]					0	0	0/↓
Lidocaine							
Normal tissue	0	↓	↓	0			
Ischemic tissue	↓↓	↑	↓↓	0			
Mexiletine	0	↓	↓	0			
Phenytoin							
Normal tissue	0	↓	↓	↑			
Ischemic tissue	↓↓	↑	↓↓	↑			
Tocainide	0	↓	↓	0			
Class IC[c]					↑	↑↑	0/↑
Encainide	↓↓	0	↓	0			
Flecainide	↓↓	0	↓	0			
Class II					0/↑	0	0/↓
Propranolol[d]	↓	↓ (Acute) ↑ (Chronic)	↓	↓↓			
Class III					↑	↑↑	↑
Amiodarone	0/↓	↑↑	0	↓			
Sotalol[e]	0	↑	0	↓			
Class IV							
Diltiazem	0	0	0	↓	↑	0	0
Verapamil	0	0	0	↓↓	↑↑	0	0

[a] Adapted from reference 22, with permission.
[b] ↑ = increase, ↓ = decrease, 0 = minimal or no effect, ↑/↓ = variable.
[c] Class I agents are subdivided into IA, IB, and IC based upon their actions on repolarization in normal ventricular tissue and their binding characteristics to the sodium channel. Class IA prolongs repolarization, class IB shortens repolarization, and class IC causes no change in repolarization.
[d] Effects occur via blockade of catecholamine-mediated effects.
[e] Sotalol also has class II or β-adrenergic blocking effects.

Class IA with Class IB Combinations

The efficacy of a IA plus IB combination has been evaluated in at least 16 studies[17,27-42] (Table 4). The rationale for using this combination is that, at fast rates of depolarization, class IB and IA agents have the additive electrophysiologic effects of decreasing conduction velocity and modifying refractoriness; IB agents may also normalize prolonged QT intervals caused by IA agents.[28] The major electrophysiologic effect of class I agents is a reduction in the maximal rate of depolarization (phase 0) via blockade of the inward sodium current. The affinity of the class I agents for the sodium channel depends on the state of the channel—resting (phase 4), open (i.e., activated, phase 0), or inactivated. The class IB agents have an equal affinity for both open and inactivated channels, whereas the class IA agents bind preferentially to activated channels.[43] Therefore, the combination of a class IA plus IB agent should have an additive effect on blocking frequency-dependent sodium channels. In addition, the class IB agents reduce the prolongation of repolarization induced by class IA drugs. A class IA plus IB combination has been used successfully in several clinical trials, the most frequently used combinations have been mexiletine with either procainamide or quinidine.

The first eight studies shown in Table 4 included an evaluation of the drug combination with a follow-up period to assess efficacy.[27-35] Short term efficacy has varied from 13% to 94%, with a trend toward lower efficacy rates when EP testing was the method of evaluation. Comparison of these studies is limited by the variable methods, definitions of successful drug therapy, and dosing regimens employed. In most of these trials, combination regimens were used only when treatment with all available single agents was unsuccessful.

There is strong evidence that using a IA plus IB combination, compared with using a drug of either class alone, causes fewer adverse effects and more favorable electrocardiographic patterns.[27,33,40,41] For example, Duff and associates[27] reported that the dose-limiting adverse effects of nausea and nervousness were experienced by only two patients (12%) receiving combination therapy, a reduction from the 81% occurrence rate when patients received mexiletine alone. Measurement of the electrocardiographic intervals in this study indicated that mexiletine, independent of dosage, had limited the quinidine-induced increases in QT_c intervals relative to baseline, theoretically decreasing the potential for a proarr-

Table 4.
Studies of Combination Therapy for Ventricular Arrhythmias

Reference No.	Method[b]	Agents[c]	Patient Population[d] *n*	No. with OHD	No. with IHD	LVEF (%)	Arrhythmia[e]	Acute Efficacy[f]: No. Patients (%)	Chronic Efficacy[g]: No. Patients (%)	Mean Follow-up (mo)
Class IA + Class IB										
27	AE	Q + M	21	NA[a]	17	NA	VT	16/17[h] (94)	10/14 (71)	18
28	EPS	Q + M	20	20	19	35 ± 13	s-VT	6/16 (37)	5/6 (83)	14
29	EPS	Q + M	89	93	78	NA	s-VT/VF	7/35 (20)	6/7 (85)	24
30	EPS/AE	Q or D + M	35	35	25	NA	PVC_{30}/s-VT/VF	NA	12/14 (85)	18
31	EPS	D or Q + DPH or T	33	29	16	NA	VT/VF	2/2 (100)	1/1 (100)	14
32	AE	PCA or D + T	20	18	12	NA	VT/VF	3/4 (75)[i]	2/4 (50)[i]	12
33	EPS	D + M	12	10	8	35	VT/VF	8/12 (66)[j]	5/7 (71)	10
34	EPS/AE	IA + M	44	42	32	42 ± 18	VT/VF	7/23 (30)[k]	5/7 (71)	7
35	EPS	IA + M	159	158	137	32 ± 15	VT/VF	48/111 (43)	50/62 (80)	19
36	EPS	Q or PCA + M	160	160	160	29	VT/VF	13/56 (23)[l]	. . .	. . .
37	EPS	Q or PCA + M	23	23	23	40	s-VT/VF	8/23 (35)	. . .	. . .
39	EPS	Q or PCA + M	76	NA	70	31 ± 14	VT/VF	21/76 (28)	. . .	. . .
17	EPS	IA + M	105	25	21	39 ± 16	PVC_{30}/VT/VF	2/15 (13)	. . .	. . .
17	AE	IA + M	105	27	22	34 ± 13	VT/VF	7/29 (24)[m]	. . .	. . .
40	AE	Q + T	14	14	7	35 ± 13	PVC_{30}/ns-VT	6/13 (46)[n]	. . .	. . .
41	AE	Q + T	20	20	20	NA	PVC_{30}/ns-VT	16/20 (80)[o]	. . .	. . .
42	EPS	IA + IB	166	166	125	41 ± 18	s-VT/VF	20/127 (16)[p]	. . .	. . .
Class II + Class I										
31	EPS	P + PCA or Q	33	29	16	NA	VT/VF	4/5 (80)	4/4 (100)	12
32	AE	P + T	20	18	12	NA	VT/VF	5/6 (83)[i]	4/6 (66)[i]	12
61	AE	N + PCA or Q	18	14	9	>30	PVC_{10}/ns-VT	5/8 (63)[q]	. . .	. . .
62	AE	P + Q	14	10	6	NA	VT	8/11 (73)[r]	. . .	. . .
46	AE	P + F	10	8	5	<50 (*n* = 5)	PVC_{10}/ns-VT	60/10 (60)[s]	. . .	. . .
47	EPS	P + Q or PCA	74	69	55	NA	VT	5/29 (17)	. . .	. . .
47	EPS	P + E	74	69	55	NA	VT	0/6 (0)	. . .	. . .
64	EMT	II + IA	54	46	33	NA	ns-VT	23/28 (82)[s]	. . .	. . .
64	AE	II + IA	54	46	33	NA	ns-VT	21/49 (43)[h]	. . .	. . .
67	EPS/TR	II + IA	20	20	17	<40	s-VT/VF	8/20 (40)	. . .	. . .

[a] NA = information not available.

[b] AE = ambulatory electrocardiography, EPS = electrophysiologic study, EMT = exercise monitored treadmill, TR = trendscription. Slash = and/or (e.g., EPS/AE = EPS or AE, or both).

[c] Q = quinidine, M = mexiletine, D = disopyramide, DPH = phenytoin, T = tocainide, PCA = procainamide, IA = quinidine or disopyramide or procainamide, IB = mexiletine or phenytoin or tocainide, P = propranolol, N = nadolol, F = flecainide, E = encainide, II = β blocker.

[d] OHD = organic heart disease; IHD = ischemic heart disease; LVEF = left ventricular ejection fraction; mean (± S.D. for some studies) of all patients in study.

[e] VT = both sustained and nonsustained ventricular tachycardia, s-VT = sustained ventricular tachycardia, VF = ventricular fibrillation, PVC_{30} = premature ventricular complexes occurring more frequently than 30/hr, ns-VT = nonsustained ventricular tachycardia, PVC_{10} = premature ventricular complexes occurring more frequently than 10/hr. Slash = and/or (e.g., s-VT/VF = s-VT or VF, or both).

[f] Acute efficacy refers to short-term drug administration with combination regimens. Except where noted, efficacy in EPS was defined as failure to induce >5 repetitive premature ventricular complexes during the stimulation protocol.

[g] Chronic efficacy refers to long-term drug administration with combination regimens. Efficacy was generally defined as survival with absence of ventricular tachycardia, ventricular fibrillation, or syncope during clinical follow-up.

[h] Complete suppression of ventricular tachycardia on 24-hour ambulatory electrocardiogram.

[i] Complete suppression of ventricular tachycardia and ventricular fibrillation, and >75% suppression of ventricular couplets and premature ventricular complexes on 24-hour ambulatory electrocardiogram.

[j] Ventricular tachycardia no longer inducible or more difficult to induce, compared with pretreatment.

[k] Ventricular tachycardia no longer inducible, or induction of well-tolerated nonsustained ventricular tachycardia.

[l] Ventricular tachycardia no longer inducible, or induction of ≤15 repetitive premature ventricular complexes in patients with baseline sustained ventricular tachycardia or ventricular fibrillation.

[m] Suppression of >80% of isolated premature ventricular complexes, 90% of ventricular couplets, and all episodes of repetitive premature ventricular complexes of three or more beats.

[n] Suppression of >70% of premature ventricular complexes and 95% of episodes of repetitive premature ventricular complexes of three or more beats.

[o] Suppression of >83% of premature ventricular complexes and all nonsustained ventricular tachycardia.

[p] Induction of ≤10 repetitive premature ventricular complexes for patients with sustained ventricular tachycardia, or induction of ≤6 repetitive premature ventricular complexes for patients with nonsustained ventricular tachycardia.

[q] Suppression of >75% of premature ventricular complexes.

[r] Absence of symptomatic ventricular tachycardia.

[s] Complete suppression of ventricular tachycardia.

hythmic event.[27] It appears that when used in combination, lower doses of each drug can be given to achieve higher efficacy and lower toxicity rates.[27,33,40,41]

The roles of EP testing and ambulatory electrocardiography in assessing clinical efficacy of class IA plus IB combinations are unclear. Kim et al.[30] conducted a nonrandomized concordance study to determine how well EP testing could identify an ineffective drug regimen. Patients with refractory s-VT or VF and frequent PVCs were treated with mexiletine either alone or in combination with a class IA agent. Only patients with persistently inducible VT and a marked reduction of PVCs during ambulatory electrocardiographic monitoring were included. Fourteen patients were discharged on a class IA plus mexiletine combination and followed for 5–37 months. Although acute EP testing predicted efficacy in only 5 of the 14 patients, 12 (85%) were free of arrhythmia recurrence during follow-up (mean = 4 mo). The authors concluded that poor results during EP testing may not predict poor clinical outcomes when initial ambulatory electrocardiography suggests drug efficacy.

Clinical trials have provided some valuable information about the electropharmacologic properties of this combination. Programmed ventricular stimulation was used to assess the efficacy of mexiletine and disopyramide, alone and in combination, in a randomized crossover study of 12 patients with VT or VF by Breithardt et al.[33] Combination therapy was effective in eight patients; in four, induction of VT was suppressed, and in the other four, the cycle length of the tachycardia was significantly prolonged. Other researchers have confirmed a prolongation of the tachycardia cycle length with this combination.[28,33,34,37,38] In most patients, a reduced rate of depolarization in ventricular tachycardia is associated with better long-term tolerance of the arrhythmia.[33,34] The combination of mexiletine and disopyramide appears to have minimal effects on ventricular refractory period and QRS duration in normal tissue. In fact, its electrical depressant effects are apparently selective for abnormal tissue at fast rates of depolarization.[28,38] Whitford et al.[35] and McGovern et al.[39] reported better success with this combination in patients with ns-VT or VF than in those with recurrent s-VT.

The combination of class IA plus IB agents may be effective in some patients with out-of-hospital cardiac arrest. In the randomized, prospective study by Mitchell et al.,[17] EP testing was compared with a noninvasive approach (24-hour electrocardiography and exercise-testing) to determine the better indicator of efficacious drug therapy. Antiarrhythmic combinations were tested when class IA and IB agents alone were ineffective. The investigators found that a combination of a class IA agent plus mexiletine was predicted to be successful in 7 of 29 (24%) patients by the noninvasive approach and in 2 of 15 (13%) by EP testing. Long-term efficacy of specific regimens was not reported. Programmed stimulation was also performed by Wilber et al.[42] in 166 survivors of out-of-hospital cardiac arrest. Serial EP tesing was performed in the 127 patients in whom ventricular arrhythmias were inducible. Success was defined as fewer than 10 repetitive PVCs during EP testing. The combination of a class IA plus IB agent successfully suppressed induction of VT in 20 of 127 trials (16%). Monotherapy with a class IA agent, class IB agent, amiodarone, or a β blocker was effective in 37, 13, 20, and 43 patients, respectively. Further studies with larger numbers of patients are needed to assess whether using a combination of a class IA plus IB agent is more effective in preventing sudden death than using a class IA agent alone. In the nonrandomized study with the longest follow-up reported, 42% of patients receiving mexiletine alone died suddenly or suffered recurrent symptomatic VT after four years; 25% of patients receiving mexiletine with a class IA agent had the same outcome.[35] The difference was not statistically significant.

The effect of the quinidine–mexiletine combination on ventricular function was studied in 14 patients with symptomatic VT.[44] A paired crossover design was used to assess ventricular function before antiarrhythmic therapy, during monotherapy with quinidine and mexiletine, and during combination therapy. Ventricular function was assessed by radionuclide ventriculography at steady state, when patients were taking the highest dosages of each drug or drug combination. The combination of quinidine and mexiletine did not affect ventricular function, either at rest or during peak exercise, in patients who did not have clinical heart failure.

These data support the contention that combination therapy with class IA plus IB agents can be effective in at least 20% of patients refractory to monotherapy with these agents (Table 4). This is a rational combination that appears to be safe and effective. When acute drug efficacy with this combination is predicted by EP testing, about 70–80% of patients will be free of arrhythmia recurrence during the next one to two years. The extracardiac toxicity experienced with combination therapy may be less than with the single agents used alone at higher dosages.[27,33,40,41] The addition of a class IB agent produces a shorter QT_c interval than that produced when a class IA agent is used alone.[27,40] Whether the incidence of proarrhythmic effects is substantially reduced by this combination should be investigated in further prospective studies.

Combinations of Class IC Agents with Other Drugs

There is some experience using the class IC agents flecainide, encainide, and propafenone in combination with class IA, II, and III agents.[45–49] Class IA and IC drugs prolong the QRS interval (reduce conduction velocity), while class IA agents prolong the JT

(QT − QRS) interval (prolong repolarization). The possibility of proarrhythmic effects caused by class IA and IC agents alone is noteworthy in patients with malignant ventricular arrhythmia, and the drug combination may cause additive undesirable electrocardiographic effects such as excessive prolongation of the QRS interval.

The efficacy of the combination of propafenone plus either procainamide or quinidine was tested in 47 patients who had frequent episodes of VT (> 10/hr) on baseline 24-hour ambulatory ECGs.[45] Thirty patients failed to respond to quinidine or procainamide and had propafenone added to their regimen. The patients received the combination for three to six weeks and then propafenone alone for one week. Each trial was evaluated by 24-hour ambulatory electrocardiography. Patients were then treated with the most effective drug regimen—either combination therapy or propafenone alone. The mean number of PVCs was lower when patients received combination therapy than when they received quinidine alone, procainamide alone, or no drug. More patients (16 of 23) had >70% suppression of PVCs and > 90% suppression of ns-VT when treated with the combination than when treated with a single drug (2 of 23). Propafenone alone appeared to be as effective as the combination regimen, but 22 of 30 patients required higher dosages during propafenone monotherapy. The addition of propafenone to quinidine or procainamide therapy caused prolongation of both the PR and QRS intervals when compared with baseline measurements, but no further QT_c interval change when compared with the interval measured during quinidine or procainamide monotherapy. Two patients (6%) experienced a probable proarrhythmic effect when propafenone was added to their regimen.

Combination therapy with a class IC plus class II agent was prospectively studied using flecainide acetate (150 mg/day) and propranolol hydrochloride (60 mg/day), alone and in combination, in a crossover study of 10 patients with benign ventricular arrhythmias.[46] The combination regimen did not have any additional antiarrhythmic effect over monotherapy when assessed by 24-hour ambulatory electrocardiography. In fact, four of the patients had episodes of VT with combination therapy; no episodes of VT were reported with flecainide alone. Similar results were found using EP testing when encainide was combined with propranolol.[47] In the flecainide–propranolol study, plasma flecainide concentration was increased by 25% during combination therapy[46]; this interaction had been reported previously.[48]

Sotalol is a promising investigational agent with class II and III properties. Gulker et al.[49] tested sotalol in combination with either propafenone or flecainide in 20 patients with arrhythmias refractory to these agents when used alone. All patients had chronic PVCs, VT, or the R on T phenomenon during baseline 24-hour ambulatory electrocardiography. The addition of oral sotalol to intravenous propafenone or flecainide resulted in a > 85% reduction in PVC occurrence in 17 of 20 (85%) patients. Based on the available studies, class IC–IA and IC–II combinations appear to be of limited utility; a class IC–sotalol combination may prove to be more useful.

Class I with Class II Combinations

Combinations of class II (β-adrenergic blocking) drugs and class I agents have been useful in treating both atrial and ventricular arrhythmias. The primary antiarrhythmic mechanism of β blockers is antagonism of catecholamine-induced electrophysiologic effects.[50] Catecholamines increase automaticity and conduction velocity and decrease the refractory period of myocardial tissue. The membrane-stabilizing effects of β blockers are negligible at the serum concentrations obtained by conventional dosing.[50,51] Studies in isolated heart preparations have shown that β blockers have an additive effect in slowing conduction when combined with class I agents.[52,53]

There is considerable evidence that long-term use of β blockers can reduce the mortality from sudden death after AMI.[54–59] This property does not appear to be specific for any one β blocker. The mechanism by which β blockers reduce mortality is not entirely known, but there is substantial evidence that the autonomic nervous system plays a critical role in the genesis of sudden cardiac death.[60]

Although β blockers have not generally been used as initial agents for malignant ventricular arrhythmias, evidence is mounting that synergistic antiarrhythmic effects can be obtained by combining β blockers with membrane stabilizing agents.[31,32,47,61–70] Most of these controlled studies evaluated efficacy after short-term therapy only, and all included some patients with coronary artery disease[61–64,67] (Table 4).

The results of several well-controlled studies indicate that the addition of a β blocker enhances the antiarrhythmic efficacy of membrane stabilizing agents.[61–63] Deedwania et al.[61] tested the efficacy of nadolol in combination with quinidine or procainamide in a double-blind placebo-controlled study. During the four-week double-blind phase, the combination was successful in five of eight patients (63%); procainamide or quinidine monotherapy was successful in 29% of patients. Mean PVC frequency was reduced by 92% with combination therapy but by only 19% with procainamide or quinidine alone. Fors and colleagues[62] added propranolol to quinidine therapy in patients with a variety of quinidine-resistant arrhythmias. A subgroup of 14 patients with paroxysmal VT was tested by 24-hour ambulatory electrocardiography while receiving propranolol alone and propranolol plus quinidine. One third of patients (3 of 9) responded to propranolol alone, while 8 of 11 (73%) responded to the combination. Bigger et al.[63] found enhanced antiarrhythmic efficacy when a β blocker was added to mexiletine therapy. Of 185 patients who received mexiletine alone, 14% responded successfully. Success was defined as a >70% reduction in PVC frequency. The same low dose of mexiletine hydrochloride (200 mg every eight hours) was used after the addition of a β blocker in 44 patients, and 30% of patients responded successfully ($p < 0.01$, combination compared with mexiletine alone).

When added to class I agents, the synergistic antiarrhythmic effect of β blockers is most pronounced during exercise. In the study by Hirsowitz et al.,[64] efficacy of this combination was evaluated by 24-hour ambulatory electrocardiography and by symptom-limited exercise testing. The study consisted of a drug-free control phase, a short-term treatment phase with β-blocking and class I agents used separately, and a short-term combination treatment phase. The combination regimen, when evaluated by ambulatory electrocardiography, abolished VT and ventricular couplets in only 43% and 20% of patients, respectively. However, the combination regimen abolished VT during exercise testing in 82% of patients who originally had exercise-induced VT during the control phase.

The results of at least three studies show prolonged survival, when compared to population averages, in patients receiving β blockers as components of combination regimens.[65-68] Although the studies were not designed to assess the effect on survival of β blockers in combination with class I agents, these findings do suggest that patients who have suffered AMI may not be the only ones to live longer because of β-blocker therapy.

There are numerous case reports of the use of β blockers in combination with class IA or IB agents. Dreifus et al.[69] described two patients with s-VT who responded to the combination of quinidine plus propranolol, although neither drug controlled the arrhythmias when used alone. Leahy et al.[70] described four patients with previous myocardial infarction and ventricular arrhythmias who were given mexiletine plus propranolol. All four had had persistent arrhythmias despite having high plasma concentrations of quinidine, procainamide, disopyramide, or phenytoin. All four patients developed adverse effects from mexiletine hydrochloride at doses of 900 or 1200 mg/day without achieving adequate arrhythmia suppression. The dosage was then reduced to a tolerable level, and propranolol hydrochloride 240 mg/day was added. All four patients experienced >80% suppression of PVCs; three of four had ns-VT abolished on ambulatory ECGs. Excellent control of ventricular arrhythmias was noted during a follow-up period (mean=17 mo).

It appears from short-term studies that β blockers in combination with class IA or IB agents are efficacious in about 60% of patients refractory to these agents used alone (Table 4). The efficacy of β blockers in combination with class IC agents has been poor.[46,47] Beta blockers are most effective in catecholamine-induced ventricular arrhythmias (i.e., those associated with exercise, with emotional stress, with the period following AMI and with congestive heart failure). There is some suggestion that, in patients with malignant arrhythmias and poor left ventricular function, β blockers in combination with class I agents may reduce the incidence of sudden cardiac death. This speculation needs confirmation by well-controlled prospective studies. Results of the ongoing timolol, encainide, sotolol trial (TEST) may help clarify the role and actions of β blockers and membrane-stabilizing agents in patients with potentially malignant ventricular arrhythmias who have had AMI.

Combinations of Class I Agents with Amiodarone

Amiodarone is usually used only for refractory malignant ventricular arrhythmias because of its potentially life-threatening toxicity. This complex agent has been tested in various drug combinations in patients who have not responded to any other mode of therapy.

The addition of a class IA agent to amiodarone therapy rarely prevents induction of s-VT yet may improve hemodynamic stability during episodes of arrhythmia by increasing the tachycardia cycle length.[71,72] In one study, 37 patients with inducible rapid VT or VF during class IA and amiodarone monotherapy were evaluated by serial EP testing.[71] Thirty-five patients had coronary artery disease and two had idiopathic congestive cardiomyopathy; the mean left ventricular ejection fraction was 32 ± 11%. After 14 days of combination therapy, s-VT became noninducible in only 2 of the 37 patients (5%). However, after the addition of procainamide the mean cycle length of induced VT increased from 283 to 352 msec ($p < 0.001$). Of the 31 patients treated with procainamide and amiodarone, 16 were hemodynamically stable during VT induction; of patients receiving amiodarone alone, 10 of 37 were stable during VT induction. Long-term therapy was assessed by randomly assigning patients to amiodarone alone (20 patients) or the combination (17 patients). Using life-table analysis, no differences in the incidence of adverse effects necessitating drug withdrawal, sudden death, or syncope were identified between the two groups. A similarly low efficacy rate (15%) with short-term therapy has been reported for amiodarone plus procainamide in another study using serial EP testing.[36]

Numerous retrospective case analyses have reported good outcomes with amiodarone in combination with class IA or IB agents. In a review of 11 cases, James et al.[73] described the use of amiodarone plus disopyramide for control of ventricular arrhythmias (n = 8) or atrial fibrillation (n = 3). All patients had failed to respond to therapy with disopyramide alone, and 9 of 11 had failed to respond to therapy with amiodarone alone. These authors reported therapeutic success (assessed clinically) with an amiodarone–disopyramide combination in six of eight (75%) patients. During the follow-up period (mean = 13 mo), only one patient required drug discontinuation and the remaining five were free of symptoms. Hoffman et al.[74] reported in a retrospective analysis that control of VT with amiodarone plus either quinidine or mexiletine was achieved in 9 of 11 patients followed for a mean of 11 months. Treatment was evaluated by 24-hour ambulatory electrocardiography, and efficacy was assessed using Lown's grading scale. Amiodarone hydrochloride 200 mg was given five times per week. The QT_c interval was <0.44 sec in three of four patients receiving amiodarone plus quinidine and <0.47 sec in all seven patients receiving amiodarone plus mexiletine. The combination of amiodarone plus mexiletine was evaluated by EP testing in nine patients with recurrent VT unresponsive to conventional therapy.[75] In two patients, amiodarone therapy alone had been unsuccessful; in seven, mexiletine therapy alone was ineffective before the combination trials. Following intravenous loading doses, patients received both mexiletine hydrochloride 600 mg and amiodarone hydrochloride 600 mg orally per day. The first three patients had complete suppression of VT within the first three days of combination therapy, although mexiletine therapy alone had previously been unsuccessful. In the other six patients, serial EP testing was performed; VT was noninducible in all six patients after seven days of therapy. During a mean follow-up period of 5.8 months, only four of nine patients continued to receive the combination without symptoms. Whether monotherapy with amiodarone or mexiletine would have been effective in the patients not given these drugs remains unknown.

Amiodarone should be used cautiously with class IA agents and only when all other forms of therapy are ineffective. Because of the delay between initiation of amiodarone therapy and achievement of a full therapeutic effect, some additional antiarrhythmic therapy is advisable during this loading phase. However, increased quinidine and procainamide concentrations have been reported following the addition of amiodarone.[76,77] At least two cases of drug-induced torsades de pointes in patients receiving amiodarone and quinidine have been reported.[77] The dosage of quinidine or procainamide should be reduced by 30–50% when amiodarone is added.[78]

Selection of Drug Therapy

The treatment of ventricular arrhythmias must be individualized, considering the patient's risk for sudden cardiac death. Horowitz and Morganroth[23] have emphasized that the selection of antiarrhythmic agents should not be considered hierarchical. Each patient must be considered his own therapeutic experiment. Individualized therapy should be based on the patient's age, medication history, and concomitant disease states. Particular attention should be placed on assessment of the patient's left ventricular function and severity of ventricular arrhythmia. Associated disease states that may influence drug selection include the sick sinus syndrome, conduction disorders, the long QT syndromes, mitral valve prolapse, recent myocardial infarction, poor left ventricular function, and renal, hepatic, and hematologic disorders.[79] The selection of antiarrhythmic agents is most commonly based on considerations of toxicity rather than comparative efficacy among the available agents.[80] The currently available antiarrhythmic drugs possess an important potential for inducing or worsening ventricular arrhythmias.[81] For example, drug-induced prolongation of the QT interval resulting in polymorphic VT (torsade de pointes) may occur in 2–3% of patients given class IA agents alone.[82,83] Proarrhythmic effects appear to be most common in patients with sustained ventricular tachyarrhythmias, compromised left ventricular function, and pre-existing conduction disturbances. The proarrhythmic potential of combination therapy has not been well studied. When combination therapy is prescribed, each agent should be used initially at low doses and the patient should be carefully monitored to assess drug safety and efficacy.

Asymptomatic patients with PVCs or ns-VT and no underlying heart disease have a long-term prognosis similar to that of the healthy U.S. population.[2] There are no data from prospective studies that conclusively support the use of antiarrhythmic agents for prevention of sudden death in patients with ns-VT.[84] Most clinicians withhold antiarrhythmic agents in patients with benign ventricular arrhythmias and direct their efforts toward reassuring the patients.

A class IA or IC agent is a reasonable first choice for patients with potentially malignant ventricular arrhythmias.[23] In patients with PVCs and ns-VT, class IC agents effectively suppress arrhythmia and cause a relatively low incidence of proarrhythmic effects.[85] However, class IC agents may be no better than class IA drugs in preventing s-VT or sudden cardiac death.[79] Tocainide and mexiletine are effective in only about 30–50% of patients with potentially malignant ventricular arrhythmia and cause toxicity requiring discontinuation in up to 20% of patients.[85] Mexiletine appears to be better tolerated and more often effective than tocainide.[85] In patients with poor left ventricular function, disopyramide and flecainide should be withheld, because of their negative inotropic effects, until other agents have been tested and found ineffective. Patients with catecholamine-induced arrhythmia may respond well to class II agents alone or in combination with membrane stabilizing agents. Combination therapy with a class IA plus IB drug is a good alternative should single agents fail. The temptation to use amiodarone in patients with benign or potentially malignant arrhythmias should be strongly resisted.[86]

In patients with malignant ventricular arrhythmias, the use of EP testing to guide drug therapy selection is recommended.[15–18] Based on results of serial drug testing, a patient-specific sequence of drug trials to assess clinical efficacy and tolerance can be employed. For those patients who are not candidates for serial EP testing, ambulatory electrocardiographic monitoring for 24–48 hours before and during drug trials and during exercise testing should be used. In general, an initial treatment sequence for patients with malignant ventricular arrhythmia could be monotherapy with quinidine and procainamide, followed by encainide or flecainide, with drug selection guided by a consideration of left ventricular function.[23] Flecainide has important negative inotropic effects and can precipitate or worsen clinical heart failure. The high incidence of proarrhythmic effects in patients with poor left ventricular function may limit the usefulness of flecainide and encainide in treating such patients. Low efficacy rates with tocainide and mexiletine may preclude their use in initial therapy. Combination therapy with mexiletine plus quinidine or procainamide should be considered when class I agents alone are ineffective. The value of adding a β blocker to class I therapy should not be underestimated. Amiodarone is usually reserved until all available agents and established combinations have proved ineffective. A combination of amiodarone plus a class I agent, used cautiously, is the last alternative if all other regimens fail. The indications for surgical intervention and implantation of cardioverter–defibrillator devices have been reviewed elsewhere.[87–89]

Conclusion

Only a few well-controlled studies have been performed that have compared the electropharmacologic effects, safety, and clinical efficacy of drug combinations with single agents. Many of the studies cited here were small or retrospective; some only reported efficacy rates incidentally. Comparative analyses are difficult because of nonuniformity in methods of monitoring and assessing efficacy, in definitions of therapeutic success, in dosing regimens and administration techniques, and in electrophysiologic stimulation protocols employed.

All of the current antiarrhythmic agents have limitations. None has been conclusively shown to prevent sudden death in patients with complex ventricular arrhythmias, with the exception of β blockers after AMI. It is not uncommon for all available antiarrhythmic agents to be ineffective or poorly tolerated when used singly. Arrhythmia control in a sizable number of refractory patients may be safely achieved by using antiarrhythmic agents with different but compatible electrophysiologic effects in combination. The most successful combinations appear to be class IA plus IB agents, and class IA agents plus β blockers. Combination regimens generally should be reserved for patients in whom single agents are ineffective or poorly tolerated. More studies that involve larger numbers of patients and are specifically designed to evaluate the efficacy, extracardiac toxicity, and proarrhythmic effects of antiarrhythmic combinations are needed.

References

1. Bigger JT. Antiarrhythmic treatment: an overview. *Am J Cardiol.* 1984; 53:8B–16B.
2. Kennedy HL, Whitlock JA, Sprague MK et al. Long-term follow-up of asymptomatic healthy subjects with frequent complex ventricular ectopy. *N Engl J Med.* 1985; 312:193–7.
3. Ruberman W, Weinblatt E, Goldberg JD et al. Ventricular premature complexes in prognosis of angina. *Circulation.* 1980; 61:1172–8.
4. Bigger JT, Fleiss JL, Kleiger R et al. The relationships among ventricular arrhythmias, left ventricular dysfunction, and mortality in the two years after myocardial infarction. *Circulation.* 1984; 69:250–8.
5. The Coronary Drug Project Research Group. Prognostic importance of premature beats following myocardial infarction: experience in the Coronary Drug Project. *JAMA.* 1973; 223:1116–24.
6. Vismara LA, Amsterdam EA, Mason DT. Relation of ventricular arrhythmias in the late hospital phase of acute myocardial infarction to sudden death after hospital discharge. *Am J Med.* 1975; 59:6–12.
7. Schulze RA, Strauss HW, Pitt B. Sudden death in the year following myocardial infarction: relation to ventricular premature contractions in the last hospital phase and left ventricular ejection fraction. *Am J Med.* 1977; 62:192–9.
8. Ruberman W, Weinblatt E, Goldberg JD et al. Ventricular premature beats and mortality after myocardial infarction. *N Engl J Med.* 1977; 297:750–7.
9. McLenachan JM, Henderson E, Morris KI et al. Ventricular arrhythmias in patients with hypertensive left ventricular hypertrophy. *N Engl J Med.* 1987; 317:787–92.
10. McKenna WJ, England D, Doi YL et al. Arrhythmia in hypertrophic cardiomyopathy. I. Influence on prognosis. *Br Heart J.* 1981; 46:168–72.
11. Unverferth DV, Magorien RD, Moeschberger ML et al. Factors influencing the one-year mortality of dilated cardiomyopathy. *Am J Cardiol.* 1984; 54:147–52.
12. Swerdlow CD, Winkle RA, Mason JW. Determinants of survival in patients with ventricular tachyarrhythmias. *N Engl J Med.* 1983; 308:1436–42.
13. Baum RS, Alvarez H III, Cobb LA. Survival after resuscitation from out-of-hospital ventricular fibrillation. *Circulation.* 1974; 50:1231–5.

14. Goldstein S, Landis JR, Leighton R et al. Characteristics of the resuscitated out-of-hospital cardiac arrest victim with coronary heart disease. *Circulation*. 1981; 64:977–84.
15. Waller TJ, Kay HR, Spielman SR et al. Reduction in sudden death and total mortality by antiarrhythmic therapy evaluated by electrophysiologic drug testing: criteria of efficacy in patients with sustained ventricular tachyarrhythmia. *J Am Coll Cardiol*. 1987; 10:83–9.
16. Podrid PJ. Treatment of ventricular arrhythmia: applications and limitations of noninvasive vs invasive approach. *Chest*. 1985; 88:121–8.
17. Mitchell LB, Duff HJ, Manyari DE et al. A randomized clinical trial of the noninvasive and invasive approaches to drug therapy of ventricular tachycardia. *N Engl J Med*. 1987; 317:1681–7.
18. Kim SG. The management of patients with life-threatening ventricular tachyarrhythmias: programmed stimulation or Holter monitoring (either or both)? *Circulation*. 1987; 76:1–5.
19. Pratt CM, Slymen DJ, Wierman AM et al. Analysis of the spontaneous variability of ventricular arrhythmias: consecutive ambulatory electrocardiographic recordings of ventricular tachycardia. *Am J Cardiol*. 1985; 56:67–72.
20. Morganroth J, Michelson EL, Horowitz LN et al. Limitations of routine long-term electrocardiographic monitoring to assess ventricular ectopic frequency. *Circulation*. 1978; 58:408–14.
21. Vaughan Williams EM. A classification of antiarrhythmic actions reassessed after a decade of new drugs. *J Clin Pharmacol*. 1984; 24:129–47.
22. Bauman JL. Cardiac drugs. In Knoben JE, Anderson PO, eds. Handbook of clinical drug data. 6th ed. Hamilton, IL: Drug Intelligence Publications, Inc.; 1988; 495–6.
23. Horowitz LN, Morganroth J. Second generation antiarrhythmic agents: have we reached antiarrhythmic nirvana? *J Am Coll Cardiol*. 1987; 9:459–63.
24. Kim SG, Seiden SW, Matos JA et al. Combination of procainamide and quinidine for better tolerance and additive effects for ventricular arrhythmias. *Am J Cardiol*. 1985; 56:84–8.
25. Duffy CE, Swiryn S, Bauernfeind RA et al. Inducible sustained ventricular tachycardia refractory to individual class I drugs: effect of adding a second class I drug. *Am Heart J*. 1983; 106:450–8.
26. Hughes B, Dyer JE, Schwartz AB. Increased procainamide plasma concentrations caused by quinidine: a new drug interaction. *Am Heart J*. 1987; 114:908–9.
27. Duff HJ, Roden D, Primm RK et al. Mexiletine in the treatment of resistant ventricular arrhythmias: enhancement of efficacy and reduction of dose-related side effects by combination with quinidine. *Circulation*. 1985; 67:1124–8.
28. Duff HJ, Mitchell LB, Manyari D et al. Mexiletine-quinidine combination: electrophysiologic correlates of a favorable antiarrhythmic interaction in humans. *J Am Coll Cardiol*. 1987; 10:1149–56.
29. DiMarco JP, Garan H, Ruskin JN. Quinidine for ventricular arrhythmias; value of electrophysiologic testing. *Am J Cardiol*. 1983; 51:90–5.
30. Kim SG, Felder SD, Waspe LE et al. Electrophysiologic effects and clinical efficacy of mexiletine used alone or in combination with class IA agents for refractory recurrent ventricular tachycardias or ventricular fibrillation. *Am J Cardiol*. 1985; 58:485–90.
31. Mason JW, Winkle RA. Electrode-catheter arrhythmia induction in the selection and assessment of antiarrhythmic drug therapy for recurrent ventricular tachycardia. *Circulation*. 1978; 58:971–85.
32. Esterbrooks D, Aronew WS, Mohinddin SW et al. Effect of tocainide on ventricular arrhythmias refractory to standard oral antiarrhythmic drugs but responsive to intravenous lidocaine. *Curr Ther Res*. 1983; 33:272–8.
33. Breithardt G, Seipel L, Abendroth RR. Comparison of the antiarrhythmic efficacy of disopyramide and mexiletine against stimulus induced ventricular tachycardia. *J Cardiovasc Pharmacol*. 1986; 3:1026–37.
34. Waspe LE, Waxman HL, Buxton AE et al. Mexiletine for control of drug-resistant ventricular tachycardia; clinical and electrophysiologic results in 44 patients. *Am J Cardiol*. 1983; 51:1175–81.
35. Whitford EG, McGovern B, Schoenfeld MH et al. Long-term efficacy of mexiletine alone and in combination with class IA antiarrhythmic drugs for refractory ventricular arrhythmias. *Am Heart J*. 1988; 116:360–6.
36. Rae AP, Greenspan AM, Spielman SR et al. Antiarrhythmic drug efficacy for ventricular tachyarrhythmias associated with coronary artery disease as assessed by electrophysiologic studies. *Am J Cardiol*. 1985; 55:1494–9.
37. Greenspan AM, Spielman SR, Webb CR et al. Efficacy of combination therapy with mexiletine and a type IA agent for inducible ventricular tachyarrhythmias secondary to coronary artery disease. *Am J Cardiol*. 1985; 56:277–84.
38. Holt G, Tchou P, Dongas J et al. Electrophysiologic effects of oral mexiletine in patients with sustained ventricular tachycardia receiving type IA antiarrhythmic agents. *PACE*. 1985; 8:302. Abstract.
39. McGovern B, Garan H, Christoduloss S et al. Treatment of refractory ventricular tachycardia with a combination of mexiletine and a class IA antiarrhythmic drug. *J Am Coll Cardiol*. 1984; 3:557. Abstract.
40. Barbey JT, Thompson KA, Echt DS et al. Tocainide plus quinidine for treatment of ventricular arrhythmias. *Am J Cardiol*. 1988; 61:570–3.
41. Kim SG, Mercando AD, Fisher JD. Combination of tocainide and quinidine for better tolerance and additive effects in patients with coronary artery disease. *J Am Coll Cardiol*. 1987; 9:1369–74.
42. Wilber DJ, Garan H, Finkelstein D et al. Use of electrophysiologic testing in the prediction of long-term outcome. *N Engl J Med*. 1988; 318:19–24.
43. Hondeghem LM, Katzung BG. Antiarrhythmic agents: the modulated receptor mechanism of action of sodium and calcium channel-blocking drugs. *Ann Rev Pharmacol Toxicol*. 1984; 24:387–423.
44. Sheldon RS, Duff HJ, Mitchell LB et al. Effect of oral combination therapy with mexiletine and quinidine on left and right ventricular function. *Am Heart J*. 1988; 115:1030–6.
45. Klein RC, Huang SK, Marcus FI et al. Enhanced antiarrhythmic efficacy of propafenone when used in combination with procainamide or quinidine. *Am Heart J*. 1987; 114:551–8.
46. Stern H, Scheininger M, Theisen F et al. Antiarrhythmic therapy with flecainide in combination and comparison with propranolol. *Drugs*. 1985; 29:77–85.
47. Ross DL, Sze DY, Keefe DL et al. Antiarrhythmic drug combinations in the treatment of ventricular tachycardia. Efficacy and electrophysiologic effects. *Circulation*. 1982; 66:1205–10.
48. Lewis GP, Holtzman JL. Interaction of flecainide with digoxin and propranolol. *Am J Cardiol*. 1984; 43(Suppl):52B–59B.
49. Gulker H, Heur H, Freking B et al. Enhanced antiarrhythmic efficacy of combined sotalol/flecainide and combined sotalol/propafenone on chronic ventricular arrhythmia. *Circulation*. 1984; 70 (Suppl II):II-444. Abstract.
50. Nixon JV, Pennington W, Ritter W et al. Efficacy of propranolol in the control of exercise-induced or augmented ventricular ectopic activity. *Circulation*. 1978; 57:115–22.
51. Woosley R, Kornhauser D, Smith R et al. Suppression of chronic ventricular arrhythmias with propranolol. *Circulation*. 1978; 60:819–27.
52. Hodess AB, Follansbee WP, Spear JF et al. Effects of a new antiarrhythmic agent, R 818, combined with oubain or propranolol on the cardiac conduction system. *Clin Res*. 1978; 26:239A.
53. Korte DW, Nash LB. Ventricular electrophysiology of quinidine–propranolol combination in the dog heart. *J Pharmacol Exp Ther*. 1976; 197:457–67.

54. Julian DG, Prescott RJ, Jackson FS et al. Controlled trial of sotalol for one year after myocardial infarction. *Lancet*. 1982; 1:1142–7.
55. β-Blocker Heart Attack Study Group. A randomized trial of propranolol in patients with acute myocardial infarction. I. Mortality results. *JAMA*. 1982; 247:1707–14.
56. The Norwegian Multicenter Study Group. Six-year follow-up of the Norwegian Multicenter Study on timolol after acute, myocardial infarction. *N Engl J Med*. 1985; 313: 1055–8.
57. The Norwegian Multicenter Study Group. Timolol-induced reduction in mortality and reinfarction in patients surviving acute myocardial infarction. *N Engl J Med*. 1981; 304:801–7.
58. Muticentre International Study. Reduction in mortality after myocardial infarction with long-term beta-adrenergic receptor blockade. *Br Med J*. 1977; 2:419–21.
59. Lichstein E, Morganroth J, Harriet R et al. Effect of propranolol on ventricular arrhythmia. The beta-blocker heart attack trial experience. *Circulation*. 1983; 67(Suppl I): 1–10.
60. Coumel P, Leclerq JF, Leenhardt A. Arrhythmias as predictors of sudden death. *Am Heart J*. 1987; 114:929–37.
61. Deedwania PC, Olukotun AY, Kupersmith J et al. Beta blockers in combination with class I antiarrhythmic agents. *Am J Cardiol*. 1987; 60:21D–26D.
62. Fors WJ, Vanderark CR, Reynolds EW. Evaluation of propranolol and quinidine in the treatment of quinidine-resistant arrhythmias. *Am J Cardiol*. 1971; 27:190–4.
63. Bigger JT Jr. The interaction of mexiletine with other cardiovascular drugs. *Am Heart J*. 1984; 107:1079–85.
64. Hirsowitz G, Podrid PJ, Lampert S et al. The role of beta blocking agents as adjunct therapy to membrane stabilizing drugs in malignant ventricular arrhythmia. *Am Heart J*. 1986; 111:852–60.
65. Lown B, Graboys TB. Management of patients with malignant ventricular arrhythmias. *Am J Cardiol*. 1977; 39:910–8.
66. Graboys TB, Lown B, Podrid PJ et al. Long-term survival of patients with malignant ventricular arrhythmia treated with antiarrhythmic drugs. *Am J Cardiol*. 1982; 50:437–43.
67. Brodsky MA, Allen BJ, Baron D et al. Enhanced survival in patients with heart failure and life-threatening ventricular tachyarrhythmias. *Am Heart J*. 1986; 112:1166–72.
68. Bigger JT Jr. Why patients with congestive heart failure die: arrhythmias and sudden cardiac death. *Circulation*. 1987; 75(Suppl IV):IV-28–IV-35.
69. Dreifus LS, Lim HF, Watanabe Y et al. Propranolol and quinidine in the management of ventricular tachycardia. *JAMA*. 1968; 204:190–1.
70. Leahey EB, Heissenbuttel RH, Giardina EV et al. Combined mexiletine and propranolol treatment of refractory ventricular tachycardia. *Br Med J*. 1980; 2:357–8.
71. Marchlinski FE, Buxton AE, Miller JM et al. Amiodarone versus amiodarone and a type IA agent for treatment of patients with rapid ventricular tachycardia. *Circulation*. 1986; 74:1037–43.
72. Waxman HL, Groh WC, Marchlinski FE. Amiodarone for control of sustained ventricular tachyarrhythmia: clinical and electrophysiologic effects in 51 patients. *Am J Cardiol*. 1982; 50:1066–74.
73. James MA, Papouchado M, Vann Jones J. Combined therapy with disopyramide and amiodarone; a report of 11 cases. *Int J Cardiol*. 1986; 13:248–52.
74. Hoffman A, Follath F, Burkhardt D. Safe treatment of resistant ventricular arrhythmias with a combination of amiodarone and quinidine or mexiletine. *Lancet*. 1983; 1:704–5.
75. Waleffe A, Mary-Rabine L, Legrand V et al. Combined mexiletine and amiodarone treatment of refractory recurrent ventricular tachycardia. *Am Heart J*. 1980; 100:788–93.
76. Saal AK, Werner JA, Greene HL et al. Effect of amiodarone on serum quinidine and procainamide levels. *Am J Cardiol*. 1984; 53:1264–7.
77. Tartini R, Steinbrunn W, Kappenberger L et al. Dangerous interaction between amiodarone and quinidine. *Lancet*. 1982; 1:1327–9.
78. Marcus FI. Drug interactions with amiodarone. *Am Heart J*. 1983; 106:924–30.
79. Dibianco R. Chronic ventricular arrhythmias: which drug for which patient? *Am J Cardiol*. 1988; 61:83A–94A.
80. Zipes DP. A consideration of antiarrhythmic therapy. *Circulation*. 1985; 72:949–56. Editorial.
81. Horowitz LW, Zipes DP, Bigger JT et al. Proarrhythmia, arrhythmogenesis or aggravation of arrhythmia—a status report, 1987. *Am J Cardiol*. 1987; 59:54E–56E.
82. Tzivoni D, Keren A, Stern S. Torsade de pointes versus polymorphic ventricular tachycardia. *Am J Cardiol*. 1983; 52:639–40. Editorial.
83. Zipes DP. Proarrhythmic effects of antiarrhythmic drugs. *Am J Cardiol*. 1987; 59:26E–31E.
84. Prystowski EN. Antiarrhythmic therapy for asymptomatic ventricular arrhythmias. *Am J Cardiol*. 1988; 61:102A–107A.
85. Woosley RL, Funck-Brentano C. Overview of the clinical pharmacology of antiarrhythmic drugs. *Am J Cardiol*. 1988; 61:61A–69A.
86. Mason JW. Amiodarone. *N Engl J Med*. 1987; 316:455–63.
87. Cox JL. The status of surgery for cardiac arrhythmias. *Circulation*. 1985; 71:413–7.
88. Reid PR, Mirowski M, Mower MM et al. Clinical evaluation of the internal automatic cardioverter-defibrillator in survivors of sudden cardiac death. *Am J Cardiol*. 1983; 51:1608–13.
89. Scheinman MM, Davis JC. Catheter ablation for treatment of tachyarrhythmias; present role and potential promise. *Circulation*. 1986; 73:10–3.

Research

Clindamycin pharmacokinetics and tissue penetration after head and neck surgery

GARY P. STOEHR, VICTOR L. YU, JONAS T. JOHNSON, EDWARD J. ANTAL, RAYMOND J. TOWNSEND, AND ROBIN WAGNER

Abstract: Penetration of clindamycin into surgical wounds was studied in 10 patients undergoing radical head and neck surgery.

Patients received one preoperative and three postoperative intravenous doses of clindamycin 600 mg. During surgery, samples of plasma and sternocleidomastoid muscle were obtained. Additional plasma samples were collected just before the fourth dose of clindamycin, just after that dose was infused, and 1, 2, 4, 6, 8, and 12 hours after dosing. Samples of wound exudate were collected at 2, 4, 6, 8, and 12 hours after the fourth dose. The muscle, plasma, and wound exudate samples were assayed for clindamycin base by a gas–liquid chromatographic method. Plasma and wound exudate samples obtained during surgery and one and eight hours after the fourth dose were assayed by a radial immunodiffusion technique for content of α_1-acid glycoprotein (AAG), the major binding protein for clindamycin. Pharmacokinetic values for plasma and wound drainage were calculated and compared.

Concentrations of clindamycin in muscle (three to six hours after the first dose) ranged from 0.6 to 5.1 µg/g; the ratio of tissue to plasma concentrations ranged from 0.24 to 0.82. The highest mean clindamycin concentration in wound drainage was 4.9 µg/mL after the fourth dose, approximately 90% of simultaneous plasma concentrations. Concentrations in wound exudate exceeded those measured in plasma four hours after the dose, and elimination from the wound was slower than from plasma. AAG concentrations in plasma increased from a mean of 89 mg/dL intraoperatively to 134 mg/dL postoperatively. AAG was present in wound exudate in concentrations that were approximately 53% of those observed in plasma.

In the dosage studied, clindamycin penetrates muscle tissue and wound exudate in concentrations that are inhibitory to oropharyngeal organisms, and drug concentrations persist longer in wound exudate than in plasma; these results support the use of clindamycin for antimicrobial prophylaxis in head and neck surgery.

Index terms: Antibiotics; Blood levels; Clindamycin; Drugs, body distribution; Excretion; Minimum inhibitory concentration; Pharmacokinetics; Tissue levels
Clin Pharm. 1988; 7:820–4

Postoperative wound infections occur in approximately three-fourths of patients who undergo radical neck surgery without the benefit of perioperative antimicrobial agents.[1] Cultures of the postoperative wounds after head and neck surgery generally show mixed flora, which may include gram-positive cocci, aerobic gram-negative rods, and anaerobic bacteria. The major pathogens appear to be the anaerobic microflora of the oropharynx.[2] The optimal prophylactic antimicrobial agent for radical neck surgery should provide coverage against streptococci, staphylococci, and those anaerobes colonizing the oropharynx. Clindamycin's antimicrobial spectrum includes these organisms, but because approximately 94% of the drug is bound to serum proteins[3] and because protein binding has been demonstrated to inhibit the penetration of some antimicrobial agents into tissue,[4]

GARY P. STOEHR, PHARM.D., is Associate Professor of Pharmacy Practice, Department of Pharmacy Practice, VICTOR L. YU, M.D., is Professor of Medicine, Department of Medicine, and JONAS T. JOHNSON, M.D., is Professor of Surgery, Department of Otolaryngology, University of Pittsburgh, Pittsburgh, PA. EDWARD J. ANTAL, PH.D., and RAYMOND J. TOWNSEND, PHARM.D., are Research Scientists, The Upjohn Company, Kalamazoo, MI. ROBIN WAGNER is Research Associate, Department of Otolaryngology, University of Pittsburgh.

Address reprint requests to Dr. Yu at the Department of Medicine, University of Pittsburgh, Scaife Hall 968, Pittsburgh, PA 15261.

Supported in part by a grant from The Upjohn Company, Kalamazoo, MI.

Copyright © 1988, American Society of Hospital Pharmacists, Inc. All rights reserved. 0278-2677/88/1101-0820$01.25.

clindamycin may appear to be a suboptimal candidate for effective antimicrobial prophylaxis.

There are few data that describe the penetration of clindamycin into surgical wounds, although Bagley et al.[5] reported that clindamycin penetrated wound fluid in patients undergoing regional lymph node dissection for treatment of a malignant tumor. Therefore, we conducted a pharmacokinetic study in patients who received clindamycin prophylaxis for oncologic head and neck surgery. The objective was to determine whether clindamycin enters muscle tissue and surgical wounds in concentrations that are inhibitory for bacterial pathogens that might cause postoperative infections. Because clindamycin is primarily bound to the acute-phase-reactant protein α_1-acid glycoprotein (AAG),[6] we were also interested in determining whether AAG is present in wound exudate and whether there is any correlation between the concentrations of AAG in plasma and wound.

Methods

The study protocol was approved by the review board of the University of Pittsburgh, and written informed consent was obtained from each patient before entry into the study. Hospitalized adult patients admitted to the oncology service of Eye and Ear Hospital of Pittsburgh for radical neck surgery were screened to determine their eligibility for entry into the study. Patients with Laënnec's cirrhosis confirmed by biopsy or with elevations of serum aminotransferases to greater than twice normal were ineligible for study. Patients with serum creatinine concentrations exceeding 2.0 mg/dL were also ineligible for the study.

Patients received 600-mg intravenous doses of clindamycin (as the phosphate salt, Cleocin Phosphate, The Upjohn Company), infused by gravity over 30–45 minutes every eight hours. The first dose was given on call to surgery, at least two hours before the beginning of the procedure. Three subsequent doses were administered every eight hours.

During the operation, simultaneous plasma and tissue samples (approximately 0.5-g sample of sternocleidomastoid muscle) were obtained. At the time of wound closure, at least one continuous-drainage catheter was placed in the deep compartment of the wound; the drains were connected to a continuous-suction reservoir device (Hemovac, Zimmer USA).

Blood samples were collected in heparin-treated tubes from an indwelling catheter, according to the following schedule: just before the fourth and final dose of clindamycin was infused, just after the dose was infused, and 1, 2, 4, 6, 8, and 12 hours after dosing. Care was taken to prevent contact between the blood and the collection tube stopper. All blood samples were immediately centrifuged, and the plasma was separated and stored at −25 °C until the time of assay.

Wound drainage was obtained by manual aspiration of the indwelling wound catheter after momentary disconnection from the suction apparatus at 2, 4, 6, 8, and 12 hours after the last clindamycin dose. Tissue and wound drainage samples were stored at −25 °C until the time of assay.

Before analysis, tissue was rinsed in 0.9% sodium chloride solution and then blotted dry to remove blood. The samples were weighed, minced, suspended in measured amounts of distilled water, and homogenized in a Polytron tissue homogenizer at 1200 rpm. Tissue, plasma, and wound drainage samples were assayed for clindamycin base, using a gas–liquid chromatographic (GLC) method with electron capture detection. The method involves an organic extraction of the sample with ethyl acetate, followed by liquid–liquid partitioning with 0.1 N hydrochloric acid and chloroform and final derivatization with heptafluorobutyric anhydride. Samples were injected onto the column, using nitrogen and helium as the carrier gases at flow rates of 35 mL/min and 2 mL/min, respectively. The limit of detection for clindamycin was 10 ng/mL, and the maximum coefficient of variation was 6.03% over the range 50 to 500 ng/mL (Unpublished data. Kaiser FE, Lednicer D, Analytical Biochemistry Laboratories, Columbia, MO, and Knuth DW, The Upjohn Company, Kalamazoo, MI). Samples were diluted with Millipore-purified deionized water to bring drug concentrations within the 20–500 ng/mL range.

Plasma samples were obtained during surgery and one and eight hours after the fourth dose of clindamycin, and wound drainage was collected two hours after the fourth dose; these samples were assayed for AAG content using a radial immunodiffusion assay technique (ICL Scientific, Fountain Valley, CA),[7] which has a coefficient of variation of less than 10% in the range of 15 to 180 mg/dL. Samples with AAG concentrations greater than 150 mg/dL were diluted 1:1 with 0.9% sodium chloride solution, and the assay was repeated.

The elimination rate constant (k) for plasma was calculated by least-squares linear regression of data points in the terminal linear phase of the log plasma concentration-versus-time curve; k was calculated in the same manner for the wound drainage. After the fourth dose, the steady-state areas under the plasma and wound drainage concentration–time curves from zero to eight hours (AUC) were determined by the trapezoidal method. Clearance (CL) was calculated by dividing the dose by the steady-state AUC and normalized using actual body weight. The elimination half-life ($t\,{}^{1}\!/_{2}$) was calculated by dividing 0.693 by k. Apparent volume of distribution (V) was calculated from the equation $V = CL/k$.[8] Differences between plasma and wound-exudate values were analyzed using a

Student's *t* test for paired data and a significance level of 0.05.

Results

Simultaneous serum and skeletal-muscle samples were obtained three to six hours after the first clindamycin dose during surgery in seven male and three female patients. Tissue concentrations of clindamycin ranged from 0.6 to 5.1 μg/g, and the ratio of tissue to plasma concentrations varied from 0.24 to 0.82 over the interval (Table 1).

The ages and weights of the patients and the individual and mean calculated pharmacokinetic values for clindamycin are given in Table 2. Figure 1 shows the mean clindamycin concentrations in both plasma and wound fluid after the fourth dose.

Table 1.
Clindamycin Concentrations in Muscle and Plasma after a Single 600-mg Dose of Clindamycin Phosphate

Patient	Time (hr) after Dose	Plasma Concentration (μg/mL)	Tissue Concentration (μg/g)	Tissue: Plasma Ratio
1	3	6.5	5.1	0.78
7	3	6.8	1.9	0.28
2	4	2.2	1.3	0.59
4	4	2.5	0.9	0.34
8	4	6.3	4.3	0.68
9	4	7.0	1.7	0.24
3	5	2.3	1.9	0.82
6	5	2.9	1.5	0.52
10	5	2.3	0.6	0.24
5	6	5.2	4.0	0.76

Wound concentrations were equal to or greater than plasma concentrations after four hours in 7 of 10 patients. The mean plasma clindamycin concentration at the end of the infusion was 25.8 μg/mL (range, 11.4 to 74.9 μg/mL). The highest observed wound concentrations ranged from 4.0 to 7.5 μg/

Figure 1. Mean ± S.D. clindamycin concentrations in plasma (O—O) and wound exudate (□—□) at steady state.

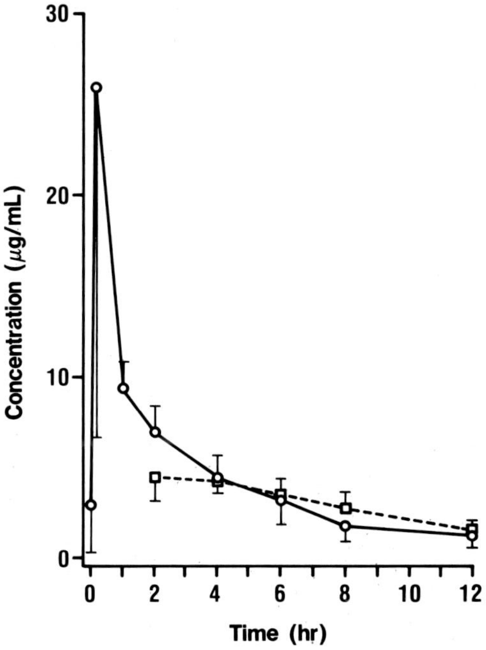

Table 2.
Patient Characteristics and Clindamycin Pharmacokinetic Data for Plasma and Wound Fluid[a,b]

Patient (Sex, Age)	Wt (kg)	Plasma Conc[c]	Plasma AUC_{0-8}	Plasma *k*	Plasma $t_{1/2}$	Plasma *V*	Plasma CL	Plasma AUC_{4-12}	Wound Conc[d]	Wound *k*	Wound $t_{1/2}$	Wound AUC_{4-12}	Wound:Plasma Ratio For AUC_{4-12}	Wound:Plasma Ratio For Conc[e]
1 (M, 64)	63.2	13.4	42.70	0.17	4.1	1.3	3.7	16.0	7.5	0.14	4.8	20.5	1.3	1.12
2 (F, 49)	75.0	44.2	58.30	0.20	3.4	0.7	2.3	14.0	5.3	0.19	3.7	18.9	1.4	0.68
3 (F, 61)	73.6	11.4	30.10	0.32	2.2	0.9	4.5	6.3	4.2	0.15	4.6	20.8	3.3	0.72
4 (M, 75)	60.0	15.4	31.30	0.16	4.3	2.0	5.3	10.9	4.5	0.16	4.2	17.0	1.6	1.05
5 (M, 75)	60.5	21.1	54.40	0.11	6.1	1.6	3.0	30.1	4.1	0.14	5.0	23.8	0.8	0.76
6 (M, 49)	65.9	23.4	43.50	0.21	3.3	1.0	3.5	15.3	4.5	0.19	3.6	18.4	1.2	1.15
7 (F, 64)	42.7	74.9	77.40	0.24	2.9	0.8	3.0	15.9	4.8	0.11	6.6	28.4	1.8	1.00
8 (M, 77)	62.7	16.2	49.50	0.15	4.6	1.3	3.2	19.9	4.0	0.09	8.0	24.3	1.2	0.95
9 (M, 59)	65.0	16.7	60.60	0.13	5.5	1.2	2.5	34.0	5.6	0.12	5.8	35.9	1.1	0.62
10 (M, 77)	79.5	21.6	48.80	0.19	3.6	0.8	2.6	22.0	4.3	0.17	4.0	25.4	1.2	0.86
Mean ±		25.8	49.66	0.19	4.0	1.1	3.4	18.44	4.9	0.15[f]	5.0	23.3[g]	1.47	0.89
S.D.		18.5	13.39	0.06	1.1	0.4	0.9	7.99	1.0	0.03	1.3	5.4	0.66	0.19

[a] Values were determined after fourth dose of clindamycin phosphate.

[b] Conc = concentration (μg/mL); AUC_{0-8} = area under the concentration–time curve from time zero to eight hours (μg · hr/mL); *k* = elimination rate constant (hr^{-1}); $t_{1/2}$ = half-life (hr); *V* = volume of distribution (L/kg); CL = clearance (mL/min/kg); AUC_{4-12} = AUC from four hours to eight hours (μg · hr/mL).

[c] Measured at the end of a 30- to 45-minute i.v. infusion of clindamycin phosphate.

[d] Highest measured concentration of clindamycin in wound fluid.

[e] Ratio of maximum clindamycin concentration in wound fluid to simultaneous plasma clindamycin concentration.

[f] Significantly different from plasma *k* ($p < 0.05$).

[g] Significantly different from plasma AUC ($p < 0.0125$).

mL (mean ± S.D., 4.9 ± 1.0 μg/mL) and the ratio of wound to plasma concentrations determined for these times was between 0.62 and 1.15 (mean ± S.D., 0.89 ± 0.19).

Elimination from wound fluid was somewhat slower than elimination from plasma ($p < 0.05$), and the mean concentration of clindamycin in the wound was 1.53 μg/mL (range, 0.95 to 2.7 μg/mL) at 12 hours, a concentration that was above the MIC for 90% of susceptible organisms (MIC_{90}).

AAG concentrations were measured in plasma during and after surgery and in wound fluid (Table 3). Plasma AAG concentrations increased significantly after surgery, from a mean intraoperative concentration of 89.0 ± 28.9 mg/dL to 134.3 ± 39.5 mg/dL eight hours after the fourth dose ($p < 0.05$). The values of AAG in plasma averaged twice those observed in wound fluid.

Table 3.
Alpha$_1$-Acid Glycoprotein (AAG) Concentrations

Patient	Plasma Concentrations (mg/dL) Intra-operative	Post-operative 1 hr Postdose[a]	Post-operative 8 hr Postdose[a]	Wound Conc 2 hr Postdose[a] (mg/dL)	Wound: Plasma Ratio[b]
1	62.7	94.6	108.0	55.4	0.58
2	78.1	126.0	141.0	98.9	0.78
3	38.4	108.0	112.0	38.4	0.35
4	62.7	90.4	86.2	45.0	0.50
5	98.9	126.0	146.0	48.4	0.38
6	112.0	156.2	141.0	62.7	0.40
7	126.0	172.4	224.0	103.0	0.60
8	98.9	156.2	148.4	59.0	0.38
9	126.0	148.4	146.0	108.0	0.73
10	86.2	86.2	90.4	51.9	0.60
Mean ±	89.0	126.4	134.3[c]	67.1	.53
S.D.	28.9	31.0	39.5	26.0	.15

[a] Time postdose = time after fourth dose of clindamycin.
[b] Ratio of wound AAG concentration, obtained two hours after the fourth dose of clindamycin, to plasma AAG concentration, obtained one hour after the same dose.
[c] Significantly greater than intraoperative concentration ($p < 0.05$).

Figure 2. Plasma versus wound clindamycin concentrations 4 to 12 hours after a steady-state dose ($n = 39$); $y = 0.7x + 1.2$; $r = 0.88$; $p < 0.005$.

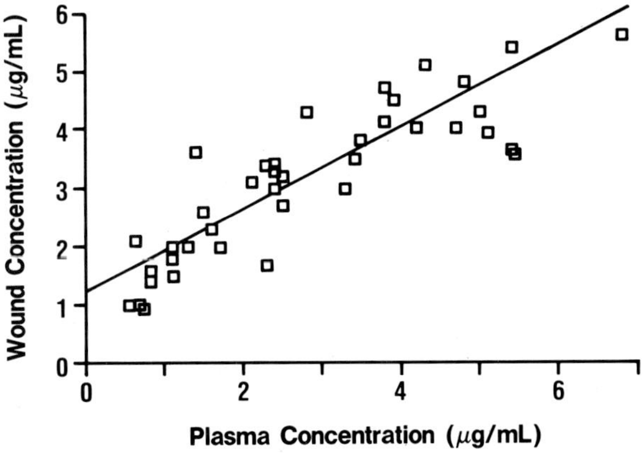

Discussion

To be effective when used prophylactically, antimicrobial agents must be active against the major pathogens responsible for postoperative infections and must be present in the wound in adequate concentrations throughout the surgical procedure, beginning with the time of incision.[9-11] Therefore, the concentrations achievable at the potential site of infection and the rate of appearance and disappearance of the drug in the wound are key factors in the selection of an appropriate prophylactic antimicrobial agent.

For gram-positive aerobic cocci and anaerobic oropharyngeal flora considered susceptible to clindamycin, the MIC_{90} is less than 0.8 μg/mL.[12] The results of this study demonstrate that clindamycin reaches concentrations in muscle tissue that exceed the MIC_{90} for the bacterial pathogens associated with postoperative infections in patients undergoing radical neck surgery. We could not measure serial muscle concentrations in order to determine the rate at which clindamycin enters muscle tissue, but it is likely that clindamycin muscle concentrations may have been higher earlier in the postinfusion period. A previous study of three patients given clindamycin before debridement of decubitus ulcers reported concentrations ranging from undetectable to 14.5 μg/g 45 to 60 minutes after a single 600-mg intravenous dose.[13]

Clindamycin concentrations measured in muscle tissue at the time of surgery, three to six hours after the dose, averaged only 52% of simultaneous plasma concentrations. There are several explanations for this observation. First, we measured muscle concentrations after only one dose, before the drug could reach steady state. We would expect muscle concentrations to increase as the drug accumulates in plasma and tissue with successive doses. Second, and most important, muscle concentrations may underestimate the concentration achieved in the interstitial compartment because antimicrobial agents are not uniformly distributed throughout intracellular and extracellular compartments.[14,15]

Since postoperative infections often originate in the wound, the concentrations of clindamycin in surgical wound exudate are clinically relevant. In this study there was a significant relationship between the concentrations of clindamycin in plasma and wound exudate ($p < 0.005$, Figure 2) for values measured from 4 to 12 hours after a steady-state dose. The correlation of clindamycin concentrations in wound fluid and plasma suggests that an increase in plasma clindamycin concentration is associated with an increase in wound exudate concentration. One would therefore expect that an increase in dose would result in a proportional increase in wound exudate concentration. Elimination of the drug from the wound was somewhat slower than from plasma, and the area under the wound fluid concentration–time curve from 4 to 12 hours was greater than the corresponding area under the plasma concentration–time curve. Coupled with the fact that clindamycin concentrations in wound exudate were still above the MIC_{90} for oropharyngeal organisms in all patients 12 hours after the fourth dose (mean concentration 1.56 μg/mL, range 0.95 to 2.7 μg/mL), these findings suggest that a higher dose administered every 12 hours should be feasible for prophylactic use in these patients. Such a regimen has the added benefit of cost savings. Future prospective studies are needed to confirm this hypothesis.

We measured AAG concentrations in both plasma and wound fluid. AAG is a major plasma binding protein for basic drugs including clindamycin,[6] and its concentration is increased by a number of pathophysiologic events such as myocardial infarction, trauma, and surgery, as well as diseases such as chronic renal failure and malignancy.[16] Increases in AAG have been postulated to affect the pharmacokinetics of several highly bound drugs.[17]

Intraoperative plasma AAG concentrations were within the normal range of 50 to 100 mg/dL in 8 of 10 patients, despite the diagnoses of malignancy in all of the patients. After surgery, AAG concentrations increased in all patients from a mean concentration of 89.0 mg/dL to a mean concentration of 134.3 mg/dL. AAG was present in wound exudate in concentrations that averaged 53% of those in plasma. It is unlikely that AAG concentrations of this magnitude are due to blood contamination of the wound exudate samples, since previous studies using similar methods have reported hematocrits in wound drainage that were less than 5%.[5,14] Thus, the presence of AAG in wound exudate would tend to increase drug movement into tissues and might provide a plausible explanation for the wound exudate penetration of clindamycin. Unbound drug that does reach interstitial fluid may bind to interstitial fluid proteins (including AAG), bind to cell membranes, or pass along the cell membrane, where it may come in contact with additional binding substances.[18] Thus, the presence of AAG in the wound could substantially modulate the effect of increased serum protein binding on clearance that might occur postoperatively. Future studies in which the free and unbound concentrations of clindamycin in plasma and wound exudate would be determined might clarify the role of AAG in clindamycin tissue penetration.

Conclusion

The results of our study support the use of clindamycin for antimicrobial prophylaxis in head and neck surgery. In the dosage studied, clindamycin penetrates muscle tissue and wound exudate in concentrations that are inhibitory to oropharyngeal organisms, and drug concentrations persist longer in wound exudate than in plasma.

References

1. Johnson JT, Yu VL, Myers EN et al. Efficacy of two third-generation cephalosporins in prophylaxis for head and neck surgery. *Arch Otolaryngol.* 1984; 110:224–7.
2. Johnson JT, Yu VL, Myers EN et al. An assessment of the need for gram-negative bacterial coverage in antibiotic prophylaxis for oncological head and neck surgery. *J Infect Dis.* 1987; 155:331–3.
3. Gordon RC, Regamey C, Kirby WMM. Serum protein binding of erythromycin, lincomycin, and clindamycin. *J Pharm Sci.* 1973; 62:1074–7.
4. Bergan T. Pharmacokinetics of tissue penetrations of antibiotics. *Rev Infect Dis.* 1981; 3:45–66.
5. Bagley DH, MacLowry J, Beazley RM et al. Antibiotic concentration in human wound fluid after intravenous administration. *Ann Surg.* 1978; 188:202–8.
6. Craig WA, Suh B, Gerber A. Enhanced protein binding of clindamycin in uremic sera: relationship to alpha 1-acid glycoprotein levels. Paper presented to 21st Interscience Conference on Antimicrobial Agents and Chemotherapy, Chicago, IL: 1981 Nov 4.
7. Mancini G, Carbonara AO, Heremans JF. Immunochemical quantitation of antigens by single radial immunodiffusion. *Immunochemistry.* 1965; 2:235–54.
8. Gibaldi M, Perrier D. Pharmacokinetics. New York: Marcel Dekker, Inc.; 1982.
9. Burke JF. The effective period of preventive antibiotic action in experimental incisions and dermal lesions. *Surgery.* 1961; 50:161–8.
10. Burke JF. Preventing bacterial infection by coordinating antibiotic and host activity: a time-dependent relationship. *South Med J.* 1977; 70 (Suppl):24–6.
11. Alexander J. Prophylaxis of experimental wound infections. *Surg Gynecol Obstet.* 1965; 120:243–8.
12. LeFrock JL, Molavi A, Prince RA. Clindamycin. *Med Clin North Am.* 1982; 66:103–20.
13. Berger SA, Barza M, Haher J et al. Penetration of clindamycin into decubitus ulcers. *Antimicrob Agents Chemother.* 1978; 14:498–9.
14. Muder RR, Yu VL, Johnson J et al. Penetration of cefoperazone into surgical wound drainage in patients undergoing head and neck surgery. *Antimicrob Agents Chemother.* 1984; 25:473–5.
15. Ryan DM, Cars O. Antibiotic assays in muscle: are conventional tissue levels misleading as indicators of the antibacterial activity? *Scand J Infect Dis.* 1980; 12:307–9.
16. Piafsky KM. Disease-induced changes in the plasma binding of basic drugs. *Clin Pharmacokinet.* 1980; 5:246–62.
17. Edwards DJ, Lalka D, Cerra F et al. Alpha-1-acid-glycoprotein concentration and protein binding in trauma. *Clin Pharmacol Ther.* 1982; 31:62–7.
18. Craig WA, Welling PG. Protein binding of antimicrobials: clinical pharmacokinetic and therapeutic implications. *Clin Pharmacokinet.* 1977; 2:252–68.

Lack of endogenous crossreactivity with three digitoxin radioimmunoassays in adults with renal insufficiency

Bruce A. Mueller, Henry I. Bussey, Daniel T. Casto, N. Kathryn Lowder, Nancy J. Sugarek, and Karl F. Cremer

Abstract: The possibility of interference by apparent digitoxin-like immunoreactive substance (DTLIS) with three radioimmunoassays was studied in patients with renal insufficiency.

From each of 25 adult patients with renal insufficiency and 25 age-matched and sex-matched control subjects with normal renal function, a single serum sample was obtained and assayed for digitoxin content by three commercially available radioimmunoassays (GammaCoat, Coat-A-Count, and the Wien assay).

Although two of the three assays found measurable concentrations, the difference in apparent digitoxin concentrations between the control subjects and those with renal insufficiency was not significant. Assay interference could not be explained on the basis of differences in age, serum creatinine concentration, or weight.

The magnitude of DTLIS interference in relation to the digitoxin therapeutic range appears to be small with the radioimmunoassays used in this study.

Index terms: Blood levels; Cardiac drugs; Digitoxin; Kidney failure; Radioimmunoassay; Sex; Tests, laboratory; Weight
Clin Pharm. 1988; 7:825–8

The utility of serum digoxin concentrations in monitoring digoxin therapy has been questioned, especially in patient populations in which assay interference is common. Digoxin-like immunoreactive substance (DLIS), an endogenous substance that is responsible for falsely high results with many of the commonly used immunoassays for digoxin, has been found in patients with renal failure.[1–8] The presence of DLIS, as well as the pharmacokinetic differences between digoxin and digitoxin, have led some clinicians to advocate digitoxin as the preferred digitalis glycoside.[9,10] Whether a digitoxin-like immunoreactive substance (DTLIS) exists and complicates digitoxin therapy has not been studied adequately. If digitoxin therapy is considered, the possible presence and degree of DTLIS interference in various patient populations needs to be identified. The objective of this study was to determine whether three commercially available digitoxin radioimmunoassays would detect more apparent digitoxin in the serum of adults with renal insufficiency than in that of adults with normal renal function.

Methods

Patient Selection. Twenty-five adult patients with renal insufficiency (Group A) and 25 age-matched and sex-matched individuals with normal renal function (Group B) were recruited during their routine clinic visits. Participants were excluded if they were pregnant or had clinically important liver disease or chronic atrial fibrillation, since digoxin-like immunoreactive substance has been reported in these populations. We wanted to eliminate these potentially complicating factors, despite the fact that we did not know whether digoxin-like immunoreactive substance would significantly interfere with the three digitoxin radioimmunoassays that we evaluated. Subjects also were excluded if they were undergoing hemodialysis or peritoneal dialysis, had been treated with a digitalis glycoside within 30 days of the study, or were being treated with any other drug known to interfere with the digitoxin assays (e.g., spironolactone, estrogens, progesterone, hydrocortisone). Inclusion in group A required a serum creatinine concentra-

Bruce A. Mueller, Pharm.D., is Assistant Professor of Clinical Pharmacy, Department of Pharmacy Practice, Purdue University, West Lafayette, IN. Henry I. Bussey, Pharm.D., is Assistant Professor, College of Pharmacy, The University of Texas at Austin, and Department of Pharmacology, The University of Texas Health Science Center at San Antonio (UTHSC). Daniel T. Casto, Pharm.D., is Assistant Professor, College of Pharmacy, The University of Texas at Austin, and Departments of Pharmacology and Pediatrics, UTHSC. N. Kathryn Lowder, Pharm.D., is Clinical Assistant Professor, College of Pharmacy, The University of Texas at Austin, and Department of Pharmacology, UTHSC. Nancy J. Sugarek, M.S.N., is Nurse Practitioner, Department of Medicine, UTHSC. Karl F. Cremer, Pharm.D., is Senior Clinical Studies Associate, IVAC Corporation, San Diego, CA.

Address reprint requests to Dr. Bussey at Clinical Pharmacy Programs, The University of Texas Health Science Center, 7703 Floyd Curl Drive, San Antonio, TX 78284-7765.

Presented in part at the Annual Meeting of the American College of Clinical Pharmacy, Philadelphia, PA, July 26, 1988.

Copyright © 1988, American Society of Hospital Pharmacists, Inc. All rights reserved. 0278-2677/88/1101-0825$01.00.

tion ≥ 2.0 mg/dL (177 μmol/L), whereas inclusion in group B required a serum creatinine concentration ≤ 1.5 mg/dL (133 μmol/L). This study was approved by the institutional review board, and all participants provided informed written consent.

Procedure. A single venous blood sample was obtained from each participant and placed in a red-topped, additive-free, silicone-coated collection tube. Samples were allowed to clot at room temperature and were then centrifuged. Two aliquots of each serum sample were then placed in plastic vials and frozen at −20 °C until the time of assay, approximately four months later. The three digitoxin radioimmunoassays used in this study were GammaCoat, lot 0932, manufactured by Dade (Cambridge, MA); Coat-A-Count, lot 171, manufactured by Diagnostic Products Corporation (Los Angeles, CA); and a digitoxin assay, lot 01537C, manufactured by Wien Laboratories (Succasunna, NJ). Coat-A-Count and GammaCoat are similar ^{125}I-based assays using tubes coated with digitoxin antibody, while the Wien assay is a ^{3}H-based assay involving a charcoal suspension step. All assays were performed in duplicate according to the manufacturers' specifications without modifications.

Samples from the Wien assay were analyzed on a Beckman beta counter (model LS 7500). A Packard Auto-Gamma Scintillation Spectrophotometer was used to analyze samples from the Coat-A-Count and GammaCoat assays. Coefficients of variation at a concentration of 10 ng/mL were less than 5% for each analytical kit. The lower concentration limit for acceptable assay performance, determined in our laboratory by measuring blank serum samples spiked with digitoxin, was 2.5 ng/mL for the Wien assay, 5.0 ng/mL for Coat-A-Count, and 7.5 ng/mL for GammaCoat.

Statistical Analysis. Differences in apparent serum digitoxin concentrations for each assay method and demographic factors between the two patient groups were compared by the Student's *t* test for unpaired data. For each assay, the number of patients in each group found to have a measurable apparent digitoxin concentration was assessed by chi-square analysis or Fisher's exact test (used when less than five subjects with measurable concentrations were noted). Within-group analysis of patient characteristics and clinical data for those subjects with measurable concentrations versus those without measurable concentrations was performed with the Student's *t* test for unpaired data. A p value ≤ 0.05 was considered significant.

Results

Profiles of the characteristics of the two patient groups are shown in Table 1. The two groups were well matched except for serum creatinine concentration. Table 2 lists the assay results for each subject in group A and each subject's age-matched and sex-matched counterpart in group B. All results are listed, regardless of whether they are below or above the lower limit for accurate measurement. Statistical analysis of the mean values was not performed, because many of the values fell below the lower concentration limit of the assay.

Table 1.
Study Patient Characteristics[a,b]

Age in Years	Weight in Kilograms	Serum Creatinine Concentration in mg/dL
Group A		
52.7 ± 17.2	73.8 ± 17.8	4.37 ± 2.0
(22–80)	(40.4–110)	(2.0–10.1)
Group B		
52.6 ± 17.2	80.7 ± 16.5	0.86 ± 0.21[c]
(21–80)	(44.9–108.6)	(0.4–1.3)

[a] Each group consisted of 16 women and 9 men.
[b] Expressed as mean ± S.D. (range).
[c] $p < 0.0005$.

The Coat-A-Count assay produced no values above the lower concentration limit (5.0 ng/mL) in either group A or group B. The GammaCoat assay yielded nine values in group B and eight values in group A above the lower concentration limit of 7.5 ng/mL. The difference between group A and group B was not significant. Results from the most sensitive assay, the Wien assay, yielded three subjects in group A but none in group B with concentration values above the lower limit of the assay (2.5 ng/mL). This difference, however, was not significant ($p = 0.11$, Fisher's exact test). An analysis of demographic factors of subjects who had measurable concentrations by the Wien assay versus those who did not have measurable concentrations by the Wien assay showed no significant differences with respect to age, serum creatinine concentration, gender, and weight.

Discussion

Evidence for the existence of DTLIS in the literature is scarce. Ebara et al.,[11] using an enzyme immunoassay, noted as much as 15 ng/mL of DTLIS in the cord blood of neonates born to mothers who were not receiving any digitalis glycoside. In a report by Bussey et al.,[12] the comparison of paired results from radioimmunoassay and fluorescence polarization digitoxin assays suggested the existence of DTLIS in a small subgroup of adults with renal insufficiency. The data from these two reports, however, provide very little information to confirm or refute the findings of this study, which failed to detect significant interference with three digitoxin assays in patients with renal insufficiency. Perhaps it is important to note that the most

Table 2.
Results of Three Digitoxin Assays[a]

Subject Pair	Apparent Digitoxin Concentration (ng/mL)					
	GammaCoat		Coat-A-Count		Wien Assay	
	Group A	Group B	Group A	Group B	Group A	Group B
1	4.2	9.2[b]	3.8	4.0	1.87	0
2	6.1	8.4[b]	3.6	3.5	0.44	0
3	6.4	6.3	3.7	3.1	3.05[b]	0
4	5.3	6.8	3.8	3.1	0.91	0
5	6.1	5.9	3.9	4.0	0.82	1.58
6	6.3	9.9[b]	3.7	3.1	1.34	0.99
7	7.2	7.3	3.5	3.1	0.83	1.59
8	5.9	6.6	3.6	3.1	2.33	1.26
9	5.7	6.4	3.4	3.2	0.74	1.41
10	7.9[b]	7.4	3.5	3.1	1.82	0.27
11	7.0	6.3	3.6	3.0	1.87	0.99
12	7.9[b]	8.0[b,c]	3.6	4.0	0.59	2.24
13	7.6[b]	6.5	3.4	3.9	2.07	0.68
14	7.0	N.D.[c]	3.4	3.1	1.61	0
15	5.6	9.1[b]	3.3	4.1	1.08	0.78
16	7.0	8.4[b]	3.4	3.1	1.53	0.54
17	5.7	5.4	4.1	3.0	0.82	1.40
18	7.8[b]	5.5	3.9	3.9	0.30	0
19	8.2[b]	7.4	4.3	3.2	0	0.58
20	6.1	6.7	4.3	3.9	2.88[b]	0
21	6.7	8.8[b]	4.2	3.2	1.47	1.21
22	7.5[b]	10.2[b]	N.D.	N.D.	N.D.	N.D.
23	7.5[b]	8.7[b]	4.2	N.D.	2.60[b]	0.72
24	6.9	6.2	4.1	3.1	0.13	0.98
25	7.7[b]	6.6	3.9	3.1	1.16	0.54
Mean ± S.D.	6.69 ± 0.97	7.72 ± 1.38	3.68 ± 0.31	3.38 ± 0.41	1.34 ± 0.85	0.74 ± 0.64

[a] Statistical analysis of means was not performed because of assay limitations.
[b] Value is above the lower concentration limit for acceptable assay performance (7.5 ng/mL, GammaCoat; 2.5 ng/mL, Wien assay).
[c] N.D. = not determined.

sensitive assay, the Wien assay, did detect apparent digitoxin serum concentrations in three subjects with renal insufficiency but none in individuals with normal renal function. Although these data failed to document the existence of DTLIS in patients with renal insufficiency, the possibility exists that the sample size was too small or that the assay sensitivity was too low to confirm the existence of DTLIS. The fact that the Wien assay did note some assay interference in group A and not in group B patients supports the latter possibility. The poorer sensitivity of the Coat-A-Count and GammaCoat assays may have precluded the detection of a small amount of DTLIS with these two assays.

GammaCoat assay yielded measurable concentrations in 8 of 25 group A patients and 9 of 25 group B subjects. Although the manufacturer[13] states that the lower concentration limit of this assay is 4.1 ng/mL, in our laboratory this limit was substantially higher (7.5 ng/mL). Although it is possible that DTLIS was actually present in large amounts in both groups A and B, it is likely that the concentrations we identified as apparent digitoxin concentrations were an extension of this assay's poor sensitivity. We have reported data from GammaCoat not because we think we found DTLIS with this assay, but because this assay did not yield credible results at lower concentrations. Laboratories that use GammaCoat should be aware that it may yield inaccurately high results in patients who are not compliant with their digitoxin regimen.

If DTLIS exists, the magnitude of assay interference becomes a clinically important question. A concentration of 3.05 ng/mL was the highest concentration detected by the most sensitive assay, the Wien assay. This is a small degree of interference relative to the therapeutic range of digitoxin (10–35 ng/mL) and is probably not clinically important. By contrast, with digoxin therapy, DLIS interference with digoxin assays can yield values within the therapeutic range of digoxin (0.8–2.0 ng/mL). If the small degree of assay interference remains unchanged with concomitant administration of digitoxin, DTLIS would be a relatively minor concern with digitoxin therapy. Such minimal assay interference is a theoretical advantage of digitoxin over digoxin and would support the contention that digitoxin is the preferred digitalis glycoside. The question of DTLIS interference in patients taking digitoxin, however, remains to be investigated. If DTLIS does exist, the degree to which it interacts with various types of assays, and the extent to which it occurs in various patient populations, are questions that warrant further assessment.

Conclusion

This study of possible DTLIS interference with three digitoxin radioimmunoassays failed to prove the existence of a crossreactive substance in serum from patients with renal insufficiency. The question of DTLIS interference with digitoxin assays should be evaluated further using various assays and other patient populations, including patients receiving digitoxin.

References

1. Graves SW, Brown B, Valdes R. An endogenous digoxin-like substance in patients with renal impairment. *Ann Intern Med*. 1983; 99:604–8.
2. Craver JL, Valdes R. Anomalous serum digoxin concentrations in uremia. *Ann Intern Med*. 1983; 98:483–4.
3. Kramer HJ, Pennig J, Klingmuller D et al. Digoxin-like immunoreacting substance(s) in the serum of patients with chronic uremia. *Nephron*. 1985; 40:297–302.
4. Oldfield PR, Singer BE, Tosel PA. Digoxin determination in the uremic patient: three immunoassays compared. *Clin Chem*. 1985; 31:1246. Letter.
5. Heazlewood VJ, Heazlewood RL, Jellett LB. An endogenous digoxin-like substance and renal failure. *Ann Intern Med*. 1984; 100:618. Letter.
6. Pleasants RA, Gadsen RH, McCormack JP et al. Interference of digoxin-like immunoreactive substances with three digoxin immunoassays in patients with various degrees of renal function. *Clin Pharm*. 1986; 5:810–6.
7. Witherspoon L, Shuler S, Alyea K et al. Digoxin-like substance in term pregnancy, newborns, and renal failure. *J Nucl Med*. 1986; 27:1418–22.
8. Yatscoff RW, Desjardina PRE, Dalton JG. Digoxin-like immunoreactivity in the serum of neonates and uremic patients, as measured in the Abbott TDx. *Clin Chem*. 1984; 30:588. Letter.
9. Storstein O, Hansteen V, Hatle L et al. Studies on digitalis. XIII. A prospective study of 649 patients on maintenance treatment with digitoxin. *Am Heart J*. 1977; 93:434–43.
10. Lukas DS. Of toads and flowers. *Circulation*. 1972; 46:1–4.
11. Ebara H, Suzuki S, Nagashima K et al. Digoxin- and digitoxin-like immunoreactive substances in amniotic fluid, cord blood, and serum of neonates. *Pediatr Res*. 1986; 20:28–31.
12. Bussey HI, Watson WA, Hawkins DW et al. Practical value of a new serum digitoxin assay. *Ther Drug Monit*. 1986; 8:90–4.
13. Baxter Travenol Diagnostics, Inc. GammaCoat (^{125}I) Digitoxin Radioimmunoassay Kit (CA-525) product information. Cambridge, MA; 1986 Jul.

Research Notes

Effect of influenza vaccine on serum concentrations of total and free phenytoin

Christopher D. Smith, Michael A. Bledsoe, Roger Curran, Lawrence Green, and Jack Lewis

Clin Pharm. 1988; 7:828–32

The Centers for Disease Control currently recommend annual vaccination of high-risk groups against influenza.[1] Residents of long-term-care facilities, such as nursing homes or facilities for the developmentally disabled, are among these groups. In addition to being at high risk of developing influenza, these residents, by virtue of the large number of maintenance medications required, are at risk of developing drug toxicities.

There are reports in the literature of influenza vaccine causing transient increases in serum theophylline concentrations.[2,3] The proposed mechanism by which the vaccine causes this elevation is suppression of the activity of the cytochrome P-450 system in the liver via interferon induction.[4,5] Many other medications are metabolized by cytochrome P-450 monooxygenase, including certain anticonvulsants.

Phenytoin, which is used in the treatment of generalized seizures and cardiac arrhythmias, is metabolized extensively by cytochrome P-450 monooxygenase.[6] Since influenza vaccines have been shown to depress cytochrome P-450 activity,[5] it would be reasonable to expect transient elevations in both total and free phenytoin concentrations after influenza vaccination. This idea is sup-

Christopher D. Smith is Clinical Staff Pharmacist, Department of Pharmacy Service, University Hospital, Seattle, WA. Michael A. Bledsoe, M.S., is Clinical Pharmacist, Department of Clinical Pharmacy; Roger Curran, M.D., is Neurologist; Lawrence Green, M.D., is Neurologist; and Jack Lewis, M.S., is Medical Director, Idaho State School and Hospital, Nampa.

Address reprint requests to Mr. Smith at the Department of Pharmacy Services, University Hospital, 1959 N.E. Pacific St., RC-32, Seattle, WA 98185.

The assistance of Patrick Gaffney, Ph.D., (statistical analysis and editorial assistance); Dan Fazzini, Ph.D.; Tom Harvey; and William Docktor, Pharm.D., and Sandra Jue, Pharm.D., (editorial assistance) is acknowledged.

Presented at the annual Western States Regional Preceptor/Resident Conference at Asilomar, Monterey, CA, April 27, 1987.

Copyright © 1988, American Society of Hospital Pharmacists, Inc. All rights reserved. 0278-2677/88/1101-0828$01.25.

ported by the findings of Jann and Fidone,[4] who concluded that total phenytoin concentrations significantly increased after influenza vaccination. Two other investigators studied this potential interaction; one found no significant change in total phenytoin concentrations,[7] and the other found a slight decrease in serum phenytoin concentrations after influenza vaccination.[8]

This study was designed to assess the effects of influenza vaccine on total and free phenytoin concentrations in an institutionalized, developmentally disabled population. The free phenytoin concentration is most indicative of both toxicity and therapeutic activity. No study to date has measured the effects of influenza vaccine on this concentration.

Methods. The case records at the Idaho State School and Hospital were reviewed to select a study group based on the following criteria: All participants were required to have been on their current medication regimen for at least eight weeks and had to be taking phenytoin sodium capsules (Dilantin, Parke-Davis) as monotherapy for seizure disorders, at clinically satisfactory concentrations, with stable seizure histories and normal aspartate aminotransferase (AST) values. Patients were excluded if they were taking other medications known definitely to interact with phenytoin,[9] if they had concurrent infections, or if they were known to be difficult blood donors because of either behavioral or physiological reasons. Out of a total of 75 patients receiving phenytoin, only eight patients qualified based on the above criteria.

Blood samples were drawn just before the morning dose, at approximately 0730, to determine trough concentrations. Participants fasted after midnight the day of blood sampling. The blood samples were drawn by the institution's medical technician and were immediately analyzed using fluorescence polarization immunoassay (TDx, Abbott Laboratories). The assay has a reported coefficient of variation of less than 5%. The lower limit of detection for total phenytoin determination is 0.5 mg/L; for free phenytoin, it is 0.02 mg/L.[10] The TDx analyzer used in this study is tested routinely by the College of American Pathologists and conforms to the coefficient of variation and lower limits of detection specified. Both total and free phenytoin concentrations were obtained from each blood sample.

Baseline data were obtained by taking two blood samples from each of the eight participants, separated by at least one week, before vaccination. All participants had been on their current dose of phenytoin for at least eight weeks, guaranteeing steady-state concentrations. No changes were made to participants' medication regimens during the study period, and acetaminophen was the only medication given as needed. Postvaccination blood samples were obtained on days 1, 2, 7, 14, and 30.

All participants received a single 0.5-mL intramuscular injection of influenza virus vaccine 1986–1987 trivalent types A and B (subvirion) containing hemagglutinin antigen of A/Chile/1/83, A/Mississippi/1/85, and B/Ann Arbor/1/86 (Wyeth Laboratories). Drug concentrations before vaccination were compared by two-way analysis of variance (ANOVA) without replication, equivalent to Student's t test for paired comparisons. Postvaccination values were compared with prevaccination mean values by use of a two-way ANOVA, using an experimentwise error rate of alpha = 0.05. This is an appropriate model for repeated testing of the same individuals.[11] Significance was defined as $p < 0.05$.

The study design was approved by the institution's human rights and advocacy committee. The institution's head administrator gave consent for each study participant, since all are wards of the state of Idaho.

Results. Table 1 summarizes the study participants' characteristics. The mean AST value was 21 U/L, with a range of 11 to 30 U/L. The mean serum albumin concentration was 4.5 g/dL, with a range of 4.3 to 4.7 g/dL. The mean age was 39 years, with

Table 1.
Study Population Characteristics

Subject No.	Serum Albumin Concentration (g/dL)	Serum AST Concentration (U/L)[a]	Age (yr)	Sex	Weight (kg)	Dose[b] (mg/kg/day)	Seizure Type[c]
1	4.7	25	25	M	83.3	4.8	II-6
2	4.5	27	33	M	75.5	5.3	II-6
3	4.5	23	46	M	71.7	6.0	IA-1i
4	4.6	11	29	M	48.8	4.1	II-6
5	4.5	30	60	F	40.0	7.5	II-6
6	4.3	13	17	M	44.8	6.7	II-6
7	4.6	11	40	M	55.3	4.7	II-6
8	4.3	29	59	F	58.8	5.1	II-6

[a] AST = aspartate aminotransferase.
[b] Phenytoin sodium capsules.
[c] International classification of epileptic seizures: II-6 = tonic–clonic seizures, IA-1i = partial seizures with focal motor symptoms.

a range of 17 to 60. Six male patients and two female patients participated in the study. The mean dose of phenytoin sodium was 5.5 mg/kg/day, with a range of 4.1 to 7.5. The characteristics of these participants closely reflected the institution's actual population, which has a mean age of 33 years and a male-to-female ratio of 3:2.

The total and free phenytoin concentrations and calculated free fractions are given in Table 2. A summary of the study means is given in Table 3. The two prevaccination readings for both total and free phenytoin concentrations were analyzed separately using a simple two-way ANOVA without replication, in this case equivalent to Student's t test for paired comparisons. Because both of the two prevaccination total phenytoin concentrations ($F = 0.43$; d.f. = 1, 7; $p > 0.05$) and the two prevaccination free phenytoin concentrations ($F = 1.07$; d.f. = 1, 7; $p > 0.05$ were found to be similar, the prevaccination baseline was defined as the mean of the first and second readings. The mean ± S.D. prevaccination total phenytoin concentration for the study population was 9.59 ± 2.21 mg/L.

Both total and free phenytoin concentrations changed significantly after vaccination. The mean ± S.D. total concentrations rose to 10.56 ± 2.40 mg/L by day 2, a significant ($p < 0.05$) change from baseline. Subsequently, total phenytoin concentrations dropped and remained at levels indistinguishable from prevaccination values. In contrast to total concentrations, free phenytoin concentrations decreased after vaccination, becoming significantly lower ($p < 0.05$) than prevaccination levels by day 14. On day 14, the mean free phenytoin concentration was 0.61 ± 0.19 mg/L (Table 3).

Analysis of the phenytoin free fraction (free concentration divided by total concentration) revealed significant reductions from baseline on days 2, 7, and 14 postvaccination. Table 3 summarizes these changes. The baseline free fraction (mean ± S.D.) was 0.084 ± 0.010 mg/L and reached a low of 0.064 ± 0.004 mg/L by day 14 postvaccination.

No changes in seizure frequency were seen during the study period. No participant suffered a seizure for at least eight weeks before the study, and no seizures were observed during the study. Based on medication administration records, no participant missed any dose of phenytoin during the study period. Acetaminophen was the only medication given as needed to the study participants, and no other changes in medication regimens were made during the study period.

Table 2.
Total Serum Phenytoin Concentrations, Serum Concentrations of Free Phenytoin, and Free Fractions

Subject No.	Variable[a]	Prevaccination[b] A	B	Mean	Postvaccination 1	2	7	14	30	Mean	C.V.[c]
1	T	11.6	11.8	11.7	11.0	12.1	12.1	11.9	12.1	11.8	4.0
	F	0.91	0.97	0.94	0.80	0.86	0.79	0.80	0.93	0.84	7.1
	FF	0.079	0.082	0.080	0.073	0.071	0.065	0.067	0.077	0.071	6.5
2	T	8.6	10.7	9.7	12.1	11.1	12.5	13.0	8.9	11.5	14.1
	F	0.79	0.83	0.81	0.91	0.83	0.93	0.79	0.60	0.81	16.2
	FF	0.092	0.078	0.084	0.075	0.075	0.074	0.061	0.067	0.071	9.0
3	T	7.5	9.4	8.45	10.9	10.7	7.6	9.4	11.7	10.1	16.0
	F	0.60	0.89	0.75	0.72	0.72	0.42	0.57	0.70	0.63	20.9
	FF	0.080	0.095	0.088	0.066	0.067	0.055	0.061	0.060	0.062	7.9
4	T	8.4	7.7	8.05	8.4	8.5	8.22	9.2	8.0	8.46	5.4
	F	0.87	0.65	0.76	0.58	0.63	0.55	0.60	0.60	0.59	5.0
	FF	0.104	0.084	0.094	0.069	0.074	0.067	0.065	0.075	0.070	6.2
5	T	7.8	8.3	8.05	8.1	8.4	7.1	7.8	8.2	7.92	6.4
	F	0.61	0.74	0.68	0.51	0.50	0.45	0.45	0.47	0.48	5.9
	FF	0.078	0.089	0.084	0.063	0.060	0.063	0.058	0.057	0.060	4.8
6	T	9.3	8.6	8.95	9.5	9.4	9.39	9.0	5.7	8.60	19.0
	F	0.69	0.69	0.69	0.64	0.63	0.60	0.58	0.40	0.57	17.2
	FF	0.074	0.080	0.077	0.067	0.067	0.064	0.064	0.070	0.067	3.8
7	T	13.5	14.5	14.0	15.5	15.5	14.6	12.2	13.5	14.26	9.9
	F	1.11	0.85	0.98	1.2	1.15	0.92	0.83	1.04	1.03	15.0
	FF	0.082	0.059	0.070	0.077	0.074	0.063	0.068	0.077	0.072	8.7
8	T	8.8	7.0	7.9	8.1	8.8	4.4	4.0	9.9	7.04	38.0
	F	0.79	0.63	0.71	0.69	0.69	0.40	0.27	0.70	0.55	36.7
	FF	0.090	0.090	0.090	0.085	0.078	0.091	0.068	0.071	0.079	12.4
Mean	T	9.4	9.8	9.6	10.5	10.6	9.5	9.6	9.8	10.0	
	F	0.80	0.78	0.79	0.76	0.75	0.63	0.61	0.68	0.69	
	FF	0.085	0.082	0.084	0.072	0.071	0.068	0.064	0.069	0.069	
C.V.	T	21.9	25.4	23.0	24.2	22.8	35.4	30.3	26.3	24.4	
	F	21.3	15.7	18.1	28.9	26.3	34.7	31.6	31.8	27.2	
	FF	11.4	13.4	12.1	10.0	8.4	15.7	6.0	10.8	8.5	

[a] T = total phenytoin concentration (mg/L), F = free phenytoin concentration (mg/L), FF = free fraction.
[b] A and B are values from two determinations.
[c] Coefficient of variation for postvaccination values.

Table 3.
Mean ± S.D. Total Serum Phenytoin Concentrations, Serum Concentrations of Free Phenytoin, and Free Fractions

Sample Time	Total Serum Phenytoin Concentration (mg/L)	F[a]	Serum Concentration of Free Phenytoin (mg/L)	F	Free Fraction	F
Baseline	9.59 ± 2.21	. . .	0.79 ± 0.14	. . .	0.084 ± 0.010	. . .
Day 1	10.45 ± 2.53	4.39	0.76 ± 0.22	0.44	0.072 ± 0.007	8.94
Day 2	10.56 ± 2.40	15.4[b]	0.75 ± 0.20	1.02	0.071 ± 0.006	15.5[b]
Day 7	9.49 ± 3.36	0.03	0.63 ± 0.22	9.13	0.068 ± 0.011	15.8[c]
Day 14	9.56 ± 2.90	0.001	0.61 ± 0.19	17.0[b]	0.064 ± 0.004	34.4[d]
Day 30	9.75 ± 2.56	0.053	0.68 ± 0.22	6.22	0.069 ± 0.006	10.9

[a] F-statistic (d.f. = 1, 7). Values on days 1, 2, 7, 14, and 30 were compared with prevaccination baseline value.
[b] $p < 0.05$.
[c] $p < 0.01$.
[d] $p < 0.001$.

Discussion. To date, there have been three published studies on the effects of influenza vaccine on total phenytoin concentrations. In 1979, Sawchuk and coworkers[8] published a study that revealed a significant reduction in total phenytoin concentrations. In 1984, Levine and Jones[7] published a study in which they found no significant change in phenytoin concentrations after influenza vaccination. However, they did see temporary increases of 46%–170% in four subjects, two of which could best be attributed to influenza vaccination. More recently, Jann and Fidone[4] observed a significant elevation in total phenytoin concentrations on day 7 postvaccination and concluded that interferon induction was the most likely explanation for this observation. Because of the small sample size, none of these studies can be viewed as conclusive.

Our study does not fully support the conclusion reached by Jann and Fidone. Although we did see a significant elevation in total phenytoin concentrations on day 2 postvaccination, this was not accompanied by a rise in concentrations of free phenytoin. If interferon induction caused substantial inhibition of cytochrome P-450 monooxygenase, both total and free phenytoin concentrations would be expected to rise. Thus, our results are unlikely to be due solely to interferon induction.

The reduction in free phenytoin concentrations was very unexpected. Because of the conservative statistical method used, only one postvaccination free phenytoin concentration was found to be significantly lower. The data, however, suggest a gradual and prolonged reduction of free phenytoin concentrations that begins almost immediately after vaccination.

Despite not seeing any changes in our study population's seizure frequency, we believe this finding has potential clinical importance. Our study group averaged less than one seizure annually before this study, so it is not surprising that a reduction in free phenytoin concentrations did not alter the seizure frequency in this group. However, if a more precarious seizure group had been studied, such as one requiring maximum doses of phenytoin or multiple drug therapy or both, an increase in seizure frequency as a result of lower free phenytoin concentrations would not be surprising. Clinicians should be aware of this potential and observe patients taking phenytoin carefully after vaccination against influenza. If an increased seizure frequency is observed, a determination of free phenytoin concentrations may be indicated. In this situation, the determination of total phenytoin concentrations alone may be misleading.

The interaction between phenytoin and the influenza vaccine is not easily explained and requires closer examination of phenytoin clearance and protein binding. Phenytoin clearance is mediated by both hepatic metabolism and renal elimination. More than 95% of phenytoin is metabolized by hepatic enzymes to various derivatives. Phenytoin is eliminated initially in the bile, and after enterohepatic circulation it is excreted in the urine. To assess the liver function of our study participants, we determined baseline AST values and performed additional measurements during the postvaccination period. No significant changes in AST values were observed, which indicates that liver function remained normal. The creatinine clearance was not determined; therefore, the possibility of altered renal elimination does exist. Changes in renal elimination, however, are unlikely to explain the observed study results because we did not observe a reduction in total phenytoin concentrations, which would be expected to accompany increased renal clearance.

Phenytoin is approximately 90% protein bound, primarily to albumin.[6,12] Changes in albumin concentrations, in particular hyperalbuminemia, could explain a reduction in free phenytoin concentrations. All prevaccination serum albumin concentrations were within normal limits (Table 1). Postvaccination albumin concentrations were not measured, so it is impossible to rule out changes in serum protein concentrations as an explanation for our findings.

Analysis of changes in phenytoin free fraction revealed significant reductions from baseline starting on day 2 postvaccination and continuing through day 14 of the study. This finding supports the idea that changes in serum protein concentrations are responsible for the reduced free phenytoin concentration. It is known that viral infections stimulate increased protein synthesis.[13] Immunization may also stimulate increased protein synthesis, which, in turn, may significantly increase serum protein concentrations. This would explain a reduction in free phenytoin concentrations without a reduction in total phenytoin concentrations. Studies examining changes in serum protein concentrations after vaccination are needed.

Another possible explanation is nonspecific induction of hepatic enzymes caused by increased protein synthesis. A study recently reported by Leppick et al.[14] looked at changes in total phenytoin concentrations in relation to febrile illness. They observed a significant reduction in total phenytoin concentrations associated with fever. They concluded that the most likely explanation was enzyme induction of the hepatic oxidative enzyme system.[14] Similarly, Sawchuk et al.[8] reported significant reductions in total phenytoin concentrations after vaccination with influenza vaccine. Unfortunately, this does not fit our findings, since we did not see significant reductions in total phenytoin concentrations and the phenytoin free fraction was significantly reduced after vaccination.

Conclusion. The initial, transient increase in total serum phenytoin concentrations that we found after influenza vaccination is probably not clinically important. Our study suggests that serum concentrations of free phenytoin are reduced after influenza vaccination and that this decrease is associated with a significant reduction in phenytoin free fraction. In those patients who exhibit increased seizures after vaccination, determination of free phenytoin concentrations may be indicated.

References

1. Centers for Disease Control. Prevention and control of influenza. *MMWR*. 1986; 35:317–23.
2. Meredith CG, Christian CD, Johnson RF et al. Effects of influenza virus vaccine on hepatic drug metabolism. *Clin Pharmacol Ther*. 1985; 37:396–401.
3. Renton KW, Gray JD, Hall RI. Decreased elimination of theophylline after influenza vaccination. *Can Med Assoc J*. 1980; 123:288–90.
4. Jann MW, Fidone GS. Effect of influenza vaccine on serum anticonvulsant concentrations. *Clin Pharm*. 1986; 5:817–20.
5. Kramer P, McClain CJ. Depression of aminopyrine metabolism by influenza vaccination. *N Engl J Med*. 1981; 305:1262–4.
6. Rall TW, Schleifer LS. Drugs used in the therapy of epilepsies. In: Gilman AG, Goodman LS, Rall TW et al., eds. The pharmacological basis of therapeutics. 7th ed. New York: Macmillan Publishing Company; 1985:446–72.
7. Levine M, Jones MW. Increased serum phenytoin concentrations following influenza vaccination. *Clin Pharm*. 1984; 3:505–9.
8. Sawchuk RJ, Rector TS, Fordice JJ et al. Effect of influenza vaccination on plasma phenytoin concentrations. *Ther Drug Monit*. 1979; 1:285–8.
9. Mangini RJ, ed. Drug interaction facts. St. Louis: Facts and Comparisons Division, J.B. Lippincott Company; 1986.
10. Abbott Laboratories Diagnostic Division. TDx systems assays manual. Irving, TX: Abbott Laboratories Diagnostics Division; 1985 Oct.
11. Sokal RR, Rohlf FJ. Biometry. 2nd ed. San Francisco: W.H. Freeman and Co.; 1981:232–71.
12. Woodbury DM. Phenytoin absorption, distribution, and excretion. In: Woodbury DM, Penry JK, Pippenger CE, eds. Antiepileptic drugs. New York: Raven Press; 1982:191–204.
13. Kits S. Viral associated and induced enzymes. *Pharmacol Ther*. 1979; 4:501–85.
14. Leppick IE, Fisher J, Kriel R et al. Altered phenytoin clearance with febrile illness. *Neurology*. 1986; 36:1367–70.

Efficacy of 0.9% sodium chloride injection with or without heparin sodium for maintaining patency of intravenous catheters in children

Thomas P. Lombardi, Berit Gundersen, Lorna O. Zammett, J. Ken Walters, and Barbara A. Morris

Clin Pharm. 1988; 7:832–6

Peripheral indwelling intravenous infusion devices (heparin locks) are often used for intermittent medication administration and blood sampling. Current standards of practice suggest that catheters should be flushed after every manipulation (i.e., medication administration or blood sampling) or at least once every eight hours to avoid clot formation in the catheter tip, catheter infiltration, or catheter-associated phlebitis.[1–5]

Heparin sodium 10 units/mL in 0.9% sodium chloride injection has been advocated as being safe and effective in maintaining the patency of such catheters and in decreasing the incidence of catheter-related phlebitis and irritation without causing unwanted anticoagulation.[1–3] This solution was used as the standard solution for flushing peripheral intravenous catheters at our institution. Higher concentrations of heparin sodium (100 units/mL) have also been used for maintaining patency of heparin locks.[4] Although this amount of heparin does not represent a substantial dosage in adults, it may have anticoagulant effects in infants or small children if used frequently.

The efficacy of such dilute solutions of heparin sodium (10 units/mL) suggests that 0.9% sodium chloride injection alone could be equally effective in maintaining catheter patency. Epperson[4] compared the efficacy of three different flushing solutions (heparin sodium 10 and 100 units/mL in 0.9% sodium chloride injection and 0.9% sodium chloride injection without heparin) in 412 adult medical and surgical patients. He found no significant differences among the three groups in rates of catheter-site loss attributable to phlebitis or any other cause. These results were confirmed by Hamilton et al.[5] in 241 adult patients. However, neither of these studies included pediatric patients.

The use of 0.9% sodium chloride injection alone, rather than heparin-containing solutions, has several potential advantages. The first is a reduction in the likelihood of medication-administration errors. The second is elimination of compatibility problems between heparin and other drugs administered through the indwelling device.[6] Third, minimizing exposure to heparin could reduce the likelihood of patients developing heparin-associated antiplatelet antibodies.[7] A last advantage would be decreased cost to the institution and the patient.

The primary goal of this study was to determine if 0.9% sodium chloride injection is as effective as heparin sodium 10 units/mL in 0.9% sodium chloride injection for maintaining patency of peripheral indwelling intravenous devices in pediatric patients. A secondary goal was to evaluate catheter patency at 48 and 72 hours by comparing sites flushed with the two study solutions. A third goal was to analyze the effect of medication administration on patency of catheters flushed with the two solutions.

Methods. Written informed consent was obtained from a parent or legal guardian before each patient's entry into the study. Oral assent was also sought from those children old enough to understand. The study was approved by the institutional review board.

The study was a nonrandomized, sequential, double-blind trial conducted on our 52-bed pediatric unit. Any patient on the pediatric unit who was between the ages of four weeks and 18 years and required a peripheral indwelling intravenous device was a candidate for the study. Patients were excluded if they were admitted to the pediatric intensive-care unit, neonatal intensive-care unit, or special-care nursery. Patients were enrolled in the study following a physician's order specifying "Heparin lock study solution as per protocol" and before placement of the catheter. All catheters were placed by trained personnel (i.v. therapists or pediatricians), according to hospital policy.

Two study solutions were used for flushing the peripheral indwelling intravenous devices: 0.9% sodium chloride injection 1 mL (solution A)[a] and heparin sodium 10 units in 0.9% sodium chloride injection 1 mL (solution B).[b] All study solutions were prepared in a laminar-airflow hood by a pharmacist using aseptic technique. Each dose was individually packaged in a 3-mL plastic syringe, given a seven-day expiration date,[8] labeled "Heparin Study Solution" (A or B), and stored on the nursing unit until used. Data were collected between April 15, 1986, and April 23, 1987. Study solutions were switched approximately every other month until all data were collected.

Each catheter was first flushed with 1 mL of 0.9% sodium chloride injection and then with 1 mL of study solution. This procedure was performed after each dose of intravenous medication administered through the catheter. Indwelling infusion devices not used for medication administration were flushed with study solution every eight hours while the catheter remained patent. For those patients receiving medication every 12 hours, the catheter was flushed after medication administration and then halfway between each scheduled dose.

The gauge and type of device and the site and time of placement were recorded by the patient's nurse or i.v. therapist. The patient's nurse or i.v. therapist also evaluated the catheter site daily and upon patient complaint. This evaluation, duration of catheter placement, and other pertinent information were recorded on a data collection form.

THOMAS P. LOMBARDI, PHARM.D., is Pediatric Clinical Pharmacy Specialist, Department of Pharmacy, Albany Medical Center Hospital, Albany, NY, and Adjunct Assistant Professor of Pharmacy Practice, Albany College of Pharmacy; at the time of this study, he was Clinical Pharmacy Fellow in Pediatric Pharmacotherapy, Department of Pharmacy Services, Hartford Hospital, Hartford, CT, and Assistant Clinical Professor, School of Pharmacy, University of Connecticut, Storrs, CT. BERIT GUNDERSEN, PHARM.D., is Assistant Professor, School of Pharmacy, University of the Pacific, Stockton, CA; at the time of this study, she was Clinical Pharmacy Fellow in Pediatric Pharmacotherapy, Hartford Hospital, and Assistant Clinical Professor, School of Pharmacy, University of Connecticut. LORNA O. ZAMMETT, PHARM.D., is Staff Pharmacist, Department of Pharmacy, Bristol Hospital, Bristol, CT; at the time of this study, she was Pediatric Clinical Pharmacist, Department of Pharmacy Services, Hartford Hospital. J. KEN WALTERS, PHARM.D., is Assistant Director of Professional Practice, Department of Pharmacy Services, Francis Scott Key Medical Center, Baltimore, MD; at the time of this study, he was Assistant Director for Clinical Pharmacy Services, Department of Pharmacy Services, Hartford Hospital, and Associate Clinical Professor, School of Pharmacy, University of Connecticut. BARBARA A. MORRIS, M.D., is Director, Pediatric Intensive Care, Department of Anesthesia and Critical Care, Children's Mercy Hospital, Kansas City, MO; at the time of this study, she was director, Pediatric Intensive Care, Department of Pediatrics, Hartford Hospital, and Assistant Professor of Pediatrics, School of Medicine, University of Connecticut.

Address reprint requests to Dr. Lombardi at the Department of Pharmacy, Albany Medical Center Hospital, 43 New Scotland Avenue, Albany, NY 12208.

Presented at the 22nd Annual ASHP Midyear Clinical Meeting, Atlanta, GA, December 9, 1987.

Copyright © 1988, American Society of Hospital Pharmacists, Inc. All rights reserved. 0278-2677/88/1101-0832$01.25.

Loss of patency was defined as inability to flush one milliliter of solution within one minute, and phlebitis was defined as inflammation of the vein leading to pain or erythema, or both. All medications administered through the catheter were recorded by a pharmacist on the data collection form.

Chi-square analysis was used to compare the heparin and sodium chloride groups; both catheter patency and catheter-site loss caused by phlebitis or infiltration were examined. Analysis included data for the entire duration of catheter patency and for 48- and 72-hour periods following catheter placement. Chi-square analysis with a Yates correction was used to compare the two groups regarding the site of placement or type or gauge of catheter.[9] Length of patency was compared between the two study groups using Student's *t* test. A p value ≤ 0.05 was considered significant.

Results. A total of 74 catheter sites (34 in the sodium chloride group and 40 in the heparin group) were evaluated. The sodium chloride group included 34 patients (23 boys and 11 girls); the heparin group included 40 patients (18 boys and 22 girls). The mean (±S.D.) age was not significantly different between the two groups (7.1 ± 6.0 years, sodium chloride group; 7.2 ± 5.5 years, heparin group). All patients had catheters placed for medication administration or for ease of intravenous access. The two groups were similar with respect to catheter placement site and type and gauge of device (Table 1). The power of the study ($1 - \beta$) to detect a significant difference in phlebitis rates at 72 hours was estimated as 0.9.

The mean duration of catheter patency between the two groups was not significantly different (Table 2). No intravenous access sites were lost because of infiltration or clot formation in the catheter. Phlebitis occurred at 7 catheter insertion sites in the sodium chloride group and at 13 insertion sites in the heparin group. A total of 54 devices (27 in each group) were discontinued for other reasons. The site of catheter placement did not affect duration of patency.

Our institution's nursing policy states that peripheral intravenous catheter sites should be changed every 72 hours; exceptions to this policy are pediatric patients and patients in whom venous access is difficult. We evaluated the data describing catheter status at 72 hours after insertion and found no significant differences in number of catheters or duration of catheter patency in any of the categories that we analyzed (Table 2).

Of the 42 devices that were discontinued before 72 hours, 69% were removed within 48 hours. This finding suggests that most pediatric patients do not retain catheters for as long as adult patients typically do. Therefore, we evaluated the data describing catheter status at 48 hours after insertion. There was no significant difference between the heparin and sodium chloride groups in either number of patent catheters or duration of catheter patency

Table 1.
Catheter Characteristics among Patients

Characteristic	No. Patients in Group: Sodium Chloride ($n = 34$)	Heparin ($n = 40$)
Catheter site		
Hand	6	15
Arm	22	22
Foot	6	3
Catheter type		
18-gauge Vicra	0	1
20-gauge Vicra	14	13
22-gauge Vicra	13	18
24-gauge Vicra	1	7
20-gauge Jelco	1	0
22-gauge Jelco	4	0
24-gauge Jelco	1	1

Table 2.
Duration of Catheter Patency

Category[a]	Sodium Chloride Group: Mean ± S.D. (hr)	*n*	Heparin Group: Mean ± S.D. (hr)	*n*
All indwelling devices	62.6 ± 42.2	34	62.6 ± 42.9	40
Devices patent ≥ 72 hr	99.0 ± 32.7	16	106.0 ± 31.5	16
Devices patent ≥ 48 hr	86.9 ± 35.9	21	88.8 ± 36.2	24
All devices removed because of phlebitis	44.3 ± 26.6	7	51.6 ± 35.5	13
Devices removed <72 hr	22.0 ± 14.0	5	30.7 ± 16.6	10
Devices removed <48 hr	22.0 ± 14.0	5	23.0 ± 5.4	8
All devices removed for reasons other than phlebitis[b]	67.3 ± 44.1	27	69.7 ± 45.1	27
Devices removed <72 hr	33.3 ± 11.6	13	35.0 ± 15.4	14
Devices removed <48 hr	24.1 ± 0.3	8	23.3 ± 8.1	8

[a] The sodium chloride and heparin groups did not differ significantly with respect to duration of catheter patency or number of catheters in any of the categories analyzed.

[b] Discontinued because no further need for i.v. access, device leaking, or device pulled out by patient.

(Table 2).

Medications administered through the intravenous devices are listed in Table 3. No patient received antineoplastic agents during the study. Only the categories of β-lactam use, use of one medication, and use of two or more medications could be analyzed statistically. There were no significant differences between the sodium chloride group and the heparin group with respect to these factors. Among those patients treated with β lactams, catheter patency was maintained for at least 48 hours in 15 of 21 (71%) patients in the sodium chloride group and in 20 of 30 (67%) in the heparin group (Table 4); the heparin and sodium chloride groups did not differ with respect to the number of patent catheters at 48 hours or the duration of patency.

Discussion. Heparin sodium 10 units in 0.9% sodium chloride injection 1 mL is a safe and effective solution advocated for flushing peripheral indwelling intravenous infusion devices. This solution has been shown to decrease the incidence of catheter-associated phlebitis without causing anticoagulation.[1-3] Others advocate the use of a flush solution with a maximum heparin concentration of 100 units/mL.[4] However, the use of heparin, in any concentration, remains controversial.

Epperson[4] found a similar incidence of phlebitis or infiltration in adults receiving heparin sodium 10 or 100 units/mL in 0.9% sodium chloride injection or 0.9% sodium chloride injection alone. These results were confirmed by Hamilton et al.[5] These findings are corroborated for pediatric patients by our report; we found no difference between groups of pediatric patients whose indwelling peripheral intravenous devices were flushed with either a heparin-containing (10 units/mL) or heparin-free solution. Although the difference was not statistically significant, there was a surprising and unexplained tendency for phlebitis to occur more often in the heparin group than the sodium chloride group.

The sequential design of this study was chosen because unit dose drug distribution services were not available on the pediatric unit at the time this study was conducted. We believed that stocking both solutions on the unit at one time would have created confusion among the staff involved in the study and may have resulted in errors in solution administration. The limitation of using a sequential trial, rather than one that is randomized, is that the study groups may differ. However, we detected no significant differences in demographic characteristics between the two treatment groups. The number of catheter sites evaluated during the study period is approximately the number of intravenous catheters placed each month on the pediatric unit. Many patients who might have been eligible for inclusion in the study had catheters in place before they were admitted to the unit.

Table 3.
Medications Administered through Catheters

Medication	No. Patients in Group: Sodium Chloride (n = 34)	No. Patients in Group: Heparin (n = 40)
β Lactams[a]	21	30
Chloramphenicol	6	3
Methylprednisolone	5	3
Aminoglycosides[b]	3	3
Aminophylline	2	3
Vancomycin	1	3
Phenobarbital	3	0
Trimethoprim–sulfamethoxazole	0	3
Others[c]	3	3
No medications	5	2
One medication	18	27
Two or more medications	11	11

[a] Ampicillin, oxacillin, cefazolin, penicillin, cefuroxime, ceftazidime, and cefoxitin.
[b] Tobramycin and gentamicin.
[c] Clindamycin, furosemide, digoxin, and diphenhydramine.

Table 4.
Duration of Catheter Patency in Patients Receiving β Lactams

Category[a]	Sodium Chloride Group Mean ± S.D. (hr)	n	Heparin Group Mean ± S.D. (hr)	n
Devices patent ≥ 48 hr	72.0 ± 17.5	15	81.4 ± 30.8	20
Devices removed <48 hr because of phlebitis	24.0 ± 0.0	3	27.2 ± 6.0	5
Devices removed <48 hr for reasons other than phlebitis[b]	31.0 ± 10.8	3	24.4 ± 4.5	5

[a] The sodium chloride and heparin groups did not differ significantly with respect to duration of catheter patency or number of catheters in any of the categories analyzed.
[b] Discontinued because of no further need for i.v. access, device leaking, or device pulled out by patient.

Factors that may alter the patency of intravenous catheters are catheter size, site of placement, and medications administered. We found no differences between the two groups with regard to these factors. A wide variety of medications was administered through the catheters; the β-lactam antimicrobials were given often enough to allow a statistical evaluation to be performed. These medications are known to be very irritating to the veins,[10] so differences between flushing solutions should be evident in a comparative analysis. No significant differences were detected in this subgroup, confirming our hypothesis that the addition of heparin was not protective against development of phlebitis.

We have also shown that pediatric patients retain intravenous catheters for shorter durations than customary institutional limits for such catheters (72 hours). This may be due to earlier discontinuation of intravenous medications or to younger patients "playing" with their intravenous catheters and causing loss of the catheter sites.

Several benefits might result from the use of heparin-free flushing solutions. First, the likelihood of medication administration errors might decrease. Since many pediatric units stock multiple concentrations of heparin solution (e.g., 10, 100, and 1000 units/mL), standard use of a heparin-free flushing solution would make less likely the use of an incorrect heparin solution and the unwanted anticoagulation or bleeding that might result.

Second, the use of heparin-free flushing solutions would allow avoidance of heparin-associated drug compatibility problems. Some commonly administered medications that may precipitate in the presence of heparin include aminoglycosides, penicillin G, vancomycin, meperidine, codeine, morphine, promethazine, and hydroxyzine.[6] In our study, 29 catheters were used to give medications that could have precipitated with heparin. Since one purpose of indwelling catheters is to ease medication administration, drug precipitation in the device must be avoided. Elimination of heparin would alleviate this concern.

A third advantage is avoidance of exposure to heparin. Thrombocytopenia attributable to development of antiplatelet antibodies has been associated with heparin exposure.[7] Although this phenomenon has not been reported to occur with exposure to dilute heparin solutions, elimination of the heparin would obviate this concern.

A final advantage is the reduced cost to the patient and institution. Based on drug acquisition and preparation (supplies and personnel) costs in our institution, heparin sodium 10 units/mL in 0.9% sodium chloride injection costs $0.82/mL, while 0.9% sodium chloride injection without heparin costs $0.03/mL. We estimate that elimination of the heparin from the flushing solution would decrease the cost of therapy for the average pediatric patient from $8.53 to $0.31. These costs are based on the average maintenance of a catheter for 2.6 days with four flushes per day. This would produce an annual cost saving of approximately $20,000 to $25,000 for our 52-bed pediatric unit.

Conclusion. Our results suggest that solutions of 0.9% sodium chloride injection with and without heparin sodium 10 units/mL are equally effective for maintaining the patency of indwelling intermittent infusion devices in children. Controlled studies in larger numbers of patients are needed to confirm these results.

---

[a] Sterile 0.9% sodium chloride for injection, McGaw Laboratories, McGaw Park, IL, lot B55001A.

[b] Sterile 0.9% sodium chloride for injection, McGaw Laboratories, lot B55001A; and heparin sodium 1000 units/mL, Elkins-Sinn, Inc., Cherry Hill, NJ, lot 115058. Final heparin sodium concentration 10 units/mL.

References

1. Hanson RL, Grant AM, Majors KR. Heparin-lock maintenance with ten units of sodium heparin in one milliliter of normal saline. *Surg Gynecol Obstet*. 1976; 142:373–6.
2. Swerling R. Normal saline or dilute heparin for heparin lock flush. *Infusion*. 1982; 6:123–4.
3. Baldwin J. Heparin locks in neonates. *ASHP Signal*. 1977; 1:1.
4. Epperson EL. Efficacy of 0.9% sodium chloride injection with and without heparin for maintaining indwelling intermittent injection sites. *Clin Pharm*. 1984; 3:626–9.
5. Hamilton RA, Plis JM, Clay C et al. Heparin sodium versus 0.9% sodium chloride injection for maintaining patency of indwelling intermittent infusion devices. *Clin Pharm*. 1988; 7:439–43.
6. Trissel LA. Handbook on injectable drugs. 4th ed. Bethesda, MD. American Society of Hospital Pharmacists, Inc.; 1985.
7. Laster J, Cikrit D. Walker N et al. The heparin-induced thrombocytopenia syndrome: an update. *Surgery*. 1987; 102:763–8.
8. Tunbridge LJ, Lloyd JV, Penhall RK et al. Stability of diluted heparin sodium stored in plastic syringes. *Am J Hosp Pharm*. 1981; 38:1001–4.
9. Schler WC. Statistics for the biological sciences. 2nd ed. Reading, MA: Addison-Wesley Publishing Co.; 1980.
10. Maddox RR, Rush DR, Rapp RP et al. Double-blind study to investigate methods to prevent cephalothin-induced phlebitis. *Am J Hosp Pharm*. 1977; 34:29–34.

Commentary

1988 Report of the Joint National Committee on Detection, Evaluation, and Treatment of High Blood Pressure: A commentary

ARTHUR A. SCHUNA

Clin Pharm. 1988; 7:837–41

I recently saw progress notes from 1972 for a patient who had been referred to our hypertension clinic. These notes indicated that this relatively young patient had been treated only with hydralazine 25 mg every four hours as needed for hypertension. I wondered how this patient would have determined when his blood pressure was high, since home blood pressure monitoring was uncommon at that time. Even if monitoring was available to him, did he check his blood pressure every four hours to determine if he needed a dose? Also, I wondered how effective this treatment was, given hydralazine's tendency to cause reflex tachycardia and sodium retention.

It is rare to see treatment plans like this one prescribed for patients we see in referral today, although it was not uncommon in the 1970s. The publication of the first report of the Joint National Committee on the Detection, Evaluation, and Treatment of High Blood Pressure, which appeared in 1977, has had a lot to do with the change in the approach to management of hypertension.[1] This initial publication outlined the "stepped-care" approach to blood pressure management, which is well known to most of us today. This approach has been widely accepted by most clinicians, yet it has been criticized in recent years. The 1988 report has attempted to address at least some of the criticisms, but debate will continue, particularly the controversy over how to manage the mildly hypertensive patient.[2]

In its first report, the Joint National Committee listed a diuretic as step 1, adrenergic inhibitors as step 2, hydralazine as step 3, and guanethidine as step 4. These recommendations took advantage of the synergistic properties of these drugs, which work at different sites to lower blood pressure. The stepped-care approach to blood pressure management also attempts to counter the various homeostatic mechanisms the body has to maintain elevated blood pressure in the resistant patient. Although β blockers were suggested as possible step 1 therapy in selected younger patients with rapid heart rates, they were not accepted at that time for general use. Acceptance of β blockers for general use as step 1 drugs would not appear until the 1984 report.[3] This occurred after the publication of several large-scale studies using β-blocker monotherapy for initial treatment of hypertension.

The 1984 report also mentioned the use of angiotensin-converting-enzyme (ACE) inhibitors and calcium-channel blockers as treatment alternatives in steps 2 through 4. These agents were too new at the time of the report to have been assigned a proper place in therapy. Captopril, the only ACE inhibitor marketed at that time, carried warnings in its package insert suggesting that, because of bone marrow and renal complications, it be used after other drugs failed. Clinical experience with captopril since that time has shown that these complications are rare when lower dosage regimens (<150 mg of captopril per day) are used and if patients with known predisposing conditions (e.g., bilateral renal artery stenoses, renal failure, connective tissue diseases) are monitored closely. In addition, ACE inhibitors are relatively free of adverse effects, such as fatigue, impotence, and reduced exercise tolerance, that affect the quality of life for many patients. Adverse effects may frequently result in decreased compliance with treatment for many patients. The use of calcium-channel blockers as antihypertensives was not well established at the time of the 1984 report.

The 1988 report differs from its predecessors in that it includes ACE inhibitors and calcium-channel blockers as alternative step 1 therapies. A greater emphasis is placed on nondrug therapies and risk factor reduction. The section dealing with individualization of treatment for special popula-

ARTHUR A. SCHUNA, M.S., is Clinical Pharmacy Coordinator, William S. Middleton Veterans Administration Hospital, and Associate Professor of Pharmacy, School of Pharmacy, University of Wisconsin, Madison.
Address reprint requests to Mr. Schuna at the Pharmacy Service, William S. Middleton Veterans Administration Hospital, 2500 Overlook Terrace, Madison, WI 53705.

Copyright © 1988, American Society of Hospital Pharmacists, Inc. All rights reserved. 0278-2677/88/1101-0837$01.25.

tions of patients and those with pre-existing conditions that may influence treatment has been expanded. In patients in whom initial therapy fails, the options for treatment are a higher dose of the same drug (within the range given in tables), addition of a second drug (the old stepped-care approach), or substitution of an alternative step 1 drug before proceeding to step 2 therapy. This approach is far more flexible than those in prior reports and takes into consideration the ever increasing antihypertensive pharmacopeia.

All of the step 1 drugs appear to be approximately equal in lowering blood pressure when used as monotherapy for hypertension. Fifty to sixty percent of patients respond to step 1 therapy. It could be argued that the recommendation of calcium-channel blockers as step 1 therapy is premature. To date, only verapamil in its sustained-release formulation has received FDA approval for hypertension. The other available calcium-channel blockers must be given at least three times daily and often more frequently to achieve sustained blood pressure control throughout the day. Sustained-release formulations of the currently available calcium-channel blockers, as well as inherently long-acting second-generation compounds, will soon be released and probably will make this treatment option more acceptable for step 1 therapy.

Given the apparently equal efficacy of these four approaches and the inability to predict in advance which treatment will work best in a given patient, how does one determine the most appropriate treatment course? In some patients, coexisting diseases or other factors help caregivers in narrowing the treatment options. But what is the best treatment choice in the patient who has mild hypertension but no complications? This is perhaps one of the biggest controversies in medicine today; some of the factors considered in making this decision deserve further comment.

Treatment of Mild Hypertension

Role of Diuretics. Diuretics have been the cornerstone of all hypertension treatment since before the first Joint National Committee Report. They are often essential as supplements to other drugs, since they prevent the secondary sodium retention that made patients resistant to other therapies available at that time. Diuretics are simple to use; their flat dose–response curve means that a low daily dose may be all that is necessary for most patients with mild hypertension. They are free of the central nervous system adverse effects associated with β blockers and other adrenergic inhibitors. They also are one of the least expensive pharmacologic treatment alternatives.

The major problems associated with diuretic use have been electrolyte and metabolic disturbances. Thiazides may lower serum potassium concentrations in as many as one third of patients treated. The risk of this complication can be reduced by having the patient take hydrochlorothiazide in a single morning dose, reduce sodium intake, and use salt substitutes (that contain potassium). Using potassium-sparing diuretics or additional potassium adds considerable expense to treatment, making alternative step 1 drugs more attractive. Thiazide diuretics may raise serum glucose concentrations in some patients predisposed to diabetes, but the effect on most patients is negligible. Thiazides increase serum uric acid concentrations, but this is usually of little consequence. An analysis of the Hypertension Detection and Follow-up Program (HDFP) data from 2068 patients treated with thiazides showed that only 15 had documented episodes of gout in five years of treatment.[4] Thiazides appear to increase serum cholesterol concentrations in short-term studies, but patients treated with the drug for longer than one year do not appear to have this increase.[5] Although it is doubtful that transient elevations of cholesterol are clinically important, some patients may have sustained elevations, which would make other treatment alternatives more appropriate. Just as we monitor serum potassium concentrations in diuretic-treated patients, monitoring of serum cholesterol concentrations is appropriate.

Thiazides have been criticized as step 1 drugs, primarily because most major treatment studies have failed to demonstrate a reduction of cardiovascular mortality in patients with diastolic blood pressures less than 95 mm Hg. At higher blood pressures thiazides do appear beneficial. Perhaps more disturbing was the finding of the Multiple Risk Factor Intervention Trial (MRFIT), which suggested that patients treated with diuretics who had pre-existing electrocardiographic abnormalities were more likely to suffer cardiovascular mortality than "usual care" patients (i.e., patients referred to their local physician for follow-up).[6] Although these findings could have occurred by chance, the question of a detrimental action of diuretic therapy has been raised. Some postulate that hypokalemia may have increased the risk of arrhythmia in these patients. Others suggest that the effect of thiazides on plasma lipids may negate any potential benefit.

The subgroup analysis of the patients with electrocardiographic abnormalities in the MRFIT trial has been criticized on several counts.[7] The investigators in the MRFIT trial admit that the findings may lack statistical power. Patients were randomized to a special intervention (SI) group or a usual care (UC) group (in which they were referred to their own physician for follow-up). Although the investigators assumed that many patients in the UC group would not be treated, the majority of patients in each group received diuretics (SI, 75%; UC, 55%). The differences in serum potassium concentrations at the last visit between patients who died of coronary artery disease and those who survived were not significant. However, there is no way to know the serum potassium concentration when the patient died. Patients treated with chlorthalidone, which is more likely than hydrochlorothiazide to induce hypokalemia, had a lower rate of cardiovascular mortality. These findings make the hypokalemia hypothesis for the MRFIT findings difficult to accept. Cholesterol concentrations in the SI group receiving diuretics were actually lower at the end of the trial, making the cholesterol hypothesis questionable. Men with electrocardiographic abnormalities in the UC group had a lower death rate than many of the other subgroups studied, which may have accounted for the statistical differences observed. The doses of diuretics used in this trial were commonly 100 mg of chlorthalidone or hydrochlorothiazide daily. These doses are higher than the 25–50 mg/day doses currently used. Analysis of the HDFP data on patients with pre-existing electrocardiographic abnormalities has failed to document a harmful effect from diuretic-based stepped-care therapy.[8] Aggressive treatment of mild hypertension resulted in reduced mortality in both the HDFP and the Australian Therapeutic Trial.[9] Although the findings of the MRFIT study should not be completely ignored, the criticisms raised about the study findings should result in questions about the validity of their findings. My conclusion is that diuretics still should have a major role in the treatment of hypertension. Convincing evidence that diuretics are detrimental is lacking, and the bad press they are receiving may not be justified. Unlike other step 1 drugs, diuretics no longer enjoy patent protection and have no corporate sponsor to promote their use.

Role of β Blockers. Beta blockers are the other most frequently used step 1 drugs. They are beneficial in patients with coexisting coronary artery disease, in whom they reduce blood pressure and prevent myocardial ischemia. In hypertensive patients who have had a recent myocardial infarction, there is evidence that β blockers may reduce the likelihood of sudden death. In patients with hypertension and migraine headaches, β blockers may also reduce the frequency of migraine attacks.

On the negative side, β blockers are frequently associated with central nervous system adverse effects, which may be severe. Claims that water-soluble β blockers are less likely to cause these problems have not been proved in double-blind clinical trials.[10,11] Beta blockers can induce bronchial constriction in patients with reversible airway disease and worsen heart failure in patients with poor left ventricular function. Beta blockers may worsen the condition of patients with Raynaud's disease or peripheral vascular disease, since these drugs result in unopposed α constriction in peripheral vessels. Beta blockers have a mild adverse effect on plasma lipids, increasing triglycerides and reducing high-density lipoproteins. This effect is apparent even in long-term studies. These detrimental effects do not appear to be associated with β blockers having intrinsic sympathomimetic properties or with the α–β blocker labetalol. However, there is no evidence that these β blockers are cardioprotective. Most trials comparing β blockers with diuretics as the primary treatment in mild hypertension have not demonstrated any differences in coronary mortality between the therapies.[12–14] Only the recently published Metoprolol Atherosclerosis Prevention in Hypertensives study suggests that β blockers reduced mortality from coronary heart disease and stroke, compared with diuretic treatment. This benefit was seen primarily among smokers.[15]

Benefit of Treatment with Diuretics and β Blockers. Despite an apparent lack of benefit from the use of diuretics and β blockers in major clinical trials involving mild hypertension, major decreases in mortality as a result of coronary heart disease and stroke have occurred since the initiation of nationwide hypertension education efforts. Stroke death rates have declined by more than 40% in the past 10 years. The cardiovascular death rate has declined 25%.[7] Other factors, such as improved diets, less smoking, and more exercise, may also contribute to lower mortality; yet, there is little question that decreased blood pressure plays some role in this reduction. The majority of these patients were treated with diuretics or β blockers.

Perhaps the failure of these trials to document benefit in the prevention of myocardial infarction is the result of study design. These studies have for the most part been done in older patients. Monitoring committees terminate studies when statistical differences in hypertensive disease endpoints are reached. The natural histories of renal and stroke complications are different, and perhaps these complications are more responsive to acute lowering of blood pressure than are atherosclerotic complications. We know that atherosclerotic vascular complications are already evident in the second decade of life and that hypertension accelerates these changes. Other factors influencing the rate of atherosclerosis include heredity, diet, other diseases (e.g., diabetes), and smoking. The impact of reducing one risk factor, mild hypertension, for the relatively short time period of a clinical trial on the adverse outcomes of atherosclerosis (coronary morbidity and mortality) is questionable. On the other hand, the reduction of stroke complications, which may be more responsive to acute lowering of blood pressure, has often resulted in the termination of these trials. The ideal study to determine the efficacy of treatment of mild hypertension would be done in younger patients without evidence of target organ damage. It is unlikely that a study such as this would be done because it would require large numbers of patients, take many years to complete, and be extremely costly. We do know that effective treatment of blood pressure reduces the likelihood of the development of left ventricular hypertrophy, congestive heart failure, progression to more severe forms of hypertension, hypertensive encephalopathy, and strokes.[9,16,17]

Role of Other Step 1 Agents. ACE inhibitors and calcium-channel blockers do not alter plasma lipids, do not cause secondary sodium retention, and are very good step 1 drugs for some patients. However, unlike thiazides or β blockers, they have not been tested in large-scale trials, and we have no evidence that they would fare any better in reducing coronary mortality. They are considerably more expensive than alternative step 1 therapy for many patients. The need for frequent dosing of nifedipine and diltiazem makes these choices less desirable in their currently available dosage forms.

Aggressive Treatment of Mild Hypertension. A recent study suggests that aggressive lowering of blood pressure in patients with coronary artery disease may be detrimental.[18] In this trial, 902 patients with diastolic blood pressures higher than 95 mm Hg were treated with atenolol as monotherapy or with other drugs if needed. Deaths from myocardial infarction were lowest when a mean treated diastolic blood pressure of 85 to 90 mm Hg was achieved and were increased if blood pressure was higher or lower than this range. Patients without coronary disease did not have increased coronary mortality when treated diastolic blood pressures were less than 85 mm Hg. This may explain the negative findings of the MRFIT study in patients with electrocardiographic abnormalities, since these patients would be more likely to have coronary artery disease. If the findings from this study are substantiated, they would suggest that other drugs may be equally detrimental if treatment is too aggressive in patients with coronary disease. A certain diastolic pressure may be necessary for patients with severe coronary disease to maintain adequate coronary perfusion; overaggressive drug therapy may reduce this perfusion.

The atenolol study raises important questions. Are we using drug therapy too aggressively? Currently, most clinicians treat patients almost by reflex action if diastolic blood pressures are greater than 90 mm Hg, often without obtaining several confirming blood pressure readings. Another factor that is often not considered is whether the patient may be experiencing office hypertension. Studies suggest that 20% of patients with mild hypertension in the office have normal blood pressure at home.[19] Should nondrug therapies such as alcohol restriction, sodium restriction, and weight reduction be used more aggressively? These measures have either no cost or a minimal cost to the patient but may pose compliance problems. These measures require the patient to take a more active role in his or her treatment than the simple act of taking medication and often require major lifestyle changes. Will any drug benefit the patient with mild hypertension and coronary disease?

Selection of Initial Treatment. Given the above concerns, what factors (other than concurrent diseases, other therapy, or demographics) need to be considered when initial therapy for a given patient with mild hypertension is chosen? Factors that may improve patient compliance must be considered. These may include ease of administration, economic factors, and the impact of treatment on quality of life. From the standpoint of ease of administration, once-daily therapy is desirable. This can be achieved with diuretics, many β blockers, enalapril and lisinopril, and sustained-release verapamil. Economic factors are an important consideration. Some of the newer step 1 options may cost 10 to 20 times as much as thiazide diuretics. Other expenses include the cost of frequent office visits needed for dosage titration for drugs with a wide dosage range (lipid-soluble β blockers, ACE inhibitors, or calcium-channel blockers) or the laboratory monitoring costs needed to maintain the various therapies (which may be more of a factor with diuretics and ACE inhibitors). Quality of life is an issue, because many treatment choices may make the patient feel worse than he or she did before treatment was started. This makes drugs that have adverse effects on the central nervous system (β blockers and other adrenergic inhibitors) less than desirable for initial therapy. Impotence is one possible complication with any antihypertensive therapy that affects quality of life. Patients need to be encouraged to take an active part in their therapy and report any changes in how they feel to their health-care providers. In turn, health-care providers need to be responsive to problems identified by the patient to ensure cooperation with the treatment regimen.

Pre-existing medical conditions may also influence the treatment choice for initial therapy. The Joint National Committee Report does an excellent job of discussing therapeutic considerations for patients with a variety of disease states and other special populations of hypertensives.

Other Changes in the Joint National Committee Report

The new Joint National Committee Report places a greater emphasis on reducing other cardiovascular risk factors and has incorporated the latest guidelines for lowering cholesterol. The role of calcium supplementation and fish oil is addressed. Although some studies suggest that calcium supplementation may have a mild effect in lowering blood pressure, the limited nature of these trials in terms of the small number of patients treated and the short duration of these studies makes it difficult to recommend this therapy at this time. The report is suitably skeptical about calcium. The evidence for the benefit of fish oil is based primarily on epidemiologic studies suggesting that populations that eat larger amounts of fish have lower rates of coronary artery disease. The use of fish oil supplements has been shown to result in lowered triglyceride levels and reduced blood-clotting ability. Whether fish oil supplementation can reduce coronary disease is not known. For this reason, the report recommends increasing the dietary intake of fish but not the routine use of fish oil supplements. Neither increased dietary fish intake nor fish oil supplements appear to affect blood pressure.

Step-down therapy (the attempt to reduce drug therapy in patients with at least one year of good blood pressure control) is given a greater emphasis in the current report. Although few patients may be completely taken off therapy for any length of time, many patients have a reduced need for medication. The least amount of drug that achieves the blood pressure treatment goal is desirable, since it reduces adverse effects and cost to the patient.

Conclusion

The 1988 Report of the Joint National Committee on Detection, Evaluation, and Treatment of High Blood Pressure incorporates many changes from its 1984 predecessor. These changes result from increased understanding about the epidemiology of hypertension and options for treatment that have evolved in the past four years. The current guidelines are far more flexible, and many new treatment options are currently recommended for initiation of therapy. Although some may criticize the continued recommendation of diuretics and β blockers for step 1 therapy, data showing that other therapies are superior are lacking at this time. Until convincing data are published demonstrating the superiority of other therapies, these criticisms are unjustified.

Despite the apparent lack of change in coronary mortality in trials using step 1 therapy for mild hypertension, we do appear to be making a major impact nationally with blood pressure treatment. There has been a decline in the incidence of myocardial infarction, congestive heart failure, ventricular hypertrophy, and stroke. These facts should not be overlooked in considering treatment.

If you have time to read only one more paper on the treatment of hypertension this year, I would recommend that you read the 1988 Joint National Committee Report. You will not find such a wealth of information presented so concisely anywhere else.

References

1. The 1977 Joint National Committee on Detection, Evaluation, and Treatment of High Blood Pressure. Report of the Joint National Committee on Detection, Evaluation, and Treatment of High Blood Pressure. *JAMA*. 1977;237:255–61.
2. The 1988 Joint National Committee on Detection, Evaluation, and Treatment of High Blood Pressure. The 1988 report of the Joint National Committee on Detection, Evaluation, and Treatment of High Blood Pressure. *Arch Intern Med*. 1988; 148:1023–38.
3. The 1984 Joint National Committee on Detection, Evaluation, and Treatment of High Blood Pressure. The 1984 report of the Joint National Committee on Detection, Evaluation, and Treatment of High Blood Pressure. *Arch Intern Med*. 1984; 144:1045–57.
4. Langford HG, Blaufox MD, Borhani NO et al. Is thiazide-produced uric acid elevation harmful?: analysis of data from the Hypertension Detection and Follow-up Program. *Arch Intern Med*. 1987; 147:645–9.
5. Moser M. Diuretics in the management of hypertension. *Med Clin North Am*. 1987; 71:935–46.
6. Multiple Risk Factor Intervention Trial Research Group. Multiple risk factor intervention trial: risk factor changes and mortality results. *JAMA*. 1982; 248:1465–77.
7. Moser M. Clinical trial, diuretics, and the management of mild hypertension. *Arch Intern Med*. 1984; 144:789–92.
8. Gifford RW, Borhani N, Krishan I et al. The dilemma of "mild" hypertension: another point of view. *JAMA*. 1983; 250:3171–3.
9. The Australian Therapeutic Trial in Mild Hypertension: report by the management committee. *Lancet*. 1980; 1:1261–7.
10. Gengo FM, Huntoon L, McHugh WB. Lipid-soluble and water soluble β-blockers: comparison of the central nervous system depressant effect. *Arch Intern Med*. 1987; 147:39–43.
11. Gengo FM, Fagan SC, de Padova A et al. The effect of β-blockers on mental performance of older hypertensive patients. *Arch Intern Med*. 1988; 148:779–84.
12. Medical Research Council Working Party. MRC trial of treatment of mild hypertension: principal results. *Br Med J*. 1985; 291:97–104.
13. The IPPPSH Collaborative Group. Cardiovascular risk and risk factors in a randomized trial of treatment based on the beta-blocker oxprenolol: the International Prospective Primary Prevention Study in Hypertension (IPPPSH). *J Hypertens*. 1985; 3:379–92.
14. Wilhelmsen L, Berglund G, Elmfeldt D et al. Beta-blockers versus diuretics in hypertensive men: main result from the HAPPHY trial. *J Hypertens*. 1987; 5:561–72.
15. Wikstrand J, Warnold I, Olsson G et al. Primary prevention with metoprolol in patients with hypertension: mortality results from the MAPHY study. *JAMA*. 1988; 259:1976–82.
16. Hypertension Detection and Follow-up Program Cooperative Group. Effect of antihypertensive medication on left ventricular hypertrophy. *Circulation*. 1981; 64(Suppl 4):322. Abstract.
17. Veterans Administration Cooperative Study Group on Antihypertensive Agents. Effects of treatment on morbidity in hypertension: II. Results in patients with diastolic blood pressure averaging 90 through 114 mm Hg. *JAMA*. 1970; 213:1143–52.
18. Cruickshank JM, Thorp JM, Zacharias FJ. Benefits and potential harm of lowering high blood pressure. *Lancet*. 1987; 1:581–4.
19. Pickering TG, James GD, Boddie C et al. How common is white coat hypertension? *JAMA*. 1988; 259:225–8.

Drug Experience

Straightforward reports of unusual drug experiences are included in this section. These may be confirmations of previously reported drug experiences or brief apparent first reports. While selected references may be cited, the purpose of a Drug Experience report is not to present an extensive review of the literature.

A related section, Grand Rounds, includes papers that are well-documented patient case reports with a thorough review of the important literature to help put the case in perspective.

Morphine concentrations in plasma, ascitic fluid, and nasogastric aspirate fluid during high-dose intravenous morphine infusion

PAUL R. HUTSON, TERRY J. BAUMANN, ROBERT R. LAVOIE, AND MICHAEL R. MULLANE

Clin Pharm. 1988; 7:842–5

Recent reports document the very high dosing requirements of selected cancer patients receiving morphine by continuous intravenous infusion.[1–3] We discuss our experience with a patient who required very high morphine infusion rates over a sustained period. Morphine concentrations in plasma, ascitic fluid, and nasogastric aspirate fluid were obtained to determine the effect of ascites or gastric suctioning on the distribution and clearance of the drug.

PAUL R. HUTSON, PHARM.D., is Assistant Professor, College of Pharmacy, University of Wisconsin at Madison; at the time of manuscript preparation, he was Assistant Professor, College of Pharmacy, University of Illinois at Chicago. TERRY J. BAUMANN, PHARM.D., is Assistant Professor, College of Pharmacy and Allied Health Professions, Wayne State University, and Clinical Coordinator of Pharmacy Service, Henry Ford Hospital, Detroit, MI. ROBERT R. LAVOIE, PHARM.D., is Assistant Director of Pharmacy for Clinical Services, Hurley Medical Center, Flint, MI; at the time this work was completed, he was Research Fellow, College of Pharmacy and Allied Health Professions, Wayne State University. MICHAEL R. MULLANE, M.D., is Instructor in Medicine, Section of Medical Oncology, College of Medicine, University of Illinois at Chicago.

Address reprint requests to Dr. Hutson at the College of Pharmacy, University of Wisconsin at Madison, 425 N. Charter St., Madison, WI 53706.

Copyright © 1988, American Society of Hospital Pharmacists, Inc. All rights reserved. 0278-2677/88/1101-0842$01.00.

Case Report. The patient was a 44-year-old white woman with metastatic papillary adenocarcinoma of the ovary. In February 1986, she was hospitalized with weakness, anorexia, postprandial nausea and vomiting, abdominal pain, and constipation. Her cancer had been diagnosed in September 1983, when she had developed ascites and a right pleural effusion. At that time, she underwent a debulking procedure with bilateral salpingo-oophorectomy, splenectomy, wedge resection of the colon, partial small bowel resection, omentectomy, and removal of the anterior abdominal wall. She had undergone a total abdominal hysterectomy in 1974 for carcinoma in situ of the cervix. After her surgery in 1983, she was plagued by progressive ascites despite cytotoxic therapy with cyclophosphamide, doxorubicin, and cisplatin, as well as trials of tamoxifen and megestrol. Her right pleural effusion eventually required sclerotherapy with tetracycline. Laparoscopy with liver biopsy showed no tumor involvement of the liver but suggested cirrhosis. Multiple sites of tumor studding were visualized on the peritoneum. Stem-cell assay of malignant cells in ascitic fluid showed resistance to fluorouracil, methotrexate, vinca alkaloids, and mitomycin. The patient was given three additional courses of cyclophosphamide and cisplatin, but she had increasing obstipation, and tumor progression was demonstrated by pelvic examination. She required frequent paracenteses to relieve her malignant ascites.

Her outpatient medications included both methadone hydrochloride (10 mg orally every six hours) and sustained-release morphine sulfate (120 mg orally every six hours) for severe pain caused by massive ascites and enlarging tumor. At the time of admission in 1986, the patient said her pain was adequately controlled. She had smoked one pack of cigarettes daily for 30 years and had consumed moderate amounts of alcohol in the past. She had no family history of cancer.

Physical examination showed active bowel sounds, with massively increased abdominal girth from ascites. There was intertriginous weeping in the lower abdomen, as well as 2+ pitting edema of the lower extremities. The rectal examination showed heme-negative stools, with an anterior rectal mass causing marked extrinsic compression.

Admission laboratory findings were remarkable

only for an unexplained hyponatremia (128 meq/L). Renal and hepatic laboratory findings were unremarkable: serum creatinine concentration 0.9 mg/dL, urea nitrogen 13 mg/dL, serum albumin 2.3 g/dL, alkaline phosphatase 193 IU/L, direct and total bilirubin 0.4 and 1.1 mg/dL, aspartate aminotransferase 48 IU/L, alanine aminotransferase 24 IU/L, and prothrombin time 12.3 seconds. A chest roentgenogram showed bilateral pleural effusions.

The patient was admitted for palliative intraperitoneal administration of cytarabine and cisplatin with intravenous sodium thiosulfate. The tumor did not respond, and continued massive ascites required repeated paracenteses. Because of total obstruction of the duodenum, a nasogastric tube with intermittent low suction was instituted. A central venous catheter, and later a Hickman catheter, was inserted to provide access for total parenteral nutrition (TPN).

Escalation of the patient's narcotic dosage was necessary during the hospitalization. Initially, the primary source of pain was the rapidly increasing ascites, which was relieved somewhat by paracenteses. Swelling of the liver capsule and bilateral lower rib pain also contributed to the patient's discomfort. She refused an epidural nerve block offered by the pain clinic.

After intravenous morphine sulfate boluses (20 mg every four hours) failed to provide adequate duration of analgesia, a continuous intravenous morphine sulfate infusion was begun at an initial rate of 3 mg/hr. Incremental escalation of the infusion rate by approximately 10% was performed by the nursing staff after a four- to six-hour assessment of pain relief. Nursing assessment included evaluating the patient's activity level and questioning as to her level of pain and her perception of the adequacy of her dose. Figure 1 demonstrates the upward titration of the morphine infusion rate.

When a rate of 32 mg/hr was reached, the pharmacy doubled the concentration to 2 mg/mL, but the change was not noticed by the nursing staff. This inadvertent doubling of the dosage to 64 mg/hr provided good analgesia and no apparent adverse effects. The patient was alert and reading when the error was discovered six hours later.

Morphine requirements later increased in a rather consistent fashion, despite repeated palliative paracenteses, suggesting a more visceral component of her pain. Her morphine sulfate requirements stabilized on day 20 at 248 mg/hr.

Informed, signed consent for testing for morphine concentrations in body fluids was obtained from the patient, after approval by the investigational review board. Samples of plasma, ascitic fluid, and nasogastric aspirate for morphine concentration determinations were collected during infusion rates of 140 and 248 mg/hr on infusion days 14 and 21, respectively. The pH of the nasogastric aspirate was not determined. Samples were centrifuged and frozen at −20 °C until assay.

Figure 1. Maximal daily morphine infusion rate (●—●) and minimum respiration rate (O—O) before and during intravenous morphine infusion. Patient received intravenous boluses of 20 mg of morphine sulfate on days −2 through 0.

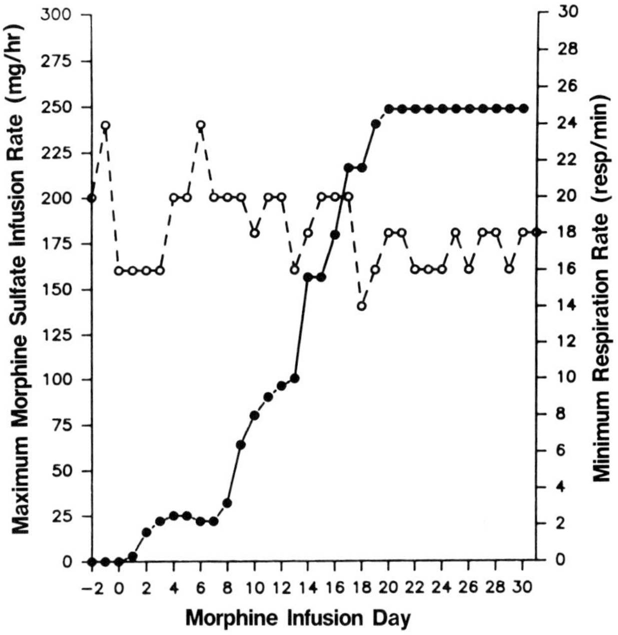

Multiple paracenteses (3.3–4.5 L over one hour) during the infusion, with rapid reaccumulation of ascitic fluid, did not require changes in the infusion rate. Although she remained bedfast, at no time during her morphine titration did the patient demonstrate serious adverse effects from the narcotic. She was not markedly sedated or hypotensive at any time, and her minimum respiration rate remained above 16/min, with one exception of 14/min (Figure 1). The patient was discharged on infusion day 31 with the same morphine infusion rate, TPN, and continuous nasogastric suction.

Although the patient was seen daily at home by a visiting nurse, some of her care was provided by a friend. At one point during the changing of the morphine infusion bag, the infusion rate was accidentally increased to deliver morphine sulfate at a rate of 1 g per hour. The patient reportedly became sleepy, but she apparently experienced no adverse effects other than recurrence of her pain when the 4 g of morphine sulfate infused unexpectedly early. Her pain remained controlled with morphine sulfate 248 mg/hr; she died two weeks after discharge.

Morphine Concentrations. At the time of analysis of specimens, morphine was extracted from the thawed body fluid samples by a double extraction method and assayed as previously described.[4] Morphine concentrations obtained at the two infusion rates are given in Table 1. Samples drawn when the infusion rate was 140 mg/hr do not represent steady state because of rapid escalation of the dose at the time. Systemic plasma clearance of morphine at 248 mg/hr was calculated by dividing the infusion rate by the plasma concentration; in Table 2, this result is compared with those from other reports.

Aspiration of an averge of 1.2 L of gastric contents daily when the infusion rate was 248 mg/hr removed an average of 6 mg of morphine, or approximately 0.1% of the amount of morphine infused each day. Paracenteses with drainage of 4 L of ascitic fluid at this infusion rate removed approximately 5 mg of morphine during each one-hour procedure.

Discussion. This case illustrates the extraordinarily high analgesic requirements of some patients with cancer. Remarkable in this patient was the complete lack of respiratory depression at any point during her inpatient titration of morphine. Only once did the respiration rate fall below 16 per minute, and no hypotension was noted. Favoring this patient's tolerance of the morphine may have been her lack of known respiratory or cardiovascular disease. Considering her lack of adequate pain relief on day 0 with 20-mg intravenous boluses of morphine sulfate every four hours, the initial infusion rate of 3 mg/hr should have been higher (120 mg per day by i.v. push = 5 mg/hr).

The morphine sulfate infusion rate of 248 mg/hr (4.8 mg/kg/hr) required for effective analgesia in this patient is not the highest that has been reported, but the final steady-state plasma concentration of 5400 ng/mL measured in our patient is, to our knowledge, the highest reported in the literature. Lo and Coleman[1] reported a case of a cancer patient who required a morphine sulfate infusion of 7.6–8.6 mg/kg/hr for pain control. Although interpatient variability in the clearance of morphine is substantial, it is likely that the plasma morphine concentration achieved in their patient was greater than those reported here. As with our patient, the infusion was well tolerated, with only minor lethargy and slowing of respirations. Other clinicians have similarly reported ranges for morphine sulfate infusion rates of 4–480 mg/hr[2] and 0.5–275 mg/hr.[3]

A comparison of morphine and heroin concentrations is made to illustrate the extremely high sustained morphine concentrations tolerated by our patient and other cancer patients treated with large intravenous doses of morphine. Postmortem plasma morphine concentrations in most cases of acute heroin overdosage have been reported to fall in the range of 100–900 ng/mL.[13,14] These comparisons suggest the possibility that toxicity of high-dose morphine may be attenuated by severe pain or opiate tolerance.

Systemic clearance of morphine has been shown to vary threefold, emphasizing the need for individual titration of the dose. The systemic clearance of morphine calculated at steady state in this patient (10.4 mL/min/kg) is slightly lower than previously reported mean values (Table 2), but it falls within the range of clearances described by other authors.[5-12] Although results of the patient's liver chemistry studies were normal, her mild cirrhosis may have decreased morphine clearance.

No change in morphine requirements occurred in our patient after large volumes of ascitic fluid were removed. Although the morphine concentra-

Table 1.
Morphine Concentrations (ng/mL)[a] during Intravenous Morphine Infusion

Fluid Sampled	Morphine Sulfate Infusion Rate (mg/hr) 140[b]	248
Plasma	1350	5400
Ascitic fluid	3000	1300
Nasogastric aspirate	1950	4950

[a] Concentration expressed as morphine base.
[b] Does not represent steady-state conditions.

Table 2.
Reported Systemic Morphine Clearance

Dosage and Route[a]	Systemic Clearance (mL/min · kg)	Subject Description	Reference
4.8 mg/kg/hr CI	10.4	44-year-old female cancer patient	Hutson et al.
0.2–4.7 mg/kg/hr CI	18.3 (11.2–24.2)[b]	4 adult cancer patients	Citron et al.[5]
0.03–0.07 mg/kg/hr CI	27.7 (22.7–36.7)	5 young male surgery patients	Sitar et al.[6]
0.02 μg/kg/hr CI	49.7 (14.5–25.6)	6 children postop	Bray et al.[7]
4 mg IVP	28.0 (18.6–34.0)	6 adult cancer patients	Sawe et al.[8]
0.1 mg/kg IVP	33.5 (18–44)	6 normal adult patients	Mazoit et al.[9]
0.1 mg/kg IVP	21.0 (11–33)	8 adult cirrhotic patients	Mazoit et al.[9]
15–25 mg IVP	17.4 (6.6–26.7)	9 adult cancer patients	Gourlay et al.[10]
10 mg IVP	14.7 (12.4–16.4)	8 healthy young male volunteers	Stanski et al.[11]
45–80 mg IVP	12.4 (9.4–14.6)	4 adult surgery patients	Stanski et al.[12]
1.0 mg/kg IVP	5.6 (3.1–10.6)	10 adult surgery patients	Stanski et al.[12]

[a] CI = continuous intravenous infusion; IVP = intravenous push.
[b] Mean (range).

tion in ascitic fluid was similar to that in plasma, the absolute amount of morphine removed was only 0.1% of the total daily dose. The amount of morphine removed by constant nasogastric suction (6 mg/day) was a similarly insubstantial amount. These findings indicate that no change in the rate of morphine infusion is necessary if nasogastric suction is discontinued or if a gastrointestinal obstruction is precipitously removed. Similarly, our data suggest that the "third-space" accumulation of morphine in massive ascites will not place the patient at risk of toxic effects from back-diffusion into the bloodstream.

A review of intravenous morphine infusions for cancer pain was recently published.[2] When a morphine infusion rate is considered inadequate, the authors recommend a 10–20% increase in rate along with an i.v. bolus of 15 to 30 mg as a loading dose at the time of each rate increase. Such boluses would likely have benefited this patient. However, when Sitar et al.[6] gave 1.0-mg/kg morphine sulfate boluses over 15 minutes to healthy men under controlled conditions, all subjects developed severe respiratory depression requiring mechanical ventilation. Morphine's short, 10-minute distribution half-life supports a splitting of the loading dose, as is done for lidocaine, to reduce the risk of opiate toxicity. Smaller (8–10 mg) i.v. boluses administered 10–20 minutes apart around the time of an increase in infusion rate are less likely to cause serious respiratory depression yet should not markedly affect the speed and degree of pain relief. Divided loading doses seem particularly prudent for home-care patients or inpatients in wards with irregular monitoring.

Citron et al.[15] have suggested criteria for monitoring toxicity in patients receiving morphine infusions. Arterial blood gas measurements are recommended for patients with preinfusion respiration rates of 20 per minute or less who manifest a $\geq$40% decrease in respiration rate accompanied by somnolence or clinical manifestations of hypoxia. Unfortunately, no clear correlation was found between changes in respiration rate and hypoxia in patients with baseline respiration rates greater than 20/min. A conservative approach would be to apply the criteria of respiration rate of 12 or less per minute with lethargy, clinical signs of hypoxia, or both, as an indication for examination of blood gases.

The use of naloxone to reverse moderate respiratory depression should be reserved for extremely somnolent or unresponsive patients. Consideration of its use must be tempered by the pain the patient will experience and the patient's overall clinical condition. Instead, when feasible, the morphine infusion should be held until the patient's mental status and respiration rate improve and then restarted at a lower rate.

Our experience with an inadvertent doubling of the infusion rate should serve as a reminder for pharmacists to explicitly inform the patient's nurse of each change of infusate concentration. Flow sheets including infusion rate, time of last rate change, morphine concentration in the i.v. bag, pain severity record, respiration rate, and mental status can contribute to the continuity of the patient's care and identify trends.

Conclusion. Assay of concurrently collected blood, gastric fluid, and ascitic fluid samples in a woman receiving morphine at a high infusion rate for chronic cancer pain did not support unusual clearance as a cause of high morphine requirements. Our data indicate that no morphine dosing changes are needed when nasogastric suctioning is begun or discontinued or in patients who have massive ascites. To corroborate these findings and to evaluate the effect of renal or hepatic dysfunction on the clearance of morphine at high infusion rates, additional studies of similar patients are desirable.

References

1. Lo SL, Coleman RR. Exceptionally high narcotic analgesic requirements in a terminally ill cancer patient. *Clin Pharm.* 1986; 5:828–32.
2. Portenoy RK, Moulin DE, Rodgers A et al. IV infusion of opioids for cancer pain: clinical review and guidelines for use. *Cancer Treat Rep.* 1986; 70:575–81.
3. DeChristoforo R, Cordon BJ, Hood JC et al. High dose morphine infusion complicated by chlorobutanol-induced somnolence. *Ann Intern Med.* 1983; 98:335–6.
4. Edwards DH, Popovski Z, Baumann TJ et al. Specific ^{125}I radioimmunoassay for morphine. *Clin Chem.* 1986; 32:157–8.
5. Citron ML, Reynolds JR, Lin WN et al. Clearance of continuous intravenous morphine for severe cancer pain. *Drug Intell Clin Pharm.* 1987; 21:981–5.
6. Sitar DS, Duke PC, Owen JA et al. Kinetic disposition of morphine in young males after intravenous loading and maintenance infusions. *Can Anaesth Soc J.* 1986; 33:145–59.
7. Bray RJ, Beeton MB, Hinton W et al. Plasma morphine levels produced by continuous infusion in children. *Anaesthesia.* 1986; 41:753–5.
8. Sawe J, Kager L, Svensson JO et al. Oral morphine in cancer patients: in vivo kinetics and in vitro hepatic glucuronidation. *Br J Clin Pharmacol.* 1985; 19:495–501.
9. Mazoit JX, Sandouk P, Zetlaoui P et al. Pharmacokinetics of unchanged morphine in normal and cirrhotic subjects. *Anesth Analg.* 1987; 66:293–8.
10. Gourlay GK, Cherry DA, Cousins MJ. A comparative study of the efficacy and pharmacokinetics of oral methadone and morphine in the treatment of severe pain in patients with cancer. *Pain.* 1986; 25:297–312.
11. Stanski DR, Greenblatt DJ, Lowenstein E. Kinetics of intravenous and intramuscular morphine. *Clin Pharmacol Ther.* 1978; 24:52–9.
12. Stanski DR, Greenblatt DJ, Lappas D et al. Kinetics of high-dose intravenous morphine in cardiac surgery patients. *Clin Pharmacol Ther.* 1976; 19:752–6.
13. Nakamura GR. Toxicologic assessments in acute heroin fatalities. *Clin Toxicol.* 1978; 13:75–85.
14. Garriott JC, Sturner WQ. Morphine concentrations and survival periods in acute heroin fatalities. *N Engl J Med.* 1973; 289:1276–8.
15. Citron ML, Johnston-Early A, Fossieck BE et al. Safety and efficacy of continuous intravenous morphine for severe cancer pain. *Am J Med.* 1984; 77:199–204.

Probable anaphylactoid reaction to a pyrethrin pediculocide shampoo

CHARLES A. CULVER, JOANNE J. MALINA, AND ROBERT L. TALBERT

Clin Pharm. 1988; 7:846–9

Infestation with head lice, pediculosis capitis, is reappearing as a common public health problem. Based on reports from the mid-1970s, a minimal annual occurrence of six million cases is projected.[1] According to epidemiologic reports, children of elementary school age have the highest incidence of infestation.[2–4]

Although infestation can occur across the spectrum of society, it predominates in the lower socioeconomic groups. Factors contributing to this prevalence include crowded conditions, bed sharing, and lower standards of hygiene.[2–4] Lack of physician accessibility to this population group probably contributes to the role self-treatment with nonprescription products has in the control of pediculosis. By one estimate, community pharmacists are asked to recommend an antilice preparation 12 times a month.[5]

Most nonprescription shampoo products available for head lice treatment have as their active ingredients natural pyrethrins (0.3%) with piperonyl butoxide (3–4%). Leading shampoo products marketed with these ingredients include A-200 Pyrinate (Norcliff Thayer, Tarrytown, NY), R & C Shampoo (Reed & Carnrick, Piscataway, NJ), Pronto (Commerce, Farmingdale, NY), and RID (Leeming, New York, NY).

Because of their superior effectiveness and less publicized toxic potential, pyrethrin with piperonyl butoxide products are becoming the preferred treatment over lindane for head lice. A recent clinical trial has shown pyrethrin products (RID, R & C Shampoo, and A-200 Pyrinate Liquid) to have lice-killing times of less than 30 minutes compared to three hours for 1% lindane shampoo (Kwell, Reed & Carnrick).[6] Piperonyl butoxide acts as a synergist to enhance the effectiveness of pyrethrin.[2] A potential problem with the use of lindane products is neurotoxicity, especially in premature infants.[7]

The natural pyrethrins are esters of chrysanthemumic acid from pyrethrum powder. Pyrethrum powder consists of dried flower extracts from chrysanthemum plants (*Chrysanthemum cinerariaefolium* Vis).[8] Because *Chrysanthemum* is in the same plant family as ragweed, a high index of cross-sensitivity exists between the two plants. Up to 40% of ragweed-sensitive patients may have a positive reaction to pyrethrum powder.[9]

The possibility of this cross-sensitivity occurring in people who are allergic to ragweed has prompted a warning in the package inserts of these products. For example, the warning heading for A-200 Pyrinate Liquid shampoo states "Not to be used by persons allergic to ragweed."

Pyrethrum has been reported to cause allergic rhinitis,[10] contact dermatitis,[8] hypersensitivity pneumonitis,[11] and chest tightness described as asthma.[10] We report a case in which a 43-year-old woman, with a history of asthma being exacerbated by insecticide sprays, molds, and ragweed, became hypotensive and unconscious after one application of A-200 Pyrinate Liquid shampoo for head lice. Periorbital edema appeared within one hour of application. Over the next nine hours the patient continued to deteriorate, finally requiring hospitalization for respiratory support. This appears to be the first case reported in the literature of an anaphylactoid reaction requiring respiratory support from the application of a pyrethrin-based product. It is unlikely that the piperonyl butoxide contained in the shampoo contributed to the reaction; piperonyl butoxide has minimal toxic effects, and hypersensitivity-type reactions have not been reported.[12]

An immunologically mediated reaction resulting from the cross-sensitivity of ragweed and pyrethrins does not appear to have occurred in this case. Therefore, we will also discuss the different mechanisms by which pyrethrins may have caused bronchoconstriction requiring respiratory support.

Case Report. At approximately 2200 on the evening before admission to the hospital, a 43-year-old white woman treated herself for head lice with A-200 Pyrinate Liquid shampoo. The patient stated that she applied the shampoo according to labeled directions, left the shampoo on her hair for 10 minutes, and rinsed after shampooing with regular shampoo. One hour after application, her eyes became "puffy," with a burning sensation.

At 0030 the day of admission, the patient summoned the emergency medical service (EMS) for treatment of her complaints. EMS personnel treated the patient by irrigating her eyes with 0.9%

CHARLES A. CULVER, PHARM.D., is Clinical Pharmacy Specialty Practice Resident in Adult Medicine, College of Pharmacy, The University of Texas at Austin, and Department of Pharmacology, The University of Texas Health Science Center at San Antonio (UTHSC). JOANNE J. MALINA, M.D., is Internal Medicine Resident, Department of Medicine, UTHSC. ROBERT L. TALBERT, PHARM.D., is Professor, College of Pharmacy, The University of Texas at Austin, and Department of Pharmacology, UTHSC.

Address reprint requests to Dr. Talbert at the Clinical Pharmacy Programs, The University of Texas Health Science Center at San Antonio, 7703 Floyd Curl Drive, San Antonio, TX 78284-7765.

Presented at the 40th Annual Seminar of the Texas Society of Hospital Pharmacists, Houston, TX, April 11, 1988.

Copyright © 1988, American Society of Hospital Pharmacists, Inc. All rights reserved. 0278-2677/88/1101-0846$01.00.

sodium chloride solution. Vital signs were as follows: blood pressure (BP), 140/88 mm Hg, sitting; pulse (P), 88 beats/minute; and respiratory rate (RR), 16 breaths/minute. The patient also reported subjective wheezing and shortness of breath, but the EMS technician attributed this to anxiety. After the irrigation, the patient's symptoms improved and EMS departed.

After the EMS departed, the patient began feeling weak, with increasing shortness of breath, for which she took one dose of terbutaline sulfate 5 mg orally. During the remaining early morning hours she was restless and could not sleep. At 0630 on the day of admission, EMS again responded because of the patient's symptoms. The patient complained of chest tightness, shortness of breath, dysphagia, numbness in the extremities, and "puffy, closed eyes." Initial vital signs were P, 120 beats/minute; RR, 20 breaths/ minute. The BP was not reported. The patient was alert and oriented to person, place, and time.

Because of the patient's progressive symptoms, EMS decided to transport the patient to the hospital for further evaluation. During EMS transport, the patient's level of consciousness deteriorated, and she became unresponsive. Therefore, oxygen was administered by face mask at 15 L/min. Vital signs at this time were BP, 118 mm Hg/palpable; P, 100 beats/minute; RR, 20 breaths/minute and labored. An electrocardiogram showed normal sinus rhythm.

The patient arrived in the emergency room at 0730. On examination the patient was unresponsive to verbal or painful stimuli. Vital signs in the emergency room were BP, 90/50 mm Hg; P, 100 beats/minute; RR, 22 breaths/minute and shallow. The only other important findings on physical examination were periorbital edema with mild injection and inflamed conjunctiva. Medications administered immediately included naloxone hydrochloride 2 mg i.v. administered twice, 50% dextrose injection 50 mL i.v., and epinephrine 0.5 mg administered twice subcutaneously. Initial laboratory data indicated a blood glucose concentration of 88 mg/dL. Endotracheal intubation was performed for airway maintenance, and 100% oxygen was administered.

Twenty minutes after arrival at the emergency room, the patient regained consciousness during the intubation procedure. The patient was then transferred to the intensive-care unit, where she remained on ventilator support for three hours. At 1030 the patient was extubated without complications. Admitting diagnoses indicated in the patient's hospital record were asthma and anaphylactoid reaction.

Medications begun in the intensive-care unit included aminophylline continuous infusion at 60 mg/hr (0.5 mg/kg/hr), albuterol sulfate inhalation solution 2.5 mg (of albuterol) every four hours via nebulizer, and methylprednisolone sodium succinate 125 mg (of methylprednisolone) i.v. every 12 hours. Intravenous medications were continued for 48 hours. After 48 hours, the patient was switched to oral sustained-release theophylline (Theo-Dur, Key Pharmaceuticals, Inc.) 400 mg every eight hours and oral prednisone 40 mg daily. Ampicillin sodium 1 g (of ampicillin) i.v. every six hours was also administered for chronic sinusitis but was discontinued after two days when sinus roentgenogram films were normal. The patient continued to improve in the hospital and was discharged four days after admission. Discharge medications were sustained-release theophylline 400 mg twice daily, a tapering dose of oral prednisone starting at 40 mg daily, and use of an albuterol metered-dose inhaler every six hours as needed.

Medical history obtained in the hospital revealed patient allergies to "sulfa drugs," perfumes, insecticide sprays, molds, ragweed, and pecan trees. The patient reported from experience only, since skin testing had never been performed. Allergic symptoms, as reported by the patient, were usually manifested by asthma attacks. The patient had had asthma since age six; oral theophylline, terbutaline, and inhaled metaproterenol had been prescribed for her condition. On admission her current regimen included oral terbutaline sulfate (5-mg tablets) and inhaled metaproterenol, both of which she took only as needed. The patient's last asthma attack had occurred five days before admission, and her last hospitalization for asthma and sinusitis had been two years previously. The patient denied exposure to ragweed before the onset of the reaction. Her medical history included the removal of nasal polyps in 1983 and 1985. The patient reported no aspirin sensitivity.

Discussion. Considering the time course of development and the failure to do an immunologic investigation, this hypersensitivity-type reaction is best described as an anaphylactoid reaction rather than anaphylaxis. Anaphylaxis is a life-threatening, immunologically mediated reaction that usually occurs within 15 minutes after exposure to the antigen.[13] The longest interval reported from exposure to the antigen to the occurrence of anaphylaxis is two to three hours.[14] There should also be laboratory evidence confirming immunoglobulin E antibody involvement for a reaction to be categorized as anaphylaxis.[15] The radioallergosorbent test (RAST) or wheal and flare skin testing can detect the presence of antigen-specific immunoglobulin E antibody.[14,16] Anaphylactoid reactions are non-antibody-mediated reactions, apparently involving the same or pharmacologically similar mediators.[17]

Anaphylaxis or anaphylactoid reactions produce clinically indistinguishable manifestations.[13] Common manifestations observed in this patient include periorbital edema, difficulty in breathing, chest tightness, hypotension, and loss of consciousness.

Hypersensitivity-type reactions such as bronchospasm, upper-airway edema, and hypotension caused by vasodilation are mediated by the release of pharmacologically active substances from the degranulation of mast cells or basophils. In a true anaphylactic reaction, cellular degranulation can be activated by the combination of antigen with immunoglobulin E antibodies on the cell surfaces of mast cells and basophils. In nonimmunologically mediated reactions, activating systems can be the complement system, the coagulation and fibrinolytic systems, and the kinin-generating systems.[13]

Pharmacologically active substances (mediators) released from mast cells or basophils include histamine, slow-reacting substance of anaphylaxis (SRS-A), eosinophilic chemotactic factor of anaphylaxis (ECF-A), leukotrienes, kinins, and prostaglandins.[13] SRS-A, an important mediator of bronchospasm in patients with extrinsic asthma, is comprised of leukotrienes C4, D4, and E4.[18] Two of these leukotrienes (C4, D4) have been shown to be 4000 times more potent than histamine on a molar basis for inducing bronchospasm in healthy humans, as evaluated by pulmonary function tests.[18]

Until recently, documentation of asthma being triggered by pyrethrum was limited to case reports from 1923 and 1930.[10] Newton and Breslin[10] have provided more recent evidence in a controlled trial in which seven patients with a history of asthma were exposed to an insecticide spray containing pyrethrin 0.3% and 1.5% piperonyl butoxide. These patients also had a positive history for chest tightness on exposure to aerosol insecticide sprays. In the trial all seven patients complained of "asthma-like" chest tightness, which lasted up to one hour after challenge. In spite of these subjective complaints, a 20% or greater decrease in forced expired volume in one second (FEV_1) occurred in only one patient. Consequently, this study provides little understanding of pyrethrin's mechanism in causing these symptoms.

The mechanism of action of pyrethrins in provoking asthma attacks remains unclear. One hypothesis may be that pyrethrin-induced epithelial damage stimulates irritant receptors to produce cough, bronchoconstriction, and hyperpnea via a vagal reflex. These irritant receptors are myelinated sensory fibers within the epithelium of the tracheobronchial tree.[10,19] Inhaled allergens can also induce β-adrenergic-receptor blockade.[20] Inhaled pyrethrins may also act likewise.

A most likely hypothesis is from evidence that nonallergic bronchial reactivity can be increased by allergen exposure. Cockcroft et al.[20] demonstrated that allergens such as ragweed can increase the reactivity of the bronchial airways to histamine. Bronchial reactivity was determined by the concentration of histamine needed to produce a 20% decrease in FEV_1. This increase in bronchial reactivity persisted for up to seven days in 7 of 13 patients. This prolonged increase in bronchial reactivity to histamine may account for the time course of symptomatology in our patient. In fact, four patients in Cockcroft's study had greater than 15% decreases in FEV_1 up to eight hours after inhalation of the allergens. Pyrethrins, like ragweed, probably are capable of stimulating an increase in bronchial reactivity to histamine.

Mitchell et al.[8] provide further evidence for this not being a cross-sensitivity reaction between ragweed and pyrethrins. These investigators reported that pyrethrins I and II are only weakly allergenic themselves, as evidenced by a negative patch test response to pyrethrin I and only a weak positive response to pyrethrin II in a patient allergic to pyrethrum. Pyrethrins I and II are mixtures of pyrethrin, clinerin, and jasmolin, the insecticidal constituents of pyrethrum. Mitchell et al. reported that the principal allergenic compound in pyrethrum, pyrethrosin, which is structurally similar to the compound in ragweed that causes sensitivity reactions, is unlikely to be present in commercially refined pyrethrum.

Nonetheless, a possible pyrethrum and ragweed cross-sensitivity existing in a patient has been reported in a case in which hypersensitivity pneumonitis occurred after repeated exposures to a pyrethrum-based insecticide (Raid, S. C. Johnson & Sons, Inc., Racine, WI).[11] After the patient was discharged, a pyrethrum-challenge test was performed. The test reproduced the pulmonary symptoms, confirming this pyrethrum and pneumonitis relationship. The patient also had a concurrent positive radioallergosorbent test to western ragweed.

In summary, the delayed development of the more severe manifestations of this reaction suggests a nonimmunologically mediated mechanism rather than classic anaphylaxis. The mechanism of pyrethrin-induced bronchospasm is yet to be clearly delinated. The most likely explanation is that the pyrethrins acted as an inhaled allergen to cause an increase in bronchial reactivity to histamine. Other possible pyrethrin actions include stimulation of irritant receptors in the tracheobronchial tree, SRS-A activation, or β-adrenergic-receptor blockade.

Conclusion. Patients who are sensitive to airborne allergens such as ragweed are susceptible to anaphylactoid reactions, manifested by severe bronchospasm and hypotension, when they are exposed to pyrethrin products. Pharmacists and other health professionals should be aware of this potential reaction, since nonprescription pyrethrin-based products are becoming the preferred treatment for head lice. Consequently, a complete patient allergy history is essential before pyrethrin-based products can be recommended for the treatment of pediculosis.

References

1. Taplin D, Castillero PM, Spiegel J et al. Malathion for treatment of *Pediculus humanus* var. *capitis* infestation. *JAMA*. 1982; 247:3103–5.
2. Rasmussen JE. Pediculosis and the pediatrician. *Pediatr Dermatol*. 1984; 2:74–9.
3. Slonka GF, McKinley TW, McCroan JE et al. Epidemiology of an outbreak of head lice in Georgia. *Am J Trop Med Hyg*. 1976; 25:739–43.
4. Billstein S, Laone P. Demographic study of head lice infestation in Sacramento County school children. *Int J Dermatol*. 1979; 18:301–4.
5. Reis L. What OTC products do pharmacists recommend in 50 categories? *Pharm Times*. 1987; 53(Sep):40–60.
6. Meinking TL, Taplin D, Kalter DC et al. Comparative efficacy of treatments for pediculosis capitis infestations. *Arch Dermatol*. 1986; 122:267–71.
7. Davies JE, Dedhia HV, Morgade C et al. Lindane poisonings. *Arch Dermatol*. 1983; 119:142–4.
8. Mitchell JC, Dupuis G, Towers GHN. Allergic contact dermatitis from pyrethrum (*Chrysanthemum* spp.). The roles of pyrethrosin, a sesquiterpene lactone, and of pyrethrin II. *Br J Dermatol*. 1972; 86:568–73.
9. Zucker, A. Investigation of purified pyrethrum extracts. *Ann Allergy*. 1965; 23:335–9.
10. Newton JG, Breslin ABX. Asthmatic reactions to a commonly used aerosol insect killer. *Med J Aust*. 1983; 1:378–80.
11. Carlson JE, Villaveces JW. Hypersensitivity pneumonitis due to pyrethrum. Report of a case. *JAMA*. 1977; 237:1718–9.
12. Rumack BH, ed. Poisindex. Vol. 57. Denver: Micromedex Inc., 1988.
13. Levy JH, Roizen MF, Morris JM. Anaphylactic and anaphylactoid reactions. A review. *Spine*. 1986; 11:282–91.
14. Stark BJ, Sullivan TJ. Biphasic and protracted anaphylaxis. *J Allergy Clin Immunol*. 1986; 78:76–83.
15. Watkins J. Anaphylactoid reactions to I.V. substances. *Br J Anaesth*. 1979; 51:51–60.
16. Wide L. Clinical significance of measurement of reaginic (IgE) antibody by RAST. *Clin Allergy*. 1973; 3:583–95.
17. Parker CW. Systemic anaphylaxis. In: Parker CW, ed. Clinical immunology. Vol. 2. Philadelphia: W. B. Saunders; 1980: 1208–18.
18. Austen KF. Tissue mast cells in immediate hypersensitivity. *Hosp Pract*. 1982; 17(Nov):98–108.
19. Empey DW, Laitinen LA, Jacobs L et al. Mechanisms of bronchial hyperreactivity in normal subjects after upper respiratory tract infection. *Am Rev Respir Dis*. 1976; 113:131–9.
20. Cockcroft DW, Ruffin RE, Dolovich J et al. Allergen-induced increase in non-allergic bronchial reactivity. *Clin Allergy*. 1977; 7:503–13.

Special offer for ASHP Members

IPA International Pharmaceutical Abstracts

International Pharmaceutical Abstracts provides information on a variety of topics ranging from drug interactions, new drugs, and investigational drugs to educational, management and reimbursement issues.

Also, *IPA* has complete coverage of the cosmetic industry publications.

IPA helps you to keep up-to-date with what's happening in pharmacy—with access to information on topics such as biopharmaceutics, drug diversion, pharmaceutical technology, and institutional practice.

This service publishes 22 abstracted/indexed issues per year, plus two semi-annual subject/author indexes. Abstracts are classified into 25 sections.

If you want to keep up with health-care literature on computers, home health care, pharmacy crime, group purchasing, drug development . . . you only need *one source of information . . . International Pharmaceutical Abstracts* is the key to these articles.

Payments to ASHP are not deductible as charitable contributions for Federal Income Tax purposes. However, they may be deductible under other provisions of the Internal Revenue Code.

Now, just $100 for a one year subscription

☐ Yes! Please enter ______ subscription(s) to *International Pharmaceutical Abstracts* at $100.00 per year ($125.00 outside the U.S.)

☐ I am enclosing $120.00 to cover overseas airmail.

☐ Enclosed is my check for $__________. (Checks must be drawn on a U.S. bank and made payable to ASHP.)

Charge $______________ to ☐ MasterCard ☐ VISA

Account #______________ Exp. __________

Signature ______________________

Name ______________________

ASHP I.D.# ______________________

Address ______________________

City ______________ State __________ Zip __________

American Society of Hospital Pharmacists
4630 Montgomery Avenue
Bethesda, MD 20814

© 1988 *American Society of Hospital Pharmacists*

Harvard Health... Pride

Clinical Pharmacist

This is a challenging opportunity in which you will perform clinical, consultative and analytical functions for HCHP clinicians and pharmacists. Your work in these areas will contribute to quality assurance activities related to the Pharmacy Program operations and drug utilization review. The qualified candidate will possess 3-5 years' experience in a clinical setting, and a degree in Pharm.D, as well as an MS or Ph.D. or equivalent Mass. licensure required.

Harvard Health provides competitive compensation and a full spectrum of benefits. Professional employees receive 3 weeks' vacation to start, 4 weeks after 2 years, and 11½ paid holidays per year. To join New England's leading HMO, send your resume to Alyce Johnson, Harvard Community Health Plan, Human Resources, 10 Brookline Place West, Brookline, MA 02146.

An Equal Opportunity Employer

Harvard Community Health Plan

Consumer Drug Digest
Revised Edition

Consumer Drug Digest, Revised Edition, is a comprehensive, authoritative guide to common prescription and non-prescription drugs . . . helping patients to understand their medications and learn what they can do to be more aware of their drug therapy.

Written in layman's language, this drug information handbook contains over 250 of the most commonly prescribed drugs, which comprise over 95% of prescriptions written in the U.S. today. ***Consumer Drug Digest*** is easy to read and use. And, it's indexed by both brand names and generic names, so it's easy to locate information.

The ***Consumer Drug Digest*** is an excellent tool for patients and for pharmacy services areas.

Order your copy today.

☐ Please send me a brochure on **Consumer Drug Digest**

Name ______________________

Address ______________________

City ____________ State ________ Zip ________

Send to: ASHP Publication Records Dept.,
4630 Montgomery Avenue, Bethesda, MD 20814

Our online databases

stand alone

in drug information.

ASHP® databases help you to locate a wide scope of drug information, including fulltext drug monographs, patient counseling information and abstracts of articles.

Drug Information Fulltext®

The DIF database contains detailed, comprehensive drug information representing over 50,000 marketed drug products.

Consumer Drug Information™

CDIF is a fulltext database with descriptions written for the patient's understanding. More than 3,000 brand name drug products are covered.

International Pharmaceutical Abstracts®

The IPA database is the practical, efficient way of locating information from over 800 pharmaceutical, medical, cosmetic and other health-related journals throughout the world. IPA's abstract/indexing system works to help you easily locate the information.

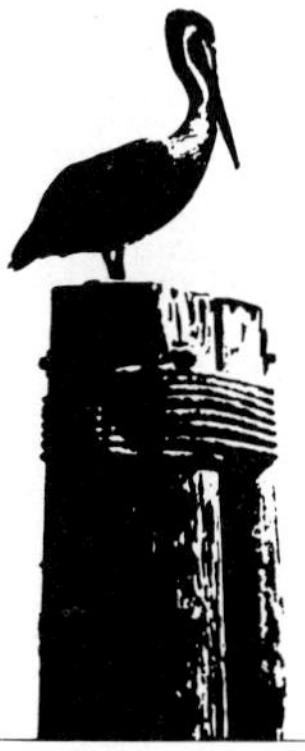

ASHP databases are available around the world through international online computer systems. For a brochure or more information, contact ASHP's Database Services at 301-657-3000, or write to:

Payments to ASHP are not deductible as charitable contributions for Federal Income Tax purposes. However, they may be deductible under other provisions of the Internal Revenue Code.

ASHP Database Services
4630 Montgomery Avenue
Bethesda, MD 20814

This space contributed as a public service.

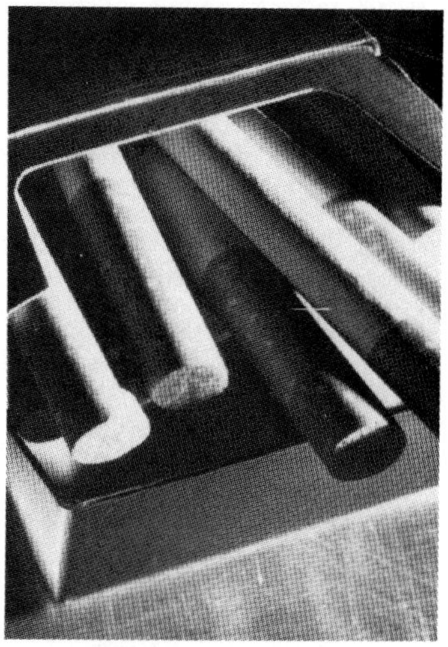

Pack of Lies.

The Great American Smokeout. Nov. 17.

AMERICAN CANCER SOCIETY®

CP Continuing Education

The ASHP Continuing Education system gives readers a self-assessment mechanism for selected articles in Clinical Pharmacy *and the* American Journal of Hospital Pharmacy. *It also allows readers to obtain continuing-education credit for these articles.*

For the purpose of CE-credit enrollment a blank answer sheet is published at the end of each installment of the column for the CE articles in that issue. An enrollee accumulates these answer sheets until the enrollment is submitted, using the form that is published in the June and December issues of Clinical Pharmacy *and in the June and December issues of the* American Journal of Hospital Pharmacy. *Any combination of tests within a 18-month period, from both* Clinical Pharmacy *and* American Journal of Hospital Pharmacy, *may be included in an enrollment. More complete details about enrollment in the system will appear in the semiannual enrollment form.*

Article 680-204-8817 (see page 795)
Qualifies for 1.0 hour of CE credit

Biological mechanisms and cardiovascular effects of omega-3 fatty acids

Learning Objectives

After studying this article, the reader should be able to

1. List the effects that the omega-3 fatty acids commonly have on very low density lipoprotein (VLDL), low-density lipoprotein (LDL), high-density lipoprotein (HDL), and triglycerides.
2. Identify variables that should be monitored when omega-3 fatty acid supplementation is instituted.
3. List at least three mechanisms by which omega-3 fatty acids may reduce the risk of coronary artery disease.
4. Differentiate the effects of a diet rich in omega-3 fatty acid versus a Western diet on prostaglandin and leukotriene formation.
5. Describe the epidemiological evidence for the use of omega-3 fatty acids to treat a variety of disease states.

Self-assessment Questions

1. Lipoprotein changes usually observed with omega-3 fatty acid administration are

   a. Increased VLDL and LDL, unpredictable HDL changes.
   b. Decreased VLDL, unpredictable LDL and HDL changes.
   c. Decreased VLDL, increased LDL and HDL.
   d. Increased HDL, unpredictable VLDL and LDL changes.

2. Greenlandic Eskimos have been found to have a higher incidence of

   a. Diabetes mellitus.
   b. Psoriasis.
   c. Acute myocardial infarction.
   d. Epilepsy.
   e. Asthma.

3. Which of the following is not a potential mechanism by which omega-3 fatty acids affect coronary heart disease?

   a. Decreased monocyte adherence to vessel endothelium.
   b. Increased blood viscosity.
   c. Increased leukotriene B_5 production.
   d. Decreased platelet aggregability.

4. A proposed mechanism for hypotriglyceridemic effects of omega-3 fatty acids is

   a. Increased VLDL synthesis in the liver.
   b. Changed VLDL molecule conformation.
   c. Decreased gastrointestinal absorption of fatty acids.
   d. Increased lipolytic enzyme activity.

5. The hypolipidemic effects of omega-3 fatty acids were not fully appreciated in early studies because

   a. Niacin consumption was not controlled.
   b. Omega-3 fatty acid preparations were rancid.
   c. Vitamin E deficiency developed.
   d. Omega-3 fatty acid preparations contained cholesterol.
   e. Doses of omega-3 fatty acids used were too small.

6. Which of the following effects is not associated with omega-3 fatty acid consumption?

   a. Thrombocytopenia.
   b. Lengthened bleeding time.
   c. Increased LDL concentration.
   d. Cataract formation.
   e. Nausea.

7. Which fish is not rich in omega-3 fatty acids?

   a. Cod.
   b. Salmon.
   c. Herring.
   d. Mackerel.

8. Substantial amounts of omega-3 fatty acids are found in all of these except

   a. Human breast milk.
   b. Chicken egg yolks.
   c. Black walnuts.
   d. Canned albacore tuna.

9. A diet enriched by omega-3 fatty acids results in an increased production of

   a. Thromboxane A_2.
   b. Leukotriene B_4.
   c. Prostacyclin.
   d. Prostaglandin I_3.

10. The ideal placebo for use in trials examining omega-3 fatty acid effects on lipids is

   a. Olive oil.
   b. Corn oil.
   c. Safflower oil.
   d. Linseed oil.
   e. A blend of oils.

Answer sheet

November 1988 ***Clinical Pharmacy***

Note: An enrollment form for the ASHP Continuing-Education System appears in the June and December issues. Please accumulate all the answer sheets you wish to use in one enrollment and submit them at one time with a completed enrollment form.

Place an X in the box(es) at the top of the column(s) corresponding to the test(s) you are taking. Darken the boxes corresponding to the correct answers.

☐
680-204-8817
1.0 hour

	a	b	c	d	e		a	b	c	d	e
1.	☐	☐	☐	☐		6.	☐	☐	☐	☐	☐
2.	☐	☐	☐	☐	☐	7.	☐	☐	☐	☐	
3.	☐	☐	☐	☐		8.	☐	☐	☐	☐	
4.	☐	☐	☐	☐		9.	☐	☐	☐	☐	
5.	☐	☐	☐	☐	☐	10.	☐	☐	☐	☐	☐

ASHP Use Only
(1.0)8817______(3)

Enhance your clinical practice skills and earn CE credit with a new self-study course from ASHP

Concepts in Clinical Pharmacokinetics

A Self-Instructional Course

Written by a trio of pharmacy professors, this book provides an orientation to pharmacokinetic concepts and procedures. It can help prepare you for pharmacokinetics courses of instruction, or serve as a handy reference and refresher course. With it you can earn up to 20 hours of ACPE-approved continuing education credit.

Input topics include:
- therapeutic drug monitoring
- compartmental models
- clearance
- volume of distribution
- loading dose
- elimination rate constant

Order your copy today!

The American Society of Hospital Pharmacists is approved by the American Council on Pharmaceutical Education as a provider of continuing pharmaceutical education.

Order Form
Concepts in Clinical Pharmacokinetics: A Self-Instructional Course (P275); 1988; approx. 150 pp; $50.00

☐ Please send me _____ copies of ***Concepts in Clinical Pharmacokinetics: A Self-Instructional Course*** (P275) at $50.00 each; 1988; 140 pp.

☐ Enclosed is my check for $__________. (Checks must be drawn on a U.S. bank and made payable to ASHP.)

☐ Enclosed is our purchase order #__________; please issue an invoice and add postage and handling.

Charge $__________ to my ☐ VISA ☐ MasterCard
Account #____________________
Exp. ________ *month/year* Signature ________________
Name ____________________
Institution ____________________
Address ____________________
City ____________ State ____ Zip ________
ASHP ID #____________________

Send to: ASHP Publications Records Dept.
4630 Montgomery Avenue
Bethesda, MD 20814

Payments to ASHP are not deductible as charitable contributions for Federal Income Tax purposes. However, they may be deductible under other provisions of the Internal Revenue Code.

© 1988 American Society of Hospital Pharmacists

Current Literature

Drug Reaction Alerts

Drug Reaction Alerts focuses primarily on serious, unlabeled reactions to new chemical entities. The citations are compiled monthly from International Pharmaceutical Abstracts, *which covers over 800 pharmacy and health-related journals worldwide. An address for reprints (when available) follows the name of the corresponding author in each citation.*

Analgesics and Antipyretics

Deakin M (Queen Elizabeth Hospital, Birmingham B15 2TH, England). Small bowel perforation associated with an excessive dose of slow release **diclofenac** sodium. *Br Med J*. 1988; 297:488–9. Case. (70-year-old man; received sustained-action diclofenac sodium 100 mg four times daily; developed perforation of ileum; uneventful recovery after surgical treatment)

Hoskin PJ, Hanks GW, White ID (Continuing Care Unit, Royal Marsden Hospital, Sutton, Surrey SM2 5PT, England). Sterile abscess formation by continuous subcutaneous infusion of **diamorphine**. *Br Med J*. 1988; 296:1605. Case. (two women with cancer pain, aged 70 and 42 years; received continuous subcutaneous injection of diacetylmorphine hydrochloride 30 mg/hr increasing to 100 mg/hr over 22 days, and diacetylmorphine hydrochloride 83.3 mg/hr increasing to 200 mg/hr, respectively; developed sterile abscesses at injection sites)

Androgens

Gately LE, Andes WA (Tulane University School of Medicine, New Orleans, LA 70112). **Danazol** and erythema multiforme. *Ann Intern Med*. 1988; 109:85. Cases. (67-year-old woman with thrombocytopenia and 49-year-old man; received danazol 600 mg/day; concomitant prednisone; developed erythema multiforme; resolution after danazol withdrawal and corticosteroid therapy)

Drugs, Adverse Reactions

Mahler JC, Perry S, Sutton B (New York Hospital–Cornell Medical Center, New York, NY). Intraurethral **cocaine** administration. *JAMA*. 1988; 259:3126. Case. (34-year-old man; injected cocaine into urethra; developed priapism, paraphimosis, disseminated intravascular coagulation, and extensive tissue necrosis; therapy with heparin, hydrocortisone, tobramycin, nafcillin, mezlocillin, blood transfusions, and surgical debridement unsuccessful; both lower legs and nine fingers amputated)

Moore B, Safani M, Keesey J (Department of Pharmacy, Memorial Medical Center, Long Beach, CA 90801). Possible exacerbation of myasthenia gravis by **ciprofloxacin**. *Lancet*. 1988; 1:882. Case. (39-year-old woman with history of myasthenia gravis; received ciprofloxacin 500–750 mg twice daily for upper respiratory tract infection; developed extreme shortness of breath and generalized weakness of limbs and neck muscles; respiratory status stabilized and strength increased after dosage reduced to 500 mg twice daily; pulmonary distress and muscle weakness recurred when dosage increased to 750 mg twice daily)

Drug Interactions

Sherman B, Panacek EA. Lactic acidosis and insulin resistance associated with epinephrine in a patient with noninsulin dependent diabetes mellitus: response. *Arch Intern Med*. 1988; 148:1879. Case. (22-year-old man with acquired immunodeficiency syndrome and ventricular tachycardia; received intravenous infusion of **isoproterenol** 4 μg/min and **insulin** 2 IU/hr; concomitant pentamidine and zidovudine; developed lactic acidosis, which worsened with increase in isoproterenol dosage; mild improvement after therapy with sodium bicarbonate 2000 meq; acidosis resolved after withdrawal of isoproterenol)

Davenport A, Will EJ, Davison AM et al. (Ironside JW, Department of Renal Medicine, St. James's University Hospital, Leeds LS9 7TF, England). Toxicity of **cyclosporin** metabolites. *Lancet*. 1988; 2:333. Case. (45-year-old woman; received erythromycin i.v. on admission and cyclosporine 400 mg and prednisolone 15 mg after renal allograft transplantation; developed neurotoxicity and died; cyclosporine concentration 120–145 ng/mL at necropsy)

Hypotensive Agents

Farraye FA, Peppercorn MA, Steer ML et al. (Rees M, Beth Israel Hospital, Harvard Medical School, Boston, MA). Acute small bowel mucosal edema following **enalapril** use. *JAMA*. 1988; 259:3131. Case. (41-year-old woman with hypertension; received single dose of enalapril 5 mg; concomitant conjugated estrogens; developed edema of mucosa and submucosa of small bowel; recovery without specific therapy; no rechallenge)

Immunosuppressive Agents

Saxen H, Heikinheimo M, Rajantie J (Aurora Hospital, Nordenskioldinkatu 20, 00250 Helsinki, Finland). Listeriosis associated with **antithymocyte globulin** treatment. *Lancet*. 1988; 2:280. Case. (nine-year-old boy with aplastic anemia; received antithymocyte globulin 20 mg/kg/day; developed septicemia and meningitis; rapid improvement after therapy with ampicillin for 10 days, and lymphocyte count rose to $2.3 \times 10^9/L$)

Bergman SM, Krane NK, Leonard G et al. (Wallin JD, Tulane University School of Medicine, New Orleans, LA 70112). **Azathioprine** and hypersensitivity vasculitis. *Ann Intern Med*. 1988; 109:83–4. Cases. (two men with renal failure, aged 32 and 56 years; received azathioprine as long-term therapy or in single doses; developed vasculitis; vasculitis resolved after azathioprine withdrawn, with one patient requiring corticosteroid treatment for two weeks; positive rechallenge)

Thyroid Drugs

Paul TL, Kerrigan J, Kelly AM et al. (Braverman LE, Division of Endocrinology and Metabolism, Department of Medicine, University of Massachusetts Medical School, Worcester, MA

01605). Long term **L-thyroxine** therapy is associated with decreased hip bone density in premenopausal women. *JAMA*. 1988; 259:3137–41. Study. (matched control; 31 premenopausal women with hypothyroidism, aged 19–41 years, compared with 31 age- and weight-matched women without bone or thyroid abnormalities; hypothyroid patients received levothyroxine 100–300 μg/day for 5–23 years; hypothyroid patients had 12.8% lower bone density at femoral neck, 10.1% lower bone density at femoral trochanter, and similar bone density in lumbar spine)

Vaccines

Nabe–Nielsen J, Walter B (Aalborg Hospital, DK-9000 Aalborg, Denmark). Unilateral deafness as a complication of the mumps, measles, and rubella vaccination. *Br Med J*. 1988; 297:489. Case. (seven-year-old girl; received **measles, mumps, and rubella vaccine**; developed unilateral deafness; no change in auditory status 11 months after vaccination)

Book Review

The Merck Manual, Fifteenth Edition

Robert Berkow, Editor-in-Chief.

Published by Merck Sharp & Dohme Research Laboratories, Rahway, NJ 07065-0900, 1987. xxvii + 2696 p. Price $21.50.

The first edition of *The Merck Manual* appeared in 1899. It was small enough to fit into a standard-sized laboratory coat pocket, weighed less than a pound, and was only 6 ¾ inches in length, 4 ½ inches in width, and ½ inch (262 pages) thick. Its principal literary contribution was in the area of rational drug therapy. In fact, the *Manual* was specifically designed to serve as an unbiased source of drug information for the general medical practitioner, "to make him at once master of the situation and enable him to prescribe exactly what his judgement tells him is needed for the occasion."

Today, in its 15th edition, the *Manual* is 8 inches long, 5 ½ inches wide, and two inches thick (2696 pages), and weighs 2 pounds, 5 ½ ounces. It has long since outgrown its original pocket-sized dimensions, but it continues to provide useful information regarding the rational treatment of common medical disorders.

The current edition of the *Manual* also serves as a helpful guide to diagnosis. There are numerous discussions of signs and symptoms, clinical procedures and laboratory tests, and technological maneuvers that aid the clinician in making a correct diagnosis.

In addition to the information provided on diagnosis and therapy, the manual provides a brief review of the etiology, pathology, incidence, and prognosis of a wide variety of medical disorders. It also contains a section on clinical pharmacology and a section on special subjects that features such topics as geriatric medicine, aids for disabled patients, nuclear medicine, and reference guides for calculating dosages for infants and children.

The Merck Manual is a well-written text that has been organized according to organ systems, etiology, and medical disciplines. It is a carefully orchestrated rendition of the words of 269 authors who revised their manuscripts at least six times before the finished product went to press. The making of a new edition of *The Merck Manual* is indeed a tedious process that now comes to fruition about every five years. Herein lies a potential weakness. The development of new diagnostic and therapeutic interventions springs forth so rapidly that textbooks with prolonged intervals between each edition are always incomplete in some areas. The 15th edition of *The Merck Manual* is no exception. For example, it bears no information about guanfacine, terazosin, lisinopril, lovastatin, the quinolone antibiotics, encainide, and flecainide, just to name a few of the newer therapeutic agents now included in our treatment armamentarium.

This inevitable deficiency notwithstanding, *The Merck Manual* remains a valuable, relatively inexpensive reference for both pharmacy students and pharmacists. It has an extensive index that contains many cross-references for medical disorders and treatments. The discussions are concise, easily understood, instructive, and helpful to the health-care practitioner who is organizing thoughts about clinical problems.

I think it is fair to say that pharmacists would prefer a more comprehensive, more frequently updated source of drug information for addressing drug therapy questions and issues. The *Manual* best serves pharmacy as a practical source of information regarding clinical presentation and diagnosis of medical disorders. Given its current dimensions, weight, and cost, *The Merck Manual* may be too big for your coat pocket, but it is not too expensive for your pocketbook.

Reviewed by David W. Hawkins, Pharm.D., UGA/MCG Clinical Pharmacy Program, The Medical College of Georgia, CN-137, Augusta, GA 30912.

Advertising Index

American Cancer Society
Institutional, 787
American College of Clinical Pharmacy
Call for Abstracts, 788
American Society of Hospital Pharmacists
Database Services, 787
ASHP Membership, 794
Concepts in Clinical Pharmacokinetics, 852
Consumer Drug Digest, 787
Handbook on Injectable Drugs, Fifth Edition, 850
International Pharmaceutical Abstracts, 849
Resource Book on Progressive Pharmaceutical Services, 793
Eli Lilly and Company
Nebcin, 789–790
Harvard Community Health Plan
Position Available, 787
Roxane Laboratories Inc., A Boehringer Ingelheim Company
Intensols, inside front cover
Marinol, inside back cover, outside back cover
San Antonio State School
Position Available, 793
St. Luke's Hospital of New Bedford
Position Available, 788
The University of Illinois at Chicago
Positions Available, 788
The Upjohn Company
Cleocin Phosphate, 783–784

CU trouble spot: IG drug administration

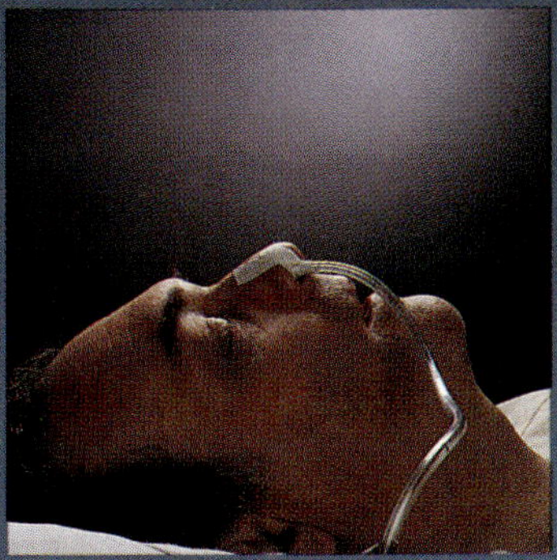

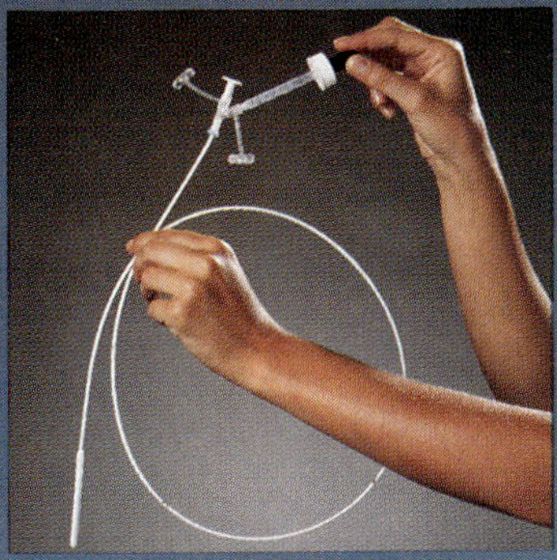

e solution is INTENSOLS™ oncentrated Oral Solutions

DEXAMETHASONE . . . . . . 1 mg/mL
PROPRANOLOL . . . . . . 80 mg/mL
PREDNISONE . . . . 5 mg/mL
DIAZEPAM . . . . 5 mg/mL

PALLIATIVE CARE AND CANCER PAIN PRODUCTS

Roxane Laboratories, Inc.
Columbus, Ohio 43216

nplifies drug ministration to sogastric patients

rsing benefits

- minates crushing tablets or dissolving apsules
- ore accurate and consistent dose
- on't clog NG tubes
- aves nursing time for more productive atient care activities

armacy benefits

- orrect dose is administered and osorbed by the patient
- ushing of sustained-release, sublingual, enteric-coated tablets is minimized
- ug/drug and acid/base interactions in ortar are avoided

sy to dispense

ach bottle comes with a calibrated opper for accurate dosing and ration. Administering directly into NG be is possible.

Ideal for patients who have difficulty swallowing tablets

- Geriatric, pediatric, and cancer patients on high or variable doses
- Mixable with soft foods or liquids; most Intensols are tasteless so they won't alter the flavor
- Easy to swallow for improved compliance

Many Intensol-formulated drugs are available

- Prednisone, dexamethasone, diazepam, propranolol, and more
- Easy to switch from injectables to orals

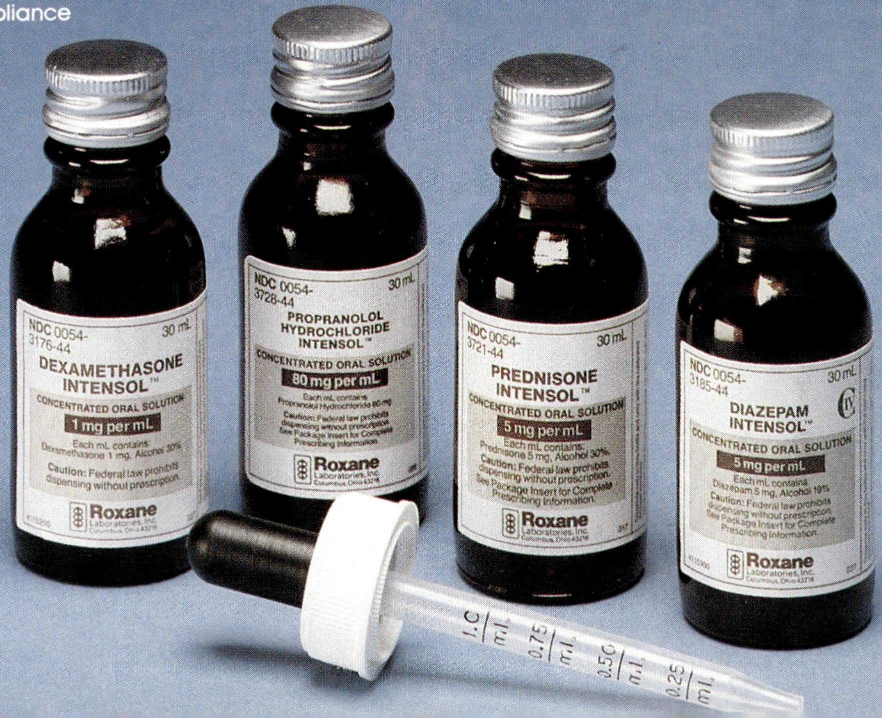

NTENSOLS™
olutions to tablet-taking problems

News

Study demonstrates efficacy of clozapine in treatment-resistant schizophrenia

Some schizophrenic patients who have not responded to treatment with conventional neuroleptic agents may improve with clozapine therapy, according to results of a recent double-blind multicenter trial comparing clozapine with chlorpromazine.[1] Previous studies have shown that clozapine is as effective as other neuroleptic agents and produces minimal extrapyramidal adverse effects; however, the drug poses a relatively high risk of agranulocytosis. Life-table analysis suggests a 2% incidence after 52 weeks of therapy. Thus, some countries have restricted use of the drug. In other countries, such as the United States, it has been available only in clinical trials or through compassionate-use protocols.

All patients recruited into the study at 16 medical centers met historical criteria for resistance to treatment and disease-severity criteria at the time of enrollment. Only those patients who did not respond to haloperidol (mean dosage, 61 mg/day) during a six-week prospective trial were randomized to the chlorpromazine or clozapine treatment groups. Benztropine mesylate (up to 6 mg/day) was administered concurrently with haloperidol and chlorpromazine. A total of 268 patients were entered into the double-blind comparison; 88% of clozapine-treated patients and 87% of chlorpromazine recipients completed the six-week drug trial.

Improvement in Brief Psychiatric Rating Scale (BPRS) scores and Clinical Global Impressions (CGI) ratings was approximately three times greater in the clozapine group. Ratings on the 30-item Nurses' Observation Scale for Inpatient Evaluation (NOSIE-30) also favored clozapine. Clozapine proved superior over a broad range of BPRS and NOSIE-30 symptom areas. Improvement was noted in 30% of clozapine recipients compared with 4% of chlorpromazine recipients. Clozapine also had a more rapid onset of activity. Mean peak daily dosages of chlorpromazine and clozapine exceeded 1200 mg and 600 mg, respectively. Hypotension and dry mouth occurred more often in the chlorpromazine–benztropine group; the clozapine group had a higher incidence of hypertension, fever, and salivation. No cases of agranulocytosis were reported, but the investigators concluded that, based on the higher relative risk with this neuroleptic agent, clozapine use should be limited to selected patients who do not respond to other treatments.

In an accompanying editorial, Marder and Van Putten[2] examined the question of who should be treated with clozapine. In their opinion, possible candidates for a trial of clozapine include schizophrenic patients with severe tardive dyskinesias; patients who respond "reasonably well" to other neuroleptics but have particularly severe extrapyramidal symptoms, particularly akathisia; and those who have not responded to other neuroleptics.

1. Kane J, Honigfeld G, Singer J et al. Clozapine for the treatment-resistant schizophrenic: a double-blind comparison with chlorpromazine. *Arch Gen Psychiatry*. 1988; 45:789–96.
2. Marder SR, Van Putten T. Who should receive clozapine? *Arch Gen Psychiatry*. 1988; 45:865–7.

Topical minoxidil approved by FDA

A topical formulation of minoxidil (Rogaine, The Upjohn Company) was approved recently by FDA for the treatment of male pattern baldness of the vertex of the scalp. Topical minoxidil was reviewed in the May 1987 issue of *Clinical Pharmacy*.

Topical application of minoxidil stimulates hair growth on the vertex of the scalp. The drug is not effective for frontal baldness, and new hair growth is not permanent. Hair loss occurs within a few months after therapy is stopped. At least four months of therapy is usually required before hair growth can be expected.

Most of the clinical trials of topical minoxidil involved men with healthy scalps and no cardiovascular disease. In these trials, changes in weight, heart rate, and blood pressure were similar with placebo and minoxidil preparations. Reactions other than dermatologic (irritant dermatitis and contact allergic dermatitis) occurred at similar frequencies in the minoxidil and placebo groups.

Minoxidil is poorly absorbed after topical application. Blood concentrations average less than 2 ng/mL with use of the 2% topical solution. It is possible that systemic effects could be achieved with application of higher-than-recommended doses to inflamed scalps in patients with higher-than-average absorption rates. Approximately 95% of systemically absorbed minoxidil is eliminated within four days after therapy is discontinued.

Continued on page 862

Certainty Sets Us Apart

Appropriate coverage during the first 48 hours of empiric antibiotic therapy is critical. And for mixed infections that may include pathogens from both sides of the spectrum—Gram-positive and Gram-negative aerobes and anaerobes—the choice of initial antibiotic therapy can make the difference between timely discharge and a potential delay in recovery.

TIMENTIN® (ticarcillin disodium/clavulanate potassium) destroys β-lactamase and destroys bacteria, thus providing 48 hours of certainty in initial antibiotic therapy.* Timentin's cross-spectrum coverage can often eliminate the need for combination antibiotic regimens—a critical reduction in cost and risk to the patient.

For significant pharmacoeconomic benefits, make the confident formulary choice: TIMENTIN®—the only I.V. clavulanate antibiotic—for 48 hours of certainty in acute empiric therapy.

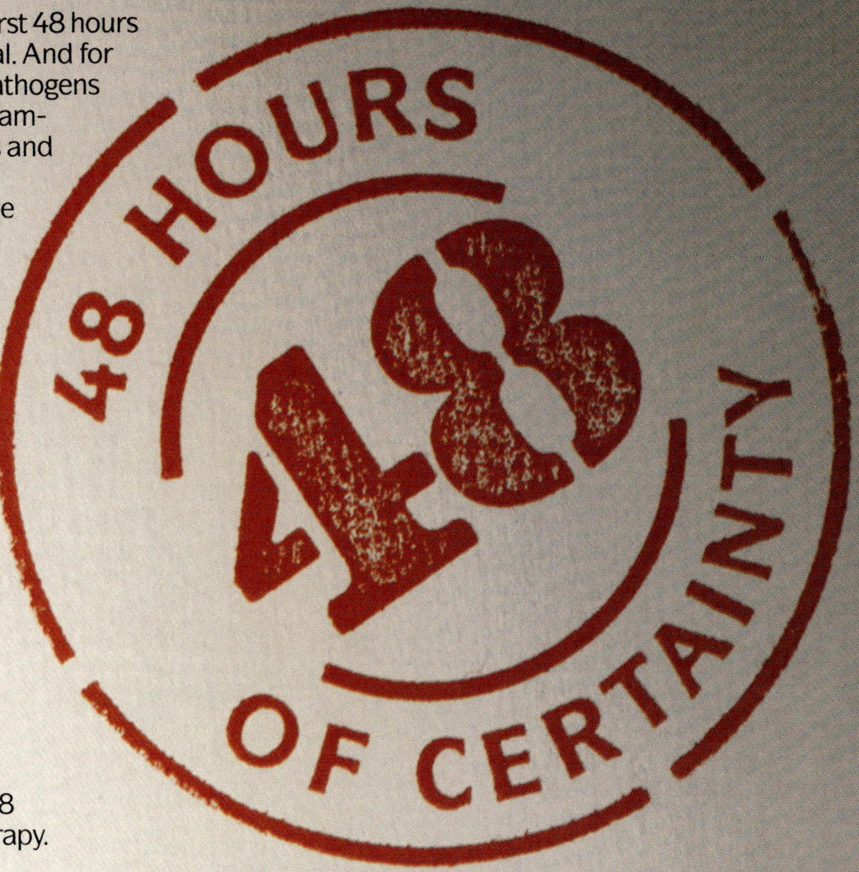

TIMENTIN®

ticarcillin disodium/ clavulanate potassium

Usual Dosage 3.1 g every 6 hours.

THE CLAVULANATES®

Beecham laboratories
BRISTOL, TENNESSEE 37620

© 1988, Beecham Laboratories.

Please see next page for brief summary of prescribing information, including dosage guidelines in gynecologic infections.

*For indicated infections due to susceptible strains of organisms.

BRIEF SUMMARY OF PRESCRIBING INFORMATION

TIMENTIN® **sterile ticarcillin disodium and clavulanate potassium** for Intravenous Administration

INDICATIONS AND USAGE: TIMENTIN® is indicated in the treatment of infections caused by susceptible strains of the designated organisms in the conditions listed below:
Septicemia: including bacteremia, caused by ß-lactamase producing strains of *Klebsiella* spp.*, *E. coli**, *Staphylococcus aureus** and *Pseudomonas aeruginosa** (and other *Pseudomonas* species*). Lower Respiratory Infections: caused by ß-lactamase producing strains of *Staphylococcus aureus, Hemophilus influenzae** and *Klebsiella* spp*. Bone and Joint Infections: caused by ß-lactamase producing strains of *Staphylococcus aureus*. Skin and Skin Structure Infections: caused by ß-lactamase producing strains of *Staphylococcus aureus, Klebsiella* spp.*, and *E. coli.** Urinary Tract Infections (complicated and uncomplicated): caused by ß-lactamase producing strains of *E. coli, Klebsiella* spp., *Pseudomonas aeruginosa** (and other *Pseudomonas* spp.*), *Citrobacter* spp.*, *Enterobacter cloacae**, *Serratia marcescens**, and *Staphylococcus aureus.** Gynecologic Infections: Endometritis caused by ß-lactamase producing strains of *B. melaninogenicus**, *Enterobacter* spp. (including *E. cloacae**), *Escherichia coli, Klebsiella pneumoniae**, *Staphylococcus aureus*, and *Staphylococcus epidermidis*.
*Efficacy for this organism in this organ system was studied in fewer than 10 infections.

While TIMENTIN is indicated only for the conditions listed above, infections caused by ticarcillin susceptible organisms are also amenable to TIMENTIN treatment due to its ticarcillin content. Therefore, mixed infections caused by ticarcillin susceptible organisms and ß-lactamase producing organisms susceptible to TIMENTIN should not require the addition of another antibiotic.

ADVERSE REACTIONS: As with other penicillins, the following adverse reactions may occur: *Hypersensitivity reactions:* skin rash, pruritus, urticaria, arthralgia, myalgia, drug fever, chills, chest discomfort, and anaphylactic reactions. *Central nervous system:* headache, giddiness, neuromuscular hyperirritability or convulsive seizures. *Gastrointestinal disturbances:* disturbances of taste and smell, stomatitis, flatulence, nausea, vomiting and diarrhea, epigastric pain. *Hemic and Lymphatic systems:* thrombocytopenia, leukopenia, neutropenia, eosinophilia and reduction of hemoglobin or hematocrit. Prolongation of prothrombin time and bleeding time. *Abnormalities of hepatic and renal function tests:* elevation of serum aspartate aminotransferase (SGOT), serum alanine aminotransferase (SGPT), serum alkaline phosphatase, serum LDH, serum bilirubin. Rarely, transient hepatitis and cholestatic jaundice–as with some other penicillins and some cephalosporins. Elevation of serum creatinine and/or BUN, hypernatremia. Reduction in serum potassium and uric acid. *Local reactions:* pain, burning, swelling and induration at the injection site and thrombophlebitis with intravenous administration. *Overdosage:* As with other penicillins, TIMENTIN in overdosage has the potential to cause neuromuscular hyperirritability or convulsive seizures. Ticarcillin may be removed from circulation by hemodialysis. The molecular weight, degree of protein binding and pharmacokinetic profile of clavulanic acid together with information from a single patient with renal insufficiency all suggest that this compound may also be removed by hemodialysis.

CONTRAINDICATIONS: TIMENTIN is contraindicated in patients with a history of hypersensitivity reactions to any of the penicillins.

WARNINGS: SERIOUS AND OCCASIONALLY FATAL HYPERSENSITIVITY (ANAPHYLACTOID) REACTIONS HAVE BEEN REPORTED IN PATIENTS ON PENICILLIN THERAPY. THESE REACTIONS ARE MORE LIKELY TO OCCUR IN INDIVIDUALS WITH A HISTORY OF PENICILLIN HYPERSENSITIVITY AND/OR A HISTORY OF SENSITIVITY TO MULTIPLE ALLERGENS. THERE HAVE BEEN REPORTS OF INDIVIDUALS WITH A HISTORY OF PENICILLIN HYPERSENSITIVITY WHO HAVE EXPERIENCED SEVERE REACTIONS WHEN TREATED WITH CEPHALOSPORINS. BEFORE INITIATING THERAPY WITH TIMENTIN, CAREFUL INQUIRY SHOULD BE MADE CONCERNING PREVIOUS HYPERSENSITIVITY REACTIONS TO PENICILLINS, CEPHALOSPORINS, OR OTHER DRUGS. IF AN ALLERGIC REACTION OCCURS, TIMENTIN SHOULD BE DISCONTINUED AND THE APPROPRIATE THERAPY INSTITUTED. **SERIOUS ANAPHYLACTOID REACTIONS REQUIRE IMMEDIATE EMERGENCY TREATMENT WITH EPINEPHRINE. OXYGEN, INTRAVENOUS STEROIDS, AND AIRWAY MANAGEMENT, INCLUDING INTUBATION, SHOULD ALSO BE PROVIDED AS INDICATED.**

PRECAUTIONS: While TIMENTIN possesses the characteristic low toxicity of the penicillin group of antibiotics, organ system functions should be assessed periodically during therapy.

Bleeding manifestations have occurred in some patients receiving ß-lactam antibiotics. These reactions have been associated with abnormalities of coagulation tests such as clotting time, platelet aggregation and prothrombin time and are more likely to occur in patients with renal impairment. If bleeding manifestations appear, TIMENTIN treatment should be discontinued and appropriate therapy instituted.

TIMENTIN has only rarely been reported to cause hypokalemia. Periodic monitoring of serum potassium may be advisable in patients receiving prolonged therapy.

Pregnancy (Category B): Reproduction studies have been performed in rats given doses up to 1050 mg/kg/day and have revealed no evidence of impaired fertility or harm to the fetus due to TIMENTIN. There are, however, no adequate and well-controlled studies in pregnant women. Because animal reproduction studies are not always predictive of human response, this drug should be used during pregnancy only if clearly needed.

DOSAGE AND ADMINISTRATION: TIMENTIN should be administered by intravenous infusion (30 min.). Usual recommended dose for systemic and urinary tract infections for average (60 kg) adults is 3.1 Gm TIMENTIN (3.1 Gm vial containing 3 Gm ticarcillin and 100 mg clavulanic acid) given every 4 to 6 hours. For gynecologic infections TIMENTIN should be administered as follows: Moderate infections 200 mg/kg/day in divided doses every 6 hours and for severe infections 300 mg/kg/day, based on ticarcillin content, in divided doses every 4 hours. For patients weighing less than 60 kg, the recommended dosage is 200-300 mg/kg/day, based on ticarcillin content, given in divided doses every 4 to 6 hours. In urinary tract infections, a dosage of 3.2 Gm TIMENTIN (3.2 Gm vial containing 3 Gm ticarcillin and 200 mg clavulanic acid) given every 8 hours is adequate. Please see official package insert for details on dosages for other patients, including those with renal insufficiency, and directions for use.

7548/G-BS ©1988, Beecham Laboratories

Beecham laboratories
BRISTOL, TENNESSEE 37620

News *Continued from page 858*

Rogaine is available as 2% minoxidil in a solution of alcohol (60% v/v), propylene glycol, and water. The recommended dosage is 1 mL of solution applied to the affected areas of the scalp twice daily. The solution is supplied in 60-mL bottles with multiple applicators (metered spray attachment, extender spray attachment, and rub-on applicator tip). The cost to the pharmacist is $42.50 per 60-mL bottle.

News Briefs

- FDA has approved use of the orphan drug **tiopronin** (Thiola, Mission Pharmacal) for use in the prevention of cysteine stone formation in selected patients with severe homozygous cystinuria; the approval provides an alternative to treatment with penicillamine.

- **A premixed dextranomer paste** (Envisan Wound Cleaning Paste, Marion Laboratories, Inc.) has been approved by FDA for use in cleaning wet ulcers and wet wounds such as venous stasis ulcers, decubitus ulcers, infected traumatic and surgical wounds, and infected burns.

- **An enteric-coated magnesium supplement** (Slow-Mag, G. D. Searle & Co.) has been introduced; each tablet contains 64 mg of elemental magnesium (as magnesium chloride).

- FDA has granted **orphan drug status to interleukin-2** (Proleukin, Cetus Corporation) for the treatment of metastatic renal cell carcinoma.

Upcoming Specialty Meetings

Thrombolysis: The Dawn of a New Era? . . . January 25–26 . . . London, England . . . contact: Penny Robinson, IBC Technical Services Ltd., Bath House, 56 Holborn Viaduct, London EC1A 2EX England.

NIH Consensus Development Conference on Therapeutic Endoscopy and Bleeding Ulcers . . . March 6–8 . . . Bethesda, MD . . . contact: Endoscopy, Office of Medical Applications of Research, National Institutes of Health, Building 1, Room 216, 9000 Rockville Pike, Bethesda, MD 20892.

International Conference on Pyridoxine . . . April 10–12 . . . Philadelphia, PA . . . contact: Conference Department, New York Academy of Sciences, 2 East 63rd Street, New York, NY 10021; 212-838-0230.

American College of Physicians . . . April 13–16 . . . San Francisco, CA . . . contact: J. R. Ball, 4200 Pine Street, Philadelphia, PA 19104; 215-243-1200.

American College of Preventive Medicine . . . April 13–16 . . . Atlanta, GA . . . contact: W. Kane, 1015 15th Street N.W., Washington, DC 20005; 202-789-0003.

American Society for Clinical Investigation . . . April 28–May 1 . . . Washington, DC . . . contact: C. R. Kahn, Joslin Diabetes Center, 1 Joslin Place, Boston, MA 02215; 609-848-1000, ext. 212.

Therapy Consultation

The Therapy Consultation *section provides brief advice, in question-and-answer format, on how to handle specific drug-therapy problems. Readers are invited to submit questions, which will be referred to a consultant for an answer. The problems should not be highly specialized or unusual, nor should they be mundane. Questions are answered briefly, based largely on the judgment and personal experience of the consultant, although selected references may be cited to substantiate the consultant's advice.*

Assistance in identifying Therapy Consultation *topics is provided by the drug information centers at the following institutions: Albert B. Chandler Medical Center and College of Pharmacy, University of Kentucky, Lexington; Arizona Health Sciences Center, Tucson; Medical College of Virginia Hospitals, Richmond; University of California Medical Center, San Diego; and University of Michigan Medical Center, Ann Arbor.*

Treatment of acute agitation in the elderly

Question: Acute episodes of agitation can occur in elderly nursing-home residents as well as in elderly patients who are hospitalized for acute medical problems. How should these episodes be treated? Is there any basis for preferentially selecting a benzodiazepine or one of the antipsychotic agents? When is intramuscular drug administration appropriate?

Answer: Acute confusion is frequently encountered in elderly patients who are admitted to nursing homes after hospitalization for acute illnesses. These episodes may actually occur anytime there is a change in the patient's environment, either a change in the physical environment (as mentioned above) or a change in familiar surroundings or routines (e.g., rearrangement of a room or a change in the normal daily pattern).

Agitation, which is one manifestation of confusion in the elderly, may be defined as "an inappropriate verbal, vocal, or motor activity that is not explained by the patient's needs or [delirium]." [1] When the activity becomes aggressive or abusive to the patient or to others despite nondrug intervention, drug therapy is appropriate. Many patients who have periods of agitation do not necessarily have a diagnosis of cognitive impairment, specifically dementia.[2]

Perhaps the best method of managing agitation is recognizing that there is a high occurrence rate during the first one to two weeks after the inciting event. Depending on the coping strategies and the cognitive status of the patient, readjustment may take four weeks or longer. Staff awareness and knowledge of the series of events and regular reorientation of the patient may obviate the need for medications. Frequently, however, especially during the initial phase of agitation, the patient's behavior is sufficiently impaired to warrant the use of medications.[3] Neuroleptics have become the mainstay for treatment of agitation in the elderly. These drugs have become the third most frequently used class of drugs in skilled-nursing homes and, in some instances, the most frequently prescribed drug class.[2]

Use of neuroleptics to control agitation has been studied in numerous uncontrolled studies and a few controlled studies.[4] Recent carefully controlled studies support earlier conclusions that neuroleptics are useful for controlling agitation, restlessness, and hostility in the elderly. No single neuroleptic or class of neuroleptics has a therapeutic advantage over another. Furthermore, not all patients will respond to therapy. When they do respond, the effect is likely to be modest, rather than striking.

When a neuroleptic is indicated, the clinician must weigh the risk-to-benefit ratio of low- and high-potency neuroleptic agents. Low-potency agents (chlorpromazine and thioridazine) commonly produce sedation and orthostatic hypotension but induce extrapyramidal symptoms infrequently. High-potency agents (haloperidol and thiothixene) are less sedating and have a low incidence of orthostatic hypotension, but they have a high incidence of extrapyramidal effects.

As a general rule, sedation is an unwanted effect since it may lead to increased confusion that may cause even more agitation. Orthostatic hypotension is undesirable because falls have been associated with antipsychotic medications and may have serious consequences. For these reasons, many clinicians prefer the high-potency neuroleptics, although they realize that older patients are more susceptible to the extrapyramidal effects. Therefore, the drug should be used in the lowest dosage and for the shortest time possible. The need for continued therapy should be evaluated at least every three months.[3] If agitation occurs only occasionally, scheduled doses of medication are not needed.

A reasonable starting dose of haloperidol is 0.25 mg orally daily. A 0.25-mg dose may be administered by mixing the oral concentrate with water or juice. The usual daily dosage ranges from 0.5 to 2 mg daily, with doses higher than 5 mg needed rarely for more severe agitation. Alternatively, chlorpromazine hydrochloride or thioridazine hydrochloride may be used, starting with 10 mg daily and slowly increasing the dose (up to 40 mg) if needed. Doses as high as 100 mg/day of the low-potency neuroleptics may rarely be needed for severe cases. Neuroleptics are frequently effective when given as a single bedtime dose; however, the daily dosage may be divided if the patient continues to experience behavioral problems or is overly sedated with a single bedtime dose. The total daily dosage should not be increased more often than every three to four days. Weekly adjustment is preferable.

If the patient is agitated to the point of being unable or unwilling to take oral medications, intramuscular therapy is indicated. Haloperidol is given in a dose of 0.25–1.0 mg i.m. (same as the oral dose). The i.m. dose of the low-potency neuroleptics (25 mg) is approximately twice the oral dose because of decreased availability after i.m. administration.

Target symptoms for which the neuroleptic agent is being used should be specified, and these symptoms should be used to monitor the effectiveness of therapy. Since cognitive impairment is a progressive process, long-term use of neuroleptics is usually not warranted. As the decline in cognition progresses, agitation becomes less common and continued use of medication is unwarranted.

Benzodiazepines have also been used to quiet disruptive behavior in the elderly. These agents are sometimes useful in controlling mild anxiety and agitation, but moderate to severe agitation is not lessened by these agents. Although no clinical differences are apparent between long- and short-acting agents, it would be prudent to use a short-acting agent to prevent drug accumulation and the resulting sequelae.

Ideally, acute confusion caused by a sudden change in environment is best managed without the use of medication. However, this is not always effective. Based on limited data, neuroleptics, if used judiciously, are the drugs of choice for control of acute agitation. It is particularly important to specify at the beginning of therapy the target symptoms for which the drug is indicated and to use these symptoms to monitor the patient's response. Furthermore, drug therapy should be started with the understanding that it is a short-term intervention, with re-evaluation of the need for therapy every three months.

1. Salzman C. Treatment of the elderly agitated patient. *J Clin Psychiatr*. 1987; 48(Suppl 5):19–22.
2. Wragg RE, Jeste DV. Neuroleptics and alternative treatments. *Psychiatr Clin N Am*. 1988; 11:195–213.
3. Raskin DE. Antipsychotic medication and the elderly. *J Clin Psychiatr*. 1985; 46(5, Sec 2):36–40.
4. Risse S. Barnes R. Pharmacologic treatment of agitation associated with dementia. *J Am Geriatr Soc*. 1986; 34:368–76.

STEVEN F. BAUWENS, PHARM.D.
Director of Clinical Services
Long Term Care Pharmaceutical Services Corp.
3002 S. Michigan Street
South Bend, IN 46614

Enhance your clinical practice skills and earn CE credit with a new self-study course from ASHP

Concepts in Clinical Pharmacokinetics

A Self-Instructional Course

Written by a trio of pharmacy professors, this book provides an orientation to pharmacokinetic concepts and procedures. It can help prepare you for pharmacokinetics courses of instruction, or serve as a handy reference and refresher course. With it you can earn up to 20 hours of ACPE-approved continuing education credit.

Input topics include:
- therapeutic drug monitoring
- compartmental models
- clearance
- volume of distribution
- loading dose
- elimination rate constant

Order your copy today!

The American Society of Hospital Pharmacists is approved by the American Council on Pharmaceutical Education as a provider of continuing pharmaceutical education.

Order Form

Concepts in Clinical Pharmacokinetics: A Self-Instructional Course (P275); 1988; approx. 150 pp; $50.00

☐ Please send me _____ copies of ***Concepts in Clinical Pharmacokinetics: A Self-Instructional Course*** (P275) at $50.00 each; 1988; 140 pp.

☐ Enclosed is my check for $__________. (Checks must be drawn on a U.S. bank and made payable to ASHP.)

☐ Enclosed is our purchase order #__________; please issue an invoice and add postage and handling.

Charge $__________ to my ☐ VISA ☐ MasterCard

Account #____________________

Exp. ________ (*month/year*) Signature ________________

Name ____________________

Institution ____________________

Address ____________________

City __________ State ____ Zip ________

ASHP ID #____________________

Send to: ASHP Publications Records Dept.
4630 Montgomery Avenue
Bethesda, MD 20814

Payments to ASHP are not deductible as charitable contributions for Federal Income Tax purposes. However, they may be deductible under other provisions of the Internal Revenue Code.

© 1988 American Society of Hospital Pharmacists

Letters

The Letters *column is a forum for rapid exchange of ideas among readers of* CP. *Liberal criteria are applied in the review of submissions to encourage contributions to this column.*

The Letters *column includes the following types of contributions: (1) comments, addenda, and minor updates on previously published work, (2) alerts on potential problems related to drug therapy or clinical research, (3) observations or comments on trends in drug therapy or clinical research, and (4) brief expressions of opinion about controversies in drug therapy or clinical research.*

Letters need not be submitted with the journal's manuscript checklist. The following conditions, however, must be adhered to: (1) the body of the letter must be no longer than two typewritten pages, (2) the use of references, tables, and illustrations should be minimized, (3) the authors' names, affiliations, and mailing addresses must be typed at the end of the letter in the format used by CP, *and (4) the entire letter (including references, tables, and authors' names) must be typed double spaced on plain white paper (not letterhead). Following acceptance of a letter, the authors are required to sign an exclusive publication statement and a copyright-transferral form.*

Hearing loss associated with muromonab-CD3 therapy

Muromonab-CD3, commonly referred to as OKT3, is effective in the treatment of acute renal allograft rejection and is under investigation for use in liver, heart, and pancreas transplants.[1-3] The most common adverse reactions experienced by patients after the first or second dose of muromonab-CD3 compose a "flu-like" syndrome of chills, fever, tachycardia, headache, nausea, vomiting, hypertension or hypotension, wheezing, and diarrhea.[4] Other less common adverse effects include acute pulmonary edema, leukopenia, hypotension, severe diarrhea, and aseptic meningitis.[5] We observed a recent case of hearing loss induced by muromonab-CD3 therapy. To our knowledge, this adverse reaction has not previously been associated with this agent.

The patient was a 43-year-old, 50-kg woman who had received a cadaveric pancreas transplant in August 1987. Since the transplant, the patient's diabetes had been controlled without insulin, and her fasting blood glucose concentrations ranged from 90 to 110 mg/dL. Her outpatient medication regimen included cyclosporine 490 mg twice daily, prednisone 17.5 mg once daily, and azathioprine 25 mg daily alternating with 50 mg daily. The woman was admitted to the University of Minnesota Hospital and Clinics in November 1987 with rising serum amylase concentrations and decreasing urine amylase concentrations; these findings were suggestive of acute pancreatitis or, more likely, acute pancreas allograft rejection.

Treatment was initiated with muromonab-CD3 5 mg. To prevent adverse reactions to muromonab-CD3, methylprednisolone 50 mg i.v., diphenhydramine 50 mg i.v., and acetaminophen 650 mg orally were administered before each dose of muromonab-CD3, and hydrocortisone sodium succinate 100 mg i.v. was administered after each dose. The dosages of the patient's usual immunosuppressive drugs were increased to cyclosporine 540 mg twice daily, prednisone 80 mg daily, and azathioprine 100 mg daily.

Within five minutes of receiving the first dose of muromonab-CD3, the patient complained of cramps in the lower back and abdomen. She also experienced tightness in the abdominal and sternal muscles. The patient's oral temperature increased to 40.2 °C from 38.0 °C. After receiving the second dose of muromonab-CD3, the patient became hypotensive with a sitting blood pressure of 68/48 mm Hg. Although the woman had an eight-year history of gradual hearing loss, she noticed a marked decrease in hearing ability in both ears following treatment with muromonab-CD3. She described the sensation as similar to being in a tunnel; she did not experience tinnitus, dizziness, or pain. Results of a pure-tone audiometry examination revealed a flat sensorineural hearing loss in the 50- to 60-dB range. At the 80-dB level, the patient complained of loudness and could not tolerate the sounds. The patient was not receiving any known ototoxic medication at the time of evaluation, but the otolaryngologist described this pattern of hearing loss as consistent with drug-induced hearing loss.

The episode of rejection resolved without further treatment after three days of muromonab-CD3 therapy. The patient tolerated the two subsequent doses of muromonab-CD3 without adverse effects but still complained of hearing difficulty. The patient's hearing ability was still diminished but had not worsened when a follow-up audiogram was performed six months after she was discharged. The evidence linking this patient's acute, nonprogressive decrease in hearing to muromonab-CD3 treatment admittedly is circumstantial. Although it is possible that hypotension played a role in this patient's hearing loss, we do not believe that hypotension could have accounted for the severity or duration of the reaction.

1. Canafax DM, Draxler CA. Monoclonal antilymphocyte antibody (OKT3) treatment of acute renal allograft rejection. *Pharmacotherapy*. 1987; 4:121-4.
2. Burke GW, Simmons RL, Canafax DM et al. Initial experiences with OKT3 for prophylaxis and treatment of rejection

Continued on page 868

Scientific Therapeutics Information, Inc

MEDICAL WRITER/EDITOR

Unique opportunities are available for clinical pharmacists in a custom medical publishing and communications company, based in New Jersey, that offers dynamic interaction with medical and marketing groups in major pharmaceutical companies. Associate- to senior-level editorial positions are available for qualified persons to plan, develop, and manage all phases of projects, including

- Educational symposia and published proceedings
- Textbooks
- Drug monographs
- In-depth drug reviews
- Journal articles

Excellent technical writing skills, a comprehensive clinical therapeutics background (Pharm.D. degree or equivalent), and drug information service experience with emphasis on medical literature analysis are required. Salary commensurate with experience; we offer a full benefits package. Send résumé and writing samples to

John A. Romankiewicz, Pharm.D.
Scientific Therapeutics Information, Inc.
505 Morris Avenue, Suite 206
Springfield, NJ 07081

EOE

Clinical Pharmacist / Pharmacologist

Texas Department of Mental Health and Mental Retardation

San Antonio State School

The 360-bed developmental disability facility is seeking a clinical pharmacist/pharmacologist. Pharm.D. required and completion of an accredited residency in clinical psychiatric pharmacy, or previous experience. Requires Texas license in pharmacy. Facility appointment and excellent fringe benefits that include no state income tax, state-paid partial social security payment, and tax deferred retirement contributions.

Interested persons should send résumé or call **Personnel Office, P.O. Box 14700, Harlandale Station, San Antonio, TX 78214; 512-532-9610.** An Equal Opportunity/Affirmative Action Employer.

Letters *Continued from page 867*

in kidney, liver and pancreas allografts. *Transplant Proc.* 1988; 20(Suppl 1):252-3.
3. Ortho Multicenter Transplant Study Group. A randomized clinical trial of OKT3 monoclonal antibody for acute rejection of cadaveric renal transplants. *N Engl J Med.* 1985; 313:337-42.
4. Norman DJ, Shield CF, Barry J et al. A U.S. clinical study of Orthoclone OKT3 in renal transplantation. *Transplant Proc.* 1987; 19:2:21-7.
5. Emmons C, Smith J, Flanigan M. Cerebrospinal fluid inflammation during muromonab-CD3 therapy. *Lancet.* 1986; 2:510-1.

Marcia Michals, Pharm.D., Psychopharmacology Resident
College of Pharmacy, Room 5.110
University of Texas at Austin
Austin, TX 78712

John P. Roberts, M.D.
Department of Surgery
Liver Transplant Service
University of California, San Francisco
533 Parnassus Avenue
San Francisco, CA 94143

Daniel Canafax, Pharm.D., Associate Professor
College of Pharmacy
Health Sciences Unit F
308 Harvard Street S.E.
Minneapolis, MN 55455

DRUG THEFT:

KNOW THE WARNING SIGNS

PREVENT IT FROM HAPPENING IN YOUR HOSPITAL

ASHP introduces "Drug Theft by Health-Care Personnel," a new two-part videotape to help you become aware of potential problems and know the warning signs.

☐ Please send me a brochure on Drug Theft Videotape

Name ______

Institution ______

Address ______

City ______ State ______ Zip ______

Send to: ASHP Marketing Services Dept.
4630 Montgomery Avenue, Bethesda, MD 20814

Propafenone: A new antiarrhythmic agent

MOSES S. S. CHOW, CYNTHIA LEBSACK, AND DANIEL HILLEMAN

Abstract: The chemical and pharmacologic properties, pharmacokinetics, drug interactions, clinical efficacy, adverse effects, and dosage of propafenone are reviewed.

Propafenone is a class IC antiarrhythmic agent that is structurally similar to the β blockers but that has only weak β-blocking and calcium-channel-blocking activity. It is well absorbed after oral administration, but systemic bioavailability is only 12% after a 300-mg dose. Among extensive metabolizers (>90% of the United States population), bioavailability seems to vary nonlinearly with dose and increases substantially with food; these effects are not seen in poor metabolizers. Elimination is primarily hepatic, with a mean elimination half-life after oral administration of 5.5 hours in extensive metabolizers and 17.2 hours in poor metabolizers. The relationship between plasma propafenone concentration and clinical response varies considerably among individual patients; therefore, plasma concentrations have limited usefulness in predicting efficacy or electrophysiologic effects.

Propafenone is effective in treating ventricular tachycardia and in suppressing premature ventricular complexes (PVCs). It is less effective in the treatment of refractory ventricular tachycardia. Concurrent administration of digoxin, warfarin, or metoprolol with propafenone has been shown to increase the serum concentrations of those three drugs, while cimetidine slightly increases the propafenone concentrations. Additive pharmacologic effect can occur when lidocaine, procainamide, and quinidine are combined with propafenone. Overall, 21% to 32% of patients experience adverse effects, with 3% to 7% of these serious enough to warrant discontinuing therapy. The most common adverse effects are dizziness or lightheadedness, metallic taste, and nausea and vomiting; the most serious adverse effects are proarrhythmic events. The initial dosage for the treatment of ventricular arrhythmias is 150 mg every eight hours for both rapid and poor metabolizers; increases should be made gradually over a three- to four-day period. For maintenance therapy, 450 to 900 mg/day orally in three or four divided doses has been shown to be effective.

Propafenone is an effective and generally well tolerated antiarrhythmic agent for the treatment of PVCs and for initial treatment of ventricular tachycardia.

Index terms: Arrhythmia; Cardiac drugs; Dosage; Drug interactions; Pharmacokinetics; Propafenone; Toxicity
Clin Pharm. 1988; 7:869–77

Cardiac arrhythmias remain a major cause of morbidity and mortality in the United States. Arrhythmias are thought to be responsible for 400,000 sudden cardiac deaths that occur each year in this country.[1] Although important advances are being made in the development of surgical techniques and implantable devices for the treatment of arrhythmias, the majority of patients with arrhythmias require treatment with antiarrhythmic drugs.

Although a large number of agents currently are available for the treatment of arrhythmias (Table 1), none of these agents has proved to be uniformly effective or safe. In fact, patients who fail to respond to or cannot tolerate any of the available marketed agents are not uncommon. Thus, new agents that can offer additional control of arrhythmia with a different adverse-effect profile are important additions.

Propafenone is one of the new antiarrhythmic agents that is close to FDA approval. (It will be available as oral tablets.) Propafenone is effective

MOSES S. S. CHOW, PHARM.D, is Director, Drug Information Services, Department of Pharmacy Services, Hartford Hospital, Hartford, CT, and Associate Professor of Clinical Pharmacy, School of Pharmacy, The University of Connecticut, Storrs. CYNTHIA LEBSACK, PHARM.D., is Clinical Research Coordinator, Cardiovascular Medicine, Sequoia Hospital District, Redwood City, CA. DANIEL HILLEMAN, PHARM.D., is Associate Professor of Medicine, Creighton Cardiac Center, Omaha, NE.

Address reprint requests to Dr. Chow at the Drug Information Center, Hartford Hospital, 80 Seymour Street, Hartford, CT 06115.

This is article **680-204-8818** in the **ASHP Continuing Education System;** it qualifies for 1.0 hour of continuing education credit. See page 911 for learning objectives and test questions.

Copyright © 1988, American Society of Hospital Pharmacists, Inc. All rights reserved. 0278-2677/88/1201-0869$02.25.

against a variety of cardiac arrhythmias but will be approved initially only for the treatment of symptomatic ventricular arrhythmias. This review provides a brief description of its chemical, pharmacologic, and pharmacokinetic properties and its clinical effects on different types of arrhythmias.

Chemical and Physical Properties

Propafenone was synthesized in 1970 by Helopharm of the Federal Republic of Germany (FRG) and later licensed by Knoll AG of FRG. It is structurally similar to the β-blocking agents; Figure 1 shows the structures of propranolol and propafenone. Propafenone is available as the hydrochloride salt, which has a molecular weight of 377.92. It is slightly soluble in water and has a pKa of 9. Propafenone occurs as a racemic mixture of D- and L-isomers and has a bitter taste.

Figure 1. Structure of propafenone compared with that of propranolol.

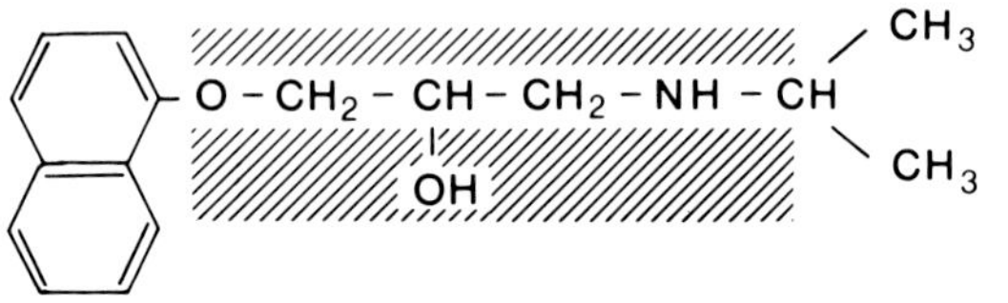

Propranolol

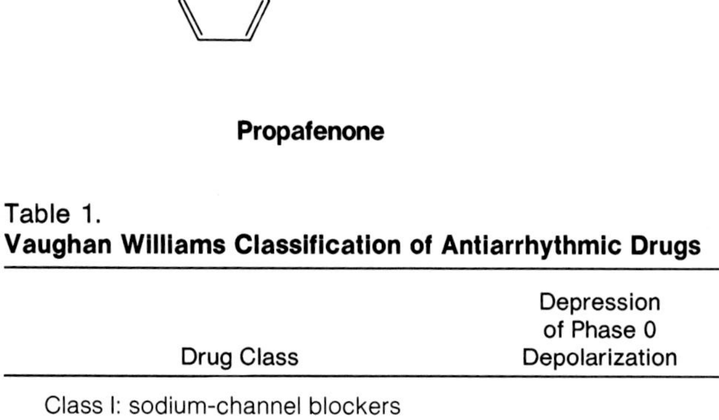

Propafenone

Pharmacology

Electrophysiologic Properties. Propafenone possesses the electrophysiologic properties of a class IC agent[2] according to the Vaughan Williams classification (Table 1). In all cardiac tissues that are normally depolarized by fast sodium current, the drug decreases the maximum rate of depolarization (phase 0 of the action potential) and the overshoot of action potential in a dose-dependent fashion. The drug lengthens AH, AV, and HV conduction times[3–7] and consequently prolongs the PR interval and QRS duration on the electrocardiogram.[4,6,7]

Another important electrophysiologic effect of propafenone is its action on accessory pathways, prolonging both conduction and effective refractory periods in both directions.[4,8,9] Thus, it appears to be effective in patients with Wolff–Parkinson–White syndrome.

The drug also has some electrophysiologic effects resembling those of class IA agents; that is, it increases the duration of the action potential at high concentrations (≥1500 ng/mL)[2] and increases the effective refractory period.[6,7] It exhibits both weak β-blocking activity (2.5% of the β-blocking potency of propranolol)[10] and calcium-channel-blocking activity (5% of the calcium-channel-blocking potency of verapamil)[11]; however, neither of these effects is probably clinically important in the majority of patients receiving low doses of propafenone.[12] In high doses (>600 mg/day) and in patients who are poor metabolizers (see Pharmacokinetics section), the β-blocking effects of propafenone may be important.[13]

Table 1.
Vaughan Williams Classification of Antiarrhythmic Drugs

Drug Class	Depression of Phase 0 Depolarization	Change in Repolarization	Drugs
Class I: sodium-channel blockers (local anesthetics)			
IA:	Moderate	Prolonged	Disopyramide, procainamide, quinidine
IB:	Weak	Shortened	Lidocaine, mexiletine, tocainide
IC:	Strong	Minimal	Encainide, flecainide, propafenone
Class II: β blockers	Moderate[a]	None	Acebutolol, propranolol
Class III	Minimal	Prolonged	Amiodarone, bretylium, *N*-acetylprocainamide,[b] sotalol[b]
Class IV: calcium-channel blockers			Diltiazem, verapamil

[a] At high concentrations.
[b] Investigational.

Hemodynamic Effects. Like other class I agents, propafenone can cause mild depression of cardiac function at therapeutic doses.[5,14] Baker et al.[14] showed that in patients with stable congestive heart failure, increasing the propafenone dosage from 300 mg to 600 mg daily did not cause a dose-related alteration of the ejection fraction. At the maximum dose of 600 mg per day, only a small change in the ejection fraction was seen (from a mean of 34.7% to 31.8% in 14 patients). Only one patient developed symptomatic heart failure associated with a decrease of the ejection fraction from 40% to 26%. Podrid and Lown[15] found that propafenone decreased the ejection fraction in patients with preexisting left ventricular dysfunction. Two patients had worsened symptoms of congestive heart failure; however, only one had to have therapy discontinued because of symptom severity. Shen et al.[5] showed that a slight depression of cardiac index and elevation of pulmonary resistance can occur after infusion of propafenone 2 mg/kg over 10 minutes followed by 2 mg/min for 30 minutes. No change in mean arterial blood pressure was noted. In patients receiving digoxin therapy, the left ventricular ejection fraction either did not change or changed slightly after a 600-mg/day oral dose of propafenone.[14,16] Thus, in patients who have depressed left ventricular function that is not fully compensated, the drug should be used with caution. If congestive heart failure worsens during propafenone therapy, the therapy should be discontinued.

Pharmacokinetics

Absorption. After oral administration, propafenone is well absorbed, with a mean peak plasma concentration observed in about two to three hours.[17] However, extensive first-pass metabolism results in systemic bioavailability of only about 12% after a 300-mg dose.[17] The systemic availability appears to vary with the dose.[13,17–19] For example, a threefold increase in the daily dosage can result in a 10-fold increase in steady-state plasma concentration[18] (Table 2). This dose-dependent bioavailability probably results from saturation of hepatic microsomal enzymes, since increased concentrations of the drug are delivered to the liver. The nonlinear relationship between dose and plasma concentration occurs in those who are extensive or rapid metabolizers of propafenone but not in those who are poor metabolizers.[13]

The bioavailability of propafenone can vary with fasting or nonfasting conditions.[20] When propafenone is administered with food, plasma propafenone concentrations are significantly higher and maximum concentrations are reached earlier. After a standard breakfast, the average increase in bioavailability is about 147%, compared with that during fasting conditions in subjects who are extensive metabolizers of propafenone (the majority of subjects in the United States population). However, there is considerable intersubject variation, and no change in bioavailability occurs in poor metabolizers. In view of these data, patients should take propafenone consistently either with or without food to ensure constant bioavailability and clinical effect.

Distribution. The distribution of propafenone follows a two-compartment model.[21] The volume of the central compartment is about 0.8 L/kg, and the volume of distribution at steady state is about 3 L/kg. The drug is most extensively distributed to the lungs, liver, and heart (in descending order); the lowest concentrations appear in the brain and in fat.[22,23] Approximately 77–89% of the drug is protein bound in human plasma.[24] The drug is bound to α_1-acid glycoproteins with two classes of binding sites, both with high affinity and low capacity.[25]

Metabolism and Elimination. Elimination of propafenone is primarily hepatic. Less than 1% of an oral dose is excreted unchanged in the urine.[17,26] There are two active metabolites, 5-hydroxypropafenone and *N*-depropyl-propafenone; concentrations of both are less than 20% that of propafenone. These metabolites have been found to be comparable to propafenone in activity and appear to be excreted in the feces (53% in 48 hours) and urine (up to 38%), based on limited human studies.[26–28] Other metabolites are present only in minor quantities.

Metabolism of propafenone is polymorphic; classification of patients as poor or extensive metabolizers is consistent with the debrisoquine metabolic phenotype.[13] More than 90% of patients have been estimated to metabolize the drug extensively; the remainder are poor metabolizers. The poor metabolizers have higher plasma propafenone concentrations than the extensive metabolizers. The

Table 2.
Nonlinear Relationship between Dosage and Plasma Concentration of Propafenone

Reference	Subjects	Dosage Change (mg)	Change in Plasma Concentration (fold)
17	Volunteers	150 to 300	2.4
		150 to 450	5.2
18	Patients	300 to 450	~2.2
		300 to 600	~5.0
		300 to 900	9.9
13	Patients		
	Extensive metabolizers	600 to 900	2.4
	Poor metabolizers	600 to 900	0.52
19	Patients	450 to 900	3.7

poor metabolizers also have much lower (undetectable) concentrations of the metabolite 5-hydroxypropafenone than the extensive metabolizers. Despite the differences in the two metabolic types, the effective dosage and frequency of antiarrhythmic response appear to be similar in both types of patients.[13]

The mean half-life of propafenone in patients after oral doses has been reported to range from 3.6 hours to 7.2 hours.[3,7,18,29] Siddoway et al.[13] reported a mean half-life of 5.5 hours in extensive metabolizers and 17.2 hours in poor metabolizers. After intravenous administration, the mean half-life was 5.0 ± 3.6 hours.[23] In patients with hepatic disease, the half-life is prolonged (mean of 14.2 hours, compared with 2.7 hours in healthy volunteers).[30] The propafenone dosage should be reduced by 50% in these patients.[30]

The reported effective plasma propafenone concentration for suppression of premature ventricular complexes has ranged from 231 to 3272 ng/mL,[19] and the reported mean concentration for suppression of induction of ventricular tachycardia during electrophysiologic studies is 1043 ± 514 ng/mL.[7] Plasma concentrations vary considerably among individual patients. Because of the wide variability in the concentration–response relationship, monitoring plasma concentrations of propafenone is of limited clinical usefulness in predicting efficacy or electrophysiologic effects.

Drug Interactions

Propafenone has been reported to interact with a number of drugs, including digoxin, warfarin, cimetidine, metoprolol, lidocaine, procainamide, and quinidine.

Drug interactions between propafenone and digoxin have been well documented.[29,31–33] After both oral and intravenous doses of digoxin, the serum digoxin concentration increased when propafenone was administered. In patients receiving propafenone 300 mg every eight hours, the serum digoxin concentration may increase as much as 136% (mean 83%) over that achieved with digoxin alone.[33] The magnitude of the increase in serum digoxin concentration appears to depend on the size of the propafenone dose.[33]

No changes in renal digoxin clearance have been observed; however, the total body clearance of digoxin decreased significantly after coadministration of propafenone.[33] The interaction is likely to be clinically important, and serum digoxin concentrations should be monitored in patients who receive this combination therapy.

In healthy volunteers, propafenone also has been reported to increase the plasma warfarin concentration (39%) and increase the prothrombin time. Therefore, when propafenone is added to warfarin therapy, the patient's prothrombin time should be monitored and the warfarin dosage should be adjusted accordingly.[34] The mechanism of interaction is probably inhibition of the oxidative pathway of warfarin metabolism. No protein-binding displacement has been observed.[34]

Concurrent cimetidine administration has been reported to slightly increase the propafenone concentration (by 20%) and change the QRS duration (from 98 ± 4 to 103 ± 3 msec).[35] These changes, however, are not likely to be clinically important.

Propafenone has been observed to increase plasma metoprolol concentrations twofold to fivefold, whereas metoprolol has no effect on plasma propafenone concentrations.[36] Propafenone also increased the duration of metoprolol's β-blocking activity. These changes may be related to a decrease in metoprolol clearance via inhibition by propafenone of the oxidative pathway. The metoprolol dosage should be reduced when propafenone therapy is added.

Combined intravenous infusion of lidocaine hydrochloride (100-mg bolus followed by an infusion of 2 mg/min) and propafenone (1 to 2 mg/kg) produced mild additive negative inotropic effects and reversed the prolongation of atrial and ventricular refractoriness produced by propafenone.[37]

Administration of propafenone in combination with either procainamide or quinidine can produce additive antiarrhythmic effects. A significant suppression of premature ventricular complexes (PVCs) after addition of propafenone was observed compared with that occurring after administration of procainamide or quinidine alone.[38]

Clinical Effects

Supraventricular Arrhythmias and Wolff-Parkinson-White Syndrome. Although propafenone will be approved initially by the FDA for treatment of ventricular arrhythmias only, its usefulness in treating supraventricular arrhythmias has been studied by a number of investigators (Table 3).[9,39–46]

In a randomized, double-blind, placebo-controlled study, Ludmer et al.[9] evaluated the safety and efficacy of intravenous propafenone in 10 patients with Wolff-Parkinson-White (WPW) syndrome and in 2 patients with concealed accessory pathways. In 11 of these patients, sustained atrioventricular nodal re-entrant tachycardia was inducible before the administration of propafenone. After infusion of propafenone 2 mg/kg over 10 minutes, the tachyardia was terminated in 10 of the 11 patients and the tachycardia slowed in the 11th patient. Before the administration of propafenone, six patients had inducible sustained atrial fibrillation and four had inducible nonsustained atrial fibrillation. After receiving propafenone, no patients had inducible sustained atrial fibrillation. The beneficial effects of propafenone in terminating re-entrant tachycardia and preventing rein-

Table 3.
Clinical Studies of Propafenone[a]

Reference	Study Design	Arrhythmia Treated	Drug Dosage	Efficacy: Effect	Efficacy: *n*
Supraventricular Arrhythmias					
9	Randomized, double-blind, placebo-controlled crossover; EPS	AV nodal re-entrant tachycardia or sustained AF	P 2 mg/kg i.v. over 10 min	Tachycardia terminated	P 10/11, Pl 0/7
42	Randomized, placebo-controlled	Atrial tachycardia (AF or A flutter)	P 2 mg/kg i.v. over 10 min	Arrhythmia converted to sinus rhythm	P 6/14, Pl 0/14
Ventricular Arrhythmias					
6	Open study; EPS	VT and/or VF	P 450–900 mg/day p.o.	VT prevented or VT rate markedly reduced	10/15
47	Open study; EPS	VT	P 900 mg/day p.o.	VT not induced Cycle length increased	5/26 21/26
7	Open study; EPS	VT	P 900 mg/day p.o.	VT not induced Nonsustained VT induced VT cycle length increased	1/16 1/16 14/26
50	Placebo-controlled, double-blind, crossover; AE	PVCs	P 900 mg/day p.o.	≥80% reduction in PVCs	P 7/12, Pl 2/12
23	Randomized, double-blind, placebo-controlled; AE	PVCs	P 450–900 mg/day p.o.	≥90% reduction in PVCs	P 7/13, Pl 0/13
51	Double-blind, placebo-controlled, crossover; AE	PVCs	P 300–900 mg/day p.o.	No. of PVCs/hr No. of paired PVCs/hr No. of VT Episodes	P 40, Pl 373 P 1, Pl 20 P 0, Pl 2
55	Double-blind, comparative (P versus D)	PVCs	P 900 mg/day p.o. D 600 mg/day p.o.	≥80% suppression of PVCs	P 5/9, D 2/9
58	Comparative (P versus Q)	PVCs	P 900 mg/day p.o. Q 1600 mg/day p.o.	≥85% suppression of PVCs	P 7/11, Q 3/10
38	Comparative (P + Q, P + Proc, Proc alone, Q alone); AE	PVCs	Maximum doses: P 900 mg/day p.o., Q 1000 mg/day p.o., Proc 50 mg/kg/day p.o.	>70% suppression of PVCs	P + Q or P + Proc 16/23, Q or Proc 2/23

[a] Placebo-controlled or comparative trials or trials using electrophysiologic studies (EPS). AE = ambulatory electrocardiography, AF = atrial fibrillation, VT = ventricular tachycardia, VF = ventricular fibrillation, PVCs = premature ventricular complexes, P = propafenone, Q = quinidine, D = disopyramide, Proc = procainamide hydrochloride, Pl = placebo.

duction of tachycardia also have been observed by Hammill et al.[39] and Shen et al.[45] in patients with WPW syndrome and atrioventricular nodal re-entrant tachycardia.

Breithardt et al.[40] studied 43 patients receiving long-term propafenone therapy for WPW syndrome or concealed accessory pathways. After treatment with propafenone for two to three years, 17 patients reported no episodes of symptomatic tachycardia and 18 patients experienced a slower, less frequent, and self-terminating tachycardia. In other studies involving small numbers of patients, excellent long-term benefits from therapy with oral propafenone also have been reported.[9,39]

Propafenone also was used to successfully treat junctional ectopic tachycardia in a small group of pediatric patients.[41] Junctional ectopic tachycardia is seen in children immediately after cardiac surgery and is not generally responsive to cardioversion.

In patients with atrial fibrillation or flutter after cardiac surgery, propafenone slowed the ventricular rate compared with placebo.[42] The drug also converted these arrhythmias to sinus rhythm in 43% of the 14 patients. No patient's arrhythmia converted to sinus rhythm after administration of placebo. In a study by Hammill et al.[43] 53% of the patients receiving long-term propafenone therapy for refractory paroxysmal atrial fibrillation had at least a 90% reduction in symptomatic episodes. Propafenone was less effective than quinidine in treating vagally dependent atrial flutter and fibrillation. However, in adrenergically dependent atrial tachycardia and fibrillation, propafenone was more effective than a β-blocker or amiodarone.[44] In this study, efficacy was determined by a decline in symptomatic episodes and 24-hour ambulatory electrocardiographic recordings.

Ventricular Arrhythmias. Propafenone has been shown to be effective in suppressing PVCs[50–

[57] and in treating various ventricular arrhythmias including nonsustained and sustained ventricular tachycardia (VT)[5-7,19,46-49] (Table 3).

Chilson et al.[6] studied 25 patients, 19 men and 6 women, with either recurrent symptomatic VT or ventricular fibrillation. The most common diagnosis of these patients was arteriosclerotic heart disease (17 patients). The remaining patients had rheumatic heart disease, primary electrical disease, cardiomyopathy, valvular heart disease, or mitral valve prolapse. Five patients continued to have episodes of nonsustained VT after treatment with propafenone and did not undergo follow-up electrophysiologic testing. Propafenone therapy was discontinued in an additional five patients because of adverse effects including nausea, paresthesias, and pleuritic chest pain. Of the 15 patients who underwent electrophysiologic testing, propafenone prevented the initiation of VT or markedly reduced the rate of tachycardia in 10 of 15 patients, and 8 of the 10 responsive patients remained free of tachycardia at follow-up. Prystowsky et al.[47] studied 26 patients in whom VT was induced by programmed electrical stimulation (PES) and obtained relatively good results with propafenone therapy. After treatment with propafenone, VT could not be initiated in five patients, and in the remaining patients the cycle length of VT increased. After discharge, 17 of these patients continued to receive propafenone therapy. The five patients in whom VT could not be induced remained free of symptomatic VT at a mean follow-up period of 11 months, and 6 of the 12 patients with inducible VT remained asymptomatic. On the other hand, in the study by Connolly et al.[7] of 16 patients with refractory VT or nonfatal cardiac arrest, the response to propafenone was not as good. All of their patients had inducible sustained VT at the time of the baseline PES study. Fourteen patients had coronary artery disease and two had cardiomyopathy. After propafenone therapy (900 mg/day), VT was not inducible in one patient, was nonsustained in one, and was harder to induce in two. In those patients whose VT was inducible, the cycle length was increased. Propafenone appeared to aggravate arrhythmias in four patients.

Propafenone's effectiveness in suppressing PVCs has been documented by a number of studies. Hodges et al.[50] evaluated propafenone in a placebo-controlled, double-blind, randomized crossover study. Based on 24-hour ambulatory electrocardiograms, PVCs were reduced ≥80% in 7 of 12 patients. After 24 months, suppression of PVCs ranged from 67% to 79% in those seven patients. These investigators found that maximum suppression of PVCs occurred with a QRS increase of 10% and that further increases in the QRS interval were not associated with improved suppression. They recommended that, because of the possibility of proarrhythmic effects of class IC drugs, it would be prudent to limit QRS increases with propafenone to 25% or less. In a similar study by Connolly et al.[18] 7 of 13 patients had a ≥90% reduction in PVCs documented by 24-hour electrocardiographic monitoring. In another trial, propafenone therapy resulted in an 85% reduction of ventricular ectopic beats as measured by 24-hour ambulatory electrocardiographic monitoring in 25 of 30 patients.[41] When propafenone therapy was tried in patients with ventricular ectopy previously refractory to a number of antiarrhythmic drugs (mean = 3.8), 30 of 45 patients responded with a ≥80% reduction of ventricular ectopic beats as measured by 24-hour recording.[52]

One long-term study recently completed by Dinh et al.[53] examined the safety and efficacy of propafenone in 37 patients with ventricular arrhythmias who had received the drug for two years. During that period more than 79% continued to respond to propafenone, one patient died suddenly, and another died of a noncardiac cause.

A number of studies have compared the use of propafenone with use of other antiarrhythmic drugs in the suppression of PVCs.[54-59] In randomized, placebo-controlled, comparative studies,[39,54-59] propafenone was found to be as effective as or better than disopyramide in suppressing PVCs. However, a higher incidence of adverse effects in patients taking disopyramide was observed. A double-blind, randomized, crossover trial with propafenone and disopyramide conducted by Libersa et al.[55] with a small number of patients found that five of nine patients treated with propafenone 300 mg every eight hours had a >80% reduction in PVCs. Only two of nine patients treated with disopyramide 200 mg three times a day had some PVC suppression. Other reports also indicate that propafenone may be more effective than disopyramide in treating ventricular ectopy.[56,57] Propafenone 300 mg three times a day was found to be as effective as quinidine 400 mg every six hours.[58]

The use of propafenone in combination with quinidine and procainamide for the treatment of frequent PVCs has been studied by Klein et al.[38] When propafenone was added to monotherapy with either procainamide or quinidine, 20 of 30 patients had a >70% reduction in PVCs as documented by 24-hour electrocardiogram recordings. They also found that propafenone was more effective than either procainamide or quinidine alone; 2 of 23 patients treated with either quinidine or procainamide versus 16 of 23 patients treated with propafenone had >70% suppression of PVCs. The combination required lower doses of each drug and resulted in fewer adverse effects than either drug alone.

Adverse Effects and Toxicity

Experience with propafenone in controlled studies suggests that it is relatively well tolerated. Overall, 21% to 32% of patients experience adverse reactions, with 3% to 7% of these serious enough to warrant discontinuing therapy. In randomized comparisons with disopyramide[54,59] and quinidine[58] in ambulatory patients with chronic ventricular arrhythmias, propafenone was found to be equal in efficacy to both agents, as well tolerated as quinidine, and better tolerated than disopyramide. The frequency of adverse reactions to propafenone is summarized in Table 4.

As with other antiarrhythmic drugs, the most serious cardiovascular reaction to propafenone is proarrhythmic events. These have been reported to occur in 6.1% of 1579 patients who participated in the initial trials of propafenone that included patients with both PVCs and serious malignant arrhythmias.[60] Most proarrhythmic events occur in patients with serious malignant arrhythmias. Podrid et al.[61] reported an incidence of 8% in such patients. In comparison, the incidence of proarrhythmic events with encainide and flecainide therapy in these patients is approximately 15% and 12%, respectively.[61] As with other class IC agents, the greatest risk of proarrhythmic events occurs in patients who have left ventricular dysfunction or malignant ventricular arrhythmias and who receive higher-than-recommended doses. Propafenone also is associated with conduction disturbance (first-degree atrioventricular block, QRS widening, and bundle branch block) in approximately 6% of patients.[62] Because propafenone is a negative inotropic agent, new or worsened congestive heart failure can occur, especially with high doses. Congestive heart failure has been reported in 2.9% of 1579 patients participating in initial trials.[60] Caution should be used when propafenone therapy is started in patients with left ventricular dysfunction, particularly those with ejection fractions of 30% or less.

Noncardiac adverse effects primarily involve the central nervous system and gastrointestinal tract.[63] The most common reactions are dizziness or lightheadedness (12% of patients), a metallic taste (8% of patients), and nausea or vomiting (10% of patients).[62] In the experience of Siddoway et al.[13] central nervous system adverse effects occur more frequently in patients who are poor metabolizers. In this patient population of 28 patients, 67% of the poor metabolizers had central nervous system adverse effects, whereas only 14% of the extensive metabolizers suffered central nervous system effects. Poor metabolizers generally had plasma propafenone concentrations of >1100 ng/mL.[13]

Table 4.
Common Adverse Reactions to Propafenone in 1579 Patients[60]

Adverse Reaction	Incidence (%)
Noncardiac	
Dizziness or lightheadedness	11.9
Nausea or vomiting	8.9
Unusual taste	8.9
Constipation	6.2
Headache	3.9
Cardiac	
Proarrhythmic events (ventricular tachycardia or premature ventricular complexes)	6.4
Conduction disturbances (atrioventricular block of intraventricular delay, or both)	5.5
New or worsened congestive heart failure	2.9

Dosage

The initial dosage of propafenone for the treatment of ventricular arrhythmias is 150 mg every eight hours for all adult patients (both rapid and poor metabolizers). This may be increased to 300 mg every 12 hours and then to 300 mg every 8 hours.[7,38,46] In general, the dosage should be increased slowly and gradually at three- to four-day intervals, and the maximum daily dosage should be 900 mg. The dosage increments should probably not be greater than 50% at each increase because of the nonlinear relationship between dose and plasma concentrations. Because plasma propafenone concentrations vary widely in patients receiving this drug, the PR interval and QRS duration should be monitored. If either is prolonged excessively (for example, >25%) during propafenone therapy, dosage should be reduced until the electrocardiogram returns to acceptable limits.

For treatment of supraventricular re-entrant tachycardia or WPW syndrome, intravenous doses of 2 mg/kg over 10 minutes have been reported to be effective and well tolerated.[9,45] (Intravenous therapy will not be generally available because only oral tablets will be approved by FDA.) For oral maintenance therapy, 450 to 900 mg daily in three or four divided doses has been shown to be effective.[9,39]

Formulary Recommendation

We recommend addition of propafenone to the hospital formulary. It is an effective antiarrhythmic agent and generally well tolerated on a long-term basis in patients who respond well to initial treatment.

Although two other class IC antiarrhythmic agents (flecainide and encainide) are already available in the United States, these agents are far from ideal. Many patients, especially those with persistent life-threatening VT, do not respond and do not tolerate these drugs well. The availability of a new agent, such as propafenone, will increase the therapeutic choices and enable better control of such arrhythmias in these patients. The addition of this drug to the hospital formulary is not expected to increase the hospital drug cost substantially.

Conclusion

Propafenone, a class IC antiarrhythmic agent, will soon be approved by the FDA for the treatment of ventricular arrhythmias. Based on the available clinical studies, propafenone is a relatively safe drug (as indicated by its adverse-effect profile and hemodynamic and pharmacokinetic properties). It is effective for the suppression of PVCs and for initial treatment of ventricular tachycardia. Like other recently approved class IC antiarrhythmics, propafenone is less effective in the treatment of refractory VT. Whether propafenone is better or more suitable than the existing class IC agents for such arrhythmias is unknown, since comparative data among these agents are limited. Based on the available data on propafenone, it appears that this new drug possesses pharmacologic properties that would make it useful for the treatment of ventricular arrhythmias, WPW syndrome, and supraventricular arrhythmias.

References

1. Myerburg RJ. Sudden cardiac death: epidemiology, causes, and mechanism. *Cardiology*. 1987; 24(Suppl 2):2–9.
2. Dukes ID, Vaughn Williams EM. The multiple models of action of propafenone. *Eur Heart J*. 1984; 5:115–25.
3. Keller K, Meyer-Estorf G, Beck OA et al. Correlation between serum concentration and pharmacological effect on atrioventricular conduction time of the anti-arrhythmic drug propafenone. *Eur J Clin Pharmacol*. 1978; 13:17–20.
4. Waleffe A, Mary-Rabine L, de Rijbel R et al. Electrophysiological effects of propafenone studied with programmed electrical stimulation of the heart in patients with recurrent paroxysmal supraventricular tachycardia. *Eur Heart J*. 1981; 2:345–52.
5. Shen EN, Sung RJ, Morady F et al. Electrophysiologic and hemodynamic effects of intravenous propafenone in patients with recurrent ventricular tachycardia. *J Am Coll Cardiol*. 1984; 3:1291–7.
6. Chilson DA, Heger JJ, Zipes DP et al. Electrophysiologic effects and clinical efficacy of oral propafenone therapy in patients with ventricular tachycardia. *J Am Coll Cardiol* 1985; 5:1407–13.
7. Connolly ST, Kates RE, Labsack CS et al. Clinical efficacy and electrophysiology of oral propafenone for ventricular tachycardia. *Am J Cardiol*. 1983; 52:1208–13.
8. Probst P, Pachinger O. The influence of propafenone on the hemodynamics of the left ventricle and atrioventricular conduction with special reference to the WPW syndrome (Ger). *Z Kardiol*. 1976; 65:212–4.
9. Ludmer PL, McGowan NE, Antman EM et al. Efficacy of propafenone in Wolff-Parkinson-White syndrome: electrophysiologic findings and long-term follow-up. *J Am Coll Cardiol*. 1987; 9:1357–63.
10. McLeod AA, Stiles GL, Shand DG. Demonstration of beta-adrenoceptor blockade by propafenone hydrochloride: clinical pharmacologic, radiological binding and adrenylate cyclate activation studies. *J Pharmacol Exp Ther*. 1984; 228:461–6.
11. Salako LA, Vaughan Williams EM, Wittig JH. Investigations to characterize a new antiarrhythmic drug, ORG6001, including a simple test for calcium antagonism. *Br J Pharmacol*. 1976; 57:251–62.
12. Cheriex EC, Krijne R, Brugada P et al. Lack of clinically significant beta-blocking effect of propafenone. *Eur Heart J*. 1987; 8:53–6.
13. Siddoway LA, Thompson KA, McAllister CB et al. Polymorphism of propafenone metabolism and disposition in man: clinical and pharmacokinetic consequences. *Circulation*. 1987; 75:785–91.
14. Baker BJ, Brodsky MA, Dinh H et al. Hemodynamic effect of propafenone and the experience in patients with congestive heart failure. *J Electrophysiology*. 1987; 1:527–35.
15. Podrid PJ, Lown B. Propafenone: a new agent for ventricular arrhythmia. *J Am Coll Cardiol*. 1984; 3:1291–6.
16. Baker BJ, Dinh H, Kroskey D et al. Effect of propafenone on ventricular ejection fraction. *Am J Cardiol*. 1984; 54:20D–22D.
17. Hollman M, Brodie E, Hotz D et al. Investigations on the pharmacokinetics of propafenone in man. *Arzneimittelforschung*. 1983; 33:763–70.
18. Connolly SJ, Kates RE, Labsack CS et al. Clinical pharmacology of propafenone. *Circulation*. 1983; 68:589–96.
19. Frabetti L, Marchesini B, Capucci A et al. Anti-arrhythmic efficacy of propafenone: evaluation of effective plasma levels following single and multiple doses. *Eur J Clin Pharmacol*. 1986; 30:665–71.
20. Axelson JE, Chan GL-Y, Kirsten EG et al. Food increases the bioavailability of propafenone. *Br J Clin Pharmacol*. 1987; 23:735–41.
21. Latini R, Marchi S, Riva E et al. Distribution of propafenone and its active metabolite, 5-hydroxypropafenone, in human tissues. *Am Heart J*. 1987; 113:843–4.
22. Schlepper M. Propafenone, a review of its profile. *Eur Heart J*. 1987; 8(Suppl A):27–32.
23. Connolly S, Lebsack C, Winkle RA et al. Propafenone disposition kinetics in cardiac arrhythmia. *Clin Pharmacol Ther*. 1984; 36:163–8.
24. Higuchi S, Urano C, Kawamura S. Determination of plasma protein binding of propafenone in rats, dogs and humans by highly sensitive gas chromatography-mass spectrometry. *J Chromatogr*. 1985; 341:305–11.
25. Gillis AM, Yee Y-G, Kates RE. Binding of antiarrhythmic drugs to be purified human α_1-acid glycoprotein. *Biochem Pharmacol*. 1985; 34:4279–82.
26. Von Philipsborn G, Gries J, Hoffman HP et al. Pharmacological studies with propafenone and its main metabolite, 5-hydroxypropafenone. *Arzneimittelforschung*. 1984; 34:1489–97.
27. Zaza A, Forster M, Danilo P et al. Electrophysiologic effects of propafenone and metabolites on canine Purkinje fibers. *Fed Proc*. 1987; 46:871. Abstract.
28. Hege HG, Kavmeier S, Weymann J. The metabolism of propafenone in man. Metabolic pattern and structure elucidation of the major metabolites in plasma, urine, and feces after oral dosing. *Eur J Drug Metab Pharmacokinet* 1984; 9:41–55.
29. Salerno DM, Granrud G, Sharkey P et al. A controlled trial of propafenone for treatment of frequent and repetitive ventricular premature complexes. *Am J Cardiol*. 1984; 53:77–83.
30. Lee JT, Yee Y-G, Dorian P et al. Influence of hepatic dysfunction on the pharmacokinetics of propafenone. *J Clin Pharmacol*. 1987; 27:384–9.
31. Belz GG, Matthews J, Doering W et al. Digoxin—antiarrhythmics: pharmacodynamic and pharmacokinetic studies with quinidine, propafenone, and verapamil. *Clin Pharmacol Ther*. 1982; 31:202–3.
32. Cardaioli P, Compostella L, DeDomenico R et al. Influenza of propafenone on the pharmacokinetics of digoxin administered by the oral route: study on healthy volunteers. *G Ital Cardiol*. 1986; 16:237–40.
33. Nolan P, Marcus FI, Erstad BL et al. Pharmacokinetic interaction between propafenone and digoxin. *J Am Coll Cardiol*. 1988; 11:168A. Abstract.
34. Kates RE, Yee Y-G, Kirsten EB. Interaction between warfarin and propafenone in healthy volunteer subjects. *Clin Phar-*

macol Ther. 1987; 42:305–11.
35. Pritchett ELC, Smith WM, Kirsten EB. Pharmacokinetic and pharmacodynamic interactions of propafenone and cimetidine. *J Clin Pharmacol.* 1988; 28:619–24.
36. Wagner F, Kalusche D, Trenk D et al. Drug interaction between propafenone and metoprolol. *Br J Clin Pharmacol.* 1987; 24:213–20.
37. Feld GK, Nademanee K, Singh BN et al. Hemodynamic and electrophysiologic effects of combined infusion of lidocaine and propafenone in humans. *J Clin Pharmacol.* 1987; 27:52–9.
38. Klein R, Huang SK, Marcus FL et al. Enhanced antiarrhythmic efficacy of propafenone when used in combination with procainamide or quinidine. *Am Heart J.* 1987; 114:551–8.
39. Hammill SC, McLaran CJ, Wood DL et al. Double-blind study of intravenous propafenone for paroxysmal supraventricular reentrant tachycardia. *J Am Coll Cardiol.* 1987; 9:1364–8.
40. Breithardt G, Borggrefe M, Wiebringhaus E et al. Effect of propafenone in the Wolff-Parkinson-White syndrome: electrophysiologic findings and long-term follow-up. *Am J Cardiol.* 1984; 54:29D–39D.
41. Garson A, Moak JP, Smith RT et al. Usefulness of intravenous propafenone for treatment of atrial tachyarrhythmias after cardiac surgery. *Am J Cardiol.* 1979; 44:298–302.
42. Connolly SJ, Mulji AS, Hoffert D et al. Randomized placebo-controlled trial of propafenone for treatment of atrial tachyarrhythmias after cardiac surgery. *J Am Coll Cardiol.* 1987; 10:1145–8.
43. Hammill SC, Wood DL, Gersh BJ et al. Propafenone for paroxysmal atrial fibrillation. *Am J Cardiol.* 1988; 61:473–5.
44. Coumel P, Leclercq JF, Assayag P. European experience with the antiarrhythmic efficacy of propafenone for supraventricular and ventricular arrhythmias. *Am J Cardiol.* 1984; 54:60D–66D.
45. Shen EN, Keung E, Huycke E et al. Intravenous propafenone for termination of reentrant supraventricular tachycardia. *Ann Intern Med.* 1986; 105:655–61.
46. Salerno DM, Granrud G, Sharkey P et al. A controlled trial of propafenone for treatment of frequent and repetitive premature complexes. *Am Heart J.* 1984; 53:77–83.
47. Prystowsky EN, Heger JJ, Chilson DA et al. Antiarrhythmic and elecrophysiologic effects of oral propafenone. *Am J Cardiol.* 1984; 54:26D–28D.
48. Heger JJ, Hubbard J, Zipes DP et al. Propafenone treatment of recurrent ventricular tachycardia: comparison of continuous electrocardiographic recording and electrophysiologic study in predicting drug efficacy. *Am J Cardiol.* 1984; 54:53D–59D.
49. Podrid PJ, Cytryn R, Lown B. Propafenone: non-invasive evaluation of efficacy. *Am J Cardiol.* 1984; 54:53D–59D.
50. Hodges M, Salerno D, Granrud G. Double-blind placebo-controlled evaluation of propafenone in suppressing ventricular ectopic activity. *Am J Cardiol.* 1984; 54:48D–50D.
51. de Soyza N, Terry L, Murphy ML et al. Effect of propafenone in patients with stable ventricular arrhythmias. *Am Heart J.* 1984; 108:285–9.
52. Hammill SC, Sorenson PB, Wood DL et al. Propafenone for the treatment of refractory complex ventricular ectopic activity. *Mayo Clin Proc.* 1986; 61:98–103.
53. Dinh H, Baker BJ, de Soyza N et al. Sustained therapeutic efficacy and safety of oral propafenone for treatment of chronic ventricular arrhythmias: a 2-year experience. *Am Heart J.* 1988; 115:92–6.
54. Rabkin SW, Boroomand-Rashti K, McKinnon J et al. Comparison of propafenone and disopyramide in the treatment of ventricular premature complexes: a randomized double blind crossover placebo controlled trial. *Can J Cardiol.* 1987; 3:105–10.
55. Libersa C, Caron J, Pladys A et al. Propafenone vs. disopyramide. A double-blind randomized crossover trial in patients presenting chronic ventricular arrhythmias. *Clin Cardiol.* 1987; 10:405–10.
56. Clementry J, Dallocchio M, Bricaud H et al. Comparative study of the therapeutic effect of propafenone and disopyramide in the oral treatment of chronic ventricular premature beats. In: Cardiac arrhythmias. Schlepper M, Olssen B, eds. Berlin: Springer-Verlag; 1983:159–69.
57. Breithardt G, Haerten K, Seipel L et al. Zur antiarrhythmischen Wirksamkeit von Disopyramide bei ventrikularer Extrasystolic und Vorhofflimmen. *Z Kardiol.* 1976; 65:713.
58. Dinh HA, Murphy ML, Baker BJ et al. Efficacy of propafenone compared with quinidine in chronic ventricular arrhythmias. *Am J Cardiol.* 1985; 55:1520–4.
59. Naccarella F, Bracchetti D, Palmieri M et al. Comparison of propafenone and disopyramide for treatment of chronic ventricular arrhythmias: placebo-controlled, double-blind, randomized crossover study. *Am Heart J.* 1985; 109:833–40.
60. Canadian official product monograph for Rythmol (propafenone hydrochloride). 1987 Oct 21.
61. Podrid PJ. Aggravation of arrhythmia by antiarrhythmic drugs. Incidence and predictors of occurrence. *Am J Cardiol.* 1987; 59:38E–44E.
62. Harron DWG, Brogden RN. Propafenone. *Drugs.* 1987; 34:617–47.
63. Siddoway LA, Roden DM, Woosley RL. Clinical pharmacology of propafenone; pharmacokinetics, metabolism and concentration-response relations. *Am J Cardiol.* 1984; 54:9D–12D.

“

Clinical Use of Antiarrhythmic Agents

While quinidine and procainamide products have been available for many decades, it was not until the late 1970s that a new antiarrhythmic drug (disopyramide) was added to the clinical armamentarium. In just the last few years, however, tocainide, mexiletine, encainide, flecainide and amiodarone have been approved and perhaps up to another half dozen antiarrhythmic agents may be available within the next few years. The sponsors of all of these new agents have increased educational and promotional programs that, in turn, have increased physicians' awareness and interest in identifying and treating patients with ventricular arrhythmias. It is now more important than ever to ask who should be treated, with what agent should a patient be treated and where should such drugs be administered initially (in-hospital or outpatient setting)?

—Morganroth J, Horowitz LN. Antiarrhythmic drug therapy 1988: for whom, how and where? *Am J Cardiol.* 1988; 62:461–5. Editorial.

”

Therapy Review

Effect of antimicrobial therapy on bowel flora

K. DALE HOOKER AND JOSEPH T. DIPIRO

Abstract: The known patterns and functions of gastrointestinal flora and antimicrobial effects on flora are described, and the clinical implications of altered bowel flora are described.

A major role of the normal endogenous intestinal flora is to inhibit gastrointestinal colonization and overgrowth by potentially pathogenic bacteria. Serious disruption of this protective mechanism may occur after the administration of various antimicrobial agents. Alteration of bacterial flora by antimicrobials is often the result of incomplete absorption after oral administration or of high concentrations in saliva, bile, or secretions from the intestinal flora. Suppression of endogeneous microflora after antimicrobial administration may permit overgrowth of pathogenic strains in the gastrointestinal tract, development or selection of antimicrobial-agent-resistant strains, and disruption of colonization resistance. The disruption of normal bowel flora can result in diarrhea, pseudomembranous colitis, and systemic infections or sepsis in immunocompromised patients. Agents that are well absorbed and have minimal biliary excretion should minimize the detrimental effects from altered flora.

The choice of an antimicrobial agent that has a narrow spectrum, is specific for the infection, is not appreciably excreted in the bile, and is completely absorbed if given orally appears to be the most appropriate practice for preventing or minimizing alteration of bowel flora.

Index terms: Absorption; Anti-infective agents; Bile levels; Diarrhea; Drug administration routes; Drugs; Enterocolitis; Excretion; Toxicity
Clin Pharm. 1988; 7:878–88

The human body accommodates literally hundreds of aerobic and anaerobic bacterial species. These bacteria play an important role in the normal functioning of the host, which becomes apparent when their numbers or balance are disrupted. Ordinarily, the composition and number of strains within the normal gastrointestinal flora remain essentially stable; however, physiologic and ecological disturbances, including antimicrobial use, may disrupt this stability. Changes in bacterial flora may result in minor clinical events such as mild diarrhea but may also be associated with more severe syndromes such as pseudomembranous colitis or systemic infections caused by fungi or resistant bacteria. The most common mechanism for alteration of microbial flora is the indiscriminate use of broad-spectrum antimicrobials, because antimicrobials do not distinguish between pathogens and commensals and therefore may dramatically alter body flora.

Drugs from a number of classes may alter bacterial flora. Antimicrobials are the most obvious offenders, but antineoplastic drugs, immunosuppressive agents, or even histamine H_2 antagonists (which promote bacterial growth by decreasing gastric acidity) may also have substantial effects on bacterial populations. Within the different classes of antimicrobials, the effects on normal flora vary considerably. Agents that achieve high concentrations in the lumen of the gastrointestinal tract and those that eradicate anaerobic bacteria tend to have the greatest effects on gut bacteria.

Disruption of bacterial flora at any body site may be important in terms of adverse events; however, alteration of bowel flora has received the most attention. The purpose of this review is to address the issues relating to alteration of gastrointestinal microflora by antimicrobials. The known patterns

K. DALE HOOKER, PHARM.D., is a Postdoctoral Research Associate, College of Pharmacy, University of Georgia. JOSEPH T. DIPIRO, PHARM.D., is Associate Professor, College of Pharmacy, University of Georgia, Athens, and Associate Clinical Professor, Department of Surgery, Medical College of Georgia, Augusta.

Address reprint requests to Dr. DiPiro at the Department of Clinical Pharmacy, CN-137, Medical College of Georgia, Augusta, GA 30912.

Copyright © 1988, American Society of Hospital Pharmacists, Inc. All rights reserved. 0278-2677/88/1201-0878$02.75.

and functions of gastrointestinal flora in the healthy individual are reviewed as a basis for examining reports of altered flora. Issues of focus for this review include the following: (1) Do alterations in gastrointestinal flora relate to adverse clinical events? (2) What characteristics of antimicrobials predict a greater effect on normal gastrointestinal flora? and (3) How may the adverse consequences of altered gastrointestinal flora be avoided or minimized?

Usual Bowel Flora

A necessary prerequisite to a discussion of alterations in bowel flora and the clinical consequences is a review of the usual character of gastrointestinal flora and the functions that are attributed to these bacteria. The most commonly isolated bacteria and approximate concentrations are summarized in Table 1. One striking observation is that the concentration of organisms varies from less than 100 bacteria per milliliter in gastric fluid to more than 1,000,000,000 organisms per milliliter or gram of colon contents. Secondly, the number of different species that can be isolated from the gastrointestinal tract is more than 100.[2,10]

Even within a given segment of the gastrointestinal tract, the concentrations of bacteria can vary with distance from the mucosal surface. In mice, *Bacteroides*, fusiforms, enterococci, and coliforms may be found in higher concentrations at the epithelial surfaces of the colon than in the lumen.[11] The complex nature of the gastrointestinal flora suggests the potential for many interactions between organisms and host.

Of the factors known to alter gastrointestinal flora, antimicrobial use will be discussed in depth. Other important factors include alterations in gastrointestinal motility, diet, altered anatomy from intestinal resection, and age. Age is important primarily in the newborn, because the gastrointestinal tract is sterile at birth. Within a few weeks after birth the gastrointestinal tract flora resembles that of adults.

With acute diarrhea, the character of intestinal flora can change dramatically. A marked reduction in anaerobes has been noted,[12,13] which is possibly related to rapid transit. If diarrhea is related to bacterial pathogens (e.g., *Vibrio cholerae, Shigella, Salmonella*, or *Escherichia coli*), high concentrations of the causative organisms are present. Also, the concentration of certain gram-negative bacilli (*Klebsiella, Enterobacter, Proteus*, and *Pseudomonas*) may also be increased with acute diarrhea.[11] With intestinal obstruction, the concentration of bacteria is increased proximal to the point of obstruction.[11]

Diet may be an important factor in determining gastrointestinal flora, although the information is conflicting. In geographic locations where diets are high in fiber and low in meat products and fat (e.g., Asian or African countries), the usual bowel flora is different from that of residents in most Western countries. Although bowel flora differs between some geographic areas, it appears relatively difficult to alter bowel flora in an individual by changing dietary habits.[14,15] The time required to effect change in bowel flora appears to be pro-

Table 1.
Usual Microflora of the Gastrointestinal Tract[a,b]

Site	Commonly Found Bacteria	Approximate Concentration (Organisms/mL)	
		Aerobes	Anaerobes
Stomach[c]	*Streptococcus, Lactobacillus*	10^0–10^2	Rare
Biliary tract	Normally sterile (*Escherichia coli, Klebsiella*, or enterococci in some patients)	0	0
Proximal small bowel	*Streptococcus* (including enterococci), *E. coli, Klebsiella, Lactobacillus*, diphtheroids	10^2	Few
Distal ileum	*E. coli, Klebsiella, Enterobacter*, enterococci, *Bacteroides fragilis, Clostridia*, peptostreptococci	10^4–10^6	10^5–10^7
Colon	*Bacteroides* spp., peptostreptococci, *Clostridia, E. coli, Klebsiella*, enterococci, *Enterobacter* (and many others)	10^5–10^8	10^9–10^{11}

[a] Reprinted from reference 1 with permission.
[b] Based on references 2–9.
[c] With achlorhydria, histamine H_2 antagonists, gastric cancer, or gastric-outlet obstruction, bacterial counts may rise to 10^5–10^7/mL.

longed.[16] Some authors note that alterations in diet have only minor effects on flora.[15]

The possible beneficial versus detrimental effects on the host have been debated since bacteria were first recognized to colonize the gastrointestinal tract. Now, most investigators believe that the usual intestinal flora are advantageous to the host because they inhibit gastrointestinal colonization by potentially pathogenic bacteria. Other roles attributed to intestinal bacteria include metabolism of the by-products of drugs and endogenous substances, which results in enterohepatic recirculation. For example, bacteria promote enterohepatic recirculation of drugs such as digoxin and morphine and substances such as estrogens, folic acid, cyanocobalamin (vitamin B_{12}), bile acids, cholesterol, and metabolites of vitamin D.[14] Also, intestinal bacteria may synthesize some vitamins such as vitamin K, cyanocobalamin, folate, pyridoxine, biotin, riboflavin, and pantothenate. The low level of vitamin production, however, suggests that this source is not important in most people.[16] Finally, the normal flora may stimulate nonspecific host immune systems that protect against potential pathogens.[17]

A few authors have summarized the possible mechanisms by which normal intestinal flora inhibit colonization by pathogenic bacteria as follows[15,17-19]:

1. The high concentration of microorganisms in the terminal segments of the gastrointestinal tract creates competition for nutrients.[15,20] Some investigators, however, question the importance of this mechanism.[21]
2. The normal intestinal flora provides limited opportunity for attachment of new organisms to gastrointestinal mucosa. Without attachment, bacteria are rapidly removed from the gastrointestinal tract.[19-21]
3. Endogenous bacteria produce bacteriocins, high-molecular-weight compounds that are antibacterial.[17,22,23,24] These substances are believed important in inhibiting potential pathogens.
4. Anaerobic and facultative bacteria produce short-chain fatty acids (acetic, propionic, and butyric) that are toxic to enterobacteria.[25-28]
5. Intestinal flora can deconjugate bile acids, which are then inhibitory to some species of pathogenic bacteria.[17]

Regardless of the mechanism by which normal intestinal bacteria inhibit colonization by pathogenic bacteria, anaerobic bacteria appear to be the most important aspect of defense, so disruption of anaerobes is likely to have physiologic consequences.[15] With normal gastrointestinal flora, an oral dose of gram-negative bacteria has little chance of colonizing the gastrointestinal tract.[29] In animal studies, the dose of *Escherichia coli* required to colonize the gastrointestinal tract decreases from about 10^7 in the presence of normal anaerobic flora to as low as 100 without anaerobic flora.[19] The term that has been applied to the inhibition of pathogenic bacteria by intestinal flora is "colonization resistance." More specifically, colonization resistance is the ability of the normal gut flora to combat colonization by extrinsic bacteria, a property that can be upset by antibiotic administration.[30] As described by van der Waaij,[19] "The anaerobes involved in this colonization resistance in the intestine appeared to live in close association with the mucosal lining of the large intestine, forming a 'living wallpaper'."

Although intestinal bacteria are usually viewed as beneficial to the host, there are some indications of detrimental effects. Endogenous bacteria may possibly act in synergy with pathogens to increase the risk of infection.[31] In immunocompromised patients, even normal intestinal flora may become pathogenic. Also, normal flora may induce immunologic tolerance to bacterial toxins.[32] Finally, intestinal bacteria may transform benign substances in the gastrointestinal tract to mutagenic substances.[14]

Features of Antimicrobial Agents That Influence Changes in Bowel Flora

The extent to which an antimicrobial agent alters the normal bowel flora is dependent on several factors, including the antimicrobial spectrum and intestinal concentration (Table 2). Narrow-spectrum antimicrobials, which have minimal effect on the anaerobic flora, appear to be less likely to disrupt the bowel flora than broad-spectrum agents. Although the antimicrobial's spectrum influences the severity of change in bowel flora, the ability to disrupt the normal bacterial composition is more often related to disposition of the antimicrobial (e.g., rate of absorption, metabolism, and routes and extent of excretion). Oral administration and biliary secretion are the two features of antimicrobial agents contributing most substantially to altered gastrointestinal flora.

Oral Administration. Antimicrobials that are poorly absorbed from the gastrointestinal tract can cause substantial alteration of the bowel flora.[18,33-35] Numerous studies have demonstrated a higher risk of ecological pressure on the intestinal flora with orally administered agents that are poorly absorbed. This has been clearly demonstrated for the tetracyclines in a comparison of doxycycline, which is well absorbed, with tetracycline hydrochloride, which is less well absorbed.[36] In addition, pseudomembranous colitis and diarrhea occurred with greater frequency in individuals receiving oral clindamycin than those receiving clindamycin intramuscularly or intravenously.[37,38] The risk of clindamycin-induced pseudomembranous colitis was three to four times greater with oral versus intramuscular or intravenous administration.[39]

A similar phenomenon has been observed with

Table 2.
Impact of Different Antimicrobial Agents on Bowel Flora and Relevant Pharmacologic Properties[a]

Antimicrobial Agent (Route of Administration)	Activity in Vitro[b]		Intestinal Concentration[c]	Emergence of Resistant Indigenous Bacterial Strains[b]		Risk for Overgrowth or Superinfection
	Aerobes	Anaerobes		Aerobes	Anaerobes	
Aztreonam (i.v.)	+++	–	Low	+	–	Low
Bacampicillin (p.o.)	++	++	Low	–	–	Low
Ciprofloxacin (p.o.)	+++	–	High	–	–	Low
Imipenem (i.v.)	+++	+++	Low	–	–	Low
Penicillin (p.o.)	–	++	Low	–	–	Low
Ampicillin + sulbactam (i.v.)	+++	+++	Moderate	–	–	Moderate
Cefoxitin (i.v.)	+++	+++	Moderate	+	+	Moderate
Doxycycline (p.o.)	++	++	Moderate	+++	+++	Moderate
Metronidazole (p.o.)	–	+++	Moderate	–	–	Moderate
Cefoperazone (i.v.)	+++	+++	High	+	+	High
Clindamycin (p.o.)	–	+++	High	–	+	High
Clindamycin (i.v.)	–	+++	High	–	+	High
Erythromycin (p.o.)	++	++	High	++	++	High
Piperacillin (i.v.)	+++	+++	High	+	+	High

[a] Adapted from reference 18 with permission.
[b] – = None, + = least, ++ = moderate, +++ = most.
[c] Concentration attributable to incomplete absorption, biliary excretion, or intestinal secretion, on the basis of data from our laboratory.

cefuroxime. When administered intramuscularly or intravenously, cefuroxime is associated with a relatively low incidence of diarrhea. However, cefuroxime axetil, the oral ester form, caused diarrhea in 50% of healthy volunteers, all of whom developed decreased fecal counts of *Bacteroides fragilis*, peptostreptococci, peptococci, *E. coli*, and enterococci.[40]

Biliary Excretion. Intramuscularly or intravenously administered antimicrobial agents or well-absorbed oral agents that are secreted in high concentrations in the saliva, bile, or intestinal mucosa can also disrupt the normal balance of microorganisms in the gastrointestinal ecosystem.[41] Cefoperazone and ceftriaxone are two examples of antimicrobials that have high biliary excretion and are commonly implicated for causing diarrhea or other undesirable effects. In several studies, it has been clearly demonstrated that these agents possess the ability to suppress both aerobes and anaerobes, resulting in overgrowth of *Clostridium difficile*, with a subsequent risk of diarrhea.[36,42] It is well recognized that in the presence of certain antimicrobial agents, *C. difficile* appears to flourish and produce a cytotoxin that has been found in the stools of the majority of patients with antibiotic-associated pseudomembranous colitis.[43] The cytotoxin, not *C. difficile*, causes the problem. The lipophilicity and molecular weight of the antimicrobial agent are the main determinants of whether an agent is likely to be secreted. Antimicrobials with a high degree of lipophilicity are found in relatively higher concentrations in the saliva and pharyngeal secretions. Generally, antimicrobial agents with high molecular weights tend to be secreted in bile.[44] Antimicrobials can substantially alter the flora, no matter how they enter the gastrointestinal tract.

Effects of Antimicrobial Agents on Bowel Flora

While suppression of endogenous bowel microflora is occasionally desirable (e.g., for preparation of the bowel for surgery), the influence of antimicrobials on the normal bowel flora is not beneficial in most cases. Antimicrobials that influence the normal microflora promote the emergence of antimicrobial-agent-resistant strains and disruption of colonization resistance.[33] Heimdahl and colleagues[44] described antimicrobial-agent-suppressed oropharyngeal and gastrointestinal flora as "a microbiological vacuum readily filled by resistant microorganisms normally excluded from this region." The consequences of altered bowel flora, both desirable and undesirable, are summarized below.

Intentional Suppression of Susceptible Microorganisms. Reduction of bacterial concentrations in the bowel before colorectal surgery is the basis for the standard surgical practice of administering a preoperative bowel preparation including an antimicrobial agent. Bacteria account for up to one third of fecal weight and pose a substantial threat of infection in patients undergoing intra-abdominal surgery.[45] Several studies have demonstrated the ability of oral neomycin–erythromycin regimens to substantially reduce the concentration of aerobic and anaerobic bacteria in the colon and rectum.[46] Neomycin reduces the aerobic bacterial count (streptococci and coliforms) but not the anaerobes. Erythromycin consistently reduces the number of anaerobic bacteria, including *B. fragilis*.[47,48]

In a Veterans Administration cooperative study of 116 patients, 13% of patients receiving preoperative oral neomycin–erythromycin developed postoperative infections, while 55% of the placebo control group acquired a postoperative infection.[49] Based on clinical studies, oral antimicrobials that suppress the aerobic and anaerobic components of bowel flora effectively reduce the incidence of septic complications after elective colon surgery.[46–49]

Overgrowth of Pathogenic Strains. Another well-recognized consequence of altered bowel flora caused by broad-spectrum antimicrobial therapy is bacterial overgrowth in the gastrointestinal tract. This occurs because commensal organisms of the bowel flora, which normally prevent colonization by pathogenic strains, are eradicated by antimicrobials.[50] The removal of selective commensal organisms allows remaining antimicrobial-agent-resistant microorganisms to flourish unopposed, leaving the host susceptible to infection and other untoward effects.[51,52] In animals, suppression of normal anaerobic microflora enhances colonization and subsequent infection by pathogenic aerobic bacteria.[33]

In a recent study by Giuliano and associates[53] comparing the effects of broad-spectrum injectable antimicrobials on the composition of intestinal microflora in humans, enterococci and yeasts were two components that were most likely to overgrow. Enterococci were more prevalent in patients treated with cefoxitin and aztreonam, while yeasts were more prevalent in subjects treated with cefoperazone and piperacillin. There was a striking relationship between the number of yeasts and the decrease in number of anaerobes during treatment with cefoperazone and piperacillin.[53]

Selection of Antimicrobial-Agent-Resistant Strains. A second potential adverse consequence on bowel flora that may be an extension of antimicrobial presence is the development or selection of antimicrobial-agent-resistant strains. This can occur with a variety of antimicrobials, including aminoglycosides,[54] tetracyclines,[55] and β-lactam antimicrobials.[56] Emergence of resistant strains involves primarily aerobic gram-negative bacilli and gram-positive cocci; however, anaerobes may also become resistant.[57]

Nord and Kager,[58] studying the impact of cefoxitin, imipenem, and aztreonam on β-lactamase production by organisms in the colon, demonstrated no significant changes in the intestinal microflora nor induction of β-lactamase with imipenem; however, cefoxitin had a significant effect on both the aerobic and anaerobic organisms, with growth of enterococci, staphylococci, resistant enterobacteria, and *Pseudomonas* spp. Beta-lactamase production occurred in all patients during treatment with cefoxitin. Aztreonam, while having no effect on the anaerobic microflora nor inducing β-lactamase, did affect the number of enterobacteria (reduced), staphylococci (increased), and enterococci (increased).[58] A marked increase in the number of resistant aerobic and anaerobic bacteria of the gastrointestinal tract has also been demonstrated with doxycycline.[33]

Disruption of Colonization Resistance. Maintaining colonization resistance in the bowel is essential to prevent colonization and overgrowth of antimicrobial-agent-resistant, potentially pathogenic bacteria or fungi.[59,60] Disruption of the anaerobic component by antimicrobial drugs permits overgrowth, which increases the risk of an iatrogenic infection. This concept of colonization resistance has been extensively documented in animal models[61–66]; however, there is less documentation that this phenomenon occurs in humans.[53,67]

Many studies have been performed to determine the effect of various antimicrobials on colonization resistance. These effects were measured in humans and animals by monitoring the acquisition of new isolates in the fecal flora and in animals by determining cecal weight. A decrease in the resistance of the digestive tract to colonization has been demonstrated with agents such as moxalactam[65]; moxalactam with tobramycin[68]; azlocillin, mezlocillin, and cefuroxime[65]; cefoxitin[67]; cefoperazone[53,69]; oral ampicillin[30,62,66]; streptomycin[62]; rifampin, cloxacillin, and penicillin V[61]; and ceftriaxone.[70]

Changes in Bowel Flora after Exposure to Various Classes of Antimicrobials

The classes of antimicrobials discussed below were selected based on the amount of published information available. Information on other classes and specific antimicrobial agents is limited. Newer antimicrobial agents were included when possible.

Aminoglycosides. Intramuscularly or intravenously administered aminoglycosides have little effect on fecal flora, presumably because of the small amount excreted in bile and because of minimal anaerobic activity.[71] In contrast, orally administered aminoglycosides usually exert a more striking effect, eliminating the aerobic fecal flora and reducing the gram-positive anaerobic flora.[71–74] Daikos et al.[72] described the emergence of resistant staphylococci and enterococci and the proliferation of yeast in the gastrointestinal tract when oral aminoglycosides were used. *Bacteroides* species are usually unaffected, although they may be reduced in some patients.[75,76]

Cephalosporins. Several studies of the first-generation cephalosporins (e.g., cephalothin, cefazolin) have demonstrated only a slight change in the fecal flora after administration.[77] Studies with second-generation cephalosporins have demonstrated that cefoxitin therapy is associated with extensive intestinal colonization with resistant strains of enterococci, clostridia, *Pseudomonas*, and *Entero-*

bacter.[56] Cefaclor, an oral second-generation cephalosporin, resulted in only minor changes in the anaerobic intestinal microflora, while the aerobic flora were unchanged. Colonization with new cefaclor-resistant strains was not observed.[78]

The potent antibacterial activity of some third-generation cephalosporins that are excreted in high concentrations in the bile has resulted in considerable changes in the normal intestinal microflora. However, ceftazidime, a drug primarily eliminated via the kidneys, was found to disrupt the gastrointestinal flora after intramuscular or intravenous administration. While ceftazidime primarily eliminated gram-negative bacilli, effects on aerobic gram-positive cocci were also seen.[50] The impact of ceftriaxone[50,70,79] and cefoperazone[69,71,80] on the microflora is evidenced by profound suppression of both aerobic and anaerobic organisms and colonization by potentially pathogenic yeast and bacteria. Moxalactam has also demonstrated marked alterations in bowel flora,[81] while cefotaxime had only a moderate influence.[79] Alteration in the normal microflora by these broad-spectrum agents has led to the development of superinfection, colitis, and diarrhea.[41]

Extended-Spectrum Penicillins. Azlocillin and piperacillin, two broad-spectrum penicillins excreted in high concentrations in the bile, are likely to induce changes in the microflora.[34,82] While overgrowth of piperacillin-resistant enterobacteria and *B. fragilis* has been observed, the incidence of *C. difficile*-induced diarrhea and colitis during and after piperacillin treatment appears to be low.[18,82] Similar results with azlocillin were obtained by Nord and associates,[34] who observed significant changes in the number of streptococci, *E. coli*, anaerobic cocci, lactobacilli, clostridia, and *Bacteroides* spp. in approximately 30% of the treated patients. There were only minor changes in the remaining patients.

Monobactams. Aztreonam, with a spectrum comparable to that of the aminoglycosides, affected only the aerobic component of the microflora in the majority of studies.[53,60,83] In a study of 20 patients undergoing colorectal surgery, prophylactic aztreonam suppressed fecal enterobacteria and increased the numbers of staphylococci.[83] In the previous study, only minor changes in anaerobes were observed.[83] In another study, the majority of isolates of *Bacteroides* spp. persisted during aztreonam administration, but three of three isolates of *B. fragilis* were eliminated.[84] As expected, yeasts persisted in six of six isolates from stool cultures during aztreonam use.[84]

Carbapenems. Few studies are available that assess the impact of imipenem on fecal flora. Nord and associates[85] determined that less than 1% of imipenem is eliminated by the fecal route and observed only minor changes in the intestinal microflora of patients receiving this drug. Welkon and associates[86] observed an increase in the number of organisms in the fecal flora that were relatively less susceptible to imipenem (such as *Enterococcus* spp. and some Enterobacteriaceae) or resistant to imipenem (such as *Candida* spp.), although no patient experienced a secondary infection as a result of the change.

Quinolones. The new orally absorbed quinolone derivatives (e.g., ciprofloxacin, norfloxacin) display activity against aerobic gram-positive and gram-negative microorganisms in the gut, especially Enterobacteriaceae and *Ps. aeruginosa*.[41,87] Activity against anaerobic bacteria, especially *Bacteroides* and *Clostridium* spp., is limited.[88] Others have reported significant suppression of enterobacteria with the use of ciprofloxacin and norfloxacin.[42,89] Rozenberg–Arska and associates[87] summarized these properties as follows: (1) ciprofloxacin had no effect on anaerobes such as *Bacteroides* spp. and *Clostridium* spp., (2) it had some effect on anaerobic gram-positive bacteria such as non-spore-forming rods and cocci, and (3) a few ciprofloxacin-resistant strains occurred, which did not contribute to colonization or infection.

The effect of norfloxacin on fecal Enterobacteriaceae has been evaluated in several studies.[89,90] Anaerobic colonic microflora (*Bacteroides*, lactobacilli, bifidobacteria, and anaerobic gram-positive cocci) were only slightly disrupted. The findings of these and additional studies[87,91,92] indicate that ciprofloxacin has a greater effect on bowel flora than does norfloxacin.

Clinical Implications of Altered Bowel Flora

Of the possible consequences that may arise as a result of antimicrobial therapy disrupting the normal gastrointestinal flora, the development of diarrhea and pseudomembranous colitis and the increased likelihood of infection in high-risk patients are of the greatest clinical importance.

Diarrhea. Diarrhea is one of the most common complications resulting from antimicrobial administration. Although nearly all broad-spectrum antimicrobials may conceivably result in diarrhea and colitis caused by *C. difficile*, the agents most often implicated are the penicillins (ampicillin), cephalosporins, lincomycin, and clindamycin.[78] The mechanisms by which antimicrobials caused diarrhea differ and include alteration in bacterial metabolism of bile acids, direct stimulation of intestinal smooth muscle,[93] and changes in intestinal water transport.[94]

The most thoroughly studied cause of antimicrobial-associated diarrhea is disruption of colonization resistance, allowing overgrowth of *C. difficile*, which may produce symptoms ranging in severity from diarrhea to fulminant pseudomembranous colitis resulting in death.[38] This serious, often life-threatening enteric disease is usually attributed to broad-spectrum antimicrobial therapy. Aronsson and associates[95] detected *C. difficile* cytotoxin in 18% of 4793 patients with antimicrobial-agent-associated diarrhea. Cephalosporins and lincosamides (clindamycin and lincomycin) were 10 to 70 times more often implicated in *C. difficile* colitis than were narrow-spectrum penicillins.[95]

Increased Risk of Infection in High-Risk Patients. Broad-spectrum antimicrobials can suppress noninvasive and potentially beneficial bowel flora that provide protection against colonization and infection by potentially pathogenic bacteria. Loss of protection caused by suppression of colonization resistance, overgrowth of bacteria, and the development of resistant bacterial strains often increases the risk of iatrogenic infection, particularly in patients with acute leukemia or in other neutropenic hosts. The endogenous microflora most commonly associated with nosocomial infections in this patient population are Enterobacteriaceae, Pseudomonadaceae, and fungi.[96]

For example, in a randomized study of 83 febrile granulocytopenic patients with cancer, broad-spectrum therapy with moxalactam and ticarcillin resulted in a significantly higher acquisition rate for yeasts and a significantly higher fungal superinfection rate (40% versus 16%) than rates associated with tobramycin and ticarcillin.[97] Patients receiving moxalactam–ticarcillin were more likely to be colonized by aerobic gram-negative bacilli, have major components of the anaerobic fecal flora eliminated, and have a higher acquisition rate for enterococci in fecal samples than patients receiving tobramycin–ticarcillin.

In a similar study, 54 febrile neutropenic patients were randomized to receive either aztreonam–tobramycin, aztreonam–cloxacillin, or moxalactam–tobramycin.[98] All regimens eliminated fecal carriage of enteric gram-negative bacilli, as demonstrated by surveillance cultures. Fecal acquisition of fungi occurred in 27% of those receiving aztreonam–tobramycin, 43% of those receiving aztreonam–cloxacillin, and 81% of those receiving moxalactam–tobramycin. Fungi were acquired at 11 (22%) of 49 sites in the aztreonam–tobramycin group, 15 (31%) of 48 sites in the aztreonam–cloxacillin group, and 28 (54%) of 52 sites in the moxalactam–tobramycin group. Fecal anaerobes were undisturbed during aztreonam–tobramycin therapy, while aztreonam–cloxacillin and moxalactam–tobramycin therapy caused mild to moderate alterations. Of these regimens, aztreonam–tobramycin recipients were least likely to acquire fungi, thus supporting the concept that colonization resistance is important in preventing fungal colonization. Other antimicrobial agents, including members of the "third-generation" cephalosporins, have also been implicated as causing overgrowth of aerobic gram-negative bacilli and *Candida* in the impaired host.[50]

Resultant infections cause substantial morbidity and mortality in the immunocompromised host. Disseminated fungal infections account for one third to one half of fatal infections in the neutropenic population.[99,100] Louie and associates[98] concluded that "since fungi and *Ps. aeruginosa* account for significant morbidity and mortality in the neutropenic host, it is probable that colonization-resistance-preserving regimens would decrease the risk of infection."

The situation is different in the immune-competent host, since intact host defense mechanisms usually confine these changes to the bowel and prevent dissemination of infection. As Louie and associates[98] stated, "although antimicrobial-induced fungal colonization of the gastrointestinal tract is a common clinical event in the nonneutropenic host, disseminated fungal infections in these patients are uncommon."

Clinical Approaches That Minimize Bowel-Flora Disruption

In general, antimicrobials are selected based on their ability to inhibit or kill known or suspected pathogens. The broad-spectrum and potent antibacterial activity of many of the newer antimicrobials are often advantageous for empiric treatment of a variety of infections. However, this must be balanced with their potential effects on the normal gut bacterial flora.

The most important method of preventing the adverse consequences of altered bowel flora is judicious use of antimicrobial agents (Table 3). Reducing exposure to antimicrobials lowers the potential for adverse influences on endogenous flora. Shortening the duration of therapy lowers the risk of many adverse effects, including those related to colonization resistance. The effect of antimicrobial dose on colonization resistance has not been ade-

Table 3.
Considerations for Preventing and Treating the Adverse Consequences of Altered Bowel Flora

- Control of antimicrobial use through prudent antimicrobial selection and administration
  - Avoidance of unnecessary antimicrobial exposure
  - Shortest possible duration of therapy
  - Avoidance of antianaerobic activity (whenever possible)
  - Substitution of narrow-spectrum agents
  - Use of well-absorbed antibiotics with minimal biliary excretion
- Treatment of consequences
  - *Lactobacillus acidophilus* for antimicrobial-agent-induced diarrhea (possibly effective)
  - Specific antimicrobial therapy for pseudomembranous colitis caused by *Clostridium difficile*
- Other measures for high-risk patients
  - Identification of high-risk patients
  - Proper precautionary measures (e.g., reverse isolation)
  - "Selective decontamination" during profound neutropenia

quately studied. Agents with broad-spectrum activity, particularly those that have antianaerobic activity, are likely to alter colonization resistance. For infections not involving anaerobes, relatively narrow-spectrum agents (for aerobic gram-positive cocci or gram-negative bacilli) would be preferable.

Other factors relating to the choice of agent may be important. Even if an agent possesses antianaerobic activity, it may have little influence on intestinal bacteria if the agent does not reach the colon. If an antimicrobial is almost completely absorbed and is not appreciably excreted in the bile, it is not likely to have a substantial effect on bowel flora.[52] Therefore, selection of agents that are well absorbed and have minimal biliary excretion should minimize the detrimental effects from alteration of colonization resistance.

Other methods have been used to minimize or reverse the effect of antimicrobials on bowel flora. The oral administration of *Lactobacillus acidophilus* has been used to treat diarrhea associated with antimicrobial use.[101] In patients with pseudomembranous colitis, fecal enemas have been used to re-establish a normal pattern of bacterial flora[102]; however, the inconvenience of this technique has limited its application. Also, it seems logical that resumption of a regular diet will assist in re-establishing normal flora; however, this has not been documented.

Finally, the adverse consequences of the alteration of bowel flora can be minimized by identification of those patients who are at greatest risk. In healthy individuals, alteration of bowel flora usually causes relatively minor problems, such as diarrhea or superficial fungal infections, although more serious conditions, such as pseudomembranous colitis, may occur. In immunocompromised patients, the consequences can be more serious. Impairment of colonization resistance may allow growth of organisms that pose a greater pathogenic potential in these patients. Establishment of gram-negative bacilli or fungi may then lead to systemic infections or sepsis. Patients at greatest risk are those with a variety of primary humoral or cell-mediated immunodeficiency diseases and those with acquired immunodeficiency disorders (e.g., transplant or neutropenic cancer patients, diabetics). Proper precautionary procedures (e.g., reverse isolation) should be followed for immunocompromised patients at high risk. In some institutions, protected environments may be selectively used.

One approach to the immunocompromised patient has been "selective decontamination."[17] Theoretically, the administration of agents that are primarily active against gram-negative bacilli and have minimal activity against anaerobic bacteria can suppress the growth of gram-negative bacilli in the bowel without inhibiting colonization resistance. Antimicrobials that have been evaluated in this setting and may be suitable for use as selective decontamination are listed in Table 4.

Table 4.
Agents That May Be Used for Selective Decontamination[103]

Agent	Reference
Aztreonam	19,60,68,84
Ceftazidime	104
Cinoxacin	61
Ciprofloxacin	87,105
Nalidixic acid	61,106–108
Norfloxacin	89,90
Polymyxin B	109
Tobramycin	110,111
Trimethoprim–sulfamethoxazole	61,97,105, 112–114

The benefits of selective decontamination are most likely to be documented in cancer patients who are neutropenic. Although a few different regimens have been shown to reduce the incidence of infection in the high-risk patient, results are not consistent, and it is uncertain whether these regimens affect survival.[106,112,113,115]

Conclusion

The normal bowel flora has a "primary" role in protecting against colonization and overgrowth of potentially pathogenic organisms. Administration of antimicrobials can cause profound changes in the normal human intestinal flora. The extent that the normal flora is altered by an antimicrobial agent is related to its pharmacokinetic properties (particularly the extent of oral absorption or biliary excretion) and antibacterial spectrum. Although the suppression of susceptible organisms may be a beneficial effect of antimicrobial therapy, it may also prove detrimental in many situations. Suppression of the endogenous flora of the gastrointestinal tract permits overgrowth of pathogenic strains, emergence of antimicrobial-agent-resistant strains, and disruption of colonization resistance. The consequences of these changes may result in (1) relatively benign diarrhea to severe pseudomembranous colitis and (2) increased risk of infections and septic conditions in immunocompromised patients. The choice of an antimicrobial agent that has a narrow spectrum, is specific for the infection, is not appreciably excreted in the bile, and is completely absorbed if given orally appears to be the most appropriate practice for preventing or minimizing these adverse consequences.

References

1. DiPiro JT, Mansberger JA, Davis JB Jr. Current concepts in clinical therapeutics: intra-abdominal infections. *Clin Pharm.* 1986; 5:34–50.
2. Finegold SM. Microflora of the gastrointestinal tract. In: Wilson SE, Finegold SM, Williams RA, eds. Intraabdomi-

nal infection. New York: McGraw-Hill Book Company; 1982:1–21.
3. Ruddell WSJ, Axon ATR, Findlay JM et al. The effect of cimetidine on gastric bacterial flora. *Lancet*. 1980; 1:672–4.
4. Drasar BS, Shiner M, McLeod GM. Studies on the intestinal flora. I. The bacterial flora of the gastrointestinal tract in healthy and achlorhydric persons. *Gastroenterology*. 1969; 56:71–9.
5. Nichols RL, Smith JW. Intragastric microbial colonization in common disease states of the stomach and duodenum. *Ann Surg*. 1975; 182:557–61.
6. Lou MA, Mandal AK, Alexander JL et al. Bacteriology of the human biliary tract and duodenum. *Arch Surg*. 1977; 112:965–7.
7. Keighley MRB. Infection and the biliary tree. In: Blumgart LH, ed. The biliary tract. New York: Churchill Livingston; 1982:219–35.
8. Gorbach SL, Nahas L, Lerner PI et al. Studies of intestinal microflora: I. Effects of diet, age, and periodic sampling of numbers of fecal microorganisms in man. *Gastroenterology*. 1967; 53:845–55.
9. Gorbach SL, Plaut AG, Nahas L et al. Studies of intestinal microflora: II. Microorganisms of the small intestine and their relations to oral and fecal flora. *Gastroenterology*. 1967; 53:856–67.
10. Moore, WEC, Holdeman LV. The human fecal flora of 20 Japanese–Hawaiians. *Appl Microbiol*. 1974; 27:961–79.
11. Gorbach SL. Intestinal microflora. *Gastroenterology*. 1971; 60:1110–29.
12. Moore WEC, Cato EP, Holdeman LV. Anaerobic bacteria of the gastrointestinal flora and their occurrence in clinical infections. *J Infect Dis*. 1969; 120:641–9.
13. Gorbach SL, Banwell JG, Chaterjee BD et al. Acute undifferentiated diarrhea in the tropics. I. Alterations in intestinal microflora. *J Clin Invest*. 1971; 50:881–9.
14. Gorbach SL. Function of the normal human microflora. *Scand J Infect Dis*. 1986; 49(Suppl):17–30.
15. Simon GL, Gorbach SL. The human intestinal microflora. *Dig Dis Sci*. 1986; 31(Suppl):147–62.
16. Hill MJ, Drasar BS. The normal colonic bacterial flora. *Gut*. 1975; 16:318–23.
17. Mackowiak PA. The normal microbial flora. *N Engl J Med*. 1982; 307:83–93.
18. Nord CE, Kager L, Heimdahl A. Impact of antimicrobial agents on the gastrointestinal microflora and the risk of infections. *Am J Med*. 1984; 76(5A):99–110.
19. van der Waaij D. Selective decontamination of the digestive tract with oral aztreonam and temocillin. *Rev Infect Dis*. 1985; 7(Suppl 4):628–34.
20. Simon GL, Gorbach SL. Intestinal microflora. *Med Clin North Am*. 1982; 66:557–74.
21. Morin S, Saheb SA, Bisaillon J-G et al. In vitro inhibition of *Neisseria gonorrhoeae* growth by strict anaerobes. *Infect Immun*. 1980; 28:776–80.
22. Sanders CC, Sanders WE. Enosin: an antibiotic produced by *Streptococcus salivarius* that may contribute to protection against infections due to group A streptococci. *J Infect Dis*. 1982; 146:683–90.
23. Sprunt K, Leidy GA, Redman W. Prevention of bacterial overgrowth. *J Infect Dis*. 1971; 123:1–10.
24. Luckey TD. Bicentennial overview of intestinal microflora. *Am J Clin Nutr*. 1977; 30:1753–61.
25. Levinson ME. Effect of colon flora and short-chain fatty acids on growth in-vitro of *Pseudomonas aeruginosa* and Enterobacteriaceae. *Infect Immun*. 1973; 8:30–5.
26. Heimdahl A, Nord CE. Effect of erythromycin and clindamycin on the indigenous human anaerobic flora and new colonization of the gastrointestinal tract. *Eur J Clin Microbiol*. 1982; 1:38–48.
27. Blacklow NR, Dolin R, Fedson DS et al. Acute infectious nonbacterial gastroenteritis: etiology and pathogenesis. *Ann Intern Med*. 1972; 76:993–1008.
28. Byrne BM, Dankert J. Volatile fatty acids and aerobic flora in the gastrointestinal tract of mice under various conditions. *Infect Immun*. 1979; 23:559–63.
29. Buck AC, Cook EM. The fate of ingested *Pseudomonas aeruginosa* in normal persons. *J Med Microbiol*. 1969; 2:521–5.
30. Van der Waaij D, de Vries–Hospers HG, Welling GW. The influence of antibiotics on gut colonization. *J Antimicrob Chemother*. 1986; 18 (Suppl C):155–8.
31. Mackowiak PA, Martin RM, Smith JW. The role of bacterial interference in the increased prevalence of oropharyngeal gram-negative bacilli among alcoholics and diabetics. *Am Rev Respir Dis*. 1979; 120:589–93.
32. Kiyono H, McGee JR, Michalek SM. Lipopolysaccharide regulation of immune response: comparisons of responses to LPS in germfree, *Escherichia coli*-monoassociated and conventional mice. *J Immunol*. 1980; 124:36–41.
33. Nord CE, Heimdahl A, Kager L et al. The impact of different antimicrobial agents on the normal gastrointestinal microflora in humans. *Rev Infect Dis*. 1984; 6(Suppl 1):270–5.
34. Nord CE, Bergan T, Aase S. Impact of azlocillin on the colon microflora. *Scand J Infect Dis*. 1986; 18:163–6.
35. Bergan T. Pharmacokinetic differentiation and consequences for normal microflora. *Scand J Infect Dis*. 1986; Suppl 49:91–9.
36. Norrby SR. Ecological consequences of broad spectrum versus narrow spectrum antibacterial therapy. *Scand J Infect Dis*. 1986; Suppl 49:189–95.
37. Tedesco FJ, Barton RW, Alpers DH. Clindamycin-associated colitis: a prospective study. *Ann Intern Med*. 1974; 81:429–33.
38. Swartzberg JE, Maresca RM, Remington JS. Clinical study of gastrointestinal complications associated with clindamycin therapy. *J Infect Dis*. 1977; 135(Suppl):99–103.
39. Tedesco FJ. Clindamycin and colitis: a review. *J Infect Dis*. 1977; 135(Suppl):95–8.
40. Wise R, Bennett SA, Dent J. The pharmacokinetics of orally absorbed cefuroxime compared with amoxycillin/clavulanic acid. *J Antimicrob Chemother*. 1984; 13:603–10.
41. Nord CE, Heimdahl A, Kager L. Antimicrobial induced alterations of the human oropharyngeal and intestinal microflora. *Scand J Infect Dis*. 1986; Suppl 49:64–72.
42. Bergan T, Delin C, Johansen S et al. Pharmacokinetics of ciprofloxacin and effect of repeated dosage on salivary and fecal microflora. *Antimicrob Agents Chemother*. 1986; 29:298–302.
43. Bartlett JG. Antibiotic-associated pseudomembranous colitis. *Rev Infect Dis*. 1979; 1:530–9.
44. Heimdahl A, Kager L, Nord CE. Changes in the oropharyngeal and colon microflora in relation to antimicrobial concentrations in saliva and faeces. *Scand J Infect Dis*. 1985; Suppl 44:52–8.
45. Jones FE, Condon RE. Infections of the colon. In: Simmons RL, Howard RJ, eds. Surgical infectious diseases; New York: Appleton–Century–Crofts; 1982:921–73.
46. Bartlett JG, Condon RE, Gorbach SL et al. Efficacy of preoperative antimicrobial preparation of the bowel. *Ann Surg*. 1972; 176:227.
47. Nichols RL. Prophylaxis for elective bowel surgery. In: Wilson SE, Finegold SM, Williams RA, eds. Intraabdominal infection. New York: McGraw-Hill Book Company; 1982; 267–85.
48. May JR, DiPiro JT. Antibiotics for preoperative bowel preparation. *Clin Pharm*. 1983; 2:299–300.
49. Clark JS, Condon RE, Bartlett JG et al. Preoperative oral antibiotics reduce septic complications of colon operations: results of a prospective, randomized, double-blind clinical study. *Ann Surg*. 1977; 186:251.
50. Bodey GP, Fainstein V, Garcia I et al. Effect of broad-spectrum cephalosporins on the microbial flora of recipients. *J Infect Dis*. 1983; 148:892–7.
51. Geddes AM. Alteration of the body flora by antibiotics—can it be avoided. *Scand J Infect Dis*. 1986; 49:131–4.
52. Van der Waaij D. Colonization resistance of the digestive

tract: clinical consequences and implications. *J Antimicrob Chemother.* 1982; 10:263–70.
53. Giuliano M, Barza M, Jacobus NV et al. Effect of broad-spectrum parenteral antibiotics on composition of intestinal microflora of humans. *Antimicrob Agents Chemother.* 1987; 31:202–6.
54. Bauernfeind A, Hörl G, Mönch V. Changes in microbial ecology by therapeutic use of aminoglycosides. *Scand J Infect Dis.* 1986; 49:106–14.
55. Heimdahl A, Nord CE. Influence of doxycycline on the normal human flora and colonization of the oral cavity and colon. *Scand J Infect Dis.* 1983; 15:293–302.
56. Mulligan ME, Citron D, Gabay E et al. Alteration in human fecal flora, including ingrowth of *Clostridium difficile*, related to cefoxitin therapy. *Antimicrob Agents Chemother.* 1984; 26:343–6.
57. Finegold SM, Mathisen GE, George WL. Changes in human intestinal flora related to the administration of antimicrobial agents. In: Hentges DJ, ed. Human intestinal microflora in health and disease. New York: Academic Press, Inc.; 1983:353–446.
58. Nord CE, Kager L. Beta-lactamase induction in the intestinal microflora during treatment with cefoxitin, imipenem, and aztreonam. *Twenty-seventh Int Cong Antimicrob Agents Chemother.* 1987; 221. Abstract 714.
59. Guiot HFL, van der Meer JWM, van Furth R. Selective antimicrobial modulation of human microbial flora: infection prevention in patients with decreased host defense mechanisms by selective elimination of potentially pathogenic bacteria. *J Infect Dis.* 1981; 143:644–54.
60. de Vries-Hospers HG, Welling GW, Swabb EA et al. Selective decontamination of the digestive tract with aztreonam: a study of 10 healthy volunteers. *J Infect Dis.* 1984; 150(5):636–42.
61. Wiegersma N, Jansen G, van der Waaij D. Effect of twelve antimicrobial drugs on the colonization resistance of the digestive tract of mice and on endogenous potentially pathogenic bacteria. *J Hyg.* 1982; 88:221–30.
62. Van der Waaij D, Berghuis JM, Lekkerkerk JEC. Colonization resistance of the digestive tract of mice during systemic antibiotic treatment. *J Hyg.* 1972; 70:605–10.
63. Wensinck F, Ruseler-van Embden JGH. The intestinal flora of colonization-resistant mice. *J Hyg.* 1971; 69:413–21.
64. Van der Waaij D, Berghuis-de Vries JM, Lekkerkerk-van der Wees JEC. Colonization resistance of the digestive tract in conventional and antibiotic treated mice. *J Hyg.* 1971; 69:405–11.
65. Van der Waaij D, Hofstra H, Wiegersma N. Effect of β-lactam antibiotics on the resistance of the digestive tract of mice to colonization. *J Infect Dis.* 1982; 146:417–22.
66. Thijm HA, van der Waaij D. The effect of three frequently applied antibiotics on the colonization resistance of the digestive tract of mice. *J Hyg.* 1979; 82:397–405.
67. Barza M, Giuliano M, Jacobus NV et al. Effect of broad-spectrum parenteral antibiotics on "colonization resistance" of intestinal microflora of humans. *Antimicrob Agents Chemother.* 1987; 31:723–7.
68. Louie TJ, Chubb H, Bow EJ et al. Effect of aztreonam plus cloxacillin, aztreonam plus tobramycin or moxalactam plus tobramycin on colonization resistance parameters during empiric therapy of febrile neutropenic episodes. *Chemioterapia.* 1985; 4(Suppl):107–9.
69. Mulligan ME, Citron DM, McNamara BT et al. Impact of cefoperazone therapy on fecal flora. *Antimicrob Agents Chemother.* 1982; 22:226–30.
70. Arvidsson A, Alvan G, Angelin B et al. Ceftriaxone: renal and biliary excretion and effect on the colon microflora. *J Antimicrob Chemother.* 1982; 10:207–15.
71. Finegold SM, Posnick DJ, Miller LG et al. The effects of various antibacterial compounds on the normal human fecal flora. *Ernaehrungsforschung.* 1965; 10:316–41.
72. Daikos GK, Kontomichalou P, Bilalis D et al. Intestinal flora ecology and oral use of antibiotics. *Chemotherapy.* 1968; 13:146–60.
73. Zintel HA. Streptomycin in peritonitis. *Am J Med.* 1947; 5:443–8.
74. Sakata H, Fujita K, Yoshioka H. The effect of antimicrobial agents on fecal flora of children. *Antimicrob Agents Chemother.* 1986; 29:225–9.
75. Reeves DS. The effect of quinolone antibacterials on the gastrointestinal flora compared with that of other antibacterials. *J Antimicrob Chemother.* 1986; 18(Suppl D):89–102.
76. Finegold SM. Interaction of antimicrobial therapy and intestinal flora. *Am J Clin Nutr.* 1970; 23:1466–71.
77. Akita H. The change in intestinal flora by administration of antibiotics. *Jpn J Infect Dis.* 1982; 56:1216–24.
78. Nord CE, Heimdahl A, Lundberg C et al. Impact of cefaclor on the normal human oropharyngeal and intestinal microflora. *Scand J Infect Dis.* 1987; 19:681–5.
79. Guggenbichler JP, Kofler J. Influence of third-generation cephalosporins on aerobic intestinal flora. *J Antimicrob Chemother.* 1984; 14(Suppl B):67–70.
80. Alestig K, Carlberg H, Nord CE et al. Effect of cefoperazone on faecal flora. *J Antimicrob Chemother.* 1983; 12:163–7.
81. Benno Y, Shiragami N, Uchida K et al. Effect of moxalactam on human fecal microflora. *Antimicrob Agents Chemother.* 1986; 29:175–8.
82. Kager L, Malmborg AS, Nord CE et al. The effect of piperacillin prophylaxis on the colonic microflora in patients undergoing colorectal surgery. *Infection.* 1983; 11:251–4.
83. Kager L, Brismar B, Malmborg AS et al. Effect of aztreonam on the colon microflora in patients undergoing colorectal surgery. *Infection.* 1985; 13:111–4.
84. Jones PG, Bodey GP, Swabb EA et al. Effect of aztreonam on throat and stool flora in cancer patients. *Antimicrob Agents Chemother.* 1984; 26:941–3.
85. Nord CE, Kager L, Philipsson A et al. Impact of imipenem/cilastatin therapy on faecal flora. *Eur J Clin Microbiol.* 1984; 3:475–7.
86. Welkon CJ, Long SS, Gilligan PH. Effect of imipenem-cilastatin therapy on fecal flora. *Antimicrob Agents Chemother.* 1986; 29:741–3.
87. Rozenberg-Arska M, Dekker AW, Verhoef J. Ciprofloxacin for selective decontamination of the alimentary tract in patients with acute leukemia during remission induction treatment: the effect on fecal flora. *J Infect Dis.* 1985; 152:104–7.
88. Edlund C, Nord CE. Comparative in vitro activities of ciprofloxacin, enoxacin, norfloxacin, ofloxacin and pefloxacin against *Bacteroides fragilis* and *Clostridium difficile*. *Scand J Infect Dis.* 1986; 18:149–51.
89. Edlund C, Bergan T, Josefsson K et al. Effect of norfloxacin on human oropharyngeal and colon microflora and multiple-dose pharmacokinetics. *Scand J Infect Dis.* 1987; 19:113–21.
90. Boerema JBJ, Olthof BJ, van Saene HKF. Effects of norfloxacin on the faecal flora in patients with complicated urinary tract infections. *Scand J Infect Dis.* 1986; 48:27–31.
91. Brumfitt W, Franklin I, Grady D et al. Changes in the pharmacokinetics of ciprofloxacin and fecal flora during administration of a 7-day course to human volunteers. *Antimicrob Agents Chemother.* 1984; 26:757–61.
92. Nord CE, Delin C, Bergan T et al. The effect of ciprofloxacin on oropharyngeal and colon microflora. *Res Clin Forum.* 1985; 7:89–94.
93. Takai A, Hirai S, Watanabe I et al. General pharmacology of cefoperazone, a new cephalosporin antibiotic. *Jpn J Antibiot.* 1980; 33:994–1018.
94. Gianella RA, Serumaga J, Walls D et al. Effect of clindamycin on intestinal water and glucose transport in the rat. *Gastroenterology.* 1981; 80:907–13.
95. Aronsson B, Möllby R, Nord CE. Antimicrobial agents and *Clostridium difficile* in acute enteric disease: epidemiological data from Sweden, 1980–1982. *J Infect Dis.* 1985; 151:476–81.
96. Clasener HAL, Vollaard EJ, van Saene HKF. Long-term

prophylaxis of infection by selective decontamination in leukopenia and in mechanical ventilation. *Rev Infect Dis.* 1987; 9:295–328.

97. Bow EJ, Louie TJ. Changes in endogenous microflora among febrile granulocytopenic patients receiving empiric antibiotic therapy: implications for fungal superinfection. *Can Med Assoc J.* 1987; 137:397–403.
98. Louie TJ, Chubb H, Bow EJ et al. Preservation of colonization resistance parameters during empiric therapy with aztreonam in the febrile neutropenic patient. *Rev Infect Dis.* 1985; 7(Suppl 4):747–61.
99. Bodey GP, Rodriguez V, Chang H-Y et al. Fever and infection in leukemic patients: a study of 494 consecutive patients. *Cancer.* 1978; 41:1610–22.
100. Hart PD, Russell E Jr, Remington JS. The compromised host and infection. II. Deep fungal infection. *J Infect Dis.* 1969; 120:169–91.
101. Gotz V, Romankiewicz JA, Moss J et al. Prophylaxis against ampicillin-associated diarrhea with a lactobacillus preparation. *Am J Hosp Pharm.* 1979; 36:754–7.
102. Bowden TA, Mansberger AR, Lykins LE. Pseudomembranous enterocolitis: mechanisms of restoring floral homeostasis. *Am Surg.* 1981; 47:178–83.
103. Fainstein V, Rodriguez V, Turck M et al. Patterns of oropharyngeal and fecal flora in patients with acute leukemia. *J Infect Dis.* 1981; 144:10–8.
104. Kemmerich B, Warns H, Lode H et al. Multiple-dose pharmacokinetics of ceftazidime and its influence on fecal flora. *Antimicrob Agents Chemother.* 1982; 24:323–38.
105. Daikos GL, Kathpalia SB, Sharifi R et al. Comparison of ciprofloxacin and beta-lactam antibiotics in the treatment of urinary tract infections and alteration of fecal flora. *Am J Med.* 1987; 82(Suppl 4A):290–4.
106. Dejace P, Klastersky J. Emergence of resistance as a consequence of antimicrobial prophylaxis in immunocompromised patients. *Scand J Infect Dis.* 1986; 49(Suppl):165–71.
107. Sleijfer DTH, Mulder NH, de Vries-Hospers HG et al. Infection prevention in granulocytopenic patients by selective decontamination of the digestive tract. *Eur J Cancer.* 1980; 16:859–69.
108. Van der Waaij D, Berghuise-de Vries JM. Selective decontamination of enterobacteriaceae species from the digestive tract in mice and monkeys. *J Hyg.* 1974; 72:205–11.
109. Emmelot CH, van der Waaij D. The dose at which neomycin and polymyxin B can be applied for selective decontamination of the digestive tract in mice. *J Hyg.* 1980; 84:331–40.
110. Van der Waaij D, Aberson J, Thijm HA et al. The screening of four aminoglycosides in the selective decontamination of the digestive tract in mice. *Infection.* 1982; 10:35–40.
111. Mulder JG, Wiersma WE, Welling GW et al. Low dose oral treatment for selective decontamination of the digestive tract: a study in human volunteers. *J Antimicrob Chemother.* 1984; 13:495–504.
112. Dekker AW, Rozenberg-Arska M, Sixma JJ et al. Prevention of infection by trimethoprim–sulfamethoxazole plus amphotericin B in patients with acute nonlymphocytic leukemia. *Ann Intern Med.* 1981; 95:555–9.
113. EORTC International Antimicrobial Therapy Project Group. Trimethoprim–sulphamethoxazole in the prevention of infection in neutropenic patients. *J Infect Dis.* 1984; 150:372–9.
114. Hargadon MT, Young VM, Schimpff SC et al. Selective suppression of alimentary tract microbial flora as prophylaxis during granulocytopenia. *Antimicrob Agents Chemother.* 1981; 20:620–4.
115. Wade JC, de Jongh CA, Newman KA. Selective antimicrobial modulation as prophylaxis against infection during granulocytopenia: trimethoprim–sulfamethoxazole vs. nalidixic acid. *J Infect Dis.* 1983; 147:624–34.

Statement of Ownership, Management, and Circulation (Required by 39 U.S.C. 3685) 1. Title of publication, Clinical Pharmacy. 1A. Publication No. 02782677. 2. Date of filing, October 1, 1988. 3. Frequency of issue, monthly. 3A. No. issues published annually, 12. 3B. Annual subscription price, $40.00. 4. Location of known office of publication, 4630 Montgomery Avenue, Bethesda, Montgomery County, MD 20814. 5. Location of the headquarters or general business offices of the publishers, 4630 Montgomery Avenue, Bethesda, MD 20814. 6. Publisher, American Society of Hospital Pharmacists, Inc., 4630 Montgomery Avenue, Bethesda, MD 20814. Editor, William A. Zellmer, 4630 Montgomery Avenue, Bethesda, MD 20814. Managing Editor, C. Richard Talley. 7. Owner, American Society of Hospital Pharmacists, Inc., 4630 Montgomery Avenue, Bethesda, MD 20814. 8. Known bondholders, mortgagees, and other security holders owning 1% or more of total amount of bonds, mortgages or other securities, None. 9. For completion by nonprofit organizations authorized to mail at special rates (Section 132.122, PSM). The purpose, function, and nonprofit status of this organization and the exempt status for federal income tax purposes have not changed during preceding 12 months. 10. Extent and nature of circulation, A. Total no. copies printed, 9,378/9,215*; B. Paid circulation, 1. Sales through dealers and carriers, street vendors and counter sales, 300/150. 2. Mail subscriptions, 7,869/7,943; C. Total paid circulation, 8,169/8,093; D. Free distribution by mail, carrier or other means, samples, complimentary and other free copies, 445/478; E. Total distribution, 8,614/8,571; F. Copies not distributed, 1. Office use, left over, unaccounted, spoiled after printing, 764/644. Returns from news agents, 0,0. G. Total, 9,378/9,215.* I certify that the statements made by me are correct and complete, signed William A. Zellmer.

*First figure, average no. copies each issue during preceding 12 months; second figure, actual no. of copies single issue published nearest to filing date.

Research Notes

Serum fibronectin and somatomedin-C as nutritional markers in adults receiving total parenteral nutrition

DOUGLAS A. POWERS, VALERIE L. FRANSE, REX O. BROWN, ANN HINSON, AND GEORGE S. M. COWAN, JR.

Clin Pharm. 1988; 7:889–93

The use of total parenteral nutrient solutions to provide safe and efficacious nutritional support to the undernourished hospitalized patient presents a formidable challenge to the clinical practitioner and the nutritional support team. Current economic conditions demand that expensive therapeutic modalities such as total parenteral nutrition (TPN) be used in the most optimal and efficient manner. Current methods of assessing the nutritional response to TPN consist of the serial assessment of body weight, anthropometric measurements, nitrogen balance, and serum concentrations of various plasma proteins. Each of these methods is associated with shortcomings that make their routine use in determining the efficacy of nutritional repletion questionable. Therefore, there remains a need to identify additional methods for evaluating nutritional efficacy in malnourished patients receiving TPN.[1] Serum fibronectin and somatomedin-C (insulin-like growth factor 1) may potentially serve as nutritional markers in malnourished patients and be used in evaluating nutritional efficacy in malnourished patients receiving TPN.

Fibronectin is a glycoprotein that has been studied extensively in immunology and appears to be a key factor in host defense mechanisms.[2,3] Fibronectin stimulates phagocytic uptake of some bacteria and other nonbacterial foreign matter in the blood. A direct correlation has been made between low serum fibronectin concentrations and organ failure in critically ill patients. Patients with sepsis, trauma, or burns have demonstrated depressed serum fibronectin concentrations.[4,5] Recent data suggest that this is due to reduced synthesis.[3] Hesselvik[6] evaluated fibronectin concentrations in 32 patients with sepsis and determined that in such patients depressed fibronectin concentrations were due to decreased hepatic synthesis rather than an increase in consumption. Additional evidence suggests that serum fibronectin may be a potentially useful marker for assessing the efficacy of nutritional intervention.[7-12]

Somatomedin-C is a growth-hormone-dependent serum growth factor that possesses a proinsulin-like structure and broad anabolic properties. It is thought to be synthesized in the liver, is a sensitive marker for nutritional status, and appears to correlate well with nitrogen balance by changing in relation to dietary intake. Somatomedin-C has potential as a marker for assessing the efficacy of nutritional intervention, and its close correlation with positive nitrogen balance makes it particularly attractive.[13-15]

This study was undertaken to characterize the serum concentrations of fibronectin and somatomedin-C sequentially during the administration of TPN to adult patients.

Methods. Adult patients requiring TPN via the central venous route for at least seven consecutive days were considered eligible for this study protocol. Patients with acute renal failure, liver failure, or congestive heart failure were excluded. Written informed consent was obtained from all patients or a responsible relative before TPN therapy was initiated. The study was approved by the institutional review boards of the Veterans Administration Medical Center and the Regional Medical Center at Memphis.

All patients were to receive nothing by mouth and received TPN in accordance with standard medical practice. Parenteral nutrition targets were defined as a nonprotein caloric intake of 150% of basal energy expenditure (BEE), calculated using the Harris–Benedict equations,[16] and attainment of nitrogen equilibrium. The nutrient solution consisted of a mixture of dextrose and crystalline

---

DOUGLAS A. POWERS, PHARM.D., is Assistant Professor of Clinical Pharmacy, Clinical Pharmacy Specialist, and Director of Nutritional Support, Veterans Administration Medical Center (VAMC), Memphis, TN. VALERIE L. FRANSE, PHARM.D., is Clinical Pharmacy Specialist, VAMC, Nashville, TN; at the time of this study, she was a clinical pharmacy resident, VAMC, Memphis. REX O. BROWN, PHARM.D., is Associate Professor of Clinical Pharmacy, University of Tennessee, Memphis, and Nutrition Support Pharmacist, Regional Medical Center at Memphis, University of Tennessee Medical Center. ANN HINSON is a clinical nurse specialist, United HealthTech Inc., Memphis, TN; at the time of this study, she was Nutritional Support Team Nurse, VAMC, Memphis. GEORGE S. M. COWAN, JR., M.D., is Associate Professor of Surgery, University of Tennessee, Memphis, and Chief of Nutritional Support, VAMC, Memphis.

Address reprint requests to Dr. Powers at the Pharmacy Service (119), Veterans Administration Medical Center, 1030 Jefferson Avenue, Memphis, TN 38104.

The assistance of David Sutherland, Pharm.D., and Rita Russel is acknowledged.

Copyright © 1988, American Society of Hospital Pharmacists, Inc. All rights reserved. 0278-2677/88/1201-0889$01.25.

amino acids, with a final concentration of 25% dextrose and 5% amino acids (50% dextrose injection 500 mL + 10% amino acids 500 mL) with the required amounts of electrolytes, vitamins, and trace elements. TPN was begun at a rate of 25–50 mL/hr and increased by 25 mL/hr/day as patient tolerance allowed until the nutritional target was attained. Intravenous fat emulsion was used as either a calorie source (daily) or a source of essential fatty acids (twice weekly). No patient received more than 2.0 g of lipid per kilogram of body weight per day. Twenty-four-hour caloric and nitrogen intake values for each patient were recorded daily.

Demographic data including age, sex, height, actual weight, major diagnosis, chronic diseases, and calculated BEE were recorded. Serum chemistries (an SMA-7 and calcium, phosphorus, magnesium, albumin, and triglyceride concentrations) were determined before TPN was begun. These studies were repeated twice weekly during TPN and as medically indicated. Serum triglycerides were used to monitor lipid tolerance. In patients who had serum triglyceride concentrations greater than 250 mg/dL during lipid infusion, the lipid dose was decreased or the lipid infusion was discontinued. Nitrogen balance (in grams) was calculated as the difference between nitrogen intake and nitrogen output (24-hour urinary urea nitrogen collection + 4 g nitrogen). These studies were performed on days 0, 4, 7, 14, and 21 of TPN.

Blood samples were drawn and the serum was harvested for somatomedin-C and fibronectin determination before the initiation of TPN and on days 4, 7, 14, and 21. Fibronectin content was measured by radial immunodiffusion (Calbiochem, La-Jolla, CA),[17] and somatomedin-C content was measured by radioimmunoassay (Nichols Institute, Los Angeles, CA).[18]

All results are expressed as mean ± S.D. Analysis of variance was used to analyze the fibronectin and somatomedin-C concentrations and nitrogen balance measurements over time. Simple linear correlation analysis was used to compare fibronectin and somatomedin-C concentrations with nitrogen balance. The a priori level of significance was $p < 0.05$.

Results. A total of 21 patients (16 men and 5 women) were studied. Information on patient characteristics and baseline serum albumin concentration and basal energy expenditure is shown in Table 1. The majority of patients were general surgery patients with various gastrointestinal abnormalities. Parenteral nutrition caloric and nitrogen intakes and nitrogen balances are shown in Table 2. During study days 4, 7, 14, and 21, there were no significant differences in nonprotein energy or protein administration. Nitrogen balance was significantly greater on days 7 and 14 versus day 0. Fourteen of twenty-one patients were in a positive nitrogen balance within the first week of TPN.

All serum samples were obtained as scheduled,

Table 1.
Patient Characteristics and Baseline Data

Patient No.	Major Diagnosis	Age (yr)	Weight (kg)	Height (cm)	BEE[a] (kcal/day)	Serum Albumin Concentration (g/dL)
1	Pancreatic cancer	60	84.5	176	1706	2.5
2	Gastric outlet obstruction	40	81.8	177	1797	3.1
3	Small-bowel resection	66	59.1	175	1341	ND[b]
4	Bleeding, upper gastrointestinal tract	89	60.4	180	1365	ND
5	Bleeding, upper gastrointestinal tract	59	128.2	178	2310	2.5
6	Pneumonia/ileus	36	72.7	175	1680	2.3
7	Pneumonia/ileus	58	103.2	180	1970	ND
8	Pneumonia/ileus	43	68.2	178	1595	ND
9	Pancreatic pseudocyst	58	80.9	188	1714	ND
10	Pneumonia/ileus	64	59.0	178	1330	ND
11	Gastric outlet obstruction	66	75.0	170	1510	3.1
12	Duodenal fistula	73	63.6	168	1280	ND
13	Bleeding, upper gastrointestinal tract	43	42.3	180	1230	ND
14	Pancreatitis	35	54.5	165	1400	2.8
15	Colorectal cancer	55	86.4	183	1850	2.4
16	Colorectal cancer	68	49.5	158	1094	3.0
17	Pancreatitis	29	52.3	162	1313	2.0
18	Cholecystitis	90	51.5	155	1005	1.3
19	Closed head injury/ileus	25	59.0	163	1517	3.2
20	Small-bowel obstruction	66	63.5	165	1252	2.9
21	Gastric outlet obstruction	25	52.3	163	1332	2.5
Mean ± S.D.		54.7 ± 18.9	68.9 ± 20.2	172 ± 9	1504 ± 313	2.6 ± 0.5

[a] Basal energy expenditure calculated from Harris–Benedict equations.
[b] Not determined.

Table 2.
Energy and Nitrogen Intake and Nitrogen Balance

Patient	Energy (kcal/kg/24 hr)				Nitrogen (g/kg/24 hr)				Nitrogen Balance (g)[a]			
No.	Day 4	Day 7	Day 14	Day 21	Day 4	Day 7	Day 14	Day 21	Day 0	Day 7	Day 14	Day 21
1	22.1	31.7	...[b]	...	0.17	0.19	...	...	−13.6	2.8	...	...
2	25.5	29.7	...	...	0.19	0.21	...	...	−10.8	10.3	...	...
3	25.3	23.3	...	...	0.23	0.21	...	...	−15.1	−3.9	...	...
4	24.9	20.7	...	...	0.16	0.13	...	...	−10.6	1.5	...	...
5	18.2	18.6	20.4	18.8	0.11	0.10	0.11	0.11	−5.6	0.9	1.4	2.8
6	31.9	27.8	...	...	0.17	0.18	...	...	−12.7	−4.5	...	...
7	19.8	19.5	...	...	0.18	0.13	...	...	−19.6	−5.6	...	...
8	33.8	31.4	33.2	...	0.19	0.20	0.21	...	−9.5	−2.7	1.6	...
9	17.5	13.7	21.6	...	0.16	0.18	0.20	...	−10.8	3.0	ND[c]	...
10	35.8	35.7	...	...	0.14	0.14	...	...	−11.6	0.7	...	...
11	30.0	30.6	27.8	28.9	0.23	0.20	0.22	0.22	−9.0	6.8	1.6	6.4
12	24.1	40.7	32.7	25.2	0.18	0.24	0.20	0.20	−14.3	3.9	3.1	ND
13	32.1	52.9	42.2	...	0.29	0.29	0.28	...	−11.8	−0.8	3.2	...
14	30.5	35.5	39.4	...	0.22	0.35	0.35	...	−10.3	5.0	ND	...
15	24.9	29.7	...	...	0.16	0.28	...	...	−11.5	8.4	...	...
16	35.7	45.4	36.2	...	0.14	0.32	0.28	...	−8.5	3.1	4.7	...
17	30.8	44.0	49.1	44.0	0.20	0.39	0.31	0.31	−7.1	6.6	10.3	8.8
18	23.0	23.1	30.7	...	0.15	0.22	0.22	...	−8.6	−1.8	ND	...
19	21.8	22.8	44.7	...	0.16	0.21	0.30	...	−17.5	−2.8	3.6	...
20	27.5	33.0	27.7	30.7	0.17	0.31	0.29	0.29	−13.2	4.0	1.5	−6.3
21	28.3	35.9	43.1	...	0.18	0.26	0.31	...	−17.5	3.6	−3.1	...
Mean	26.8	30.7	34.5	29.5	0.18	0.23	0.25	0.23	−11.9	1.8	2.8	2.9
± S.D.	± 5.5	± 9.8	± 8.9	± 9.3	± 0.04	± 0.08	± 0.06	± 0.08	± 3.5	± 4.4[d]	± 3.4[d]	± 6.6

[a] Nitrogen balance on day 4 was determined in two patients only; values are not reported.
[b] Administration of nutrient solution was discontinued before the indicated day.
[c] Not determined.
[d] Significantly different from value on day 0.

except for 10 patients on day 4. Serum fibronectin concentrations increased significantly during the treatment period, and a significant increase was observed on days 4, 7, 14, and 21 compared with day 0 (Table 3). Serum somatomedin-C concentrations increased significantly on day 4 and fell thereafter; no significant difference was found between days 7, 14, and 21 compared with day 0 (Table 3). Nitrogen balance correlated poorly with both somatomedin-C concentrations and fibronectin concentrations.

Changes in serum fibronectin and somatomedin-C concentrations for anabolic (positive nitrogen balance) and catabolic (negative nitrogen balance) patients on days 0, 7, and 14 were compared. Serum fibronectin concentrations increased significantly between days 0 and 7 in the 14 patients who were anabolic on day 7 (253 ± 106 versus 348 ± 133 μg/mL). In the nine patients who were anabolic on day 14, the serum fibronectin concentrations increased significantly between days 0 and 14 (225 ± 117 versus 362 ± 132 μg/mL). The seven catabolic patients on day 7 also demonstrated a significant increase in serum fibronectin concentrations between days 0 and 7 (181 ± 105 versus 323 ± 91 μg/mL). Only one patient was catabolic on day 14, and the serum fibronectin concentration increased from 342 to 530 μg/mL between days 0 and 14. There was no difference in fibronectin concentration changes between anabolic and catabolic patients.

The 14 anabolic patients on day 7 demonstrated a slight but nonsignificant increase in somatomedin-C concentrations between days 0 and 7 (0.8 ± 0.3 versus 1.0 ± 0.5 units/mL). The somatomedin-C concentrations in the nine anabolic patients on day 14 increased from 0.8 ± 0.3 units/mL to 1.1 ± 0.3 units/mL between days 0 and 14 ($p = 0.054$). The seven catabolic patients on day 7 demonstrated a significant increase in somatomedin-C concentrations between days 0 and 7 (0.8 ± 0.3 versus 1.9 ± 1.4 units/mL). The somatomedin-C concentrations increased from 0.8 to 1.3 units/mL in the one catabolic patient on day 14. Between groups, the catabolic patients demonstrated a significantly greater increase in somatomedin-C on day 7 compared with the anabolic group.

Discussion. In this study, we found fibronectin to be a sensitive marker for nutritional repletion. Somatomedin-C was found to be a sensitive marker of nutritional repletion early during TPN (day 4); the concentration returned to baseline thereafter. The patients studied responded well to TPN, attaining nitrogen equilibrium within the first week in 14 of 21 cases.

Studies including serum concentrations of fibronectin have recently been reported in the nutrition literature.[7-12] Scott et al.[7] demonstrated a significant decrease in serum fibronectin in 18 healthy obese subjects after 7 days of a 21-day fast.

Table 3.
Serum Concentrations of Fibronectin and Somatomedin-C on Days 0, 4, 7, 14, and 21

	Fibronectin (μg/mL)[a]					Somatomedin-C (units/mL)[b]				
Patient No.	Day 0	Day 4	Day 7	Day 14	Day 21	Day 0	Day 4	Day 7	Day 14	Day 21
1	308	428	439	472	. . .[c]	1.1	1.3	0.8	1.2	. . .
2	387	540	494	. . .	. . .	0.8	0.8	0.8	. . .	. . .
3	158	173	229	. . .	. . .	1.3	2.0	1.4	. . .	. . .
4	272	246	204	. . .	. . .	1.2	1.0	0.8	. . .	. . .
5	165	ND[d]	407	387	397	0.9	ND	1.4	1.5	1.2
6	123	387	397	. . .	. . .	0.7	5.2	4.8	. . .	. . .
7	397	ND	346	. . .	. . .	0.9	ND	0.7	. . .	. . .
8	219	390	310	375	. . .	0.8	1.8	2.1	1.5	. . .
9	230	472	387	366	. . .	0.8	0.5	0.5	0.6	. . .
10	97	189	85	. . .	. . .	0.8	1.4	1.6	. . .	. . .
11	417	439	461	577	552	0.9	1.0	0.8	1.1	1.3
12	188	237	263	221	237	1.1	1.3	1.9	0.9	1.8
13	69	266	439	283	. . .	0.4	1.9	1.9	0.6	. . .
14	200	ND	266	. . .	. . .	0.5	ND	0.4	. . .	. . .
15	109	ND	175	. . .	. . .	0.8	ND	0.7	. . .	. . .
16	390	ND	390	490	. . .	1.0	ND	1.0	1.5	. . .
17	283	ND	492	480	544	0.3	ND	0.4	0.7	0.5
18	161	ND	182	219	. . .	0.3	ND	0.4	0.5	. . .
19	143	ND	361	219	. . .	1.0	ND	1.7	1.0	. . .
20	147	ND	300	234	211	0.4	ND	0.7	1.2	0.9
21	342	ND	507	530	. . .	0.8	ND	1.6	1.3	. . .
Mean	229	342[e]	340[e]	373[e]	388[e]	0.8	1.7[e]	1.3	1.0	1.1
± S.D.	± 109	± 124	± 119	± 129	± 162	± 0.3	± 1.3	± 1.0	± 0.4	± 0.5

[a] Normal = 300–400 μg/mL.
[b] Normal = 0.34–1.9 units/mL (men), 0.45–2.2 units/mL (women).
[c] Administration of nutrient solution was discontinued before the indicated day.
[d] Not determined.
[e] $p < 0.05$ compared with day 0.

Five days of refeeding resulted in normalization of serum fibronectin concentrations. Likewise, Howard et al.[8] reported a 20–25% decrease in plasma concentrations of fibronectin in 12 healthy subjects after five days of starvation. Refeeding with a normal diet in six subjects restored plasma fibronectin concentrations to normal; however, refeeding with a low carbohydrate diet raised plasma concentrations to only 82% of normal in the other six subjects. McKone et al.[9] observed a 30% or greater increase in serum fibronectin concentrations above baseline in six hospitalized patients during TPN therapy.[9] The two patients who died had increases in serum fibronectin concentrations of 15% or less during TPN. The caloric and nitrogen intakes, however, were not described in this study. In a study by Horowitz et al.,[10] eight healthy subjects were starved for 10 days and then refed with central TPN for 10 days. Serum fibronectin concentrations decreased significantly after starvation and increased significantly to slightly above baseline after TPN. In a study by Sandstedt et al.,[11] 12 malnourished patients and 9 women with anorexia nervosa demonstrated a significant increase in serum concentrations of fibronectin after two to three weeks of TPN. Interestingly, six well-nourished patients did not have a significant increase in serum concentrations of fibronectin after TPN. When changes in serum fibronectin concentrations were compared with nitrogen balance measurements in a group of 27 heterogeneous patients, a relatively poor correlation was found.[12] Fibronectin concentrations did, however, increase significantly in most patients after one week of nutritional support. Results are difficult to interpret, because the nutritional therapy was not described in more than one half of the patients.[12]

Our data mirror that of previous studies supporting fibronectin as a marker of nutritional intervention. Significant increases were seen as early as four days after initiation of parenteral nutrition and were sustained throughout the course of nutritional intervention. Fibronectin synthesis appears to be a high priority in malnourished adults receiving TPN. This is supported by the significant increase in serum concentrations observed soon after refeeding is begun. An increase in serum fibronectin concentrations was observed in both anabolic and catabolic patients.

Studies evaluating the utility of serum somatomedin-C as a marker of nutritional support have been reported. Isley and coworkers[13] found that serum somatomedin-C concentrations decreased significantly in five healthy subjects who were starved for five days. During another study period, refeeding these subjects an energy–protein-deficient diet resulted in a further decline in somatomedin-C concentrations.[13] Underman et al.[14] have reported somatomedin-C concentrations of 38% of normal in 28 patients with evidence of protein-calorie malnutrition. Refeeding six of these patients with parenteral or enteral nutrition resulted in a mean increase of 181% in serum somatomedin-C concentrations.[14] Clemmons et al.[15] reported six undernourished patients who received vigorous nutritional support and demonstrated profound nitrogen accretion.[15] Somatomedin-C concentrations in these patients increased from a mean of 0.67 units/mL at baseline to 1.8 units/mL after 10 days of nutritional support. In our study, serum somatomedin-C concentrations rose markedly from baseline to day 4 but then declined by day 7 to a level that was higher than, yet not significantly different from, baseline, where it remained throughout the study period. The observation that serum somatomedin-C concentrations increase significantly early in nutritional intervention with TPN and then decline was also reported by Clemmons et al.; however, in the study by Clemmons et al., the somatomedin-C concentrations remained significantly higher than baseline levels. However, the patients in the study by Clemmons et al. were unstressed and they had positive nitrogen balances by the second or third day of nutritional repletion. This fact may explain the difference in results between studies.

The significant increase in serum somatomedin-C concentrations observed on day 7 in catabolic patients compared with anabolic patients may be explained by at least two factors. First, the significant increase in somatomedin-C concentrations seen on day 7 in the catabolic group was principally due to the dramatic rise observed in a single patient. Second, although the increase in somatomedin-C concentrations observed in the anabolic group approached significance, more patients may have been required to attain significance in this group. Therefore, based on our data, the utility of somatomedin-C as a nutritional marker in adults receiving TPN requires further study.

Conclusion. The results of this study support the potential utility of serum fibronectin concentrations as a marker of response to nutritional intervention in patients receiving total parenteral nutrition. The use of serum somatomedin-C concentrations as a nutritional marker requires further study. Additional studies are needed to elucidate the usefulness of serum fibronectin as a measure of nutritional response as it correlates to clinical outcome.

References

1. Grant JP. Nutritional assessment in clinical practice. *Nutr Clin Pract*. 1986; 1(1):3–11.
2. Mosher DF. Physiology of fibronectin. *Ann Rev Med*. 1984; 35:561–75.
3. Russell BA, Peake PW, Brown MA et al. Human fibronectin metabolism. *J Clin Invest*. 1985; 76:143–8.
4. Scovill WA, Saba TE, Blumenstock FA et al. Opsonic alpha 2 surface binding glycoprotein therapy during sepsis. *Ann Surg*. 1978; 188:521–9.
5. Lanser ME, Saba TE, Scovill WA. Opsonic glycoprotein (plasma fibronectin) levels after burn injury: relationship to extent of burn and of sepsis. *Ann Surg*. 1980; 192:776–82.
6. Hesselvik JF. Plasma fibronectin levels in sepsis: influencing factors. *Crit Care Med*. 1987; 15:1092–7.
7. Scott RL, Sohmer PR, MacDonald MG. The effect of starvation and repletion on plasma fibronectin in man. *JAMA*. 1982; 248:2025–7.
8. Howard L, Dillon B, Saba TM et al. Decreased plasma fibronectin during starvation in man. *J Parenter Enter Nutr*. 1984; 8:237–44.
9. McKone TK, Davis AT, Dean RE. Fibronectin: a new nutritional parameter. *Am Surg*. 1985; 51:336–9.
10. Horowitz GD, Groeger JS, Legaspi A et al. The response of fibronectin to differing parenteral caloric sources in normal man. *J Parenter Enter Nutr*. 1985; 9:435–8.
11. Sandstedt S, Cederblad G, Larsson J et al. Influence of total parenteral nutrition on plasma fibronectin in malnourished subjects with or without inflammatory response. *J Parenter Enter Nutr*. 1984; 8:493–6.
12. Kirby DF, Marder RJ, Craig RM. The clinical evaluation of plasma fibronectin as a marker for nutritional depletion and repletion and as a measure of nitrogen balance. *J Parenter Enter Nutr*. 1985; 9:705–8.
13. Isley WL, Underwood LE, Clemmons DR. Dietary components that regulate serum somatomedin-C concentrations in humans. *J Clin Invest*. 1983; 71:175–82.
14. Underman TG, Vazquez RM, Slas AJ et al. Nutrition and somatomedin. XIII. Usefulness of somatomedin-C in nutritional assessment. *Am J Med*. 1985; 78:228–34.
15. Clemmons DR, Underwood LE, Dickerson RN et al. Use of plasma somatomedin-C/insulin-like growth factor I measurements to monitor the response to nutritional repletion in malnourished patients. *Am J Clin Nutr*. 1985; 41:191–8.
16. Rosa AM, Shizgal HM. The Harris Benedict equation reevaluated: resting energy requirements and the body cell mass. *Am J Clin Nutr*. 1984; 40:168–82.
17. Saba TM, Blumenstock FA, Shah DM et al. Reversal of fibronectin and opsonic deficiency in patients. *Ann Surg*. 1984; 199:87–96.
18. Furlanetto RW, Underwood C, Van Wyk JJ et al. Estimation of somatomedin-C levels in normals and patients with pituitary disease by radioimmunoassay. *J Clin Invest*. 1977; 60:648–57.

Predicting human-albumin replacement dosages in hypoalbuminemic patients receiving total parenteral nutrition

DANA J. REID, REX O. BROWN, KATHRYN L. VEHE, DOUGLAS A. POWERS, AND R. WAYNE LUTHER

Clin Pharm. 1988; 7:894–7

Current medical practice supports the provision of nutritional support to selected hospitalized patients who are unable to meet their nutritional needs through consumption of adequate foodstuffs. Patients who do not have functioning or accessible gastrointestinal tracts often require total parenteral nutrition (TPN). Frequently, patients who require TPN are hypoalbuminemic and receive supplemental human albumin.[1–4] Hypoalbuminemia, whether caused by malnutrition or a metabolic disorder, can have profound effects on the maintenance of the intravascular volume. Therefore, patients with this disorder may receive albumin infusions in an attempt to raise the plasma colloid oncotic pressure and normalize the volume status. Normal plasma oncotic pressure often allows provision of sufficient fluid volume to meet the patient's energy and amino acid needs. Maintenance of a normal serum albumin concentration (SAC) is also desirable because SACs have been inversely correlated with hospital morbidity and mortality.[5–9]

Because administration of human albumin is expensive, empiric, and controversial, a method of determining the amount of human albumin required to safely meet a predetermined endpoint would optimize administration and possibly result in considerable financial savings to the hospital. The purpose of this study was to use a previously published predictive equation to determine human-albumin replacement dosages[10] and then to compare the SAC after replacement with the predicted SAC.

Methods. From July 1987 to December 1987, consecutive adult patients from three hospitals in a major medical center who were hypoalbuminemic and required central TPN were considered for entry into the study. Central TPN was administered in accordance with standard medical practice.[11,12] Hypoalbuminemia was defined as an SAC of <3.0 g/dL. Patients were excluded if they had acute renal failure, severe liver failure, thermal injury, nephrotic syndrome, or a protein-losing enteropathy. Any patient weighing less than 45 kg or more than 100 kg also was excluded. Demographic data including sex, height, weight, age, major diagnosis, and chronic diseases were recorded for each patient. Each patient was assessed for sepsis or bacterial pneumonia during the study period. Patients who had a positive blood culture, fever, and leukocytosis were presumed to have sepsis. A positive sputum culture, fever, and leukocytosis were used to identify patients with pneumonia.

Patients were assigned a desired SAC by a table of random numbers. The desired SACs were either 3.1, 3.2, 3.3, 3.4, or 3.5 g/dL. A replacement dosage of human albumin was then calculated from a regression equation ($y = 0.003x + 0.33$) that has been previously published.[10] The albumin replacement dosage was calculated by $x = (y - 0.33)/0.003$ where y is the desired change in SAC (desired SAC − initial SAC) and x is the number of grams of human albumin to be replaced during concurrent administration of central TPN. Human albumin was added to TPN in doses of 12.5 or 25 g per liter until the total replacement dosage was infused. Then the human albumin was removed from the TPN solution, and SAC was measured the next morning between 5 and 7 a.m. SACs were measured by the bromocresol green method.[13] The desired SAC was then compared with the SAC measured after the completion of the albumin infusion.

Nitrogen balance was determined once for each patient during the administration of the human-albumin replacement dosage. Nitrogen intake was calculated by adding the grams of protein infused as crystalline amino acids to protein ingested orally and dividing by 6.25. Infused human albumin was not included in the calculation of nitrogen intake. Nitrogen output was calculated by adding 4 to the grams of urea nitrogen measured during a 24-hour urine collection.[14]

All data are expressed as mean ±S.D. The ability of the regression equation to determine a dosage of human albumin that would result in a predetermined SAC was assessed by the mean prediction error (a measurement of bias) and the root mean squared prediction error (a measurement of preci-

DANA J. REID, PHARM.D., is Clinical Pharmacy Resident, Department of Clinical and Institutional Pharmacy, Medical University of South Carolina, Charleston; at the time of this study, she was a Doctor of Pharmacy student, College of Pharmacy, University of Tennessee, Memphis. REX O. BROWN, PHARM.D., is Associate Professor of Clinical Pharmacy, College of Pharmacy, University of Tennessee, Memphis, and Nutrition Support Pharmacist, Regional Medical Center at Memphis, University of Tennessee Medical Center. KATHRYN L. VEHE, PHARM.D., is Nutrition Support Fellow and Instructor of Clinical Pharmacy, University of Tennessee, Memphis. DOUGLAS A. POWERS, PHARM.D., is Assistant Professor of Clinical Pharmacy and Clinical Pharmacist, VA Medical Center, Memphis. R. WAYNE LUTHER, M.D., is Associate Professor of Surgery, College of Medicine, University of Tennessee, Memphis.

Address reprint requests to Dr. Brown at the Department of Clinical Pharmacy, College of Pharmacy, University of Tennessee, Memphis, 26 South Dunlap, Memphis, TN 38163.

Copyright © 1988, American Society of Hospital Pharmacists, Inc. All rights reserved. 0278-2677/88/1201-0894$01.00.

sion).[15] Measured and predicted SACs were compared using a paired Student's *t* test. The a priori level of significance was $p < 0.05$.

Results. Fifty-five patients were considered eligible for the study and received central TPN with added human albumin after calculation of the replacement dosage. Thirteen patients were excluded after entrance to the study for the following reasons: died before the human albumin replacement dosage was infused (four patients); had TPN discontinued before the human albumin replacement dosage was infused (four patients); did not meet the body weight criteria (three patients); received more human albumin than the calculated replacement dosage (one patient); or did not receive a SAC measurement after receiving the replacement dosage (one patient). This left 42 available patients, whose major diagnoses appear in Table 1. These patients also had a variety of chronic diseases, which included hypertension (seven patients), end-stage renal failure (two patients), congestive heart failure (two patients), diabetes mellitus (two patients), and chronic obstructive pulmonary disease (two patients).

The mean age and weight of the patients were 55.1 ± 15.1 years and 70.9 ± 14.7 kg, respectively. There were 34 men and 8 women. The mean energy and protein doses administered during TPN were 29.1 ± 5.7 kcal/kg/day and 1.6 ± 0.5 g/kg/day, respectively. The mean of 40 calculated nitrogen balances in 40 patients during TPN and human albumin replacement was 1.2 ± 4.0 g/day. The two patients with chronic renal failure received hemodialysis three times per week and did not have nitrogen balance meaurements calculated. The mean human-albumin dosage was 235 ± 106 g administered over 7.0 ± 2.9 days.

The mean initial SAC was 2.3 ± 0.4 g/dL for the 42 patients. The mean desired randomized SAC was 3.4 ± 0.1 g/dL, and the observed SAC after human-albumin administration was 3.4 ± 0.3 g/dL ($p > 0.05$). Follow-up SACs (three to seven days after administration of human albumin was discontinued) were available for 19 patients. The mean observed SAC in the 19 patients was 3.4 ± 0.3 g/dL (immediately after supplementation), whereas the mean follow-up SAC was 3.4 ± 0.4 g/dL. Table 2 lists the initial, desired, and observed SACs of the 42 patients and the percent error. The mean prediction error (bias) was −0.02 g/dL (95% confidence interval, −0.1 to 0.06), and the root mean squared prediction error (precision) was 0.24 g/dL

Table 1.
Major Diagnoses of the Study Patients

Diagnosis	No. Patients
Trauma	10
Blunt	7
Penetrating	3
General surgical condition	23
Gastrointestinal surgery	12
Pancreatitis	8
Extremity amputation	2
Splenectomy	1
Gynecological cancer	3
Cervical	1
Ovarian	1
Endometrial	1
Liver transplants	2
General medical condition	4
Peritonitis	1
Stomatitis	1
Pneumonia	1
Myocardial infarction/ileus	1

Table 2.
Serum Albumin Concentrations (Initial, Desired, and Observed) after Administration of Human Albumin

Patient No.	Serum Albumin Concentration (g/dL)			% Error[a]
	Initial	Desired	Observed	
1	2.4	3.4	3.3	2.9
2[b]	2.8	3.5	3.2	8.6
3[b]	2.2	3.2	3.3	(3.1)[c]
4[b]	2.5	3.3	3.0	9.1
5[b]	1.7	3.5	3.2	8.6
6	2.7	3.3	3.0	9.1
7[b]	1.7	3.4	3.5	(2.9)
8	2.4	3.1	3.4	(9.7)
9	2.0	3.3	3.1	6.1
10	2.7	3.3	3.6	(9.1)
11	2.7	3.1	3.0	3.2
12	2.1	3.5	3.7	(5.7)
13	2.6	3.4	3.3	2.9
14	2.1	3.5	3.4	2.8
15	2.7	3.5	3.7	(5.7)
16	2.3	3.3	3.1	6.1
17[b]	2.8	3.2	3.6	(12.5)
18[b]	2.1	3.5	3.4	2.8
19	1.7	3.4	3.6	(5.9)
20[b]	2.6	3.5	3.1	11.4
21	2.3	3.4	3.2	5.9
22	2.1	3.5	3.3	5.7
23	2.6	3.5	3.2	8.6
24	2.4	3.5	3.8	(8.6)
25	2.6	3.5	3.5	0
26	2.1	3.2	3.2	0
27	2.0	3.4	3.7	(8.8)
28	2.2	3.5	3.7	(5.7)
29	1.8	3.3	3.2	3.0
30	1.6	3.2	3.1	3.1
31[b]	2.4	3.5	3.3	5.7
32	2.7	3.2	3.5	(9.4)
33	2.8	3.3	3.4	(3.0)
34[b]	2.2	3.4	3.1	8.8
35[b]	1.5	3.1	3.0	3.2
36	2.8	3.4	3.6	(5.9)
37	2.2	3.4	3.8	(11.8)
38	2.4	3.3	3.6	(9.1)
39	2.9	3.5	3.8	(8.6)
40	2.6	3.4	3.7	(8.8)
41[b]	1.9	3.1	3.0	3.2
42	2.3	3.3	3.8	(15.1)

[a] Calculated as the product of [(concentration desired − concentration observed)/concentration desired] × 100.
[b] Patient with pneumonia or sepsis.
[c] Parentheses denote negative variance.

(95% confidence interval, 0.19 to 0.29).

For the 12 patients in the study with sepsis or pneumonia (Table 2), the mean initial SAC was 2.2 ± 0.4 g/dL. The mean desired SAC was 3.4 ± 0.2 g/dL and the mean observed SAC after replacement was 3.2 ± 0.2 g/dL ($p > 0.05$) in these patients.

Discussion. Concurrent administration of human albumin and TPN is controversial. The expense of TPN support can double with the addition of human albumin. Usually human albumin is administered empirically in the TPN solution or as a separate infusion with no established endpoint. Without an established endpoint, human-albumin infusion can be continued indefinitely. Our results show that this prospective dosing method can accurately predict the appropriate human-albumin dosage for achieving the desired SAC. Because the 95% confidence interval for the mean prediction error (−0.10 to 0.06 g/dL) includes zero, we fail to reject the null hypothesis that bias equals zero. With bias equal to zero, we have an accurate equation that neither underpredicts nor overpredicts systematically the dosage of human albumin required to achieve a desired SAC. The precision of our equation gives us an estimate of the magnitude of the typical error. Using the regression equation to calculate albumin dosages, we expect to reach an SAC within 0.2 to 0.3 g/dL above or below our target. By calculating the human-albumin dosage in advance and giving it as 12.5- or 25-g increments, a predetermined number of supplemented liters can be prescribed. There would be little need to check the SAC until the human-albumin replacement dosage was infused completely. Also, by gradually increasing the SAC, one avoids intravascular fluid overload and the potential for congestive heart failure and pulmonary edema that may accompany rapid infusions.

Hardin et al.[16] reported that 13 patients who were studied retrospectively received human albumin concurrently with TPN using an albumin replacement formula with an assumed volume of distribution. This study demonstrated that the targeted SAC was reached after the calculated dosage was administered over 24 to 72 hours.[16] Our study prospectively calculated an albumin dosage for 42 patients. The dosage calculation was derived from a regression equation developed in a previous study.[10] The replacement dosage was administered in daily doses of 25 to 37.5 g over a period of five to nine days.

The 19 patients for whom follow-up SACs were available maintained their SACs after completion of the human-albumin replacement dosage; however, this represents only one half of the study population. When adequate energy and protein are not administered concurrently with human albumin, the albumin will be catabolized for energy and the increase in SAC will be transient. Although this effect is unproven, administration of adequate nutritional support appears to protect the human albumin from degradation. Our data support this speculation, since the patients generally attained nitrogen equilibrium as measured by nitrogen balance. The equation used in this study tended to underpredict the dosage of albumin for patients who had pneumonia or sepsis. This underprediction can most likely be explained by the redistribution of albumin observed in the septic state (movement into the interstitial space) and the net decrease in endogenous albumin synthesis. Hepatic synthesis of acute-phase reactant proteins (e.g., C-reactive protein, α_1-acid glycoprotein, ceruloplasmin) takes priority during the septic state. Also, the hypermetabolism that accompanies sepsis may have raised energy expenditure beyond the amount of energy that our patients received. In this case some of the administered human albumin or crystalline amino acids probably would have been used for energy.

The concurrent administration of human albumin with TPN remains controversial; however, some recent data support this practice.[17,18] Ford et al.[17] recently demonstrated that gastrointestinal tolerance to enteral feedings in hypoalbuminemic pediatric patients improved markedly after exogenous administration of human albumin. Brown et al.[18] reported significantly less hospital morbidity in hypoalbuminemic patients who received human albumin plus TPN when compared with a group receiving just TPN. It is not clear, however, whether the expense associated with human-albumin administration is justified by the decrease in morbidity. Because many institutions probably will continue to administer human albumin with TPN, methods to optimize the administration of this expensive supplement seem warranted.

Conclusion. The regression equation tested in this study can be used to calculate the albumin replacement dosage required by hypoalbuminemic patients who are to receive TPN. The formula may slightly underpredict the replacement dose in septic patients.

References

1. Grant JP. Handbook of parenteral nutrition. Philadelphia: W. B. Saunders Company; 1980:103.
2. Dudrick SJ, Mac Fayden BV, Ionchon EA et al. Parenteral nutrition techniques in cancer patients. *Cancer Res.* 1977; 37:2440–50.
3. Mirtallo JM, Schneider PJ, Ruberg RL. Albumin in TPN solutions: potential savings resulting from prospective review. *J Parenter Enter Nutr.* 1980; 4:300–2.
4. Louie N, Niemiec PW. Parenteral nutrition solutions. In: Rombeau JL, Caldwell MD, eds. Parenteral nutrition. Philadelphia: W. B. Saunders Company; 1986:272–305.
5. Warnold I, Lundholm K. Clinical significance of preoperative nutritional status in 215 noncancer patients. *Ann Surg.* 1984; 199:299–305.
6. Apelgren KN, Rombeau JL, Twomey PL et al. Comparison of nutritional indices and outcome in critically ill patients. *Crit Care Med.* 1982; 10:305–7.
7. Randle NW, Hubert-Hartmann K, Mulheran LC. Serum al-

bumin levels: relationship to length of hospital stay. *Hosp Pharm.* 1984; 19:802–5.
8. Anderson CF, Wochos DN. The utility of serum albumin values in the nutritional assessment of hospitalized patients. *Mayo Clin Proc.* 1982; 57:181–4.
9. Buzby GP, Mullen JL, Matthews DC et al. Prognostic nutritional index in gastrointestinal surgery. *Am J Surg.* 1980; 139:160–6.
10. Brown, RO, Bradley JE, Luther RW. Response of serum albumin concentrations to albumin supplementation during central total parenteral nutrition. *Clin Pharm.* 1987; 6:222–6.
11. Anon. Guidelines for use of total parenteral nutrition in the hospitalized adult patient. *J Parenter Enter Nutr.* 1986; 10:441–5.
12. Shanbhogue LK, Chawals WJ, Weintraub M et al. Parenteral nutrition in the surgical patient. *Br J Surg.* 1987; 74:172–80.
13. Doumas SP, Watson WA, Briggs HG. Albumin standards and the measurement standards of serum albumin with bromocresol green. *Clin Chim Acta.* 1971; 31:89–96.
14. Blackburn GL, Bistrian BR, Maini BS et al. Nutritional and metabolic assessment of the hospitalized patient. *J Parenter Enter Nutr.* 1977; 1:11–22.
15. Sheiner LB, Beal SL. Some suggestions for measuring predictive performance. *J Pharmacokinet Biopharm.* 1981; 9:503–12.
16. Hardin TC, Page CP, Schwesinger WH. Rapid replacement of serum albumin in patients receiving total parenteral nutrition. *Surg Gynecol Obstet.* 1986; 163:359–62.
17. Ford EG, Jennings M, Andrassy RJ. Serum albumin (oncotic pressure) correlates with enteral feeding tolerance in the pediatric surgical patient. *J Pediatr Surg.* 1987; 7:597–9.
18. Brown RO, Bradley JE, Bekemeyer WB et al. Effect of albumin supplementation during parenteral nutrition on hospital morbidity. *Crit Care Med.* 1988; (in press).

Lack of correlation between objective indicators and clinical-response scores during antimicrobial therapy for acute pulmonary exacerbations of cystic fibrosis

JOHN A. BOSSO AND KAY B. WALKER

Clin Pharm. 1988; 7:897–901

Cystic fibrosis is the most common lethal inherited disease in the white population. Inherited through an autosomal recessive mode, it has an incidence of 1 in 2000 live births in Caucasians in the United States.[1] Pulmonary disease is responsible for the vast majority of morbidity and mortality in patients with cystic fibrosis.[2] As pulmonary disease progresses over time, affected patients require ever-increasing medical intervention, including hospitalization for respiratory therapy and antimicrobial therapy. Patients are frequently hospitalized for acute pulmonary exacerbations. Acute pulmonary exacerbations have been defined by Rubio[3] as the presence of five or more of the following findings: increased productive cough; changes in volume, appearance, or color of sputum; increased respiratory rate or dyspnea; progressive physical findings on chest auscultation; new infiltrates on chest roentgenograms; deterioration of pulmonary function test results; decreased appetite and weight loss; fatigue and decreased exercise tolerance; fever; emergence of a new pathogen in sputum cultures; and presence of increasing numbers of granulocytes or more immature granulocytes. These respiratory exacerbations are often associated with bacterial pathogens such as *Pseudomonas aeruginosa, Pseudomonas cepacia, Staphylococcus aureus,* and *Haemophilus influenzae.* The objective evaluation of response to antimicrobial therapy in cystic fibrosis is difficult. Many investigators have reported an apparent lack of correlation between clinical-response scores and presumed objective indicators normally used to assess response to treatment with antimicrobial agents in patients with infectious diseases.[4–10]

A number of methods traditionally have been used to assess response to antimicrobial therapy in cystic fibrosis. These have included various clinical "scoring systems," which are used to quantitate the patient's clinical condition. Although such systems may include some objective data, they also include observations that may reflect subjectivity on the part of the observer or rater, such as evaluations of exercise tolerance and appetite. Nonetheless, such scoring systems seem to correlate fairly well with the clinician's impression of the patient's condition. Objective observations or determinations that are traditionally used to diagnose and monitor infectious diseases also have been used to assess response to therapy in patients with cystic fibrosis. These include sputum culture (with identification and quantitation of pathogens), white blood cell count and differential in peripheral blood, erythrocyte sedimentation rate, chest roentgenogram, and tests of pulmonary function. The value or reliability of such tests has been questioned by various authors.[4,5,11] Because traditional markers of infectious disease may not correlate well with clinical response, some clinicians and investigators have questioned the therapeutic role of antimicrobial agents in this condition. Further, if such tests are indeed not useful indicators of response, their use makes little economic sense.

JOHN A. BOSSO, PHARM.D., is Professor of Clinical Pharmacy, Department of Pharmacy Practice, College of Pharmacy; Adjunct Professor of Pediatrics, Division of Clinical Pharmacology, Department of Pediatrics, School of Medicine; and Director, Clinical Pharmacology Research Program, Intermountain Cystic Fibrosis Center, University of Utah, Salt Lake City. KAY B. WALKER, M.D., is Assistant Professor of Pediatrics, Division of Allergy and Immunology, Department of Pediatrics, School of Medicine, University of Utah, Salt Lake City.

Address reprint requests to Dr. Bosso at the College of Pharmacy, University of Utah, Salt Lake City, UT 84112.

Copyright © 1988, American Society of Hospital Pharmacists, Inc. All rights reserved. 0278-2677/88/1201-0897$01.25.

Table 1.
Description of Antimicrobial Studies

Study	No. Patients	Mean Age (years)	Antimicrobial Therapy[a]	Mean No. Days of Therapy (range)	Scoring System	Scoring Times (days)
Bosso et al.[12]	27	13.5	Aztreonam 200 mg/kg/day	12.5 (7–19)	Beaudry	First, every 7, last, FU[b]
					Clinical	First, every 5, last
Bosso and Black[13]	16	23.6	Ciprofloxacin 750 mg b.i.d.	17.5 (7–35)	Kercsmar	First, every 7, last, FU
Bosso and Black[14]	15	14.1	Aztreonam 200 mg/kg/day	17.2 (11–29)	Beaudry	First, every 7, last, FU
	15	14.7	Tobramycin[c] plus azlocillin 350 mg/kg/day	14.8 (8–22)	Clinical	First, every 5, last
Bosso et al.[15]	12	22.9	Ciprofloxacin 750 mg b.i.d.	13.4 (7–21)	Kercsmar	First, every 7, last, FU
	13	23	Tobramycin[c] plus azlocillin 350 mg/kg/day	12.5 (6–18)		

[a] Ciprofloxacin was given orally as the hydrochloride salt; aztreonam, tobramycin sulfate, and azlocillin were given intravenously.
[b] FU = follow-up (7–14 days after completion of therapy).
[c] Tobramycin dosage was varied to produce peak serum concentrations of 8–10 μg/mL and trough concentrations of <2 μg/mL.

The purpose of this study was to identify any strong correlations between clinical-response scores and objective measures of response to determine which of the latter could be recommended as monitoring tools.

Methods. Response data from 106 courses of antimicrobial therapy for acute pulmonary exacerbations were analyzed. These data were derived from four previously completed antimicrobial trials[12-15] and thus may be more complete and inclusive than those collected during routine hospitalization and treatment. These studies included two open-label, noncontrolled studies, one with aztreonam and the other with ciprofloxacin, and two open-label, controlled studies, one comparing aztreonam with tobramycin plus azlocillin and the other comparing ciprofloxacin with tobramycin plus azlocillin. All studies were completed in the same institution. The four studies involved 27, 16, 30, and 25 patients, respectively. (The published report of the study comparing ciprofloxacin with tobramycin plus azlocillin included data on 20 of the 25 study participants.) More detailed information regarding the nature of these studies is presented in Table 1. All patients were experiencing acute pulmonary exacerbations (as defined by Rubio[3]) requiring hospitalization and treatment with antimicrobial agents. Patients with allergies to the study antimicrobial agents or with renal or hepatic impairment were excluded from participation. The only other antimicrobial agents used in these trials were dicloxacillin and nafcillin, which were given to patients whose sputum cultures showed *Staph. aureus* in the two aztreonam studies. Patients also received respiratory therapy, vitamins, and enzyme replacement therapy.

One or two of three different clinical scoring systems were used in these studies: that of Kercsmar et al.,[16] that of Beaudry et al.,[17] and a third

Table 2.
Clinical Scoring Systems

Response Indicator	Method: Kercsmar[16]	Clinical[a]	Beaudry[17]
General condition	+		
Temperature	+		+
Activity/exercise tolerance	+		
Appetite	+		
Chills		+	
Heart rate	+		+
Respiratory rate	+	+	+
Respiratory effort	+	+	+
Cyanosis			+
Cough	+	+	+
Sputum production	+	+	+
Sputum character	+		
Chest examination	+	+	
P_{CO_2}	+		
P_{O_2}	+		
White blood cell (WBC) count	+		
Immature WBC count	+		

[a] The clinical scoring system incorporates some of these response indicators into the general categories of consolidation/pleural effusion, decreased pulmonary function, and symptoms related to bronchitis rather than evaluating them separately.

(referred to in the tables as "clinical score"), a general method used to evaluate lower-respiratory-tract infections. Each of these systems incorporates various signs and symptoms from physical examination and patient history (e.g., appetite, exercise tolerance); the Kercsmar system also incorporates peripheral white blood cell count and differential. A numerical value is assigned to each observation to arrive at a quantitative score. The indicators evaluated (and rated) with each of these clinical scoring methods are presented in Table 2. In all four studies, the rater was one of two individuals. In the case of the Kercsmar system, points (total number possible = 100) are deducted based on the severity of the finding, whereas with the other two systems, points (total number possible = 21 for the Beaudry system and 24 for clinical score system) are added based on severity. Thus, a higher score indicates improvement with the Kercsmar system, whereas the opposite is true with the other two systems.

Other measures of response included peripheral white blood cell count and differential, pathogen density in sputum (colony-forming units/milliliter of sputum), chest roentgenogram scores (scored by the method of Brasfield et al.[18]), and the following pulmonary function test values: forced vital capacity (FVC), forced expiratory volume in one second (FEV_1), maximal midexpiratory flow (FEF_{25-75}), and forced expiratory flow at 75% exhaled FVC (FEF_{75}). Since these data were derived from a number of previously completed clinical trials, not all values were available for all patients included. The two patient groups included in each of the two controlled studies were comparable with respect to age and disease severity. In addition, no differences in response to antimicrobial therapy were noted between the group receiving the study drug (aztreonam or ciprofloxacin) and the group receiving the control regimen (tobramycin plus azlocillin).

For the purposes of this analysis, absolute and percentage changes (pretherapy to end of therapy) in the clinical scores and the other measures of response were tested for statistically significant correlations ($p \leq 0.05$) using Spearman's correlation.

Results. All courses of antimicrobial therapy were associated with a positive response to treatment that was matched by a concomitant change in clinical score reflecting improvement. Overall, the other measures of response also changed with therapy (Table 3). It should be noted, however, that changes were not always in a positive direction (indicating improvement) and that the standard deviations for these changes were large, perhaps because of the heterogeneous nature of our patient population in terms of disease severity. Of particular note are the observations that white blood cell counts and pathogen (*Ps. aeruginosa*) counts in sputum increased in some patients in the face of apparent clinical improvement.

A number of statistically significant correlations were noted between clinical score (usually the Kercsmar system) and other response indicators (Table 4). These significant correlations were, for the most part, limited to those between changes in pulmonary function test values and changes in Kercsmar clinical score, although changes in chest roentgenogram scores did correlate to a significant degree with changes in the Beaudry clinical score. Changes in white blood cell count or differential, pathogen density in sputum, and chest roentgenogram score did not correlate with changes in the Kercsmar clinical score. In the cases of significant correlations, the correlation coefficients (r) were often small enough that the clinical usefulness of these relationships may be questioned.

Table 3.
Mean Change in Response Indicators

Response Indicator	n	Mean ± S.D. Change
Clinical score	53	−4.85 ± 2.45 points
% Clinical score	55	−37.57 ± 14.04
Beaudry score	55	−4.18 ± 2.29 points
% Beaudry score	55	−64.15 ± 26.75
Kercsmar score	49	13.74 ± 9.18 points
% Kercsmar score	49	28.53 ± 25.12
White blood cell count	100	−2.89 ± 3.59 × 10^3/cu mm
% Bands	101	−1.74 ± 6.23
Pseudomonas aeruginosa count	91	−2.68 ± 3.65 log colony-forming units/mL
% *Ps. aeruginosa* count	91	−33.82 ± 45.18
FVC	79	4.85 ± 11.10 % predicted
% FVC	79	8.50 ± 19.62
FEV_1	79	6.24 ± 8.53 % predicted
% FEV_1	79	15.60 ± 22.63
FEF_{25-75}	79	5.63 ± 13.70 % predicted
% FEF_{25-75}	79	28.40 ± 44.95
FEF_{75}	79	5.56 ± 12.60 % predicted
% FEF_{75}	79	32.02 ± 67.09
CXR score	58	1.36 ± 1.93 points
% CXR score	58	10.83 ± 18.07

[a] FVC = forced vital capacity, FEV_1 = forced expiratory volume in one second, FEF_{25-75} = maximum midexpiratory flow, FEF_{75} = forced expiratory flow at 75% exhaled FVC, CXR = chest roentgenogram.

Table 4.
Correlations between Changes in Clinical Scores and Other Response Indicators[a]

Clinical Scoring System	Response Indicator	n	r	p[b]
Kercsmar	FVC	44	0.327	0.030
% Kercsmar	FVC	44	0.363	0.015
Kercsmar	% FVC	44	0.357	0.017
% Kercsmar	% FVC	44	0.416	0.005
Kercsmar	FEV_1	44	0.444	0.003
% Kercsmar	FEV_1	44	0.388	0.009
Kercsmar	% FEV_1	44	0.456	0.002
% Kercsmar	% FEV_1	44	0.461	0.002
Kercsmar	FEF_{25-75}	44	0.463	0.002
% Kercsmar	FEF_{25-75}	44	0.358	0.017
Beaudry	CXR score	24	−0.529	0.008
Beaudry	% CXR score	24	−0.493	0.014

[a] Abbreviations: n = number of paired observations; r = Spearman's correlation coefficient; FVC = forced vital capacity; FEV_1 = forced expiratory volume in one second; FEF_{25-75} = maximum midexpiratory flow; FEF_{75} = forced expiratory flow at 75% exhaled FVC; CXR = chest roentgenogram.

[b] Only statistically significant ($p \leq 0.05$) correlations are included.

Discussion. The results of this study verify informal observations and conclusions that a number of typically monitored response indicators do not correlate with apparent clinical response to antimicrobial therapy for acute pulmonary exacerbations of cystic fibrosis. Of the various measures of response studied, only pulmonary function tests correlated to a significant degree with clinical-response scores, as quantitated by the Kercsmar scoring system. Changes or lack thereof in traditional markers of infectious disease (such as white blood cell count and differential and pathogen density in sputum), and thus response to antimicrobial therapy, do not appear to correlate with clinical-response scores. This amplifies the debate concerning the usefulness of treating cystic fibrosis patients with antimicrobial agents. If such response indicators do not change concomitantly with the clinical condition, the antimicrobial agent apparently has no effect.

A recent study by Gold et al.[19] suggested that antimicrobial therapy may not be necessary in mild to moderate pulmonary exacerbations. In this randomized, placebo-controlled study, no difference in response was observed between ceftazidime- or placebo-treated patients. Response was defined as changes (improvements) in vital signs, cough, dyspnea, pulmonary function test results, chest roentgenogram, body weight, appetite, pathogen density in sputum, and peripheral white blood cell count. Although the methods and conclusions of this study have been criticized,[20] it is probably safe to assume that antimicrobial therapy is not always necessary in all patients for all pulmonary exacerbations.

A number of factors acting singly or in combination probably account for the occurrence of an acute pulmonary exacerbation. These may include acute viral infections, air pollutants, allergens, and, of course, bacterial infection. Thus, one may assume that therapy with antimicrobial agents will not always benefit the patient. However, there is little question that chronic or acute bacterial infection or colonization of the airways contributes both directly and indirectly to the lung pathology observed in cystic fibrosis. As a result, it seems logical to conclude that antimicrobial therapy should benefit patients with those conditions. Because pulmonary exacerbations are treated with a number of different modalities (chest physiotherapy, bronchodilators, exercise therapy, nutritional intervention, and antimicrobial agents), and because no study to date has included an "antimicrobial agent only" treatment group, it is difficult to assess how antimicrobial agents affect response. The fact that typical markers of infection do not correlate with clinical response only confounds the picture further.

One may conclude from our results that such measures as pathogen density in sputum, chest roentgenograms, and peripheral white blood cell counts are of little use in monitoring response to therapy with antimicrobial agents in cases of acute respiratory exacerbations of cystic fibrosis. Their use, therefore, may represent an ineffective use of health-care dollars. This does not imply that such tests are useless, however; they should still be expected to yield informative diagnostic results. It is their repeated use during a course of therapy that apparently should be avoided. Further, if it had been feasible to classify patients according to disease severity (by pulmonary function data that were not available for all patients analyzed in this study), additional statistically significant correlations might have occurred for one or more patient groups with milder disease. For example, it may be that the appearance of pulmonary infiltrates and their subsequent disappearance with therapy are more readily apparent in patients without the permanent roentgenogram changes associated with severe disease. Our results and conclusions also should be tempered with the knowledge that, in our patients, the disease severity and nature of the antimicrobial therapy (monotherapy versus combination treatment, duration of therapy) varied. If such characteristics had been standardized, better correlations might have been seen.

Other objective measurements are obviously needed, both for evaluation of antimicrobial therapy during routine hospitalizations and for formal efficacy trials of antimicrobial agents. A recent study by Smith et al.[11] suggests that sputum DNA content and total protein concentrations may be reliable and objective markers of infection or inflammation. Thus, serial measurement of these indicators may be a reasonable way to monitor therapy. In their study, changes in sputum DNA, total protein, and albumin content and quantitative microbiology of sputum were studied in relation to clinical improvement. Changes in sputum DNA and protein correlated with clinical improvement, as did changes in quantitative microbiology. Albumin concentrations in sputum did not change with treatment. We did not find a correlation between changes in quantitative microbiology of sputum and clinical change, which is consistent with the report of Reed et al.[21] In fact, we found that sputum pathogen density often increases in the face of clinical improvement. A recent article by Glass et al.[22] reported that serum C-reactive protein is a reliable marker of acute or impending pulmonary exacerbation and that serial measurement of this marker is a useful way to monitor response to therapy.

Conclusion. A number of markers traditionally used to evaluate efficacy of antimicrobial agents in the treatment of pulmonary exacerbations of cystic fibrosis do not correlate with clinical-response scores. These tests cannot be recommended for routine monitoring of patients with this condition. The search for objective response indicators that correlate with clinical-response scores—such as sputum DNA, total protein, and C-reactive protein—should continue.

References

1. Steinberg AG, Brown DC. On the incidence of cystic fibrosis of the pancreas. *Am J Hum Genet.* 1960; 12:416–24.
2. Mischler EH. Treatment of pulmonary disease in cystic fibrosis. *Semin Respir Med.* 1985; 6:271–84.
3. Rubio TT. Infection in patients with cystic fibrosis. *Am J Med.* 1986; 81(Suppl 1A):73–7.
4. Nelson JD. Management of acute pulmonary exacerbations in cystic fibrosis: a critical appraisal. *J Pediatr.* 1985; 106:1030–4.
5. Smith AL. Antibiotic therapy in cystic fibrosis: evaluation of clinical trials. *J Pediatr.* 1986; 108:866–9.
6. Govan JRW, Doherty C, Glass S. Rational parameters for antibiotic therapy in patients with cystic fibrosis. *Infection.* 1987; 15:300–8.
7. Cullen RET, McCrae WM, Govan JRW et al. Ceftazidime in cystic fibrosis: clinical, microbiological and immunological studies. *J Antimicrob Chemother.* 1983; 12(Suppl A):369–75.
8. Krilov LR, Blumer JL, Stem RC et al. Imipenem/cilistatin in acute pulmonary exacerbations of cystic fibrosis. *Rev Infect Dis.* 1985; 7(Suppl 3):S482–S489.
9. Gold R, Overmeyer A, Knie B et al. Controlled trial of ceftazidime vs. ticarcillin and tobramycin in the treatment of acute respiratory exacerbations in patients with cystic fibrosis. *Pediatr Infect Dis.* 1985; 4:172–7.
10. Reed MD, Stern RC, O'Brien CA et al. Randomized double-blind evaluation of ceftazidime dose ranging in hospitalized patients with cystic fibrosis. *Antimicrob Agents Chemother.* 1987; 31:698–702.
11. Smith AL, Redding G, Doershuk C et al. Sputum changes associated with therapy for endobronchial exacerbation in cystic fibrosis. *J Pediatr.* 1988; 112:547–54.
12. Bosso JA, Black PG, Matsen JM. Efficacy of aztreonam in pulmonary exacerbations of cystic fibrosis. *Pediatr Infect Dis J.* 1987; 6:393–7.
13. Bosso JA, Black PG. Efficacy of ciprofloxacin in patients with cystic fibrosis. *Drug Intell Clin Pharm.* 1988; 22:551–3.
14. Bosso JA, Black PG. Controlled trial of aztreonam vs tobramycin and azlocillin for acute pulmonary exacerbations of cystic fibrosis. *Pediatr Infect Dis J.* 1988; 7:171–6.
15. Bosso JA, Black PG, Matsen JM. Ciprofloxacin versus tobramycin plus azlocillin in pulmonary exacerbations in adult patients with cystic fibrosis. *Am J Med.* 1987; 82(Suppl 4A):180–4.
16. Kercsmar CM, Stern RC, Reed MD et al. Ceftazidime in cystic fibrosis: pharmacokinetics and therapeutic response. *J Antimicrob Chemother.* 1983; 12(Suppl A):289–95.
17. Beaudry PH, Marks MI, McDougall D et al. Is anti-*Pseudomonas* therapy warranted in acute respiratory exacerbations in children with cystic fibrosis? *J Pediatr.* 1980; 97:144–7.
18. Brasfield D, Hicks G, Soong S et al. The chest roentgenogram in cystic fibrosis: a new scoring system. *Pediatrics.* 1979; 63:24–9.
19. Gold R, Carpenter S, Heurter H et al. Randomized trial of ceftazidime versus placebo in the management of acute respiratory exacerbations in patients with cystic fibrosis. *J Pediatr.* 1988; 111:907–13.
20. Wood RE. What is a "pulmonary exacerbation" in cystic fibrosis? *J Pediatr.* 1988; 111:841–2.
21. Reed MD, Goldfarb J, Crenshaw D. Lack of correlation between clinical response and sputum quantitative cultures in patients with cystic fibrosis (CF) treated with ciprofloxacin. Paper presented to the 27th Interscience Conference on Antimicrobial Agents and Chemotherapy. New York, NY: 1987 Oct 6.
22. Glass S, Hayward C, Govan JRW. Serum C-reactive protein in assessment of pulmonary exacerbations and antimicrobial therapy in cystic fibrosis. *J Pediatr.* 1988; 113:76–9.

Additive and synergistic bactericidal activity contributed by desacetylcefotaxime during cefotaxime therapy

EMORY S. MOORE, MAYRA JIMENEZ, STEVEN L. BARRIERE, MARISA L. CIMINO, AND F. ROBERT FEKETY

Clin Pharm. 1988; 7:901–5

Cefotaxime (CTX) is a broad-spectrum cephalosporin that undergoes metabolism in vivo to a desacetyl metabolite. The metabolite is active in vitro against many of the same bacteria as cefotaxime but retains only 1/4 to 1/16 the activity of the parent compound.[1–3] Approximately 40–60% of an administered dose of CTX is converted to desacetylcefotaxime (dCTX), and the remainder is excreted in the urine as unchanged drug.[4] After intravenous administration in patients with normal renal function, the elimination half-life of CTX is approximately one hour, and the apparent half-life of the metabolite is 1.5–2.6 hours.[5] Because of differing elimination half-lives, the ratio of the serum concentrations of CTX and dCTX observed after i.v. administration of CTX changes over time.

In vitro synergy between CTX and dCTX has been observed against a variety of aerobic and anaerobic bacteria using a variety of testing methods, most commonly the checkerboard method.[1–3,6] In one study using fixed concentrations of CTX and its metabolite, synergy and partial synergy were observed in more than 70% of isolates tested, but antagonism was found against strains of *Morganella morganii* and *Proteus vulgaris*.[2]

EMORY S. MOORE, PHARM.D., is Assistant Professor, Clinical Division, College of Pharmacy, The University of Texas, Austin; at the time of this study, he was Pharmacokinetics Resident, Department of Pharmacy Services, University of Michigan Hospitals, Ann Arbor. MAYRA JIMENEZ, PHARM.D., is Clinical Pharmacist, Department of Pharmacy, Veterans Administration Medical Center, Miami, FL; at the time of this study, she was a Doctor of Pharmacy candidate at the College of Pharmacy, University of Michigan, Ann Arbor. STEVEN L. BARRIERE, PHARM.D. is Clinical Specialist, Infectious Diseases, Department of Pharmaceutical Services, and Adjunct Associate Professor of Medicine and Pharmacology, University of California, Los Angeles. MARISA L. CIMINO is Laboratory Technician and F. ROBERT FEKETY, M.D., is Division Chief, Division of Infectious Diseases, Department of Internal Medicine, University of Michigan Hospitals, Ann Arbor.

Address reprint requests to Dr. Barriere at the UCLA Medical Center, Room A4-215 CHS, Los Angeles, CA 90024.

Supported in part by a grant from Hoechst-Roussel Pharmaceuticals.

Presented at the 1986 American College of Clinical Pharmacy Annual Meeting, Chicago, IL, July 28, 1986.

Copyright © 1988, American Society of Hospital Pharmacists, Inc. All rights reserved. 0278-2677/88/1201-0901$01.25.

The synergistic activity noted in vitro may have important implications in certain clinical situations. The in vivo antimicrobial activity of CTX therapy (which includes the activity of both CTX and dCTX) may be greater than would be predicted by current in vitro susceptibility testing methods, which consider only the activity of the parent compound. Also, since concentrations of the metabolite are proportionally greater at the end of a typical dosing interval (trough), the in vivo trough antimicrobial activity of both parent and metabolite may be greater than anticipated if only the concentration of the parent compound were considered.

In most in vitro studies, synergy between CTX and dCTX has been examined using fixed concentrations of each drug. Because of the differing and changing ratios of drug concentrations found in vivo, the results of such studies may have limited clinical relevance.

Reller[7] administered cefotaxime 1 g i.v. to healthy volunteers and assayed serum concentrations of CTX and dCTX at six time points (from 15 minutes to four hours) after drug infusion. The serum bactericidal titers of each sample were measured against a strain of *Escherichia coli* (minimum bactericidal concentration (MBC) for CTX = 0.03 μg/mL), *Bacteroides fragilis* (MBC for CTX = 4.0 μg/mL), and *Staphylococcus aureus* (MBC for CTX = 2.0 μg/mL). These values were compared with the serum bactericidal titers (SBTs) of simulated serum samples that were spiked with an equal amount of parent CTX and lacked dCTX. Additive and synergistic killing were defined as, respectively, a twofold or a fourfold or greater increase in the SBT. When the SBT results were examined, no enhanced activity against the strain of *E. coli* or *Staph. aureus* was observed in the patient samples that contained both CTX and dCTX, compared with the simulated samples containing CTX only. However, when dCTX concentrations were at least 50% of the CTX concentration, additive and synergistic killing were seen against the strain of *B. fragilis.*

The purpose of this investigation was to determine the contributions and interactions of the parent drug CTX and its metabolite dCTX in providing bactericidal activity early in i.v. CTX therapy (non-steady-state). To accomplish this, selected strains of Enterobacteriaceae, which were additively or synergistically inhibited by CTX and dCTX in vitro and representative of pathogens commonly found in clinical medicine, were used to determine and then compare the in vivo bactericidal activity of each drug alone and the activity of CTX and dCTX combined.

Methods. To select three strains of Enterobacteriaceae appropriate for this study, 20 serum-resistant clinical isolates from the infectious disease laboratory were tested by standard microtiter dilution for susceptibility to CTX and dCTX.[8] Further, checkerboard technique was performed in duplicate to select for the in vitro presence of additive or synergistic inhibition and killing by the combination of the two drugs.[6] For this checkerboard test, additive and synergistic interactions were defined as at least a twofold or a fourfold decrease, respectively, in the minimum inhibitory or bactericidal concentration of the drugs in combination, compared with those seen with each drug alone.

Based on these results (Table 1), one isolate each of *Proteus mirabilis, E. coli,* and *Klebsiella pneumoniae* were selected. The isolates determined to meet these specific selection criteria were found to have MICs for CTX of ≤0.125, with dCTX susceptibilities being twofold to tenfold less. As determined by this in vitro test, all isolates selected were either additively or synergistically killed by the combination of CTX and dCTX (Table 1). The *Proteus* strain was shown to be inhibited and killed additively by the combination, whereas the *Escherichia* and *Klebsiella* strains were shown to be inhibited and killed synergistically by the combination.

As an indicator of the in vivo antimicrobial activity observed at the initiation of cefotaxime therapy, the bactericidal activities of CTX with dCTX and that of CTX and dCTX alone were determined by performing SBTs using a microtiter dilution test.[9] To simulate patient samples, stock solutions of CTX sodium standard powder (lot RP 6088) and dCTX sodium standard powder (batch 2111 3Na) (Hoechst–Roussel Pharmaceuticals, Somerville, NJ 08876) were prepared in pooled human serum and diluted to produce three sets of simulated patient samples.

Table 1.
Minimum Inhibitory Concentrations of Cefotaxime (CTX), Desacetylcefotaxime (dCTX), and a Combination of the Two Drugs (CTX–dCTX) against Test Isolates[a]

Test Isolate	MIC (μg/mL) CTX	dCTX	CTX–dCTX[b]	Interpretation of Results
Escherichia coli	≤0.125	≤1.25	≤0.031, ≤0.31	Synergistic
Proteus mirabilis	≤0.031	≤0.031	≤0.008, ≤0.008	Additive
Klebsiella pneumoniae	≤0.031	≤0.125	≤0.008, ≤0.031	Synergistic

[a] In all instances, minimum bactericidal concentrations were identical to minimum inhibitory concentrations.
[b] CTX concentration, dCTX concentration.

Set A of simulated patient samples contained both CTX and dCTX in concentrations that approximated those typically observed early in therapy after a single i.v. bolus dose of CTX 2 g (as opposed to those observed midtherapy at steady-state conditions). Concentrations of CTX and dCTX employed in these simulated patient samples (Table 2) were representative of typical concentrations obtained at one, two, four, and six hours in patients with normal renal function after an initial (single) dose of cefotaxime.[7,10-13] When specific concentrations after a 2-g i.v. bolus dose were not available, these were extrapolated from pharmacokinetic values calculated after a 1-g i.v. bolus dose.

Set B of simulated patient samples, technically unobtainable in an actual clinical setting, contained only the parent compound, CTX, at the same concentrations as found in set A described above, yet contained no metabolite. Set C, also unobtainable in actual CTX therapy, contained only the metabolite, dCTX, at the same concentrations found in set A but contained no parent drug. Solutions were not analyzed to confirm final drug concentrations.

As an indicator of the in vivo antimicrobial activity observed at the initiation of cefotaxime therapy in the clinical setting, SBTs were performed on set A of the simulated patient samples. As an indicator of the in vivo antimicrobial activity of each drug individually, SBTs were determined for sets B and C. Following standard methodology for SBT testing, the simulated patient serum sample for each time point was added to the first well of the microtiter tray and diluted serially from 1:1 (undiluted sera) to 1:512 with Mueller–Hinton broth containing approximately 10^5 colony-forming units of each organism, to create a final volume of 200 μL.[9] Trays were incubated for 24 hours at 35 °C. After 24 hours, 5 μL of broth from wells with no growth was subcultured onto agar plates and incubated to determine whether killing had occurred. SBTs were recorded as the highest dilution of antibiotic tested that killed at least 99.9% of organisms after 24 hours of subculture incubation. SBTs were run in duplicate for all three sets and repeated four times. The reported SBT was that titer most often observed in the above test.

Table 2.
Concentrations of Cefotaxime (CTX) and Desacetylcefotaxime (dCTX) in Patients with Normal Renal Function after I.V. Bolus Administration of Cefotaxime 2 g

Time (hr)	Concentration (μg/mL) CTX	dCTX	Ratio
1	50	8	6.25
2	15	8	1.9
4	3	3	1
6	0.5	1	0.5

SBTs at Each Time Point. In the first method of evaluation, SBTs were used to examine the relative bactericidal activity of each compound and the interactions between CTX and dCTX at each point in the dosing interval. In comparing SBTs, a fourfold difference was required for significance because of this test's inherent variability. At each time point, antagonistic, indifferent, or additive or possibly synergistic activity was evaluated by comparing the SBTs of the CTX–dCTX combination (set A) versus the SBTs of CTX alone (set B) and dCTX alone (set C). Indifference was defined as a twofold difference or no difference in the SBT seen with the combination (set A) and the most active drug alone (set B or C). Additive or possibly synergistic interactions between the drugs in combination were defined as a fourfold or greater increase in the SBT of set A compared with the SBT of the most active drug alone (set B or C). Antagonism was defined as at least a fourfold decrease in the SBT of the drugs in combination (set A) compared with the SBT of the most active drug alone (set B or C).

The AUBC Test. In a second method, the interaction between CTX and dCTX over the entire dosing interval was evaluated by comparing the total area under the bactericidal titer curve (AUBC) for the drugs in combination (set A) versus the AUBC for CTX alone (set B), the AUBC for dCTX alone (set C), and their sum (sets B and C). The inverse of the titers for each drug alone and the combination were plotted versus time, and the AUBCs were calculated using the trapezoidal rule.[14] Since a method of statistical comparison for AUBC values was lacking, the values generated for CTX and dCTX alone (sets B and C) were simply compared with the AUBC values for set A (containing both drugs) to discern what contribution dCTX makes to CTX therapy and to define what interactions exist over the entire dosing interval. In the AUBC method, finding the AUBC for the drugs in combination (set A) to be less than the AUBC of the most active drug alone (in most cases CTX) would indicate possible antagonism. Indifference would be suggested by an AUBC for the drugs in combination (set A) approximately equal to that for the most active drug alone. An additive effect would be suggested if an AUBC for the drugs in combination (set A) was approximately equal to the sum of the AUBC for CTX alone plus the AUBC for dCTX alone (AUBC of set B and AUBC of set C). Possible synergy would be suggested when the AUBC for the drugs in combination (set A) was found to be much greater than the sum of the AUBC for CTX alone plus the AUBC for dCTX alone (AUBC of set B and AUBC of set C).

The comparative clinical utility of these two methods—the comparison of SBTs at each time point and the comparison of AUBCs—in examining and meaningfully describing the contribution of each agent to the total bactericidal activity expected during CTX therapy, and the antimicrobial interactions between CTX and dCTX, was also considered.

Results. *SBTs at Each Time Point.* The average SBTs against the three organisms for serum containing CTX alone were all at least 1:256 one hour after the dose, declining to 1:16 or less at six hours after the dose. The average SBTs for dCTX alone were lower than those for the parent drug (1:64 or less) at one hour after the dose, yet their decline at a rate slower than the SBTs of parent drug resulted in SBTs similar to those of the parent drug at six hours after the dose.

Evaluation of the SBTs at each time point shows that at one, two, and four hours after the dose, the SBTs for the CTX–dCTX combination (set A) were typically similar to that of the parent drug alone (set B), indicating that the metabolite, despite showing additive or synergistic activity by in vitro checkerboard tests, contributes little or nothing to the total antimicrobial activity early in the dosing interval compared with the parent drug. At the final six-hour time point, the SBTs for the metabolite alone (set C) indicate that it contributed bactericidal activity similar to that associated with the parent alone (set B). Also, the SBTs for the combination (set A) showed synergistic activity in two of three isolates. The third isolate, that of *E. coli*, which had a higher dCTX MIC, showed probable indifference at the six-hour time point (Table 3). This suggests that the additive or synergistic activity observed in in vitro checkerboard tests may be evident clinically when the in vivo bactericidal activity of CTX and the bactericidal activity of its metabolite are similar, as is found at the end of a dosing interval. This method of evaluating SBT results was believed to be more clinically meaningful for an antibiotic such as CTX, the relatively short half-life of which may result in less-than-optimal end-of-interval antimicrobial activity; however, its metabolite may enhance this activity. The twofold variability of the SBT test affected its utility only slightly.

The AUBC Test. In using the AUBC test to determine the interaction of CTX and dCTX over the entire simulated dosing interval, the following results were observed (Table 4). By our established definitions, the interaction against *P. mirabilis* ap-

Table 3.
Serum Bactericidal Titers (SBTs) for Simulated Samples

Time point (hr)	SBT[a] CTX	dCTX	CTX–dCTX	Interaction	Relative Contribution to Bactericidal Activity during Therapy
Escherichia coli					
1	1:256	1:8	1:256	Indifferent	CTX is primary agent
2	1:128	1:4	1:128	Indifferent	CTX is primary agent
4	1:16	1:4	1:32	Indifferent	CTX is primary agent
6	1:4	1:2	1:8	Indifferent	CTX is primary agent
Proteus mirabilis					
1	1:≥512	1:64	1:256	Indifferent	CTX is primary agent
2	1:≥512	1:32	1:≥512	Indifferent	CTX is primary agent
4	1:128	1:32	1:128	Indifferent	CTX is primary agent
6	1:16	1:16	1:64	Additive or possibly synergistic	Both agents contribute
Klebsiella pneumoniae					
1	1:≥512	1:64	1:≥512	Indifferent	CTX is primary agent
2	1:256	1:64	1:≥512	Indifferent	CTX is primary agent
4	1:128	1:16	1:128	Indifferent	CTX is primary agent
6	1:8	1:8	1:32	Additive or possibly synergistic	Both agents contribute

[a] CTX = cefotaxime alone, dCTX = desacetylcefotaxime, CTX–dCTX = combination of cefotaxime and desacetylcefotaxime.

Table 4.
Results of AUBC Analysis for Simulated Samples

Organism	AUBC[a] CTX	dCTX	Sum of CTX and dCTX	CTX–dCTX	Interpretation of Results[b]
Escherichia coli	484	24	508	520	Activity of dCTX may be additive
Proteus mirabilis	1568	192	1760	1344	Activity of dCTX appears antagonistic
Klebsiella pneumoniae	1160	200	1360	1568	Activity of dCTX may be synergistic

[a] CTX = cefotaxime, dCTX = desacetylcefotaxime, CTX–dCTX = combination of cefotaxime and desacetylcefotaxime.
[b] See text for discussion of AUBC results.

pears slightly antagonistic, but this finding is solely due to the twofold dilution difference at the one-hour postdose time point. Because of the low AUBC for dCTX against the *E. coli* isolate, it is difficult to assess by our criteria whether the combination of CTX and dCTX exhibited indifference against the organism or whether there was additive killing. The combination of CTX and dCTX exhibited some possible synergy against the *K. pneumoniae* isolate. The AUBC test, although useful in past evaluations of antimicrobial activity over an entire dosing interval, proved less useful than comparing SBTs at each time point. It minimized the importance of end-of-interval bactericidal activity, because the trapezoidal rule "overweighted" the initial high titers. It was also clear in this analysis that the twofold variability of the SBT test (e.g., 1:256 versus 1:≥512) interfered with the AUBC test and thus limited its utility.

Conclusion. As evidenced by an examination of SBTs at each time point in a dosing interval, despite an in vitro test that indicated a beneficial antimicrobial interaction between CTX and dCTX, it appears that early in the dosing interval for patients with normal renal function when parent drug concentrations are very high, the presence of dCTX provides little additional in vivo antimicrobial activity against these isolates. However, the SBTs observed at the six-hour time point suggest that dCTX possesses a similar degree of bactericidal activity to the parent drug, and that, in support of the in vitro test, the drugs in combination may act additively or synergistically to provide enhanced bactericidal activity against selected strains of Enterobacteriaceae. Such activity may, in some cases, allow extension of the standard dosing interval typically based solely on the activity of the parent drug. Further information may be gained by considering the contributions of the metabolite and its interactions with the parent drug at concentrations found at steady state.

References

1. Jones RN, Barry AL, Thornsberry C. Antimicrobial activity of desacetyl cefotaxime alone and in combination with cefotaxime: evidence of synergy. *Rev Infect Dis.* 1982; 4(Suppl):366–73.
2. Neu NC. Antibacterial activity of desacetylcefotaxime alone and in combination with cefotaxime. *Rev Infect Dis.* 1982; 4(Suppl):374–8.
3. Wise R, Wills PJ, Andrews JM et al. Activity of the cefotaxime (HR756) desacetyl metabolite compared with those of cefotaxime and other cephalosporins. *Antimicrob Agents Chemother.* 1980; 17:84–6.
4. Reeves DS, White HA, Bahari D et al. Human metabolism of cefotaxime. *J Antimicrob Chemother.* 1980; 6(Suppl A):93–101.
5. Ings RMJ, Fillastre JP, Godin M et al. The pharmacokinetics of cefotaxime and its metabolites in subjects with normal and impaired renal function. *Rev Infect Dis.* 1982; 4(Suppl):379–91.
6. Krogstad DJ, Moellering RC. Antimicrobial combinations. In: Lorian V, ed. Antibiotics in laboratory medicine. 2nd ed. Baltimore: Williams and Wilkins; 1986:537–95.
7. Reller LB. Interaction of cefotaxime and desacetylcefotaxime against pathogenic bacteria. Assessment with the serum bactericidal test. *Diagn Microbiol Infect Dis.* 1984; 2(Suppl):55–61.
8. Thrupp LD. Susceptibility testing of antibiotics in liquid media. In: Lorian V, ed. Antibiotics in laboratory medicine. 2nd ed. Baltimore: Williams and Wilkins; 1986:93–148.
9. Edberg SC. The measurement of antibiotics in human body fluids: techniques and significance. In: Lorian V, ed. Antibiotics in laboratory medicine. 2nd ed. Baltimore: Williams and Wilkins; 1986:381–476.
10. Matzke GR, Abraham PA, Halstenson CE et al. Cefotaxime and desacetyl cefotaxime kinetics in renal impairment. *Clin Pharmacol Ther.* 1985; 38:31–6.
11. Neu HC, Aswapoke P, Fu KP et al. Cefotaxime kinetics after intravenous and intramuscular injection of single and multiple doses. *Clin Pharmacol Ther.* 1980; 27:677–85.
12. Plouffe JF, Perkins RL, Fass RJ et al. Cefotaxime: pharmacokinetics and in vitro antibacterial activity of serum and urine in normal human volunteers. *Chemotherapy.* 1983; 29:73–9.
13. Quintiliani R, Nightingale CH, Tilton R. Comparative pharmacokinetics of cefotaxime and the role of desacetylcefotaxime in the antibacterial activity of cefotaxime. *Diagn Microbiol Infect Dis.* 1984; 2(Suppl):63–70.
14. Barriere SL, Ely E, Kapusnik JE et al. Analysis of a new method for assessing activity of combinations of antimicrobials: area under the bactericidal activity curve. *J Antimicrob Chemother.* 1985; 16:49–59.

Pharmacokinetic Monitoring of Drug Enantiomers

". . . many drug enantiomers have different pharmacological properties in man and there seems to be substantial intersubject variation in the ratios of the concentration of the individual drug enantiomers in plasma of man. Both conditions have already been demonstrated for verapamil, propranolol and possibly tocainide. In the future, more examples will more than likely be demonstrated. If therapeutic drug monitoring is proposed for these drugs, it probably is a good idea for individual drug enantiomer plasma levels to be determined and correlated with effect to see if any extra clinical benefit is gained by this additional analytical step.

—Drayer DE. Problems in therapeutic drug monitoring: the dilemma of enantiomeric drugs in man. *Ther Drug Monit.* 1988; 10:1–7."

Drug Experience

Straightforward reports of unusual drug experiences are included in this section. These may be confirmations of previously reported drug experiences or brief apparent first reports. While selected references may be cited, the purpose of a Drug Experience report is not to present an extensive review of the literature.

A related section, Grand Rounds, includes papers that are well-documented patient case reports with a thorough review of the important literature to help put the case in perspective.

Use of conjugated estrogens to control gastrointestinal tract bleeding in two patients with chronic renal failure

SHIV SETH AND TERESA M. GEIER

Clin Pharm. 1988; 7:906–9

One of the major complications of uremia is coagulation abnormalities.[1,2] Gastrointestinal bleeding has many potential causes in patients with chronic renal failure and has been a subject of extensive research.[3,4] The abnormalities in coagulation include platelet dysfunction, prolongation of bleeding time, and other unknown phenomena that lead to a generalized hemorrhagic diathesis in patients with renal failure. Other gastrointestinal mucosal lesions such as gastritis and duodenitis occur with increased frequency in these patients. Zuckerman and coworkers,[2] in a study of 482 patients, showed that angiodysplasia was the most frequent source of bleeding in patients with renal failure, while peptic ulcer disease was the most likely source of recurrent bleeding in patients without renal failure.

SHIV SETH, PH.D., is Clinical Pharmacist, Department of Pharmacy, The Ohio State University Hospitals, Columbus. TERESA M. GEIER, M.S., is Assistant Director, Department of Pharmacy, Broward General Medical Center, Ft. Lauderdale, FL.

Address reprint requests to Dr. Seth at the Department of Pharmacy, The Ohio State University Hospitals, 410 West 10th Avenue, Columbus, OH 43210-1228.

The assistance of William H. Bay, M.D., is acknowledged.

Copyright © 1988, American Society of Hospital Pharmacists, Inc. All rights reserved. 0278-2677/88/1201-0906$01.00.

Cryoprecipitate rich in factor VIII and von Willebrand factor has been shown to decrease bleeding time in uremia and has been used to prevent extensive bleeding during surgical procedures.[5,6] The biggest drawback has been the heterogeneity of the product and the risk of hepatitis, acquired immunodeficiency syndrome, and other blood-borne diseases. Desmopressin (1-deamino-8-D-arginine vasopressin), a synthetic derivative of antidiuretic hormone that causes the release of autologous von Willebrand factor, has also been effective in treating bleeding in uremia.[7–9] The fact that bleeding time is corrected by pregnancy[10] and an increase in blood levels of estrogen in women with von Willebrand's disease led to uncontrolled and controlled trials using high-dose conjugated estrogens and an estrogen–progesterone combination to control bleeding in uremia.[11–13] The mechanism of action of estrogens in controlling bleeding has not been elucidated. Conjugated estrogens have also been used to treat hereditary hemorrhagic telangiectasia.[14] Resective surgery[15] and electrocoagulation of these lesions have been unsuccessful because of their tendency to recur and the difficulty in identifying all of the lesions. We used high-dose estrogen therapy for uncontrolled bleeding in two patients with chronic renal failure.

Case 1. A 68-year-old white woman who had bright red blood from the rectum was admitted to University Hospitals on September 16, 1987. She had chronic renal failure as a result of hypertension and congestive heart failure. Her medical history included repair of an abdominal aortic aneurysm and left nephrectomy. She also had aortic insufficiency. During an admission eight months previously for weakness, nausea, and vomiting, a colonoscopy for evaluation of diarrhea showed no lesions. Her abdomen was soft and nontender, with active bowel sounds. Her admission medications included prazosin, furosemide, and nitroglycerin patches for control of high blood pressure; ranitidine for possible gastritis; and calcium carbonate for control of serum phosphate levels. Her admission laboratory data showed a white blood cell count of 9.1×10^3/cu mm; hemoglobin, 5.7 g/dL; hematocrit, 16.2%; platelets, 210,000/cu mm; prothrombin time (PT), 9.5 seconds; partial thromboplastin time (PTT), 30 seconds; BUN, 76 mg/dL; and serum creatinine concentration, 3.7

mg/dL. Her vital signs were pulse, 90 beats/minute; respiratory rate, 20 breaths/minute; temperature, 36.9 °C; and blood pressure, 134/90 mm Hg. Urinalysis was unremarkable. The bleeding time was 14 minutes (normal range, 3–8 minutes). The patient was transfused with two units of packed red blood cells. On September 17 her hemoglobin improved to 8.5 g/dL and her hematocrit reached 24.6%. The patient continued to bleed through her rectum. The next day an esophagogastroduodenoscopy showed duodenitis but no active bleeding. A colonoscopy showed a few flecks of blood in the cecum but no mucosal lesions. A bleeding scan performed by labeling the patient's own blood (10 mL) with technetium and reinfusing the blood back into the patient confirmed the lesion to be proximal to the cecum. She received a transfusion of two units of packed red blood cells, and on September 20 her hemoglobin reached 11 g/dL and her hematocrit, 31%. The patient was not receiving hemodialysis. Therapy with conjugated estrogens (Premarin, Wyeth-Ayerst) 0.6 mg/kg i.v. (infused over 30 minutes) daily for five days was begun on September 20. Her bleeding stopped after the second dose, and results of a guaiac test for blood in the stool were negative. Bleeding time after the fourth dose was 7.0 minutes. Her hemoglobin and hematocrit stabilized around 12–12.6 g/dL and 33.1–36.9%, respectively, over the next week, and she was discharged. Laboratory test results and blood pressure measurements during her stay in the hospital are summarized in Table 1. The patient was treated with furosemide, nitroglycerin patches, calcium carbonate, ranitidine, and prazosin during hospitalization, and these medications were continued after discharge.

Case 2. A 58-year-old black woman came to University Hospitals on December 5, 1987; she had had dizziness, bloody diarrhea, and abdominal pain for two days. She had been admitted to the hospital several times intermittently during the last six months. The patient had chronic renal failure as a result of hypertension and was maintained on hemodialysis. She had a history of peptic ulcer disease and now had bloody diarrhea and hematochezia. The patient denied dysuria and hematuria and had no masses on physical examination. Her vital signs were normal except for marked orthostatic hypotension, as follows: pulse, 100 beats/minute; temperature, 37.2 °C; blood pressure, 140/90 (supine) and 95/60 (upon standing). Urinalysis showed cloudy urine. Results of a blood culture were negative, but a urine culture showed growth of *Gardnerella vaginalis*. Prophylactic therapy with ceftazidime (started on admission) for urinary tract infection was discontinued on December 12 and changed to metronidazole 500 mg orally three times per day. Her admission laboratory data were as follows: white blood cell count, 16.0 × 10^3/cu mm; red blood cell count, 2.2 million/cu mm; hemoglobin, 2.7 g/dL; hematocrit, 8.0%; platelets, 192,000/cu mm; PT, 10.9 seconds; PTT, 35 seconds; BUN, 135 mg/dL; and serum creatinine concentration, 9.0 mg/dL. Two days before admission, her hemoglobin was 8.7 g/dL. Her bleeding times on December 9 and 12 were 10 and 15 minutes, respectively. She received a transfusion of nine units of packed red blood cells, and on December 7 her hemoglobin rose to 7.0 g/dL and her hematocrit reached 20.4%.

Her workup for bleeding included esophagogastroduodenoscopy, superior and inferior mesenteric angiography, and colonoscopy. She had red blood in her duodenum and mild gastritis. Angiography was nonconclusive. A bleeding scan with technetium-labeled blood showed increased uptake in the descending colon. Colonoscopy showed bleeding on the right side of the colon, with no mucosal lesions. Stools were still grossly bloody. On December 9, a repeat esophagogastroduodenoscopy showed two arteriovenous malformations along the anterior surface of the body of the stomach. Hemocoagulation was attempted but was unsuccessful. The patient still had bloody stools and complained of diffuse tender abdominal pain. By December 12 she had received 27 units of packed red blood cells and had undergone one colonos-

Table 1.
Laboratory Test Results and Blood Pressure Measurements for Patient 1 during Hospitalization

Item	September 16	17	18	19	20	21	22	23
BUN (mg/dL)	76	71	77	70	73	69	67	73
Serum creatinine conc (mg/dL)	3.7	3.2	3.6	3.8	4.1	3.7	3.5	4.1
Platelets (×10^3/cu mm)	210	135	120	123	107	...	...	...
Prothrombin time (seconds)	9.5	9.5	9.5	9.6	9.7	9.2	...	9.6
Partial thromboplastin time (seconds)	30	31	31	30	32	28	...	31
Blood pressure (mm Hg)	150/90	190/80	180/84	170/70	182/70	160/70	168/70	144/70

copy, three esophagogastroduodenoscopies, two bleeding scans, and two angiograms, and the bleeding site could not be located.

Therapy was begun with conjugated estrogens (Premarin) 60 mg i.v. (infused over 30 minutes) daily for five days (December 13–17). In three days, her hemoglobin improved from 6.3 to 8.5–10.5 g/dL, and her hematocrit rose from 18.5% to 24–29.3% (determinations of hemoglobin and hematocrit were done every eight hours). On December 15, her abdominal pain improved, her hemoglobin and hematocrit stabilized, and results of a guaiac test for blood in the stool were negative. Results of a workup for disseminated intravascular coagulation were negative. Laboratory test results during this admission are summarized in Table 2.

Her medications during the hospital course and after discharge included clonidine, nifedipine, aluminum hydroxide antacid, ranitidine, furosemide, calcium carbonate, calcitriol, metolazone, and extended-release potassium chloride capsules. The patient was discharged on December 17.

Discussion. Uncontrolled bleeding is a major complication of uremia in patients with chronic renal failure and renal transplant patients.[2] The pathophysiological distribution of these lesions is generally limited to the lower colon and small bowel in patients with chronic renal failure. Despite endoscopy, colonoscopy, bleeding scans, and superior and inferior mesenteric angiographic studies, we were not successful in locating the source of gastrointestinal bleeding in our patients. Both patients were also poor surgical risks, necessitating a medical approach to the bleeding problems. Laboratory values that are helpful in daily monitoring of these patients include hemoglobin and hematocrit, bleeding time, and guaiac testing of nasogastric fluid aspirate and stool. Our patients had normal PTs and PTTs. Bleeding time has been shown to increase in uremic patients.[5,6] Although measurement of bleeding time involves complex interactions of the vascular wall, the circulating platelets, plasma coagulation proteins, and red blood cells,[16] this is the only test result that has been shown to improve with estrogen therapy. Bleeding time was abnormal in the above two cases.

Treatment of bleeding in uremic patients remains unsatisfactory and empirical. Although surgical management, electrocautery, laser therapy, and sclerotherapy have been recommended, precise identification of the bleeding site in cases of active gastrointestinal bleeding is difficult, and the recurrent bleeding rate is still high.[15] Dialysis has reduced the frequency of bleeding caused by uremia, and platelet transfusions may produce transient improvement in hemostasis.[17] Cryoprecipitate[5] and desmopressin[6–9] have been used to treat bleeding in uremic patients. Cryoprecipitate is a product obtained when plasma is frozen and then thawed at 4 °C. It is enriched in factor VIII, fibrinogen, fibronectin, and small amounts of all plasma constituents.[18,19] It is used in the treatment of hemophilia A, von Willebrand's disease, and hypofibrinogenemia. Janson et al.[5] have shown it to be effective in controlling uremic bleeding. The effect of cryoprecipitate lasts for only 12 to 18 hours. Cryoprecipitate is a biological product of variable activity. The quality of the product depends on the amount of factor VIII and von Willebrand factor multimers present. Highly purified cryoprecipitate may have lower amounts of von Willebrand factor because of degradation, resulting in less effective response in uremic patients. Larger von Willebrand factor multimers are effective in shortening the bleeding time.[20]

Desmopressin (1-deamino-8-arginine vasopressin) causes the release of von Willebrand factor multimers from storage sites into the plasma.[21] In a prospective, controlled study by Mannucci et al.,[7] 12 uremic patients who had prolonged bleeding times were given desmopressin (0.3 μg/kg), which resulted in shortened bleeding times in all the patients except one. The factor VIII:C activity, von Willebrand factor antigen, and von Willebrand functional activity increased after the desmopressin infusion. The only disadvantage associated with desmopressin was that the effect was transient and reached a peak in most patients between one and four hours. The most likely explanation

Table 2.
Laboratory Test Results for Patient 2 during Hospitalization

Item	December 5	6	7	8	9	10	11	12	13	14	15
BUN (mg/dL)	135	147	131	124	124	115	109	109	110	95	92
Serum creatinine conc (mg/dL)	9.0	8.8	7.8	6.9	6.9	6.3	6.0	6.0	5.6	5.4	5.3
Platelets (×10³/cu mm)	. . .	192	157	124	111	75	96	62	73	90	90
Prothrombin time (seconds)	10.9	10.9	11.1	10.9	10.8	11.2	11.2	11.6	10.6	10.1	10.4
Partial thromboplastin time (seconds)	35	35	33	34	32	37	36	36	31	28	28

for the beneficial effect of desmopressin is an increase and redistribution of von Willebrand multimers in the patients. The mechanism of action may involve release of the von Willebrand factor stored in the endothelial cell after desmopressin binds to the endothelial receptor. Long-term use of desmopressin in uremic bleeding has not been studied; it could be a potentially useful therapy, since desmopressin produces very few adverse effects.

Several uncontrolled trials[11-13] of estrogen to control bleeding in uremic patients have been done since the first observation that estrogen levels and factor VIII are increased in pregnant women with von Willebrand's disease.[10] Liu et al.[11] used intravenous conjugated estrogens in six uremic patients to control bleeding over a period of 6 to 10 days. The bleeding time decreased, and the bleeding stopped in their patients. The cumulative dose of conjugated estrogens over this period was 95-325 mg. Our schedule was chosen after examination of data from the studies of Liu et al.[11] and Livio et al.[12] We gave the cumulative dose of 3 mg/kg in divided doses over three to five days. In a double-blind crossover study in six uremic patients of the effect of estrogen on bleeding time and other variables in serum, Livio and coworkers[12] were not able to elucidate the mechanism of action of estrogens in their study. They did not detect any changes in the levels of von Willebrand factor or in multimeric structure after infusion of estrogen. Since the only demonstrable change after estrogen administration is decreased bleeding time, estrogen may prove to be an important tool in controlling bleeding episodes when long-lasting effects are desired. In our experience, i.v. conjugated estrogens stabilized the hemoglobin and hematocrit dramatically. The adverse effects of conjugated estrogens remain a major concern. Minor adverse effects include nausea, vomiting, loss of libido, and gynecomastia. Major complications include thromboembolic disease and the risk of malignancy. We are not aware of any efficacy study done on long-term use of estrogen in patients with renal failure.

Conclusion. Our experience and other published case reports suggest that conjugated estrogens may be useful for controlling gastrointestinal tract bleeding in patients who have chronic renal failure.

References

1. Deykin D. Uremic bleeding. *Kidney Int*. 1983; 24:698–705.
2. Zuckerman GR, Cornette GL, Clouse RE et al. Upper gastrointestinal bleeding in patients with chronic renal failure. *Ann Intern Med*. 1985; 102:588–92.
3. Rabiner SF. The effect of dialysis on platelet function of patients with renal failure. *Ann NY Acad Sci*. 1972; 201:234–42.
4. Livio M, Benigni A, Remuzzi G. Coagulation abnormalities in uremia. *Semin Nephrol*. 1985; 5:82–90.
5. Janson PA, Jubelirer SJ, Weinstein MJ et al. Treatment of the bleeding tendency in uremia with cryoprecipitate. *N Engl J Med*. 1980; 303:1318–22.
6. Steiner RW, Coggins C, Carvelho ACA. Bleeding time in uremia: a useful test to assess clinical bleeding. *Am J Hematol*. 1979; 7:107–17.
7. Mannucci PM, Remuzzi G, Pusineri F et al. Deamino-8-D-arginine vasopressin shortens the bleeding time in uremia. *N Engl J Med*. 1983; 308:8–12.
8. Watson AJS, Keogh JAB. Effect of 1-deamino-8-D-arginine vasopressin on the prolonged bleeding time in chronic renal failure. *Nephron*. 1982; 32:49–52.
9. Shapiro MD, Kelleher SP. Intranasal deamino-8-D-arginine vasopressin shortens the bleeding time in uremia. *Am J Nephrol*. 1984; 4:260–1.
10. Caldwell DC, Williamson RA, Goldsmith JC. Hereditary coagulopathies in pregnancy. *Clin Obstet Gynecol*. 1984; 28:53–72.
11. Liu YK, Kosfeld RE, Marcum SG. Treatment of uraemic bleeding with conjugated estrogen. *Lancet*. 1984; 2:887–90.
12. Livio M, Mannucci PM, Vigano G et al. Conjugated estrogens for the management of bleeding associated with renal failure. *N Engl J Med*. 1986; 315:731–5.
13. Bronner MH, Pate MB, Cunningham JT. Estrogen-progesterone therapy for bleeding gastrointestinal telangiectasias in chronic renal failure. *Ann Intern Med*. 1986; 105:371–4.
14. Vase P, Lorentzen M. Histological findings following estrogen treatment of hereditary haemorrhagic telangiectasia: a controlled double-blind investigation. *J Laryngol Otol*. 1983; 97:427–9.
15. Richardson JD, Max MH, Flint LM Jr et al. Bleeding vascular malformations of the intestine. *Surgery*. 1978; 84:430–6.
16. Livio M, Marchesi D, Remuzzi G et al. Uremic bleeding: role of anemia and beneficial effect of red cell transfusions. *Lancet*. 1982; 2:1013–5.
17. Di Minno G, Martinez J, McKean ML et al. Platelet dysfunction in uremia: multifaceted defect partially corrected by dialysis. *Am J Med*. 1985; 79:552–9.
18. Johnson AJ, Aronson DL, William WJ. Preparation and clinical use of plasma and plasma fractions. In: Williams WJ, Beutler E, Ersley AJ et al., eds. Hematology, 2nd ed. New York: McGraw-Hill; 1977:1561–83.
19. Pool JG, Hershgold EJ, Pappenhagen AR. High potency antihemophilic factor concentrate prepared from cryoglobulin precipitate. *Nature*. 1964; 203:312.
20. Weinstein MJ, Deykin D. Comparison of factor VIII related von Willebrand factor proteins prepared from human cryoprecipitate and factor VIII concentrate. *Blood*. 1979; 53:1095–1105.
21. Ruggeri ZM, Mannucci PM, Lombardi R et al. Multimeric composition of factor VIII/von Willebrand factor following administration of DDAVP: implications for pathophysiology and therapy of von Willebrand's disease subtypes. *Blood*. 1982; 59:1272–8.

ASHP Report

Acknowledgment to reviewers—October 1, 1987, to September 30, 1988

This year, 160 manuscripts were submitted for publication consideration to *Clinical Pharmacy*, including papers solicited by the editors. Approximately 53% of the papers received were ultimately accepted. During this same period, we received critiques from 260 reviewers who evaluated the merit of *Clinical Pharmacy* submissions. Readers are indebted to these reviewers, who contributed their time in this advisory capacity. Their efforts have helped maintain the high standards of *CP*. Several referees reviewed more than one paper during the year, and their extra contributions are especially appreciated.

Wendy G. Abe
Stephen C. Adams
William A. Agostinucci
Brian Alldredge
Barbara Ameer
Philip O. Anderson
Graciela M. Armayor
Patricia R. Audet
Elaine M. Bailey
Robert T. Bailey, Jr.
Jan N. Bair
Donald Baker, Jr.
Carol E. Balmer
Joseph A. Barone
Steven L. Barriere
Larry A. Bauer
Carol L. Beck
Sue Beck
Rosemary R. Berardi
Maria Bergamo
Roger Berlin
Karen E. Bertch
Joseph S. Bertino, Jr.
Kathryn V. Blake
Robert A. Blouin
William S. Bond
John A. Bosso
Michael B. Bottorff
Bradley A. Boucher
David Bourne
Susan K. Bowles
Diane M. Brundage
Michael E. Burton
Nicole Busch
Henry I. Bussey
D. L. Calhoun
Ronald Callahan
Peggy Carver
Daniel T. Casto
Mary H. H. Chandler
Frank C. Chenella
Moses S. S. Chow
Karen Church
Michael A. Clotz
James C. Cloyd
Emily B. Cochran
Patricia A. Colaizzi
Brian Crabtree
James C. Cradock
Richard E. Crass
A. Cremos
Lynn M. Crismon
William R. Crom
Burke A. Cunha
Larry H. Danziger
Joseph F. Dasta
Robin Davis
Robert G. Deeter
Jeffrey C. Delafuente
C. L. DeVane
Roland N. Dickerson
Joseph T. DiPiro
Paul L. Doering
Robert T. Dorr
Marsha Driscoll
Michael N. Dudley
George E. Dukes, Jr.
Frederic E. Eckhauser
David J. Edwards
Thomas R. Einarson
Catherine E. Emory
Larry Ereshefsky
Rebecca S. Finley
John F. Flaherty
Courtney Fletcher
Thomas S. Foster
David W. Fuhs
Peter Gal
John G. Gambertoglio
Richard H. Gannon
William R. Garnett
James C. Garrelts
Lorne K. Garrettson
Mark Garrison
Cynthia J. R. Gelman
Jamie T. Gilman
Thomas M. Gilman
Howard M. Glazer
W. Manford Gooch III
William R. Good
Richard Gorman
David A. Graves
Nina M. Graves
Terri Graves
Jeffrey A. Green
Laurence Green
David R. P. Guay
Sally K. Guthrie
Lawrence J. Hak
Robert A. Hamilton
Monty Hampton
Philip D. Hansten
Richard Helms
John D. Hirsh
Dennis M. Hoffman
Beverly J. Holcombe
K. D. Hooker
Alan W. Hopefl
John R. Horn
Paul R. Hutson
Robert J. Ignoffo
A. Lane Ilersich
Thomas E. Imhoff
Ann L. Janer
Michael Jann
Douglas D. Janson
John W. Jenne
Curtis A. Johnson
Mary Johnston
Randy P. Juhl
Joan E. Kapusnik
James A. Karboski
Michael Katz
David J. Kazierad
Gregory L. Kearns
James H. Keller
H. William Kelly
John M. Kessler
Debbie Khachikian
Ujjaini Khanderia
Richard Kingston
Betty J. Kinzie
Edward B. Kirsten
Wendy Klein-Schwartz
Frank J. Kohout
Wayne A. Kradjan
Edward P. Krenzelok
James J. Kresel
Thomas Krol
Peggy G. Kuehl
Robert J. Kuhn
Ken Kulig
James LaBraico
Dustan G. Labreche
Richard L. Lalonde
Victor Lampasona
Phillip G. Lange
Ghassem E. Larijani
Sherri Larson
Alan H. Lau
Leo M. Lawless
Richard D. Leff
Marc Levin
Susan Lisby-Sutch
Larry M. Lopez
Virgil S. Lucas, Jr.
Patricia Lurvey
Ray R. Maddox
Henry J. Mann
C. Randall Marchanks
Sabrina Martiny
Kenneth L. Massey
Neil Massoud
Vince Mattaliano
Gary R. Matzke
Elizabeth C. Mauer
William W. McCloskey
Paula McGibbon
James M. McKenney
Kathleen McNeil Teasley
Frederick L. Meister
Donald M. Miller
Lucinda G. Miller
Carol H. Millette
Jim Minor
Timothy Mirando
Jay M. Mirtallo
Michael A. Montwill
Kevin Moores
John Mucenski
John E. Murphy
Milap C. Nahata
Michele F. Naylor
David E. Nix
Jean K. Noguchi
Paul E. Nolan, Jr.
Bernadette O'Brien
Julie Oki
Keith M. Olsen
Brian G. Ortmeier
Julie P. Owens
Norma J. Owens
Joseph A. Paladino
Roy Parish
Dale A. Pastel
John M. Patrias
J. Herbert Patterson
Vaughn W. Payne
Mitchell Pelter
John Penta
Karen Petros
Stephanie J. Phelps
John A. Pieper
Karen I. Plaisance
Roy A. Pleasants
Ron E. Polk
Charles D. Ponte
William R. Porter
John R. Powell
Randall A. Prince
Randy D. Pryka
Anna Przybylo
Robert P. Rapp
Michael D. Reed
Larry A. Robinson
John H. Rodman
Keith A. Rodvold
Mary B. Ross
John C. Rotschafer
Ronald J. Ruggiero
Jean A. Rumsfield
Michael J. Rybak
Rosalie Sagraves
Jan Sahai
Francine R. Salamone
Reuven Sandyk
William T. Sawyer
Debra Sayler
Arthur A. Schuna
Richard Segal
Stanley M. Shaw
Steven L. Sheaffer
Jill Shwed
Judith L. Siegel
John K. Siepler
Richard L. Slaughter
Gary E. Sloskey
Robert A. Smaglia
Ralph E. Small
Catherine A. Sohn
John C. Somberg
William J. Spruill
Clinton F. Stewart
Gary P. Stoehr
Robert J. Straka
Maureen Sullivan
Dennis P. Swanson
Robert L. Talbert
Jon J. Tanja
Jerry W. Taylor
Scott L. Traub
Peter H. Vlasses
Paul C. Walker
Lynda Welage
Roger White
Terry D. Wilson
Cindy J. Wordell
Bradley G. Wulf
Darwin Zaske
Karin E. Zenk

CP Continuing Education

The ASHP Continuing Education system gives readers a self-assessment mechanism for selected articles in Clinical Pharmacy *and the* American Journal of Hospital Pharmacy. *It also allows readers to obtain continuing-education credit for these articles.*

For the purpose of CE-credit enrollment a blank answer sheet is published at the end of each installment of the column for the CE articles in that issue. An enrollee accumulates these answer sheets until the enrollment is submitted, using the form that is published in the June and December issues of Clinical Pharmacy *and in the June and December issues of the* American Journal of Hospital Pharmacy. *Any combination of tests within a 18-month period, from both* Clinical Pharmacy *and* American Journal of Hospital Pharmacy, *may be included in an enrollment. More complete details about enrollment in the system will appear in the semiannual enrollment form.*

Article 680-204-8818 (see page 869)
Qualifies for 1.0 hour of CE credit

Propafenone: A new antiarrhythmic agent

Learning Objectives

After studying this article, the reader should be able to

1. Describe the electrophysiologic and hemodynamic effects of propafenone.
2. Compare and contrast the pharmacokinetics of propafenone in extensive and poor metabolizers of the drug.
3. List the drugs that have been reported to interact with propafenone.
4. List the arrhythmias that have been treated successfully by propafenone.
5. List important cardiac and noncardiac adverse effects of propafenone.

Self-assessment Questions

For each question there is one best answer only.

1. Propafenone is structurally related to the

   a. β-blocking agents.
   b. Calcium-channel blockers.
   c. Cardiac glycosides.
   d. Angiotensin-converting-enzyme inhibitors.

2. According to the Vaughan Williams classification system for antiarrhythmic agents, propafenone is a

   a. Class Ia agent.
   b. Class Ic agent.
   c. Class II agent.
   d. Class III agent.

3. Systemic availability of propafenone after oral administration is

   a. Approximately 90%.
   b. Dose dependent in extensive metabolizers.
   c. Not affected by administration with food.
   d. Dose dependent in poor metabolizers.

4. What percentage of the population metabolizes propafenone rapidly?

   a. Less than 10%.
   b. 50%.
   c. 75%.
   d. More than 90%.

5. The difference in metabolic phenotype influences all of the following except the

   a. Effective dose.
   b. Half-life of propafenone.
   c. Incidence of adverse central nervous system effects.
   d. Concentration of propafenone and its metabolites in plasma.

6. Propafenone has been reported to increase the serum concentrations of

   a. Cimetidine only.
   b. Phenytoin and cimetidine.
   c. Digoxin, warfarin, and metoprolol.
   d. Warfarin only.

7. Clinical trials indicate that propafenone will be useful in treating

   a. Sustained and nonsustained ventricular tachycardia.
   b. Wolff–Parkinson–White syndrome.
   c. Supraventricular arrhythmias.
   d. Alternatives a and b only are correct.
   e. All of the above alternatives are correct.

Continued on page 912

Help your patients use their medicines effectively, with ASHP's

Revised

Medication Teaching Manual, 4th Edition and Medication Teaching Manual Disk File

ASHP's **Medication Teaching Manual**—in print and on disk—is regarded by many professionals as one of the best tools for counseling patients about the proper use of their medicines. Drug monographs supply information on uses, administration, side effects, precautions and storage.

The fourth edition includes:

- 319 updated monographs
- Special dietary instructions
- A special section with cancer chemotherapy drugs

The **Medication Teaching Manual** is also available on IBM*-compatible diskettes. The disk file lets you:

- Print out or view monographs
- Incorporate monographs into an existing pharmacy or hospital computer system
- Customize monographs for patient education programs

(For further information on the disk file, call or write: Renato Cataldo, ASHP, 4630 Montgomery Avenue, Bethesda, MD 20814; 301/657-3000)

No matter what your role in the health-care arena, the **Medication Teaching Manual** and versatile Medication Teaching Manual Disk File can help you educate patients about their medicines. And that can only improve patient cooperation in the health management process.

*IBM is a registered trademark of International Business Machines Corporation.

Order Form

Medication Teaching Manual, Fourth Edition; 428 pp; softbound; $30.00 Medication Teaching Manual Disk File; includes five 5¼″ floppy diskettes and a copy of the printed **Medication Teaching Manual**; $195.00

Please send me ________ copies of the **Medication Teaching Manual** (P253) at $30.00

Please send me ________ copies of the Medication Teaching Manual Disk File (PL33) at $195.00

☐ Enclosed is my check for $________ (Checks must be drawn on a U.S. bank and payable to ASHP.)

☐ Enclosed is our purchase order #________. Please issue an invoice and add postage and handling.

Charge $________ to my ☐ VISA ☐ MasterCard

Account #________________ Exp. ________________ month/year

Signature ________________

Name ________________

Institution ________________

Address ________________

City ________________ State ________ Zip ________

ASHP ID# ________________

Send to:
ASHP Publications Records Dept.
4630 Montgomery Avenue
Bethesda, MD 20814

Payments to ASHP are not deductible as charitable contributions for Federal Income Tax purposes. However, they may be deductible under other provisions of the Internal Revenue Code.

© 1988 American Society of Hospital Pharmacists

CP Continuing Education *Continued from page 911*

8. The most serious cardiac adverse reaction to propafenone is

   a. New or worsened congestive heart failure.
   b. Conduction disturbance.
   c. Proarrhythmia.
   d. Hypotension.

9. The most common noncardiac adverse effect of propafenone is

   a. Dizziness or lightheadedness.
   b. Elevation of liver function test values.
   c. Visual disturbances.
   d. Nervousness and tremor.

10. The usual starting dosage of propafenone for the treatment of ventricular arrhythmias is

    a. 300 mg once daily.
    b. 100 mg twice daily.
    c. 150 mg every eight hours.
    d. 300 mg every eight hours.

Answer sheet

December 1988 *Clinical Pharmacy*

Note: An enrollment form for the ASHP Continuing-Education System appears in the June and December issues. Please accumulate all the answer sheets you wish to use in one enrollment and submit them at one time with a completed enrollment form.

Place an X in the box(es) at the top of the column(s) corresponding to the test(s) you are taking. Darken the boxes corresponding to the correct answers.

☐
680-204-8818
1.0 hour
a b c d e

1. ☐☐☐☐
2. ☐☐☐☐
3. ☐☐☐☐
4. ☐☐☐☐
5. ☐☐☐☐
6. ☐☐☐☐
7. ☐☐☐☐☐
8. ☐☐☐☐
9. ☐☐☐☐
10. ☐☐☐☐

ASHP Use Only
(1.0)8818________(3)

ASHP CE instructions and enrollment form

Instructions

1. The system is flexible. You may select any combination of tests from the *American Journal of Hospital Pharmacy* and *Clinical Pharmacy* to give you the number of credits you need.
2. An Answer Sheet is published at the end of each installment of the CE column. An Enrollment Form is published in the June and December issues of *AJHP* and *CP*.
3. Complete only one Enrollment Form, but note on the form all the tests you are taking. Staple together all answer sheets for one enrollment.
4. Tests included in one enrollment must have been published within the past 18 months. Once a particular test is included in an enrollment, it may not be included in a subsequent enrollment.
5. The passing score on each test is 70%. Within four weeks of receiving your enrollment, ASHP will mail you a CE letter or notify you that certain tests were failed. Failed tests may be retaken only one time, without additional cost. There are no refunds for failed tests.
6. ASHP is approved by the American Council on Pharmaceutical Education as a provider of continuing pharmaceutical education (Provider Number 680-204). (The following states recognize ACPE-approved providers: AK, AR, AZ, CA, DE, FL, IA, ID, IL, IN, KS, KY, LA, MA, ME, MI, MN, MO, MS, MT, NE, NH, NM, NV, OH, OR, PA, RI, SD, TN, WA, and WY [also Puerto Rico].) Most states that recognize ACPE-approved providers will accept credit earned through journal CE programs; however, since some states have restrictions on the number of credit hours or CE units they will accept toward the total requirement, it is advised that readers check with their respective state board of pharmacy if they are uncertain about the board's regulations.
7. Send your Enrollment Form, Answer Sheet(s), and check (made payable to ASHP) to:

ASHP CE
American Society of Hospital Pharmacists
4630 Montgomery Avenue
Bethesda, MD 20814

Enrollment Form

Name____

Address______________________________________

City____________________ State__________ Zip________

Tests included in this enrollment must have been published within the past 18 months.

Test Number	*Hours of Credit*

(Write additional numbers and hours on a separate sheet and attach it to this form.)

Total hours ________
Total fee($) enclosed ________

Fee Schedule
$5.00/hour
$20.00 minimum/enrollment

Current Literature

Drug Reaction Alerts

Drug Reaction Alerts focuses primarily on serious, unlabeled reactions to new chemical entities. The citations are compiled monthly from International Pharmaceutical Abstracts, *which covers over 800 journals. An address for reprints (when available) follows the name of the corresponding author in each citation.*

Anabolic Agents

Tennant F (Community Health Projects Medical Group, West Covina, CA 91790), Black DL, Voy RO. Anabolic steroid dependence with opioid-type features. *N Engl J Med.* 1988; 319:578. Case. (23-year-old man with three-year history of taking anabolic steroids for body building; for two months, received **methandrostenolone** 75 mg and **methenolone acetate** 150 mg by injection every other day, and **oxandrolone** 20 mg/day and **oxymetholone** mg/day orally; received naloxone; developed nausea, chills, headache, and dizziness within 15 minutes, and increases in diaphoresis, piloerection, pulse rate, and blood pressure lasting four hours; treated with clonidine for six days; withdrew from treatment)

Antivirals

Hargreaves M, Fuller G, Costello C et al. (Gazzard B, Department of Medicine and Hematology, St. Stephen's Hospital, London SW10 9TH, England.) **Zidovudine** overdose. *Lancet.* 1988; 2:509. Case. (34-year-old man with acquired immunodeficiency syndrome; received zidovudine 200 mg every four hours for two weeks, took overdose of zidovudine 20 g; on admission, blood zidovudine concentration 185 μmol/L and zidovudine metabolite concentration 114 μmol/L; no development of leukopenia, thrombocytopenia, abnormal liver function tests, or abnormal electrolyte concentrations; zidovudine withdrawn, patient remained well)

Cardiac Drugs

Carmichael AJ, Paul CJ (Skin Hospital, Birmingham B15 1BR, England). Vasculitic leg ulcers associated with **diltiazem**. *Br Med J.* 1988; 297:562. Case. (59-year-old man with heart failure; received diltiazem 60 mg three times daily for three months; concomitant valproate sodium, aspirin, methyldopa, metoprolol, nifedipine, and isosorbide dinitrate; developed vasculitic rash and leg ulcers; resolution of ulcers after local treatment and withdrawal of diltiazem)

Salerno DM (Division of Cardiology, Hennepin County Medical Center, 701 Park Avenue South, Minneapolis, MN 55415), Fifield J, Krejci J et al. **Encainide** induced hyperglycemia. *Am J Med.* 1988; 84:39–44. Study. (23 patients with arrhythmias; received encainide; four patients developed five episodes of hyperglycemia requiring insulin therapy; encainide withdrawn; insulin requirements decreased, hypoglycemic reactions to insulin in two patients)

Drug Interactions

Ben-Ari J, Eisenstein B, Davidovits M et al. (Stark H, Pediatric Nephrology Unit, Beilinson Medical Center, 49 100 Petah Tikva, Israel.) Effect of **erythromycin** on blood **cyclosporine** concentrations in kidney transplant patients. *J Pediatr.* 1988; 112:992–3. Cases. (two 10-year-old children with renal transplants; received cyclosporine and erythromycin; developed acute elevation in plasma cyclosporine concentrations and reversible renal dysfunction)

Gupta SK (Department of Pharmacy, University of Manchester, Manchester M13 9PL, England), Bakran A, Johnson RW et al. **Erythromycin** enhances the absorption of **cyclosporine.** *Br J Clin Pharmacol.* 1988; 25:401–2. Study. (six patients with renal transplants; received cyclosporine 5 mg/kg orally and 3.5 mg/kg intravenously on separate days before and during three-day course of erythromycin 500 mg four times daily; plasma cyclosporine concentrations higher than control when oral cyclosporine given with erythromycin, but no different from control when intravenous cyclosporine given with erythromycin)

Jarosinski PF (Pharmacy Department, National Institutes of Health, Building 10, Room 1N-257, 9000 Rockville Pike, Bethesda, MD 20892), Moscow JA, Alexander MS et al. Altered **phenytoin** clearance during intensive chemotherapy for acute lymphoblastic leukemia. *J Pediatr.* 1988; 112:996–9. Case. (10-year-old boy receiving phenytoin for epilepsy; received **methotrexate**, **leucovorin calcium**, **vincristine sulfate**, **asparaginase**, **daunorubicin hydrochloride**, **mercaptopurine**, and **prednisone** for acute lymphoblastic leukemia; required escalation of phenytoin dosage to 17 mg/kg/day to maintain therapeutic trough concentration; phenytoin requirement returned to baseline when induction therapy completed, rose again with first maintenance cycle of chemotherapy)

Kerin NZ (Section of Cardiovascular Disease, Department of Medicine, Sinai Hospital of Detroit, 6767 West Outer Drive, Detroit, MI 48235), Blevins RD, Goldman L et al. Incidence, magnitude, and time course of the **amiodarone–warfarin** interaction. *Arch Intern Med.* 1988; 148:1779–81. Cases. (eight patients with heart disease, aged 39–70 years; received amiodarone hydrochloride 200–400 mg/day and warfarin sodium; concomitant propranolol, chlorpropamide, digoxin, furosemide, prednisone, clonidine, sucralfate, dipyridamole, metoprolol, and levothyroxine sodium; mean maximum increase in prothrombin time 44% during first two weeks of amiodarone therapy; warfarin sodium dosage decreased by 33–35% after four or eight weeks of amiodarone therapy, with six patients having prothrombin times within 15% of baseline and two patients having prothrombin times greater than 15% over baseline)

Robson RA (Department of Clinical Pharmacology, Flinders Medical Center, Bedford Park 5042 SA, Australia), Miners JO,

Birkett DJ. Selective inhibitory effects of **nifedipine** and **verapamil** on oxidative metabolism: effects on **theophylline**. *Br J Clin Pharmacol.* 1988; 25:397–400. Study. (nine patients; received theophylline 125 mg every eight hours for four days, with subsequent administration of theophylline plus nifedipine 20 mg every 12 hours for four days, and then theophylline plus verapamil 80 mg every eight hours for four days; compared with control, theophylline clearance reduced 9% by nifedipine and 14% by verapamil)

Drugs, Adverse Reactions

Elliott AT (Western Infirmary, Glasgow G11 6NT, Scotland), Murray T, Mackie RM et al. Severe reaction to diphosphonate: implications for treatment of Paget's disease. *Br Med J.* 1988; 297: 592–3. Case. (47-year-old woman; received single dose of **medronate disodium** for bone scan; developed vasculitis and erythema multiforme; eruption resolved after four weeks of treatment with topical clobetasol propionate twice daily)

Revell P, Nicholson F, Pearson TC (St. Thomas's Hospital, St. Thomas's Campus, London SE1 7EH, England). Granulocytopenia caused by **fusidic acid**. *Lancet.* 1988; 2:455. Case. (18-year-old man with osteomyelitis; received fusidic acid; concomitant floxacillin; developed reversible agranulocytosis)

Roth D (University of Miami School of Medicine, Division of Nephrology, R-126, P.O. Box 016960, Miami, FL 33101), Alarcon FJ, Fernandez JA et al. Acute rhabdomyolysis associated with **cocaine** intoxication. *N Engl J Med.* 1988; 319:673–7. Cases. (39 patients, mean age 30.8 years, with cocaine intoxication and acute rhabdomyolysis; of 13 patients developing acute renal failure, 7 developed disseminated intravascular coagulation, 11 developed severe hepatic dysfunction, and 6 died; all patients without renal failure survived)

Drugs, Availability

Nishimura LY, Armstrong EP, Plezia PM (Department of Pharmacy Practice, College of Pharmacy, University of Arizona, Tucson, AZ 85721) et al. Influence of enteral feedings on **phenytoin sodium** absorption from capsules. *Drug Intell Clin Pharm.* 1988; 22:130–3. Study. (randomized crossover; six subjects; received single doses of phenytoin sodium 400 mg in capsules alone or with second of 10 hourly 100-mL enteral feedings of Ensure; no significant difference between doses in area under plasma concentration–time curves from 0 to 48 hours; relative bioavailability of phenytoin with enteral feedings 101.7%)

Our online databases

stand alone

in drug information.

ASHP® databases help you to locate
a wide scope of drug information,
including fulltext drug monographs,
patient counseling information
and abstracts of articles.

Drug Information Fulltext®

The DIF database contains detailed, comprehensive drug information representing over 50,000 marketed drug products.

Consumer Drug Information™

CDIF is a fulltext database with descriptions written for the patient's understanding. More than 3,000 brand name drug products are covered.

International Pharmaceutical Abstracts®

The IPA database is the practical, efficient way of locating information from over 800 pharmaceutical, medical, cosmetic and other health-related journals throughout the world. IPA's abstract/indexing system works to help you easily locate the information.

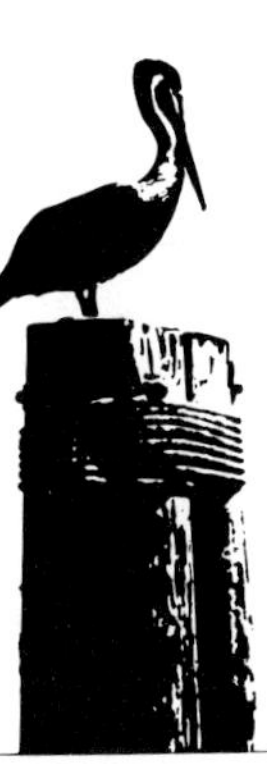

ASHP databases are available around the world through international online computer systems. For a brochure or more information, contact ASHP's Database Services at 301-657-3000, or write to:

Payments to ASHP are not deductible as charitable contributions for Federal Income Tax purposes. However, they may be deductible under other provisions of the Internal Revenue Code.

ASHP Database Services
4630 Montgomery Avenue
Bethesda, MD 20814

Books Received

Books are listed as soon as received; selected books may be reviewed in Book Reviews in subsequent issues.

Pharmacotherapy: A Pathophysiologic Approach, edited by Joseph T. DiPiro, Robert L. Talbert, Peggy E. Hayes et al. Published by Elsevier Science Publishing Co., Inc., 655 Avenue of the Americas, New York, NY 10010, 1989. xx + 1730 p. Price $75.

Principles of Medicinal Chemistry, Third Edition, by William O. Foye. Published by Lea & Febiger, 600 South Washington Square, Philadelphia, PA 19106-4198, 1989. xiii + 925 p. Price $49.50.

USAN and the USP Dictionary of Drug Names. Published by the United States Pharmacopeial Convention, Inc., 12601 Twinbrook Parkway, Rockville, MD 20852, 1988. 744 p. Price $74.95 per copy (1 to 24 copies), $55.60 per copy (25 to 99 copies), additional discounts on larger quantities.

Advertising Index

American Society of Hospital Pharmacists
- ACCRUE, inside back cover
- ASHP Membership, inside front cover
- Clinical Pharmacy, outside back cover
- Concepts in Clinical Pharmacokinetics, 866
- Database Services, 915
- Drug Theft (videotape), 868
- Medication Teaching Manual, 912

Beecham Laboratories
- Timentin, 861–862

Eli Lilly and Company
- Tazidime, 863–864

Roxane Laboratories, Inc., A Boehringer Ingelheim Company
- Intensols, 857

San Antonio State School
- Position Available, 868

Scientific Therapeutics Information, Inc.
- Positions Available, 868

The Upjohn Company
- Cleocin Phosphate, 859–860

Index to Volume 7

The index to Volume 7 is composed of three parts: a subject index, an author index, and an advertising index.

The subject index is made up mainly of terms constructed by *International Pharmaceutical Abstracts*. The *IPA* index is an alphabetical, open-ended, controlled-vocabulary index that makes use of standardized headings. (The primary index terms for major articles are listed routinely in *Clinical Pharmacy* as "index terms" after abstracts.) *IPA* covers all authored papers and editorials in *Clinical Pharmacy*, as well as selected letters and news reports. The subject index also notes all regular columns and, under the respective column headings, the titles of items in the "Editorials," "Therapy Consultation," "Letters," and "Book Reviews" sections and the titles of individual stories in "News." The subject index also contains, under the heading "Correction Notices," the title and issue of publication of items for which corrections were printed, as well as the page numbers on which the corrections appear.

Issue	*Pages*
January	1–80
February	81–162
March	163–246
April	247–330
May	331–406
June	407–482
July	483–556
August	557–630
September	631–706
October	707–780
November	781–854
December	855–928

Subject Index

A

Absorption
anti-infective agents; oral, effects, GI flora, review, 878
fluconazole; ketoconazole malabsorption, 622
guanfacine hydrochloride; review, 187
ketoconazole; effects, food, gastric pH, 228; malabsorption, fluconazole absorption, 622
quinidine sulfate; interactions, atropine, combination, diphenoxylate, 139
theophylline; interactions, sucralfate, lack, 58
Acetaminophen
concomitant therapy, 528, 867
poisoning; therapy, acetylcysteine administration, 563; toxicity, pediatrics, 391
Acetylcysteine; toxicity; side effects, administration routes, 563
Acetylcysteine sodium; therapy; acetaminophen poisoning, pediatrics, 391
Achlorhydria; ketoconazole; availability, 228
Acids, fatty; mechanism of action; 3-omega, antilipemic effects, 795
Acquired immunodeficiency syndrome
amphotericin B and flucytosine; cryptococcal meningitis therapy, 528
anti-infective agents; toxicity, neutropenia, 398
antituberculars; mycobacterium infections therapy, pediatrics, 545
flucytosine and amphotericin B; cryptococcal meningitis therapy, 528
ganciclovir; retinitis therapy, approval denials, 86
nutrition; parenteral, Kaposi's sarcoma, 536; parenteral, therapy, 512
pentamidine isethionate; *P. carinii* pneumonia therapy, 501
therapy; opportunistic infections, 511; *P. carinii* pneumonia, 514
trimetrexate; treatment IND, *P. carinii* pneumonia, 337
Acyclovir
excretion; hemofiltration, 198
toxicity; neutropenia, AIDS, 398
Additives; injections; phenytoin, i.v. infusion, 219
Administration
Food and Drug Administration; approval process, 166
policies and procedures; adverse reactions, vaccines, DHHS regulations, 489; FDA, generic equivalency, 334
Admixtures, see **Additives, injections**
Adolescents; aspirin; toxicity, Reye's syndrome, FDA labeling regulations, 639
Adrenergic agents, see **Sympathomimetic agents**
Adsorbents; diarrhea; infectious, therapy, review, 746
Adverse reactions, see **Drugs, adverse reactions**
Advertising Index, 80, 162, 246, 330, 406, 482, 556, 630, 706, 780, 854, 915
Age
geriatrics; digoxin blood levels, radioimmunoassay, 449
patients; glipizide pharmacokinetics, 224
pediatrics; anticonvulsant blood levels, binding, 688; parenteral nutrition, review, 351
AIDS, see **Acquired immunodeficiency syndrome**
Albumin human; dosage; hypoalbuminemia, equations, prediction, 894
Albuterol; anaphylaxis; therapy, pyrethrins adverse reactions, 846
Allergies
antihistamines; combined therapy, H_1 and H_2 antagonists, 422
phenytoin; pseudolymphoma, mycosis fungoides, 153
pyrethrins; adverse reactions, anaphylaxis, 846
sodium bisulfite; anaphylaxis, preservatives, injections, 269
Alopecia; minoxidil; topical solutions, FDA approvals, 858
Alteplase
approvals; FDA, 85
comparison, streptokinase; myocardial infarction therapy, 469, 473
Aluminum hydroxide; concomitant therapy, 906
Alzheimer's disease; tacrine; clinical studies, FDA attitudes, 337
Amino acids; nutrition; parenteral, pediatrics, review, 351
Aminoglycosides
dosage schedules; changes, prediction, models, 681
excretion; hemofiltration, 198
gentamicin; injections, preservatives, adverse reactions, 269; pharmacokinetic calculations, blood level errors, 307
gentamicin sulfate; administration, CRIS, minibags, 303
pharmacokinetics; critical patients, variations, 207; monitoring, cost–benefit analysis, 608
therapy, 385
tobramycin; cystic fibrosis therapy, response indicators, 897; urine levels computer programs, 792
tobramycin sulfate; i.v. administration systems, 367; pharmacokinetics, i.v. administration systems, 374
Aminophylline
anaphylaxis; therapy, pyrethrins adverse reactions, 846
asthma; therapy, theophylline half-life, 620
Amiodarone; arrhythmia; combined therapy, review, 808
Amphotericin B
and flucytosine; cryptococcal meningitis therapy, AIDS, 528
candidiasis; oral, therapy, mouthwashes, 70
therapy; review, 424
Ampicillin; therapy, 37
Ampicillin sodium; combination, sulbactam sodium; therapy review, 37
Analgesics and antipyretics
acetaminophen; overdose, toxicity, pediatrics, 391; poisoning, acetylcysteine administration, 563
aspirin; toxicity, Reye's syndrome, labeling regulations, 639
morphine sulfate; body distribution, ascites, 842
Analysis;
drugs; blood, urine levels, TDx assay, 792
theophylline; blood levels, tests comparison, 462
Anaphylaxis
epinephrine; therapy, interactions, 493
pyrethrins; adverse reactions, 846
sodium bisulfite; adverse reactions, preservatives, injections, 269
Androgens; anemia; therapy, kidney failure, 117
Anemia
sodium bromate; toxicity, poisoning, pediatrics, 68
therapy; kidney failure, 117
Anesthetics; midazolam; electric countershock, 423
Anesthetics, local; stomatitis; therapy, 14
Angina pectoris
bepridil; therapy, 97
nicardipine; therapy, 97
Angiotensin-converting enzyme inhibitors
and nicardipine or nitrendipine; hypertension therapy, 97
hypertension; therapy, protocols, 837
Anthelmintics; ivermectin; distribution, developing countries, 11
Antiarrhythmic drugs, see **Cardiac drugs**
Antibiotics
aztreonam; cystic fibrosis therapy, response indicators, 897
β-lactam; catheter patency, phlebitis, pediatrics, 832; comparision, aminoglycosides, therapy, 385
cefotetan; comparisons, therapy, selection, 285
cefoxitin; comparisons, therapy, selection, 285
clindamycin; body distribution, muscle, wound, 820; toxicity, phlebitis, catheter flushes, 439
diarrhea; infectious, therapy, review, 746
moxalactam; comparisons, therapy, selection, 285
stomatitis; therapy, 14
sulbactam sodium, combination, ampicillin sodium; therapy, 37
teicoplanin; review, 647
vancomycin; blood level monitoring, costs, 18; comparison, metronidazole, pseudomembranous enterocolitis, 93; excretion, hemofiltration, 198
vancomycin hydrochloride; toxicity, phlebitis, i.v. administration, 720; toxicity, red-man syndrome, 184
Antibodies; monoclonal; theophylline blood level monitoring, 462
Anticoagulants; heparin sodium; and sodium chloride, catheter patency, 832; comparison, sodium chloride, catheter flushes, 439
Anticonvulsants
midazolam hydrochloride; status epilepticus therapy, 322
phenobarbital; excretion, hemofiltration, 198
phenobarbital sodium; status epilepticus therapy, 322
phenytoin; adverse reactions, mycosis fungoides, 153; blood levels, binding, pediatrics, 688; interactions, influenza vaccines, 828
phenytoin sodium; status epilepticus therapy, 322; therapy, i.v. infusion, 219
valproic acid; blood levels, binding, pediatrics, 688

Antidepressants
clomipramine hydrochloride; obsessive–compulsive disorder, treatment IND, 638
fluoxetine hydrochloride; therapy, 169
Antidiabetic agents; glipizide; pharmacokinetics, geriatrics, 224
Antidiarrheal agents
atropine sulfate, combination, diphenoxylate hydrochloride; interactions, quinidine absorption, 139
therapy; review, 746
Antidotes
acetylcysteine; toxicity, administration routes, 563
acetylcysteine sodium; therapy, acetaminophen poisoning, pediatrics, 391
Antiemetics; metoclopramide hydrochloride; bolus vs. infusion, cisplatin toxicity, 454
Antifungals
amphotericin B; oral candidiasis therapy, mouthwashes, 70
amphotericin B and flucytosine; cryptococcal meningitis therapy, AIDS, 528
fluconazole; blood levels, ketoconazole malabsorption, 622
flucytosine and amphotericin B; cryptococcal meningitis therapy, AIDS, 528
ketoconazole; availability, effects, food, pH, 228; malabsorption, fluconazole absorption, 622
review, 424
stomatitis; therapy, 14
Antihistamines
cimetidine; and H_1 antagonists, therapy, allergies, 422
cromolyn sodium; aphthous stomatitis therapy, 334
diphenhydramine; and epinephrine, therapy, anaphylaxis, 269; neuroleptic malignant syndrome therapy, 697
diphenhydramine hydrochloride; therapy, metoclopramide toxicity, 454; therapy, red-man syndrome, 616
therapy; vancomycin toxicity, red-man syndrome, 184
Anti-infective agents
acquired immunodeficiency syndrome; opportunistic infections therapy, 511
ciprofloxacin; cystic fibrosis therapy, response indicators, 897
ciprofloxacin hydrochloride; FDA approvals, 7
eflornithine; *P. carinii* pneumonia therapy, AIDS, 514
metronidazole; pseudomembranous enterocolitis therapy, 93; resistance , *T. vaginalis*, therapy, 718
pentamidine isethionate; *P. carinii* pneumonia therapy, AIDS, 501, 514
toxicity; effects, GI flora, review, 878; neutropenia, AIDS, 398
trimethoprim; combined therapy, *P. carinii* pneumonia, 514
Anti-Infective Drug Products Advisory Committee; ganciclovir; FDA approval denials, 86
Anti-inflammatory agents
diclofenac sodium; FDA approvals, 785
ibuprofen; cimetidine, ranitidine hydrochloride, lack, 317
prednisone; toxic epidermal necrolysis therapy, 766
sulindac; adverse reactions, toxic epidermal necrolysis, 766
Antilipemic agents
fish oil; effects, mechanism, 795
gemfibrozil; hypercholesterolemia, combined therapy, 21
hypercholesterolemia; therapy, controversy, 592, 604, 605
lovastatin; hypercholesterolemia therapy, review, 21
niacin; hypercholesterolemia, combined therapy, 21
Antimanic agents; lithium carbonate; interactions, tetracycline, blood levels, 314
Antineoplastic agents
breast neoplasms; NCI protocols, 560
cisplatin; toxicity, metoclopramide administration rate, 454
mitoxantrone; review, 574
tamoxifen; early breast neoplasms therapy, 640
Antiprotozoals; trimetrexate; treatment IND, *P. carinii* pneumonia, 337
Antithyroid drugs; sodium iodide I 131; Graves' disease therapy, theophylline half-life, 620
Antituberculars
mycobacterium infections; combined therapy, pediatrics, 545
rifampin; toxicity, red-man syndrome, 616
Antivirals
acyclovir; excretion; hemofiltration, 198
ganciclovir; FDA approval denials, 86
Anxiolytics, sedatives, and hypnotics; diazepam; overdose, diagnosis, flumazenil, 614
Aromatic elixir; vehicles; leucovorin administration, 52
Arrhythmia
bepridil; therapy, 97
cardiac drugs; combined therapy, review, 808
procainamide hydrochloride; sustained action, generic equivalency, 135
propafenone; therapy, review, 869
verapamil; therapy, administration routes, dosage conversion, 791
Arthritis; diclofenac sodium; rheumatoid, therapy, FDA approvals, 785
Ascites; morphine; body distribution, 842
Aspirin; toxicity; Reye's syndrome, FDA labeling regulations, 639
Atropine sulfate; combination, diphenoxylate hydrochloride; interactions, quinidine, absorption, 139
Availability, drugs, see **Drugs, availability**
Azathioprine; concomitant therapy, 867
Azlocillin; cystic fibrosis; therapy, response indicators, methodology, 897
Aztreonam
comparison, aminoglycosides; therapy, 385
cystic fibrosis; therapy, response indicators, methodology, 897

B

Benzodiazepine antagonists; flumazenil; diagnosis, diazepam overdose, 614
Benztropine; and diphenhydramine; neuroleptic malignant syndrome therapy, 697
Bepridil; review, 97
Bile levels
anti-infective agents; effects, GI flora, review, 878
cefmetazole; body distribution, 467
Binding
anticonvulsants; blood levels, pediatrics, 688
bepridil; protein, 97
nicardipine; protein, 97
nitrendipine; protein, 97
phenytoin; interactions, influenza vaccines, 828
quinidine; serum proteins, temperature effects, 142
Bioavailability, see **Drugs, availability**
Biotechnology; research; pharmaceutical industry, survey, 713
Blood; transfusions; anemia therapy, kidney failure, 117
Blood levels
acetaminophen; overdose, toxicity, pediatrics, 391
albumin human; hypoalbuminemia, equations, dosage prediction, 894
aminoglycosides; dosage changes, prediction, models, 681; pharmacokinetics monitoring, cost benefit, 608; pharmacokinetic variations, critical patients, 207
cefmetazole; distribution, 467
cholesterol; measurement, standards, 260
clindamycin; body distribution, 820
creatinine; clearance estimation, nutrition disorders, 62
digitoxin; inteference, digitoxin-like substance, 825
digoxin; false positive, tests comparison, 444; interactions, bepridil, nicardipine and nitrendipine, 97; radioimmunoassay, 449
drugs; computer programs, TDx assay, 792
fibronectin; parenteral nutrition markers, 889
fluconazole; absorption, ketoconazole malabsorption, 622
generic drugs; equivalency, FDA regulations, 334
gentamicin; CRIS, comparison, minibag administration, 303; errors, effects, pharmacokinetic calculations, 307
glipizide; pharmacokinetics, geriatrics, 224
guanfacine hydrochloride; review, 187
ibuprofen; interactions, cimetidine, ranitidine, lack, 317
ketoconazole; effects, food, pH, 228; malabsorption, fluconazole absorption, 622
leucovorin; and metabolites, 52
lithium; tetracycline interactions, 314
methyltetrahydrofolate; leucovorin metabolites, 52
mezlocillin sodium, comparison, ticarcillin disodium; pharmacokinetics, dosage, 380
morphine; body distribution, ascites, 842
phenytoin; binding, pediatrics, 688; interactions, influenza vaccines, 828; i.v. therapy, 219
potassium; relation, dosage, 150
procainamide hydrochloride; sustained action, generic equivalency, 135
quinidine; serum free fractions, temperature effects, in vitro, 142
quinidine sulfate; interactions, atropine, combination, diphenoxylate, 139
somatomedin-C; parenteral nutrition markers, 889
theophylline; interactions, sucralfate, lack, 58; interference, pentoxifylline, metabolites, 457; tests comparison, 462
ticarcillin disodium, comparison, mezlocillin sodium; pharmacokinetics, dosage, 380
tobramycin; i.v. administration systems, 367; pharmacokinetics, i.v. administration systems, 374
valproic acid; binding, pediatrics, 688
vancomycin; monitoring, costs, 18
Book Reviews, 78, 161, 244, 406, 628, 705, 779, 854
Avery's Drug Treatment: Principles and Practice of Clinical Pharmacology and Therapeutics, Third Edition, 161
Basic Clinical Pharmacokinetics, Second Edition, 779
Cancer Chemotherapy by Infusion, 78
Cardiovascular Drug Therapy, 244
Clinical Pharmacokinetics: The MCQ Approach, 780
Drug Treatment of the Rheumatic Diseases, Third Edition, 244
Drug Use in Respiratory Disease, 406
Guide to Planning and Managing Multiple Clinical Studies, 162
Immunology, Immunopathology, and Immunity, 705
Manual of Antibiotics and Infectious Diseases, Sixth Edition, 629
The Merck Manual, Fifteenth Edition, 854
Pharmacokinetics and Pharmacodynamics: Research and Analysis, 245
Pharmacology in Medicine: Principles and Practice, 245
Problems in Pediatric Drug Therapy, Second Edition, 246
Psychotropic Drug Handbook, 5th Edition, 628
Therapeutic Pharmacology, 705
Books Received, 80, 162, 246, 330, 482, 556, 630, 706, 780, 915
Breast neoplasms
mitoxantrone; therapy, review, 574
tamoxifen; therapy, early stage, 640
therapy; NCI protocols, 560
Bromocriptine; and dantrolene sodium; neuroleptic malignant syndrome therapy, 697
Bronchodilators; ipratropium bromide; review, 670

C

Calcitriol; concomitant therapy, 906
Calcium antagonists; hypertension; therapy, protocols, 837
Calcium carbonate; concomitant therapy, 906
Calculations
creatinine; clearance estimation, nutrition disorders, 62
dosage; albumin, equations, prediction, 894; drugs, hemofiltration, 198; phosphorus, supplementation, 123
gentamicin; pharmacokinetics, blood level errors, 307
Caloric agents; nutrition; parenteral, pediatrics, review, 351
Cancer drugs, see **Antineoplastic agents**
Candidiasis
amphotericin B; oral, therapy, mouthwashes, 70
fluconazole; therapy, ketoconazole malabsorption, 622
ketoconazole; malabsorption, fluconazole therapy, 622
Cardiac drugs
arrhythmia; combined therapy, review, 808
bepridil; review, 97
digitoxin; interference, digitoxin-like substance, 825
digoxin; interactions, bepridil, nicardipine and nitrendipine, 97; radioimmunoassay, interference, lack, 449
diltiazem hydrochloride; effects, glucose tolerance, 235
diltiazem hydrochloride, comparison, verapamil hydrochloride; hypertension therapy, 129
nicardipine; review, 97
nitrendipine; review, 97
procainamide hydrochloride; sustained action, generic equivalency, 135
propafenone; arrhythmia therapy, review, 869
quinidine; serum free fractions, temperature effects, 142
quinidine sulfate; interactions, atropine, combination, diphenoxylate, 139
verapamil; administration routes, dosage conversion, 791
verapamil hydrochloride, comparison, diltiazem hydrochloride; hypertension therapy, 129
Catheters; intravenous; dressing changes, effects, infections, 88; flushing, sodium chloride, heparin, 832; heparin vs. sodium chloride flushes, 439; phlebitis, i.v. administration methods, 760

Cefmetazole; tissue levels; bile, gallbladder, 467
Cefmetazole sodium; body distribution; bile, gallbladder levels, 467
Cefotaxime
interactions; desacetylcefotaxime, metabolites, synergism, 901
toxicity; neutropenia, AIDS, 398
Cefotetan; comparison, cefoxitin, ceftizoxime, moxalactam; therapy, selection, 285
Cefoxitin; comparison, cefotetan, ceftizoxime, moxalactam; therapy, selection, 285
Ceftizoxime; comparison, cefotetan, cefoxitin, moxalactam; therapy, selection, 285
Centers for Disease Control; protocols; polio immunization, 169
Central nervous system stimulants; tacrine; clinical studies, FDA attitudes, 337
Cephalosporins
cefmetazole sodium, distribution; gallbladder, 467
cefotaxime; interactions, desacetylcefotaxime, metabolites, synergism, 901
ceftizoxime; comparison, antibiotics, therapy, 285
comparison, aminoglycosides; therapy, 385
comparison, ampicillin sodium, combination, sulbactam sodium; therapy, 37
excretion; hemofiltration, 198
toxicity; phlebitis, catheter flushes, 439; phlebitis, i.v. administration, 760
Chloramphenicol; Rocky Mountain spotted fever; therapy, 109
Chloramphenicols
chloramphenicol; Rocky Mountain spotted fever, 109
chloramphenicol sodium succinate; Rocky Mountain spotted fever, 109
Chloramphenicol sodium succinate; Rocky Mountain spotted fever; therapy, 109
Cholesterol; blood levels; measurement, standards, 260
Chromatography, liquid; theophylline; interference, pentoxifylline, metabolites, 457
Cimetidine
and antihistamines; combined therapy, allergies, 422
comparison, famotidine; therapy, review, 271
interactions; ibuprofen, lack, 317
Ciprofloxacin; cystic fibrosis; therapy, response indicators, methodology, 897
Ciprofloxacin hydrochloride; approvals; FDA, 7
Cisplatin
concomitant therapy, 842
toxicity; metoclopramide prophylaxis, 454
Clearance, see **Excretion**
Clindamycin
body distribution; muscle, wound levels, 820
toxicity; phlebitis, catheter flushes, 439
Clinical Pharmacy
acknowledgment to reviewers, October 1, 1987–September 30, 1988, 910
procedure for submission of manuscripts to journals published by the American Society of Hospital Pharmacists, 73
statement of ownership, management, and circulation, 888
Clinical studies
aminoglycosides; pharmacokinetics monitoring, cost benefit, 608
methodology; sample size selection, 694
tacrine; Alzheimer's disease, FDA attitudes, 337
Clofazimine; mycobacterium infections; combined therapy, pediatrics, 545
Clomipramine hydrochloride; obsessive–compulsive disorder; treatment IND, FDA approvals, 638
Clonidine
comparison, guanfacine hydrochloride; hypertension therapy, review, 187
concomitant therapy, 906
transdermal; withdrawal, rebound hypertension, geriatrics, 772
Clonidine hydrochloride; oral; therapy, transdermal clonidine withdrawal, 772
Combined therapy
amphotericin B and flucytosine; cryptococcal meningitis therapy, AIDS, 528
antihistamines; H_1 and H_2 antagonists, allergies, 422
anti-infective agents; toxicity, neutropenia, AIDS, 398
antituberculars; mycobacterium infections, pediatrics, 545
breast neoplasms; NCI protocols, 560
bromocriptine and dantrolene sodium; neuroleptic malignant syndrome, 697
calcium antagonists; hypertension, 97
cardiac drugs; arrhythmia, review, 808
dantrolene sodium and bromocriptine; neuroleptic malignant syndrome, 697
dapsone and trimethoprim; *P. carinii* pneumonia, AIDS, 514
flucytosine and amphotericin B; cryptococcal meningitis therapy, AIDS, 528
heparin sodium and sodium chloride; catheter patency, pediatrics, 832
lovastatin; hypercholesterolemia, 21
sodium chloride and heparin sodium; catheter patency, pediatrics, 832
trimethoprim and dapsone; *P. carinii* pneumonia, AIDS, 514
Commentaries, 239, 385, 469, 592, 694, 837
Committees
Anti-Infective Drug Products Advisory Committee; FDA, ganciclovir approval denials, 86
Joint National Committee on Detection, Evaluation and Treatment of High Blood Pressure; 1988 hypertension protocols, 837
Complexes
diphtheria toxoids and *Haemophilus* b polysaccharide vaccines; FDA approvals, 169
Haemophilus b polysaccharide vaccines and diphtheria toxoids; FDA approvals, 169
Compounding
amphotericin B; solutions, oral candidiasis therapy, 70
Elliot's B solution; diluents, intrathecal injections, 265
neomycin sulfate; FDA labeling regulations, 490
Computers
gentamicin; models, blood level errors, 307
programs; urine levels, TDx assay, 792
Concentration; vancomycin hydrochloride; toxicity, phlebitis, i.v. administration, 720
Contraindications
fat emulsions; neonates, hyperbilirubinemia, review, 351
isotretinoin; FDA labeling regulations, pregnancy, 490
pyrethrins; allergies, 846
Correction Notices, 269
Effect of two cimetidine regimens on prothrombin time and warfarin pharmacokinetics during long-term warfarin therapy (Jun 1987 Research Note), 269
Encainide and flecainide: two class 1c antiarrhythmic agents (Nov 1987 Continuing Education), 269
Cost-effectiveness, see **Economics, cost-benefit analysis**
Costs
alteplase, 85
alteplase, comparison, streptokinase; myocardial infarction therapy, 469
blood levels; theophylline, tests comparison, 462
cefotetan; comparison, antibiotics, selection, 285
cefoxitin; comparison, antibiotics, selection, 285
ceftizoxime; comparison, antibiotics, selection, 285
ciprofloxacin hydrochloride, 7
metronidazole, comparison, vancomycin; pseudomembranous enterocolitis therapy, 93
moxalactam; comparison, antibiotics, selection, 285
nutrition; parenteral, therapy, AIDS, 512
somatrem, comparison, somatropin recombinant; growth disorders therapy, 239
somatropin recombinant, comparison, somatrem; growth disorders therapy, 239
streptokinase, comparison, alteplase; myocardial infarction therapy, 469
vancomycin; blood level monitoring, 18
vancomycin, comparison, metronidazole; pseudomembranous enterocolitis therapy, 93
CP Continuing Education, 75, 158, 241, 326, 402, 478, 552, 624, 702, 775, 851, 911
Creatinine; clearance; estimation methods, nutrition disorders, 62
Cromolyn sodium; stomatitis; aphthous, therapy, 334
Current Literature, 77, 160, 243, 329, 405, 481, 555, 627, 704, 778, 853, 914
Cyclophosphamide; breast neoplasms; combined therapy, 560
Cyclosporine; concomitant therapy, 867
Cystic fibrosis; anti-infective agents; therapy, response indicators, methodology, 897
Cytarabine; concomitant therapy, 842
Cytotoxic agents, see **Antineoplastic agents**

D

Dantrolene sodium; and bromocriptine; neuroleptic malignant syndrome therapy, 697
Dapsone; and trimethoprim; *P. carinii* pneumonia therapy, AIDS, 514
Data collection; Pharmaceutical Manufacturers Association; biotechnology, genetic engineering research, 713
Density; gentamicin sulfate; injections, CRIS administration, 303
Department of Health and Human Services; regulations; reports, adverse reactions, vaccines, 489
Depression; propranolol; toxicity, 146
Desacetylcefotaxime; interactions; cefotaxime, metabolites, synergism, 901
Developing countries; ivermectin; distribution, onchocerciasis therapy, 11
Devices
catheters; heparin vs. sodium chloride flushes, 439
CRIS; gentamicin administration, comparison, minibags, 303
infusion pumps; piston cassette, nitroprusside pharmacodynamics, 214; tobramycin administration, accuracy, 367; tobramycin pharmacokinetics, 374
syringe pumps; tobramycin administration, accuracy, 367; tobramycin pharmacokinetics, 374
Dexamethasone
concomitant therapy, 454
tests, laboratory; depression, propranolol toxicity, 146
Dextrose
alone and with sodium chloride; diluents, gentamicin administration, CRIS, 303
anaphylaxis; therapy, pyrethrins adverse reactions, 846
DHPG, see **Ganciclovir**
Diabetes mellitus; diltiazem hydrochloride; effects, glucose tolerance, 235
Diagnosis; overdose; diazepam, flumazenil effects, 614
Dialysis; peritoneal; bromate poisoning, therapy, 68
Diarrhea
anti-infective agents; toxicity, effects, GI flora, review, 878
therapy; infectious, review, 746
Diazepam; overdose; diagnosis, flumazenil, 614
Diclofenac sodium; approvals; FDA, 785
Dicloxacillin; cystic fibrosis; therapy, response indicators, methodology, 897
Digitoxin; blood levels; interference, kidney failure, 825
Digoxin
blood levels; false positive, tests comparison; 444; radioimmunoassay, 449
interactions; bepridil, nicardipine and nitrendipine, blood levels, 97
Digoxin-like factor; interference; false-positive digoxin tests, 444; lack, radioimmunoassay, digoxin levels, 449
Digoxin-like immunoreactive substance, see **Digoxin-like factor**
Diltiazem hydrochloride
comparison, verapamil hydrochloride; hypertension therapy, 129
effects; glucose tolerance, 235
Diluents
dextrose; alone and with sodium chloride, gentamicin administration, 303
injections; intrathecal, 265
sodium chloride and dextrose; gentamicin administration, CRIS, 303
Water for Injection; gentamicin administration, CRIS, 303
acetylcysteine; GI side effects, 563
3,7-Dimethyl-1-(5-hydroxyhexyl) xanthine; interactions; theophylline, blood level assays, 457
Diphenhydramine
and benztropine; neuroleptic malignant syndrome therapy, 697
and epinephrine; therapy, sodium bisulfite allergies, 269
concomitant therapy, 528, 867
Diphenhydramine hydrochloride; therapy; metoclopramide toxicity, 454; red-man syndrome, rifampin toxicity, 616
Diphenoxylate hydrochloride; combination, atropine sulfate; interactions, quinidine, absorption, 139
Diphtheria toxoids; and *Haemophilus* b polysaccharide vaccines; conjugates, FDA approvals, 169
Disopyramide; arrhythmia; combined therapy, review, 808
Diuretics
and nicardipine or nitrendipine; hypertension therapy, 97
furosemide; bromate poisoning therapy, 68
hypertension; therapy, protocols, 837
DLIS, see **Digoxin-like factor**
Dosage
albumin human; hypoalbuminemia, equations, dosage prediction, 894
alteplase; myocardial infarction therapy, 85
aminoglycosides; pharmacokinetics monitoring, cost–benefit, 608; pharmacokinetic variations, critical patients, 207

aminophylline; theophylline half-life, hypothyroidism, 620
amphotericin B; cryptococcal meningitis therapy, AIDS, 528
antifungals; review, 424
cardiac drugs; arrhythmia, combined therapy, 808
cimetidine, comparison, famotidine; review, 271
ciprofloxacin hydrochloride, 7
clonidine; withdrawal, transdermal, geriatrics, 772
diclofenac sodium, 785
diltiazem hydrochloride, comparison, verapamil hydrochloride; low vs. high, hypertension, 129
drugs; hemofiltration, 198; nutrition disorders, 62
enalaprilat; hypertension therapy, FDA approvals, 416
estrogens conjugated; GI hemorrhage therapy, kidney failure, 906
famotidine, comparison, cimetidine, ranitidine; review, 271
fluoxetine hydrochloride, 169
guanfacine hydrochloride; hypertension therapy, review, 187
ipratropium bromide, 670
lisinopril; therapy, 659
lovastatin; hypercholesterolemia therapy, review, 21
metronidazole; *T. vaginalis* resistance, therapy, 718
mezlocillin sodium, comparison, ticarcillin disodium; high, low, pharmacokinetics, 380
midazolam; anesthetics, electric countershock, 423
minoxidil; alopecia therapy, 858
mitoxantrone; review, 574
morphine sulfate; body distribution, ascites, 842
muromonab-CD3; toxicity, aseptic meningitis, 721
nizatidine; duodenal ulcer therapy, 560
omeprazole; therapy, review, 725
overdose; acetaminophen, toxicity, pediatrics, 391; diazepam, diagnosis, flumazenil, 614; pentoxifylline, interference, theophylline assays, 457
pentamidine isethionate; *P. carinii* pneumonia therapy, 501
phenytoin sodium; seizures, i.v. infusion, 219
phosphorus; hypophosphatemia therapy, 123
polio vaccines; ACIP protocols, 169
potassium; supplements, equivalency, 150
propafenone; review, 869
psychotherapeutic agents; agitation therapy, geriatrics, 865
ranitidine, comparison, famotidine; review, 271
rifampin; toxicity, red-man syndrome, 616
somatrem, comparison, somatropin recombinant; growth disorders therapy, 239
somatropin recombinant, comparison, somatrem; growth disorders therapy, 239
teicoplanin; review, 647
ticarcillin disodium, comparison, mezlocillin sodium; high, low, pharmacokinetics, 380
tobramycin; pharmacokinetics, i.v. administration systems, 374
vancomycin; blood level monitoring, costs, 18
verapamil; conversion, i.v., oral, 791
verapamil hydrochloride, comparison, diltiazem hydrochloride; low vs. high, hypertension, 129

Dosage forms
clonidine; transdermal, withdrawal, hypertension, 772
potassium; wax matrix, equivalency, 150

Dosage schedules
acetaminophen; chronic, overdose, toxicity, pediatrics, 391
aminoglycosides; changes, prediction, models, 681; toxicity, 385
cefotaxime; metabolites, synergism, 901
gentamicin; pharmacokinetic calculations, blood level errors, 307
vancomycin hydrochloride; toxicity, red-man syndrome, 184

Dressings; catheters; changes, effects, infections, phlebitis, 88

Drug administration
acetylcysteine; oral, nasogastric, GI side effects, 563
enalaprilat; hypertension therapy, FDA approvals, 416
gentamicin sulfate; CRIS, comparison, minibags, 303
injections; push, comparison, piggyback, phlebitis, 760
intermittent; heparin vs. sodium chloride flushes, 439
mitoxantrone; review, 574
pentamidine isethionate; *P. carinii* pneumonia therapy, 501
phenytoin sodium; i.v. infusion, 219
self-medication; acetaminophen overdose, toxicity, pediatrics, 391; pyrethrins adverse reactions, 846
sodium nitroprusside; piston infusion pumps, pharmacodynamics, 214
teicoplanin, 647

Drug administration rate
metoclopramide hydrochloride; bolus vs. continuous, cisplatin toxicity, 454
midazolam hydrochloride; continuous i.v. status epilepticus therapy, 322
vancomycin hydrochloride; toxicity, phlebitis, i.v., 720; toxicity, red-man syndrome, 184

Drug administration routes
acetylcysteine; i.v., oral, protocols, 563
ampicillin sodium, combination, sulbactam sodium; oral, i.v., 37
anti-infective agents; oral, effects, GI flora, review, 878
intrathecal; injections, diluents, 265
leucovorin calcium; oral, i.m., i.v., pharmacokinetics, 52
metronidazole; oral, intravaginal, *T. vaginalis* resistance, 718
metronidazole, comparison, vancomycin; pseudomembranous enterocolitis therapy, 93
phosphorus; oral, i.v., hypophosphatemia therapy, 123
psychotherapeutic agents; agitation therapy, geriatrics, 865
vancomycin, comparison, metronidazole; pseudomembranous enterocolitis therapy, 93
vancomycin hydrochloride; i.v., toxicity, phlebitis, 720
verapamil; arrhythmia, i.v., oral, dosage conversion, 791

Drug administration sites
anti-infective agents; i.v., toxicity, phlebitis, 760
vancomycin hydrochloride; i.v., toxicity, phlebitis, 720

Drug administration systems; tobramycin sulfate; pumps, minibags, accuracy, 367; pumps, minibags, pharmacokinetics, 374

Drug distribution
ivermectin; developing countries, onchocerciasis therapy, 11
somatropin recombinant; costs, 239

Drug interactions
alpha blockers and epinephrine; hypotension, 493
antifungals; review, 424
atropine sulfate, combination, diphenoxylate hydrochloride and quinidine sulfate; absorption, 139
calcium antagonists and digoxin; blood levels, 97
cefotaxime and desacetylcefotaxime; synergism, 901
cimetidine and ibuprofen; pharmacokinetics, lack, 317
desacetylcefotaxime and cefotaxime; synergism, 901
digoxin and calcium antagonists; blood levels, 97
3,7-dimethyl-1-(5-hydroxyhexyl) xanthine and theophylline; interference, blood level assays, 457
epinephrine and alpha blockers; hypotension, 493
epinephrine and tranquilizers; hypotension, 493
famotidine; review, 271
food and ketoconazole; absorption effects, 228
glutamic acid hydrochloride and ketoconazole; absorption effects, 228
ibuprofen and cimetidine; pharmacokinetics, lack, 317
ibuprofen and ranitidine hydrochloride; pharmacokinetics, lack, 317
influenza vaccines and phenytoin; blood levels, 828
ketoconazole and food; absorption effects, 228
ketoconazole and glutamic acid hydrochloride; absorption effects, 228
lithium carbonate and tetracycline hydrochloride; blood levels, 314
pentoxifylline and theophylline; interference, blood level assays, 457
phenytoin and influenza vaccines; blood levels, 828
propafenone; review, 869
quinidine sulfate and atropine sulfate, combination, diphenoxylate hydrochloride; absorption, 139
ranitidine hydrochloride and ibuprofen; pharmacokinetics, lack, 317
sucralfate and theophylline; pharmacokinetics, 58
tetracycline hydrochloride and lithium carbonate; blood levels, 314
theophylline and 3,7-dimethyl-1-(5-hydroxyhexyl) xanthine; interference, blood level assays, 457
theophylline and pentoxifylline; interference, blood level assays, 457
theophylline and sucralfate; pharmacokinetics, 58
tranquilizers and epinephrine; hypotension, 493

Drug Reaction Alerts, 77, 160, 243, 329, 405, 481, 555, 627, 704, 778, 853, 914

Drugs
generic; equivalency, FDA regulations, 334
latentiated; sultamicillin, 37
new; FDA approvals, 1987, 166; topical minoxidil, FDA approvals, 858
orphan; FDA approvals, 1987, 253
reconstitution; diluents, intrathecal injections, 265; gentamicin administration, CRIS, 303
selection; alteplase, streptokinase, myocardial infarction therapy, 469, 473; antifungals, review, 424; anti-infectives, effects, GI flora, 878; extended spectrum antibiotics, 285; somatrem, somatropin recombinant, equivalency, 239

Drugs, adverse reactions
muromonab-CD3; sensorineural hearing loss, 867
phenytoin; pseudolymphoma, mycosis fungoides, 153
pyrethrins; anaphylaxis, 846
sodium bisulfite; anaphylaxis, preservatives, injections, 269
sulindac; toxic epidermal necrolysis, 766

Drugs, availability
bepridil; review, 97
leucovorin calcium; oral, i.m., i.v., 52
ketoconazole; effects, food, pH, 228
nicardipine; review, 97
nitrendipine; review, 97
procainamide hydrochloride; sustained action, generic equivalency, 135
quinidine sulfate; interactions, atropine, combination, diphenoxylate, 139

Drugs, body distribution
aminoglycosides; pharmacokinetic variations, critical patients, 207
cefmetazole; gallbladder levels, 467
clindamycin; muscle, wound, 820
glipizide; pharmacokinetics, geriatrics, 224
guanfacine hydrochloride; review, 187
leucovorin; and metabolites, administration routes, 52
morphine; ascites, nasogastric fluid levels, 842
tobramycin; pharmacokinetics, i.v. administration systems, 374

Drugs, investigational; investigational new drugs; clomipramine, obsessive–compulsive disorder, protocols, 638; trimetrexate, *P. carinii* pneumonia therapy, 337

Drug withdrawal; clonidine; transdermal, rebound hypertension, 772

Duration of action; midazolam; anesthetics, electric countershock, 423

E

Economics; cost–benefit analysis; aminoglycoside pharmacokinetics, monitoring, 608; hypercholesterolemia therapy, controversy, 592; parenteral nutrition, AIDS, 512; vancomycin blood level monitoring, 18

Editorials, 511
Infectious complications of AIDS, 511
What is the role of parenteral nutrition in AIDS? 512

Eflornithine; pneumonia; *P. carinii*, therapy, AIDS, 514

Electrolytes; potassium; dosage, relation, blood levels, 150

Elimination, see **Metabolism**

Elliot's B solution; diluents; intrathecal injections, 265

EMIT, see **Immunoassay, enzyme multiplied**

Enalaprilat; hypertension; therapy, FDA approvals, 416

Enterocolitis
anti-infective agents; pseudomembranous, toxicity, GI flora, 878
metronidazole; pseudomembranous, therapy, 93
vancomycin, comparison, metronidazole; pseudomembranous, therapy, 93

Epidermal necrolysis; sulindac; toxic, adverse reactions, 766

Epilepsy; anticonvulsants; blood levels, binding, pediatrics, 688

Epinephrine
anaphylaxis; therapy, pyrethrins adverse reactions, 846
and diphenhydramine; therapy, sodium bisulfite allergies, 269
interactions; alpha blockers, tranquilizers, hypotension, 493

Equations
clearance; creatinine, estimation, nutrition disorders, 62
dosage; albumin, hypoalbuminemia, prediction, 894

Equivalency; leucovorin calcium; oral, i.m., i.v., 52

Equivalency, generic
potassium; supplements, 150
procainamide hydrochloride; sustained action. 135
regulations; FDA, 334

Equivalency, therapeutic
alteplase, comparison, streptokinase; myocardial infarction therapy, 469, 473
cefotetan; comparison, antibiotics, selection, 285
cefoxitin; comparison, antibiotics, selection, 285
ceftizoxime; comparison, antibiotics, selection, 285
moxalactam; comparison, antibiotics, selection, 285
somatrem, comparison, somatropin recombinant; growth disorders, 239
somatropin recombinant, comparison, somatrem; growth disorders, 239
streptokinase, comparison, alteplase; myocardial infarction therapy, 469, 473
Errors
clinical studies; tacrine, Alzheimer's disease, FDA attitudes, 337
tests, laboratory; cholesterol blood levels, measurement, 260
Errors, medication
acetaminophen; overdose, toxicity, pediatrics, 391
diazepam; overdose, diagnosis, flumazenil, 614
gentamicin; blood levels, pharmacokinetic calculations, 307
Erythropoietin; anemia; therapy, kidney failure, 117
Escherichia coli; resistance; mezlocillin, ticarcillin, dosage, 380
Esophagitis; omeprazole; peptic, therapy, review, 725
Estrogens conjugated; hemorrhage; GI, therapy, kidney failure, 906
Ethambutol hydrochloride; mycobacterium infections; combined therapy, pediatrics, 545
Ethics; clinical studies; sample size selection, 694
Excretion
aminoglycosides; pharmacokinetic variations, critical patients, 207
anti-infective agents; bile, effects, GI flora, review, 878
clindamycin; muscle, wound levels, 820
creatinine; clearance estimation, nutrition disorders, 62
drugs; hemofiltration, 198
glipizide; pharmacokinetics, geriatrics, 224
guanfacine hydrochloride; review, 187
leucovorin; and metabolites, administration routes, 52
mezlocillin sodium, comparison, ticarcillin disodium; pharmacokinetics, 380
nicardipine; review, 97
nitrendipine; review, 97
quinidine sulfate; interactions, atropine, combination, diphenoxylate, 139
ticarcillin disodium, comparison, mezlocillin sodium; pharmacokinetics, 380

F

Famotidine; comparison, cimetidine, ranitidine; therapy, review, 271
Fat emulsions; nutrition; parenteral, pediatrics, review, 351
Filtration; hemo-; kidney failure, drug dosages, 198
Fish oil; effects; lipids, mechanism, 795
Flow; rates; piston cassette infusion pumps, 214
Fluconazole; blood levels; ketoconazole malabsorption, 622
Flucytosine
and amphotericin B; cryptococcal meningitis therapy, AIDS, 528
therapy; review, 424
Flumazenil; therapy; diagnosis, diazepam overdose, 614
Fluorouracil; breast neoplasms; combined therapy, 560
Fluoxetine hydrochloride; therapy, 169
Food; interactions; ketoconazole, absorption, 228
Food and Drug Administration (U.S.)
alteplase; approvals, 85
approvals; diclofenac, 785; new drugs, 1987, 166
ciprofloxacin hydrochloride; approvals, 7
clomipramine hydrochloride; obsessive–compulsive disorder, treatment IND, 638
enalaprilat; approvals, injections, 416
ganciclovir; approval denials, 86
Haemophilus b polysaccharide vaccines; conjugates, approvals, 169
isotretinoin; labeling regulations, contraindications, pregnancy, 490
minoxidil; topical solutions, approvals, 858
neomycin sulfate; labeling regulations, 490
nizatidine; approvals, 560
orphan drugs; approvals, 1987, 253
polio vaccines; approvals, 1987, 169
regulations; aspirin, Reye's syndrome, labeling, 639; generic equivalency, 334; trimetrexate, treatment IND, pneumonia, 337
tacrine; attitudes, clinical studies, Alzheimer's disease, 337
5-Formyltetrahydrofolate, see **Leucovorin**
Furosemide
concomitant therapy, 906
therapy; bromate poisoning, 68

G

Ganciclovir; approvals; denials, FDA, 86
Gastrointestinal drugs
cimetidine; interactions, ibuprofen, lack, 317
cimetidine, comparison, famotidine; therapy, review, 271
famotidine, comparison, cimetidine, ranitidine; therapy, review, 271
nizatidine; FDA approvals, 560
omeprazole; therapy, review, 725
ranitidine; excretion, hemofiltration, 198
ranitidine, comparison, famotidine; therapy, review, 271
ranitidine hydrochloride; interactions, ibuprofen, lack, 317
sucralfate; interactions, theophylline pharmacokinetics, 58
Gemfibrozil; and lovastatin; hypercholesterolemia, combined therapy, 21
Genetic engineering; research; pharmaceutical industry, survey, 713
Gentamicin
blood levels; CRIS, comparison, minibag administration, 303
injections; preservatives, sodium bisulfite, adverse reactions, 269
pharmacokinetics; calculations, blood level errors, 307
toxicity; neutropenia, AIDS, 398
Gentamicin sulfate; administration; CRIS, comparison, minibags, 303
Geriatrics
clonidine; withdrawal, rebound hypertension, 772
digoxin; blood levels, radioimmunoassay, 449
glipizide; pharmacokinetics, 224
psychotherapeutic agents; psychomotor agitation therapy, 865
Glipizide; pharmacokinetics; geriatrics, 224
Glucose tolerance tests; diltiazem hydrochloride; effects, 235
Glutamic acid hydrochloride; interactions; ketoconazole, absorption, 228
Gonorrhea; ampicillin sodium, combination, sulbactam sodium; therapy, 37
Graves' disease; sodium iodide I 131; therapy, effects, theophylline half-life, 620
Growth disorders
somatrem, comparison, somatropin recombinant; equivalency, 239
somatropin recombinant, comparison, somatrem; equivalency, 239
Guanfacine hydrochloride; review, 187
Guidelines, treatment, see **Protocols**

H

***Haemophilus* b polysaccharide vaccines;** and diphtheria toxoids; conjugates, FDA approvals, 169
***Haemophilus influenzae*;** immunizations; conjugated vaccines, FDA approvals, 169
Hair preparations; sodium bromate; poisoning, pediatrics, 68
Half-life
acetaminophen; overdose, toxicity, pediatrics, 391
aminoglycosides; pharmacokinetic variations, critical patients, 207
glipizide; pharmacokinetics, geriatrics, 224
leucovorin; and metabolites, administration routes, 52
mezlocillin sodium, comparison, ticarcillin disodium; pharmacokinetics, dosage, 380
theophylline; hypothyroidism, 620; interactions, sucralfate, lack, 58
ticarcillin disodium, comparison, mezlocillin sodium; pharmacokinetics, dosage, 380
Haloperidol; toxicity; neuroleptic malignant syndrome, therapy, 697
Health care; home; parenteral nutrition, AIDS, 536
Hearing loss; muromonab-CD3; sensorineural, adverse reactions, 867
Heart arrest; epinephrine; therapy, interactions, 493
Hemorrhage; estrogens conjugated; GI, therapy, kidney failure, 906
Hemorrheologic agents; pentoxifylline; interactions, theophylline, blood level assays, 457
Hemostatics; estrogens conjugated; GI hemorrhage therapy, kidney failure, 906
Heparin sodium
and sodium chloride; catheter patency, pediatrics, 832
comparison, sodium chloride; catheter flushes, 439
Hoffmann-La Roche; isotretinoin; FDA labeling regulations, 490
Home health care, see **Health care, home**
Hospitals; intensive-care units; dosage schedules, prediction, models, 681
Hydrocortisone; concomitant therapy, 528
Hydrogen ion concentration; ketoconazole; effects, availability, 228
Hyperalimentation, see **Nutrition, parenteral**
Hyperbilirubinemia; fat emulsions; neonates, contraindications, review, 351
Hypercholesterolemia
acids, fatty; 3-omega, mechanism, 795
lovastatin; therapy, review, 21
therapy; controversy, 592, 604, 605
Hypertension
clonidine; toxicity, withdrawal, transdermal patches, 772
diltiazem hydrochloride, comparison, verapamil hydrochloride; therapy, 129
enalaprilat; therapy, FDA approvals, 416
guanfacine hydrochloride; therapy, review, 187
sodium nitroprusside; piston infusion pumps, pharmacodynamics, 214
therapy; crisis, review, 582; 1988 protocols, changes, 837
verapamil hydrochloride, comparison, diltiazem hydrochloride; therapy, 129
Hypophosphatemia; therapy, 123
Hypotensive agents
clonidine; transdermal, withdrawal, toxicity, geriatrics, 772
clonidine, comparison, guanfacine hydrochloride; review, 187
clonidine hydrochloride; oral, therapy, transdermal clonidine withdrawal, 772
enalaprilat; therapy, FDA approvals, 416
guanfacine hydrochloride; review, 187
lisinopril; therapy, 659
methyldopa, comparison, guanfacine hydrochloride; review, 187
propranolol; toxicity, depression, 146
sodium nitroprusside; piston infusion pumps, pharmacodynamics, 214
therapy; hypertensive crisis, review, 582; 1988 protocols, changes, 837
Hypothyroidism; theophylline; half-life, 620

I

Iatrogenic diseases, see **Drugs, adverse reactions**
Ibuprofen; interactions; cimetidine, ranitidine hydrochloride, lack, 317
Imipenem; comparison, aminoglycosides; therapy, 385
Immunization
Haemophilus influenzae; conjugated vaccines, FDA approvals, 169
influenza; interactions, phenytoin, 828
polio; inactivated vaccines, FDA approvals, 169
Immunoassay
enzyme multiplied; theophylline, interference, pentoxifylline, metabolites, 457
fluorescence; theophylline, interference, pentoxifylline, metabolites, 457
fluorescence polarization; false-positive digoxin blood levels, 444
fluorometric enzyme; false-positive digoxin blood levels, 444
Immunogenicity
somatrem, comparison, somatropin recombinant, 239
somatropin recombinant, comparison, somatrem, 239
Immunosuppressive agents
methylprednisolone; therapy, pyrethrins adverse reactions, 846
muromonab-CD3; adverse reactions, hearing loss, 867; toxicity, aseptic meningitis, 721
prednisone; therapy, pyrethrins adverse reactions, 846
Industry, pharmaceutical; research; biotechnology, genetic engineering, survey, 713
Infections; therapy; opportunistic, AIDS, 511
Influenza vaccines; interactions; phenytoin, blood levels, 828
Infusion devices, see **Devices, infusion pumps**

Injections
acetylcysteine; investigational protocols, U.S., 563
enalaprilat; hypertension therapy, FDA approvals, 416
gentamicin; adverse reactions, preservatives, 269
gentamicin sulfate; administration, CRIS, minibags, 303
intrathecal; diluents, 265
intravenous; toxicity, phlebitis, administration methods, 760
tobramycin sulfate; i.v. administration systems, 367; i.v. administration systems, pharmacokinetics, 374
vancomycin hydrochloride; toxicity, red-man syndrome, 184
verapamil; i.v., oral, dosage conversion, 791
Institutional Review Boards; clinical studies; role, sample size selection, 694
Intravenous therapy
anti-infective agents; toxicity, phlebitis, administration methods, 760
catheters; dressing changes, effects, infections, 88; flushing, sodium chloride, heparin, 832; heparin vs. sodium chloride flushes, 439
Investigational drugs, see **Drugs, investigational**
Ipratropium bromide; review, 670
Iron; anemia; therapy, kidney failure, 117
Iron preparations; iron; anemia therapy, kidney failure, 117
Isoniazid; mycobacterium infections; combined therapy, pediatrics, 545
Isotretinoin; labeling; FDA regulations, contraindications, pregnancy, 490
Ivermectin; onchocerciasis; distribution, developing countries, 11

J

Joint National Committee on Detection, Evaluation and Treatment of High Blood Pressure; reports; hypertension therapy, protocols, 837

K

Ketoconazole
availability; effects, food, gastric pH, 228
blood levels; malabsorption, fluconazole absorption, 622
therapy; review, 424
Kidney failure
digitoxin; interference, digitoxin-like substance, 825
estrogens conjugated; chronic GI hemorrhage therapy, 906
filtration; hemo-, drug dosages, 198
Kidney failure
sodium bromate; acute, toxicity, poisoning, pediatrics, 68
therapy; anemia, 117

L

Labeling
aspirin; toxicity, Reye's syndrome, FDA regulations, 639
isotretinoin; FDA regulations, contraindications, pregnancy, 490
neomycin sulfate; FDA regulations; 490
streptokinase; myocardial infarction therapy, 85
Laboratories; errors; cholesterol blood levels, measurement, 260
Laws; National Childhood Vaccine Injury Act; adverse reactions reports, 489
Letters, 18, 95, 269, 423, 497, 570, 720, 792, 867
Anabolic steroid use as an AIDS risk factor, 95
Applicability of phenytoin predictive formulas to long-term-care facility residents, 497
Aseptic meningitis associated with muromonab-CD3 therapy, 721
Diminishing bioavailability of oral leucovorin calcium, 721
Hearing loss associated with muromonab-CD3 therapy, 867
Magnesium gluconate can be used as oral supplement, 269
Midazolam sedation and amnesia in elective cardioversion, 423
Notice to readers, 18
Phlebitis associated with vancomycin therapy, 720
Routine monitoring of serum vancomycin concentrations: the answer lies in the middle, 18
Sodium thiosulfate unproven as bromate antidote, 570
Status of injectable calcium antagonists, 497
Storing extra calibration curves in the TDx assay system, 792
Suspected gentamicin allergy could be sulfite sensitivity, 269
Wanted: insightful authors of review articles, 95
Leucovorin
blood levels; and metabolites, administration routes, 52
breast neoplasms; combined therapy, 560
Leucovorin calcium; pharmacokinetics; oral, i.m., i.v., 52
Leukemia; mitoxantrone; therapy, review, 574
Levothyroxine sodium; hypothyroidism; therapy, effects, theophylline half-life, 620
Lisinopril; review, 659
Lithium; blood levels; tetracycline interactions, 314
Lithium carbonate; interactions; tetracycline, blood levels, 314
Liver diseases; effects; false-positive digoxin blood levels, 444
Lovastatin; hypercholesterolemia; therapy, review, 21
Lung diseases; ipratropium bromide; obstructive, therapy, 670
Lymphoma; mitoxantrone; therapy, review, 574

M

Management, see **Administration**
Manufacturers
new drugs; FDA approvals, 1987, 166
orphan drugs; FDA approvals, 1987, 253
Marketing
diclofenac sodium; FDA approvals, 785
minoxidil; topical solutions, FDA approvals, 858
new drugs; FDA approvals, 1987, 166
nizatidine; FDA approvals, 560
Matrices; wax; potassium, supplements, equivalency, 150
Mechanism of action
acids, fatty; 3-omega, antilipemic effects, 795
antifungals; review, 424
fluoxetine hydrochloride, 169
guanfacine hydrochloride; review, 187
lovastatin; hypercholesterolemia therapy, review, 21
pentamidine isethionate; *P. carinii* pneumonia therapy, 501
sulbactam; β-lactamase inhibition, review, 37
teicoplanin; review, 647
Meningitis
amphotericin B and flucytosine; cryptococcal, therapy, AIDS, 528
flucytosine and amphotericin B; cryptococcal, therapy, AIDS, 528
muromonab-CD3; aseptic, toxicity, 721
Meperidine; concomitant therapy, 528
Merck; ivermectin; distribution, developing countries, 11
Metabolism
cefotaxime; interactions, desacetylcefotaxime, synergism, 901
guanfacine hydrochloride; review, 187
leucovorin; pharmacokinetics, 52
nicardipine; review, 97
nitrendipine; review, 97
pentoxifylline; metabolites, interference, theophylline, blood level assays, 457
verapamil; i.v., oral, dosage conversion, 791
Methionyl human growth hormone, see **Somatrem**
Methodology
albumin human; hypoalbuminemia, equations, dosage prediction, 894
aminoglycosides; monitoring, cost–benefit analysis, 608
anticonvulsants; blood level monitoring, pediatrics, 688
clinical studies; sample size selection, 694
creatinine; clearance estimation, nutrition disorders, 62
cystic fibrosis; therapy, response indicators, 897
digoxin; blood levels, false positive, 444; blood levels, interference, digoxin-like factor, 449
dosage schedules; changes, prediction, models, 681
gentamicin; computer models, blood level errors, 307
nutrition; parenteral, fibronectin, somatomedin-C, markers, 889
quinidine; serum free fractions, temperature effects, in vitro, 142
Methotrexate; breast neoplasms; combined therapy, 560
Methylcellulose; conjunctivitis; therapy, toxic epidermal necrolysis, 766
Methyldopa; comparison, guanfacine hydrochloride; hypertension therapy, review, 187
Methylprednisolone
anaphylaxis; therapy, pyrethrins adverse reactions, 846
concomitant therapy, 867
5-Methyltetrahydrofolate, see **Methyltetrahydrofolate**
Methyltetrahydrofolate; metabolites; leucovorin, blood levels, 52
Metoclopramide hydrochloride; vomiting; prophylaxis, cisplatin toxicity, 454
Metolazone; concomitant therapy, 906
Metronidazole
enterocolitis; pseudomembranous, 93
resistance; *T. vaginalis,* therapy, 718
Mexiletine; arrhythmia; combined therapy, review, 808
Mezlocillin sodium; comparison, ticarcillin disodium; dosage, pharmacokinetics, 380
Miconazole; therapy; review, 424
Midazolam; anesthetics; electric countershock, 423
Midazolam hydrochloride; status epilepticus; continuous i.v. therapy, 322
Minerals; phosphorus; hypophosphatemia therapy, 123
Minimum inhibitory concentration; clindamycin; muscle, wound levels, 820
Minoxidil; alopecia; topical solutions, FDA approvals, 858
Mitoxantrone; review, 574
Models
dosage schedules; changes, prediction, 681
pharmacokinetics; calculations, gentamicin blood level errors, 307
Morphine; body distribution; ascites, nasogastric fluid levels, 842
Morphine sulfate; dosage; high, body distribution, 842
Mouthwashes
amphotericin B; oral candidiasis therapy, 70
stomatitis; therapy, 14
Moxalactam; comparison, cefotetan, cefoxitin, ceftizoxime; therapy, selection, 285
Muromonab-CD3
adverse reactions; sensorineural hearing loss, 867
toxicity; aseptic meningitis, 721
Mycobacterium infections; antituberculars; combined therapy, pediatrics, 545
Mycosis fungoides; phenytoin; adverse reactions, pseudolymphoma, 153
Myocardial infarction
alteplase; therapy, FDA approvals, 85
alteplase, comparison, streptokinase; therapy, equivalency, 469, 473
streptokinase; therapy, labeling indications, 85
streptokinase, comparison, alteplase; therapy, equivalency, 469, 473

N

Nafcillin
cystic fibrosis; therapy, response indicators, methodology, 897
toxicity; neutropenia, AIDS, 398
Naloxone; anaphylaxis; therapy, pyrethrins adverse reactions, 846
National Cancer Institute; protocols; breast neoplasms, adjuvant therapy, 560
National Childhood Vaccine Injury Act; drugs, adverse reactions; reports, procedures, DHHS regulations, 489
Negroes; diltiazem hydrochloride; effects, glucose tolerance, 235
Neomycin sulfate; regulations; labeling, FDA, 490
Neuroleptic malignant syndrome; tranquilizers; toxicity, therapy, 697
Neutropenia; anti-infective agents; toxicity, AIDS, 398
News, 7, 85, 166, 253, 334, 413, 488, 560, 634, 710, 785, 858
Biotechnology-based drug products grow in importance, 713
CDC advises on detection and control of antibiotic-resistant *Neisseria gonorrhoeae,* 88
CDC updates influenza recommendations for 1988–89 season, 713
Conference for health-statistics data users set, 419
Design of future thrombolytic studies explored by speaker, 786
Distribution of ivermectin for onchocerciasis announced by Merck, 11
Efficacy of *Haemophilus influenzae* vaccine reassessed,

12
Efficacy of intravenous streptokinase after myocardial infarction confirmed; labeled indications expanded, 85
Experimental antineoplastic regimen granted treatment IND status, 264
FDA amends standards for nonsterile neomycin sulfate to specify oral use only, 490
FDA approves marketing of diclofenac, 785
FDA approves marketing of second fluoroquinolone, ciprofloxacin, 7
FDA approves treatment IND protocols for selegiline and pentostatin, 786
FDA approves treatment IND protocol for trimetrexate, 337
FDA challenges Alzheimer's disease study findings, 337
FDA divides drugs and biologics evaluation unit, 11
FDA issues consumer warning, announces crackdown on bogus Retin A products, 714
FDA requires new, permanent Reye's syndrome warning on aspirin products, 639
FDA requires stronger warnings, imposes no limits on isotretinoin use, 490
FDA's drug review process is focus of attention in 1987; agency approves 27 new products, 166
Focus of new FDA division is AIDS, opportunistic infections, 337
Fourth histamine antagonist, nizatidine, reaches U.S. market, 560
Future applications of biotechnology explored by ACCP speakers, 710
Ganciclovir shows promise against cytomegalovirus, but data are insufficient for approval recommendation, 86
Guidelines for authors of biomedical journal articles revised, 413
Guidelines issued on treatment of pediatric bacterial meningitis, 638
Immunization of younger children possible with new *Haemophilus influenzae* vaccine, 169
Information sheets for institutional review boards available from FDA, 419
Marketing of intravenous enalaprilat approved by FDA, 416
More potent inactivated poliovirus vaccine approved by FDA; CDC to review vaccination policies in 1988, 169
National Cancer Institute announces new study findings on breast-cancer treatment, 560
National committee recommends greater flexibility in stepped-care treatment of hypertension, 488
New AIDS reference service available through National Library of Medicine, 714
News Briefs, 12, 176, 264, 340, 420, 562, 639, 717, 786, 862
Overview of studies shows benefit of perioperative heparin use, 562
Panel cites deficiencies in cholesterol testing, urges national laboratory standardization, 260
Papers sought for National Conference on High Blood Pressure Control, 714
Pediatrics academy issues recommendations on use of *Haemophilus influenzae* type b conjugate vaccine, 634
Periodic dressing changes of peripheral venous catheter sites not indicated, study shows, 88
Preliminary findings suggest APSAC reduces mortality after myocardial infarction, 416
Preliminary study suggests role for clonidine in smoking cessation, 560
Primary prevention study finds cardiovascular benefit with aspirin therapy, 253
Procedures for reporting childhood-vaccine injuries announced, 489
Recombinant tissue-plasminogen activator approved by FDA, 85
Record number of orphan drug designations granted in 1987, 253
Reimbursement for contraception counseling, initial pregnancy test included in isotretinoin program, 786
Report supports FDA's bioequivalence evaluation criteria, advocates more stringent statistical testing, 334
Research fellowships and grants offered for 1988–1989, 12
Rule on nonprescription first-aid antibiotics finalized by FDA, 176
Second AIDS vaccine enters clinical trials, 264
Serotonin-uptake inhibition accounts for activity of new antidepressant, 169
Studies refute efficacy of corticosteroids in severe sepsis, 11
Studies suggest possible role for sucralfate in critically ill patients, 172
Study demonstrates efficacy of clozapine in treatment-resistant schizophrenia, 858
Study finds similar reperfusion rates with intravenous APSAC and intracoronary streptokinase in acute myocardial infarction, 634
Study shows gemfibrozil reduces risk of coronary heart disease, 86
Study shows photoaged skin improves with topical tretinoin, 263
Study suggests added benefit from combined aspirin–streptokinase therapy after myocardial infarction, 785
Study suggests limited role for comprehensive toxicology testing in drug overdoses, 337
Study suggests role for trimetrexate in AIDS-associated *Pneumocystis carinii* pneumonia, 7
Study supports previous findings of colchicine activity in primary biliary cirrhosis, 714
Topical minoxidil approved by FDA, 862
Upcoming Specialty Meetings, 12, 92, 176, 264, 340, 420, 490, 562, 639, 717, 788, 858
Wider use of clomipramine approved by FDA, 638

Niacin; and lovastatin; hypercholesterolemia, combined therapy, 21
Nicardipine; review, 97
Nicotinic acid, see **Niacin**
Nifedipine
comparison, nicardipine, nitrendipine, 97
concomitant therapy, 906
Nitrendipine; review, 97
Nitroglycerin; concomitant therapy, 906
Nizatidine; ulcers; duodenal, FDA approvals, 560
Nomograms; creatinine; clearance estimation, nutrition disorders, 62
Nutrition
diet; hypercholesterolemia therapy, controversy, 592, 604; hypertension therapy, protocols, 837; oral, phosphorus, hypophosphatemia therapy, 123
parenteral; fibronectin, somatomedin-C levels, markers, 889; hypoalbuminemia, albumin dosage prediction, 894; Kaposi's sarcoma, AIDS, 536; pediatrics, review, 351; therapy, AIDS, 512
Nutrition disorders; creatinine; clearance estimation, 62

O

Obsessive-compulsive disorder; clomipramine hydrochloride; treatment IND, FDA approvals, 638
OKT3, see **Muromonab-CD3**
Omeprazole; ulcers; therapy, review, 725
Onchocerciasis; ivermectin; therapy, distribution, developing countries, 11
Opiate antagonists; naloxone; therapy, pyrethrins adverse reactions, 846
Oral rehydration compound; diarrhea; infectious, therapy, review, 746
Osteoarthritis; diclofenac sodium; therapy, FDA approvals, 785

P

Package inserts; streptokinase; labeling indications, myocardial infarction, 85
Parenterals, see **Injections**
Patches transdermal; clonidine; withdrawal, rebound hypertension, geriatrics, 772
Patient care; aminoglycosides; pharmacokinetics monitoring, cost benefit, 608
Pediatrics
acetaminophen; overdose, toxicity, 391
antituberculars; mycobacterium infections, combined therapy, 545
aspirin; toxicity, Reye's syndrome, FDA labeling regulations, 639
Haemophilus b polysaccharide vaccines; conjugates, FDA approvals, 169
heparin sodium and sodium chloride; catheter patency, 832
nutrition; parenteral, review, 351
phenytoin; blood levels, binding, 688
rifampin; toxicity, red-man syndrome, 616
Rocky Mountain spotted fever; therapy, 109
sodium bromate; poisoning, 68
sodium chloride; alone and with heparin, catheter patency, 832
somatrem, comparison, somatropin recombinant; growth disorders, equivalency, 239
somatropin recombinant, comparison, somatrem; growth disorders, equivalency, 239
valproic acid; blood levels, binding, 688
Pediculicides; pyrethrins; adverse reactions, anaphylaxis, 846
Penicillins
ampicillin sodium, combination, sulbactam sodium; therapy review, 37
cystic fibrosis; therapy, response indicators, methodology, 897
mezlocillin sodium, comparison, ticarcillin disodium; dosage, pharmacokinetics, 380
ticarcillin disodium, comparison, mezlocillin sodium; dosage, pharmacokinetics, 380
toxicity; phlebitis, catheter flushes, 439; phlebitis, i.v. administration, 760
Pentamidine isethionate; pneumonia; *P. carinii*, therapy, AIDS, 501, 514
Pentoxifylline; interactions; theophylline, blood level assays, 457
Perphenazine; toxicity; neuroleptic malignant syndrome, therapy, 697
Pharmaceutical Manufacturers Association; data collection; biotechnology, genetic engineering research, 713
Pharmacokinetics
alteplase, 85
aminoglycosides; critical patients, variations, 207; monitoring, cost–benefit analysis, 608
antifungals; review, 424
bepridil; review, 97
cefmetazole; bile, gallbladder levels, 467
cefotetan; comparison, antibiotics, selection, 285
cefoxitin; comparison, antibiotics, selection, 285
ceftizoxime; comparison, antibiotics, selection, 285
clindamycin; muscle, wound levels, 820
consultation; dosage changes, prediction, models, 681
diclofenac sodium, 785
drugs; blood, urine levels, computers, 792
fluoxetine hydrochloride, 169
gentamicin; calculations, blood level errors, 307
glipizide; geriatrics, 224
guanfacine hydrochloride; review, 187
ibuprofen; interactions, cimetidine, ranitidine, lack, 317
ipratropium bromide, 670
leucovorin; oral, i.m., i.v., 52
lisinopril, 659
lovastatin; review, 21
mezlocillin sodium, comparison, ticarcillin disodium; high, low dosage, 380
minoxidil; topical solutions, 858
mitoxantrone; review, 574
morphine; ascites, nasogastric fluid levels, 842
moxalactam; comparison, antibiotics, selection, 285
nicardipine; review, 97
nitrendipine; review, 97
nizatidine, 560
omeprazole; review, 725
pentamidine isethionate; review, 501
phenytoin; interactions, influenza vaccines, 828
propafenone; review, 869
sucralfate; interactions, theophylline, 58
sulbactam; review, 37
teicoplanin; review, 647
theophylline; interactions, sucralfate, 58
ticarcillin disodium, comparison, mezlocillin sodium; high, low dosage, 380
tobramycin; i.v. administration systems, 374
Phenobarbital; excretion; hemofiltration, 198
Phenobarbital sodium; status epilepticus; therapy, 322
Phenytoin
adverse reactions; pseudolymphoma, mycosis fungoides, 153
blood levels; binding, factors, pediatrics, 688; i.v. administration, 219
interactions; influenza vaccines, blood levels, 828
Phenytoin sodium
seizures; therapy, i.v. infusion, 219
status epilepticus; therapy, 322
Phlebitis
catheters; toxicity, heparin vs. sodium chloride flushes, 439
cephalosporins; toxicity, i.v. administration methods, 760
heparin sodium and sodium chloride; catheter patency, pediatrics, 832
intravenous therapy; dressing changes, effects, lack, 88
penicillins; toxicity, i.v. administration methods, 760
sodium chloride; alone and with heparin, catheter patency, 832
vancomycin hydrochloride; toxicity, i.v. administration, 720
Phosphates; hypophosphatemia; therapy, 123

Phosphorus; hypophosphatemia; therapy, 123
Pituitary hormones
somatrem, comparison, somatropin recombinant; equivalency, 239
somatropin recombinant, comparison, somatrem; equivalency, 239
Plasminogen human tissue-type activator, see **Alteplase**
Pneumonia
pentamidine isethionate; *P. carinii*, therapy, AIDS, 501
therapy; *P. carinii*, AIDS, 514
trimetrexate; treatment IND, *P. carinii*, AIDS, 337
Poisoning; sodium bromate; hair-waving preparations, pediatrics, 68
Policies and procedures, see **Administration**
Polio vaccines; approvals; FDA, 1987, 169
Potassium; dosage; supplements, equivalency, 150
Potassium bicarbonate; concomitant therapy, 906
Potassium chloride; equivalency, generic; supplements, 150
Prazosin; concomitant therapy, 906
Prednisone
anaphylaxis; therapy, pyrethrins adverse reactions, 846
breast neoplasms; combined therapy, 560
concomitant therapy, 867
epidermal necrolysis; toxic, therapy, 766
Pregnancy; isotretinoin; contraindications, FDA labeling regulations, 490
Preservatives; sodium bisulfite; adverse reactions, anaphylaxis, 269
Procainamide; arrhythmia; combined therapy, review, 808
Procainamide hydrochloride; sustained release; generic equivalency, availability, 135
Prolactin inhibitors; bromocriptine; and dantrolene, neuroleptic malignant syndrome therapy, 697
Propafenone; arrhythmia; therapy, review, 869
Propranolol; toxicity; depression, 146
Proteins; nutrition; parenteral, pediatrics, review, 351
Protocols
acetylcysteine; i.v., oral, acetaminophen poisoning, 563
breast neoplasms; therapy, NCI recommendations, 560
cardiac drugs; arrhythmia, combined therapy, 808
clomipramine hydrochloride; obsessive-compulsive disorder, treatment IND, 638
hypotensive agents; 1988, changes, 837
polio vaccines; ACIP, changes, 169
trimetrexate; treatment IND, *P. carinii* pneumonia, 337
***Pseudomonas* infections**
aminoglycosides; therapy, 385
ampicillin sodium, combination, sulbactam sodium; resistance, 37
Psychomotor-agitation; psychotherapeutic agents; therapy, geriatrics, 865
Psychotherapeutic agents; psychomotor agitation; therapy, geriatrics, 865
Pyrethrins; adverse reactions; anaphylaxis, 846

Q

Quinidine
arrhythmia; combined therapy, review, 808
blood levels; free fractions, temperature effects, 142
Quinidine sulfate; interactions; atropine, combination, diphenoxylate, 139

R

Race; Negroes; diltiazem effects, glucose tolerance, 235
Radioimmunoassay
digitoxin; interference, digitoxin-like substance, 825
digoxin; false-positive blood levels, 444; interference, lack, digoxin-like factor, 449
Ranitidine
comparison, famotidine; therapy, review, 271
concomitant therapy, 906
excretion; hemofiltration, 198
Ranitidine hydrochloride; interactions; ibuprofen, lack, 317
Rational therapy
hypercholesterolemia; review, 592, 604, 605
nutrition; parenteral, AIDS, 512
r-DNA somatropin, see **Somatropin recombinant**
Reconstitution, see **Drugs, reconstitution**
Regulations
Department of Health and Human Services; vaccines, adverse reaction reports, 489
enalaprilat; FDA approval, 416
Food and Drug Administration; alteplase approvals, 85; approvals, *Haemophilus* b conjugated vaccine, 169; aspirin, Reye's syndrome, labeling, 639; ciprofloxacin approvals, 7; clomipramine treatment IND, 638; ganciclovir approval denials, 86; generic drugs, equivalency, 334; marketing approvals, diclofenac, 785; new drug approvals, 1987, 166; nizatidine approvals, 560; orphan drug approvals, 1987, 253; topical minoxidil, approvals, 858; trimetrexate, treatment IND, 337
isotretinoin; FDA, labeling, contraindications, pregnancy, 490
neomycin sulfate; labeling, FDA, 490
Replacement solutions
dextrose; therapy, pyrethrins adverse reactions, 846
oral rehydration compound; infectious diarrhea therapy, review, 746
Reports; Joint National Committee on Detection, Evaluation and Treatment of High Blood Pressure; 1988 protocols, changes, 837
Research; industry, pharmaceutical; biotechnology, genetic engineering, survey, 713
Resistance
antifungals; review, 424
metronidazole; *T. vaginalis*, therapy, 718
mezlocillin sodium, comparison, ticarcillin disodium; *E. coli*, dosage, 380
ticarcillin disodium, comparison, mezlocillin sodium; *E. coli*, dosage, 380
Respiratory smooth-muscle relaxants
aminophylline; theophylline half-life, hypothyroidism, 620; therapy, pyrethrins adverse reactions, 846
theophylline; blood levels, tests comparison, 462; excretion, hemofiltration, 198; interactions, pentoxifylline, metabolites, blood levels, 457; interactions, sucralfate, 58
Respiratory-tract infections; ampicillin sodium, combination, sulbactam sodium; therapy, 37
Retinitis; ganciclovir; therapy, FDA approval denials, 86
Reye's syndrome; aspirin; toxicity, FDA labeling regulations, 639
Rifabutin; mycobacterium infections; combined therapy, pediatrics, 545
Rifampin; toxicity; red-man syndrome, pediatrics, 616
Ringer's injection lactated
concomitant therapy, 68
diluents; intrathecal injections, 265
Rocky Mountain spotted fever; therapy, 109

S

Sarcoma; nutrition; Kaposi's, parenteral, AIDS, 536
Seizures; phenytoin sodium; therapy, i.v. infusion, 219
Sex; patients; catheters, patency, 439; digitoxin radioimmunoassay, kidney failure, 825
Shampoos; pyrethrins; adverse reactions, anaphylaxis, 846
Silver sulfadiazine; epidermal necrolysis; toxic, therapy, 766
Skeletal-muscle relaxants; dantrolene sodium; and bromocriptine, neuroleptic malignant syndrome therapy, 697
Skin and mucous membrane preparations
isotretinoin; FDA labeling regulations, contraindications, 490
silver sulfadiazine; toxic epidermal necrolysis therapy, 766
Smooth-muscle relaxants; benztropine; neuroleptic malignant syndrome therapy, 697
Sodium bicarbonate; concomitant therapy, 68
Sodium bisulfite; adverse reactions; preservatives, gentamicin injections, 269
Sodium bromate; toxicity; poisoning, hair-waving preparations, pediatrics, 68
Sodium chloride
alone and with heparin sodium; catheter patency, pediatrics, 832
and dextrose; diluents, gentamicin administration, CRIS, 303
comparison, heparin sodium; catheter flushes, 439
diluents; intrathecal injections, 265
injections; phenytoin, i.v. admixtures, 219
Sodium iodide I 131; Graves' disease; therapy, effects, theophylline half-life, 620
Sodium nitroprusside; hypertension; crisis, therapy, review, 582; piston infusion pumps, pharmacodynamics, 214
Sodium thiosulfate
concomitant therapy, 842
therapy; bromate poisoning, 68
Solutions; amphotericin B; oral candidiasis therapy, 70
Solutions, ophthalmic; methylcellulose; conjunctivitis therapy, toxic epidermal necrolysis, 766
Somatrem; comparison, somatropin recombinant; growth disorders, equivalency, 239
Somatropin recombinant; comparison, somatrem; equivalency, 239
Spectinomicin; comparison, ampicillin sodium, combination, sulbactam sodium; therapy, 37
Spondylitis; diclofenac sodium; ankylosing, therapy, FDA approvals, 785
Standards; cholesterol; blood levels, measurement, 260
Status epilepticus
midazolam hydrochloride; continuous i.v. therapy, 322
phenobarbital sodium; therapy, 322
phenytoin sodium; therapy, 322
Stomatitis
antineoplastic agents; toxicity, therapy, 14
cromolyn sodium; aphthous, therapy, 334
Streptococcal infections; aminoglycosides; therapy, 385
Streptokinase
comparison, alteplase; myocardial infarction therapy, 469, 473
myocardial infarction; therapy, labeling, 85
Streptomycin; mycobacterium infections; combined therapy, pediatrics, 545
Sucralfate
interactions; theophylline, pharmacokinetics, 58
stomatitis; therapy, 14
Sulbactam; therapy; review, 37
Sulbactam sodium; combination, ampicillin sodium; therapy review, 37
Sulfamethoxazole; combination, trimethoprim; *P. carinii* pneumonia therapy, AIDS, 514; toxicity, neutropenia, AIDS, 398
Sulfonamides; sulfamethoxazole, combination, trimethoprim; *P. carinii* pneumonia therapy, AIDS, 514
Sulfones; dapsone; and trimethoprim, pneumonia therapy, AIDS, 514
Sulindac
adverse reactions; toxic epidermal necrolysis, 766
concomitant therapy, 772
Sultamicillin; therapy, 37
Surgical supplies; administration sets; i.v. tobramycin, accuracy, 367
Surgical wound infection; antibiotics; selection, therapy, prophylaxis, 285
Sustained-action medications
lithium carbonate; interactions, tetracycline, 314
nicardipine; review, 97
nitrendipine; review, 97
procainamide hydrochloride; generic equivalency, 135
Sympatholytic agents
alpha blockers; interactions, epinephrine, hypotension, 493
beta blockers; and nicardipine or nitrendipine, hypertension, 97; combined therapy, arrhythmia, 808; hypertension therapy, protocols, 837
Sympathomimetic agents
albuterol; therapy, pyrethrins adverse reactions, 846
epinephrine; and diphenhydramine, therapy, anaphylaxis, 269; therapy, pyrethrins adverse reactions, 846
Syringe pumps, see **Devices, syringe pumps**

T

Tablets; clonidine hydrochloride; therapy, transdermal clonidine withdrawal, 772
Tacrine; Alzheimer's disease; clinical studies, FDA attitudes, 337
Tamoxifen; breast neoplasms; adjuvant therapy, 560; therapy, early stage, 640
Taste; palatability; acetylcysteine, administration, 563
Teicoplanin; review, 647
Temperature; quinidine; effects, free fractions, in vitro, 142
Teratogenicity; isotretinoin; FDA labeling regulations, contraindications, 490
Tests, laboratory
Acculevel; theophylline blood levels, 462
cholesterol; blood levels, measurement, standards, 260
digitoxin; interference, digitoxin-like substance, 825
digoxin; false positive, comparison, 444; radioimmunoassay, interference, lack, digoxin-like factor, 449
quinidine; free fractions, temperature effects, 142
Seralyzer; theophylline blood levels, 462
theophylline; blood levels, comparison, 462; interference, pentoxifylline, metabolites, 457

urine levels; computer programs, TDx assay, 792
Vision; theophylline blood levels, 462
Tetracycline; Rocky Mountain spotted fever; therapy, 109
Tetracycline hydrochloride
interactions; lithium, blood levels, 314
Rocky Mountain spotted fever; therapy, 109
Tetracyclines
tetracycline; Rocky Mountain spotted fever, 109
tetracycline hydrochloride; interactions, lithium, blood levels, 314; Rocky Mountain spotted fever, 109
Theophylline
blood levels; monoclonal antibody tests comparison, 462
excretion; hemofiltration, 198
half-life; effects, hypothyroidism, 620
interactions; pentoxifylline, metabolites, blood level assays, 457; sucralfate, pharmacokinetics, 58
Therapy Consultation, 14, 93, 184, 265, 344, 422, 493, 563, 640, 718, 791, 865
Catecholamine selection for vasopressor-dependent patients, 493
Choice of diluents for intrathecal drug administration, 265
Conversion from oral to intravenous verapamil therapy, 791
Management of vancomycin-induced "red-man syndrome," 184
Metronidazole for pseudomembranous colitis, 93
Topical cromolyn sodium for recurrent aphthous ulcers, 344
Treatment of acetaminophen overdose when oral acetylcysteine therapy is not tolerated, 563
Treatment of acute agitation in the elderly, 865
Treatment of metronidazole-resistant cases of vaginal trichomoniasis, 718
Treatment of stomatitis associated with antineoplastic-drug therapy, 14
Use of H_2 histamine antagonists in allergic disorders, 422
Use of tamoxifen in stage I breast cancer, 640
Thioridazine; toxicity; neuroleptic malignant syndrome, therapy, 697
Thrombolytic agents
alteplase; FDA approvals, 85
alteplase, comparison, streptokinase; myocardial infarction therapy, 469, 473
streptokinase; labeling indications, myocardial infarction, 85
streptokinase, comparison, alteplase; myocardial infarction therapy, 469, 473
Thyroid drugs; levothyroxine sodium; therapy, effects, theophylline half-life, 620
Ticarcillin; toxicity; neutropenia, AIDS, 398
Ticarcillin disodium; comparison, mezlocillin sodium; dosage, pharmacokinetics, 380
Time; sampling; gentamicin blood levels, errors, 307
Time studies; theophylline; blood levels tests comparison, 462
Tissue levels
cefmetazole; gallbladder, 467
clindamycin; muscle, postoperative prophylaxis, 820
Tissue plasminogen activator, see **Alteplase**
Tobramycin
blood levels; i.v. administration systems, 367
cystic fibrosis; therapy, response indicators, methodology, 897
pharmacokinetics; i.v. administration systems, 374
urine levels; computer programs, TDx assay, 792
Tobramycin sulfate; administration systems; minibags, pumps, accuracy, 367; minibags, pumps, pharmacokinetics, 374
Topical preparations
cromolyn sodium; aphthous stomatitis therapy, 334
minoxidil; alopecia therapy, FDA approvals, 858
pyrethrins; adverse reactions, anaphylaxis, 846
Toxicity
see also **Drugs, adverse reactions**
acetaminophen; overdose, pediatrics, 391
acetylcysteine; side effects, i.v., oral, 563
acids, fatty; 3-omega, side effects, 795
alpha blockers and epinephrine; hypotension, 493
alteplase; side effects, 85
alteplase, comparison, streptokinase; side effects, 469
aminoglycosides; pharmacokinetics monitoring, cost benefit, 608; side effects, dosage schedules, 385
amphotericin B; side effects, mouthwashes, lack, 70
ampicillin sodium, combination, sulbactam sodium; side effects, 37
antifungals; review, 424
anti-infective agents; effects, GI flora, review, 878; neutropenia, AIDS, 398
antineoplastic agents; stomatitis, therapy, 14
aspirin; Reye's syndrome, FDA labeling regulations, 639
bepridil; side effects, 97
cardiac drugs; side effects, combined therapy, 808
catheters; phlebitis, heparin vs. sodium chloride flushes, 439; phlebitis, infections, dressing changes, 88
cefotetan; comparison, antibiotics, side effects, 285
cefoxitin; comparison, antibiotics, side effects, 285
ceftizoxime; comparison, antibiotics, side effects, 285
cephalosporins; phlebitis, i.v. administration methods, 760
cimetidine, comparison, famotidine; side effects, 271
ciprofloxacin hydrochloride; side effects, 7
cisplatin; metoclopramide administration rate, 454
clonidine; withdrawal, rebound hypertension, 772
diazepam; overdose, diagnosis, flumazenil, 614
diclofenac sodium; side effects, 785
diltiazem hydrochloride, comparison, verapamil hydrochloride; side effects, 129; effects, glucose tolerance, 235
epinephrine and alpha blockers or tranquilizers; hypotension, 493
erythropoietin; side effects, 117
famotidine, comparison, cimetidine, ranitidine; side effects, 271
flucytosine; bone marrow suppression, 528
fluoxetine hydrochloride, 169
ganciclovir; side effects, approval denials, 86
guanfacine hydrochloride; side effects, review, 187
ipratropium bromide; side effects, 670
isotretinoin; FDA labeling regulations, contraindications, pregnancy, 490
lisinopril; side effects, 659
lithium carbonate; interactions, tetracycline, 314
lovastatin; side effects, review, 21
metoclopramide hydrochloride; extrapyramidal effects, administration rate, 454
midazolam; side effects, electric countershock, 423
mitoxantrone; review, 574
moxalactam; comparison, antibiotics, side effects, 285
muromonab-CD3; aseptic meningitis, 721
nicardipine; side effects, 97
nitrendipine; side effects, 97
nizatidine; side effects, 560
nutrition; parenteral, AIDS patients, 512; parenteral, pediatrics, review, 351
omeprazole; review, 725
penicillins; phlebitis, i.v. administration methods, 760
pentamidine isethionate; side effects, AIDS, 501, 514
phenytoin sodium; side effects; i.v. infusion, 219
potassium; side effects, 150
propafenone; side effects, review, 869
propranolol; depression, 146
psychotherapeutic agents; side effects, geriatrics, 865
ranitidine, comparison, famotidine; side effects, 271
rifampin; red-man syndrome, pediatrics, 616
sodium bromate; poisoning, pediatrics, 68
sodium iodide I 131; hypothyroidism, theophylline half-life, 620
somatrem, comparison, somatropin recombinant; immunogenicity, 239
somatropin recombinant, comparison, somatrem; immunogenicity, 239
streptokinase, comparison, alteplase; side effects, 469
sulbactam; side effects, review, 37
sulfamethoxazole, combination, trimethoprim; side effects, AIDS, 514
teicoplanin; side effects, 647
theophylline; half-life, hypothyroidism, 620
tranquilizers and epinephrine; hypotension, 493
tranquilizers; neuroleptic malignant syndrome, 697
vancomycin hydrochloride; phlebitis, i.v. administration, 720; red-man syndrome, 184
verapamil hydrochloride, comparison, diltiazem hydrochloride; side effects, 129
Tranquilizers
haloperidol; toxicity, neuroleptic malignant syndrome, 697
interactions; epinephrine, hypotension, 493
perphenazine; toxicity, neuroleptic malignant syndrome, 697
thioridazine; toxicity, neuroleptic malignant syndrome, 697
Transplantation
pancreas; rejection therapy, muromonab-CD3 adverse reactions, 867
renal; muromonab-CD3 toxicity, aseptic meningitis, 721
Trichomonas vaginalis
metronidazole; resistance, high dose therapy, 718
resistance; metronidazole, therapy, 718
Trimethoprim
and dapsone or sulfamethoxazole; *P. carinii* pneumonia therapy, AIDS, 514
combination, sulfamethoxazole; toxicity, neutropenia, AIDS, 398
Trimetrexate; pneumonia; FDA treatment IND, AIDS, 337

U

Ulcers
cimetidine, comparison, famotidine; therapy, review, 271
famotidine, comparison, cimetidine, ranitidine; therapy, review, 271
nizatidine; duodenal, FDA approvals, 560
omeprazole; gastric, peptic, therapy, review, 725
ranitidine, comparison, famotidine; therapy, review, 271
United States; industry, pharmaceutical; research, biotechnology, genetic engineering, 713
United States Public Health Service; Advisory Committee on Immunization Practices; polio immunization guidelines, 169
Urinary-tract infections; ampicillin sodium, combination, sulbactam sodium; therapy, 37
Urine levels
creatinine; clearance estimation, nutrition disorders, 62
drugs; computer programs, TDx assay, 792

V

Vaccines
adverse reactions; reports, DHHS regulations, 489
Haemophilus b polysaccharide; conjugates, FDA approvals, 169
influenza; interactions, phenytoin, blood levels, 828
polio; FDA approvals, 1987, 169
Valproic acid; blood levels; binding, factors, pediatrics, 688
Vancomycin
blood levels; monitoring, costs, 18
comparison, metronidazole; pseudomembranous enterocolitis therapy, 93
excretion; hemofiltration, 198
Vancomycin hydrochloride; toxicity; phlebitis, i.v. administration, 720; red-man syndrome, 184
Vehicles; water; sterile, amphotericin B oral solutions, 70
Verapamil; arrhythmia; therapy, administration routes, dosage conversion, 791
Verapamil hydrochloride; comparison, diltiazem hydrochloride; hypertension therapy, 129
Vitamins
anemia; therapy, kidney failure, 117
leucovorin calcium; pharmacokinetics, oral, i.m., i.v., 52
Volume; injections; small, gentamicin administration, CRIS, 303
Volume of distribution, see **Drugs, body distribution**
Vomiting; metoclopramide hydrochloride; prophylaxis, cisplatin toxicity, 454

W

Water; vehicles; sterile, amphotericin B oral solutions, 70
Water for Injection
diluents; gentamicin administration, CRIS, 303
vehicles; leucovorin administration, 52
Waxes; matrices; potassium supplements, equivalency, 150
Weight
patients; digitoxin radioimmunoassay, kidney failure, 825; hypertension therapy, protocols, 837
pediatrics, parenteral nutrition, review, 351
World Health Organization; ivermectin; distribution programs, developing countries, 11

Z

Zollinger-Ellison syndrome; omeprazole; therapy, review, 725

Author Index

A

Adams, Marijke H. Therapeutic evaluation of omeprazole, 725
Agostinucci, William A. Continuous i.v. infusion versus multiple bolus doses of metoclopramide for prevention of cisplatin-induced emesis, 454
Alvarado-Hughes, Mariela see Burch, Kelly J., 239
Angaran, David M. Status of injectable calcium antagonists (letter), 497
Antal, Edward J. see Stoehr, Gary P., 820
Appleman, Maria D. see Ito, Matthew K., 467
Ast, Dan see Garrelts, James C., 720, 760
A'Zary, Edward see Baker, Brian A., 135

B

Bailey, David see Blake, Kathryn V., 391
Baker, Brian A. Comparative bioavailability of two oral sustained-release procainamide products, 135
Banning, Jon W. Book review, 245
Barone, Joseph A. see Lelawongs, Parichat, 228
Barriere, Steven L. Aminoglycosides: a reassessment of their therapeutic role, 385
Barriere, Steven L. Infectious complications of AIDS (editorial), 511
Barriere, Steven L. see also Deeter, Robert G., 380
Barriere, Steven L. see also Moore, Emory S., 901
Barson, William J. see Fan-Havard, Patty, 616
Bartels, David Association between depression and propranolol use in ambulatory patients, 146
Bartkowski, Henry see Fan-Havard, Patty, 616
Bauer, Larry A. see Kobayashi, Kelly A., 224
Bauman, Jerry L. Conversion from oral to intravenous verapamil therapy (Therapy Consultation), 791
Bauman, Jerry L. see also Schoen, Marieke Dekker, 791
Baumann, Terry J. see Hutson, Paul R., 842
Bauwens, Steven F. Treatment of acute agitation in the elderly (Therapy Consultation), 865
Beck, Diane E. Predicting need for pharmacokinetic consultation follow-up using discriminant analysis, 681
Benson, John M. Clinical use of systemic antifungal agents, 424
Berardi, Rosemary R. Comparison of famotidine with cimetidine and ranitidine, 271
Berk, Steven I. see Lau, Alan H., 62
Berne, Thomas V. see Ito, Matthew K., 467
Bickley, Susan K. Drug dosing during continuous arteriovenous hemofiltration, 198
Blake, Kathryn V. Death of a child associated with multiple overdoses of acetaminophen, 391
Bledsoe, Michael A. see Smith, Christopher D., 828
Bodenheimer, Monty M. see Baker, Brian A., 135
Bolinger, Ann M. see Levin, Robert H., 545
Bosso, John A. Lack of correlation between objective indicators and clinical-response scores during antimicrobial therapy for acute pulmonary exacerbations of cystic fibrosis, 897
Boyce, Eric G. Simulated effect of gentamicin assay errors on calculated pharmacokinetic values, 307
Bradley, Edwin L. see Beck, Diane E., 681
Brandell, Renée Treatment of oral candidiasis with amphotericin B solution, 70
Brown, John M. see Pleasants, Roy A., 367
Brown, Rex O. see Powers, Douglas A., 889
Brown, Rex O. see also Reid, Dana J., 894
Bucci, Kathryn K. see McClain, Walter J., 95
Burch, Kelly J. Selection of a human growth hormone product, 239
Burki, N. K. see Clifton, G. Dennis, 462
Burton, Michael E. see Hill, Donald P. Jr., 780
Bussey, Henry I. see Mueller, Bruce A., 825

C

Canafax, Daniel M. see Joy, Martha E., 721
Canafax, Daniel M. see also Michals, Marcia, 867
Cantral, Kimberly A. Effect of sucralfate on theophylline absorption in healthy volunteers, 58
Carver, Peggy L. Treatment of metronidazole-resistant cases of vaginal trichomoniasis (Therapy Consultation), 718
Casto, Daniel T. see Mueller, Bruce A., 825
Cerra, Frank B. see Fuhs, David W., 207
Cerra, Frank B. see also Mann, Henry J., 214
Chase, Sandra L. see Brandell, Renée, 70
Chenella, Frank C. see Ito, Matthew K., 467
Chessman, Katherine Hammond see Kamper, Claudia A., 109
Chester, Michael I. S. see Johnson, Curtis A., 117
Chow, Moses S. S. Propafenone: a new antiarrhythmic agent, 869
Chrymko, Margaret M. see Munoz, Dee Marie, 303
Cimino, Marisa L. see Moore, Emory S., 901
Clay, Carol see Hamilton, Robert A., 439
Clifton, G. Dennis Accuracy and time requirements for use of three rapid theophylline assay methods, 462
Cochran, Emily B. Parenteral nutrition in pediatric patients, 351
Cohen, Ira A. Effect of pentoxifylline and its metabolites on three theophylline assays, 457
Cohen, Ira A. see also Johnson, Cary E., 620
Cohn, John R. see Brandell, Renée, 70
Colaizzi, John L. see Lelawongs, Parichat, 228
Colburn, Pamala see Carver, Peggy L., 718
Collette, David R. see Murphy, John E., 779
Connolly, Brigid see Fankhauser, Martha P., 314
Converse-Swastek, Kathleen see Cohen, Ira A., 457
Cooke, L. Evans Phenytoin-induced pseudolymphoma with mycosis fungoides manifestations, 153
Cornish, Laura A. Guanfacine hydrochloride: a centrally acting antihypertensive agent, 187
Cowan, George S. M. Jr. see Powers, Douglas A., 889
Cremer, Karl F. see Mueller, Bruce A., 825
Crisp, Catherine B. Continuous infusion of midazolam hydrochloride to control status epilepticus, 322
Culver, Charles A. Probable anaphylactoid reaction to a pyrethrin pediculocide shampoo, 846
Cunha, Burke A. see Salamone, Francine R., 501
Curran, Roger see Smith, Christopher D., 828

D

Dahl, Stephen L. Book review, 244
De Vito, Joseph see Steffan, Richard, 722
Deeter, Robert G. Pharmacokinetic and pharmacodynamic comparison of mezlocillin and ticarcillin, 380
Dela Cruz, Francine G. Efficacy of individualized phenytoin sodium loading doses administered by intravenous infusion, 219
Delafuente, Jeffrey C. Use of H_2 histamine antagonists in allergic disorders (Therapy Consultation), 422
DesChamps, Mary see Hollifield, John W., 129
Dickson, Brian see Hollifield, John W., 129
Dinonno, Emelie B. see Agostinucci, William A., 454
DiPiro, Joseph T. Use of cephalosporins with enhanced antianaerobic activity for treatment and prevention of anaerobic and mixed infections, 285
DiPiro, Joseph T. see also Hooker, K. Dale, 878
Dorson, Peter G. Book review, 628
Drew, Richard H. Use of fluconazole in a patient with documented malabsorption of ketoconazole, 622
Drinka, Paul J. Applicability of phenytoin predictive formulas to long-term-care facility residents (letter), 497

E

Eble, Melody see Koeller, Jim, 574
Edwards, Deborah L. see Lue, Jane N., 66

F

Fan-Havard, Patty Histamine-like reaction after a single intravenous dose of rifampin, 616
Fankhauser, Martha P. Evaluation of lithium-tetracycline interaction, 314
Farringer, John A. see Beck, Diane E., 681
Fekety, F. Robert see Deeter, Robert G., 380
Fekety, F. Robert see also Moore, Emory S., 901
Finley, Rebecca S. Book review, 78
Fischer, James H. see Dela Cruz, Francine G., 219
Fitzsimmons, William E. see Ponzillo, John J., 139
Franse, Valerie L. see Powers, Douglas A., 889
Frisolone, Julie False-positive serum digoxin concentrations determined by three digoxin assays in patients with liver disease, 444
Fuhs, David W. Intrapatient variation of aminoglycoside pharmacokinetics in critically ill surgery patients, 207
Fuhs, David W. see also Mann, Henry J., 214

G

Gallis, Harry A. see Drew, Richard H., 622
Gannon, Richard H. see Agostinucci, William A., 454
Gannon, Richard see also Crisp, Catherine B., 322
Garnett, William R. see Small, Ralph E., 766
Garrelts, James C. Phlebitis associated with vancomycin therapy (letter), 720
Garrelts, James C. Postinfusion phlebitis after intravenous push versus intravenous piggyback administration of antimicrobial agents, 760
Geier, Teresa M. see Seth, Shiv, 906
Gelb, Adrian W. see Ume, Emeka O. C., 614
Gelwan, Jeffrey see Frisolone, Julie, 444
Gill, Mark A. see Ito, Matthew K., 467
Gill, Mark A. see also Noguchi, Jean K., 37
Glasser, Michael see Bartels, David, 146
Gleckel, Louis see Baker, Brian A., 135
Golub, Grant R. see Agostinucci, William A., 454
Gonzalez, Edgar R. Catecholamine selection for vasopressor-dependent patients (Therapy Consultation), 493
Goodman, Robert P. see Jones, Barbara J., 235
Graves, David A. Book review, 245
Gray, James see Hollifield, John W., 129
Green, Elaine R. see Munoz, Dee Marie, 303
Green, Jeffrey A. Thrombolysis for acute myocardial infarction: is proof of a reduction in mortality critical to drug selection? 473
Green, Laurence Choice of diluents for intrathecal drug administration (Therapy Consultation), 265
Green, Lawrence see Smith, Christopher D., 828
Guarnieri, Joseph see Lelawongs, Parichat, 228
Guerrero, Rawley M. Diagnosis and treatment of neuroleptic malignant syndrome, 697
Gundersen, Berit see Lombardi, Thomas P., 832
Gutierrez, Manuel L. see McGuire, Brian W., 52

H

Hamid, Imtiaz see Krichbaum, Daniel W., 423
Hamilton, Robert A. Heparin sodium versus 0.9% sodium chloride injection for maintaining patency of indwelling intermittent infusion devices, 439
Hardin, Thomas C. see Cooke, L. Evans, 153
Harris, Steven C. see Verme, Catherine N., 142
Hasegawa, Guy R. Nicardipine, nitrendipine, and bepridil: new calcium antagonists for cardiovascular disorders, 97
Hauptman, Stephen P. see Wordell, Cindy J., 514
Hawkins, David W. Book review, 854
Healey, Walter J. see Fankhauser, Martha P., 314
Helms, Richard A. see Cochran, Emily B., 351
Hendeles, Leslie see Blake, Kathryn V., 391
Hendrickson, Dan J. see Cooke, L. Evans, 153
Heseltine, Peter N. R. see Ito, Matthew K., 467
Heusner, James J. see Hollifield, John W., 129
Hewett, Mary K. see Roohk, Bonita L., 150
Hill, Donald P. Jr. Book review, 780
Hilleman, Daniel E. Book review, 244
Hilleman, Daniel see also Chow, Moses S. S., 869
Hinson, Ann see Powers, Douglas A., 889
Hollifield, John W. Comparison of equal-weight oral dosages of verapamil hydrochloride and diltiazem hydrochloride in patients with mild to moderate hypertension, 129
Hooker, K. Dale Effect of antimicrobial therapy on bowel flora, 878
Hopefl, Alan W. What is the role of parenteral nutrition in AIDS? (editorial) 512
Horn, John R. see Kobayashi, Kelly A., 224
Hsuan, Alice T. M. see Lelawongs, Parichat, 228
Hunt, Bernard A. see Clifton, G. Dennis, 462
Hutson, Paul R. Morphine concentrations in plasma, ascitic fluid, and nasogastric aspirate fluid during high-dose intravenous morphine infusion, 842

I

Ito, Matthew K. Intraoperative serum, bile, and gallbladder-wall concentrations of cefmetazole in patients undergoing cholecystectomy, 467

J

Janson, Douglas D. Parenteral nutrition in the management of gastrointestinal Kaposi's sarcoma in a patient with AIDS, 536
Jimenez, Mayra see Moore, Emory S., 901
Johnson, Cary E. Book review, 406
Johnson, Cary E. Sodium thiosulfate unproven as bromate antidote (letter), 572
Johnson, Cary E. Theophylline toxicity after iodine 131 treatment for hyperthyroidism, 620
Johnson, Cary E. see also Cohen, Ira A., 457
Johnson, Cary E. see also Lloyd, Charles W., 123
Johnson, Cary E. see also Lue, Jane N., 66
Johnson, Curtis A. Pathophysiology and treatment of the anemia of renal failure, 117
Johnson, Jonas T. see Stoehr, Gary P., 820
Johnson, Steven M. see Stephenson, David W., 317
Jones, Barbara J. Effects of diltiazem hydrochloride on glucose tolerance in persons at risk for diabetes mellitus, 235
Joy, Martha E. Aseptic meningitis associated with muromonab-CD3 therapy (letter), 721
Jungnickel, Paul W. see Cantral, Kimberly A., 58

K

Kamper, Claudia A. Rocky Mountain spotted fever, 109
Kanter, Michele Z. see Dela Cruz, Francine G., 219
Karnes, H. Thomas see Stephenson, David W., 317
Katz, Norman L. Book review, 706
Kearney, Thomas E. see McElwee, Newell E., 570
Khanderia, Ujjaini Metronidazole for pseudomembranous colitis (Therapy Consultation), 93
Kinzie, Betty J. Treatment of stomatitis associated with antineoplastic-drug therapy (Therapy Consultation), 14
Kirkwood, Craig F. see Adams, Marijke H., 725
Kitrenos, Jack G. see Munoz, Dee Marie, 303
Klamerus, Karen J. see Zeller, Frederick P., 18
Knauft, Frederic see Crisp, Catherine B., 322
Kobayashi, Kelly A. Glipizide pharmacokinetics in young and elderly volunteers, 224
Koeller, Jim Mitoxantrone: a novel anthracycline derivative, 574
Kosnik, Edward see Fan–Havard, Patty, 616
Kradjan, Wayne A. see Kobayashi, Kelly A., 224
Krichbaum, Daniel W. Combination drug therapy for ventricular arrhythmias, 808
Krichbaum, Daniel W. Midazolam sedation and amnesia in elective cardioversion (letter), 423
Kubajak, Carol Ann M. see Fuhs, David W., 207

L

Labreche, Dustan G. Reassessment of the value of lowering serum cholesterol: questioning the wisdom of widespread intervention, 592
Lackner, Thomas E. Endogenous digoxin-like immunoreactivity in elderly patients with normal serum creatinine concentrations, 449
Larijani, Ghassem E. see Norris, Mark C., 162
LaRocca, Joanne see Garrelts, James C., 720, 760
Lau, Alan H. Estimation of creatinine clearance in malnourished patients, 62
Lau, Brad W. C. see Lackner, Thomas E., 449
Lavoie, Robert R. see Hutson, Paul R., 842
Lebsack, Cynthia see Chow, Moses S. S., 869
Leese, Philip T. see McGuire, Brian W., 52
Legendre, Robert see Lelawongs, Parichat, 228
Leikin, Jerrold B. see Dela Cruz, Francine G., 219
Lelawongs, Parichat Effect of food and gastric acidity on absorption of orally administered ketoconazole, 228
Leon, Ann L. see Mann, Katherine V., 670
Levin, Robert H. Treatment of nontuberculous mycobacterial infections in pediatric patients, 545
Lewis, George P. see Ponzillo, John J., 139
Lewis, Jack see Smith, Christopher D., 828
Lindon, James L. see Fankhauser, Martha P., 314
Lloyd, Charles W. Management of hypophosphatemia, 123
Lombardi, Thomas P. Efficacy of 0.9% sodium chloride injection with or without heparin sodium for maintaining patency of intravenous catheters in children, 832
Lowder, N. Kathryn see Mueller, Bruce A., 825
Ludden, Thomas M. see Verme, Catherine N., 142
Lue, Jane N. Bromate poisoning from ingestion of professional hair-care neutralizer, 66
Luther, R. Wayne see Reid, Dana J., 894

M

Malina, Joanne J. see Culver, Charles A., 846
Mann, Henry J. Effect of infusion pump fill-stroke flow interruption on response to sodium nitroprusside in surgical patients, 214
Mann, Henry J. see also Fuhs, David W., 207
Mann, Katherine V. Treatment of acetaminophen overdose when oral acetylcysteine therapy is not tolerated (Therapy Consultation), 563
Mann, Katherine V. Use of ipratropium bromide in obstructive lung disease, 670
Martin, Robert S. see Agostinucci, William A., 454
May, J. Russell see DiPiro, Joseph T., 285
McClain, Walter J. Anabolic steroid use as an AIDS risk factor (letter), 95
McCloskey, William W. see Mikolich, Dennis J., 269
McElwee, Newell E. Sodium thiosulfate unproven as bromate antidote (letter), 570
McGuire, Brian W. Pharmacokinetics of leucovorin calcium after intravenous, intramuscular, and oral administration, 52
McGuire, Brian W. see also Steffan, Richard, 722
McKenna, William R. see Pleasants, Roy A., 367, 374
McKenney, James M. Lovastatin: a new cholesterol-lowering agent, 21
McKenney, James M. Reassessment of the value of lowering serum cholesterol: the questions are when and how to treat, not whether to treat, hypercholesterolemia, 605
McKenney, James M. see also Jones, Barbara J., 235
McLarty, Jerry W. How many subjects are required for a study? 694
McPherson, Mary Lynn Neutropenia associated with oral acyclovir and multiple antibacterial agents in a patient with acquired immunodeficiency syndrome, 398
Mechlinski, Witold see Lelawongs, Parichat, 228
Meister, Fred L. see Roohk, Bonita, L., 150
Melby, Michael J. Book review, 161
Michals, Marcia Hearing loss associated with muromonab-CD3 therapy (letter), 867
Michals, Marcia L. see also Joy, Martha E., 721
Mikolich, Dennis J. Suspected gentamicin allergy could be sulfite sensitivity (letter), 269
Miles, Michael V. Predictability of unbound antiepileptic drug concentrations in children treated with valproic acid and phenytoin, 688
Miller, Jan see Drinka, Paul J., 497
Miller, Jane L. Future applications of biotechnology explored by ACCP speakers (News), 710
Monsour, Howard P. see Cantral, Kimberly A., 58
Moore, Emory S. Additive and synergistic bactericidal activity contributed by desacetylcefotaxime during cefotaxime therapy, 901
Morris, Barbara A. see Lombardi, Thomas P., 832
Mueller, Bruce A. Biological mechanisms and cardiovascular effects of omega-3 fatty acids, 795
Mueller, Bruce A. Lack of endogenous crossreactivity with three digitoxin radioimmunoassays in adults with renal insufficiency, 825
Mullane, Michael R. see Hutson, Paul R., 842
Munar, Myrna Y. Use of tamoxifen in stage I breast cancer (Therapy Consultation), 640
Munoz, Dee Marie Delivery of gentamicin by a controlled-release infusion system versus a minibag system, 303
Murphy, John E. Book review, 779
Murray, Kim M. see Noble, Teresa A., 659
Mylotte, Joseph M. see Munoz, Dee Marie, 303

N

Nahata, Milap C. see Benson, John M., 424
Nahata, Milap C. see also Fan–Havard, Patty, 616
Nix, David E. Storing extra calibration curves in the TDx assay system (letter), 792
Noble, Teresa A. Lisinopril: a nonsulfhydryl angiotensin-converting enzyme inhibitor, 659
Noguchi, Jean K. Sulbactam: a β-lactamase inhibitor, 37
Nolan, Paul E. Jr. Thrombolysis for acute myocardial infarction: does a greater incidence of reperfusion justify preferential use of an agent? 469
Norris, Mark C. Book review, 162
Nostrant, Timothy T. see Berardi, Rosemary R., 271

O

Opheim, Kent see Kobayashi, Kelly A., 224
Ostrosky, John D. see Adams, Marijke H., 725

P

Pal, Somnath see Frisolone, Julie, 444
Paone, Robert P. see Ponzillo, John J., 139
Parr, Michael D. Book review, 705
Parvin, Curtis see Lackner, Thomas E., 449
Peace, Karl E. see Hollifield, John W., 129
Pellechia, Crescens see Frisolone, Julie, 444
Peloquin, Charles A. see Nix, David E., 792
Perfect, John R. see Drew, Richard H., 622
Peterie, Jerry D. see Garrelts, James C., 720, 760
Phelps, Stephanie J. see Cochran, Emily B., 351
Phelps, Stephanie J. see also Kamper, Claudia A., 109
Plaisance, Karen I. see McPherson, Mary Lynn, 398
Pleasants, Roy A. Accuracy of tobramycin delivery by four i.v. infusion methods, 367
Pleasants, Roy A. Effect of four intravenous infusion methods on tobramycin pharmacokinetics, 374
Plis, Jeannine M. see Hamilton, Robert A., 439
Polk, Ron E. Management of vancomycin-induced "red-man syndrome" (Therapy Consultation), 184
Ponzillo, John J. Effect of diphenoxylate with atropine sulfate on the bioavailability of quinidine sulfate in healthy subjects, 139
Powell, J. Robert see Pleasants, Roy A., 367, 374
Powers, Douglas A. Serum fibronectin and somatomedin-C as nutritional markers in adults receiving total parenteral nutrition, 889
Powers, Douglas A. see also Reid, Dana J., 894
Prosser, Theresa see Lau, Alan H., 62
Pryka, Randy D. Teicoplanin: an investigational glycopeptide antibiotic, 647
Pugh, Carol B. see Boyce, Eric G., 307

R

Rajasekharaiah, Kusuma see Stephenson, David W., 317
Rayment, Carolyn M. see Ponzillo, John J., 139
Reid, Dana J. Predicting human-albumin replacement dosages in hypoalbuminemic patients receiving total parenteral nutrition, 894
Reynolds, John R. see Baker, Brian A., 135
Roberts, John P. see Michals, Marcia, 867
Rodman, John H. Wanted: insightful authors of review articles (letter), 95
Rodvold, Keith A. Aminoglycoside pharmacokinetic monitoring: an integral part of patient care? 608
Rodvold, Keith A. see also Pryka, Randy D., 647
Roohk, Bonita L. Comparison of 16-meq and 20-meq daily potassium supplement regimens, 150
Rossi, Joseph G. Diminishing bioavailability of oral leucovorin calcium (letter), 721
Rotschafer, John C. see Pryka, Randy D., 647
Rotschafer, John C. see also Rodvold, Keith A., 608
Rumsfeld, John A. see Roohk, Bonita L., 150
Rumsfield, Jean Topical cromolyn sodium for recurrent aphthous ulcers (Therapy Consultation), 344

S

Sahai, Jan Management of cryptococcal meningitis in patients with AIDS, 528
Salamone, Francine R. Update on pentamidine for the treatment of *Pneumocystis carinii* pneumonia, 501
Salamone, Francine R. see Suarez, Jeanette, 746
Sawyer, William T. see Pleasants, Roy A., 367, 374
Sayers, Jeffrey F. B. Routine monitoring of serum vancomycin concentrations: the answer lies in the middle (letter), 18
Scavone, Joseph M. see Ponzillo, John J., 139
Schaaf, Larry J. see Cantral, Kimberly A., 58
Schauer, Peter K. see Agostinucci, William A., 454
Schmidt, Gary R. Rebound hypertension after discontinuation of transdermal clonidine, 772
Schoen, Marieke Dekker Conversion from oral to intravenous verapamil therapy (Therapy Consultation), 791
Scholtz, Jean M. see Munar, Myrna Y., 640
Schuna, Arthur A. 1988 Report of the Joint National Committee on Detection, Evaluation, and Treatment

of High Blood Pressure: a commentary, 837
Schuna, Arthur A. see also Schmidt, Gary R., 772
Seth, Shiv Use of conjugated estrogens to control gastrointestinal tract bleeding in two patients with chronic renal failure, 906
Shifrar, Kenneth A. see Guerrero, Rawley M., 697
Shimasaki, Robert see Sayers, Jeffrey F. B., 18
Sia, Luisa L. see McGuire, Brian W., 52
Small, Ralph E. Sulindac-induced toxic epidermal necrolysis, 766
Small, Ralph E. see also Stephenson, David W., 317
Smith, Christopher D. Effect of influenza vaccine on serum concentrations of total and free phenytoin, 828
Smith, Dale F. Jr. see Garrelts, James C., 720, 760
Snead, O. Carter III see Miles, Michael V., 688
Sorsby, Stephen see Lue, Jane N., 66
Spyker, Daniel A. see Hollifield, John W., 129
Steffan, Richard Diminishing bioavailability of oral leucovorin calcium (letter), 722
Stephenson, David W. Effect of ranitidine and cimetidine on ibuprofen pharmacokinetics, 317
Stoehr, Gary P. Clindamycin pharmacokinetics and tissue penetration after head and neck surgery, 820
Stokstad, E. L. Robert see McGuire, Brian W., 52
Stonich, Terry see Lau, Alan H., 62
Stumpf, Janice L. Drug therapy of hypertensive crises, 582
Suarez, Jeanette Management and prevention of bacterial diarrhea, 746
Sugarek, Nancy J. see Mueller, Bruce A., 825
Swanson, Patrick see Bartels, David, 146
Sylvan, Lawrence see Hamilton, Robert A., 439
Sylvia, Lynne M. see Frisolone, Julie, 444

T

Talbert, Robert L. Reassessment of the value of lowering serum cholesterol: defending cholesterol-reduction efforts, 604
Talbert, Robert L. see also Culver, Charles A., 846
Talbert, Robert L. see also Mueller, Bruce A., 795
Tankanow, Roberta M. see Berardi, Rosemary R., 271
Teasley, Kathleen M. see Janson, Douglas D., 536
Thorn, Michael D. see Miles, Michael V., 688
Tietze, Karen J. see Mann, Katherine V., 670
Townsend, Raymond J. see Stoehr, Gary P., 820

U

Ume, Emeka O. C. Reversal of iatrogenic diazepam overdose with flumazenil, 614

V

Valdes, Roland Jr. see Lackner, Thomas E., 449
Vehe, Kathryn L. see Reid, Dana J., 894
Verme, Catherine N. Effect of temperature on in vitro measurement of quinidine free fraction, 142
Voeks, Susan K. see Drinka, Paul J., 497

W

Wagner, Robin see Stoehr, Gary P., 820
Walker, Kay B. see Bosso, John A., 897
Walters, J. Ken see Lombardi, Thomas P., 832
Wang, Arthur see Bartels, David, 146
Wesolowicz, Laurie see Cohen, Ira A., 457
West, Mark E. see Clifton, G. Dennis, 462
Williams, Dennis M. see Pleasants, Roy A., 367, 374
Willis, Hayes E. see Stephenson, David W., 317
Wong, Harry Magnesium gluconate can be used as oral supplement (letter), 269
Wood, Francis Jr. see Kobayashi, Kelly A., 224
Wood, John H. see Stephenson, David W., 317
Wordell, Cindy J. Treatment of *Pneumocystis carinii* pneumonia in patients with AIDS, 514
Wright, Jackson T. Jr. see Jones, Barbara J., 235

Y

Yellin, Albert E. see Ito, Matthew K., 467
Yu, Victor L. see Stoehr, Gary P., 820

Z

Zammett, Lorna O. see Lombardi, Thomas P., 832
Zeller, Frederick P. Notice to readers (letter), 18
Zenk, Karin E. Book review, 246
Zhanel, George G. Book review, 629
Zientek, Gary M. see Blake, Kathryn V., 391
Zokufa, Humphrey see Rodvold, Keith A., 608

Advertising Index

A

American Cancer Society
Institutional, 850
American College of Clinical Pharmacy
Call for Abstracts, 788
9th Annual Meeting, 266, 404
American Institute of the History of Pharmacy
Institutional, 556, 719
American Red Cross
Institutional, 159
American Society of Hospital Pharmacists
ACCRUE, Dec IBC
ASHP Membership, 723, 794, Dec IFC
Clinical Pharmacy, 13, 183, Dec OBC
Concepts in Clinical Pharmacokinetics, 625, 852, 866
Consumer Drug Digest, 564, 703, 722, 850
Database Services, 410, 487, 850, 915
Drug Theft (videotape), 868
Handbook on Extemporaneous Formulations, 76, 330
Handbook on Injectable Drugs, 420, 489, 626
International Pharmaceutical Abstracts, 849
Medication Teaching Manual, 912
Pharmacy Management Curriculum, 409, 499
Pocket Guide to Injectable Drugs, 17
Positions Available, 79, 264
Resource Book on Progressive Pharmaceutical Services, 629, 777, 793

B

Baxter Healthcare Corporation, MultiPlex Systems Division
Multiplex Fluid Management System, 571, 573, Oct IFC
Beecham Laboratories
Ticar, 20, 96, 186, 325, 350
Timentin, 170–172, 258–260, 338–340, 414–416, 494–496, 861–862
Bristol Bay Area Health Corporation, Kanakanak Hospital
Position Available, 719

C

Council for Aid to Education
Institutional, 266

H

Harvard Community Health Plan
Position Available, 850

K

Knoll Pharmaceuticals
Rythmol, 270

L

Lederle Laboratories, A Division of American Cyanamid Company
Clindamycin Phosphate, 561
Leucovorin Calcium, Nov IFC
Lemmon Company
Clindamycin, 724
Epitol, 345
Eli Lilly and Company
Nebcin, 261–262, 335–336, 417–418, 491–492, 641–642, 789–790
Tazidime, 167–168, 255–256, 411–412, 565–566, 715–716, 863–864
Lorex Pharmaceuticals
Position Available, 643

M

M. D. Anderson Cancer Center
Positions Available, 554
Merieux Institute, Inc.
Multitest CMI, 19, 185, 349, 633
Miami Valley Hospital
Position Available, 479

O

Owen Healthcare, Inc.
Positions Available, 717

P

Partnership for a Drug-Free America
Institutional, 257, 569

R

Rezayat Medical Services
Positions Available, 346
Roxane Laboratories Inc., A Boehringer Ingelheim Company
Computer Program, 263, 419
Intensols, Jan IFC, 87, 165, 333, 421, 500, 559, Sep IFC, 709, 787, 857
Marinol, Jan IBC, OBC; Mar IBC, OBC; May IBC, OBC; Jul IBC, OBC; Aug IBC, OBC; Sep IBC, OBC; Nov IBC, OBC

S

San Antonio State School
Position Available, 793, 868
Scientific Therapeutics Information, Inc.
Positions Available, 868
E. R. Squibb & Sons, Inc.
Azactam, 3–6, 177–180, 249–252
St. Luke's Hospital of New Bedford
Position Available, 788
State University of New York at Buffalo
Position Available, 564
Stuart Pharmaceuticals, Division of ICI Americas Inc.
Cefotan, 8–10; 89–91; Feb IBC, OBC; 173–175; Apr IBC, OBC; 341–343; Jun IBC, OBC; Aug IBC, OBC; 635–637; Oct IBC, OBC

U

U.S. Public Health Service
Positions Available, 346, 477, 498
The University of Alabama Hospital
Positions Available, 719
University of Alberta
Position Available, 644
The University of Illinois at Chicago
Positions Available, 717, 788
University of North Carolina at Chapel Hill
Positions Available, 242, 644
University of Washington
Position Available, 572
The Upjohn Company
Cleocin Phosphate, 15–16, 83–84, 181–182, 267–268, 347–348, 485–486, 567–568, 645–646, 711–712, 783–784, 859–860

V

Veterans Administration Medical Center (Bronx)
Positions Available, 328
Veterans Administration Medical Center (Syracuse)
Position Available, 94, 644

W

Washington State University
Positions Available, 556
Witikar Saudi Arabia Ltd.
Positions Available, 479
Wyeth Laboratories
Tubex, Feb IFC, Mar IFC, Apr IFC, May IFC, Jun IFC, Jul IFC, Aug IFC